NEONATAL WEIGHT CONVERSION FROM POUNDS TO GRAMS

Lbs.	Ounces 0	1	2	3	4	5	6	7	8	9	10	11	12	13	14	15
0	—	28	57	85	113	142	170	198	227	255	283	312	340	369	397	425
1	454	482	510	539	567	595	624	652	680	709	737	765	794	822	850	879
2	907	936	964	992	1021	1049	1077	1106	1134	1162	1191	1219	1247	1276	1304	1332
3	1361	1389	1417	1446	1474	1502	1531	1559	1588	1616	1644	1673	1701	1729	1758	1786
4	1814	1843	1871	1899	1928	1956	1984	2013	2041	2070	2098	2126	2155	2183	2211	2240
5	2268	2296	2325	2353	2381	2410	2438	2466	2495	2523	2551	2580	2608	2637	2665	2693
6	2722	2750	2778	2807	2835	2863	2892	2920	2948	2977	3005	3033	3062	3090	3118	3147
7	3175	3203	3232	3260	3289	3317	3345	3374	3402	3430	3459	3487	3515	3544	3572	3600
8	3629	3657	3685	3714	3742	3770	3799	3827	3856	3884	3912	3941	3969	3997	4026	4054
9	4082	4111	4139	4167	4196	4224	4252	4281	4309	4337	4366	4394	4423	4451	4479	4508
10	4536	4564	4593	4621	4649	4678	4706	4734	4763	4791	4819	4848	4876	4904	4933	4961
11	4990	5018	5046	5075	5103	5131	5160	5188	5216	5245	5273	5301	5330	5358	5386	5415
12	5443	5471	5500	5528	5557	5585	5613	5642	5670	5698	5727	5755	5783	5812	5840	5868
13	5897	5925	5953	5982	6010	6038	6067	6095	6123	6152	6180	6209	6237	6265	6294	6322
14	6350	6379	6407	6435	6464	6492	6520	6549	6577	6605	6634	6662	6690	6719	6747	6776
15	6804	6832	6860	6889	6917	6945	6973	7002	7030	7059	7087	7115	7144	7172	7201	7228

Comprehensive Neonatal Nursing

A PHYSIOLOGIC PERSPECTIVE

Comprehensive Neonatal Nursing

A PHYSIOLOGIC PERSPECTIVE

SECOND EDITION

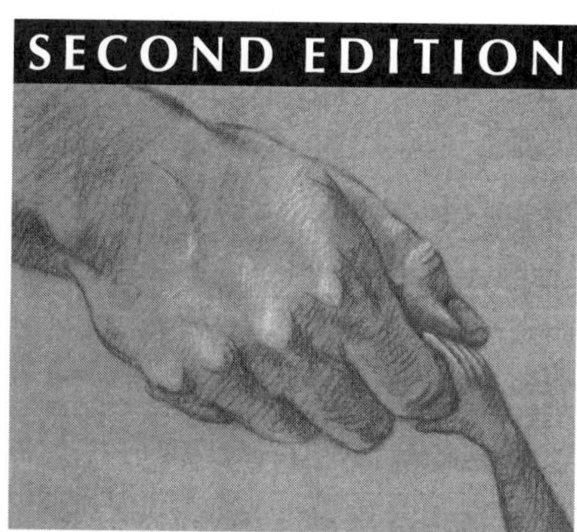

Carole Kenner, D.N.S., R.N.C., F.A.A.N.
Professor and Department Head
Parent Child Health Nursing
University of Cincinnati
Cincinnati, Ohio

Judy Wright Lott, D.N.S., R.N.C., N.N.P.
Associate Professor
College of Nursing and Health
University of Cincinnati
Cincinnati, Ohio

Ann Applewhite Flandermeyer, Ph.D., R.N.C.
Assistant Director, Clinical Services
Kendle Research
Cincinnati, Ohio

W.B. SAUNDERS COMPANY
A Division of Harcourt Brace & Company
Philadelphia ▪ London ▪ Toronto ▪ Montreal ▪ Sydney ▪ Tokyo

W.B. SAUNDERS COMPANY
A Division of Harcourt Brace & Company

The Curtis Center
Independence Square West
Philadelphia, Pennsylvania 19106

Library of Congress Cataloging-in-Publication Data

Comprehensive neonatal nursing: a physiologic perspective / [edited by] Carole Kenner, Judy Wright Lott, Ann Applewhite Flandermeyer.—2nd ed.

p. cm.

Includes index.

ISBN 0–7216–6535–7

1. Infants (Newborn)—Diseases—Nursing. I. Kenner, Carole. II. Lott, Judy Wright. III. Flandermeyer, Ann Applewhite. [DNLM: 1. Neonatal Nursing. 2. Infant, Newborn, Diseases—nursing. WY 157.3 C737 1998]

RJ253.C66 1998 618.92′01—dc21

DNLM/DLC 97-703

COMPREHENSIVE NEONATAL NURSING: A PHYSIOLOGIC PERSPECTIVE ISBN 0–7216–6535–7

Printed in the United States of America.

Last digit is the print number: 9 8 7 6 5 4 3

Contributors

Cynthia Margaret Acree, M.S.N., N.N.P.
Clinical Nurse Specialist, Neonatal Intensive Care, Miami Valley Hospital, Dayton, Ohio
Neonatal Transport

Stephanie Rockwern Amlung, M.S.N., Ph.D.
Research Associate, Institute for Nursing Research, College of Nursing and Health, University of Cincinnati, Cincinnati, Ohio
Neonatal Thermoregulation

Helen Archer-Dusté, M.S.N., R.N.
Kaiser Foundation Health Plan, San Francisco, California
Ethical Aspects of Perinatal Care

Vicky L. Armstrong, M.S.N, R.N.C.
Clinical Nurse Specialist, Perinatal Outreach Program, Children's Hospital, Columbus, Ohio
Regionalization of Care

Gail A. Bagwell, M.S.N., R.N.
Clinical Nurse Specialist/Case Manager, Children's Hospital, Columbus, Ohio
Regionalization of Care; Assessment and Management of the Transition to Home

Kathy Bergman, M.S.N., R.N.C., C.C.E.
Faculty, Department of Nursing, Xavier University, Cincinnati, Ohio
Fetal Therapy

Susan M. Berns, M.S.N., R.N.C., N.N.P.
Volunteer Clinical Faculty, University of Cincinnati; Neonatal Nurse Practitioner, Good Samaritan Hospital, Cincinnati, Ohio
The Changing Family Unit

Kim Bivens, M.S.N., R.N., C.N.S.
Trauma Clinical Nurse Specialist, Children's Hospital Medical Center, Cincinnati, Ohio
Assessment and Management of Endocrine Dysfunction

Susan Tucker Blackburn, Ph.D., R.N.C., F.A.A.N.
Professor, Department of Family and Child Nursing, University of Washington, Seattle, Washington
Assessment and Management of Neurologic Dysfunction; Assessment and Management of Neonatal Neurobehavioral Development

Susan M. Broughton, R.G.N., R.M., G.D.M.S., B.H.Sc.(Hons), P.G.Dip.Ed.
Midwifery Lecturer, Division of Midwifery, School of Human and Health Sciences, The University of Huddersfield, West Yorkshire, England
Sibling Adaptation to the Neonate

Lois A. Brown, M.S.N., R.N.C., N.N.P.
Neonatal Nurse Practitioner, Riverside Methodist Hospitals, Columbus, Ohio, Good Samaritan Hospital, Cincinnati, Ohio
The Changing Family Unit

Kimberly S. Burton, R.N.C., B.S.N.
Clinical Nurse III, Regional Center for Newborn Intensive Care, Children's Hospital Medical Center, Cincinnati, Ohio
Assessment and Management of Endocrine Dysfunction

Joyce Butler, M.S.N., R.N.C., N.N.P.
Neonatal Nurse Practitioner Coordinator, The University of Mississippi Medical Center, Jackson, Mississippi
Assessment and Management of Musculoskeletal Dysfunction

Waldemar A. Carlo, M.D.
Professor of Pediatrics and Director, Division of Neonatology, School of Medicine, University of Alabama at Birmingham; Director, Newborn Nurseries, University of Alabama Medical Center and the Children's Hospital of Alabama, Birmingham, Alabama
Assessment and Management of Respiratory Dysfunction

Javier Cifuentes, M.D.
Instructor in Pediatrics, University Hospital, Pontificia Universidad Catolica de Chile, Santiago, Chile
Assessment and Management of Respiratory Dysfunction

Marguerite Degenhardt, M.S., R.N., N.D.
Lisle, Illinois
Assessment and Management of Metabolic Dysfunction

Sergio DeMarini, M.D.
Attending Physician, Division of Neonatology, Ospedale Civile, Udine, Italy
Fluids, Electrolytes, Vitamins, and Trace Minerals: Basis of Ingestion, Digestion, Elimination, and Metabolism

Edward F. Donovan, M.D.
Professor of Pediatrics, University of Cincinnati Medical Center; Attending Staff, University of Cincinnati Hospital, Children's Hospital Medical Center, Cincinnati, Ohio
New Technologies Applied to the Management of Respiratory Dysfunction

Donna A. Dowling, Ph.D., M.N., R.N.
Assistant Professor of Nursing, Frances Payne Bolton School of Nursing, Case Western Reserve University, Cleveland, Ohio
Nutrition: Physiologic Basis of Metabolism and Management of Enteral and Parenteral Nutrition

Kathleen M. Driscoll, J.D., M.S., B.S.N., R.N.
Associate Professor, College of Nursing and Health, University of Cincinnati, Cincinnati, Ohio
Legal Aspects of Perinatal Care

Jody Farrell, B.S.N., R.N.
Coordinator, Fetal/Neonatal Care, Pediatric Surgery, University of California, San Francisco, San Francisco, California
Fetal Therapy

Dianne M. Felblinger, M.S.N., Ed.D., R.N.
Associate Professor, College of Nursing and Health, University of Cincinnati, Cincinnati, Ohio
Effects of Labor on the Fetus and Neonate

Linda Sturla Franck, Ph.D., R.N.
Assistant Professor, School of Nursing, University of California, San Francisco; Nursing Research Coordinator, Pediatric Clinical Research Center, University of California, San Francisco, San Francisco, California
Collaborative Research in Neonatal Nursing; Identification, Management, and Prevention of Pain in the Neonate; Computer Technology Use in Neonatal Nursing

Vivian Gamblian, M.S.N., R.N.
President, Gamblian Enterprises, Inc. (Healthy Homecomings), Plano, Texas
Assessment and Management of Endocrine Dysfunction

Lynda Hutt Hall, M.N., R.N.C., N.N.P., P.N.P.
Nursing Faculty Consultant, University of Phoenix, Phoenix, Arizona
Home Care

Jeanne Harjo, R.N.
Staff Nurse, Clinical Nurse III, Children's Hospital, Cincinnati, Ohio
Diagnostic Tests and Laboratory Values; The Surgical Neonate

Judith S. Harmon, M.S., R.N., C.F.N.P.
Adjunct Faculty, College of Nursing, Grand Canyon University, Phoenix, Arizona; Women and Infants' Health and Certified Family Nurse Practitioner, Samaritan Family Health Center, Payson, Arizona
High-Risk Pregnancy

Rosanne C. Harrigan, Ed.D., C.P.N.P., F.A.A.N.
Dean and Professor, University of Hawaii at Manoa, Honolulu, Hawaii
Neonatal Nursing and Its Role in Comprehensive Care; Collaborative Practice in the Neonatal Intensive Care Unit

Kathleen Haubrich, M.S.N., R.N.C.
Assistant Professor, Department of Nursing, Miami University, Hamilton, Ohio; Clinical Nurse, Obstetrical Special Care Unit, University of Cincinnati Medical Center, Cincinnati, Ohio
Assessment and Management of Auditory Dysfunction

James L. Haywood, M.D.
Associate Professor of Pediatrics, School of Medicine, University of Alabama at Birmingham; Medical Director, Newborn Intensive Care Unit, Children's Hospital of Alabama, Birmingham, Alabama
Assessment and Management of Respiratory Dysfunction

Carol Hetteberg, M.S.N., R.N.
Assistant Professor of Clinical Nursing, College of Nursing and Health, University of Cincinnati, Cincinnati, Ohio
Human Genetics

Marcia A. Hilse, M.S.N., R.N.
In Vitro Fertilization Coordinator, Center for Human Reproduction, Glenview, Illinois
Human Genetics

Diane Holditch-Davis, Ph.D., R.N., F.A.A.N.
Associate Professor, School of Nursing, University of North Carolina at Chapel Hill, Chapel Hill, North Carolina
Neonatal Sleep–Wake States

Lori J. Howell, M.S., R.N.
Clinical Associate, University of Pennsylvania School of Nursing; Program Manager, Surgery Advanced Practice Nurse Program, The Center for Fetal Diagnosis and Treatment, Philadelphia, Pennsylvania
Fetal Therapy

Maribeth Inturrisi, M.S.N.
Associate Professor, Department of Family Health Care Nursing, School of Nursing, University of California, San Francisco; Clinical Nurse Specialist (Obstetrics), UCSF Medical Center, San Francisco, California
Fetal Therapy

Nia Johnson-Crowley, M.N., R.N.
Doctoral Candidate, Educational Psychology, Department of Education, University of Washington, Seattle, Washington
Systemic Assessment and Home Follow-Up: A Basis for Monitoring the Neonate's Integration Into the Family Unit

Karen Katz, R.N.C., N.N.P., M.S.N.(C)
MSN-CNS Student, Beth-El College of Nursing, Colorado Springs, Colorado; RNC, NNP Level II Nursery, Columbia North Suburban Medical Center, Thornton, Colorado; RNC, NNP–Locum Tenens, Innovative Health Care, Inc., Denver, Colorado
Neonatal Assessment

Charlotte A. Kenreigh, Pharm.D.
Manager, Clinical Education and Training, Merck-Medco Managed Care, L.L.C., Columbus, Ohio
Principles of Neonatal Drug Therapy

Caroline Hoell Kistler, M.S.N., R.N.C., N.N.P.
Adjunct Clinical Instructor, Neonatal Nurse Practitioner Program, College of Nursing Health, University of Cincinnati; Neonatal Nurse Practitioner, Family Birthing Center, Jewish Hospital Kenwood, Cincinnati, Ohio
Assessment and Management of Endocrine Dysfunction

Tracey A. Kleeman, M.S.N., R.N.C., N.N.P.
Envision Group, Inc., Cincinnati, Ohio
Assessment and Management of Endocrine Dysfunction

Joanne McManus Kuller, M.S.N., R.N.
Assistant Clinical Professor, School of Nursing, University of California, San Francisco, San Francisco, California; Education Resource Specialist, Children's Hospital Oakland, Oakland, California
Assessment and Management of Integumentary Dysfunction

Rita Maria Kunk, M.S.N., R.N.C.
Neonatal Nurse Practitioner, Winchester Medical Center, Winchester, Virginia
Neonatal Transport

Linda Lefrak, M.S., R.N., N.N.P.
Assistant Clinical Professor, University of California, San Francisco, San Francisco, California; Assistant Clinical Professor, School of Nursing, University of Illinois, Chicago, Illinois; Neonatal Clinical Nurse Specialist, Children's Hospital, Oakland, California
Nutrition: Physiologic Basis of Metabolism and Management of Enteral and Parenteral Nutrition; Iatrogenic Complications of the Neonatal Intensive Care Unit

Denise Lucas, M.S.N., R.N.C.
Staff Nurse, Labor and Delivery, Bethesda Hospital, Cincinnati, Ohio
Collaborative Research in Neonatal Nursing

Carolyn Houska Lund, M.S.N., R.N., F.A.A.N.
Assistant Clinical Professor, School of Nursing, University of California, San Francisco, San Francisco, California; Assistant Clinical Professor, School of Nursing, University of Illinois, Chicago, Illinois; Neonatal Clinical Nurse Specialist and ECMO Coordinator, Intensive Care Nursery, Children's Hospital, Oakland, California
Assessment and Management of Integumentary Dysfunction

Linda L. McCollum, Ph.D., R.N.C., C.N.N.P.
Regional Education Coordinator, Emory Regional Perinatal Center, Emory University School of Medicine; Adjunct Clinical Faculty, Nell Hodgson Woodruff School of Nursing, Emory University, Atlanta, Georgia
Resuscitation and Stabilization of the Neonate; Assessment and Management of Gastrointestinal Dysfunction

Lisa M. Moles, M.S.N., R.N., C.P.N.P.
Pediatric Nurse Practitioner, Division of Cardiothoracic Surgery, Children's Hospital Medical Center, Cincinnati, Ohio
New Technologies Applied to the Management of Respiratory Dysfunction

Jane A. Nichols, M.Ed.
Coordinator of Bereavement Services, Children's Hospital Medical Center of Akron, Akron, Ohio
Bereavement: The State of Having Suffered a Loss

Elaine Nishioka, M.S.N., R.N., C.P.N.P.
Pediatric Nurse Practitioner, Healthy Steps Specialist, Eastover Pediatrics, Presbyterian Healthcare System, Charlotte, North Carolina
Neonatal Assessment

Susan H. Pedersen-Ryckman, M.S.N., R.N., P.N.P.
Visiting Assistant Professor, Miami University, Oxford, Ohio; Pediatric Nurse Practitioner, Cardiac Care Center, Children's Hospital Medical Center, Cincinnati, Ohio
Hepatic and Renal Transplantation in Infants and Children

Dennis Perez, Ph.D.
Staff Psychologist, University of Illinois at Chicago, Chicago, Illinois
Neonatal Nursing and Its Role in Comprehensive Care; Collaborative Practice in the Neonatal Intensive Care Unit

Cynthia Prows, M.S.N., R.N.
Adjunct Instructor of Clinical Nursing, College of Nursing and Health, University of Cincinnati; Clinical Nurse Specialist, Human Genetics Department, Children's Hospital Medical Center, Cincinnati, Ohio
Assessment and Management of Endocrine Dysfunction

Linda L. Rath, M.S.N.
Assistant Professor, University of Texas Medical Branch, Galveston, Texas; Adjunct Clinical Instructor, University of Texas Health Science Center–Houston, Houston, Texas
Fluids, Electrolytes, Vitamins, and Trace Minerals: Basis of Ingestion, Digestion, Elimination, and Metabolism

Madeline Ross, M.S.N., C.R.N.P., C.N.S.
Manager, Clinical Specialist Group, Ohmeda, Inc.; Consultant for NICU, Brookwood Medical Center; Neonatal Nurse Practitioner, NNP Services of Alabama, Birmingham, Alabama
Assessment and Management of Respiratory Dysfunction

Frederick C. Ryckman, M.D.
Associate Professor of Surgery, University of Cincinnati; Director, Pediatric Transportation, Children's Hospital Medical Center, Cincinnati, Ohio
Hepatic and Renal Transplantation in Infants and Children

Jonathan E. Schwartz, M.D.
Neonatal Fellow, Children's Hospital Medical Center, Cincinnati, Ohio; Staff Neonatologist, Neonatal Associates of Jacksonville, Jacksonville, Florida
New Technologies Applied to the Management of Respiratory Dysfunction

Nancy Shaw, M.S.N., R.N., N.N.P.
Auxiliary Faculty, University of Utah; Neonatal Nurse Practitioner, Primary Children's Medical Center, Salt Lake City, Utah
Assessment and Management of Hematologic Dysfunction

Sheila M. Southwell, M.S.N., M.B.A.
Director of Patient Care Services, Pediatrics, Sinai Hospital of Baltimore, Baltimore, Maryland
Ethical Aspects of Perinatal Care

Frances Strodtbeck, D.N.S., R.N.C., N.N.P.
Coordinator, Neonatal Nurse Practitioner Program, Rush University College of Nursing; Neonatal Nurse Practitioner, Rush–Presbyterian–St. Luke's Medical Center, Chicago, Illinois
Assessment and Management of Ophthalmic Dysfunction

Catherine Jursich Theorell, M.S.N., R.N.C., N.N.P.
Associate Professor, Neonatal Nurse Practitioner Program, University of Illinois, Chicago, Illinois
Assessment and Management of Metabolic Dysfunction; Diagnostic Imaging

Janet L. Thigpen, M.N., R.N.C., C.N.N.P.
Clinical Associate, Nell Hodgson Woodruff School of Nursing, Emory University; Neonatal Nurse Practitioner, Division of Neonatal Medicine, Department of Pediatrics, Emory University School of Medicine, Atlanta, Georgia
Assessment and Management of Gastrointestinal Dysfunction

Reginald C. Tsang, M.B.B.S.
Professor of Pediatrics, University of Cincinnati; Associate Chairman, Pediatrics, Executive Director, Children's Center for Bone Research and Health, University of Cincinnati/Children's Hospital Medical Center, Cincinnati, Ohio
Fluids, Electrolytes, Vitamins, and Trace Minerals: Basis of Ingestion, Digestion, Elimination, and Metabolism

Kathleen A. VandenBerg, M.A.
Director, Infant Development Program NICU, Director, Stanford NIDCAP Training Center, Division of Neonatal and Developmental Medicine, Department of Pediatrics, Stanford University School of Medicine, Palo Alto, California
Assessment and Management of Neonatal Neurobehavioral Development

Linda Timm Wagner, Pharm.D.
Senior Manager, Clinical Practice and Education, Merck-Medco Managed Care, L.L.C., Columbus, Ohio
Principles of Neonatal Drug Therapy

Elizabeth Elder Weiner, Ph.D., R.N.
Professor, College of Nursing and Health, Director, Center for Academic Technologies, University of Cincinnati, Cincinnati, Ohio
Computer Technology Use in Neonatal Nursing

Tina Leigh Weitkamp, M.S.N.
Associate Professor of Clinical Nursing, College of Nursing and Health, University of Cincinnati; Staff Nurse, Mercy Hospital–Anderson, Cincinnati, Ohio
Effects of Labor on the Fetus and Neonate

Vignettes

Heidi Campbell, B.S.N., R.N.
Program Manager, Transport Team, Children's Hospital Medical Center, Cincinnati, Ohio

Cynthia Stone DeAngelis, M.A., C.C.C.
Speech-Language Pathologist, The Christ Hospital, Cincinnati, Ohio

Joyce M. Dohme, M.S.N., R.N.C., P.N.P.
Pediatric Nurse Practitioner, School-Based Health Care, West End Health Center, Cincinnati, Ohio

Sandy Heim, R.N.
Special Care and Transitional Nurseries, The Christ Hospital, Cincinnati, Ohio

Judith A. Hostiuck, M.S.N., R.N.C.
Manager, Perinatal Services, Family Birthing Center, Jewish Hospital–Kenwood, Staff Nurse, University Hospital, Inc., Cincinnati, Ohio

Marianne McGraw, M.S.N., R.N.
Neonatal Nurse Practitioner, The Christ Hospital, Cincinnati, Ohio

Vicky Merritt, B.S.N., R.N.
Assistant Patient Care Manager, Post-Partum Mother/Baby Unit, The Christ Hospital, Cincinnati, Ohio

Dee Overbeck, M.S.N., R.N.
Neonatal Nurse Practitioner, Good Samaritan Hospital, Cincinnati, Ohio

Robin Roe, M.A., R.N.
Speech Pathology, The Christ Hospital, Cincinnati, Ohio

Lisa Spangler-Torok, M.S.N., R.N.
Doctoral Candidate, University of Cincinnati; Assistant Professor, Thomas More College, Crestview Hills, Kentucky; Clinical Nurse, Regional Center for Newborn Intensive Care, Children's Medical Center, Cincinnati, Ohio

Kathleen Spiering, M.S.N., R.N., C.N.N.P.
Neonatal Nurse Practitioner, Mercy Hospital–Anderson, Cincinnati, Ohio

Dan Wells, B.S., R.R.T.
Outreach Education Coordinator, Neonatal/Pediatric Transport Team, Children's Hospital Medical Center, Cincinnati, Ohio

Pamela P. White, M.S.N., R.N.
Lecturer, Indiana University Southeast, New Albany, Louisiana

Foreword

Advances in management and treatment of newborns, in knowledge of their capabilities and development, and in care of high-risk newborns and the need to extend support to families caring for smaller and sicker newborns have challenged health care providers in many ways. First, there is the need to keep abreast of advances in knowledge regarding care of newborns and support of their families. Equally important are the need to keep abreast of legal and public policy issues surrounding their care and the need for research to further improve care to this vulnerable group. To accomplish this, textbooks for nurses caring for newborns and their families require both a comprehensive approach to care and a thorough discussion of problem areas of management and treatment. This book has both.

The authors address the breadth of issues in neonatal care, including high-risk pregnancy; the changing family unit; sibling reactions to the newborn; neonatal development; home follow-up of neonates; and legal, ethical, and research issues. The impact of health care reform on neonatal care is addressed throughout the text. Although the breadth of content of the chapters is extensive, the text also covers major problems in depth, including respiratory, cardiovascular, metabolic, and gastrointestinal dysfunction, to name but a few. Such breadth and depth will be an invaluable aid to clinicians providing care to neonates and their families and to educators preparing others to do so. The editors are to be applauded for contributing such an effort to the field of neonatal care.

DOROTHY BROOTEN, PH.D., R.N., F.A.A.N.
Professor and Assistant Dean of Research
Frances Payne Bolton School of Nursing
Case Western Reserve University
Cleveland, Ohio

Preface

Trends in neonatology encompass the survival of very low birth weight premature infants and infants with multiple, severe congenital anomalies. Maternal risk factors have changed over the past decade. For example, more infants of mothers with chronic illnesses such as diabetes or sickle cell anemia or who are products of in vitro fertilization are found in the neonatal units today. More infants in neonatal intensive care units (NICUs) have been substance-exposed or are born to mothers with other risk factors such as delayed childbearing or childhood cancers. Often neonatal survival of these at-risk infants depends on the use of high-level technology. Extracorporeal membrane oxygenation (ECMO), surfactant administration, liquid ventilation, nitric oxide administration, high-frequency jet ventilators, dialysis, organ transplantation, and other heroic measures are rapidly becoming more commonplace.

A neonatal nurse is faced with a tremendous need for accurate, comprehensive information. This nurse must have a thorough understanding of normal physiology as well as the pathophysiology of disease processes. The neonatal nurse must be knowledgeable about associated risk factors, genetics, critical periods of development, principles of nutrition and pharmacology, and current neonatal research findings. The concepts of a family-centered approach to nursing care are important, too. All these elements form the solid foundation for assessment, planning, and implementation of comprehensive neonatal nursing care.

In the 1990s, the nurse's role has broadened to include added responsibilities, felt at both the staff and the advanced practice levels. For the purposes of this book, two definitions of advanced practice are being used. They are the National Association of Neonatal Nurses' (NANN) definitions of clinical nurse specialist and neonatal nurse practitioner (NANN, Position Statement, 1990).

Clinical Nurse Specialist

The clinical nurse specialist (CNS) is a registered nurse with a master's degree who, through study and supervised practice at the graduate level, has become expert in the defined clinical area of nursing. The CNS provides for the diagnosis and treatment of human responses to actual or potential health problems of patients and their families within the specialized area through direct patient care and clinical consultation. In addition, the CNS may act in an educational, research, liaison, or leadership role to promote optimal nursing care for the patients served.

Neonatal Nurse Practitioner

The neonatal nurse practitioner (NNP) is a registered nurse with clinical expertise in neonatal nursing who has received formal education with supervised clinical experience in the management of sick newborns and their families. The NNP manages a caseload of neonatal patients with consultation, collaboration, and general supervision from a physician. Utilizing the extensive knowledge of pathophysiology, pharmacology, and physiology acquired, the NNP exercises independent or intradependent (in collaboration with other health professionals) judgment in the assessment, diagnosis, and initiation of certain delegated medical processes and procedures. As an advanced practice neonatal nurse, the NNP is additionally involved in education, consultation, and research at various levels.

At the present time, the blurring of these two roles is being discussed. It has been proposed, but certainly not fully accepted, that a more appropriate term would be advanced practice nurse, or APN. This change is emotion-laden, because although those involved in both practice and education have felt the difference was necessary in the past, with health care reform, it appears to be more critical for advanced practice nurses to work together rather than have a dichotomous title.

The neonatal staff nurse role, although not as broad and comprehensive as the advanced practice roles, still requires accurate and thorough assessment skills, excellent ability to communicate with other health professionals and patients' families, and a broad understanding of physiology and pathophysiology upon which to base management decisions. It requires highly developed technical skills as well as critical decision-making. With health care delivery changes, it also requires supervision of ancillary personnel and an informed delegation of certain patient-oriented tasks. These changes require the staff nurse to possess even better assessment skills and sound knowledge of physiology and pathophysiology than in the past, because some decision-making will be done in concert with other, less highly trained personnel.

Purpose and Content

The second edition of this book again provides a comprehensive examination of neonatal nursing management from a physiologic and pathophysiologic approach appropriate for any health professional concerned with neonatal care. For the advanced practitioner and neonatal staff nurse, it provides a complete physiologic and embryologic foundation for each neonatal system. It includes medical, surgical, and psychosocial care, because the collaborative management approach is absolutely imperative to the well-being of the neonate and family. Appropriate diagnostic tests and their interpretation are included in each system chapter. There is extensive use of research findings in the chapters to round out practice strategies and demonstrate rationale for clinical decision-making. Complete references for more in-depth reading are found at the end of each chapter so that the reader may pursue more specific information on a topical area. Use of tables and illustrations to support material that is presented in the narrative portions is sure to be another help to the practicing neonatal nurse.

The thread of collaborative management is interwoven throughout the text. Foundational topics such as genetics, physiologically critical periods of development, nutrition, and parenting are included, as are topics of recent interest such as iatrogenic complications, neonatal pain, use of computers in nursing, and neonatal AIDS. Research agendas are found in each of the chapters to serve as reminders that practice decisions need to be grounded in research findings rather than in tradition. These reflect new trends or those areas that still need research. Now more than ever, nursing must examine patient outcomes and nurse outcomes in order to meet the demands for providing cost-effective and high-quality care. Research is critical to support both the art and science of neonatal care. Whenever possible, the contributors remind the reader of areas in need of further study. Vignettes are found at the beginning of many chapters that are concerned with assessment and management of a specific neonatal problem. These case studies are intended to represent excellence in neonatal nursing care. They pull together common content of their representative chapters and highlight how nursing care should proceed if it is to be more holistic and less task-oriented.

Many of the chapters in the first edition ended with the nursing process tools to document patient outcomes. However, these have been replaced in many institutions by computerized forms. Most institutions are attempting some form of critical pathway for documentation of patient process and outcomes. Examples of critical pathways are included to help validate data collection points for research and care defining points to track progress, and to determine patient care and nursing care costs. If your institution has not attempted to develop a critical pathway, there is a table in the Appendix that highlights the steps in readying a unit and staff for this work.

This book is not a quick reference but provides comprehensive in-depth discussions along with detailed physiologic principles and collaborative management strategies. It provides a sound basis for safe and effective neonatal care.

The book begins with a discussion of general areas of neonatal nursing: the collaborative role of nursing in comprehensive neonatal care, the ethical and legal considerations, and the need for neonatal research. Next the content focuses on the family: the changing family unit and the siblings' adaptation to a new family member. Bereavement and chronic sorrow are discussed, because a happy ending is not always possible in perinatal and neonatal nursing. Human genetics is introduced, and the impact of environmental influences on the developing fetus is discussed. This provides the transition into discussion of the high-risk pregnancy, the effects of labor on the fetus, and other perinatal topics of regionalization of care and neonatal transport. The text then deals with more specific neonatal topics, starting with stabilization, thermoregulation, and assessment. This edition includes the most up-to-date information from the American Heart Association's Neonatal Resuscitation Program. Each organ system is discussed in depth, beginning with the respiratory system, including its complications and new technologies, followed by assessment of and management strategies for the cardiovascular system; nutrition and the gastrointestinal system; and metabolic, endocrine, immunologic, hematopoietic, neurologic, musculoskeletal, genitourinary, integumentary, auditory, and ophthalmic systems. Monitoring of biophysical parameters, diagnostic imaging, and diagnostic text and laboratory values represent the section of the text that highlights the evaluative measures used by practitioners to identify the neonatal problem and its progress. A section on new technologies and special topics follows these chapters. This section addresses such areas as new advances in fetal therapy and surgery, the surgical neonate, neonatal pain, neonatal AIDS, iatrogenic complications of the NICU, the drug-exposed neonate, use of computers in neonatal nursing, and specific procedures used by neonatal nurses. The final group of chapters covers the discharge phase. Topics include systematic assessment and home follow-up, neonatal behavior, assessment and management of neonatal behavior, the transition to home, and, finally, home care.

In this edition, each of the chapters and sections has been updated to include the newest techniques, such as the latest trends in fetal therapy; progress with the mapping of human genes; use of computers, including Internet connections opening up global neonatal care issues for examination and discussion; inclusion of the latest issues in health care reform and its impact on nursing care; and the latest research findings appropriate to each of the sections.

To provide depth to these topical areas, physicians, nurses, infant developmental specialists, and other health professionals concerned with neonatal care from across the country and around the world were used as contributors in both editions. The attempt was made not only to tap the experts in the neonatal field but to have them represent as wide a geographic area as possible. We hope that the broad geographic distribution both of contributors and of the manuscript reviewers will help to minimize the effect of regional differences in clinical practice as reflected in the text.

CAROLE KENNER, D.N.S., R.N.C., F.A.A.N.
JUDY WRIGHT LOTT, D.S.N., R.N.C., N.N.P.
ANN APPLEWHITE FLANDERMEYER, PH.D., R.N.C.

Acknowledgments

This book has been a major undertaking, one of which we are all most proud. It would not have been possible without the support of many people who worked in many hidden ways. First we would like to thank our former nursing editor Ilze Rader for her assistance, encouragement, and support during this seemingly never-ending process. Her suggestions, along with the critiques of the first edition's nursing editor, Thomas Eoyang, have made a big difference in the polishing of this work.

We are truly grateful to our contributors, who in the midst of their very busy lives took on one more project. For those who stuck with us through a second edition, we are especially indebted. We want to thank the new contributors for their willingness to share their expertise. We certainly recognize the time commitment that was made. We believe that because of their efforts wc have been able to bring together the best knowledge of the true neonatal experts.

We would also like to thank our many reviewers for the constructive comments. Without these suggestions, a book that represents a national perspective would not have been possible. We want to thank the nurses of many of the nurseries in Cincinnati, especially Children's Hospital Medical Center, Good Samaritan Hospital, The Christ Hospital, Bethesda Hospital, Jewish Hospital, Mercy Hospital–Anderson, and University Hospital, for contributing vignettes and suggestions or reading sections of chapters in order to improve the integrity of the manuscript. We would also like to acknowledge the help of an editor friend, Sonnie Choto, who was visiting from Africa during the first and second editions (her visits were perfectly timed) and agreed to turn part of her holidays into working vacations to do some revisions. We would like also like to acknowledge Kathleen Pompa's contribution in reviewing galley and page proofs.

Finally, but certainly not least, we would all like to acknowledge the support and encouragement of our families: Les and Betty Kenner; Bill, Tam, and Blake Lott; and Brian, Christina, and Rebecca Flandermeyer. Their strength and positive thoughts have kept us going throughout these many months.

We want to thank our readers, who have validated the need for this text. Without your support there would be no need for a second edition.

NOTICE

Nursing is an ever-changing field. Standard safety precautions must be followed, but as new research and clinical experience broaden our knowledge, changes in treatments and drug therapy become necessary or appropriate. The editors of this work have carefully checked the generic and trade drug names and verified drug dosages to ensure that the dosage information in this work is accurate and in accord with the standards accepted at the time of publication. Readers are advised, however, to check the product information currently provided by the manufacturer of each drug to be administered to be certain that changes have not been made in the recommended dose or in the contraindications for administration. This is of particular importance in regard to new or infrequently used drugs. It is the responsibility of the treating physician, relying on experience and knowledge of the patient, to determine dosages and the best treatment of the patient. The editors cannot be responsible for misuse or misapplications of the material in this work.

THE PUBLISHER

Contents

UNIT ONE

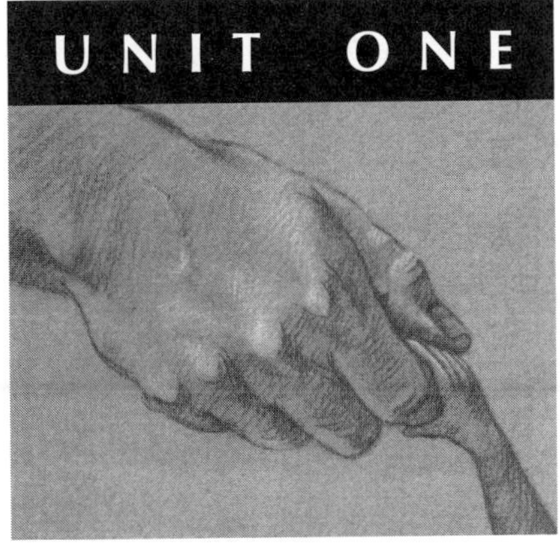

Neonatal Nursing Care: A Collaborative Practice Arena

While [Emily] was working to gain weight, Leslie said the other NICU nurses cheered her on with friendly teasing. When she crossed the hundred-pound Rubicon, one nurse, Wanda, began calling her Fats. The mood was intense here in K9. It was crowded, and the working conditions were far from luxurious. The nurses, too, went through their highs and lows, as each of their babies improved or faltered. A foul humor here could poison the air in an instant. Instead these women coped with the inherent adversities of their situation by pulling together. Never mind the respect with which they treated each other—and that was enormous. The camaraderie they had developed was truly remarkable.

ELIZABETH MEHREN
Born Too Soon

CHAPTER 1

Neonatal Nursing and Its Role in Comprehensive Care

ROSANNE C. HARRIGAN DENNIS PEREZ

RESEARCH AGENDA

Explore the developmental stages of the neonatal nurse and identify strategies that promote development

Determine whether a relationship exists between credentialing and neonatal outcomes

Determine whether the cost of care is dependent on qualifications of neonatal care providers

Determine whether nursing management influences the outcomes of neonatal care

The purpose of this chapter is to describe the role of the neonatal nurse in the delivery of comprehensive neonatal health care. The discussion focuses on (1) the developmental aspects of neonatal nursing roles in comprehensive care; (2) the contributions of neonatal nurse practitioners and specialists to the advancement of neonatal care; (3) the issues related to the practice, credentialing, and education of neonatal nurses; and (4) the effect of nursing management on neonatal outcomes.

Neonatal nursing practice consists of at least three elements: (1) implementing nursing therapy, (2) collaborating with other health care providers, and (3) assisting with medical care. The interrelationship of these three components centers on improving or maintaining the health of the neonate and the family. Nursing therapy consists of assessment, planning, intervention, and evaluation of newborns and their families to provide developmentally appropriate environments, physical care, feeding, and parent care. Neonatal nursing care is protective, generative, and nurturing in nature and focuses on the needs of neonates as embodied persons rather than as biologic systems.

Protective nursing services encompass early identification and evaluation of risk factors. The neonatal nurse uses specific screening tools to identify problems and then initiates appropriate action and referral. The nurse provides anticipatory guidance and teaching for the family in relation to the neonate's health and developmental status. *Generative nursing activities* incorporate developing new behaviors and modifying environments or roles to help parents and neonates adjust to their developmental and health needs. *Nurturing nursing* behaviors provide surveillance of physiologic variables, infant comfort, and family education about the infant's health and illness. Neonatal nurses are also involved in research, developing linkages with other hospitals' services, interaction with community-based follow-up programs, and the education of other neonatal care providers.

ROLE OF THE NEONATAL NURSE

The proliferation of the neonatal positive pressure respirator in the 1970s and the development of the neonatal intensive care unit (NICU) forever changed the practice environment of the nursery. An environment that was once filled with the lusty cries of healthy newborns became a space-age life-support station for infants who previously would not have survived. The skills required of a neonatal nurse have continued to evolve since the mid-1970s, to the point that the cost of an orientation to a beginning role in neonatal intensive care usually exceeds $8000 (S. Swanson, 1991, personal communication). Generic-level nursing programs (associate, diploma, and baccalaureate levels) currently contain very little preparation in the knowledge and skills necessary for practice in the NICU. In fact, the Maternal Infant Core Competency Project, completed in 1986, suggested that generic nursing programs focus primarily on cognitive content related to management of low-risk infants. Content related to the care of high-risk neonates was deemed the responsibility of continuing and graduate education.

The neonatal staff nurse is often confronted with a role for which she or he is not prepared, at either the cognitive or the psychomotor level. Of growing concern is the demand for new graduates, soon after entry into a system, to deliver collaborative care that requires the competence of an expert socialized practitioner (Sherwen, 1990).

One result of changes since the 1980s in medical education is that residents spend progressively less time in the NICU. This diminished rotation means that they have less time to become proficient in common procedures such as endotracheal intubation; thus interns often complete the NICU rotation without ever intubating an infant. Funds for the continuing education of neonatal nurses at all levels of career development are also reported to be diminishing. The impact of managed care on neonatal nursing roles has not been clearly delineated in the literature. However, neonates are being discharged earlier than ever, and there is an emerging need for home care nurses that possess and maintain neonatal management competencies. There is even a need for the provision of high-tech care in the home, where nurses do not have the personnel or equipment back-up found in hospital settings. 

DEVELOPMENTAL ASPECTS OF NEONATAL NURSING PRACTICE

Neonatal Nursing Care Providers

Beginning Practitioners

When the neonatal nurse joins the staff of a NICU, many challenges await. The nurse must learn to perform at least some of the care delivery tasks competently. She or he must also learn which elements of the role are critical and which require the majority of attention. Tasks must be accomplished through the use of both formal and informal communication channels. In addition, the nurse must perform while being observed, for indications of competence and future potential.

Because the new NICU nurse lacks experience and others on the staff do not know how much they can rely on the new nurse's judgment, direct supervision of the new nurse is essential. In other words, the new nurse must begin by helping a more seasoned nurse preceptor with an assignment (Perez, 1981).

Early work assignments should be routine. However, it is important for the entry-level neonatal nurse not to be tied only to work that is tedious and detailed. She or he should be expected to show some initiative. Central activities of this role include helping, learning, and following directions. The entry-level neonatal nurse is a dependent practitioner. Home care nurses who manage neonates must spend a portion of their orientation in the NICU to experience this developmental stage and acquire associated competencies before accepting responsibility for the sick newborn in the home.

Technicians

The primary theme in the second developmental stage for neonatal nurses is independence. Transition is accomplished by establishing a reputation as a technically competent professional who can work independently to produce designated patient outcomes. This nurse looks forward to having primary responsibility for a small number of patients. The nurse no longer requires close supervision on the specific methods used to get her or his job done. At this stage, the nurse's technical skills are expected to have evolved to a high level. In fact, it is often a time when the nurse establishes an area of subspecialization, an area of practice in which expertise is recognized by the unit (Perez, 1981). Establishment of this expertise forms the basis for a productive and successful career. This level of expertise is optimal for the home-care nurse.

Peer relationships take on a great deal of importance during this stage of development. The nurse continues to be a subordinate but begins to rely less on the preceptor for direction. Transitions can be difficult because changes in attitudes and behavior are necessary on the part of the supervisor as well as the nurse.

To complete the developmental tasks associated with this stage, the nurse must go beyond dependence and begin to develop personal ideas or views on what is required in a given situation. Individual standards of performance begin to develop, as does an awareness of a professional value system (Dalton & Thompson, 1971).

Developing confidence in personal judgment is a difficult but necessary transition. Often the neonatal nurse takes a supervisory position during this stage, long before she or he has become established as a competent professional. Administrative staff or personnel may conspire with individual nurses to move them into management too soon. Management opportunities can be very attractive economically, but they involve a high degree of risk (France & McDowell, 1983). First-line managers can never be effective if they are unable to understand the technical aspects of the work that they supervise. Lack of technologic expertise undermines the manager's self-confidence as well as the trust and confidence of her or his staff. Successful achievement of developmental tasks associated with this stage is extremely important in the process of long-term career development. Many nurses remain in this stage throughout their careers, making a substantial contribution to the well-being of infants and experiencing a high degree of professional satisfaction (Perez, 1981).

Communicators and Translators of Neonatal Nursing Care Practices

During this stage, nurses begin to take responsibility for influencing, guiding, directing, and developing the skills of other people and are ready to become full members of the collaborative practice team. Nurses also broaden their interest and begin to involve themselves in professional activities at the regional and national levels. Many return to school for additional education or a graduate degree. Nurses interact with others outside the unit for the benefit of those on the unit.

The nurse begins to act as an informal mentor as an outgrowth of her or his personal esteem as a competent clinician. More work is expected because of the nurse's evolving capabilities; thus the nurse needs assistance if expectations are to continue to be met. The nurse accomplishes the work by seeking the assistance of parents and other health professionals for both the detail work and the development of personal ideas about neonatal care. In this way, the nurse becomes a mentor for those who help with the implementation of the role; in turn, she or he is mentored by more experienced nurses. The nurse may also become innovative during this stage. Unit staffs begin to contact this informal mentor nurse for suggestions on how to solve problems. At this developmental stage, the nurse becomes involved and influential in more than individual work: The nurse influences other nurses. The most common role initiated during this stage is that of manager or supervisor. The nature of relationships must change significantly in this new role. The nurse must begin to be sensitive to the needs of other nurses and assume responsibility for collaboration with a variety of disciplines (Perez, 1981). In addition, interpersonal skills in setting objectives, delegating, supervising, and coordinating must be developed.

At this point, the neonatal nurse has responsibilities to people at both higher and lower levels within the organization. The nurse must learn to cope with divided loyalties and with being in the middle. This situation requires developing confidence in the ability to produce results and helping others do the same. At this level, the neonatal nurse must be able to assist others in developing confidence by providing guidance and freedom. She or he must learn to experience success through the accomplishments of others. A delicate balance must be developed between providing direction for others and allowing them the freedom to explore and develop their skills.

The neonatal nurse must be psychologically willing to take responsibility for the output of another. At this level, responsibility is owed to the patient, the patient's family, and other providers. Technical skill must be maintained in this stage or the nurse will soon stagnate and be unable to keep up with other competitors.

Shapers and Generators of Neonatal Care Delivery Systems

Some nurses move onto another developmental stage. These nurses become shapers. They interface and negotiate with key segments of the NICU organization, developing new ideas, procedures, or services that lead to new areas of activity for the staff or directing the resources of the organization toward specific goals. The nurse at this developmental stage formulates policy and initiates and approves new programs (Perez, 1981). Intense relationships outside the organization are developed. Skills needed to influence outcomes such as personnel selection, resource allocation, and organizational design must be learned. Such neonatal nurses must be able to form alliances and take strong positions without feeling personal enmity toward people who have differing positions.

The concept of career stages for neonatal staff nurses has both pragmatic and theoretical implications for the NICU. Neonatal nurses are provided a framework for predicting the consequences of short-term career decisions. Managers are afforded a framework for predicting the consequences of their management decisions and for establishing unit structures that promote the development of neonatal nurses' knowledge and skills and enhance the outcomes of collaborative neonatal care. The implications of expecting nurses to demonstrate practice competencies before they have been developmentally achieved are clear.

Career stages also assist nurses in planning what needs to occur and how much time will be needed if they want to move onto another stage, and they assist the NICU staff in developing a structure that promotes career development (Harrigan, 1995). Career stages also provide a viable structure for the development of a career ladder.

ADVANCED NEONATAL NURSES PRACTICE: EXTENDED AND EXPANDED NEONATAL NURSING ROLES

Since the 1970s, there has been a national effort toward improving the outcome of care for high-risk neonates. The development of effective NICUs has increased the demand for experienced personnel available on a 24-hour basis in order to manage emergency neonatal problems. To help meet this demand, the American Academy of Pediatrics (AAP) in 1977 recommended the use of neonatal nurse practitioners in the NICU (Harper, Little, & Sia, 1982). This endorsement of the practitioner's role was based in part on concerns about a potentially excessive exposure of the pediatric house officer to NICUs during residency training. In order to maintain a well-balanced residency training program and an appropriate time commitment to newborn intensive care, it was believed by the AAP that extended-role nurses could adequately meet the demands for a portion of the personnel requirements. However, more recent concern about the need for cost containment has slowed the emergence of this role. In a number of settings, neonatologists have become concerned about the impact advanced practice neonatal nurses may have on their job security.

The employment of neonatal nurse practitioners who would be responsible for the medical management of patients required a redefinition of the traditional bounds of nursing practice. The scope of nursing practice in this role extends into the realm of medical practice and increases the need for collaborative planning of neonatal care.

No data are available to suggest that the practice of neonatal nurse practitioners is any less efficacious than that of physician providers. However, in general, few data are available, and the data that are available are from studies with very small samples. In addition, in these investigations, the practice of nurses was compared with that of student physicians (Johnson, Jung, & Boros, 1979). One fact is clear from a review of the literature: Investigations to date have evaluated the dependent component of these nursing roles—that is, their extended role into neonatal medicine—and not their expanded role in nursing or their overall impact on the cost of achieving defined care outcomes.

The concept of expanded and extended roles in nursing is not new. In fact, the development of nursing specialization is currently in its sixth decade. The term *extended role* was first used when nurse practitioners and physicians' assistants were referred to as physician extenders. *Extended-role practices* refers to the performance of practices previously considered medical; *expanded practice* refers to refinement and innovation within nursing. The difference between these two terms is more than semantic. In the past, much of the practice of the practitioner has been in the extended role, whereas that of the specialist has been primarily in the expanded nursing role. However, practice is changing, and recognition of the importance of both these roles and the blurring of the distinction between medical and nursing practices has contributed to the merging of these roles and incorporation of both components into the interdependent advanced practice of neonatal nursing (Bates, 1970). There is, beyond a doubt, an intense professional interest in and a recognized social need for the leadership of enterprising nurses and the availability of financial resources to support these roles. Trotter and Danaher (1994) completed a descriptive evaluation of the advanced practice role and reported that both professionals and families were very satisfied with the clinical skills, knowledge base, and contributions to patient care that neonatal nurse practitioners provided.

The practitioner in the extended role has a legacy: nursing is a practicing profession. The practitioner and specialist roles have provided alternative developmental paths that lead not to administration but to advanced neonatal nursing practice. This exceedingly important aspect tends to be underplayed. Expanded and extended practice roles have provided an incredibly significant clinical renaissance, a quiet revolution within nursing that has helped the profession not only to survive and keep pace with technology and practice demands but also to progress and strengthen itself despite dramatic and far-reaching changes in health care. Nurse practitioners and clinical specialists have turned advanced neonatal nursing into a complex, highly technologic enterprise.

Three activities of advanced practitioners have contributed to the improvement of neonatal care: (1) innovation and refinement of practice, (2) acceptance of control of neonatal nursing practice, and (3) development of a research basis for practice. A review of literature reveals that the publication of research has significantly increased since the 1970s (Perez-Woods, 1991). The same is true of books on neonatal nursing. Of interest is that the majority of authors are clinically prepared neonatal nurses and that many have been educated as practitioners and specialists.

Nurse specialists and practitioners have extended the boundaries of neonatal nursing practice in relation to both independent and dependent functions and have developed innovative forms of service. Nurse practitioners and specialists have established consultation and practice services, thus demonstrating independence and autonomy in a visible way to the public. The nursing profession has always been ambivalent about specialized practice. On the face of it, specialization suggests that what the ordinary nurse does can be done better by a more educated nurse. "A nurse is a nurse is a nurse" has for almost a century been a blinding myth in a profession having the widest possible heterogeneity in demographic, educational, and other characteristics of its members. The profession has been unwilling to determine what level of education is needed to deliver competent neonatal nursing care. Discussion within the American Nurses Association (1991) suggests that specialist and practitioner roles will be merged. The previous ambivalence, uncertainty, and lack of clarity about specialization and the advanced practice of neonatal nursing are giving way to a valuing and commitment to the contributions of advanced practice nurses. Nurses are beginning to value each other as they view the impact of work redesigning and the use of assistive personnel on patient management (McCanless, 1994). Neonatal nurses are demanding that their tiny patients receive care from nurses.

Advanced practitioners of nursing have a responsibility to the profession and to society to know the field of neonatal nursing extremely well. In addition, advanced practice neonatal nurses have a responsibility to know a great deal about neonatal medicine. Together with neonatal nurse researchers, nurse practitioners and specialists work at mastering knowledge of practice at the boundaries of nursing's domains. It is mastery over this domain that yields public confidence in neonatal nurses. The term *specialist* is preferable to the term *practitioner* because all nurses currently in neonatal nursing are practitioners. However, advanced practitioners require additional competencies to perform the practitioner role (Spitzer, 1978). The current hodgepodge of titles for practitioners with very different types of competencies is confusing to the public. Regrettably, and perhaps to our profession's detriment, virtually all titles in the range of possibilities have been used in both certification and postgeneric licensure laws on neonatal nursing.

Because of this ambivalence, we have often sought expedient measures and overlooked long-term consequences. We have gone with the flow rather than deciding on a position on the basis of reason, logic, or long-established tradition and then staying with it. Managed care and the implementation of care paths and care maps require that neonatal nurses move away from a process focus and develop an outcome-oriented practice focused on improving the outcomes of neonatal care (Harrigan, 1995). Common ground between the health professions is emerging and serves as the foundation of neonatal health care.

PRACTICE AND CREDENTIALING OF NEONATAL NURSES

There should be a relationship among the certification standards, requirements and options, and titles and content of curricula used to prepare advanced practitioners of nursing. Students as well as the public have the right to know whether the certification will be available and under what auspices and whether there is an acceptable level of congruence between program content and certification requirements. Legislation to control the development of advanced practice in neonatal nursing should not be sought. This control is a responsibility of the professional organization, and it has been accepted by the National Association of Neonatal Nurses (NANN, 1994).

The public also has a right to reasonable expectations about the competencies of nurse providers of neonatal care. This right is based on a social contract that the profession has with society. The profession turns to the public for economic resources in order to carry out its socially delegated mandate. In return, the public needs to know the nature of specialized services to be provided by neonatal nurses to meet the needs of society. The broadening field of practice of the neonatal nurse, authorized by society, carries with it the profession's responsibility for maintaining high educational standards. The credibility and trustworthiness of all neonatal nurses are compromised when any nurse or specialist decides to call herself or himself an advanced practitioner without having the credentials or skills and knowledge deemed appropriate by the profession. To represent oneself falsely to the public is indeed a gross violation of the public trust. The hallmark of an expert neonatal nurse is knowing the limits of her or his professional knowledge and recognizing the scope of practice. The profession has a responsibility to inform the public about advanced practitioners in neonatal nursing, and advanced practitioners have a responsibility to put before the public useful health information that they derive from their work. Employers have a right to know whether a nurse who claims to be a specialist is indeed so qualified, and they have a responsibility to verify credentials of neonatal nurse specialists.

The goals and norms of science are not identical to those of neonatal nurses. Scientists work primarily to accumulate a body of knowledge that can help us understand and explain the world around us. Neonatal nurses are primarily engaged in the delivery of care to newborns and the improvement of this care, and today these activities involve technology. The scientists' work is guided by the professional code of conduct (Donaldson & Crowley, 1978). Although scientists and neonatal nurses may have similar perspectives, the relative importance of criteria that they use to assess data may be different, depending on whether the goal is to develop a body of knowledge or to solve a health-related problem. Both nurses and scientists develop knowledge as they attempt to explain phenomena. An understanding of science is necessary both for the nurse who is to contribute to the body of scientific knowledge and for the nurse who is going to use the information that is produced.

Expert neonatal nurses must (1) be able to use appropriate knowledge, (2) have sufficient expertise to evaluate the knowledge for its appropriateness in improving the quality of life, and (3) contribute to the development of a body of knowledge relevant to neonatal health care (Sherwen, 1990). These goals will never be possible unless the neonatal nurse is competent in both a technical and a theoretical sense. Thus the education of neonatal nurses should occur in a graduate realm. Graduate programs to prepare neonatal nurse specialists must be committed to welding the practitioners' primary focus on the application of available knowledge with the scientists' interest in the expansion of knowledge. Neonatal nurses must be prepared to empirically investigate the adequacy of a statement's plausibility or the relevance of predictive factors associated with treatment approaches. Neonatal nurse research specialists are needed to conduct research and communicate the emerging scientific foundation for neonatal nursing practice.

Standardization of education on the master's level also provides a service to the profession by gaining educational parity with other health care professions (e.g., social work, pharmacy). Policy makers are very aware of formal educational credentials. When the advanced practice nurse possesses a "universal degree," such as the master's of science, it adds credibility to negotiating issues surrounding scope of practice such as prescriptive authority and third-party payment.

Hickey (1996) indicated that advanced practice graduate education must change to meet the new health care era. The areas that must be included or, if present, strengthened in this education are biologic sciences, computer literacy, clinical reasoning, health policy, and financial management. How does this translate to what the neonatal advanced practice nurses' educational program needs to be? It means that physiology, pathophysiology, genetics, fetal development, developmental physiology, and pharmacology must be considered essential elements of graduate education. These will underlie the art and science of nursing in scientific principles. Along with this scientific basis come the skills of critical thinking and application to neonatal care management. Further skills are needed in the politics of nursing. These include a very keen awareness of political health care issues/legislation that affects care and the profession of nursing. Financial management skills are also necessary to move the profession forward, to justify the nursing outcomes and their cost effectiveness, and to contribute meaningfully to the continuous quality improvement of neonatal care, including nursing's part of the total care package. Computer skills are necessary to keep abreast of changes in the education, practice, and research concerning neonatal care. They are also necessary to document what nursing does and what impact nursing has on neonatal outcomes. According to Hickey (1996, p. 357), this educational process should parallel the career paths for nurses (delineated earlier in this chapter). This type of thinking about neonatal nursing and its education is new but one that presents much potential for future growth.

CONCLUSION

Several important issues have been discussed in this chapter: the developmental aspects of neonatal nursing roles, the ambivalence among neonatal nurses about allowing better educated nurses to be called specialists, the merging of extended and expanded neonatal nursing roles into an advanced practice focus for neonatal nursing, the responsibility of students and practitioner to understand the basis for credentialing within the specialty, and the education of neonatal nurses for advanced practice. Five groups of neonatal nurses have been identified: *providers* of neonatal nursing care, *communicators* or managers of neonatal nursing practice, *translators* of research data into useful practice information, *generators* of knowledge for neonatal nursing practice, and *chapters* of policy related to neonatal health care. Today neonatal nursing is adapting to, as well as promoting, changes in the management of the health of the fragile infants for whom we care. Neonatal nursing management skills are needed both within the NICU as well as in home-care delivery systems. Neonatal nurses are in a unique position in this regard because of the significant impact they have on the family. Neonatal nursing roles will continue to evolve; we should therefore be flexible, systematic, and cogent in making practice decisions along the way.

REFERENCES

American Nurses Association (1991). *The American nurse.* Kansas City, MO: Author.

Bates, B. (1970). Doctor and nurse: Changing roles and relations. *New England Journal of Medicine, 283*(3), 129–134.

Dalton, G., & Thompson, P. (1971). Accelerating obsolescence of older engineers. *Harvard Business Review, 8,* 57–68.

Donaldson, S. K., & Crowley, D. M. (1978). The discipline of nursing. *Nursing Outlook, 26*(2), 113–120.

France, M. H., & McDowell, C. (1983). A systematic career development model: An overview. *Canadian Vocational Journal, 19*(1), 31–34.

Harrigan, R. C. (1995). Health care reform: Impact of managed care on perinatal and neonatal care delivery and education. *Journal of Perinatal Neonatal Nursing, 8*(4), 47–58.

Harper, R. G., Little, G. A., & Sia, C. G. (1982). The scope of nursing practice in level III neonatal intensive units. *Pediatrics, 70*(6), 875–878.

Hickey, J. V. (1996). Advanced practice nursing: Moving into the 21st century in practice, education, and research. In J. V. Hickey, R. M. Ouimette, & S. L. Venegoni (Eds.). *Advanced practice nursing: Changing roles and clinical application* (pp. 349–360). Philadelphia: J. B. Lippincott.

Johnson, P. J., Jung, A. L., & Boros, S. J. (1979). Neonatal nurse practitioners: Part 1. A new expanded nursing role. *Perinatology/Neonatology,* January–February, 34–36.

McCanless, L. L. (1994). Work redesign in the neonatal intensive care unit: Role development and training from an education perspective. *Journal of Perinatal Neonatal Nursing, 8*(3), 69–82.

NANN (1994). *Position Statement on Advanced Practice Nursing, NANN.* Petaluma, CA: National Association of Neonatal Nurses.

Perez, R. (1981). *Protocols for perinatal nursing practice.* St. Louis: C. V. Mosby.

Perez-Woods, R. (1991). *Data based publications in maternal-child health.* Unpublished manuscript. (University of Hawaii, 2528 The Mall, Honolulu, HI)

Sherwen, L. (1990). Interdisciplinary collaboration in perinatal/neonatal health care. A worthwhile challenge. *Journal of Perinatology, 10*(1), 1–2.

Spitzer, W. O. (1978). Pediatric nurse practitioners. *New England Journal of Medicine, 298*(3), 163–164.

Trotter, C., & Danaher, R. (1994). Neonatal nurse practitioners: A descriptive evaluation of an advanced practice role. *Neonatal Network, 13*(1), 39–47.

CHAPTER 2

Collaborative Practice in the Neonatal Intensive Care Unit

ROSANNE C. HARRIGAN DENNIS PEREZ

RESEARCH AGENDA

Identify and test strategies to promote collaborative practice

Explore the impact of the physical environment on neonatal staff interactions

Test the impact of collaborative case management on neonatal outcomes

The neonatal intensive care unit (NICU) has improved the prognosis for the critically ill newborn, particularly the low-birth-weight infant. This unique environment has brought together sophisticated technology and highly trained personnel, including physicians, nurses, laboratory technicians, respiratory therapists, and social workers. Today the environment of the NICU has moved into the home, necessitating distance collaborative management strategies to ensure optimal outcome achievement from home-care providers. The disciplined, professional group working in the high-technology environment of the home or NICU must develop a harmonious, collaborative spirit to achieve its aim: improving the welfare of the very fragile newborn and the newborn's family. The development of a collaborative spirit is a significant challenge in this paradoxical environment, in which the source of greatest stress and greatest satisfaction is the same: caring for desperately ill infants. Development of collaborative relationships can be both a satisfying and a productive experience.

The purpose of this chapter is to explore the concept of collaborative practice in achieving neonatal management outcomes. Collaborative practice is the delivery of care to patients and their families by using the resources of a variety of health care providers. Collaborative practice involves a group of individuals with different skills who work together to provide care (Temkin-Greener, 1983). Lamb and Napodano (1984) added that each person contributes to the decision-making process. The family also contributes to the decision-making, inasmuch as it is an integral part of the decision-making process (Aradine & Hansen, 1970). The concept of collaboration does not assume that the contribution of each member of the group of providers is equal, but it does acknowledge that each profession has something unique and important to contribute to the well-being of the infant and family. In addition, collaborative practice requires that professionals have mature role competence and highly developed technologic expertise. The ability of professionals to explicate their role and communicate their expertise to others while participating in strategic planning is essential (Aradine & Hansen, 1970; Leininger, 1971). The physician is not the overall authority in a collaborative approach (Aradine & Hansen, 1970). Leadership is decentralized, flexible, and problem-oriented (Ames & Perrin, 1980; Aradine & Hansen, 1970; Leininger, 1971; Shumaker & Goss, 1980; Temkin-Greener, 1983).

Collaborative care requires that outcome goals and care maps or critical pathways be established for the major health problems and developmental needs experienced by the neonate and family. Today, management outcomes focus both on care in the NICU and on management at home. Strategies to achieve these goals are then identified in the form of a care map or critical pathway. (For more information on the development and use of critical pathways, see the Appendix.) The implementation and modification of the plan are coordinated by a designated case manager. A case manager is an expert practitioner who serves to coordinate formal and informal health services for an individual child and family (Gilles, 1991; Hickey, 1996). Identification of a case manager is essential because families experience significant anxiety during this period, and a consistent relationship with a consistent health care provider such as a case manager assists with communication and reduces anxiety. Case managers are also responsible for the consistency, efficiency, and timeliness of neonatal management (Harrigan, 1995).

In this chapter, the factors associated with the development of collaborative practice environments are described, and the strategies known to promote collaborative practice are explored.

CREATING THE CONTEXT

Collaborative practice environments are based on the belief that the results of the collaborative efforts of a group of dedicated professionals are greater than the results achieved by each of the professionals acting independently. Collaborative practice environments result from the communication and cooperation among health care professionals (Aminu, 1985). Such professionals recognize that the collective effort of a number of talented professionals is needed to achieve neonatal outcomes efficiently and consistently. Because of the variety of backgrounds and experiences that each professional brings to the care of the neonate, there are more ideas, skills, and information with which to seek solutions. In order for collaboration to occur, dedicated, cooperative professionals are needed (Aminu, 1985).

It is also essential to view the developmental context in which collaboration occurs. The context includes what the professionals bring to the care of the neonate and what they have to contribute. Professional development is influenced by interactions with others in the caregiving environment. Growth is influenced by the environmental and personal context within the unit. The developmental context is evolutionary and consists of a combination of factors specific to the situation and point in time. There are philosophical, structural, and dynamic correlates of contexts that support collaboration.

Philosophical Correlates

Collaborative care environments require dedication on the part of professional providers to the process of identifying their values concerning patient care. The process used to define shared values requires professionals to recognize their own value system, gain a better understanding of themselves, and compare their beliefs with those of other providers. Ethical conflicts that exist are identified and discussed (Erlen, 1994). There is opportunity for compromise, resolution, or refinement; making the decision to leave the system is also an option.

The development of collaborative practice goals requires constancy. Constancy is the consistent implementation of principles as the basis for clinical decision-making related to goal achievement. Consistency is needed for the development of trust, which is a basic element of collaboration. For example, in order for a collaborative health care team to function effectively, there must be general agreement on the basic concepts of professional practice (Aradine & Hansen, 1970). This agreement includes an understanding not only of one's own profession but also of a colleague's profession. This understanding is important because there are areas that are unique to each profession and areas that overlap with other professions (Aradine & Hansen, 1970). For example, both a nurse and a psychologist may provide emotional support to a neonate's family, but their responsibilities concerning the administration of medication would not overlap (although nurses and physicians may have overlapping responsibilities in this area). Shared values are represented in the individualization of a critical path or care map to a specific unit. (See the Appendix for examples of critical pathways.)

Development of constancy is compromised in units in which there are frequent nursing staff turnover; many rotating house staff, students, and faculty; and weak leadership. A significant investment of time is needed in order to reveal personal attitudes, clarify value systems, and develop trusting relationships. In a collaborative practice environment, additional time is also necessary to develop an understanding of the attitudes and values of others. Value conflicts often arise during the development or refinement of care maps or critical pathways. The consensus that evolves provides the foundation for the selection of principles that reflect unit values and goals that do not conflict with the beliefs of any individual staff member. The use of collaborative partnerships between service and academia for mediation may be of assistance in resolving conflicts (Organek & Hegedus, 1993).

The principles also serve as a basis for the evaluation of patient care outcomes to be achieved by the unit staff. In mature collaborative systems, the principles and goals are written and formalized. Oral communication of outcome goals is no longer the norm (Harrigan, 1995); today, collaborative development of written care maps is the norm.

Philosophical belief systems are continuously evolving and are subject to change. Changes can be the result of the addition of new staff with values and beliefs different from those of the current staff, changes in the values and beliefs of the current staff, changes in the patient care environment, or changes in care models (i.e., managed care). Ongoing opportunity should be provided for input from new unit staff as well as for expression of the changing views of continuing staff members and administrators. Opportunity for participation should be available for all disciplines involved with outcome achievement, especially in managing long-term patient care outcome goals (Miller, Mutton, & Williams, 1993). Affirmation of identified belief systems at designated intervals is highly desirable.

Structural Correlates

Both physical and organizational aspects of the neonatal care system structure have an impact on the nature of the collaborative practice environment. Five aspects of the physical environment—the location of the equipment used to provide care, the locations of offices of leadership personnel, the location of communication equipment, communication flow patterns, and traffic flow patterns—are of primary concern. Characteristics of the organization of medical, nursing, and allied health staff also have the potential to affect collaboration. The organization of the perinatal system or managed care network, as well as cultural characteristics of families, should be considered. Several investigations have related personnel stress and burnout with structural and organizational factors (Consolvo, Brownewell, & Distefano, 1989; Rosenthal, Schmid, & Black, 1989). Nurses were often socialized into systems in which they lacked power to develop health care delivery patterns and were sheltered from the impact of health care decisions because of the place they held in the system structure. Passive acceptance of new care models such as managed care will only cause further problems associated with this role (Harrigan, 1995). Failure to provide data-based documentation of the value-added outcomes associated with professional nursing will result in diminished nursing resources within provider systems (Harrigan, 1995).

Physical factors such as the location of the offices of both nurse and physician leadership personnel can significantly affect availability and involvement with collaboration. The clinical specialist with an office on, rather than off, the unit is far more likely to be a collaborator. The use of space planners has significantly improved the flow of interactions on NICUs. In numerous NICUs across the country, however, the NICU staffs are separated both physically and organizationally. Although early discharge and referral to home care are now the norm, well-developed structures for collaborative planning and communication between the NICU staff and home-care agencies are rare.

In the NICU at Foster McGaw Hospital in Chicago, placement of all equipment and supplies and a communication system at the bedside of individual infants has improved collaborative decision-making. Although such anecdotal reports abound, little research has been done to study the impact of physical environments in the NICU on the interactions of staff. Well-designed studies focusing on the impact of physical space on caregiving would be of significant value to the profession. Literature from other fields, such as business, certainly confirms the importance of space design on the development of human interactions. In some NICUs, overcrowding is a significant barrier to collaboration. Space planning should include consideration of the caregiving physical environment, work flow patterns, location of offices for leadership personnel, and physical equipment for communication.

The organization of medical and nursing services can reveal a great deal about the probability of developing collaborative practice in the neonatal care system. Organizational structures that are centralized and hierarchical provide the greatest challenge for collaboration, whereas those that allow for decentralized decision-making are the best (Aradine & Hansen, 1970). Collaboration requires that each individual's ability to contribute to clinical decision-making be recognized (Sherwen, 1990). Collaborative practice is not a team for which the coach makes all the calls. Evaluation of the organizational structures and decision-making norms used by each group concerned with the patient outcomes in the neonatal care system is an important element of developing collaboration. The questions raised are as follows: are the groups committed to collaboration, and are the values, attitudes, and goals proposed by the members of the groups reflected in the organizational structure chosen to manage the group? Concern regarding the use of hierarchical models and residual concerns about territoriality have prohibited the development of organizational structures that integrate neonatal care services. Investigation of integrated organizational structures through the use of controlled research designs is warranted. Organizational models that are fully integrated and evaluated by use of quantitative measures of quality are needed. Successful collaborative systems require efficiency and recognized quality service at a low price. Systems must also be responsive to customers. High standards of care will be the hallmarks of successful competitors, and innovative structures to monitor, measure, and manage clinical performance will be the norm (Harrigan, 1995).

Organizational structures of groups of care providers are not static entities. They often reflect the developmental status of the group. Groups move from dependent centralized organizational structures to participative, self-directed, decentralized structures as they mature. However, stress caused by the demands of care provision staff turnover or availability can alter the organizational structure preferred by a group. As in other aspects of human development, organizational development occurs in stages, and stress may cause a return to an earlier stage of development. It is time for the discipline of nursing to experiment with new models of patient care management and to create cultures that embrace collaborative patient care management, continuous quality improvement, or the like. For the first time in the delivery of health care in the United States, there is a premium associated with prevention and a profit associated with realigned incentives (Harrigan, 1995). Rewards will be provided to those who can eliminate operational efficiencies and inappropriate caregiving practices. Collaborative structures are no longer just desirable; they are required. Regionalized perinatal system structures are disappearing and being replaced by systems that include primary care providers, home-care services, and specialty services. Financing is needed to develop neonatal home-care providers capable of managing technology, case finding, and provision of social support (Cooke, Schwartz, & Gagnon, 1989).

Once an evaluation of the organizational structure of each professional group providing service on the unit has occurred, identification of similarities, differences, and the potential for collaboration is possible. Believe it or not, collaboration does not work for all units. Collaboration requires a commitment to interdependence. Many professions function within primarily autonomous or primarily dependent types of organizational structures. Adherence to these types of organizational structures is not compatible with collaborative practice. Organizational characteristics that suggest successful collaboration include (1) low staff turnover (you must know someone in order to collaborate with her or him); (2) adequate numbers of staff; (3) decentralized decision-making; and (4) delegation of authority of caregiving to small groups of staff for a cohort of patients (Sherwen, 1990). The most important factor for effective team functioning is a clear understanding of the different roles of health care professionals (Beckhard, 1972; Nagi, 1975). This understanding may also be the most difficult area in the development of a health care team because the exact roles of health care professionals are difficult to define in terms of their unique aspects. As mentioned earlier, different health care professionals often perform the same tasks because of overlapping skills. Systems that are needed include interdisciplinary community-based planning; integrated structure and accountability; integrated data collection, documentation, and evaluation; and innovative approaches to financing (March of Dimes Birth Defects Foundation, 1993).

Dynamic Correlates

Both professional and personal dynamics must be considered within the collaborative context. Professional dynamics that project mutual support, respect for persons, and the recognition of the contribution that each group provides to patient outcomes encourage collaboration. These professional characteristics are usually reflections of personal qualities that the individual brings to the caregiving setting. It is unusual for a person to portray one set of values and attitudes as a professional and another set of values on a personal level. Evaluation of a potential staff member's values and beliefs can do a great deal to assist with the development of collaborative care environments. Concern with merely filling a vacancy with a qualified nurse or physician often prevents recognition of the potential impact of a values conflict on the dynamics of the group. Exploration of an applicant's value system should be an essential component of the interview process. No matter how brilliant the applicant, values conflicts can alter and potentially destroy a collaborative practice environment.

The evolution of collaborative practice is a developmental process. A new staff member focuses primarily on technical aspects of care and after 6 to 9 months begins to develop a notion of self as a professional provider in the NICU and often believes that she or he knows more than other professionals and parents about what is appropriate for an individual infant. During this developmental stage, the nurse has difficulty interacting with others and is not amenable to a collaborative mode of professional practice. However, transition to the communicator level of development soon occurs (see Chapter 1, Neonatal Nursing and Its Role in Comprehensive Care). The nurse in the first developmental stage (technician) practices in a dependent role, whereas during the second developmental stage, practice is characterized by independence and at times counterindependence. Territoriality is an additional characteristic of the second stage of professional development. This stage may persist for 1 to 2 years. During the first two developmental stages, professionals function best in associate care roles. Full participation in a collaborative care environment is difficult.

Collaborative practice requires participation from experienced neonatal staff: those who are at the expert or contracted clinician level of development. At this level, professionals are able to identify their roles clearly, specify their limitations, and accept responsibility for implementing their role. Managers must have a vision of the ingredients needed to form a successful collaborative group and of the patient care goals to be achieved. The developmental process that is required before successful collaborative practice environments can be achieved needs to be anticipated. The expertise of experienced staff is needed to assist with the socialization of new members to the collaborative professional group.

DEVELOPING A VISION

There are four major factors associated with the development of a vision of a collaborative practice environment: (1) realistic role expectations; (2) acceptance of responsibility; (3) recognition of limitations; and (4) resolution of territoriality.

Mature clinicians with experience in the delivery of neonatal care develop an understanding of the contributions and limitations of all the different care providers. It is unfortunate that most nurses are not socialized into their role in collaborative care environments, in which mutual respect and role competence of the different types of care providers can be appreciated. Often the preceptor of the neonatal nurse is another staff nurse who is not ready to mentor. The development of collaborative care environments requires that managers appreciate the impact of socialization and mentorship on the development of professional values and attitudes. Internships or fellowships in collaborative practice settings assist with the development of realistic role expectations, as does the opportunity to be associated with mature, experienced practitioners. Collaborative practice is a role more appropriate for the experienced neonatal nurse (expert or contracted clinician). Nurses at the technical or surrogate parent level of development have significant difficulty with this role.

Once role expectations have been identified, responsibility for the role assumed must be accepted. This acceptance of responsibility is not as easy as it may seem. Collaborative practice roles are demanding and require a commitment that may extend beyond the traditional assigned scheduled shift. Traditional scheduling systems for patient management by nurses can be a barrier to collaboration because professionals must be present when they are needed by a particular newborn and family. In NICUs in which flexibility cannot be accommodated, a traditional case manager system may not be appropriate. Unit-based case managers have been tried with varying degrees of success. This model of care requires further exploration.

Collaborative practice requires that the expert practitioner recognize her or his limitations. Trust between members of the collaborative practice group is dependent on the ability of group members to indicate when they are in over their heads and in need of the expertise of another professional. Collaboration is dependent on the ability of members of the group to recognize the expertise that they have to contribute and to acknowledge their limitations. Collaboration would be unnecessary if the skill of any one member of the group was sufficient to achieve the identified patient care goals.

Territoriality is a characteristic of most professional disciplines. Territoriality begins where the boundaries of a profession become clear. Collaboration requires that lines that box professions in separate containers be removed from time to time to achieve the best interests of the patient. Territoriality is also characteristic of environments in neonatal care systems in which there are few truly expert or contracted clinicians and many new group members. Most new members of a profession have been effectively socialized to believe that they have an independent practice mode and that dependency on others is a sign of weakness rather than a sign of strength. Learning to be interdependent takes time and trust. Mature, experienced clinicians can trust others in their group to provide care, recognizing that they can seek assistance of other group members whenever it is needed. Nursing must reduce its focus on autonomy and develop a power structure within an integrated organizational system.

COMMUNICATING VISION

In NICUs in which there is a constant change in staff (e.g., university medical centers), collaboration is possible only when there are empowering visionary health care professionals. Empowerment is the process of making staff believe that they can do their job and that what they do makes a difference. Visionary care providers must communicate their vision by using metaphors that are understandable to all members of the group. Each individual member of the group must be helped to value her or his contribution toward the achievement of patient care goals for the infants and their families. The neonatal care system is a challenging and often frustrating work environment, in which socialization of new staff members must include not only unit policies and procedures but also incorporation of a vision, reflecting care goals for the unit. This socialization process takes at least a year, and expectations that a staff member will be a productive member of a collaborative practice group before this time are unreasonable. Socialization of new staff members is a responsibility for the most mature members of the collaborative practice group. The socialization experience should also include experience with all system components, including the home care.

Visionary care providers are responsible for the empowerment of the infants and their families as well as members of the staff. Parents and community involvement in the care of high-risk neonates is essential for the achievement of both short-term and long-term developmental goals for these infants. The family established the primary value system for the infant. Families must learn that they have significant contributions to make to the fragile humans for whom we care (Aradine & Hansen, 1970). In the neonatal care system, in which parents and staff are bombarded with information, the role of assertive health care professionals is to integrate information and facts into meaningful knowledge.

Collaboration reflects the communication of a vision, a vision so clear to the members of the staff that all are committed to the same goals as the infant and family. This commitment is made within an environment in which values and attitudes are shared. Approaches to the care of infants are consistent, and families believe that they play an important and valued role in management.

CONCLUSION

Collaboration is the commitment of an entire group of care providers to shared values, approaches to care, and treatment goals. Collaborative care assumes that a group of disciplined professionals is present, each with a unique contribution to make to the well-being of the neonate and family. Collaboration is the result of a developmental process through which the visions of talented health care professionals are communicated to the group and shared values and goals are developed. Collaborative practice demands responsibility and recognition of limitations from mature, expert clinicians. Collaborative practice is the practice model of choice for delivery of services to fragile, sick newborns in the highly technical intensive care unit and to their vulnerable families.

REFERENCES

Ames, A., & Perrin, J. M. (1980). Collaborative practice: The joining of two professionals. *Journal of the Tennessee Medical Association, 73*(8), 557–560.

Aminu, J. (1985). Teaming up for better health. *Social Science and Medicine, 21*(12), 1349–1353.

Aradine, C. R., & Hansen, M. F. (1970). Interdisciplinary teamwork in family health care. *Nursing Clinics of North America, 5*(2), 211–222.

Beckhard, R. (1972). Organizational issues in the team delivery of comprehensive health care. *Milbank Memorial Fund Quarterly, 50*(3), 287–316.

Consolvo, C. A., Brownewell, V., & Distefano, S. M. (1989). Profile of the hardy NICU nurse. *Journal of Perinatology, 9*(3), 334–337.

Cooke, S. S., Schwartz, S. M., & Gagnon, D. E. (1989). *Perinatal partnership: An approach to organizing care in the 1990s.* Princeton, NJ: Robert Wood Johnson Foundation.

Erlen, J. A. (1994). Ethical dilemmas in the high-risk nursery: Wilderness experiences. *Journal of Pediatric Nursing, 9*(1), 21–26.

Gilles, C. (1991). Nonsurgical management of the infant with gastroesophageal reflux and respiratory problems. *Journal of the American Academy of Nursing Practice, 3*(1), 11–16.

Harrigan, R. C. (1995). Health care reform: Impact of managed care on perinatal and neonatal care delivery and education. *Journal of Perinatal Neonatal Nursing, 8*(4), 47–58.

Hickey, J. V. (1996). Advanced practice nursing: Moving into the 21st century in practice, education, and research. In J. V. Hickey, R. M. Ouimette, & S. L. Venegoni (Eds.). *Advanced practice nursing: Changing roles and clinical application* (pp. 349–360). Philadelphia: J. B. Lippincott.

Lamb, G. S., & Napodano, R. J. (1984). Physician–nurse practitioner interaction patterns in primary care practices. *American Journal of Public Health, 74*(1), 26–29.

Leininger, M. (1971). This I believe: About interdisciplinary health education for the future. *Nursing Outlook, 19*(12), 787–791.

March of Dimes Birth Defects Foundation. (1993). *Toward improving the outcome of pregnancy: The 1990s and beyond.* White Plains, NY: Author.

Miller, M., Mutton, C., & Williams, B. F. (1993). Collaborative experiences for NICU and early childhood education personnel. *Neonatal Network, 12*(7), 37–42.
Nagi, S. Z. (1975). Teamwork in care in the U.S.: A sociological perspective. *Milbank Memorial Fund Quarterly/Health and Society, 53*(1), 75–91.
Organek, N., & Hegedus, K. (1993). Advanced practice: A model for neonatal/perinatal and women/child nursing. *AACN Clinical Issues in Critical Care Nursing, 4*(4), 631–636.
Rosenthal, S. L., Schmid, K. D., & Black, M. M. (1989). Stress and coping in a NICU. *Research in Nursing and Health, 12*(4), 257–265.
Sherwen, L. (1990). Interdisciplinary collaboration in perinatal/neonatal health care. A worthwhile challenge. *Journal of Perinatology, 10*(1), 1–2.
Shumaker, D., & Goss, V. (1980). Toward collaboration: One small step. *Nursing and Health Care, 1*(4), 183–185.
Temkin-Greener, H. (1983). Interprofessional perspectives on teamwork in health care: A case study. *Milbank Memorial Fund Quarterly/Health and Society, 61*(4), 641–657.

CHAPTER 3

Ethical Aspects of Perinatal Care

SHEILA M. SOUTHWELL HELEN ARCHER-DUSTÉ

RESEARCH AGENDA

What are the family's views on perinatal medicine?

What are the nurse's views on ethical issues in perinatal medicine?

Examine both the parents' and the nurse's attitudes and views on perinatal ethics

What is the impact of health care reform on ethical issues facing neonatal nurses?

VIGNETTE

The diagnosis of fetal hypoplastic left ventricle was made at 36 weeks' gestation by sonogram and confirmed by intrauterine echocardiogram. The parents (the Ps) were fully apprised of the options available. They later told me that they did not make any decisions because they hoped the medical diagnosis would be wrong. It is a common phenomenon for parents to hold on to hope despite significant medical evidence.

Baby Matthew was born by repeat C-section 3 weeks later. Except for his pale, dusky color in room air, this big ($10\frac{1}{2}$-lb.), vigorous baby looked as if he might have fulfilled his parents' secret hope. After an initial bonding period with his family, Matthew was transferred to the special care nursery (SCN) for assessment and cardiology consultation.

Vital signs: pulse, 146 with a loud murmur; respiratory rate, 68. Breath sounds were clear. Initial pulse oximeter reading was 88; concurrent arterial blood gases: pH, 7.29; PCO_2, 57; PO_2, 36; and BE, 0. BPs: equal in all four extremities. Hematocrit and blood glucose were within normal limits.

Mr. P and grandparents arrived at the SCN as soon as the C-section was over. All were solemn and concerned. They touched and talked to Matthew and asked appropriate questions of the staff. The cardiologist arrived and conducted a full assessment, including echo- and electrocardiograms. During the long assessment, Matthew appeared to pink up as he sucked on his pacifier. Matthew's mother arrived at the SCN by stretcher during his testing. She held him and seemed relieved by his appearance. "I've been worrying about you," she said to him as she gently outlined his facial features with one fingertip.

After Mrs. P and family settled in her room, the cardiologist and I (primary nurse) arrived for a conference. The cardiologist showed drawings of a normal heart and blood circulation and then compared it with Matthew's heart and circulation. "Matthew has aortic atresia, meaning the ascending aorta did not develop correctly, along with a very tiny and weak left ventricle. He cannot live very long." "But he looks so good," his mother said wearily. "Yes, he does, because his body is being supplied in this way"—the cardiologist drew some arrows to illustrate blood flow from the right ventricle through the pulmonary arteries to an open duct. "This is tremendous work for the heart, so it cannot keep this up for too long." The cardiologist went on to discuss three treatment options: (1) heart transplantation, which would require long distance transport to an appropriate facility; (2) a series of three Norwood operations, to be done during the first year of life, with low chances of survival; and (3) no surgery, which means the baby would probably live several days to weeks.

The Ps had heard all this before, so they had few questions. There were several moments of silence. Matthew's mother began to cry. I comforted her. Matthew's father took a deep breath, squared his shoulders, and spoke, "We have pondered this decision for the past month. We wished all the tests would be proven wrong when . . . ." His voice trailed off. "But as they were correct, we chose for no surgery to be done. The other options show few survivors, and we cannot put him through all that pain if there is little hope of success." The physician and I assured the family that the staff would make Matthew comfortable and be available to answer questions and concerns. Mother wanted to have her son in her room as much as possible for their few short days together. I encouraged Mr. P to stay with his family at the hospital.

I brought Matthew to his mother's room and cared for them that day and throughout the week. I assisted her with breastfeeding and newborn care. As the days went by, Matthew remained pale pink, sometimes slightly dusky with exertion. Otherwise he acted as if nothing was unusual. Mother–infant attachment was progressing normally. She sometimes laughingly referred to him as "Mr. Sleep-and-Eat." And yet she talked of the inevitability of his death. Sometimes she cried; sometimes she was resigned. She asked how it would happen, so I described some of the obvious signs and symptoms of congestive heart failure and hypoxia. Even after a short separation, she would question staff about any changes in his condition. The options were discussed and rediscussed by the family. They always came back to their original decision, because the options were painful and virtually hopeless.

Five days passed, and Mrs. P was discharged from the hospital. She wanted to take her son home: "I just can't leave him here. I have to be with him when his time comes." The cardiologist affirmed that Matthew did not require hospital care and that he would be discharged at the parents' request. Mr. P voiced concern about their 4-year-old daughter's response to the baby and his inevitable death.

I discussed sibling response to an infant's death. The Ps described their child's developmental level, and we discussed possible perceptions of death and the necessary preparation for their older child. The Ps indicated that they felt their daughter would be able to cope, given appropriate preparation. I wrote a care plan that included preparation, degree of participation in the actual death, follow-up care, and a referral for siblings who grieve. The Ps seemed enthusiastic about taking Matthew home. "I've got to put the crib up," Mr. P smiled. It seemed there was comfort in being able to parent his baby, even for a short time.

The Ps felt comfortable with infant care. They felt nighttime help was necessary. They did not want Matthew to be alone. I arranged for night care. The Ps left the hospital as any other family that afternoon: mother holding baby, father toting bags and flowers, and a sibling dancing in front of the wheelchair all the way to the car.

I called the next day, and Mrs. P reported that things were going well. I received the same report several days later. When Matthew was 9 days old, he began to have shortness of breath and dyspnea with feeding. His condition deteriorated until he expired in his mother's arms 2 days later. I kept in touch with the family throughout this time, during the funeral, and afterward. Their daughter responded as anticipated, and the parents felt that the care plan helped them assist her in understanding and coping skills. At my last contact with them, the Ps expressed conviction that the whole experience had been handled in the best possible way. They strongly believed in their treatment decision: they had done the right thing for Matthew. Still, they would have given anything to have changed the outcome.

Joyce M. Dohme

The practice of neonatal nursing requires expertise in clinical decision-making, collaboration, and ethical problem-solving. Neonatal intensive care units (NICUs) are a relatively new feature in the critical care arena and are characterized by complex, sometimes competing, perspectives. The technologic and scientific advances that led to the development of NICUs have engendered the key questions identified by the nurse: reproductive technologies, prenatal evaluation and intervention, withholding and withdrawing of life support, fetal versus maternal rights, and access to care concerns. In this milieu, the role of the professional nurse is essential in collaboration with other health care professionals to ensure that the interests of the neonate and the neonate's family are safeguarded.

The purpose of this chapter is to provide the nurse with an overview of ethical principles, an awareness of recurring issues in neonatal care, and the tools with which to approach decision-making. It is not an exhaustive exploration of the topics; use of the recommended readings and sources is encouraged.

A HERITAGE OF ADVOCACY

The heritage of the nursing profession is one of caring and advocacy. Although the profession has evolved greatly since the 1960s, these primary values remain intact. Nursing is the application of a distinct body of knowledge and skill in the care of human beings. It is a humanistic experience and therefore has its own moral tradition. Styles (1982) described it this way: "I believe in nursing as a humanistic field, in which the fullness, self-respect, self-determination, and humanity of the nurse engage the fullness, self-respect, self-determination, and humanity of the client" (p. 61).

Articulation of these values is evident in the early publications of organized nursing and in early literature. The American Nurses' Association's (ANA's) contemporary *Code for Nurses* is derived from the original (1893) Florence Nightingale Pledge (Gretter, 1956):

> I solemnly pledge myself before and in the presence of this assembly, to pass my life in purity and to practice my profession faithfully.
>
> I will abstain from whatever is deleterious and mischievous, and will not take or knowingly administer any harmful drug.
>
> I will do all in my power to maintain and elevate the standard of my profession; and will hold in confidence all personal matters committed to my keeping, and all family affairs coming to my knowledge in the practice of my calling.
>
> With loyalty will I endeavor to aid the physician in this work and devote myself to the welfare of those committed to my care.

The concepts and language of the *Code for Nurses* (Table 3–1) make explicit the direct relationship and obligations of the nurse to the patient. The code embodies abiding concern for the four

TABLE 3–1 Code for Nurses

1. The nurse provides services with respect for human dignity and the uniqueness of the client, unrestricted by considerations of social or economic status, personal attributes, or the nature of health problems.
2. The nurse acts to safeguard the client's right to privacy by judiciously protecting information of a confidential nature.
3. The nurse safeguards the client and the public when health care and safety are affected by the incompetent, unethical, or illegal practice of any person.
4. The nurse assumes responsibility and accountability for individual nursing judgements and actions.
5. The nurse maintains competence in nursing.
6. The nurse exercises informed judgment and uses individual competence and qualifications as criteria in seeking consultation, accepting responsibilities, and delegating nursing activities to others.
7. The nurse participates in activities that contribute to the ongoing development of the profession's body of knowledge.
8. The nurse participates in the profession's efforts to implement and improve standards of nursing.
9. The nurse participates in the profession's efforts to establish and maintain conditions of employment conducive to high-quality nursing care.
10. The nurse participates in the profession's effort to protect the public from misinformation and misrepresentation and to maintain the integrity of nursing.
11. The nurse collaborates with members of the health professions and other citizens in promoting community and national efforts to meet the health needs of the public.

Reprinted with permission from American Nurses' Association. (1985). *Code for Nurses with Interpretive Statements.* Kansas City, MO: Author.

root ethical principles of autonomy, nonmalfeasance, beneficence, and justice.

The second document serving as a cornerstone of nursing's ethical belief system is the ANA's *Nursing: A Social Policy Statement* (1980, 1995). This masterwork delineates the distinct contract between the nursing profession and society:

> Nursing, like other professions, is an essential part of the society out of which it grew and with which it has been evolving. Nursing can be said to be owned by society, in the sense that nursing's professional interest must be and must be perceived as serving the interests of the larger whole of which it is a part (ANA, 1980, p. 3).

The ANA's *Standards for Clinical Practice* (1991) state that the nurse's decisions and actions on behalf of clients are determined in an ethical manner. Together the *Code for Nurses*, the *Social Policy Statement*, and the *Standards for Clinical Practice* provide the mandate for nurses' participation in ethical deliberations.

Neonatal nursing is largely practiced in an organizational context. Much has been written about the professional-bureaucratic conflict and interprofessional conflict experienced by the professional nurse (Ashley, 1976; Benne & Bennis, 1959; Corwin, 1961; Etzioni, 1969; Grissum & Spengler, 1976; Hall, 1982; Jacox, 1978; Mauksch, 1976; Seward, 1969; Vollmer & Mills, 1966; Wandelt et al., 1981). Fralic (1983) summarized this role confusion: "The organization sees the professional as a resource to be utilized—the professional sees the organization as a resource to be used while accomplishing professional and personal goals" (p. 662). When organizational goals are in conflict with professional intentions, moral distress can result. The relationship between nursing and medicine has further compounded this role conflict. Traditionalists see only the dependent component of nursing practice, leading to a lack of collaboration, unhealthy interpersonal dynamics, and dissonance in decision-making. If the nurse is viewed exclusively as an agent of the physician or the institution, the nurse cannot fulfill a primary obligation to the public.

This positioning of nursing in the organizational matrix may be viewed as a disadvantage. The autonomous, risk-taking nurse may feel vulnerable in an environment that expects obedience and codified behavior. It is a mutual responsibility of nurses in both clinical and leadership roles to institute organizational elements that preserve and sustain the relationship of the nurse to the client. The *Standards for Accreditation* of the Joint Commission for Accreditation of Healthcare Organizations (JCAHO; 1995) require institutional mechanisms for resolution of ethical conflicts. Of equal importance is the development of nurses' skills in ethical deliberation. All too frequently, communication issues and interpersonal behaviors are misidentified as ethical concerns. Appropriate structures might include clinical ethics rounds, a formal mechanism for the identification and resolution of ethical questions, an administrative–medical staff coalition that recognizes the key value of nursing's participation in ethical decision-making, and joint-practice committees and peer support groups (Edens et al., 1990). The implementation of such a professional practice model in a given nursing unit provides structural and behavioral assurance of the viability of nursing's primary accountability to the client.

CLINICAL ETHICS

Clinical ethics has frequently been equated with medical ethics. This misconception is based on the notion that the nurse–client relationship is secondary to the physician–client relationship. As the previous discussion affirms, the scope of clinical ethics is larger and incorporates the problems and situations that nurses encounter in the independent and collaborative domains of practice.

The terms *ethics* and *morality* are commonly used interchangeably. The concepts are distinct but interrelated. Morality is established by consensus and conveys a sense of a common social tradition or acceptable behaviors. Ethics is the area of intellectual contemplation beyond the simple acceptance of social norms (Fowler, 1987).

The field of ethics has its roots in theology and philosophy and is a complex, specialized area of study. It is divided into two major categories: nonnormative, which includes metaethics and descriptive ethics, and normative ethics. Metaethics is concerned with the inquiry into the meaning, logic, and semantics of ethics. The work is not immediately applicable to everyday situations but is of scholarly significance. Descriptive ethics is the examination of the values of subgroups of society and the development of human moral reasoning. Metaethics and descriptive ethics are nonnormative; they do not prescribe behaviors (Fowler, 1987). Normative ethics is the exploration of ethical norms or standards and their application to the human world.

Two key elements constitute normative ethics: norms of obligation and norms of moral value. Norms of obligation specify duties of obligations for human behavior. Two schools of thought discuss these obligations. Teleologists assert that an action can be judged right or wrong by the consequences of the action as measured against a specific end that is sought. The common illustration of teleologic thought is utilitarianism: "the greatest possible balance of values over disvalue for all persons who would be affected" (Beauchamp & Childress, 1983, p. 20). This perspective is also defined as goal-based or outcome-based reasoning: the best good for the most people. Deontologic thought affirms that the intrinsic quality of the action determines its rightness or wrongness. A set of rules serves as the foundation for decision-making. These rules are universally applicable and recognize individuals as persons of absolute worth. This approach is also known as duty-based reasoning (Fowler, 1987). An example of this decision-making is found in Figure 3–1.

Norms of moral values identify that which is good or bad in humans. Norms of nonmoral values analyze that which is good or bad in things. Together, norms of obligation and norms of moral values compose the field of normative ethics. The application of normative ethics to specific issues, cases, or situations is called *applied ethics*. The *Code for Nurses* is an example of applied ethics. It establishes a normative standard for a specific professional group.

Root Principles

Four root principles of ethical decision-making have been described by multiple scholars: autonomy, nonmalfeasance, beneficence, and justice (Beauchamp & Childress, 1983; Fowler, 1987). From these root principles, other ethical rules are derived, including accountability, veracity, integrity, confidentiality, and fidelity.

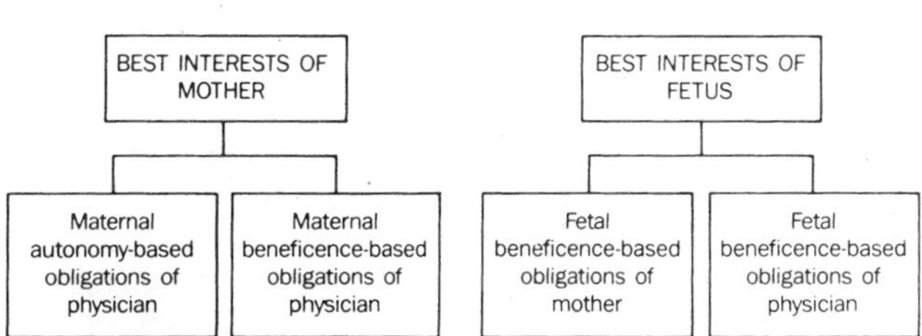

FIGURE 3–1. Moral obligations in obstetrical care. (From Chervenak, F. A., & McCullough, L. B. [1985]. Perinatal ethics: A practical method of analysis of obligations to mother and fetus. *Obstetrics and Gynecology, 66*[3], 443. Reprinted with permission from the American College of Obstetricians and Gynecologists.)

The application of these principles to ethical questions can assure the nurse of acceptable and appropriate intervention.

The concept of *autonomy* implies self-governance: the ability to be one's own person without constraints from others. Three issues are related to the principle of autonomy: advocacy, competence, and informed consent. The principle does not apply to persons who are not in a position to act independently, such as the fetus/neonate or an individual judged to be incompetent by standard intellectual, psychological, and physiologic appraisal (Beauchamp & Childress, 1983). Respect for the individual's autonomy and advocacy to remove constraints is an inherent role of the nurse. The client who chooses not to proceed with a recommended medical plan may freely do so; the nurse safeguards this decision by ensuring that coercive efforts are not used to alter the client's chosen path.

The notion of informed consent is derived from the principle of respect for autonomy. There are four key elements to informed consent: Disclosure of accurate information and assurance that the information is comprehended by the receiving party constitute the two information elements; determination of voluntary participation without coercion and the competence of the individual to make an autonomous decision are the two consent elements. Informed consent must be secured whenever the purpose of the intervention is questionable, the risks are significant, and the procedure is physically or psychologically intrusive. Threats to any of these elements must result in a modification of the consenting procedure. The nurse would inform the involved parties of the need to ensure consent and would suggest means by which informed consent could specifically be ensured. Such means might include additional information, language interpretation, visual aids, and a second description from another practitioner.

The second root principle is *nonmalfeasance*. It is defined as the responsibility not to inflict harm (Beauchamp & Childress, 1983). Implicit in this definition is the obligation to prevent actual or potential harm and to act in a prudent, thoughtful manner. Nonmalfeasance focuses on the notions of risk–benefit analysis and detriment–benefit analysis. The first addresses the harm associated with a given procedure, and the latter emphasizes the consequences of the intervention. The questions that arise regarding the appropriateness of aggressive intervention are determined with evaluation of these two factors. Conditions that would override the duty to treat include pointless treatment, burdens outweighing benefits, and quality-of-life factors.

The concept of double effect encompasses the balancing of doing harm and doing good. It is used "to support claims that an act having harmful effects is not always morally prohibited" (Beauchamp & Childress, 1983, p. 113). Rather, the harmful effect is viewed as indirect or merely unforeseen and is therefore not the intended outcome of a given action. Four conditions must be met for the principle of double effect to be used to support the idea that the action is not morally prohibited (Beauchamp & Childress, 1983):

1. The action itself must be good or at least morally indifferent.
2. The individual must intend only the good effect and not the evil effect.
3. The evil effect cannot be a means to the good effect.
4. There must be a favorable balance between the good and evil effects of the action.

Beneficence, the third root principle, is the process of actively promoting good and preventing or removing harm. It is an underlying premise of all health profession codes. Three areas of balance must be explored. First, the risk of paternalism—acting on behalf of an autonomous person without her or his participation in the decision—is a prevalent threat to autonomy in the name of beneficence. Second, acting on behalf of one party may cause conflict with the duty to others. For example, focusing on the interests of the fetus may preclude one's duty to the mother. Third, one must consider the limits of beneficence: when is not proceeding with interventions actually acting in the best interests of the client? The withholding or withdrawing of treatment reflects this consideration.

The last root principle is *justice:* acting justly by giving what is due or owed to the entitled person (Beauchamp & Childress, 1983). The major issue in prenatal care that invokes contemplation of this principle is the allocation of scarce resources. A lack of consensus regarding the standards to be used in determining distribution of resources is a highly visible and much debated aspect of contemporary health care. Shall we allocate resources on the basis of equal share, individual need, individual effort, societal contribution, or merit? Such questions are asked in individual cases when patients are actively placed into and out of NICUs, follow-up programs, state financial aid programs, and specialized health and education systems depending on eligibility criteria.

The interwoven aspects of ethics and the law must be considered because both influence behaviors and practices of the clinician. An ethically correct position may not be legally sustained; conversely, a decision may be legally sound but morally reprehensible. The law focuses on minimum standards for societal behavior. Ethics emphasizes a desirable, deliberate, maximized course of action. Both fields drive changes in the other, and it is a nursing responsibility to participate in the societal forums for resolution and change. The *Code for Nurses* states, "The nurse collaborates with members of the health professions and other citizens in promoting community and national efforts to meet the health needs of the public" (ANA, 1985).

In the following sections, the multitude of ethical issues contemplated by the neonatal nurse are considered.

REPRODUCTIVE TECHNOLOGIES

Changing demographics, new technologic capabilities and a reduction in the fertility rate in the United States have caused an explosion in reproductive technologies.

In Vitro Fertilization and Gamete Intrafallopian Transfer

In vitro fertilization (IVF) and gamete intrafallopian transfer (GIFT) are two technologies that have been developed since 1985 to permit conception by couples in whom infertility has been caused by endometriosis, ovulatory dysfunction, cervical abnormalities, diethylstilbestrol (DES) exposure of the woman in utero (Pace-Owens, 1988), or some types of male infertility and for whom pelvic surgery to restore fertility has failed. Both procedures involve drug-induced ovarian stimulation and ovulation induction, followed by laparoscopy for egg recovery. Transfer of sperm and egg into the fallopian tube takes place at the time of egg recovery in the GIFT procedure. In IVF, fertilization and incubation of the embryo take place in the laboratory, with transfer to the uterus 44 hours later. Intrinsically, these procedures have raised few ethical questions. A review (Hastings Center, 1987) summarized 85 reports of the various official bodies of 20 countries, and without exception, IVF was found to be acceptable by these bodies. The only document that objected to IVF was the Instruction on the Respect for Human Life in Its Origins for the Doctrine of the Faith of the Vatican (Donum Vitae).

Often during the IVF and GIFT procedures, many more eggs are produced than can be safely returned in one cycle. In the past, the three or four "best" eggs or embryos would be selected for transfer and the rest donated or discarded. More recently, excess embryos have been frozen, to be thawed and transferred in a later cycle. The benefits of such a procedure (Bonnicksen, 1988) are purported to be

1. Less waste of embryos.
2. Decreased risk of multiple pregnancy (because excess embryos could be saved rather than several embryos' being transferred in the first cycle).
3. Opportunity for patient recovery from the stress of a hyperstimulation cycle before transfer.
4. Theoretical increased chance of implantation during future "normal" unstimulated cycles.
5. Decreased morbidity risk as a result of decreased need for stimulated cycles and laparoscopies.
6. Decreased cost, because drug stimulation and frequent ultrasonograms and blood tests are unnecessary.

These benefits are presumed but not proved. It is not clear that in the average IVF cycle enough "good" excess embryos would be retrieved and survive freezing and thawing to make the cost of freezing and storage outweigh the cost of future drug cycles. Reimbursement for such procedures and the consequences to the couple from delayed anticipation are other concerns. Ethical and legal questions focus on what happens if the family unit is disrupted by death or divorce. Case law and professional codes of ethics are beginning to establish societal answers to these questions (American Fertility Society: Ethics Committee, 1994a, 1994b; Annas, 1989, 1991; Capron, 1992; Robertson, 1988, 1989). Legislative and other policy options lag behind technologic capabilities.

Selective Reduction

A possible outcome of IVF and GIFT is multiple pregnancy. During any one cycle, at least three or four embryos may be transferred, on the assumption that this will increase the chance of one successful implantation. If more than two embryos implant at a time, a triplet or larger pregnancy will result. Such pregnancies carry substantial physiologic, psychological, and financial consequences for both mother and fetuses, such as toxemia, prematurity, long-term hospitalization, and increased risks of mortality and morbidity (Berkowitz et al., 1988; Evans et al., 1988; "Selective Fetal Reduction," 1988); the chance of adverse outcome is directly proportional to the number of fetuses (Berkowitz et al., 1988). Such pregnancies create an ethical dilemma: should the woman attempt to carry such a high-risk pregnancy as far as possible, knowing that the lives and well-being of all the fetuses are jeopardized, or should she agree to selective fetal reduction? Selective termination (abortion) of some of the fetuses is accomplished by ultrasonogram-guided lethal cardiac injection.

This situation represents a choice between doing nothing, thereby chancing great harm to all concerned, and doing intentional harm to some in order to benefit a few survivors. Selective termination, when performed, is usually in the form of reduction to two fetuses, so that if anything should happen to one of the remaining fetuses, the pregnancy would not be a total loss. The incidence of spontaneous miscarriage of the remaining fetuses after this procedure is unknown (Berkowitz et al., 1988).

Extraconjugal Gametes

Increasingly, reproductive technologies employ the contributed gamete of a party outside of the primary couple. Many ethical and legal quandaries are associated with this approach (Jones, 1992): Does it violate the religious and moral covenant of marriage? Does it distort the genealogy of the conceived child? Does it offer an advantageous option to intractable male factor infertility, or is it ideal in preventing the passing on of an undesirable gene from one parent? Does it commercialize organ/gamete donation?

In Vitro Surrogacy

In this form of surrogacy, IVF is used to implant an embryo formed from the primary couple's gametes into a third party's uterus. This approach is considered largely experimental, and many authors recommend rigid and scrupulous delineation of candidate selection, provider relationships, legal contracts, and monitoring of the process (American Fertility Society: Ethics Committee, 1994a, 1994b).

Surrogacy

The surrogate supplies the egg and the uterus and is inseminated (directly or artificially) by the prospective father's sperm. The American Fertility Society stipulates that this should be regarded as a clinical experiment. Little discussion of this approach, usually negotiated privately between parties, appears in the clinical literature. Societal and legal questions abound (American Fertility Society Ethics Committee, 1994a, 1994b).

PRENATAL TESTING AND TREATMENT

Diagnostic Assessments

Diagnostic assessments of the fetus and its well-being are commonplace. Ultrasound screening has become routine in many obstetrical practices, and many fetal anomalies are detected by such serendipitous means rather than by surveillance needed because of a risk factor (Elias & Annas, 1983). Ultrasonographic and echocardiographic machines assist in prenatal diagnosis of the most complex structural and functional congenital defects. The well-being of at-risk fetuses can be monitored with serial ultrasonography by calculation of the biophysical profile, nonstress tests, and contraction stimulation tests.

Amniocentesis—the withdrawing and analysis of amniotic fluid—is used to diagnose congenital problems (Johnson & Godmilow, 1988). Once used primarily to pinpoint defects that were either incompatible with life (anencephaly) or synonymous with certain (although maybe only mild) retardation (trisomy 21) in order to facilitate termination of defective pregnancies, many of the problems now detectable may be amenable to therapy. Some centers offer earlier testing than others (at less than 14 weeks' gestation) (Johnson & Godmilow, 1988). Prenatal screening of maternal serum levels of human chorionic gonadotropin, unconjugated estriol, and alpha-fetoprotein may be useful in reducing the rate of unnecessary amniocentesis in women 35 years of age or older (Haddow et al., 1994).

Chorionic villus sampling (CVS) is a procedure that tests fetal tissue at an earlier point in gestation (9 to 12 weeks) to provide the same data available by amniocentesis (except alpha-fetoprotein levels) (Wapner & Jackson, 1988). The advantage of CVS is its earlier timing, inasmuch as abortion at that time should be less complex, less dangerous, and less expensive than the second-trimester abortion available after amniocentesis. Its disadvantages include slightly greater risks of procedure failure and of fetal loss than those of amniocentesis (Rhoads et al., 1989).

The field of human genetics is replete with ethical issues, ranging from the advances of the Human Genome Project (U.S. Department of Health & Human Services, 1990) to the ideal prenatal decisions of a particular family unit to the new capability for embryo genetic diagnosis (Bonnicksen, 1992). The application of ethical principles to clinical practice and research is essential to practitioners in the neonatal specialty (see Chapter 9, Human Genetics).

Genetic counseling is indicated ethically before any use of prenatal diagnosis. The goal is to educate patients and prepare them for the choices they must make during the informed-consent process of prenatal diagnosis. Informed consent and genetic counseling are interdependent (Fletcher & Evans, 1992, p. 765).

Intrapartum Monitoring

Intrapartum fetal heart rate and contraction monitoring is a standard practice for the majority of deliveries. Because monitoring offers continuous indication of the fetus's tolerance of labor and the intrauterine environment, it holds obvious advantages over intermittent auscultation in detecting fetal distress. Certain fetal heart rate patterns in response to uterine contractions have been recognized as indicative of fetal difficulties (Hill & Volpe, 1994).

Studies have not demonstrated any prognostic value of continuous monitoring (Rosen & Dickinson, 1993). In some cases of supposedly "ominous" tracings, the infants have turned out healthy and vigorous (Blooston, 1989). Acting on those tracings resulted in cesarean sections that would not otherwise have been done and that increased morbidity for the mother. The chance of litigation in such cases may be lessened if the infant is actually born with a problem.

Frequency of monitoring of the fetus of very low birth weight varies among practitioners. Factors considered in the decision to monitor include

1. Interventions to be taken if data were available.
2. Intentions of the parents.
3. Maternal risks associated with the interventions.

Fetal Research and Fetal Cell Transplants

The concept of in utero diagnosis and treatment of structural and functional fetal anomalies has become a reality (American Academy of Pediatrics Committee on Bioethics, 1988). Some of these treatments, such as intrauterine transfusions for erythroblastosis fetalis, have been accepted as standard therapy effective in correcting harmful fetal defects and contributing to beneficial outcomes. Others, such as in utero surgical correction of congenital diaphragmatic hernia, are relatively new (Harrison, 1993; Harrison et al., 1990; Twomey, 1989). For the purpose of this discussion, all forms of therapy aimed at minimizing, ameliorating, or correcting fetal defects of structure or function, including actual surgery, are considered as a group.

Large numbers of fetal defects can now be detected by the early diagnostic assessment tools. Appropriate intervention is based on the type of defect. Abnormal fetuses first have to be identified. Careful evaluation of extent and context of the defect must be done, including identifying coexisting malformation, the type of treatment needed, and the establishment of a reasonable expectation of a positive outcome after treatment (Elias & Annas, 1983; Murray, 1985).

For the mother, the procedural risks of preterm labor, uterine damage, hemorrhage, and infection must be weighed against the benefits of the therapy to the fetus and to the parents. For the fetus, the risks of procedural failure or further harm caused by the procedure must be weighed against the possibilities of correction or amelioration of the malformation (Fletcher & Evans, 1992). Factors to be considered in the decision (Elias & Annas, 1983; Murray, 1985) include

1. Severity of the malformation.
2. Predictable consequences of survival and quality of life with or without the treatment.
3. Invasiveness of the procedure.
4. Standard versus experimental treatment.
5. Effects of failure and side effects of the procedure.
6. Threat of premature labor.

REPRODUCTIVE AND PRENATAL ISSUES

Maternal-Fetal Conflict

The development of methods to assess and treat the fetus has opened up a whole new arena of conflicts between maternal and fetal rights and interests. From the point of view of many practitioners, the fetus has now become the other patient in the obstetrical encounter, a patient who is separate from the mother in terms of interests, rights, and outcomes. Out of this perception comes a sense that the practitioner has some degree of ethical obligation toward the fetus that may preempt his or her maternal-based obligations (Nelson, 1992; Ruddick & Wilcox, 1982). Although there continues to be some debate in the literature, most legal/ethical authorities agree on the following principles (Francoeur, 1985; Mahowald, 1992; Nelson, 1992; Strong, 1992; Twomey, 1989):

1. The fetus has not achieved full personhood in the legal and moral sense, which means that its rights are of lesser consideration than those of individuals who are persons.
2. The legal/moral status of the fetus increases throughout gestation.
3. The point of viability of the fetus is a legal marker that may influence its legal/moral status.
4. The status of a fetus is never equal to that of a newborn.
5. The mother's status always exceeds that of the fetus.
6. Harm or benefit caused by an act of commission (i.e., coercive treatment) requires more proof for justification than does that caused by an act of omission (i.e., withholding treatment).
7. Fetal rights and maternal/practitioner obligation toward the fetus increase if the treatment is standard (nonexperimental) and has a proven large benefit to the fetus and a minimal (or no) risk to the mother.
8. Maternal/practitioner obligations toward the fetus increase if significant harm will result from nontreatment.
9. Maternal obligations toward the fetus increase after she has chosen to carry the pregnancy past the legal cutoff for abortion; she has then assumed responsibility for the well-being of the future child.
10. Practitioners may have additional obligations toward the fetus that increase with advancing gestation, but they are not as strong as their maternal obligations.
11. Fulfillment of maternal/practitioner obligations toward the fetus should not be coerced or enforced by legal means (Fig. 3–2).

The legal/moral case against practitioners' seeking legal intervention on behalf of the fetus when the mother refuses treatment is strong. Fletcher (1981) and Nelson (1992) identified the following objections to coercive treatment:

1. Patient confidentiality is breached.
2. It is counter to the medical standard of adult freedom of choice.
3. Coercion is introduced into the practitioner–patient relationship.
4. Due process rights of the mother are often violated.
5. The fetus's legal status is ambiguous at best.
6. Bodily integrity and privacy values are violated.
7. Dangerous elasticity exists in the standards used to justify forced intervention.
8. Undesirable consequences of forced intervention can occur.
9. Equal protection statutes and fairness values are violated because nonpregnant persons are not subject to same standards used to justify intervention.
10. Existing legal precedents are ambiguous.

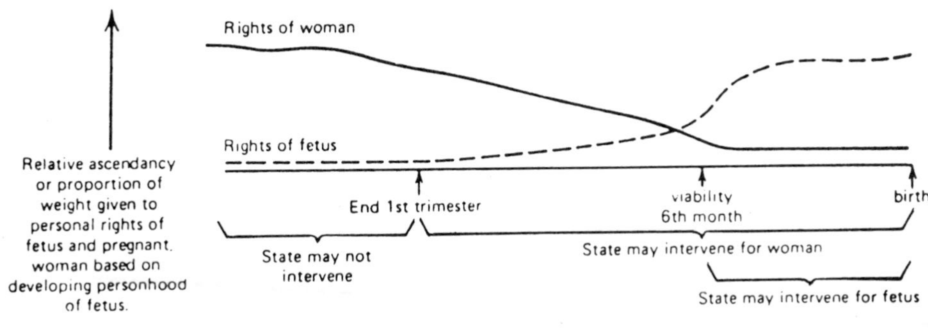

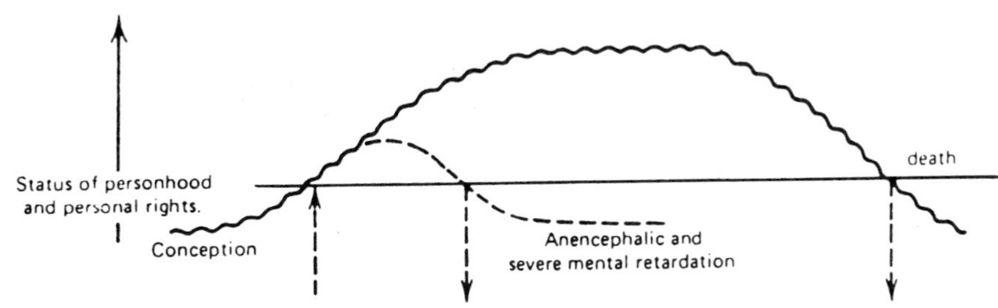

FIGURE 3–2. Relative comparison of fetal and maternal rights over span of pregnancy. (From Francoeur, R. T. [1985]. From then to now: The evolution of bioethical decision making in perinatal intensive care. In C. C. Harris & F. Snowden [Eds.], *Bioethical frontiers in perinatal intensive care* [p. 26]. Natchitoches, LA: Louisiana State University Press. Reprinted with permission.)

11. The potential for significant diagnostic inaccuracies exists with regard to fetal medical status and well-being.
12. Legal responsibility for treatment-caused harm is not well established.

Both the Board of Trustees of the American Medical Association (1990) and the American College of Obstetricians and Gynecologists Committee on Ethics (1990) have issued standards regarding physicians' seeking legal interventions in cases of maternal-fetal conflict:

1. The physician's role is to fully inform, educate, counsel, and advise but not to coerce.
2. Procedures unwanted by the pregnant woman should not be performed.
3. Recourse to the courts to resolve conflicts is almost never warranted.
4. Maternal autonomy takes precedence over fetal rights.

In conclusion, the legal/moral status of the fetus and the resultant obligations of the mother and practitioners to promote fetal well-being are still argued. However, although each situation must be thoroughly reviewed individually, some general evaluative principles are established. In addition, most experts agree that in most maternal-fetal conflict situations, maternal autonomy is the prevailing principle and compelling evidence that the fetus's rights should override the mother's rights would be required in order for the mother's autonomy to be overruled.

Chervenak and McCullough (1985) proposed a schema (see Fig. 3–1) to categorize maternal and practitioner obligations on the basis of both maternal and fetal autonomy and beneficence considerations. Because the fetus has not achieved full personhood status, fetal autonomy is not an issue. However, maternal autonomy and beneficence may conflict with fetal beneficence obligations, particularly in situations of maternal refusal of treatment that might benefit the fetus. Because any fetal therapy must be done by invading the mother's body to some degree, maternal autonomy–based obligations are threatened. If the therapy is of benefit to the fetus and/or if nontreatment will cause harm to the fetus, maternal refusal of the treatment threatens fetal beneficence-based obligations.

Underlying this schema is the concept of relative maternal and fetal rights. Most authorities agree that both entities have some rights and that these rights vary in degree and in terms of relative dominance at different times in the pregnancy (Elias & Annas, 1983; American Academy of Pediatrics Committee on Bioethics, 1988; Mahowald, 1992; Murray, 1985; Nelson, 1992; Ruddick & Wilcox, 1982). More recent literature argues that because the fetus is not autonomous, maternal rights cannot be fully overridden, but that fetal rights have become an increasingly more significant consideration with advancing gestation, which may modify maternal considerations (Mahowald, 1992; Nelson, 1992).

Chervenak and McCullough's (1985) schema provides a framework for the three possible ethical positions regarding maternal autonomy–fetal beneficence conflicts (Mahowald, 1992):

1. The pregnant woman's autonomy has priority.
2. Beneficence toward the fetus has priority.
3. Beneficence toward both patients shows respect for the pregnant woman's autonomy.

These positions can be used to analyze and evaluate conflict situations. Support for each position in a particular situation can be determined by weighing the obligations involved in the situation according to Chervenak and McCullough's (1985) schema. Such an exercise is helpful for providing a complete analysis of all factors from all perspectives, but it is not intended to result in one correct answer.

The first position, giving priority to maternal autonomy, has several legal/ethical foundations (Mahowald, 1992). First, there is a need to be consistent with previous legal standards for similar health care situations. This position maintains that pregnant women should not be treated differently from other adults with regard to their rights to free and informed consent to medical treatment. The right of nonpregnant adults to refuse unwanted treatment is accepted by the legal and medical communities and by society at large. Even if their decision is contrary to medical advice that is based on well-recognized standards, it is respected as the choice of a competent adult. This position holds that pregnant women should be given equal consideration.

Second, the law and society's norms support the right to privacy and protection against unwanted bodily invasion for nonpregnant persons, even when the treatment or procedure is life-saving or would greatly benefit another person. Blood transfusions for adult Jehovah's Witnesses and enforced organ donation are examples of these situations in which there are an overwhelming number of precedents against legal intervention. Enforced treatment of a pregnant woman is equated to these situations, and this position again holds that pregnant women should be treated equally.

Third, current views on the legal/moral status of the fetus (see previous section for discussion) also support this position. Because the fetus has not attained full personhood status in either a legal or a moral sense, maternal autonomy rights are always more powerful than fetal considerations.

The problem with this position comes from its either-or orientation that denies the ability to weigh and compare relative degrees of obligation to the mother *and* fetus. As a result, this stance can result in an incomplete examination of the problem and cause everyone involved to be treated equally badly, without resolving the conflict. Mahowald (1992) suggested that the degrees of harm and benefit of treatment and the fluctuating levels of obligation must be factored into the analysis in order to give a more accurate picture of the issues in an individual situation.

The second position, giving priority to fetal beneficence, has its roots both in the Hippocratic injunction to do good or, at least, do no harm and in the ethical root principles of beneficence, nonmalfeasance, and justice. As discussed in the beginning of this chapter, the principle of justice supports an obligation to those who are in greatest need. For example, the practice of triage in emergency medicine is based on this principle: prioritizing limited resources on the basis of need and chance of success. The fetal beneficence position argues that the practitioner has an obligation to protect and/or benefit the viable fetus (after the deadline for legal abortion has passed) that can override both maternal autonomy-based and maternal beneficence-based obligations (Mahowald, 1992). The argument for this position has four points:

1. Having carried the pregnancy past the legal cutoff for abortion, the mother has committed herself to act in ways that promote a good outcome for the fetus.
2. The fetus is vulnerable and in need of protection. In the absence of maternal consent, it is the obligation of some other entity (health care practitioners or the state) to provide this protection.
3. The technologic capability exists to treat and support the viable fetus.
4. The fetus has more years to lose than the mother because of its expected longer life span.

The problems with this position are many (Mahowald, 1992). First, using viability as an ethical marker is a problem with regard to assessing degrees of vulnerability. One could successfully defend the position that the previable fetus is more vulnerable than the viable fetus, because it cannot exist separately from the mother and therefore is more in need of protection. However, the law has clearly supported the mother's decision-making rights over fetal rights in the previable period.

Second, this position does not make a clear distinction between decisions about ends and decisions about means. The mother is being used as the means for the end benefit of another without her consent. Legal/ethical precedence does not support this use.

Third, the implied maternal commitment to pregnancy may not always have been a completely free, conscious choice, and given additional information, the mother may choose to change her mind.

Fourth, the existence of technologic support for the fetus does not make its usage obligatory, especially when that usage creates additional ethical questions.

Fifth, this position, by giving precedence to fetal rights, ignores the ambiguous legal/moral status of the fetus.

The third position gives precedence to maternal autonomy as long as that decision does not force the practitioner to violate obligations of beneficence toward both the mother and the fetus (Mahowald, 1992). This position is based on the argument that practitioners should not be forced to render treatment that would put them in the position of acting in ways that would be medically inappropriate or acting on the basis of unreliable clinical judgment and therefore to violate established standards. For example, coerced cesarean delivery for complete placenta previa would be justified under this position because maternal autonomy is overridden by concerns for both maternal and fetal beneficence (Chervenak & McCullough, 1985). Maternal refusal of this treatment is argued to put both fetus and mother at risk for harm and would compel the practitioner to act in a manner contrary to accepted medical standards.

There are four problems with this position. First, it violates the mother's right to privacy. Second, it enables the mother to be used as a means to another's ends. Third, refusal of one method of treatment does not necessarily constitute asking to be treated in a way that is medically inappropriate; it is merely refusal of one aspect or modality of care. The mother may accept other aspects of care that are appropriate. Fourth, the law does not compel practitioners to seek legal action in such cases, even when harm may result; nor does it provide any sanction for not doing so.

In conclusion, these three positions are meant as guides to assist with analysis of conflict situations in order to more thoroughly evaluate all aspects. No one position is the right answer, but the situation can be evaluated simultaneously from all three perspectives to ensure an in-depth analysis that will aid in decision-making.

Maternal Brain Death

With the advent of life-support techniques, another ethical problem involving conflicting maternal and fetal interests has surfaced: maintaining the vital functions of the body of a brain-dead mother for the sake of her fetus (Dillon et al., 1982; Field et al., 1988). The main ethical question is whether extraordinary care for the mother is justified in order to save the fetus. The important points are as follows:

1. Maternal/fetal interests and practitioner obligations. How does maternal brain death change the health care practitioner's obligations to the mother and fetus? Because she meets the universally accepted criteria for death, the mother could be said to have no further interests beyond her earlier expressed desires to bear a healthy child (Siegler & Wikler, 1982). Her autonomy has ended with her loss of brain function. Obligations toward the fetus involve the obligation to rescue an endangered life, as long as there are minimal risks to the rescuer (Field et al., 1988).
2. Benefit to the fetus. A fetus close to or beyond the point of viability benefits from the maintenance of maternal life functions for even a short period of time, increasing the chances of intact survival by prolonging gestation as long as possible. A previable fetus may benefit from this support, although it is more questionable, but there is also the possibility of harm (Dillon et al., 1982; Field et al., 1988). Even if life support measures are successful for awhile, deterioration of the mother's body may force preterm delivery if the fetus is viable but at a gestational age when the risk of extrauterine death or serious morbidity is high. Also, the effects on the fetus of treatment to maintain a "normal" intrauterine environment, especially drugs for hypotension, for infection, and for correcting metabolic aberrations, are unknown. The technical feasibility of maintaining the mother for a prolonged length of time is questionable. There have been case reports of successful long-term maintenance (Field et al., 1988), but other experts claim that treatment of the mother is useful only for 2 to 4 weeks, after which physiologic deterioration results in spite of support measures (Dillon et al., 1982). In the end, the best interests of the individual fetus are important but do not entail a standardized response.

3. Cost. Maintaining the mother's body for a long period of time can be very costly and can still lead to a neonatal death or to the delivery of a premature infant who requires costly care.
4. Brain death. Because these women meet the criteria for brain death, maintaining their bodies causes some ambivalence about the brain death standard (Siegler & Wikler, 1982). Are these women fatally ill but living patients who will die when life support is withdrawn? Or are they cadavers who retain artificially supported life function? This distinction is important for consent purposes, especially in cases in which the mother's next of kin refuses treatment (Veatch, 1982). If the mother is considered still living, a court order could be obtained to override next of kin's refusal when the benefit to the fetus is considered strong enough to justify such action. If the mother is considered to be dead, next of kin refusal could be overridden only if the mother had previously agreed to donation of her organs in the event of her death, since the use of her dead body is covered under the Uniform Anatomical Gift Act. If she had not previously given such permission, a court order could probably not be obtained, because there is no precedent for legally granting access to a dead body, even to save another's life. Also, consent for treatment must be given by the *mother's,* not the fetus's, next of kin.

Maternal Chemical Dependency

With chemical dependency on the rise, there has been increasing interest in whether pregnant women have the right to choose to use substances that are known to cause damage and addiction in their infants. This conflict is between the interests of the fetus and the autonomy of the mother. Chemically dependent mothers have been prosecuted for child abuse, both successfully and unsuccessfully, and their infants or fetuses have been made wards of the state (Blooston, 1989). The relevant considerations are as follows:

1. The reliability of predictions of fetal harm and the seriousness of harm. Some substances, such as alcohol, cocaine, and heroin, are known to cause serious fetal harm (Flandermeyer, 1987). The effects of many other drugs are unknown.
2. The personhood of the fetus and encroachment on maternal autonomy. Is the fetus a person with rights, especially the right not to be harmed? Does this right override the mother's right to make her own choices about her lifestyle? Current legal and ethical literature (Mahowald, 1992; Nelson, 1992) continues to support maternal autonomy over fetal rights and confirms the lack of personhood of the fetus. Court decisions have been inconsistent.
3. The consequences of forced treatment. How can a physician's recommendation or a court order to a mother not to take a substance that could harm her fetus be enforced? Who is responsible for the newborn's defects? Who will be responsible for the infant's care? Will this type of enforcement in these "worst" cases, with beneficence to the fetus as its object, lead to other restrictions on maternal behavior for lesser problems? What are the obligations to which a woman agrees when she plans to carry a pregnancy to term?

Jehovah's Witnesses

Jehovah's Witnesses have definite objections to blood transfusions for both religious and medical reasons. They are deeply religious people who believe that Biblical passages, although not stated in medical terms, rule out the transfusion of whole blood, red blood cell plasma, and platelets and white blood cells. However, their religious understanding does not absolutely prohibit the use of components such as albumin, immune globulins, and hemophiliac preparations; each witness must decide individually whether he or she can accept these (Dixon & Smalley, 1981). Keeping God's approval and having a good conscience are very important to Jehovah's Witnesses, religiously and psychologically, and they ask that others respect these sincere aspirations. Jehovah's Witness parents believe God's promise that those who are obedient to Him have the hope of everlasting life on earth restored to a paradise. They want this inheritance for their children also. Nevertheless, they do not adhere to so-called faith healing and are certainly not opposed to the practice of medicine. They seek medical care for themselves and their children and ask physicians to use alternatives to blood.

Jehovah's Witnesses believe that blood removed from the body should be disposed of, so they do not accept autotransfusions of predeposited blood. Techniques for intraoperative collection or hemodilution that involve blood storage are objectionable to them. However, many Jehovah's Witnesses permit the use of dialysis and heart-lung equipment (non-blood-prime) as well as intraoperative salvage in which the extracorporeal circulation is uninterrupted; the physician should consult with the individual patient as to what his or her conscience dictates.

Jehovah's Witnesses are trying to work with and improve communications with health care providers. They want cooperation, not confrontation. With this in mind, they have taken steps to help health care providers accommodate Jehovah's Witness patients. In more than 100 major U.S. cities, Hospital Liaison Committees of Jehovah's Witnesses are active in meeting with physicians, medical societies, risk managers, and nurses. Coordinated by the Hospital Information Services Department at the Jehovah's Witnesses national headquarters in Brooklyn, the members of those local committees have been trained to work as intermediaries to help avoid conflict whenever possible. Each Committee maintains directories of cooperative doctors for purposes of consultation and possible transfer. The local liaison committees, under the oversight of the national office, are ready to provide help not only to Jehovah's Witness families, but also to doctors, risk managers, hospitals, and nurses.

Because the practice of blood transfusion is well accepted as an efficacious treatment, there is a well-established legal precedent of overriding parental refusal in the case of an infant endangered after birth. But what about the fetus, whose separate personhood status is not as well established? The relevant considerations in deciding to overrule parental refusal by court order are (1) the reliability and seriousness of fetal harm without transfusion; (2) the efficacy and fetal benefits of transfusion; (3) the personhood status of the fetus; (4) the magnitude of encroachment on maternal autonomy; and (5) the risks to the mother.

The courts have ordered maternal and intrauterine transfusions to benefit the fetus, establishing a precedent that the fetal benefits outweigh the mother's rights (Ganiats et al., 1981; Kolder et al., 1987). However, more recent literature has questioned the legal and ethical basis of such orders (Mahowald, 1992; Nelson, 1992). Objections to coerced intervention include concerns about equal protection under the law for pregnant women, privacy rights, and use of the pregnant woman as the means to another's end. A detailed discussion can be found elsewhere in this chapter.

NEONATAL ISSUES

Once the fetus is born as a viable neonate, new ethical issues arise. The neonate, now separated from dependence on the mother's body, becomes more of an independent, individual entity, although its claim to full personhood rights is still hotly debated. Lebacqz (1986), Erlen and Frost (1991), and Erlen (1994) described the decision-making process and experience of professionals and parents in the NICU as a wilderness experience characterized by uncertainty, uncharted territory, choosing paths that lead nowhere, becoming hopeful and despairing.

The problems associated with ethical decision-making for the neonate are many (Berseth, 1987; Coulter, 1987; "Imperiled Newborns," 1987):

1. Dependent patient. Newborns, because they cannot make their wishes known and cannot do things for themselves, are necessarily dependent on others for their care and for decisions about what care is appropriate.
2. Uncertainty. Decision-making in the treatment of infants is fraught with uncertainty, both medical (unclear diagnosis and prognosis) and moral (expected benefits of treatment unclear). This uncertainty is the product of many factors.
   a. The biologic variability of individual patients causes varied responses to treatment.
   b. Rapid technologic advancements provide many options of treatment.
   c. There is a lack of information about the efficacy of neonatal intensive care technologies and postnursery interventions. Clinical trials are often not done because of ethical problems concerning withholding possibly effective treatment from control infants and because of medical traditions of uncontrolled expansion of new technology.
   d. The decisions are inconsistent because of incomplete data and unclear and conflicting value systems.
   e. Skills of practitioners vary, and the benefits of a treatment may vary with them.
   f. Parent follow-through with continued treatment varies.
   g. Interaction between health care practitioners and parents in making decisions is prone to distortion from biases, communication problems, and the values clarification process inherent in the decision-making.
3. Potential treatment-induced harm.
4. Lack of available treatment options for survivors. NICU survivors often require prolonged support, although the services and economic support needed are not available in many communities.
5. Lack of consistent treatment guidelines. There is an absence of established, agreed-upon guidelines for treatment.
6. Cost. NICU care continues to be expensive; costs are rapidly increasing as a result of the use of many high-technology treatments, prolonged hospitalizations, and follow-up support for damaged survivors. Government and insurance reimbursements often underestimate cost and length of stay.
7. Emotions. There is a highly emotional context in which any decisions are made.
8. Pluralism. Neonates come from diverse ethnic, cultural, and spiritual backgrounds.
9. Brain death. There are no accepted definitions and criteria for the documentation of brain death in neonates (American Academy of Pediatrics Committee on Bioethics, 1988; Ashwal et al., 1991).

Uncertainty

Uncertainty is dealt with by the use of one of three strategies for decision-making ("Imperiled Newborns," 1987; Rhoden, 1986; Todres et al., 1988). These strategies are designed to save infants whose lives would be tolerable (i.e., a quality of life not completely debilitated or in a vegetative state) and not save those whose lives would not be tolerable, including infants who would not have been treated had their poor outcomes been known. Two of the strategies actively try to minimize the worst possible outcome and are called "maximin" strategies.

The first strategy is the statistical approach. This strategy is used by practitioners to whom the worst possible outcome is the survival of infants who would not have been treated if their poor outcome had been known. This strategy bases treatment decisions on the statistical probability of poor outcome. It is used in some countries, such as Sweden, in which infants below a certain birth weight (750 g in Sweden) are not treated. The advantage of this approach is that it eliminates agonizing decisions over individual cases, because standards are agreed upon in advance, and it permits equitable and just intervention for each case. The disadvantages are significant. First, decisions are only as good as the statistics on which they are based, and such statistics are variable. Second, this strategy can result in the loss of more potentially salvageable survivors than is necessary. Third, the role of parents in decision-making is minimal. Last, the strategy is simplistic and ignores the complexities of individual ethical dilemmas.

The second strategy is the "wait-until-near-certainty" approach. For proponents of this approach, widely used in the United States, death is the worst outcome. This approach gives the infant the benefit of the doubt when choosing treatment, unless the inevitability of death or serious brain damage is clear. The advantages of this approach are respect for individual life and the lack of agonizing over discontinuing treatment of viable infants. However, parents are left out of decision-making, because the option not to treat is offered only in extreme cases. This approach ignores concerns about quality of life and therefore represents vitalism (to be described). It ignores the probability of outcomes in that it operates on certainty alone. It does not consider the suffering that sustaining life can cause to patient, parent, and society.

The third strategy is the individualized prognosis approach. This approach, used in Great Britain, does not attempt to anticipate the worst possible outcome but instead involves initiating treatment in borderline cases and then frequently reevaluating whether to continue treatment on the basis of reassessments of its efficacy and the probabilities of death or impairment. It does not require certainty to withdraw treatment, and it attempts to minimize both survival of severely damaged infants and death of potentially healthy infants. Its advantages include a wide variation in treatment decisions that address individual variabilities, more parental involvement in decisions, and confrontation of the realities of moral and medical uncertainty. Its disadvantages are, first, a possibility of failure to correlate prognostic criteria with a substantive standard in order to decide how much impairment warrants withholding treatment. Second, criteria that allow withholding treatment in too many cases may be adopted. Third, practitioners may unduly influence parents to follow their recommendations, rather than permitting parental independence. Fourth, practitioners may inflate the predictive value of the criteria or fail to revise criteria to reflect medical advances.

Along with a strategy, substantive standards of judgment for treatment must be chosen, against which the strategies are measured ("Imperiled Newborns," 1987). The first are sanctity-of-life standards. An extreme form of this type is vitalism, in which the continuation of life is viewed as the greatest good. Another view is the "medical indications" policy, under which the sanctity of life is upheld but treatment may be withheld if the infant is judged to be dying or the treatment is medically contraindicated. These criteria uphold nondiscrimination principles against handicapped infants and "medical benefit" principles, which hold that treatment should be beneficial to the patient on the basis of "reasonable medical judgment." This view is typified in the U.S. Department of Health and Human Services' "Baby Doe" regulations (Carter, 1993; Moreno, 1987), which state that treatment should be effective in "reasonable medical judgment" and can be withheld or withdrawn only if (1) the infant is chronically and irreversibly comatose; (2) the provision of such treatment would merely prolong dying and not be effective in ameliorating or correcting all the infant's life-threatening conditions or would otherwise be futile in terms of the survival of the infant; or (3) the provision of such treatment would be virtually futile in terms of the survival of the infant and the treatment itself under such circumstances would be inhumane.

The second standards are those relating to quality of life. These standards focus on social worth, in which the quality of life is measured by its degree of benefit or burden to others, primarily parents and society. Drawbacks are the potential for abuses in judging someone's worth only by his or her impact on other lives and the lack of accepted evaluation criteria of what constitutes well-being (U.S. Department of Health & Human Services, 1985).

The third is the "acceptable life" standard, which evaluates whether the infant's probable outcome would give her or him an acceptable life. The problem with this standard is the lack of consensus about what is "acceptable."

The fourth is the "best interests" standard, in which choices are based on what is in the best interest of the infant from the infant's perspective. Treatment can be withheld if the infant is dying, the treatment is medically contraindicated, or continued life would be "worse than death," involving continual pain and suffering. The difficulties with this standard are many. First, it is a problem for a normal adult to try to imagine what a damaged infant could consider in its best interests. Second, because this standard holds that pain and suffering are evil and benefit consists of abolishing or ameliorating them, this standard, when used in extreme cases, can mean that the absence of pain is the only morally relevant consideration. The focus is on the absence of burdens rather than the presence of benefits (Arras, 1984). However, in the absence of any human capabilities, how can these infants be said to have any "best interests" to consider?

The fifth is the "relational potential" standard, which considers the presence or absence of distinctly human capacities and therefore deals with moral complexities. Without the capacity to think, communicate, love, and otherwise participate in relationships with other humans, an infant's best interests may not be served by initiating or continuing treatment.

Infants of Very Low Birth Weight

The extremely premature infant has a very uncertain medical and moral status. Although statistics on mortality and morbidity are available for groups of infants, outcomes for individual infants are impossible to predict. Improvements in survival have made uncertain the benefits and harm of neonatal intensive care, the limits of viability, and reliable prognoses (Allen et al., 1993; Klebanov et al., 1994; McCormick et al., 1984, 1990; Ross et al., 1990). Statistical and wait-until-near-certainty approaches invariably err on both sides, allowing the deaths of viable infants or the rescue of defective infants. The individualized prognostic approach seems reasonable for this group but leaves open the possibility of many anguishing decisions that are inevitably based on unknowns; calculations based on "best interests" or future "relational potential" are guesses at best. However, as time goes on, probabilities can be used to make predictions (Allen et al., 1993; Davis, 1993; Hack & Fanaroff, 1989; Jain et al., 1992; Kitchen et al., 1991; Landwirth, 1993; Synnes et al., 1994).

Initiation and Withdrawal of Life Support

The difficulties in deciding to withdraw treatment have made some health care practitioners either reluctant to start treatment, for fear that it cannot be stopped later, or committed to continuing treatments that have proved useless or even harmful. However, ethicists agree that there is no moral difference between withholding and withdrawing treatment. Some authorities have also suggested that there is no legal difference (Elias & Annas, 1983; President's Commission for the Study of Ethical Problems in Medicine and Biomedical and Behavioral Research, 1983a, 1983b).

The problems with not accepting the option of withdrawing useless or harmful treatment are many ("Imperiled Newborns," 1987):

1. Prolongation of death with its burden of suffering and economic cost can result.
2. Some treatments need to be tried before their benefit can be documented. If they are not beneficial, withdrawal is based on better information than the withholding would have been.
3. Withdrawing is usually discussed with the family, whereas withholding may not be.
4. The inability to withdraw treatment once it has been initiated may prevent initiation of that treatment to an infant who would otherwise benefit.

Anesthesia and Analgesia

In the past, anesthesia and analgesia were not often given to infants undergoing surgery. Two rationales were given for this practice. The first was the prevention of intraoperative hypotension associated with anesthetic use ("Neonatal Anesthesia," 1987). Today, with increased knowledge of neonatal physiologic response to stress, improved intraoperative monitoring capabilities, and greater anesthetic control, hypotensive episodes are uncommon (Berry & Gregory, 1987; Robinson & Gregory, 1981). Second, neonates were thought to have insufficiently developed neurologic systems to perceive or recall painful experiences (Anand & Hickey, 1987). Accepted theory was that newborns had neither the integration of cortical function to perceive and remember pain nor the maturity of myelination of neural pathways to transmit painful stimuli to the brain. However, as illustrated in Figure 3–3 (Anand & Hickey, 1987), even preterm newborns are now known to have the anatomic and functional maturity of the nervous system to transmit and perceive pain.

Newborns demonstrate physiologic responses to pain similar to or greater than those of adults (Anand & Hickey, 1987). Increases in heart rate and blood pressure, wide variability in transcutaneous or pulse oximeter oxygen saturation readings, palmar sweating, and release of stress hormones have been documented as indicators of pain responses in neonates. Behavioral changes in response to pain, such as motor responses, facial expressions, changes in crying tones and patterns, and alterations in sleep-wake cycles, attention, orientation, irritability, quieting ability, and feeding schedules have also been studied (Anand & Hickey, 1987; Bell, 1994).

As a result of this evidence, most practitioners now accept that withholding anesthesia from neonates would be unethical because its benefits outweigh any potential harm and because doing nothing certainly causes harm (Bell, 1994; Friedrich et al., 1995).

Invasive Technologies

Highly invasive technologies are now being used for neonates with previously fatal maladies. Extracorporeal membrane oxygenation (ECMO) is now in widespread use for neonates with respiratory failure, among whom the mortality rate was previously 50 to 80 percent. ECMO involves temporary cardiopulmonary bypass to provide adequate oxygenation without the barotrauma caused by mechanical ventilation.

Neonatal heart transplantation is being performed for neonates with hypoplastic left heart syndrome, a congenital heart defect that is fatal, usually within the first few days or weeks of life. The donors have sometimes been anencephalic infants, creating other ethical problems that are considered in the next section.

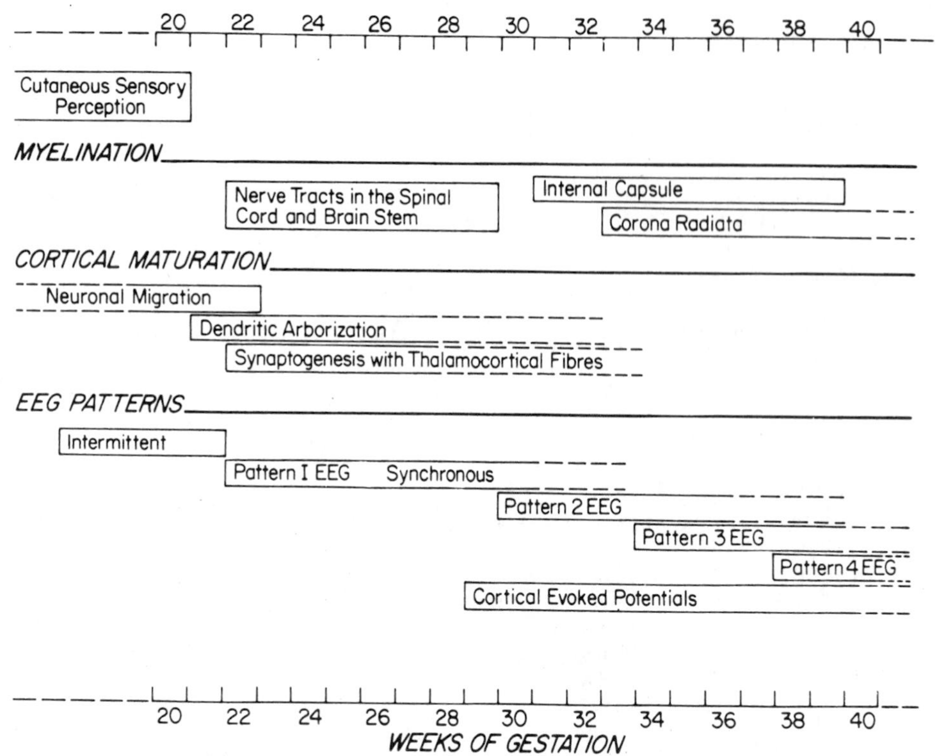

FIGURE 3–3. Schematic diagram of the development of cutaneous sensory perception, myelination of the pain pathways, maturation of the fetal neocortex, and electroencephalographic patterns in the human fetus and neonate. (From Anand, K. J. S., & Hickey, P. R. [1987]. Pain and its effects in the human neonate and fetus. *New England Journal of Medicine, 31*[721], 1322. Reprinted with permission.)

These two technologies share certain characteristics that highlight the ethical dilemmas involved (Elliott, 1991):

1. Lack of experimental clinical studies. Although some animal experimentation has been done, neither of these technologies has been subjected to controlled experimental studies to compare harms and benefits, usually because of perceived ethical and legal problems in study design, primarily informed consent and the withholding of efficacious treatment (Bartlett et al., 1985; Miké et al., 1993). Because the technologies are new, long-term effects are unknown (Fink et al., 1989; Schumacher et al., 1989; Steinhorn et al., 1989; Walsh-Sukys et al., 1994; Zach et al., 1990). Treatment has been offered to these neonates either on historically based predictions or as a "rescue" alternative to certain death (Bartlett et al, 1985; Miké et al, 1993; O'Rourke et al., 1989). Informed consent is difficult under these circumstances. With imminent death as the alternative, few parents would not consent, but health care practitioners are unable to provide much information on benefits, harm, and prognosis on which parents can base their decisions (Lantos & Frader, 1990).
2. Experimental or standard therapy. When do these treatments cease to be experimental and become accepted, standard treatment? Some practitioners assert that use of ECMO is so widespread that it should no longer be considered experimental (Bartlett et al., 1985). As interventions become standard therapy, parental choice to accept or refuse such treatment becomes restricted. Parents become obligated to seek and agree to treatment in the "best interest" of their child.
3. Outcomes. Even while the use of an invasive technology is becoming widespread and popular, advances in standard therapy may improve outcomes to the point where the efficacy of the treatment is essentially equal (Walsh-Sukys et al., 1994). However, the aggressive, mostly invasive approach is often entrenched by this time.
4. Selection of recipients. Many factors influence the selection of candidates for new therapies: geographic proximity, parental intention, financial resources, clinical criteria, research protocols, and resource availability.
5. Societal obligations. Innovative technologies are frequently costly and initially are available to only a few candidates. Should the financial, human, and technologic resources be invested instead in clinical services that could benefit a larger number of patients?

Miké and associates (1993) proposed an ethics of evidence as an approach to medical uncertainty with standards for creation, assessment, and communication of evidence. This approach balances the need to develop and communicate the best possible scientific evidence for all medical decisions with the need to come to terms with the unavoidable, irreducible nature of uncertainty.

The Anencephalic Infant

With the perfection of surgical techniques, the transplantation of hearts, kidneys, and livers into infants is possible. Infants with organs that are nonfunctional as a result of developmental defects, disease, or pre- or postnatal damage can be saved from certain death by such transplants. Among children less than 2 years of age awaiting transplantation, 30 to 50 percent die before the organ becomes available. The United Network for Organ Sharing reported in 1990 that 320 children less than 5 years of age were waiting for organ transplants (Holzgreve & Beller, 1992). The problem is the limited supply of organs. Because of size limitations, only organs from infants can usually be used, and the number of infants who die under circumstances that would preserve their organs for transplantation is limited. To increase the supply of organs, it has been suggested that anencephalic infants be used as donors because their life span is short and their death inevitable. Anencephaly is a congenital defect in which the cranium is absent and the cerebral cortex is virtually absent. Use of such infants' organs not only would be an advantage to the recipients but also has been proposed as helpful to parents of anencephalic infants as a means of salvaging good out of their misfortune (Holzgreve et al., 1987). An estimated 1050 anencephalic infants are born each year, although this number could be reducible to less than 100 per year as a result of prenatal detection of the condition and early abortion (Botkin, 1988; Holzgreve & Beller, 1992). Of those who go on to delivery, many are inappropriate as donors because of intrauterine growth retardation, premature birth, short survival time, and associated malformations of organs (Holzgreve & Beller, 1992). Nonetheless, the supply of organs would be substantially increased above the present levels by the use of anencephalic infants as donors (Botkin, 1988).

The difficulty in this practice lies in the determination of death. According to the Uniform Anatomical Gift Act, gifts of vital organs can be given only after the donor has been declared legally dead (Capron, 1987; Byrne et al., 1993; Ivan, 1988). The legal definition of death provided by the Uniform Determination of Death Act is irreversible cessation of either (1) cardiorespiratory function or (2) whole brain function, including cerebral and brain stem function. Anencephalic infants who are not stillborn do not meet either of these criteria. Brain death determination in newborns is fraught with problems and depends on (1) establishment of cessation of all brain functions by clinical and laboratory criteria and (2) demonstration that cessation of function is irreversible by determining cause, excluding reversible conditions, and documenting that cessation persists for an appropriate period of observation (Volpe, 1987). Table 3–2 documents the criteria used.

The problems with using these determinations are both developmental and experimental. Many of the critical functions assessed are either developing or recently developed. Electroencephalographic patterns of even normal infants are in the process of evolution. There is a lack of validation that meeting the laboratory criteria demonstrates brain death, inasmuch as some infants who have met those criteria have later recovered function. It is unknown whether a reversible injury can cause total but transient loss of electrocerebral activity (Stumpf et al, 1990; Volpe, 1987).

Each of the proposed solutions to these problems has its own drawbacks (Churchill & Pinkus, 1990; Fost, 1988; Shinnar & Arras, 1989; Walters, 1991):

1. Waiting for traditional cardiorespiratory death to occur. Under this method, there is a good chance that organs will be damaged in the death process, becoming unsuitable for transplantation. Success with transplantation of organs from anencephalic infants is highest when maximal life support of the infant begins immediately at birth (Holzgreve & Beller, 1992). Legal questions regarding the long-term viability of anencephalic infants and the appropriateness of continued life support were also raised in the 1992 case of Baby K (Annas, 1994).
2. Maintaining cardiorespiratory support until brain death occurs. The problems with this approach are four: the uncertainty that brain death will occur; the difficulty of confirmation that brain death will occur; the treatment of the anencephalic infant only as a means to benefit another; and the further emotional stress on the parents, in that parents may be too overwhelmed by the situation to grieve until the infant actually dies (American Academy of Pediatrics Committee on Bioethics, 1992).
3. Redefining brain death as death of brain tissue required for higher level functioning for anencephalic infants to allow them to be pronounced dead at birth (Shinnar & Arras, 1989). This approach leaves a door open to future redefinitions of death, including for other groups of individuals. It also would now include patients in a persistent vegetative state, not just anencephalic infants (American Academy of Pediatrics Committee on Bioethics, 1992).
4. Redefining anencephalic infants as infants in a special "brain absent" category who are the same as dead (Kohrman, 1994). The objections to this approach are many: There is the chance for misdiagnosis, because there is a range of anencephaly that merges with other conditions; the anencephalic infant is being redefined solely as a utilitarian means to obtain donors; and using this argument for justifying using anencephalic infants for organ donation may lead to looser regulations about organ donors—the "slippery slope" argument (American Academy of Pediatrics Committee on Bioethics, 1992).
5. Abandoning the "dead donor" rule, thereby allowing procurement of organs from live anencephalic infants before death is pronounced. The argument in favor of this approach is that anencephalic infants, being unable to establish meaningful human interactions, do not have full personhood status and have no best interests or rights to protect (Capron, 1987). But there are also other questions. Are these infants conscious and therefore capable of suffering? Can they experience pain? To what types of respect and treatment are they entitled, and are they overruled by the needs of the recipient (American Academy of Pediatrics Committee on Bioethics, 1992; Shewmon, 1988)?

The American Academy of Pediatrics Committee on Bioethics

TABLE 3–2 Criteria for Brain Death Determination in Infants

I. History. Proximate cause of coma to ensure absence of remediable or reversible conditions.
II. Physical examination.
  1. Coma and apnea must coexist.
  2. Absence of brain stem function.
    (a) Midposition or fully dilated pupils that are unresponsive to light.
    (b) Absence of spontaneous eye movement induced by oculocephalic and oculovestibular testing.
    (c) Absence of movement of bulbar musculature, including facial and oropharyngeal muscles (corneal, gag, cough, sucking, rooting reflexes absent).
    (d) Respiratory movements absent with patient off the respirator.
  3. Not significantly hypothermic or hypotensive for age.
  4. Flaccid tone and absence of spontaneous or induced movements, excluding spinal cord events.
  5. Results remain consistent with brain death throughout the observation and testing period.
III. Observation period. For 7 days to 2 months old: two exams and EEGs separated by at least 48 hours.
IV. Laboratory testing.
  1. EEG: 30 minutes using standardized techniques for brain death determinations.
  2. Angiography: lack of visualization of cerebral circulation.

EEG, electroencephalogram.
From American Academy of Pediatrics Task Force in Brain Death in Children. (1987). Guidelines for the determination of brain death in children. *Pediatrics, 80,* 298–300. Reprinted with permission.

(1992) concluded that in light of the current lack of data, any attempt to use these infants' organs should be classified as experimental and constrained by the usual ethical and regulatory principles applicable to research using human subjects (p. 1116). The American Medical Association Council on Ethical and Judicial Affairs concluded in 1995 that it is ethically permissible to consider the anencephalic neonate as a potential organ donor, although still alive under the current definition of death only if key criteria were met. Unfortunately, what these key criteria are is up for interpretation at each institution and within the context of individual cases.

ROLE OF PARENTS IN CLINICAL DECISION-MAKING

The determination of a proxy decision-maker for the infant is of importance in neonatal intensive care. Desirable characteristics of such persons are as follows: (1) They should advance the infant's best interests; (2) they should be involved in present or future care of the infant; (3) they should have knowledge of the infant's medical problems; and (4) they should be comprehensive and impartial in their evaluations ("Imperiled Newborns," 1987).

Obviously no one person, health care practitioner or parent, has all these characteristics. Parents should be involved, especially when quality-of-life standards are used. They have traditional legal and moral authority over the child, and they have to live with the consequences of any decisions. What should be the role of health care practitioners? Health care practitioners need to ensure that parental interests do not override respect for the best interests of the child. There is a strong possibility for conflict of interest by health care practitioners, however, because no consensus about treatment policies exists and because the goals for treatment, research, and education can be mutually exclusive. Health care practitioners can be advisors to the parents, giving them accurate information with which to make decisions and triggering appropriate outside intervention when parental decisions are inappropriate for the medical condition of the infant (Pinch & Spielman, 1990). Infant Care Review Committees, encouraged by the 1984 Child Abuse Amendments (Baby Doe laws) and Infant Ethics Committees, recommended by the President's Commission for the Study of Ethical Problems in Medicine and Biomedical and Behavioral Research (1983a, 1983b) and the American Academy of Pediatrics, can also provide assistance to practitioners and parents in decision-making (Levine-Ariff, 1989).

Disagreements can arise between practitioners and parents regarding the choice of therapies, and the issues of parental autonomy, informed consent, and the proven efficacy of the therapy emerge (Harrison, 1986; Lee et al., 1991). Many therapies used on newborns have been introduced without controlled clinical trials to document efficacy, benefit, or adverse effects (Silverman, 1987). Benefits are often documented only by anecdotes, historical data, and clinical experience. Many things about newborn physiology, the natural history of their diseases, and the possible effects of treatment are unknown. The use of therapies is often mandated over parental objection. Conversely, if a parent insists on treatment that practitioners believe to be futile for the infant, can the parent's wishes be overridden? The wishes of the parents often stand in this case, especially if payment is available for such treatment. Recent legal decisions reaffirm this role of parents.

A conference of parents and professionals convened by Harrison (1993) has published the Principles for Family-Centered Neonatal Care:

1. Family-centered neonatal care should be based on open and honest communication between parents and professionals on medical and ethical issues.
2. To work with professionals in making informed treatment choices, parents must have available to them the same facts and interpretation of those facts as the professionals have, including medical information presented in meaningful formats, information about uncertainties surrounding treatments, information from parents whose children have been in similar medical situations, and access to the chart and rounds discussions.
3. In medical situations involving very high rates of mortality and morbidity, great suffering, and/or significant medical controversy, fully informed parents should have the right to make decisions regarding aggressive treatment for their infants.
4. Expectant parents should be offered information about adverse pregnancy outcomes and be given the opportunity to state in advance their treatment preferences if their baby is born extremely prematurely or critically ill.
5. Parents and professionals must work together to acknowledge and alleviate the pain of infants in intensive care.
6. Parents and professionals must work together to ensure an optimal environment for babies in the NICU.
7. Parents and professionals should work together to ensure the safety and efficacy of neonatal treatments.
8. Parents and professionals should work together to develop nursery policies and programs that promote parenting skills and encourage maximum involvement of families with their hospitalized infants.
9. Parents and professionals must work together to promote meaningful long-term follow-up for all high-risk NICU survivors.
10. Parents and professionals must acknowledge that critically ill newborns can be harmed by overtreatment as well as by undertreatment, and they must insist that laws and treatment policies be based on compassion. They must work together to promote awareness of the needs of NICU survivors with disabilities to ensure adequate support for them and their families. They must also work together to decrease disability through universal prenatal care.

CLINICAL RESEARCH

The advances made since the 1960s in neonatal care have resulted largely from the clinical research conducted by health care professionals. The advent of continuous positive airway pressure, the discovery of surfactant and the development of exogenous surfactant, the refinement of open heart surgery techniques, the analysis of touch and "kangaroo care," neonatal organ transplantation, ECMO, and the understanding of neonatal behavioral and motor development all are outcomes of basic science and applied research. The primary purposes of research are to describe phenomena, evaluate the efficacy of interventions, and confirm anecdotal clinical impressions. Also since the 1960s, society has more clearly defined the acceptable criteria for clinical research, including mechanisms of approval, subject population selection, benefit–risk analysis for the subjects, overall value and utility of the research, and informed consent methods for subjects or their surrogates. All clinical research now requires institutional review board approval and supervision (National Commission for the Protection of Human Subjects, 1978). The Belmont Report (1983) identifies three tasks in the protection of human subjects: informed consent, risk–benefit assessment, and selection of subjects. The key ethical concerns are to ensure that informed consent takes place without coercion, to provide for subject safety and benefit, and to maintain subject privacy, anonymity, and confidentiality.

The use of fetal tissue for transplantation into another human to treat various diseases and for laboratory research has become possible and has generated much ethical controversy. Fetal tissue, because of its rapidly dividing cells, has been useful in the laboratory for studying Alzheimer's disease, cancer, and acquired immunodeficiency syndrome (AIDS). Because of its capacity to divide and possibly to differentiate after transplantation, fetal adrenal and nervous tissue has been transplanted into patients with Parkinson's disease and has relieved symptoms, probably owing to its ability to produce dopamine ("Fetuses and Parkinsonism," 1988). Fetal islet cells that have been transplanted into diabetic patients produce insulin in the host (Robertson, 1988). The Federal government, through legislation and executive order, has established restrictions and standards for the use of fetal tissue (Verklan, 1993).

As the discussion of ECMO clinical trails revealed, the ethics of neonatal clinical research are complex. Randomization of patients out of potentially life-saving experimental modalities is poorly regarded by society. Conversely, concluding that interventions are effective with inadequate provisions for a control group is a methodologic threat. Lilford (1992) concluded that "clinical trials involve a compromise between micro- and macroethics. Utilitarians favor randomized trials because more people outside the trial stand to lose from acceptance of an inferior treatment than do those inside the trial who are allocated to an inferior treatment arm" (p. 844). The countervailing view suggests that the burden sustained by the individual patient in the trial is unethical, regardless of the benefit to the greater good.

Ethical questions of reproductive technology are key areas for nursing inquiry. From a unique perspective in the decision-making milieu, the nurse can identify critical questions for study:

1. The rights of the child contrasted with the rights of the family when the child is chronically ill.
2. The role of social support systems in the decision-making process and its consequences.
3. The relative obligations of society to the child and family.
4. The varying perceptions of health care professionals tackling a common ethical question.
5. The organizational implementation of the *Code for Nurses* in perinatal and neonatal centers.
6. The emotional consequences for families participating in the withdrawal of life support from the neonate.
7. The impact of religious and moral values on families' decision-making.
8. The evaluation of consent procedures in a given setting for the key elements of informed consent.
9. The identification of local community needs and the allocation of resources.
10. The impact of education in clinical ethics on the nurses' subsequent involvement in and comfort with decision-making.
11. The evaluation of various models for collaborative ethical decision-making.
12. The description of a given population's position on anencephalic organ donation.
13. The longitudinal studies of survivors' outcomes correlated with decision-making methods used during their intensive care hospitalization.
14. The emotional response and decision outcome of particular families considering withholding or withdrawing life support.

RESOURCE ALLOCATION

The allocation of increasingly scarce resources for health care is a growing concern in the United States. It is apparent that we can no longer do all that we want to do as a nation and, indeed, that the methods and purposes of resource allocation are themselves flawed. Nowhere is the question of justice and cost–benefit analysis more evident than in the perinatal and neonatal area. Numerous macroallocation studies have examined the value of prenatal care and neonatal intensive care and the impact on client outcomes (Berki & Schneier, 1987; Institute of Medicine, 1985; McCormick et al., 1984; McManus, 1983; Phibbs et al., 1981; Wise et al., 1988). Repeatedly the investigators have concluded that primary prevention enhances outcome for clients (ANA, 1987; Institute of Medicine, 1985; Meis et al., 1987; Moore et al., 1986; Poland et al., 1987; Strain, 1993). Rapidly changing health care markets, financing arrangements, and integrated systems change previous assumptions regarding prenatal/neonatal and neonatal services (Gehl & Erlen, 1993; Kohrman, 1994; Newacheck et al., 1994; Perrin et al., 1994). Access to care, both prenatal and pediatric, remains a primary obstacle for many of the nation's citizens (Murphy, 1986; National Commission for Reducing Infant Mortality, 1988; President's Commission for the Study of Ethical Problems in Medicine and Biomedical and Behavioral Research, 1983a, 1983b; Vladeck, 1981). Changes in health care financing to a capitation system rather than a fee-for-service system may exaggerate access to care issues, leading to more ethical dilemmas for nurses. Why? Because in a capitated system there is a lifetime cost expenditure proposed through a continuum of care; once this cap is reached, what happens to the patient and family? No one is sure. Another part of this reform is the confusion over who can go to which hospital, practitioner, or physician for which service—thus some patients avoid health care until there is a crisis. Fifty-six million Americans now belong to health maintenance organizations (HMOs) (Hammonds, 1996b).

In relation to neonatal nursing and ethics, the prediction is that more high-risk mothers and infants will be seen until the health care environment stabilizes and there will be more dictates from organizations as to what services can be provided, on the basis of dollar amounts and not necessarily patients' needs. In the NICU, early discharges are a reality regardless of whether the infants and mothers are ready. Legislation is pending in approximately 25 states regarding early discharges for healthy mothers and infants, but where is the legislation to protect the NICU population (Hammonds, 1996a)? This legislative movement has ethical implications for neonatal nurses and needs close monitoring.

ETHICAL DECISION-MAKING

Myriad models for ethical decision-making have been developed. The reader is encouraged to review the work of Fromer (1981), Jonsen and colleagues (1992), Thompson and Thompson (1981), and Veatch and Fry (1987). The application of their models may be helpful in the resolution of individual clinical issues.

Of greater value, however, is the skill of being conversant with the four root principles and the *Code for Nurses* in their application to a particular circumstance. In this way, the individual permutations and peculiarities of the situation can be considered thoughtfully and an intellectually rigorous and ethically grounded decision can be reached (Bailey, 1986).

The following case studies are presented to review the process of problem resolution, not to suggest a prescriptive manner for handling seemingly similar situations. The nurse must approach each ethical question or problem with the same individualization that one uses in planning clinical care. The problem-solving method includes these steps: identification of the problem, identification of the involved parties, description of the problem, generation of alternatives, analysis of the alternatives, selection of the best alternatives, and execution of the decision.

CASE 1

A 24-year-old, gravida 1, para 0, Jehovah's Witness presented to the hospital with premature rupture of membranes at 28 weeks' gestation. She was not in labor. The fetus was discovered to be in the breech position. The mother had a history of idiopathic thrombocytopenic purpura and was severely anemic and thrombocytopenic on admission. Over the next 24 hours, there were indications of infection, including maternal fever and increased white blood cell count and fetal tachycardia. The obstetricians recommended cesarean section delivery for maternal and fetal indications but wanted to administer transfusions before surgery in order to lower maternal risk. The mother refused transfusions on religious grounds, and the obstetricians felt they could not safely operate without transfusion therapy.

1. What is the ethical question of this case?
2. Who should be involved in the decision-making process?
3. Who has the right to the final decision?
4. What ethical principles are primarily involved in this deliberation?
5. What are the threats to maternal autonomy? To fetal beneficence? What factors would one consider in evaluating the ethical risk to the fetus and the mother and the subsequent weighting of each risk?
6. What obligation does the mother have to the fetus?
7. What obligation and subsequent action does the nurse have to the mother? To the medical team?
8. What are the ethical consequences of each potential course of action?

CASE 2

A 36-year-old, gravida 1, para 0, American woman, married to a Saudi Arabian, presented in labor at 36 weeks' gestation. She had had two previous ultrasonograms that were interpreted as normal, and she had refused amniocentesis for prenatal diagnosis. The infant's father had returned to Saudi Arabia before delivery, and the mother planned to emigrate with the infant after birth.

At delivery the male infant was found to have amniotic band disruption complex, an in utero breaking of the amnion that caused it to wrap around body parts and restrict their normal growth and development. He had a midfacial cleft involving the left orbit, nose, palate, and lip. He had only one skull bone (right parietal). The rest of the brain was covered only by dura, without leakage of cerebrospinal fluid. He also had a Dandy-Walker malformation of the brain, a posterior fossa cyst causing hydrocephalus and neurologic deficit. He had minor amputation of the ends of some fingers. Other organs were intact on ultrasound evaluation. On the second day of life, the infant developed severe, life-threatening apnea and bradycardia episodes. The nurse caring for the patient seeks to clarify the infant's resuscitation ("code") status. The nurse should consider the following questions:

1. Who should be involved in the decision-making process?
2. What are the ethical questions raised in this case?
3. What ethical principles are germane to this deliberation?
4. What potential course of action can be identified? What are the ethical and clinical consequences of each?
5. What informational factors would need to be reviewed with the parents?
6. What legal precedence has been established relative to the treatment plan?

CONCLUSION

Inherent in the practice of nursing is the practice of ethical behavior. In an increasingly complex environment, the nurse must identify ethical concerns and actively intervene in their resolution. Consistent, thoughtful application of the root principles and the *Code for Nurses* can assure the nurse of personal and professional integrity. It is an accountability that society expects.

REFERENCES

Allen, M. C., Donohue, P. K., & Dusman, A. E. (1993). The limit of viability—Neonatal outcome of infants born at 22 to 25 weeks' gestation. *New England Journal of Medicine, 329*(22), 1597–1601.

American Academy of Pediatrics Committee on Bioethics. (1988). Fetal therapy: Ethical considerations. *Pediatrics, 81*(6), 898–899.

American Academy of Pediatrics Committee on Bioethics. (1992). Infants with anencephaly as organ sources: Ethical considerations. *Pediatrics, 89*(6), 1116–1119.

American Academy of Pediatrics Task Force on Brain Death in Children. (1987). Guidelines for the determination of brain death in children. Report of special task force. *Pediatrics, 80*(2), 298–300.

American College of Obstetricians and Gynecologists Committee on Ethics. (1990). Patient choices: Maternal-fetal conflict. *Women's Health Issues, 1*(1), 13–15.

American Fertility Society: Ethics Committee. (1994a). Ethical considerations of assisted reproductive technologies. *Fertility and Sterility, 46*(3, Suppl. 1), 1S–94S.

American Fertility Society: Ethics Committee. (1994b). Ethical considerations of assisted reproductive technologies. *Fertility and Sterility, 62*(5), 1S–119S.

American Medical Association Council on Ethical and Judicial Affairs. (1995). The use of anencephalic neonates as organ donors. *Journal of the American Medical Association, 273*(20), 1614–1618.

American Nurses' Association. (1980). *Nursing: A social policy statement.* Kansas City, MO: Author.

American Nurses' Association. (1985). *Code for nurses with interpretive statements.* Kansas City, MO: Author.

American Nurses' Association. (1987). *Access to prenatal care: Key to preventing low birth weight.* Kansas City, MO: Author.

American Nurses' Association. (1991). *Standards for clinical nursing practice.* Washington, DC: Author.

American Nurses' Association. (1995). *Nursing: A social policy statement.* Washington, DC: American Nurses Publishing.

Anand, K. J. S., & Hickey, P. R. (1987). Pain and its effects in the human neonate and fetus. *New England Journal of Medicine, 317*(2), 1321–1329.

Annas, G. J. (1989). A French homunculus in a Tennessee court. *Hastings Center Report, 19*(6), 20–22.

Annas, G. J. (1991). Crazymaking: Embryos and gestational mothers. *Hastings Center Report, 21*(1), 35–38.

Annas, G. J. (1994). Asking the courts to set the standard of emergency care—The case of Baby K. *New England Journal of Medicine, 330*(21), 1542–1545.

Arras, J. D., (1984). Toward an ethic of ambiguity. *Hastings Center Report, 14*(2), 25–33.

Ashley, J. A. (1976). *Hospitals, paternalism and the role of the nurse.* New York: Teachers College Press.

Ashwal, S., Caplan, A. L., Cheatham, W. A., et al. (1991). Session IX: Social and ethical controversies in pediatric heart transplantation. *Journal of Heart & Lung Transplantation, 10*(5, Part 2), 860–876.

Bailey, C. F. (1986). Withholding or withdrawing treatment on handicapped newborns. *Pediatric Nursing, 12*(6), 413–416.

Bartlett, R. H., Roloff, D. W., Cornell, R. G., et al. (1985). Extracorporeal circulation in neonatal respiratory failure: A prospective randomized study. *Pediatrics, 76*(4), 479–487.

Beauchamp, T. L., & Childress, J. F. (1983). *Principles of biomedical ethics.* New York: Oxford University Press.

Bell, S. G. (1994). The national pain management guideline: Implications for neonatal intensive care. *Neonatal Network, 13*(3), 9–17.

Benne, K. D., & Bennis, W. (1959). Role confusion and conflict in nursing. *American Journal of Nursing, 59*, 196–198.

Berkowitz, R. L., Lynch, L., Chitkara, V., et al. (1988). Selective reduction of multifetal pregnancies in the first trimester. *New England Journal of Medicine, 318*(16), 1043–1047.

Berki, S. E., & Schneier, N. B. (1987). Frequency and cost of diagnosis-related group outliners among newborns. *Pediatrics, 79*(6), 874–881.

Berry, F. A., & Gregory, G. A. (1987). Do premature infants require anesthesia for surgery? *Anesthesiology, 67*(3), 291–293.

Berseth, C. L. (1987). Ethical dilemmas in the neonatal intensive care unit. *Mayo Clinic Proceedings, 62*(1), 67–72.

Blooston, G. (1989, February). Fetal frontier. *Savvy Woman*, pp. 68–71, 101.

Board of Trustees of the American Medical Association. (1990). Legal interventions during pregnancy. *Journal of the American Medical Association, 264*(20), 2663–2670.

Bonnicksen, A. (1992). Genetic diagnosis of human embryos. *Hastings Center Report, 22*(4, Special suppl.), S5–S11.

Bonnicksen, A. L. (1988). Embryo freezing: Ethical issues in the clinical setting. *Hastings Center Report, 18*(6), 26–30.

Botkin, J. R. (1988). Anencephalic infants as organ donors. *Pediatrics, 82*(2), 250–256.

Byrne, P. A., Evers, J. C., & Nilges, R. G. (1993). Anencephaly—Organ transplantation? *Issues in Law & Medicine, 9*(1), 23–31.

Capron, A. M. (1987). Anencephalic donors: Separate the dead from the dying. *Hastings Center Report, 17*(1), 5–9.

Capron, A. M. (1992). Parenthood and frozen embryos. *Hastings Center Report, 22*(5), 32–33.

Carter, B. S. (1993). Neonatologists and bioethics after Baby Doe. *Journal of Perinatology, 13*(2), 144–150.

Chervenak, F. A., & McCullough, L. B. (1985). Perinatal ethics: A practical method of analysis of obligations to mother and fetus. *Obstetrics and Gynecology, 66*(3), 442–446.

Churchill, L. R., & Pinkus, R. L. B. (1990). The use of anencephalic organs: Historical and ethical dimensions. *Milbank Quarterly, 68*(2), 147–169.

Corwin, R. G. (1961). Role conception and career aspiration: A study of identity in nursing. *Sociological Quarterly, 2*, 69–86.

Coulter, D. L. (1987). Neurologic uncertainty in newborn intensive care. *New England Journal of Medicine, 316*(14), 840–844.

Davis, D. J. (1993). How aggressive should delivery room cardiopulmonary resuscitation be for extremely low birth weight neonates? *Pediatrics, 92*(3), 447–450.

Dillon, W. P., Lee, R. V., Tronolone, M. J., et al. (1982). Life support and maternal brain death during pregnancy. *Journal of the American Medical Association, 248*(9), 1089–1091.

Dixon, J. L., & Smalley, M. G. (1981). Jehovah's Witnesses: The surgical/ethical challenge. *Journal of the American Medical Association, 246*(21), 2471–2472.

Edens, M. J., Eyler, F. D., Wagner, J. T., & Eitzman, D. V. (1990). Neonatal ethics: Development of a consultative group. *Pediatrics, 86*(6), 944–949.

Elias, S., & Annas, G. J. (1983). Perspectives on fetal surgery. *American Journal of Obstetrics and Gynecology, 145*(7), 807–812.

Elliott, S. J. (1991). Neonatal extracorporeal membrane oxygenation: How not to assess novel technologies. *The Lancet, 337*(8739), 476–478.

Etzioni, A. (1969). *The semiprofessions and their organization.* New York: Free Press.

Erlen, J. A. (1994). Ethical dilemmas in the high-risk nursery: Wilderness experience. *Journal of Pediatric Nursing, 9*(1), 21–26.

Erlen, J. A., & Frost, B. (1991). Nurses perceptions of powerlessness in influencing ethical decisions. *Western Journal of Nursing Research, 13*(3), 397–407.

Evans, M. I., Fletcher, J. C., Zador, I. E., et al. (1988). Selective first-trimester termination in octuplet and quadruplet pregnancies: Clinical and ethical issues. *Obstetrics and Gynecology, 71*(3, Part 1), 289–296.

Fetuses and parkinsonism. (1988). *Nature, 332*, 667.

Field, D. R., Gates, E. A., Creasy, R. K., et al. (1988). Maternal brain death during pregnancy. *Journal of the American Medical Association, 260*(6), 816–822.

Fink, S. M., Bockman, D. E., Howell, C. G., et al. (1989). Bypass circuits as the source of thromboemboli during extracorporeal membrane oxygenation. *Journal of Pediatrics, 115*(4), 621–624.

Flandermeyer, A. A. (1987). A comparison of the effects of heroin and cocaine abuse upon the neonate. *Neonatal Network, 6*(3), 42–48.

Fletcher, J. C. (1981). The fetus as patient: Ethical issues. *Journal of the American Medical Association, 246*(7), 772–773.

Fletcher, J. C., & Evans, M. I. (1992). Ethics in reproductive genetics. *Clinical Obstetrics and Gynecology, 35*(4), 763–782.

Fost, N. (1988). Organs from anencephalic infants: An idea whose time has not yet come. *Hastings Center Report, 18*(5), 5–10.

Fowler, M. D. (1987). Introduction to ethics and ethical theory. In M. D. Fowler & J. Levine-Ariff (Eds.), *Ethics at the bedside: A source book for the critical care nurse* (pp. 24–38). Philadelphia: J. B. Lippincott.

Fralic, M. F. (1983). Developing the head nurse role—A key to survival in nursing administration. In N. L. Chaska (Ed.), *The nursing profession: A time to speak* (pp. 659–670). New York: McGraw-Hill.

Francoeur, R. T. (1985). From then to now: The evolution of bioethical decision making in perinatal intensive care. In C. C. Harris & F. Snowden (Eds.), *Bioethical frontiers in perinatal intensive care* (pp. 19–37). Natchitoches, LA: Northwestern State University Press.

Friedrich, J. B., Young, S., Gallagher, D., et al. (1995). Where does it hurt? An interdisciplinary approach to improving the quality of pain assessment and management in the neonatal intensive care unit. *Nursing Clinics of North America, 30*(1), 143–159.

Fromer, M. J. (1981). *Ethical issues in health care.* St. Louis: C. V. Mosby.

Ganiats, T. G., Norcross, W. A., Schneiderman, L. J., et al. (1987). Intrauterine transfusion: Ethical issues involving a Jehovah's Witness mother. *Journal of Family Practice, 24*(5), 467–472.

Gehl, M. B., & Erlen, J. A. (1993). An ethical dilemma in the neonatal intensive care unit: Providing due care. *Journal of Perinatology, 13*(1), 50–54.

Gretter, L. (1956). The Florence Nightingale Pledge. In L. R. Seymer (Ed.), *A general history of nursing* (4th ed., p. 317). New York: Macmillan.

Grissum, M., & Spengler, C. (1976). *Womanpower and health care.* Boston: Little, Brown.

Hack M., & Fanaroff, A. A. (1989). Outcomes of extremely-low-birth-weight infants between 1982 and 1988. *New England Journal of Medicine, 321*(24), 1642–1647.

Haddow, J. E., Palomki, G. E., Knight, G. J., et al. (1994). Reducing the need for amniocentesis in women 35 years or older with serum markers for screening. *New England Journal of Medicine, 330*(16), 1114–1118.

Hall, R. H. (1982). The professions, employed professionals and the professional association. In *Professionalism and the empowerment of nursing* (pp. 1–15). Papers presented at the 53rd convention of the American Nurses' Association, Washington, DC, June 25–July 1, 1982. Kansas City, MO: American Nurses' Association.

Hammonds, K. H. (1996a, January 8). Newborn babies, bawling moms. *Business Week*, p. 40.

Hammonds, K. H. (1996b, January 8). The patient is stable—for now. *Business Week*, p. 102.

Harrison, H. (1986). Neonatal intensive care: Parents' role in ethical decision making. *Birth, 13*(3), 165–175.

Harrison, H. (1993). The principles of family-centered neonatal care. *Pediatrics, 92*(5), 643–650.

Harrison, M. R., Adzick, N. S., Longaker, M. T., et al. (1990). Successful repair in utero of a fetal diaphragmatic hernia after removal of herniated viscera from the left thorax. *New England Journal of Medicine, 322*(22), 1582–1584.

Hastings Center. (1987). Ethics and the new reproductive techniques: An international review of committee statements. *Hastings Center Report, 17*(Suppl. 3).

Hill, A., & Volpe, J. J. (1994). Neurologic disorders. In G. B. Avery, M. A. Fletcher, & M. G. MacDonald (Eds.), *Neonatology: Pathophysiology and management of the newborn* (4th ed., pp. 1117–1138). Philadelphia: J. B. Lippincott.

Holzgreve, W., & Beller, F. K. (1992). Anencephalic infants as organ donors [Review]. *Clinical Obstetrics & Gynecology, 35*(4), 821–836.

Holzgreve, W., Beller, F. K., Buchholz, B., Hansmann, M., & Kohler, K. (1987). Kidney transplantation from anencephalic donors. *New England Journal of Medicine, 316*(17), 1069–1070.

Imperiled newborns. (1987). *Hastings Center Report, 17*(6), 5–32.

Institute of Medicine. (1985). *Preventing low birth weight.* Washington, DC: National Academy Press.

Instruction on the Respect for Human Life in Its Origins for the Doctrine of the Faith of the Vatican. *Donum Vitae.*

Ivan, L. P. (1988). Brain death in the infant and what constitutes life. *Transplant Proceedings, 20*(4, Suppl. 5), 17–25.

Jacox, A. (1978). Professional socialization of nurses. In N. L. Chaska (Ed.), *The nursing profession: Views through the mist.* New York: McGraw-Hill.

Jain, L., Ferre, C., Vidyasagar, D., et al. (1992). Cardiopulmonary resuscitation of apparently stillborn infants: Survival and long term outcome. *Journal of Pediatrics, 118*(5), 778–782.

Joint Commission for the Accreditation of Healthcare Organizations. (1995). *Accreditation Standards.* Chicago, IL: Author.

Jones, H. W. (1992). Assisted reproduction. *Clinical Obstetrics and Gynecology, 35*(4), 749–757.

Jonsen, A. R., Siegler, M., & Winslade, W. J. (1992). *Clinical ethics: A practical approach to ethical decisions in clinical medicine.* New York: McGraw-Hill.

Johnson, A., & Godmilow, L. (1988). Genetic amniocentesis at 14 weeks or less. *Clinical Obstetrics and Gynecology, 31*(2), 408–417.

Kitchen, W. H., Doyle, L. W., & Ford, G. W. (1991). Changing two-year outcome of infants weighing 500–999 gms at birth: A hospital study. *Journal of Pediatrics, 118*(6), 938–943.

Klebanov, P. K., Brooks-Gum, J., & McCormick, M. C. (1994). Classroom behavior of very low birth weight elementary school children. *Pediatrics, 94*(5), 700–708.

Kohrman, A. F. (1994). Financial access to care does not guarantee better care for children. *Pediatrics, 93*(3), 506–508.

Kolder V. E. B., Gallagher, J., & Parsons, M. D. (1987). Court-ordered obstetrical interventions. *New England Journal of Medicine; 316*(19), 1192–1196.

Landwirth, J. (1993). Ethical issues: Pediatric and neonatal resuscitations. *Annals of Emergency Medicine, 22*(2), 502–507.

Lantos, J. D., & Frader, J. (1990). Extracorporeal membrane oxygenation and the ethics of clinical research in pediatrics. *New England Journal of Medicine, 323*(6), 409–413.

Lebacqz, K. (1986). Focus on the NICU. Imperiled in the wilderness. *Second Opinion, 2,* 26–31.

Lee, S. K., Penner, P. L., & Cox, M. (1991). Comparison of the attitudes of health care professionals and parents toward active treatment of very low birth weight infants. *Pediatrics, 88*(1), 110–114.

Levine-Ariff, J. (1989). Institutional ethics committees: A survey of children's hospitals. *Issues in Comprehensive Pediatric Nursing, 12*(6), 447–461.

Lilford, R. J. (1992). The substantive ethics of clinical trials. *Clinical Obstetrics and Gynecology, 35*(4), 837–845.

Mahowald, M. B. (1992). Maternal-fetal conflict: Positions and principles. *Clinical Obstetrics and Gynecology, 35*(4), 729–737.

Mauksch, H. O. (1976). The organizational context of nursing practice. In F. David (Ed.), *The nursing profession: Five sociological essays* (pp. 109–137). New York: John Wiley & Sons.

McCormick, M. C., Gortmaker, S. L., & Sobol, A. M. (1990). Very low birth weight children: Behavioral problems and school difficulties in a national sample. *Journal of Pediatrics, 117*(5), 687–693.

McCormick, M. C., Shapiro, S., & Starfield, B. (1984). High-risk young mothers: Infant mortality and morbidity in four areas in the United States. *American Journal of Public Health, 74*(1), 18–23.

McManus, M. (1983). *The role of Medicaid in delivering prenatal care to low-income women.* Unpublished manuscript, available from the Institute of Medicine, Washington, DC.

Meis, P. J., Ernest, J. M., Moore, M. L., et al. (1987). Regional program for prevention of premature birth in northwestern North Carolina. *American Journal of Obstetrics and Gynecology, 157*(3), 550–556.

Miké, V., Krauss, A. N., & Ross, G. S. (1993). Neonatal extracorporeal membrane oxygenation (ECMO): Clinical trials and the ethics of evidence. *Journal of Medical Ethics, 19*(4), 212–218.

Moore, T. R., Origel, W., Key, T. C., & Resnik, R. (1986). The perinatal and economic impact of prenatal care in a low-socioeconomic population. *American Journal of Obstetrics and Gynecology, 154*(1), 29–33.

Moreno, J. D. (1987). Ethical and legal issues in the care of the impaired newborn. *Clinics in Perinatology, 14*(2), 345–360.

Murphy, E. K. (1986). Health care: Right or privilege? *Nursing Economics, 4*(2), 66–68.

Murray, T. H. (1985). Ethical issues in fetal surgery. *American College of Surgeons Bulletin, 70*(6), 6–10.

National Commission for the Protection of Human Subjects. (1978). *Report and recommendations: Institutional review boards.* Washington, DC: U.S. Department of Health, Education and Welfare.

National Commission for Reducing Infant Mortality. (1988). *1988 Report.* Washington, DC: Author.

Nelson, L. J. (1992). Legal dimensions of maternal-fetal conflict. *Clinical Obstetrics and Gynecology, 35*(4), 738–748.

Neonatal anesthesia. (1987). *Pediatrics, 80*(3), 446.

Newacheck, P. W., Hughes, D. C., Stoddard, J. J., & Halfon, N. (1994). Children with chronic illness and Medicaid managed care. *Pediatrics, 93*(3), 497–500.

O'Rourke, P. P., Crone, R. K., Vacanti, J. P., et al. (1989). Extracorporeal membrane oxygenation and conventional medical therapy in neonates with persistent pulmonary hypertension of the newborn: A prospective randomized study. *Pediatrics, 84*(6), 957–963.

Pace-Owens, S. (1988). Gamete intrafallopian transfer (GIFT). *Journal of Obstetric, Gynecologic, and Neonatal Nursing, 18*(2), 93–97.

Perrin, J. M., Kahn, R. S., Bloom, S. R., et al. (1994). Health care reform and the special needs of children. *Pediatrics, 93*(3), 504–506.

Phibbs, C. S., Williams, R. L., & Phibbs, R. H. (1981). Newborn risk factors and costs of neonatal intensive care. *Pediatrics, 68*(3), 313–321.

Pinch, W. J., & Spielman, M. L. (1990). The parents' perspective: Ethical decision making in neonatal intensive care. *Journal of Advanced Nursing, 15*(6), 712–719.

Poland, M. L., Ager, J. W., & Olson, J. M. (1987). Barriers to receiving adequate prenatal care. *American Journal of Obstetrics and Gynecology, 157*(2), 297–303.

President's Commission for the Study of Ethical Problems in Medicine and Biomedical and Behavioral Research. (1983a). *Deciding to forgo life-sustaining treatment.* Washington, DC: U.S. Government Printing Office.

President's Commission for the Study of Ethical Problems in Medicine and Biomedical and Behavioral Research. (1983b). *Securing access to health care.* Washington, DC: U.S. Government Printing Office.

Rhoads, G. G., Jackson, L. G., Schlesselman, S. E., et al. (1989). The safety and efficacy of chorionic villus sampling for early prenatal diagnosis of cytogenetic abnormalities. *New England Journal of Medicine, 320*(10), 609–617.

Rhoden, N. K. (1986). Treating Baby Doe: The ethics of uncertainty. *Hastings Center Report, 16*(4), 34–42.

Robertson, J. A. (1989). Resolving disputes over frozen embryos. *Hastings Center Report, 19*(6), 7–12.

Robertson, J. A. (1988). Rights, symbolism, and public policy in fetal tissue transplants. *Hastings Center Report, 18*(6), 5–12.

Robinson, S., & Gregory, G. A. (1981). Fentanyl-air oxygen anesthesia for ligation of PDA in preterm infants. *Anesthesia and Analgesia, 60*(5), 331–334.

Rosen, M. G., & Dickinson, J. C. (1993). The paradox of electronic fetal monitoring: More data may not enable use to predict or prevent infant neurologic morbidity. *American Journal of Obstetrics & Gynecology, 168*(3), 745–751.

Ross, G., Lipper, E. G., & Auld, P. M. (1990). Social competence behavior problems in premature children at school age. *Pediatrics, 86*(3), 391–397.

Ruddick, W., & Wilcox, W. (1982). Operating on the fetus. *Hastings Center Report, 12*(5), 10–14.

Schumacher, R. E., Weinfield, I. J., & Bartlett, R. H. (1989). Neonatal vocal cord paralysis following extracorporeal membrane oxygenation. *Pediatrics, 84*(5), 793–796.

Selective fetal reduction. (1988). *The Lancet, 2*(8614), 773–775.

Seward, J. F. (1969). Professional practice in a bureaucratic structure. *Nursing Outlook, 17*(12), 58–61.

Shewmon, D. A. (1988). Anencephaly: Selected medical aspects. *Hastings Center Report, 18*(5), 11–19.

Shinnar, S., & Arras, J. (1989). Ethical issues in the use of anencephalic infants as organ donors. *Neurologic Clinics, 7*(4), 729–743.

Siegler, M., & Wikler, D. (1982). Brain death and live birth. *Journal of the American Medical Association, 248*(9), 1101–1102.

Silverman, W. A. (1987). Human experimentation in perinatology. *Clinics in Perinatology, 14*(2), 403–416.

Steinhorn, R. H., Isham-Schopf, B., Smith, C., & Green, T. (1989). Hemolysis during long-term extracorporeal membrane oxygenation. *Journal of Pediatrics, 115*(4), 625–630.

Strain, J. E. (1993). Update on the American Academy of Pediatrics activities to achieve universal access to health care for all children. *American Journal of Disease of Children, 147*(5), 526–528.

Strong, C. (1992). An ethical framework for managing fetal anomalies in the third trimester. *Clinical Obstetrics & Gynecology, 35*(4), 792–802.

Stumpf, D. A., & the Medical Task Force on Anencephaly. (1990). The infant with anencephaly. *New England Journal of Medicine, 322*(10), 669–674.

Styles, M. M. (1982). *On nursing: Toward a new endowment.* St. Louis: C. V. Mosby.

Synnes, A. R., Ling, E. W. Y., Whitfield, M. F., et al. (1994). Perinatal outcomes of a large cohort of extremely low gestational age infants (twenty-three to twenty-eight completed weeks of gestation). *Journal of Pediatrics, 125*(6), 956–960.

The Belmont Report. (1983). *The Belmont Center Report.* Baltimore: National Commission of Human Subjects Biomedical and Behavioral Research.

Thompson, J. B., & Thompson, H. O. (1981). *Ethics in nursing.* New York: Macmillan.

Todres, I. D., Guillemin, J., Grodin, M. A., & Batten, D. (1988). Life-saving therapy for newborns: A questionnaire survey in the state of Massachusetts. *Pediatrics, 81*(5), 643–649.

Twomey, J. G. (1989). The ethics of in utero fetal surgery: A possible threat to the autonomy of pregnant women? *Nursing Clinics of North America, 24*(4), 1025–1032.

U.S. Department of Health & Human Services. (1985). Child abuse and neglect prevention and treatment program. *Federal Register, 50,* 14878–14892.

U.S. Department of Health & Human Services. (1990). *Understanding our genetic inheritance: The U.S. human genome project: The first five years, FY 1991–1995.* Washington DC: U.S. Government Printing Office.

Veatch, R. M. (1982). Maternal brain death: An ethicist's thoughts. *Journal of the American Medical Association, 248*(9), 1102–1103.

Veatch, R. M., & Fry, S. T. (1987). *Case studies of nursing ethics.* Philadelphia: J. B. Lippincott.

Verklan, M. T. (1993). The ethical use of fetal tissue for transplantation and research. *Journal of Advanced Nursing, 18*(8), 1172–1177.

Vladeck, B. C. (1981). Equity, access, and the costs of health services. *Medical Care, 19*(12), 69–80.

Vollmer, H., & Mills, D. (1966). *Professionalization.* Englewood Cliffs, NJ: Prentice-Hall.

Volpe, J. J. (1987). Brain death determination in the newborn. *Pediatrics, 80*(2), 293–297.

Walsh-Sukys, M. C., Bauer, R. E., Cornell, D. J., et al. (1994). Severe respiratory failure in neonates: Mortality and morbidity rates and neurodevelopmental outcomes. *Journal of Pediatrics, 125*(1), 104–110.

Walters, J. W. (1991). Anencephalic infants as organ sources. *Bioethics, 5*(4), 326–341.

Wandelt, M. A., Pierce, R. M., & Widdowson, R. R. (1981). Why nurses leave nursing and what can be done about it. *American Journal of Nursing, 81*(1), 72–77.

Wapner, R. J., & Jackson, L. (1988). Chorionic villus sampling. *Clinical Obstetrics and Gynecology, 31*(2), 328–344.

Wise, P. H., First, L. R., Lamb, G. A., et al. (1988). Infant mortality increase despite high access to tertiary care: An evolving relationship among infant mortality, health care, and socioeconomic change. *Pediatrics, 81*(4), 542–548.

Zach, T. L., Steinhorn, R. H., Georgieff, M. K., et al. (1990). Leukopenia associated with extracorporeal membrane oxygenation in newborn infants. *Journal of Pediatrics, 116*(3), 440–444.

CHAPTER 4

Legal Aspects of Perinatal Care

KATHLEEN M. DRISCOLL

RESEARCH AGENDA

What do nurses know about perinatal law or investigations programs?

What effect do legal concerns about practice have on the actual nursing care rendered?

What is the relationship between adverse outcomes and caregiver preparation?

What is the relationship between legal and ethical concerns in relationship to "do not resuscitate (DNR)" orders?

What is the impact of legal issues on parental rights in the transport of neonates to a neonatal intensive care unit (NICU)?

Three decades ago, nurses in newborn care settings depended largely on vision and intuition as tools of assessment. Technology in the newborn unit consisted of nasogastric tube feedings, an occasional intravenous infusion, and monitoring infant response to oxygen levels. Nursing policy and procedure manuals listed in litany format the "right way" to carry out nursing activities. Following the litany meant meeting the standard of care.

In the 1960s, there was no risk management director to examine medication procedures or suggest mandatory training sessions for the use of new equipment. In fact, the risk manager did not exist because the risk of institutional financial loss through a malpractice suit was practically nil. Health care consumers simply did not sue providers of care. First, no health care consumer felt comfortable suing individual physicians and nurses whom they viewed as doing their best toward the consumer's benefit. Second, although clearly all care was not provided as a matter of charity, hospitals were still generally insulated from suit under the doctrine of charitable immunity.

Thirty years ago, the term *nursing intervention* would have been viewed as a foreign phrase. Why not? The term carries the implication that outcomes should be examined. True, the term *evaluation* was part of the nursing process schema, but only the most forward-thinking nurse extended the evaluation of nursing activities to measurable outcomes that indicated consumer adaptation to health problems. Nurses thought that providing quality care was a "given." Examination of quality via quality assurance or quality improvement incorporated into a total quality management program was not done.

For most nurses, the law three decades ago was a societal institution having little to do with nursing as a profession. The exception was periodic licensure renewal, which reminded nurses that a law governed the scope of their practice. Entire courses, parts of every course in nursing curricula, and continuing education programs were not devoted to legal aspects of nursing practice as they are today.

Today, nurses often appear obsessed with the potential for legal challenge to their practice through negligence or malpractice litigation. In light of this concern about lawsuits, the first part of this chapter discusses the legal elements of negligence; sources for nursing standards of care; the process of litigation, including the role of the expert witness; risk management, emphasizing communication and documentation; and the counterpart of risk management, quality assurance and improvement.

The law also touches perinatal and neonatal intensive care nursing in other ways. In the 1960s, family involvement in infant care meant showing up to hold the infant. Bonding was a concept in its own infancy. Decision-making about the use of life-sustaining measures was deferred to the expertise of the physician. Even for the physician, the range of treatment choices was limited when compared with the armamentarium of life-sustaining measures available today. Decision-making was a private experience. Ethics committees did not scrutinize the process. The law was not waiting to intrude on the process.

In the past, nurses might have observed that some infants responded more positively to some measures than did others. Few would have identified those observations as a component of the first stage of the research process—identifying a research problem—let alone raise questions about when research should be carried out on infants and who should consent to such research.

In the 1960s, transplant technology was a futuristic idea. No nursery nurse viewed the anencephalic infant as a source of organs. Watson and Crick were breaking the DNA code. Few nurses thought about a critical scientific breakthrough leading to testing for genetic disorders, nor did nurses think that the DNA breakthrough would create the potential for parents to consider interrupting a pregnancy to prevent bringing a disabled or dying child into the world. Certainly no nurse thought that a child would bring an action for his or her own wrongful life.

Substance abuse was drinking too much on social occasions, not the cause of fetal alcohol syndrome. Cocaine addiction was rare, not a rising health care concern. Smoking was socially acceptable, even if it was a noxious, smelly habit. Not until the late 1960s was this habit found to be related to low birth weight and stillborn infants. Smoke was not viewed as a toxic substance related to respiratory disorders of infants. Certainly no one raised the question of mothers or fathers abusing fetuses through exposure to these substances.

The law touched neonates in some ways. The federal government provided funds to increase levels of maternal and child health. States provided some financial support for the health care of disabled children. State regulations for nurseries dictated the distance between nursery beds and guidelines for isolation of infants with infectious diseases. The nurse who was aware of these state and federal activities thought of funding and regulations as social goods, not the arm of the law intruding into the management of health care. Furthest from the nurse's mind was under what circumstances neonatal care should be provided and who should pay for that care. The day of the third-party arbiter of care and payment was far distant.

In view of these technologic and social developments, the second part of this chapter focuses on law as society's response to these developments. Law embodies social policy. This part of the chapter also examines decisions about the use of life-sustaining measures for infants, research on infants, the use of anencephalic infants as organ donors, lawsuits involving the prenatal discovery of genetic disorders, the issue of fetal abuse, state and federal regulation of care delivery, and cost issues. Responses the neonatal nurse might make to these legal concerns are identified.

Law consists of case, statutory, and regulatory laws. Each type of law balances competing perspectives to establish guidelines for relationships among individuals and groups in a society. Law acts as both a dispute resolution mechanism and a social policy tool. The concept of law as a dispute resolution mechanism is the central theme of the first part of this chapter. The concept of law as a social policy tool underpins the second part.

LAW AS A DISPUTE RESOLUTION MECHANISM

Elements of Negligence

In law, a negligence suit may be brought when careless, as opposed to intentional, acts of an individual bring about harm to a person to whom one has a duty of care. For example, a driver will be successfully sued under the legal theory of negligence if he or she carelessly proceeds through a stop sign and collides with another vehicle, injuring its occupants. The driver has violated his or her duty of care for the persons in the car coming in the opposite direction. The four legal elements necessary to prove negligence are present in this situation. They are (1) duty, (2) breach of duty, (3) injury, and (4) causation. Litigation results when the presence of these elements is disputed.

The process of litigation is an attempt by plaintiff and defendant to get a disinterested third party—a judge or a jury—to believe a particular version of the facts. The plaintiff seeks monetary damages. The defendant seeks exoneration.

If parents sue the nurse in neonatal practice, they must show that the nurse owed the neonate a duty of care. Demonstration of employment by a health care facility, assignment to the NICU, and provision of direct or even supervisory care to the particular infant establishes the nurse's duty of care. The plaintiff must then show breach of that duty of care. Evidence of deviation from the expected standard of care through an action or omission establishes breach of duty.

Violation of the standard of care must then be causally tied or connected to the actual injury. This connection is not always easy. For example, it may be difficult to prove that an already brain-damaged infant suffered additional damage as a result of deviation from the expected standard of care during a cardiac arrest. It is important to recognize that injury must always occur to prove negligence. For example, medication errors that result in no harm to an infant eliminate the possibility of legal liability in a negligence suit.

Malpractice Versus Negligence

Malpractice is professional negligence. The law uses the term *malpractice* to describe negligence by individuals who violate a standard of care that can be known only by virtue of education in a field. Negligence that is not malpractice violates a standard of care that a lay person would know.

Because NICU nursing is a specialized area of practice, it would be rare for a nurse to deviate from the standard of care in such a way that a lay jury could understand the deviation without some explanation. The implications of medication errors, equipment misuse, and fluid and oxygen administration misjudgments are not readily understood by lay persons. However, a lay person would not need an expert witness to explain that leaving a side rail down on the crib of a normal 3-month-old child is a negligent act. Therefore, nurses can both commit malpractice and be negligent.

Statutes of Limitations

Statutes of limitations are laws that set time frames during which certain legal actions must be brought. The policy purpose of the statutes is to prevent stale claims; that is, claims that have lost their credibility because information bases and persons knowledgeable about events are long removed from the event precipitating the suit. The time frames set in the statute are intended to provide sufficient time for plaintiffs to discover injuries and bring suit, while assuring potential defendants that they are not at risk forever.

As a result of the medical malpractice insurance crisis of the 1970s, many states shortened the statute of limitations for bringing a negligence action against physicians and some other licensed health care professionals, most often dentists and podiatrists. Nurses are not generally included in these malpractice statutes. Neither are health care facilities. Nurses who are employees of health care facilities fall under their longer statute of limitations. If sued personally, the longer period also applies to nurses. Statutes of limitations vary from state to state.

Statutes of limitations are even more extended for nurses in neonatal practice. Actions against nurses in neonatal nursing practice can be brought even beyond the ordinary statutory time limitation because the law has recognized that an injustice may occur if parents do not bring an action on behalf of their child during the usual statutory time frame. The remedy for this potential injustice is to permit individuals to bring actions on their own behalf within the ordinary statutory time frame after they reach the age of majority. For example, a child injured as a result of breach of the standard of care in a NICU has until age 18 years plus the usual statutory time frame for bringing an action. A 1-year statute of limitations for physician suits would leave liability open through the child's reaching age 19 years. A 3-year statute of limitations for hospitals would leave liability open through the child's reaching age 21 years. Statutes of limitations for neonatal care also vary from state to state. Nurses in neonatal practice should be aware of the time frames for the states in which they practice.

Professional Liability Insurance

The long period over which suits may potentially be brought by persons cared for as infants in a NICU has implications for professional liability (malpractice insurance) coverage. There are two types of professional liability coverage. One is called claims-made coverage and the other is called occurrence coverage.

Claims-made coverage pays damages only for claims brought during the period in which the policy is in force. Thus any claim in negligence brought during the policy period, even if the event occurred many years in the past, is covered. Occurrence coverage provides for claims brought many years after the precipitating event has occurred, even though the nurse no longer carries professional liability insurance.

Claims-made policies are advantageous to the insurer because the insurer receives premiums in an amount judged sufficient to cover claims during a certain period. Occurrence policies are advantageous to the nurse because he or she does not have to continue insurance coverage after ceasing to work or on retirement. Nurses should examine their professional liability policies to determine whether coverage is the claims-made or occurrence type. If coverage is the claims-made type, nurses should make arrangements to purchase a *tail* policy, which takes effect after the original policy period ends. The nurse should continue coverage through the duration of the statute of limitations—for an infant as long as 21 years.

Nurses are often informed by health care facility employers that they do not need to carry personal professional liability insurance coverage. The reason given is that facilities purchase insurance to cover the negligent acts or omissions of their employees. Although health care facilities are generally well meaning in proffering this advice (in terms of saving nurses' money), they ignore the probably minor but real risk that the nurse may practice independently outside the facility setting. Inappropriate advice to a neighbor or inappropriate care to an injured child on a scout troop outing while acting as a medical support person could result in a malpractice suit. There is also the remote possibility that damages awarded might exceed hospital policy limits, and the plaintiff could then tap the nurse's personal assets. Personal professional liability insurance serves as insulation for the nurse from loss of personal possessions through negligence or malpractice suits.

Nurses should know that professional liability insurance does not insulate their assets from intentional acts. A nurse who defames a parent, threatens a parent, or deliberately harms an infant is not protected. This lack of protection is the case even if criminal charges have not been upheld before a civil suit is brought.

Standard of Care

Today, the higher acuity level, the more complex nursing judgments, and the exceptional vulnerability of the neonatal client raise the likelihood of lawsuits. The anxiety associated with fear of potential legal liability for practice, however, can be positively channeled by increasing one's focus on professional accountability. Accountable professionals practice prudently and reasonably based on their education and experience. Knowing and practicing nursing according to current standards helps ensure that a legal challenge to one's practice can be successfully defended.

Note that in Table 4–1 professional accountability can also be defined as carrying out the nursing process. Legal accountability is then defined by giving a positive orientation to the legal elements of negligence. Nursing documentation provides evidence of both professional accountability and legal accountability.

Nursing is an integral and valued aspect of neonatal care. Care is a close-knit effort that principally involves nurses and physicians. Pegalis and Wachsman (1986) quote from the 1979 edition of *Nelson's Textbook of Pediatrics* that "the most important factor in the successful care of premature infants is the skill, experience, and number of nursing staff. It's the responsibility of the physician to insist on an optimal amount of expert nursing" (p. 334). Professional and facility standards of practice should reflect this important alliance of professionals.

Sources for the Standard of Care

How does the neonatal nurse know what the standard of care is at any given point in time? The nurse can look to various sources.

TABLE 4–1 Relationship of Professional and Legal Accountability

Professional Accountability		Legal Accountability
	D	
	O	
	C	
	U	
Assessment	M	Duty
Planning	E	Fulfilled
Implementation	N	Causes
Evaluation	T	Benefits
Revision	A	
	T	
	I	
	O	
	N	

The American Nurses' Association uses the nursing process as a generic approach to guide nursing decision-making (American Nurses' Association, 1993). Thus an attorney representing a plaintiff wants to know if the nurse assessed the infant's status, planned and carried out care, evaluated that care, and made appropriate revisions. Table 4–1 takes this approach to accountability.

Specialty professional associations may provide more specific guidelines to practitioners in the neonatal area. These are updated by professional consensus mechanisms based on changing knowledge in the field. The National Association for Neonatal Nurses (NANN), for example, has Neonatal Nursing Transport Standards and Guidelines (NANN, 1994) and Standards of Care for Neonatal Nursing Practice (NANN, 1993). Table 4–2 provides an example of how the standard of care has evolved over time in relation to oxygen administration in neonates. The level of oxygen administered has changed over time as research has refined levels that achieve a therapeutic result but generally avoid complications such as retinopathy of prematurity. It is the nurse's responsibility to be aware of these changing standards. The development and widespread distribution of guidelines in neonatal care set by professional associations such as the American Academy of Pediatrics/American College of Obstetricians and Gynecologists (1992) are among the influences that have led states to recognize standards of care as being national rather than local in origin. Other influences have included ready accessibility of information about care in professional journals as well as the need for adherence to national standards in order to receive accreditation through the Joint Commission on Accreditation of Healthcare Organizations (JCAHO). Attendance at continuing education programs in the specialty area, referring to recognized texts when questions about care arise, and keeping abreast of state licensing standards also keep the nurse current in practice.

Health care facilities have a corporate duty of care (Darling v. Charleston Community Memorial Hospital, 1965). Thus they have a responsibility to ensure conditions of employment that permit meeting the expected standard of care in areas like NICUs. Plaintiffs look at the hospital's responsibility to meet JCAHO accreditation standards by examining hospital policy and procedure. Policy and procedure manuals should reflect these current standards of care. An example of a standard that must be met is ensuring that staff understand the function and operation of new equipment.

Standards should be thought of as general guidelines to practice. More important, however, is that any nurse be able to defend any action or inaction in relation to care of the neonate as reasonable and prudent. This defense means that the nurse must not only be able to identify what is regarded as the current general standard of care but also must have a rationale for decision-making that adjusts care to the specific individual. For exam-

TABLE 4–2 Evolution of the Standard of Care for Oxygen Administration to Neonates

1942	Retrolental fibroplasia recognized as cause of blindness in newborns, especially premature infants
1948	American Academy of Pediatrics: Supports administration of oxygen to all premature infants and infants suffering asphyxia or respiratory distress Suggested oxygen levels 50 percent
1954	Report of cooperative study links retrolental fibroplasia to oxygen administration
1956	American Academy of Pediatrics: Recommends oxygen levels not to exceed 40 percent Needed additional oxygen to be obtained from supplemental source Oxygen to be prescribed rather than routinely administered Independent confirmation of oxygen levels using oxygen analyzer every 4 hours
1971	Focus on oxygen tension in blood (up to 100 mm Hg) rather than oxygen administration levels Term infants to be administered oxygen only to abolish cyanosis Calibration of oxygen analyzer daily
1977	Oxygen tension dropped to 50 mm Hg
1983	American Academy of Pediatrics and American College of Obstetrics and Gynecology: Oxygen 50 to 90 mm Hg Calibration of oxygen analyzers every 8 hours
1988	Oxygen 50 to 80 mm Hg

Compiled from American Academy of Pediatrics/American College of Obstetricians and Gynecologists. (1983). *Guidelines for perinatal care*. Elk Grove Village, IL: Author; Lewis, S. M. (1986). *OB/GYN malpractice*. New York: John Wiley & Sons; Lewis, S. M. (1991). *OB/GYN malpractice* (Cum. Suppl.). New York: John Wiley & Sons; Pegalis, S. E., Wachsman, H. F. (1986). *American law of medical malpractice* (Vol. 3). Rochester, NY: Lawyers Co-Operative Publishing; Pegalis, S. E., Wachsman, H. F. (1990). *American law of medical malpractice* (Cum. Suppl.). Rochester, NY: Lawyers Co-Operative Publishing.

ple, the general standard of practice may be to administer certain fluids at specific rates depending on the weight and maturity of the infant. This general standard does not excuse the nurse from failing to adjust the rate downward—even halting fluid administration—and seeking consultation in the event that the infant begins to show signs of fluid overload.

Changing Nursing Care Delivery Standards of Care

The redesign of nursing care delivery systems to include the use of unlicensed assistive personnel to perform nursing care most recently reserved to licensed staff is cause for concern about patient safety. Echoing the quote in Nelson's text, nurses believe successful neonatal care depends on the "skill, experience, and number of (licensed) nursing staff." Although skill, experience, and numbers are, no doubt, critical components of quality and certainly safety in care, finding a proper staffing mix in the face of changing interventions, changing reimbursements, and changing delivery sites is not so certain. In the face of these changes, caution is in order.

First, staffing mix changes should be piloted in individual facilities using not only patient satisfaction but also clinical outcomes as measures of quality and safety. Developing such measures is not easy. Care must be taken to assure that the clinical outcomes measured have a relationship to staffing changes. For example, in the face of earlier discharges, the research design may call for home visits after patient discharge to determine if infant and mother health outcomes are similar to those seen in the past. If an increase in postpartum infections is found, was the difference due to the use of unlicensed assistive personnel or some other change in perinatal care?

An example of morbidity and mortality associated with early discharge includes problems of dehydration in infants with first-time breastfeeding mothers. New mothers who had no health care professionals to evaluate their infant and assist with breastfeeding sometimes got into trouble with their infants over the first several days at home. As a result of changed discharge policies, infants were discharged before their mothers' milk came in and the breastfeeding routine had been established. Nationally it has been reported that some of these infants became dehydrated, with reports of death as well as infants who had to undergo amputation of extremities secondary to emboli associated with severe dehydration. There have been reports of seizures linked to hyponatremia and dehydration as well.

Second, before delegating care to unlicensed assistive personnel the nurse must be aware of the education and experience of the unlicensed assistive personnel. Facilities have the responsibility for developing policies to ensure transmission of this vital information to staff nurses. Records of unlicensed assistive personnel education, both of content and competency, must be retained (Ohio Board of Nursing, 1995).

Third, the nurse must keep in mind that he or she cannot delegate patient assessment and *therefore the judgment calls changing nursing care plans and collaborating with other providers*. Because redesign increases the number of patients for whom the nurse is responsible, some reliance on unlicensed assistive personnel for information about patient status is inevitable. Consistency in patient care teams is one risk management approach to ensure that necessary information is transmitted from unlicensed assistive personnel to nurses. Consistent teams have knowledge of each member's strengths and weaknesses and can adjust for these differences to ensure patient safety. Cross-trained personnel from other units should be used with discretion, as they disrupt team consistency and pose a potential risk to patient safety.

At the national level, the American Nurses' Association has called for nurses to act as advocates in alerting the public to unsafe staffing conditions (American Nurses' Association, 1995a). Concurrently, the American Nurses' Association has called for an increasing focus on the quality of care research (American Nurses' Association, 1995b). At the state level, nursing boards are moving to regulate unlicensed assistive personnel under their nursing standards authority. Ohio is an example (Ohio Board of Nursing, 1995, August).

Steps in the Litigation Process

Suppose a nurse's practice does come under scrutiny in a lawsuit. What are the steps in the litigation process?

The first ingredient of a malpractice suit is a parent or, as indicated previously, the neonate who has now achieved the age of majority and is unhappy with the result of his or her care as a neonate. The disaffected parent or former patient who perceives that caregivers may be responsible for a functional disability will seek out an attorney. The attorney usually first seeks the advice of an expert in the field to determine whether the plaintiff has sufficient cause to initiate a suit. This first step means that the attorney needs to obtain the consent of the client to get copies of the patient's records, find an expert, and have the expert review the record.

Medical records are critical to the conduct of a lawsuit. They are admissible in evidence as the business records of the health care facility and, as such, are accorded the presumption of being a true record of events. Any evidence that records have been tampered with immediately raises questions about the credibility of both the defendant institution and any nurse involved.

If the presence of the legal elements of negligence can be

ascertained from a reading of the records, the attorney files a complaint in the appropriate court of law. Simultaneously, the attorney serves the defendant with a copy of the complaint. The defendant hospital notifies its insurance carrier of the suit. The carrier notifies its defense law firm of the need for an answer to the complaint. Response must occur within a specified time. The statutory rules of civil procedure govern the period for receiving this answer. An answer offers the opportunity to state a defense to the action. The answer may be accompanied simply by a motion to dismiss the action for failure to state the legal elements of a claim. The plaintiff may then have an opportunity to reply to the answer. If the defendant's answer has been accompanied by a motion to dismiss the complaint, the plaintiff will defend against the motion in a court proceeding that does not involve a jury.

After these actions, if the lawsuit moves forward, attorneys for both sides will seek to find out more about the circumstances surrounding the case. In legal language, this is termed the *period of discovery.* It consists of gathering information from both parties—for example, information about the injury or harm suffered by the plaintiff and about the standard of care in the defendant institution. This information gathering may be accomplished through written questions to both parties, called *interrogatories,* and by obtaining depositions (sworn oral statements) from persons involved in care and perhaps also from expert witnesses.

The discovery period has several purposes. First, it helps both lawyers prepare for trial. Second, during this time grounds for settlement may be established if liability becomes clear or the defense cannot muster a case sufficient to win at trial. Third, facts may unfold that clearly favor either the plaintiff or the defendant, thus permitting that party to move for a summary judgment. Settlement of a lawsuit can occur at any time prior to a trial or even while a trial is in session. Motions for directed verdicts can end litigation if following presentation of evidence, a party views the evidence as favorable to their case. In rare instances, the judge may even reverse a judgment arrived at by a jury.

A trial is a formal process used to present a case. Attorneys for both sides have the opportunity to select jurors from a group of persons summoned for jury duty. Following jury selection, plaintiff and defense attorneys make opening statements about what they intend to demonstrate in their side of the case. The formal presentation of testimony then occurs, with the plaintiff presenting first and the defendant second.

Both witnesses of fact and expert witnesses generally testify at trial. The witness is first questioned by the attorney for the side the witness is representing, and then the opposing attorney cross-examines the witness. Redirect examination may follow, particularly when a witness' credibility has been undermined and the attorney for the side the witness represents wishes to "rehabilitate" the witness. Depositions taken prior to trial may be used in lieu of in-person testimony when a witness has died or is out of reach (e.g., out of the country). Witnesses testifying in person will want to review their depositions prior to trial so that their testimony does not conflict. Conflicting testimony is a source for destroying the credibility of a witness.

After the presentation of both the plaintiff's and the defendant's cases, attorneys make closing statements. After the judge's instructions on the law, the jury considers all trial testimony to arrive at a verdict. In civil cases, the verdict reflects that a preponderance, or greater weight, of the evidence was determined to be in favor of the winning party.

Verdicts may be appealed. Appellate courts generally defer to trial courts on matters of fact because appellate courts deal only with the written transcripts of a trial. Appellate court judges lack the benefit of observing the nonverbal communication of a trial witness. Thus a person who appeals on the weight of the evidence has a heavy burden to bear. Appellate courts are more likely to rule on issues such as whether the trial judge instructed the jury correctly as to the application of the law.

In trials, judges are responsible for the application of the law—hence the importance of their instruction to juries—and juries are responsible for applying the facts. Although parties in civil cases do have a right to a jury trial, in some instances agreement may be reached to try a case before a judge alone. The judge then rules on both the law and the facts.

Expert Witnesses

Expert witnesses supply opinions about the standard of practice in similar situations. They differ from witnesses of fact who supply "presence at the scene" knowledge—actual knowledge of the particular set of circumstances that has led to litigation. The expert witness's knowledge of the particular facts is limited to a reading of the medical record. The more clearly the record reveals that the nurse practiced according to the standards of care current at the time of the situation in question, the more beneficial the expert witness can be to the nurse's defense.

Nurses who act as expert witnesses must have practice experience in the area in which they are testifying as well as be knowledgeable about that area of practice. Juries have discretion in the weight they accord the evidence provided by an expert witness.

Testifying as an expert witness for the defendant offers the opportunity to act as an advocate for the nurse who is arguably not negligent. Testifying as an expert witness for the plaintiff offers the opportunity to act as an advocate for the harmed person. Testifying as an expert witness also affords the opportunity to act as an advocate for society. This occurs when the expert, on reviewing a record, determines that negligence has not occurred. In such an instance, the forthright report of the expert prevents the misuse of societal resources in an action not worthy of pursuit.

A nurse acting as an expert witness is entitled to charge for the service. The nurse should expect to be prepared by the attorney for the party represented. This preparation includes discussion about the line of questioning to be expected from both attorneys. Strategies for establishing credibility as a witness should be discussed. Some of these include remaining calm despite the opposing attorney's attempt to shake the nurse's self-confidence, asking that ambiguous questions be repeated, answering only what is asked, and acknowledging the jury's presence both by looking at the jury and by using language that the jury can understand.

MANAGEMENT OF RISK

The nurse in the NICU is at risk for lawsuit in a number of areas but can take measures to reduce exposure to this risk. Areas of particular concern are assessment, medication and fluid administration, equipment use, resuscitation, oxygen administration, and discharge planning with parents.

Individual Nursing Practice and Management of Risk

A total systems assessment by the nurse is critical. As the caregiver closest to the neonate, the nurse is best positioned to make and act on observations that reflect a deviation in the neonate's system functions. The nurse reduces risk when he or she promptly records deviations and takes and records appropriate actions. Appropriate actions may include changes in care under protocol or seeking consultation from another appropriate provider—a more experienced staff nurse, the nurse manager, a clinical specialist or nurse practitioner in the field, or the responsible physician. Nurses should take care that when following protocols they do not fail to take into consideration infant responses that are not covered by the protocol. "Cookbook" responses, to the extent that they are "knee-jerk" rather than thoughtful reactions, are not good practice.

Today's monitoring equipment reduces the risk of providing too much fluid, but the possibility of human error remains in the initial rate-setting process. Familiarity with usual quantities of fluids for infants of various weights is critical to determine whether an order for fluid has been miswritten or misinterpreted. Guidelines to reduce risks associated with fluid administration are similar to those for administering pharmacologic agents: "right time, right dose, right route, right medication, and right person" should be checked and rechecked. The infant patient, not just the equipment, requires constant assessment for reaction to fluid administration.

Nurses have an obligation to raise questions with the infant care team when they suspect that a new drug may be causing adverse reactions. This type of teamwork can lead to the timely withdrawal of a drug from the market. The withdrawal of the vitamin E preparation E-Ferol is an example (Schorr, 1984).

The use of high-technology equipment has made life easier for the nurse. However, the nurse must have sufficient working knowledge of equipment operation to recognize equipment malfunction. Risk management in this case requires that the nurse leave the repair of malfunctions to trained persons. Faulty equipment altered by hospital personnel to make it work voids the manufacturer's strict liability for a defective product when harm occurring to an infant can be attributed to the equipment. Moreover, equipment must be used as directed by the manufacturer for its stated purpose. Equipment used for other than its intended purpose makes the facility rather than the manufacturer liable for any infant harm attributed to the equipment's use.

Resuscitation events require careful documentation of both the sequence of events that precipitated resuscitation efforts and the sequence of interventions occurring during those resuscitation efforts. Assigning an individual to document the sequence of resuscitation efforts is critical to establishing the standard of care that was followed should questions later arise. Similarly, oxygen support for infants requires meticulous documentation to demonstrate that oxygen levels were commensurate with need and finely tuned to the infant's developmental stage.

As care patterns move infants home quickly, nurses become more vulnerable to suits rooted in communication failure. Parents who have not adequately understood and practiced complicated technologic care—and even the seemingly low technology of breastfeeding—bring suit if their child suffers harm because of their lack of understanding or ability to provide care. Clear documentation of teaching that includes evidence of both parent understanding and practice opportunities serves in the nurse's defense. Written instructions and follow-up home visits are additional risk management measures for these situations.

Communication and Documentation

Communication and documentation are the linchpins of professional practice. Risk management literature indicates that the value of communication as a risk management tool cannot be overemphasized (Kraus, 1986).

Verbal and written communication skills make possible a team approach to neonatal care. In turn, effective team efforts increase the chances for the most positive yet realistic outcomes for neonate and family. Timely and clear communication among nurse, physician, and family acknowledges and values the roles of each in the care of the infant. Communication with family serves the added purpose of warding off misunderstandings that could lead to later lawsuits. In the situation noted earlier, the nurse observes signs of fluid overload and promptly takes action to reduce volume flow and report his or her observations to the responsible physician. These actions, as well as further interventions on the infant's behalf, should be shared with the family by the infant care team. Discussion of the infant's adverse response to normal fluid flow, which may relate to compromised cardiac or renal function, is critical.

As the business record of the health care facility, the medical record is the enduring evidence of the activities of assessment, planning, implementation, and evaluation of the neonate's care. Documentation should provide not only evidence of this nursing process but also documentation of the time and content of communication among nurses, physicians, and the family of the neonate. Interventions that reflect new professional thought or a more conservative standard of care than usual deserve a notation indicating their rationale. For example, giving oxygen at minimally therapeutic levels is a conservative approach to treatment. More aggressive therapy might increase those levels for an infant whose respiratory response is judged marginal, even though the risk of damage to the retinal nerve is raised. Rationale for the decision to stay the course at minimal oxygen levels or to increase the level should appear in the record. Physician progress notes should reflect the physician's rationale. The nurse's notes should reflect his or her discussion with the physician and other nurses and the subsequent treatment decisions and nursing interventions.

Documentation ideally occurs contemporaneously with nursing actions. Practically speaking, however, notes may be written a few hours subsequent to nursing care events. Observations might, for example, be charted immediately on a checklist form, but narrative notes might be written later. Attorneys understand that this is the reality of nursing practice.

Insertion of information some time subsequent to the shift on which an event has occurred also takes place. Such additions, known as late entries, are acceptable practice. The underlying reason for their acceptance is that it is better to have pertinent data that is admissible as evidence. If not present in the record, data may be inadmissible as evidence because the person reporting an event may not have actually witnessed the occurrence. Such information would be termed hearsay because of the witness's lack of firsthand knowledge. By precluding hearsay as evidence, legal procedure acknowledges that the truth is best known by a person who was at the scene of an event.

Documentation is the legal evidence of professional accountability. Assessments, interventions, evaluations and re-evaluations, and communications not documented are presumed not to have occurred. Without documentation, the nurse who asserts at deposition or trial that an activity occurred can expect a deserved assault on his or her credibility.

Truth-telling

Truth-telling ranks high on the list of risk management techniques. Truth-telling may not avoid lawsuits, but it can mitigate damages and serve to establish the reputation of the health care facility as being a caring provider.

Truth-telling becomes a concern when some harm has occurred to the neonate because of the negligent action or inaction of a nurse or other provider. First, on discovery of the incident, measures should be instituted to remediate or minimize the harm. Second, institutions may absorb the cost of care for the extra procedures required by the harm that has occurred. These two steps can minimize the actual monetary damages suffered by the neonate and the neonate's family. A forthright explanation to the family about the event and corrective actions that have been taken then serves to dispel the commonly held perception that wrongdoers cover up their errors. For example, failure to discover immediately the incorrect placement of a chest tube because of a delay in obtaining an x-ray film to check its location can result in severe compromise of the infant. Use of truth-telling as a risk management tool would involve explanation of the erroneous placement to the family. The health care facility would also absorb the cost of the second placement and any additional care required because of the error.

Incident Reports

Incident or variance reports detail occurrences that pose a risk of monetary loss for a health care facility. A lawsuit need not occur for this financial loss to be realized. As in the example of the misplaced chest tube, loss may occur because the cost of additional care is voluntarily absorbed. Not only neonates but also family, visitors, and staff can experience injury or risk of injury. It is critical to sound risk management that incident reports be filed not only when actual injury has occurred but also when potential for injury exists to any of these persons.

Malfunctioning equipment that has the potential for, but may not yet have caused, injury is a good example of the type of information included in this potential risk category. Consistent failure to communicate or respond to communication in a timely manner about changes in patient status by nurses and other providers also falls into this category. Even a highly effective risk management program cannot achieve zero risk, but incident reports can afford facility administrators the opportunity to identify areas of actual and potential risk so that steps can be taken to reduce such risk by changing practices or altering the environment.

Incident reports involving neonates should mirror descriptions found in the medical record. These reports should contain *facts* surrounding the event. Conclusory or blaming statements should be absent from the report. The report should reflect the facts of the incident and the steps taken to assess and alleviate any actual injury that might have occurred. Incident reporting systems should require professionals not only to disclose their own mistakes but also to report those of peers. The filing of an incident report should not be mentioned in the record.

A risk management maxim is that the incident reporting system should be separate from the system for nursing staff evaluation. Incident reports are an administrative tool providing the opportunity for adjustments to systems involved in delivering care in order to enhance the safety of clients, visitors, and staff. The incident reporting system itself should afford the opportunity for those involved to discuss the incident at the unit level as a health care delivery team. Occasion for discussion should provide opportunities to suggest strategies for avoiding similar incidents in the future. Staff evaluation, in contrast, focuses on the individual rather than on the system. The perception that incident reports are used for staff evaluation rather than system change will deter nurses from completing incident reports, thus reducing their effectiveness as a risk management tool.

However, a series of incident reports involving one nurse and separate types of errors or multiple instances of the same type of error cannot be ignored in a performance review. Otherwise, the facility runs the risk of being charged with failing to fulfill its corporate duty of care to staff with competent nurses. Thus, although good reason exists for keeping the incident reporting system and staff evaluation systems parallel, it would be poor corporate practice to make their separation a policy with no exceptions.

Incident reports can, of course, be used to foster professional growth as opposed to discipline. This opportunity occurs when incident reports reveal that a nurse needs additional guidance in planning work or avoiding distraction in an emergency situation. Incidents may be precipitated by management practices that result in chronic insufficient staffing or by a nurse whose errors stem from a substance abuse problem. These examples are susceptible to strategies that do not place at issue the competence of the nurse. Staffing can be redesigned. Participation in a peer assistance program can assist the substance-abusing nurse in achieving recovery and renewed practice.

Incident reports can direct management's attention to concerns other than personnel. Faulty equipment has been mentioned earlier. Concerns about whether particular drugs are hazardous to employee health or patient health, or both, may initially derive from incident reports. Management has responded with protective measures for the use of cytotoxic drugs with equipment, supplies, and institutional policies and procedures that provide directives for protective behaviors. The use of universal precautions for handling body fluids is a response to a new infectious agent. Because personnel who fail to use precautions put themselves and patients at risk for acquiring human immunodeficiency virus (HIV), they should be identified in the incident reporting system. Consistent failure to use precautions should also be cause for disciplinary action because it violates the standard of care.

Incident reports not only afford opportunities for management to take appropriate corrective actions to reduce risks but also serve the useful purpose of prompting an immediate investigation following the occurrence of an incident, when memories are still fresh and the facts surrounding the incident are likely to be reported accurately. Should a lawsuit ensue, this timely follow-up can be valuable in preparing a case. The incident reporting and claims investigation process may then become the work product of the hospital attorney and thus be immune from plaintiff scrutiny during the discovery period under the rule of attorney work product privilege.

Accessibility of the incident report to the plaintiff's attorney does, however, vary from state to state and even from circumstance to circumstance. Sharing an incident report can be viewed as disadvantageous to the defendant because the plaintiff's attorney will attempt to show that the incident report was filed solely in anticipation of a lawsuit rather than for effective risk management. Conversely, when incident reports are subject to the discovery rule, they can also serve to enhance the credibility of the defendant when facts on incident report and medical record match.

Ideally, neonatal nurses should view incident reports as an extension of their ethical obligation to safeguard the health and safety of clients (American Nurses' Association, 1984). This obligation requires an extension of the concept of *client* to include not only the neonate and family but also facility staff and visitors. In the process of fulfilling this professional ethical obligation, the nurse also fulfills the obligation to the facility to assist it in meeting its corporate legal duty to provide a safe environment.

Quality Programs

Quality assurance and improvement and total quality management programs can be thought of as the proactive counterpart of risk management efforts. Early efforts at quality assurance took the form of audits of nursing care. Audits sought to determine whether the complete nursing process was applied in relation to nursing problems. This audit was process-oriented quality assurance. If the steps were present, quality was present. Patient satisfaction surveys have also long been used as measures of quality. Rather than measure actual clinical care, however, they have focused on environmental conditions such as waiting times and staff courtesy. More recently, quality improvement programs have set goals and then defined indicators to measure goal achievement. In a neonatal setting, this might include maintaining optimal respiratory status for infants. An indicator might be defined in percentages of infants having cyanotic extremities—one would look for a low rate after the first few days of life. Focus is also shifting to longer term outcomes of care—for example, how many infants successfully move into a normal pattern of development after a time in a NICU. The JCAHO is currently using the term *continuous quality improvement* to reflect health care facility quality aims.

What implications do quality programs have for neonatal nursing practice? First, they suggest that nurses need to examine their interventions to determine whether they improve infant functional outcomes. Second, as data about the relationship of interventions and outcomes are generated, quality programs will generate new standards of care. Plaintiff's attorneys in the future will ask their expert witnesses in what percentage of cases a positive outcome could be expected in a given situation. Studies of the relationship of restraint use to the prevention of falls are beginning to yield these data for elderly clients. In NICUs, nurses can study different approaches to teaching parents infant care and measure levels of success associated with each approach. The emphasis on quality offers the nurse and nursing the opportunity to forge a stronger link between practice and outcome.

SOCIAL AND PUBLIC POLICY CONCERNS IN PERINATAL CARE

Decision-Making in Infant Care

The issue of deciding treatment is different for children than it is for adults. Infants in particular have no experience with life, nor for that matter can they speak for themselves in relation to choice of treatment. Parents, as the natural guardians of children, are presumed to act in the child's best interests in making choices about treatment. By providing information, health care providers should assist parents in the decision-making process. Unfortunately, providers sometimes may personally be at ethical or clinical odds with parental choices. These situations can generate legal action in the form of case, statutory, and regulatory laws.

Situations that give rise to legal action generally involve choice of treatment or the use of life-sustaining measures. Informed consent, including the signing of a specific informed consent form, is sought for invasive procedures that carry serious risks as well as benefits. Treatments that are within the usual course of care, such as measurement of weight, feeding, bathing, and observation of physiologic systems function, are part of the general consent to care signed by parents on the infant's admission to a health care facility. This section first reviews the formal consent procedure. It then discusses the use of life-sustaining measures for infants, focusing on the evolution of law in response to the Baby Doe cases.

Informed Consent

Neonates may need surgical intervention (to correct defects), invasive diagnostic procedures, and invasive treatment procedures. Does the nurse in these situations have a legal role in the informed consent process? Yes, but the legal role is generally limited to witnessing the consent form signed by the parents or legal guardian of the infant. By law, the responsibility for obtaining informed consent for treatments belongs to the physician. Ideally, in fact, the physician witnesses the signing of the consent form. This practice has the advantage of placing the parents and physician together at a time when discussion regarding care could take place. Thus the nurse is not legally responsible for ascertaining whether the parents' consent is truly informed. Arguably, however, she is ethically responsible.

Information about the procedure to be undertaken, who will do the procedure, its benefits and risks, and alternatives to the procedure—including no treatment—must be shared with the consenting persons by the physician. Ethically, the physician should explain interventions so that the decision makers are rationally persuaded to agreement. Rational persuasion occurs when the decision maker arrives at the same conclusion as the advisor but bases the decision on the acceptance of reasoning presented by the advisor and concurred with according to the value system of the decision maker. With rational persuasion, the decision maker feels free to make a truly personal choice. This approach differs from manipulation, which occurs when the decision maker simply assumes the values of the physician and follows the physician's suggestion. *Rational persuasion* also differs from *coercion*, which occurs when the decision maker feels subjugated to the physician and powerless to choose. When coercion occurs, the decision maker keeps his or her own value system but goes along with the physician because he or she feels compelled to do so (Benjamin & Curtis, 1992).

Although the nurse does not have a legal duty to obtain informed consent, he or she can play an important risk management role by accompanying the physician to the conference with the family at which consent to treatment is discussed. The role of observer places the nurse in a position to augment or clarify the family's understanding of the procedure when they have had time to reflect on, and possibly become confused about, the physician's explanations. Knowledge of the content of the informed consent conversation can assist the nurse in supporting the family in their choices—that is, play an advocate role—even when those choices may differ from the sincere and well-meaning recommendations of the medical establishment. The nurse is never, however, in a position to initiate medical recommendations or comment on medical prognoses. When parents or other surrogate decision makers exhibit concern about prognoses, the nurse needs to reinvolve the physician in the consent process. Medical recommendations or discussion of prognoses by the nurse could easily become the basis of charges of practicing medicine without a license.

Obtaining informed consent is a process. Lack of informed consent can also be the reason for a malpractice action. The occurrence of an undisclosed material risk—a risk that could cause reasonable decision makers to refuse the procedure—can result in suit. Flores v. Flushing Hospital and Medical Center (1985) is a case in point. The family in that case was not told that the risks of providing oxygen to the premature neonate included blindness. They later sued both hospital and physicians.

Legal Legacy of Baby Doe

When withholding or withdrawing care from a disabled newborn becomes an issue, social policy introduces further constraint on the decision maker. A 1982 case precipitated public outcry against the parents' nontreatment decision for a newborn with Down syndrome and esophageal fistula (Indiana *ex rel.* Infant Doe v. Monroe Circuit Court, 1982). With nutrition and treatment withheld, the child died. Brown and colleagues (1986) chronicled the evolution of the public policy response to that decision.

First, then-President Ronald Reagan issued a memorandum to the Secretary of the U.S. Department of Health and Human Services stating that federal law prohibited discrimination, including the withholding of medical treatment, on the basis of disability. Richard Schweiker, who was Department of Health and Human Services Secretary at the time, followed up with a notice to health care providers that emphasized the applicability of Section 504 of the Rehabilitation Act of 1973 (47 Federal Register 26,027, 1982).

About a year later, the Department of Health and Human Services issued regulations titled "Interim Final Rules" or "Baby Doe Regulations." The regulations required the posting in delivery, maternity, pediatric, and nursing units of a notice stating: "Discriminatory failure to feed and care for handicapped infants in this facility is prohibited by federal law" (48 Federal Register 9630, 1983). The regulation required inclusion of two accompanying statements in each posting. The first was to indicate that Section 504 applied to the treatment of disabled newborns. The second statement contained instructions for any citizen to call a Department of Health and Human Services hotline if they had any knowledge of a severely defective newborn being denied food or customary medical care on the basis of a disability. The regulations were subsequently challenged and defeated because they had bypassed the Federal Administrative Procedures Act for promulgating regulations (American Academy of Pediatrics v. Heckler, 1983).

Following legal defeat of the Baby Doe Regulations, the Department of Health and Human Services moved to issue "Proposed Rules," which restated the requirement of the Interim Final Rules while adding a provision that state child protective service agencies would develop and carry out procedures to prevent medical neglect of severely defective infants (48 Federal Register 30,846, 1983). Response to the rules was overwhelmingly positive: more than 16,000 responses from the public favored the rules. Nonetheless, the rules were criticized by provider organizations. The American Academy of Pediatrics proposed the establishment of infant care review committees. The American Medical Association vehemently opposed all federal intrusion into treatment decisions. Following the comment period, the Department of Health and Human Services issued "Final Rules," reflecting a compromise of smaller notice requirements and areas of display where only nurses and other medical professionals would see them (49 Federal Register 1622, 1984). Sanction for violation of the rules was the withdrawal of financial aid to states under the Child Abuse Prevention and Treatment Act.

Subsequently, the Final Rules were defeated. Their defeat followed the decision of the U.S. Court of Appeals for the Second Circuit in United States v. University Hospital (1984)—the Long Island Baby Jane Doe case—in which the parents chose to follow a conservative course of treatment for their spina bifida–afflicted child. The basis for the defeat of the rules was that Congress never intended the Rehabilitation Act to apply to decisions affecting medically defective newborns (Bowen v. American Hospital Association, 1986).

However, in the midst of legal controversy surrounding the Final Rules, Congress in 1984 chose to amend the Child Abuse Prevention and Treatment Act. Rules enacted under these amendments expanded the definition of child abuse to include "withholding medically indicated treatment" as the

> . . . failure to respond to the infant's life-threatening conditions by providing treatment (including appropriate nutrition, hydration and medication) which, in the treating physician's or physicians' reasonable medical judgments will be most likely to be effective in ameliorating or correcting conditions. (45 Code of Federal Regulations S 1340.15 (b) (2), 1985)

The rules reflected the balance in the Child Abuse Amendments "between the need for an effective program and the need to prevent unreasonable governmental intrusion" (49 Federal Register 14,879, 1984).

The Child Abuse Amendments tie federal funding to implementation of procedures designed to prevent instances of medical neglect, including withholding medically indicated treatment. The rules promulgated under the Child Abuse Amendments stress that infant care review committees are permissive rather than mandatory. Right-to-life constituencies are assured that decisions regarding treatment are not based on quality-of-life criteria.

It is important to note that the Child Abuse Amendments exempt three categories of infants from their provisions. These are reflected in the rules and include the following:

> . . . when, in the treating physician's or physicians' reasonable medical judgment, (A) the infant is chronically and irreversibly comatose; (B) the provision of such treatment would (i) merely prolong dying, (ii) not be effective in ameliorating or correcting all of the infant's life threatening conditions, or (iii) otherwise be futile in terms of survival of the infant; or (C) the provision of such treatment would be virtually futile in terms of survival of the infant and the treatment itself under the circumstances would be inhumane. (45 Code of Federal Regulations S 1340.15 (b) (2), 1985)

Under no circumstances is it permissible to withhold appropriate nutrition, hydration, and medication.

Brown and associates (1986) note these rules: (1) clarify when life-sustaining treatment may be withheld from a defective newborn; (2) affirm the parents or guardians as decision makers; (3) clarify the standard for decision makers; and (4) clarify the standard for decision-making as the best interests of the infant.

Brown and associates also note that, as in the defeated rules promulgated under Section 504 of the Rehabilitation Act, sanctions for violating the rules do not affect the decision makers but rather affect state funding. However, states choosing not to seek federal funding for child abuse are not bound by the regulations. States adopting the federal amendments give state protection agencies the exclusive rights to bring suit on behalf of the defective infant.

Feldman and Murray (1984) reviewed the legislative activity that occurred in several states in the early 1980s concerning disabled newborns. By December 1983, 19 states had considered legislation. Seven states took action, with five passing legislation and two enacting resolutions. Not surprisingly, the states addressed issues of treatment needs and the administration of nutrition and hydration in a manner similar to the federal Child Abuse Amendments.

Concerns about the use of life-sustaining measures with infants continue. Fairfax Hospital in Virginia requested a declaratory judgment that withholding a ventilator from an anencephalic infant when the infant suffered respiratory distress would not violate state or federal law. Both district and circuit courts found withholding the ventilator support would violate the Emergency Medical Treatment and Active Labor Treatment Act (1986) (*In the Matter of Baby K*, 1993; *In the Matter of Baby K*, 1994; Capron, 1994). The Supreme Court declined to hear the case. With ventilator support when needed, the child lived to be 2½ years old.

In another case (Baby Ryan, cited in Capron [1995]), when parents sought a court order for life support for what physicians considered a futile situation, the hospital countered with a child abuse complaint against the parents. The child lived.

Treatment decisions are not made lightly. For every treatment issue reaching a court, many more issues are resolved through negotiation (Spielman, 1995). The occasional court decision simply adds to the framework within which those individual negotiations occur.

Research on Infants and Children

Nurses may find themselves conducting or participating in research conducted on neonates. Federal law establishes criteria for conduct of research on children according to varying degrees of risk (45 Code of Federal Regulations S 46.404–46.407, 1983). Familiarity with the provision of regulations guiding research is critical to the nurse assuming an advocacy role for the child.

There are four categories of risk:

1. Research not involving greater than minimal risk.

2. Research with greater than minimal risk but representing the prospect of direct benefit to the individual subjects.
3. Research involving greater than minimal risk and no prospect of direct benefit to individual subjects.
4. Research not otherwise approvable that presents an opportunity to understand, prevent, or alleviate a serious problem affecting the health or welfare of children.

The regulations in all four categories call for assent of children capable of participating in the decision-making process, with consent coming from parents or guardians. Clearly assent does not apply to neonates. The second category, greater than minimal risk with possible benefit to subjects, requires that the risk be justified by the anticipated benefit and that the anticipated benefit be at least as favorable to the subjects as available alternatives. The third category, greater than minimal risk with no prospect of direct benefit, is approvable if (1) the risk is only a minor increase over minimal risk; (2) the intervention presents experiences commensurate with what the subjects might experience in their actual or expected medical, dental, psychological, social, or educational situations; and (3) the intervention is likely to yield generalizable knowledge of vital importance for the understanding or amelioration of the subject's disorder or condition. Prior to approval of the fourth category of research, the Secretary of the Department of Health and Human Services must consult with a panel of experts and afford opportunity for public review. Following this review procedure, the research must satisfy either the conditions for the first three categories of risk or (1) be determined to present a reasonable opportunity of further understanding, prevention, or alleviation of a serious problem affecting the health or welfare of children (the category purpose); (2) be conducted in accordance with sound ethical principles; and (3) fulfill the necessary consent requirements.

Had the federal research regulations been in place in 1953, the infant plaintiff in a New York case might not have had cause to bring a lawsuit (Burton v. Brooklyn Doctors Hospital, 1982). Burton was born 2 days after the beginning of a national study known as the Cooperative Study of Retrolental Fibroplasia and the Use of Oxygen. The infant (Burton) was in good condition, and initial higher oxygen levels were later reduced by a resident physician. Later, however, another resident physician drastically increased the oxygen level as part of Burton's random assignment in the study. The assignment of the infant to increased oxygen levels in his "good condition" was ethically questionable. Although retinopathy of prematurity might be regarded as a "serious problem affecting the health and welfare of children," one might argue that present requirements for review of the study by a panel of experts as well as public review might have resulted in a modification of the study design to exclude infants in "good condition." Of course, one might also argue, from a justice or utilitarian perspective, that the time involved in the current review process might have resulted in more infants suffering injury because dissemination of study results would have occurred later than 1954. In this case, however, the plaintiff did recover damages because the court found that the informed consent of the parents for oxygen administration should have been obtained because the treating physician's own study revealed that increased oxygen was dangerous for a healthy infant. Administration of the oxygen thus exposed the child to an unwarranted risk.

Only federally funded research falls under the law. However, many institutional review boards (IRBs) apply federal regulations to all research projects conducted within the institution. The IRBs review research proposals to ensure protection for human subjects under the regulations. Nurses working in institutions in which the review of human subjects does not apply to privately funded research may consider acting as advocates for children when research would violate the ethical tenets of the federal regulations. Nurse researchers who sit on IRBs bring the voice of the profession to board deliberations.

Organ Donation for Neonates

Frequently, infants could benefit from whole-organ transplants. Unfortunately, the availability of suitable organs for infants is even more limited than it is for adults. One approach to resolving the scarcity has been using anencephalic infants as donors. Waiting until the natural death of the anencephalic infant precludes using organs for transplant because in the process of dying, vital oxygen delivery and blood flow to organs are increasingly compromised. What then are the legal vehicles that might be used for anencephalic donors, and what ethical problems do such donations raise?

One legal approach is the use of a state's Uniform Anatomical Gift Act. All states have passed this type of legislation. Acts permit living adult donors to elect to donate one of a paired organ. The acts also provide for an individual to designate organ donation on his or her driver's license in the event of death. Amendments might be made to these acts permitting parents to act as decision makers regarding donation of their anencephalic child's organs. This first approach avoids the larger societal concerns raised by the second approach; that is, amending acts that define death by adding a new category of anencephalic infant. Physiologically, anencephalic infants do not meet the criteria for brain death because brain stem function exists and therefore mechanical support for breathing via a respirator is generally unnecessary.

The development of brain death statutes actually originated with the need for transplantable organs as successful organ transplantation became a reality. Nonetheless, societal consensus does not currently exist to broaden brain death definitions. This lack of consensus is principally because right-to-life groups would argue that the definition of anencephalic infants and persons in persistent vegetative states as "brain dead" would be one more step down a slippery slope leading to our society's condoning active euthanasia (Capron, 1987; Cranford, 1988). The Baby K case mentioned earlier in relationship to the Baby Doe regulations illustrates the reluctance of two federal courts to begin forging such a trail.

Paliokas (1989) suggested that this need not be the case if statutes are specifically tailored to deal with anencephaly. Statutory safeguards against abuse would include (1) guidelines for establishing accurate diagnosis, (2) voluntary choice by the parents prior to birth, (3) review of each situation and the parental decision by a panel of legal and health professionals, and (4) court review when parents and panel body disagree. Policy statements in the statutes would emphasize their purpose as preservation of the child's dignity through minimization of any extraordinary medical interventions that simply prolong the dying process. In this respect, they would mirror current law, discussed earlier, regarding the treatment of disabled newborns.

Capron (1987) discussed ethical problems associated with both approaches. First, amending anatomical gift or definition of death acts may set a poor precedent because similarly situated persons—the comatose, demented, or severely retarded—might also then be considered as sources for the harvest of organs. Second, if the rationale for the use of anencephalic infants is that they are nonpersons because they will never be able to interact meaningfully with other persons, one might then destroy an anencephalic infant without being charged with homicide. In contrast, if anencephalic infants are recognized as persons, is it right to use one person as a means to save the life of another? This approach violates Kantian ethical principles, which do not permit the use of persons as a means to an end.

Capron suggested that the better alternative, in the ethical and legal sense, is to maintain both anatomical gift acts and definition of death statutes in their current form. He proposed, instead, that the medical profession work toward achieving approaches to maintaining anencephalic infant organs in a state viable for transplant when brain death does eventually occur.

Nurses working in NICUs should discuss these ethical and legal issues. Discussion and resultant understandings will put neonatal nurses in a better position to support not only the parents of a dying anencephalic infant but also those parents who wish to donate their anencephalic infant's organs and who are precluded from doing so by the current state of the law.

Litigation Surrounding Pregnancy

Nurses working in NICUs should be aware of wrongful pregnancy, wrongful birth, and wrongful life lawsuits. The reason for this is that nurses may need to support parents who feel wronged when negligently performed sterilization surgery results in a pregnancy, when pregnancy is misdiagnosed, or when parents are uninformed of infant defects that might have resulted in their electing abortion. In all instances, there is pecuniary damage to the families involved.

Courts have denied wrongful pregnancy claims on policy grounds, arguing that allowing the cause of action would generate fraudulent claims (Rieck v. Medical Protective Co. of Fort Wayne, Ind., 1974). Other courts have allowed damages for emotional distress of the mother, loss of consortium (loss of the companionship and services of husband and wife in marriage), and hospital and medical expenses associated with the pregnancy (Boone v. Mullendore, 1982). Most courts have denied costs of raising the healthy child on the basis that the child provides emotional benefit to the parents. This benefit rule, strictly followed, requires that the court ascribe a value to the benefit of having a child against the financial damage suffered by the family as the result of his or her birth (Restatement of Torts 2d, S 920, 1991). More recently, however, the Massachusetts and Wisconsin high courts have permitted costs for raising a healthy child (Burke v. Rivo, 1990; Marciniak v. Lundborg, 1990).

Wrongful birth actions occur when the parents of a severely defective infant allege that the opportunity to choose to terminate or continue the pregnancy was lost because the physician failed to advise the parent of risk of defect or the means (genetic counseling or amniocentesis) available to determine potential or actual defects. In a 1979 case, Berman v. Allan, parents of a Down syndrome child alleged that the obstetrician had not met the standard of care because of a failure to alert the 38-year-old woman of the availability of amniocentesis. Parents recovered damages for mental and emotional anguish but did not recover the cost of child rearing. The court saw the disabled child as still being a benefit to the parents and, therefore, the obstetrician was not found liable to the parents for child rearing expenses.

In wrongful life lawsuits, the defective child seeks compensation for the burdens of a life that would not have been desired had a choice been available. Courts are reluctant to classify actions as "wrongful life" for two reasons: (1) there is no fundamental right to be born normal and whole and (2) there is a problem valuing the life versus the nonlife the plaintiff states would have been desired (Becker v. Schwartz and Park v. Chessin, 1978; Elliott v. Brown, 1978). In California, Washington, and New Jersey, courts have resolved these difficulties by awarding the child only special damages—the cost of special care—rather than general damages that include pain and suffering. The courts have reasoned that special damages are congruent with what parents might recover in wrongful birth actions and that the actual injured party should not be in a lesser position than the parents for receiving damage awards. Courts have viewed not awarding damages for pain and suffering as consistent with the difficulty of determining the value of nonlife over life with disabilities (Harbeson v. Parke-Davis, 1983; Procancik v. Cillo, 1984; Turpin v. Sortini, 1982).

Nurses working in perinatal care may see potential plaintiffs in all these categories. The extension of compensation for wrongful pregnancy and wrongful birth claims affirms in law society's concern for the cost of raising disabled children and the mental and financial distress to parents and their other children caused by physician failure to adhere to the standard of care.

Perinatal Maternal Substance Abuse

Treatment

Increasingly, neonatal nurses care for infants suffering ill effects as a result of maternal drug abuse. Thus nurses should be aware of the policy issues raised by suggestions that the definition of child abuse be extended to include fetal abuse or that the mother be viewed as a criminal guilty of delivering drugs to a minor.

One in 10 births in 1988 was a cocaine-exposed infant, and societal outrage is clearly evident (Curriden, 1990). Curriden cites an *Atlanta Constitution* survey of 1500 individuals; it found that 71 percent were in favor of criminal penalties for women who abused illegal drugs during pregnancy and a surprising 45 percent were in favor of prosecution of women who used only tobacco or alcohol.

Until recently, however, the law has been satisfied to find women who abuse drugs during pregnancy in violation of child protective laws only. A common practice has been to wait until the child is born and then immediately move for child protective agencies to assume custody. Child protective laws generally do not involve criminal charges. Their policy goal is reunification of families. The law directs that this be achieved through development and implementation of reunification plans that call for the development of parental skills and, in the case of substance-abusing parents, successful completion of drug rehabilitation programs. A South Carolina court found legal authority lacking for a child abuse and neglect charge against a mother who used cocaine while pregnant. The court noted that in passing the law, the legislature did not intend to include "fetus" in the definition of "child" (Tolliver v. South Carolina, 1992).

Parents are not, of course, immune from criminal charges. For example, when children are left alone and uncared for by adults for long periods, the parents may be charged with child endangerment. Neglect and abuse can rise to a criminal level. Recently, however, in response to growing public concern prosecutors have begun to bring criminal charges against drug-abusing pregnant women. The women have been charged under a number of criminal statutes: delivering cocaine to a newborn child through the umbilical cord, involuntary manslaughter, and criminal neglect (Curriden, 1990). Jennifer Johnson, who was charged with delivering drugs to her child during the period after delivery and before the umbilical cord was cut, was found guilty by lower Florida courts (Key case on pregnant women and drug abuse going to trial, 1991). The Florida Supreme Court overturned the decision (Jos et al., 1995).

How does the law look at the fetus? An Ohio lower court case has chronicled the typical evolution of state law in response to this question (*In re* Ruiz, 1986). Common law, or case law, had for centuries recognized live birth as the prerequisite for legal protection. In the middle 20th century, however, negligence law recognized separate recovery in damages for the child when a viable unborn child was injured prenatally and was born alive (Williams v. Marion Rapid Transit, Inc., 1949). No longer was recovery in damages limited to the mother. Ohio law, and other state law, later recognized not only negligence but also wrongful death actions for injuries suffered in utero if the child was born alive and later died (Jasinsky v. Potts, 1950). A 1959 appellate court decision, Stidam v. Ashmore (1959), held that a wrongful death action—an action brought by the estate after death as opposed to a negligence action brought by the plaintiff when alive—existed even if a viable fetus was stillborn. In 1985, the Ohio Supreme Court ratified this approach (Werling v. Sandy, 1985). In the Ruiz case, the mother used drugs during pregnancy, and the issue was whether the unborn fetus might be considered a child under the child abuse statute. The court found that the state had a "compelling interest" in the welfare of children under Roe v. Wade (1973) at the point of viability and that therefore the child abuse and neglect statutes should apply. The potential deprivation of liberty for the defendant has led courts to defer to legislatures the task of defining the viable fetus as the victim under criminal law.

Jos and colleagues (1995) reported the development of an institutional policy at the Medical University of South Carolina that threatened criminal sanction if drug-abusing pregnant women failed to seek drug counseling and prenatal care. The policy applied only to women attending university clinics, not private obstetrical patients. In September 1994, the university discontinued the policy after encountering multiple legal difficulties. Dropping the policy was the condition of settlement in a suit brought by the Civil Rights Division of the Department of Health and Human Services. Several women jailed under the policy have brought a class action lawsuit. In addition, the Federal Office of Protection from Research Risks deemed the policy experimentation conducted without IRB approval and deferred renewal of the University's Multiple Project Assurance for at least 1 year.

The Illinois legislature has criminalized drug abuse under its child protective legislation. The legislative response occurred when a prosecutor dropped involuntary manslaughter charges against a drug-abusing mother because case law supporting the charges was insufficient. The legislative response was to make the state's Child Abuse Act applicable to newborns. More specifically, the Illinois Infant Neglect and Controlled Substances Act of 1989 makes it a felony to "inflict or create a substantial risk of physical injury to a newborn infant by means of illegal drug use by the mother during pregnancy" (Curriden, 1990).

In general, those who support criminalization of prenatal substance abuse prefer accomplishing this under child protective statutes. They argue that this does not preclude the development of social policy supportive of substance abuse education and increasing the availability of drug abuse treatment centers to pregnant women (Robertson, 1989). On the other side, however, are those who argue that despite the symbiotic relationship of fetus and mother, the woman's right to choose her individual personal behaviors should be legally inviolate. According to this viewpoint, any attempt to criminalize a woman's behavior during pregnancy would be a violation of her fundamental rights. Beyond legalism and on a more practical level, opponents of criminalization argue that any threat of prosecution discourages substance abusers from seeking prenatal care and from providing accurate information to health care providers. Like their counterparts who support criminalization, advocates for women's rights suggest that the moral and proper approach is to increase the availability of health care services to pregnant women in general, including access to drug abuse treatment. The American Civil Liberties Union and the American Public Health Association take the women's rights approach (Key case on pregnant women and drug abuse going to trial, 1991; Paltrow, 1989). Jos and colleagues (1995) noted that the American Medical Association, the American Academy of Pediatrics, the American College of Obstetrics and Gynecology, the American Society of Addiction Medicine, and the American Nurses' Association find criminal sanction inconsistent with the role of the health care provider as caregiver.

The effects of prenatal drug abuse are pervasive. Drug-addicted children, whose learning problems persist throughout life, may not be productive citizens. Thus, ultimately, because of the scope of the abuse problem, our society's productivity can become impaired. Nurses delivering perinatal care should scrutinize the issues and be ready to move forward with proposed programs as well as develop new approaches to respond to this serious societal concern. Awareness of state and federal laws and societal resources applicable to this concern is key to formulation of any health care facility policy.

Research

In addition to questions of how the law should *treat* the alcohol- or drug-abusing mother, or mothers who abuse both, there is also the question of how the law should protect *research* subjects who participate in drug and alcohol abuse studies. Generally the nurse researcher must separate the research role from the clinician role. However, in studying maternal drug and alcohol abuse, a potential legal and ethical conflict arises when the researcher must decide, "Does the confidentiality of the research relationship override the obligation of the nurse to report child abuse and neglect?"

From a legal perspective, the answer is, "It depends." In 1988, Congress legislated confidentiality protection in section 301(d) of the Public Health Service Act (1988). Although researchers generally are ethically required to protect confidentiality, the act provides specific protection from being compelled to identify subjects in any federal, state, or local civil, criminal, administrative, legislative, or other proceeding. Specifically the act provides that the Secretary of the Department of Health and Human Services:

> . . . may authorize persons engaged in biomedical, behavioral, clinical, or other research (including research on mental health, including research on the use and effect of alcohol and other psychoactive drugs) to protect the privacy of individuals who are the subject of such research by withholding from all persons not connected with the conduct of such research the names or other identifying characteristics of such individuals." (Section 301 (d))

Thus, if a subject is prosecuted for child abuse, the nurse researcher need not testify that the subject was participating in a study on drug and alcohol abuse. If the researcher is unaware of the circumstances that led to the charges there is *no dilemma.* However, what if the nurse researcher's observations of the subject, the children, and the environment lead to a judgment that child neglect or abuse is occurring? Should the researcher regard the child neglect and abuse reporting laws as having more weight than the confidentiality protection? The answer is *yes.* How does the researcher know this?

Researchers seeking confidentiality protection apply for confidentiality certificates for alcohol and drug abuse research through the National Institute on Alcohol Abuse and Alcoholism or the National Institute on Drug Abuse. For other biomedical research, confidentiality certificates must be sought through the Office of the Assistant Secretary for Health. The coverage and limitations of the certificate of confidentiality should be explained as part of the informed consent process of the research study. Although neither the Public Health Service Act nor regulations based on the act specifically state that reporting laws take precedence, according to the Department of Health and Human Services Policy for Communicable Disease Reporting to the Centers for Disease Control and Prevention, the reporting laws do. The policy requires that in the research informed consent process, potential subjects be advised of the child neglect and abuse law reporting exception to confidentiality. Further, subjects must understand that confidentiality applies only to those data collected for research purposes. Thus observations that suggest child neglect or abuse may fall outside the scope of the research data. Overall, when child neglect or abuse becomes a concern, researchers should work cooperatively with local authorities (personal communication, Lura Abbott, NIAAA, October 24, 1995).

When the researcher has both a treatment and research relationship with a subject, care must be taken to keep research and treatment data separate. Research data are reported in the aggregate or the subject's identity is masked. Thus, confidentiality is assured. Federal privacy protection applies to records of persons treated for drug and alcohol abuse problems (Comprehensive Alcohol Abuse and Alcoholism Prevention, Treatment and Rehabilitation Act, The Drug Abuse Office and Treatment Act, 1988). Under certain circumstances, information from these records must be revealed. Circumstances include court order, child abuse, medical emergency, or informed consent from the affected person. The researcher must be careful when reporting research data that treatment information is not inadvertently disclosed.

Financing and Delivery of Perinatal Care

In a 1987 article, MacPherson discussed public policy as the choices made by governments and noted that social policy consists of both the guiding principles adopted and the actions pursued by societies and their governments. Health care policy then is one type of social policy. Thus the individualism that fosters competitiveness and self-interest in American society cannot help but result in health care policies that "tend to promote structured inequalities" (MacPherson, 1987, p. 3).

Although the aged can "spend down" to Medicaid levels to obtain long-term care, families with working parents can become bankrupt paying for the level of care that American society considers standard for neonates with intensive care needs. Health insurance has its dollar limits, which can be spent on a single child. Individuals who are working but do not have health insurance simply reach bankruptcy more quickly. Both individual and societal productivity may be curtailed when a working parent must drop out of the work force to meet the needs of a disabled child. Intensive care that goes unpaid results in higher health care costs in another area to balance the deficit. In today's world, however, with the limits on reimbursement from third-party payers, shifting such hospital costs is becoming more difficult.

The complexity of private and public reimbursement systems for health care is itself a contributor to continually escalating health care costs. Estimates assign as much as 10 percent of health care costs to administering reimbursement systems. Furthermore, states find increasing percentages of their Medicaid dollars allocated to the elderly, with little left over for the care of those in poverty, including children. Serious ethical dilemmas are posed for legislatures in the face of these resource constraints. Legislatures face the dilemma of how to obtain the most societal benefit for their investment of government dollars. Mitchell (1985) discussed the critical importance of looking at perinatal outcomes when deciding approaches to funding. The state of Oregon has recently made headlines as it takes drastic steps to reform its Medicaid reimbursement system to support the collective good for those in need of health care. First, it declined to pay for organ transplants. More recently, the state reviewed other payments and ranked 28 days of neonatal care as essential. Needed additional care does not fall in the "essential" category. The Oregon legislature has made explicit its concern that it fund care that has long-term individual and societal benefit (Dougherty, 1991; Hadorn, 1991).

Even before health care costs reached 14 percent of the gross national product and national health care reform failed, states began to seek waivers to reform their Medicaid systems. Congress is currently wrestling with Medicare reform and Medicaid funding, so many waivers are still on hold (General Accounting Office, 1995). In the meantime, managed care is gradually assuming dominance in the health care system.

The neonatal nurse must become knowledgeable about the issues concerning the financing and delivery of neonatal care and become involved in proposed solutions. Involvement translates into citizen–nurse action that demands and then supports legislation that strikes a just balance among primary, secondary, and tertiary care needs. Activity in political campaigns, personal and written contacts with federal and state legislators, and testifying at legislative hearings are ways in which nurses can become involved in these issues. The nurse's role should not end at the legislative level. State and federal agencies develop rules not only for implementing payment mechanisms but also for guiding the standard of care in neonatal settings. Nurses are free to comment on rules proposed by federal agencies, which are published in the Federal Register, and on state agency rules, which appear in hearing notices published in newspapers and are sent to interested parties. Making sure that political candidates, members of state legislatures, and executive agency staff know that you are a nurse and a member of a professional association in nursing is key to assuring that political involvement as a citizen is also viewed by those persons as involvement as a nurse (Kenner, 1995).

CONCLUSION

Although nurses have an obligation to meet the current standard of nursing perinatal care in their own practice setting, they should view their practice as extending to concern about, and activity in relation to, the broader social policy concerns encompassing the delivery of perinatal care. Thus the range of the nurse's professional life should include being part of the discourse—both in the employment setting and in society at large—about the impact of technologic change and social concerns on nursing education, practice, and research.

REFERENCES

American Academy of Pediatrics v. Heckler, 561 F. Supp. 395 (D.D.C. 1983).

American Academy of Pediatrics/American College of Obstetricians and Gynecologists. (1992). *Guidelines for perinatal care* (3rd. ed.). Elk Grove Village, IL: Author.

American Nurses' Association. (1984). *Code for nurses with interpretive statements.* Kansas City, MO: Author.

American Nurses' Association. (1991). *ANA standards of clinical nursing practice*. Washington, DC: Author.

American Nurses' Association. (1993). *ANA standards for nursing practice.* Washington, DC: Author.

American Nurses' Association. (1995a). *Nursing report card for acute care settings: A tool for protecting our patients, February 2, 1995.* Washington, DC: Author.

American Nurses' Association. (1995b). *Summary of the Lewin-VHI, Inc. Report: Nursing report card for acute care settings, February 2, 1995.* Washington, DC: Author.

Becker v. Schwartz and Park v. Chessin, 46 N.Y. 2d 401, 386 N.E. 2d 807 (1978).

Benjamin, M., & Curtis, J. (1992). *Ethics in nursing* (3rd ed.). New York: Oxford University Press.

Berman v. Allan, 80 N.J. 421, 404 A.2d 8 (1979).

Boone v. Mullendore, 416 So.2d 718 (Al. 1982).

Bowen v. American Hospital Association, 106 S. Ct. 2101 (1986).

Brown, H., Dent, M., Dyer, L.M., et al. (1986). Special project: Legal rights and issues surrounding conception, pregnancy, and birth (Baby Doe: The controversy surrounding withholding treatment from severely defective newborns). *Vanderbilt Law Review, 39,* 687–718.

Burke v. Rivo, No. SJC-5162 (Mass. S. Ct., March 1, 1990).

Burton v. Brooklyn Doctors Hospital, 88 A.D.2d 217, 452 N.Y.S.2d 875 (1982).

Capron, A.M. (1987). Anencephalic donors: Separate the dead from the dying. *Hastings Center Report, 17*(1), 5–9.
Capron, A. M. (1994). At law—medical futility: Strike two. *Hastings Center Report, 24*(5), 42–43.
Capron, A. M. (1995). Baby Ryan and virtual futility. *Hastings Center Report, 25*(2), 20–21.
Cranford, R.E. (1988). The persistent vegetative state: The medical reality (getting the facts straight). *Hastings Center Report, 18*(2), 27–32.
Curriden, M. (1990). Holding mom accountable. *American Bar Association Journal, 76*(3), 50–53.
Darling v. Charleston Community Memorial Hospital, 33 Ill.2d 326, 211 N.E.2d 253 (1965), *cert. denied,* 383 U.S. 946 (1966).
Dougherty, C.J. (1991). Supplement: Setting health care priorities: Oregon's next steps. *Hastings Center Report, 21*(3), 1–9.
Elliott v. Brown, 361 So.2d 546 (Al. 1978).
Emergency Medical Treatment and Active Labor Treatment Act of 1986, 42 U.S.C. S 1395 dd.
Feldman, E., & Murray, T. (1984). State legislation and the handicapped newborn: A moral and political dilemma. *Law, Medicine & Health Care, 12*(5), 156–163.
Flores v. Flushing Hospital and Medical Center, 109 A.D.2d 198, 490 N.Y.S.2d 770 (1985).
45 C.F.R. S 46.404–46.407 (1983).
45 C.F.R. S 1340.15 (b) (2) (1985).
47 Fed. Reg. 26,027 (1982).
48 Fed. Reg. 9630 (1983).
48 Fed. Reg. 9818 (1983) (to be codified in 45 C.F.R. S 46.404–46.407).
48 Fed. Reg. 30,846 (1983).
49 Fed. Reg. 1622 (1984).
49 Fed. Reg. 14,879 (1984).
General Accounting Office. (1995). *Medicaid restructuring approaches leave many questions* (GAO Publication No. GAO/HEHS-95–103). Washington, DC: U.S. General Accounting Office.
Hadorn, D.C. (1991). Supplement: The Oregon priority-setting exercise: Quality of life and public policy. *Hastings Center Report, 21*(3), 10–16.
Harbeson v. Parke-Davis, 98 Wash.2d 460, 656 P.2d 483 (1983).
Indiana *ex rel.* Infant Doe v. Monroe Circuit Court, No. 482–5140 (Ind. Apr. 16, 1982), *cert. denied,* 464 U.S. 961 (1982).
In the matter of Baby K, 832 F. Supp. 1022 (E.D. Va 1993); *In the matter of* Baby K, 16 F.3d 590 (4th Cir. 1994), *cert. denied,* 115 U.S. 91 (1994).
In re Ruiz, 27 Ohio Misc.2d 31 (Ct. Comm. Pleas 1986).
Jasinsky v. Potts, 153 Ohio St. 529 (1950).
Jos, P. H., Marshall, M. F., & Perlmutter, M. (1995). The Charleston policy on cocaine use during pregnancy: A cautionary tale. *The Journal of Law, Medicine & Ethics, 23,* 120–128.
Kenner, C. (1995). Use of professional associations for political action. *Journal of Perinatal and Neonatal Nursing,* 9(1), 78–88.
Key case on pregnant women and drug abuse going to trial. (1991, October). *The Nation's Health,* pp. 1, 20.
Kraus, G.P. (1986). *Health care risk management: Organization and administration.* Owings Mills, MD: National Health Publishing.
Lewis, S.M. (1986). *OB/GYN malpractice.* New York: John Wiley & Sons.
Lewis, S.M. (1991). *OB/GYN malpractice (cum suppl).* New York: John Wiley & Sons.
MacPherson, K.I. (1987). Health care policy, values, and nursing. *Advances in Nursing Science,* 9(3), 1–11.
Marciniak v. Lundborg, No. 88–0088 (Wisc. S. Ct., January 16, 1990).
Mitchell, R.G. (1985). Child health: Objectives and outcome of perinatal care. *Lancet,* 2(846), 931–933.
National Association for Neonatal Nurses. (1993). *Standards of care for neonatal nursing practice.* Petaluma, CA: Author.
National Association for Neonatal Nurses. (1994). *Neonatal nursing transport standards and guidelines.* Petaluma, CA: Author.
Ohio Board of Nursing. (1995, August). Notice of hearing to establish parameters for the delegation of certain nursing tasks by registered nurses to licensed practical nurses and by licensed nurses to trained unlicensed persons in all settings, including dialysis centers (rules 4723-13-01 through 4723-13-10).
Paliokas, K.L. (1989). Anencephalic newborns as organ donors: An assessment of "death" and legislative policy. *William and Mary Law Review, 31,* 197–239.
Paltrow, L. (1989, August). Fetal abuse: Should we recognize it as a crime? No. *American Bar Association Journal, 75*(8), 39.
Pegalis, S.E., & Wachsman, H.F. (1986). *American law of medical malpractice* (Vol. 3). Rochester, NY: Lawyers Co-Operative Publishing.
Pegalis, S.E., & Wachsman, H.F. (1990). *American law of medical malpractice (cum suppl).* Rochester, NY: Lawyers Co-Operative Publishing.
Procancik v. Cillo, 478 A.2d 755 (N.J. S. Ct. 1984). Restatement of Torts 2d, S 920 (1991 App.).
Public Health Service Act, S 301(d), 42 U.S.C. S 241(d), as added by Public Law No. 100–607, S 163 (November 4, 1988).
Restatement of Torts 2d, S920 (1991).
Rieck v. Medical Protective Co. of Fort Wayne, Ind., 64 Wis.2d 514, 219 N.W.2d 242 (1974).
Robertson, J. (1989). Fetal abuse: Should we recognize it as a crime? Yes. *American Bar Association Journal, 75*(8), 38.
Roe v. Wade, 410 U.S. 113 (1973).
Schorr, B. (1984, May 7). Firm didn't disclose vitamin E item was linked to infant deaths, FDA says. *The Wall Street Journal,* p. 6.
Spielman, B. (1995). Bargaining about futility. *The Journal of Law, Medicine & Ethics, 23,* 136–142.
Stidam v. Ashmore, 109 Ohio App. 431, 11 O.O.2d 383 (1959).
The Comprehensive Alcohol Abuse and Alcoholism Prevention, Treatment and Rehabilitation Act of 1970 (42 U.S.C. S 290dd-3) (1988).
The Drug Abuse Office and Treatment Act of 1972 (42 U.S.C. S 290ee-3) (1988).
Tolliver v. South Carolina, 90-CP-23-5178 (Cir. Ct. Mannin County, S.C. 1992).
Turpin v. Sortini, 643 P.2d 954 (Cal. S. Ct. 1982).
United States v. University Hospital, 729 F.2d 144 (2d Cir. 1984).
Vaughn, V.C., III, & McKay, R.J. (1979). *Nelson textbook of pediatrics* (11th ed.). Philadelphia: W.B. Saunders.
Werling v. Sandy, 17 Ohio St. 3d 45 (1985).
Williams v. Marion Rapid Transit, Inc., 152 Ohio St. 114 (1949).

CHAPTER 5

Collaborative Research in Neonatal Nursing

LINDA STURLA FRANCK   CAROLE KENNER   DENISE LUCAS

RESEARCH AGENDA

What types of research questions are being addressed by neonatal nurses?

How are patient outcomes linked to nursing research?

What is the current status of neonatal nursing research?

What is an effective method of airway management?

What effect does nonnutritive sucking have on oxygenation?

What effect does temperature stability have on oxygenation and neonatal well-being?

What is the cost comparison between advanced-practice neonatal nurses and other health professionals rendering the same service?

What is the effectiveness of hospital-based infant developmental intervention programs on physiologic outcomes? (Kachoyeanos, 1995, 1996)

(See Table 5–1 for additional current neonatal nursing research questions.)

Practitioners, educators, and dedicated researchers can find a fertile ground for conducting neonatal research in the neonatal intensive care unit (NICU) or in neonatal follow-up settings. Neonatal nursing is an area that has evolved quickly, resulting in the use of techniques, equipment, and interventions that are not always research-based. Rather, many of the techniques are based on traditions, unsubstantiated methods, or trial-and-error approaches that have not been scientifically validated.

Substantiating neonatal nursing and neonatal care requires collaboration with other nurses and individuals in the health professions. The clinical nurse is often the first to recognize and identify neonatal care problems. With the guidance and assistance of other nurses, nurse specialists, and physicians, a collaborative investigation may be used to explore the problem. The combination of expertise from multiple disciplines can make a highly effective team.

Research is a formal, systematic inquiry or examination of a given problem. The outcome or goal of research is to discover new information or relationships, or to verify existing knowledge. The pursuit may be somewhat different in the academic setting, where the investigation of hypothetical propositions about the presumed relationships among natural phenomena is concerned with theory development. Other, less formal definitions of research focus on understanding an event by logically relating it to other events. Some types of research attempt to predict events by relating them empirically to antecedents in time. Other types of research attempt to control or manipulate an event or procedure to determine the impact on other phenomena.

The focus of this chapter is on linking neonatal nursing practice and research. We discuss the identification of clinical problems amenable to research, different types of research designs, and the research process. The use of consultation and collaboration for successful practice-based research is presented. Finally, the practical aspects of initiating a research project and using research findings in clinical practice are discussed.

WHY DO RESEARCH?

Using the research process to discover new information or to confirm empirical knowledge allows for the growth and evolution of nursing practice. Without research, nursing care would be based simply on tradition. The practice of nursing would change slowly and grow little because things would be done the way they have always been done. The failure to conduct research regarding neonatal care has taught us some sobering lessons. Judgments of efficacy based on observation of small numbers of infants only or of treatments based on the principle "if a little is good, more is better" have resulted in significant morbidity and mortality for neonates. Misuses of oxygen therapy, chloramphenicol, and vitamin E are examples (Jain & Vidyasagar, 1989). From these experiences, the use of clinical research trials to evaluate new therapies scientifically prior to widespread application has become more common in neonatal care.

The research process also provides a vehicle for challenging accepted routines and theories. Nurses caring for neonates frequently identify issues for which there is inadequate scientific information on which to base clinical judgments. Nurses in the clinical setting are often in the best position to identify and articulate research questions and to carry out research studies that improve the delivery of nursing care. The types of questions posed by clinical nurses range from basic physiologic mechanisms to comparisons of efficacy between different caregiving techniques to identification and description of new phenomena. Table 5–1 lists topics of current research interest for neonatal nurses.

Many of these research questions are derived from the concern about the prevention of iatrogenic complications of treatments. Others emerge from systematic observation of clinical phenomena or from frustration with current practices. The nursing profession also demands research to address social issues and that research contributes to the overall societal health needs (Mercer, 1984).

TABLE 5–1 Some Current Neonatal Nursing Research Questions

Skin Care
How can epidermal damage from tape removal be reduced?
Can the permeable skin of preterm infants be used to deliver medication?
How can the barrier properties of the skin be improved to prevent infection and water loss?

Nutrition
How can breast feeding practices be promoted among mothers of premature infants?
What are the most effective methods of delivering formula to ill infants (e.g., continuous versus intermittent)?
Is weight gain improved with demand versus scheduled feeding?
How can intravenous access be improved and complications minimized?
What is the effect of non-nutritive sucking on neonatal weight gain?

Instruments and Procedures
What is the best method for collecting urine?
Which scale provides the most accurate weight?
Which device provides the most accurate measure of temperature?
What is the effect of routine care tasks such as suctioning on cerebral blood flow velocity?

Effect of the Environment
What is the impact of light, noise, and handling on infants in the NICU?
What is the appropriate level of stimulation for preterm infants?

ECMO
Is the initial training and ongoing education of ECMO specialists sufficient to maintain emergency management skills?
What are the long-term effects of ECMO's use?

Endotracheal Tube Stabilization and Maintenance
How can slippage of the endotracheal tube within the trachea be measured?
How can movement of the endotracheal tube be minimized?

Management of Pain
How can neonatal pain be assessed?
When is pharmacologic treatment appropriate?
Are there long-term consequences of unrelieved pain experienced in the neonatal period?
What is the most effective method for weaning the infant from analgesics?

Thermoregulation
Which techniques are most effective in minimizing insensible water loss and maintaining thermoregulation in the extremely premature infant?

Positioning
Which positions are most effective in promoting optimal oxygenation and in minimizing postural deformities?
Should all infants be turned every 2 hours?
Under what conditions is the prone position linked to sudden infant death syndrome?

Effects of Cocaine
How is the behavior of a cocaine-exposed infant different from that of the nonexposed infant?
What is the appropriate level of environmental stimulation for these infants?

Effective Parent Teaching Techniques
What are the most effective teaching methods for instructing parents in the care of their newborn?
Is computer-assisted instruction effective?
What kind of posthospital follow-up is most helpful to parents of infants who are released from the NICU?

Staff Education
What is the most effective method of orientation of new NICU nurses?
How should formal classroom teaching and clinical preceptorship be integrated?
Are self-paced learning modules an effective teaching methodology for neonatal nurses?
Can neonatal nurses use expert systems to support decision-making?

Delivery of Nursing Care
What is the most effective model for delivery of nursing care in the NICU?
Can nonprofessional staff be used in the NICU to support the professional nurse?
Does the use of critical pathways facilitate "costing out" nursing services?

Retention of Nurses in the Critical Care Setting
What are the factors that increase job satisfaction for nurses working in the NICU?
How do NICU nurses cope with stress?
What factors increase the likelihood that nursing jobs will be retained?

NICU, neonatal intensive care unit; ECMO, extracorporeal membrane oxygenation.

The following questions, adapted from Fleming (1984), should be considered when selecting a research problem:

1. Is the problem important to the discipline of nursing?
2. Is the problem of interest to the investigator?
3. Does the problem reflect patterns of human behavior in interaction with the environment in critical life situations?
4. Does the problem reflect processes by which health status is affected?
5. Is the problem an ethical one?
6. Is the problem feasible to research?

The research process may appear intimidating at first, but it is not difficult to learn. Very simply, research is a method of problem-solving similar to the nursing process itself.

REVIEW OF THE LITERATURE

One of the first steps in the research process is review of the literature. The main purpose of this review is to bring together data and theories that pertain to the topic of interest. The relationships between the concepts and the major issues are uncovered, and the gaps or potential flaws in the current knowledge are identified. In essence, the review of the literature provides a logical step toward the formulation of the research question. The review also helps to formulate the research questions or hypotheses and direct the methodology or design of the study. Perhaps the question can be answered after the review. If not, the review of the literature will allow the practitioner to identify what has been studied, what suggestions on the same topic other researchers have made about further research, and what instruments for measuring variables have been used or developed.

The next step is to explore appropriate methods for answering the question. The nature of the question dictates or determines the level of inquiry. The methodology, however, can vary depending on the conceptual framework guiding the inquiry.

RESEARCH METHODS AND DESIGN

"The best design is the one that will best answer a specific research question" (Oberst, 1985, p. 51). The phenomenon of interest to neonatal nurses and the need to produce data that are clinically based and can direct clinical practice may necessitate a variety of research approaches (Meier, 1983).

Defining the Level of Inquiry

The level of inquiry is considered by many as occurring on a continuum. Brink and Wood (1989) identify three levels of nurs-

TABLE 5–2 Levels of Research Inquiry

Purpose or End Sought			
To become familiar with phenomena; to gain new insights; to formulate a more specific research problem or research hypothesis. (Use research questions or objectives.)	To portray accurately incidence, distribution, and characteristics of a group or situation. (Do not usually begin with specific hypotheses; use research questions or objectives.)	To investigate relationships between variables. (Begin with specific hypotheses.)	To test hypotheses of causal relationships between variables.
(Explore)	(Describe)	(Explain-predict)	(Control)
	Descriptive research (Pre-experimental research)		
Survey research (normative or status studies)			
	Correlational and ex post facto research (Relational studies)		
			Experimental and quasi-experimental research
Independent Variables			
Independent variables (x) not controlled (manipulated) by investigator			
"Variables" investigated termed *characteristics*		"Variables" investigated called *independent variables* Active independent variables (x) controlled (manipulated) by investigator	

ing research: (1) exploratory-descriptive, (2) comparative, and (3) experimental. To determine the appropriate level of inquiry, the researcher must answer the following questions:

1. *Why* is the study being done (to test a hypothesis, to build theory, to generate new knowledge, to answer clinical questions)?
2. *What* is to be studied or tested?
3. *Who* is the investigation about?
4. *How* are the data to be gathered (retrospectively, as in a chart review, or prospectively, now and in the future as in a longitudinal study)?
5. *Where* is the research study to take place?

For an overview of the levels of research inquiry, see Table 5–2.

Exploratory-Descriptive Inquiry

If the purpose of the research is to become more familiar with phenomena, to gain new insights, or to formulate a more specific research problem or hypothesis, the research is exploratory. If the purpose is to portray accurately the incidence, distribution, and characteristics of a group or situation, the research is descriptive.

Exploratory or descriptive research studies can be either qualitative or quantitative. Quantitative studies use numbers to categorize data. The data are reported via descriptive statistics such as frequencies, actual numbers, and percentages. Qualitative studies categorize and describe data according to patterns, themes, and categories of response at a nominal or naming level. Ethnographers, for example, attempt to describe characteristics of certain groups by qualitative methods (Fetterman, 1989). The data from these qualitative studies are analyzed through content analysis, reporting the categories or themes found. The sample may or may not be random. The subjects most likely are selected based on availability and for a specific purpose. The data are collected through either unstructured or semistructured methods. Some exploratory-descriptive studies use triangulation, or a combination of quantitative and qualitative methods. Many neonatal nursing studies have been conducted at this level of research, but more comparative and predictive studies are appearing in the literature (Sherwen & Toussie-Weingarten, 1983). Examples of descriptive research include (1) survey research, (2) developmental studies, and (3) case studies (Table 5–3).

Comparative Studies

Comparative studies involve more structure than do exploratory-descriptive studies, and the samples are usually randomized or stratified. The design may compare or correlate groups of subjects (Brink & Wood, 1989). These studies compare one group with another for the purpose of describing the differences or similarities between groups. Survey methods are often used to determine the prevalence of a certain variable (e.g., attitudes or incidence). Examples are described in Table 5–4.

Experimental Studies

The "gold standard" of experimental research is the randomized clinical trial. In this most rigorous of research designs, care-

TABLE 5–3 Descriptive Research

Survey research (status studies or normative studies)	The purpose of survey research is to explore and describe the phenomenon of interest. The researcher gathers data from a large group of persons, often by mail or personal interview. The data generally are collected at one point in time. Survey research cannot investigate relationships between variables or generalize about those relationships (i.e., determine cause and effect). Examples include follow-up studies, parent opinion surveys, and needs assessments.
Developmental studies	Developmental studies include longitudinal studies such as trend studies and cohort and panel studies. Data are collected at several points in time. Other examples are documentary analysis and follow-up studies.
Case studies	Case studies have the same purpose as survey and development studies. In contrast to surveys, case studies use smaller samples but have greater depth of inquiry. Case study research often involves direct observation or interviews. Examples include single-subject research and small single social units such as a family. These studies are often qualitative in nature, using techniques such as naturalistic inquiry, phenomenology, and ethnography.

TABLE 5–4 Comparative Research

Correlational studies	Compare two or more different characteristics from *the same group of individuals.* These studies cannot demonstrate cause and effect. They can only demonstrate how characteristics vary together, or are associated, and how well one can be predicted from knowledge of the others. *Concurrent* correlational studies show a relationship that is drawn from the same point. An example is the relationship between Apgar scores and gestational age. *Predictive* correlational studies use certain characteristics to predict other characteristics. An example is using gestational age to predict risk for respiratory distress syndrome.
Ex post facto research	This is a type of relational study, often called *causal-comparative research,* which also does not establish causality. A relational study (explain-predict) may substitute for an experimental study. It uses naturally occurring treatment or subjects that have been self-selected at the level of the independent variable. In this type of study, the researcher is looking for natural "cause" without researcher manipulation of the independent variables (treatment). The dependent variable is observed first. The principal reasons are sought, and alternative (rival explanations) are enumerated and tested. An example would be the relationship between parent satisfaction with open visiting hours in the NICU and parent perceptions of the hospital experience after discharge.

NICU, neonatal intensive care unit.

fully controlled, prospective, blind trials can definitively establish risks and benefits of new treatments, minimizing bias and error (Chalmers, 1990). This method of clinical research is not without controversy, however. Ethical, financial, and social factors are often involved in decisions to introduce new treatments (Fetter et al., 1989). The rigorous requirements for controlled evaluation of all new therapies may fail to acknowledge these clinical realities. The introduction of extracorporeal membrane oxygenation (ECMO) therapy in the NICU exemplifies the complex issues clinicians face in determining the need for and adequacy of clinical trials to determine benefits and risks of new therapies (Lantos & Frader, 1990).

When experimental designs are used, the ethics of clinical research require that the investigator maintain a genuine state of uncertainty regarding the merits of one treatment over another (Freedman, 1987). This state of equipoise is often difficult to achieve, particularly if the clinicians have a strong belief regarding the efficacy of one of the study treatments (Korn & Baumrind, 1991). Therefore, study treatments must be randomized to minimize or eliminate bias. Education concerning the statistical dangers of making decisions based on studies with insufficient sample size should assist all involved (other clinical staff and parents) in recognizing the merit of suspending judgment until all the data are collected. Criteria can be established to ensure that a study is not conducted longer than is necessary when clear benefit or harm becomes evident early on. This type of experimental research is summarized in Table 5–5.

Mixed Research Designs

The use of a combination of research designs is acceptable in today's research arena. Brink and Wood (1989) suggested that historical research, meta-analysis, epidemiologic research, instrument development, evaluative research, and philosophical research are examples of mixed designs.

Historical Research

Historical research is just coming into its own in nursing. Sarnecky defines this type of research as "a process of examining data from the past, integrating it into a coherent unity and putting it to some pragmatic use for the present and future" (Sarnecky, 1990, p. 2). It uses previously recorded information to draw conclusions about past events and suggests present and past implications. Secondary analysis may also fall into this category because it represents the use of either secondary sources for information or a reexamination of previously collected data (Stewart, 1984). An advantage to this method of data analysis is that it is cost-effective and allows the researcher to explore another research question that was not asked in the original study or studies (Gleit & Graham, 1989). False inferences resulting from lack of random assignment, incomplete information, and inherent group differences are risks of this design (Grant, 1985).

Meta-Analysis

Another form of research is meta-analysis. By definition, it is a large analysis of pre-existing data. The rationale is that studies that focus on a particular phenomenon using very small samples cannot be generalized to the population at large from which the samples were drawn unless the results are combined. Meta-analysis uses data from many previously conducted studies that are related to a particular phenomenon of interest in order to determine the effect of the variable of interest (Hunter et al., 1982). In some respects, this type of analysis is collaborative in nature because it usually crosses lines of disciplines. Some nurse scientists, however, feel that nurses should focus on more discrete types of studies that are aimed at solving clinical problems or at least have direct clinical application (Moody, 1990a). Meta-analysis offers the possibility of integrating findings from many studies, thus yielding more significant and usable results (Moody, 1990b).

Epidemiologic Research

Epidemiologic research has attracted much attention because the tracking of certain diseases, such as acquired immunodefi-

TABLE 5–5 Experimental Research

Experimental studies (general type)	The purpose of experimental research is to probe cause and effect ("if . . . then") and to establish causality. The researcher deliberately manipulates a treatment (independent variable) to see if it causes a change in response (dependent variable). This is the highest-level, most structured type of research. In quasi-experimental studies, subjects may be assigned to treatment or a control group. The researcher may be aware of the treatment even if randomly assigned. True experiments use random assignment with the researchers blind to group assignment, treatment, or both.
Randomized clinical trials (one type of experimental study)	These studies establish the risks and benefits of treatment modalities. *Example:* the efficacy of surfactant therapy given as compared with conventional respiratory support in the low birth weight neonate.

ciency syndrome (AIDS), has significant public health implications. These studies are concerned with documenting the natural history, determining prevalence, and longitudinally following the evolution of phenomena. The objective of epidemiologic studies is "the distribution and determinants of health and disease in the human population groups" (Meininger, 1990, p. 201). Although this type of research has historically been more medical in nature, many nurses are becoming interested in epidemiologic methods to guide nursing interventions toward the promotion or restoration of health.

Instrument Development

Instrument development is a common nursing research design. It reflects the need for reliable and valid instruments to measure nursing phenomena. This type of research may be conducted at any level of inquiry (Brink & Wood, 1989). Qualitative methods may be used to establish content validity of a pre-existing or newly developed instrument (Tilden et al., 1990). Instrument development takes considerable time and effort and may be a lifelong program of research itself if a valid and reliable instrument is truly developed.

The focus group is a method used to identify items that should be included in questionnaires (Kingry et al., 1990). Focus groups usually consist of 10 to 12 people from similar backgrounds with regard to the research area of interest. The group's homogeneity is desired so that the participants can generate ideas on a similar topic, such as the use of extracorporeal membrane oxygenation in the NICU and ethical dilemmas facing neonatal nurses.

Evaluative Research

Evaluative research has been conducted in education for many years. Nurses have become more involved in these types of studies as quality assurance–quality improvement or total continuous quality improvement programs and the need for documentation of client outcomes or nursing care costs have grown. Nurse educators use evaluation methods in revising nursing curricula, providing documentation for National League for Nursing accreditation visits, as do nurse specialists in providing in-service education and community workshops. These studies may be qualitative and concerned with why a program works (Marshall & Rossman, 1989); quantitative, focusing on describing changes; or experimental, with an emphasis on establishing cause and effect relationships. Outcome-based research is a priority for the National Institutes of Health (NIH). It is also part of the Joint Commission for Accreditation of Healthcare Organizations (JCAHO) visits. In part this is due to the mandate by third-party payers to have a validation that the treatment, procedure, and nursing care is cost-effective and appropriate according to outcome (Kachoyeanos, 1995, 1996). Research is a method of justifying neonatal nursing's role in care, "costing out" services, and validating patient outcomes. Patient outcome research teams are part of the initiative outlined by the Agency for Health Care Policy and Research (AHCPR), which is concerned with patient care guideline development.

Philosophical Research

Philosophical research asks value questions. This type of research is more likely to be qualitative in nature, focusing on individual or cultural values and beliefs. Studies that address value questions can be most useful when nurses are concerned about how a group or individual may view a philosophical or ethical dilemma such as discontinuation of life support or the use of anencephalic infants for donor organs.

Replicating Studies

Nurses in particular often feel that replicating or repeating a study is "cheating" and of no value. This feeling could not be further from the truth. Studies need to be repeated to support the findings from the original study. Replication lends credibility to previous results and allows the findings to be generalized. Researchers should provide accurate, detailed descriptions of how the research was performed so that it can be replicated by others.

Replication also provides an opportunity to learn from the experience of others—that is, to analyze what was done right as well as what was done wrong so that more accurate, precise studies can be designed. If a study that is replicated fails to produce the same results, it may mean that practice has changed, the study's original sample differs from the new sample, the methods in one or both studies were faulty, or the hypothesized relationships do not exist. In such cases, further exploration is needed. Replication of studies is an easy way to begin to learn the research process and is often less frustrating for the beginning researcher who does not feel capable of designing an original study.

RESEARCH TEAM COMPOSITION

The decision regarding the composition of the research team should be based on the type of research to be carried out, the expertise needed to conduct a credible study, the type and amount of funds available to support the research, and the time that is expected to be needed to complete the study. The team may be a single investigator or a group of investigators.

Single Investigator Versus Coinvestigators

Single Investigator

There are advantages and disadvantages to conducting a research project as an individual. The single investigator has complete control of the project, conducts the project according to his or her own schedule, and is not dependent on others for information about the progress of the project. One of the disadvantages is that there is no one to help bear part of the research burden. Tasks such as writing the proposal, collecting data, and analyzing data can be facilitated through the use of a team. A single investigator may also be more vulnerable to bias.

Coinvestigators

Bringing others in to help share the burden of research can be helpful and time-saving. Sharing knowledge and expertise has the potential for making a better project. The blend of an academician and clinician is often helpful in keeping theory in perspective while remaining based in reality in the clinical setting. Collaborative studies using professionals from other disciplines can give breadth to a project (Lyons et al., 1990). The use of a collaborative model can improve resources for research because funds from the different disciplines can be sought. Some funding sources give preference to collaborative research teams.

However, working in a group is not always easy. It requires cooperation and often compromise on the project's purpose or plan. It is unrealistic to assume that there will be an equal distribution of work in such a collaborative effort; it does not often occur. Thus before entering into a collaborative venture, the group should outline precisely what tasks each member is to assume and the responsibilities and authorship credits throughout the project (Hanson, 1988; Stevens, 1986). A contract may prevent misunderstandings during the project and prevent communication problems that may jeopardize the entire project's completion. During the proposal development stage, a time schedule for completion of each member's part of the project as well as a target for completion of the entire project should be established. If insurmountable problems arise among the members of the team, the principal investigator must decide how to proceed with the project, shifting responsibilities, replacing team members, or halting the project.

DEVELOPING THE RESEARCH PROJECT

Identifying Hypotheses

The purpose of the research project will dictate the form of the specific objectives. Not all research investigations will have hypotheses. In descriptive studies, research questions direct the investigation, whereas in experimental studies, specific hypotheses are tested. The hypothesis is a statement of the expected differences to be found in the study; it is usually phrased in the negative (null hypothesis): "There will be no difference in heart rate variability in an infant when suction is performed via an endotracheal tube adapter as compared with standard procedure." On the basis of the hypothesis, the investigator then sets out to test the stated relationship.

Defining Variables

Variables are those concepts that are of interest to the researcher. They include the concepts under investigation that are to be manipulated by the researcher (the independent variables) and those that are dependent on the effect (the dependent variables). Situational (or influencing or confounding) variables are those concepts that relate to the situation or case under study. They may influence or exert an effect on the variables of interest, but they may or may not be controlled for in the study's design. For instance, a research study that is concerned with transition of infants from the NICU to the home may have as an independent variable the caring for an infant following discharge from the hospital from a level III nursery into the home. The dependent variables are the responses to the caring for the infant after discharge from the hospital to the home. The situational or influencing variables are those that may influence parental responses to having and caring for the infant at home. These may include birth order of the infant, previous experience with a NICU, and length of time the mother and infant were separated.

All variables must be conceptually (operationally) defined. An operational definition tells how the variables are to be measured. The operational definition for the dependent variables in the example given previously would be: (1) informational needs: knowledge, instruction, or information that is necessary for parents to provide care and cope with the transition from hospital to home and (2) grief and fear about ultimately losing the infant and loss of the ideal child. Operational definitions lead the researcher to seek appropriate instruments to measure the variables.

Selecting Research Instruments

Techniques or instruments used to measure the dependent variable or variables, or outcomes, must be described according to:

1. Validity: Does the instrument measure what it purports to measure?
2. Reliability: Does the instrument provide consistent measures?
3. Suitability–utility: Is the instrument appropriate for the setting and subjects?
4. Sensitivity: Is the instrument sensitive enough to measure the phenomenon?
5. Specificity: Is the instrument specific enough to measure only the phenomenon?

If a well-established instrument is used, the instrument's validity and reliability in previous investigations must be addressed. If the investigator is developing an instrument, validity and reliability must be established. To establish validity and reliability, the instrument must be pilot-tested. A pilot test is a test run on a very small sample. This trial will provide the researcher with data to identify problems with the instrument, awkward wording of questions, or other methodologic problems that need to be corrected prior to implementation of the full project. A detailed description of how the pilot test was conducted, the number of subjects, and their characteristics should be documented by the investigator.

If interviews or observations are used to gather data, inter-rater and intrarater reliability must be established. Inter-rater reliability refers to consistent measurement across *several* observers, whereas intrarater reliability refers to consistent measurements on different occasions with the *same* observer. There are a number of ways to conduct inter- and intrarater reliability to ensure that there is consistency in the variable being measured.

Defining the Study Sample

The next step of the research project is to define the study sample. For example, if one wished to investigate respiratory procedures in preterm infants, the investigators would need to define the age, sex, and specific characteristics of the population of infants from which the sample will be selected for the study. In this case, the sample might be selected from the population of all premature infants less than 37 weeks of gestation. Sample selection may be established in relation to exclusion criteria as well, for example, all infants except those on mechanical ventilation. The researcher must be able to explain why the population is appropriate for the proposed investigation. However, it is seldom feasible to study the entire target population; therefore, the researcher is left with the accessible population (e.g., all infants in a given nursery).

After the researcher determines the population and its characteristics, the specific methods for obtaining the subjects should be explained. The investigator needs to plan ahead to determine what will be done about subjects who decline to participate, drop out, or do not participate in all parts of the study. For example, what will be done about incomplete questionnaires or ones with obvious response sets, less than truthful responses, or unanswered items.

Power Calculations

The exact number of subjects necessary to achieve statistical significance in experimental investigations can be predicted by the use of power analysis. To calculate the number of subjects needed for a given investigation, a brief review of the two types of statistical error, alpha and beta, is needed. Alpha, or a type I, error refers to the rejection of the null hypothesis when in fact it is true. Beta, or a type II, error refers to failure to accept the alternative hypothesis when in fact it is true. The "power" of a statistical test is an important concept. The more powerful the test, the less likely one is of committing a type II error. To apply the concept of power to an investigation, three aspects need to be considered: (1) alpha level, (2) sample size, and (3) effect size. Knowledge of two of the three parameters will enable the investigator to calculate the missing value. Therefore, if one has determined the alpha level and if a previous investigation will give parameters for estimating the effect size, the overall estimate for sample size can be calculated mathematically. A good description of the procedure can be found in Kraemer and Thiemann (1987) and in Polit and Sherman (1990). There are also some statistical packages or computer software that will perform power calculations for the researcher who knows the alpha level, sample size, and effect size desired.

Setting

Investigations that focus on the neonate can occur in a variety of settings, including the nursery (level I, II, or III). Research that is focused on the parents may take place in the delivery room, the nursery, the home, or the follow-up clinic.

Most nursing research studies will be conducted in the field versus the laboratory setting. The term *field* refers to the world at large or a more natural setting. The laboratory setting may be used for quasiexperimental or experimental designs, such as nurses conducting physiologic research or research using animal models.

Regardless of the setting, the investigator needs to be very specific in describing the setting in which the study is conducted. Specificity in the description of the setting allows for others to replicate the study in the future.

Developing a Support Network

Whether one is conducting an investigation as the sole principal investigator or as part of a collaborative effort, clinical research is not an individual activity. High-quality research is most commonly the product of dialogue with experts and critique by colleagues. Of primary importance to the success of the project is the development of a support network. There are aspects of the research project that one will tackle with enthusiasm, whereas other aspects will be put off or never completed. Whether one works alone or in a collaborative effort, a support network in which one receives assistance with refocusing on the goal, problem-solving, or motivation eases the road to completion of the project.

Consultation

Although a basic understanding of the entire research process is needed by all members of a research team, each member may contribute specific, unique expertise. The word *statistics* often freezes the potential researcher. Statistical consultation is an excellent example of using special expertise in the conduct of a research project to improve its scientific merit. Data cannot and should not be turned over to a statistician without consultation. The researcher must clarify with the statistician what is to be accomplished from the analysis; otherwise the study's results may be erroneous.

In a university setting, statistical consultants can be found in many departments, including biology, medicine, nursing, psychology, and sociology. Graduate students are often assigned the task of data entry and statistical analysis. The services of students can assist with the mechanics of data analysis but do not constitute and should not substitute for consultation with a statistician. Hospitals sometimes have statisticians within their own research departments, especially if they are involved in experimental or laboratory research.

Developing the Proposal

Clearly identifying the elements that are expected in the proposal helps keep the development stage to a minimum. If a funding agency is to be involved, it may have a specific format for submission (Tornquist & Funk, 1990). Often this format is different from the proposal that will be submitted for institutional review.

Funding

There are many sources of funds available for research: local foundations, corporations, managed care or health maintenance organizations, university funding agencies, professional organizations such as the National Association of Neonatal Nurses or Association of Women's Health, Obstetrical and Neonatal Nurses, local chapters of Sigma Theta Tau, and the March of Dimes Birth Defects Foundation. The single most important item to determine prior to writing a proposal is the funding priorities of the agency. A critical element is the credentials needed by the principal investigator in order to qualify for funds. Some institutions require that a researcher be employed at that institution; other institutions require that a potential recipient of funds have a doctorate degree. See Table 5–6 for a list of potential funding sources.

ETHICAL CONSIDERATIONS

The topic of medical ethics and consideration for the patient goes back to Hippocrates. The guiding principle was "first do no harm." During World War II, prisoners in Nazi camps were often subjects of experiments. They were exposed to altitude changes and extreme cold to see what their physiologic response would be. They were injected with the malaria and typhus viruses without consideration about personal harm. These subjects had no rights to refuse and often died as a result of the experimentation (National Commission for the Protection of Human Subjects of Biomedical and Behavioral Research, 1979).

Once the war was over, the Nuremberg trials were held. From these trials came a code of ethics to protect human subjects. The articles of the Nuremberg Tribunal of 1948 outlined what came to be known as the Nuremberg codes. This document was the First International Code of Research Ethics. It set the standards for research and described the need for informed consent. The responsibilities of the researcher were also highlighted. The code suggested that animal trials be performed prior to experimentation on human subjects. It further suggested that the researcher be scientifically expert and have some knowledge of the area in which the research is to be conducted. Furthermore, every subject was to have the right to withdraw at any time during a study.

It was not until the early 1960s in the United States that informed consent was mandated by Congress and the federal government. In 1964, the World Medical Association Declaration of Helsinki (revised in 1975) was an international attempt to provide ethical guidelines related to the use of humans in experiments. Following the first Helsinki Declaration, the Surgeon General in 1966 issued a policy statement on the protection of human subjects. During the same year, the American Medical Association published *Guidelines for Clinical Investigation*. The American Nurses' Association's "Human Rights Guidelines for Nurses in Clinical and Other Research" followed in 1975. These documents represent only broad guidelines about the conduct of general research and are not legally binding in and of themselves. They do not specify individual cases or situations.

The National Research Act of 1974 established the National Commission of Human Subjects of Biomedical and Behavioral Research. Institutional review boards (IRBs) were then established. The commission was to look at the ethical underpinnings of research, specifically the boundaries between practice and

American College of Health Care
8120 Woodmont Ave., Suite 200
Bethesda, MD 20814
1-301-652-8384

American Foundation for the Blind
15 W. 16th Street
New York, NY 10011
1-212-620-2000

American Red Cross
17th and D Streets, NW
Washington, DC 20006
1-202-737-8300

American Speech-Language-Hearing Association
10801 Rockville Pike
Rockville, MD 20852
1-301-897-5700

Association of Women's Health, Obstetric, and Neonatal Nurses (AWHONN)
Program Abstracts/Research Guidelines
Department of Education and Research
700 14th Street, N.W., Suite 600
Washington, DC 20005-2019
1-202-662-1600
1-202-737-0575 (FAX)
Deadline first week November of 1 year
Selection announced by January 15 of following year

Directory of Biomedical and Health Care Grants 1989-90-Fourth Edition
Oryx Press
For more information: The Editors, GRANTS
2214 North Central at Encanto
Phoenix, AZ 85004-1483
1-602-254-6156

(Lists grant title, restrictions, requirements, application-renewal data, and sponsor information, grant description, funding amount, and catalogue of federal domestic assistance page number.)

Grants Magazine: The Journal of Sponsored Research and Other Programs
Plenum Publishing Corporation
233 Spring Street
New York, NY 10013

National Association of Neonatal Nurses (NANN)
Foundation for Nursing Education and Research (FNER)
1304 Southpoint Blvd. Suite 280
Petaluma, CA 94954-6859
1-707-762-5588
1-707-762-0401 (FAX)
Deadline Fall and Spring

National Guide to Foundation Funding in Health
The Foundation Center
Found in the University of Cincinnati Health Sciences Library or similar libraries

NIH Extramural Programs
U.S. Department of Health and Human Services
Public Health Service
National Institutes of Health
Office of Extramural Research and Training
9000 Rockville Pike
Bethesda, MD 20205

National Institute of Nursing Research (NINR)
Director, Division of Extramural Programs
1-301-496-0523

National Cancer Institute
1-301-427-8898

National Institute of Diabetes and Digestive and Kidney Diseases
1-301-496-7277

National Institute of Child Health and Human Development
1-301-496-1848

Sigma Theta Tau International
Honor Society of Nursing
550 West North Street
Indianapolis, IN 46202
1-317-634-8171
1-317-634-8188 (FAX)

Sigma Theta Tau International/American Association of Diabetes Educators
American Association of Diabetes Educators
Education and Research Foundation
444 N. Michigan Avenue, Suite 1240
Chicago, IL 60611-3901
1-312-644-AADE
1-312-644-4411 (FAX)
Deadline: October 1

Sigma Theta Tau International/Glaxo New Investigator Grant
Sigma Theta Tau International
Deadline: October 1

Sigma Theta Tau International/Mead Johnson Nutritionals Perinatal Research Grant
Sigma Theta Tau International
Deadline: June 1

Sigma Theta Tau International/American Association of Critical Care Nurses (AACN) Critical Care Grant
AACN
101 Columbia
Aliso Viejo, CA 92656-1491
1-800-899-AACN
Deadline: June 1

Sigma Theta Tau International Small Research Grant
Sigma Theta Tau International
Deadline: March 1

Sigma Theta Tau International/American Nurses Foundation Grant
American Nurses Foundation
600 Maryland Avenue, S.W., Suite 100 West
Washington, DC 20024-2571
1-202-554-444
Deadline: May 1

Society of Pediatric Nurses
Corinne Barnes Research Award
Research Committee
2170 South Parker Road, Suite 350
Denver, CO 80231-2902
1-800-723-2902
Deadline: February 1

The Foundation Center
Publications Catalog
79 Fifth Avenue, Department NC
New York, NY 10003
1-212-620-4230
1-800-424-9836

*This list is only a small sample of potential sources. Deadlines are subject to change. Other good sources are local chapters of professional organizations, corporations, university and hospital foundations.

research, risks and benefits, selection of subjects, and informed consent. They convened at the Belmont Center in Baltimore, Maryland. They encouraged debate among the membership to consider if research could be performed without human subjects and to consider whether research is really necessary. These two questions are considered today by IRBs when research proposals are reviewed.

In 1979, the commission issued the *Belmont Report*. This report outlined three guiding principles for research: (1) respect for persons, (2) beneficence, and (3) justice. Respect incorporates the idea that subjects are autonomous agents who can think clearly and make choices for themselves. If they cannot choose for themselves, they need special protection. This principle of special protection applies to children, the unborn, the poor or disadvantaged, the mentally retarded, or psychiatric and mental health clients who are considered mentally disabled. Respect also involves treating all subjects fairly and openly. All information, then, must be given through informed consent, which is implemented by the researcher by explaining the nature of the study, checking the understanding of the subject about his or participation in the study, offering the right to withdraw at any time during the research, and ensuring freedom from coercion (i.e., no penalty will be attached if the potential subject refuses to participate or withdraws before the study ends). Respect includes privacy and confidentiality of information that the investigator obtains during the study's course.

The second principle outlined by the Belmont Report is beneficence, which involves the validation of trust and respect. Again, this goes back to the principle of "first do no harm." Researchers as well as IRB members must realize that there may be risks that are unforeseen. Many of the medications and treatments that are currently used in practice may have long-range side effects that will not be recognized for years to come. The same holds true for research experimentation; however, the cost versus benefit as currently known must be considered. The following question must be asked: What are the currently known risks? The IRB and researcher share equal responsibility in protecting the human subject against untoward risks. The nature and scope of the risks must be weighed against the benefits of the study. There must be agreement that the clinical trial will be stopped when the results are obvious.

The third ethical principle is justice, which is concerned with whether the risks are distributed equitably. This principle also guides the adjustment of protocols as problems are identified or more information becomes available, such as a recently discovered side effect of a treatment that makes an arm of the research protocol dangerous to continue. Any adjustment in the protocol for protection of the human subjects must go back to the IRB for approval.

Review and approval of proposals must take place before the involvement of human or animal subjects can occur. This review may be by a committee within a department or it may occur within an institution such as a hospital or a university. These reviews generally involve the departments of nursing, neonatology, and perinatology. They look at the merit of the design, feasibility, coherence with the institution's mission, and the use of human subjects. The primary purpose of any review is the protection of the subjects involved in the study. In some institutions, review of the scientific merit of a study occurs separately from the review of the human subjects, whereas in others, these two objectives are combined.

INSTITUTIONAL REVIEW BOARDS

IRBs were developed to ensure the rights and welfare of research subjects. Only three states—New York, Missouri, and Virginia—outline the exact composition of their IRBs according to state and federal statutes. In general, these committees are multidisciplinary, including scientists, nonscientists, and lay public representatives. Each institution conducting research does not have to have its own board, but it must have access to one. Some institutions have human ethics committees to safeguard the rights of clients. If a research proposal is to be reviewed for which no one on the committee has expertise, an outside expert can be brought in for review to discuss the appropriateness of the protocol and whether any side effects of the treatment or research have been overlooked. Outside experts do not vote on the project, however.

The review process can benefit the researcher as well as the subjects because the committee can see problems that the researcher might not have thought of before. One problem with the review process is that the researcher is sometimes not available to answer questions directly. Not all IRBs require the researcher's presence at the review meeting.

The basic concern regarding neonatal research is that the patient cannot speak and give informed consent. Parents sometimes feel vulnerable and unable to refuse a request for participation in research by the caregiver of their infant (Cunningham & Hutchinson, 1990). It is then up to the collaborative health care team and the IRB to safeguard the neonates and their families. They must weigh the risks and benefits as well as the ethics of the proposed research. An informed consent process is the method of operationalizing the process of protection of human subjects. The basic elements are:

- An understandable explanation of the study and its procedures
- An explanation of any risk or discomfort to be encountered by a subject
- Identification of the cost versus the benefits of participation in the study
- Assurance that the researcher will be available to answer the subject's questions
- Assurance of confidentiality of information obtained
- Assurance of the right to withdraw from the study at any time during the project

The function of the IRB, then, is to review, approve, disapprove, or request revision of research protocols for the purposes of protecting human subjects and upholding the ethical principles of research. The actual review consists of examining the risks to the subjects in relation to the potential benefits. It also ensures that selection of subjects is equitable and not discriminatory in nature. The informed consent is scrutinized for the previously mentioned basic elements and for readability. Today, the average United States citizen reads at less than a seventh grade level. Many committees are suggesting that a fourth- to fifth-grade reading level be used for informed consent. This reading level is sometimes difficult to achieve because risk managers within institutions often dictate that legal language be incorporated into the informed consent. It is then up to the researcher or whoever is obtaining the informed consent to determine the level of comprehension of the potential subject. The researcher must also assure the IRB that the data collection will be monitored to determine if and when a research protocol should be terminated.

In some institutions, studies that involve minimal risk to subjects may be expedited or reviewed by a subcommittee rather than the full IRB. Survey research, retrospective chart reviews, and examination of data collected as part of clinical care, such as diagnostic specimens, may not require informed consent of the subjects.

The issues surrounding informed consent continue to change as questions arise about ethics and ethical decision-making. Genetic research, organ procurement, the use of anencephalic infants as organ donors, organ transplantation, as well as some behavioral research are all raising new concerns that IRBs must consider.

An issue recently raised at a nursing conference was whether there should be an international code for nursing research, since more nursing research is being conducted. The Nuremberg Codes and Helsinki Declaration are more medically focused. This is the question: Is there a need for a different set of guidelines, or does nursing research still fall within the same considerations as research within any other discipline? It is a question worth considering because more nurses with master's and doctoral degrees are conducting psychosocial and physiologic research. Another issue being raised by nurses is why physician permission is needed to study the physician's patient and the patient's family. This issue is one that implies ownership of clients by the physicians and is not easily resolved.

Protocols for government funding must also be reviewed and approved by local IRBs. By 1991, almost $40 million was allocated for the National Institute for Nursing Research (NINR) (Sharp, 1991). This money is only a portion of the $8.3 billion appropriated to the NIH overall (Sharp, 1991). Therefore, nursing research, although gaining monies, still represents only a small portion of the funding. One of the concerns about the current 104th Congress is the threat to cut monies for the Nursing Education Act and to the NINR (ANA Conference Call, May, 1995).

GETTING INVOLVED IN RESEARCH

Neonatal nurses can become involved in research in a variety of ways. One effective method to gain knowledge about the research process is to become involved in a colleague's project. As a research subject (e.g., in a research survey) or a collector of research data, the nurse has an opportunity to observe and participate in the research process. Many reports can now be found in the clinical literature describing the accomplishments and obstacles of implementing unit-based research projects with staff nurse participation (Rizzuto et al., 1990; Welch et al., 1990).

Another method of participating in the research process is to perform secondary analysis on data that were collected to answer another research question. Often answers to other research questions can be extracted from a single data base without having to collect new data. Caution, however, must be used in the design of secondary analysis studies to minimize threats to validity and reliability inherent in the method (Grant, 1985).

Quality assurance and quality improvement activities often lead to the design and conduct of research. Nurses are often introduced to issues related to objective data collection through quality assurance audits. Issues of clinical consequence identified through quality assurance screening can lead to the articulation of research questions.

Research principles can also be used in the evaluation of new procedures, protocols, and products. Evaluation is often an integral part of NICU nursing, but it is performed subjectively. Using research methodology to perform evaluation promotes scientific objectivity.

Obstacles to Involvement in Research

The reluctance of nurses to become involved in research generally stems from two basic obstacles: lack of knowledge and lack of resources. Both of these can be overcome. To address these issues effectively, nurses must receive education regarding the research process, have the opportunity to participate in research projects (in data collection or as subjects), and participate with colleagues in sessions to stimulate the formulation of questions from their clinical experience. One can begin by asking the question "why?" of every NICU nursing practice.

Lack of resources, including time, money, and consultation, can be difficult to address. In many institutions, the conduct of nursing research is still viewed as a frill and not central to the delivery of patient care. In such a setting, nurses wishing to conduct research may initially need to invest their own time and even money. However, once the research process has demonstrated clinical relevance, additional resources are often made available. Collaboration with colleagues within the institution, schools and universities, and industry can enhance resources.

Using Research to Change Neonatal Nursing Practice

Completion of a research study is not the end of the research process. A key step that is often neglected is the dissemination of the information obtained. This dissemination serves two purposes: (1) the sharing of information learned so that others may benefit and (2) the promotion of critical dialogue among professionals related to the study design, results, and interpretation. Sharing research results can take place through presentations, posters, and abstracts at professional meetings and through publication in peer-reviewed journals. Many resources are available to guide the publication of research findings.

Becoming a Critical Consumer of Research

As previously stated, the nurse must be a critical reader of research articles. A rigorous critique of research should also be carried out before trying to use the findings in a practice situation. Table 5–7 lists questions to consider when critically reviewing research studies. This critique can be applied to lay reports in local newspapers or magazines as well. The reader should also consider who funded the project. If, for instance, a drug company supported the research and the findings are favorable, good questions to ask are: Was the research biased by the funding source? or Have the findings been replicated by outside agencies? In addition, in brief reports look to see if the conclusions drawn are erroneous or if they address intervening variables that might also be affecting the research outcomes. Ideally, studies should be replicated to make certain that the results will hold true in a different setting or with a new subject pool, or both. Replication with similar findings lends credibility to the results. No single study's results should be accepted at face value without consideration of the potential biases.

Conducting clinical research is not a requirement or expectation of every neonatal nurse. However, being a critical consumer of research is a priority. The next decade will bring an increase in research with possible application to the nursing care of neonates. Each nurse caring for neonatal patients must first maintain an awareness of the research literature by keeping up to date with the professional journals. Implementation of research innovations has been shown to be correlated with the reading of professional journals and attendance at research seminars (Luckenbill-Brett, 1987). Unfortunately, research findings may be applied without critical review (Perez-Woods & Tse, 1990). Haller and colleagues (1979) proposed the following criteria for determining whether research is ready for use in practice: (1) evaluation of the scientific merit of the study concerning validity, reliability, generalizability, and statistical significance; (2) replication of findings to provide greater confidence in reliability and validity of results; and (3) determination of any potential risk to patients. When reviewing research literature, one must keep in mind that negative findings can be as important to practice as positive results. However, there is a tendency not to publish negative findings.

Goode and associates (1987) identified the following process for using research findings in practice: (1) identify problems occurring in the clinical area; (2) gather information from research studies that adds knowledge regarding the problem; (3) assure that nurses have adequate knowledge to critique research studies and understand their implications; (4) determine if the research is relevant to the patients and setting in which it is to

TABLE 5–7 General Criteria for Evaluating a Research Report

Step 1: Research Problem
1. Is the problem clearly and concisely stated?
2. Is the problem adequately narrowed down into a researchable problem?
3. Is the problem significant to nursing?
4. Is the relationship of the identified problem to previous research clear?

Step 2: Literature Review
1. Is the literature review logically organized?
2. Does the review provide a critique of the relevant studies?
3. Are the gaps in knowledge about the research problem identified?
4. Are important relevant references omitted?

Step 3: Theoretical or Conceptual Framework
1. Is the theoretical framework easily linked with the problem, or does it seem forced?
2. If a conceptual framework is used, are the concepts adequately defined and are the relationships among these concepts clearly identified?

Step 4: Research Variables
1. Are the independent and dependent variables operationally defined?
2. Are any extraneous or intervening variables identified?

Step 5: Hypotheses
1. Is a predicted relationship between two or more variables included in each hypothesis?
2. Are the hypotheses clear, testable, and specific?
3. Do the hypotheses logically flow from the theoretical or conceptual framework?

Step 6: Sampling
1. Is the sample size adequate?
2. Is the sample representative of the defined population?
3. Is the method for selection of the sample appropriate?
4. Are the sample criteria for inclusion into the study identified?
5. Is there any sampling bias in the chosen method?

Step 7: Research Design
1. Is the design adequately described?
2. Does the research design control for threats in internal and external validity of the study?
3. Are the sample criteria for inclusion into the study identified?
4. Are the reliability and validity of the measurement tools adequate?

Step 8: Data Collection Methods
1. Are the data collection methods appropriate for study?
2. Are the data collection instruments described adequately?
3. Are the reliability and validity of the measurement tools adequate?

Step 9: Data Analysis
1. Is the results section clearly and logically organized?
2. Is the type of analysis appropriate for the level of measurement for each variable?
3. Are the tables and figures clear and understandable?
4. Is the statistical test the correct one for answering the research question?

Step 10: Interpretation and Discussion of the Findings
1. Are the interpretations based on the data obtained?
2. Does the investigator clearly distinguish between actual findings and interpretations?
3. Are the findings discussed in relation to previous research and to the conceptual-theoretical framework?
4. Are unwarranted generalizations made beyond the study sample?
5. Are the limitations of the results identified?
6. Are implications of the results for clinical nursing practice discussed?
7. Are recommendations for future research identified?
8. Are the conclusions justified?

From Beck, C.R. (1990). The research critique: General criteria for evaluating a research report. *Journal of Obstetric, Gynecologic, and Neonatal Nursing, 19*(1), 18–22. Reprinted with permission.

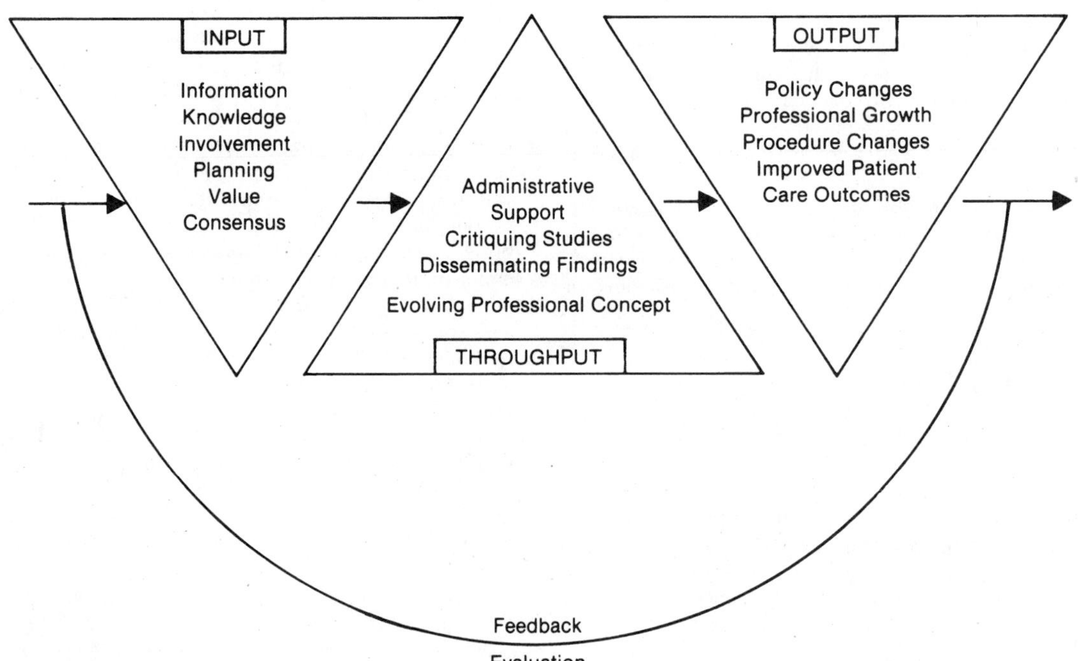

FIGURE 5–1. A systems theory model for using new research-based knowledge. (From Goode, C. J., Lovett, M. K., Hayes, J. E., & Butcher, L. A. [1987]. Use of research based knowledge in clinical practice. *Journal of Nursing Administration, 17*[12], 15. Reprinted with permission.)

be used; (5) devise ways to transform knowledge so that it can be used in clinical practice; (6) determine what patient outcomes are expected; (7) provide education that is needed to get the practice change implemented; and (8) evaluate and adjust or modify the new practice protocol as additional knowledge is available. The authors proposed a systems model for using research-based knowledge in the clinical setting (Fig. 5–1). Through the use of such models, neonatal nursing practice will be both validated and challenged, leading to improved quality of patient care.

CONCLUSION

Research must not be thought of as a discrete activity within neonatal nursing but rather as a way of thinking and an approach to each nursing encounter. Meier stated that "the evolving issue is not whether research in nursing is essential but rather how data that is crucially needed to guide clinical practice can be attained through systematic investigation" (Meier, 1983, p. 16). Neonatal nurses, by virtue of their relatively new and rapidly evolving practice and their exposure to the research process, are in an excellent position to demonstrate the integration of research and clinical practice.

REFERENCES

ANA Conference Call. (May, 1995). *Call with Nursing Organization Liaison Forum (NOLF) officers or representatives.*

Beck, C. T. (1990). The research critique: General criteria for evaluating a research report. *Journal of Obstetric, Gynecologic, and Neonatal Nursing, 19*(1), 18–22.

Brink, P. J., & Wood, M. J. (Eds.). (1989). *Advanced design in nursing research.* Newbury Park, CA: Sage Publications.

Chalmers, T. C. (1990). A belated randomized control trial. *Pediatrics, 85,* 366–369.

Cunningham, N., & Hutchinson, S. (1990). Neonatal nurses and issues in research ethics. *Neonatal Network, 8*(5), 29–48.

Fetter, M. S., Feetham, S. L., D'Apolito, K., et al. (1989). Randomized clinical trials issue for researchers. *Nursing Research, 38*(2), 117–120.

Fetterman, D. M. (1989). *Ethnography: Step by step* (Applied Social Research Methods Series, Vol. 17). Newbury Park, CA: Sage Publications.

Fleming, J. W. (1984). Selecting a clinical nursing problem for research. *Image: Journal of Nursing Scholarship, 16*(2), 62–64.

Freedman, B. (1987). Equipoise and the ethics of clinical research. *New England Journal of Medicine, 317,* 141–145.

Gleit, C., & Graham, B. (1989). Secondary data analysis: A valuable resource. *Nursing Research, 38*(6), 380–381.

Goode, C. J., Lovett, M. K., Hayes, J. E., & Butcher, L. A. (1987). Use of research based knowledge in clinical practice. *Journal of Nursing Administration, 17*(12), 11–18.

Grant, A. (1985). Do computers help or hinder the clinical evaluation of alternative treatments in perinatal medicine? *American Journal of Perinatology, 2*(3), 242–244.

Haller, K. B., Reynolds, M. A., & Horsley, J. (1979). Developing research based innovation protocols: Process, criteria, and issues. *Research in Nursing and Health, 2,* 45–51.

Hanson, S. M. (1988). Collaborative research and authorship credit: Beginning guidelines. *Nursing Research, 37*(1), 49–52.

Hunter, J. E., Schmidt, F. L., & Jackson, G. B. (1982). *Meta-analysis: Cumulating research findings across studies* (Studying Organizations: Innovations in Methodology, 4). Newbury Park, CA: Sage Publications.

Jain, L., & Vidyasagar, D. (1989). Iatrogenic disorders in modern neonatology. *Clinics in Perinatology, 16*(1), 255–273.

Kachoyeanos, M. K. (1995). Opportunities in outcome evaluation research. *American Journal of Maternal Child Nursing, 20*(4), 223.

Kachoyeanos, M. K. (1996). The current state of research in MCH nursing. *MCN; American Journal of Maternal Child Nursing, 21*(1), 13.

Kingry, M. J., Tiedje, L. B., & Friedman, L. L. (1990). Focus groups: A research technique for nursing. *Nursing Research, 39*(2), 124–125.

Korn E. L., & Baumrind, S. (1991). Randomized clinical trials with clinician preferred treatment. *Lancet, 337,* 149–152.

Kraemer, H. C., & Thiemann, S. (1987). *How many subjects? Statistical power and analysis in research.* Newbury Park, CA: Sage Publications.

Lantos, J. D., & Frader, J. (1990). Extracorporeal membrane oxygenation and the ethics of clinical research in pediatrics. *New England Journal of Medicine, 323,* 409–413.

Luckenbill-Brett, J. L. (1987). Use of nursing practice research findings. *Nursing Research, 36*(6), 344–349.

Lyons, N. B., Stein, M. B., Blackburn, S., et al. (1990). Too busy for research? Collaboration: An answer. *American Journal of Maternal Child Nursing, 15*(2), 67–68, 70, 72.

Marshall, C., & Rossman, G. B. (1989). *Designing qualitative research.* Newbury Park, CA: Sage Publications.

Meier, P. (1983). Research methodologies in neonatal nursing. *Neonatal Network, 2*(2), 16–22.

Meininger, J. C. (1990). Epidemiologic designs. In P. J. Brink & M. J. Wood (Eds.), *Advanced design in nursing research* (pp. 201–222). Newbury Park, CA: Sage Publications.

Mercer, R. T. (1984). Nursing research: The bridge to excellence in practice. *Image: Journal of Nursing Scholarship, 16*(2), 47–51.

Moody, L. E. (1990a). *Advancing nursing science through research* (Vol. 1). Newbury Park, CA: Sage Publications.

Moody, L. E. (1990b). *Advancing nursing science through research* (Vol. 2). Newbury Park, CA: Sage Publications.

National Commission for the Protection of Human Subjects of Biomedical and Behavioral Research. (1979). *The Belmont Report: Ethical principles and guidelines for the protection of human subjects of research* (DHEW Publication No. [OS] 78-0013 and No. [OS] 78-0014). Washington, DC: U.S. Government Printing Office.

Oberst, M. T. (1985). Integrating research and clinical practice roles. *Topics in Clinical Nursing, 7*(2), 45–53.

Perez-Woods, R., & Tse, A. M. (1990). Research attitudes, activities, competencies, and interest of NANN members. *Neonatal Network, 8*(5), 57–59.

Polit, D. F., & Sherman, R. E. (1990). Statistical power in nursing research. *Nursing Research, 39*(6), 365–369.

Rizzuto, C., Lough, M. E., & Palange, K. (1990). Unit-based research in critical care nursing. *Dimensions of Critical Care Nursing, 9*(3), 170–176.

Sarnecky, M. T. (1990). Historiography: A legitimate research methodology for nursing. *Advances in Nursing Science, 12*(4), 1–10.

Sharp, N. (1991). $40 million for nursing research: Is it enough? *Nursing Management, 22*(2), 22–23.

Sherwen, L. N., & Toussie-Weingarten, C. (1983). *Analysis and application of nursing research: Parent–neonate studies.* Monterey, CA: Wadsworth Health Sciences Division.

Stevens, K. R. (1986). Authorship: Yours, mine and ours. *Image: Journal of Nursing Scholarship, 18*(4), 151–154.

Stewart, D. W. (1984). *Secondary research: Information sources and methods* (Applied Social Research Methods Series, Vol. 4). Newbury Park, CA: Sage Publications.

Tilden, V. P., Nelson, C. A., & May, B. A. (1990). Use of qualitative methods to enhance content validity. *Nursing Research, 39*(3), 172–175.

Tornquist, E. M., & Funk, S. G. (1990). How to write a research grant proposal. *Image, 22*(1), 44–51.

Welch, J. A., Dye, J. S., Games, C., et al. (1990). Staff nurses' experience as co-investigators in a clinical research project. *Pediatric Nursing, 16*(4), 364–367, 396.

GENERAL REFERENCES

Barnard, K. E. (1985). MCN keys to research. *American Journal of Nursing.* Reprints (1-800-223-2282).

Code of federal regulations, title 45 public welfare. (1983, March 8). Washington, DC: Department of Health and Human Services, National Institutes of Health Office for Protection from Research Risks.

Federal policy for the protection of human subjects: Notice and proposed rules, part II. (1988, November 10). *Federal Register, 53*(218), 45660–45682.

Final regulations amending basic HHS policy for the protection of human research subjects, part X. 45 CFR part 46. (1981, January 26). *Federal Register, 46*(16), 8366–8392, 8949–8980.

Herxheimer, A. (1988). The rights of the patient in clinical research. *Lancet, 2,* 1128–1130.

Miller, D. C. (1991). *Handbook of research design and social measurement* (5th ed.). Newbury Park, CA: Sage Publications.

National Research Act Public Law 93-348, July 12, 1974.
Tanner, C. A. (1987). Evaluating research for use in practice: Guidelines for the clinician. *Heart and Lung, 16*(4), 424–431.
Wilson, H. S., & Hutchinson, S. A. (1996). *Consumers guide to nursing research.* Albany, NY: Delmar Publishers.

QUALITATIVE RESEARCH REFERENCES

Kirk, J., & Miller, M. L. (1986). *Reliability and validity in qualitative research.* Beverly Hills, CA: Sage Publications.
Lincoln, Y. S., & Guba, E. G. (1985). *Naturalistic inquiry.* Beverly Hills, CA: Sage Publications.
Miles, M. B., & Huberman, A. M. (1984). *Qualitative data analysis: A source book of new methods.* Beverly Hills, CA: Sage Publications.
Munhall, P. L., & Oiler, C. J. (1986). *Nursing research: A qualitative perspective.* Norwalk, CT: Appleton-Century-Crofts.
Norris, C. M. (1982). *Concept clarification in nursing.* Rockville, MD: Aspen Publications.
Weber, R. P. (1985). *Basic content analysis.* Beverly Hills, CA: Sage Publications.

UNIT TWO

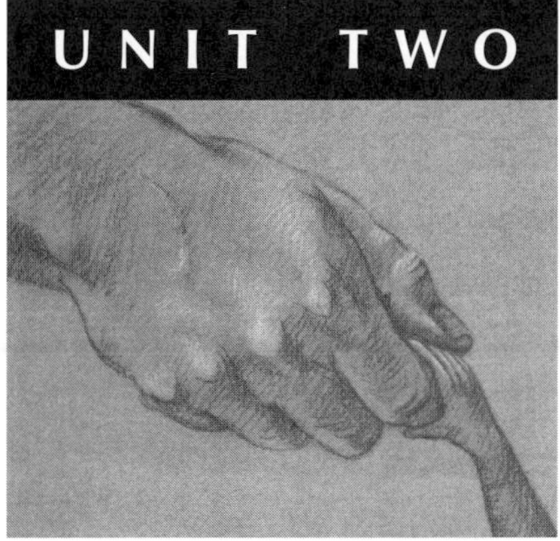

Family Dynamics

So obviously, in caring for these babies, Leslie and her nursing associates had to be equally adept at dealing with the parents. They had to juggle the egos of the doctors with the anxieties of the mothers and fathers. Working so closely with the parents, Leslie came to know them very well. She warned me early on about the stress that a long hospital stay with a small, sick child can put on a marriage. "It's a terrible strain," she said. "There really isn't any way around it."

Soon Leslie and I struck a pact. "You may not always like what I have to say, but I promise I'll be straight with you," she said. "If things look bad, I'll tell you." She vowed she would offer no false hopes. "When I get worried," she said, "I'll let you know." I knew instinctively that she could be trusted. In this crazy labyrinth of a hospital, she would be an ally for me and, most of all, for Emily.

ELIZABETH MEHREN
Born Too Soon

CHAPTER 6

The Changing Family Unit

SUSAN M. BERNS LOIS A. BROWN

■ **RESEARCH AGENDA**

Determine the effect that having a neonate in the neonatal intensive care unit (NICU) has on the adaptation of the family to their new role as parents.

How do parent and staff perceptions differ regarding having an infant in the NICU?

Determine whether the parental locus of control affects how they respond to the "change" of having a new infant who requires specialized neonatal care.

What types of social supports help the parents assume their new role in the NICU?

Change is the most certain event in life. A moment of reflection on our own lives would validate that elements of change affect our daily existence in varying degrees. A couple experiencing the birth of an infant faces many changes. Some variations in lifestyle occur in the areas of employment, financial security, daily activities, relationships with others, and role. The change in life role has a major impact on a parent.

This chapter explores role theory as it relates specifically to parenting. Factors that influence parenting behaviors include personal experiences, medical and nursing staff expectations, environmental conditions, and peer relationships. These factors can either promote or interfere with the development of an intact family unit. A critically ill newborn complicates the learning of parenting skills. The chapter concludes with strategies that optimize the functioning of the family unit during the NICU experience and promote the discharge of intact families after the crisis has resolved.

ROLE THEORY

Role theory appeared in the literature around 1930. As a broad term, *role theory* represents a collection of concepts, subtheories, and research that addresses certain aspects of social behavior. Over the years, role theory has developed to include two major theoretical perspectives: symbolic interaction and social structural role (Hardy & Conway, 1988). Both use role as a basic concept in an attempt to explain social order.

The symbolic interaction theory relates to individuals who create and construct their personal environment as they interact with, shape, and adapt to their own social environment. These individual behaviors aid in constructing the meaning of roles.

In contrast, social structural role theory has a broader base. It focuses on how society, social structure, and other social systems shape and determine an individual's behavior. Roles are social facts with patterned behaviors that develop over time, predetermined by social forces (Hardy & Conway, 1988).

The term *role* has diverse use. One definition of role is overt and covert goal-directed patterns of behavior that result from individuals interacting with, shaping, and adapting to their social environment (Thomas & Biddle, 1979). Roles are dynamic, interactional, and reciprocal relationships among individuals. Thus values, attitudes, and behaviors influence these relationships (Linton, 1945).

Examples of roles include sick, student, and maternal roles. Reciprocal relationships include the physician-nurse and parent-child roles. Each of these roles has specific behaviors and expectations placed on them by society; these expectations guide individuals as to when, where, and how they are to perform the role.

Each role also has specific demands. An individual learns these demands by maturing and advancing through the stages of the life cycle: (1) adolescence, (2) adulthood, (3) marriage and parenthood, and (4) middle and old age (Hardy & Conway, 1988). A person responds to the demands of a role differently based on his or her maturity and life cycle stage. For example, one would anticipate that a single, adolescent girl would perform her maternal role differently than would a married, adult woman.

Role theory identifies seven problems associated with roles: (1) role ambiguity, (2) role conflict, (3) role incongruity, (4) role overload, (5) role underload, (6) role overqualification, and (7) role underqualification. These terms are defined in Table 6–1.

TABLE 6–1 Role Problems

Role ambiguity	Vagueness, lack of clarity of role expectations
Role conflict	Role expectations are incompatible
Role incongruity	Self-identity and subjective values are grossly incompatible with role expectations
Role overload	Too much expected in time available
Role underload	Role expectations are minimal and underuse abilities of the role occupant
Role overqualification	Role occupant's motivation, skills, and knowledge far exceed those required
Role underqualification	Role incompetence; role occupant lacks the necessary resource (commitment, skill, knowledge)

Data from Hardy, M., Conway, U. (1988). *Role theory: Perspectives for health professionals (2nd ed.).* Norwalk, CT: Appleton & Lange.

These problems are responsible for producing role stress and strain. Role stress is defined as either internal or external pressure that generates role strain. Subsequently, feelings of frustration, tension, or anxiety are produced in either the individual or the reciprocal partners (Hardy & Conway, 1988).

ROLE CHANGE

When problems occur with a role, a person may need to modify or completely change roles. As an individual changes roles and learns a new role, the required behavioral changes can be stressful. However, not changing roles results in intrapersonal and interpersonal role conflict and leads to further stress and anxiety.

The working mother is an example of role conflict and role overload problems. She struggles with her dual professional and maternal roles. A decision to quit work and devote all her time to mothering may contribute to a lack of self-worth or identity. A decision to continue both roles may generate feelings of guilt because she feels she is neglecting her family's needs. Reducing her work hours is a behavioral change she may use to allow more time for her family. Thus she receives the positive reinforcement of employment, while having more time for family and her maternal role. If she does not modify her roles, she experiences further stress and anxiety.

Role change involves several steps to be effective. Such change develops through gradual, continuous, and dynamic processes based on the person's and relevant other's needs (Hall-Johnson, 1986). The steps to successful role change include identifying the role of the relevant other, identifying expectations of the new role, developing abilities for it, taking on the new role, and modifying it (Hall-Johnson, 1986). Figure 6–1 is a model for the role change process.

PARENTAL ROLE

Certain behaviors that are specific for both mother and father define the role of the parent. Several factors influence these behaviors: cultural background, personality, previous parenting and life experiences, the degree of attachment to the infant, and the expectations the parents have of themselves and the infant.

The situation in which one must parent also influences behaviors. For parents faced with a crisis state, there is a need to modify their role and adapt to the necessary changes. Role and behavior changes can produce considerable stress, especially if these changes occur abruptly.

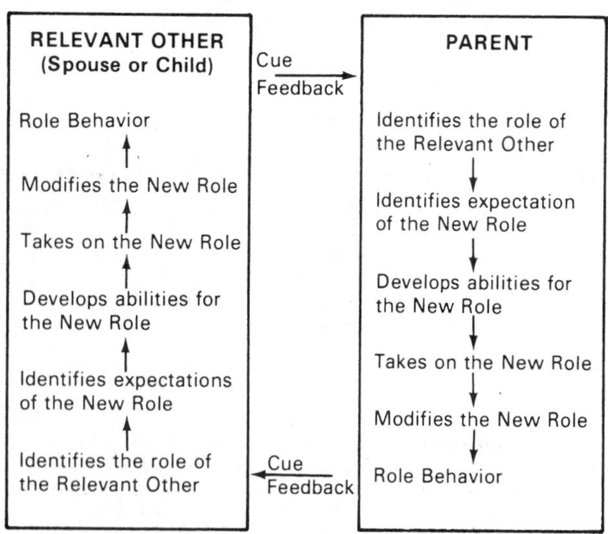

FIGURE 6–1. Model of the role change process. (From Hall-Johnson, S. [1986]. *Nursing assessment and strategies for the family at risk* [2nd ed., p. 392]. Philadelphia: J. B. Lippincott. Reprinted with permission.)

Parents suffering from mental or physical illness or those who are chemically dependent can have limited coping abilities and social supports. Single, adolescent, or first-time parents are also at a disadvantage. They can lack maturity and coping skills as the result of limited life experiences and social support systems. These situations may inhibit the development of the parent-infant relationship and thus impair parenting behaviors.

Infant-related factors can also interfere with parental attachment and subsequent parenting behaviors. An example is an infant born with a congenital anomaly. Many of these infants will be mentally or physically disabled for a lifetime, which interferes with the parents' expectations of their infant. An anomaly that is visible is particularly difficult for parents because society places such emphasis on appearance. An infant with an easily correctable anomaly is tentatively accepted by society until the anomaly is corrected. A visible, noncorrectable anomaly has a greater impact on the parents.

Another situation that may interfere with parenting attachment and behaviors is one in which the child has a life-threatening or terminal illness. Parents may "hold back" their feelings for the child to save themselves from pain if the child dies. This inability to attach to their infant may also interfere with the parenting experience.

At any birth, the nurse must identify adaptive and maladaptive parenting behaviors. Adaptive behaviors indicate that both the infant's and parent's needs are met, and thus the parent-child relationship can be established. Mothers and fathers have different ways of expressing their parental roles based on gender differences alone.

Tables 6–2 and 6–3 identify potential mothering and fathering behaviors that the nurse can use in assessing adaptive versus maladaptive behaviors. These are guidelines and must be adapted to each parent based on the specific situation.

Parenting During Crisis

Taking on the parenting role is a major life task for a couple. The crisis of a critically ill newborn in an NICU compounds the stress of that task. Whether the family unit attains growth from a positive resolution of this crisis or splinters following a maladaptive adjustment largely depends on the quality of support by the nursing staff (Edwards & Allen, 1988).

Parents' Reactions

Crisis can be defined as an upset in steady state. It is a period of disequilibrium precipitated by an inescapable demand to which the person is temporarily unable to respond adequately (Kaplan & Mason, 1960). The birth of a critically ill infant represents two types of crisis for parents. The birth of any infant is a developmental crisis, a natural transitional phase in the lives of a couple. When the infant is premature or ill, parents experience an accidental and unexpected crisis. The meaning of the event for the family and the resources available to deal with the event are variables that determine the scope of the crisis.

Families of the premature or sick newborn react in different and individual ways. Some common characteristics include anxiety, guilt, fear, resentment, and anger. During the illness of a sick newborn, the parents must face many charged issues. Two such issues are the loss of the perfect child they have anticipated and a fear that their infant may die (Mahan et al., 1982).

Within our cultural background, excitement and preparations surround the birth of a child. Parties help families celebrate the

TABLE 6–2 Potential Adaptive and Maladaptive Mothering Behaviors According to Situation

Adaptive	Maladaptive
Delivery	
Attempts to position head to see infant as soon as delivered and while infant is on warming table.	Does not position head to see baby. Stares at ceiling.
When shown infant:	When shown infant:
Smiles.	Frowns.
Keeps eyes on infant, looking at all parts exposed.	Stares at baby without expression.
Attempts en face position.	Does not assume en face position.
Uses fingertip touch on face and extremities.	Does not touch baby.
Asks to hold baby.	Does not ask to hold baby. Declines offer to hold.
Partially opens blanket to see more of infant.	If infant is placed in her arm, lies still, and does not touch or stroke face or extremities. May not look at infant.
Talks to baby.	Does not talk to baby.
Asks questions about baby.	Asks few or no questions.
Makes positive statements about baby: "She is so cute." "He is so soft!"	Makes no comments or makes only negative statements: "She looks awful." "He's ugly."
May cry out of joy or relief that infant is normal or of desired sex.	May cry, appearing unhappy or depressed.
May smile and cry at the same time. (To differentiate from crying out of disappointment, note facial expressions and verbal statements.)	When asked why she is crying, states being disappointed in baby.
Expresses satisfaction with or acceptance of sex of infant: "We really wanted a girl, but it is more important that he is healthy." "I can't believe, a boy, at last!"	Expresses dissatisfaction with sex of baby: "Not another girl. I should have known better than to have tried again for a boy." "I don't even want to see him." May use profanity when told sex.
Predominant affect—appears pleased and happy.	Predominant affect—appears sad, angry, or expressionless.
Suddenly decides she wants to breastfeed.	Suddenly decides against breastfeeding.
First Week	
Initially uses fingertips on head and extremities. Progresses to using fingers and palm on infant's trunk. Eventually draws infant toward her, holding infant against her body.	Uses fingertip touch, without progressing to palm on trunk or drawing infant toward her body.
Snuggles infant to neck and face.	Does not hold infant to neck or face.
Makes spontaneous movements, kissing, stroking, rocking.	Makes few or no spontaneous movements with infant.
Attempts to establish eye contact by moving infant, assuming en face position, or shielding infant's eyes from light.	Does not use en face position or attempt to establish eye-to-eye contact.
Handles and holds baby at times other than when giving direct care.	Handles only as necessary to feed or change diapers.
Talks to infant.	Does not talk to infant.
Smiles at baby frequently—changes affect appropriately, such as when infant cries.	Rarely smiles at baby, or smiles all the time without change in affect.
Makes many specific observations of infant: "Her eyes look like they might turn brown." "One foot turns in just a bit."	Makes no observations. Makes few observations that are either general or negative.
Discusses infant's characteristics, attempting to relate them to others in the family: "He has my ears, but his daddy's chin." "She really doesn't look like either of us, she just looks like herself."	Does not discuss infant's characteristics in relation to characteristics of family members.
With a positive manner, uses animal characteristics to describe baby: "She is just like a cuddly little kitten." "His hair feels like down."	In a negative or hostile manner, uses animal characteristics to describe baby: "She looks awful, just like a drowned rat." "He looks like an ape to me."
Asks questions about caring for infant discharge.	Asks no questions about care.
First Few Weeks (if infant remains hospitalized after mother is discharged)	
Calls every 1–2 days.	Calls less frequently than every other day, or not at all.
Visits minimum of twice a week.	Visits less frequently than twice a week, or not at all.
Visits minimum of 30 minutes.	Visits for less than 30 minutes.
Asks specific questions about infant's condition.	Asks no specific questions. Asks few questions. Asks inappropriate questions.
Spends most of visit looking at and handling infant.	Spends most of visit observing unit activities and other infants (this may be normal behavior for the first one or two visits); has little or no interaction with infant during visits.
Becomes involved with care when encouraged and supported by staff.	When encouraged by staff to participate in care, refuses, terminates visit, or does only minimal care.
Although visits are frequent and last longer than 30 minutes, makes statements about missing infant (e.g., expresses that she misses infant at home or that she wishes she could visit more often and stay longer).	Makes no statements about missing infant, or states she misses infant at home and wishes she could visit more often, but comments are not validated by frequent or lengthy visits.
Expresses reluctance to terminate visit.	Leaves nursery with little hesitation.

Table continued on following page

TABLE 6–2 Potential Adaptive and Maladaptive Mothering Behaviors According to Situation *(Continued)*

Adaptive	Maladaptive
First Few Weeks (Continued) (if infant remains hospitalized after mother is discharged)	
Waits until infant is asleep before leaving; touches or talks to baby just before leaving; may stand outside window and look at baby before leaving unit.	Frequently asks nurse to complete feeding or to change and settle infant.
First Months	
Holds infant close to her body.	Does not hold infant securely against body.
Supports infant's trunk and head in position of comfort.	Head and body of infant are not well supported.
Muscles in arms and hands are relaxed and conform to curvature of infant's body.	Shoulder, arm, and hand muscles appear tense; hands and fingers do not conform to infant's body.
During feedings, holds infant in well-supported position against her body.	Holds infant away from body during feedings, or props infant or bottle.
Positions during feeding so eye-to-eye contact can occur.	Position during feeding prevents eye-to-eye contact.
Minimizes talking to infant while he or she is sucking.	Continues talking to infant during feeding even though infant is distracted and stops sucking.
Refers to infant using given or affectionate name.	Refers to infant in impersonal way (e.g., "the baby," "she," or "it").
Plays with infant at times unrelated to direct care.	Handles infant mainly during caretaking activities.
When infant is in infant seat, playpen, or crib, frequently interacts with him or her.	Leaves infant for long periods in infant seat, playpen, or crib, interacting only after infant becomes fussy.
Places infant, when awake, in an area where he or she can observe and interact with others.	Leaves infant, when awake, alone for long periods of time in bedroom or isolated area.
Occasionally leaves infant with someone else.	Frequently leaves baby with someone else, or refuses to leave baby with someone else.
Uses discretion in selecting baby sitter and provides instructions on baby's routines, likes, and dislikes.	Does not use good judgment in selecting baby sitter; provides inadequate or no instructions for care.
Provides infant with routine well-baby care.	Fails to provide infant with well-baby care, seeking medical assistance only after problems, or keeps all appointments, and makes additional phone calls or additional visits to physician or emergency room for imagined or insignificant problems.
Carries out medical plan for management of specific problems or conditions (e.g., thrush, anemia, or ear infection).	
Remains close to infant during physical examinations, and attempts to soothe baby if he or she becomes distressed.	Remains seated at a distance from the examination table; does not soothe infant during examination; frequently arranges for someone else to take infant for medical appointments.
Makes positive statements about mothering role.	Makes negative statements about mothering role.

Modified from Hall-Johnson, S. (1986). *Nursing assessment and strategies for the family at risk* (2nd ed., pp. 22–24). Philadelphia: J.B. Lippincott. Reprinted with permission.

anticipation of a new infant. Parents spend much time imagining what this child will look like and dreaming about the joys of parenting. The couple experience disappointment when the infant or pregnancy is not as anticipated. They may feel a sense of isolation from other couples who have had a normal pregnancy or infant. They may even have feelings of isolation from each other. The inability to produce a healthy infant or protect the infant from the invasive and painful environment necessary to sustain the infant's life may produce feelings of inadequacy.

Parents must reconcile their idealized image of the child with the actual infant. There is not only mourning for the loss of the perfect child that was expected but also anticipatory grief for the infant whose life is now in jeopardy (Olshansky, 1962) (see Chapter 8, Bereavement). The birth of a sick or premature infant puts parents in a state of disequilibrium. Mothers of premature infants have the work of pregnancy cut short and are unprepared for birth. If the mother felt ambivalent about pregnancy, she may feel the infant's illness is punishment for those emotions.

Many parents of sick newborns go through identifiable stages of emotional reactions (Drotar et al., 1975). The initial response is usually one of overwhelming shock, characterized by irrational behavior, crying, and feelings of helplessness and despair (Mahan et al., 1982). Many families have difficulty with organization because their lives have been disrupted by the unexpected birth.

Parents may then experience feelings of guilt for the premature delivery or for the illness of the sick infant. Self-blame often characterizes these feelings: "If only I had stayed home that day I noticed the spotting." Parents may try to escape the situation by denial: "It will all be fine in just a few days."

Intense feelings of resentment and anger follow denial. Parents may direct these feelings at themselves, the infant, members of the health care team, God, or even at each other as parents. They can also experience feelings of ambiguity. They may fear the infant's physical and mental outcome. Thus, they avoid emotional involvement to protect themselves from the pain of potential loss.

A lessening of the intense emotional reactions and an increased ability to begin caring for their infant's emotional and physical needs are characteristic of adaptation. Reorganization is the final stage (Drotar et al., 1975). At this time, parents come to terms with their infant's problems. This process may take a few days to several months. Unfortunately, in some cases it may never be successfully resolved.

Factors that Affect Parenting Skills

Certain factors affect the ability to acquire parenting skills during the NICU experience. Parents are unable to attach and detach at the same time. These two tasks are incongruent. Parents need time to detach or grieve for the lost perfect child before they can begin to attach to the ill infant.

Physical, mechanical, and psychological or emotional barriers are obstacles to parents faced with the NICU environment (Griffin, 1990; Hall-Johnson, 1986). Some investigators have developed

TABLE 6–3 Potential Adaptive and Maladaptive Fathering Behavior

Time-Situation	Adaptive	Maladaptive
Touches child	Freely, uses whole hand	Infrequent, uses fingertips, rough
Holds child	Holds close to body, relaxed posture	Holds distant from body, unrelaxed
Talks to child	Positive manner, tone; uses appropriate language, speech, content	Uses curt, loud, inappropriate language or content
Facial expression	Makes eye contact, expresses spectrum of emotions	Makes limited eye contact, little change in expression
Listens to child	Active listener, gives feedback	Is inattentive or ignores child
Demonstrates concern for child's needs	Active, involves others, seeks information	Indifferent, asks few questions
Aware of own needs	Expresses feelings about self in relation to child	Gives no expression about self
Responds to child's cues	Responds promptly to verbal, nonverbal cues	Has limited awareness and response
Relaxed with child	Posture, muscle tone relaxed	Posture rigid, tense, fidgets
Disciplines child	Initiates reasonable, appropriate discipline	Does not initiate or uses measures that are too severe or too lax
Spends time with, visits child	Routinely, utilizes time so that child is involved	Has no routine, no emphasis on child during time spent
Plays with child	Uses appropriate level of play, active, both enjoy	Uses appropriate play, no obvious enjoyment
Gratification after interaction with child	Father states, appears gratified	Gives no statement or display of gratification
Initiates activity with child	Frequently	Infrequently
Seeks information and ask questions about child	Concerned, asks frequent, appropriate questions	Asks few questions, needs prompting
Responds to teaching	Positive, reinforces instructor, seeks more information	Has little interest
Knowledge of child's habits	Is knowledgeable	Has little knowledge
Participates in physical care	Feeds, bathes, dresses child	Allow others to perform tasks
Protects child	Aware of environmental hazards, actively protects	Protective behaviors not exhibited
Reinforces child	Gives verbal-nonverbal responses to child's positive behaviors	Does not notice or acknowledge child's behavior
Teaches child	Initiates teaching	No teaching
Verbally communicates with mother about child	Uses positive, frequent verbal encounter	Gives negative, infrequent communication
Verbally and nonverbally supports mother	Demonstrates support; reassures, touches, guides	Support not obvious
Mother supports father, father responds	Gives positive response	Responds negatively, no response
Speaks of other children	Responds when asked, initiates	Shows no interest, no initiation

From Hall-Johnson, S. (1986). *Nursing assessment and strategies for the family at risk* (2nd ed., p. 46). Philadelphia: J.B. Lippincott. Reprinted with permission.

a parental stressor scale for the parent with an infant in the NICU. Its purpose is to measure parental perceptions of stressors that are inherent to the NICU environment (Miles et al., 1993). If the nurse can properly identify the stressors for each individual family, he or she has the opportunity to assist the family in decreasing those stressors and to promote adaptation for the family unit. The nurse, however, is still potentially the principal barrier to parenting in the NICU, since he or she is the gatekeeper of the infant (Griffin, 1990).

Mothers and fathers react to stress and grief in different ways. A father can become engrossed in work and not share feelings with the mother. A father often tries to be strong for the mother and may become protective, shielding the mother from painful information. The mother may view the husband's stoic behavior as cold and unfeeling. Both may have difficulty discussing the child because of guilt feelings. Normal postpartum blues can increase the mother's sensitivity and her depression. She may cry for no real reason and feel embarrassed at irrational behavior. Existing weaknesses in a relationship may be magnified. Parents are separated at this time, and there may be fear that their relationship will fall apart. Lack of communication can lead to isolation and feelings of resentment. They may make assumptions about the other's feelings. Misconceptions can form. These misconceptions, along with gender differences in coping, can continue for a lifetime if not recognized in this neonatal period, especially if there is a developmental disability involved (Heaman, 1995).

Other stressors in the family—such as financial concerns, illness of other family members, and marital stress—complicate the situation. Coping abilities during previous crises can predict how parents will cope with the current crisis. Maintaining a support system and using community resources and professional assistance are ways of dealing with the crisis.

Certain personality types thrive on stress and deal effectively with any crisis. Others are unable to deal with even the smallest crisis. The family's expectations for itself and this new child affect parenting skills. Finally, the couple draws on childhood experience for parenting role models.

PARENT AND STAFF EXPECTATIONS

When parents have a sick infant in an NICU, they have certain expectations. They expect excellent medical and nursing care. Throughout the illness, parents expect accurate and timely information. At the same time, they expect to be involved in decision-making about their infant's care. The medical and nursing staff, working as a team and being supportive of each other, instill confidence in the parents. The parents also benefit from communication that includes information about their infant and involvement in the decisions related to care (Gilbert & Harmon, 1986).

Medical and nursing staff have expectations. Sometimes their expectations of infant or parents are unrealistic. The staff may expect parents to visit more often. Other responsibilities, travel distance, or financial burden may prevent more frequent visits. The staff may expect the infant to nipple-feed more often or be weaned from oxygen faster. It can be distressing to parents if they believe that the medical staff is not pleased with their infant's progress, even though this attitude may not have been verbalized. Therefore, incongruities in actions as well as information should be avoided.

PROMOTING PARENTING IN THE NEONATAL INTENSIVE CARE UNIT

A major nursing goal in the NICU is to optimize parenting skills and discharge an intact family unit. There are different ways to ease parental anxiety during the NICU experience. Open visiting policies, especially 24-hour visiting, give parents more opportunities to be with their infant while allowing them to deal with other responsibilities. Restricted visiting may imply that the staff is hiding details about their infant's condition. Unrestricted access to their infant allows the bonding and parenting process to begin.

The attachment process begins at birth. With a sick or premature infant, this process is delayed until the parents can establish eye contact and begin touching their infant (Klaus & Kennell, 1983). Bonding is enhanced by allowing the parents to touch and hold the infant as soon as his or her condition allows.

The preterm neonate's physical appearance, disorganized behavioral responses, and variable physiologic response to touch can produce much anxiety in the parents as they attempt to interact with their infant (Edwards & Saunders, 1990; Harrison et al., 1990). Using a semistructured interview technique, a recent study of mothers of premature infants found that mothers interact most often by talking and touching their infants and felt that their infants responded through body activity, eye opening, and orientation (Oehler et al., 1993). Since only about half of the mothers in this study were able to monitor their infants' activity and use it as a guide for any further interaction, it continues to be important that the bedside nurse, who is well versed in what the sick or premature infant will tolerate, share this information with the parents. Knowledge regarding an infant's inability to respond or tolerate eye contact or parental voice cues is vital for parents to understand; otherwise parents may misinterpret cues or detach from their infant. It is also important for the nurse to teach parents to recognize an infant's distress signals (such as hiccups, apnea, cyanosis, bradycardia, or mottling) so that parents know how to gauge their interactions with their infant.

External stimuli in the NICU must be controlled. Unnecessary stimuli aggravate the infant's already overwhelmed immature nervous system. Also, loud monitor alarms and excessive staff noise can be upsetting and unnerving to parents. A quiet and comforting atmosphere with decreased lighting helps calm parents (see Chapter 50, Assessment and Management of Neonatal Development). Achieving a balance between the high-technology environment and the need of parents to touch their infant frequently helps foster parental self-confidence. This balance must be a priority for neonatal nurses (Kowalski et al., 1996).

"Kangaroo care" is a "high-touch" avenue for promoting parenting, and it aids in the recovery of ill newborns. Kangaroo care, or skin-to-skin holding, of even the sickest infants has been documented in the literature to provide many benefits, including decreased oxygen requirements, longer quiet sleep periods, and shortened hospitalization (Drosten-Brooks, 1993). During kangaroo care, the infant is held next to the parent's chest. A covergown is put on backward with the opening in the front to allow the infant to be snuggled next to the chest, with the gown providing a cover over the infant. (For more information on environmental factors and how they affect neonatal development, see Chapter 50, Assessment and Management of Neonatal Development.) Parents using kangaroo care can provide a warm bed with a heartbeat. Besides the benefits to neonates, there are also benefits to parents, including early bonding, increased confidence in parenting skills, and a sense of control; parents start to have a sense of confidence that their infant is well cared for and may survive (Gale et al., 1993; Ludington-Hoe & Golant, 1993). Staff may resist kangaroo care fearing that intravenous lines or endotracheal tubes could become dislodged or that problems could occur while the infant was underneath the parent's clothes and they would be blamed. Gale and associates (1993) found that nurses were reassured about skin-to-skin holding when the neonatal development nurse stayed at the bedside with the parent and that the infant was returned to the bed immediately if there were any signs of compromise. Nurses who were able to observe this technique first were less resistant as well, and after seeing the benefits to the infants and the limited problems, many nurses became supporters of kangaroo care. Established protocols and education of both staff and parents also helps with the transition to kangaroo care in the nursery.

If an infant is being transferred to another hospital, parents need time to view their infant. This brief viewing decreases inaccurate fantasies about the neonate and promotes bonding and attachment behaviors. Occasionally, the mother's condition is unstable and she cannot visit the NICU soon after delivery. Instant pictures can be taken and given to the mother as soon as possible.

Many hospitals use volunteer "cuddlers" for the stable infants in the NICU. Cuddling, singing, patting, and rocking are some of the soothing activities these volunteers provide for infants at times when the nursing staff have other duties or when the infants' parents are not available. Many parents find it comforting to know that these "cuddlers" assist in consoling their infants while they are separated.

Throughout the illness, parents need accurate and timely information about the infant's condition. Shellabarger and Thompson (1993) have identified specific information parents feel they need regarding their infant. That information should be direct and honest and should not be contradictory. Parents also appreciate the use of drawings and diagrams when their infant's condition is being explained to them and they appreciate being encouraged by staff to ask questions. Presenting this information with some optimism allows the family some hope. Ideally, the information should be presented to both parents at the same time. It should be expressed in simple terms with short explanations. The parents are under much stress, and this information is unfamiliar. Facts may have to be repeated several times before they are absorbed. Parents need a clear understanding of the information provided to make informed decisions about their infant's care. Medical information from a primary caregiver, such as a neonatal nurse practitioner or primary physician, provides consistency.

Families need information about visiting hours, unit policies, equipment, procedures, and treatments their infant is receiving. Direct telephone access allows an update from their nurse or physician at all times. After verbal communication, written information helps parents remember important facts.

The number of nursing or medical personnel in surgical outfits and interacting with parents can be overwhelming. Therefore, introductions by name and position are important, and personnel should wear name tags to help families identify the staff members. Many institutions have adopted the primary nursing concept. Families often feel more secure knowing one nurse directs their baby's nursing care throughout the hospitalization; thus a trusting relationship can be established. A friendly approach opens communication and demonstrates openness and approachability. The primary nurse can act as liaison between the family and the health care team. This liaison function ensures that information about the infant's current condition, any changes in condition, and long-term outcomes for the infant are communicated to the family. This liaison function becomes essential if the infant is ever transported back to a community hospital. Parents need to know what to expect at that hospital and to understand that the agency can now handle the infant who was once too sick for them. Otherwise, parental mistrust of the community hospital may develop (Page & Lunyk-Child, 1995).

Staff attitudes are an important part of the development of positive parenting. Staff behaviors and attitudes can inhibit or encourage parenting skills. Conflict about parenting roles can exist between parents and staff. This conflict may escalate into a struggle for control. Parents may view the staff as acting as the infant's parents or the infant as belonging to the staff because the staff provide most of the care. The staff's pet names for the neonate further reinforce parents' fears. Nursing staff can help the family by encouraging them to personalize the infant's care. Bringing in clothes, toys, and pictures of other family members and making cassette tapes of family voices are ways parents contribute to caretaking.

It is also necessary to identify inappropriate nursing behaviors and correct them (Griffin, 1990). This identification can be facilitated by educating the nursing staff regarding the parenting process. The education can be initiated during orientation of new staff members and reinforced at intervals with continuing education workshops on the subject.

Adequate nursing staff can also promote parenting in the NICU. Overworked nurses can be frustrated and stressed, becoming overwhelmed with their own anxieties. These feelings may impede their ability to interact calmly and therapeutically with a fragile family unit. Nursing management considerations should include provision for adequate staffing to allow nurses the time and emotional energy necessary to meet the needs of parents in crisis (Griffin, 1990). Patient assignments should be evaluated not only for the technical care an infant requires but also for the psychosocial demands of the family.

Caretaking is a normal part of parenting. However, parents of sick or premature infants have been deprived of time to prepare psychologically and develop their caretaking skills (Goldson, 1979). If the staff never allows the family to become involved in caretaking tasks, parents may feel inadequate or resent the nurses. Positive reinforcement builds self-confidence in parenting abilities. Assessment of readiness to participate in caretaking activities is important (Fig. 6–2).

As the nurse prepares the parents for their infant's discharge from the NICU, it is important that the parents feel prepared to care for their infant. Kenner and Lott (1990) suggest these key techniques to prepare parents properly:

1. Give constructive criticism.
2. Encourage parents to verbalize their concerns and emotions.
3. Provide parents with information specific to their infant's care or condition.
4. Clarify information parents have received from other channels.
5. Point out the positive aspects of the infant, including how he or she responds to the parents.
6. Keep the channels of communication open by remaining nonjudgmental.

A complete discussion related to discharge needs can be found in Chapter 51, Assessment and Management of the Transition to Home.

Parent networking can be a vital tool for promoting parenting. Knowing that other families have survived this crisis can be reassuring. Support groups generally are helpful; however, they are not appropriate for every situation. Some couples need counseling. The primary nurse plays a key role in assessing signs that the family is not coping and needs therapeutic counseling. Support groups or counseling helps families look at problems objectively and learn alternative behavior for adaptive coping (Mahan et al., 1982).

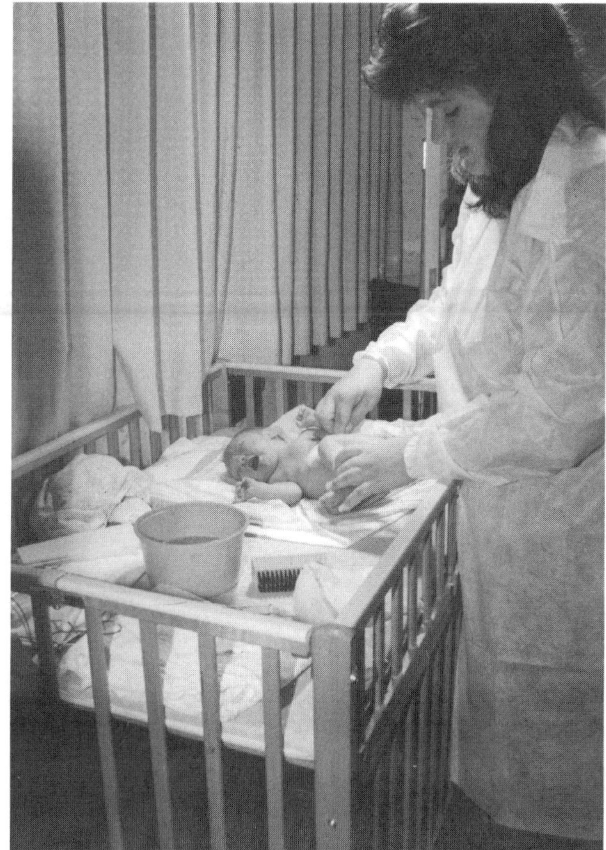

FIGURE 6–2. Participation in infant care promotes self-confidence and supports the development of parenting skills.

The nurse can assist parents in identifying additional means of support. Ideally, parents should be permitted to define their "family" as needed to provide support during this crisis, allowing them to visit as unit policy dictates. Grandparents, siblings, extended family, neighbors, and friends may constitute this group.

Grandparents may be a source of support in some instances. They may be forced into an uncomfortable role by seeing their own child in pain without a way to relieve that pain. Grandparents may also relive their own birthing experiences, which may result in associated anxieties and not allow them to provide support for parents. Extended family members may be more helpful if there is discord between grandparents and the nuclear family.

Siblings have needs as they are an important part of this new infant's life. Sibling visits may help relieve anxieties and make the birth a reality. The siblings' roles and needs are discussed in detail in Chapter 7, Sibling Adaptation to the Neonate.

Friends of the family can be an asset if they are effective listeners. They can offer to provide transportation for the mother and child care for siblings or take over meals and housekeeping chores to help alleviate family responsibilities. Just making telephone calls to other friends and family to update them on the infant's condition can be a great relief for the family.

Social workers involved early in the hospital stay provide parents with an objective person and contact with community resources. Families are reluctant to verbalize dissatisfaction with their child's care to nursing staff. Social workers can help parents express concerns without fear of retaliation against their child.

Clergy provide spiritual support for a family. Families often turn to religion for comfort and support at a time of crisis. It is

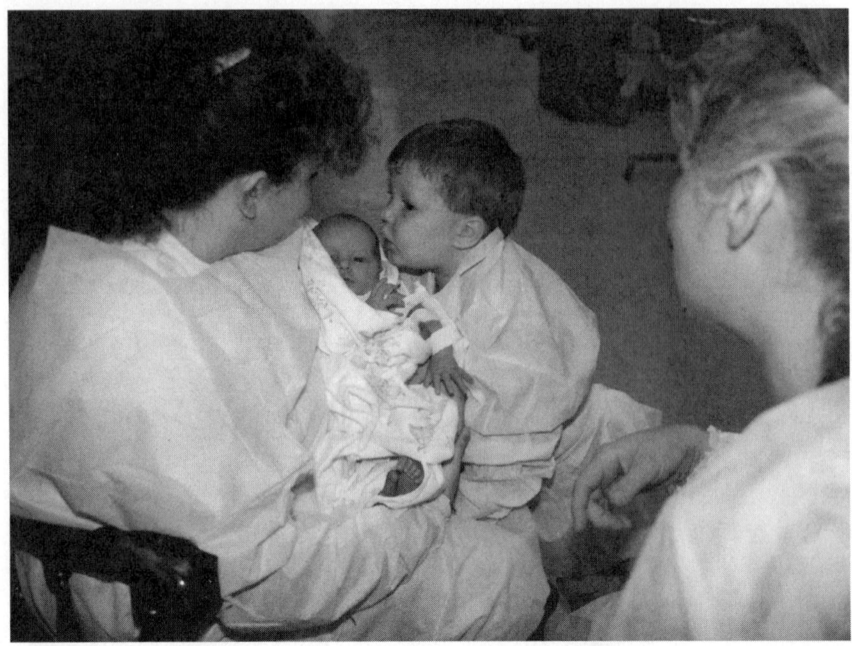

FIGURE 6–3. The ultimate goal of the nurse is to ensure the integration of the infant into the changing family unit.

important to offer parents privacy with the clergy to exercise their religious freedom.

Parents can be given one last boost in confidence by allowing them to room-in with sick newborns prior to discharge. Parents feel secure knowing that nursing staff is close by if they are needed. This process also allows parents the assurance that they can care for their babies adequately.

CONCLUSION

The birth of any infant produces tremendous changes in the lives of the parents. Normal adaptation can be complicated by the birth of a premature, critically ill infant or an infant with congenital anomalies. Without adequate coping strategies or resources for the parents, this crisis could produce much role stress and strain, which ultimately can weaken or destroy the family unit. The nurse plays an integral role in guiding the family to appropriate resources and support services. By promoting adaptive rather than maladaptive roles, the nurse can ensure an intact family unit after the crisis (Fig. 6–3).

REFERENCES

Drosten-Brooks, F. (1993). Kangaroo care: Skin-to-skin contact in the NICU. *MCN; American Journal of Maternal Child Nursing, 18*(5), 250–253.

Drotar, D., Baskiewicz, A., Irvin, N., et al. (1975). The adaptation of parents to the birth of an infant with a congenital malformation: A hypothetical model. *Pediatrics, 56*(5), 710–717.

Edwards, K. A., & Allen, M. E. (1988). Nursing management of the human response to the premature birth experience. *Neonatal Network, 6*(5), 82–86.

Edwards, L. D., & Saunders, R. B. (1990). Symbolic interaction: A framework for the care of parents of preterm infants. *Journal of Pediatric Nursing, 5*(2), 123–128.

Gale, G., Franck, L., & Lund, C. (1993). Skin-to-skin (kangaroo) holding of the intubated premature infant. *Neonatal Network, 12*(6), 49–57.

Gilbert, E. S., & Harmon, J. S. (1986). *High-risk pregnancy and delivery.* St. Louis: C. V. Mosby.

Goldson, E. (1979). Parents' reaction to the birth of a sick infant. *Children Today, 8*(4), 13.

Griffin, T. (1990). Nurse barriers to parenting in the special care nursery. *Journal of Perinatal Neonatal Nursing, 4*(2), 56–57.

Hall-Johnson, S. H. (1986). *Nursing assessment and strategies for the family at risk: High-risk parenting.* Philadelphia: J. B. Lippincott.

Hardy, M., & Conway, M. E. (1988). *Role theory: Perspectives for health professionals* (2nd ed.). Norwalk, CT: Appleton & Lange.

Harrison, L. L., Leeper, J. D., & Yoon, M. (1990). Effects of early parent touch on preterm infants' heart rates and arterial oxygen saturation levels. *Journal of Advanced Nursing, 15*(8), 877–885.

Heaman, D. J. (1995). Perceived stressors and coping strategies of parents who have children with developmental disabilities: A comparison of mothers with fathers. *Journal of Pediatric Nursing: Nursing care of Children and Families, 10*(5), 311–320.

Kaplan, D. N., & Mason, E. A. (1960). Maternal reactions to premature birth viewed as an acute emotional disorder. *American Journal of Orthopsychiatry, 30,* 539–552.

Kenner, C., & Lott, J. W. (1990). Parent transition after discharge from the NICU. *Neonatal Network, 2*(6), 31–37.

Klaus, M. H., & Kennell, J. H. (1983). *Bonding: The beginnings of parent-infant attachment.* St. Louis: C. V. Mosby.

Kowalski, K., MacMullen, N., Stifter, J., et al. (1996). The high-touch paradigm: A 21st century model for maternal-child nursing. *MCN; American Journal of Maternal Child Nursing, 21*(1), 43–51.

Ludington-Hoe, S. M., & Golant, S. K. (1993). *Kangaroo care.* New York: Bantam Books.

Linton, R. (1945). *The cultural background of personality.* New York: Appleton-Century.

Mahan, C. K., Krueger, J. C., & Schreiner, R. L. (1982). The family and neonatal intensive care. *Social Work in Health Care, 7*(4), 67–78.

Miles, M. S., Funk, S. G., & Carlson, J. (1993). Parenteral stressor scale: Neonatal intensive care unit. *Nursing Research, 42*(3), 148–152.

Oehler, J. M., Hannan, T., & Catlett, A. (1993). Maternal views of preterm infants' responsiveness to social interaction. *Neonatal Network, 12*(6), 67–74.

Olshansky, S. (1962). Chronic sorrow: A response to having a mentally defective child. *Social Case Work, 43,* 190–193.

Page, J., & Lunyk-Child, O. (1995). Parental perceptions of infant transfer from an NICU to a community nursery: implications for research and practice. *Neonatal Network, 14*(8), 69–71.

Shellabarger, S., & Thompson, T. (1993). The critical times meeting parental communication need throughout the NICU experience. *Neonatal Network, 12*(2), 39–45.

Thomas, E., & Biddle, B. (1979). Basic concepts for classifying the phenomena of role. In B. Biddle & E. Thomas (Eds.), *Role theory: Concepts and research.* New York: John Wiley & Sons.

CHAPTER 7

Sibling Adaptation to the Neonate

SUSAN M. BROUGHTON

RESEARCH AGENDA

How does a sibling adapt to having a critically ill brother or sister?

How do siblings adapt to a neonatal death?

How do siblings adapt over time to having a premature or critically ill brother or sister?

How well does a sibling visitation program prepare and assist the siblings in integrating the sick neonate into the family unit?

Siblings have a variety of responses to a newborn's arrival in the home, especially after a lengthy hospitalization. Family routines are disrupted by a "normal" birth and are further disturbed by an admission to the neonatal intensive care unit (NICU) and then again at the time of discharge. Siblings may feel displaced while parents are visiting the ill infant. Often, siblings are left with babysitters when they have rarely had experience with caretakers outside of immediate family. Fathers may be uncertain about what their family role is, and so they embrace their familiar work role and spend more time on the job. Thus, routines are disrupted, and parents are less available for their other children. These feelings may result in a variety of acting-out experiences. The following is an example of a family's response to the homecoming of a new brother who had been in the NICU.

VIGNETTE

John Jones was born at 33 weeks' gestation, and the nurses described him as a typical preemie with RDS and intermittent apnea and bradycardia. He required CPAP for several days and then hood oxygen for a week. After being weaned to room air, he was moved to the transitional nursery, where he stayed for another week until he mastered sucking, swallowing, and breathing. John's mother visited often. Mrs. Jones kept John supplied with breast milk and the latest drawings from his two sisters, Suzie (aged 6) and Becky (aged 4). John's father visited once in a while on his way home from work but did not take an active role in caretaking. He said that he was afraid to hold John but would once John got bigger and stronger. John was a cuddly little guy who had an uneventful recovery and was discharged after 3 weeks in the NICU.

Several days before discharge, John's mother confided in his primary nurse that she was about at the end of her rope because her husband was working longer hours and her daughters were acting out in ways they had never before done. Becky had demonstrated regression behaviors of bed-wetting and thumb-sucking. She had also found her blanket, which had been forgotten long ago. Becky was particularly close with her mother, and after her mother's daily visit to the NICU, Becky hit her mother, crying, "I hate you! I wish the baby would go away!" Mrs. Jones said that when she tried to console Becky, she ran and hid under her bed, crying, "Leave me alone, you only love that baby." If that wasn't bad enough, Suzie had begun waking up with stomachaches and refusing to go to school. Suzie had always loved her teacher and classmates and now was frequently in trouble for misbehaving in class. When Mrs. Jones would make Suzie go to school, she would cry, "I hate that baby and would like to run him over with daddy's car!" Mr. Jones had withdrawn from family life and was spending long hours at work. Mrs. Jones was beside herself.

The nurse was able to reassure Mrs. Jones that the behaviors of her husband and daughters were typical. Although this reassurance didn't immediately alter the situation, at least Mrs. Jones could know that many families respond to NICU hospitalization in this way and that, given time, the family would reestablish equilibrium. Mrs. Jones was encouraged to take the weekend off from her NICU visiting routine. She was able to spend a couple of special days with her daughters and engage her husband in life outside the worries of the NICU.

However, this did not provide Mrs. Jones with emotional support or help with her feelings of being overwhelmed and depressed. The nurse was able to listen to her concerns and then put her in touch with a parent organization that had been formed to help support families through the transition home. The parent organization offered peer support from parents who had been through the experience. They were also able to help Mrs. Jones place the experience in its proper perspective.

The girls had enjoyed their weekend together and were in a better frame of mind for the homecoming. Peer support helped Mrs. Jones so that she could in turn be available to her family. John was about ready for discharge and had progressed normally. Once John was home, Mrs. Jones included the girls in the baby's routine as much as possible by asking them to get his diapers and having them feed their dollies while she fed John. Suzie brought pictures of John to school for show and tell, and after Mrs. Jones called to speak to the teacher to explain the disruptions at home, Suzie gradually quit misbehaving. Becky continued to have problems with thumb-sucking and bed-wetting for several months while John was incorporated into the family and while a new family routine established.

Ann Flandermeyer

The birth of a new baby precipitates a family upheaval and the need for realignment of relationships and positions within the family constellation (Raphael-Leff, 1991). Becoming a sibling is known to be a stressful or "crisis" experience for young children and can have an effect on their mental, emotional, and social development (Spero, 1993).

The birth of a preterm or critically ill neonate who requires intensive care constitutes a further crisis for parents and consequently disrupts the equilibrium of the family system. Parents are reported to experience feelings of anxiety, grief, fear, anger, and guilt in response to the unanticipated events (Lindsay et al., 1993; Newman & McSweeney, 1990). Siblings are also affected and may experience helplessness, powerlessness, guilt, and anger in addition to the disruption of their daily routines and separation from their parents (Kenner, 1988). The siblings may feel very alone as their worried parents are preoccupied with the newborn baby. Siblings feel like the "forgotten family member" at the very time that they need attention (Trause & Irvin, 1983).

Addressing the needs of families of hospitalized patients has gained acceptance and support among nurses since the advent of the concept of family-centered care (Ahmann, 1994; Bass, 1991; Hegedus & Madden, 1994; Kenner, 1990; Lindsay et al., 1993; Plaas, 1994). Researchers have recognized the need for families of NICU patients to have increased psychosocial support and understanding during the crisis of hospitalization (Affleck et al., 1989; Kowalski et al., 1996; Lindsay et al., 1993; McKim et al., 1995; Vasquez, 1995; Zahr, 1991). All members of the family, parents and siblings, may exhaust their coping strategies and feel unsupported by those who are usually available emotionally and physically. The philosophy of family-centered care in a NICU is reported to encourage not only parent participation but involvement of the well sibling or siblings in the family process (Shea-McAleavey & Janusz, 1991). This involvement allows children to see their new sibling and to feel a part of the family process. Feelings of isolation may engender fantasies of what is taking place in the NICU. It is easier to cope with reality than with what can be imagined at any age.

Today, increasing numbers of hospitals are allowing participation of children at siblings' birth, siblings' contact with the infant at birth, sibling contact with the infant on the postpartum unit, and sibling visiting in intensive care nurseries (Murphy, 1993; Shea-McAleavey & Janusz, 1991). For nurses facing these challenges, the philosophy of family-centered care can provide a firm foundation in striving toward excellence in the practice of caring for children and families (Ahmann, 1994).

The development of a sibling–infant bond is vital in establishing and enhancing the relationship within the family unit (Newman & McSweeney, 1990). Holistic care surrounding childbirth may set up patterns or pathways that dramatically affect subsequent family interactions (Sherr, 1995). This chapter discusses a sibling's adaptation to the sick neonate.

SIBLING ADAPTATION: A REVIEW

Sibling relationships have often been viewed from a Freudian perspective, which emphasizes the concepts of sibling rivalry and displacement of the older child (Bank & Kahn, 1980; Kayiatos et al., 1984; Neubauer, 1982). Studies addressing changes in interactional patterns between the mother and firstborn (Dunn & Kendrick, 1981; Kendrick & Dunn, 1982) identify competition for and separation from maternal affection as factors that influence interaction between the older sibling and the newborn infant. The older child, previously the center of parental attention, is "dethroned" by the arrival of a new child (Wolterman, 1990). Leon (1990) suggested that it is very common for children to feel as if the birth of a brother or sister is a stress. The birth causes a competition for the mother's attention even when the new baby is healthy.

This Freudian framework has led researchers to focus on the negative aspects of sibling responses to the newborn with an emphasis on reducing jealousy and negative behavior (Fortier et al., 1991; Murphy, 1993). Faller and Ratcliffe (1993) argued that sibling attachments differ from general sociability and are independent of parental attachments. Lamb (1978) noted that sibling interactions that are initiated by the newborn have the potential for greater influence on infant development than do the parental interactions.

Psychoanalytic authors have emphasized that siblings are not only rivals but potential playmates, allies, teachers, and friends, fulfilling important object-related roles and narcissistic needs (Colonna & Newman, 1983; Provence & Solnit, 1983). The sibling relationship can be rich, intense, and uniquely endowed by the young participants themselves (Raphael-Leff, 1991).

Studies of siblings and newborns have focused almost exclusively on the period encompassing late pregnancy, the birth, and the early months and years after. Studies of preschool firstborn siblings reported that the most common initial reactions to the birth of a new baby are hostility and rivalry with the infant, rage and possessiveness toward the mother, increased attention-seeking behaviors, and often regression to bed-wetting, thumb-sucking, baby talk, and use of pacifiers and diapers by younger children (Raphael-Leff, 1991).

Increased engagement in fantasy play has been reported as children negotiate the stressful transition to becoming a sibling. Kramer and Schaefer-Hernan (1994) reported that children who, with few problems, accepted their siblings experienced a suppression in fantasy immediately after their siblings' birth; thus, a temporary disruption in fantasy play may indicate adaptive coping. Anderberg (1988) examined the attachment process of siblings during initial encounters with the newborn and during interviews with parents. The children were found to interact more with their mothers, which corroborates earlier research findings from Legg and colleagues (1974) and Marecki and associates (1985). The sequence of touching did vary between the school-age and preschool groups; younger children tended to touch the newborn's head most commonly, whereas the older children touched the extremities first.

Gottlieb and Mendelson (1990), in a study of 50 families with firstborn daughters, found that the firstborn's involvement with the newborn was associated with corresponding types of parental support. In some cases, parental support promoted the adjustment of the firstborn child, and in others, the needs of the firstborn shaped the parental support.

More recently, research studies have refuted the negative Freudian aspects of sibling response to the newborn. Gullicks and Crase (1993), examining parents' expectations and observations of their firstborn children's behavior before and after the birth of their second child, indicated that parents generally expected more negative behavior than they actually observed. The findings of Faller and Ratcliffe (1993), who described development of early interaction between siblings, indicated that positive sibling relationships may be the norm rather than the exception. The literature reveals evidence that indicated that reactions to the new arrival vary according to the family constellation, emotional development of the older siblings, the age gap between them, and the sex of each sibling.

SIBLING VISITATION TO THE NEONATAL INTENSIVE CARE UNIT

Today, sibling visitation in the hospital after delivery of a newborn has become common practice. However, limited research has examined the consequences of permitting and prohibiting sibling visiting in the NICU despite the argument that sibling involvement is consistent with the concept of family-centered perinatal care.

Earlier studies of NICU sibling visitation programs provided valuable descriptive data on the responses of siblings to the sick neonate. Ballard and colleagues (1984) reported that the NICU visits provided an opportunity for the older child to see, touch, and talk to the newborn sibling. This exposure was reported to help the children integrate the reality of the experience, prepare for the possible loss of the newborn, and in some cases reverse regressive behavior that had begun during the newborn's hospitalization.

A program addressing siblings' needs on the NICU was strongly supported by parents in a study by Troy and associates (1988). The development of a therapeutic play program involved the siblings in the NICU nursery environment and maintained the concept of family-centered care when siblings accompanied their parents on the hospital visits. Newman and McSweeney (1990) conducted a two-phase descriptive study designed to identify practices that fostered sibling involvement in the NICU. After interviews with national experts in neonatology, three factors were identified: (1) recognition of sibling's needs; (2) organization of sibling involvement programs; and (3) positive staff attitudes. The NICU head nurses further identified common themes within their unique programs that centered on families, the NICU atmosphere, and the promotion of sibling activities. A liberal visiting policy was recognized in all the units, promoting the concept of family-centered care and providing parents, siblings, and grandparents with the opportunity to be supportive together (Newman & McSweeney, 1990). The findings of this study, however, focused on two areas of limitation: The results reflected the perceptions of providers and not necessarily of the parents or siblings, and the exemplary NICUs, all being level III units in teaching hospitals, may have been associated with higher levels of technology and consequently different practices or policies on family visiting.

A Sibling Behavior Scale was developed by Wolterman (1990) for studying behavior in siblings after visitation to a NICU. The data suggested that siblings who were involved in the program demonstrated fewer overall negative behavior patterns than did siblings who were not involved. The preschool-age siblings who visited the NICU appeared to be more interested in the environment, whereas school-age siblings wanted to touch and hold the new baby. Wolterman (1990) found that NICU visitations give the siblings an opportunity to have a "sense of history" from this early exposure to the baby. They will remember when they first saw the baby and be able to reflect on this experience the rest of their lives. Although not intended to focus on the parent–child relationship, this study highlighted the importance of the NICU visitation's becoming a total family experience.

The need for sibling education classes in the NICU is currently recognized. Speck and colleagues (1993) evaluated a NICU sibling education and visitation program implemented by nurses practicing in a 60-bed NICU. Parents commented that the program encouraged family cohesiveness by allowing all family members to visit the infant together more frequently than the sibling visitation policy allowed. Parents also believed that it was important that siblings learned about the baby and the equipment in the NICU. In order to provide new learning experiences for siblings who attend sibling classes, a variety of additional books and craft activities, consistent with meeting the program's objectives, have been incorporated since its inception. Results of a hospital-based sibling preparation class, reported by Spero (1993), supported these findings, substantiating that the classes helped ease the siblings' transition and increased parents' awareness of the crisis potential for the older children.

PERINATAL SIBLING LOSS

The impact of perinatal loss on surviving and subsequent siblings have largely been unexplored (Leon, 1990). Children who lose a brother or sister have specific psychological needs. All too often, siblings do not receive sufficient attention, as health care workers usually focus on the bereaved parents (Sherr, 1995).

Raphael-Leff (1991) reported that a common parental reaction to perinatal death is protection of the dead baby's siblings from their own feelings. Parents hid their grief or attempted to be cheerful in their presence. There is surprisingly little written about the impact of the death of a baby on an older sibling. Studies of sibling loss have focused on the intensification of guilt in the surviving children. The guilt centers on the magical thinking of the toddler and preschool-age children, who wished the baby dead and got their wish. The older children's guilt is usually over their survival versus the baby's, especially if they never wanted the new baby in the family.

Davids (1993) described a clinical study of a young boy in Freud's developmental period of latency who struggled to come to terms with the painful loss of his baby brother. The study describes his sensitivity to his mother's sad moods and how he felt deprived of the usual emotional availability of his parents, who were preoccupied with their own grief and mourning. This psychological absence of his parents constituted a second loss.

Although it was previously held that very young children were unable to mourn, psychoanalytic investigations have shown that when accurate information is given and family permission is granted to grieve within a secure pre- and postloss environment, mourning is evident as early as the age of 3 (Bowlby, 1980). Raphael-Leff (1991) emphasized that young children may be undergoing reactions to the separation from their mother during the birth and, in addition, go through a mourning process for the baby who never came home or the one they knew so very briefly—a process that may be exacerbated by feelings of real guilt. For older children, the levels of meaning vary depending on family factors, age, developmental and cognitive abilities of the child, individual circumstances, and subsequent life circumstances (Sherr, 1995).

Van Eerdewegh and associates (1982), in a study of bereaved children, found an increase in general symptoms. These included moods, bouts of sadness, crying and irritability, many reports of sleep difficulties, reduction in appetite, withdrawn social behavior, temper episodes, and bed-wetting. Family adaptation to the loss determines the level of discussion, understanding, explanation, and help that a child receives at the time of bereavement.

IMPLICATIONS FOR PRACTICE

Nurses have a unique opportunity to support the development of positive sibling relationships in the NICU environment. Evolving models of comprehensive care can no longer overlook or delegate the care and needs of the whole family. Research on families of NICU neonates demonstrates parental desires for family-centered approaches to care. Siblings are an integral part of any family, and their adjustment or lack of adjustment to the birth of newborn greatly affects the well-being of the whole family. Their adjustment to the once-sick newborn needs further exploration.

CONCLUSION

When the birth of a sibling is further complicated by the baby's being ill or at risk, professionals caring for the baby are in a position to reassure parents that siblings will respond to the neonate in various ways on the basis of the child's personality, age, and interests. Parents are helped by professional reassurance that siblings cannot help feeling angry and displaced by the baby. Parent's capacity to accept their older children's competitive feelings and yet continue to love the older children helps the children to integrate ambivalence. Support through this ambivalence facilitates acceptance of the baby and the baby's incorporation into the family.

Increasing parents' knowledge about promoting positive sibling relationships through parentcraft education programs may influence the parents' attitudes, thereby enhancing the future sibling relationship. In response to consumer demand, many hospitals have implemented sibling visitation and educational programs. The preparation can help deal with the realities of this experience.

Special attention from the NICU staff can help siblings to feel recognized, supported, and appreciated during this time of stress. Encouraging the sibling to gently touch and talk to the infant and allowing gifts of toys or even a drawing of themselves to be kept with the baby are activities that may foster attachment and ongoing connection with the newborn.

The death of a sibling usually has profound and lasting effects on surviving children. Surviving siblings, however young, may need some evidence that the baby existed: a visit to see the ill newborn in the incubator, a photograph, or a chance to participate in the funeral. Regardless of the age of the child, it seems that the level of care offered in its place is crucial in determining the psychological and life adjustment of the bereaved child. Nurses need to be alert to the range and depth of childhood reactions.

Many research findings discussed here are invaluable in guiding NICU nurses in promoting and facilitating effective sibling interactions and positive involvement between the sick neonate and the siblings. Providing the appropriate environment in which to assist the siblings in coping with the profound changes that affect the sibling bond is also recommended, in order to help the siblings fully integrate this major event into their young lives.

REFERENCES

Affleck, G., Tennen, H., Rowe, J., et al. (1989). Effects of formal support on mothers' adaptation to the hospital to home transition of high risk infants: The benefits and costs of helping. *Child Development, 60*(2), 488–501.

Ahmann, E. (1994). Family centered care: Shifting orientation. *Pediatric Nursing, 20*(2), 113–117.

Anderberg, G. (1988). Initial acquaintance and attachment behavior of siblings with the newborn. *Journal of Obstetric, Gynecologic, and Neonatal Nursing, 17*(1), 49–54.

Ballard, J., Maloney, M., Shank, M., & Hollister, L. (1984). Sibling visits to a newborn intensive care unit: Implications for siblings, parents and infants. *Child Psychiatry and Human Development, 14*(4), 203–214.

Bank, S., & Kahn, M. (1980). Freudian siblings. *Psychoanalytic Review, 67*, 493–504.

Bass, L. (1991). What do parents need when their infant is a patient in the NICU? *Neonatal Network, 10*(4), 25–33.

Bowlby, J. (1980). *Attachment and loss* (Vol. 3). New York: Basic Books.

Colonna, C,. & Newman, L. (1983). The psychoanalytic literature on siblings. *Psychoanalytic Study Child, 38*, 285–309.

Davids, J. (1993). The reaction of an early latency boy to the sudden death of his baby brother. *Psychoanalytic Study of the Child, 48*, 277–292.

Dunn, J., & Kendrick, C. (1981). Interaction between young siblings: Association with the interaction between mother and firstborn child. *Developmental Psychology, 17*, 336–343.

Faller, H., & Ratcliffe, L. (1993). Sibling visitation: How far should the pendulum swing? *Journal of Pediatric Nursing, 8*(2), 92–99.

Fortier, J., Carson, V., Will, S., & Shubkagel, B. (1991). Adjustment to a newborn: Sibling preparation makes a difference. *Journal of Obstetric, Gynecologic, and Neonatal Nursing, 20*(1), 73–79.

Gottlieb, L., & Mendelson, M. (1990). Parental support and firstborn girls: Adaptation to the birth of a sibling. *Journal of Applied Developmental Psychology, 11*(1), 29–48.

Gullicks, J., & Crase, S. (1993). Sibling behavior with a newborn: Parent expectations and observations. *Journal of Obstetric, Gynecologic, and Neonatal Nursing, 22*(5), 438–444.

Hegedus, K., & Madden, J. (1994). Caring in a neonatal intensive care unit: Perspectives of providers and consumers. *Journal of Perinatal and Neonatal Nursing, 8*(2), 67–75.

Kayiatos, R., Adams, J., & Gilman, B. (1984). The arrival of a rival: Maternal perceptions of toddlers' regressive behaviors after the birth of a sibling. *Journal of Nurse-Midwifery, 29*(3), 205–213.

Kendrick, C., & Dunn, J. (1982). The arrival of a sibling. *Health Visitor, 55*, 155–157.

Kenner, C. (1988). The forgotten siblings. In C. Kenner, J. Harjo, & A. Brueggemeyer (Eds.), *Neonatal surgery: A nursing perspective* (p. 67). Orlando, FL: Grune & Stratton.

Kenner, C. (1990). Caring for the NICU parent. *Journal of Perinatal and Neonatal Nursing, 4*(3), 78–87.

Kowalski, K., MacMullen, N., Stifter, J., et al. (1996). The high-touch paradigm: A 21st century model for maternal-child nursing. *MCN: American Journal of Maternal Child Nursing, 21*(1), 43–51.

Kramer, L., & Schaefer-Hernan, P. (1994). Patterns of fantasy play engagement across the transition to becoming a sibling. *Journal of Child Psychology and Psychiatry and Allied Disciplines, 35*(4), 749–767.

Lamb, M. E. (1978). The development of sibling relationships in infancy: A short term longitudinal study. *Child Development, 49*(4), 1189–1192.

Legg, C., Sherick, I., & Wadland, W. (1974). Reaction of preschool children to the birth of a sibling. *Child Psychiatry and Human Development, 5*(1), 3–39.

Leon, I. (1990). *When a baby dies: Psychotherapy for pregnancy and newborn loss*. New Haven, CT: Yale University Press.

Lindsay, J. K., Roman, L. A., DeWys, M., et al. (1993). Creative caring in the NICU: Parent to parent support. *Neonatal Network, 12*(4), 37–43.

Marecki, M., Wooldridge, P., Dow, A., et al. (1985). Early sibling attachment. *Journal of Obstetric, Gynecologic, and Neonatal Nursing, 14*(5), 418–423.

McKim, E. M., Kenner, C., Flandermeyer, A., et al. (1995). The transition to home for mothers of healthy and initially healthy newborns. *Midwifery, 11*, 184–194.

Murphy, S. (1993). Siblings and the new baby: Changing perspectives. *Journal of Pediatric Nursing, 8*(5), 277–288.

Neubauer, P. B. (1982). Rivalry, envy, and jealousy. *Psychoanalytic Study of the Child, 37*, 121–142.

Newman, C. B., & McSweeney, M. E. (1990). A descriptive study of sibling visitation in the NICU. *Neonatal Network, 9*(4), 27–31.

Plaas, K. (1994) The evolution of parental roles in the NICU. *Neonatal Network, 13*(6), 31–33.

Provence, S., & Solnit, A. J. (1983). Development-promoting aspects of the sibling experience. Vicarious mastery. *Psychoanalytic Study of the Child, 38*, 337–351.

Raphael-Leff, J. (1991). *Psychological process of childbearing*. London: Chapman & Hall.

Shea-McAleavey, C. E., & Janusz, H. B. (1991). Sibling visitation—A plan for change. *Dimensions of Critical Care Nursing, 10*(4), 218–222.

Sherr, L. (1995). *The psychology of pregnancy and childbirth*. Oxford, UK: Blackwell Science.

Speck, L., Miller, B., & Rohrs, K. (1993). Sibling education: Implementing a program for the NICU. *Neonatal Network, 12*(4), 49–52.

Spero, D. (1993). Sibling preparation classes. *AWHONNS: Clinical Issues in Perinatal and Women's Health Nursing, 4*(1), 122–131.

Trause, M., & Irvin, N. (1983). Care of the sibling. In M. Klaus & J. Kennel (Eds.), *Bonding*. St. Louis: New American Library.

Troy, P., Wilkinson-Faulk, D., Smith, A. B., & Alexander, D. A. (1988). Sibling visiting in the NICU. *American Journal of Nursing, 88*(1), 68–70.

Van Eerdewegh, M. M., Bieri, M. D., Parrilla, R. H., & Clayton, P. J. (1982). The bereaved child. *British Journal of Psychiatry, 140*, 23–29.

Vasquez, E. (1995). Creating paths: Living with a very-low-birth-weight infant. *Journal of Obstetric, Gynecologic, and Neonatal Nursing, 24*(7), 619–624.

Wolterman, M. C. (1990). *Validation of an instrument to study behaviors in siblings following sibling visitation on a neonatal intensive care unit.* Unpublished doctoral dissertation, University of Cincinnati, College of Education, Cincinnati, OH.

Zahr, L. (1991). Correlates for mother-infant interaction in premature infants from low socioeconomic backgrounds. *Pediatric Nursing, 17*(3), 259–264.

CHAPTER 8

Bereavement: The State of Having Suffered a Loss

JANE A. NICHOLS

RESEARCH AGENDA

What is the impact of a neonatal loss on siblings?

What is the impact of grief and loss of a neonate on grandparents?

Examine the case managers' or primary nurses' response to loss and pending loss.

How does the grief process differ according to gender?

VIGNETTE

Mrs. Q is a 30-year-old gravida 4, with one earlier miscarriage and two living children at home. She was admitted to the hospital at 41 + weeks' gestation for an induction. At 1:48 A.M., baby Patricia Q was born to a delighted set of parents. The obstetrician noted the infant's change in color as the cord was clamped and cut. Assessment showed a limp blue baby with some respiratory effort and spontaneous movement. None of our resuscitative measures had a positive impact. The x-ray indicated a large left diaphragmatic hernia with hypoplastic lungs.

While we worked on the baby, the obstetrician and labor nurses stayed with the family, offering support and information about the resuscitation. The parents were grave and silent; the mother was intermittently tearful. At intervals the father paced into the hallway, as if he had to shake off his feeling of helplessness. The neonatologist informed the family about the defect and the hopelessness of the situation. The parents agreed to stop all life support and asked to hold their baby.

After the neonatologist stopped the life support, I wrapped the baby in warm blankets and took her to her parents. Glenda scooped her up and ran her fingers over her daughter's facial features. She explored all of Patricia's body parts. When she finished, she held the baby tightly and sobbed. Scott held his wife and baby and gazed intently into Patricia's face, as if to memorize it. They decided that she looked like her mother. I stayed with them to give support and took some instant pictures of them together when the time seemed right.

A clergyman arrived to baptize Patricia as she lay in her father's arms. Fifteen minutes later she died. They held her for a little while longer, whispering, "We love you. We will never forget you." I took formal photographs and got Patricia's footprints. I recorded her length and weight on the crib card, then collected her bracelet and cap. I placed her baptismal record in the packet along with one of the blankets. I notified the grandparents to come to the hospital, as the Qs had requested. I also arranged for meals for them.

When family members arrived, they wished to see Patricia again. I wrapped the baby in warm blankets and, after preparing them for what they would see, brought her to their room. The grandparents were initially uncomfortable, peering at the baby but declining to hold her. They were eventually able to hold Patricia for a while. When they were ready, I took Patricia, prepared her body, and transported her to the morgue.

The next day I visited the Qs in their room and gave them the packet of mementos. I prompted them to discuss the experience and their feelings about it. They seemed ready to discuss funeral arrangements, so we reviewed the different disposition options. I gave them several referrals and numbers of funeral directors. I helped them sign the necessary documents.

We resumed the discussion the next day. We explored their feelings further and discussed the grief response they would experience: characteristics, duration, and gender-specific differences. This was a time of honesty and mutual discovery for them. We discussed their support network, and I gave them referrals for a peer support group. We discussed the normalcy of grief. I did point out several uncommon signs that would indicate that they might need some help in working through it: prolonged lack of sleep, inability to complete basic activities of daily living after several weeks have elapsed, prolonged lack of interest in eating, marital discord, or obsessive thoughts of dying or committing suicide. The Qs were concerned about the response of their other children, ages 3 and 5, so we reviewed children's perceptions and grief response based on their developmental level. I recommended that the Qs share their feelings with their children and invite the children to share theirs with the parents. Finally, I gave the parents my phone number and encouraged them to call me if they had questions or just wanted to talk.

I checked with the Qs at home 1 week after the mother's discharge and found that although the parents were physically and emotionally exhausted, they were receiving support from friends and relatives. I checked with them again 2 weeks after Patricia's death and spent a long time talking with Glenda about her feelings. Although Scott was quiet and didn't want to talk about the baby, Glenda wanted to talk about her all the time.

Scott contacted me 2 weeks later and said he was worried about Glenda because she cried much of the time and didn't want to do anything but talk about the baby. Assessment revealed that Glenda was grieving appropriately, so I reminded him that individuals grieve differently and progress at different rates through their grief work. He seemed relieved and did share some information about his feelings. He had gone back to work and after the first several days found that it helped him to "get back to business" and concentrate on something else. He questioned whether he should force Glenda to get involved in some out-of-the-house project to "get her mind off the baby." I discouraged this suggestion, and encouraged him to be patient, keeping communication open about their feelings. I prompted him to encourage Glenda to contact the support group for bereaved parents. Sometimes a mother finds it helpful to talk to another mother who has had a similar experience. Fathers sometimes find it difficult to understand the mother's tenacity in her grief work, because his issues and experience are different from hers.

I called the Qs 2 weeks later, and Glenda reported that she had contacted the support group. The Qs had attended a group meeting and found it very supportive. Glenda stated that their grief experience seemed similar to that of many couples at the meeting. She felt encouraged by assertions that it does get easier and that the grief work would end in time. She also said she had been afraid she would forget Patricia and was reassured by the other mothers that this would not happen. Glenda felt that they would continue to attend the meetings. She agreed to contact me if she felt the need in the future.

Joyce M. Dohme

In the past, when an infant was born prematurely or critically ill, parents were advised to keep the child warm, nourish him or her with drops from an infant feeder, and wait to see what would happen. Parents of just two or three generations ago tell stories of nestling their child in a wicker laundry basket placed by the stove as they maintained the prayerful vigil over life and death. If the child lived, they felt blessed. If death came, the child was buried in the family plot.

More recently, well-intended but misinformed professionals separated parents, especially the mother, from their dying infant because it was feared "they couldn't take it." With the child removed from the family and isolated in the hospital, death could be denied and avoided. There was no vigil. It was considered genteel for family and friends to pretend that nothing had happened.

Today, the vigil is again kept. We have rediscovered the wisdom of old that parents *can* "take it." We still keep infants warm and feed them by the drop. We still wait to see. The vigil now takes place in a specialized care center, amid lights, beeps, bustle, and machines.

In the last three decades, with the development of regionalized neonatal intensive care units (NICUs) and the increased focus on perinatal health care, there have been exciting advances in the treatment of critically ill infants. Nevertheless, infant death still occurs. When it does, the health care team is called on to offer comfort and relief to parents as well as to assist them in beginning their grief work. To do so, the caregiver needs an understanding of the grief process and the issues unique to newborn death in addition to interpersonal nursing skills that are already in place. This chapter discusses the grief process within the context of theoretical models and their clinical application.

THEORETICAL EXPLANATIONS OF BEREAVEMENT

Bereavement is the state of having suffered a loss. Grief is an individual's response to the loss. Models of grief provide a theoretical framework for describing responses to loss.

On examination of the various grief models, one finds that each has the potential to contribute to our understanding of parental grief following neonatal death. Although these models have implications for explaining grief following perinatal death, such linkages have not been empirically tested. It is beyond the scope of this chapter to review the models of grief in depth; however, some of the key contributors and elements of their work that may pertain to bereaved parents of neonates are introduced. The models are introduced separately, yet it should be kept in mind that they overlap considerably.

Early models of grief were based primarily on the study of widowhood, that is, conjugal bereavement (Bowlby, 1980; Gorer, 1965; Parkes, 1970a, 1970b). At one time, it was generally accepted that all grief was alike. Some theorists still hold this view. However, Rando (1986) disagrees. "We can no longer afford to ignore the distinct needs of different types of bereavement . . . the loss of a child [will] be experienced much differently than the loss of a spouse" (pp. xii–xiii).

Psychodynamic models were heavily influenced by Freud (1959) and focused on grief as a dilemma resulting from the process of relinquishing a beloved object. Freud observed somatic distress in grievers, as well as a lack of interest in the outside world, an apparent loss of capacity to love, and painful dejection. Lindemann (1944), who conducted the first empirically based study of grief, found that the daily activities of the bereaved changed significantly and that the duration of grief seemed to depend on one's willingness to mourn. Lindemann coined the term *grief work* to describe the mourning process. He characterized grief work as emancipation from the bondage of the deceased, readjustment to the environment in which the deceased is missing, and the formation of new relationships. Most studies of grief have built on Lindemann's ideas.

Attachment models are rooted in the belief that attachment behavior is instinctive and that attachments are essential to human behavior. The goal of attachment behavior is to maintain effectual bonds; if the bonds are threatened, the individual seeks to preserve them. Bowlby (1980), a leading proponent of attachment theory, identified four phases of mourning or detachment: (1) the numbing phase, (2) the yearning and searching phase, (3) the phase of disorganization and despair, and (4) the phase of reorganization.

Building on attachment theory, Marris (1974), in his Pulitzer Prize winning book *Loss and Change,* maintained that everyone experiences many losses and that loss evokes a search for meaning. To find meaning, he said, individuals need to perceive a climate of safety and the opportunity for continuity. In general, sociobiologic models consider grief to be an evolutionary process that functions to ensure the survival of the human group and the species. Raphael (1983) shared this point of view because it provides a purpose for pain and loss.

Cognitive and behavioral grief models suggest that the bereaved must first relinquish their assumptions about the world and the deceased, and then they must develop a new set of assumptions. Parkes and Weiss (1983) recognized that grief is not a state but rather a process of cognitive restructuring. This process consists of three major components: (1) preoccupation with thoughts of the person who died, (2) painful repetitious recollection of the loss experience, and (3) attempts to make sense of the loss. They noted that the newly bereaved (i.e., persons suffering from acute grief) may require assistance in making even the simplest decisions and need time to reorganize their lives. Parkes and Brown (1972) also suggested that bereavement is similar to a physical injury that heals gradually—possibly bringing new strength, as with a mended bone, but with the possibility of complications.

Engel (1961) viewed grief as an illness that impairs functioning and produces suffering with its own group of symptoms. Illness models may have special value in that they recognize loss as a factor in the onset of illness. Therefore, grief can be considered a legitimate concern of the health care domain.

The newest model to emerge is the holistic model, which builds heavily on models of stress and earlier theories. In recent years, as more attention has been given to the mind–body connection (Stillion, 1986), many clinicians have focused on grieving as a holistic process that requires the involvement of the whole person—physical, mental, emotional, and spiritual—in meeting the challenges of living through grief. In their book *Ended Beginnings*, Panuthos and Romeo (1984) review the holistic approach to healing:

> We must understand the integrated relationship between the body, mind, heart, and soul. In the most simple sense, what we sow in the mind (or heart or soul), we reap in the body...in other words, mind, emotions, and body (and, we believe, spirit as well) are a unified system; if one is affected, so are the others (pp. 80–81).

Holistic models include the belief that not only do supportive interventions facilitate a griever's return to homeostasis but also may promote growth.

The contributions of Elisabeth Kubler-Ross, although eclectic, can best be characterized as holistic. Kubler-Ross' pioneering work can be credited with popularizing the public discussion of dying and death.

Kubler-Ross (1969) studied the emotional responses of terminally ill adult patients as they anticipated their own deaths. These reactions are generally assumed to be similar to the patterns of individuals who are bereaved. The five-stage model of grief developed by Kubler-Ross is her most frequently cited contribution to the literature. She identified the stages of denial, anger, bargaining, depression, and acceptance. Over the years, many have mistakenly come to view the five-step model as a predictive, developmental model in which the second stage cannot occur unless the first stage is completed, and so on. Although the stages provide a useful framework, they should not be seen as a fixed formula or recipe for grieving. The erroneous belief that the five stages are prescriptive in nature has fostered unrealistic expectations about grief on the part of both grievers and caregivers.

Another of Kubler-Ross's major contributions was to re-establish death as a natural part of life and to recognize that most dying patients wish to discuss their impending death. This is believed to be true for most family members who are preparing for the death of a loved one as well. They welcome the opportunity to discuss their situation.

NATURE OF GRIEF

Drawing from examples in the neonatal setting, an overview of grief is presented to help the caregiver grasp its comprehensive nature. Grief is a natural human response to any loss, whether the loss is real, perceived, threatened, or anticipated. We experience many losses, for example, loss of health, loss of resources, loss of innocence, loss of independence, loss of feeling, and so on. Grief may accompany any loss, not just death. Furthermore, individuals may grieve when a loss is only threatened. From this standpoint, any parent with a child in the NICU may exhibit a grief response if their infant's condition worsens.

Acute Phase

Acute grief is the initial phase of mourning. During this time, responses are likely to be intense and the sense of loss all-consuming. The self-centered nature of acute grief is such that the fact of death is at the center of the griever's reality. He or she can barely think of anything else.

This has several implications. Caregivers cannot rely on the griever to unselfishly engage in a mutual relationship. Similarly, the parents cannot rely on each other. The myth that "they have each other" tends to be true only in the very early days of bereavement, if at all. For instance, couples may be most supportive of each other immediately following the death. However, soon after the funeral one can observe the parents grieving separately, unable to offer each other support. Couples may benefit from being forewarned about this possibility as well as being advised on what to do about it.

The nature of acute grief also has implications for the surviving children of bereaved parents. The parents may be so consumed by grief that their parenting skills become seriously compromised. In this manner, surviving children may temporarily experience the loss of their parents. Special arrangements may be needed; children should not be removed from their parents (for young children need the reassurance of their parents' presence), but in-home child care should be provided.

Individualistic Aspects

Grief is highly individualized. It is unique to each person and to each circumstance. Almost everything that goes into making individuals unique also goes into making their grief unique. Researchers have identified numerous factors that combine to determine how a person might respond to a loss. Factors identified by Worden (1982, 1991a, 1991b) include the strength of attachment there had been between the deceased and the survivor and the degree of ambivalence in their relationship, the mode of death, and personality factors such as the sex, age, and coping skills of the survivor. In addition, Worden (1991a, 1991b) cited the kinds of life crises in the survivor's past, how they were handled, and what they meant to the individual, as well as a variety of social variables such as the presence of supportive persons and the uses of rituals. Rando (1984) added other determinants of how one might respond to a death, including the individual's level of maturity, cultural and ethnic factors, the circumstances of the death itself, and whether or not death was expected.

Recognizing these variables and how they affect a particular person's grief helps us understand that there is no right or wrong response to loss. Caregivers cannot legitimately judge a griever's reaction. In an effort to avoid the tendency for parents to be critical of each other, they need to be informed that divergent responses to grief are to be expected. Parents need to know that the grieving process can place their relationship under a severe strain and that they might be burdened by the threat of an additional loss, their partnership.

Holistic Description

Grief is more than just being sad. Holistically, individuals are affected by profound loss in each dimension of their being. Shock waves reverberate through the griever physically, mentally, emotionally, and spiritually. In turn, each dimension interacts with the others to affect the whole being (Marris, 1974; Rando, 1984; Schneider, 1984; Wolfelt, 1992).

Physical effects of grief can include tension, headaches, and a feeling of "emptiness" in the pit of one's stomach, as well as changes in sleeping, eating, energy level, and sex drive, to mention only a few. Bereaved mothers of newborns frequently report an aching in their arms, presumably for the baby they cannot hold. Recognizing that these are natural reactions that can serve an adaptive function, caregivers might take a cue from behavioral medicine and look first to natural ways of attaining relief, such as mild exercise, walking, deep breathing, and the use of relaxation techniques. If physical problems persist, medical intervention is appropriate. For example, although inability to sleep well might serve some short-term psychological need, it is likely that prolonged sleeplessness interferes with effective coping. Small amounts of sleep medication prescribed by a physician may be appropriate.

Cognitive reactions to loss are particularly frightening to grievers because they may fear they are going crazy. Cognitive responses center around a preoccupation with what has been lost (Lindemann, 1944; Parkes, 1970a, 1970b). Parents spend considerable time reviewing the details of the pregnancy, birth, life, and death of their infant. Other mental reactions include dreaming about the infant, an inability to accept the reality of the death, confusion and disorganization, and disruption of short-term memory. Parents need to be assured that these reactions are common and normal.

Cognitive functioning tends to be either scattered or fixed. For this reason, grievers are encouraged to postpone life-altering decision-making until their thinking has cleared. For example, immediately after his baby's death, one father, over his wife's protests, decided to get a vasectomy to ensure that he and his wife would never have to endure a similar painful experience again. Months later he was grateful that he had been persuaded to postpone such a permanent decision. After the emotional pain had subsided and his thinking had cleared, both he and his wife very much wanted another child.

There is a wide range of emotional response to death. Feelings do not follow a particular order. Some feelings are more intense and pervasive than others. In the beginning, there may be numbness or a lack of feelings. Although numbness almost always goes away, it may be followed by feelings of helplessness, fear, jealousy, anger, abandonment, betrayal, depression, or relief, among others. Some parents have expressed anger at the infant for leaving them. Others feel cheated, guilty, or responsible. New mothers often report feeling betrayed by their bodies.

A given person does not experience all the possible feelings. In addition, different individuals have different feelings. For example, one mother asked, "When will the guilt come?" She needed to be reassured that she did not need to make herself have feelings that were not present simply because they appeared in the list of potential responses.

There has been a tendency for some caregivers to consider certain emotional responses as more appropriate than others. For instance, sadness could be viewed as being more appropriate than anger. Although the expression of some feelings may be easier to witness than others, feelings associated with grief are not inherently right or wrong, appropriate or inappropriate. All related feelings need to be experienced and eventually released as the griever moves toward recovery.

Spiritual responses are, perhaps, the least studied of all the responses to death. It is the spiritual aspect of grief that encompasses the possibility of personal growth and enriched relationships through grief (Coles, 1990; Rando, 1984; Schneider, 1984; Tatelbaum, 1980). Although spiritual issues are widely acknowledged as a component of grief, especially by those who espouse the hospice philosophy of care, responding to them has been primarily relegated to the clergy. Yet every bedside neonatal nurse has heard the questions: Why has this happened? Why has it happened to *me*? What have I done to deserve this? What kind of a God lets a little baby suffer? Sometimes spiritual issues are expressed as anger directed at the church or God. Frequently, there are feelings of betrayal and abandonment.

Some clinicians have noted that spiritual issues tend to surface sooner in the grief process of parents than following the more timely deaths of older individuals. Even if he or she has no theological training, the alert caregiver need not defer the search for understanding to religious experts. The nurse's role is not to provide answers but to facilitate the process of learning. The same therapeutic listening skills that are typically used by nurses can be employed to encourage parents to explore spiritual questions and to reach an understanding that satisfies their queries. The caregiver has the skills to assist parents in coming to their own conclusions.

Finally, it may be tempting to offer comfort with a simple "It is God's will." However, far from being comforting, this response provokes anger in many parents and signals to them that this caregiver is blaming God. It is more appropriate to simply acknowledge and facilitate the griever's personal search for meaning.

PROCESS OF MOURNING

Grief Work

Grief work, or mourning, is the active process that individuals engage in to heal the wound of grief. The goal of grief work is to enable the survivor to remember everything about the infant—the pregnancy, the delivery, the life, the death, the aftermath, and so forth—without pain (Lindemann, 1944). When this is accomplished, the infant takes his or her rightful place in the family history, neither forgotten nor given excessive importance. Many parents fear that the goal of grief work is to forget the infant, and being unwilling to forget, they resist complete grieving. It is beneficial for parents to make the distinction between remembering without pain and forgetting.

The four tasks of grief work are accepting the reality of loss, working through the pain of grief, adjusting to the environment in which the deceased is missing, and emotionally relocating or repositioning the deceased and moving on with life (Worden, 1991a, 1991b). These tasks help clarify the therapeutic role of the caregiver in the grieving process. For example, viewing the body is thought to facilitate parents coming to terms with the reality of a death.

A major deterrent that prevents individuals from engaging in the work of grief is the natural tendency to avoid pain (Gorer, 1965). However, sooner or later the issues of grief must be faced. Contrary to the conventional wisdom that "time heals all wounds," unresolved issues of grief do not go away on their own. Instead, they linger and can become a destructive force that threatens parents' physical, mental, emotional, and spiritual well-being (Bowlby, 1980; Clayton, 1974). Grief may be anticipated, delayed, or prolonged; however, eventually the grief work will be done.

Behaviors that individuals use to ease their pain, relieve their feelings, and progress through their grief work can be called *coping behaviors.* These behaviors include withdrawal, denial, confrontation, expression of feelings, avoidance, distraction, blame of self or others, seeking additional information, and reframing. Many professionals have tended to overlook the uses of some of these behaviors. Again, the issue is not whether the behavior is right or wrong, the issue is whether the behavior is effective. Some methods work better in the short term; others are more effective in the long term. For example, during acute grief some parents find comfort and relief by visiting their child's grave on a weekly basis. Most report that this routine eventually becomes draining. The criteria used to assess the merit of a particular coping behavior are (1) whether it helps and (2) whether it is harmful to oneself or others.

Duration of Grief

How long does grief take? Thanatologists (individuals who study dying, death, and bereavement) agree that the resolution of grief takes time. As reported in the literature, the period of mourning varies greatly because grief is so personalized and is influenced by numerous factors. Further, researchers have not agreed on the definition of grief resolution, and measuring it has also been problematic (Davidson, 1977; Gorer, 1965; Kalish, 1977; Shneidman, 1977). Thanatologists can agree, however, that the resolution of grief takes more than time. It also takes courage and effort to accomplish the tasks associated with grief, to remember the deceased eventually without the associated negative feelings, and to get on with one's life. For this, each person has his or her own timetable, which needs to be respected.

Sometimes the circumstances of loss are such that acute grief appears to continue indefinitely. *Chronic sorrow,* as it is called, seems to be most prevalent in response to violent, unexpected deaths. It is often seen following deaths of children with whom the parent was in a dependent and irreplaceable relationship (Rando, 1984). Similarly, some parents of chronically ill children have reported an ongoing intense sadness and anger. Parents can use chronic grief as a way of controlling and punishing others and to receive secondary gain. Clinicians are well aware that chronic grievers are very difficult to assist. Nurses should refer these parents to a specialist (Rando, 1993).

Peppers and Knapp (1980), in their studies on mothers' reactions to newborn death, describe a phenomenon called *shadow grief.* This is "that portion of grief which mothers tuck away and which appears from time to time. It is something—a burden—they carry for the rest of their lives" (p. 47). This form of grief can be distinguished from chronic sorrow and generally is not debilitating to those who experience it.

GRIEVING THE LOSS OF A NEWBORN

Additional factors come together in unique ways when a newborn infant dies. The circumstances under which death occurs can further complicate and alter parental grieving. Perhaps the most common circumstance is the one in which a mother goes into premature labor, knowing its danger, and the infant is born, lives a few days, and then dies.

There are other situations. There is the special grief of the parents of twins, when one infant dies and the other precariously lives; when one dies and the other dies later; or when one dies and the other thrives. Parents who have experienced several previous perinatal losses may have "rehearsed" for the present experience. Infertile couples may lament two losses: the infant who has died and the death of their dream to be natural parents. Grandparents who suffer the loss of their grandchild also must endure seeing their child in pain. Parents who have contributed to the death of their infant through the use of drugs or the presence of sexually transmitted disease may run the risk of being alienated from NICU care.

There is the ongoing sorrow of parents whose infant does not die but who does not fully live either. Weary grief occurs when an infant lives for many months before succumbing. Delayed maternal grief may occur in a mother who has suffered an obstetrical-related critical illness and could not participate in the events following birth and death. Historical, unresolved grief may affect the bereaved mother who experienced childhood abuse or a previous abortion. There is the hidden, disenfranchised grief of staff members.

In each of these situations, parents, family members, and health professionals experience grief differently. The goal in each case is to incorporate the specifics of the situation into the caregiver's response (Borg & Lasker, 1981).

Grief can be further complicated when loss is uncertain, when death is negated, or when social support is inadequate. Neonatal intensive care separates a mother from her infant. In many instances, death occurs before the mother or father has had time to visit and see the infant for themselves. Particularly in these cases, the infant may not seem real to the parents, much less the infant's death. Parents report that it is difficult to accept that their child lived and died. They have difficulty identifying who or what they have lost. Reality may be dream-like. This lack of focus does not mean that parents will not grieve; it means that grieving may be more difficult and less concrete unless steps are taken to sharpen the image.

There is a common misconception that parents have only a minimal emotional investment in their newborn infant and will not grieve for one who died so soon. The reality is that throughout the pregnancy both parents have bonded physically, emotionally, and spiritually with the infant to varying degrees (Klaus & Kennell, 1976). They have invested in hopes, wishes, and dreams for their child. This is a part of what is lost when their infant dies.

Our society has generally taken the attitude that a dead infant is replaceable (Ilse & Furrh, 1988). In addition, family and friends may have had little opportunity to become attached to the infant and therefore do not recognize his or her value. Thus, family and friends may underestimate the impact of the death of a newborn. Believing that nothing important has happened, individuals in the support network often minimize the parents' grief because if a loss is considered inconsequential, grieving is not expected. These misconceptions can leave parents isolated and without social support.

Hospital policies and community traditions can promote the denial of the infant's worth. Examples include hospital policies that allow the institution to dispose of the body for parents; hospital policies that move grieving mothers from obstetrical to surgical recovery units; friends who remove preparations for the infant from the home before the mother's return from the hospital; the tendency to minimize or omit funeral rituals for infants; and newspaper policies that prohibit the printing of death announcements for stillborn or newborn infants. Each of these circumstances may inadvertently convey the subtle message "Nothing important has happened" and thus minimize a parent's loss.

The fact that an infant is born gravely ill and in need of technical care may deprive parents of activities normally associated with having a new infant. The long-awaited opportunity to hold, cuddle, nurse, or gaze at their infant is interrupted by NICU care. Members of the extended family are denied the opportunity to greet the new family member. Pictures are not taken. Celebrations are postponed. Birth announcements are not sent. Many bereaved parents need the opportunity to parent, if only symbolically.

When death occurs shortly after birth, it may be extraordinarily burdensome for the mother. Weary from the effort to deliver her child, the mother may be unusually weakened and vulnerable. Her body is flooded with hormones that may alter her mood; moreover, she may be experiencing the aftereffects of anesthetics. In addition, the presence of breast milk is a painful reminder that there is no baby. Mothers may need information on how to reduce lactation. If the mother is still confined to the hospital, regulations, particularly in regard to visiting, may need to be relaxed to accommodate her special needs. Perhaps new policies, specific to the situation, should be developed.

Finally, newborn death is an infrequent event in the life cycle of families, and as such, it typically produces unusually high stress. It is an experience for which few role models exist. Parents do not know what to expect. Caregivers, not knowing what to say or how to offer comfort, may say nothing and may even avoid the parents. Family and friends may join the conspiracy of silence. Thus, parents frequently find themselves alienated and misunderstood. Each of the factors mentioned can complicate parental grief.

We know that when a newborn dies, parents grieve (Benfield et al., 1976). When they grieve, they deserve support, care, consideration, empathy, and understanding. They may need to be encouraged to grieve. Significant others can be informed about the parents' need to grieve and how to help facilitate the process.

GENDER DIFFERENCES

Clinical observation and survey research suggest that fathers and mothers grieve in different ways and for different lengths of time (Benfield & Nichols, 1979; Helmrath & Steinitz, 1978; Pine & Brauer, 1986). These differences are probably the result of gender-related factors. Social, psychological, and physiologic factors appear to play a role in the different patterns of grieving for men and women (Staudacher, 1991). In general, fathers of newborns who die display fewer grief responses and exhibit them for shorter periods than do the mothers of these newborns (Gardner & Merenstein, 1986). For instance, in 1979, 115 bereaved parents of newborn infants were asked, "When did you experience a sense of release from the emotional pain caused by your baby's death?" (Benfield & Nichols, 1979). Only 18 percent of the mothers, but 44 percent of the fathers, reported that they felt release at the end of 6 months. Fathers who have experienced this sense of emotional release tend to join the ranks of family and friends who presume that the mother should also be over it by that time. Consequently, mothers may either fear that something *is* wrong with them or think that the reason the father adjusted sooner is because he did not love the infant as much as she did. This adjustment difference can lead to confusion and resentment (Pappas & McCoy, 1996).

When offering ongoing support to bereaved parents, it is important for the caregiver to recognize that there can be gender-related differences. It may also be useful to inform the couple that these differences are to be expected and to explore with parents alternative reasons why a mother might grieve for a longer time, reasons that are unrelated to the amount of love the father had for their infant.

One possibility is that mothers are often more attached to newborns simply because they have had a constant physical connection with the baby during pregnancy (Klaus & Kennell, 1976). A second possible reason is one that fathers themselves have offered. Fathers have reported that although they grieve the loss of their infant, they are consoled by the fact of the mother's survival. Third, when a child dies, each parent loses someone different (Rando, 1986). Each parent had his or her own set of dreams and expectations, which died with the child. Fourth, in keeping with traditional gender role explanations, some have speculated that men do not complete their grief sooner but that they simply deny or avoid their feelings. This reasoning has not been documented and may be counterproductive as a basis for understanding and healing. An alternative to this, and just as plausible, is that men might employ more effective, but less obvious, coping styles than do women.

Another potential cause for lengthier grieving among mothers may be that they are not comforted sufficiently. In our culture, appropriate or not, women primarily are ascribed the role of nurturing and consoling. When a woman is bereaved, who comforts her? Who "mothers" the mother? It is likely that young husbands need coaching in this area, or perhaps a substitute comforter can be found.

A final explanation considers the activity level of men and women following the birth and death of an infant. Mothers often remain in the hospital, out of the mainstream, passive and isolated. Fathers, in contrast, are frequently called on to calm the mother, speak with physicians, notify family members, make funeral arrangements, and so on. Although these activities may be difficult, they may also have a cathartic, therapeutic effect and thus facilitate the grief work.

EFFECTS ON SIBLINGS

Other children in the home may also be affected by the death of a newborn. Even very young children sense that something is wrong. Whether siblings grieve the death of their newborn brother or sister is an issue that has not been addressed empirically. Theorists generally concur that children do grieve, although their grief may be different from adult grief (Rosen, 1986). Although there are few studies on the impact of perinatal loss on other children in the family, we can draw on studies of the effects of the death of older children (Ross-Alaolmolki, 1990). This literature is fraught with methodologic shortcomings. It remains for researchers and clinicians alike to refine our understanding of the experiences and capacities of bereaved siblings.

Certainly the responses of siblings are influenced by their ability to conceptualize death, as well as the meaning they attach to the loss (Weiner, 1970). These factors are related to age and cognitive development (Kastenbaum, 1967; Koocher, 1981; Piaget, 1929) and are shaped by social and cultural influences and by the child's experience with illness and loss (Bluebond-Langner, 1978). In this way, the concept of death continuously evolves and varies with each child. Both caregivers and parents need to be mindful of the individuality of each child when planning interventions.

An equally important factor that affects children's responses to the death of their newborn sibling is the way in which their parents cope. Parental instability and vulnerability affect the children. Grollman (1967) points out that children cannot cope with death unless their parents can. Parents naturally model behavior for their children. In addition, if parents are withdrawn and remote, the children may suffer a significant secondary loss, the functional loss of their parents (Dowden, 1995).

The responses of children may include feelings of guilt because of the resentment they felt when parents were visiting the sick infant. Others may express anger at the parents for allowing the child to die (Binger et al., 1969). They may respond to the pain around them by trying to alleviate it. Older children may react to the realization that this could happen to them. Some have reported concerns about what to tell their friends. Preliminary results based on the Harvard Child Bereavement Study (Worden, 1991a, 1991b) indicate that many children are concerned with two additional issues: "Did I cause the death?" and "Who will care for me?"

Although there are conflicting reports in the literature about the long-term effects of sibling loss, clinicians concur on several practical interventions (Goldman, 1994; Grollman, 1967; Huntley, 1991; Ilse, 1982; LaTour, 1983; Schwiebert & Kirk, 1982). Resist the temptation to try to protect the child from pain. Help the child understand in terms he or she can comprehend. Be honest and do not tell stories that have to be changed as the child grows up. Answer all questions, even if the answer is "I don't know." Educate the child and let him or her decide whether to visit the hospital, attend the funeral, and so on. Involve the child and make her or him feel important. Help the child find ways to say hello and goodbye. To the extent possible, maintain a family structure so that children can anchor themselves. Spend time alone with the child. Let the child be alone. Stay connected through touch. Encourage children to be with peers with whom they may talk more freely.

Dowden (1995) in a study of children aged 3 to 7 years who had lost a sibling found that sibling grief is often ignored. Her findings indicate that children must be given permission to grieve. They need to share in their parents' grief and not be closed out of the process. Each child grieves in his or her own way and this must be supported by the family, teachers, and health professionals. Story telling and drawing are excellent tools to help with the grieving process.

Another aspect of siblings and death has to do with the loss of an infant to sudden infant death syndrome. If there are subsequent children, the parents may be afraid that this child too will die. There is a somewhat increased risk for such a recurrence (Hunt, 1995). However, the subsequent child may suffer from the parents anticipatory grief—anticipating the worst for this child. As the child grows older, he or she may be overprotected or suffer a sibling grief reaction to an infant that he or she never knew, as a result of picking up cues from the parents. The parents must be helped to recognized their effect on the child and their child's grief response if the family is to develop positive coping skills.

NURSE'S ROLE WHEN A BABY IS DYING

When one begins to work with bereaved parents, the work may seem overwhelming. How does the clinician begin to offer care and consolation? How does one know what will be helpful, and to which parent, and at what time? The obvious answer is that there is no recipe. There is no certain, absolute formula. The circumstances in which the infant died, combined with each parent's experience, produces a personalized, unique grief experience to which the caregiver is called on to respond. We do our best to create the optimal conditions in which the work can be done and then we listen intently and take cues from the parents as to what is helpful and useful to them (Hutti, 1988). We proceed with caution, care, and abundant respect as we venture to work with human beings who may be at the most vulnerable point of their lives.

This process is the same approach nurses take when caring for themselves. Sometimes I am asked to discuss "care for the caregiver" issues separately. In this chapter, I have not distinguished between bereaved parent and bereaved caregiver. All may benefit from the suggestions that are offered here.

Although examples given in this discussion are confined to death that occurs in the NICU, caregivers should be aware that the death could take place in other settings. Possibilities include returning the infant, before or after death, to the hospital of birth, especially if the mother is still confined; sending the infant home to die; or arranging for the infant and parents to stay at a Ronald McDonald House. Each of these choices has its own potential difficulties and advantages, which should be carefully considered before the option being offered to parents.

Decision-Making

Several researchers have indicated that the mode of death can significantly affect the grief response (Rando, 1984; Worden, 1982, 1991a, 1991b). This difference may be particularly true for parents of neonates when decisions to limit care have been made. As technologic advances continue, parents and caregivers are increasingly faced with moral and ethical decisions regarding continuation or termination of curative care for critically ill newborns. Making a decision to shift to palliative care can be complex and highly sensitive (Duff, 1979). Since palliative care often results in death, the decision-making process may also complicate parental grief and is part of bereavement care. Communication is crucial. Provided with advice and recommendations, most parents are capable of discussing their infant's care and reaching a satisfying decision (Benfield et al., 1978; VanPutte, 1988). Some NICU bereavement programs have developed a multidisciplinary team, with active nurse participation, to assist in family-oriented decision-making (Siegel et al., 1985).

Physical Environment

Perhaps the simplest task is that of promoting an optimal physical environment. The goal is to create an atmosphere in which parent–infant interaction and intimacy can be maximized while a neonate is dying. Specifics can be further identified by parents, but it could encompass offering privacy, maintaining a minimum of interruptions and confusion, minimizing distractions, and maximizing the opportunity for normalcy. Since death is so intimate and most NICUs are so public, an immediate concern is to create privacy for infant and parents (Siegel et al., 1985). Ideally, a separate room with home-like furnishings that is large enough to accommodate family and friends would be situated in or near the NICU. If the infant must remain in the NICU, the caregiver could use a screen or his or her body, if need be, to shield the family from public scrutiny. An individual's need for privacy may include time alone, as well as time for the couple away from the extended family. Not all parents want to be alone with their infant. The easiest way to assess this need is to ask.

Comfort and Relief

As the time of death approaches, the nurse's role is to offer physical, mental, emotional, and spiritual comfort and relief to the infant and family. In preparation, it may be helpful for the nurse to take a brief moment consciously to "switch gears," to shift mentally from curing and caring toward comfort and caring. As much as possible, the nurse should dismiss himself or herself from other obligations and turn full attention to the task at hand. In many ways, the nurse uses himself or herself as a therapeutic tool (Gardner, 1985) during this extraordinarily intimate time. (For a listing of dilemmas facing the caregiver, see Table 8–1 and Nichols, 1982.)

The nurse must assess the current response of each person who is present and respond to them in kind. Touch should be firm and steady. Words should be clear, gentle, and simple. A focus on the child and parents should be maintained. Other things are not important now.

Downey and associates (1995) conducted one of the few reported studies on NICU nurses' responses to dying neonates. They found that nurses, no matter how seasoned, experience feelings of powerlessness and helplessness as the death approaches and intense sorrow when the death actually occurs. These nurses (59 nurses in a midwestern NICU) reported physical-psychological symptoms of "chronic fatigue, decreased interest in exercise, irritability, and being overcritical" (Downey et al., 1995). Specific interventions that help the nurses and families get through the grieving process are needed.

TABLE 8–1 Dilemmas of Care

1. A difficult burden is placed on the caregiver who is asked, in addition to other tasks, to be supportive to others. A caregiver will fail in efforts to be supportive, unless he or she also receives nurturing and supportive care.
2. There will be times when caregivers have nothing left to give. This is to be expected. If caregivers expect too much of themselves, they will live in guilt for not having done enough. Harm can be done by offering what cannot be fulfilled.
3. Care is shaped by expectation. If the griever defines support in a different way than the caregiver does, the parent will not recognize specific behaviors as being supportive and thus will continue to experience his or her pain alone.
4. Sometimes parents do not accept support. Sometimes they choose to receive support only from a particular caregiver. If so, the caregiver is apt to feel shut out and uncertain about his or her skills.
5. How far can or should a caregiver go to accommodate the bereaved? If the caregiver's values differ greatly from those of the parent, what is the caregiver's highest responsibility in light of knowing that value conflicts often arise at a time when the parent may need nurturing and support the most?
6. There is always some hostility directed back at the supportive caregiver. After all, the caregiver is the person who sees the parents when they feel weak, exposed, and vulnerable. To parents, the caregiver may symbolize the unpleasant reality of the death of their child.

Specific Interventions

Worden (1991a, 1991b) provides 10 principles a nurse can use to assist individuals with their grieving:

1. Help the survivor actualize the loss.
2. Help the survivor identify and express feelings.
3. Assist adjustment to living without the deceased.
4. Facilitate emotional withdrawal from the deceased.
5. Provide time to grieve.
6. Interpret "normal" behavior.
7. Allow for individual differences.
8. Provide continuing support.
9. Examine defenses and coping styles.
10. Recognize one's limitations and know when to refer to a specialist.

These principles can be translated into specific interventions that may help bring a newborn's short life and death into focus and facilitate the grieving process. These responses may help make the infant real, suggest that his or her life had dignity, and that he or she was valued (also see Appendix).

- Encourage parents to name the infant. Know the name and use it.
- Speak openly and candidly about the infant.
- Put a signal marker developed by the institution on the mother's hospital door if she is still there when the infant dies. This symbol, whose significance is known only to staff, alerts individuals entering the room of the infant's outcome (Cooney, 1995).
- Be supportive of the need to recall memories of the pregnancy, labor, delivery, and events in the nursery, as well as fantasies and expectations revolving around the infant.
- Create memories by providing occasions for parents to see, touch, hold, talk to, give something to, bathe, sing to, or in other ways parent their child before or after death, even if the infant is deformed.
- Arrange to take the infant to the mother if she desires to see him or her and cannot come to the NICU.
- Prepare the family for any change in the infant's appearance since their last visit.
- Remove the tubes, if possible, and bathe the infant.
- Dress the infant in clothing that allows parents easy exploration so that they can see the infant for themselves. Wrap the infant in a fresh blanket.
- Provide tangible mementos: a lock of hair, the hospital bracelet, footprints, pictures or videotapes (Johnson et al., 1985), birth and death certificates, a death notice, the infant's blanket. Cooney (1995) reports that homemade blankets that are used to present the baby to parents often serve as good momentos of their infant's existence.
- Help grievers clarify the nuances of feeling.
- Encourage funeral rituals and disposition of the body that are in keeping with family and cultural values and serve as an opportunity to gain closure.

Not all parents want or choose these options, which should be presented to couples in a neutral manner (Nichols, 1986). Parents need not be coerced into choosing any option. The choice of each parent should be accepted and supported. The needs and desires of each survivor should be respected individually and collectively to the extent possible. For example, the mother who prefers to wait in the lobby should be supported as much as the father who chooses to hold the dying neonate.

The nurse should ask each parent whether he or she wants to be with the child; ask whether other family members should be included, even if the child has already died; and listen, really listen. The nurse should listen for clues parents give as to what would be helpful. Parents often know what is best for them. However, they may defer to outside authorities, may discount their own ideas, or may be too timid to make a request directly. Cues often surface with comments that begin with, "I just wish I could...." or "If only...." For example, sometimes a parent may sigh wistfully and say, "My baby never got to be in the sunshine." When possible, the caregiver should accommodate these needs.

The nurse should answer questions and respond to comments gently, simply, and truthfully. Grievers are very vulnerable, and vulnerable individuals can easily detect insincerity. We risk distancing ourselves or "having the curtain drawn" if we are less than honest. If there is a question for which there is no answer, the nurse should say so.

Baptism is a concern that frequently comes up during this time. Of the religious denominations that observe the sacrament of baptism, most believe that the rite is theologically unnecessary for the salvation of newly born infants or stillborns; however, there are differences of opinion (Windau & Dewitt, 1988; Zumbro Valley Medical Society, 1978). Find out whether baptism is important to the parents. If a member of the clergy is not available to perform the rite, the nurse may administer the sacrament or ask the parents or grandparents if they would like to do it. Many fathers have regarded this as one practical role they can fulfill.

After the infant has died, there are opportunities to offer practical assistance that is comforting. The nurse should ask who will notify the rest of the family and help parents determine which funeral home they will contact. Do the parents have a ride home? Is there someone they want to stay with them the first night? If parents prefer to make these contacts themselves, they should be encouraged to do so. It should be remembered that parents react to the death of their child in a wide variety of ways. Some want to take charge, as though to gain some control over their lives; others are more passive.

Unusual Requests

Sometimes parents make requests that are out of the ordinary. Davidson (1977) said, "As long as requests are not life-threatening, we can be helpful by quietly encouraging the mourner to explore openly." He continued, "When survivors are thwarted in their attempts to grieve honestly, they are forced to grieve less honestly, by unconscious means." In *Some Babies Die* (Down, 1986), Dr. Peter Barr put it another way: "The aim of the team is to enable people to fulfill what they need from the experience. We aren't into telling people what they should or shouldn't do or feel or think."

It is appropriate to consider unusual requests, yet one may need some direction when deliberating. To remain neutral when contemplating an unusual request, the caregiver needs to resist the urge to reply, "Why?" and replace it with "Why not?" The following questions can guide the decision-making process:

1. What is the worst thing that could happen?
2. What would be done about that?
3. Is the request in line with reality? The reality is a child lived, and a child died.

For example, one father, a medical resident, asked to attend his infant's postmortem examination—certainly an unusual request. The request was considered according to the guidelines. Unquestionably, the request was in touch with the reality of death. He was cautioned about what to expect, including the cool room temperature and odor of formaldehyde; the fact that the pathologists would be discussing his baby as a scientific specimen, not as his infant; and the nature of the incisions that are made during autopsy. It was believed that the worst that could happen would be that the man might faint or that the pathology team might be uncomfortable with his presence. The resident was instructed that he would have to be seated, smelling salts were available, and the pathology team was informed of the plan. Accompanied by a caregiver, the grieving father attended his infant son's autopsy. After a few moments, he decided to leave.

The point about unusual requests is that caregivers have no real way of knowing what is useful to a particular parent's grieving. It is known, however, that overprotection can be harmful and can add to suffering (Kubler-Ross, 1969). The choice, with certain safeguards, can and should be theirs.

Leave-Taking

Parting with the infant's body can be a delicate time for parents. It literally signifies "letting go." Although it may not be the last time they see their infant (some parents have the opportunity to see their child again if a funeral is held), the separation at the hospital symbolically signals what will come and what must be. It is a sensitive transition and requires as much grace and tenderness as the caregiver can muster. Parents may need time; they must not be rushed. Some may return moments later, just to see their child one more time. Some may choose to accompany the body to the funeral home. These would not be unusual requests.

It is crucial that caregivers understand that they cannot make the grief go away. This is often one of the most difficult concepts a caregiver has to face. Many are accustomed to "fixing" almost any hurt. That is what nurses are trained to do. Attempts to "fix it," however, can be perceived by parents as an attempt to minimize their grief. We cannot take their grief away, nor can we eliminate or contain the pain. It takes restraint to witness a mother's or father's pain without attempting to mend their wounds, and that is what we are called on to do.

Funerals

Many parents have reported emotional distress when they have not been given options as to the final disposition of their infant. In particular, many mothers have expressed anger that they were excluded from planning and attending the funeral service.

Funerals offer parents many psychological, social, and spiritual benefits (Imber-Black & Roberts, 1992), including reinforcement of the reality of death, opportunity for catharsis and receiving comfort, and reaffirmation of one's religious beliefs (Irion, 1976). For the bereaved family of a newborn, the funeral may also provide an opportunity to introduce their beloved infant to the rest of the family so that they, too, can acknowledge the reality of his or her existence. An infant's funeral can be a therapeutic experience for survivors (Nichols & Doka, 1991). As such, the funeral can be thought of as a worthy bereavement tool. Some caregivers, however, have been hesitant to encourage funerals for infants because of their desire to protect parents from additional expenses. Yet it has long been the custom among funeral directors in the United States to provide infant funerals at a minimal charge. Caregivers may want to investigate funeral costs in their community so that they can provide accurate information and guidance.

Finally, families generally report that they are deeply touched when NICU personnel send a personal note of sympathy, call the family, or attend the funeral. For many infants, the members of the NICU staff were the individuals who knew them best, and parents may have come to regard staff as kin.

Posthospital Care

The caregiver's role need not end once the family leaves the NICU. Comprehensive bereavement care should be available throughout the mourning process (Table 8–2). Ryan and colleagues (1991) advocate the use of a comprehensive checklist to ensure continuity of care before and after discharge. During the process, as feelings emerge, parents continue to need empathy and quiet support. The goals of ongoing care are to increase the reality of the loss, deal with expressed and latent effects, overcome various impediments to readjustment, assist parents in making a healthy emotional withdrawal from the baby, and help them feel comfortable reinvesting in other relationships (Worden, 1982, 1991a, 1991b). This time is ideal for offering comfort and relief and, when one can, informing, instructing, challenging, and guiding the parents to move on.

Miscellaneous Issues

Eventually, parents come face to face with difficult issues—issues of real or imagined guilt, issues about God and church and the fact that life is not fair, issues about afterlife and learning to relate to their child in new ways, issues about the lessons they learned from their child and how backward it is that a child should teach parents and how it is not supposed to be that way, issues about iatrogenic causes of death, issues about friends and family who were not adept at demonstrating their care and concern, issues about how their mate's grief differs from theirs and how scary that is and what to do about it, issues about the "stone-cold" spot in their heart and how they do not want it to melt, and issues from old losses that have not been resolved previously.

These concerns and myriad others are apt to surface during bereavement. Many involve more concrete matters. For instance, holidays, anniversaries, and birthdays are likely to be stressful. Although most parents report that the dread of these events seems to be worse than the occasion itself, parents may benefit from being alerted so that they can prepare for the event. Each of these issues must be gently and honestly considered to the extent that the parent is willing to explore them. Regardless of the situation at hand, caregivers should make an effort to tailor their suggestions to the individual's needs. By using therapeutic listening skills and exploring creative alternatives, the likelihood of making satisfying and practical recommendations is improved.

One example comes from a mother who said, "I just wish people would realize he was a part of our family and quit pretending otherwise!" How could she help make that happen? She decided to cross-stitch a small sampler that included her child's full name, the dates of his birth and death, and the words "He is a part of us always. We will never forget." The sampler now hangs on the living room wall along with the school pictures of the woman's other children. She reported that the activity brought closure to this issue.

Suggestions for Caregiving for Parents

The following ideas may be helpful to parents, depending on the issues they confront. After the funeral, it may be cathartic for parents to write notes of appreciation, to send out birth and death announcements, to prepare an album of memories, or to express themselves through poetry or other art forms. Some parents find it helpful to assist in the design of their child's grave marker or to visit and tend to the grave; others do not. Some dismantle the nursery immediately; others find solace in sitting in the room. Some find relief by holding and rocking a substitute object, often a teddy bear; others do not. Some are comforted by the presence of other babies or of pregnant women; others are upset by them.

Furthermore, parents often need to be reminded to take care of themselves and each other and not to expect too much too quickly. They should be encouraged to avoid alcohol, drugs, and junk food; to eat properly; to drink plenty of water; and to take brisk walks (Limbo & Wheeler, 1986). The use of massage and therapeutic touch (Krieger et al., 1979; Leduc, 1989; Macrae,

TABLE 8–2 Comprehensive Regional NICU Bereavement Program

Open Communication and Visiting
Throughout the baby's stay in the NICU, parents are offered benefit from frequent, truthful, accurate information about their child, his or her condition, diagnosis, treatment, and prognosis. There is a toll-free WATS line and 24-hour open visiting for parents and four other significant people of their choosing. Siblings may visit with permission.

Parent Participation in Decision-making
The health care team provides information and recommendations regarding continued care for the infant when considering a shift from curative to palliative care.

Opportunity to be Present, to Focus on the Baby
Opportunities for parents to be present, to see, touch, or hold their infant are routinely offered near-death, at-death, and after-death. A hospice room is provided in the NICU.

Opportunity to Discuss Autopsy and Funeral Options
When possible, caregivers discuss with parents the desirability, purpose, and method of autopsy, as well as review funeral, burial, and cremation options and how to proceed.

Parent Information Packet
Before taking their final leave from the hospital, parents are given a specially designed packet of materials which is meant to carry the message that the NICU community continues to care and support parents. The packet is not comprehensive, but rather is aimed at bridging the gap between the day of death and connection with other bereavement resources. It was designed with parent input and includes information regarding the purpose of autopsies and funerals, a description of grief and its hazards, suggestions on how to tell children who will be affected by the death of this baby, and annotated bibliography, tips for handling holidays and anniversaries, and a listing of community services. The packet also includes a letter of sympathy from the staff and a remembrance book containing mementos of the baby.

Parent-Centered Follow-up Conference
All parents are invited, both verbally and by letter, to return for a follow-up conference with the attending neonatologist and bereavement consultant. The purpose of the conference is to review the baby's condition and care, review autopsy findings if an autopsy was performed, discuss implications for future pregnancies, discuss other parent concerns, and consider bereavement issues.

Private Consultation
Both long-term and short-term consultation with a designated staff member is available for parents, grandparents, and siblings.

Telephone and Written Support
For crisis support, a toll-free number is available for parents who reside a long distance from the hospital. Parents who prefer to express feelings and experiences by writing a letter, poem, or song are responded to in kind.

Parent-to-Parent Support
Staff members cooperate with autonomous parent groups which are available for men and women who find it helpful to talk face-to-face with other parents who have experienced the death of their infant.

Resource Referral
Staff members seek to maintain an up-to-date listing of community resources throughout the region that have expertise in assisting bereaved parents. Linkage to funeral directors at the time of death can be a useful procedure. A hospital-maintained family library houses many grief-related books.

Holiday Remembrance Service
The holidays can be difficult times for bereaved parents. NICU staff members coordinate a holiday observance for parents in which the memory of each deceased child is honored.

Education and Research
Members of the NICU staff are available to each other and to community, educational, professional, and religious groups to inform them about issues of neonatal death. Caregivers are reminded of the need for ongoing research since many questions remain unanswered.

Courtesy of Children's Hospital Medical Center of Akron (Ohio). Used with permission.

1988) may also be indicated. As this chapter has described, grief affects all levels of human existence. If all levels are affected, healing must likewise take place on all levels—physical, emotional, mental, and spiritual. In addition to the traditional forms of talk-counseling, group therapy, and providing information, other forms of assistance can be offered.

Providing effective feedback to caregivers can have therapeutic results. Dr. Irwin Weinfeld, neonatologist at Toledo (Ohio) Hospital, has suggested that if a letter is to be the vehicle of communication to caregivers (for praise or criticism), the letter should be addressed to the chief executive officer of the hospital so that it can be read by many as it "trickles down" the system. In this way, it can carry more influence.

If parents find their feelings are frozen, the technique called *toning*, described by Keyes (1964), can be employed to enable them to begin to express their grief ("get the sounds moving"). Toning, or tonal vibration, is the use of sound with breath. Essentially, one simply squares off the body, drops down the jaw, and lets out whatever sounds come forth. Parents, then, can be encouraged to find a safe place and tone the wails, screams, and moans associated with grief.

We can work with mental attitudes. In particular, we can seek to replace self-inflicted negative affirmations ("I can't handle this" or "I'm losing it") with positive affirmations, such as "I *will* get through this." We can use forgiveness affirmations to assist the griever in releasing negative connections with caregivers, family members, or self.

We can make use of the near-death experience literature, some of which is now more than 20 years old (Moody, 1975; Morse, 1990). In this literature, dying is described as peaceful, safe, and compelling. This description is comforting to many parents.

Progressive relaxation or guided relaxation with or without music may ease sleeplessness, as well as the troubled soul. Deep conscious breathing can be used to release pent-up emotion and calm the body. Boerstler (1982) describes a technique that focuses on specific breathing patterns to establish deep muscle relaxation and a more peaceful emotional state in grievers.

Finally, some have found expression and release and ways to remember their child through symbolic ritual (Feinstein & Mayo, 1990). Symbolic rituals are common activities such as dancing, singing, or building, which take on special meaning when related to the infant. Thus, they become therapeutic experiences that offer a sense of control, that touch deeply, and that express inner feeling (Rando, 1984). One father volunteered his time and craftsmanship to help restore an ancient sailing vessel. He dedicated this activity to his son's memory and achieved a sense of closure.

CONCLUSION

When an infant dies, parents grieve. When they grieve, they deserve our support and skilled caring. Because nurses are present before, during, and after a child's death, they are in a unique position to provide individualized bereavement care. The most important qualities of bereavement care are being supportive and providing opportunities through which parents are allowed to experience the fullness of the situation.

Acknowledgments

I am grateful to D. Gary Benfield, M.D., neonatologist, whose attitudes, openness, inquiry, collaboration, efforts, and faith in me have made my work possible. I am also indebted to Deb Miller, M.A., Kent State University, whose assistance has been invaluable.

This work was supported in part by the Ohio Department of Health, Maternal and Child Health Grant 523-E8.

REFERENCES

Benfield, D. G., Leib, S. A., & Reuter, J. (1976). Grief response of parents after referral of the critically ill newborn to a regional center. *New England Journal of Medicine, 294*(18), 975–978.

Benfield, D. G., Leib, S. A., & Vollman, J. H. (1978). Grief response of parents to neonatal death and parent participation in deciding care. *Pediatrics, 62*(2), 171–177.

Benfield, D. G., & Nichols, J. A. (1979). Parent grief response to newborn death. Unpublished raw data.

Binger, C. M., Ablin, A. R., Feuerstein, R. C., et al. (1969). Childhood leukemia: Emotional impact on patient and family. *New England Journal of Medicine, 280*(8), 414–418.

Bluebond-Langner, M. (1978). *The private worlds of dying children.* Princeton, NJ: Princeton University Press.

Boerstler, R. W. (1982). *Letting go.* Watertown, MA: Associates in Thanatology.

Borg, S., & Lasker, J. (1981). *When pregnancy fails.* Boston: Beacon Press.

Bowlby, J. (1980). Loss, sadness and depression. In J. Bowlby (Ed.), *Attachment and loss* (Vol. 3). New York: Basic Books.

Clayton, P. J. (1974). Mortality and morbidity in the first year of widowhood. *Archives of General Psychiatry, 30*(6), 747–750.

Coles, R. (1990). *The spiritual life of children.* Boston: Houghton Mifflin.

Cooney, J. K. (1995). A blanket that eases the pain of loss. *American Journal of Maternal-Child Nursing, 20*(1), 57.

Davidson, G. W. (1977). Death of a wished for child: A case study. *Death Education, 1,* 265–275.

Dowden, S. (1995). Young children's experience of sibling death. *Journal of Pediatric Nursing, 10*(1), 72–79.

Down, M. L. (Producer). (1986). *Some babies die* [Videotape]. Berkeley, CA: University of California, Extension Media Center.

Downey, V., Bengiamin, M., Heuer, L., & Juhl, N. (1995). Dying babies and associated stress in NICU nurses. *Neonatal Network, 14*(1), 41–46.

Duff, R. S. (1979). Guidelines for deciding care of critically ill or dying patients. *Pediatrics, 64*(1), 17–23.

Engel, G. L. (1961). Is grief a disease? A challenge for medical research. *Psychosomatic Medicine, 23,* 18–22.

Feinstein, D., & Mayo, P. E. (1990). *Rituals for living and dying.* New York: Harper Collins.

Freud, S. (1959). Mourning and melancholia. In J. Riviere (Trans.), *Collected papers* (Vol. 4). New York: Basic Books.

Gardner, D. (1985). Presence. In G. M. Bulechek & J. C. McCloskey (Eds.), *Nursing interventions.* Philadelphia: W. B. Saunders.

Gardner, S. L., & Merenstein, G. B. (1986). Helping families deal with perinatal loss. *Neonatal Network, 5*(2), 17–33.

Goldman, L. (1994). *Life and loss: A guide to help grieving children.* Muncie, IN: Accelerated Development.

Gorer, G. (1965). *Death, grief, and mourning.* London: Cresset.

Grollman, E. A. (1967). *Explaining death to children.* Boston: Beacon Press.

Helmrath, T. A., & Steinitz, E. M. (1978). Death of an infant: Parental grieving and the failure of social support. *Journal of Family Practice, 6*(4), 785–790.

Hunt, C. E. (1995). Sudden infant death syndrome and subsequent siblings. *Pediatrics, 95*(3), 430–432.

Huntley, T. (1991). *Helping children grieve.* Minneapolis: Augsburg.

Hutti, M. H. (1988). A quick reference table of interventions to assist families to cope with pregnancy loss or neonatal death. *Birth, 15*(1), 33–35.

Ilse, S. (1982). *Empty arms.* Long Lake, MN: Wintergreen Press.

Ilse, S., & Furrh, C. B. (1988). Development of a comprehensive follow up care plan after perinatal and neonatal loss. *Journal of Perinatal and Neonatal Nursing, 2*(2), 23–33.

Imber-Black, E., & Roberts, J. (1992). *Rituals for our times.* New York: Harper Collins.

Irion, P. (1976). The funeral and the bereaved. In V. R. Pine, A. Kutscher, D. Peretz, et al. (Eds.), *Acute grief and the funeral.* Springfield, IL: Charles C Thomas.

Johnson, S. M., Johnson, J., Cunningham, J. H., & Weinfeld, I. J. (1985). *A most important picture.* Omaha, NE: Centering Corp.

Kalish, R. A. (1977). Dying and preparing for death: A view of families. In H. Feifel (Ed.), *New meanings of death.* New York: McGraw-Hill.

Kastenbaum, R. (1967). The child's understanding of death: How does it develop? In E. A. Grollman (Ed.), *Explaining death to children.* Boston: Beacon Press.

Keyes, L. E. (1964). *Toning: The creative power of voice.* Marina del Rey, CA: DeVorss & Co.

Klaus, K., & Kennell, J. H. (1976). *Maternal-infant bonding.* St. Louis: C. V. Mosby.

Koocher, G. P. (1981). Children's conceptions of death. In R. Bibace & M. E. Walsh (Eds.), *Children's conceptions of health, illness, and bodily functions.* San Francisco: Jossey-Bass.

Krieger, D., Peper, E., & Ancoli, S. (1979). Therapeutic touch. *American Journal of Nursing, 79*(4), 660–662.

Kubler-Ross, E. (1969). *On death and dying.* New York: Macmillan.

LaTour, K. (1983). *For those who live: Helping children cope with the death of a brother or sister.* Omaha, NE: Centering Corp.

Leduc, E. (1989). The healing touch. *American Journal of Maternal-Child Nursing, 14*(1), 41–43.

Limbo, R. K., & Wheeler, S. R. (1986) *When a baby dies: A handbook for healing and helping.* LaCrosse, WI: Resolve Through Sharing and LaCrosse Lutheran Hospital.

Lindemann, E. (1944). Symptomatology and management of acute grief. *American Journal of Psychiatry, 101,* 141–149.

Macrae, J. (1988). *Therapeutic touch.* New York: Alfred A. Knopf.

Marris, P. (1974). *Loss and change.* New York: Random House.

Moody, R. A., Jr. (1975). *Life after life.* Atlanta: Mockingbird Books.

Morse, M. (1990). *Closer to the light.* New York: Villard Books.

Nichols, J. A. (1982, May). *On supportive care.* Paper presented at the Fifth Annual Symposium of Ethical Dimensions in Medicine, Akron, OH.

Nichols, J. A. (1986). Newborn death. In T. A. Rando (Ed.), *Parental loss of a child.* Champaign, IL: Research Press.

Nichols, J. A., & Doka, K. J. (1991). No more rosebuds. In K. J. Doka (Ed.), *Death and spirituality.* Amityville, NY: Baywood Publishing.

Panuthos, C., & Romeo, C. (1984). *Ended beginnings.* South Hadley, MA: Bergin & Garvey.

Pappas, D. J. H., & McCoy, M. C. (1996). Grief counseling. In J. A. Kuller, N. C. Chescheir, & R. C. Cefalo (Eds.), *Prenatal diagnosis and reproductive genetics* (pp. 70–76). St. Louis: C. V. Mosby.

Parkes, C. M. (1970a). The first year of bereavement. A longitudinal study of the reaction of London widows to the death of their husbands. *Psychiatry, 33*(4), 444–467,

Parkes, C. M. (1970b). "Seeking" and "finding" a lost object: Evidence from recent studies of the reaction to bereavement. *Social Science and Medicine, 4*(2), 187–201.

Parkes, C. M., & Brown, R. J. (1972). Health after bereavement. A controlled study of young Boston widows and widowers. *Psychosomatic Medicine, 34*(5), 449–461.

Parkes, C. M., & Weiss, R. (1983). *Recovery from bereavement.* New York: Basic Books.

Peppers, L. G., & Knapp, R. J. (1980). *Motherhood and mourning.* New York: Praeger.

Piaget, J. (1929). *The child's conception of the world.* London: Routledge & Kegan-Paul.

Pine, V. R., & Brauer, C. (1986). Parental grief: A synthesis of theory, research, and intervention. In T. A. Rando (Ed.), *Parental loss of a child.* Champaign, IL: Research Press.

Rando, T. A. (1984). *Grief, dying, and death: Clinical interventions for caregivers.* Champaign, IL: Research Press.

Rando, T. A. (Ed.). (1986). *Parental loss of a child.* Champaign, IL: Research Press.

Rando, T. A. (1993). *Treatment of complicated mourning.* Champaign, IL: Research Press.

Raphael, B. (1983). *The anatomy of bereavement.* New York: Basic Books.

Rosen, H. (1986). *Unspoken grief.* Lexington, MA: Lexington Books.

Ross-Alaolmolki, K. (1990). Coping with family loss. In M. J. Craft & J. A. Denehy (Eds.), *Nursing interventions for infants and children.* Philadelphia: W. B. Saunders.

Ryan, P. F., Coté-Arsenault, D., & Sugarman, L. L. (1991). Facilitating care after perinatal loss: A comprehensive checklist. *Journal of Obstetric, Gynecologic, and Neonatal Nursing, 20*(5), 385–389.

Schneider, J. (1984). *Stress, loss, and grief.* Baltimore: University Park Press.

Schwiebert, P., & Kirk, P. (1982). *When hello means goodbye.* Portland: Oregon Health Sciences University.

Shneidman, E. S. (1977). The college student and death. In H. Feifel (Ed.), *New meanings of death.* New York: McGraw-Hill.

Siegel, R., Rudd, S. H., Cleveland, C., et al. (1985). A hospice approach to neonatal care. In C. A. Corr & D. M. Corr (Eds.), *Hospice approaches to pediatric care.* New York: Springer.

Staudacher, C. (1991). *Men and grief.* Oakland, CA: New Harbinger Publications.

Stillion, J. M. (1986). The demise of dualism: Toward a convergence of brain research and therapy. *Death Studies, 10*(3), 313–329.

Tatelbaum, J. (1980). *The courage to grieve.* New York: Harper & Row.

VanPutte, A. W. (1988). Perinatal bereavement crisis: Coping with negative outcomes from prenatal diagnosis. *Journal of Perinatal and Neonatal Nursing, 2*(2), 12–22.

Weiner, J. M. (1970). Reaction of the family to the fatal illness of the child. In B. Schoenberg, A. Corr, D. Peretz, & A. Kutscher (Eds.), *Loss and grief: Psychological management in medical practice.* New York: Columbia University Press.

Windau, V., & Dewitt, P. J. (1988). Emergency baptism by nurses in an NICU: Answering a spiritual need. *Neonatal Network, 7*(1), 57–62.

Wolfelt, A. (1992). *Understanding grief.* Muncie, IN: Accelerated Development.

Worden, J. W. (1982). *Grief counseling and grief therapy.* New York: Springer.

Worden, J. W. (1991a). *Grief counseling and grief therapy* (rev. ed.). New York: Springer.

Worden, J. W. (1991b). *Childhood bereavement study.* Address presented at the annual conference of the Association of Death Education and Counseling, Duluth, MN.

Zumbro Valley Medical Society, Medicine & Religion Committee. (1978). *Religious aspects of medical care: A handbook of religious practices of all faiths* (2nd ed.). St. Louis: The Catholic Hospital Association.

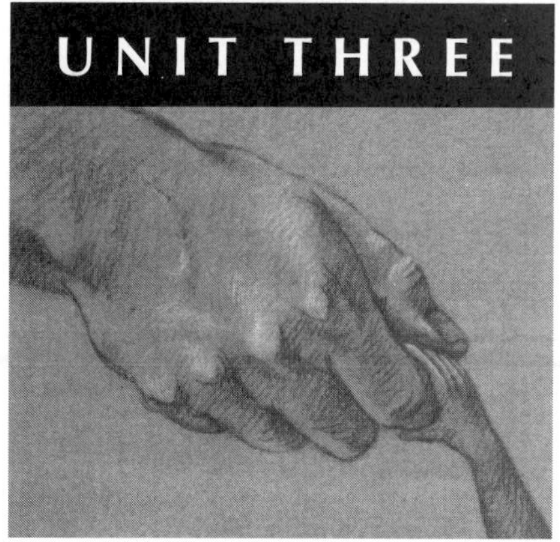

The Prenatal Environment: Maternal-Fetal Interactions

Leslie's regular days off had happened to fall in the first few days after Emily was born. In her absence, Emily had had a different nurse each day. They all seemed highly capable. They were patient, well-informed, and universally gracious. Nevertheless, I welcomed the prospect of continuity and consistency in the person of Leslie. Emily would remain her charge throughout her stay on K9, Leslie said. If and when we moved across the hall to the well-baby nursery, or next door, where the even weller babies were, Leslie would go, too. It was great news for many reasons. Leslie was just about my age. She was smart, with a master's degree and 5 years of teaching in the New York City public schools before turning to nursing. She'd spent 11 years at the hospital, all of it right here in the NICU. "Right from the beginning I knew that was where I belonged," she said. "I knew this was where I wanted to work."

Most of all, she radiated equal and enormous quantities of competence and confidence. Her shift started at 7 A.M., and by the time I arrived at 8, Leslie knew all about Emily's chart, and she had talked to some of the young pediatric residents who had been on duty these last few days. This impressed me, and made me feel less like a modular patient. Leslie was clearly a responsible professional who took her job seriously, but she also telegraphed a sense of warmth and concern. She cared about her job, and about doing it well, and she also cared about people.

ELIZABETH MEHREN
Born Too Soon

CHAPTER **9**

Human Genetics

CAROLE KENNER MARCIA A. HILSE CAROL HETTEBERG

RESEARCH AGENDA

Determine the impact of a referral to a genetics counselor on parent–child interaction.

What factors influence a family's decision to seek genetics counseling?

What genetic factors influence the susceptibility to diseases such as cancer later in life?

What are the client's or family's educational needs?

What are nurses' genetic educational needs?

Determine the quality of genetics-based nursing services and their impact on families' needs.

Determine the need for revision or expansion of care to incorporate genetic aspects through the use of outcome-based criteria.

VIGNETTE

After a difficult pregnancy, Mrs. Z delivered a 5 lb, 10 oz daughter by emergency C-section. Apgars were 8 and 9. When a period of bonding with her parents was completed, Baby Z was transferred to the nursery. During the assessment, the nurse noted characteristics that might indicate Down syndrome. The infant had a wide, flat face with low-set ears and widely spaced eyes. Epicanthal folds were not present. Her tongue protruded slightly. One simian crease was found, and her fifth fingers hooked inward. No murmur was present. Examination of the feet revealed a wide space between the great and second toes bilaterally. Neurologic exam indicated decreased muscular tone. Other findings were normal.

Around 6 hours of age, Baby Z became cyanotic. She quickly improved with 100 percent blow-by O_2. She was transferred to the special care nursery because of concern about the possibility of congenital cardiac defects. An intensive assessment was performed: oxygen challenge test, chest x-rays, electro-, and echocardiograms were done. Meanwhile, the O_2 was decreased to 26 percent to keep the infant pink. On review, the cardiologist determined that Baby Z had a small patent ductus arteriosus and foramen ovale, with left-to-right shunting. The pediatrician informed the parents that their baby possibly had Down syndrome and a genetics specialist needed to be consulted. The anxious parents arrived at the special care nursery. I encouraged them to touch her.

"She doesn't look different to me," Mrs. Z stated. "Why do the doctors think she has Down syndrome?" I gently showed them the characteristics. The parents listened intently. "Can she have those things and still be normal?" they questioned. "Yes, she can be completely normal. Your doctor called for a genetics consult because these combined characteristics *may* indicate Down syndrome. The specialist will examine your baby, talk to you to get a family history, and draw blood to analyze the chromosomes. Only by chromosome analysis can he absolutely diagnose Down syndrome. Usually that takes several days to several weeks," I informed them. After a genetics consult, it was fairly certain that Baby Z's chromosomes would indicate Down syndrome. The genetics specialist carefully explained what this meant chromosomally, physically, and mentally. He answered the parents' questions and was supportive, but the news was very distressing. After the specialist left, I found them both with swollen, red faces and teary eyes. I then sensed it was time to hear how they felt about all this. Their grief poured out. Grief for (1) the perfect baby they didn't have; (2) the physical care and financial burden they must assume (and didn't want); (3) their baby's handicap and changed quality of life compared with what they expected; (4) their older children, who now had a sister with Down syndrome; and (5) all the decisions made regarding, and in the course of, this pregnancy (the decision not to have prenatal testing, the decision to smoke, even the decision to become pregnant was grieved).

Today I listened, accepted what they said without correction, and supported them. This interaction was hard for me because Mr. Z expressed much anger; he slammed his fist down, paced about, and was forceful in his verbalizations. Anger was the only way he knew to deal with his feelings of helplessness and unfairness. "We must be terrible parents to think this about our baby," Mrs. Z confided. I let them know that these feelings were normal and that they needed to verbalize and share them before they could begin the task of parenting their daughter. I gave them a book about infants with Down syndrome and some information from the local Down Syndrome Association chapter. I told them that I'd be caring for their baby tomorrow and would talk to them again. I returned the next day and outlined my agenda: expectations for growth and development, capabilities and limitations, programs and agencies, early intervention, and future considerations. They indicated their interest. My first topic was one that is difficult to talk about, but the information is necessary in order for parents to fully consider and exercise their options. "I am not making assumptions about your willingness or ability to parent this baby. There is the option of adoption. If you feel you cannot parent or accept her into your home, there is a very active adoption service for Down syndrome children. Many people welcome the opportunity to parent, and these babies never wait very long for a set of willing parents." They thought about this surprise information. "I want her, but I can't speak for you. We have to do it together, " Mrs. Z said to her husband. He sat down on his wife's bed, held her hands, and intently searched every detail of her face. After several moments, he turned to me and said, "We're going to take her home. She's our daughter."

The adoption option presents a turning point. Parents become empowered and give up their previous status as victims. Before the option is revealed, parents deal mostly with their disappointment and grief. Adoption brings the possibility of choice to them. Parents consider whether they can or want to parent this baby. They mobilize to make a conscious decision that parenting a baby with Down syndrome is their choice, or that it is not. Having exercised this choice, the parents approach the situation with resolution and the determination of being self-directed. Empowerment changes the parents' role definition for themselves, their baby, and all involved.

I emphasized that every child is an individual and has different potential to develop. The goal is to see their child on the continuum of possibilities, not as a member of a distinct, handicapped subgroup. We discussed the importance of developmental stimulation and early intervention programs. I referred them to the Down Syndrome Association chapter. It is a resource for information on programs, parent support, toys and activities, and counseling about the future, including education and vocational training, financial planning, and adult care. Fathers show concerns about these topics early.

The Zs were worried about their other children's responses, so we talked about how they should meet their sister. Baby Z went home at 1 week of age, stable and breastfeeding well. Her parents had already contacted the Down Syndrome Association chapter.

To inform parents about Down syndrome, the nurse has the obligation to have current, factual information. As recently as 25 years ago, the standard of care was institutionalization. We are still learning about the capabilities of these children.

Joyce M. Dohme

It is estimated that more than 12 million Americans have at least one recognizable genetic problem (Cummings, 1994). These problems range from gross abnormalities that impair physical or mental function to minor irritations and inconveniences that may result from insufficient production or utilization of one nonspecific, noncritical enzyme. With the accessibility of new methods of genetic analysis at the molecular level, it is likely to be determined that all individuals are less than perfect genetically.

Today's nurses and other health care professionals are becoming increasingly aware of the vast and complex role genetics and patterns of inheritance play in determining health and maintaining homeostasis. Not only are congenital physical defects and errors in metabolism associated with heritable gene variations and aberrations, but increased susceptibility to pathologic conditions that develop long after birth, such as cancer and coronary artery disease, also appear to have a genetic basis. These genetic variations may have causative or permissive roles in the development of defects and disease. With the Human Genome Project's continued success at mapping genes and designating their exact loci on specific chromosomes, the possibilities for future testing and genetic intervention are limitless (Raff, 1994a). It is essential for all health professionals to have a good grasp of genetic information (Raff, 1994b). Nurses are involved in assisting the genetic testing procedures and educating families and other health professionals about genetic abnormalities, and some are involved in genetic counseling (Foresman, 1994).

Long before deoxyribonucleic acid (DNA) was discovered or any of the intracellular contents of cells were known, scientists noted that the basic traits of certain organisms were passed down to succeeding generations with varying degrees of constancy. This observation was noted not only among humans and other "higher order" species of animals but also among plants and simple forms of animal life. In general, the physical characteristics of offspring usually resembled the physical characteristics of the parent organism. This fact was explained as a basic "mixing" of maternal and paternal characteristics in the formation of a new individual or new generation. More difficult to explain was how a child could resemble or have a specific characteristic found only in a more remote family member, such as a great grandmother or an uncle, rather than in one of the parents. Gregor Mendel, a 19th century botanist, in observing variation in heritable characteristics over many generations among plants, proposed a mechanism that essentially involved the varying "strength" of some characteristics to explain variation in patterns of inheritance. Even at this point, no one cell structure was identified as responsible for the transmission of these patterns of inheritance.

During the late 19th century, biologists discovered small "chromatic elements" within the nucleus of a cell that stained differently from other cell components. In addition, these elements were present only at specific times in the cell cycle. These elements were called *chromosomes.* Later, scientists (interpreted by Dunn, 1965; Wolf, 1976) speculated on the function of chromosomes.

It was determined that chromosomes were composed of homologous pairs that split longitudinally during cell division. Chromosomes were thought to be responsible for mendelian heredity. One half of each pair of chromosomes was derived from the maternal gamete and the other half of each pair of chromosomes was derived from the paternal gamete (interpreted by Dunn, 1965; Wolf, 1976).

In 1914 it was noted that chromosomes disappeared during the interphase of the cell cycle only to reappear at mitosis in the same number and with the same morphologic features as at the previous mitosis. As a result of these observations, chromosome formation was speculated to be an organized process from one cell generation to another and not merely a result of random meshing of nuclear material.

It was observed that when there were abnormally shaped or an abnormal number of chromosomes that subsequent development was abnormal. Thus, it was hypothesized that chromosomes were the carriers of heredity and that aberrations in chromosomes (both numeric aberrations and structural aberrations) would subsequently result in aberrant development. Normal functioning of cells and whole organisms was dependent on an equilibrium of this genetic material.

Even though these concepts were proposed more than 70 years ago, testing was limited by the dearth of cytogenetic and molecular genetic technologic advances until relatively recent times. Cytogenetic advancements occurred first and led to a means of diagnosing some specific genetic abnormalities. The early cytogenetic work increased the precision and clinical application of molecular genetic advancements.

CELL BIOLOGY

Because the genetic and epigenetic events that determine which characteristics or traits are inherited and expressed occur at the cellular and subcellular levels, it is important to understand the basic components of all cells and how they function. The following is a brief discussion of cell structure and function.

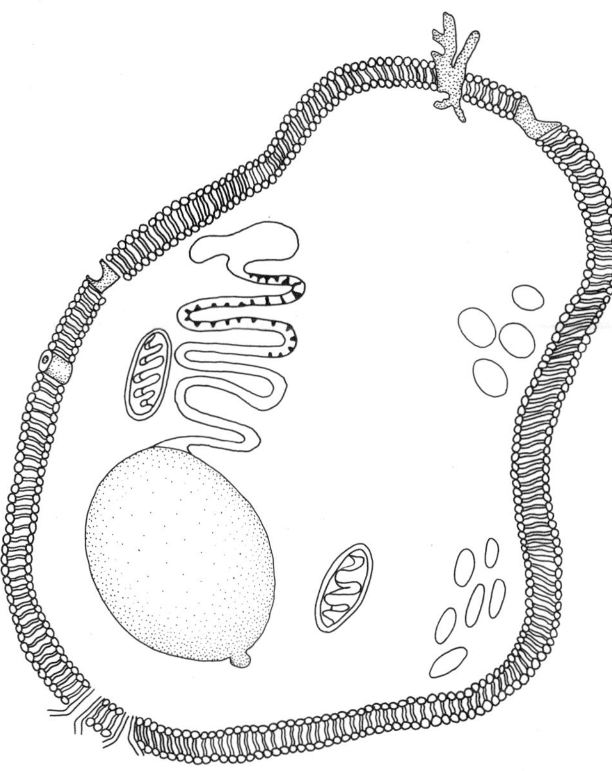

FIGURE 9–1. Cellular structures.

Figure 9–1 presents cellular structures common to most mammalian cells.

Plasma Membrane

All mammalian cells are surrounded by a plasma membrane (plants have cell walls). This membrane is composed of phospholipids, molecules of cholesterol, and molecules of protein. The arrangement and proportion of these substances differ from cell type to cell type, although the basic structure of the plasma membrane remains the same. The phospholipids are arranged in a double layer termed the *phospholipid bilayer* (Fig. 9–2). In the formation of the bilayer, the phosphate heads of the phospholipids are on the exterior surfaces of the membranes, and the fatty acid tails or lipid portions of the phospholipids intercalate with each other in the interior of the plasma membrane. Cholesterol molecules and protein molecules are interspersed to varying degrees throughout the membrane.

The phospholipids serve a barrier function for the cell, preventing intracellular substances from being lost to the extracellular environment and preventing unnecessary substances from the extracellular environment from entering the cell. The cholesterol molecules change the pliability of the membrane and serve as a mechanism to permit substances to pass through the membrane in either direction. The proteins within and through the membrane confer specificity on the membrane. The proteins serve as (1) receptors for specific substances, (2) antigenic determinants (cell recognition elements), and (3) specific enzymes required for various intracellular functions.

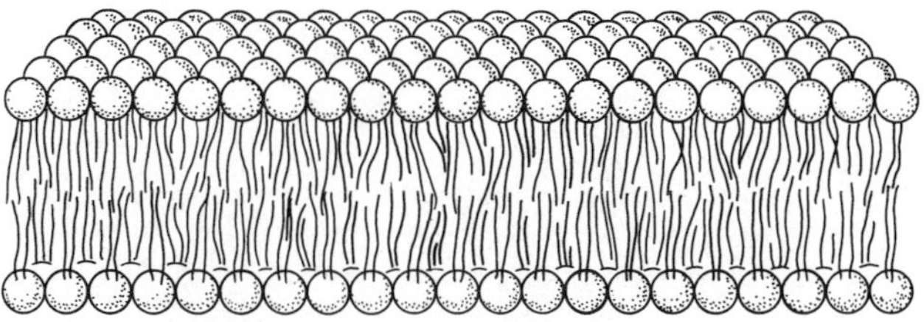

FIGURE 9–2. Phospholipid bilayer.

Intracellular Structures

Cytoplasm

The cytoplasm (also called *cytosol, intracellular fluid*) is the fluid portion of a cell surrounded by the plasma membrane. Cytoplasm does not include the fluid inside the nucleus and other various organelles; it is composed primarily of water. This fluid contains enough solute particles (mainly electrolytes and proteins) to maintain the cytoplasm in a isotonic state in relation to most other body fluids. For most cells, the cytoplasmic pH is close to neutral.

Mitochondria

Mitochondria, which are often called intracellular "power plants," are present in nearly all cells. Mitochondria assist the cell in converting fuel substances (mostly glucose) into chemical energy substances (mostly adenosine triphosphate). Chemical energy substances are necessary for the cells to perform active work (such as phagocytosis, generation of action potentials, and synthesis of specific hormones and enzymes). The number of mitochondria present in a given cell type is in direct proportion to the biologic activity and rate of metabolism of that cell. For example, mature red blood cells perform only passive actions and have few if any mitochondria. More biologically active cell types, such as hepatocytes (liver cells) and skeletal muscle, contain huge numbers of mitochondria per cell.

Endoplasmic Reticulum

The endoplasmic reticulum is actually a system of small vesicles and tubules made from plasma membrane materials. In most cells, this system is attached to the nucleus directly. The purpose of the endoplasmic reticulum is to serve as a "factory" for the synthesis of various proteins made by that cell. In addition to synthesizing the proper protein, other mechanisms within the endoplasmic reticulum "finish" the protein by attaching appropriate nonprotein substances (such as sugars or lipid groups) in the proper place to increase the new protein's biologic activity.

Golgi Vesicles

Golgi vesicles (also known as the *Golgi complex, apparatus,* or *body*) are also necessary for the proper production of proteins. The proteins synthesized within the endoplasmic reticulum are seldom complete when they leave it. These newly synthesized proteins are transported to the Golgi vesicles, where it appears that further processing or finishing of the proteins occurs. In addition, if a specific protein is to be used in parts of the body other than the cell that synthesized it, the Golgi vesicle prepares the protein to leave the cell by packaging it in a plasma membrane so that the protein's membrane can fuse with the cell's plasma membrane, allowing the protein to separate from the cell and plasma membrane by "budding off."

Cytoskeletal Elements

The cytoskeletal elements are contractile structures within the cell that help the cell achieve and maintain its ultimate shape and assist the cell in movement. All cells must move to some degree. Some cells actually change location from one part of the body to another. Other cells change position within a specific tissue area. For cells that divide, the process of cell division is dependent on having the cell change its shape and pull apart. All these movements and processes require contraction and relaxation of cytoskeletal elements. There are at least three different categories of cytoskeletal elements; microtubules and microfilaments are the most common. Although nearly all cells contain all categories, cells vary in the amount and distribution of cytoskeletal elements they contain.

Lysosomes

Lysosomes are specialized organelles that contain enzymes capable of degrading proteins, lipids, and nucleic acids. Because these enzymes would work indiscriminately throughout the cell if they were free in the cytoplasm and could destroy important cellular structures, lysosomes serve as a confinement area for the degradative enzymes. Although only some leukocytes (white blood cells) have the specific function of phagocytosis with degradation of engulfed materials, most cells require some lysosomes to remove normal cellular debris and maintain homeostasis.

Nucleus

The nucleus consists of genetic material (primarily DNA), nucleoli, and nucleoplasm surrounded by a nuclear membrane or envelope with a structure similar to that of the plasma membrane. Normal cells in the reproductive resting state contain only one nucleus. Because the nucleus contains all the cell's genetic material, only cells with a nucleus are capable of cell division. Proper function of this organelle is critical for individual cell function and propagation. Because the products of one cell type may influence the development and activity of another cell type, impaired nuclear function of one cell type can have widespread deleterious effects for the whole organism.

MOLECULAR GENETICS

Why do cells have and need genetic material? The nucleus of a cell contains the DNA that holds the codes or patterns for construction of every protein made by every cell within the body. It is important to remember that all hormones, factors, and enzymes synthesized by the human body are composed partially or entirely of protein. Examples of these protein substances include insulin, interferon, thyroxine, interleukin-2, trypsin, lactase, lipase, and myeloperoxidase, to name only a few. The controlling factors for cell development and function are the genes. A gene is a specific segment of DNA that contains codes for the pattern or plan for a specific gene product (a protein).

All cells make substances that are used for the normal "housekeeping" duties of the cell. In addition, some cells make at least one specific substance that leaves the cell and either is used by other cells or controls the activity of other cells. All these substances are proteins, and the processes involved in making these proteins are termed *protein synthesis.* This process can occur only if the specific segment of DNA (the gene) that contains the coding pattern for a protein is present to direct the actual synthesis of the protein.

DNA is composed of two very long chains (strands) of interlocking nucleotides. Each nucleotide is composed of a molecule of any one of the following four bases: adenine (A), guanine (G), thymine (T), and cytosine (C). Adenine and guanine are purine bases; thymine and cytosine are pyrimidine bases. These bases are attached to a five-carbon sugar (a pentose arrangement called a ribose) that is connected to a phosphate group (Fig. 9–3).

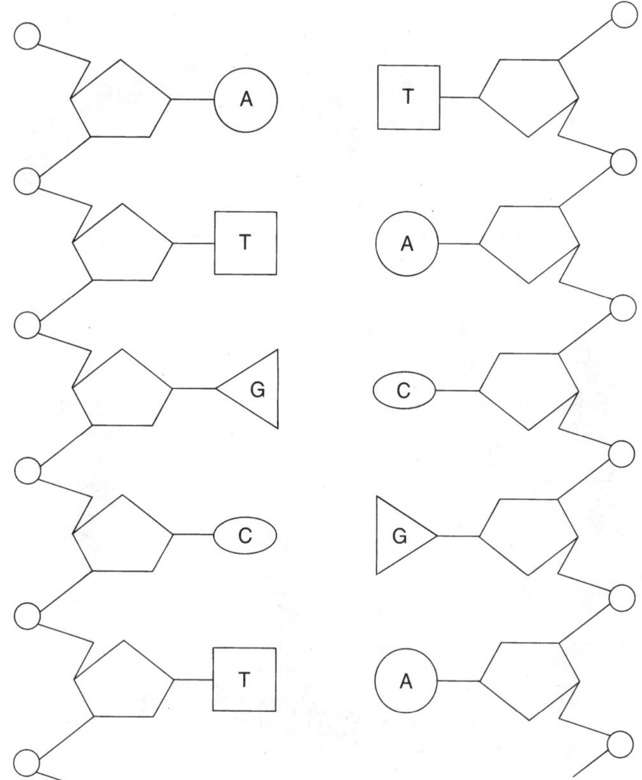

FIGURE 9–3. Nucleotide: four bases and five-carbon sugar with a phosphate group.

The phosphate groups actually provide the linkage between the individual bases so that long strands are formed. Thus, the phosphate connections are the actual "backbone" of the DNA strand.

In humans, DNA does not exist as a single strand. Instead, the DNA is double-stranded in an "antiparallel" arrangement. The two strands are not directly physically connected. Rather, there are a number of relatively weak ionic forces that hold the two strands in close proximity. These ionic forces are different for the two groups of bases, and these differences are responsible for adenine always pairing with thymine (and vice versa) and guanine always pairing with cytosine (and vice versa). Thus, the two strands of DNA are lined up together and are composed of interacting bases that form *base pairs.* Because the bases are specific in their attractions, the two strands of DNA are complementary to each other in terms of their nucleotide sequence. Therefore, if the sequence of one DNA strand is known, it is possible to predict with accuracy the sequence of the complementary DNA strand.

5′ 3′
A—T
C—G
C—G
G—C
T—A
T—A
T—A
A—T
C—G
C—G
T—A
G—C
G—C
3′ 5′

Antiparallel (complementary) double strands

C—G
G—C
T—A
A—T

Examples of base pairs

In its native state during the reproductive resting state of the cell (G_0), the double-stranded DNA has a loosely coiled helical arrangement. At various times in the cell cycle, the DNA becomes more tightly packed together. This packing together involves further coiling of the DNA at well-regulated intervals around protein substances called *histones* so that the DNA has an appearance similar to that of beads on a string. The complex of DNA wound around each histone is called a *nucleosome*. In addition to the histone proteins that come into close contact with the DNA at specific points in the strand and at certain times in the cell cycle, there are other nonhistone proteins that also are associated with the DNA. During cell division, the DNA must become even more tightly packed together to form dense structures called *chromosomes*. Each chromosome is composed of a relatively large section of DNA containing many genes.

The basic structure of chromosomes is presented in Figure 9–4. Most of the current nomenclature used to describe specific areas or features of chromosomes is derived from the 1971 Paris Conference of the International Human Genetics Congress.

Chromatids are the two long structures making up the two longitudinal halves of the chromosome present during metaphase of cell division. Chromatids on the same chromosome are called *sister chromatids*. The point at which the two sister chromatids are joined together is called the *centromere*. Many chromosome features are described in relation to the centromere. The portions of the chromatids above the centromere are shorter than the portions below the centromere and are called the *p arms* (or the "short" arms). The portions of the chromosomes below the centromere are called the *q arms* (or the "long" arms). The distal ends of the chromosome are called the *telomeres* or the *terminals*.

Normally, human beings have 46 chromosomes (23 different pairs) in all cells except mature red blood cells and the mature sex cells (sperm and ova). This number is called the *diploid number* (2N) of chromosomes for humans and constitutes the genome or the complete set of human genes. Of the 23 pairs, 22 pairs are autosomal chromosomes (autosomes), which code for and regulate somatic cell development and function. One pair of chromosomes constitutes the sex chromosomes, which code for and regulate sexual development and function. Mature red blood cells contain no nucleus and therefore have no chromosomes. Mature sex cells (gametes) have only 23 chromosomes (half of each pair). This number is known as the *haploid number* (1N) of chromosomes for humans.

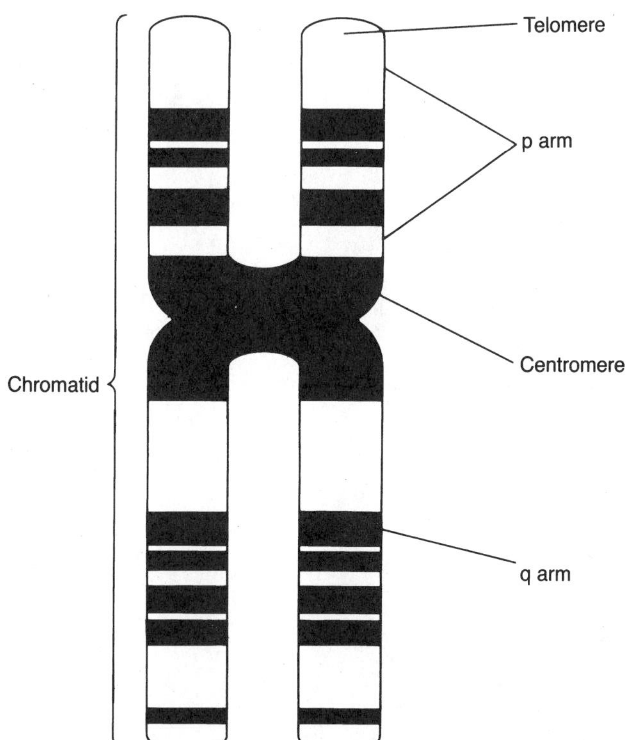

FIGURE 9–4. Basic structure of chromosomes (giemsa-banded chromosome 11).

The constitutional chromosomes of an individual can be studied through a process called *chromosome analysis (karyotyping)*, which can be performed on dividing cells only. This process involves obtaining a sample of sterile, living tissue that is capable of relatively rapid cell division. Most frequently, blood lymphocytes or skin fibroblasts are used for this purpose. The tissue is incubated with nutrient fluids at 37°C for several hours to several days to encourage more cells to enter the reproductive cycle and proceed to the mitotic phase. The dividing cells are artificially trapped in the metaphase stage of mitosis, fixed with preservative, placed on microscope slides, stained, and evaluated under the microscope.

After these preparatory steps, chromosome analysis is carried out through examination of karyotypes. Microscope photographs of metaphase chromosomes are made. From these photographs the chromosomes are karyotyped—grouped in sequences of pairs according to the size of the chromosome pairs and the positions of the centromeres (Fig. 9–5). Each group begins with the largest pair of chromosomes that has the centromeres most centrally located. Subsequent chromosome pairs are ordered according to descending size and more distally located centromeres. Analysis of this type of karyotype can determine numeric chromosome aberrations. This type of chromosome analysis is haphazard because specific individual chromosomes cannot be identified precisely by this method.

A more accurate chromosome analysis is obtained when standard cytogenetic techniques are combined with the process of banding. Giemsa banding (G-banding) is the most common of the banding techniques for chromosome analysis. This process involves exposing the fixed slides to a proteolytic enzyme (usually trypsin), which selectively digests areas of the chromosome, and then staining the slide. The areas in which protein is digested do not take up the stain and leave a white space (negative band) on the chromosome. The areas in which protein is not digested do take up the stain and leave a dark area (positive band) on the chromosome. As a result of this process, each chromosome pair has a unique banded or striped appearance, which permits absolute identification of specific chromosomes (Fig. 9–6). Chromosome analysis that uses banding techniques can accurately identify structural chromosome abnormalities within individual chromosomes, as well as numeric chromosome abnormalities. Even this technique has severe limitations because the smallest chromosome area that can be observed under standard light microscopy contains at least 10,000 base pairs. It is known that many genetic disorders involve deletions or rearrangements of genes much smaller than 10,000 base pairs.

Each human develops as a result of one haploid egg fertilized by a single haploid sperm. The result of this union is a single cell containing the entire human genome, 23 pairs of chromosomes, half of each pair from the maternal gamete (egg or ovum) and the other half of each pair from the paternal gamete (sperm). For successful development of this one-cell organism to the complete human being, cell division by duplication is necessary. Duplication divisions occur through the process of mitosis.

Mitosis

Mitosis permits a duplication division of one cell to form two daughter cells identical to each other and identical to the original

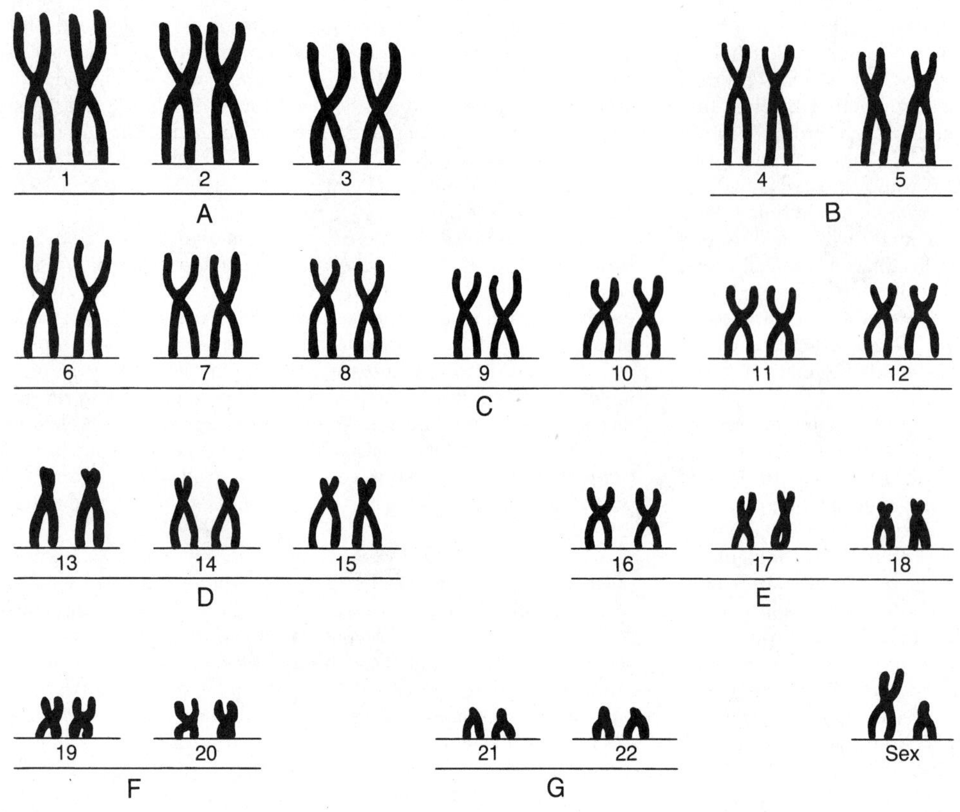

FIGURE 9–5. Karyotype of chromosome pairs.

FIGURE 9–6. Giemsa-banded karyotype. (Courtesy of Chin Ho, The Hospital for Sick Children, Toronto.)

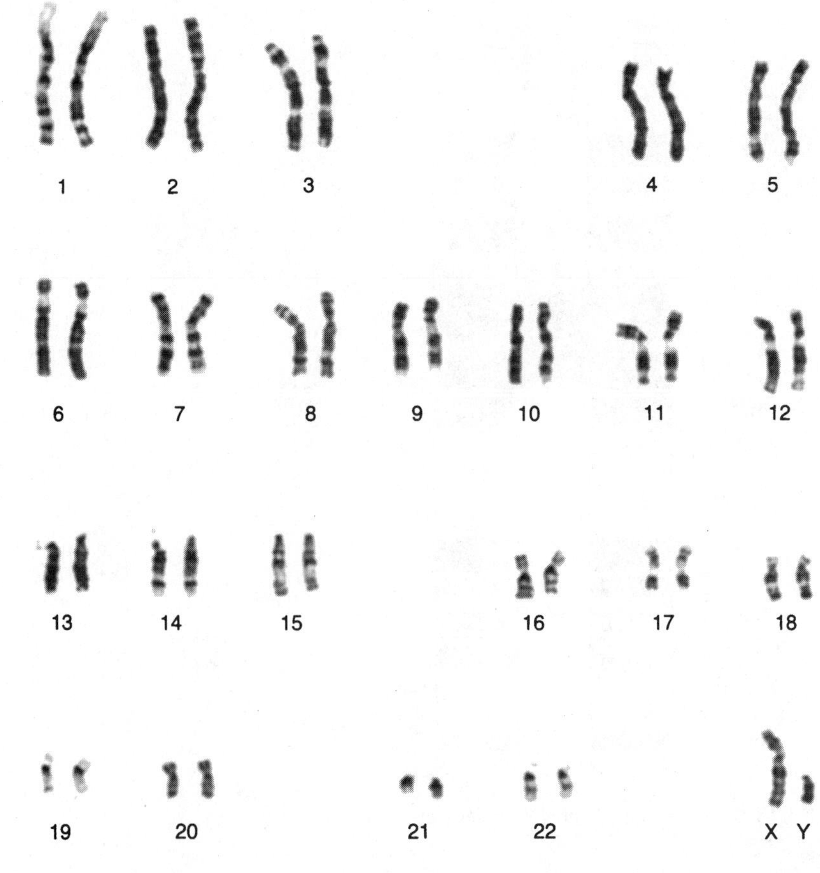

cell. The complete process of cellular reproduction, including actual mitosis, is outlined in Figure 9–7 and involves four phases, which collectively are called the *cell cycle.* The primary purpose of the processes involved in mitosis is to ensure that each daughter cell precisely inherits the exact human genome. Although the process of mitosis usually results in an equal division of all cellular structures and contents for the two daughter cells, it is absolutely essential for function that the genetic material inherited by each daughter cell be identical to that of the original cell. Therefore, a critical phase of cell division is the phase of DNA synthesis.

The cell cycle is actually a model depicting various activities that cells must accomplish for a successful cell division that results in high-fidelity duplication. It is important to remember that the cell cycle refers only to the reproductive cycle of a cell and does not take into consideration the cell's total life cycle. After development is complete, most cell types do not spend much time in the actual reproductive cycle. Rather, they exist as functional cell citizens that are performing all their specific and appropriate duties except reproduction. This nonreproductive state is termed G_0. Normal cells leave this state and enter the reproductive cycle only if (1) they are a specific cell type that is capable of cell division (some cells, such as neurons, skeletal muscle cells, and cardiac muscle cells do not divide after development is complete) and (2) that particular cell type is needed for normal growth or replacement of dead or damaged cells.

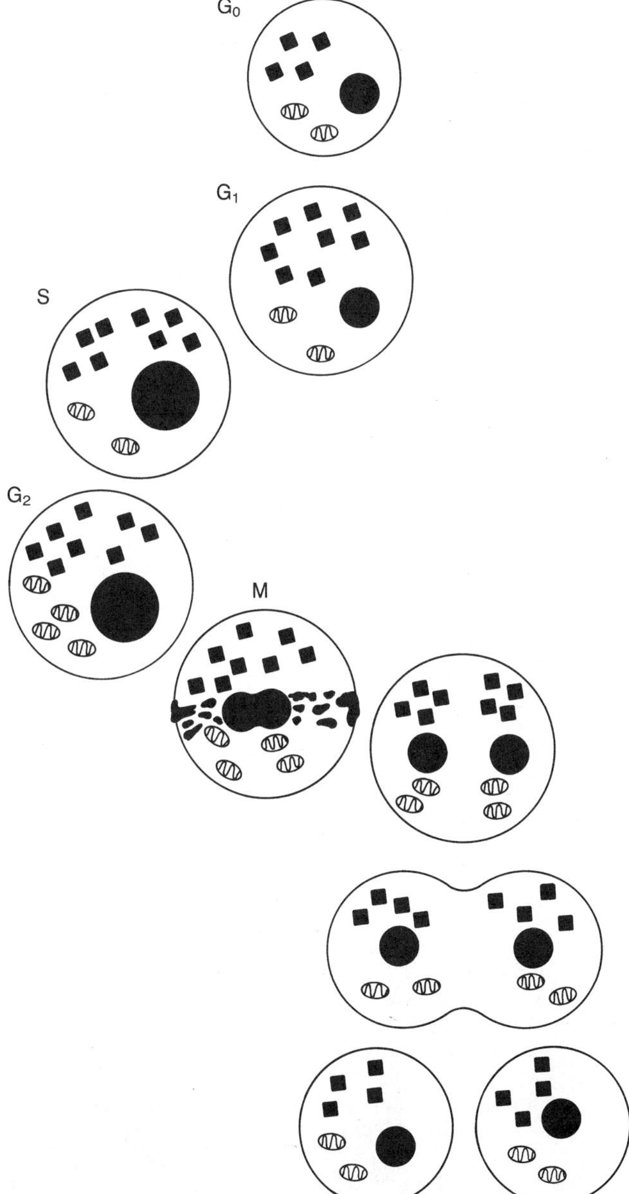

FIGURE 9–7. Four phases of cellular reproduction: cell cycle.

G_1 Phase

On entering the G_1 phase of the cell cycle, the cell has committed to divide, and this is an irreversible step for normal cells. At this time the cell takes on added nutrients to form energy substances needed for the strenuous processes involved in actual cell division. In addition, the cell increases the fluid and membrane contents in order to accommodate the needs of two cells.

S Phase

For each daughter cell to inherit the proper human genome, the DNA content of the original cell must first duplicate itself. The process of making more DNA to form a new cell is called *DNA synthesis* (S phase of the cell cycle) and occurs entirely within the nucleus. The new DNA is made by using the original strands of DNA as models or templates. The original strands of DNA temporarily loosen from the tight helical arrangement. The loosened strands separate into two single strands so that each single strand can be used as a template for the new DNA (Fig. 9–8). A series of enzymes is required for this process. The steps in this process involve having the DNA relax, unwind from the histones, and straighten out the helix slightly. An additional enzyme enters the straightened area and separates the two strands over a limited area. Another enzyme enters and prevents the two strands from rejoining. A different enzyme attaches itself to one strand, travels down the strand (from the 5′ to 3′ direction), "reads" the base sequence of this strand, and forms a new strand of DNA that is complementary to the one being read.

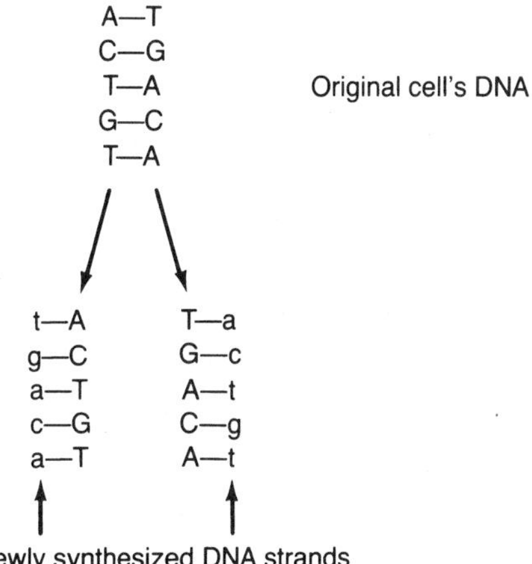

This process is called the "semiconservative" mode of DNA synthesis because it results in two identical double helices, each containing one original strand of DNA and one newly created strand of DNA. After the strands of DNA have been duplicated (replicated), they pack back down into supercoiled chromosomes and line up so that they are ready to be pulled apart (split) during the M phase of the cell cycle. This splitting permits the two sets of DNA to become part of two new cells instead of just one cell.

G_2 Phase

The G_2 phase of the cell cycle is characterized by intense protein synthesis. The cell is synthesizing all the enzymes and

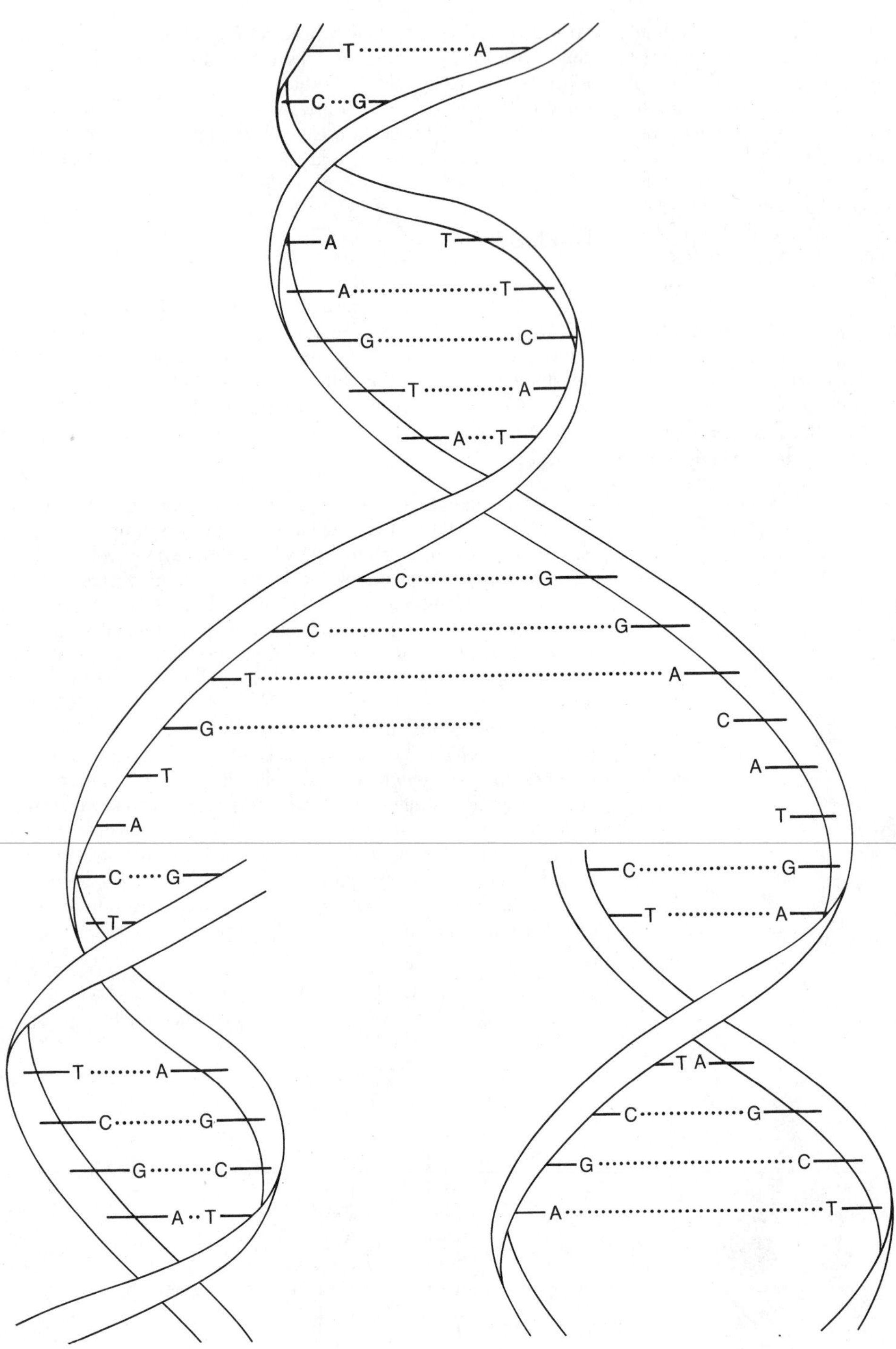

FIGURE 9–8. DNA synthesis.

other complexes necessary to carry out the actual division of the cell as well as those proteins that are needed for the regular "housekeeping" duties of the cell. In addition, increased amounts of various organelles are synthesized to meet the needs of two future cells.

M Phase

The actual part of the cell cycle in which two new cells are formed from the original cell is called mitosis and is the only time when the DNA is organized into chromosomes. This phase is further divided into subphases (Fig. 9–9).

From the time that the cell's DNA is duplicated in S phase through the G_2 phase, the cell's nucleus is said to be in interphase. The DNA during interphase is loosely coiled into nucleosomes and is widely dispersed throughout the nucleus. Only the nucleolus and two centrioles are distinguishable under standard light microscopy (see Fig. 9–9*A*). At this time the two centrioles each begin to form a daughter centriole. As the cell leaves the G_2 phase and begins the M phase, the DNA begins to condense. In early prophase, long spaghetti-like strands of newly formed chromosomes are discernible (see Fig. 9–9*B*). Throughout prophase, the DNA continues to condense until recognizable chromosomes are present. Later in prophase, the centrioles move to

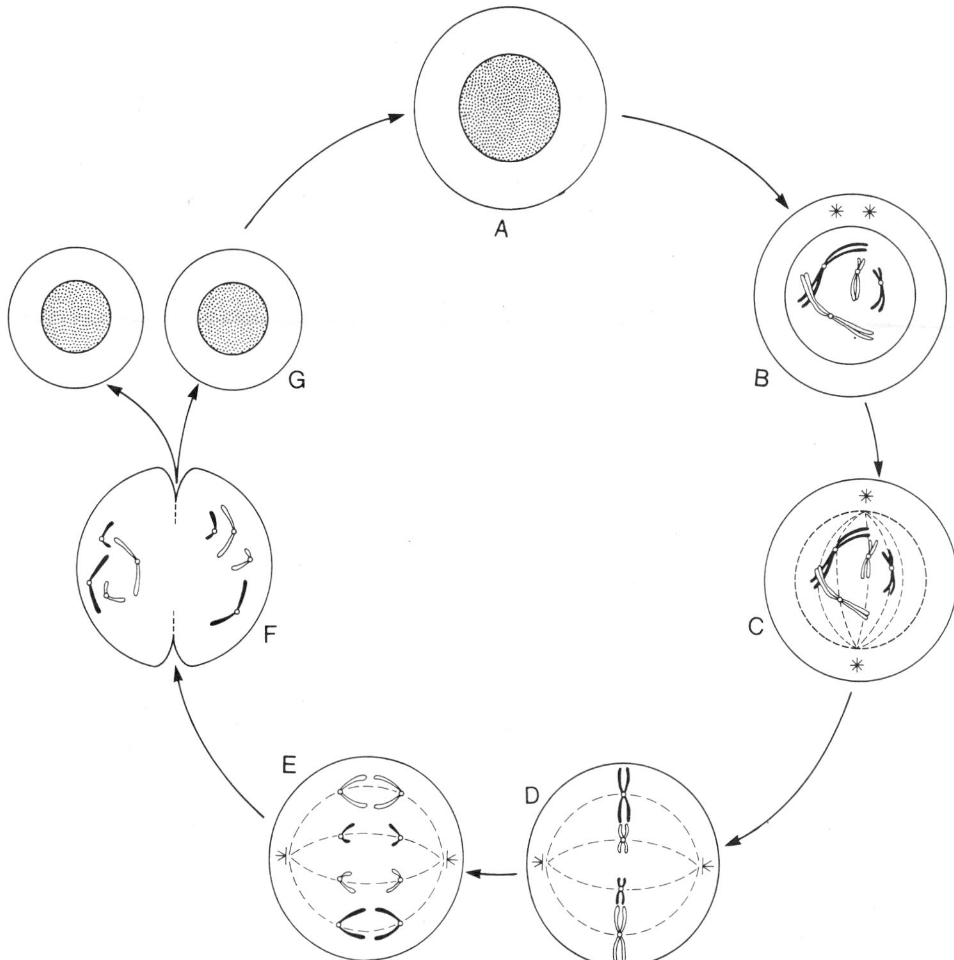

FIGURE 9–9. Mitosis. Diagrammatic representation, showing only two chromosome pairs. *A*, Interphase; *B*, prophase; *C*, prometaphase; *D*, metaphase; *E*, anaphase; *F*, telophase; *G*, interphase. For further details, see text. (From Thompson, M.W., McInnes, R.R., & Willard, H.F. [1991]. *Thompson & Thompson genetics in medicine* [5th ed., p. 22]. Philadelphia: W.B. Saunders. Reprinted with permission.)

opposite poles of the cell and begin to synthesize spindle fibers. During prometaphase, these spindle fibers attach to the kinetochores of chromosomes on or near the centromeres, and the nuclear membrane begins to disintegrate (see Fig. 9–9*C*). During metaphase of mitosis, the chromosomes are at their most compact and most readily visible structural forms. The chromosomes line up in the middle of the cell along the equatorial plane (see Fig. 9–9*D*). At this point the cell enters anaphase of mitosis, during which the two sister chromatids of each chromosome are pulled apart toward the pole to which each is attached (see Fig. 9–9*E*). This process is called *nucleokinesis,* indicating that the nucleus has moved and separated into two nuclei within the one cell. Under normal conditions, the chromosomes separate in such a way that the two daughter cells receive genetic components identical to each other and identical to the originating cell. The spindle fibers continue their pulling motion, and the cell begins cytokinesis, or the separation of the single cell body into two separate cell bodies each with one nucleus. Cytokinesis is completed during telophase of mitosis, and at this time the DNA begins to loosen from the compacted chromatids (see Fig. 9–9*F*). When the nuclear material is completely dispersed throughout the nucleus with only the centrioles and nucleolus discernible, the two new daughter cells are in interphase (see Fig. 9–9*G*).

During early embryonic development, the initial fertilized egg with 46 chromosomes undergoes many duplication divisions resulting in a large, hollow ball of cells (blastocyte), each with the same amount and organization of genetic material in its nucleus and exactly the same appearance and function. Although individual genes can undergo mutations after conception that result in altered gene expression, the actual genetic fate of this future human being, determined at the time of conception, is irreversible and cannot be changed.

At this point, these early embryonic cells are called undifferentiated because none of these cells has yet taken on the specific appearance (morphologic characteristics) and function or functions of the mature cell type it will eventually become. Obviously something has to change during the course of development, because normal human infants are not born as large balls of undifferentiated cells.

Between 8 and 10 days after conception, the human embryonic cells initiate the steps to become differentiated. In response to an unknown signal or signals, each cell commits itself to a specific maturational outcome. At the time of commitment, the cell has not taken on any differentiated features or functions, but it now positions itself within a group that will eventually take on specific morphologic characteristics and functional behavior. The process of commitment involves turning off specific genes that regulated and directed the early rapid growth and turning on other individual specific genes that control the expression of specific differentiated functions.

It is critical to remember that all differentiated somatic cells (body cells, not including sex cells) retain all the genes in the human genome. At one time the differences in appearance and function between cell types was explained by suggesting that different cells actually "lost" those genes that it did not need and retained only the genes that it required to reproduce itself and perform its special functions. We now know that this is not the way differentiation occurs and is maintained. Instead, all cells

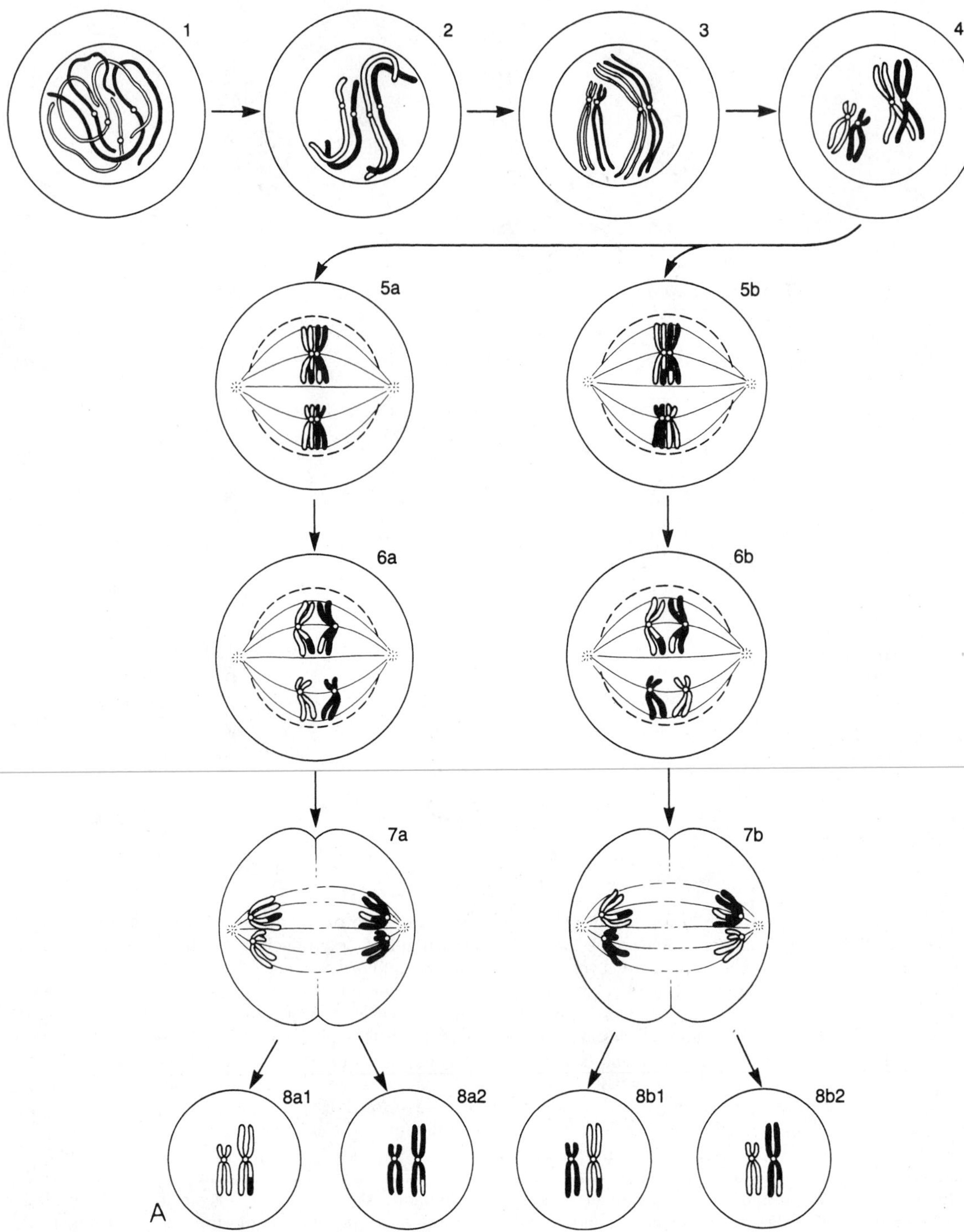

FIGURE 9–10. *A,* Meiosis I.

(excluding the sex cells) retain all genes. However, genes are selectively expressed or repressed in different cell types. For example, the gene for insulin is present in all cells; however, only in the beta cells of the pancreas is the insulin gene allowed to be expressed or "turned on" to meet the body's need for insulin production. There is nothing wrong with the insulin genes located in other cell types (such as in skin cells or skeletal muscle cells), but because the special functions of these other cells do not include the production of insulin, the insulin gene in these other cells is maintained in a repressed or "turned off" state. This turning off of early embryonic genes appears to be accomplished through the activity of special repressor genes that function solely to repress the activity of the early embryonic genes so that they can no longer be freely expressed.

Meiosis

The early embryonic cells that are destined to become mature sex cells undergo a somewhat different process to achieve maturation than do somatic cells. Early in development, the committed sex cells continue to undergo mitotic cell divisions in order to

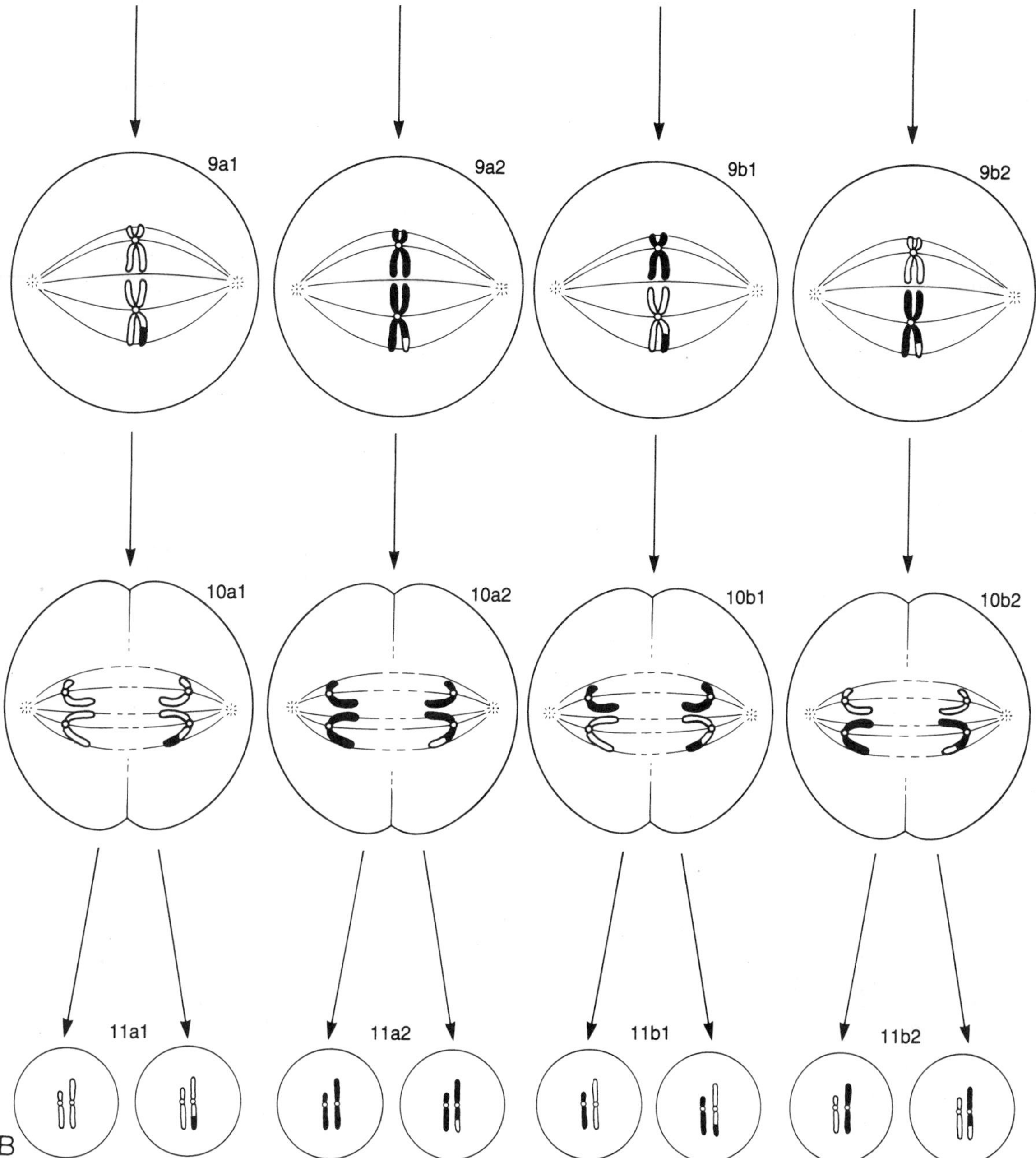

FIGURE 9–10 *Continued B,* Meiosis II. (From Thompson, M.W., McInnes, R.R., & Willard, H.F. [1991]. *Thompson & Thompson genetics in medicine* [5th ed., pp. 24, 25]. Philadelphia: W. B. Saunders. Reprinted with permission.)

increase their overall numbers. The cells resulting from these mitotic divisions continue to be diploid. Before the sex cells can completely mature, however, they must reduce their chromosome complement to the haploid rather than the diploid number through meiotic cell division.

Meiosis is the form of cell division that reduces the genetic complement of the cells by half, an actual reduction division that is different from the duplication division of mitosis. The result of meiosis is the production of new daughter cells that are identical to each other (in terms of their autosomes) but different from the originating cell. This process is necessary for gametogenesis, the final formation of sex cells. In order to accomplish this feat, the entire process of meiosis involves two completely separate series of cell divisions, one stage of which closely resembles a mitotic cell division. As a result of meiosis, four haploid cells are formed from a single diploid precursor sex cell.

As the precursor gametes (sex cells) prepare to become haploid gametes, each diploid precursor undergoes one round of DNA replication (synthesis), just as mitotic cells do in the S phase of mitosis. At this point in the process, the diploid precursor cell is now tetraploid (4N) with twice the normal number of chromosomes (92) (Fig. 9–10).

The cell now enters prophase of the first meiotic division. Each chromosome has two sister chromatids joined only at the centromere. Early in prophase, or meiosis I, the chromosomes condense and coil up, and the homologous pairs of chromosomes form a synapse. During synapse the homologous pairs of chromosomes associate with each other, lying side by side to form a tetrad with four chromatids. Because they are in such close proximity and because they are not yet compacted completely, there is some "crossing over" of genetic material both from the chromatids on the same chromosome (sister chromatids) and from the chromatids on the homologous pair (non-sister chromatids). Many genes are located on each chromatid. This crossing over of genetic material from non-sister chromatids has the effect of randomly "reshuffling" the maternally and paternally derived genes within the chromatids of homologous pairs, producing a wide variety of new combinations.

All the autosomes undergo this reshuffling process during synapse. The sex chromosomes have only a few limited exchanges at the telomeres. This limitation of exchanges is necessary because the chromatids of the X and the Y chromosomes are different, each with unique areas. By not exchanging unique areas, the integrity of the sex chromosomes is maintained. In this way, the species continues with only two sexes.

After synapse, the two centrioles within the cell move to opposite poles on the nucleus and begin to form spindles. The synaptic pairs of chromosomes further condense and move to the equatorial plane of the nucleus, where metaphase of meiosis I begins. This metaphase stage of meiosis is similar to metaphase in mitosis. The newly created spindles attach to the centromeres of the chromosomes. Contraction of the spindles causes whole chromosomes to be separated from chromosome pairs, but the newly reorganized chromatids of each chromosome remain together (anaphase I). At this point, dysfunction occurs as the chromosomes form dyads or pairs of sister chromosomes, and the cell completes cytokinesis so that two new cells with 46 chromosomes each are formed. However, because of the crossing over that occurred during synapse and because the new chromosomes randomly assort into pairs, the two newly created cells do not contain the identical gene complement of the precursor sex cell that began the process of meiosis. The new combination of chromosomes cannot be equally separated by maternal and paternal origin. Although the two new cells each contain 22 pairs of autosomes and one pair of sex chromosomes, it is possible that some of the pairs are composed wholly of maternally derived chromosomes, others are composed wholly of paternal chromosomes, and still others may be composed of varying combinations of maternal and paternal genetic material.

These two cells, which contain 46 chromosomes each (two copies of each chromatid), now spend some time in interphase before completing meiosis. The amount of time spent in interphase varies, with secondary oocytes remaining considerably longer in interphase (years) than do secondary spermatocytes. No further duplication or synthesis of DNA occurs in these cells.

Meiosis is completed after the second meiotic division. In meiosis II, the two new interphase diploid cells created in meiosis I enter prophase and begin condensing their DNA so that chromatids are formed. The centrioles within each of the two nuclei separate to opposite poles and form spindles that attach to the centromere of each chromosome. The cells now enter metaphase as the nuclear membrane begins to disintegrate.

The chromosomes in each of the two cells move to the equatorial plane and line up. The spindles separate the chromatids. Each pair of chromosomes has four chromatids. When these chromatids separate, one chromatid from each chromosome is segregated to each new daughter cell. Therefore, each daughter cell receives two chromatids from each pair of chromosomes. However, because the four chromatids segregate independently to the two daughter cells, there is no guarantee that each daughter cell will receive a chromatid from each chromosome of the chromosome pair. It is highly likely that for some chromosome pairs, the daughter cell will inherit two chromatids from one chromosome of a pair and none from the other chromosome.

The result of the entire process of meiosis is the formation of four haploid gamete cells from one diploid precursor sex cell. The crossing over of genetic material from homologous pairs of chromosomes during synapse with random assortment of chromatids in meiosis I, followed by independent segregation of chromatids in meiosis II has some intriguing consequences. It is possible that even though all gametes descended from the same clone of precursor sex cells and have identical genetic constitutions, the reshuffling of paternal and maternal whole genes and alleles (recessive as well as dominant) can result in hundreds or even thousands of possible minor variations in the genetic makeup of gametes. With this possibility, the astounding fact is not that sometimes siblings do not resemble each other but rather that they ever do look alike.

PROTEIN SYNTHESIS

All cells that make some protein have in their DNA the code for that protein, the actual gene for that protein. The unique DNA pattern (gene) for that specific protein is first converted into a piece of ribonucleic acid (RNA). RNA is similar to DNA, but instead of containing thymine (T), RNA contains uracil (U).

Proteins are formed by linking individual nitrogen units called amino acids together in a linear strand. There are 22 different amino acids. Each amino acid has a unique three-base code sequence, called a codon, which identifies the DNA and RNA pieces specific for that amino acid. Some amino acids have only one codon, whereas others have as many as four different (but closely related) codons. For example:

Specific Amino Acid	**RNA Codon**
Methionine	AUG
Alanine	GCU, GCC
Valine	GUU, GUC, GUA, GUG
Phenylalanine	UUU, UUC

The total number of amino acids in a specific protein and the exact order in which they are connected together help determine the nature and activity of the protein. The making of protein, protein synthesis, is similar to some of the steps in DNA synthesis, although carried out on a smaller scale.

Central Dogma

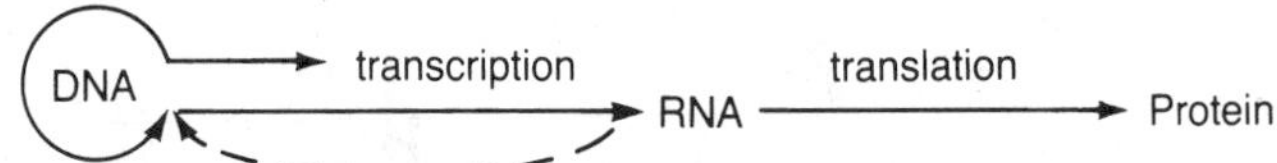

When a cell decides that it is time to make a specific protein (e.g., insulin), the cell must loosen the area of DNA that contains the amino acid code (gene) for insulin. The DNA in the region of the gene to be read loosens and unwinds slightly from the histones, using enzymes that are similar to those involved in DNA synthesis. Once the appropriate area of DNA is unwound and the two strands are separated and held open, a special RNA enzyme binds to the gene area of the DNA and reads it. When the enzyme recognizes a "start" signal, it moves along the strand and synthesizes a new strand of RNA complementary to the gene area of the DNA. When the enzyme reaches the end of the gene sequence, there will be a "stop" signal that tells the enzyme to stop making new RNA. The newly created RNA strand moves away from the gene. The DNA closes back together and re-coils in the normal helical formation. This new piece of RNA is called messenger RNA (mRNA or sometimes just the "message") because it contains the special coded pattern sequence (the message) for building the specific protein (in this case, insulin) (see diagram at top of page 99).

```
DNA sense  C–A–G–T–A–C–C–A–A–G–T–G–A–T–C–T–G–C
antisense  G–T–C–A–T–G–G–T–T–C–A–C–T–A–G–A–C–G
                                 transcription with
                                 RNA polymerase
mRNA       G–U–C–A–U–G–G–U–U–C–A–C–U–A–G–A–C–G
```

After the mRNA has been transcribed from the gene areas of the DNA, it moves from the nucleus to the cytoplasm. In an active cell, the message becomes very busy here in conjunction with two other types of RNA. A lot of individual amino acids are present inside the cytoplasm, waiting to be properly lined up and hooked together to form a protein. This process is called *translation*. There are also substances called ribosomes, which are made of special bunches of ribosomal RNA, along with yet another type of RNA called *transfer RNA* (tRNA).

Transfer RNAs are adapter molecules that assist in bringing the correct amino acid into the lineup at the proper time. Each tRNA can carry or hold only one amino acid at a time, and the tRNA has an anticodon that is complementary to that specific amino acid's codon. Therefore, because each tRNA can bind to only 1 of the 22 different amino acids, there must be at least 22 different types of tRNA.

In the cytoplasm, the ribosome attaches to the mRNA strand and begins to move along the strand, "reading" the strand as it moves along. When a three-base code is read and interpreted by the ribosome as a specific codon for a specific amino acid, the ribosome allows the tRNAs to come in and attempt to match their anticodons to the codon. When the correct tRNA matches up with the codon on the mRNA, that tRNA releases its amino acid and allows the amino acid to bind to the growing protein strand. This process is repeated all the way down the mRNA until all the correct amino acids are lined up and hooked together in the right order to make the specific protein.

PATTERNS OF INHERITANCE

General rules or concepts concerning the inheritance of specific traits governed by single genes were established by Gregor Mendel and others before gene composition was determined. Much of the preliminary information was obtained through observation and manipulation of many generations of plant reproduction; however, these concepts also appear generally accurate for the transmission of some human traits.

Mendelian Laws of Gene Expression

Mendel's work explained the concept of dominant traits and recessive traits. His observations of different types of garden peas led Mendel to determine that specific varieties of peas had unique traits. For example, one variety of peas always produced wrinkled seeds when fertilized with pollen from the same pea type, whereas another variety of peas always produced smooth seeds when fertilized with pollen from its same pea type. Modeling out this information yielded the following table, in which P_1 indicates the original parent generation, F_1 indicates the first-generation offspring or progeny, F_2 indicates the second-generation offspring or progeny, F_3 indicates the third-generation offspring or progeny, and so forth for succeeding generations. Each generation of progeny was fertilized with pollen from the same generation.

Generation	Smooth Seeds	Wrinkled Seeds
P_1	smooth × smooth	wrinkled × wrinkled
	↓	↓
F_1	all smooth seeds	all wrinkled seeds
	↓ self-pollination	↓ self-pollination
F_2	all smooth seeds	all wrinkled seeds
	↓ self-pollination	↓ self-pollination
F_3	all smooth seeds	all wrinkled seeds
	↓ self-pollination	↓ self-pollination
F_4	all smooth seeds	all wrinkled seeds

When Mendel experimented with cross-pollination (crossbreeding) of pea varieties, the inheritance of the traits came out differently than expected. The following model depicts Mendel's results of using a smooth pea variety fertilized with the pollen of a wrinkled pea variety.

P_1	smooth × wrinkled
F_1	all smooth seeds self-pollination
F_2	smooth and wrinkled seeds (3:1 smooth:wrinkled ratio)

Mendel's explanation for this observation was that the trait for seed texture was determined by the inheritance of a pair of hereditary elements, now known as gene alleles (allele is any possible alternative form of a gene) and that variation existed in the relative "strength" of these two elements. This variation in strength resulted in variable expression of the trait when the pair of hereditary elements was mixed (heterogeneous). When both parent seeds had the same hereditary element or genotypes (homogeneous), all the offspring in succeeding generations have the same appearance or phenotype of the expression of that element. For homogeneous pairs, the phenotypes and the genotypes were identical. When the parent seeds were heterogeneous for a particular hereditary element, the first-generation offspring expressed only the stronger or dominant element even though both elements were present in all offspring. In this situation, the appearance or phenotype was different from the genotype (the appearance of the peas in the F_1 generation was smooth even though the hereditary elements for texture of these peas consisted of one gene allele for smooth texture and one gene allele for wrinkled texture).

The mixed appearance of the peas in the second self-fertilized generation led Mendel to determine that the hereditary element (gene allele) for smooth texture was dominant and the hereditary element for wrinkled texture was recessive. Dominant traits could be expressed in the phenotype when the genotype for that trait was either homogeneous or heterogeneous, but recessive traits could be expressed in the phenotype only when the genotype for that trait was homogeneous.

Further experimentation with cross-pollination of plants led to the determination of codominance or incomplete dominance. In cross-pollinating red roses with white roses in the parental generation, Mendel predicted that only the dominant color trait would be expressed in the F_1 generation, with both colors being expressed in the F_2 generation (in a 3:1 ratio). Because red was a stronger, bolder color, Mendel expected that the first-generation flowers from this cross-pollination would all be red. Instead, the roses in the first-generation progeny were all pink, indicating that the gene for red and the gene for white were equally dominant. Roses in the second generation of this cross-pollination were red, pink, and white in a 1:2:1 ratio. Thus in codominance, the phenotype accurately expresses the genotype. Red roses must have two red gene alleles (homogeneous), pink roses must have one red gene allele and one white gene allele (heterogeneous), and white roses must have two white gene alleles (homogeneous).

These mendelian rules for patterns of inheritance apply only to those traits or characteristics that are regulated by a single gene with multiple possible alleles. The relationship between genotype and phenotypic expression as well as predictability can be explained with the use of the Punnett square. This model involves plotting the known maternal genotype for one or more specific traits against the known paternal genotype for the same specific trait or traits (Fig. 9–11). The example provided in Figure 9–11 uses blood type. The allele for type O blood is recessive, and the alleles for either type A or type B blood are dominant.

The mother in Figure 9–11*A* is phenotypically and genotypically type O (OO); the father is phenotypically and genotypically type B (BB). The expected genotypes for all first-generation offspring is BO, with the expressed phenotype for all first-generation offspring being type B blood.

The mother in Figure 9–11*B* is phenotypically and genotypically type O (OO), and the father is phenotypically and genotypically heterozygous (BO). The expected expression and genotypes for the first-generation offspring of this mating would be 50 percent heterozygous (BO) with a type B phenotype and 50 percent homozygous (OO) with a type O phenotype.

In Figure 9–11*C*, the mother and father are both phenotypically type B and genotypically heterogeneous (BO). The expected phenotypes and genotypes for the first-generation offspring of this mating would be type B (25 percent homozygous [BB] and 50 percent heterozygous [BO]) and 25 percent type O (homozygous OO). Therefore, two parents expressing type B blood can produce a child with type O blood if they are both genotypically heterozygous for that blood type.

In Figure 9–11*D*, the mother and father both express type O blood. Because the alleles for type O blood are recessive, the presumed genotype for this pair is OO, with the expected phenotypes and genotypes in all the first-generation offspring being type O homozygous (OO). According to mendelian patterns of inheritance, it is not possible for parents with a type O phenotype to produce a child with type B blood. However, two type O parents have (rarely) produced a child with blood type B (with absolute parentage established by tissue typing and the presence of identifying polymorphic chromosomes). One explanation for this phenomenon is incomplete penetrance of a dominant trait. In such a situation, one of the phenotypically type O blood parents could have a BO genotype, but in that parent the type B blood allele did not completely penetrate and therefore did not get expressed. Because the B gene was present, it was able to be transmitted to the offspring, in whom penetrance was complete and the gene expressed.

A

Mother		O	O
Father	B	BO	BO
	B	BO	BO

B

Mother		O	O
Father	B	BO	BO
	O	OO	OO

C

Mother		B	O
Father	B	BB	BO
	O	BO	OO

D

Mother		O	O
Father	O	OO	OO
	O	OO	OO

FIGURE 9–11. Punnett squares of single-gene traits.

Patterns of Traits Inherited by Single-Gene Transmission

A trait may be controlled by a single gene (regardless of whether that single gene is dominant or recessive). The chromosomal locations of some genes have been specifically identified or mapped on human chromosomes; the exact location of many genes have not yet been identified. Even without establishing the chromosome location, it is possible to determine how the gene for a specific trait is transmitted. By looking at how that trait is expressed through multiple generations of a family, specific patterns emerge that indicate whether that gene is dominant, recessive, located on an autosomal chromosome, or located on one of the sex chromosomes. This information can be elucidated without identification of the specific gene through the use of pedigree analysis. Determining inheritance patterns for a specific trait makes it possible be more accurate in predicting the risk for any one individual of transmitting that trait or characteristic.

The pedigree is a schematic drawing of a family history, which allows a pictorial representation of patterns of inheritance over many generations. When analyzing a pedigree, the answers to the following specific questions are noted:

1. Is any pattern of inheritance present or does the trait appear sporadic?
2. Is the trait transmitted equally or unequally to males and females?
3. Is the trait present in every generation or does it skip a generation?
4. Do only affected individuals have children affected with the trait or can unaffected individuals also have children who express the trait?

Figure 9–12 shows a variety of typical pedigrees for a number of inherited traits. Pedigree construction as a part of history taking provides the following advantages:

1. It facilitates note taking, increasing the accuracy of the

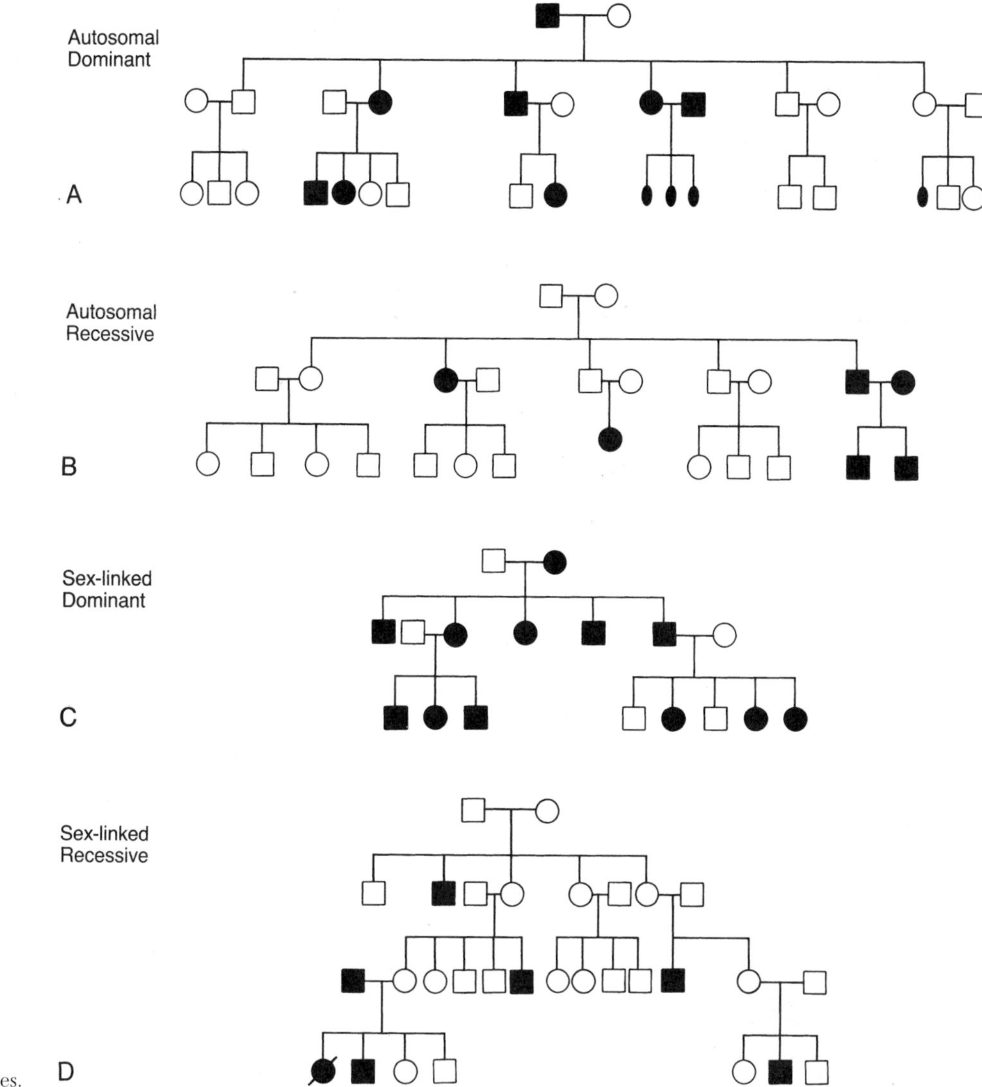

FIGURE 9–12. Pedigrees.

history taking and serving as a means to organize collected information.

2. It serves as a means of communication, allowing sharing of information that has been collected by one member of the health care team with other professionals working with the individual or family so that information is not repeated.
3. It provides a means for professionals working with an individual or family to visualize and validate the relationships of affected individuals within a family scope. Creating a visual image of relationships may assist family members in clarifying who is or is not a blood relative of an affected individual.
4. It facilitates emergence of patterns of inheritance for a specific trait within a specific family.
5. It enhances analysis of gene expression and transmission of more than one trait through linkage studies.
6. It helps to identify individuals at risk within a kinship more accurately (who, once identified, can have examination or counseling).

Construction of a pedigree involves the use of a symbol key (some symbols vary with region, institution, and organization). A typical key for pedigree construction and analysis is presented in Figure 9–13. The pedigree is usually started with the *proband* (also known as the *prepositus*), the individual who draws medical (genetic) attention to the family. Usually the proband is indicated with an arrow.

The four types of inheritance patterns associated with single-gene controlled traits include autosomal dominant, autosomal recessive, sex-linked dominant, and sex-linked recessive. Each inheritance pattern for single-gene controlled traits is characterized by specific defining criteria.

Traits With an Autosomal Dominant Pattern of Inheritance

Autosomal dominant single-gene traits require that the gene controlling the trait is located on an autosomal chromosome and is usually expressed even when the gene is present on only one chromosome of a chromosome pair. The pedigree in Figure 9–12*A* depicts a typical autosomal dominant pattern of inheritance that meets all the defining criteria:

1. The trait appears in every generation with no skipping. When the trait is a result of a new mutation (de novo), this criterion is demonstrated only in the branch of the pedigree stemming from the person who first exhibited the new mutation.

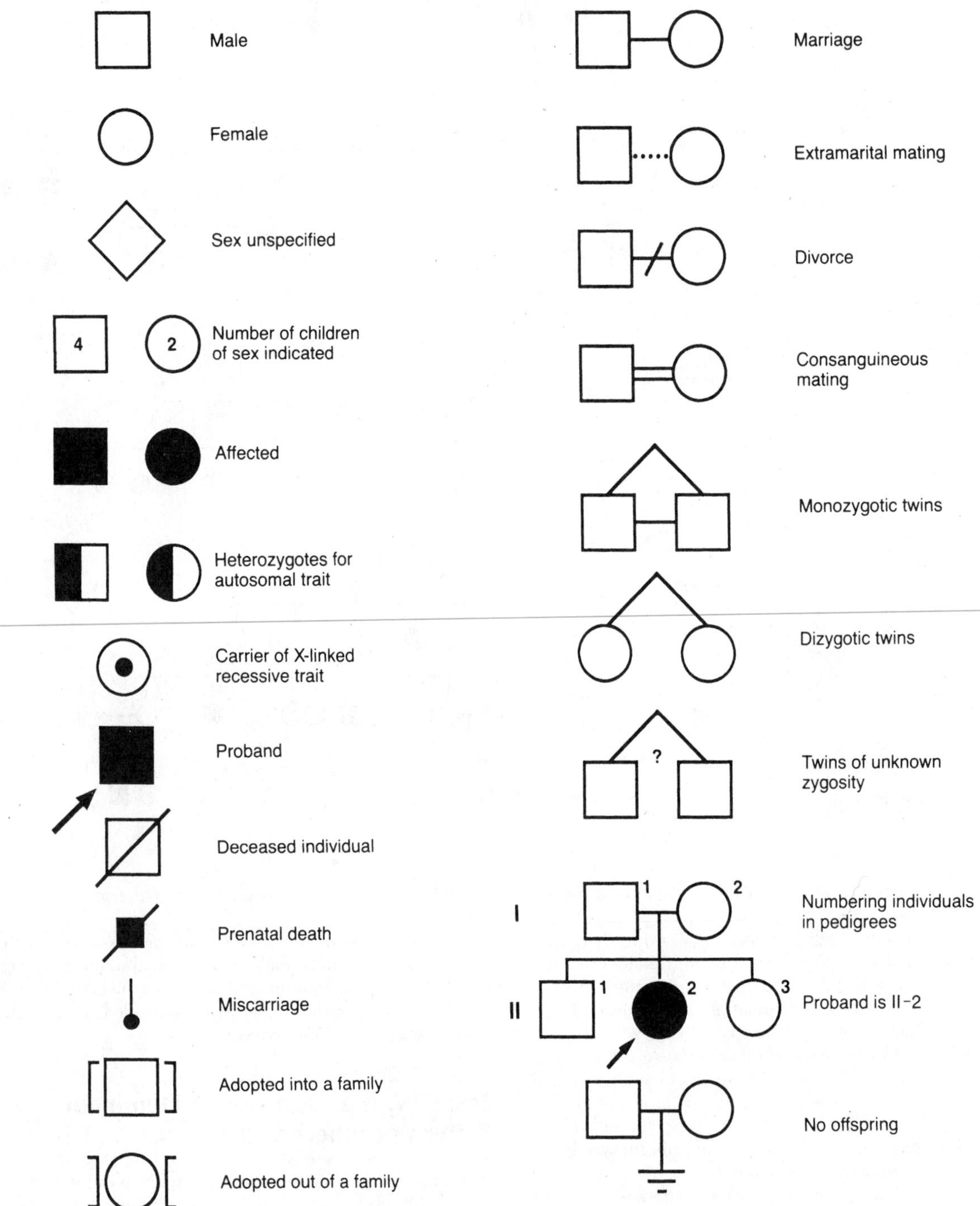

FIGURE 9–13. Key for pedigree construction and analysis. (From Thompson, M.W., McInnes, R.R., & Willard, H.F. [1991]. *Thompson & Thompson genetics in medicine* [5th ed., p. 55]. Philadelphia: W. B. Saunders. Reprinted with permission.)

2. The risk for affected individuals to have affected children is 50 percent with each pregnancy.
3. Unaffected individuals do not have affected children; therefore, their risk is 0 percent.
4. The trait is found equally in males and females.

Autosomal dominant patterns of inheritance are associated with many normal variations in body structure, such as brown eye color, widow's peak hairline, and curly hair. In addition, this pattern of inheritance has been demonstrated in a variety of genetically transmitted problems, including achondroplasia, familial hypercholesterolemia, Huntington's disease, dentinogenesis imperfecta, brachydactyly, allergic hypersensitivity, Marfan's syndrome, and familial hypercalcemia.

Traits With an Autosomal Recessive Pattern of Inheritance

Autosomal recessive single-gene traits require that the gene controlling the trait be located on an autosomal chromosome and that the trait can be expressed only when the gene is present on both chromosomes of a chromosome pair. The pedigree in Figure 9–12*B* depicts a typical autosomal recessive pattern of inheritance that meets all the defining criteria:

1. The trait appears in alternate generations of any one branch of a kinship.
2. The trait or characteristic usually first appears only in siblings (progeny of unaffected parents) rather than in the parents themselves.
3. Approximately 25 percent of a kinship is affected and expresses the trait.
4. The children of an affected father and an affected mother are always affected (risk is 100 percent for each pregnancy). Two affected individuals cannot have an unaffected child.
5. Unaffected individuals who are carriers (have the gene on only one chromosome of a chromosome pair) and do not express the trait themselves can transmit the trait to their offspring if their mate either is also a carrier or is affected. The risk of a carrier having a child who expresses the trait is 25 percent with each pregnancy when the carrier is married to another carrier, 50 percent with each pregnancy when the carrier is married to an affected individual, and 0 percent with each pregnancy when the carrier is married to a noncarrier. The risk of the unaffected carrier having a child who is a carrier for the trait is 50 percent with each pregnancy.
6. The trait is found equally in males and females.

Autosomal recessive patterns of inheritance are associated with many normal characteristics and variations in body structure and function, such as blue eye color, straight hair, and the Rh-negative blood type. In addition, this pattern of inheritance has been demonstrated in a variety of genetically transmitted conditions, including albinism, sickle cell anemia, cystic fibrosis, phenylketonuria, Tay-Sachs disease, Hurler's syndrome, Bloom's syndrome, Fanconi's anemia, galactosemia, and hyperextensible thumb.

For some of these diseases, the carrier has no symptom of the trait, and in other conditions the carrier does not express the full-blown condition but may express a more mild form when predisposing environmental or personal events are present. For example, carriers of sickle cell anemia may have some sickling of their red blood cells under conditions of extreme hypoxia, although the sickling is never as severe or widespread as it is in the person who is homozygous for sickle cell anemia.

Sex-Linked Patterns of Inheritance

Some genes are present only on the sex chromosomes. The Y chromosome appears to have few genes that are not also present on the X chromosome. However, the X chromosome has many single genes that do not appear to be present elsewhere in the human genome. Thus, for all intents and purposes, the discussion of sex-linked patterns of inheritance is really a discussion of X-linked patterns of inheritance.

Because there is an unequal distribution of X chromosomes between males and females (1:2, respectively), there is an accompanying unequal distribution of the X-linked chromosome genes between the two sexes. Males have only one X chromosome and are said to be hemizygous for any gene on the X chromosome. As a result, X-linked recessive genes have a dominant expressive pattern of inheritance in males and a recessive expressive pattern of inheritance in females. This difference in expression occurs because males do not have a second X chromosome to balance the expression of any recessive gene on the first X chromosome.

Dominant Patterns

Sex-linked (X-linked) dominant single-gene traits require that the gene controlling the trait be located on only one of the X chromosomes in order for the trait to be expressed. The pedigree in Figure 9–12*C* depicts a typical sex-linked dominant pattern of inheritance that meets all the defining criteria.

The most common known X-linked dominant problem is hypophosphatemia. Examination of the pedigree demonstrates that this condition meets the following defining criteria:

1. There is no carrier status; all individuals with the gene are affected.
2. Female children of affected males are all affected (risk is 100 percent), whereas the male children of affected males are unaffected (risk is 0 percent). Therefore, the overall risk of an affected male having affected children is 50 percent for each pregnancy, since the probability of having a female is also 50 percent. It is the inheritance of the trait by female offspring of affected males that defines the problem as X-linked dominant, since the inheritance pattern among the offspring of affected females identically resembles an autosomal dominant pattern.
3. The trait appears in every generation.
4. For homozygous females, the risk of having an affected child is 100 percent with each pregnancy, and offspring of both sexes are affected equally. For heterozygous females, the risk of having an affected child is 50 percent with each pregnancy, and children of both sexes are equally at risk.
5. In the general population, X-linked dominant problems affect twice as many females as males, but heterozygous females usually express a more mild form of the problem than do the hemizygous males.

Recessive Patterns

Sex-linked (X-linked) recessive single-gene traits are among the most well defined inherited health problems. This pattern of inheritance requires that the gene controlling the trait be present on both of the X chromosomes in order for the trait to be fully expressed in females (females must be homozygous for the trait) and on only one of the X chromosomes in order for the trait to be expressed in males (males must be hemizygous). The pedigree in Figure 9–12*D* depicts a typical sex-linked recessive pattern of inheritance that meets all the defining criteria:

1. Expression or incidence of the trait is much higher among males in a kinship (and in the general population) than among females.
2. The trait cannot be transmitted from father to son because the father contributes only the Y chromosome to his son's sex chromosome pair.

3. Transmission of the trait is from father to all daughters (who are all carriers but either do not express any of the trait or express it in a very mild form).
4. Female carriers have a 50 percent risk (with each pregnancy) of transmitting the gene to their offspring. Female offspring inheriting the trait are carriers, and male offspring inheriting the trait are affected.

Sex-linked recessive inheritance patterns may be responsible for normal variation of some secondary female sex characteristics. In addition, this pattern of inheritance has been associated with a variety of disorders including hemophilia (A and B), Duchenne muscular dystrophy, ichthyosis, Lesch-Nyhan syndrome, color blindness and, probably, fragile X syndrome. For some of these disorders, females who are heterozygous for the gene have no overt symptoms of the disorder (such as color blindness), whereas for other disorders, female heterozygotes do express some mild aberrations (increased bleeding tendency with carriers of hemophilia, mild retardation in fragile X syndrome). Few females expressing homozygosity for these disorders have been found. It is probable that the homozygosity leads to such a severe disorder that it is lethal in embryonic or early fetal life.

Multifactorial Inheritance

Some single-gene traits have a consistently predictable pattern of gene expression that follows strict mendelian law for patterns of inheritance and degree of expression in affected individuals. Other single-gene traits have a relatively high level of variability (especially autosomal dominant traits), with no established reason for this variation of expression. Some proposed theories include the concept of evolution. This concept suggests that developmental interactions over time (generations) may modify the response of the individual to an abnormal gene. Another theory is that although a particular trait may be the result of the expression of one gene, other genes may act in concert to regulate the activity and expression of that one gene. This theory suggests that in order for the expression of an aberrant gene to cause severe problems, a regulating gene or genes must also have abnormal expression.

In addition to variation in the expression of single genes, it is now known that a single gene may be responsible for the expression of many effects that appear unrelated. This concept is known as *pleiotropy* and probably involves changes or aberrations in regulatory genes rather than in structural genes. One example of pleiotropy is Marfan's syndrome. This syndrome is transmitted as an autosomal dominant trait, but the expression involves a variety of aberrations in unrelated tissue types. These aberrations include excessive growth of long bones, the presence (or predisposition to the development of) an aortic aneurysm, and severe nearsightedness.

Some heritable problems are associated with more than one gene. For example, congenital deafness is an outcome associated with a variety of abnormal genes, although not all of the genes have to be abnormal for deafness to result. A possible explanation for this phenomenon is that ear development and hearing involve complex structures and functions that require the input of many genes working in concert for proper development during embryonic and fetal life. An aberration in any one of these genes may result in a failure of one specific aspect of development that leads to overt deafness, although the exact mechanism causing the deafness is different for each gene aberration. Therefore, more than one factor can cause the aberrant development. When more than one gene is responsible for a specific characteristic or trait, the trait is said to be controlled through polygenic expression. Other examples of developing tissues that require polygenic expression for normal development and that can develop abnormally if any of the required genes is not normal include cleft palate and neural tube defects.

CHROMOSOMAL ABERRATIONS

As discussed earlier in this chapter, chromosomes are formed during the metaphase of mitosis from tightly packed, supercoiled DNA. Each chromosome contains hundreds of genes. Detectable aberrations of any chromosome can result in aberration in the structure or expression of one or more genes (Moore et al., 1994).

Numeric Aberrations

The normal diploid number of human chromosomes at metaphase of mitosis is 46—that is, 23 pairs. Some individuals have missing or extra whole chromosomes. This type of aberration usually is the result of abnormal or delayed disjunction during meiosis I or meiosis II in gamete formation. Thus, instead of resulting in the formation of all gametes that each contain 23 chromosomes, some gametes have 24 chromosomes, some have 22 chromosomes, and some have 23 chromosomes. When a 24-chromosome gamete is united with a 23-chromosome gamete of the opposite sex during fertilization, the resulting new individual has 47 chromosomes. One chromosome set contains three copies of a chromosome instead of the normal two copies. This situation is termed a *trisomy*. When a 22-chromosome gamete from one parent is united with a 23-chromosome gamete of the other parent during fertilization, the resulting new individual has 45 chromosomes. One chromosome set contains only one copy of a chromosome instead of the normal two copies. This situation is termed a *monosomy*. Whenever the individual has more or fewer chromosomes than normal, some malformations and abnormal developmental processes are expressed. Nondisjunction is most commonly associated with advanced maternal age at the time of conception, presumably as a result of primary oocytes spending years in prophase of meiosis I. However, nondisjunction can occur at any age.

In theory, nondisjunction can occur within any chromosome pair. However, in examining the chromosomes of individuals who survive into the fetal period, it is apparent that nondisjunction of some chromosome pairs must lead to embryolethal consequences. The most common chromosomal aberration found among all conceptuses is a missing X chromosome—Turner's syndrome (45,XO). Evidently most conceptuses with a chromosome constitution of 45,XO do not survive beyond the embryonic period. The most common chromosomal aberration observed among newborns is trisomy 21 (Down syndrome) (47,XX or XY, +21). Other syndromes of trisomy that can be observed among newborns include trisomy 13, trisomy 15, trisomy 18, and sex chromosome trisomies (47,XXX; 47,XXY; 47,XYY). Trisomy 16 has been identified in embryonic and early fetal wastage, but this abnormality does not usually lead to a fully developed individual. Autosomal monosomes may be conceived but rarely survive to the stage of birth, although monosomy 21 has been reported among newborns.

All individuals with autosomal trisomies experience some degree of mental retardation. In addition, each trisomy is associated with a specific set of abnormalities, malformations, and unique developmental patterns. This is why although individuals with trisomy share heritable characteristics in common with their normal family members (such as hair color and texture, skin tone, eye color, and so on), many structural features in these individuals tend to resemble other nonrelated individuals who have the same trisomy.

Individuals with missing or extra whole sex chromosomes tend to be intellectually normal and have fewer recognizable physical malformations when compared with individuals with autosomal numeric aberrations. Somewhat controversial is the concept that these individuals have behavioral patterns that are not completely normal, such as attention deficit problems and other learning disorders.

Table 9–1 indicates the malformations and developmental deviations associated with the five most common syndromes of numeric chromosomal aberrations.

Structural Aberrations

Structural aberrations can occur in either of two ways. Parts of chromosomes can break off and either become lost or attach themselves to other chromosomes, an actual translocation of chromosome material from one chromosome to another. Also, one whole chromosome can become joined to another whole chromosome, a translocation of chromosomes called *robertsonian translocation.*

When chromosomes are broken and translocated to other chromosomes, the total amount of chromosome material may be balanced (normal) or unbalanced (abnormal). If the total amount of chromosome material present in the individual's cells is normal (balanced), even though it is not located in the usual positions, the individual is phenotypically normal. Problems do not arise until this individual reproduces. Because some of this individual's gametes are not normal (i.e., not balanced) as a result of random assortment and independent segregation of chromatids during gametogenesis, the person is at risk for having chromosomally unbalanced and abnormal offspring. This individual should be referred for genetic counseling. The same situation is true for individuals with robertsonian translocations. As long as the normal amount of chromosome material is present in all the individual's cells, the individual is phenotypically normal, even though chromosome locations might be abnormal.

PRENATAL TESTING AND SCREENING

For some heritable conditions, prenatal screening is available to determine whether or not a fetus is affected. The issue of prenatal diagnosis is complex. Many of the tests are expensive, carry some degree of risk to the pregnancy, and cannot always provide conclusive results. Tests may be performed directly on fetal cells or indirectly on products synthesized by the fetus, or by imaging.

Fetal Ultrasonography

Fetal ultrasonography involves the use of high-frequency sound waves that are reflected differently in various media and in tissues of different densities. With computer enhancement, ultrasonography can provide a relatively detailed image of the embryo and fetus. Interpretation of the images produced has been refined to such a degree that even minor structural aberrations can be detected. Ultrasonography is frequently used in locating the placenta, cord, embryo or fetus, amniotic fluid pockets, and other associated structures before engaging in diagnostic procedures that are more invasive. Fetal ultrasonography can provide information regarding fetal age, the amount of amniotic fluid present, and a variety of structural abnormalities. Among the many abnormalities that can be identified with fetal ultrasonography are the following:

Neural tube defects (spina bifida, encephaloceles, microcephaly, anencephaly, hydrocephaly)
Skeletal dysplasia (fractures, disproportions, bowing)
Gastrointestinal anomalies (gastroschisis, atresias, tracheoesophageal fistulas)
Congenital heart disease (coarctation of the aorta, transposition of the great vessels) (echocardiograms can be performed in conjunction with ultrasonography to determine chamber and

TABLE 9–1 Characteristics of Common Chromosomal Syndromes

Trisomy 21 (Down Syndrome)
Mental retardation
Skeletal muscle hypotonia
Broad, flat face
Epicanthal folds
Widely spaced eyes
Brushfield spots on irises
Low-set ears
Thick, protruding, and furrowed tongue
Short neck with redundant skin folds
Simian crease on palmar surface
Clinodactyly of the fifth finger
Rocker-bottom feet
Wide separation between first and second toes
Frequent cardiac cushion defects

Trisomy 13 (Trisomy D)
Profound mental retardation
Central nervous system malformations
Polydactyly
Cardiac defects
Malformations of the eye (all types)
Urogenital defects
Cleft lip and palate
Clenched fists
Rocker-bottom feet

Trisomy 18
Mental retardation
Failure to thrive
Skeletal muscle hypertonia

Trisomy 18 *(Continued)*
Prominent occiput
Micrognathia
Low-set, malformed ears
Clenched fists
Simian creases on palmar surfaces
Hypoplastic nails
Rocker-bottom feet
Cardiac defects

Monosomy X (Turner's syndrome)
Short stature
Short neck with some webbing attached to shoulders
Low hairline with hair on neck growing in an upward slant
Broad, shield-like chest
Widely spaced nipples
Inability to fully pronate lower arms
Lack of secondary sex characteristics
Streaked gonad with gonadal dysgenesis

Klinefelter's Syndrome (47,XXY)
Tall stature
Broad hips
Small external male genitalia
Lack of facial hair
Lack of male pubic hair distribution
Infertility

valvular abnormalities, hypoplastic ventricles, and septal defects)
Genitourinary problems (horseshoe kidneys, polycystic kidneys, exstrophy of the bladder, Potter's syndrome, among others)
Cystic hygromas

Advantages. Fetal ultrasonography is noninvasive, readily available, and relatively inexpensive. The procedure can be performed at any stage of pregnancy and can be repeated to determine changes over time.

Disadvantages. Only two proposed disadvantages are associated with fetal ultrasonography. Although the sound waves are presumed to be harmless, little is known about the long-term effects and possible damage these waves can inflict on developing tissues. In addition, the images are subject to misinterpretation when viewed by physicians with inadequate training or skill. The relatively low cost of ultrasonography equipment, coupled with increased patient demand for its use, has caused many private physicians to incorporate ultrasonography routinely in their practices, and many of these physicians have not had special training in its use and interpretation.

Tests on Fetally Derived Cells

A wide variety of tests can be performed directly on fetally derived cells. The most common methods of obtaining fetal cells are through amniocentesis and chorionic villus sampling.

Chromosome Analysis by Amniocentesis

Amniocentesis is an invasive procedure in which the amniotic cavity is accessed under sterile conditions through the abdominal wall of the mother. This procedure is usually performed in conjunction with fetal ultrasonography to minimize the risks of puncturing vital fetal structures with the relatively large-bore amniocentesis needle. The ideal gestational age for safe amniocentesis is 16 weeks after conception has occurred. At this time, there is considerable amniotic fluid, and the fetus is capable of shedding many viable cells. Once the needle is in place, approximately 20 ml of amniotic fluid is withdrawn. Some viable fetal cells will be present in the fluid.

Usually there are not enough fetal cells to ensure an adequate sample size for most tests. Therefore, it is necessary to place these cells on a slide or culture plate and cultivate them in tissue culture, increasing the number of cells to ensure an adequate sample size.

The amniotic fluid is centrifuged under sterile conditions. The dense cells separate from the fluid and migrate to the bottom of the tube. These cells are gently transferred from the tube to tissue culture plates or flasks into which nutrient medium is added. The cells are incubated for 3 to 10 days. When the cells have undergone sufficient mitoses to increase the original number of cells by at least a factor of 10, most tests for abnormal conditions can be accomplished. The most common tests performed include chromosome analysis, enzyme analysis, tests for the presence or absence of a specific product, and examination of genes through the use of molecular probes.

When sufficient fetal cells are present in the cultures, a substance is added to trap cells in metaphase of mitosis (the stage during which chromosomes are visible). The cells are harvested and the chromosomes analyzed.

Advantages. The major advantage of chromosome analysis by amniocentesis for prenatal screening is accuracy. These techniques have been refined to such a degree that identification of even relatively small structural aberrations (such as the interstitial deletion of chromosome 11, and the small deletion on chromosome 15 associated with Prader-Willi syndrome) is possible.

Disadvantages. There are numerous disadvantages of chromosome analysis by amniocentesis. One disadvantage is the amount of time involved for a complete analysis—from 1 to 3 weeks. The procedure itself is labor-intensive and expensive (approximately $1000.00), and not all insurance providers cover the cost of this test. Because amniocentesis is an invasive technique, the complication of infection is possible. In addition, it is possible that the needle penetrating maternal tissues can become contaminated with maternal cells and these cells may be cultured instead of fetal cells. Thus, the results of the chromosome analysis may reflect maternal chromosome constitution rather than fetal chromosomal constitution. A small percentage of women have gone into premature labor following amniocentesis. Although the risk of this complication is low, it is still possible.

Chromosome Analysis by Chorionic Villus Sampling

Chromosome analysis can also be performed on fetally derived tissues obtained through chorionic villus sampling. This technique involves removing a piece of tissue from the growing placenta after its location has been identified through ultrasonography. The needle can be inserted either through the cervical os (more common method) or by transabdominal puncture. This procedure can be performed during the first trimester, as early as 9 to 10 weeks' gestation.

Advantages. The major advantage is timing. The chorionic villi are rapidly dividing cells, and because a large number of cells are obtained by the sampling technique, chromosome analysis can be completed in 1 to 3 days.

Disadvantages. At the current state of this technique, the major disadvantage is concerned with accuracy. These preparations are not yet as refined as chromosome analysis by amniocentesis, and although numeric aberrations are easily identified by chorionic villus sampling, small structural aberrations may be missed. Possible complications of this procedure include infection and spontaneous abortion. There is also a disadvantage of possible material contamination. This contamination can result in faulty test results. There have been concerns about the procedure causing fetal anomalies or damage but there has been no research to support these fears.

Enzyme Analysis

Some genetic metabolic diseases are caused by a deficiency of a specific enzyme in the fetus. Often, these children are born normal because maternal enzymes crossed the placenta and performed the specific function in the fetus. However, when the child is born, maternal enzymes can no longer be used, and whatever pathway is affected by the missing or inactive enzyme begins to demonstrate abnormal build-up of products or abnormal metabolism.

Fetal cells cultured for several weeks away from maternal enzyme influences can express the same metabolic abnormalities that the child would show after birth. Enzyme analysis of the cells or culture fluid, or both, can determine whether a specific enzyme is present at all or whether it is present in normal concentrations. Some of the genetic metabolic problems that can be identified through enzyme analysis of fetal cells include Tay-Sachs disease, Hurler's syndrome, metachromatic leukodystrophy, galactosemia, and homocystinuria.

Disadvantages. The disadvantages of these screening procedures involve (1) the sampling technique and (2) the possibility of laboratory error. The sampling techniques of amniocentesis or chorionic villi sampling have already been discussed. Laboratory errors with false-positive and false-negative results do happen and are more likely to occur at laboratories with less experience in performing these analyses.

Molecular Probes

In some cases, the actual gene associated with a specific problem has been identified, and molecular probes complementary to the gene have been made. These probes can be used to determine whether the gene is present in the fetal cells. It is not necessary to have dividing fetal cells to use molecular probes, although a sufficient volume of cells is necessary. In some cases, enough fetal cells can be obtained at amniocentesis or chorionic villus sampling so that the test can be performed directly on the DNA of the tissue. At other times, a greater volume of fetal cells is required, and it is necessary to grow the fetal cells in culture first before the DNA can be extracted and probed.

Some molecular probes are commercially available, so testing is more available and less costly. Genetic metabolic diseases for which there are molecular probes commercially available include cystic fibrosis, hemophilia B, Huntington's disease, retinoblastoma, sickle cell anemia, and thalassemia. Molecular probes for other genetic metabolic diseases are not commercially available, and the tests can be performed only in certain university research centers. These genetic metabolic diseases include Duchenne muscular dystrophy, hemophilia A, Lesch-Nyhan syndrome, neurofibromatosis, and phenylketonuria.

Disadvantages. The major disadvantages for these prenatal screening tests are sampling-related (as stated previously) and test-specific. These tests are expensive and not completely perfected (increased risk of false-positive and false-negative results).

Alpha-Fetoprotein

Alpha-fetoprotein (AFP) is normally synthesized in measurable quantities only during embryonic and fetal life. In the early embryo, the yolk sac synthesizes AFP. Later this function is picked up by the fetal liver and gastrointestinal cells. AFP is present in fetal blood and some extracellular fluids and serves the same function that albumin does in human blood after birth. Because fetal and maternal circulations are integrated, substances made by the fetus that are small enough move down their concentration gradients into maternal serum. In addition, AFP is present in fetal urine, so it is also present in amniotic fluid. The synthesis of AFP is well regulated, and the pattern of normal amniotic fluid levels specific to gestational age is known. Variation from this normal pattern is associated with some developmental problems.

AFP can be measured in the amniotic fluid (requires amniocentesis) or in maternal serum. The accuracy of both levels requires exact identification of gestational age at the time the fluid or serum is obtained.

AFP levels are considered elevated if they are at least twice the value of the mean for that specific gestational age. The most common problem associated with elevated AFP levels is an open neural tube defect (the open tube provides a means for extra AFP to leak into the amniotic fluid).

Lower than normal AFP levels also have been associated with fetal developmental problems, although this phenomenon shows more variability. The most common condition consistently associated with low AFP values is Down syndrome (although this phenomenon is not consistent enough to be used as the only screen for Down syndrome). Other conditions associated with a low AFP level include gestational diabetes and spontaneous abortion.

Advantages. For open neural tube defects, AFP determination is a reliable screening mechanism with a direct relationship between degree of elevation and degree of neural tube defect (highest levels are associated with anencephaly). Other advantages of this test are that it is relatively inexpensive (usually less than $50.00) and widely available with a fast turnaround time.

Disadvantages. The test for AFP levels can produce false-positive and false-negative results. False-positive results are associated with inaccurate dating of the pregnancy, twin pregnancy, Turner's syndrome, fetal distress, and intrauterine fetal demise. The value may be falsely elevated if fetal blood is accidentally sampled during the procedure.

Triple-Marker Screen

The triple-marker screen, or triple screen, is prenatal testing that is more sensitive for aneupoloidy than is AFP by itself (Coulson et al., 1996). It is capable of detecting changes in the maternal AFP, human chorionic gonadotropin (hCG) and unconjugated estriol (uE_3). These are particularly useful in detecting conditions such as trisomies. The same factors that can affect AFP levels, of course, can cause inaccurate results in the triple screen—that is, wrong esimated dates of confinement and multiple gestations (twins). Low levels of AFP, uE_3, and hCG indicate possible trisomy 18, whereas high levels of hCG with low levels of AFP and uE_3 are found with Down syndrome (Coulson et al., 1996).

The triple-marker screen is performed between 15 and 20 weeks of gestation. If there is an abnormality found, it should be followed by ultrasonography for confirmation of a problem. The exact mechanism involved in the alteration of AFP and hCG levels when there is a chromosomal problem is not known. It is speculated to be related to a problem with the fetal liver (Coulson et al., 1996).

Advantages. The triple-marker screen is noninvasive and yet more sensitive than most other screening tests for Down syndrome, with a 60 percent detection rate (Coulson et al., 1996).

Disadvantages. The triple-marker screen must be corrected for maternal age and weight. AFP levels in particular can be lower in overweight women if there is not a correction made for this factor. This finding is probably due to an increased maternal blood volume (Coulson et al., 1996). A low AFP value is also found in insulin-dependent diabetics and must be corrected. Ethnic differences are also noted in black women who have a 9 to 15 percent higher AFP level than their white counterparts (Coulson et al., 1996). Smoking is also known to result in an increase in AFP levels but a lowering of the hCG and uE_3 levels. No correction for this condition is advocated but should be considered.

NURSE'S ROLE IN GENETICS

Genetics is a complex topic and touches on many aspects of perinatal and neonatal nursing. It involves prenatal screening and diagnosis, assistance with infertility testing and intervention, diagnosis of congenital syndromes and associations and metabolic disease, identification of reproductive hazards in the workplace and the surrounding environment for the professional as well as the lay public, identification of congenital problems secondary to substance abuse, and fetal therapy and surgery and the neonatal implications following such procedures (Jones, 1994; Wright, 1994). For neonatal nurses, knowledge about critical periods of development, prenatal testing procedures, and long-term neonatal outcomes is essential. Why should neonatal nurses be concerned with this information? What is the neonatal nurse's role in genetics?

Over the past 25 years, advances in genetic knowledge, resulting especially from the findings from the Human Genome Project, coupled with technologic advances, have made prenatal screening and diagnosis available as part of conventional prenatal care. Genetic disease and congenital anomalies occur in 3 to 5 percent of liveborn children and make up 25 to 50 percent of pediatric hospital admissions and 10 percent of adult hospital admissions (Hall, 1987; Jones, 1988; Weatherall, 1985; Zacharias, 1990).

A positive family history for a disorder as well as identification with ethnic, racial, or age groups at risk for genetic conditions may encourage couples to seek prenatal testing. Carrier status screening is available for many disorders such as cystic fibrosis, hemophilia, and sickle cell and thalassemia trait or disease. There have been 370 disorders identified. A woman who is a carrier of an X-linked disorder has a 50 percent chance of passing the affected gene to her child. This could have devastating results, such as severe mental retardation in fragile X syndrome or muscular degeneration and death as in Duchenne muscular dystrophy (Jones, 1994).

Prenatal testing is performed through either maternal-fetal tissue cell or fluid analysis or through the use of ultrasonography to visualize the fetus and detect major structural abnormalities. Fetal echocardiography and Doppler blood flow studies are being widely used to determine congenital malformations, fetal distress, or circulatory problems in high-risk pregnancies (Robinson & Linden, 1993). Fetal tissue cells obtained through chorionic villus sampling at 9 to 11 weeks' gestation, or by amniocentesis at 14 to 17 weeks' gestation (amniocentesis is being performed as early as 12½ weeks gestation) can be analyzed for chromosomal and single-gene defects and for the detection of enzyme deficiencies (Cohen, 1984; Lemons & Brock, 1990).

Maternal serum and amniotic fluid analysis allows screening for proteins such as AFP. High levels of AFP may point to the presence of an open neural tube defect in the fetus. Testing amniotic fluid for the presence of acetylcholinesterase and using ultrasonography for fetal visualization has helped identify 90 percent of normal pregnancies with an elevated AFP (Cohen, 1984).

Elevated AFP levels may also indicate (1) multiple pregnancy, (2) underestimated fetal gestational age, (3) open body defects such as omphalocele, (4) Rh disease, (5) threatened miscarriage or fetal death, and (6) other conditions such as polycystic kidneys, Turner's syndrome, sacrococcygeal teratoma, and Meckel's syndrome (Lemons & Brock, 1990).

Recent studies demonstrate that low levels of AFP may point to a fetus with Down syndrome. According to Gabbe and colleagues (1986), there is a three- to sevenfold increase in risk over that determined for maternal age (Lemons & Brock, 1990).

Genetic abnormalities can also be sought by retrieving blood samples for DNA testing via percutaneous umbilical blood sampling. This procedure is usually performed using ultrasonographic visualization after 16 weeks' gestation; it involves the collection of a fetal blood sample for DNA analysis. This type of testing also enables the detection of fetal coagulopathies and hemoglobinopathies (Lemons & Brock, 1990; Robinson & Linden, 1993). An important aspect of prenatal screening and testing is awareness of preconceptual and postconceptual reproductive hazards.

Reproductive hazards are a concern for professionals and the public. Neonatal nurses are questioning their own reproductive hazards in the workplace. Handling chemotherapeutic or antineoplastic agents, giving aerosolized medications such as ribavirin (Prows, 1989), and exposure to viruses such as cytomegalovirus, rubella, toxoplasmosis, herpes simplex, acquired immunodeficiency syndrome (AIDS), and hepatitis have all been linked with possible birth defects (Williamson et al., 1988). It is estimated that one in three conceptions will end in spontaneous abortion, a congenital malformation, or a genetic dysfunction. The exact cause in about 60 percent of the cases will be unknown (Brent, 1987), but reproductive hazards probably play an important role in these statistics.

Antibiotics, anticonvulsants, antineoplastic agents, and other medications have been implicated as reproductive hazards (Conover, 1994; Shortridge, 1990). Anesthetic gases and organic solvents are suspected to affect fetal development. Although not proved, studies have consistently shown the potential for fetal malformations and increased fetal loss among women operating room personnel (American Society of Anesthesiologists, 1974; Cohen et al., 1971; Letts & Wilkinson, 1985; Williamson et al., 1988). This finding was supported by Saurel-Cubizolles and associates (1994) in a study of pregnancy outcomes among operating room nurses. The highest incidence of either spontaneous abortions or birth defects was when there was a combination of exposure to anesthetic gases and antineoplastic agents or tobacco, or a combination of these substances. Neonatal nurses are sometimes exposed to one or more of these agents.

Lifestyle factors such as smoking, alcohol consumption, long hours of work, and stress place neonatal nurses at risk for reproductive and pregnancy complications. Physical agents such as ionized radiation, microwaves, and heat are potential reproductive risks for nurses (Williamson et al., 1988). Nutritional status is also a factor because poor nutrition decreases the efficiency of the immune system (Shortridge, 1990). Because a large number of neonatal nurses are of childbearing age, they must be aware of the role genetics and genetic influences play in their own health. Monitoring their own reproductive health and being knowledgeable about reproductive risks is certainly a part of the nurse's role in genetics (Kenner, 1991). This knowledge can then be applied to practice with neonates and their families.

Through education, the public is becoming more aware of the potential reproductive risks that may be encountered in everyday life. For example, isotretinoin (Accutane), a drug released in 1982 for the treatment of severe acne, is known to cause miscarriages and birth defects if used during or within 1 month of becoming pregnant. Anomalies reported to be associated with the use of isotretinoin are hydrocephaly, microcephaly, small and malformed ears, severe congenital heart defects, and cleft palate (Effective medication, 1984; Schardein, 1985). The mutagenic effects of the drug occur during the early weeks of pregnancy, frequently before a woman knows she is pregnant. The effects are of special concern for teenagers, who are often risk takers and are not knowledgeable about the harmful fetal-neonatal effects of using street drugs, tobacco, or alcohol or practicing huffing (use of inhalant breathing in of substances) during a pregnancy. With the high rate of teenage pregnancy today, this ultimately may have a major impact on the future genetic well-being of children in the United States.

The number of alcohol and substance abusers is growing, as is the number of birth defects. Approximately 1 in 20 women in the United states is considered to be an alcoholic (Nurses Association of the American Association of Obstetrics and Gynecology [NAACOG], 1989).

Fetal alcohol syndrome and fetal alcohol effects are growing problems today. The incidence of fetal alcohol syndrome and fetal alcohol effects in the United States is estimated at one to three cases per 1000 births (Smitherman, 1994). Frequently the diagnosis is not made until later in life in relation to learning disabilities and developmental delays (Cohen, 1984). Signs of fetal alcohol syndrome may include (1) prenatal or postnatal growth retardation; (2) central nervous system involvement such as neurologic abnormalities, developmental delays, or intellectual deficits; and (3) dysmorphologic facial features, which may include microcephaly, microphthalmia or short palpebral fissures, poorly developed philtrum, thin upper lip, or flattened maxillary area (Cohen, 1984).

It is estimated that 4 to 6 million individuals in the United States today are regular cocaine users. It is estimated that 1 in 10 pregnant women uses cocaine, and the rate is significantly higher in some urban areas (Lynch & McKeon, 1990).

It is difficult to show a cause-and-effect relationship between cocaine use in pregnancy and specific birth defects because so many of these women are heavy smokers, coffee drinkers, multiple drug users, and have poor nutritional status and receive little prenatal care. Therefore, cocaine is said to be associated with rather than the direct cause of poor maternal, fetal, and neonatal findings. Two cases of anomalies that have been reported in association with cocaine use in pregnancy include severe ocular malformation and Turner's syndrome with bilateral foot defects (Schardein, 1985).

The neonatal nurse may be the first health care professional to identify an infant who is a victim of substance abuse. Knowledge in this field may enable a nurse to obtain early interventional care for mother and child to decrease the debilitating effects of substance abuse on the family (see Chapter 45, The Drug-Exposed Neonate).

The nurse may be involved preconceptually with families who have past histories of risky behaviors or other families who for some unknown reason have had little success at becoming pregnant. The use of assisted reproductive technologies for in vitro fertilization is having an impact on the field of genetics as never before (Jones, 1994; Lewis, 1994). This technology not only has had a significant impact on the achievement of successful pregnancies but also has helped develop techniques that allow health professionals to perform sophisticated prenatal genetic testing. The opportunity for earlier prenatal diagnosis than chorionic villus sampling is available through the use of preconceptual and preimplantational genetics. Gamete analysis is possible through micromanipulation of the oocyte and aspiration of the first polar body after the first meiotic division. If the polar body containing the abnormal gene for a single-gene disorder (such as cystic fibrosis) is found in a heterozygous woman, the woman can be assured that the remaining oocyte will carry the normal gene (Bombard & Naef, 1993; Jones, 1994). Preimplantational embryo biopsy can be performed by extracting a single cell from the eight-cell embryo at 72 hours of growth and testing it for Y-specific DNA in the case of some X-linked disorders or for other genetic disorders such as Tay-Sachs or cystic fibrosis. This technique would enable only unaffected embryos to be transferred (Bombard & Naef, 1993; Jones, 1994).

The specialty of genetics as a nursing major or option at the master's level is a growing field being pursued by some neonatal nurses. The advanced practitioner with added genetic knowledge is on the cutting edge of the new technologies. This nurse is also in the midst of some of the most intense ethical and legal dilemmas facing neonatal nurses. For example, fetal therapy and surgery is now possible for a variety of conditions. However, the question is raised, "Should the therapy or surgery be performed and who should decide?"

Potentially lethal cardiac arrhythmias of the fetus identified in utero have been successfully treated with medications such as digoxin, propranolol, and quinidine (Ho, 1988; Lingman et al., 1980; Spinnato et al., 1984). This fetal treatment has helped to decrease the number of resulting cases of cardiac failure, hydrops fetalis, and intrauterine death (Ho, 1988) (see Chapter 38, Fetal Therapy).

Conditions such as hydrocephaly, obstructive uropathy, congenital diaphragmatic hernia, gastroschisis, and omphalocele have been successfully treated surgically during fetal life (Ho, 1988; Pediatric surgeons, 1984). Certain guidelines have been established as criteria for fetal surgery: (1) the elimination of the presence of a genetic condition that might be lethal or complicate in utero treatment; (2) careful selection of fetal patients made by a multidisciplinary team involved in the prenatal care and "natural history" of the fetal defect; (3) commitment by the family for involvement and long-term care; and (4) the family's understanding that the treatment is experimental (Ho, 1988) (see Chapter 38, Fetal Therapy). More neonatal nurses are going to see these types of neonates come into their units as fetal therapy and surgery centers spread across the country.

Assessment of the neonatal skin may reveal a genetic problem. A whole area of genetics called *genodermatosis* focuses on genetic skin disorders (Spitz, 1996). Genetic diseases such as Turner's syndrome, Marfan's syndrome, Sturge-Weber syndrome, epidermolysis bullosa, and phenylketonuria are just a few examples of dysfunctions that have skin or dermatologic manifestations. Although not conclusive, these manifestations give the nurse another "genetic" clue of a complex neonatal problem.

Consumers want health professionals to be knowledgeable about these treatments and the long-term prognoses for their infants. Families expect nurses to help them prepare for these treatments and to understand the emotions and trauma involved.

The field of genetics puts emphasis on prevention. The aim is to reduce the long-term complications associated with a disorder. Prevention also includes the "family of the future." There is a need to identify the diagnosis of the proband (the affected individual) as well as to determine the risks to other family members and offspring. The hope is to prevent illness from occurring and to avoid complications that might result in chronic illness or hospitalization.

Community-based screening programs can be cost-effective if sickle cell or Tay-Sachs disease, for example, is detected preconceptually. Fetuses with neural tube defects may be delivered at a tertiary care center where immediate care is available, thus decreasing cost, preventing injury to the neonate, and allowing treatment to begin immediately after birth.

Where does nursing fit into all of this? A nurse with a subspecialty or a major in genetics may act as a genetic counselor to inform the family of their genetic risks, to provide nondirective information, and to provide support during the initial diagnosis and through follow-up. However, the holistic nature of nursing, which takes in the biopsychosocial needs, extends beyond just counseling measures as they are often defined. It includes a broader perspective of care. The six roles of the professional nurse—advocate, practitioner, collaborator, investigator, educator, and leader—are all essential in working with clients and families with genetic and congenital disorders.

Families that are identified through prenatal testing or at the birth of their child as having a genetic problem are shocked by the news. They experience a grief reaction. Loss of the "perfect child" triggers grief and begins the mourning over the unfulfilled expectations of their fantasy child. The nurse can support the family in assimilating the information that is being given by other disciplines. This response can turn into chronic sorrow as grief is prolonged (see Chapter 8, Bereavement: The State of Having Suffered a Loss) Without psychological support and intervention, the family's grief may eventually interfere with their ability to carry out their daily responsibilities (Olsen, 1994). The nurse can help the family recognize the normalcy of such a reaction and can anticipate its occurrence when planning care.

The nurse can also act as an advocate for the family and refer them to community resources such as genetics clinics, family support groups, or specialized home health care services. Access to care issues are also an important aspect of advocacy for these families (Mackta & Weiss, 1994; Prows, 1992). They need to mobilize themselves psychologically in order to use these community supports. Such mobilization is difficult when grief has taken away hope and the ability to move forward. Without active intervention and professional support, many of these families will not progress beyond this stage of immobility. Health professionals must recognize this need early in care to be most effective with intervention.

As specialization and technology improves in health care, the professional often appears to the family as an expert that is too busy or too highly knowledgeable to answer the seemingly less important questions or concerns. Can our efficiency and knowledge as practitioners actually become barriers to communication? Owing to our expertise, we are valued as important to care, but if we do not make ourselves accessible to the family or investigate their concerns, many of these concerns or misconceptions will not be verbalized. Parents sometimes express the feeling that the physician or genetics counselor is too focused on the person with the disorder to be bothered with their other questions (Olsen, 1994). These feelings are not usually shared with the health professional at the time. The nurse involved in follow-up, especially community-based follow-up, often senses these feelings. Collaboration and a sharing of information are needed if the family is to receive holistic care. The family may need referral to a support group (Mackta & Weiss, 1994). There will be a need for referrals for assessment of developmental disabilities so that early intervention can be started (Ross, 1994). Use of the nursing process enables us to identify the needs of the family not addressed by other disciplines (Prows, 1992).

Positive family histories for certain familial or genetic conditions are often identified in community-based health care. A familial problem can also be identified in an inpatient setting or in any type of care unit. Pedigree analysis can be a useful investigative tool in the prevention or detection of a familial problem. Subtle changes in expressivity of a genetic disorder may be detected if this tool is used to obtain and document a family history. Visual charts are more likely to be looked at than are several written pages. This timesaving technique is especially important with shortened hospital stays and fewer personnel, because less time is spent in actually reading charts. A pedigree analysis might also be the key to more aggressive treatment or follow-up on information that might otherwise not be identified. It may also form the basis of health education and teaching, in which the nurse is often involved.

It should also be evident that the educator and collaborator roles do not stop with the immediate client population but must extend to the community at large. There is a tremendous need for interpretation of the information that is being received by the public. A day does not go by that television or newspapers do not have an item that relates to genetics. This information must be clarified, and a nurse with a specialized knowledge in genetics can carry out this public education effectively. Other health professionals who lack this specialized knowledge will also need education about recent genetic developments. Outreach education is an important aspect of nursing practice. Nurses as educators and leaders provide role modeling for mentoring of their peers. They may lead others into formal education in the genetics field and can provide accurate and timely information to nursing and the public.

The neonatal nurse who is involved in community-based follow-up is one type of nurse that is in special need of updated genetic information. Prenatal screening, newborn screening, and early identification of genetic, congenital, or familial problems often occur in this practice setting. This nurse is also involved in the treatment of the actual disease, such as phenylketonuria or cystic fibrosis, and must help educate the family as to the need for compliance with treatment and for continued follow-up care (White et al., 1995). The nurse should also be aware of community resources, both for the lay public and the professional, that provide treatment, support, and education of such medical-genetic disorders.

The genetic clinical nurse specialist or the neonatal nurse involved with neonates and families experiencing genetic problems must use this knowledge in the area of nursing research. This research might include epidemiologic studies following the natural history of a disease or the environmental factors that may be involved as well as qualitative studies that describe the perceptions of families (Kenner & Berling, 1990). The Midcourse Review of Healthy People 2000 objectives by the U.S. Department of Health and Human Services (1995) has revised one of the objectives to address incidence rates and screening for neural tube defects specifically. Educational studies may include a client's or family's knowledge of their specific disease entity. What are their educational needs? What are the educational needs of nurses regarding their knowledge of genetics? Evaluative studies may also be conducted to determine the quality of genetic-based nursing services and their impact on families' needs. Evaluation of nursing care based on outcome criteria is also essential for determining the need for revision or expansion of this care.

Nursing research may potentially have an impact on the morbidity and mortality of patients. Development of protocols and standards based on nursing research findings may be instrumental in significantly decreasing long-term complications of the very low birth weight infant. Developmental supportive environmental studies, the impact of positive parent–infant interaction, and aspects of skin care for this population have all been linked with decreased morbidity of the very low birth weight group (Becker, 1989).

Despite the positive aspects of nursing practice and research outcomes, there is the problem of ethical dilemmas arising in genetics. "An ethical dilemma consists of conflicting moral obligations, rights, or claims" (NAACOG, 1987, p. 2). Technologic advances frequently precede ethical considerations and decision-making. Issues of maternal versus fetal rights are arising when it comes to fetal therapy and surgery. Whose rights take precedence? Tort liability of wrongful birth and death cases are becoming more common in the judicial system. Fetal abuse cases regarding cocaine ingestion during pregnancy are also occurring more frequently (Jones, 1988; Landwirth, 1987; Pennticuff, 1994). These ethical and legal considerations only add to the concerns nurses face today (Ott, 1995). These dilemmas may cause "burnout" related to stress in the workplace. The end result is fewer nurses staying in neonatal nursing (see Chapters 3, Ethical Aspects of Perinatal Care, and 4, Legal Aspects of Perinatal Care). The American Nurses' Association Center for Ethics and Human Rights just completed a 2-year grant project funded by the Ethical, Legal and Social Implications (ELSI) Branch of the National Center for Human Genome Research at NIH. The product was a publication entitled "Managing Genetic Information: Implications for Nursing Practice" (Scanlon & Fibison, 1995). This publication presents guidelines for nursing practice, including disclosure of genetic information, informed consent, and confidentiality issues surrounding genetic testing.

Collaboration with other disciplines is essential to keeping abreast of the most current information. There is a critical need for the blending of neonatal nursing with sound genetic knowledge. This blending might even increase the retention of nurses in the field.

The American Nurse (American Nurses' Association, 1989) stated that an important aspect of retention was finding the right niche. Nursing provides many opportunities in and of itself. The field of genetics is open to neonatal nurses, and the clinical application of genetic knowledge can clear new avenues for advancement. Finding the right niche becomes easier when the possibilities are considered. Genetics with its rapidly evolving knowledge base challenges nurses to explore new types of practice.

CONCLUSION

This chapter described the general principles of genetics. It described its application in the clinical area and nursing's role in the genetic revolution.

REFERENCES

American Nurses Association (1989, November/December). *The American Nurse.* Kansas City, MO: The American Nurses' Association.

American Society of Anesthesiologists, Ad Hoc Committee on the Effect of Trace Anesthetics on the Health of Operating Room Personnel. (1974). Occupational disease among operating room personnel. *Anesthesiology, 41*(4), 321–340.

Becker, A. (1989, November/December). Forum: RN cites impact of research on morbidity of infants. *The American Nurse,* p. 10.

Bombard, A. T., & Naef, R. W. (1993). Reproductive genetics for couples older than 40 years of age. *Obstetrics and Gynecology Clinics of North America, 20*(2), 279–297.

Brent, R. L. (1987). Environmental factors in the causation of birth defects. In M. M. Kaback & L. J. Shapiro (Eds.), *Frontiers in genetic medicine: Report of the 92nd Ross Conference on Pediatric Research* (pp. 13–23). Columbus, OH: Ross Laboratories.

Cohen, E. N., Bellville, J. W., & Brown, B. W. (1971). Anesthesia, pregnancy, and miscarriage: A study of operating room nurses and anesthetists. *Anesthesiology, 35*(4), 343–347.

Cohen, F. L. (1984). *Clinical genetics in nursing practice.* Philadelphia: J. B. Lippincott.

Conover, E. (1994). Hazardous exposures during pregnancy. *Journal of Obstetric, Gynecologic, and Neonatal Nursing, 23*(6), 524–532.

Coulson, C. C., Katz, V. L., & Kuller, J. A. (1996). Triple-marker screening for aneuploidy. In J. A. Kuller, N. C. Chescheir, & R. C. Cefalo (Eds.), *Prenatal diagnosis and reproductive genetics* (pp. 84–95). Philadelphia: J. B. Lippincott.

Cummings, M. R. (1994). *Human heredity: Principles and issues* (3rd ed.). New York: West Publishing.

Dunn, L. (1965). *A short history of genetics.* New York: McGraw-Hill.

Effective medication for severe acne documented as cause of birth defects. (1984). *Occupational Health Nursing, 32*(10), 556–557.

Foresman, I. (1994). Evolution of the nursing role in genetics. *Journal of Obstetric, Gynecologic, and Neonatal Nursing,* 23(6), 481–486.

Gabbe, S., Niebyl, J. R., & Simpson, J. L. (1986). *Obstetrics: Normal and problem pregnancies.* New York: Churchill Livingstone.

Hall, J. G. (1987). Impact of genetic disease on pediatric health care. In M. M. Kahack & L. J. Shapiro (Eds.), *Frontiers in genetic medicine: Report of the 92nd Ross Conference on Pediatric Research* (pp. 1–7). Columbus, OH: Ross Laboratories.

Ho, E. (1988). The unborn patient. *Nursing Times, 84*(5), 38–40.

Jones, S. L. (1988). Decision making in clinical genetics: Ethical implications for perinatal nursing practice. *Journal of Perinatal and Neonatal Nursing, 1*(3), 11–23.

Jones, S. L. (1994). Assisted reproductive technologies: Genetic and nursing implications. *Journal of Obstetric, Gynecologic, and Neonatal Nursing, 23*(6), 492–497.

Kenner, C. (1991). Genetic risks and other hazards for the NICU nurse. *Neonatal Network, 10*(1), 37-40, 49–51.

Kenner, C., & Berling, B. (1990). Nursing in genetics: Current and emerging issues for practice and education. *Journal of Pediatric Nursing, 5*(6), 370–374.

Landwirth, J. (1987). Fetal abuse and neglect: An emerging controversy. *Pediatrics, 79*(4), 508–514.

Lemons, P. K., & Brock, M. J. (1990). Prenatal diagnosis and congenital disease: Role of the clinical nurse specialist. *Neonatal Network, 9*(3), 15–22.

Letts, D. J., & Wilkinson, W. E. (1985). A teaching guide for employees exposed to waste anesthetic gases. *Occupational Health Nursing, 33*(2), 76–78.

Lewis, R. (1994). *Human genetics: Concepts and applications.* Dubuque, IA: Wm. C. Brown Communications, Inc.

Lingman, G., Ohrlander, S., & Ohlin, P. (1980). Intrauterine digoxin: Paroxysmal treatment of fetal tachycardia. *British Journal of Obstetrics and Gynaecology, 87*(4), 340–342.

Lynch, M. L., & McKeon, V. A. (1990). Cocaine use during pregnancy. *Journal of Obstetric, Gynecologic, and Neonatal Nursing, 19*(4), 285–292.

Mackta, J., & Weiss, J. O. (1994). The role of genetic support groups. *Journal of Obstetric, Gynecologic, and Neonatal Nursing, 23*(6), 519–523.

Moore, K. L., Persaud, T. V. N., & Shiota, K. (1994). *Color atlas of clinical embryology.* Philadelphia: W. B. Saunders.

Nurses Association of the American Association of Obstetrics and Gynecology (NAACOG). (1987). *OGN Nursing Practice Resource: Ethical Decision Making in OGN Nursing Practice.* Washington, DC: Author.

NAACOG. (1989, October). Caring for cocaine's mothers and babies. *NAACOG Newsletter, 16*(10), 1, 4–6.

NAACOG. (1984). Pediatric surgeons focus on congenital defects. *AORN Journal, 39*(2), 195-196.

Olsen, D. G. (1994). Parental adjustment to a child with genetic disease: One parent's reflections. *Journal of Obstetric, Gynecologic, and Neonatal Nursing, 23*(6), 516–518.

Ott, B. B. (1995). The human genome project: An overview of ethical issues and public policy concerns. *Nursing Outlook, 43*(5), 228–231.

Pennticuff, J. (1994). Ethical issues in genetic therapy. *Journal of Obstetric, Gynecologic, and Neonatal Nursing, 23*(6), 498–501.

Prows, C. A. (1989). Ribavirin's risks in reproduction—how great are they? *MCN; American Journal of Maternal Child Nursing, 14*(6), 400–404.

Prows, C. A. (1992). Utilization of genetic knowledge in pediatric nursing practice. *Journal of Pediatric Nursing, 7*(1), 58–62.

Raff, B. S. (1994a). The genome project. *Journal of Obstetric, Gynecologic, and Neonatal Nursing, 23*(6), 488–491.

Raff, B. S. (1994b). Nursing and genetics for the 21st century. *Journal of Obstetric, Gynecologic, and Neonatal Nursing, 23*(6), 477–480.

Robinson, A., & Linden, M. G. (1993). *Clinical genetics handbook* (2nd ed.). Boston: Blackwell Scientific Publications.

Ross, L. J. (1994). Developmental disabilities: Genetic implications. *Journal of Obstetric, Gynecologic, and Neonatal Nursing, 23*(6), 502–505.

Saurel-Cubizolles, M. J., Hays, M., & Estryn-Behar, M. (1994). *Work in operating rooms and pregnancy outcomes among nurses. International Archives of Occupational and Environmental Health, 66*(4), 235–241..

Scanlon, C., & Fibison, W. (1995). *Managing genetic information: Implications for nursing practice.* Washington, DC: American Nurses' Association.

Schardein, J. L. (1985). *Chemically induced birth defects* (pp. 713–716, 772–774). New York: Marcel Dekker, Inc.

Shortridge, L. (1990). Advances in the assessment of the effect of environmental and occupational toxins on reproduction. *Journal of Perinatal and Neonatal Nursing, 3*(4), 1–11.

Smitherman, C. H. (1994). The lasting impact of fetal alcohol syndrome and fetal alcohol effect on children an adolescents. *Journal of Pediatric Health Care, 8*(3), 121–126.

Spinnato, J. A., Shaver, D. C., Flinn, G. S., et al. (1984). Fetal supraventricular tachycardia in utero therapy with digoxin and quinidine. *Obstetrics and Gynecology, 64*(5), 730–735.

Spitz, J. L. (1996). *Genodermatoses: A full-color clinical guide to genetic skin disorders.* Baltimore: Williams & Wilkins.

U.S. Department of Health and Human Services. (1995). *Healthy people 2000: A midcourse review.* Washington, DC: Author.

Weatherall, D. J. (1985). *The new genetics in clinical practice* (2nd ed., p. 36). New York: Oxford University Press.

White, K. R., Munro, C. L, & Pickler, R. H. (1995). Therapeutic implication of recent advances in cystic fibrosis. *MCN; American Journal of Maternal Child Nursing, 20*(6), 304–308.

Williamson, K. M., Turner, J. G., Brown, K. C., et al. (1988). Occupational health hazards for nurses—Part II. *Image, 20*(3), 162–168.

Wolf, U. (1976). Theodore Boveri and his book "on the problem of the origin of malignant tumors." In J. German (Ed.), *Chromosomes and cancer.* New York: John Wiley & Sons.

Wright, L. (1994). Prenatal diagnosis in the 1990's. *Journal of Obstetric, Gynecologic, and Neonatal Nursing, 23*(6), 506–515.

Zacharias, J. F. (1990). The new genetics. *Journal of Obstetric, Gynecologic, and Neonatal Nursing, 19*(2), 122–128.

CHAPTER **10**

Fetal Development: Environmental Influences and Critical Periods

JUDY WRIGHT LOTT

RESEARCH AGENDA

How can we optimize the environment for the best fetal development?

What is the relationship between specific environmental hazards and fetal waste and the impact on critical periods of development?

What is the relationship between genetic factors and environmental influences on fetal development?

EARLY FETAL DEVELOPMENT

The process of human development begins with the fertilization of an ovum (female gamete) by a spermatocyte (male gamete). The fusion of the ovum and sperm initiates a sequence of events that causes the single-celled zygote to develop into a new human being. During the 38 to 42 weeks of gestation, there are dramatic growth and development that are unequaled during any other period of life. In this chapter, the major events of prenatal development are described, and critical development periods for the major organ systems are identified. A brief review of the events beginning with fertilization is included, but the reader is referred to an embryology text for a more thorough account. Human genetics is discussed in Chapter 9, Human Genetics.

Fertilization

Approximately 200 to 500 million sperm are deposited in the posterior fornix of the vagina during ejaculation. The large numbers of spermatozoa are necessary to increase the chances for conception because the spermatozoa must traverse the cervical canal, the uterus, and the uterine (fallopian) tubes to reach the ovum. The usual site of fertilization is in the ampulla, the widest portion of the uterine tubes, which is located near the ovaries. Sperm are propelled by the movement of the tails and are aided by muscular contractions of the uterus. The spermatozoa must undergo two physiologic changes in order to penetrate the corona radiata and zona pellucida, the barriers around the secondary oocyte. The first change is capacitation, an enzymatic reaction that removes the glycoprotein coating from the spermatozoa and plasma proteins from the seminal fluid. Capacitation takes approximately 7 hours, and it usually occurs in the uterus or uterine tubes. The acrosome reaction occurs when a capacitated sperm passes through the corona radiata. The acrosome reaction results in structural changes that cause fusion of the plasma membranes of the sperm and the oocyte. Progesterone released from the follicle at ovulation stimulates the acrosome reaction. Three enzymes are released from the acrosome to facilitate entry of the sperm into the ovum. Hyaluronidase allows the sperm to penetrate the corona radiata. Trypsin-like enzymes and a zona lysin digest a pathway across the zona pellucida.

Approximately 300 to 500 spermatozoa survive the journey and actually reach the ovum. When a spermatozoon comes into contact with the ovum, the zona pellucida and the plasma membrane fuse so that entry by other sperm is prevented. After penetration by a single sperm, the oocyte completes the second meiotic cell division, resulting in the haploid number of chromosomes (22,X) and the second polar body. The chromosomes are arranged to form the female pronucleus.

As the spermatozoon moves close to the female pronucleus, the tail is detached and the nucleus enlarges to form the male pronucleus. The male and female pronuclei fuse, resulting in a diploid cell called the *zygote.* The zygote contains 23 autosomes and one sex chromosome from each parent (46,XX or 46,XY). The genetic sex of the new individual is determined at fertilization by the contribution of the father. The male parent (XY) may contribute either an X or a Y chromosome. If the spermatozoon contains an X chromosome, the offspring is female (46,XX). If the spermatozoon receives one Y chromosome, the offspring is male (46,XY). Individual variation is the result of random or independent assortment of the autosomal chromosomes.

Cleavage

Mitotic cell division occurs after fertilization as the zygote passes down the uterine tube, resulting in the formation of two blastomeres (Fig. 10–1). The cells continue to divide, increasing in number, although decreasing in size. The term *cleavage* is used to describe the mitotic cell division of the zygote (Fig. 10–2). When the number of cells reach approximately 16 (usually on the third day), the zygote is called a *morula,* because of its resemblance to a mulberry. The zygote reaches the morula stage at approximately the time it enters the uterus. The morula consists of groups of centrally located cells called the *inner cell mass* and an outer cell layer. At this stage the individual cells are called blastomeres. The outer cell layer forms the trophoblast, from which the placenta develops. The inner cell mass, called the *embryoblast,* gives rise to the embryo.

After the morula penetrates the uterine cavity, fluid enters through the zona pellucida into the intercellular spaces of the inner cell mass. About the fourth day after fertilization, the fluid-filled spaces fuse, forming a large cavity known as the blastocyst

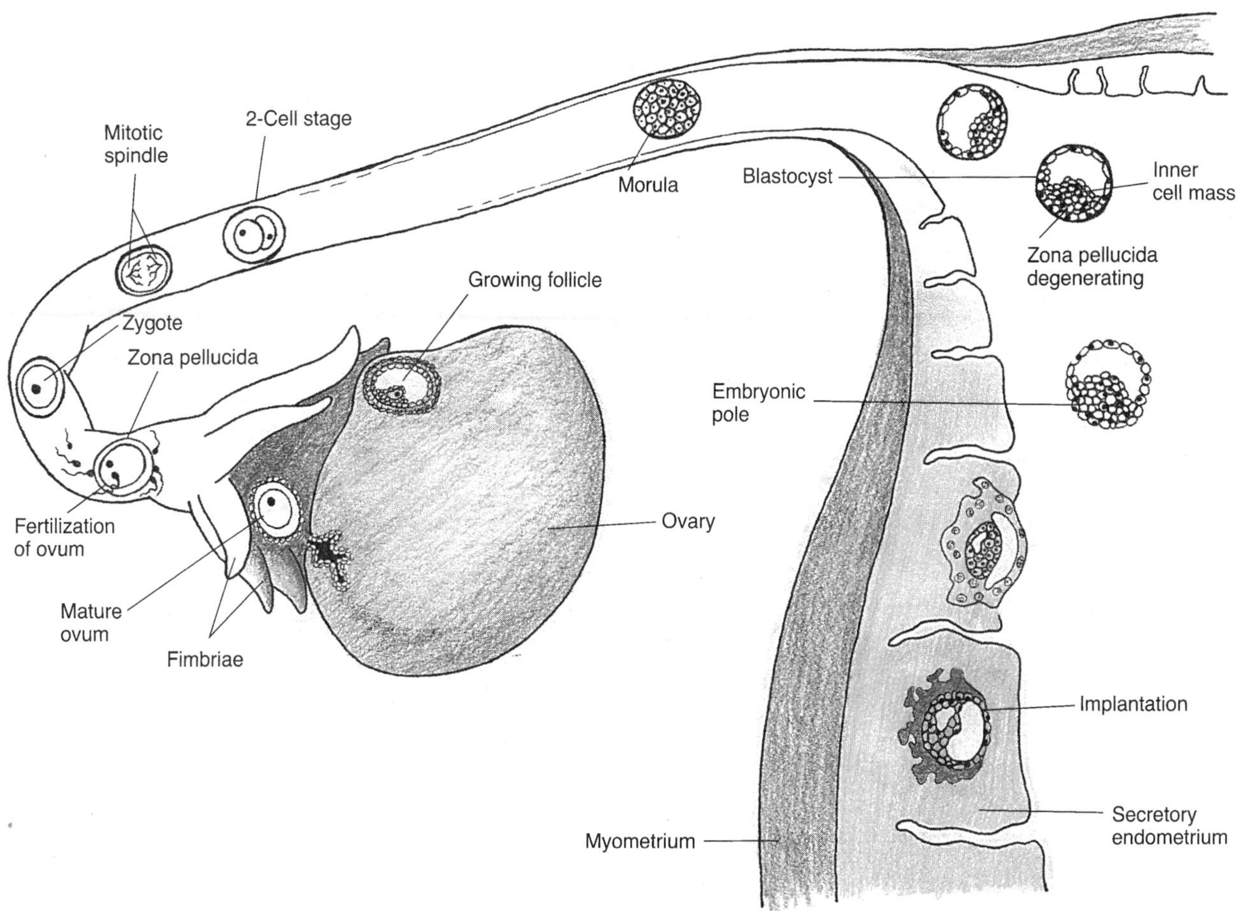

FIGURE 10–1. Fantastic voyage: from fertilization to implantation. The journey through the fallopian tubes takes approximately 4 days. During this time, mitotic cell division occurs. Implantation occurs on about day 9 through day 12.

cavity. The morula is now called the *blastocyst*. The trophoblast forms the wall of the blastocyst, and the embryoblast projects from the wall of the blastocyst into the blastocyst cavity. The blastocyst is nourished by the uterine secretions until implantation occurs.

Implantation

Degeneration of the zona pellucida occurs on about the fifth day after fertilization, allowing the blastocyst to attach to the endothelium of the endometrium on about the sixth day. The trophoblasts then secrete proteolytic enzymes that destroy the endometrial endothelium and invade the endometrium. Two layers of trophoblasts develop. The inner layer is made up of cytotrophoblasts, and the outer layer is composed of syncytiotrophoblasts. The syncytiotrophoblast has finger-like projections that produce enzymes capable of further eroding the endometrial tissues. By the end of the seventh day, the blastocyst is superficially implanted (Fig. 10–3).

Formation of the Bilaminar Disk

Implantation is completed during the second week. The syncytiotrophoblast continues to invade the endometrium and becomes embedded. Spaces in the syncytiotrophoblast called *lacunae* fill with blood from ruptured maternal capillaries and secretions from eroded endometrial glands. This fluid nourishes the embryoblast by diffusion. The lacunae give rise to the uteroplacental circulation. The lacunae fuse to form a network that then becomes the intervillous spaces of the placenta. The endometrial capillaries near the implanted embryoblast become dilated and eroded by the syncytiotrophoblast. Maternal blood enters the lacunar network and provides circulation and nutrients to the embryo. Maternal-embryonic blood circulation provides the developing embryo with nutrition and oxygenation and removes waste products before the development of the placenta. The primary chorionic villi form at about the same time. These finger-like projections of the chorion develop into the chorionic villi of the placenta.

The inner cell mass differentiates into two layers: the hypoblast (endoderm), a layer of small cuboidal cells, and the epiblast (ectoderm), a layer of high columnar cells. The two layers form a flattened, circular bilaminar embryonic disk. The amniotic cavity is derived from spaces within the epiblast. As the amniotic cavity enlarges, a thin layer of epithelial cells that act as a roof covers the amniotic cavity.

During the development of the amniotic cavity, other trophoblastic cells form a thin extracoelomic membrane, which encloses the primitive yolk sac. The yolk sac produces fetal red blood cells. Other trophoblastic cells form a layer of mesenchymal tissue, called the *extraembryonic mesoderm,* around the amnion and primitive yolk sac.

Isolated coelomic spaces in the extraembryonic mesoderm fuse to form a single, large, fluid-filled cavity surrounding the amnion and yolk sac, with the exception of the area where the amnion is attached to the chorion by the connecting stalk. The primitive yolk sac decreases in size, creating a smaller secondary yolk sac.

Two layers of extraembryonic mesoderm result from the forma-

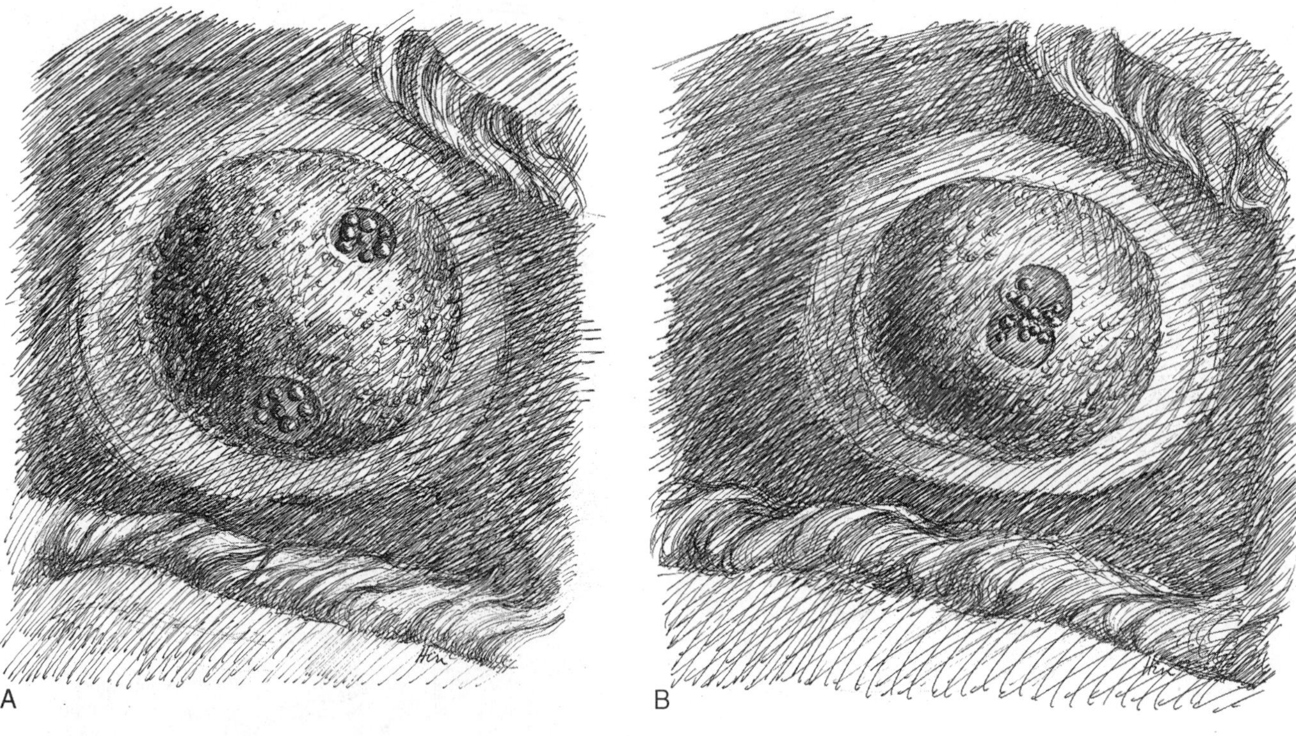

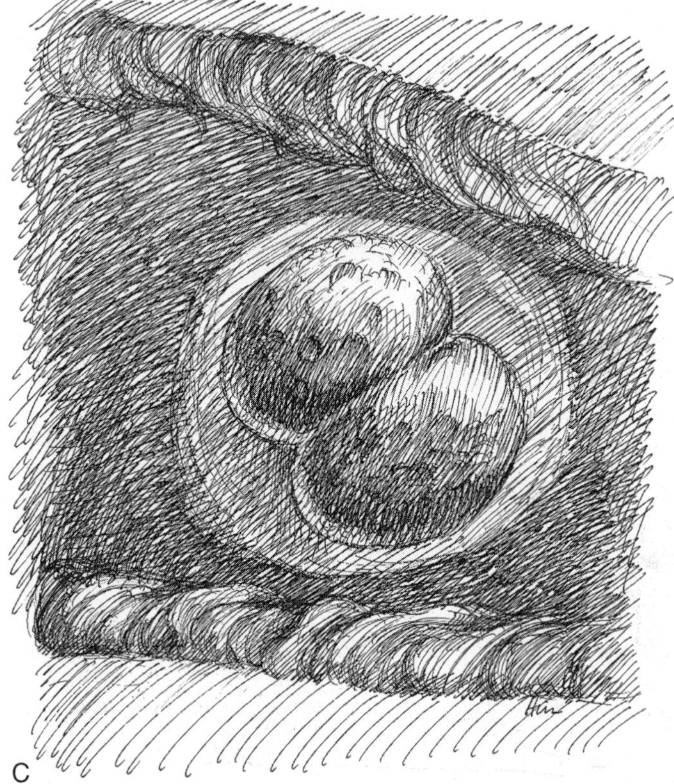

FIGURE 10–2. Stages of cell division: Cleavage. *A*, Zygote; *B*, zygote undergoing first cleavage; *C*, two-cell blastomere state.

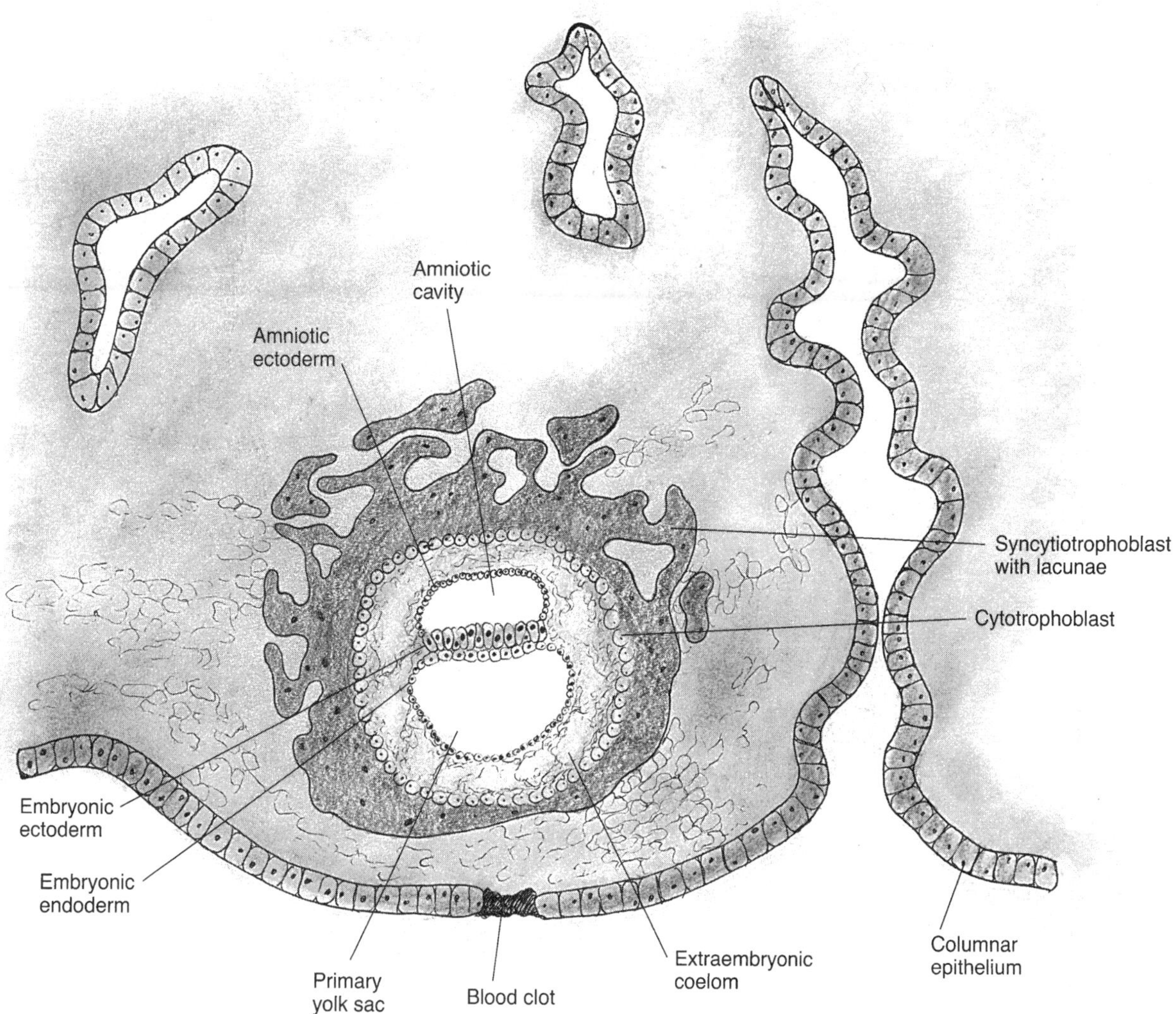

FIGURE 10–3. Cross section of a blastocyst at 11 days. Two germ layers are present. The trophoblast has differentiated into the syncytiotrophoblast and the cytotrophoblast.

tion of the extraembryonic cavity. The extraembryonic somatic mesoderm lines the trophoblast and covers the amnion, and the extraembryonic splanchnic mesoderm covers the yolk sac. The chorion is made up of the extraembryonic somatic mesoderm, the cytotrophoblast, and the syncytiotrophoblast. The chorion forms the chorionic sac, in which the embryo and the amniotic and yolk sacs are located.

By the end of the second week, there is a slightly thickened area near the cephalic region of the hypoblastic disk, known as the *prochordal plate*, which marks the location of the mouth.

Formation of the Trilaminar Embryonic Disk: The Third Week of Development

The third week of development is marked by rapid growth, the formation of the *primitive streak*, and the differentiation of the three germ layers, from which all fetal tissues and organs are derived (Fig. 10–4).

Gastrulation

Gastrulation is the process by which the bilaminar disk is expanded to a trilaminar embryonic disk. It is the most important event that occurs during early fetal formation. This event affects all the rest of embryologic development. During the third week, epiblast cells separate from their original location and migrate inward, forming the mesoblast, which spreads cranially and laterally to form a layer between the ectoderm and the endoderm called the *intraembryonic mesoderm*. Other mesoblastic cells invade the endoderm, displacing the endodermal cells laterally, forming a new layer, the embryonic ectoderm. Thus, the hypoblastic ectoderm produces the embryonic ectoderm, embryonic mesoderm, and the majority of the embryonic endoderm. These three germ layers are the source of the tissues and organs of the embryo.

Primitive Streak

On days 14 to 15, a groove and thickening of the ectoderm (epiblast), called the *primitive streak*, appear caudally in the center of the dorsum of the embryonic disk. The primitive streak results from the migration of ectodermal cells toward the midline in the posterior portion of the embryonic disk. The primitive groove develops in the primitive streak. When the primitive streak begins to produce mesoblastic cells that become intraembryonic mesoderm, the epiblast is referred to as the *embryonic ectoderm* and the hypoblast is referred to as the *embryonic mesoderm*.

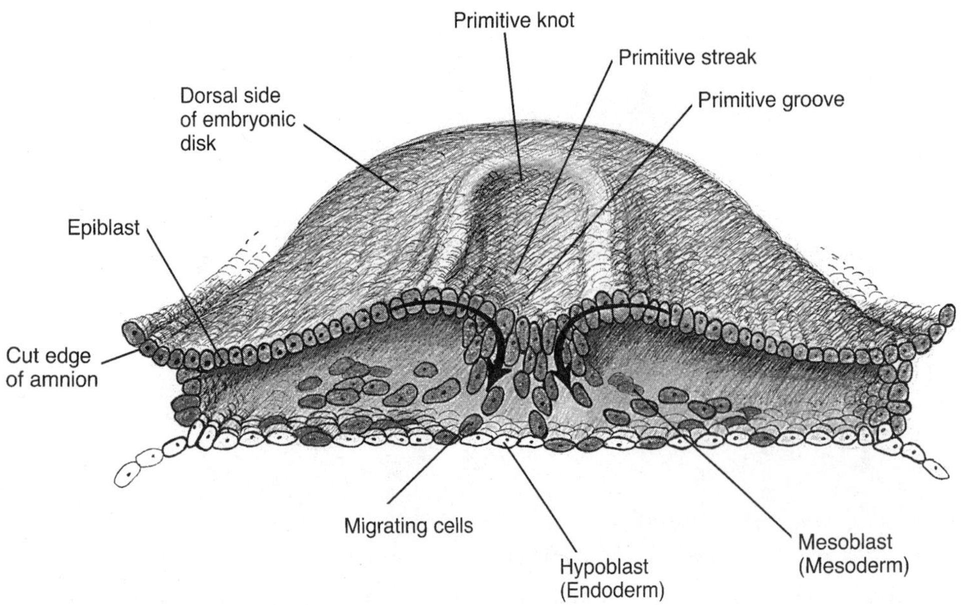

FIGURE 10–4. Formation of the trilaminar embryonic disk: gastrulation. During gastrulation, the bilaminar embryonic disk is changed to a trilaminar embryonic disk, consisting of the epiblast (ectoderm), hypoblast (endoderm), and mesoblast (mesoderm).

Notochordal Process

Cells from the primitive knot migrate cranially and form the midline cellular *notochordal process*. This process grows cranially between the ectoderm and the endoderm until it reaches the prochordal plate, which is attached to the overlying ectoderm, thus forming the oropharyngeal membrane. The cloacal membrane, caudal to the primitive streak, develops into the anus.

The primitive streak produces mesenchyme (mesoblasts) until the end of the fourth week. The primitive streak does not grow as rapidly as the other cells, making it relatively insignificant in size when compared with the other structures that continue to grow. The primitive streak or remnants of the primitive streak may persist and develop into a sacrococcygeal teratoma.

The *notochord* is a cellular rod that develops from the notochordal process. The notochord is the structure around which the vertebral column is formed. It forms the nucleus pulposus of the intervertebral bodies of the spinal column (Fig. 10–5).

Neurulation

Neurulation is the name given to the process by which the neural plate, neural folds, and neural tube are formed. The developing notochord stimulates the embryonic ectoderm to thicken, forming the neural plate. The neuroectoderm of the neural plate gives rise to the central nervous system. The neural plate develops cranial to the primitive knot. As the neural plate elongates, the neural plate gets wider and extends cranially to the oropharyngeal membrane. The neural plate invaginates along the central axis to form a neural groove with neural folds on each side. The neural folds move together and fuse, forming the neural tube (Fig. 10–6). The neural tube detaches from the surface ectoderm, and the free edges of the ectoderm fuse, covering the posterior portion of the embryo. With formation of the neural tube, nearby ectodermal cells lying along the crest of each neural fold migrate inward, invading the mesoblast on each side of the neural tube. These irregular, flattened masses are called the *neural crest*. This structure's cells give rise to the spinal ganglia, the ganglia of the autonomic nervous system, and a portion of the cranial nerves. Neural crest cells also form the meningeal covering of the brain and spinal cord and the sheaves that protect nerves. The neural crest cells contribute to the formation of pigment-producing cells, the adrenal medulla, and skeletal and muscular development in the head.

Development of Somites

Another important event of the third week is the development of somites. During formation of the neural tube, the intraembryonic mesoderm on each side thickens, forming longitudinal columns of paraxial mesoderm. At about 20 days, the paraxial mesoderm begins to divide into paired cuboidal bodies known as somites. The somites give rise to most of the skeleton and associated musculature and much of the dermis of the skin. The somites develop in a craniocaudal sequence. In all, 42 to 44 somites develop, although only 38 develop during the "somite" period. These somite pairs can be counted and give an estimate as to fetal age before a crown–rump measurement is possible.

Intraembryonic Cavity

One other significant process is the formation of the intraembryonic cavity. This stucture first appears as a number of small spaces within the lateral mesoderm and the cardiogenic mesoderm. These spaces combine to form the intraembryonic cavity; it is horseshoe-shaped and lined with flattened epithelial cells. These cells eventually line the peritoneal cavity. The intraembryonic cavity divides the lateral mesoderm into the parietal (somatic) and visceral (splanchnic) layers. It gives rise to the pericardial cavity, the pleural cavity, and the peritoneal cavity.

PLACENTAL DEVELOPMENT AND FUNCTION

The rudimentary maternal-fetal circulation is intact by the fourth week of gestation. Growth of the trophoblast results in numerous primary and secondary chorionic villi, covering the surface of the chorionic sac until about the eighth week of gestation. At about the eighth week, the villi overlying the conceptus (decidua capsularis) degenerate, leaving a smooth area (smooth chorion). The villi underlying the conceptus (decidua basalis) remain and increase in size, producing the chorion frondosum, or fetal side of the placenta.

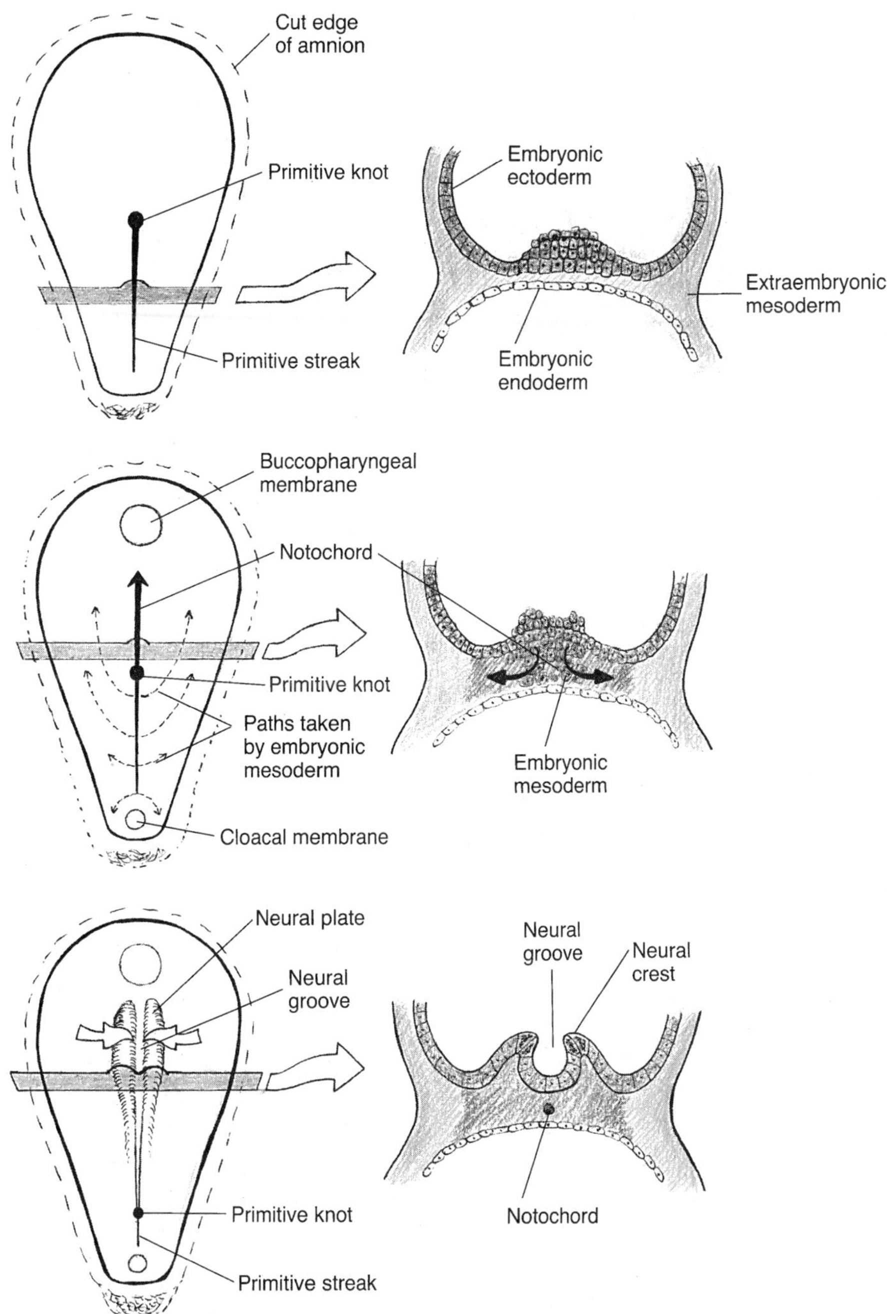

FIGURE 10–5. Formation of primitive streak, primitive knot, notochord, and neural groove.

The maternal side of the placenta is made up of the chorion and the chorionic villi. On implantation of the conceptus, maternal capillaries of the decidua basalis are ruptured, causing maternal blood to circulate through the developing fetal placenta (chorion frondosum). As growth and differentiation progress, extensions from the cytotrophoblast invade the syncytial layer and form a cytotrophoblastic shell, surrounding the conceptus and chorionic villi. This shell is continuous but has communications between maternal blood vessels in the decidua basalis and the intervillous spaces of the chorion frondosum. The latter is attached to the maternal side of the placenta (decidua basalis) by the cytotrophoblastic shell and anchoring villi. The placenta is mature and completely functional by 16 weeks of development (Fig. 10–7). If the corpus luteum begins to regress prior to the 16th week and fails to produce enough progesterone (the hormone responsible for readying the uterine cavity for the pregnancy), the pregnancy is aborted because the placenta is not capable of supporting the pregnancy on its own until about this time.

Placental-Fetal Circulation

A simple ebb and flow circulation occurs in the embryo, yolk sac, connecting stalk, and chorion by 21 days of gestation. By 28 days, unidirectional circulation is established. Deoxygenated fetal blood leaves the fetus via the umbilical arteries and enters the capillaries in the chorionic villi, in which gaseous and nutrient exchange takes place. Oxygenated blood returns to the fetus through the umbilical veins. At first there are two arteries and two veins, but eventually only two arteries and one vein remain, owing to degeneration of one of the veins. If only one artery is

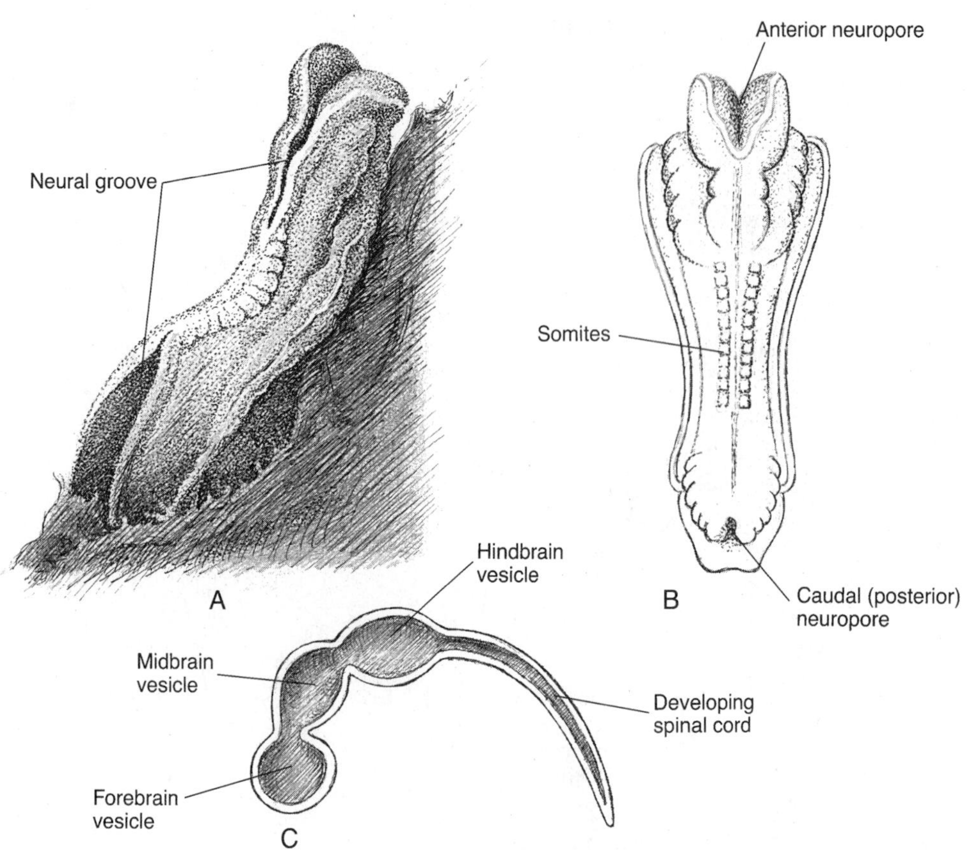

FIGURE 10–6. Formation of the neural tube. *A*, Neural groove; *B*, closure of the neural tube almost completed; *C*, dilation of the neural tube forms the forebrain, midbrain, and hindbrain.

present, a congenital anomaly, especially a renal one, should be suspected.

Placental Function

Normal growth and development of the embryo are dependent on adequate placental function. The placenta is responsible for oxygenation, nutrition, elimination of wastes, production of hormones essential for maintenance of the pregnancy, and transport of substances. The placenta synthesizes glycogen, cholesterol, and fatty acids, which provide nutrients and energy for early fetal development.

Transport across the placental membrane occurs primarily through simple and facilitated diffusion, active transport, and pinocytosis. Oxygen, carbon dioxide, and carbon monoxide cross the placenta through simple diffusion. The fetus is dependent on a continuous supply of oxygenated blood flowing from the placenta.

Water and electrolytes cross the placenta freely in both directions. Glucose is converted to glycogen in the placenta as a carbohydrate source for the fetus. Amino acids move readily across the placental membranes for protein synthesis in the fetus. Free fatty acids are transferred across the placenta by pinocytosis. There is limited or no transfer of maternal cholesterol, triglycerides, and phospholipids. Water- and fat-soluble vitamins cross the placenta and are essential for normal development (Moore & Persaud, 1993).

The placenta produces and transports hormones that maintain the pregnancy and promote growth and development of the fetus. Chorionic gonadotropin, a protein hormone produced by the syncytiotrophoblast, is excreted in maternal serum and urine. The presence of human chorionic gonadotropin is used as a test for pregnancy. Human placental lactogen, also a protein hormone produced by the placenta, acts as a fetal growth-promoting hormone by giving the fetus priority for receiving maternal glucose.

Steroid hormones are also produced by the placenta. Progesterone is produced by the placenta throughout gestation and is responsible for maintaining the pregnancy. Estrogen production by the placenta is dependent on stimulation by the fetal adrenal cortex and liver.

Placental transport of maternal antibodies provides the fetus with passive immunity to certain viruses. IgG antibodies are actively transported across the placental barrier, providing humoral immunity for the fetus. IgA and IgM antibodies do not cross the placental barrier, placing the neonate at risk for neonatal sepsis. However, failure of IgM antibodies to cross the placental membrane explains the lower incidence of a severe hemolytic process in ABO blood type incompatibilities when compared with Rh incompatibilities. The latter result when an Rh-negative mother has an Rh-positive fetus. If the mother is sensitized to the Rh-positive fetal blood cells, IgG antibodies are produced by the mother. IgG is transferred from the maternal to fetal circulation, and hemolysis of fetal red blood cells occurs.

The placenta is selective in the transfer of substances across the placenta; however, this selectivity does not screen out all potentially harmful substances. Viral, bacterial, and protozoal organisms can be transferred to the fetus through the placenta. Toxic substances such as drugs and alcohol can also be transferred to the fetus. The effects of these substances depend on the stage of gestation and type and duration of exposure, as well as the interaction of these and other factors, such as nutrition.

EMBRYONIC PERIOD: WEEKS 4 THROUGH 8

The embryonic period lasts from the beginning of gestational week 4 through the end of week 8. All major organ systems are

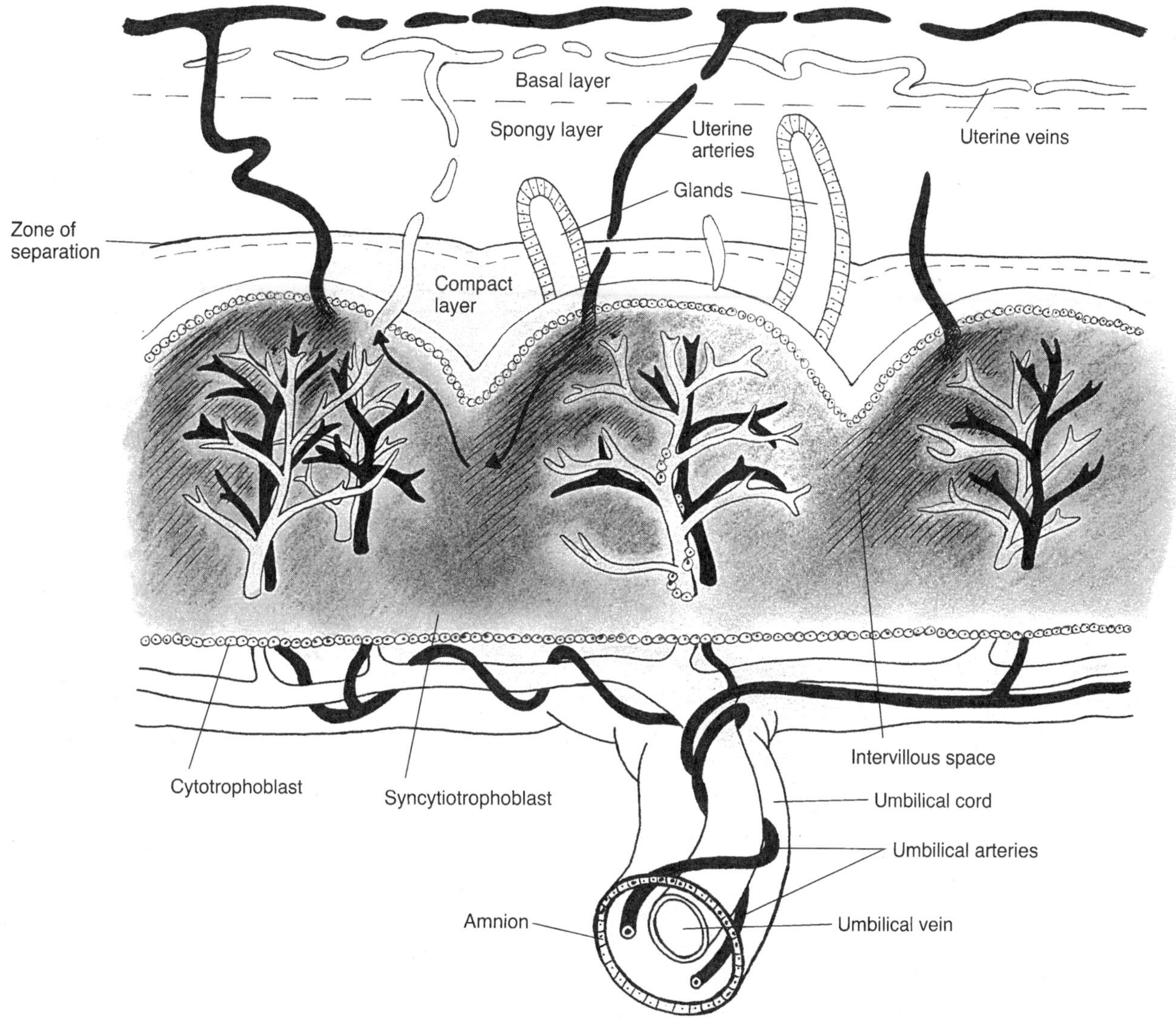

FIGURE 10–7. Formation of the placenta. The fetal and maternal sides of the placenta. Separation of the placenta from the uterus occurs at the site indicated by the black line labeled "Zone of separation."

formed during this period. The shape of the embryo changes as the organs develop, taking a more human shape by the end of the eighth week. The major events of the embryonic period include the folding of the embryo and organogenesis (Fig. 10–8).

Folding of the Embryo

In the trilaminar embryonic disk, the growth rate of the central region exceeds that of the periphery so that the slower growing areas fold under the faster growing areas, forming body folds. The head fold appears first, as a result of craniocaudal elongation of the notochord and growth of the brain, which projects into the amniotic cavity. The folding downward of the cranial end of the embryo forces the septum transversum (primitive heart), the pericardial cavity, and the oropharyngeal membrane to turn under onto the ventral surface. After the embryo has folded, the mass of mesoderm cranial to the pericardial cavity, the septum transversum, lies caudal to the heart. The septum transversum later develops into a portion of the diaphragm. Part of the yolk sac is incorporated as the foregut, lying between the heart and the brain. The foregut ends blindly at the oropharyngeal membrane, which separates the foregut from the primitive mouth cavity (stomodeum).

The tail fold occurs after the head fold as a result of craniocaudal growth progression. Growth of the embryo causes the caudal area to project over the cloacal membrane. During the tail folding, part of the yolk sac is incorporated into the embryo as the hindgut. After completion of the head and tail folding, the connecting stalk is attached to the ventral surface of the embryo, forming the umbilical cord.

Folding also occurs laterally, producing right and left lateral folds. The lateral body wall on each side folds toward the median plane, causing the embryo to assume a cylindrical shape. During the lateral body folding, a portion of the yolk sac is incorporated as the midgut. The attachment of the midgut to the yolk sac is minimal after this fold develops. After folding, the amnion is attached to the embryo in a narrow area in which the umbilical cord attaches to the ventral surface.

Organogenesis: Germ Cell Derivatives

The three germ cell layers (ectoderm, mesoderm, and endoderm) give rise to all tissues and organs of the embryo. The germ cells follow specific patterns during the process of *organogenesis*. The main germ cell derivatives are listed in Table 10–1.

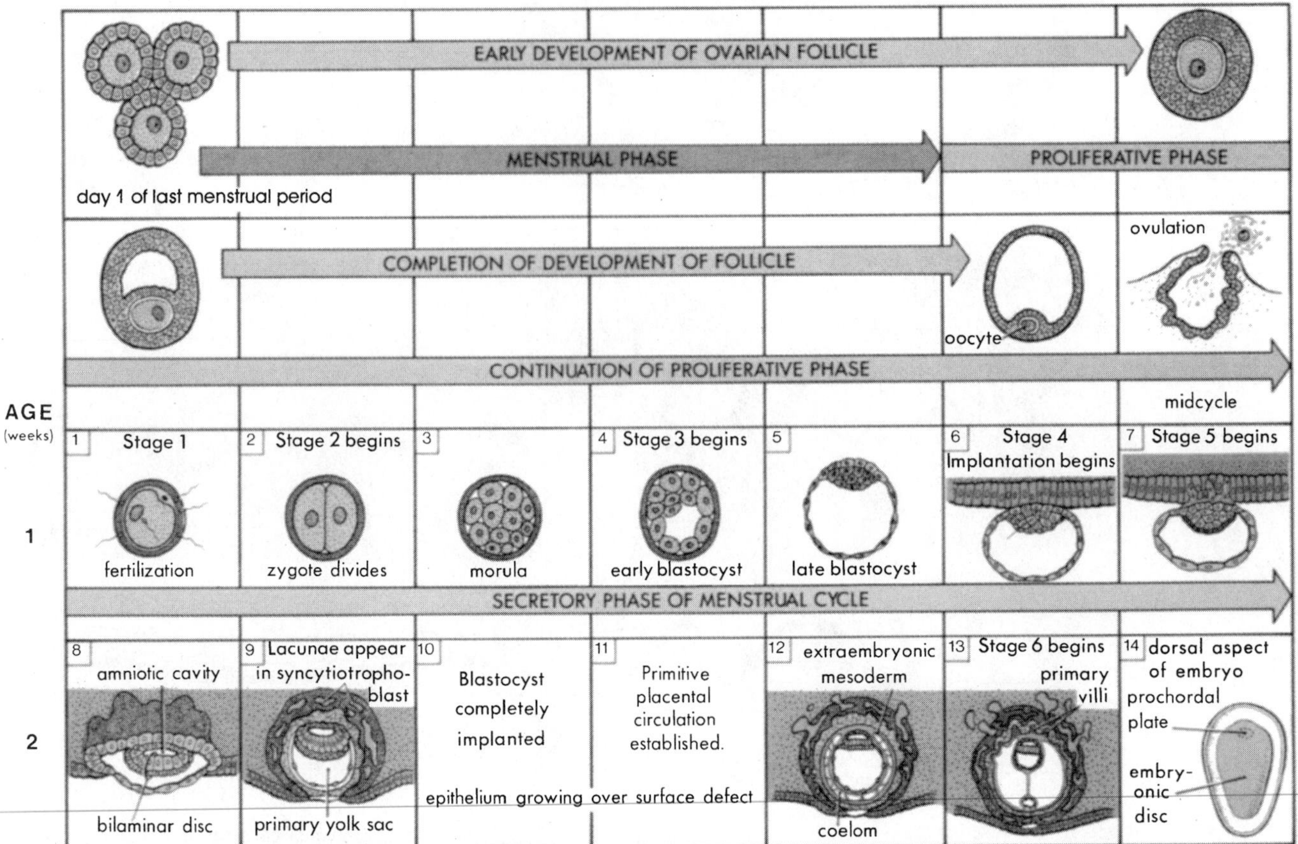

FIGURE 10–8. Critical periods of development. (From Moore, K. L., & Persaud, T. V. N. [1993]. Before we are born: Essentials of embryology and birth defects, 4th ed., pp. 2–5. Philadelphia: W. B. Saunders. Reprinted with permission.)

The development of each major organ system is discussed separately. The embryonic period is the most critical period of development because of the formation of internal and external structures. The critical periods of development for the organs are also discussed in the section on specific organ development.

FETAL PERIOD: WEEK 9 THROUGH BIRTH

The *fetal period* begins at the start of the ninth week of gestation and extends through the duration of the pregnancy. It

TABLE 10–1 Germ Cell Derivatives

Ectoderm	Mesoderm	Endoderm
Central nervous system (brain, spinal cord) Peripheral nervous system Sensory epithelia of eye, ear, and nose Epidermis and its appendages (hair and nails) Mammary glands Subcutaneous glands Teeth enamel Neural crest cells Spinal, cranial, and autonomic ganglia cells Nerve sheaths of peripheral nervous system Pigment cells Muscle, connective tissue, and bone of branchial arch origin Adrenal medulla Meninges	Cartilage Bone Connective tissue Striated and smooth muscle Heart, blood, and lymph vessels and cells Gonads Genital ducts Pericardial, pleural, and peritoneal lining Spleen Cortex of adrenal gland	Epithelial lining of respiratory and gastrointestinal tracts Parenchyma of tonsils, thyroid, parathyroid, liver, thymus, and pancreas Epithelial lining of bladder and urethra Epithelial lining of tympanic cavity, tympanic antrum, and auditory tube

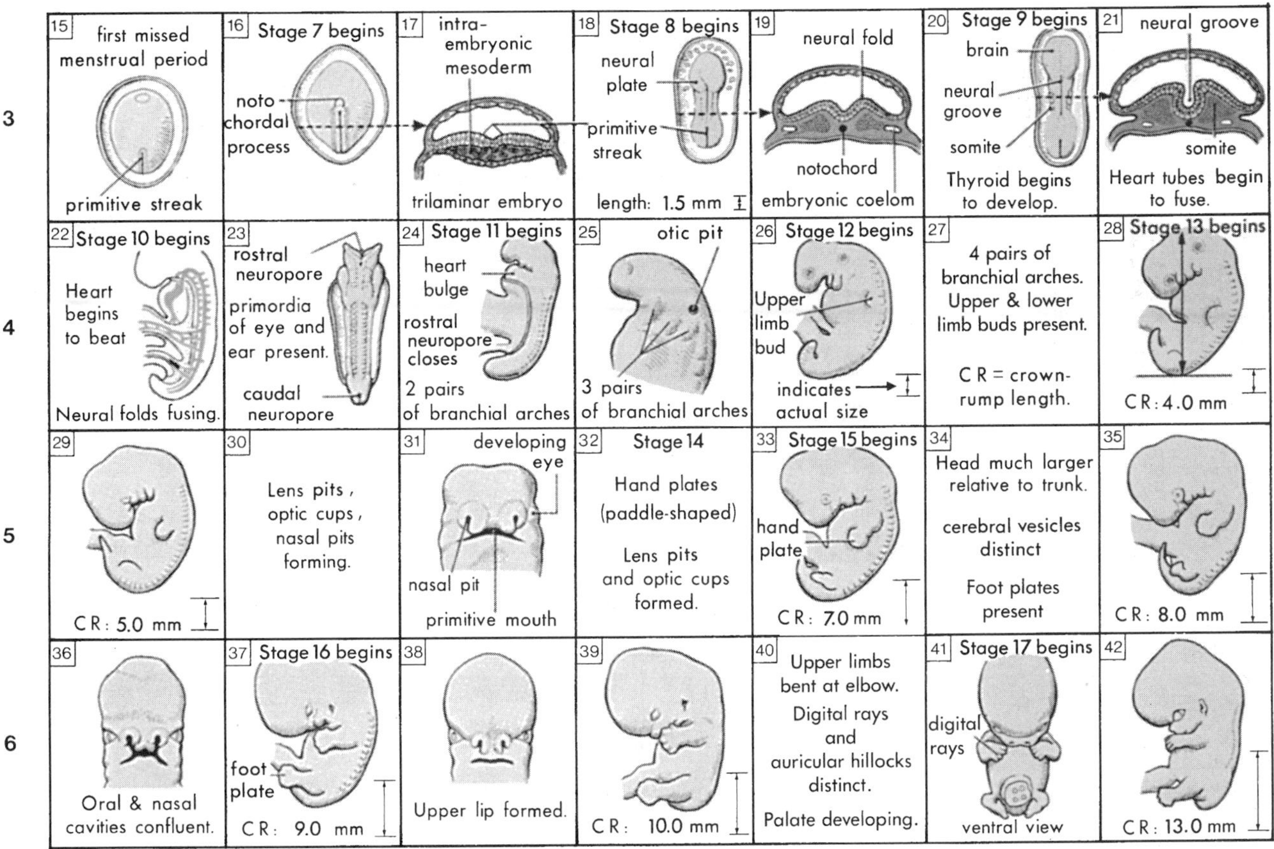

TIMETABLE OF HUMAN PRENATAL DEVELOPMENT
7 to 38 weeks

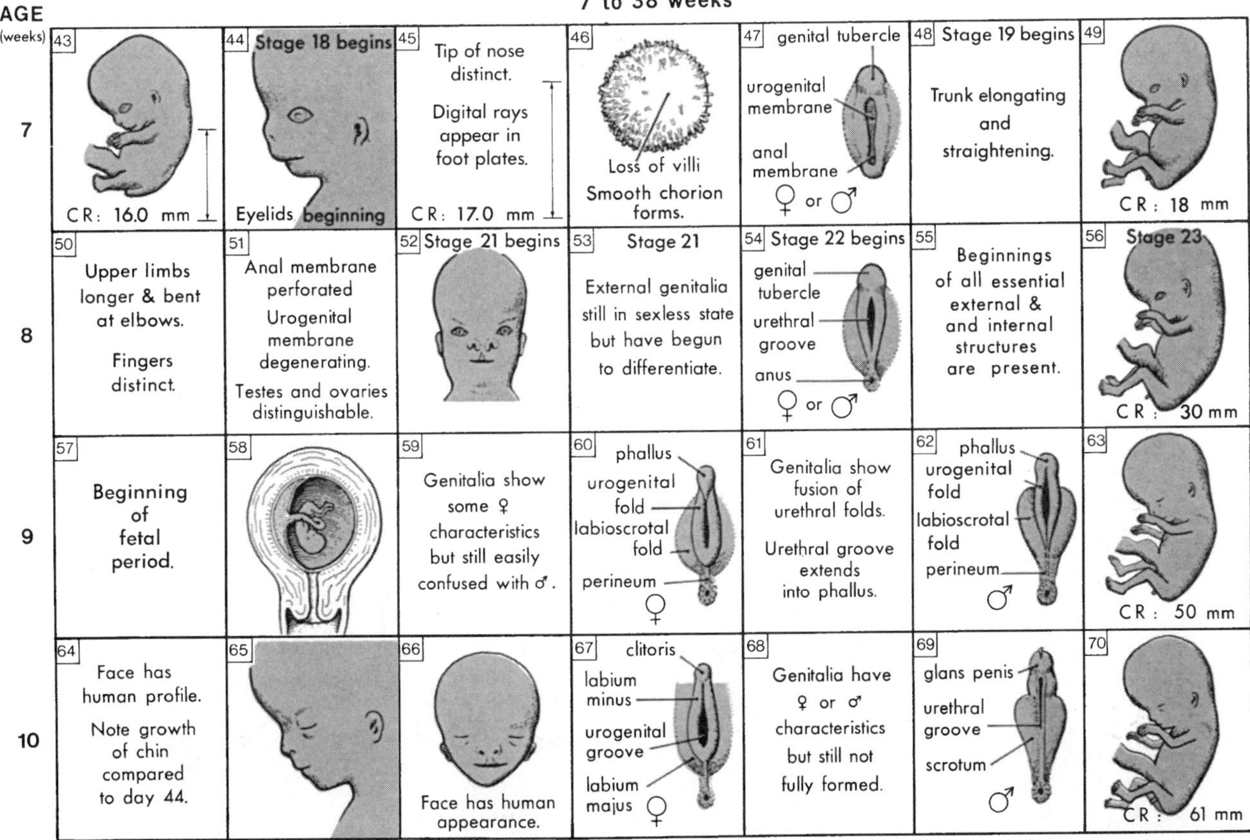

FIGURE 10–8 *See legend on opposite page*

Illustration continued on following page

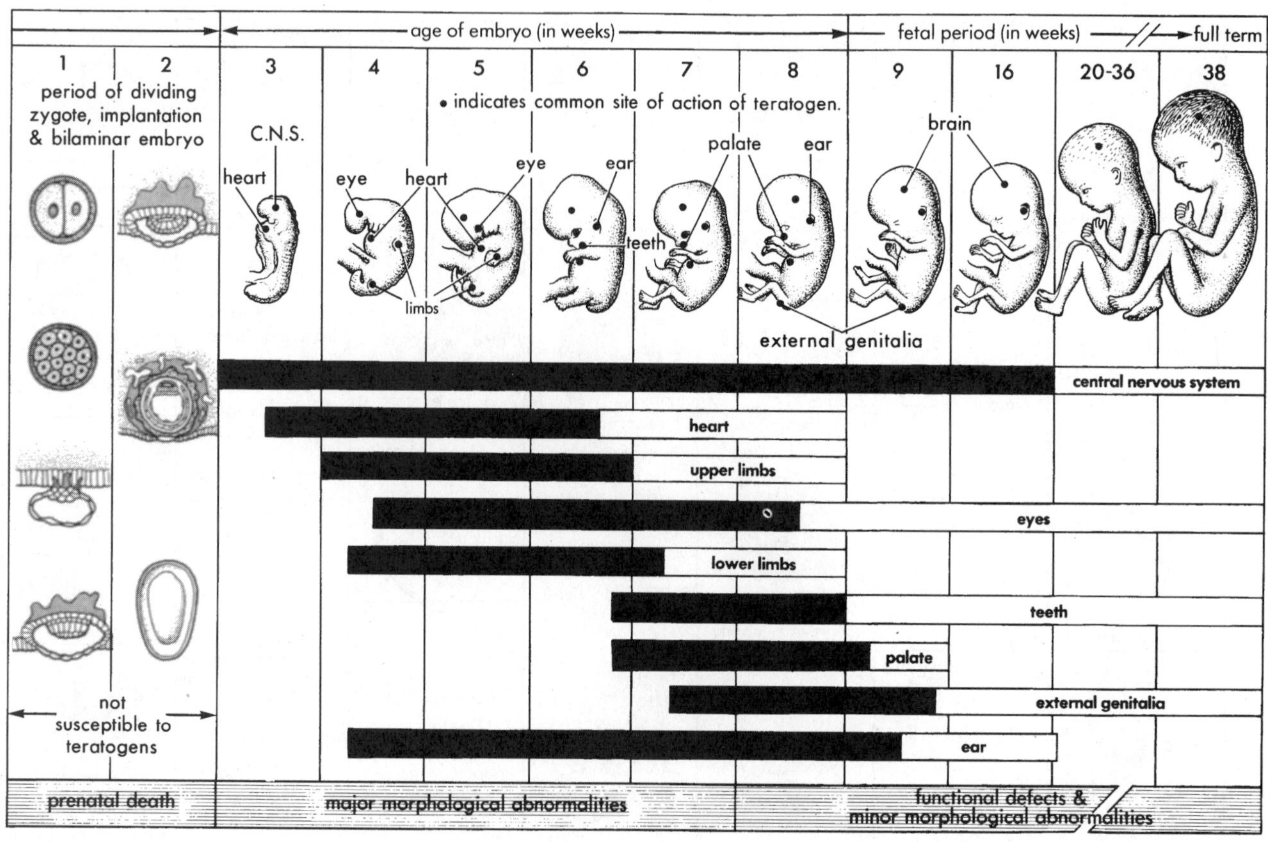

The Fetal Period

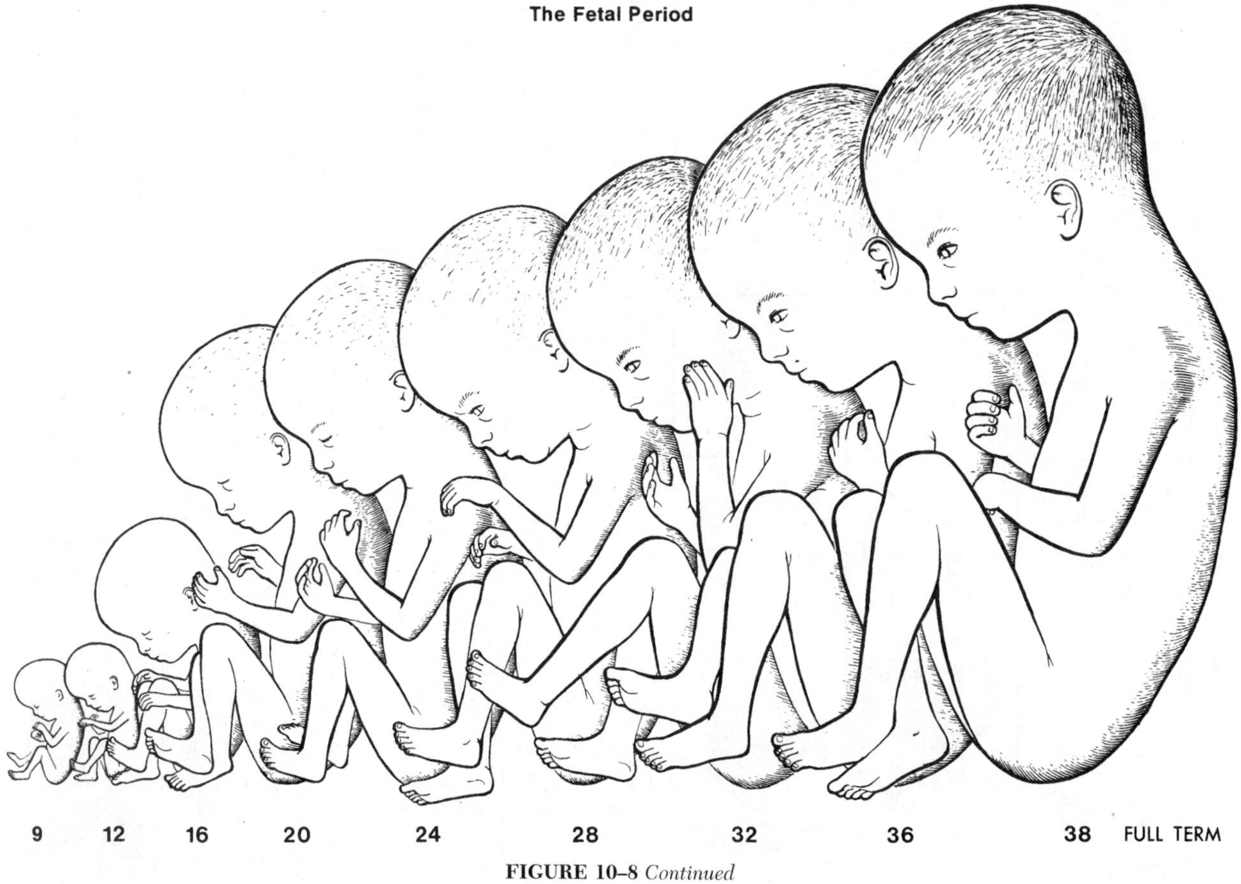

9 12 16 20 24 28 32 36 38 FULL TERM

FIGURE 10–8 *Continued*

TABLE 10–2 Three Periods of Fetal Development

Period 1 Pre-embryonic period	Extends from the fertilization of the ovum to the formation of the embryonic disk with three germ layers—week 1 through week 3.
Period 2 Embryonic period	Period of rapid growth and differentiation; formation of major organ systems occurs—week 4 through week 8.
Period 3 Fetal period	Further growth and development of organ systems—extends from week 9 to week 40 (term).

Data from Moore, K. L. (1989). *The developing human* (4th ed.). Philadelphia: W. B. Saunders.

is characterized by further growth and development of the fetus and the organs formed during the embryonic period. Other changes that occur include the appearance of vernix caseosa, lanugo, and scalp hair. The eyelids open at about 24 to 26 weeks' gestation. The fetus has the potential for survival at approximately 24 weeks, but the preterm newborn experiences many difficult physiologic adjustments for intact survival. Closer to term, subcutaneous fat is deposited, giving the skin a smooth, firm, plump appearance and texture. The last part of the fetal period provides preparation for transition to the extrauterine environment.

The fetus is at less risk for structural defects caused by teratogenic factors than is the embryo. However, there is still a risk for functional impairment of existing structures. This risk is addressed in the section on environmental factors. Changes in specific organs or organ systems during the fetal period are discussed in the section on the development of specific organs. For a summary of prenatal development, see Table 10–2.

DEVELOPMENT OF SPECIFIC ORGANS AND STRUCTURES

Nervous System

The origin of the nervous system is the neural plate, which arises as a thickening of the ectodermal tissue about the middle of the third week of gestation. The neural plate further differentiates into the neural tube and the neural crest. The neural tube gives rise to the central nervous system. The neural crest cells give rise to the peripheral nervous system (Fig. 10–9).

The cranial end of the neural tube forms the three divisions of the brain: the forebrain, the midbrain, and the hindbrain. The cerebral hemispheres and diencephalon arise from the forebrain; the pons, cerebellum, and medulla oblongata arise from the hindbrain. The midbrain makes up the adult midbrain.

The cavity of the neural tube develops into the ventricles of the brain and the central canal of the spinal column. The neuroepithelial cells lining the neural tube give rise to nerves and glial cells of the central nervous system.

The peripheral nervous system consists of the cranial, spinal, and visceral nerves and the ganglia. The somatic and visceral sensory cells of the peripheral nervous system arise from neural crest cells. Cells that form the myelin sheaths of the axons, called *Schwann cells,* also arise from the neural crest cells.

Cardiovascular System

The fetal cardiac system appears at about 18 to 19 days of gestation, and circulation is present by about 21 days. The cardio-

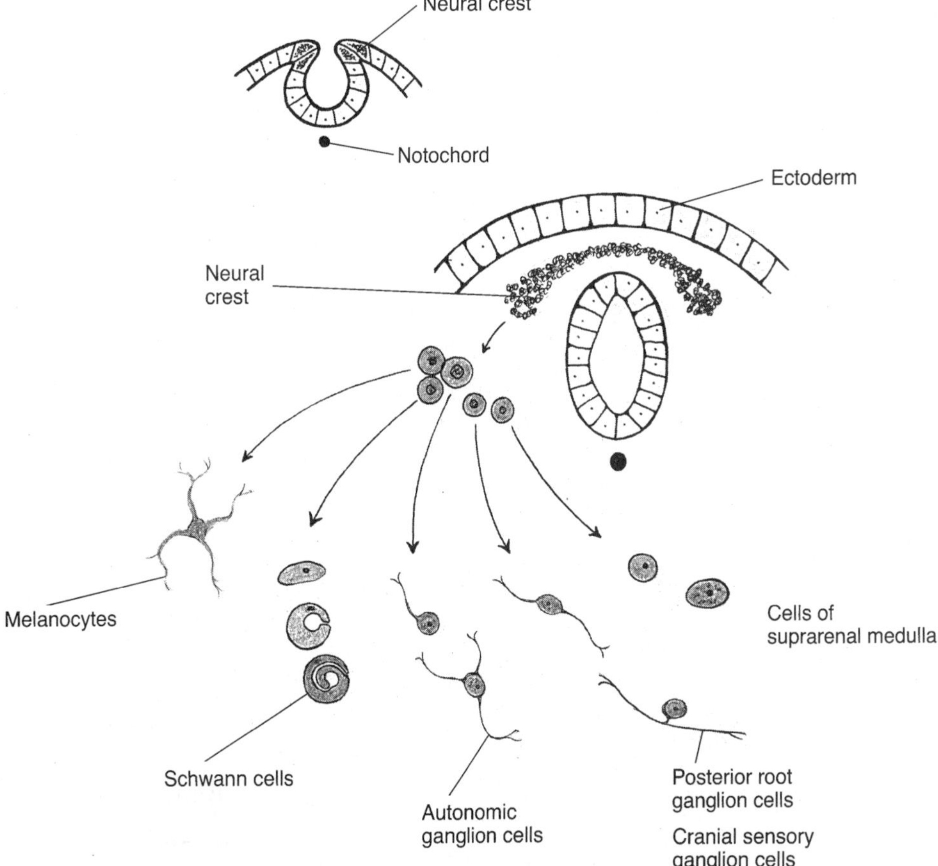

FIGURE 10–9. Differentiation of the nervous system. The cells of the neural crest differentiate into the cells of the ganglia, Schwann cells, and the cells of the suprarenal medulla and melanocytes.

vascular system is the *first* organ system to function in utero. The heart and blood develop from the middle layer (mesoderm) of the trilaminar embryonic disk. Tissue from the lateral mesoderm migrates up the sides of the embryonic disk, forming a horseshoe-shaped structure that arches and meets above the oropharyngeal membrane. With further development, paired heart tubes form, which then fuse into a single heart tube (Fig. 10–10). The vessels that make up the vascular system throughout the body develop from mesodermal cells that connect to each other, with the developing heart tube and the placenta. Thus, by the end of the third week of gestation, there is a functional cardiovascular system.

As the heart tube grows, the folding of the embryonic disk results in the movement of the heart tube into the chest cavity. The heart tube differentiates into three layers: the endocardial layer, which becomes the endothelium; the cardiac jelly, which is a loose tissue layer; and the myoepicardial mantle, which becomes the myocardium and pericardium.

The single heart tube is attached at its cephalic end by the aortic arches and at the caudal end by the septum transversum. The attachments limit the length of the heart tube. Continued growth results in dilated areas and bulges, which become specific components of the heart. First, the atrium, ventricle, and bulbus cordis can be identified. The sinus venosus and truncus arteriosus follow. To accommodate continued growth, two separate bends in the heart occur. It first bends to the right to form a U shape, and the next bend results in an S-shaped heart. The bending of the heart is responsible for the typical location of cardiac structures (Fig. 10–11).

Initially, the heart is a single chamber. Partitioning of the heart into four chambers occurs from the fourth to sixth weeks of gestation. The changes that cause the partitioning of the heart occur simultaneously. The atrium is separated from the ventricle by endocardial cushions, which are thickened areas of endothelium that develop on the dorsal and ventral walls of the open area between the atrium and ventricle. The endocardial cushions fuse with each other to divide the atrioventricular canals into right and left atrioventricular canals.

Partitioning of the atrium occurs through invagination of tissue toward the endocardial cushions, forming the septum primum. As the septum primum grows toward the endocardial cushions, it becomes very thin and perforates. The perforation becomes the foramen ovale. The septum primum does not fuse completely with the endocardial cushions; it has a lower portion that lies beside the endocardial cushions. Overlapping of the septum primum and the septum secundum forms a wall if the pressure in both atria are equal. In utero, the pressure on the right side is increased, allowing blood to flow across the foramen ovale from the right side of the heart to the left side (Fig. 10–12).

The ventricle is also partitioned by a septum, which is membranous and muscular. The muscular portion of the septum develops from the fold of the floor of the ventricle. With blood flowing through the atrioventricular canal, ventricular dilation occurs on either side of the fold or ridge, causing it to become a septum. The membranous septum comes from ridges inside the bulbus cordis. These ridges, continuous into the bulbus cordis, form the wall that divides the bulbus cordis into the pulmonary artery and the aorta. The bulbar ridges fuse with the endocardial cushions to form the membranous septum. The membranous and muscular septa fuse to close the intraventricular foramen, resulting in two parallel circuits for blood flow. The pulmonary artery is continuous with the right ventricle, and the aorta is continuous with the left ventricle (Fig. 10–13).

The blood flowing through the bulbus cordis and truncus arteriosus in a spiral causes the formation of ridges. The ridges fuse to form two separate vessels that twist around each other once. Thus, the pulmonary artery exits the right side of the heart and is in the left upper chest; the aorta exits the left side of the heart and is located close to the sternum.

The pulmonary veins grow from the lungs to a cardinal vein plexus. Concurrently, a vessel develops from the smooth wall of the left atrium. As the atrium grows, the pulmonary vein is

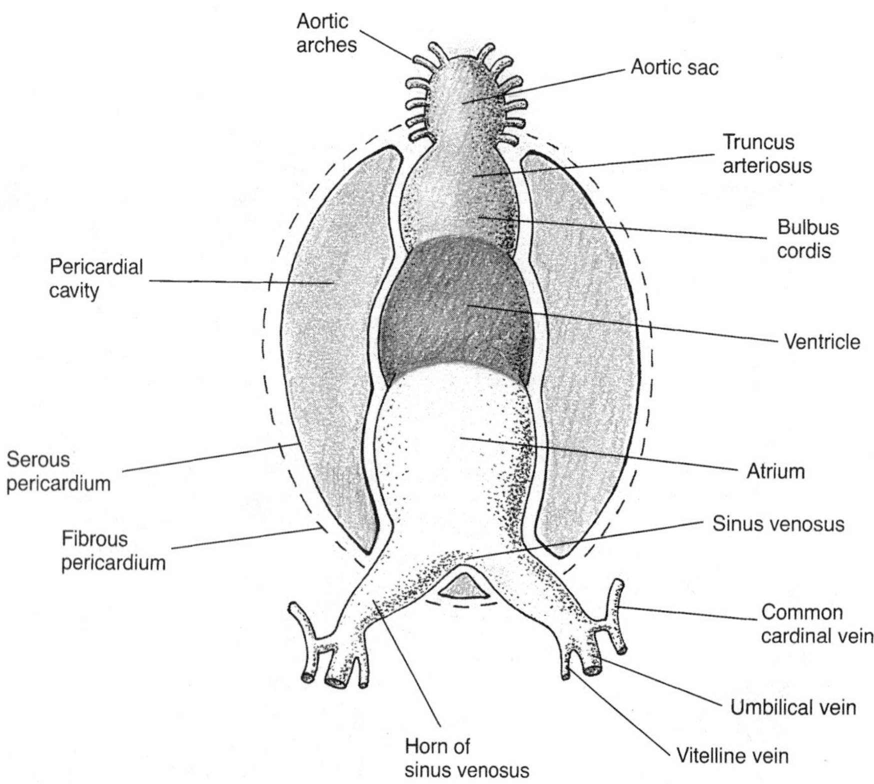

FIGURE 10–10. Formation of the single heart tube. The appearance of the single heart tube inside the pericardial cavity. Note that the atrium and sinus venosus are outside the pericardial cavity.

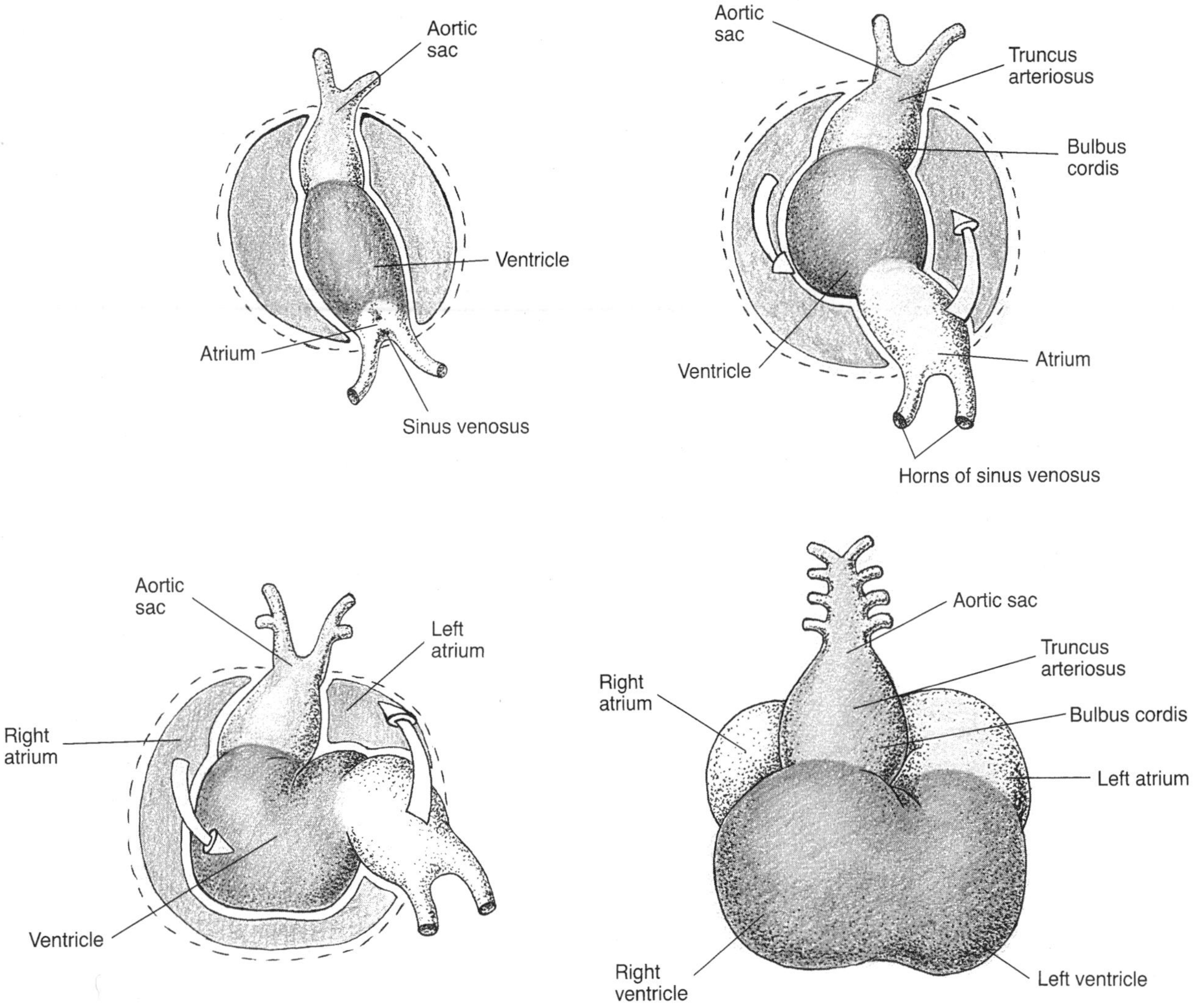

FIGURE 10–11. Bending of the heart tube inside the pericardial cavity. The bending of the heart tube brings the atrium into the pericardial cavity. The sinus venosus is taken into the right atrium and the coronary sinus.

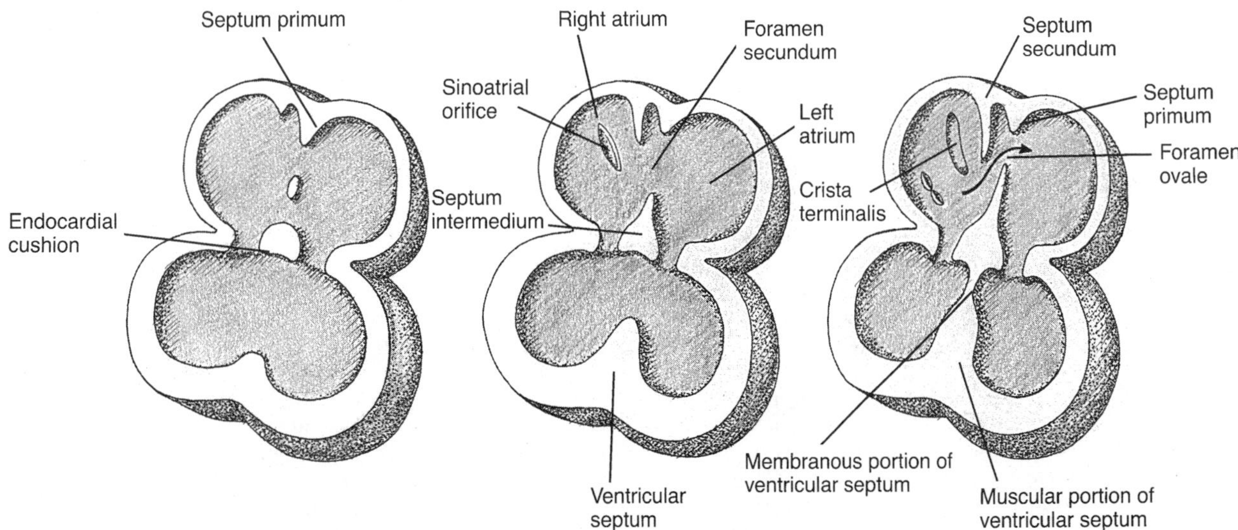

FIGURE 10–12. Partitioning of the atrium. The partitioning of the atrium into the right and left atria through septation.

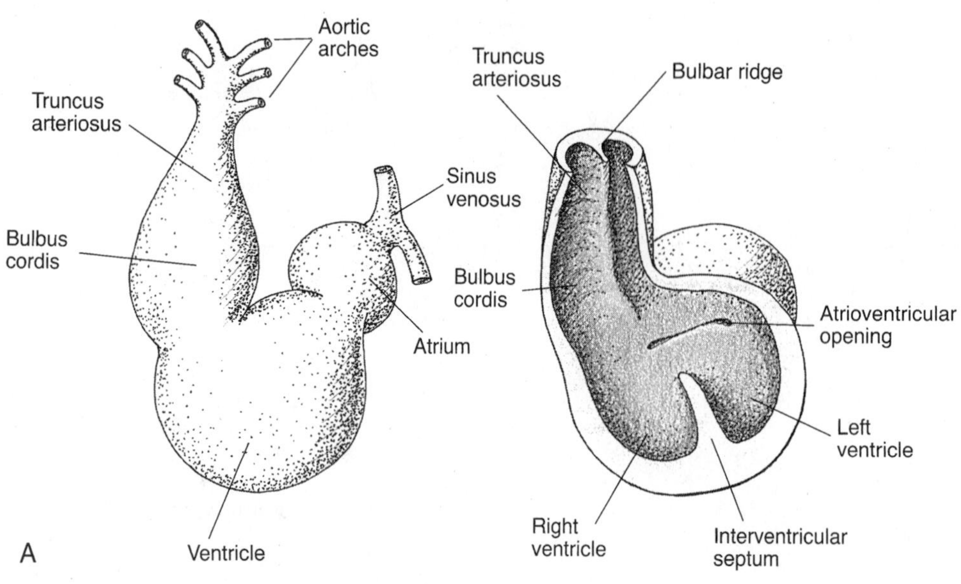

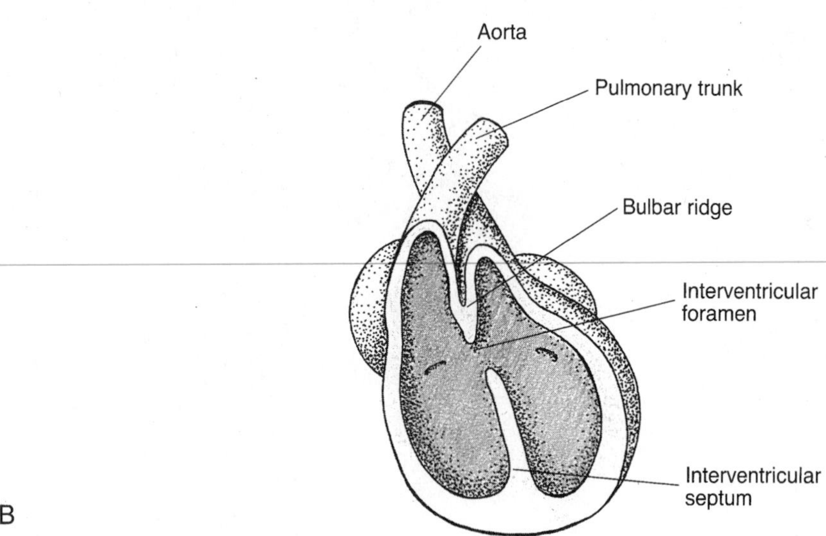

FIGURE 10–13. Partitioning of the ventricles. *A*, Five chambers are present in the heart at 5 weeks' gestation. *B*, At 6 weeks the bulbus cordis has been taken into the ventricles and the interventricular septum has partitioned the ventricles into right and left sides.

incorporated into the atrial wall. The atrium and its branches give rise to four pulmonary veins that enter the left atrium. These pulmonary vessels, connected to the plexus of the cardinal vein, provide a continuous circulation from lung to heart.

The pulmonary and aortic valves (semilunar valves) develop from dilations within the pulmonary artery and aorta. The ebb and flow circulation through these structures causes them to hollow out to form the cusps of the valves. The tricuspid and mitral valves develop from tissue around the atrioventricular canals that thicken and then thin out on the ventricular sides, forming the valves (Fig. 10–14).

Respiratory System

The development of the respiratory system is linked to the development of the face and the digestive system. The respiratory system is composed of the nasal cavities, nasopharynx, oropharynx, larynx, trachea, bronchi, and lungs (Fig. 10–15).

Development of the lungs occurs in four overlapping stages, which extend from the fifth week of gestation until about 8 years of life. The stages are listed in Table 10–3. With a term birth, the normal respiratory system functions immediately. For adequate functioning of the respiratory system, there must be a sufficient number of alveoli, adequate capillary blood flow, and an adequate amount of surfactant produced by the secretory epithelial cells or the type II pneumatocytes. It is the surfactant that prevents alveolar collapse and aids in respiratory gas exchange. Research is under way to examine the use of multidose surfactant instillations after birth in premature infants. This research is an attempt to prevent long-term complications of respiratory distress. Use of liquid ventilation is another area of research; it is aimed at decreasing surface tension and increasing gas exchange.

Muscular System

The muscular system develops from mesodermal cells called myoblasts. Striated skeletal muscles are derived from myotomal mesoderm (myotomes) of the somites. The majority of striated skeletal muscle fibers develop in utero. Almost all striated skeletal muscles are formed by 1 year of age. Growth is achieved by an increase in the diameter of the muscle fibers, rather than the growth of new muscle tissue. Smooth muscle fibers arise from the splanchnic mesenchyme surrounding the endoderm of the

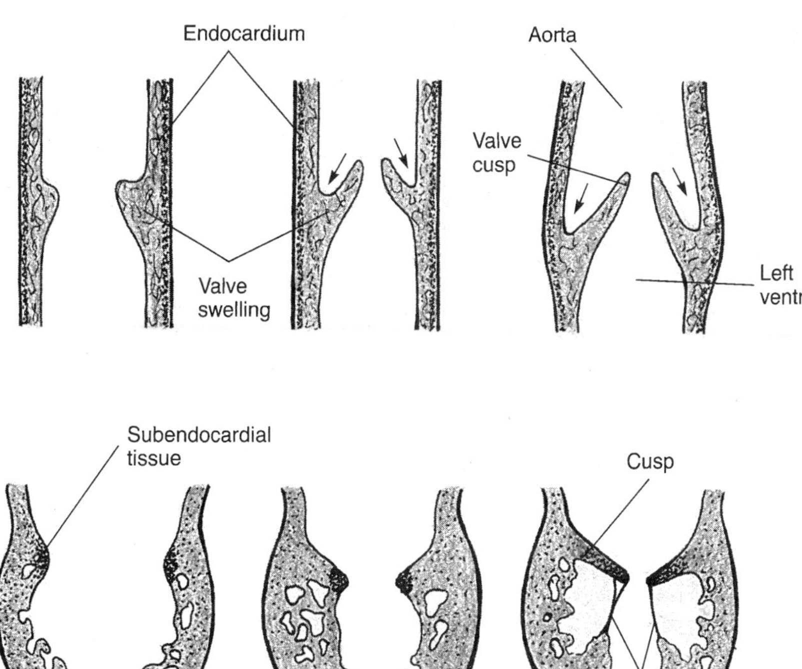

FIGURE 10–14. Formation of the heart valve. *A,* Formation of the semilunar valves of the aorta and the pulmonary artery. *B,* Formation of the cusps of the atrioventricular valves.

primitive gut. Smooth muscles lining vessel walls of blood and lymphatic systems arise from somatic mesoderm.

As smooth muscle cells differentiate, contractile filaments develop in the cytoplasm, and the external surface is covered by an external lamina. As the smooth muscle fibers develop into sheets or bundles, the muscle cells synthesize and release collagenous, elastic, or reticular fibers (Fig. 10–16).

Cardiac muscle develops from splanchnic mesenchyme from the outside of the endocardial heart tube. Cells from the myoepicardial mantle differentiate into the myocardium. Cardiac muscle fibers develop from differentiation and growth of single cells rather than fusion of cells. Cardiac muscle growth occurs through the formation of new filaments. The Purkinje fibers develop late in the embryonic period. These fibers are larger and have fewer myofibrils than do other cardiac muscle cells. The Purkinje fibers function in the electrical conduction system of the heart.

TABLE 10–3 Stages of Lung Development

Stage 1 Weeks 5–7	***Pseudoglandular Period*** Development of the conducting airway
Stage 2 Weeks 13–25	***Canalicular Period*** Enlargement of the bronchial lumina and terminal bronchioles Vascularization of lung tissue Development of respiratory bronchioles and alveolar ducts Development of a limited number of primitive alveoli
Stage 3 Week 24–Birth	***Terminal Sac Period*** Development of primitive pulmonary alveoli from alveolar ducts Increased vascularity Type II pneumatocytes begin to produce surfactant by about 24 weeks
Stage 4 Late fetal period until about 8 years of age	***Alveolar Period*** Pulmonary alveoli formed by thinning of terminal air sac lining One eighth to one sixth of adult number of alveoli present at term birth Number of alveoli increase until age 8 years

Skeletal System

The skeletal system develops from mesenchymal cells. In the long bones, condensed mesenchyme forms hyaline cartilage models of bones. By the end of the embryonic period, ossification centers appear, and these bones ossify by endochondral ossification. Other bones, such as the skull bones, are ossified by membranous ossification in which the mesenchyme cells become osteoblasts (Fig. 10–17).

The vertebral column and the ribs arise from the sclerotome compartments of the somites. The spinal column is formed by the fusion of a condensation of the cranial half of one pair of sclerotomes with the caudal half of the next pair of sclerotomes.

The skull can be divided into the neurocranium and the viscerocranium. The neurocranium forms the protective covering around the brain. The viscerocranium forms the skeleton of the face. The neurocranium is made up of the flat bones that surround the brain and the cartilaginous structure, or chondrocranium, that forms the bones of the base of the skull. The neurocranium (chondrocranium) is made up of a number of separate cartilages, which fuse and ossify by endochondral ossification to form the base of the skull.

Gastrointestinal System

The gastrointestinal system is primarily derived from the lining of the roof of the yolk sac. The primitive gut, consisting of

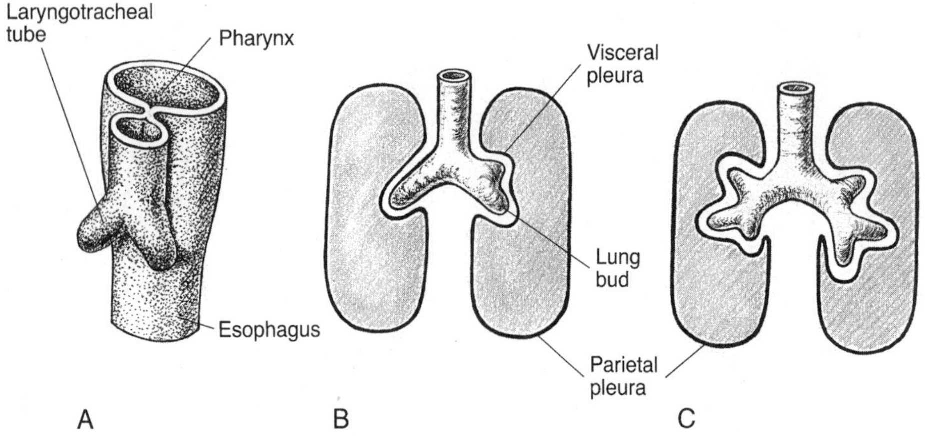

FIGURE 10–15. Development of the pulmonary system. *A*, The laryngotracheal groove and tube have formed; the margins of the laryngotracheal groove fuse, forming the laryngotracheal tube. *B*, Invagination of the lung buds into the intraembryonic cavity. *C*, Division of the lung buds into the right and left mainstem bronchi.

the foregut, midgut, and hindgut, is formed during the fourth gestational week (Fig. 10–18).

The structures that arise from the foregut include the pharynx, esophagus, stomach, liver, pancreas, gallbladder, and part of the duodenum. The esophagus and trachea have a common origin, the laryngotracheal diverticulum. A septum, formed by the growing tracheoesophageal folds, divides the cranial part of the foregut into the laryngotracheal tube and the esophagus. Smooth muscle develops from the splanchnic mesenchyme that surrounds the esophagus. The epithelial lining of the esophagus, derived from the endoderm, proliferates, partially obliterating the esophageal lumen. The esophagus undergoes recanalization by the end of the embryonic period.

The stomach originates as a dilation of the caudal portion of the foregut. The characteristic greater curvature of the stomach results because the dorsal border grows faster than the ventral border. As the stomach develops further, it rotates in a clockwise direction around the longitudinal axis.

The duodenum is derived from the caudal and cranial portions of the foregut and the cranial portion of the midgut. The junction of the foregut and midgut portions of the duodenum is normally distal to the common bile duct.

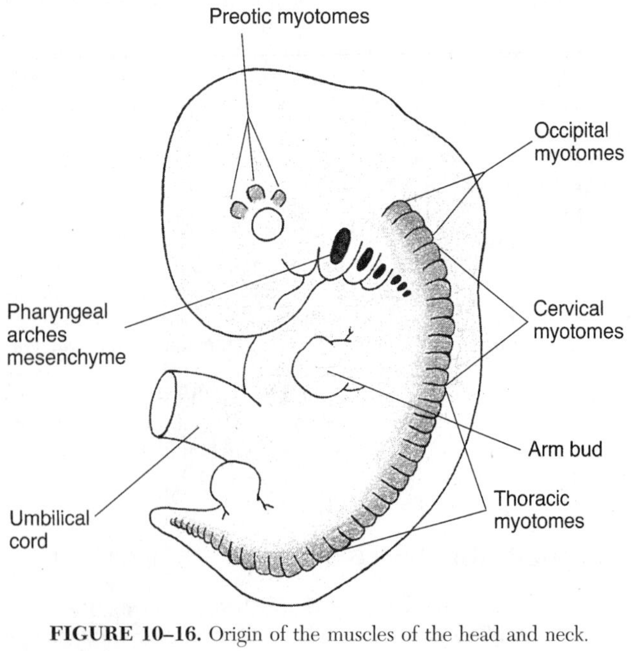

FIGURE 10–16. Origin of the muscles of the head and neck.

The liver, gallbladder, and biliary ducts originate as a bud from the caudal end of the foregut. The liver is formed by growth of the hepatic diverticulum, which grows between the layers of the ventral mesentery, forming two parts. The liver forms from the largest, cranial portion. Hepatic cells originate from the hepatic diverticulum. Hematopoietic tissue and Kupffer cells are derived from the splanchnic mesenchyme of the septum transversum. The liver develops rapidly and fills the abdominal cavity. The liver begins its hematopoietic function by the sixth gestational week.

The smaller portion of the hepatic diverticulum forms the gallbladder. The common bile duct is formed from the stalk connecting the hepatic and cystic ducts to the duodenum. The pancreas is derived from the pancreatic buds that arise from the caudal part of the foregut.

The structures that are derived from the midgut include the remainder of the duodenum, the cecum, the appendix, the ascending colon, and the majority of the transverse colon.

The intestines must undergo extensive growth during the first weeks of development. The liver and kidneys occupy the abdominal cavity, restricting the space available for intestinal growth. The phenomenal growth of the intestines is accommodated through a migration out of the abdominal cavity via the umbilical cord. A series of rotations occurs before the intestines return to the abdomen. The first rotation is counterclockwise, around the axis of the superior mesenteric artery. At about the tenth week, the intestines return to the abdomen, undergoing further rotation. When the colon returns to the abdomen, the cecal end rotates to the right side, entering the lower right quadrant of the abdomen.

The cecum and appendix arise from the cecal diverticulum, a pouch that appears in the fifth week of gestation on the caudal limb of the midgut loop (Fig. 10–19).

The hindgut is that portion of the intestines from the midgut to the cloacal membrane. The latter structure consists of the endoderm of the cloaca and the ectoderm of the anal pit. The cloaca is divided by the urorectal septum. As the septum grows toward the cloacal membrane, folds from the lateral walls of the cloaca grow together, dividing the cloaca into the rectum and upper anal canal dorsally and the urogenital sinus ventrally.

By the end of the sixth week, the urorectal septum fuses with the cloacal membrane, forming a dorsal anal membrane and a larger ventral urogenital membrane. At about the end of the seventh gestational week, these two membranes rupture, forming the anal canal.

Urogenital System

The development of the urinary and genital systems is closely related. The urogenital system develops from the intermediate mesoderm, which extends along the dorsal body wall of the

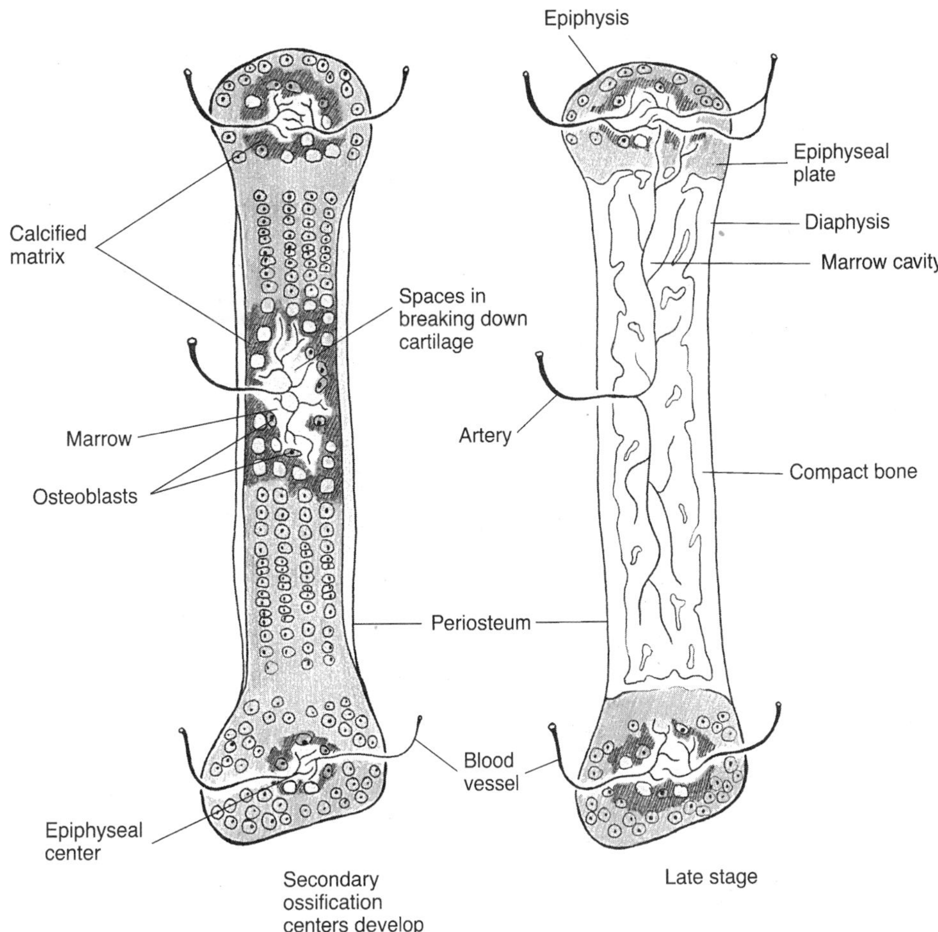

FIGURE 10–17. Endochondral ossification of bones.

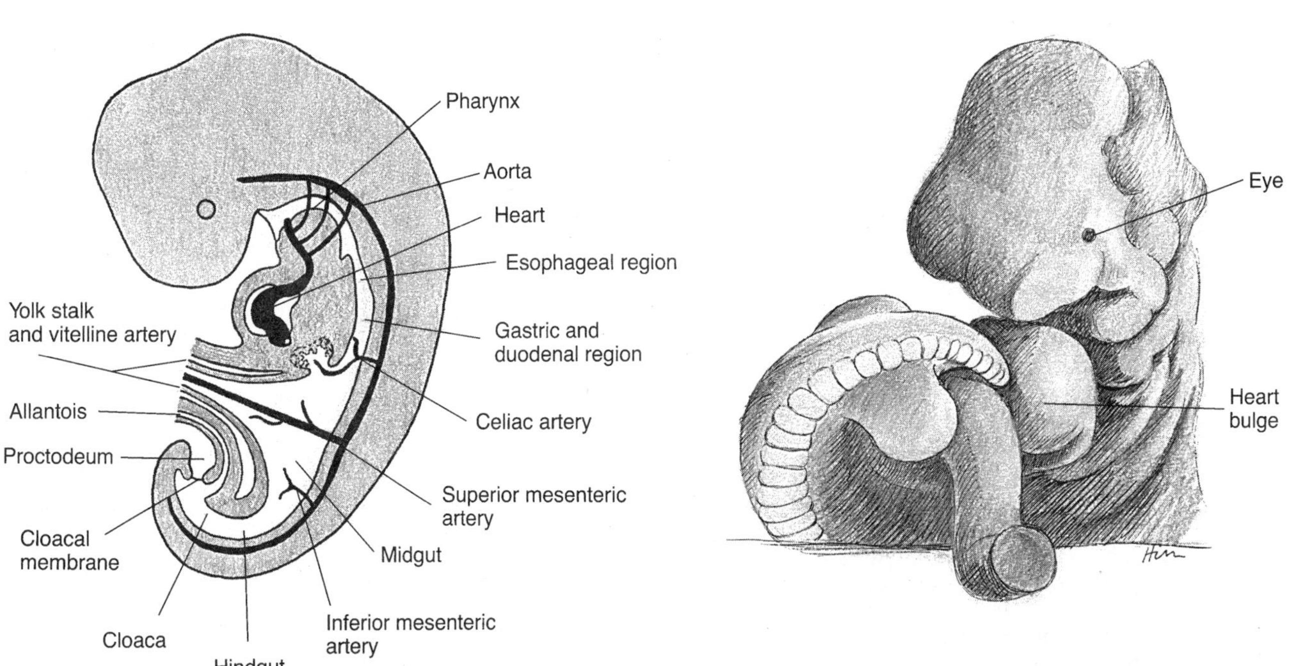

FIGURE 10–18. The primitive gut. The early gastrointestinal system present in an embryo at about 4 weeks' gestation.

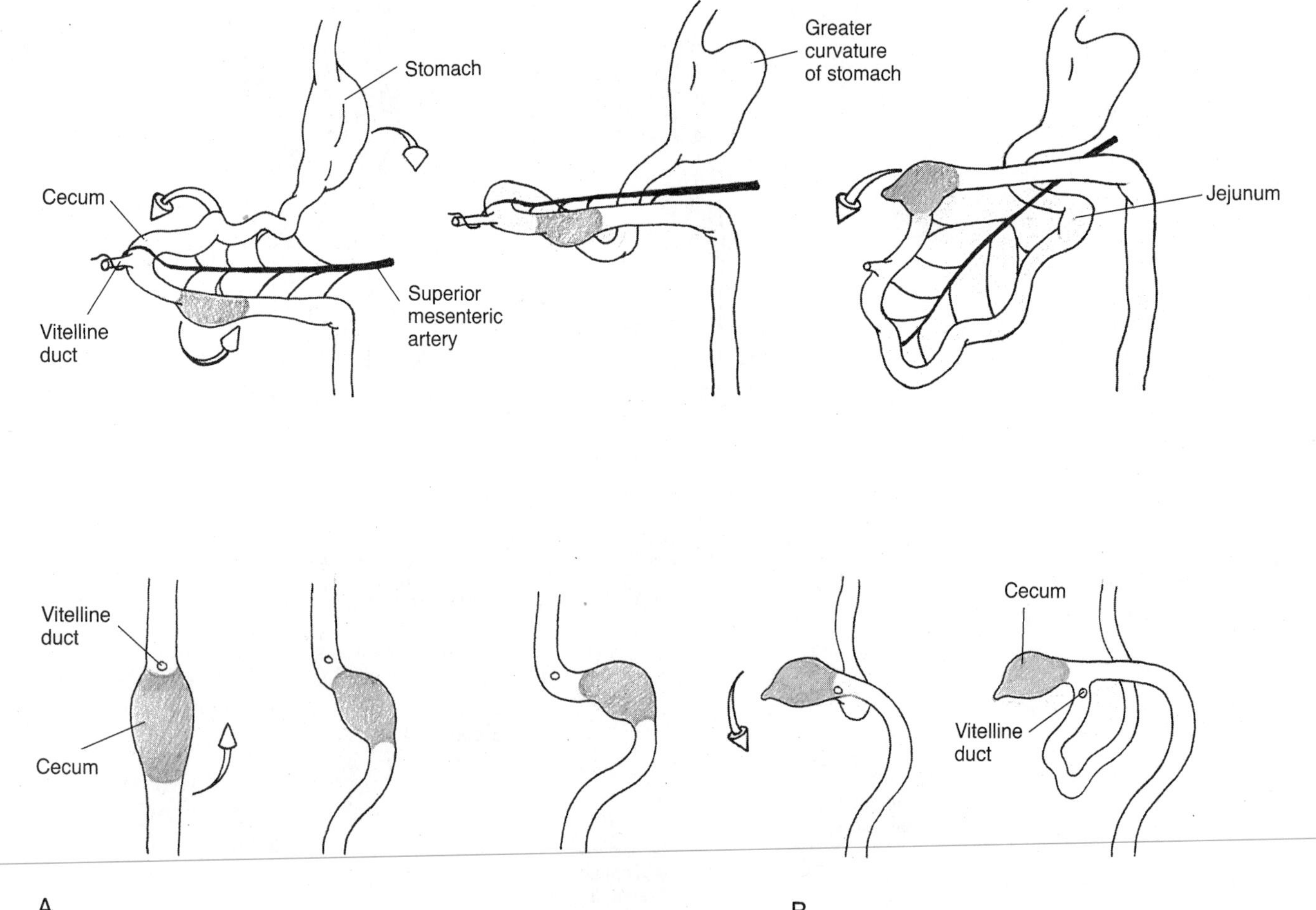

FIGURE 10–19. Migration and rotation of the midgut. *A,* Counterclockwise 90-degree rotation of midgut loop and "herniation" into extraembryonic cavity. *B,* Counterclockwise 180-degree rotation of midgut loop on return to the abdominal cavity.

embryo. During embryonic folding in the horizontal plane, the intermediate mesoderm is moved forward and is no longer connected to the somites. This mesoderm forms the urogenital ridge on each side of the primitive aorta. Both the urinary and genital systems arise from this urogenital ridge. The area from which the urinary system is derived is called the *nephrogenic cord.* The genital ridge is the area from which the reproductive system is derived.

There are three stages of development of the kidney: the pronephros, the mesonephros, and the metanephros. The pronephros, a nonfunctional organ, appears in the first month of gestation and then degenerates, contributing only a duct system for the next developmental stage. The mesonephros uses the duct of the pronephros and develops caudally to the pronephros (Fig. 10–20). The mesonephros may function in urine formation during the development of the metanephros. The mesonephros degenerates by the end of the embryonic period. Remnants of the mesonephros persist as genital ducts in males or vestigial structures in females. The metanephros appears in the fifth week of gestation and becomes the permanent kidney. The metanephros begins to produce urine by about the 11th week of gestation.

The urinary bladder and the urethra arise from the urogenital sinus and the splanchnic mesenchyme. The caudal portion of the mesonephric ducts is incorporated into the bladder, giving rise to the ureters.

Although the genetic sex of the embryo is determined at conception, the early development of the genital system is indistinguishable until the seventh week of gestation. Beginning in the seventh week, the gonads begin to be differentiated. The ovaries and the testes are derived from the coelomic epithelium, the mesenchyme, and the primordial germ cells.

Development of female sexual organs occurs in the absence of hormonal stimulation precipitated by the H-Y antigen gene carried on the Y chromosome. If the Y chromosome is present, testes develop; otherwise, ovaries develop.

CONGENITAL DEFECTS

Congenital defects or anomalies are structural or anatomic abnormalities present at birth. Congenital defects vary in severity and location, ranging from minor insignificant defects to major organ system defects. Congenital defects are attributed to genetic or chromosomal abnormalities or to maternal or environmental factors. Most congenital defects result from an interaction between genetic and environmental factors. This type of transmission of defects is categorized as multifactorial inheritance.

The generally reported incidence of significant congenital defects is about 2 to 3 percent. The actual incidence is higher because some defects are not apparent at birth. The incidence of all defects (including both minor and major defects) is approximately 14 percent. Almost 20 percent of all perinatal deaths are caused by congenital defects.

Congenital defects caused by single-gene disorders and chromosomal abnormalities are discussed in Chapter 9, Human Ge-

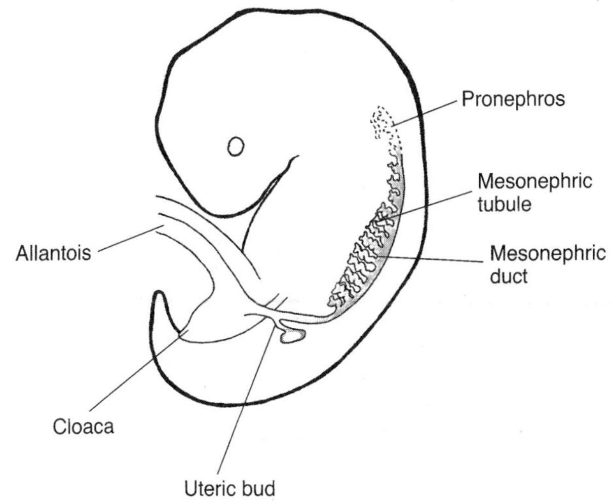

FIGURE 10–20. Development of the kidney. The locations of the pronephros and mesonephros.

netics. The influence of the environment on embryonic development is discussed in this section.

Moore and Persaud (1993) listed six mechanisms that can cause congenital defects: (1) too little growth, (2) too little resorption, (3) too much resorption, (4) resorption in the wrong location, (5) normal growth in an abnormal position, and (6) overgrowth of a tissue or structure. Embryonic organs are most sensitive to noxious agents during a period of rapid cell growth and differentiation. Damage to the primitive streak at about 15 days of gestation could cause severe congenital malformations of the embryo because of its role in the production of intraembryonic mesoderm, from which all connective tissue is formed. Biochemical differentiation occurs before morphologic differentiation, so organs or structures are sensitive to the action of teratogens before they can be identified.

Critical Periods of Human Development

Environmental influences during the first 2 weeks after conception may prevent successful implantation of the blastocyst and cause abortion of the embryo. The most sensitive period for the embryo is the period of organogenesis, especially from day 15 to day 60. Each organ has a critical period during which its development is most likely to be adversely affected by the presence of teratogenic agents (see Fig. 10–8 for critical periods for each major organ system).

Teratogens

Teratogens are agents that may adversely affect embryonic development. About 7 percent of all congenital defects are caused by exposure to teratogenic agents. Known teratogenic agents include drugs or other chemicals, radiation, and infectious organisms. Very few agents have been proved teratogenic, primarily owing to the risks to humans that make scientific study difficult. Some agents have been tested on animal models; however, caution must be used when extrapolating these findings to humans. Some agents have been identified as teratogenic after exposure to the agent resulted in an increased incidence of defects (Kenner, 1991). The limited knowledge about safety of all substances makes it prudent for women to avoid all potential teratogens prior to conception and during pregnancy.

Drugs and Chemicals

Drugs and chemicals account for about 2 to 3 percent of congenital defects. Few drugs are known to be teratogenic; however, no drug can be considered completely safe. Therefore, all drugs should be avoided unless the benefit of taking the drug outweighs potential risks. Drugs of various classifications have been identified as being teratogenic (Kuller, 1990).

Alcohol has been associated with congenital defects, which include craniofacial abnormalities, limb deformities, and cardiovascular defects. Associated abnormalities include growth deficiency and mental retardation. The term *fetal alcohol syndrome* is used to describe the cluster of defects characteristic of maternal ingestion of alcohol. There is no level of alcohol consumption that can be considered safe; therefore, it is recommended that alcohol be avoided throughout the perinatal period (Baraitser & Winter, 1996; Eliason & Williams, 1990).

Certain antibiotics have been identified as teratogens. Tetracycline is deposited in the embryo's bones and teeth, leading to a brown discoloration to the teeth and diminished growth of the long bones. Antituberculosis agents, such as streptomycin and dihydrostreptomycin, have been associated with hearing deficits and damage to cranial nerve VIII. Sulfonamides have been associated with an increased incidence of kernicterus in the newborn. Currently, the safest antibiotic for use in pregnant women appears to be penicillin. This drug has not been associated with an increased incidence of congenital defects.

Several anticonvulsant drugs have been implicated in the presence of congenital defects (Sanders, 1996). The use of phenytoin may cause craniofacial defects, nail and digital hypoplasia, intrauterine growth retardation, microcephaly, and mental retardation. Other anticonvulsant drugs that have been identified as teratogens include trimethadione (Tridione) and paramethadione (Paradione). The defects include fetal facial dysmorphia, cardiac defects, cleft palate, and intrauterine growth retardation.

Warfarin, an anticoagulant, can cause craniofacial abnormalities, optic atrophy, microcephaly, and mental retardation. Other anticoagulants, although not specifically teratogenic, cross the placental barrier and may lead to hemorrhage in the fetus. Heparin does not cross the placental barrier and is used for anticoagulation in pregnant women.

Antineoplastic agents are particularly teratogenic. Aminopterin and methotrexate have both been associated with major congenital malformations, especially central nervous system defects. Antineoplastic drugs may be harmful to health care workers exposed to them during routine nursing interventions. Women who are pregnant or trying to conceive should not administer antineoplastic agents (Shortridge, 1990).

Antipsychotic and antianxiety agents are also suspected teratogenic agents. Phenothiazine and lithium have been linked to congenital defects. Diazepam (Valium), meprobamate, and chlordiazepoxide may cause congenital defects. Diazepam is associated with an increased incidence of cleft lip with or without cleft palate.

Hormonal agents are also implicated in the incidence of congenital defects. Androgenic agents (progestins) may cause masculinization of female fetuses. Diethylstilbestrol (DES), a synthetic estrogen used to prevent abortion in the 1940s and 1950s, has been found to cause an increased incidence of vaginal and cervical cancer in female children exposed to the drug in utero. Additionally, there are associated abnormalities of the reproductive system, often causing reproductive dysfunction (Sadler, 1995). Cortisone has been shown to cause cleft palate in animal models but has not been implicated as a factor in cleft palate in human newborns.

Social or recreational drugs are highly suspected of contributing to congenital defects. Drugs such as lysergic acid diethylamide (LSD) have been associated with limb abnormalities and central nervous system abnormalities. Other drugs that may be teratogenic include phencyclidine and marijuana. "Crack" cocaine, a relative newcomer to the social drug inventory, has been associated with congenital abnormalities (Kennard, 1990). The tendency of drug abusers to use multiple drugs, combined with their poor nutritional habits and lack of prenatal care, makes it difficult to establish the effects of the drugs individually (Kenner, 1991).

Miscellaneous drugs from other categories that are suspected of leading to congenital defects include propylthiouracil and potassium iodide, which are associated with neonatal goiter and mental retardation. Amphetamines are associated with oral clefts and heart defects. Salicylates (aspirin), the most commonly used medication during pregnancy, may be harmful to the fetus if taken in large amounts. Retinoic acid (vitamin A) is teratogenic in high doses in humans (Kenner, 1991). Isotretinoin, a drug used to treat acne, causes craniofacial abnormalities, cleft palate, thymic aplasia defects, and neural tube defects.

Environmental chemicals such as pollutants, fungicides, food additives, and defoliants have been suspected of causing congenital defects. There is the most support for the claim that mercury produces neurologic manifestations similar to those seen in cerebral palsy, blindness, and mental retardation (Sadler, 1995). Although there is little evidence to prove that other environmental agents are teratogenic, no data prove that environmental chemicals are not dangerous. Therefore, pregnant women should avoid exposure to potentially toxic chemicals. Unfortunately, because of their many uses it is difficult to recognize exposure to potentially hazardous products.

Radiation

Exposure to high levels of ionizing radiation can result in microcephaly, skull defects, spina bifida, blindness, and cleft palate. Studies of the outcomes of women who were pregnant during the atomic bombing of Hiroshima and Nagasaki showed that 28 percent had abortions, 25 percent had liveborns who died within 1 year, and 25 percent of the survivors gave birth to children with central nervous system disorders (Sadler, 1995).

There is no established "safe" level for radiation. The severity of the defect depends on the duration and timing of exposure. There is no evidence that the small amount of radiation required for modern x-ray studies is harmful; however, caution is used to minimize the exposure to the fetus.

Infectious Agents

Three viral agents have been positively identified as teratogenic to the developing fetus: rubella, cytomegalovirus (CMV), and herpes simplex. There is a 15 to 20 percent incidence of congenital malformations in newborns of women who have had rubella in the first trimester of pregnancy. The typical malformations include heart defects, deafness, and cataracts (Lott, 1994).

CMV is thought to be the most commonly occurring viral infection of the human fetus. CMV in early embryonic development probably results in spontaneous abortion. CMV infection during the second or third trimester may cause microcephaly and microphthalmia (Lott, 1994).

Herpes simplex infection of the fetus primarily occurs late in the pregnancy, commonly during delivery. Congenital abnormalities in fetuses infected prior to delivery include microcephaly, microphthalmia, retinal dysplasia, and mental retardation.

Maternal infection with *Toxoplasma gondii*, a protozoal parasite, can cause hydrocephalus, cerebral calcification, microphthalmia, and ocular defects. *T. gondii* can be contracted from undercooked meat, by handling feces of infected cats, or from the soil.

Untreated primary maternal infections of *Treponema pallidum*, the microorganism that causes syphilis, results in serious fetal infection, but adequate treatment kills the organism, preventing serious defects. Syphilis can lead to congenital deafness and mental retardation if untreated (Lott, 1994).

Other viral agents have been implicated as causes of congenital malformations. Such malformations have been reported following maternal infection with mumps, varicella, echovirus, coxsackievirus, and influenza virus. The incidence of congenital malformations following these infections is suspected to be low (Sadler, 1995). (For further information on viral agents, see Chapter 27, Assessment and Management of Immunologic Dysfunction). One other factor has recently been identified as being teratogenic: hyperthermia. It may be the causative factor in congenital defects associated with viral agents, because of the fever produced by the agents. Hyperthermia can also be caused by maternal use of hot tubs or saunas.

CONCLUSION

This chapter has outlined the critical periods of development. It has described the more common congenital problems that may be seen in the neonatal intensive care unit resulting from developmental dysfunction in utero.

REFERENCES

Baraitser, M., & Winter, R. M. (1996). *Color atlas of congenital malformation syndromes.* St. Louis: C. V. Mosby.

Eliason, M. J., & Williams, J. K. (1990). Fetal alcohol syndrome and the neonate. *Journal of Perinatal and Neonatal Nursing, 3*(4), 64–72.

Kennard, M. J. (1990). Cocaine use during pregnancy: Fetal and neonatal effects. *Journal of Perinatal and Neonatal Nursing, 3*(4), 53–63.

Kenner, C. (1991). Genetic risks and other hazards for the NICU nurse. *Neonatal Network, 10*(1), 37-40, 49–51.

Kuller, J. M. (1990). Effects on the fetus and newborn of medications commonly used during pregnancy. *Journal of Perinatal and Neonatal Nursing, 3*(4), 73–87.

Lott, J. W. (1994). *Neonatal infection: Assessment, diagnosis, and management.* Petaluma, CA: NICU Ink.

Moore, K. L., & Persaud, T. V. N. (1993). *Before we are born: Basic embryology and birth defects* (5th ed.). Philadelphia: W. B. Saunders.

Sadler, T. W. (1995). *Langman's medical embryology* (7th ed.). Baltimore: Williams & Wilkins.

Sanders, R. C. (Ed.). (1996). *Structural fetal abnormalities: The total picture.* St. Louis: C. V. Mosby.

Shortridge, L. A. (1990). Advances in the assessment of the effect of environmental and occupational toxins on reproduction. *Journal of Perinatal and Neonatal Nursing, 3*(4), 1–11.

CHAPTER 11

High-Risk Pregnancy

JUDITH S. HARMON

RESEARCH AGENDA

Are some cesarean births related to nursing care, independent of physician management?

If some cesarean births are related to nursing care, what are the nursing behaviors and interventions that are absent in cesarean and present in vaginal birth outcomes?

How do the costs and outcomes of antepartal home care nursing compare with those of uterine home monitoring devices?

Does the fetus play a role in the initiation of labor?

Do tocolytic agents or bed rest or both prolong the pregnancy and effectively stop premature labor?

What is the experience of women given tocolytics or put on bed rest for premature labor?

What are the risk factors for developing a high-risk pregnancy?

VIGNETTE

The request came during a quiet time in our NICU. "Could you come out and talk to one of our mothers? She's 30 weeks and has severe pregnancy-induced hypertension [PIH]. The OB is planning to deliver her this afternoon. She's expressing a lot of concern about the baby." Marla O was a 28-year-old Afro-American primigravida with a history of chronic hypertension, treated with medication for the past 3 years. The antihypertensive was discontinued early in the pregnancy owing to normalization of Marla's BP. She had begun to show the classic signs of PIH at 30 weeks: edema of the hands, rise in blood pressure, and 3+ urine protein. Her OB had admitted her at that time. Treatment consisted of bed rest with 2-hour vital signs, deep tendon reflexes and continual fetal heart assessment q 4 hours, betamethasone 12 mg q 24 hours $\times$ 2 doses, $MgSO_4$ IV at 3 g/hour, urine protein with each void, I & O q void, and labs including uric acid, ALT, AST, Hgb, HCT, PT, PTT, and platelet count. During her 2-day hospitalization, Marla's condition stabilized; uric acid increased and platelet count was 78,000. Fetal heart baseline rate was in normal range with some 10 $\times$ 10 beat accelerations; however, an ultrasound indicated asymmetrical growth retardation. Marla was reassured, as betamethasone had been administered and her baby was in the "steroid window" for lung maturity.

Review of the OB's progress notes indicated increasing BP and deterioration in laboratory studies and a planned delivery as soon as Marla was stable. Orders detailed a 4-g $MgSO_4$ loading dose to infuse over 15 minutes, followed by a 2-g/hour infusion of a solution of 40 g $MgSO_4$ in 500 ml of fluid. A 2-mg IV bolus of hydralazine was ordered. Continuous fetal monitoring was ordered. Marla was placed on 10L/min O_2 by face mask. A urinary catheter was inserted, and I & O q.h. until delivery was to be reported to the physician. Vital signs were ordered for q 15 minutes. Lab tests included CBC, creatinine, uric acid, serum Mg levels, coagulation studies, liver enzymes, and type and crossmatch. The cervix was noninducible, so a C-section with a general anesthesia and pediatrician in attendance was planned. I concluded my chart review and entered Marla's room. Her nurse stood at her bedside. She introduced me. "This is Susan, from the newborn nursery. She's an expert with babies that are born early. She can answer your questions." She smiled and winked at me, then went about her work. Marla didn't smile. "Thank you for coming. I'm only 30 weeks along, and my doctor wants to deliver me today because of my preeclampsia. I know my baby isn't ready to be born yet, but my doctor says it's safer than to leave her inside. I'm scared about what might happen to her."

I sat at the bedside for quite some time, explaining some general expectations for a 30-week, intrauterine growth–retarded infant of a severely preeclamptic mother. I emphasized that anticipation and readiness were the keys to a good start for her baby, and that we would attend the delivery to provide for her infant's needs from the very first minute of life. I told her that the baby would look small because of her prematurity and that she may need some help with breathing effectively. I reassured her that, given her progressive preeclamptic condition, the baby may be better prepared to breathe on her own than another infant of the same gestational age. I described her probable needs for warmth, fluids, and special feeding and the way we would care for each of these needs. I described the possible problem of polycythemia, which is common in infants of PIH mothers. Marla listened intently to the information. She stated that she felt less worried. "Will you come to my delivery?" she asked. "I'll try," I smiled. "I'm here until 7 this evening. Get your BP fixed before that, and I promise I'll be there." Marla laughed. Late that afternoon I attended Marla's delivery. Her baby girl was small for 30 weeks' gestation, and her head looked large in proportion to her body, owing to the asymmetrical growth retardation. Cord pH was 7.10 at time of birth. Respirations were slow to start. Positive pressure ventilation with 100 percent O_2 was initiated immediately. The pulse was greater than 100 beats per minute from the start. Neonatal acidemia was treated aggressively, and within 5 minutes, her respiratory effort was adequate enough to downgrade the positive pressure to blow-by oxygen. I wrapped Baby O and showed her to her mother.

We then transported Baby O to the NICU. Within 40 minutes, we had weaned her O_2 to 28 percent. Respiratory effort was slightly labored; rate, 48. Blood gases were normal. Admitting lab tests indicated polycythemia (central HCT, 68) and hypoglycemia (blood glucose, 28). $D_{10}W$ was hung, an umbilical line was placed, and a partial exchange transfusion was done.

Baby O progressed with few complications. She was weaned from O_2 to room air at 8 days of age. Small-volume diluted formula feedings by gavage were begun on day 3 of life. Feedings progressed slowly over 2 weeks to full-strength oral feedings.

Marla spent 2 more days on the intensive care regimen. During this time, she was restricted to bed rest. I was caring for her infant, so I brought Baby O to see her mother once each day, including O_2 tank and paraphernalia. I provided footprints, pictures, and progress reports several times a day. Marla was sleepy and disoriented because of the $MgSO_4$. Each time I visited her she said, "Tell me about my baby again. Is she all right?" Marla spent 10 days in the hospital recovering from her operative delivery and PIH and HELLP syndrome. She was discharged on day 11, looking and feeling much better than the day I had met her. The edema was resolved, her BP was back within her prepregnancy limits, and her renal function was returning to normal. Marla visited the NICU frequently and was taught basic baby care. At 4 weeks of age, Marla took "Miracle" home, weighing 4½ lb and eating like a champion.

Joyce M. Dohme
Judith S. Harmon

Perinatal nursing is developing at a rapid pace. The expanded knowledge in this field has resulted in a greater emphasis on identification of maternal risk factors, early preventive and therapeutic treatment, patient education, and transport of undelivered women after stabilization of maternal conditions. This chapter provides an overview of common maternal complications and their potential deleterious effects on the fetus and neonate.

MATERNAL-FETAL UNIT

Placenta

From the beginning of cell division and the formation of the morula, certain cells are destined to form the placenta. As the morula passes through the fallopian tube, it becomes the blastocyst. The outer layer of the blastocyst is called the *trophoblast*. Trophoblasts invade the maternal endometrium, forming three layers of cells that send out finger-like projections called villi. Implantation of the villi requires that the lining of the uterus, or endometrium, be richly supplied with nutritive substances (Gilbert & Harmon, 1997).

Previous scarring from incisions into the uterus or from infection in the lining may adversely affect where implantation takes place. Typically, the placenta implants in the posterior portion of the fundus of the uterus. If the placenta implants in the lower portion of the uterus or does not implant securely, bleeding and separation may occur in the third trimester.

The placenta serves four main organ or system functions:

1. As a fetal lung or respiratory function for exchange of oxygen and carbon dioxide through a process of simple diffusion dependent on an adequate uteroplacental blood flow and moving from the side of greater concentration to the side of lesser.
2. As a fetal kidney for the metabolic side of acid–base balance, regulating the excretion of wastes and electrolyte balance.
3. As a fetal gastrointestinal tract for storage and release of nutrients, based on fetal need.
4. As a fetal skin for temperature control.

Circulation of essential components to and from the fetus is dependent on a number of factors. The surface area of the placenta—specifically, the integration of the villi—dictates the amount and rate of diffusion of necessary nutrients and other biochemical components. Depending on gestation from the 20th week on, approximately 400 to 700 ml of maternal blood flows through the uterus. Approximately 80 percent of this blood flow goes into the intervillous space. There, in the "lake" surrounding the "peninsula"-like villi, the maternal blood, through villous tissue, exchanges nutrients and oxygen for wastes and carbon dioxide. Nutrients are stored in the placenta and released upon the fetus' need, independent of blood flow or concentration.

The umbilical cord, or life line to the fetus, is normally made up of two arteries and one vein encased in Wharton's jelly. The umbilical cord delivers biochemical components to and from the fetus. Because the placenta functions as the fetal lung, the arteries carry the relatively unoxygenated blood from the fetus to the placenta, whereas the vein carries reoxygenated blood from the placenta to the fetus. The arteries are firmer walled than is the vein, and thus the vein, or the more oxygenated blood flow, constricts more easily. Under healthy circumstances, all blood flow to the uterus and through the placenta is a low-pressure system through widely dilated vessels. Therefore, maternal disease and pregnancy complications that affect the mother's cardiac or vascular systems inevitably have an impact on nutrition and ultimately on oxygen and carbon dioxide exchange across the placental membrane to the fetus.

Amniotic Fluid

The amnion is a membranous sac that surrounds the fetus. As the sac enlarges, it gradually sheathes the umbilical cord. Most of the fluid contained within the sac is initially derived from maternal blood. Later, the fetus contributes to the quantity by excreting urine into the amniotic fluid. Amniotic fluid is also normally swallowed by the fetus and absorbed into the gastrointestinal (GI) tract.

Certain fetal or maternal conditions may affect the quantity of amniotic fluid. Fetal renal malfunctions may lead to less amniotic fluid, whereas GI anomalies may result in greater amniotic fluid. Certain maternal conditions, especially nutritional deficiencies, are often associated with a smaller placenta and lower amniotic fluid volume. These factors, in turn, can lead to nutritional growth retardation of the fetus. The most common occurrence of decreased amniotic fluid is with postterm pregnancy, in which both fetal and maternal contribution to the volume is reduced.

Amniotic fluid has a number of functions:

1. It permits symmetrical growth and development.
2. It prevents adherence of the amnion to the embryo.
3. It cushions the fetus against jolts by distributing any impacts the mother may receive.
4. It helps to control fetal body temperature by maintaining a relatively constant temperature.
5. It enables the fetus to move freely, thus aiding musculoskeletal development.

6. It protects the umbilical cord.
7. It provides antimicrobial protection.

These functions may be impaired in the presence of oligohydramnios or polyhydramnios (Creasy & Resnik, 1994; Gilbert & Harmon, 1997; Moore & Persaud, 1993).

Maternal Nutrition

Maternal nutrition plays a significant role in fetal well-being, as well as in the prevention and treatment of high-risk pregnancies. A 25 percent deficit in needed calories and protein can interfere with the synthesis of DNA. As a result, during the first 2 to 3 months of pregnancy, a deficit in nutrients can have teratogenic effects or lead to spontaneous loss. After 2 to 3 months, a maternal nutritional deficit can impede fetal growth, resulting in smallness for gestational age or in small brain growth. These infants may be unable to attain their optimum potential in stature, intellect, and future health.

Specific maternal nutritional deficiencies can have deleterious effects on the fetus. Protein, 75 to 100 g daily, is important in supporting embryonic-fetal cell growth, in promoting necessary increased maternal blood volume, and possibly in facilitating prevention of pregnancy-induced hypertension (PIH). To prevent maternal anemia, which affects oxygenation and neonatal red blood cell mass, an adequate maternal intake of iron, folic acid, and vitamins B_6 and B_{12} is needed. Supplemental iron of at least 300 mg in maternal stores is necessary for the fetus to draw upon.

During pregnancy, the diet should contain 30 to 50 mg of zinc each day. Zinc is found in such foods as nuts, meats, whole grains, legumes, and dairy products. A deficiency of zinc during pregnancy increases the risk of premature rupture of membranes and preterm labor. This deficiency may be the result of a related deficiency in the antimicrobial properties of the amniotic fluid as well.

Alterations in sodium intake can also pose problems in pregnancy. Restricted sodium intake of less than 2.5 g per 24 hours can impede adequate maternal blood volume increase, which in turn can activate the renin-angiotensin-aldosterone cycle and lead to vasoconstriction. Excess sodium intake can also cause vasoconstriction through an increased sensitivity of the blood vessel wall to angiotensin.

To meet the growing needs of the fetus for maternal storage of fat and protein, an increase of 300 to 500 calories per day above normal caloric requirements is required. The formation and storage of fat and lean body tissue act as a reserve for the fetus during the last part of pregnancy, as well as provide an energy source for labor, delivery, and lactation. Intake of harmful substances such as alcohol, tobacco, and illegal drugs interferes with adequate absorption of nutrients by the fetus and the mother (Gilbert & Harmon, 1997).

MATERNAL HEALTH AND EFFECTS ON THE FETUS

Postterm Pregnancy

Incidence

Postterm pregnancy has long been reported in humans. Postmaturity in the fetus is the second leading cause of intrapartum asphyxia. Approximately 10 percent of all pregnancies continue 14 or more days beyond term. Of these, 20 to 40 percent result in postmature neonates, among whom the perinatal mortality rate is three times that of term newborns. Mortality rates show that 35 percent of the deaths occur antepartum, 47 percent intrapartum, and 18 percent in the neonatal period (Creasy & Resnik, 1994).

Etiology

It has been widely accepted that the postmature neonate is affected because of some degree of placental insufficiency; however, this does not explain the prolongation of pregnancy past term. The actual onset of labor appears to be explained by alterations in estrogen:progesterone ratios; these substances ultimately release prostaglandins from the uterine muscle through contractions. Prostaglandins, in turn, pave the way for release of oxytocin to increase the intensity of the contractions. Maternal oxytocin is released because of stimulation from increased mature fetal adrenocortical activity (Gilbert & Harmon, 1997).

Pathophysiology

As gestation advances, the placenta begins to age after 36 weeks by laying down fibrinoid material on the surface of the villi. Beginning at about 42 weeks, the surface area of the placenta that is available for oxygen and carbon dioxide exchange is diminished. In addition, a decreased quantity of amniotic fluid is formed by diminished maternal blood flow. Thus the fetus is at risk for both uteroplacental insufficiency and cord entrapment (Gilbert & Harmon, 1997).

Signs and Symptoms

A number of obstetrical warning signs can alert to potential postterm problems. These include (1) maternal weight loss of greater than 2 pounds per week; (2) oligohydramnios of less than 300 ml; (3) meconium-stained amniotic fluid; (4) advanced bony maturation of fetal head; and (5) prolonged labor (Gilbert & Harmon, 1997).

Fetal and Neonatal Effects

The effects of postterm pregnancy on the fetus and neonate include (1) failure of growth; (2) dehydration; (3) dry, cracked, wrinkled, parchment-like skin as a result of reduction of subcutaneous fat; (4) long, thin arms and legs; (5) advanced hardness of skull; (6) absence of vernix and lanugo; (7) skin maceration, especially in folds; (8) brownish-green discoloration of the skin; and (9) increased appearance of alertness (Gilbert & Harmon, 1997).

The postmaturity syndrome is considered to be an imbalance between continued placental capacity to function and fetal nutritive and respiratory demands.

Antepartum Complications

1. Failure of growth.
2. Cord accident.
3. Hypoxia manifested by decreased fetal movement, late deceleration with contraction stress testing, or absent long- and short-term variability on fetal heart rate (FHR) monitoring strips.

Intrapartum Complications

1. Increase in cesarean birth rate as a result of lack of cephalic molding and high arrest of fetal head or as a result of fetal response to labor stressors.
2. Intrauterine fetal hypoxia caused by placental insufficiency or cord compression.
3. Traumatic vaginal birth.

Treatment

At between 40 and 42 completed weeks of gestation, decisions regarding intervention in the pregnancy should be made. If the physician and the pregnant woman elect to continue the pregnancy and await the onset of labor, antepartum FHR monitoring tests are ordered. These may be biweekly nonstress tests, contraction stress tests, amniotic fluid volume indices, biophysical profiles, or some combination of these.

The medical management also includes decisions regarding delivery time and route. With careful antepartum FHR monitoring and a fetus who is continuing to show well-being in utero, the pregnancy can continue uninterrupted until 42 weeks. At that time, a trial induction is usually opted for so that advanced rapid placental aging is less likely to adversely affect the outcome. Induction is usually preceded either by prostaglandin gel ripening of the cervix or immediately by oxytocin drip. Careful FHR and maternal monitoring during the intrapartum period improves the outcome, but a cesarean birth is more likely if the fetus does not tolerate labor or if the mother does not progress in labor (Creasy & Resnik, 1994).

Nursing Management

Prenatal care should include careful collection of data for accurate dating, such as the following (Gilbert & Harmon, 1997):

1. First day of last menstrual period.
2. Conception preceded by normal menses.
3. Ultrasonogram dating before 20 weeks.
4. First felt fetal movement between 18 and 20 weeks.
5. Doptone FHR monitoring at 12 to 13 weeks; fetoscope FHR monitoring at 18 to 19 weeks.
6. Fundal height growth rates at 22 weeks not varying by 3 cm or more from the number of weeks of gestation.

As the woman approaches 40 weeks, history of previous pregnancies should be reassessed for increased risk. Factors that increase risk are

1. Previous postterm delivery.
2. Previous cesarean birth for failure to progress.
3. Previous unexplained stillbirth before estimated date of confinement. Begin this reassessment before 40 weeks' gestation.
4. Decreased fetal movement in patient doing daily counts.
5. Maternal weight loss greater than 2 to 3 pounds in 1 week without identified cause.
6. Hard, bony fetal head palpated at symphysis with no early cervical changes.

The pregnant woman should be educated and evaluated according to needs for fetal movement daily counts. Usually four kicks per hour is adequate. The woman should be educated regarding any FHR monitoring. The purpose of challenging fetal well-being should be understood, as well as interpretation of good, bad, and equivocal results. She should be prepared for the potential of a cesarean birth.

Intrapartum care should include

1. Careful review of all dating information and general health history.
2. Knowledge about any FHR monitoring results.
3. Fundal height evaluation with position and engagement and Leopold's maneuver to estimate fetal size, presentation, and position.
4. Careful electronic FHR monitoring or intermittent auscultation to rule out FHR patterns of cord compression or insufficient uteroplacental transfer of oxygen. If nonreassuring patterns are identified, prompt independent treatment is expected by the nurse and should include
   a. Turning patient to left side or from side to side.
   b. Improving maternal circulating volume with intravenous fluid challenge (usually with lactated Ringer's solution).
   c. Discontinuing labor stimulation, if used.
   d. Administering oxygen at 8 to 10 L by face mask.
   e. Notifying physician or midwife.
   f. Preparing for expeditious delivery if condition is not improved within 30 minutes.
5. Suction equipment if meconium is in the amniotic fluid.

Preterm Delivery

Incidence

Preterm delivery occurs in 8 to 10 percent of all live births in the United States. Despite current therapies for halting preterm labor, this incidence has remained unchanged for the past 25 years. Preterm delivery accounts for 75 to 80 percent of all neonatal morbidity and mortality (Gilbert & Harmon, 1997).

Etiology

The exact etiology of preterm labor has continued to elude health professionals. We have, however, learned to screen for risk factors. Risk factors fall into four main categories: past medical and pregnancy history, current pregnancy history, socioeconomic factors, and daily habits and lifestyle (Gilbert & Harmon, 1997). Medical and pregnancy history factors that contribute to a risk for preterm labor or preterm delivery or both include (1) conditions such as diabetes, hypertension, renal disease, heart disease, or systemic lupus erythematosus; (2) more than two spontaneous or elective abortions; (3) previous preterm labor or preterm delivery or both (increasing the likelihood of repetitive preterm labor or preterm delivery or both by 40 percent); (4) diethylstilbestrol (DES) exposure; and (5) uterine anomalies. The current pregnancy may reveal problems that may lead to preterm labor or preterm delivery or both, such as (1) abruptio placentae; (2) placenta previa; (3) preeclampsia or PIH; (4) multiple gestation; (5) urinary tract infection; (6) febrile illness; (7) abdominal or cervical surgery; and (8) small stature or weight (<5 feet or <100 pounds). Socioeconomic factors that contribute to risk of preterm labor or delivery include (1) employment outside the home; (2) less than 12th-grade education; (3) single mother; (4) less than 17 or more than 39 years old; (5) late prenatal care; (6) poor nutritional resources; and (7) two or more toddlers in the home. Daily habits or lifestyles that may contribute to preterm labor include (1) smoking more than half a pack of cigarettes per day; (2) substance use and abuse (nicotine, alcohol, cocaine, heroin, and so forth); (3) long commute to health care or work; (4) inadequate rest during the day; and (5) poor nutritional habits.

Pathophysiology

Preterm events may trigger preterm labor. Examples include (1) increased estrogen in relation to progesterone; (2) increased stretch of uterine muscle, leading to release of arachidonic acid; (3) fetal stress, leading to increased fetal cortisol; (4) increased amounts of prostaglandins; and (5) increased maternal oxytocin (Gilbert & Harmon, 1997).

Signs and Symptoms

The definition of preterm labor consists of the following occurrences between 20 and 37 weeks of gestation: (1) painless or mildly uncomfortable contractions; (2) more than four contractions per hour; (3) contractions longer than 30 seconds in duration; and (4) contractions leading to cervical changes.

The signs and symptoms of preterm labor may vary from specific to vague complaints, and reports by the pregnant woman include the following: (1) low abdominal cramping or pressure; (2) rhythmic "tightening" and relaxation of the abdomen; (3) low backache; (4) tingling down the thighs; (5) increase in or "watery" vaginal discharge; (6) brownish or pink vaginal discharge; (7) diarrhea with or without abdominal cramping; and (8) "feeling bad" (Gilbert & Harmon, 1997).

Fetal and Neonatal Effects

In general, preterm labor in and of itself is not harmful to the fetus. Exceptions occur when preterm labor leads to increased stress on the fetus, such as cord compression with contractions or diminished blood supply that exceeds the fetal-placental ability to compensate.

Preterm delivery, especially before 32 completed gestational weeks, causes significant neonatal morbidity and fatality. The usual and most significant problem is related to lung immaturity, resulting in the inability of the neonate to perform the vital respiratory functions, even with technology.

Hypoxia, in turn, leads to intracranial bleeds, necrotizing enterocolitis, and other serious system failures. Neonates can experience serious birth injuries, lifetime disabilities and intellectual compromise, and death (Gilbert & Harmon, 1997).

Treatment

A number of tocolytic drugs (labor suppressants) are available to halt preterm labor. Two problems must be solved before these can be effective: (1) maternal identification of the early signs and symptoms and (2) health care providers' timely response to clients' reports of signs and symptoms.

Some of the tocolytic agents available are magnesium sulfate ($MgSO_4$); beta-sympathomimetics (terbutaline, ritodrine); prostaglandin inhibitors (indomethacin, ibuprofen); and calcium channel blockers. The first two agents are accepted methods of halting labor; the latter two are still experimental. All appear to be effective if signs and symptoms are detected, reported, and responded to in early stages of preterm labor.

Other adjunct treatment, such as cervical cerclage and early bed rest or restricted activities, also helps. They are, however, dependent on early access to health care, acceptability of that health care, and adequate screening (Creasy & Resnik, 1994; Gilbert & Harmon, 1997).

Cortisol has also been administered as an adjunct when successful halting of labor is doubtful. It is theorized that at between 28 and 32 weeks, cortisol stimulates a cascade of events that stabilizes lecithin, stimulating production of fetal surfactant and therefore promoting lung function. Cortisol has been widely researched, with diverse opinions about its efficacy (Creasy & Resnik, 1994; Obstetrics and Gynecology Supplement, 1990).

Medical management may also include the use of home uterine contraction monitors or terbutaline pumps for subcutaneous infusion therapy. Neither of these have proved effective without professional nursing care and education of the client (Obstetrics and Gynecology Supplement, 1990).

Nursing Management

Nurses can have a major role in improving the preterm delivery rate. Early prenatal care should be accessible and acceptable to all pregnant women. Nurses working in maternity clinics and offices should implement creative programs that meet the needs of the population being served for both accessibility and acceptability. Once into the health care system, all pregnant women should be systematically screened for the previously discussed risk factors. In addition, all pregnant women should be educated about the physical signs of preterm contractions and how to use their hands to self-detect rhythmic abdominal tightening. Finally, they should be taught and supported in self-advocacy when reporting self-detected signs and symptoms of preterm labor (Gilbert & Harmon, 1997; Obstetrics and Gynecology Supplement, 1990).

Third-Trimester Bleeding

The two major sources of third-trimester bleeding are placental adherence or implantation problem. These may result in placental abruption or placenta previa.

Incidence

The risk of placental abruption is 0.5 to 2.5 percent; the risk of recurrence in subsequent pregnancies is increased to 5.6 percent. The risk of placenta previa is 0.5 percent. Multigravidas have a slightly higher risk of placenta previa, and the risk of recurrence increases fivefold (Creasy & Resnik, 1994; Gilbert & Harmon, 1997).

Etiology

The actual cause of placental abruption is unknown. Conditions associated with abruption (Gilbert & Harmon, 1997) are

1. PIH or chronic hypertension, present in 4 percent of patients.
2. Maternal age over 35 years.
3. Multiparity of more than five pregnancies.
4. Previous abruption; risk is increased 10 percent after one abruption and 25 percent after two abruptions.
5. Trauma from a direct blow to the abdomen or needle puncture during an amniocentesis.
6. Short umbilical cord.
7. Folic acid deficiency.
8. Cigarette smoking, cocaine use, and polysubstance abuse, causing vasoconstriction of spiral arterioles and leading to decidual necrosis.

The cause of placenta previa is also unknown. It is frequently associated with factors that cause uterine scarring or interfere with blood supply to the endometrium. Predisposing factors are (1) abortion, (2) cesarean birth, (3) increased parity, (4) prior previa, (5) uterine infection, (6) closely spaced pregnancies, (7) uterine tumors, (8) multiple pregnancy, and (9) maternal age over 35 years.

Pathophysiology

Theoretically, abruption of the placenta is thought to occur when the spiral arterioles, which nourish the decidua (endometrium) and the placenta, begin the process of degeneration. As necrosis takes place, the blood vessels rupture and bleed into the site, leading to separation of the placenta as pressure of the bleeding increases. Abruption may occur at the marginal edges of the placenta, outward to the edges. An abruption is classified, by the quantity of the surface involved, as mild (less than 15 percent), moderate (15 to 60 percent), or severe (greater than 60 percent) (Creasy & Resnik, 1994; Gilbert & Harmon, 1997).

Signs and Symptoms

Signs and symptoms of placental abruption include (1) uterine tenderness or rigidity and low back pain; (2) dark red vaginal bleeding; (3) fetal symptoms of stress; and (4) maternal signs of shock and disseminated intravascular coagulation (DIC). Signs and symptoms of placenta previa rarely occur before the early third trimester. The initial onset of symptoms is usually mild, and their recurrence is unpredictable. The signs and symptoms of previa include (1) painless bleeding, usually bright red and initially slight in amount; (2) high presenting fetal part; and (3) subsequent recurrences of bleeding in increasingly significant amounts and associated signs of fetal stress (Gilbert & Harmon, 1997).

Fetal and Neonatal Effects

The major effects of third-trimester bleeding on the fetus are related to inadequate oxygen–carbon dioxide exchange via the placenta, the potential maternal imperative for premature delivery, or a combination of factors (Gilbert & Harmon, 1997).

Treatment

Treatment of placental abruptions or placenta previa depends on three major factors: severity of blood loss, fetal maturity, and fetal well-being. When bleeding is mild and ceases readily and the fetus is immature without evidence of being distressed, expectant management is chosen. This plan (Creasy & Resnik, 1994) includes

1. Hospitalization; bed rest for at least 72 hours.
2. Close observation for bleeding.
3. Continuous FHR monitoring.
4. Maternal red blood cell replacement as necessary.
5. No maternal vaginal examinations.
6. Preparation for cesarean birth; vaginal birth is not safe for mother or infant in the presence of continual abruption or partial or complete placenta previa.
7. Discharge to home, undelivered, only if bleeding subsides and ceases, or, if placenta previa is present, it is incomplete; provide instructions for bed rest with restricted activity and preterm labor prevention.

Fetal maturity needs to be assessed to determine the risks and benefits of prolonging the pregnancy with a compromised uteroplacental unit. If fetal well-being is compromised by maternal bleeding, emergency cesarean section is indicated.

Nursing Management

Nursing care (Gilbert & Harmon, 1997) consists of

1. Assessment:
   a. Risk screening in early prenatal care.
   b. FHR monitoring for presence, absence, or compromise of fetal well-being in the presence of maternal bleeding.
   c. Visually inspecting and quantifying maternal blood loss.
   d. Rapid change in fundal height or maternal vital signs or both in association with abdominal or back pain.
2. Intervention:
   a. If bleeding is life-threatening to mother or distressing to fetus or both, prepare for emergency delivery, usually by cesarean birth.
   b. If management is to be expectant, educate mother for prevention of preterm labor.
   c. Prepare parents for potential preterm delivery.

Hypertensive Disorders of Pregnancy

The Committee on Terminology of the American College of Obstetricians and Gynecologists has developed a classification of the various hypertensive states in pregnancy:

1. PIH:
   a. Gestational hypertension: development of hypertension after 20 weeks' gestation without proteinuria; blood pressure normotensive within 10 postpartum days.
   b. Preeclampsia: development of hypertension with or without edema after 20 weeks' gestation or early postpartum.
   c. Eclampsia: development of convulsions or coma in a preeclamptic patient.
   d. Superimposed preeclampsia or eclampsia in a patient with chronic hypertension.
2. Concurrent hypertension and pregnancy (CHP): chronic hypertension that develops before pregnancy or before 20 weeks' gestation and is not associated with pregnancy.
3. HELLP syndrome is a complex of symptoms described as a severe forerunner of PIH that has a sudden onset and is diagnosed from signs and symptoms of *h*emolysis, *e*levated *l*iver enzymes, and *l*ow *p*latelets.

Incidence

Approximately 6 to 30 percent of all pregnant women have hypertensive disorder. A primigravida is six times more likely than a multigravida to develop PIH. PIH is five times more prevalent in the lower socioeconomic groups. Other factors associated with a higher incidence of PIH include (1) family history, (2) diabetes, (3) multiple gestation, (4) polyhydramnios, (5) persistent hypertension, (6) hydatidiform mole, and (7) RH incompatibility (Gilbert & Harmon, 1997).

Etiology

The etiology of PIH is largely unknown. Four theories are widely accepted to be associated with PIH: nutritional deficiency, immunologic deficiency, genetics, and uterine ischemia. For example, women with a protein/sodium-poor diet, a suppressed immune system, a family history positive for genetic dysfunction that might lead to vascular changes or hypertension, or signs of uterine ischemia are at risk for developing PIH.

Pathophysiology

In PIH disorders, there is an increased vascular sensitivity to angiotensin II. This increase in sensitivity occurs before the onset of hypertension. When the normal pregnancy-related resistance to angiotensin II is lost, blood vessel spasms occur, causing vasoconstriction and a rise in blood pressure.

Blood flow to most organs is decreased, especially that to the uterus, placenta, kidneys, liver, and brain, impairing their function by 40 to 60 percent. Impaired blood flow results in pathophysiologic changes (Creasy & Resnik, 1994) such as

1. Decreased uterine and placental blood flow, resulting in premature, exaggerated degeneration of the placenta. Uterine activity is increased.
2. Decreased blood supply to the kidney and reduced glomerular filtration rate, causing degenerative changes in the glomerulus, which cause
   a. Sodium and water retention.
   b. Decreased serum albumin and decreased plasma colloid osmotic pressure.
   c. Fluid shifts and generalized edema.

3. Decreased blood supply to the liver, impairing liver function.
4. Decreased blood supply to the eyes, with retinal arteriolar spasms and blurred vision.
5. Loss of fluid from blood vessels in the brain, leading to cerebral edema and hemorrhages.
6. Damage to blood vessel wall, occurring with progression of the disease. Platelets, fibrinogen, immunoglobulin, and components of complement are deposited at the damaged sites, and DIC occurs.

Signs and Symptoms

The two cardinal signs of PIH are proteinuria and blood pressure of 140/90 or greater on two occasions within 6 hours or an increase of 50 mm systolic or 15 mm diastolic or both over the baseline blood pressure (Gilbert & Harmon, 1997).

Fetal and Neonatal Effects

Perinatal mortality related to PIH usually ranges from 1 to 8 percent; if allowed to progress to eclampsia or HELLP syndrome, however, the incidence is as high as 35 percent. The majority of perinatal losses are directly related to placental insufficiency, resulting in intrauterine fetal demise or early neonatal death in an already compromised premature infant.

Placental insufficiency in PIH usually leads to some degree of nutritional intrauterine growth retardation. The fetus is asymmetrically affected, in that head size is close to normal for gestation but general body size and fat deposition are decreased. This nutritional deprivation causes the fetus to be more vulnerable to the effects of labor contractions and other stressors. During antepartum or intrapartum monitoring, the fetus is more likely to show signs of fetal stress when oxygen and carbon dioxide exchange is mildly compromised over a shorter period of time.

Growth retardation of the fetus is more often associated with decreased amounts of amniotic fluid as well. Therefore, any repetitive occlusion of the umbilical cord during contractions, or with fetal movement, may cause stress. Signs of fetal stress with FHR monitoring (Gilbert & Harmon, 1997) may include

1. Tachycardia: rate above 160, or more than 20 beats per minute rise from previous baseline.
2. Absence of long- or short-term variability.
3. Late decelerations with or without cord compression (variable decelerations), tachycardia, or absent long- or short-term variability.

Treatment

The only cure for PIH is delivery. Because the fetus may be at higher risk from prematurity or because the maternal condition is unstable, or both, treatment is aimed at stabilizing the maternal condition and reducing immediate risks to the fetus.

Because the maternal intravascular volume is depleted through loss of intravascular fluid into interstitial tissue, absolute bed rest facilitates optimal use of existing intravascular volume. Other treatment varies in relation to antepartum, intrapartum, or postpartum complications.

Antepartum. Treatment is directed at improving maternal status to gain gestational time for the fetus. Treatment (Creasy & Resnik, 1994) consists of

1. Pharmacologic treatment of maternal hypertension with drugs such as hydralazine, alpha-methyldopa, clonidine, or sodium nitroprusside. There has been long-term experience with the use of hydralazine for rapid response to hypertension and with alpha-methyldopa for long-term effects.
2. Intermittent evaluation of fetal well-being through contraction stress or nonstress tests or biophysical profiles.
3. Ultrasound evaluation for growth of fetus every 2 to 3 weeks.
4. High-protein maternal diet (>100 g per day).
5. Monitoring of maternal laboratory studies—that is, uric acid, platelets, liver enzymes, and clinical signs—for worsening disease.

Diuretics and severe sodium restriction currently have no place in the treatment of PIH and, in fact, may worsen the disease. Likewise, long-term expectant management is not likely to result in improved maternal or fetal status and is therefore not practiced in most centers (Creasy & Resnik, 1994).

Intrapartum. Treatment is aimed at obtaining and maintaining immediate stabilization of the mother and then delivering the premature or mature fetus. Stabilization (Creasy & Resnik, 1994) consists of

1. Pharmacologic therapy for prevention of central nervous system irritability with intravenous magnesium sulfate and treatment of maternal hypertension above 160/100 with hydralazine or other fast-acting antihypertensives.
2. Plasma volume expanders, which may be used as a temporary therapy.
3. A delivery route based on whether labor can be induced (cervical ripening), gestation of the fetus, and fetal tolerance to stress of labor. A surgical delivery may not be safe for a woman with signs of DIC or HELLP syndrome because of the potential for hemorrhage. On the other hand, continuing the pregnancy through labor may not be tolerated by the fetus or may progress to eclampsia in the mother with HELLP syndrome, because of diminished clotting factors; an epidural may be contraindicated because of increased potential epidural space bleeding. Therefore, a surgical delivery with general anesthesia would be the best choice.

Nursing Management

Assessment

1. Fetal: Monitor for signs of antepartum fetal stress intermittently during the antepartum period with contraction stress tests or nonstress tests or continuously during the intrapartum period.
2. Maternal: Monitor blood pressure and laboratory studies.

Intervention

1. Treat signs of fetal stress with maternal bed rest in left lateral position. Provide oxygen therapy and prevent volume depletion.
2. Administer antihypertensives intravenously only in conjunction with continuous FHR monitoring.
3. Educate pregnant women identified at risk for developing PIH to recognize and report early signs and symptoms.

Diabetes in Pregnancy

In pregnancy, diabetes is classified according to White's classification system (Gilbert & Harmon, 1997). This classification system was originally intended to prognosticate neonatal outcome. It has since been modified; it is now used primarily to make decisions for timing fetal surveillance and to evaluate for maternal complications.

The classifications are as follows:

Class A_1: gestational onset, normal fasting blood glucose level; necessitates diet control.

Class A_2: gestational onset, abnormal fasting blood glucose levels; necessitates insulin therapy.
Class B: onset after age 20, necessitates insulin therapy.
Class C: onset after age 10, less than 10 years' duration, no vascular complications; necessitates insulin therapy.
Class D: onset before age 10 or greater than 10 years' duration or early vascular complications; necessitates insulin therapy.
Class F: renal changes; necessitates insulin therapy.
Class R: renal and retinal changes; necessitates insulin therapy.
Class H: heart complications, often over age 35 with early age onset of diabetes, 50 percent obstetrical maternal mortality; necessitates insulin therapy.
Class T: postrenal transplantation; necessitates insulin therapy.

Incidence

Diabetes exists in 1 to 2 percent of all pregnancies. Women can readily be screened for gestational onset with a 50-g glucola load and a 1-hour post–blood glucose study. Levels above 120 to 140 mg are then evaluated for the requirement of insulin with a 3-hour glucose tolerance test that yields two or more abnormal results or when fasting blood glucose levels rise above 110 mg percent while the patient is treated with diet.

Etiology

Diabetes exists when insufficient amounts of effective insulin are produced by the beta cells in the islets of Langerhans in the pancreas. Pregnancy has been likened to a diabetogenic state because of increases in metabolism of protein, fat, and carbohydrate, necessitating additional insulin. The increased production of estrogen, progesterone, human placental lactogen (HPL), and cortisol produces an antagonistic effect on insulin that is produced or taken exogenously. Women at risk for developing gestational-onset diabetes (Gilbert & Harmon, 1997) are

1. Over age 35 years.
2. Chronically hypertensive.
3. Obese.
4. Multigravidas with a previous unexplained stillbirth, more than two or three spontaneous miscarriages, a previous macrosomic infant, especially if larger than 9 pounds, at term.
5. Women with a strong, positive family history of diabetes or a history of frequent vaginal monilial infections or current history of glucosuria.

Pathophysiology

During the first trimester, alterations in maternal metabolism foster the rapid cell division and organ differentiation in the embryo. As a result, thyroid function enhances an increased metabolic rate, which results in increased need for protein and fat stores and rapid glucose use. Therefore, there is commonly a decreased need for insulin, which may be further complicated by decreased food intake in the presence of early pregnancy nausea and vomiting.

The placenta begins to function as its own endocrine organ in the second trimester, producing increasing amounts of estrogen, progesterone, HPL, and cortisol. These hormones work antagonistically against the effectiveness of insulin to carry glucose into cells. The pancreas must produce increased amounts of insulin to overcome the antagonistic effects of the four hormones. If it is unable to do so, glucose builds up in the maternal blood stream, and metabolism is diverted to an anaerobic route. Amino acids and fats are burned in excess during anaerobic metabolism, leading eventually to ketoacidemia in the mother. Because the normal fetal pH is lower and derived solely from the maternal blood in the intervillous space, fetal acidemia is likely.

Excess glucose from maternal circulation is used and stored in the placenta. As the fetus draws on the glucose, the fetal pancreas is stimulated to produce increased amounts of insulin. The increased fetal insulin acts as a growth promoter, causing the fetus to grow large and depositing increased amounts of body adipose tissue.

As a vascular organ, the placenta is vulnerable to the vascular complications of maternal diabetes. It may age earlier or faster, or it may not develop sufficiently to supply the fetus with adequate blood supply. The placenta may also swell with added fluid, resulting in poor diffusion of necessary substrates, carbon dioxide, and oxygen (Gilbert & Harmon, 1997).

Effects on the Fetus and Neonate

The following fetal effects are possible:

1. Interference with DNA–RNA transfer as a result of maternal high blood glucose before and at the time of conception. This effect probably explains the high incidence of neonatal congenital heart defects, lethal and nonlethal neurologic malformations, GI defects, and renal polycystic disease.
2. Increased, rapid fetal body growth.
3. Decreased fetal brain growth.
4. Decreased fetal body growth.

The following neonatal effects are seen (Creasy & Resnik, 1994; Gilbert & Harmon, 1997):

1. Hypoglycemia in the transitional period because of high insulin production but loss of maternal glucose supply.
2. Hyperbilirubinemia from increased "glucose-saturated" fetal hemoglobin and breakdown of this in the early neonatal period.
3. Hypercalcemia, hypokalemia, and other abnormalities in electrolytes.
4. Increased incidence of cesarean birth.
5. Increased incidence of traumatic vaginal birth, usually from shoulder dystocias.
6. Neonatal respiratory distress syndrome even after 36 weeks. High maternal blood glucose, high placental glucose storage, high placental production of cortisol, low fetal production of cortisol, and low surfactant production lead to decreased lung maturity at expected gestation.

Treatment

Medical treatment of a pregnancy complicated by diabetes is aimed at maintenance of euglycemia before conception and throughout the entire pregnancy. Euglycemia requires a careful balance of diet, insulin, and activity (Creasy & Resnik, 1994):

1. Diet of 1800 to 2400 calories, consisting of four to six meals made up of 50 percent complex carbohydrate, 30 percent fat, and 20 percent protein.
2. Insulin, when required, in a split-dose regimen, usually consisting of some combination of regular and intermediate insulin based on a prospective regulation of blood glucose levels between 60 and 150 mg percent.
3. Activity schedule that does not vary much from day to day or week to week.

A careful evaluation of maternal estimated date of delivery is required before fetal surveillance parameters can be ordered. In general, this estimate is made with an early prenatal examination, history, and ultrasound confirmation. Further early maternal evaluation for diabetic vascular complications in insulin-dependent diabetes may include glycosylated hemoglobin, 24-hour urine tests for protein and creatinine, recent eye examination, and electrocardiogram.

Antepartum fetal surveillance includes

1. Maternal serum alpha-fetoprotein measurement to screen for neural tube defects.
2. Ultrasound evaluation between 15 and 20 weeks' gestation for congenital developmental problems.
3. Ultrasound evaluation for growth rate, usually between 26 and 30 weeks and near expected delivery (37 to 38 weeks).
4. Amniocentesis for fetal lung maturity at the time of the last ultrasound evaluation.
5. Fetal movement counts daily, biweekly nonstress tests, weekly contraction stress tests, weekly ultrasound biophysical profile evaluation, or some combination of testing weekly. These may begin anytime after 25 weeks and before 38 weeks, depending on fetal risk and maternal complications.

Intrapartum management usually consists of an insulin drip for an insulin-dependent labor patient. If laboring for an anticipated vaginal birth, continuous FHR monitoring should be evaluated for the onset of signs of fetal stress.

Nursing Management

Antepartum Assessment

1. Maternal educational needs.
2. Fetal assessment with evaluation of fetal movement counts, nonstress tests, or contraction stress tests.
3. Maternal complications of polyhydramnios, PIH, urinary tract infections, or preterm labor, or persistent abnormal blood glucose levels.

Antepartum Intervention

1. Education of the pregnant woman and her support system for
   a. Dietary management.
   b. Blood glucose determination four to six times daily.
   c. Insulin injections and changes in dosage.
   d. Activity schedule and modification.
   e. Effects of diabetes and pregnancy on self and fetus.
   f. Reason for testing for maternal and fetal complications.
2. Support and assistance with time management and financial stressors from increased testing.

Cardiac Disease and Pregnancy

Cardiac disease has four classifications:

Class I: asymptomatic.
Class II: symptomatic with increased exercise.
Class III: symptomatic with normal exercise.
Class IV: symptomatic at rest.

Although a patient's classification does not change for the worse with pregnancy, the increased workload on the heart may increase symptoms by one or two classifications (Gilbert & Harmon, 1997).

Incidence

The incidence of cardiac disease in pregnancy varies from 0.5 to 2.0 percent. Rheumatic fever is responsible for about 50 percent and congenital heart disease in the mother for the other half.

Etiology

Cardiac disease in pregnancy may take one of several forms: rheumatic fever, valve deformities, congenital heart disease, congestive cardiomyopathies, or cardiac dysrhythmias. Several conditions may predispose pregnant women to a greater than 50 percent mortality rate: Marfan's syndrome with aortic arch dissection; primary pulmonary hypertension, or Eisenmenger's syndrome; and diabetes complicated by heart disease.

Pathophysiology

When the heart fails as an efficient pump, blood volume is shunted to essential organ systems in the body. During pregnancy, the heart that is complicated by heart disease may be unable to respond efficiently to the increased circulating volume. As blood is shunted to essential organs for the mother, it may bypass the growing uterus, placenta, intervillous space, and thus the fetus to some extent.

Effects on the Fetus and Neonate

The fetus or neonate may suffer adverse effects as a result of decreased maternal placental blood flow, including diminished fetal body growth, diminished brain growth, and higher incidence of fetal wastage and pregnancy loss.

During the intrapartum period, the fetus may be stressed beyond capacity to demonstrate its ability to withstand labor. Signs of fetal stress may include deceleration patterns such as late decelerations because of insufficient uteroplacental blood flow or variable decelerations because of insufficient amniotic fluid to protect the umbilical cord from compression.

The neonate, if delivered prematurely for maternal reasons, has the additional difficulties of premature birth. If congenital heart disease is present in the mother, there is an increased risk of congenital heart abnormalities in the neonate as well (Gilbert & Harmon, 1997).

Fetal Assessment

Antepartum

1. Ultrasonography for growth rate.
2. Nonstress or contraction stress tests, biophysical profiles, or some combination of these on a weekly or biweekly basis after 26 weeks' gestation.

It is important to try to prevent development of associated maternal complications such as anemia or severe preeclampsia, which might further compromise fetal well-being.

Intrapartum

1. Carefully monitored labor for problems with maternal cardiac preload or afterload, often with central-line hemodynamic invasive monitoring.
2. Continuous FHR monitoring, often with the pregnant woman on her left side with oxygen therapy.
3. Shortened and assisted second stage of labor, usually with epidural anesthesia/analgesia to reduce pain and cardiac workload as well as preload. Because pain is complex interaction of physiologic and psychological aspects, the management requires pharmacologic agents and good communication. The latter may include cognitive management by thorough explanations of what is anticipated to happen next (Lowe, 1996).

Urinary Tract Disease in Pregnancy

Urinary tract infection (UTI) occurs in 4 to 7.5 percent of childbearing women. Approximately 30 percent of pregnant women with untreated asymptomatic bacteriuria develop pyelonephritis during pregnancy.

The organisms usually responsible for UTI are *Escherichia coli*, staphylococci, or streptococci. The inflammation occurring in bladder or renal tissue may result in fever and increased prostaglandin production. Increase in prostaglandin production predisposes a pregnant woman to preterm labor and thus the fetus to preterm delivery. If maternal sepsis occurs, fetal fever and potential infection from amnionitis often occur.

Renal disease in pregnancy is infrequently the result of diabetic glomerulonephritis or maternal connective tissue disease, especially if end-stage renal disease has occurred. In general, women with end-stage renal disease do not ovulate. When they do become pregnant, there is high fetal wastage because of increased urea by-products in the maternal blood stream and thus in the amniotic fluid. The fetus, as a result, grows poorly and often succumbs to the hostile maternal environment.

UTIs and fever must be treated with appropriate antibiotics therapeutically or prophylactically or both. Treatment of renal disease, which may temporarily worsen in pregnancy in response to increased renal blood flow and work, is usually aimed at clearing maternal blood of ureal wastes. Most recently, some success has been reported with the modality of continuous ambulatory peritoneal dialysis for end-stage renal disease in pregnancy (Gilbert & Harmon, 1997).

Nursing Management

Nursing management for UTI is primarily aimed at prevention of infection, reinfection, and preterm labor. This management is best accomplished through prenatal education regarding the need for (1) increased oral fluids to 6 to 8 oz per waking hour; (2) perineal hygiene with cleaning front to back and urinating after intercourse; (3) recognition of early signs of preterm labor; and (4) reporting of early signs of infection and preterm labor.

MATERNAL TRANSPORT

Many states have regionalized care for newborns and pregnant women. Some states still do not. There are three possible levels of care facilities (Gilbert & Harmon, 1997):

Level I: cares for low-risk pregnant women and their healthy newborns.

Level II: cares for moderate-risk pregnant women likely to deliver newborns without need for ventilatory assistance as well as low-risk pregnant women and their newborns.

Level III: cares for high-risk pregnant women likely to deliver high-risk newborns requiring specialized high-technologic care and for moderate- and low-risk pregnant women and their newborns.

Identification of Need

A level III perinatal service must be able to provide services for all mothers and neonates, have research support, and be able to compile, analyze, and evaluate regional data. It is desirable to have a level III regionalized center available and centrally located in relation to several level I and II facilities. Transport equipment and educated team members should be accessible within a reasonable time. Ideally, maternal transport should occur, because the mother is the best incubator. The availability of research and resources makes this a more likely reality in a level III facility than in a level I or II facility.

Population

Assignment of maternity patients into high-risk and low-risk categories is useful in defining patient acuity and determining staffing patterns. Determinations of staffing requirements should be related to patient acuity, numbers, staff education and experience, and facility resources.

Equipment

State-of-the-art monitoring equipment should be available for monitoring fetal well-being in a level III center. This monitoring includes antepartum and intrapartum FHR monitoring, as well as ultrasonography. Immediate cesarean delivery should be available within the delivery suites and ideally within the labor, delivery, and recovery areas. Antepartum maternal care requiring invasive hemodynamic monitoring should be a technical resource.

Evaluation or Maternal-Fetal Stabilization

Ideally, the fetus is best incubated maternally until fetal lung maturity is determined. Certain maternal conditions such as HELLP syndrome, connective tissue disease, and cardiac compromise may unbalance the risk:benefit ratio in such a way that delivery of a premature infant would result in the best neonatal outcome. These decisions are best made when sophisticated maternal and fetal surveillance techniques are available and level III nursery facilities can be used. Stabilization occurs when that ratio is weighted toward either better-off delivered or better-off undelivered. Depending on the maternal or fetal condition and the treatment modalities available, the decision may take hours or days (Gilbert & Harmon, 1997).

Care During Transport

Fixed-wing, helicopter, and ground transport should all be options for maternal transport from level I or II facilities to level III centers. Teams composed of qualified staff, nurse, and physician should be ready to respond to the need for transport. Fetal monitoring equipment should be used when appropriate during transport. Therefore, transport staff must have education and experience in labor and delivery care of high-risk mothers and neonates (Gilbert & Harmon, 1997).

LEGAL ISSUES

Obstetrical litigation continues to lead in major medical malpractice cases. The four elements necessary for successful litigation are duty, breach of duty, causation, and proven damage. Duty is the particular relationship that arises when a hospital, nursing staff, and physician agree to assume the care of a particular patient. Breach of duty occurs when the minimum agreed-upon standard of care is not met by one or more members of that group. Causation is shown when the breach of duty has a direct link to the proven cause of the actual damages. Damages are generally physical and often lasting. (See Chapter 4, Legal Aspects of Perinatal Care.)

Professionals practicing high-risk obstetrics place themselves and their patients at high risk (Gilbert & Harmon, 1997) when

1. Staff fails to keep current in knowledge and skills.
2. There is poor risk identification for mother or neonate.
3. New or unexpected complications are not anticipated and planned for.
4. Families are not included in the decision-making process and are therefore uninformed about risks and consequences.
5. Consultation is not sought when it was clearly available.

In the long run, the best defense is always to consider the risk:benefit ratio to the mother and unborn infant. Professional behavior demands that the caregiver advocate for clients who are unable to do so themselves, by safeguarding the client from harm that may result from the unsafe, illegal, or unethical conduct of others.

CONCLUSION

This chapter has presented a brief overview of the most common maternal high-risk conditions and the effects on fetus and neonate. It has presented information in a manner to help neonatal nurses understand how the neonate comes to need special care.

REFERENCES

Creasy, R., & Resnik, M. (1994). *Maternal fetal medicine: Principles and practice.* (3rd ed.) Philadelphia: W. B. Saunders.

Gilbert, E., & Harmon, J. (1997). *Manual of high risk pregnancy and delivery.* St. Louis: Mosby–Year Book.

Lowe, N. K. (1996). The pain and discomfort of labor and birth. *Journal of Obstetric, Gynecologic, and Neonatal Nursing, 25*(1), 82–92.

Moore, K. L., & Persaud, T. V. N. (1993). *Before we are born: Basic embryology and birth defects* (4th ed). Philadelphia: W. B. Saunders.

SUGGESTED READINGS

Abdella, T. (1991). *PIH and H.E.L.L.P. syndrome and preeclampsia.* Presented at the Special Delivery Deviations from the Norm Workshop, Phoenix.

Alexander, G. R., Weiss, J., Hulsey, T. C., & Papiernik, E. (1991). Preterm birth prevention: An evaluation of programs in the U.S. *Birth, 18*(3), 160–169.

American College of Obstetricians & Gynecologists (ACOG). (1988). Premature rupture of membranes. *ACOG Technical Bulletin,* No. 115. Washington, DC: Author.

American College of Obstetricians & Gynecologists (ACOG) (1990a). Prevention of isoimmunization. *ACOG Technical Bulletin,* No. 147. Washington, DC: Author.

American College of Obstetricians & Gynecologists (ACOG), (1990b). Management of isoimmunization. *ACOG Technical Bulletin,* No. 148. Washington, DC: Author.

Barton, J., & Sibae, B. (1991). Care of the pregnancy complicated by H.E.L.L.P. syndrome. *Obstetrics and Gynecology Clinics of North America, 18*(2), 165–179.

Burlew, B. (1990). Managing the pregnant patient with heart disease. *Clinics in Cardiology, 13*(11), 757–762.

Elliott J. P., O'Keeffe, D. F., Schon, D. A., & Cherem, L. B. (1991). Dialysis in pregnancy: A critical review. *Obstetrical and Gynecological Survey, 46*(6), 319–324.

Freda, M., Damus, K., & Merkatz, I. (1991). What do pregnant women know about preventing preterm birth? *Journal of Obstetrics, Gynecologic, and Neonatal Nursing, 20*(2), 140–145.

Friedman, S. (1991a). Pathophysiology of preeclampsia. *Clinics in Perinatology, 18*(4), 661–681.

Friedman, S., Bernstein, M. S., & Kitzmiller, J. L. (1991b). Pregnancy complicated by collagen vascular disease [Review]. *Obstetrics and Gynecology Clinics of North America, 18*(2), 213–234.

Grimes, D., & Schuly, K. (1992). Randomized controlled trials of home uterine activity monitoring: A review and critique. *Obstetrics and Gynecology, 79*(1), 137–142.

Heppard, M., & Garite, T. (1992). *Acute obstetrics: A practical guide,* St. Louis: Mosby–Year Book.

Keohane, N., & Lacey, L. (1991). Preparing the woman with gestational diabetes for self care. *Journal of Obstetric, Gynecologic, and Neonatal Nursing, 20*(3), 189–193.

Lavery, P. (1990). Placenta previa. *Clinical Obstetrics and Gynecology, 33*(3), 414–421.

Lockwood, C. (1990). Placenta previa and related disorders. *Contemporary Obstetrics/Gynecology, 35*(1), 47–68.

Maikranz, P., & Katz, A. (1991). Acute renal failure in pregnancy. *Obstetrics and Gynecology Clinics of North America, 18*(2), 333–343.

Nurses Association of the American College of Obstetricians and Gynecologists (NAACOG). (1991). *Standards for the nursing care of women and newborns* (4th ed.). Washington, DC: Author.

Steel, J., Johnston, F. D., Hepburn, D. A., & Smith, A. F. (1990). Can prepregnancy care of diabetic women reduce the risk of abnormal babies? *British Medical Journal, 301*(6760), 1070–1074.

Walker, J. (1991). Hypertensive drugs in pregnancy. *Clinics in Perinatology, 18*(4), 845–873.

Wallenburg, C., Dekker, G. A., Makovitz, J. W., & Rotmans, N. (1991). Effect of low dose aspirin on vascular refractoriness in angiotensin sensitive primigravida women. *American Journal of Obstetrics and Gynecology, 164*(5, Pt 1), 1169–1173.

York, R., Brown, L. P., Swank, A., et al. (1990). Diabetes mellitus in pregnancy: A clinical review. *Journal of Perinatology, 10*(3), 285–293.

CHAPTER 12

Regionalization of Care

GAIL A. BAGWELL VICKY L. ARMSTRONG

■ **RESEARCH AGENDA**

Compare neonatal morbidity and mortality rates for cases in which maternal versus neonatal transport were used for similar conditions.

Is there a correlation between length of stay, neonatal morbidity, and readmissions and those neonates kept in level II nurseries in comparison with those transferred to level III nurseries?

What is the impact of the trend toward deregionalization on neonatal morbidity and mortality rates?

Is the use of back transfers a financial benefit to hospitals? To parents?

Explore the reasons back transfers are used (this study could be done from an administrative and parental perspective).

What are the effects of regionalization on parent–infant interaction?

In the late 1970s, guidelines describing a regionalized system of perinatal care were published. Hospitals were divided into three levels, each level having defined capabilities. Factors that influenced the level of designation were (1) number of deliveries per year, (2) location, (3) training level of physicians and nurses, and (4) availability of ancillary support systems (The National Foundation—March of Dimes, 1976). The goal in developing a regionalized system was to guarantee availability and accessibility of quality care for those in need and the economic delivery of that care (Ryan, 1975).

American health care delivery changed during the 1980s and 1990s. The growth of health maintenance organizations (HMOs), the implementation of diagnosis-related groups (DRGs) in certain states, changes in Medicaid and third-party reimbursement, and a staffing crisis led to a deterioration in perinatal regional care in some areas. Within regions, hospitals began competing for patients rather than cooperating to provide optimal care (Allison-Cooke et al., 1988).

This chapter reviews the development of the regionalized system and delineation of levels of care. It outlines the responsibilities of the nursery staff at each level and the staff's role within the system. The chapter concludes with a discussion of the challenges facing the regionalized system approach to care and the steps being taken to adapt the system for the future.

DEVELOPMENT OF THE REGIONALIZED SYSTEM

During the first half of the 20th century, infant mortality rates decreased steadily worldwide. From 1950 to 1965, mortality rates continued to fall in western nations; in the United States, however, rates did not fall significantly. Barriers such as race, poverty, geographic location, and cultural and physical isolation kept high-risk pregnant women and infants from medical care. Research showed that persons at high risk, socially and medically, were least likely to receive the necessary medical care. When these people received appropriate care, their outcomes improved. This relationship was demonstrated during World War II, when more than 1,450,000 women and infants received medical care through the Emergency Maternity and Infant Care Program for armed forces' dependents. Perinatal and infant mortality rates improved. The program was discontinued in 1949, and a coincidental rise in mortality rates began in 1950.

As the medical community learned of the multiple causes affecting infant mortality, it began to change the delivery of perinatal care. High-risk maternal and neonatal care had a positive influence on mortality rates. Neonatal transport provided new access to intensive care nurseries.

The American Medical Association (AMA) Committee on Maternal and Child Care began holding conferences on infant mortality in 1966. Its focus was on identifying high-risk infants, the organization and delivery of high-risk care, problems of prematurity, need for perinatal research, education, and staffing requirements. In 1968, the Canadian Department of Health and Welfare stated, "Hospital delivery is provided to ensure that all resources are available to take care of any deviations from normal which might endanger the mother or her baby." The department also stated, "When the high risk mothers and their babies are recognized and their problems anticipated it is considered valuable to ensure their care in the hospitals with the most appropriate facilities even though this may require referral to another institution" (Meyer, 1980).

The AMA supported the development of regional perinatal programs outlined in the 1971 Policy Statement on Centralized Community or Regionalized Perinatal Care. The AMA, together with the American Academy of Family Physicians (AAFP), the American Academy of Pediatrics (AAP), and the American College of Obstetricians and Gynecologists (ACOG), formed the Committee on Perinatal Health. The committee had the task of developing guidelines for a regional perinatal care system.

In 1976, the committee, supported by The National

Foundation—March of Dimes, published *Toward Improving the Outcome of Pregnancy: Recommendations for the Regional Development of Maternal and Perinatal Health Service*. The committee determined that a "systems approach" would meet the objective of providing optimal care for the women and infants within a region. The committee defined regionalization as the development, within a geographic area, of a coordinated, cooperative system of maternal and perinatal health care in which, by mutual agreements between hospitals and physicians and on the basis of population needs, the degree of complexity of maternal and perinatal care that each hospital is capable of providing is identified so as to accomplish the following objectives: quality care to all pregnant women and newborns, maximal utilization of highly trained perinatal personnel and intensive care facilities, and assurance of reasonable cost effectiveness (The National Foundation—March of Dimes, 1976).

According to the recommendations, a region would serve a population with 8000 to 12,000 live births per year. Within each region, a medical center with over 2000 deliveries yearly would be designated a level III, or tertiary, center. These hospitals would care for pregnant women and infants at highest risk. Level II centers would serve as the referral center for hospitals that provided less specialized services. Level II hospitals would provide routine care and have capabilities to handle most obstetrical complications and short-term neonatal intensive care.

Level I hospitals would serve a small population and provide care for uncomplicated deliveries and healthy newborns. Personnel would be trained to recognize obstetrical and neonatal emergencies and to give competent care in these situations.

Across the United States, the committee's recommendations were acted upon and regional systems were developed. The ACOG and AAP adopted the recommendations.

The National Foundation—March of Dimes had already determined a relationship between perinatal events and crippling diseases of infants. The National Foundation committed administrative and financial support to the committee, financed projects to raise community awareness about the need for perinatal care, and designed educational programs for both pregnant women and health professionals.

The Robert Wood Johnson Foundation, a philanthropic organization, supported the committee's recommendations and financed eight regional programs (National Demonstration Program) for a 5-year period. The Foundation's goal was to evaluate the feasibility of the regional approach and its effect on improving health care. Evaluation of this National Demonstration Program found that (1) in both funded regions and comparison areas, the neonatal mortality rates decreased sharply over the decade of the 1970s, and (2) the centralization of high-risk deliveries appeared so widespread that the special effect of the Foundation program could not be detected (McCormick et al., 1985).

In 1989, the AAP and ACOG requested the March of Dimes to reconvene the Committee on Perinatal Health to make further recommendations for regional development (Little, 1993). The document, *Toward Improving the Outcome of Pregnancy: The 90s and Beyond (TIOP II)* (Committee on Perinatal Health, 1993), moves from a discussion of the past and current climate of care through indicators of the problem to key recommendations considered to be essential for improving the outcome of pregnancy (Little, 1993).

IMPACT OF REGIONALIZATION ON NEONATAL MORTALITY

A result of the development of the neonatal intensive care unit (NICU) and improved obstetrical care is the decline in neonatal mortality. The improvement in mortality rates must be examined by inspecting birth weight at delivery. The greatest impact is seen on the survival rates of extremely low birth weight (ELBW) neonates, or infants who weigh 750 to 1000 g at delivery. In 1960, the mortality rate of ELBW infants was 90 percent. Today, more than two thirds of infants born weighing between 750 and 1000 g survive. ELBW infants born at level I and II centers and then transferred to a level III center have a lower rate of survival. There is a large variation in the reported survival rates of infants born weighing less than 750 g. The chance of survival improves when these infants are delivered at level III centers (U.S. Congress, Office of Technology Assessment [OTA], 1987). Also, empirical studies indicate that tertiary level units provide more effective care for infants of very low birth weight (Perkins, 1993).

Although the benefit of concentrating high-risk deliveries at level III and designated level II perinatal centers can be seen in improved survival rates, some physicians are reluctant to transfer their high-risk patients. The reasons given for this reluctance are (1) financial issues, (2) the competition among hospitals to attract patients by offering a full complement of services, and (3) a lack of agreement by the obstetrician or pediatrician of the ELBW infant's viability.

The voluntary cooperation of hospitals, physicians, and health officials to regionalize services had a positive impact on infant survival rates. Even today, the technology to determine at birth which handicaps, if any, ELBW infants will incur is not available. The opportunity for survival and normal development is influenced by the place of delivery (OTA, 1987). The mortality rate among ELBW infants increases for those born at a level I or II hospital. When possible, a high-risk pregnant woman should be transferred to a level III hospital before delivery. To increase survival chances and influence a positive developmental outcome, ELBW infants should be transferred to a level III NICU after stabilization following delivery (Powers & McGill, 1987). Changes are being implemented to continue the success of perinatal regionalization. The issues influencing the future of the program are explored later in this chapter.

THREE LEVELS OF PERINATAL CARE

In 1976, the Committee on Perinatal Health recommended that the delivery of perinatal care be divided into three levels. For the regionalized system to function effectively, a coordinated communication network was established within each region.

Level I hospitals were responsible for recognizing high-risk mothers and neonates and coordinating either their referral or their transport to a higher level of care. Level II hospitals had the Level I hospital responsibility but also had intensive care facilities, usually used to care for sick neonates with a moderate degree of illness (Freeman & Poland, 1992). The level III hospital was responsible for the provision of comprehensive perinatal care services of all risk categories. A method of obtaining consultation and arranging maternal or neonatal transports was outlined. *TIOP II* calls for modifying the current system from being defined as levels to being identified as basic, specialty, and subspecialty perinatal centers. Currently, however, the original levels of care still essentially exist.

Outreach education programs were implemented by the level III centers for the smaller hospitals. The purpose of outreach was to educate perinatal personnel in recognizing high-risk conditions and to educate them in handling obstetrical and neonatal emergency complications when immediate transport was not possible (Burkett, 1989).

The committee set guidelines for establishing a regionalized system and the responsibilities for hospitals at each level. The committee's framework was designed, not as a standard of care, but rather as an achievable goal of improving the outcome of pregnancy (The National Foundation—March of Dimes, 1976).

There is no defined national standard by which to determine

the difference between level II and level III care. In some states, individual hospitals classify their level of care; in others, the state sets the perinatal designation (OTA, 1987). The descriptions of care outlined below are those of the committee. Table 12–1 outlines the responsibilities for each level of care according to the AAP's *Guidelines for Perinatal Care.*

Level I

These facilities are located in communities with small populations, either suburban or rural. Because of their low number of births per year and their smaller economic base, these hospitals are responsible for managing uncomplicated maternal and newborn care. They must be able to give competent emergency care in unexpected situations. A strength of the level I facility is its ability to recognize potential high-risk situations and provide both primary and preventive care or consultation and/or referral to an appropriate center.

The level I hospital has a formal relationship with the regional level III center. This relationship supports a method of consultation and communication and of patient transport between the two. The level I hospital participates in an educational program to train its personnel in neonatal resuscitation and in stabilization of patients for transport. Infants can be transferred back to the community hospital from a level II or III center after the acute illness is resolved. The community hospital promotes the infant's growth and development in a family-centered environment.

Level II

A wide variation in the abilities of level II units exists, depending on the medical specialists and support services available in each institution. Level II facilities offer services for uncomplicated maternal and neonatal patients and are competent in handling certain obstetrical and neonatal complications (Fig. 12–1). When needed specialists and services are not available, patients are transferred to the level III center.

A pediatrician with neonatal expertise directs the medical care in the special care nursery. The nursing staff is skilled in caring for sick infants and communicating effectively with the infant's parents. Infants either transported to or delivered at the level III center can be transferred back to the level II nursery when their condition has stabilized. The level II unit participates in collaborative educational programs with the level III center. If the appropriate services are available, the level II unit can serve as the referral site for level I nurseries in the region.

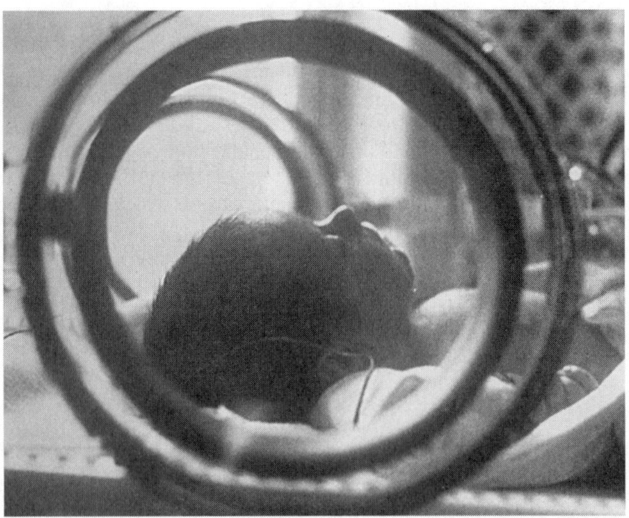

FIGURE 12–1. Level II neonate requiring close supervision. (Courtesy of March of Dimes Birth Defects Foundation.)

TABLE 12–1 Role Definitions in a Regional Perinatal Network*

Level I
Manage uncomplicated perinatal care
Identify patients at risk and initiate maternal and fetal transport
Provide emergency care and stabilization for unexpected complications
Provide patient and community education
Collect and evaluate patient data
Level II
Provide all services of level I facility
Identify and treat select high-risk maternal and neonatal problems
Initiate and receive maternal-fetal and neonatal transport
Provide education for allied health personnel
Level III†
Provide all services of level I and II facilities
Identify and treat all maternal and perinatal problems
Coordinate and accept perinatal and neonatal transports
Conduct research and evaluate outcomes
Provide education within the region
Direct system management

*Transport of neonates occurs to and from all facilities.

†Level III NICUs located in children's hospitals may not offer services of level I and II facilities.

Adapted from American Academy of Pediatrics. (1992). *Guidelines for perinatal care* (3rd ed.). Washington, DC: American Academy of Pediatrics and American College of Obstetricians and Gynecologists. Used with permission.

Level III

Level III facilities serve as the region's referral sites for the most high-risk maternal and neonatal patients and provide routine obstetrical and newborn care. These institutions offer a full complement of consultants and ancillary services to care for their patients. Many children's hospitals have intensive care and specialized resources for neonates. The children's hospital is an appropriate referral site but should not be used as the sole level III facility in the region.

The level III NICU has an equipped and trained team and is available around the clock for neonatal transport. A similar team may be available for transporting high-risk maternity patients. The team provides management and treatment during transport. It is also responsible for educating personnel at the referring hospital.

The level III unit is responsible for instituting a continuing education program for the region. The regional center, often affiliated with an educational institution, serves as an educational training center for health care professionals. Perinatal personnel throughout the region may come to the level III center to gain experience in caring for critically ill mothers and infants (Fig. 12–2).

Nurses in the NICU have expertise in caring for the sickest neonates. They understand the physiology, the disease processes, and the necessary monitoring equipment. Communication with the infant's parents and offering emotional support are essential skills for the NICU staff. This staff includes respiratory therapists, nutritionists, occupational and physical therapists, pharmacists, early intervention specialists, and perinatal social workers with expertise in working with neonates and their parents.

COORDINATING THE REGIONAL SYSTEM

Coordination of services and communication among institutions and personnel within the region is essential for the success of the

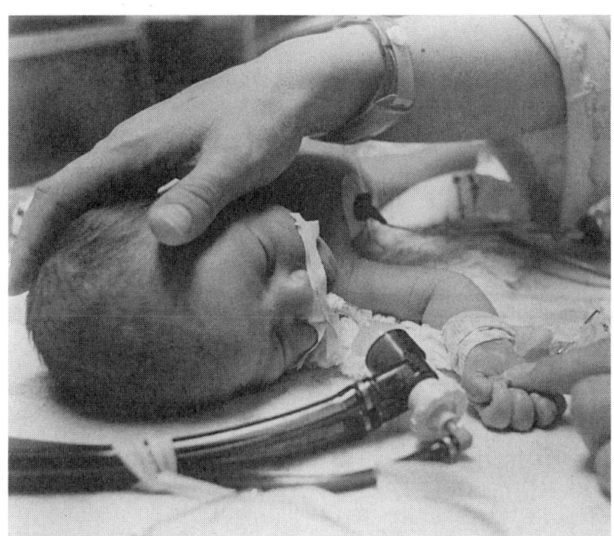

FIGURE 12–2. Level III neonate requiring high-technology care. (Courtesy of March of Dimes Birth Defects Foundation.)

system. All those involved must be aware of their responsibilities and roles within the system; they must have a working knowledge of how the system functions. Medical and nursing personnel, health departments, third-party payers, and consumer groups participate in the planning of delivery care within each region (The National Foundation—March of Dimes, 1976).

To foster communication and continuity of care, interhospital conferences are held. These meetings provide the referring hospital with information on patients transferred to the regional center and information on learning opportunities (Fickeissen, 1986). The conferences give community physicians the chance to participate in case management and to learn the steps in obtaining consultations and patient transfers.

Evaluation of perinatal care plays an appropriate role in assessing whether the provision of care has been effective. Evaluation should include a perinatal data program (1) to help monitor outcome, (2) to identify problem areas that require improvement, and (3) to use for comparative studies.

ROLE OF OUTREACH EDUCATION

To ensure quality care for patients within the region, outreach education programs have been developed by the regional centers to assess educational needs, educate and train health care providers, implement and evaluate the program, collect and analyze perinatal data, provide patient follow-up to referral hospitals, and provide continuity of communication among hospitals. Education and training programs include physiologic and technical information and a psychological component on the emotional issues of high-risk care and ways to promote parent–infant bonding in a crisis situation. These educational programs focus on meeting the goals of the regional approach (Scoblic, 1989). The impact of the outreach programs is seen in the improvement of care and the decrease of mortality and morbidity in the region (Jones & Modica, 1989).

FACTORS INFLUENCING PATIENT TRANSFER

The transport of sick neonates from their birth hospital to a perinatal center is a direct result of the regionalization system (Fig. 12–3). There is continuing argument about the advantages and disadvantages of neonatal transport after delivery versus maternal transport before delivery. Studies that reported no significant differences between the mortality rates of premature infants transferred to level III centers after delivery and those of infants born in level III centers may have a built-in bias, because the most critically ill and premature infants may not survive long enough to be transferred to a NICU and premature infants with no morbidity are not always transferred (OTA, 1987). Studies show a decrease in mortality when high-risk mothers are transferred to perinatal centers before delivery. There is minimal difference between the survival rates of infants born after antenatal transport and those of deliveries scheduled at the referral center.

There exist both physical and financial barriers that prevent the transfer of patients to perinatal centers. Competition between hospitals, especially in urban areas, may be a reason for level II hospitals not to refer their patients to the level III center. Hospitals use their ability to provide services for the entire family to attract clients; in addition, it provides continuity of care and promotes maternal-infant bonding. Childbirth may be the first experience that a family has with hospitalization. Hospitals want to develop a continuing relationship with the family, and a maternal or neonatal transport to a neighboring hospital for needed services can threaten this relationship (OTA, 1987). In addition to competition issues, the technology of neonatal intensive care is no longer the exclusive preserve of heavily funded academic centers (Gagnon et al., 1988). The ease of technology transfer, the surplus of neonatologists and ancillary neonatal personnel, and reimbursement issues have enabled level II NICUs to be

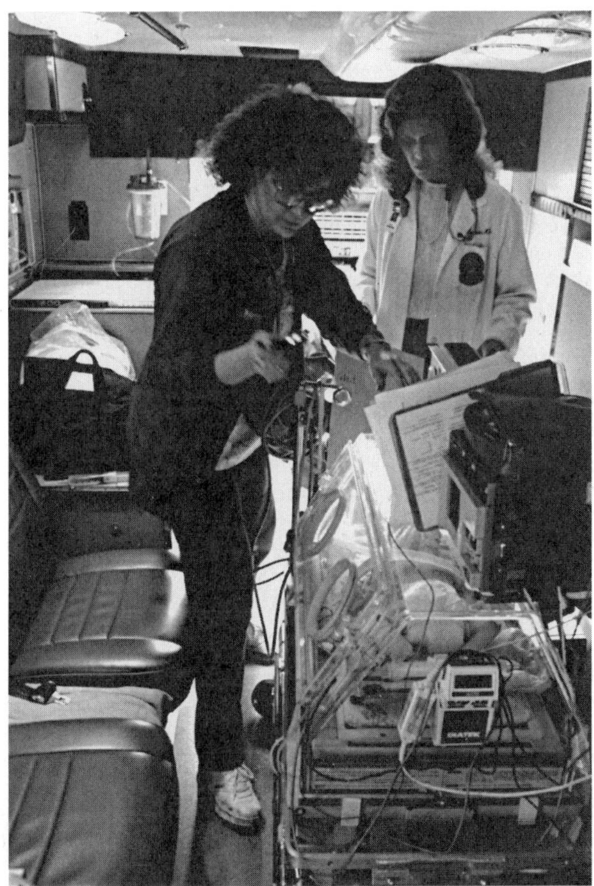

FIGURE 12–3. Transporting a neonate for high-technology care. (Courtesy of March of Dimes Birth Defects Foundation.)

established. Moreover, with the availability of skilled neonatal nursing staff to respond quickly to neonatal emergencies, the liability risks of hospitals and the medical staff have decreased (Chiu & Brennan, 1992). A physician's decision to transfer a patient can also be influenced by the risk of nonpayment or loss of payment. Medicaid reimbursement for obstetrical care is more than 30 percent lower than reimbursement from a private paying patient. Obstetricians have been slower than other physicians to accept Medicaid patients (OTA, 1987). When the level III hospital is university-affiliated and has a closed medical faculty, nonfaculty obstetricians do not have admitting privileges. These physicians risk loss of payment by transferring patients to such a facility.

Other factors that can affect the transfer of patients to a level III center include (1) a lack of bed space, (2) unavailability of the needed resources, and (3) unavailability of the needed equipment (e.g., extracorporeal membrane oxygenation [ECMO]). If one of these cases arises, the level III center should help the referring hospital find another institution to which to transfer the infant and should assist with medical management of the infant over the phone until transfer. Finally, the Joint Commission on Accreditation of Healthcare Organizations (JCAHO), although responsible for reviewing the operation guidelines of the NICU, does not have authority over access to treatment. Some NICUs were created under an individual state certificate-of-need legislation. The state does not have continuing authority over the operation of neonatal services once the certificate of need is granted. Institutions that received federal funding for construction and renovation under the 1946 Hill-Burton Act must provide charity care for patients who cannot pay. The Consolidated Omnibus Budget Reconciliation Act, enacted in March 1986, prohibits Medicare-participating hospitals from denying treatment to or transferring a woman in labor.

BACK TRANSFER

When the demand for NICU beds exceeds availability, the results are overcrowding and transport to level III centers far from the delivery site (Jung & Bose, 1983). Returning convalescing infants to their community hospital—back transfer—has multiple benefits.

Back transfer strengthens the referral system in the region by promoting communication and mutual trust among hospitals. Because the capabilities of level I and II hospitals vary, it is important to learn each nursery's capabilities along with its limitations. This information can be ascertained by the level III transport team during their transport calls. The level III nursery can match the appropriate level I or II nursery to the infant's continuing care needs when this information is available (Jung & Bose, 1983).

An efficient back-transfer program helps eliminate an acute shortage of NICU beds. Planning ahead for an infant's return transfer to the community hospital optimizes the management of NICU beds in a shortage crisis (Croop & Kenner, 1990).

The back transfer of infants also promotes the sharing of fiscal responsibility within the region. Per-day costs are higher in the NICU than in the level I or II nursery, and the occupancy of critical care beds by convalescing infants is not an effective use of NICU resources. Transferring convalescing infants improves the efficacy of use of level I and II beds and provides the hospital with a financial benefit of additional patient days.

The staff of the community hospital is able to maintain its expertise and skills by caring for back-transferred infants. The result is an increase in pride and an investment in accountability in the care of these infants. In the less hectic environment of the nursery, the staff can focus on teaching the family how to care for the infant. Having the infant closer to the family allows for regular visits and greater involvement in the infant's care. The local physician can become involved with both infant and family sooner, which facilitates the transfer of trust from the level III center to the local community hospital.

A successful back-transfer program depends on the involvement of personnel in both the transferring and receiving hospitals and the preparation of the family. A state's public health code and the receiving hospital's infection control policy must be understood before planning the back transfer. If the hospital has an isolation protocol, the family should be informed of the policy, to alleviate a last-minute surprise before the transfer.

The financial issues surrounding back transfer need to be clear before the transport is arranged. Parents may refuse a transfer if they are unable to pay or if the third-party payer is unwilling to reimburse them for the transfer.

It is the responsibility of the physician in the level III to define the medical criteria for transfer and to communicate the infant's care plan to the community physician. The community physician must agree to accept the infant and provide the medical supervision required. The physician at the level III provides the community physician with ongoing support and communication.

The NICU nursing staff has a major responsibility in the success of the program; they can identify infants who are ready for transfer. It is the level III center staff's responsibility to communicate the infant's nursing care needs, family needs, and any potential problems to a designated key contact on the receiving nursery staff. The communication between the nurses of both hospitals helps to strengthen collegiality throughout the region.

The social workers in both hospitals must communicate to assure the family of the available resources—physical, emotional, and financial—at the community hospital. This communication helps ease the family's transition to the new institution.

Family involvement and preparedness are essential to the success of the back transfer. The idea of back transfer should be presented when the infant or mother is initially transferred to the level III. Back transfer should be presented as a positive step: a milestone for the infant. The family must be reassured that the infant is well enough for transfer and that the transfer is a safe procedure. It is important for the family to understand that policies and procedures may differ in the community hospital and that different methods are acceptable. The family should be encouraged to visit the community hospital and become acquainted with the staff before the infant's transfer.

The attitude of the level III staff toward back transfer is a major force in the success or failure of the program (Croop & Kenner, 1990). Communicating confidence in and commitment to back transfer, along with support for the parents, helps to overcome the separation anxiety experienced by family and staff. The benefits of back transfer are sabotaged when the level III staff communicates uncertainty and lack of confidence in the community hospital to the parents (Gates & Shelton, 1989).

There are disadvantages in the back-transfer program. The potential for incomplete transfer of information exists with the change in care provider. This communication failure can cause a disruption in the infant's continuing care (Croop & Kenner, 1990). A family's problems with the changes in care providers, policies, and procedures are lessened when the actions just discussed are followed.

The level III NICU faces two main disadvantages when all convalescing infants are back transferred: (1) There is less of an opportunity to learn to provide convalescent care, and (2) caring for less critical infants provides both relief from intensive care nursing and enjoyment for the nursing staff.

For the regionalized system to function as designed, the transfer of patients must complete a circle. Level I and II nurseries rely on the level III centers for sophisticated perinatal services. Level III centers, in turn, depend on level I and II centers for needed resources to care for the convalescing infant and family (Grassi, 1988).

CHALLENGES TO REGIONALIZATION

The primary goal set by the Committee on Perinatal Health was to improve patient outcomes. To accomplish this task, the committee recommended the regional structure for providing care. Inherent in the proposed regional system was a sense of altruism and the sharing of patients by physicians to benefit the patients at risk.

Toward Improving the Outcome of Pregnancy (The National Foundation—March of Dimes, 1976) outlined a regional concept but provided few details for implementation. The plan was to develop exemplary systems that would function as role models for others. Across the country, regional systems were organized, influenced by the geographic area represented, the personnel involved, and the political climate.

The health care environment has undergone dramatic changes since the implementation of regionalized care. Changes in the prospective reimbursement to hospitals in the 1980s affected the altruism and sharing inherent in regional systems and led to competition for patients. As a result, regional perinatal systems are breaking down.

The three levels of neonatal care established by the Committee on Perinatal Health have become blurred in the current environment. Level I nurseries are upgrading their services to level II. The widest range of services provided is found in level II nurseries, many of which provide services of a level III NICU. With the advances in technology and services and the wide variation in levels of care, the traditional regional concept has become outdated (Allison-Cooke et al., 1988).

The prospective reimbursement to hospitals was altered with the introduction of DRGs. DRGs classify patients on the basis of principal diagnosis, age, surgical procedure, comorbidities, complications, and discharge status. Reimbursement to a hospital is relatively fixed according to a patient's classification. DRG reimbursement for Medicare patients began in 1983; a number of states followed, using DRGs for reimbursement of Medicaid patients. Blue Cross and some other national and regional commercial payers also implemented DRG reimbursement.

Neonatal care is contained in Major Diagnostic Category 15: Newborns and Other Neonates with Conditions Originating in the Perinatal Period. This category is broken down into the seven classifications listed and described in Table 12–2.

Studies of infants transferred within the regional network showed that DRGs did not acknowledge differing levels of neonatal care or transport systems. As the federal DRG stood, regional systems would be disrupted.

TABLE 12–2 Major Diagnostic Category 15: Newborns and Other Neonates With Conditions Originating in the Perinatal Period

Diagnosis-Related Group	Description
385	Neonates—died or transferred
386	Extreme immaturity (<1000 g), neonate
387	Prematurity with major problems
388	Prematurity without major problems
389	Full-term neonate with major problems
390	Neonates with other significant problems
391	Normal newborns

Adapted from Lagoe, R. J., Milliren, J. W., & Baader, M. J. (1986). Impact of selected diagnosis-related groups on regional neonatal care. *Pediatrics, 77*, 627–632. Reproduced by permission of *Pediatrics*.

Reimbursement policies favored level I nurseries with shorter patient stays. Level II and III nurseries would be discouraged from returning stable neonates to level I nurseries, creating a potential for overcrowding of NICUs and lack of available level III resources (Lagoe et al., 1986).

To maintain established regional networks, many states modified the federal DRGs to increase reimbursement for neonatal care. Although Medicaid reimbursement does not have a serious impact on perinatal regionalization, it does affect ambulatory services, with a lesser reimbursement for obstetricians, creating a barrier to accessible care.

Competition among hospitals for patients is the largest threat to existing regional networks. The increase in multihospital systems has made it difficult for one hospital to serve as the referral site within a defined region. This has led to the creation of new perinatal systems and the elimination of existing ones.

When insurance coverage is provided through HMOs and preferred provider organizations (PPOs), access is limited to contracted hospitals. Contracts, and hence transport patterns, are decided by the administrators of provider organizations, not by the physicians. In the past, physicians established professional relationships within the region, and patients were often transferred along the lines of those relationships.

The changing health care environment of the 1980s created a competitive atmosphere that has led to the breakdown of traditional regional alliances. The goal of decreasing perinatal mortality has been accomplished. The future of regionalized care is uncertain (Allison-Cooke et al., 1988).

THE FUTURE OF REGIONALIZATION

The effects of a changing health care environment has resulted in a decreased commitment to regional networks and an expansion in the services hospitals offer to be more competitive in the marketplace (Jones & Modica, 1989). These "threats to the perinatal system point to the need for individual hospitals and health care agencies to reexamine the part they play in providing service to women, infants, and families" (Scoblic, 1989).

In a 3-year study, the National Perinatal Information Center examined the changes in regional networks during the 1980s and the steps needed to adapt the networks for the 1990s. Members of the perinatal community, including some members of the original Committee on Perinatal Health, met to discuss and outline a structure for the future delivery of perinatal care. Key findings from the study included (1) general deterioration of perinatal regionalization in many areas; (2) frequent replacement of cooperation by competition among hospitals; (3) blurring of differences in levels of care, with a general escalation of services to higher levels; (4) upgrading of neonatal programs, regardless of whether the number of high-risk infants is sufficient either to maintain skill levels or to be cost effective; and (5) factors in health care environments (such as HMOs, multihospital systems, prospective payment and malpractice liability) that are influencing and changing the delivery of perinatal care (Allison-Cooke et al., 1988).

The goals outlined by the Committee on Perinatal Health in *Toward Improving the Outcome of Pregnancy* (The National Foundation—March of Dimes, 1976) have been reached. Changes in the health care environment, most notably competition among hospitals for patients, has weakened the regional systems developed in the 1970s. The future of perinatal regional care is in jeopardy. A broad-based Committee on Perinatal Health reconvened to analyze current definitions of care, identify problems with the existing system, and modify it to function through the 1990s and beyond. There has been a shift in the focus of perinatal care from hospital-based care to overall health care awareness. Emphasis must be placed on preventative health care, education and counseling, the goal being quality health care that is accessible to all and economically efficient for the provider. Because of this shift, the new committee on Perinatal Health focused on four key areas: (1) care before and during pregnancy; (2) care during birth and beyond; (3) data, documentation, and evaluation; and (4) financing (Committee on Perinatal Health, 1993, p. III). Recommendations for improving the outcome of pregnancy that were developed from the four key areas are described in Table 12–3. A recommendation from this committee is that the three levels of inpatient perinatal care be modified, enhanced, and promoted (Committee on Perinatal Health, 1993). Three types of perinatal centers have been defined as basic, specialty, and subspecialty. Basic perinatal centers provide basic inpatient care for pregnant women and newborns without complications; management of perinatal emergencies, including neonatal resuscitation; leadership in early risk identification before and at birth; consultation or referral for high-risk patients; and public and professional education (Committee on Perinatal Health, 1993; Maloni et al., 1996). Specialty perinatal centers provide management for certain high-risk pregnancies, including maternal referrals from basic care enters; services for newborns with selected complications, particularly those who are moderately ill; and appropriate continuing education (Committee on Perinatal Health, 1993). Subspecialty perinatal centers provide inpatient care for maternal and fetal complications; a NICU equipped to treat critically ill neonates; follow-up medical care of NICU graduates; consultation and referral arrangements with other hospitals (including transport arrangements); educational opportunities; a perinatal data base; and evaluation activities (Committee on Perinatal Health, 1993).

CONCLUSION

The development of regional systems for providing perinatal care came in response to increasing perinatal mortality rates after World War II. Health care professionals recognized that to lower mortality rates, high-risk care for mothers and infants had to be made accessible.

In 1976, a regional design was outlined by the Committee on Perinatal Health, and regional models were implemented across the United States. These regional systems varied according to their geographic location, but all operated with a spirit of altruism to reach the goal of improving the outcome of pregnancy.

That goal has been accomplished. Perinatal mortality rates have decreased, as a direct result of accessible high-risk care (OTA, 1987). The regional approach is now threatened by a rapidly changing health care environment. Competition for patients has replaced the sharing of patients that existed between professional colleagues. Existing regional networks are being modified; some have deteriorated completely.

As we enter the 21st century, the regional approach, with

TABLE 12–3 Key COPH Recommendations Essential for Improving the Outcome of Pregnancy

Health Promotion and Health Education
In collaboration with families and health professionals, every school (K–12) should develop and implement a plan for comprehensive school health education that includes age-appropriate reproductive health information.

Reproductive Awareness
New strategies to reach each man and woman of childbearing age with reproductive awareness messages should be implemented. All health providers should employ reproductive health screening to reduce risks.

Structure and Accountability
Perinatal regions should be well defined to ensure accountability for care of a total population. State and regional Perinatal Boards should be established with the authority and responsibility for ensuring, providing or coordinating nonclinical activities such as planning, monitoring access, data collection, and provider education.

Preconception and Interconception Care
Risk reduction should be emphasized and family planning counseling and services routinely available. Preconception or interconception visits annually, as well as a prepregnancy planning visit, should become standard components of care.

Ambulatory Prenatal Care
Early risk assessment, followed by appropriate care, consultation or referral, must be a universal and ongoing component of prenatal care; medical and social services may be needed.

Inpatient Perinatal Care
Three levels of perinatal care defined in the 1970s should be modified, enhanced, and promoted; three types of facilities should be recognized: basic, specialty, and subspecialty perinatal centers, with all facilities integrated into networks of care.

Infant Care
Perinatal services must extend through the first year of life, with access to pediatric care and a regular source of care for all infants. Early intervention services should be structured to include appropriate care for infants with complex problems and integrated into the regionalized system.

Improving the Availability of Perinatal Providers
State and regional Perinatal Boards should assess need, develop and improve the supply and distribution of perinatal providers. Strategies should include supports and incentives to encourage qualified providers to deliver perinatal care.

Date, Documentation, and Evaluation
Every state should have a perinatal data program to facilitate accountability and to provide information for monitoring the system and perinatal outcome, including population-based and clinical data.

Financing Perinatal Care
Any health care reform plan should include a benefit package that meets the unique needs of pregnant women and infants, and a process for updating the benefit package to add effective new interventions. Financing mechanisms should be determined for nonclinical services and used to support perinatal system structures.

From Committee on Perinatal Health (COPH). (1993). *Toward improving the outcome of pregnancy: The 90's and beyond.* March of Dimes Birth Defect Foundation, pp. III & IV. Used with permission of copyright holder.

three distinct levels of care, faces a challenge for survival. New approaches for the delivery of perinatal care have been outlined. The new committee has evaluated the positive aspects of their original work along with the needs of today's perinatal population and has designed an approach for the 21st century.

REFERENCES

Allison-Cooke, S., Schwartz, R. M., & Gagnon, D. E. (1988). *The perinatal partnership: An approach to organizing care in the 1990s.* (Project No. 12129). Providence, RI: National Perinatal Information Center.

American Medical Association. (1971). *Policy statement on centralized community or regionalized perinatal care.* Chicago: Author.

Burkett, M. E. (1989). The tertiary center and health department in cooperation: The Duke University experience. *Journal of Perinatal and Neonatal Nursing, 2*(3), 11–13.

Chiu, T., & Brennan, L. (1992). University neonatal centers and level II centers compatibility. Jackson experience. *Journal of the Florida Medical Association, 79*(7), 464–468.

Committee on Perinatal Health. (1993). *Toward improving the outcome of pregnancy: The 90s and beyond.* White Plains, NY: March of Dimes Birth Defect Foundation.

Croop, L., & Kenner, C. (1990). Protocol for reverse neonatal transports. *Neonatal Network, 9*(1), 49–53.

Fickeissen, J. L. (1986). Interhospital perinatal nursing transport conferences. *Neonatal Network, 5*(3), 45–48.

Freeman, R. K., & Poland, R. L. (Eds.) (1992). *Guidelines for perinatal care* (3rd ed.). Elk Grove Village, IL: American Academy of Pediatrics.

Gagnon, D., Allison-Cooke, S., & Schwartz, R. M. (1988). Perinatal care: The threat of deregionalization. *Pediatric Annals, 17*(7), 447–452.

Gates, M., & Shelton, S. (1989). Back-transfer in neonatal care. *Journal of Perinatal and Neonatal Nursing, 2*(3), 39–50.

Grassi, L. C. (1988). Life, money, quality: The impact of regionalization on perinatal/neonatal intensive care. *Neonatal Network, 6*(4), 53–59.

Jones, D. B., & Modica, M. M. (1989). Assessment strategies for the outreach educator. *Journal of Perinatal and Neonatal Nursing, 2*(3), 1–9.

Jung, A. L., & Bose, C. L. (1983). Back transport of neonates: Improved efficiency of tertiary bed utilization. *Pediatrics, 71*(6), 918–922.

Lagoe, R. J., Milliren, J. W., & Baader, M. J. (1986). Impact of selected diagnosis-related groups on regional neonatal care. *Pediatrics, 77*(5), 627–632.

Little, G. A. (1993). Toward improving the outcome of pregnancy, 1993: Perinatal regionalization revisited. *Pediatrics, 92*(4), 611–612.

Maloni, J. A., Cheng, C.-Y., Liebl, C. P., & Maier, J. S. (1996). Transforming prenatal care: Reflections on the past and present with implications for the future. *Journal of Obstetric, Gynecologic, and Neonatal Nursing, 25*(1), 17–23.

McCormick, M. C., Shapiro, S., & Starfield, B. H. (1985). The regionalization of perinatal services. *Journal of the American Medical Association, 253*(6), 799–804.

Meyer, H. B. (1980). Regional care for mothers and their infants. *Clinics in Perinatology, 7*(1), 205–221.

The National Foundation—March of Dimes. (1976). *Toward improving the outcome of pregnancy: Recommendations for the regional development of maternal and perinatal health services.* White Plains, NY: Committee on Perinatal Health.

Perkins, B. B. (1993). Rethinking perinatal policy: History and evaluation of minimal volume and level of care standards. *Journal of Public Health Policy, 14*(3), 299–319.

Powers, W. F., & McGill, L. (1987). Perinatal market penetration rate. A tool to evaluate regional perinatal programs. *American Journal of Perinatology, 4*(1), 24–28.

Ryan, G. M. (1975). Toward improving the outcome of pregnancy. Recommendations for the regional development of perinatal health services. *Journal of Obstetrics and Gynecology, 46*(4), 375–384.

Scoblic, M. A. (1989). The clients of outreach. *Journal of Perinatal and Neonatal Nursing, 2*(3), 59–68.

U.S. Congress, Office of Technology Assessment (OTA). (1987). *Neonatal intensive care for low birthweight infants: Costs and effectiveness* (OTA-HCS-38). Washington, DC: U.S. Government Printing Office.

CHAPTER 13

Neonatal Transport

CYNTHIA MARGARET ACREE   RITA MARIA KUNK

RESEARCH AGENDA

How do nurse-managed transport outcomes compare with the outcomes for transports coordinated by other health professionals?

Compare patient outcomes and transport costs for neonates with the same medical diagnoses who are transferred via ground and air.

What are parents' perceptions of the transport process?

How are decisions made regarding reverse transport—is it for cost-effective use of bed space, for parent–infant interaction, or both?

How accurate are patient monitoring devices while en route?

What is the feasibility of the use of high-technologic treatment modalities during transport (e.g., ECMO, nitric oxide)?

What is the impact of managed care contracts on decisions about neonatal transport?

VIGNETTE

In a regional system for neonatal care, some delivery hospitals do not have a focus on providing high-tech or long-term neonatal care. They depend on the expertise and back-up from regional referral centers that specialize in critical neonatal care. The crucial link between the delivery hospital and the referral center is the multidisciplinary team. This team is responsible for the safe transport of the infant. This system requires excellent communication and teamwork between the two staffs. The management in the first few minutes after birth can have tremendous influences over the quality of the infant's life. The following case demonstrates use of the transport team's expertise in influencing an infant's outcome.

It was 0200 when I was awakened by the sound of my pager. There was a very sick baby at a local hospital, and the transport team was needed as quickly as possible. No information regarding the infant was given by the referral hospital except that we were needed for a 36-week-gestation male, weighing 3.2 kg. In less than 1 hour, the team, consisting of a nurse, a physician, and a respiratory therapist, rushed into the referral hospital, only to find a very gray, limp, apparently lifeless infant in a radiant warmer. The nursery staff were busy working on the infant, but to no avail. After one look at this infant, we all agreed that the problem might be cardiac disease, since there appeared to be more than respiratory distress. The infant's initial arterial blood gases were as follows: pH, 7.02; Pco_2, 48; Pao_2, 38; base excess, –14. Vital signs were as follows: HR, 180; RR, 80; peripheral BP, 45/29 in the upper right arm; temperature, 36.8°C. Unconsciously, our priorities of airway, breathing and circulation were formed, and immediately the transport physician and respiratory therapist intubated the infant as I, the transport nurse, quickly started two IVs for access. A bolus of 5% albumin was given for volume, and the infant was started on prostaglandins (PGE). Sodium bicarbonate was started for acidosis, a glucose level was obtained, and $D_{10}W$ was started. Blood pressure remained low, necessitating dopamine to be started. X-ray revealed tube placement to be correct and showed a large heart, confirming in our minds a cardiac defect of some type, most probably a left obstructive outflow lesion. After initial systematic stabilization of the infant, a hat was placed on the infant's head and pictures were taken before the infant was loaded into the incubator. Monitoring was accomplished, and along with the E.T. tube, IVs, and the infant's poor color, it was a very frightening sight. The visit to the family was brief because the infant remained in critical condition. As we brought the infant to the mother's room, tears came streaming down her face as she begged us to "just go"; she wanted her baby to live. She reached her hand into the incubator and touched the infant's foot and began crying, asking us to "please take care of my baby." Empathy was communicated, and the photos and information about the regional center were given to the mother. The father was also encouraged to touch the infant as we began to move out of the room. Once inside the ambulance, we quickly switched power and oxygen over to the ambulance's supply, and we were ready to go. We were not out of the parking lot before the heart rate precipitously dropped to 30 beats per minute and the infant stopped breathing while on CPAP. Chest compressions were started, the PGE dose was doubled, and the respiratory management was evaluated. One round of epinephrine was given, and the heart rate began to stabilize. Now we felt it was time to begin our trip back to the regional center. With lights and sirens all the way, we quickly returned to the regional center for newborn intensive care. Report was called to the unit while we were still en route. They were prepared for our arrival. Upon arrival, the transition of care went smoothly. After observing that the infant was stable in the hands of the new caregivers, a phone call was made to the parents to update them on the infant's condition. Although not all transports are as critical as this one, it is important for the transport team to always be ready to respond to a critical need and to be prepared for the worst possible scenario, in hopes that it will not occur. Equipment should always be checked and ready to roll out the door at a moment's notice. Lines of communication should be outlined in advance so that response to a call can be facilitated as quickly as possible. Team members often work closely in stressful situations and often develop a strong trust in each other's abilities to handle critical situations. Many times we know instinctively what each will do in a particular situation. Transport teams are highly skilled and experienced in physical assessments as well as certified and experienced in many different technical procedures. Along with all the education, experience, and qualifications come the most important components to being a member of a transport team: compassion and understanding. No matter how critical the situation, the fears, concerns, and feelings of the family need to be taken into consideration, and empathy for their crisis should be conveyed.

Dee Overbeck
Heidi Campbell
Dan Wells

The uterus is the natural and best means of transport for the fetus. At birth, the fetus leaves the uterus and the safety of the intricate physiologic environment that meets its every need. In the event of an unexpected outcome, health professionals are faced with the challenge of meeting the complex needs of the compromised neonate. If the neonate is born in a location without the resources to fulfill these special needs, transportation of the neonate to a hospital with necessary resources becomes an additional challenge.

Neonatal transport has evolved into a sophisticated, dynamic process that is essential for providing optimal perinatal and neonatal care. This chapter reviews the development of the transport process, the effect of regionalization, and various transport models. It presents a detailed framework of an incoming transport, the impact of the transport process, posttransport information exchange, alternative types of transport, financial considerations, and legal issues. The chapter concludes with a discussion of how the constantly changing health care environment will affect the transport process in the future.

HISTORICAL PERSPECTIVE

Written reports of the transport of sick individuals can be traced back to Biblical times, in the Gospel; in Luke 5:18–19, a paralytic was brought on a mat to Jesus, who, according to the physician Luke, was the great healer (Salyer & Masi-Lynch, 1995).

Before the invention of the wheel, individuals in need of medical assistance were carried on animals and by family members and friends (Chou & MacDonald, 1989). The wheel was then used in wagons created for patient transport. Wars and resulting casualties were the primary stimuli for the development of ambulance systems in the 1400s through modern times (Chou & MacDonald, 1989). The Vietnam War was the major impetus for the development of effective helicopter evacuation and transport. During the Crimean War, Florence Nightingale brought to the public's attention the neglect of the sick and wounded by the British army (Hackel, 1987). In 1834, a basic form of the ambulance was used in England (Hart, 1978). In the mid-1800s, the United States army recognized the benefits of an organized ambulance service. The Red Cross was formed in Europe in 1864, encouraging an organized method of rescuing the wounded from the various battlefields during the Civil War (Chou & MacDonald, 1989).

The first electric ambulance was used in 1899 at the Michael Reese Hospital in Chicago; it was capable of traveling at a speed of up to 16 miles per hour (Chou & MacDonald, 1989). Neonatal ground transport started in the early 1900s with the use of horse-drawn carriages to transport premature neonates to regional centers (Hackel, 1987). This type of early transport was developed by a French physician, Martin Couney, who wanted to display premature infants in London at a public exhibition (Chou & MacDonald, 1989). British hospitals would not permit their infants to be used for exhibition, but they did not forbid others from being exhibited. Dr. Couney decided to transport French infants across the English Channel by boat. The infants were transported in washbasins containing pillows and hot-water bottles to keep them warm and comfortable (Chou & MacDonald, 1989). By 1933, when Dr. Couney came to the United States with his exhibition, he had developed an ambulance for the transport of infants (Chou & MacDonald, 1989). One of his sources of neonates was the Chicago Premature Station. In 1948, an organized transport service was developed in New York City. The neonates were transported via a hand-carried aluminum incubator with hot-water bottles and a portable cylinder of oxygen (Chou & MacDonald, 1989) (Figs. 13–1 and 13–2). The average times were just over 2 hours for transport and 27 minutes for travel time, at a cost of $48.62. They experienced good outcomes, even with neonates who weighed less than 1000 g (Chou & MacDonald, 1989).

In the 1960s and 1970s, the need for the regionalization of newborn intensive care became evident. Regions were demarcated and hospitals were given "level of care" designations (level I, II, or III) according to the resources available to them. Regional centers were developed to provide state-of-the-art care with well-trained staff and the highest technology and services available. This was a means of providing cost-effective use of health care dollars, inasmuch as not all hospitals needed to replicate equipment and services that would not be used on a regular basis. The transport team evolved out of the need to take high-technology care to the neonates and the need to bring neonates to regional centers when the care they required was beyond the scope of the birth hospital. Such transports necessitated personnel who were skilled in caring for critically ill neonates.

Despite the efforts of regionalization and the focus on improving technology, the mortality and morbidity statistics in the United States have not significantly improved. The second edition of *Toward Improving the Outcome of Pregnancy* (March of Dimes

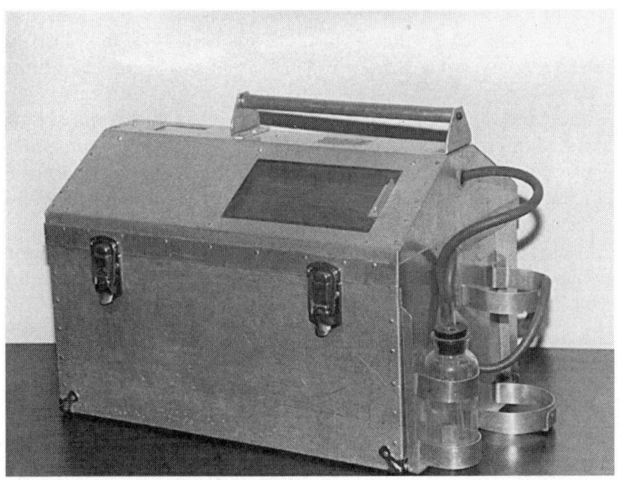

FIGURE 13–1. Transport incubator of the 1950s. (Incubator from the collection of Dr. Irwin Light. Photograph courtesy of T. L. Marcus.)

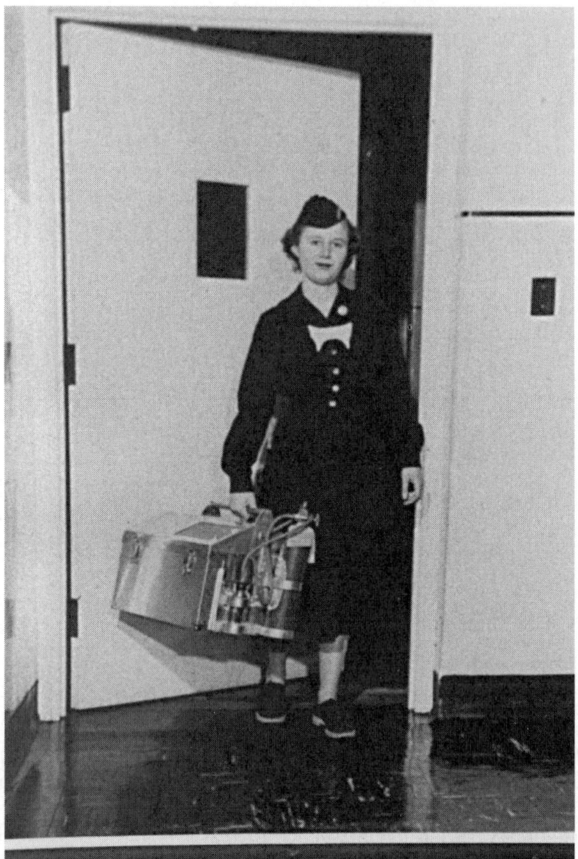

FIGURE 13–2. Transport nurse of the 1950s. (Photograph from the collection of Dr. Paul Perlstein. Courtesy of T. L. Marcus.)

Birth Defect Foundation, 1993) recommends addressing the need for more of an emphasis on dealing with the causal root of the problem of infant mortality or morbidity. There is advocation for prevention and the development of collaborative services to meet the needs of the consumer in the community. A more academic approach is used in meeting health professionals' needs in the community through the provision of education, data collection, research, and evaluation with regard to infant outcomes when transport is and is not used. Ideally, the transport team can readily support the changing needs of perinatal clients with their unique contributions.

Likened only to the advent of diagnosis-related groups (DRGs), the current focus on financial concerns in order for institutions to survive is making history. Nationwide many institutions are merging and developing alliances that are changing regional perinatal health care. With some regions and states eliminating their certificate-of-need process for justifying the need for maternity beds, institutions will add maternity beds to become more diversified and to generate more revenue, potentially increasing the needs for both maternal and neonatal transports. The transport team can ideally provide an educational liaison with new community perinatal health care professionals to optimize care and improve outcomes. For more information on regionalization, see Chapter 12, Regionalization of Care.

NATIONAL STANDARDS AND GUIDELINES

Nationally recognized guidelines for Neonatal Transport have been established by both the American Academy of Pediatrics (AAP) (1993) and the National Association of Neonatal Nurses (NANN) (1994). Transport systems developed according to guidelines will be more responsive to the need for rapid access, will be better able to ensure delivery of high-quality care, and will function more safely and efficiently. The following areas are addressed by the guidelines:

- Organization and administration of a team
- Education and competency of team members
- Quality care
- Support of parents whose infants require transport
- Quality improvement
- Communications
- Safety
- Medicolegal issues
- Vehicles, equipment, and medications
- Outreach education

Professionals interested in forming a team, ensuring adherence to a basic national standard, developing team competencies, or establishing a sound quality improvement program will find these references a valuable resource. Examples of specific treatment protocols for neonatal transport have also been published for such conditions as persistent pulmonary hypertension, sepsis, and intestinal obstruction (MacDonald & Miller, 1989).

TRANSPORT TEAM MODELS

Composition

Transport team composition varies from institution to institution, depending on the number of transports per year, the acuity of the patient population, the medicolegal climate, and the availability of funding and personnel. Some hospitals that transport infrequently pull staff from the newborn unit in the event of a transport. However, other facilities may require a highly trained independent team to meet their transport needs. With the emphasis on cross-training and cost effectiveness, an increasing number of dedicated teams are also transporting pediatric, adult, or obstetric patients. Regardless of whether the team is composed of emergency medical technicians, paramedics, respiratory therapists, registered nurses, neonatal nurse practitioners, physician assistants, or physicians, it must function as a unit. The registered nurse plays an integral role by being a consistent member of any transport team. The collaborative team approach is essential for the survival of any transport program. Each team member must acknowledge the abilities, limitations, and scope of licensures for each person who participates in the transport process.

Qualifications

Hospitals, infants, and families are best served by careful selection of transport team members. An assessment of the applicants' qualifications should be based on, but not limited to, the following characteristics as cited in the NANN (1994) guidelines:

- Educational and experiential background
- Technical and clinical competence
- Leadership skills
- Critical thinking skills
- Proficient communication and interpersonal skills
- Appreciation of public/community relations

The best transport team members are skilled and creative at making critical decisions and being patient advocates. They are also diplomatic and effective communicators, realizing their roles as ambassadors in the community and acknowledging the contribution of all players in the transport process.

Team members must also be able to physically tolerate confined spaces, motion, and vibration. Teams performing air transport often have weight restrictions. The ideal team member is flexible enough to function professionally and effectively in any setting.

Orientation

The orientation of new transport team members varies according to the knowledge and experience of each candidate. After input from the new candidate is considered, an individualized needs assessment should be completed to determine exactly which didactic and practical experiences are needed to prepare the potential team member for transporting intensely ill neonates. Then both the person responsible for transport orientation and the new team member can develop an individualized orientation plan. The plan should be detailed enough to provide structure and yet flexible enough to enable revision as needed. Education and experience is gained most effectively in a one-on-one preceptor relationship. This preceptor can and should utilize fellow team members as resources in their particular area of skill such as procedural or therapeutic communication skills. The program should be structured to encourage increasing independence, including building of rapport with current team members and allowing for independent study time. After orientation, the new member should have his or her schedule matched with that of a veteran team member to aid in the completion of the transition. Scheduled evaluations with the preceptor and coordinator helps ensure progress and address individual challenges or needs. Evaluations are also a time to commend and encourage unique skills that the new member may bring to the team. Content areas of orientation and competency should include the following, many of which are cited in the NANN (1994) guidelines:

- Neonatal Resuscitation Program and or Pediatric Advanced Life Support Course
- Maternal health factors as they affect the neonate
- Neonatal assessment
- Interpretation of laboratory and diagnostic data
- Thermoregulation
- Advanced airway management
- Medications and fluid therapy
- Assessment and treatment of neonatal disorders and diseases
- Therapeutic communication for handling crises
- Customer-oriented public relations
- Documentation of care and of process
- Setting up the transport
- Problem solving and setting of priorities
- Transport policies and procedures
- Team performance improvement
- Safety
- Equipment and monitoring
- Medicolegal concerns
- Flight physiology
- Expectations of team member's participation in the work team

Continuing Education/Outreach Education

Continuing education is a vital part of any transport program. Orientation and precepting should just be the beginning of a continuous education process for all transport team members. Continuing education helps to create a dynamic transport program that stimulates both personal and professional growth among team members and improves the quality of care that they deliver. Because transport team members often function in an environment of limited access to expert resources, they should plan the time and funds to educate themselves to be as expert as possible for the work that they must do.

Team education days planned by the team members are essential for addressing learning needs, practicing skills, demonstrating competencies, and accomplishing required learning. When speakers are recruited, it is essential that they address the topic specifically as it relates to the mobile intensive care environment.

Maintaining certification in neonatal resuscitation is nationally recognized and can be used as a check on competency for the team members. Specialty certifications should also be encouraged. By achieving certification, team members reinforce their knowledge base and attain recognition among their peers.

Competency checks of transport skill and knowledge can be creatively designed to provide bursts of fun and challenging learning. Checkpoints of learning should take place throughout the year. Group activities at team meetings, individual challenges by mail, and team office visual aids are all options. Connolly and associates (1992) emphasized the importance of open case review of transports with the medical director. Case reviews allow team members to gain an understanding of a variety of issues and to explore alternative methods of problem solving.

Attendance at national conferences benefits the team in many ways. In addition to supplying new knowledge, it provides a chance for the team to consider new ideas, view new equipment, establish resource contacts, and talk with transport experts.

Some team members learn best by teaching others. Referral hospitals consistently request outreach education. Team members participating in outreach education learn by researching their topics and by listening to the comments and anecdotes of the referral hospital staff. Team members also discover a great deal about adult learning principles and audiovisual presentation. Delivering a well-developed lecture in a referral hospital helps to strengthen community ties and improve the quality of care throughout the region.

All continuing education must be documented. Individual documentation is important for license renewal, performance evaluations, professional liability protection, and maintenance of specialty certification.

Although an essential component of any transport program, the educational modalities mentioned do not replace actual transport experience. Actual transport experiences on a frequent basis are necessary and invaluable as a teaching tool. Theory must be applied to practice in these situations for true adult learning.

COMMUNICATION

To function effectively, transport team members must be master communicators. They must understand the communication principles, know how to enhance the process, and be able to troubleshoot all potential barriers. Typical barriers include distraction, individual perceptions, time pressures, unfamiliar jargon, anxiety, and ego-protective defense mechanisms (Lancaster, 1982).

The most valuable and important characteristic of communication for team members is flexibility. As it was very appropriately stated on behalf of nursing's invaluable contribution to patient care, "Blessed are the flexible, for they shall change the earth!" (Curtin, 1995, p. 8). Transport members must speak clearly and concisely with the dispatch center. In the next moment, information sharing must be accomplished in an efficient and respectful manner with the referral hospital staff. Between team members, unspoken nonverbal cues with phrases of clarification often characterize the communication during the stabilization for transport. Crisis communication skills with parents require yet another set of skills that are called upon quickly and adjusted to each individual situation. Plans of care are based on the information that the transport team members bring and share with the receiving institution. Virtually every aspect of the transport process is completely dependent on each individual's ability to communicate effectively.

Communication Within the Team

Communication between team members is vital to the function and survival of a safe and effective transport program. Methods for sharing information on equipment readiness and repair, prescheduled transports, hospital memoranda, team meetings, and decisions are critical to daily operations. Checklists, erasable boards, communication books, and voice mail can all be used. Digital pagers worn at all times can display messages requesting help for simultaneous transports, changing needs, or reminders of meetings and educational offerings.

Exercises and education in team building, conflict resolution, and awareness of communication styles with coworkers are an increasingly valuable area of focus for continuing education. More teams are beginning to function in a participative management framework that requires these skills.

Interpersonal communication among members is complex. The team often has close-knit, family-like relationships. Respect for one another's skills and appreciation of individual styles are necessary in well-functioning teams.

The Communication Center

A central dispatch or coordinating center for centralizing information flow is needed, especially for busy programs or if the institution is involved in other types of transport. The person receiving the calls is aware of available resources and can obtain contact phone numbers and initial information needed to mobilize, thereby avoiding "on-hold" waiting by referral staff who need to continue stabilizing an infant.

Experienced personnel—often the team member, the neonatologist, or the charge nurse—completes the referral call to ensure stabilization of the patient until the team arrives. Some units choose to establish a designated "hotline" within the unit. Although communication algorithms (Table 13–1) may vary the opportunity for expert consultation and rapid team mobilization are the optimal goals for this portion of the transport process.

TABLE 13–1 Communication Algorithm

I. Take transport call
   A. Obtain required information for admission to obtain a *complete* picture of the infant's status.
   B. Assess the urgency or tone of the call—comfortable or hysterical.
   C. Verbally assist in stabilizing infant or ask physician to do so (if you are not comfortable or do not have the time).
   D. Document all instructions given.

II. Take responsibility for notifying the appropriate people (or ask the clerk to call).
   A. The attending physician or fellow covering the floor will determine:
      1. If transport is appropriate.
      2. Who needs to go on transport (RN-only runs must have attending physician's permission except for reversals).
         a. If MD needed: Monday through Friday 8 A.M. to 5 P.M.—second fellow or transport fellow for month will accompany team.
            Monday through Friday 8 A.M. to 5 P.M. and Saturday through Sunday 8 A.M. to 8 A.M. next morning—neonatal fellow or attending physician on call for transport.
      3. What mode of transportation is to be used.
         a. Ambulance. Document time call was made.

From Transport Department, Children's Hospital Medical Center, Cincinnati, OH. Reprinted with permission.

Communication of the Team With Others

Communication and rapport with the referral hospital can have a significant impact on patient outcome and on the relationship between the referral and level III hospitals. Each specializes in what they do most often; each wants a smooth transfer process, and each works for a good patient outcome. A climate of respect assures all parties involved that their input is valued and the information they provide will be accepted nonjudgmentally. The respect must be genuine; otherwise, nonverbal signals belie underlying judgments.

Effective communication can be further impaired when two people perceive the same information differently. In addition, time pressures caused by health care professionals' desire to resuscitate, stabilize, and transport sick neonates as quickly as possible can limit their ability to send, receive, and validate information.

Transport team members are viewed as representatives of the care and quality of their institution. They must assume the responsibility of continually improving the quality of their communication skills and their neonatal skills. Personnel who are pulled onto the team for a transport without receiving communication training may benefit from a review of basics or team-led cues.

MOBILIZATION OF THE TEAM

The plan to mobilize the team must be devised in a manner that ensures the most efficient response time possible. It is generally accepted that the time should be 30 minutes or less. This time is measured from the time the referral hospital begins the call to the time the team leaves the tertiary center. Information sharing, notifications, mobilization of team members, checking availability of ground or air vehicles, and movement of equipment and personnel all must take place within these 30 minutes. Each hospital must investigate its own problems within this process. Documenting times and process problems are typically parts of a quality check performed by transport teams.

The occurrence of delays should be investigated. Would having a hospital-owned ambulance help? When is the physician not in house? Can on-call team members drive directly to the referral institution? Can the mode of transport and team composition be determined in the first 2 minutes of the referral call so that mobilization can begin? Can the referral hospital fax information?

Extremely critical transports may require alterations in the usual mobilization process. Communication becomes critical as certain responsibilities are delegated and usual patterns are changed. Preplanning for such an event helps clarify what is acceptable to all parties and what is best for the patient.

MODES OF TRANSPORT

A variety of modes of transport are being used by transport teams throughout the country. Many teams have access to ground transport via ambulance or to air transport via aircraft, including helicopters, small propeller planes, medium-sized fixed-wing planes, Lear jets, and large commercial aircraft. The decision to use one mode of transport instead of another depends on the distance to be traveled, traffic and weather conditions, the terrain, the patient's condition and diagnosis, crew and vehicle availability, cost effectiveness, and the number of people to be transported. Each mode of transport is associated with a unique set of advantages and disadvantages. Thus, making a choice about which transport vehicle is most appropriate is a complex decision. Each institution should have predetermined guidelines, policies, and lines of authority in order to prevent a delay in response time related to the decision-making process.

In general, transport teams typically use some means of ground transport if traveling within a 100-mile radius. Very little time is saved by flying within this range because of the arrangements that must be made for loading, unloading, and ground transport from the landing site to the hospital. Helicopter transports have been found to be most advantageous when used for transports over distances between 100 and 250 miles (Merenstein & Gardner, 1993). Because helicopters can typically land close to the hospital, time is not lost on ground transport at each end of the flight. Any transport over a distance greater than 250 miles usually requires the use of some type of fixed-wing aircraft.

Traffic and weather conditions must be taken into consideration when a transport is planned. Traffic conditions have an obvious impact on the amount of time that it takes to travel a given distance. Even though a referral hospital may be only 20 miles from the receiving hospital, a decision may be made to transport by helicopter if bumper-to-bumper rush hour traffic is likely to prolong ground transportation profoundly. On the other hand, ground transport may be the mode of choice for a 200-mile run if there is poor visibility at flying altitudes. The decision to fly in inclement weather should be left strictly up to the pilot, who should not be aware of, and therefore potentially influenced by, the condition of the patient. If weather conditions are severe, the best choice may be to postpone the transport until it is considered safe for both the infant and the transport team to travel.

A patient's diagnosis or condition is another consideration that must be reviewed when a preferred mode of transport is chosen. If the patient is in need of immediate resuscitation efforts, it is unlikely that any mode of transportation will be able to respond quickly enough to prevent long-term sequelae or even death. Therefore, phone consultation should be provided while the team is en route, and outreach education should be delivered year-round. It is also important to consider the effect that certain modes of transport may have on the infant. The condition of an infant with severe barotrauma may only worsen at high altitudes. The infant may also have a defect that requires specialized care and may benefit by procedures performed at certain hospitals that lie outside the region. More long-distance transports can be anticipated as hospitals establish "Centers of Excellence." Consequently, the nature of the infant's condition is an important aspect to be reviewed when a transport is planned.

Crew and vehicle availability can have an impact on the decision-making process. All transport vehicles are certain to require some time for maintenance, repair, and inspection. In addition, the Federal Aviation Administration (FAA) has specific guidelines concerning the number of flight hours a pilot can have in a given period of time. Many aircraft have restrictions regarding the number of passengers who can be safely carried. Therefore, the guidelines developed to ensure safe transport practice may serve to limit the possible transport modes available at any given time.

At a time when cost containment is considered essential for the survival of most institutions, expenditures generated by various modes of transport certainly have an impact on the decision-making process. Ground transportation is typically the least expensive way to travel, whereas helicopter transports tend to be even more expensive than Lear jet travel in some regions.

Once all these factors have been taken into consideration, a review of the advantages and disadvantages of each type of vehicle should be explored. Ambulance travel provides a more stable environment, in which temperature is controlled more easily, pressure is not an issue, and space confinement is not as drastic. In addition, it is easy to stop and perform any necessary procedures that must be done while en route. The obvious advantages of helicopter transport are the speed of travel and the ability to avoid obstacles. Disadvantages of helicopter travel include cost, noise level, the inability to control temperature, changes in vibration and pressure, risk of fatal accident, severe space restrictions, and team members' concern about flying. The benefits of flying in a medium-sized fixed-wing aircraft include a relatively unlimited range, and a more controlled environment. A major disadvantage of fixed-wing flight is the additional time that it takes to make arrangements, which include the need for ground transport to or from the hospitals at both ends of the trip.

For a transport vehicle to be considered for transport use, it must first meet all safety standards set, provide a means to secure all equipment and supplies, have power and gas sources, ensure available back-up, be clean and well maintained, and have access to some form of communication network. Once an institution has determined which transport vehicles meet these criteria, the decision to choose one mode over another becomes specific to each transport.

To prevent inconsistent decision-making and delayed response times, hospital policies and guidelines should be outlined in advance. The complex decision of choosing the best mode of transport is often a judgment call made by the transport personnel preparing for an impending transport.

EQUIPMENT

In the mobile intensive care environment of transport, the skills of the team and the equipment they carry become the critical basics of getting from one place to another in an optimal state. Certain essential pieces of equipment must be maintained to be ready and dedicated solely for transport purposes (AAP, 1993, p. 79).

All transports should have available a light transport incubator (Fig. 13–3), monitoring equipment, suction, air and oxygen with blender, a ventilator, and infusion pumps. Monitoring electrocardiogram (ECG), respirations, temperature, oxygen saturation, blood pressure, and ventilation all must be possible with a basic transport equipment. A stethoscope and a mobile phone should also be considered part of the durable equipment.

Equipment should be chosen to be durable, lightweight, and portable as well as capable of performing the advertised functions. The equipment must be durable enough to function in adverse environmental conditions to withstand motion, temperature, and pressure changes. Flights, narrow doorways, lifting, and maneuvering necessitate consideration of the weight and dimensions of the equipment.

Battery capability takes on a new importance, as does AC/DC conversion ability. All equipment should be able to stand alone

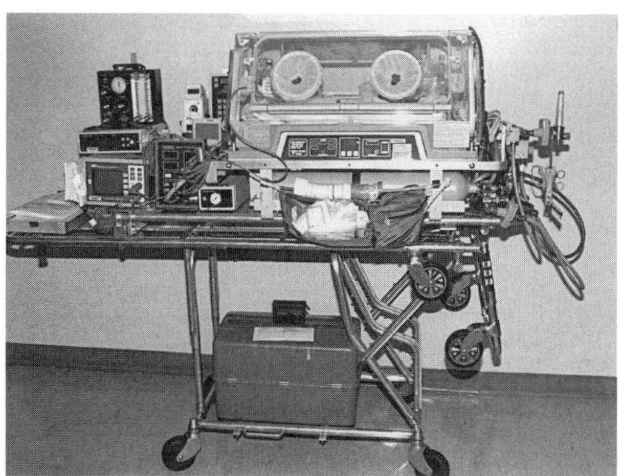

FIGURE 13–3. Incubator of the 1990s. (Equipment from Children's Hospital Medical Center, Cincinnati, OH. Photograph courtesy of T. L. Marcus.)

for twice the anticipated transport time (AAP, 1993). Even then, teams carry a manual back-up, always preparing for the unexpected.

The clinical engineering department can help with decisions on equipment but also on compatibility and securability of all pieces. Equipment built with attachments for securing, Velcro, tiedown straps, and individually designed securing measures all help ensure the safety of patient and the team as well as protect expensive equipment. The biomedical department should test and maintain equipment on a regular schedule. They also are most qualified to determine whether replacement parts are readily available and whether warranty and maintenance contracts are adequate.

Original and replacement purchase of durable medical equipment requires forethought. Advice from established teams or persons familiar with the equipment newly on the market can prove invaluable. With the budgetary constraints affecting practically every facet of health care, equipment priorities must be set and cost–benefit analysis determined. Planning to replace the most expensive equipment items every 5 to 10 years avoids unexpected emergency purchases.

Once the transport team has acquired the equipment that it has determined to be essential for an effective transport program, team members must be responsible for maintaining the entire transport unit in a state of readiness. At the beginning of each shift and after the completion of each transport, the equipment should be checked to determine that it is functioning correctly, has adequate battery power, and remains securely mounted to the incubator. Many teams have discovered that an equipment checklist is the best way to ensure that each team member takes responsibility for equipment preparation and upkeep. In addition, many teams find that appointing one member to be responsible for handling equipment repair, concerns, and follow-up is an effective means of problem solving. Figure 13–4 is an example of an equipment checklist from a level III regional referral center in the Midwest.

Week of___/___/___

DURABLE EQUIPMENT LIST	Monday	Tuesday	Wednesday	Thursday	Friday	Saturday	Sunday
2 Phones							
3 Cameras							
Medication Frig. T = 36–46 degrees F							
1 Pedi Stretcher							
1 Flight Stretcher							
#1 Isolette							
#2 Isolette							
#3 Isolette							
3 Neo-Med Boxes / 2 Pedi-Med Boxes							
1 Flight Bag							
2 Pedi-Airway Bags							
1 Airway Bag							
1 C-Line Bag							
1 Pedi-Immobilizer							
1 Head-Block							
3 Car Seats							
7 Monitors: 2 Spacelabs 3 Ivy 1 Escort 1 Lifepak 8							
10 Pumps: 3 Siemens 7 Baxters							
6 Suctions: 2 Laerdol 4 Vacu-Aide							
3 TCM's							
5 Chart Boxes							
3 Oximeters / 8 Oximeter Batteries							
1 Vent Tube + Humid.							
5 Ivac Thermometers							
1 Manual BP							
1 Dinemap BP							
1 Zoll Defib / Access.							
Change Defib. Battery							
1 O_2 Tank / Reg / Carrier							
1 Air Tank / Reg / Carrier							
Full Tanks							
Initials							

Comments:

CE = CLINICAL ENGINEERING
CP = CENTRAL PROCESSING

FIGURE 13–4. Equipment list. This list should be updated regularly. (From Transport Department, Children's Hospital Medical Center, Cincinnati, OH. Reprinted with permission.)

SUPPLIES

To be adequately prepared, the transport team must determine which supplies are needed to care for their particular patient population. At minimum, transport teams should be equipped with supplies for oxygen delivery, ventilation, airway maintenance, resuscitation, blood sampling, intravenous insertion, pharmacologic administration, chest tube and umbilical line placement, nutrition and fluid support, gastric decompression, wound dressing, and thermoregulation. In addition, unusual diagnoses or circumstances may require items that must be readily available and added at the time of transport. These may include narcotics and chest tube drainage supplies. Additional completely stocked supply bags prevent delays in the event of closely spaced transport calls (Fig. 13–5). Each supply bag should be stocked with the same supplies and organized in exactly the same manner so as to quickly retrieve supplies as needed. A checklist serves to organize and ensure complete supplies. A small disposable lock should be used to secure the container. Figure 13–6 is an example of a supply box checklist used by a transport team in the Midwest.

ROLE OF TRANSPORT PERSONNEL

The roles of the numerous types of transport personnel vary tremendously from state to state. The way in which a team member practices may depend on the individual's knowledge base, level of formal education, and level of experience and on state regulations, hospital policies, predetermined job descriptions, and team composition. Ideally, all transport personnel would be capable of providing holistic care for the neonate. If everyone were cross-trained to deliver all care to the neonate, the infant would never be forced to depend on any one individual for a successful transport. However, there are legal constraints that prevent some transport personnel from independently providing all of the care that may be needed. Consequently, it is imperative that the transport members function as a team, wherein each member provides quality care within the legal constraints designated by the position that he or she holds.

All team members should be informed about the job descriptions for each type of health professional that could potentially serve on the transport team to avoid confusion. The job descriptions and decision-making authority may change, depending on the composition of the team. In addition, most job descriptions are written from a broad perspective and can be perceived differently by everyone who reads them. Consequently, clearly defining each transport team member's role requires practice. The team needs to go on transports together regularly to establish a method of delivering care that is within the legal boundaries of each position, is efficient, and provides the best quality of holistic neonatal care.

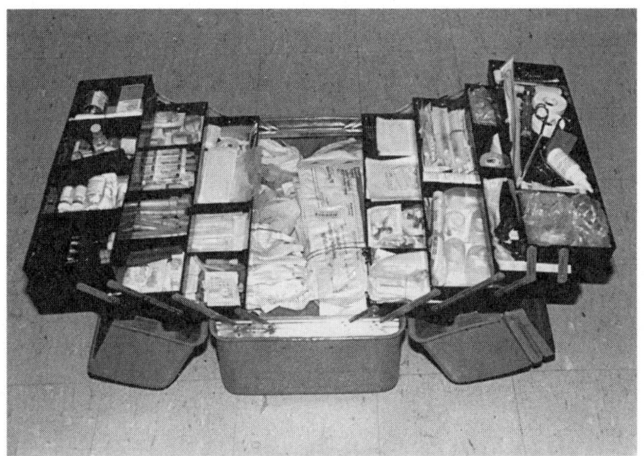

FIGURE 13–5. Transport supply box. (Equipment from Children's Hospital Medical Center, Cincinnati, OH. Photograph courtesy of T. L. Marcus.)

SAFETY ISSUES

The following safety issues, as cited by NANN (1994), should be of primary importance throughout the transport process. Safety policies, procedures, training, and monitoring must be ongoing and updated to ensure a high level of safety awareness among all team members. Teams may choose to appoint their own safety officers to provide accountability for this critical area. Securing or restraining of the patient, team members, and equipment is a critical basic of personal safety. Considerations such as adequate lighting in the mobile environment cannot be taken for granted. Team familiarity with safety features of vehicles and training for "mock accidents" are also important in the mobile care environment. In dangerous weather, the safety of the team and infant must be a top priority. Equipment and vehicles must meet safety standards and be kept safe and operational through regularly scheduled maintenance. Vehicles and aircraft must also meet guidelines set by the FAA and the U.S. Department of Transportation. Teams performing air transports should also follow guidelines established by the Association of Air Services and professional specialty organizations. Fitness and crew fatigue are issues that individual teams need to address through scheduling, policy, or other creative solutions.

Keeping current with the new safety guidelines and equipment and reviewing safety standards makes the team member perhaps the most valued resource for a smooth and safe patient transport. Training and use of body mechanics, hearing protection, and universal blood and body fluid precautions keep each team member safer. Attention to safety of the patient environment, including equipment, vehicle, and travel conditions, helps ensure patient safety.

THE TRANSPORT PROCESS

Assessment

The assessment of a neonate before transport begins with the gathering of subjective data from referral hospital staff via telephone or fax machine. The amount of helpful information varies from basic to comprehensive, depending on the staff of the referral hospital. Objective assessment begins when the team arrives and does a system-by-system, head-to-toe examination. Cardiovascular assessment includes color, perfusion, capillary refill, quality of peripheral pulses, liver boundaries, precordial activity, heart sounds, rate, and rhythm. Respiratory assessment includes color, rate, rhythm, use of accessory muscles, presence of grunting, retracting, flaring of nares, presence and quality of breath sounds, air exchange, and verification of airway patency. Neurologic assessment includes muscle tone, reactivity to stimuli, reflexes, fontanelles, quality of cry, and level of comfort at rest. Gastrointestinal and genitourinary assessment includes abdomen, genitalia, and history and specifics of meconium and urine output. Head-to-toe assessment includes gestational age, body and bone structure, nutritional status, skin, and extremities.

The treatment plan depends on the abnormalities found and the degree of neonatal compromise. Laboratory and radiographic data are helpful adjuncts to care when the degree to which the neonate is compromised is assessed. Routine laboratory values include complete blood count (CBC) with hematocrit, hemoglobin, and differential blood count; blood cultures, if there is a

NEONATAL PANIC BOX CHECKLIST

			(TOP LEFT #1, continued)
	TOP RIGHT #1		Normal Saline for Injec., 2 ea.
	Transilluminator, 1 ea.		Sterile Water 20 ml., 2 ea.
	Magills, 1 sm.		Aquamephyton, 1 ea.
	Laryngoscope, 1 sm. 1 lrg. blade		Sodium Bicarb. 4.2%, 4 ea.
	Batteries, AA, 2 ea.		Epinephrine 1:10,000, 2 ea.
	Blade Bulbs, 4 sm.		Dopamine 200 mg., 1 ea.
	1/2 Inch Adhesive Tape, 1 ea.		Heparinized Saline, 2 ea.
	4.0 Silk, 2 ea. (curved)		Phenobarb 65 mg/ml, 2 ea.
	Dacron Tape, 1 ea.		Narcan 1 mg/ml, 1 ea.
	Lubafax, 3 ea.		
	Benzoin, 1 Bottle or 4 strips		MIDDLE LEFT #2
	Cotton applicators, 4 ea.		Specimen tubes, Green, Purple, Peach, 2 ea.
	Oral airways, 000-0, 1 ea.		Lancets, 2 ea.
	Preemie and Newborn Masks, 1 ea.		Safety Pins & Rubber Bands
	N.S. Vials, 2 ea.		Labels
	Plasmanate 50 ml., 2 ea.		1- & 3-cc Syringes
	X-mas Tree adapter, 1		Miscellaneous Gauge Needles
			Filter Needles, 3 ea.
	MIDDLE RIGHT #2		Butterflies, #23, 25, 27 g, 2 ea.
	500 ml Mapleson With T-Piece, 1 ea.		
	Green O2 Tubing, 2 ea.		
	Stylet, 1 sm.		MIDDLE LEFT #3
			Stopcocks, 2 ea.
	BOTTOM RIGHT #3		Angiocaths, #16–22g, 3 ea., #24, 6 ea.
	Restraints, 2 ea.		PRN Adapter, 1 ea.
	IV Cups, 3 ea.		Sims Tip, 2 ea.
	Razor, 1 ea.		Alcohol Pads
	Transpore Tape 1", 1 ea.		Interlink Ext. Tubing, Inj. Site, 1
	Dermaclear Tape 1/2", 1 ea.		
	Micropore Tape 1", 1 ea.		BOTTOM LEFT #4
	Micropore Tubing, 1 ea.		Penthanol Pins, 2 ea.
	Preemie Armboards, 2 ea.		Tape Measure, 1 ea.
	Infant Armboards, 2 ea.		Referral and Transfer Consent, 1 ea.
	T-piece Ext. Sets, 2 ea.		Tegaderm, 2 ea.
			IV Extension Tubing, 1 ea.
	TOP LEFT #1		Toppers
	Ampicillin 250 mg., 2 ea.		Y-Adapters, 1
	Gentamycin 80 mg., 1 ea.		

Lock # ____________ Date Filled __________ Name ______________________________

FIGURE 13–6. Neonatal panic box checklist. This list should be updated regularly. (From Transport Department, Children's Hospital Medical Center, Cincinnati, OH. Reprinted with permission.)

setup for sepsis; blood glucose; and an arterial or capillary blood gas measurement. Routine radiographs include an anteroposterior (AP) view of the chest and abdomen. Data from lateral views may also be necessary. Physical assessment and laboratory and radiology results are valuable in establishing a data base for determination of future treatment decisions.

Planning

Planning is vital to successful transport. Pretransport planning must consider desired optimal patient outcomes. Transport care can be at the beginning of any of the neonatal critical path or care maps that are developed to direct and monitor care. (See the Appendix for sample critical pathways.) It includes not only patient and family needs but also logistics, communications, equipment, and vehicles. "Ten golden rules of transport" convey the importance of planning (Tharp, 1985, p. 164):

1. Plan ahead.
2. Transports are palliative, not curative.
3. Any treatment can only be as good as the diagnosis for which it is administered.
4. Some hospitals are better hospitals than others.
5. If it is possible for a sick person to become sicker, he or she probably will.
6. Big problems are simply small problems that you have not anticipated.
7. "Probably" is good enough when the "usual" or normal sequence of events occurs.

	BOTTOM SECTION
	Alcohol/Betadine Swabs, 3 ea.
	Bulb Syringe, 1 ea.
	Chest Tubes, 10–16 Fr., 2 ea.
	Culture Bottle, 1 ea.
	D5W, 50 ml Bag, 1 ea.
	ET Tubes, 2.5–4.0, 2 Soft, 1 Hard
	Hat and Bottles, 1 set
	Heimlich Valve, 1 ea.
	Laerdal With Reservoir, 1 ea.
	Manometer, 1 ea.
	Mucus Trap, 1 ea.
	N.S., 1 bag
	Needle Aspiration Kit, 1 ea.
	Oximeter Probes, Purple/Orange, 1 ea.
	Repogle, 10 Fr., 1 ea.
	Suction Caths, 5/6–10 Fr., 2 ea.
	Syringes, 6, 12, 35-cc, Leur, 4 ea. 35-cc Cath Tip, 2 ea.
	Syringes With Needles, 1 & 3 cc, 4 ea.
	Umbilical Caths, 3.5–8 Fr., 2 ea.
	Vaseline Gauze, 1 pack
	Veno/Thoro Pack, 1 ea.
	Quick Connectors 02/Air

FIGURE 13–6 *See legend on opposite page*

8. No transport unit is ideal for every patient.
9. Nothing lasts forever: oxygen/air, battery power.
10. Some days are better than others. No matter what you do, the outcome will be poor.

The plan of care for the patient and family must be individualized and appropriate for the setting, how far the team and patient are from the regional center, and the mode of transport that is being used. Planning is a dynamic process that changes moment to moment on the basis of the patient's response. Protocols can serve as a resource from which to begin.

Implementation

If resuscitation is required, it is accomplished as quickly as possible. The main objectives of resuscitative efforts are to verify and maintain a patent airway, to provide effective oxygenation and ventilation, and to ensure that circulation is adequate to meet metabolic demands. Necessary neonatal resuscitation must begin immediately, even before Apgar scores are determined. Those scores and other evaluation measures were originally designed to assess the success of extrauterine adaptation and with full-term babies. The American Heart Association (AHA) and AAP have established a Neonatal Resuscitation Program (NRP) and have made it available to health care workers for guidance in achieving these objectives (ACOG & AAP, 1988; Chameides, 1990; Bloom & Cropley, 1994). The program focuses on resuscitation in the delivery room; the same principles can be applied to resuscitation in the transport process. There is also an AAP program for Pediatric Advanced Life Support (PALS) that focuses on the more complex issues that a transport team may be faced with, such as line placement, airway adjuncts, and synchronized cardioversion for the infant who is compromised as a result of supraventricular tachycardia. The course provides valuable resuscitation information. Guidelines for neonatal resuscitation are updated and published in the *Journal of the American Medical Association* approximately every 5 to 6 years. One such publication is due out in 1997–1998. (For more information, see Chapter 15, Resuscitation and Stabilization of the Neonate.)

The process of stabilization is important and often determines the degree of success of the transition to extrauterine life and transport. Time spent in seeking stabilization is vital to ensure optimal care for the neonate during the transport process. The transport team minimizes the time spent at the referral hospital in the stabilization process. Ideally, appropriate stabilization has occurred before the team arrives. The transport team completes procedures and provides care to prevent complications during the transport process and to achieve the highest level of stability for each infant. The process of stabilization includes

- Airway—assessed, secured, supported
- Respiratory effort—assessed, assisted/supported
- Ventilation—assessed, assisted/supported
- Oxygenation—assessed, facilitated
- Circulation—assessed, supported
- Acidosis—assessed, corrected
- Temperature—assessed, supported
- Glucose levels—assessed, supported
- Medications—need assessed, administered
- Nasogastric or orogastric tubes—need assessed, placed
- All other special interventions—need assessed, completed

Stabilization is accomplished according to the patient's need. Measures to be taken before transport, such as intubation or umbilical line or chest tube placement, will be determined by how well the patient is adapting, the trend of the disease process, patient's age, time, distance, and mode of transport. Procedures are better performed in a hospital than in an ambulance at the side of the road or in a helicopter descended for an emergency landing in a cornfield. Whitfield and Buser (1993) suggested that once the mobile intensive care team has arrived, the status of the patient is likened to that of being admitted to the regional center, and there is no need to rush care and departure except under extenuating circumstances. They studied 1757 neonatal transports completed over a 3-year period and found stabilization time to be an average of 89 ± 45 minutes, the median time being 80 minutes. This time includes the time spent with parents, which is an essential part of their program (Whitfield & Buser, 1993). Care should be modified according to the patient's condition and what type of transport vehicle the transport team is using. Working toward providing a developmentally supportive environment during transport as much as possible may help decrease the stress of the transport process. Use of appropriate positioning, water mattresses, ear protection, pacifiers, and minimal stimulation precautions may help to decrease the negative stimulation during this stressful process. During the transport process, all aspects of care require constant monitoring, assessment and support, correction, intervention, and evaluation.

Patient Response to the Transport Process

The nursing process is useful in determining the neonate's response to illness and to interventions during the transport process. There is frequently a knowledge deficit regarding the neonate's previous history and subtle signs of compromise. This deficit, compounded with the dynamics of the situation, provides a challenge for the team.

The transport team must focus on how each neonate may uniquely respond to the transport process. The neonate's response depends on how tolerant she or he is of stimulation and movement and how capable of adapting to the transport process. With stimulation and the use of reserve energy for metabolism, there is often an increase in oxygen consumption that the neonate may not be able to tolerate. Some neonates may need sedative and paralytic agents to decrease the ability to respond to stress. Other neonates may improve or deteriorate during the transport process as a result of manipulation and intervention. In addition, responses to the different modes of transport vary and are unpredictable. It is important to stress in outreach education the necessity of referring critically ill neonates to a regional center as soon as possible.

Transition Into the Neonatal Intensive Care Unit

No transport can be considered complete until the infant is settled into a new bed at the receiving hospital and the admitting team of health care professionals has received a complete written and verbal report. To ensure a smooth transition, the admitting team must have a recent report of the infant's status and a reasonable estimated time of arrival. This type of communication can best be facilitated by the use of a mobile phone or two-way radio en route. However, if verbal contact cannot be established en route, the transport team should call the receiving hospital just before their departure from the referral hospital and provide the admitting team with the necessary information.

Upon arrival at the receiving hospital, the transport team should establish that the bed has been prewarmed and that all of the necessary equipment and supplies are available. Once it has been determined that the admitting team is adequately prepared for the arrival of the new infant, transport team members should prepare for the transfer of the infant from the incubator to the bed provided by the unit. Admitting nurses often prefer to weigh the infant before transferring him or her into the new bed. The transport team knows best whether the infant is stable enough to be weighed first. Consequently, the transport team members are responsible for making decisions about the most effective way to transfer the infant.

Once the decisions have been made and the infant and the equipment have been transferred to the new bed, the admitting team should take responsibility for getting the infant attached to all of the necessary equipment. Unless the infant needs to have immediate intervention, the transport team should begin giving a thorough, chronologic history of both the mother's pregnancy and the infant's hospital course. Any additional insights that the transport team has noted should be shared. In addition, a social history should be reported. It is important for the admitting team to know whether the mother is planning to breastfeed, whether the family has a social support network, or whether visitors can be expected. Once the infant has been settled and stabilized as much as possible, the report has been given, and questions have been answered, the transport team members may leave the bedside to restock their equipment and complete their charting. Not until all written reports are completed and placed in the chart can the transition be considered complete. It is helpful to the mother and referral hospital staff for a call to be placed to the mother and nursery to inform them of how the transport was tolerated, the infant's current status, and plans for care, as well as answering any last-minute questions.

Documentation

A thorough, accurate documentation is not only the most crucial form of communication in the transport process; it is also a medicolegal necessity and an essential quality improvement tool. Written transport documents are the only permanent records of the entire transport process. Consequently, the documentation process should begin as soon as contact has been made between the referral hospital and the receiving hospital. All verbal interaction between the referral hospital staff, the transport team, the receiving hospital staff, and the infant's family must be meticulously recorded. The infant's status, the care provided, and the infant's response to that care must be thoroughly and accurately documented. In addition, the names of all the personnel involved in the care, stabilization, and transport of the infant must be noted. The mode of transport, as well as a list of problems or concerns that may have occurred, should also be recorded.

The forms used to record the transport process vary from institution to institution. Each transport team should create its own checklists and flowsheets that specifically meet its needs. Because hospital policies, patient population, and transport styles vary, the forms used to document the process also vary. Also, if the transport team is not directly involved in the creation of the flowsheets, it is essential that they at least provide valuable input into their development. The flowsheets need to be designed in a manner that provides adequate space for narrative, allows for individualized charting, and simplifies the charting process without omitting valuable information or requiring redundant documentation. It is possible that as transport programs continue to grow and develop, the flowsheets may require review and revision. Figure 13–7 is an example of a flowsheet used for incoming transports in a tertiary center in the Midwest. Regardless of the format chosen within an institution, it is essential that all forms of documentation used for the transport process become a legal part of the infant's chart. Ideally, the team can collaborate so there is only one document for the entire process, one that includes a history, a physical examination summary, a transport summary, a flowchart of vital signs and interventions, the consent, and orders. Ideally, charting by exception can be completed, and abnormalities, patient tolerance of the transport process, and parental reaction can be elaborated upon in a succinct manner.

Appropriate documentation should also be maintained by the transport team when alternative types of transports are performed or assistance within the hospital setting is rendered. Transport teams may find that a separate flowsheet for reverse transports or test runs is more efficient and practical. Figure 13–8 is an example of a flowsheet designed specifically for alternative types of transports. This form is made in triplicate so that the receiving hospital, the referral hospital, and the transport team each have a copy. If there is no form designated for documenting a specific transport function, team members must be aware of how to chart it on the hospital's standard flowsheets. All transport functions must be thoroughly and accurately documented on an appropriate form that is a legal part of the chart.

Any information or action not documented in the infant's chart is not considered in the legal arena. Regardless of the number of eyewitnesses available, if an action is not charted, it is considered not done. Consequently, the legal ramifications of incomplete or inaccurate documentation are great. With the rise in the number of lawsuits being filed against health care professionals, meticulous documentation has become a medicolegal necessity.

Documentation is also a vital part of any quality improvement program. Throughout the entire transport process, beginning with the first phone contact made by the referral hospital until the infant has been smoothly transferred and settled into the new bed space at the receiving hospital, the transport team must meticulously pay attention to time. Recording the exact time that every action or communication takes place is particularly crucial in view of outcome standards and quality assurance issues such as response times, resuscitation techniques, and problem solving. In addition, a transport program needs good record keeping in order to maintain accurate transport statistics, which are an essential part of any quality improvement program.

To ensure documentation accuracy for both legal and quality assurance purposes, charting should be completed within 8 to 12 hours after the transport. Documenting during and immediately after each transport would be the most likely way to maintain accurate record keeping. However, back-to-back transports often make immediate charting impossible. Every attempt should be made to complete all transport documentation as soon as possible after each transport.

Without an appropriate documentation format established for every transport function, thorough and accurate record keeping may be compromised. Without a permanent, written account of the entire transport process and the quality of patient care, the legal security of the health care professionals and the maintenance of a quality transport program might be in jeopardy.

IMPACT OF THE TRANSPORT PROCESS

Referral Hospital Staff

The referral hospital staff at times has a forewarning of an impending delivery of a high-risk neonate who requires care beyond the scope provided by the referral hospital. When this is the case, a mother may be transported to a level III care center, or arrangements may be made for a neonatal transport team to attend the delivery or to arrive shortly thereafter. Unexpected pregnancy outcomes, however, can be stressful events for the staff in the referral hospital nursery. The nursery nurses are called upon to meet the challenge of providing one-to-one nursing care for the intense stabilization period for a compromised neonate while maintaining care for the remaining patients in the nursery. This staffing pattern is usually not planned for in routine staffing numbers, and colleagues must pick up additional nursing assignments as well as help in providing care for a compromised neonate. There may also be requests from the regional center's physician, by phone or in person, for a nurse to perform procedures that are infrequently experienced but related to the care of the critically ill neonate, which add stress to an already stressful situation.

The neonate who initially does not meet transport criteria at birth but becomes progressively ill causes another stressful situation for the referral hospital because the amount of time for which the nurses at the referral hospital are responsible for the neonate is not predictable. The attending physician may not be present or available for continual care demands. The nursing staff must carefully monitor the status of the compromised neonate and report changes as necessary. In an emergency, nursery nurses may have to call in physicians not specializing in neonatology to intubate a baby or aspirate a tension pneumothorax.

The referral staff should look upon these experiences as opportunities for growth and development in the area of intense neonatal care. From these experiences, protocols may be developed to guide staff through the next similar scenario. Different circumstances may prove to be opportunities to request outreach education from the regional center with regard to a certain problem or diagnosis that would help prepare staff for the care of the next critically ill neonate delivered in the referral hospital.

The referral hospital staff acts as a liaison to communicate with both the transport team and the family. It is ideal to assign one individual to work with and support the family during this dynamic time (Frischer & Gutterman, 1992). Communication with the family, especially the mother, is especially important. The referral hospital staff and the transport team should collaborate closely regarding care and progress of the neonate before and after the time of admission to the regional center.

If it is feasible, the mother of the transported baby should be moved to a floor without newborns to help alleviate the emptiness that the mother without her baby feels when she hears other babies crying or sees another mother with a baby. The referral staff also need to assist the mother in the beginning of her grief work over the loss of the perfect child by letting her know that her feelings of sadness and depression are normal for the situation that she is going through. Nursing care for the mother should also focus on elevating self-esteem, helping her to fully understand the situation to the best of her ability, providing strategies for dealing with other family members and friends, and understanding the myriad of information and new technology that she has been and will be exposed to during her child's stay in the neonatal intensive care unit (NICU) (Olds et al., 1994).

Family

When transport of a neonate is required, the involved family members must not be left out of the plan of care, because they are the individuals who are going to be caring for the neonate after discharge from the regional center. In some cases the need for transport is planned, but in most cases it is unplanned and can be very stressful for the affected family.

Parents are often either in crisis or in a stage of grief over the loss of the perfect child at the time they are informed that their neonate needs to be transported. Consequently, they may not remember what was said to them during the time of explanation about prognosis and impending transport. To assist in developing a therapeutic communication style with the parents, the team can introduce themselves and begin the questioning portion of interaction with the parents by congratulating them and asking whether they have chosen a name for their infant. This communication style lets the parents know that the neonate is being considered as a special individual. The stress of the event can also prevent the parents from grasping the details of the medical diagnosis and plan of care for their neonate at the birth hospital and the regional center. Therefore, there is a need to emphasize the diagnoses and plan of care more than one time.

Having preprinted information to leave with the parents in a parent information packet can assist in the education of parents regarding diagnoses and the policies and procedures of the regional center. The packet can also include simple maps, telephone numbers, lists of medical and nursing terminology, information on breastfeeding, and booklets on the care of the neonate. Regional centers may also have videotapes available for the parents to view the type of environment that their child is going into and that they will be visiting. The informational need of the parents at the time of transport are tremendous. If the infant is to be transported by air, needs may center on the patient's condition, why the patient has to be flown, where the patient is going to be admitted, and whether they can see the patient before the flight (Fultz et al., 1993). Other informational needs include mode of travel, length of time of transport, care during transport, who can accompany the transport, regional center visiting and phoning policies, names of individuals caring for the patient, type of care to be rendered, costs involved, insurance coverage, directions to reach the center, and accommodations for parents (Davis & Hawkins, 1985).

All the responses of parents are unique. Transport is a significant event in the lives of each. Nurses must be nonjudgmental when a parent reacts dramatically to what is seen as a minor problem. Parents do not have the experience level that health care professionals have in the care of the compromised neonate (Kenner & Gunderson, 1988).

It should be a routine practice of a transport team to stop by the mother's room so that the parents can see and touch the neonate. This may be the first time that the neonate is seen and perhaps the last time the neonate is seen alive by the parents and family. When compromised neonates are born, they are quickly whisked away from the parents at the delivery room table for the initiation of resuscitative efforts. The parents remember their child's quick removal from them and their inability to begin the attachment process. Seeing the neonate, whom they could only imagine until birth, assists the parents with closure of the pregnancy. Leaving an instant-developing photograph of the neonate with the parents is an added courtesy; it can become a keepsake

Children's Hospital Medical Center

NEONATAL TRANSPORT FLOWSHEET

__________ Date
__________ Referring Hospital
__________ Age
__________ Gestational Age
__________ Weight
__________ Apgars
__________ Referring Physician

Consent . . . . Y N
Placenta . . . . Y N
Chart / X-Rays . . . . Y N
Mothers / Cord Blood . . Y N

	Temps		Assessment									Vent Settings						TCM		Blood Gases				SX	Other		CIRC ✓		Comments
Time	Set Pt. / A/R	Isol / Skin	HR	RR	GFR	BP	MAP		Color	Cap Refill	Activ	Mode	FiO_2	Pip / Peep	Rate	Insp Time / Flow	Temp	O_2 Sat	TC PO_2 / TC CO_2	Site	PH / CO_2	O_2 / HCO_3	BE / O_2 Sat	ET / NP	Alarms On / IV Site	Chem Strip	Site / Color	Temp / Cap Refil	

KEY:
PINK . . . . . . P
PALE . . . . . . W
MOTTLED . . . . . . M
DUSKY . . . . . . D
ACROCYANOTIC . . A
JAUNDICED . . . J
CYANOTIC C
RUDDY . . . . . R

RESP EFFORT:

	0	1	2
GRUNTING	NONE	AUDIBLE & STETH.	AUDIBLE
FLARING	NONE	MINIMAL	MARKED
RETRACTING	NONE	MINIMAL	MARKED

ACTIVITY:
ACTIVE . . . . A
ACTIVE c̄ CARE . . . . . . AS
LETHARGIC L
PARALYZED . . . . P
(+) DRUG INDUCED . . P+
IRRITABLE I
TWITCHY . . . . T

SEIZURES . . . . S
FLACCID . . . . . F
SEDATED . . . . M

MODE:
NASOTRACHEAL . . . . . NT
ORO TRACHEAL . . . . . OT
HEAD HOOD . . . . HH
NASOPHARYNGEAL . . . NP
BLOW BY . . . . BB
HAND BAG . . . . HB

CIRC ✓:

	1	2	3	4
COLOR	PINK	PALE	DUSKY	RED
TEMP	WARM	COOL	COLD	HOT
CAP FILL	<3 SEC	>3 SEC	ABSENT	
SITE	UAC	UVC	RADIAL LINE	

FIGURE 13–7 *See legend on opposite page*

MOST RECENT LAB VALUES TIME	Na / K	Ca / Bili	Cl / CO_2	WBC / RBC	HCT / Hgb	Poly / Band	Lymph / Seg	Plt / Gluc		PH / CO_2	O_2 / HCO_3	BE

CULTURES	YES	NO	COMMENTS
URINE			
BLOOD			
CSF			
NP			
SPUTUM			
WOUND			
OTHER			

MEDICATIONS

TIME	DRUG	DOSE & SITE

INTAKE		IV FLUIDS		BLOOD PRODUCTS				
SOLUTION		SOLUTION		SOLUTION		SOLUTION		TOTAL
Rate / Site	Total	Rate / Site	Total	Rate / Site	Total	Rate / Site	Total	

OUTPUT				
UA	NG / Emesis	Stool / Wound	CT #1 / CT #2	Total

FLOW CHARTING

PROCEDURE CHECKLIST

	Time	Site/ Size	Init.
INTUBATION			
IV, UAC, UVC, ART			
NG INSERTION			
CT PLACEMENT			
X-RAY			
DRESSING			
OTHER			

Signatures	Title/Initials
1)	
2)	
3)	
4)	

FIGURE 13–7. Neonatal transport flowsheet. (From Transport Department, Children's Hospital Medical Center, Cincinnati, OH. Reprinted with permission.)

Children's Hospital Medical Center

PROCEDURE RUNS/REVERSE TRANSPORT FLOWSHEET

DATE:

NAME: AGE: WEIGHT:

TRANSPORT FROM: TO: METHOD:

MEDICAL DIAGNOSIS/HISTORY:

ALLERGIES:

RECENT EXPOSURES:

ISOLATION PRECAUTIONS:

I.D. BAND LOCATION:

NURSING NOTES/ASSESSMENT:

Time	Vital Signs										Respiratory Adjuncts					ALARM ON	Suction		IV Site	Comments:
	Tap / Rte	P	R	BP	MAP	tcPO₂ / CO₂	O_2 Sat	Color	Act.	Cap Refill	Mode	FiO_2	Rate / CPAP	PIP / Pump	Flow / IT		ET	NP / OP	✓	

MSCL. (Meds, IVF (rate & total), TX, P.O. Intake, etc.)

KEY:

ROUTE:
O - Oral
A - Axillary
R - Rectal
S - Skin

COLOR:
P - Pink
D - Dusky
L - Pale
J - Jaundiced
R - Ruddy
M - Mottled

Active........A
Active c̄ Care........AS
Lethargic........L
Paralyzed........P
(+) Drug Induced........P+
Sedated........M

Irritable........I
Twitchy........T
Seizures........S
Flaccid........F

MODE:
NC - Nasal Cannula
HH - Head Hood
TC - Trach Collar
OT - Orotracheal
T - Trach
FM - Face Mask
BB - Blowby
NP - Nasopharyngeal
NT - Nasotracheal

Report Called By: Time: Given To:

Personnel: Nurse: Respiratory Therapist: Physician:

Received By: Unit: Personnel: Time:

FIGURE 13–8. Procedure runs/reverse transport flowsheet. (From Transport Department, Children's Hospital Medical Center, Cincinnati, OH. Reprinted with permission.)

for the parents until they can actually see their infant at the regional center.

If the neonate has any abnormalities, they should be pointed out to the parents, because the defects are usually not as severe as the parents had imagined them to be during pregnancy or at the time of delivery. Positive features can also be pointed out at this time to encourage the parents to look at the whole infant, as opposed to only his or her defects.

The parents' responses to the event depend on what other events are going on in their lives and the effectiveness of their coping strategies. Parents need to be encouraged to call and visit, with their other children if possible, as often as they can. They also need to be involved in care as is feasible, and breastfeeding can be encouraged if a mother has expressed an interest in doing so and the infant is stable enough to be fed. Mothers can be given information on the pumping and storage of breast milk. This information gives the mother something to do for her neonate during this time, when she may feel the loss of her maternal caretaking role. The parents should be encouraged to seek as much support for themselves as they need and be informed of the support services at the regional center. Parents and family should be advised of the stress associated with these events and encouraged to ask questions and to ask for help as needed. No family should be expected to handle this crisis situation on their own. Working with families is in some cases the most difficult part of the transport. Concerns over the patient and the limited resources of battery, oxygen, and air prevail as the team works to support and inform the family of the current status and plans for care (Frischer & Gutterman, 1992).

POSTTRANSPORT INFORMATION EXCHANGE

After the transport is completed and care is transferred to the receiving team of health care workers, it is good practice and professional courtesy to phone the birth hospital. This call is helpful to the referral hospital staff, because they are working with the mother and family that are left behind after the transport. These mothers and families are often in crisis or in a stage of grief or shock at the time of transport and are eager for information. The referral hospital staff, pediatrician, and obstetrician need as much information as possible to assist in facilitating communication between the referral and the receiving hospitals.

Staff at the birth hospital should call, as well as encourage parents to call, the regional center as much as can be accepted by the regional center nursery. As information concerning condition and treatment is relayed to the birth hospital and the parents, the birth hospital staff can help the parents gain greater understanding of the care and condition of the neonate as well as potentially establish community resources for the family.

Weekly contact should be maintained with the birth hospital by phone or letter or both in order to keep everyone informed of progress or deterioration. A primary nursing follow-up letter can be done by the transporting nurse. An initial follow-up letter is ideally given within 24 hours, followed by reports weekly and monthly and upon discharge. These reports prove to be especially helpful when a neonate is reverse transported after recovery from the acute stage of illness.

Multidisciplinary mortality and morbidity conferences can be scheduled on a regular basis between referral hospitals and the regional center to facilitate information exchange and learning. Outreach education can also be a means of development and growth in optimizing the care for the compromised neonate.

ALTERNATIVE TYPES OF TRANSPORT

The main focus of this chapter is the incoming neonatal transport. The emphasis placed on this particular type of transport is appropriate because stabilizing and transporting intensely ill neonates will most likely remain the first priority of transport teams across the country. However, as a result of the dramatically changing health care environment of the 1990s, the skills and expertise of the transport team members may be called upon for transporting patients both within and outside the hospital for procedures.

International Transports

International transports provide one of the biggest challenges for a transport coordinator and team. Planning must begin as soon as possible in order to ensure that all the logistic details are meticulously worked out, such as finances arranged; airline or aircraft arranged; visas or passports updated; an accepting physician and hospital located; transfer notes, radiographs, and progress notes copied to be sent with the patient; ground transport arrangements determined for use upon arrival of the team at the destination; and equipment to be used by the team cleared through the airline or aircraft. Commercial airlines need to know the exact voltage and amperage of all carry-on equipment. There may be a limitation on when the equipment may be used. If special medications or special formula is required for the patient, documentation is needed to clear customs, depending on the country of origin. Some commercial airlines require a written physician's statement regarding the documentation of patient stability for the transport. If oxygen will be in use or on standby, a prescription is required, and the order must be placed as far in advance as possible. The airlines cannot provide heat or humidification for needed oxygen.

Supplies must be packed and arranged to be as accessible as possible. If a team is staying at the location of the referral hospital or another patient transfer site, lodging must be arranged. Currency must be exchanged. Special customs that are culture specific should be followed. Transports across time zones necessitate special attention to times and dates involved. The pay rate and reimbursement policy for expenses for extended transports must be prearranged with participating team members. Communications must be arranged for the transport process. The need for translators must also be considered. In addition to these guidelines for international transport, it is beneficial to ask questions concerning each specific situation.

A care conference should be arranged as soon as the transport is approved. At this time, the patient and family can meet the team with the primary nurse or care manager. Plans, idiosyncrasies in care, and specific likes and dislikes can be discussed. Diversional or developmental activities can be planned.

One cannot plan too much when considering the health and well-being of the team, patient, and parents as they travel, at times, halfway around the world. Planning is the key to success.

Reverse Transports

A reverse transport (back transport, back transfer) is the return of a previously ill neonate from a tertiary NICU to another level I, II, or III nursery for intermediate or convalescing care or both. Many institutions have found that the reverse transport process is therapeutic, cost effective (Phibbs & Mortenson, 1992), and safe. In addition, reverse transport provides improved efficiency of tertiary bed utilization, facilitates parent–infant interaction, and improves relations with referral hospitals. Consequently, many institutions have found that reverse transports make up approximately 20 to 30 percent of the total number of transports being performed per year. Therefore, reverse transport has become an essential part of the regionalization process and will continue to be a vital part of the care offered by tertiary care centers across the country.

Like the incoming transport process, reverse transport must be performed consistently according to a well-designed plan. Without a consistent practical approach, reverse transporting can become an unsafe, chaotic process. However, with the assistance of a protocol, a reverse transport can effectively meet the expectations and needs of all parties involved. A thorough protocol should address five key populations: the health care professionals at the tertiary care center, the health care professionals at the referral hospital, the transport team, the patient, and the family. To work together, many teams find that they are participating in an increasing number of alternative types of transports. As previously discussed, many hospitals have increased the number of reverse transports being performed.

To work together effectively, all parties need to follow a unified approach. The protocol at the end of this chapter is just one proposed method for ensuring a successful transition from the tertiary care unit to the referral nursery. It is divided into three categories: psychosocial and parent concerns, interprofessional concerns, and transport procedure. Kuhly and Freston (1993) described the 3-day transitional period during which the parents realize the extent of the crisis associated with back transport. Anticipatory guidance helps parents and includes sharing of specific transport information, discussing changes that the parents will experience, and empowering parents in making decisions for their infant. By consistently performing reverse transports according to a well-designed protocol, hospitals, families, and health care professionals can continue to benefit from the reverse transport process.

Intrahospital and Interhospital Test Runs and Interhospital Transfers

It is not uncommon for hospital personnel to request the expertise of transport team members when an intensely ill patient needs to be moved either within or outside the institution for a specific test procedure. In most institutions, the transport team is considered a valuable resource for all staff members who need to stabilize, monitor, and move patients from one site to another. Transport team members tend to be more familiar with the hospital policies and procedures that affect the transport process, as well as the equipment, supplies, and personnel needed to ensure a safe transport. Most important, transport team members are valued for their creative, critical decision-making and problem-solving abilities. Hence, it is sensible to use the skills and expertise of the team members for transporting patients both within and outside the hospital for procedures.

Postmortem Transports

A postmortem transport occurs when a mother remains hospitalized at the birth hospital and is unable to come to hold her dead or dying infant at the tertiary center. Transport of the infant to the mother is requested, not for medical reasons, but to provide an important first step in the grieving process. Most parents desire the opportunity to see their dying infant before the life support is removed or further treatment now considered futile is denied. Extent of further life support is decided, consent is obtained, and the parents are reminded that the infant could possibly die en route.

Several aspects of postmortem transports require special consideration. Changing the mindset from acute life-saving measures to the baby's comfort and the family's grief influences most aspects of the transport. The team composition often changes. Team members who originally transported or who have the best skills in care of the dying may be especially requested to participate. The unit physician or nurse who cared for the infant often accompanies the team to answer parents' questions about the uniqueness or response of their baby. "What went wrong? Will it happen again? Did you try everything? Was it something I did"? are questions that parents ask. Clergy may also accompany and help to answer questions such as "Why me? Why did God do this?" They are also a resource for funeral arrangements. Often, the parents appreciate a close family member or friend who can ride along so that someone they know is with the baby should the baby die en route.

The deposition of the body and the paperwork associated with a death cause other considerations. Sometimes, the infant's body is left at the birth hospital, and the hospital handles postmortem needs. This process can best be accomplished if no autopsy is planned, if the family physician is able to come to pronounce death and complete paperwork, and if the birth hospital is familiar with handling this situation. More often, the transport team returns the infant's body to the tertiary center, where paperwork, postmortem care, and an autopsy are performed. The team should allow as much time as the parents need, including completely private time with their infant. The postmortem unit personnel should be aware and arrange care to support this. If a physician does not accompany the team, the nurse should note time and document assessment, especially the absence of vital signs. On return, the physician can confirm and pronounce death.

Financial reimbursement for such a transport may also become an issue. Some insurance companies do pay, considering it part of the care of the infant. Many that do not can be persuaded to pay, in view of the circumstances. When insurance companies refuse to pay, hospitals can choose to provide this compassionate service at no cost. Because postmortem transports are not a frequent occurrence, investigating what works in a particular system and establishing a protocol are prudent. The transport team is often regarded as a resource for the many considerations it takes to make this transport effective for all.

THE BUSINESS OF TRANSPORT

The business of transport provides the support structure for a viable quality team. Administrative support, reimbursement, leadership, staffing, quality improvement, and program evaluation are key areas that, when functioning smoothly, allow the skilled team member to provide optimal care.

Administrative Support for a Transport Team

Transport is an expensive service that involves personnel, equipment, and vehicles. Hospitals are increasingly evaluating the cost versus benefit of transport services. Administration generally focuses on costs that are quantitative and more easily measured. Benefits of a transport service are qualitative and relate to patient outcomes. There are, however, few objective quantitative studies on the effect of transport on patient outcome or length of stay (Brimhall, 1995a).

Transport teams are low revenue producers, especially in comparison with the expense of 24-hour staffing, advanced training, and equipment purchases. However, the cost of staffing the team may be looked upon as the cost of doing business, inasmuch as the transport team services the hospital and community in the transport of patients that can potentially stay in the hospital for months.

Administrators do understand the importance of a first-rate team for their image in the community. They also respond to the competitive need to maintain market position and the customer needs and requests for service. Level III nurseries not located in a delivery hospital often depend almost entirely on transport services to bring their patients to their institutions.

Reimbursement

Reimbursement for transport services varies tremendously. Contracts and alliances affect both patient costs and transport fees. General guidelines are also changing as the United States moves increasingly toward managed health care and capitation.

Precertification is increasingly requested. Some teams offer to help families with this necessity. Letters of medical necessity may be needed, as may a cost analysis justifying transfer of a patient to another institution. These issues can be prepared for on planned transports, especially for reverse transports or transports for planned surgeries, if advance notice occurs during the insurance companies' business hours. Most often however, precertification is not possible when stabilization and transfer of a critically ill neonate is needed. In those cases, it is helpful to understand a region's general guidelines.

Land ambulance is the most inexpensive and generally the first choice. If land ambulance is contraindicated by environmental factors, extreme distances, or the patient's medical condition, air ambulance can be considered. Team members should be aware of travel time and costs of ground, fixed wing, and helicopter services in their area so that the mode most appropriate to patient need is utilized. Those reviewing documentation should be able to ascertain necessity for transfer and choice of the receiving hospital. Choice of the receiving hospital is influenced by proximity, by services offered, and possibly by the insurance alliance of "preferred" hospitals.

Private insurance companies generally provide the best reimbursement. Coverage varies widely according to the plan. Requests for increased reimbursement that are based on special need can often be made, usually by a physician describing the medical necessity. Medical reimbursement is much lower and varies from state to state, with a preference for land ambulance.

The billing system for the patient also varies. The hospital's patient accounts department, the ambulance company, and the transport team itself may also be involved. This process should be reviewed to meet both customer and provider needs. The team members' role is often to gather financial information from the referral hospital so that charges can be billed.

Staffing/Pay Issues

Providing 24-hour and multiple coverage for simultaneous transport is a challenge for every team. Is the team unit based and pulled from unit staffing or dedicated to transport services? How many teams are in house or on call? Is the transport team large enough to provide flexibility in staffing but small enough to maintain each member's transport expertise?

In making decisions about team availability, the following should be considered: Volume and timing of transports, average length of transports, response time, needs for non–transport time, and maintenance of transport skills.

Both the Commission on Accreditation of Air Medical Services (CAAMS) and the National Flight Nurses Association (NFNA) address the need for adequate rest of team members to help ensure optimal performance. Individual work schedules are planned to minimize work-related fatigue. Team members should also receive adequate food and fluid even during the busiest times. Fatigue and stress cannot always be self-determined, and scheduling to provide physical and mental rest can be perhaps the most significant contribution to team performance. Pay can be hourly or salary. Team members are often called upon to respond to patient needs on their off-time or by taking many on-call hours. Pay or compensation should match their efforts. However, additional pay for hazardous duty or extended practice is becoming less common.

Leadership

Transport team members are often considered mavericks that are confident, skilled, and stimulated by challenges. How does one lead such a group of individuals? Most programs have a manager whose specific responsibility is for transport.

Teams are, however, often well suited for the self-directed work team approach. The work of the team is initiated, developed and accomplished by team members. The program manager can then take the role of a coach, providing stability and guidance as a contact person as well as tracking the coordination of efforts.

Performance Improvement/Program Evaluation

The intent of any transport quality improvement program is to monitor and improve patient care in a cost-effective manner. Availability, accessibility, responsiveness, and effectiveness of the team are key issues (AAP & ACOG, 1992). Because care is often provided for just a few hours, short-term outcome and patient response should be the focus of clinical indicators (Steenson & Erdman, 1989). Indicators should be established for high-volume, high-risk, and problem-prone transports.

The quality and effectiveness of patient care are tied closely to the quality and effectiveness of the transport team processes. Indicators tracking safety, competency, response times, unusual events, and communication help to highlight areas for improvement. Figure 13–9 provides a summary of quality indicators on neonatal transport. Staffing patterns may be changed to accommodate high-volume times for transports. New equipment may be purchased or training recommended.

Also important to quality is the customer's definition of quality. Major customers include the patient, the family, and referral personnel. Questionnaires directed to parents and referral hospitals provide valuable feedback regarding team presentation, explanations, and interactions. Focus groups meeting with referral hospital personnel can give the team feedback on consumer service and learning needs that have become apparent. Customer input should be reflected in the team's plan to improve services.

A data collection system to track indicators should be built into the team documentation or into a team process that is easy for team members to complete. Problems occurring on a transport run should be documented immediately after transport, as should response times. Computers can be a valuable aid to recording and reporting data. Having all team members trained to master a user-friendly program increases involvement and accountability for quality of patient care.

LEGAL ISSUES

Many questions of legal responsibility and liability are raised by the unique circumstances of critical care transport. The dynamic acuity level of the patient, the dual responsibility of the transport team and the referral hospital, and the provision of care in unusual settings often with limited resources confuse the issues of duty and proximate cause (Brimhall, 1987).

Historically, statutes and regulations have addressed first-response teams and ambulance services. Regulations have not been issued for the critical care transport teams, whose composition and function differ significantly from those of the first-response teams. Most critical care transport teams are hospital based, have mixed composition and skill sets, have a higher level of physician supervision, and transport more critically ill patients.

A few main principles underlie the framework for legal protection of a neonatal transport team (Brimhall, 1995b). First, the team member is a member of an institution, often the tertiary

Quality Indicators on Neonatal Transport

INDICATOR	APPLICATION
Intervention	Airway security
	ETT size and placement
	ETT placement confirmation
	Medication appropriateness and documentation
	IV access obtained and patent
	Vital sign assessment and documentation
	Neutral thermal environment
	Vital assessment upon arrival
Data collection and documentation	Compliance with policy and procedure
Timeliness of care	Response time
	Patient preparation time
Safety	Patient secured per procedure
Education	Training standards are met
Staffing	Staffing is comprehensively met
Professional competence	Prerequisite license and certification
	Continuing education met and documented
	Team effectiveness
Utilization review	Team composition per protocol
	Carrier selection per protocol
	Equipment use per protocol
	Procedure use per protocol
	Severity of illness versus appropriateness of orders
Unusual events reviewed	CPR during transport
	Mortality during transport
Customer's needs	Referring hospital staff competence
	Dispatch calls per protocol
	Follow-up calls per protocol
Program sucess/marketing	Referral demographics
	Revenue and billing projections

FIGURE 13–9. Quality indicators for neonatal transport. (From Dunn, N. [1995]. Quality management strategies in interfacility transport. In *Current concepts in transport: Neonatal obstetric, pediatric, and administrative, Administration Subsection* [7th ed.]. Columbus, OH: Ross Laboratories. Reprinted with permission.)

medical center. The medical director defines, authorizes, and insures team members in performance of all duties. Second, the transport team functions under the direction of an appropriate physician who approves protocols and is involved in quality improvement activities. Finally, it is important to realize that each individual assumes professional accountability for his or her actions. Accurate assessment and critical care thinking are expected of the professional nurse. Each state has a nurse practice act that should be reviewed and may limit the scope of care (Brimhall, 1987).

Critical care transport teams are protected in two ways. First and foremost, the team must provide appropriate and quality care. Training, experience, and updated protocols are imperative. Developing quality and safety indicators helps track the effectiveness of training and of the team processes. In times of financial constraints, decreasing time for training and quality improvement activities risks increased liability and undesired patient outcomes.

Second, team members functioning as agents of the institution must conform to defined protocols to operate within the chain of command (Brimhall, 1987). Medical supervision must be available and used appropriately. Team members who do not perform within the scope of their employment or follow team protocols are legally liable for their actions. Standardized resuscitation guidelines are currently available in the *Neonatal Nursing Transport Standards and Guidelines* (NANN, 1994), which also defines appropriate care that should be evident in each individual team's protocols. It is the adherence to these protocols and standards that constitute the second area of legal protection for team members. Often the question regarding provision of care across state lines is raised. The most important license is professional licensure in the state of employment (Brimhall, 1995b).

The dual responsibility of the transport team and referral hospitals also influences legal liability. The Consolidated Omnibus Reconciliation Act (COBRA) regulations generally affect referring hospitals more than transport teams. The Act requires that the hospital evaluate all patients presenting to the hospital with emergency conditions, determine appropriate care, stabilize, and obtain informed consent to transfer (Youngberg, 1992).

The transport process usually begins with the referral call requesting transfer services to deliver the neonate to the regional center. At this point the responsibility of the regional center begins for the neonate and increases to a more equal responsibility as both the team and the referral staff provide care just before the team's departure from the referral hospital. Team responsibility peaks once they are en route with the neonate and continues until transfer of care to the staff of the receiving institution is completed (Brimhall, 1995b).

Informed consent is a basic requirement for treatment, and treatment without consent constitutes battery. A signed and witnessed consent form generally includes agreement to treatments and admission to the hospital, excluding surgery, and should specify the mode of transport and name of the receiving institution. A common situation that raises questions of consent is that of a legal minor teenage mother's providing consent. States vary in laws on the treatment of minors. Emancipated minors, able to sign a consent form, are those who are self-reliant, living apart from their parents, and are financially self-supporting. Mature minors are deemed competent if they are of sufficient intellect and maturity to appreciate the benefits and risks of and alternatives to the proposed medical care (AAP, 1993). Cautious teams have both teenage mothers and one of their parents sign the consent form for transport. They also avoid signatures of fathers when the mothers are unwed or before responsibility is accepted on a signed birth certificate. Another situation is the unavailability of an ill or sedated mother who is unable to sign the consent form. In emergency situations, both public policy and law support the assumption of implied consent for medical care. The responsible physician must document that an emergency situation exists, that treatment is for the patient's benefit, and that there is an inability to obtain express consent.

Choosing not to transport an infant because of presumed nonviability or futility of transfer and treatment raises both legal and ethical questions. In most cases, the duty is to transport until these issues can be discussed by all involved parties and the patient's condition becomes more clearly defined. If the patient is not transported, documentation of condition, parental wishes, and all considerations leading to this decision is essential.

Nearly every nurse has heard, "In God we trust, all others must document." Documentation, always critical legally, takes on an added importance for nurses functioning in more autonomous, expanded roles in a variety of settings. Because cases of legal negligence often take years to reach the trial phase, team members should be attentive to complete and accurate documentation that is usually the only way to review and corroborate testimony related to the care provided. Documentation could well be the sole factor that establishes or disproves negligence. Development of documentation forms that promote critical documentation areas is important. Nurses are often aware of the need for documenting actual care given. Transport members must also include documentation of referral call advice, times of arrival and departure, and any delays in arriving at the referral institution. Identification of the patient, summarizing the patient's condition initially, and transfer of care to the receiving institution are also noteworthy elements.

A focus on quality, training, and documentation of both care and process reduces legal risk. When high-quality care is provided and patients have positive outcomes, the liabilities associated with transport are negligible (Youngberg, 1992).

FUTURE TRENDS

The future of neonatal transport is most likely to be influenced by cost–benefit analysis as it relates to patient outcomes rather than by technologic advances as it has been in the past. Current health reform is changing the paradigms of who provides care, where care is provided, and which care is considered appropriate.

Basic service parameters are undergoing very little change (Chester, 1995). Stabilization protocols are even more standardized as guidelines are published or information is rapidly shared on computer information highways.

The transported neonatal population is changing as the maternal transports increase. Fewer preterm infants are transported because more mothers make it to delivering hospitals that can also care for ventilated and ill preterm infants. Surfactant replacement therapy at referral hospitals has also influenced the need for transport to tertiary centers. In addition, capitation may influence where care can be provided with tertiary care for acute phases of illness and with intermediate nurseries for convalescent care. Maternal transports may not continue to increase if managed care contracts change the regionalizaton process. Mothers may be kept at outlying hospitals and the infants transported only when there is a postdelivery problem. Only time will tell.

Technologic advances continue to produce increasingly sophisticated equipment, to monitor the most delicate of vital signs even though the equipment is very lightweight and transportable. The future of most sophisticated treatments, including on-the-road extracorporeal membrane oxygenation, nitric oxide, and liquid ventilation will depend on improving patient outcomes, including cost–benefit concerns.

More likely is increased use of complex information systems for documentation, dispatch, stabilization advice, data input, tracking of the transport process, patient outcomes, and communication between institutions. A national data base is already being developed. Researchers and clinicians request information currently on the Internet. Faxing patient information, which currently is increasingly more common, may be replaced by relaying information from one computer to another by modem.

Team composition is also changing. Although there is a trend toward more designated teams whose members are strictly dedicated to transport, the number of members can be expected to be downsized. With cross-training, the job description may resemble less that of a registered nurse, respiratory therapist, or paramedic and more likely to resemble a blended role with many common skill sets. Teams are increasingly physician referred rather than physician based. Research is supporting comparable patient outcomes in nonphysician transport of intubated pediatric patients (Beyer et al., 1992). Tertiary care physicians will be less available as the emphasis on prevention and wellness increases. Use of certified nurse practitioners versus an expanded-role registered nurse varies, depending on state practice acts and regional preferences and resources.

The high cost of air transport in comparison with ground transport is already causing a shift to increased usage of ground transport and prompting a more critical look at when air transport is truly appropriate and for which conditions. Ground transport services are also experiencing the effect of mergers as private companies vie for contracts and as some hospitals decide whether it is or is not cost effective to have their own ambulance service.

To date, response time of 20 to 30 minutes to mobilize a team remains unchanged. Some teams may be expected to find a way to break this paradigm also.

Budget reductions are likely to affect all areas of neonatal care. Patient care hours are most likely to be supported, and training and daily operations will most likely be trimmed. However, teams around the country continue to place strong emphasis on education and training of team members. There is concern that administrators may not understand the unique challenges of transport and the critical importance of trained, skilled personnel in settings with limited resources. Teams will continue to be challenged in evaluating the effectiveness of their methods of training as well as all team processes to prove their value in the age of health care reform (Chester, 1995).

CONCLUSION

This chapter has provided an overview of, but by no means an exhaustive look at, the transport team and the transport process. Whenever a critically ill neonate is taken into a constantly moving and dynamic environment, the situation provides a great challenge to the caregiver. The challenge is to complete each transport, making it better than the one before. The ultimate goal is a collaborative team approach to optimize patient and family outcomes in a cost-effective and compassionate manner.

PROTOCOL FOR THE REVERSE TRANSPORT OF A STABLE NEONATE

PSYCHOSOCIAL/PARENT CONCERNS

Intervention

1. Mention the possibility of reverse transport when initially transferring the neonate (particularly for families coming from distant hospitals and for mothers who will have extensive hospitalizations).

Rationale

1. With early exposure to the concept of reverse transporting, parents are assured that the process is a routinely performed health care option. Having realistic expectations and goals helps decrease stress and foster acceptance.
2. Transport the patient back as soon as possible to ensure a convalescence of at least 2 weeks at the referral hospital.
3. Bose and associates (1985) found that this is the optimal length of stay to ensure cost effectiveness. The earlier the infant can be moved closer to home, the sooner parent–infant interaction can benefit.
4. All health professionals should convey confidence and support for the process of reverse transporting when addressing the parents. Assure the parents that they may call the nursing and medical staff for advice or information at any time and that the health care professionals at the referral center are capable of caring for their baby.
5. There must be a transfer of confidence and trust to the referral hospital staff.
6. If possible, some parents should, if they wish, meet the referral hospital staff and tour the nursery before the infant's reverse transport.
7. Familiarizing parents with their new surroundings makes it easier for them to cope with the transition by reducing their fear of the unknown.
8. Explain to the parents that there are often many correct ways to perform the same procedure.
9. Telling parents to anticipate variations in care makes them less anxious when they witness a familiar procedure being performed in a different way.
10. Assess the parents' current level of knowledge regarding the reverse transport process. Anticipate the knowledge needed, and plan accordingly. The parents may be experiencing anticipatory grief.
11. The family's informational needs must be met in order to decrease anxiety by eliminating fear of the unknown. Anticipatory grief is the fear that the infant will eventually die.
12. Tell the parents exactly what time to expect their infant to arrive at the referral hospital. It is also helpful to give them the name of the admitting nurse if possible.
13. Parents often feel less anxious if they know when their infant is arriving, so that they can be present.
14. Include the parents as central figures in the team caring for their infant from the time of admission until transfer. Let them know that their input and views are highly valued.
15. When parents feel that their opinions count, they feel more in control, cope better, and experience less anxiety.
16. First and foremost, always be an advocate for the infant and family.
17. The responsibility of all health professionals should always be to consider the patient and family first.
18. All health care professionals should continually assess and document the parents' verbal and nonverbal reactions before, during, and after the reverse transport process.
19. If health professionals remain sensitive to parental responses, plans can be made to better meet their needs.
20. Reassure parents that their feelings of anxiety are normal. Acknowledge their fears and concerns.
21. Parents will have less stress and cope better if they know that what they are experiencing is normal.
22. Assess the social supports available to the family and encourage their use. Tell parents what is available within the community (such as social support groups, La Leche League, equipment supply pharmacies, etc.).
23. Psychosocial support is essential during periods of high stress.
24. Provide the parents and the referral hospital with a form for a written evaluation of the reverse transport process. This evaluation should be open-ended so that individualized, honest responses may be elicited.
25. Feedback enables the tertiary care center and the transport department to refine the reverse transport process. Open-ended responses provide more concrete information about specific concerns.

INTERPROFESSIONAL CONCERNS

Intervention

1. The patient's primary nurse, neonatal nurse practitioner, and attending physician should maintain an ongoing discussion about whether the patient can become a candidate for a reverse transport and about a potential estimated time for reversal. This information should be promptly shared with parents, and their response should be addressed.

Rationale

1. These collaborative discussions help ensure that all parties have similar goals and expectations. Those involved will be well informed of future plans.
2. The transport team and attending neonatal physician at the tertiary center can use the region's outreach education coordinator as a resource person when determining whether a particular outlying hospital has the resources to care for a certain infant.
3. This step is important to the process of deciding whether an infant is stable enough for transport.
4. Ultimately, it will be the collaborative decision of the receiving hospital, the attending and private physicians, the primary nurse at the tertiary center, and the charge nurse at the referral hospital to determine whether and when a patient is eligible to undergo reverse transport.
5. When the ultimate responsibility for decision-making is designated, confusion can be eliminated.
6. Have a transport team representative participate in routine NICU discharge rounds.
7. Attending rounds heightens awareness of impending reverse transports.
8. All health professionals should keep all lines of communication open and encourage verbalization.
9. Good communication skills help establish and maintain therapeutic relationships.

PROTOCOL FOR THE REVERSE TRANSPORT OF A STABLE NEONATE *(Continued)*

TRANSPORT PROCEDURE

Intervention

1. Parental consent must be obtained. If phone consent is obtained, there must be a witness. When consent is obtained, the mode of transport must be indicated.

Rationale

1. Because parents should not be hearing about their infant's reverse transport for the first time when consent is being obtained, getting permission should be just a necessary formality.
2. At the earliest possible time, the transport team should be notified about the possibility of the reverse transport.
3. Preplanning often ensures a safer, smoother, more effective transport process.
4. Check and document that the NICU physician has requested permission from the private physician to reverse transport the infant. Establish that the infant's medical report has been verbally delivered.
5. Confirming that a medical report has been given ensures the infant of physician coverage upon arrival at the referral hospital. This procedure helps prevent confusion, especially when pediatricians practice in large groups.
6. Once consent from both the private physician and attending NICU physician has been obtained, the transport nurse calls the referral hospital nursing staff and requests permission to reverse transport the infant to the referral nursery. An estimated time of arrival should be given, as should a complete patient profile and history.
7. Transferring information from one health care team to another decreases stress and enables staff members to prepare for the transport.
8. A checklist should be created and placed in the chart of infants who might be reverse transported.
9. The list reminds staff of all the tasks that must be accomplished before the infant's discharge.
10. Determine the safest and most cost-effective mode of transportation for each infant. Make arrangements as early as possible in accordance with contractual agreements between institutions.
11. The reverse transport process must be a practical option.
12. On the basis of each patient's status and health care needs and any pre-existing hospital policies, determine the appropriate transport team composition (i.e., transport respiratory therapist, transport registered nurse, neonatal nurse practitioner, or physician).
13. Having different health care professionals represented provides the infant with a well-rounded, effective team.
14. Determine which equipment and supplies are needed to safely monitor, protect, and care for the infant en route.
15. Being prepared for the unexpected is the key to safe transporting.
16. Reverse transporting a patient with a complex history and complicated plan of care requires a care conference. The referral hospital staff, parents, and any potential caregivers should be present.
17. This conference helps meet the informational needs of the referral hospital and the parents. In addition, the parents have an opportunity to offer their input, which decreases stress by giving them a sense of control. The parents are reassured that the referred hospital is informed and prepared for the transition.
18. The referral hospital should receive a copy of all the pertinent parts of the patient's chart. This includes nursing notes, progress notes, recent laboratory values, physician orders, drug administration record, nursing process tool, discharge teaching records, follow-up needs, and any other pertinent records. In addition, it may be appropriate to send a copy of the infant's latest chest x-ray film or other recent special procedure results.
19. Documentation of transfer is an important step in meeting the information needs of the referral hospital.
20. On the day of the reverse transport, the nursing and physician staff of the referral hospital should receive an updated review of the patient's status and an estimated time of arrival.
21. Stress is decreased by reassuring the referral hospital that they are adequately prepared for the infant's arrival.
22. All personal items as well as any special supplies (i.e., special formula, colostomy supplies) should be transported with the infant.
23. Transporting interim supplies decreases the likelihood that the infant's care will be interrupted.
24. Upon arrival at the referral hospital, the transport team should give a thorough history and report to the nurse who admits the infant. Any questions should be answered, and a phone number should be given to staff so that they can call for additional information, if necessary.
25. Stress is decreased when staff members know that they have a resource person whom they can contact.
26. Transport personnel share the responsibility of 24-hour patient status reports to the referral hospital, the obstetrician, and the pediatrician upon admission to the level III unit. Weekly updates are also mailed until the infant is 6 months old. After this time, only a discharge summary or expiration notice is required. Variations in this written communication schedule can be arranged.
27. The written communications ensure that the informational needs of all health care professionals involved are met.
28. Long-distance transports (especially flights) should be arranged at least 24 hours in advance, if possible.
29. Preplanned transports are safer, smoother, and more efficient. There is less anxiety when adequate time is allotted.
30. Infants considered infectious are not transferred until their status has changed.
31. The spread of infection must be prevented.
32. When possible (especially for flights), preapproved insurance reimbursements should be arranged.
33. Parental anxiety will be decreased when financial matters are taken care of ahead of time. Insurance companies are unlikely to refuse support when financing is prearranged.
34. When there is no insurance coverage or financial means to pay for the reverse transport, the tertiary care center must determine whether it is willing to absorb the cost of the transport.
35. There is still a potential savings to the institution if it absorbs the cost of the transport rather than keeping the infant in an NICU. Many families also have no further insurance coverage or have never had the financial means to pay for the initial hospitalization. In this instance, it is the prerogative of the hospital of origin to accept or reject the readmission of this infant.
36. Reverse transports should not be scheduled after 5 P.M. on weekdays and should be avoided on weekends and holidays.
37. Transferring patients at a time when staffing is not optimal increases stress.

From Croop, L., & Kenner, C. (1990). Protocol for reverse neonatal transports. *Neonatal Network*, 9(1), 49–53. Reprinted with permission.

REFERENCES

American Academy of Pediatrics. (1993). *Task Force on Interhospital Transport: Guidelines for air and ground transport of neonatal and pediatric patients*. Elk Grove, IL: Author.

American College of Obstetrics and Gynecology & American Academy of Pediatrics. (1988). *Guidelines for perinatal care* (2nd ed.) Elk Grove, IL: Author.

American Academy of Pediatrics & American College of Obstetrics and Gynecology. (1992). *Guidelines for perinatal care* (3rd ed., pp. 35–45). Elk Grove, IL: Author.

Beyer, A. J., Land, G., & Zaritsky, A. (1992). Nonphysician transport of intubated pediatric patients: A system evaluation. *Critical Care Medicine, 20*(7), 961–966.

Bloom, R. S., & Cropley, C., 1994. *Textbook of neonatal resuscitation.* Elk Grove Village, IL: American Academy of Pediatrics and American Heart Association.

Bose, C., Lapine, R., & Jung, A. (1985). Neonatal back-transport: Cost effectiveness. *Medical Care, 23*(1), 14–19.

Brimhall, D. (1987). Medicolegal aspects of neonatal transport. *Journal of Perinatal and Neonatal Nursing, 1*(2), 77–82.

Brimhall, D. (1995a). Developing administrative support for transport. In M. S. Trautman (Ed.), Proceedings from *Current concepts in transport: Neonatal, obstetric, pediatric and administrative, Administrative Subsection* (7th ed.). Columbus, OH: Ross Laboratories.

Brimhall, D. (1995b). Legal aspects of transport. In M. S. Trautman (Ed.). Proceedings from *Current concepts in transport: Neonatal, obstetric, pediatric and administrative, Administrative Subsection* (7th ed.). Columbus, OH: Ross Laboratories.

Chameides, L. (Ed.). (1990). *Textbook of neonatal resuscitation.* Dallas: American Heart Association.

Chester, G. (1995). Neonatal ground transports–1994. A four year evaluation of previous study. In M. S. Trautman (Ed.) *Current concepts in transport, Administrative Subsection* (7th ed., pp. 150–151). Columbus, OH: Ross Laboratories.

Chou, M. M., & MacDonald, M. G. (1989). Landmarks in the development of patient transport systems. In M. M. MacDonald & M. K. Miller (Eds.), *Emergency transport of the perinatal patient* (pp. 2–31). Boston: Little, Brown.

Connolly, H. V., Fletcho, S., & Hageman, J. R. (1992). Education of personnel involved in the transport program. *Critical Care Clinics, 8*(3),481–491.

Curtin, L. (1995). Blessed are the flexible. *Nursing Management, 26*(3), 8.

Davis, D. H., & Hawkins, J. W. (1985). High risk maternal and neonatal transport: Psychosocial implications for practice. *Dimensions in Critical Care Nursing, 4*(6), 368–379.

Frischer, L., & Gutterman, D. L. (1992). Emotional impact on parents of transported babies. Considerations for meeting parents' needs. *Critical Care Clinics*, 8(3), 649–660.

Fultz, J. H., McKee, J. L., Zalaznik, F. R., & Kidd, P. S. (1993). Air medical transport: What the family wants to know. *Air Medical Journal, 12*(11–12), 431–435.

Hackel, A. (1987). An organizational system for critical care transport. *International Anesthesiology Clinics, 25*(2), 1–13.

Hart, H. (1978). The conveyance of patients to and from the hospital, 1720–1850. *Medical History, 22,* 397–407.

Kenner, C., & Gunderson, L. P. (1988). Parent care: Anticipatory guidance for the neonate and family. In C. Kenner, J. Harjo, & A. Brueggemeyer (Eds.), *Neonatal surgery: A nursing perspective* (pp. 57–78). Orlando, FL: Grune & Stratton.

Kuhly, J. E., & Freston, M. S. (1993). Back transport: Exploration of parents' feelings regarding the transition. *Neonatal Network, 12*(1), 49–56.

Lancaster, J. (1982). Communication as a tool for change. In J. Lancaster & J. Lancaster (Eds.), *Nurse as a change agent* (pp. 109–132). St. Louis: C. V. Mosby.

MacDonald, M., & Miller, M. (Eds.). (1989). Emergency transport of the perinatal patient. Boston: Little, Brown.

March of Dimes Birth Defects Foundation. (1993). *Toward improving the outcome of pregnancy: The 90's and beyond.* White Plains, NY: Author.

Merenstein, G., & Gardner, S. (1993). *Handbook of neonatal intensive care* (3rd ed.). St. Louis: C. V. Mosby.

National Association of Neonatal Nurses. (1994). *Neonatal nursing transport standards and guidelines*. Petaluma, CA: Author.

Olds, S. B., London, M. L., & Ludwig, P. A. (1994). *Maternal-newborn nursing: A family centered approach* (5th ed.). Menlo Park, CA: Addison-Wesley.

Phibbs, C. S., & Mortenson, L. (1992). Back transporting infants from neonatal intensive care units to community hospitals for recovery care: Effect on total hospital charges. *Pediatrics, 96*(No. 1, Pt. 1), 22–26.

Salyer, J. W., & Masi-Lynch, J. (1995). Respiratory care during the transport of infants and children. In S. L. Barnhart & M. P. Czervinske (Eds.), *Perinatal and pediatric respiratory care* (pp. 637–657). Philadelphia: W. B. Saunders.

Steenson, M., & Erdman, T. S. (1989). A comprehensive quality assurance structured transport system: A qualitative and quantitative approach to improving patient care. *Journal of Nursing Quality Assurance*, 3(4), 64–71.

Tharp, P. (1985). Patient care in the transport environment: Experience and problem solving. In *Proceedings of the Sixth Annual Conference on Critical Care Transport* (p. 164). San Francisco, CA: Contemporary Forums.

Whitfield, J. M., & Buser, M. K. (1993). Transport stabilization times for neonatal and pediatric patients prior to interfacility transfer. *Pediatric Emergency Care, 9*(2), 69–71.

Youngberg, B. J. (1992). Medical-legal considerations involved in transport of critically ill patients. *Critical Care Clinics*, 8(3), 501–514.

UNIT FOUR

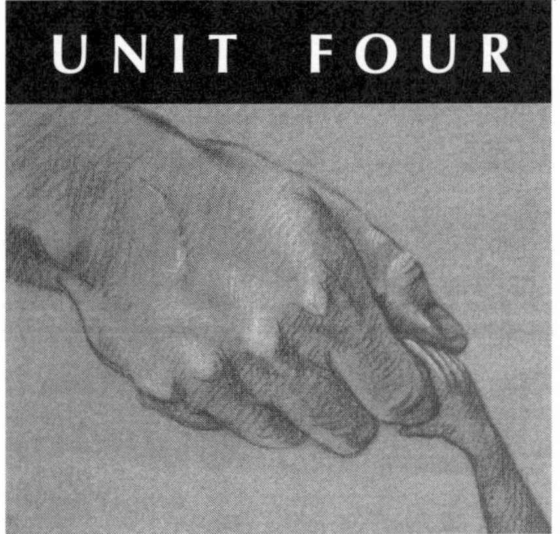

The Intrapartal Environment: Maternal-Child Interactions

The nurses reminded us that we could telephone the unit for information about Emily whenever we wanted. In fact, I soon discovered that an entry called "social" on Emily's daily progress chart made note of every visit or telephone call. "Mom visited, played with baby," it might say. Or "No visits, no phone calls." Even if the latter notation occurred on the all-night shift, I felt chastised and vowed to be a more attentive mother.

ELIZABETH MEHREN
Born Too Soon

CHAPTER 14

Effects of Labor on the Fetus and Neonate

DIANNE M. FELBLINGER TINA LEIGH WEITKAMP

RESEARCH AGENDA

What factors influence fetal well-being during the intrapartal period?

How does fetal monitoring affect neonatal morbidity and mortality rates?

Which factors alter the accuracy of fetal monitoring?

While providing care for the pregnant mother, nurses have also demonstrated concern for the welfare of the fetus too. Since the 1980s, reliable methods of fetal assessment have evolved. During this time, nurses have also become increasingly cognizant that regardless of whether the pregnancy has progressed within normal parameters or has been complicated, labor and delivery place the greatest stress on the fetus and have the highest potential for inducing fetal distress (Polin & Frangipane, 1986).

The human body has a tremendous capacity to remain resilient during the stress of the labor period, but efforts to determine the various factors related to fetal stress and distress during labor have escalated. The advent of fetal monitoring has provided nurses with a wealth of knowledge regarding fetal status, so that when this general state of normalcy gives way to a more critical or complicated labor scenario, the nurses are able to provide care immediately as indicated. This chapter provides an overview of the effects that labor can have on the fetus and how to monitor fetal well-being during the intrapartal period.

FETAL DEVELOPMENT AND FETAL MONITORING

With implantation of the blastocyst into the decidua, the placenta begins to develop. As the trophoblast grows, it develops into two layers: the cytotrophoblast and the syncytiotrophoblast. The syncytiotrophoblast forms the primitive uteroplacental circulation through erosion of the maternal blood vessels of the decidua, resulting in the formation of the intervillous space. The intervillous space allows for transfer of oxygen (O_2) and nutrients from the maternal circulation to the fetal circulation and the return of carbon dioxide (CO_2) and waste products to the maternal circulation. By the end of the second week of development, chorionic villi begin to form. During the third week there is rapid growth, resulting in an increase in the surface area for maternal and fetal circulation. Chorionic villi cover the entire surface of the chorionic sac until the eighth week, at which time those on the decidua capsularis stretch and gradually disappear, giving the chorion a smooth appearance. The chorionic villi attached to the decidua basalis increase rapidly in size and complexity and are known as the villous chorion. The placenta is formed from both fetal (villous chorion) and maternal (decidua basalis) portions, which are held together by stem villi or anchoring villi.

Blood leaving the fetus through the umbilical arteries enters and moves through the placental arteriocapillary-venous network to the chorionic villi, where it comes in contact with the placental membrane, and gas and nutrient exchange occurs. The O_2 and nutrients then reach the fetus through the umbilical vein.

During pregnancy, the maternal and fetal circulations are separated by the placental membrane. Until midpregnancy this membrane consists of four layers: syncytiotrophoblast, cytotrophoblast, connective tissue, and endothelium from the fetal capillary. As the pregnancy progresses, the cytotrophoblast disappears, and the syncytiotrophoblast thins out to approximately 1 μm thick (Moore & Persaud, 1993).

Oxygenated blood enters the intervillous space though the ends of the eroded maternal spiral arteries of the decidua basalis. The maternal blood pressure forces the maternal blood toward the placental membrane, allowing for exchange of gases and metabolic products. These products cross the placental membrane through simple diffusion, facilitated transport, active transport, pinocytosis, and bulk flow (Table 14–1). Factors that affect the rate of transfer include molecular size, electrical charge, lipid solubility, placental size, placental blood flow, level of saturation, and metabolism of the substance by the mother, fetus, and placenta. Waste products from the placenta cross the placental barrier into the maternal circulation rapidly (Moore, 1989; Moore & Persaud, 1993).

The development of the fetal cardiovascular system begins in the wall of the yolk sac during the third week of gestation. Primitive fetal blood begins to be formed in the wall of the yolk sac during the third week. Blood vessels from the yolk sac connect with those in the connecting stalk and chorion to form the

TABLE 14–1 Placental Transport

Type of Transport	Substance
Simple diffusion	Water, electrolytes, carbon dioxide, anesthetic gases, free fatty acids
Facilitated transport	Glucose, galactose, oxygen
Active transport	Amino acids, calcium, iron, iodine, water-soluble vitamins, glucose
Pinocytosis	Albumin, gamma globulins, fat-soluble vitamins
Bulk flow	Water

primitive cardiovascular system. As the development progresses, the blood travels throughout the entire fetus in a unique pattern.

The umbilical vein divides as it enters the fetus, and a small amount of the blood circulates through the liver and then empties into the inferior vena cava. The majority of the blood entering the fetus bypasses the liver through the ductus venosus and enters the inferior vena cava. From the inferior vena cava, the blood enters the right atrium and passes through the foramen ovale into the left atrium, left ventricle, and aorta. From the aorta, the blood travels to the head and upper extremities or to the trunk and lower extremities. Blood returning from the head enters the superior vena cava and then the right atrium and right ventricle. From the right ventricle, a small amount of blood enters the pulmonary circulation; the majority of the blood enters the pulmonary artery through the ductus arteriosus, flowing to the descending aorta and to the placenta through the two umbilical arteries.

Formation of the heart occurs at 18 or 19 days of gestation, when the cardiogenic cords appear and lay the foundation of the endocardial heart tube. Heart pulsations begin as peristaltic waves forcing blood through the tube at day 22. As the fetal heart develops, the beating of the heart comes under control of the sinoatrial node, which sets the heart rate. Normal fetal heart rate (FHR) is 120 to 160 beats per minute (bpm). As in the adult, both the sinoatrial and atrioventricular nodes are under the influence of the vagus nerve. Stimulation of the vagus nerve results in a decrease of the FHR. Sympathetic stimulation of the heart occurs when norepinephrine is released by the fetus, resulting in an increase in the fetal blood pressure and heart rate. This increase is often counteracted through stimulation of the baroreceptor found in the internal and external carotid arteries that stimulates the vagus and glossopharyngeal nerves.

As the fetal heart develops, the sinoatrial node controls the rhythm. Normal FHR is 120 to 160 bpm. The FHR is regulated by the parasympathetic and sympathetic branches of the autonomic nervous system along with baroreceptor and chemoreceptors. The parasympathetic nervous stimulation results in a decreased heart rate. This system is responsible for producing long-term and short-term variability in heart rate. Sympathetic nervous system stimulation results in an increase of the heart rate and myocardial contraction. The chemoreceptors respond to changes in oxygen and carbon dioxide levels. Baroreceptors increase the FHR in response to an increase in blood pressure. This increase is often counteracted through stimulation of the baroreceptor found in the internal and external carotid arteries that in turn stimulates the vagus and glossopharyngeal nerves, resulting in a decrease in FHR and blood pressure.

Fetal Heart Rate

Auscultation of the FHR with use of a fetoscope is possible between 16 and 20 weeks' gestation. Use of a Doptone unit allows for auscultation of the fetal heart once the uterus has ascended above the pelvic bone, usually after 12 weeks' gestation. The fetal heart is heard loudest through the fetus's back. As the fetus matures and reaches term, the back is easily identified through use of the Leopold maneuvers.

Baseline Fetal Heart Rate

Baseline FHR is defined as the FHR between contractions for at least a 10-minute period. This does not include periodic changes. Most fetuses have a baseline FHR of 120 to 160 bpm at term.

The term or postterm fetus may have a baseline FHR as low as 110 bpm. The lower heart rate is a result of maturation of the neurologic system.

Fetal Bradycardia

Fetal bradycardia is an FHR of less than 120 bpm for 10 minutes or more. It may be further defined as moderate or marked bradycardia. *Moderate* bradycardia is an FHR of 100 to 119 bpm; *marked* bradycardia is an FHR of less than 100 bpm; and *severe* bradycardia is an FHR of less than 70 bpm. Maternal causes of fetal bradycardia include ingestion of anesthetics or oxytocic agents, hypotension, position, hypothermia, and systemic lupus erythematosus. Fetal causes include prolonged cord compression, prolapse of the umbilical cord, congenital cardiac conduction and structural defects, hypothermia, fetal hypoxia, and continuous pressure on the fetal head during descent (terminal or end-stage bradycardia). A continuous FHR of 100 to 120 bpm in a term or postterm infant may be due to a mature parasympathetic system.

Fetal Tachycardia

Fetal tachycardia is an FHR of greater than 160 bpm for 10 or more minutes. *Moderate* tachycardia is an FHR of 160 to 179 bpm, and *severe* tachycardia is an FHR greater than 180 bpm. Rates of more than 180 bpm have been associated with fetal hypoxia. Other causes of tachycardia are often unknown; however, known causes include extreme prematurity, maternal hyperthermia, fetal or maternal infection, fetal or maternal anemia, beta-sympathomimetic drug ingestion, drugs that inhibit vagal response (atropine, hydroxyzine, and phenothiazine), inotropic drugs, maternal anxiety, hyperthyroidism, chronic hypoxia, fetal cardiac anomalies, fetal heart failure, supraventricular tachycardia, and excessive fetal activity.

Variability

Variability results from interaction between the sympathetic and parasympathetic nervous systems. For variability to occur, an unimpaired autonomic nervous system, a medulla oblongata, and a heart must be present. The interplay of the sympathetic and parasympathetic systems is then communicated to the medulla and the heart and recorded as variability on the fetal tracing. This interplay is more evident as the fetus matures. The changes between each beat or between the R-waves are known as short-term variability. Short-term variability is mostly influenced by the parasympathetic system, which innervates both the sinoatrial and atrioventricular nodes. Short-term variability is evaluated only through the use of internal electronic fetal monitoring and is noted as being present or absent. Long-term variability is seen as larger changes or cyclic changes occurring over a 2- to 10-minute period and is influenced more by the sympathetic system than by the parasympathetic system. Evaluation of long-term variability can occur only with internal electronic fetal monitoring. Long-term variability (Fig. 14–1) is an indicator of fetal wellness and is evaluated in the following manner (Adelsperger et al., 1993):

Decreased or minimal: 0 to 5 bpm
Average: 6 to 25 bpm
Marked or saltatory: >25 bpm

The presence of decreased or minimal variability mandates evaluation of possible causes. Fetal anomalies, maternal medications, and fetal behavioral states all can decrease variability. Interventions to correct decreased variability include position changes, hydration, changes in breathing techniques, stress reduction methods, and discontinuation of oxytocin. Marked or saltatory variability may result from a sympathetic response to an acute hypoxic episode, possible interventions to correct this include position change, hydration, oxygen, stress-reduction methods, and discontinuation of oxytocin or tocolytic agents.

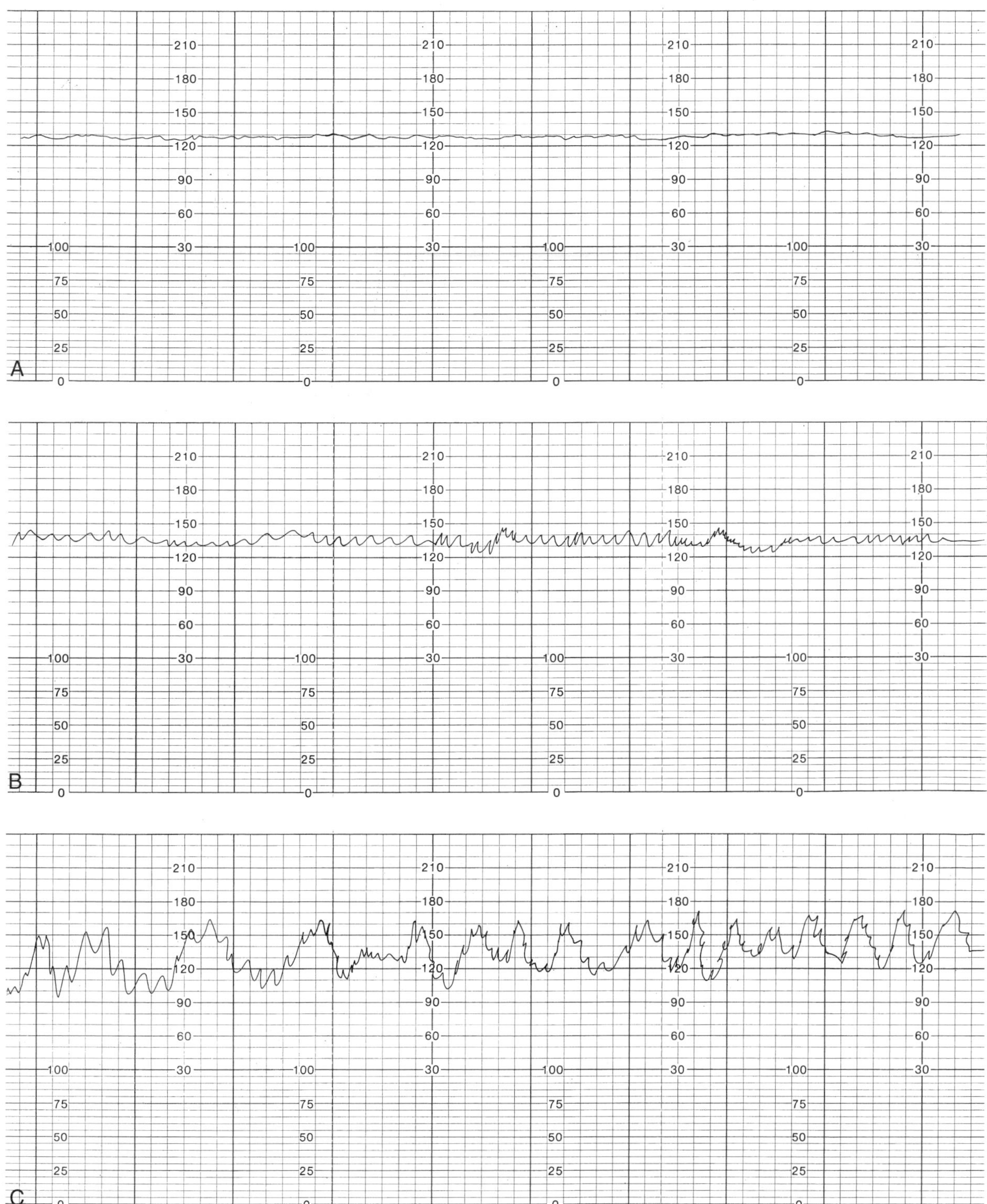

FIGURE 14–1. Variability in fetal heart rate. *A,* Decreased or minimal variability. *B,* Average variability. *C,* Marked or saltatory variability.

Variability of the FHR is affected by many things, including prematurity, severe fetal tachycardia, maternal drug ingestion (analgesic, hypnotic, and parasympathetic blocking agents), deep fetal sleep, fetal hypoxia, congenital anomalies, anencephaly, and fetal acidosis.

Periodic Heart Rate Changes

Periodic changes are changes that occur in the baseline FHR during a contraction or as a result of a contraction. The two types of periodic changes are accelerations and decelerations. Accelerations are sudden increases in the FHR and are usually associated with fetal movement that lasts less than 10 minutes. Accelerations are a result of the beta-adrenergic sympathetic nervous system and indicate an intact nervous system. Most accelerations are reassuring signs. However, repetitive uniformly shaped accelerations may be an early response to mild hypoxia resulting from cord compression. Decelerations are abrupt decreases in the FHR usually lasting less than 10 minutes and often associated with fetal stress and hypoxia. A deceleration is evaluated in relation to its timing in a uterine contraction and general shape.

FHR dysrhythmias are irregularities in the FHR, usually a result of electrical firing within the heart that causes ectopic or premature beats. These are best detected with the use of a fetoscope, because irregularities often appear as artifacts with external monitoring.

Accelerations

Accelerations of the FHR occur with stimulation of the sympathetic nervous system. Accelerations appear as an increase in the FHR above the baseline and may resemble the shape of uterine contractions when they are present or after fetal movement. The onset of an acceleration depends on the stimulus and may be a result of spontaneous movement, stimulation of the fetal scalp, abdominal palpation, fundal pressure, or uterine contractions or a result of mild umbilical cord compression. (For an example of accelerations, see Fig. 14–2.)

Decelerations

Early Decelerations. These occur as a result of pressure, usually on the fetal head, which stimulates the vagus nerve, resulting in a decrease in FHR; recovery occurs once the pressure is removed from the head. When these are visualized, they appear to be a mirror image of the contraction pattern. The deceleration starts early in the contraction, peaks at about the acme of the contraction, and then returns to baseline by the time the contraction is complete. Shape is uniform in early decelerations, and variability is present. The decrease in FHR typically does not drop below 110 bpm or more than 20 bpm from the baseline rate. The depth of the deceleration increases as the length of contraction increases. Early decelerations are usually seen during active labor as the fetus is descending into and through the pelvis and are frequently seen with cephalopelvic disproportion. Treatment of early decelerations begins with the identification of the pattern and assessment of fetal status. (For an example of early decelerations, see Fig. 14–3.)

Late Decelerations. Late decelerations are a result of uteroplacental insufficiency. Uteroplacental insufficiency occurs when gas exchange is restricted anywhere between the uterus, placenta, and fetus, resulting in fetal hypoxia. When late decelerations are a result of decreased maternal circulation, the underlying cause can include pregnancy-induced hypertension (PIH), diabetes, anemia, cardiac disease, respiratory disease, or regional anesthesia. When impaired uterine circulation results in late deceleration, the cause is often related to hyperstimulation of the uterine musculature from oxytocin or prostaglandin stimulation. Placental gas exchange is often jeopardized by a decrease in the placental area or increased distance between the fetal capillaries and the maternal blood supply. Placental problems usually arise from a small placenta, as seen with intrauterine growth retardation, or from separation of part of the placenta, as seen with premature separation of the placenta or placenta previa; postmaturity, malformations, and placental fibrin deposits and calcification also decrease the surface area. Women with histories of diabetes, collagen diseases, herpes, poor nutrition, smoking, multiple gestations, and PIH experience late decelerations.

When uteroplacental insufficiency results in a Po_2 of less than 19 mm Hg, the fetus is hypoxemic and the FHR falls (Edelstone, 1984). The actual cause of the decreasing heart rate is not clearly understood but is thought to be related to one or more

1. Chemoreceptor stimulation.
2. Catecholamine release from the adrenal glands.
3. Direct depression of the heart rate.
4. Intrinsic myocardial conduction interference (Gimovsky & Caritis, 1982).

In addition, uteroplacental insufficiency results in a secondary chemoreceptor response and drop in fetal blood pressure. This decrease in fetal blood pressure produces an alpha-adrenergic response as a result of catecholamine release from the adrenal glands. Fetal blood vessels then constrict, causing fetal hypertension and stimulation of the baroreceptor to decrease the heart rate. Simultaneously, the initial hypoxia stimulates the parasympathetic nervous system and vagus nerve, which further lowers FHR. As the contraction decreases in intensity, the blood flow throughout the uterine musculature increases, and oxygen delivery to the fetus is increased.

Even though late decelerations indicate a decrease in placental perfusion, the presence of short-term variability, long-term variability, spontaneous accelerations, and a baseline FHR between 120 to 160 bpm is a reassuring sign (Tournaire et al., 1980).

Late decelerations have a smooth, uniform appearance and occur after the contraction has begun, usually around the acme of the contraction. The lowest point of the deceleration generally comes well after the acme, and return to baseline is gradual, after uterine resting tone has returned to normal. Heart rate decreases

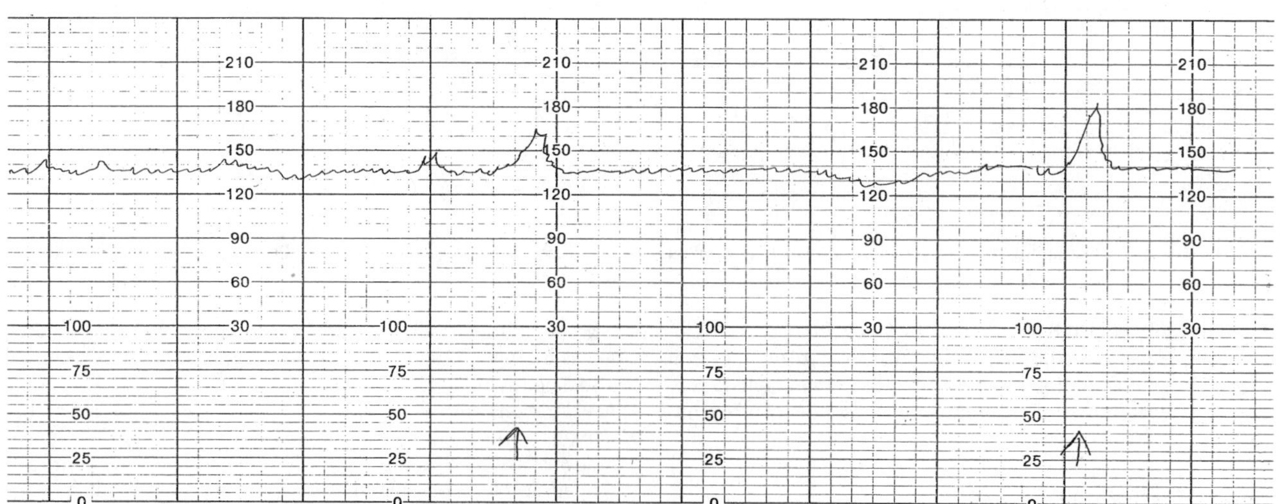

FIGURE 14–2. Acceleration in fetal heart rate.

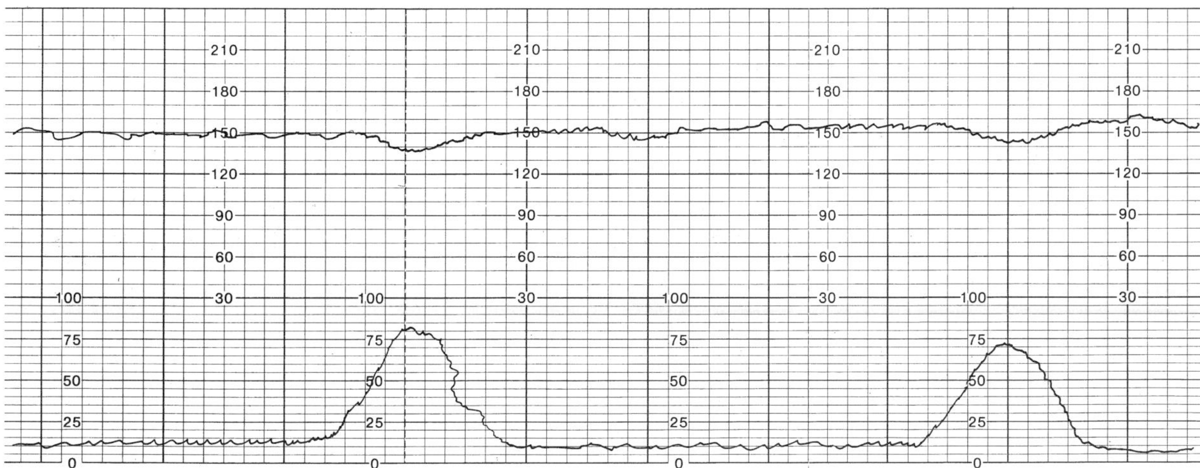

FIGURE 14–3. Early deceleration in fetal heart rate.

by 5 to 30 bpm and is usually maintained above 100 bpm. Late decelerations are often seen with a loss of variability and a rising baseline FHR (Fig. 14–4).

Treatment of late decelerations involves increasing the uterine blood flow and gas exchange. The methods used depend on possible causes and current maternal status; correcting maternal hypotension (increasing intravenous fluids), decreasing uterine stimulation (stopping or decreasing oxytocic medication or the administration of tocolytic agents), position changes, or administration of oxygen by tight face mask. Other interventions may include checking for a prolapsed cord and insertion of an internal spiral electrode and an intrauterine pressure gauge in order to obtain an accurate picture of the FHR pattern, uterine activity, and relationship of the deceleration to uterine activity and possible amnioinfusion. In addition, the physician or nurse-midwife should be notified, and the actions should be documented.

Variable Decelerations. Variable decelerations are usually the result of umbilical cord compression and result in patterns of FHR decrease that differ in size, duration, and shape from contraction to contraction. Variable decelerations occur in approximately half of all labors and are most common during the second stage of labor (Freeman, 1979). The duration and depth of the deceleration are directly related to the fetal hypotension, hypoxia, and hypertension that result (Edelstone, 1984). The onset of the deceleration is usually rapid; outset differs in relation to the contraction. If mild cord compression occurs and only the umbilical vein is compressed, the result is mild hypoxia with fetal hypotension (Murray, 1988). This condition stimulates the baroreceptor and chemoreceptor, resulting in an increase in the heart rate. With compression of the umbilical arteries, fetal hypertension results, owing to the alpha-adrenergic response, followed by a vagal response. The accelerations that occur with the compression of the umbilical vein are seen as transient increases in the FHR before and just after the deceleration and are called *shoulders*. Recovery of the baseline FHR is usually rapid, as the pressure of the contraction decreases. These decelerations may be U-, V-, or W-shaped, with a rapid drop in the FHR (Fig. 14–5).

Repeated hypoxic episodes that stress the fetus can result in overshoots. Overshoots are smooth accelerations that follow a variable deceleration lasting more than 20 seconds and are predictive of decompensation. Overshoots are thought to be a result of catecholamine release by the fetal adrenal glands.

Treatment of variable decelerations involves changing the maternal position in hopes of relieving the pressure on the umbilical cord. Oxygen is administered by a tight face mask if the pattern continues or becomes more severe. A fluid bolus is given to increase the maternal vascular bed. Uterine activity is decreased through discontinuing or decreasing oxytocic agents if previous actions do not improve the fetal status. A spiral electrode may

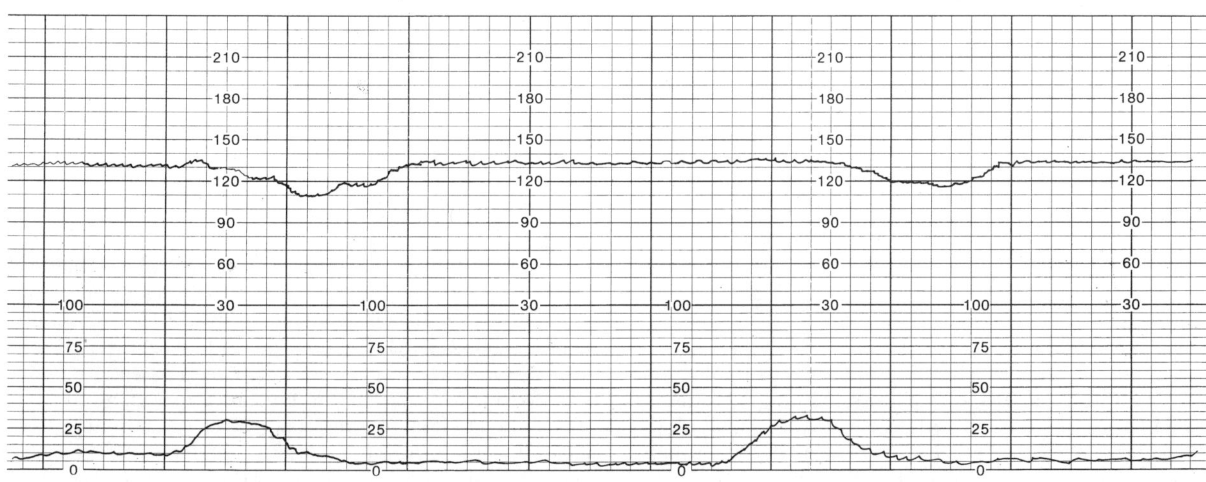

FIGURE 14–4. Late deceleration in fetal heart rate.

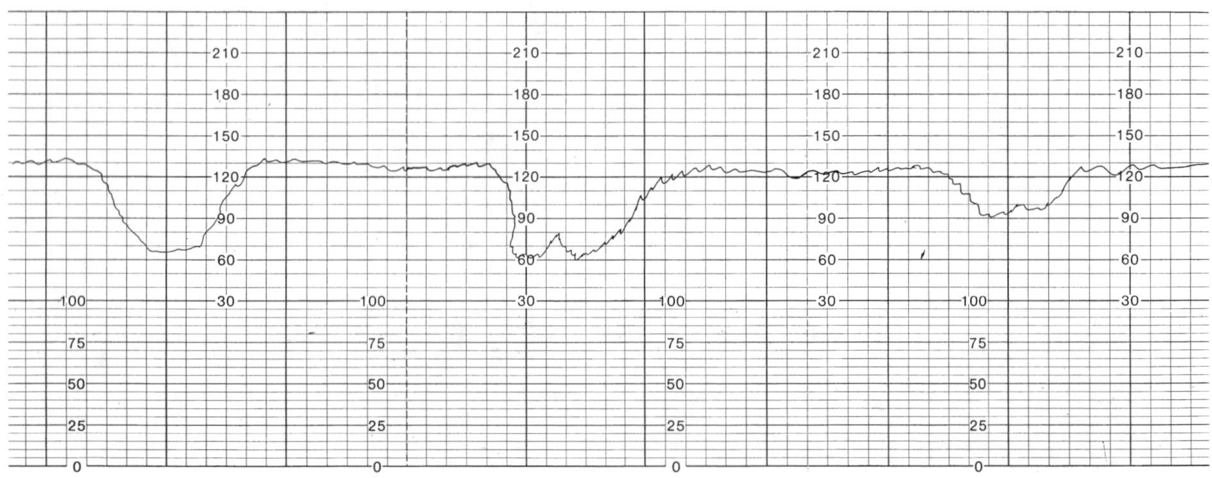

FIGURE 14–5. Variable deceleration in fetal heart rate.

also be applied to increase the quality of the monitor strip. An amnioinfusion may also be done. The physician or nurse-midwife should be notified, and appropriate documentation should be recorded.

During antepartal and intrapartal periods, the fetus is susceptible to hypoxia. Hypoxia can be present in either an acute or a chronic form. When it is acute, decelerations appear on the fetal monitor. If chronic hypoxia exists, fetal growth is diminished. To evaluate for chronic hypoxia, a biophysical profile is obtained. This profile consists of five parameters: reaction to a nonstress test, fetal breathing motions, gross fetal body movements, fetal body tone, and volume of amniotic fluid (Murphy, 1990). It is explained in detail later in this chapter.

PLACENTAL FACTORS CONTRIBUTING TO FETAL DISTRESS DURING LABOR

The placenta plays a very important role throughout the pregnancy. Numerous placental factors can directly or indirectly cause fetal distress during labor. Maternal perfusion of the placenta may be decreased, or fetal uptake from the placenta may be decreased. Both these factors affect the fetal outcome of the labor process.

Decreased Maternal Perfusion of the Placenta

Decreased maternal perfusion of the placenta can be caused by such factors as (1) hypotension, (2) hypertension, (3) abruptio placentae, and (4) hypertonic contractions. Any of these factors has the potential to adversely affect the maternal-fetal dyad. Therefore, the nurse must constantly assess for these factors. They may be indicative of a decrease in maternal-placental perfusion during the labor process.

Hypotension

Hypotension can manifest itself in conjunction with numerous situations, such as (1) maternal blood loss, (2) drug ingestion or exposure, and (3) position changes, such as placement of the mother in the supine position for administration of anesthetic agents. Any of these complications has the ability to adversely affect fetal well-being.

Maternal Blood Loss

Maternal blood loss, or obstetrical hemorrhage, has been documented as one of the leading causes of maternal mortality. Except for pregnancies that have been linked to abortive outcomes, postpartum hemorrhage has been shown to be connected to 50 percent of hemorrhagic deaths (Kaunitz et al., 1985). Third-trimester bleeding complicates approximately 3.8 percent of all pregnancies and may be a potentially life-threatening situation (Creasy & Resnik, 1994). Conditions that may manifest in relation to obstetrical hemorrhage include cesarean section, obstetrical lacerations, uterine atony, retained placenta, uterine inversion, and, more rarely, placenta accreta. The nurse must be able to manage any of these potentially dangerous situations.

The goals for management of these situations that can result in hypotension and consequent hemorrhagic shock are generally twofold. The primary goal is the immediate restoration of the blood volume and the oxygen-carrying capacity. The second goal is to be aware of the specific nursing care needs of the patient that are related to the condition directly causing the hemorrhage. Stabilization of the patient is of paramount importance (Creasy & Resnik, 1994). Without the stabilization of the mother, the effects of blood loss on the fetus have the potential to be ominous. Uteroplacental insufficiency can result in the inability of the fetus to exhibit a life-sustaining physiologic response. The fetal response to acute blood loss is similar to the maternal reaction: Hypoxemia and acidosis result in bradycardia, vasospasm, and the initial shunting of blood to vital organs. As the maternal condition progresses and these compensatory mechanisms are no longer adequate, brain damage and fetal demise may occur (May & Mahlmeister, 1994).

Drug Ingestion and Exposure

Exposure to certain drugs may have hypotensive effects on the mother and thus may adversely affect the fetus in utero. The nurse caring for the patient must be aware of the pharmacologic action of any drugs that the patient receives during hospitalization, as well as the action of any drugs that the patient has taken before admission. Medications known to have hypotensive effects include ritodrine, magnesium sulfate, and narcotic substances.

Ritodrine (Yutopar) and terbutaline are often given as tocolytic agents in an effort to arrest labor. Because these drugs cross the placenta, the nurse must be aware of their effects on both the mother and the fetus. These drugs may result not only in a decrease in maternal blood pressure but also in an increase in maternal and fetal heart rates. Another drug that is used for its tocolytic effect and that has a depressant effect on myometrial contractility is magnesium sulfate ($MgSO_4$). $MgSO_4$ may also be given for the treatment of preeclampsia. The nurse must be aware that $MgSO_4$ has the ability to alter blood pressure as a result of splanchnic dilatation and that severe maternal hypotension may occur. A decrease in FHR may also occur when $MgSO_4$ is administered to the mother. In addition to maternal and fetal effects, the neonatal toxic effects of maternal $MgSO_4$ administration are generally minimal; however, decreased muscle tone and drowsiness may occur in the newborns whose mothers receive $MgSO_4$ for tocolysis.

Narcotic substances, particularly in conjunction with anesthesia administration, may cause respiratory depression and hypotensive episodes in the laboring patient. Whether these substances are administered in therapeutic doses in a controlled labor setting or ingested by a drug-addicted mother before admission, the nurse needs to be aware that there is generally a rapid placental transfer of these drugs. Narcotic addiction during pregnancy may lead to premature delivery, stillbirth, or addiction in infants, who may experience neonatal abstinence reactions. The nurse caring for the drug-addicted mother must understand that the narcotic-exposed infant may demonstrate severe withdrawal symptoms in utero, at birth, or during the 10- to 15-day period immediately after birth. Some drug-exposed infants experience subacute withdrawal for 4 to 6 months after birth. Because of the potential for depressant and hypotensive effects of therapeutic narcotic administration and the magnitude of the complications associated with illicit maternal use of these drugs, the nurse must be alert to the potential impact that these drugs have on the mother, the fetus, and the infant.

Maternal Position Changes During Labor

In addition to the effects of drugs, the relative position of the mother during the labor and delivery process may affect the hypotensive state of the mother and thus the response of the fetus. It has been generally well documented that the supine position is not ideal for the mother in labor. Supine positioning of the mother alters cardiac output via compression of the aorta and the venae cavae, thus adversely affecting the circulatory response of the fetus. As an alternative, the laboring mother generally is placed in the left lateral recumbent position to avoid a hypotensive state. When a supine hypotensive syndrome occurs, the accompanying maternal decreased cardiac output may be harmful to the fetus. There may be an accompanying decrease in uterine arterial pressure that could be especially detrimental to the fetus if it occurs concomitantly with extensive blood loss or with anesthesia administration during delivery.

Hypertension

In addition to assessment for hypotension, the nurse must also be aware of the presence of an existing or an impending hypertensive state during labor. Hypertension may manifest itself in numerous situations, such as (1) in patients with chronic hypertension, (2) in preeclampsia, and (3) in connection with the intake of certain drugs. Hypertension has the potential to compromise placental function and thus can adversely affect fetal health. Infants of all hypertensive women should be treated and monitored as being potentially at high risk. Intrauterine growth retardation and perinatal mortality are more prevalent among pregnancies of hypertensive women (Tervila et al., 1973).

Ideally, this condition is documented early in the pregnancies of women who have a history of chronic hypertension. Early recognition of this chronic state allows time for adequate blood pressure monitoring and also provides baseline data that later helps the nurse to differentiate the chronic hypertensive state from a superimposed state of preeclampsia. The nurse must understand that the fetal effects of these two hypertensive states are different. The perinatal mortality rates of infants of women with superimposed preeclampsia have been noted to be higher than those of infants of women in whom the hypertension exists alone (Lin et al., 1982). The decidual vessels of women with mild to severe hypertension may exhibit changes similar to those noted in the renal arterioles of women with an extensive history of hypertension (Robertson et al., 1967). Decreased uteroplacental perfusion secondary to this change is at least additive and perhaps synergistic with the decidual vascular changes of preeclampsia. These additional decidual vascular changes may also be associated with the higher rate of abruptio placentae in women with superimposed preeclampsia. Creasy and Resnik (1994, p. 834) noted that "Preeclampsia also has been seen earlier in pregnancies of hypertensive women than in the pregnancies of normotensive women." In view of the difficulties that arise in the recognition and treatment of superimposed preeclampsia, all infants of hypertensive women should be considered at risk, and their nursing care should be planned accordingly.

To treat the patient with PIH, the nurse must first be aware of the classic triad of symptoms associated with the physiologic changes that accompany PIH. These symptoms include

Hypertension that is defined as any of the following: blood pressure of 140/90, an increase in systolic pressure of 30 mm Hg over baseline nonpregnancy levels, or an increase in diastolic pressure of 15 mm Hg above baseline nonpregnancy levels.

Proteinuria: 0.5 g/L in a 24-hour period or a dipstick reading of +1 or +2. Proteinuria is usually the last symptom to occur.

Edema: clinically evident swelling or a sudden, rapid weight gain in the second or third trimester; nondependent edema of the hands and face is significant.

For the developing fetus, PIH is often seen in conjunction with intrauterine growth retardation and an increase in the rate of preterm delivery among the surviving infants (May & Mahlmeister, 1994). The nurse must assess for uterine growth in relation to gestational age by the use of McDonald's measurements (fundal heights). The nurse must also be familiar with the results of the mother's ultrasound examination, nonstress test, and amniocentesis. The understanding of the effects of hypertension on the fetus can aid the nurse in the development of an individualized plan of care for the mother and the fetus during the prenatal and the labor periods.

The ingestion of certain drugs may also result in an untoward hypertensive effect on the mother and thus adversely affect fetal health. Stimulants such as cocaine, amphetamines, and methamphetamines may induce an increase in maternal heart and respiratory rates and may elevate blood pressure. Cocaine may diffuse across the placenta and decrease placental blood flow. Fetal gas and nutrient exchange is hampered. Cocaine-exposed infants have an increased incidence of impaired fetal growth, premature birth, and neonatal seizures (see Chapter 45, The Drug-Exposed Neonate.) Because many mothers who use illicit substances may be polydrug users, the nurse must be capable of assessing the infant for multiple indications of maternal substance use or abuse. The infant may exhibit signs of central nervous system hyperirritability, gastrointestinal disturbance, respiratory distress, and vague autonomic symptoms (Finnegan, 1986).

Abruptio Placentae

Decreased maternal perfusion of the placenta is also related to the presence of abruptio placentae, the separation of the normally implanted placenta before the birth of the fetus (Creasy & Resnik, 1994).

Abruption of the placenta may also contribute to fetal distress during labor. The decreased perfusion of the placenta may result in untoward fetal effects. Although not every case of abruptio placentae results in fetal death, there are three major causes of fetal demise related to abruptio placentae: fetal anoxia, neonatal prematurity, and fetal exsanguination. The neonatal intensive care unit (NICU) nurse needs to be aware that an abruption occurring before 28 weeks lessens the fetus's chance for survival. More than 20 percent of births resulting from abruption occur between 28 and 32 weeks' gestation, and these neonates present a challenge in nursing care (Blair, 1973).

The method and timing of delivery and consequently the labor period of the patient with abruptio placentae are of paramount concern to the nurse. The factors that affect the progression of the labor period are related to fetal gestational age, maternal condition, and the status of the cervix. If the gestational age is early and the abruption is only mild, an observational approach is acceptable. In the absence of maternal complications or fetal compromise, the nurse may cautiously administer tocolytic agents with an ongoing assessment of maternal and fetal status. Early pregnancy may be prolonged with careful ongoing assessment for signs of abruptio placentae. Abruptio placentae may manifest with concealed or apparent hemorrhage. When hemorrhage is concealed, the nurse sees no vaginal bleeding but must be alert for the presence of sudden, pronounced uterine or abdominal pain, a rapid increase in rigidity or size of the uterus, absence of fetal heart tones, and signs of acute fetal distress. When hemorrhage is present, the nurse also assesses for bright red or dark clotted vaginal bleeding. Uterine tonicity may also increase, and the uterus may fail to relax between contractions. Abruptio placentae may progress to the point of hypovolemia and shock secondary to the hemorrhage state, and disseminated intravascular coagulation may also occur.

When the placental separation is moderate or severe, the nurse must be ready to prepare the patient for delivery. In the event of fetal demise, vaginal delivery is indicated as a means of decreasing the chance of maternal morbidity. If the fetal heart tracing is within normal parameters and the uterus relaxes between contractions, the mother may be prepared for a vaginal delivery. If intravenous oxytocin is used to augment uterine activity, extreme caution must be exercised, because uterine response may be unpredictable and the threat of uterine rupture is increased.

If the fetus is alive but shows signs of acute fetal distress, immediate cesarean section is indicated. Signs of fetal distress may include changes in FHR (tachycardia, bradycardia), late decelerations, and decreasing or absent variability. The rate of fetal death secondary to abruption has been estimated as 1 in 420 deliveries (Creasy & Resnik, 1994). Of the infants of mothers with grade II or grade III placental separation, 33 percent survive, although survival is accompanied with an increased risk of neurologic damage (Bobak & Jensen, 1993).

Hypertonic Contractions

In addition to hypotension, hypertension, and abruptio placentae, hypertonic contractions may also be related to decreased maternal perfusion of the placenta. Hypertonic contractions may occur in conjunction with (1) excessive oxytocin administration and (2) precipitous labor.

Under usual conditions, oxytocin is released from the posterior lobe of the pituitary gland. Intravenous oxytocin may also be used to augment the labor process. Synthetic oxytocin preparations, such as Pitocin, act on the uterine muscle to stimulate uterine contractions. Pitocin is a powerful drug and must be used judiciously. When oxytocin is administered, there is a risk of stimulating abnormally strong or tetanic uterine contractions secondary to uterine overstimulation. The use of an intravenous infusion pump is necessary to ensure safe administration of Pitocin. The nurse must be alert for signs of fetal distress and must be cognizant of the possibility of uterine rupture. The fetus must be monitored constantly, and the internal uterine pressure monitor is used as indicated. If signs of hypertonicity are evident, the nurse should immediately discontinue the oxytocin infusion and notify the physician. Hyperstimulation of the uterus may result in the following complications (May & Mahlmeister, 1994): (1) fetal distress related to impaired uteroplacental perfusion, (2) abruption of the placenta, (3) amniotic fluid embolism, (4) cervical laceration or uterine rupture, and (5) neonatal trauma. The nurse must be aware of these complications and assess the patient for the risk and benefit to the patient and her fetus.

Precipitous labor may also result from a pattern of unusually strong and frequent uterine contractions. Precipitous labor generally lasts less than 3 hours before the spontaneous delivery of the fetus. The fetus may pass quickly through the pelvis because of a relatively low resistance of the maternal tissue. Factors that may signal the possibility of precipitous labor include multiparity, large bony pelvis, soft and pliable genital tissue, small fetus in vertex position, previous precipitous labor, or cocaine abuse (May & Mahlmeister, 1994). The fetus may survive a precipitous labor if there is little resistance to fetal descent and if there is adequate placental perfusion. If the fetus experiences chronic distress, however, the fetal status may deteriorate during a precipitous delivery because perfusion is decreased by uterine hypermobility. If any bony or soft tissue resistance to the delivery occurs, there may also be trauma to the fetal head upon descent. There is also the possibility of neonatal aspiration and hypothermia in any unassisted birth situation. The nurse must be alert to these risk factors and carefully monitor the labor progress of the mother at risk for precipitous labor. The mother's contractions, cervical dilatation, and effacement, as well as the fetal station and presentation, must be continually assessed. The consistent attention of the nurse during the labor period is of grave importance to the safe delivery of the fetus in this situation.

Decreased Fetal Uptake From the Placenta

Decreased fetal uptake from the placenta may also cause or contribute to fetal distress during labor. A decrease in fetal uptake may occur in situations such as umbilical cord compression and fetal anemia.

Umbilical Cord Compression

Partial, brief compression of the umbilical cord may occur during the first stage of labor and may be evidenced by the presence of variable decelerations on the electronic fetal monitor. A change in maternal position, such as turning the mother from side to side, may eliminate or lessen the compression pattern. Maternal vital signs must be closely monitored.

During the second stage of labor, compression may occur during fetal descent. Variable decelerations are associated with fetal complications only when these heart rate changes are severe or prolonged. Repeated stress diminishes fetal oxygen reserve. Fetal depression occurs when the nuchal cord is tight. Severe variable decelerations may result in fetal acidosis. Fetal pH blood is sampled, and oxygen is administered to the mother at 8 to 10 L/minute by face mask. Severe, persistent fetal bradycardia with recurrent or diminished variability after a uterine contraction may indicate cord compression and the need for immediate delivery. The nurse must possess the skill needed to react swiftly while concomitantly displaying a supportive demeanor for the patient and her family. Intrauterine amnioinfusion may be attempted in order to relieve cord compression, particularly in selected cases of oligohydramnios or premature rupture of membranes. Amnioinfusion involves the administration of a warmed normal saline solution into the uterus via a hollow intrauterine pressure catheter. The complications of this procedure include uterine overdistention and an increase in the uterine resting tonus. Continuous fetal and maternal monitoring is essential during this procedure (Murray, 1988).

Fetal Anemia

Another factor that can cause or contribute to fetal distress during labor is hemolytic disease of the newborn: fetal anemia (erythroblastosis fetalis, nonimmune hydrops). Fetal anemia may occur in relation to Rh incompatibility. Rh is a factor that is genetically determined. Rh disease is present when the mother is Rh negative, the father is Rh positive, and the fetus is Rh positive. When fetal Rh positive red blood cells come in contact with the mother's circulating blood, an antigen-antibody response may be stimulated. In general, the mother becomes sensitized during her first pregnancy, and the Rh positive fetus of a subsequent pregnancy is affected. Rh positive antibodies are produced, are transferred across the placenta, and subsequently attach to the fetal red blood cells. The fetal red blood cells are then destroyed. In response to the red blood cell destruction, the fetus produces many immature red blood cells—a condition known as erythroblastosis fetalis. In the most severe form of the disease, known as hydrops fetalis, the fetus may become severely anemic. Although this condition is not as common today as it was in years past, the complications can be devastating. Ascites and generalized edema may develop. One half of these fetuses become hydropic between 20 and 34 weeks' gestation; the other half, between 34 and 40 weeks. Hydrops fetalis is not due to fetal heart failure, nor is the fetus hypervolemic or in heart failure at birth. Heart failure may develop after birth. Hepatic enlargement and hepatocellular damage are the more likely etiologic factors (Creasy & Resnik, 1994). Although there is evidence of severe anemia in most hydropic fetuses, the nurse must also be aware that some may present with hemoglobin levels well above 7 g per 100 ml. (See Chapter 28, Assessment and Management of Hematologic Dysfunction, for a complete discussion.)

During labor, the mother who is Rh negative should be cross-matched for Rh immunoglobulin to be given after the delivery. If there is some degree of erythroblastosis present in a sensitized mother, the labor nurse and the neonatal team need to work together during the delivery. The infant is transfused with Rh negative blood soon after determination of the hemoglobin, hematocrit, and blood type. The hydropic infant will likely be transferred to the NICU for follow-up. The nurse must be cognizant of the needs of both the infant and the family and make every effort to explain the rationale for the infant's care in a supportive manner. The explanation needs to be given in terms that the family can comprehend, and it will often need to be repeated soon after delivery and again before discharge. Because of the stress of the labor and delivery and the effects of any medication during delivery and the postpartum period, the mother, regardless of educational level, may need to have the explanation repeated. Providing written information or explanations to the mother and another family member helps the family process the information.

ADMINISTRATION OF ANESTHETIC AGENTS DURING LABOR

During labor, the pain of the contractions is difficult for many women to tolerate. Beginning with Queen Victoria in the late 1800s, pain control during childbirth became accepted. Since that time, many drugs and methods of pain control have been used. Almost all medications that are administered to the mother cross through the placenta and enter the fetal circulation. The type of drug, maternal dose, route, and fetal age all play a role in the effect that the drug has on the fetus. Today rarely are pain-controlling drugs administered orally during labor because of the decreased absorption from the maternal gastrointestinal tract. Because of the decreased gastrointestinal activity, some institutions routinely administer an agent to increase the pH of the stomach in the event that maternal aspiration would occur. These drugs have minimal if any effect on the fetus during the labor process (Pedersen, 1990).

During labor, either anesthetic or analgesic agents may be administered. The purpose of the analgesic agent is to diminish pain sensation and thereby increase the pain threshold. If an anesthetic is administered, it not only provides analgesia but also inhibits pain perception and increases muscle relaxation. If an analgesic agent is administered, a drug from one of the following classifications is usually given: sedative, ataractic (tranquilizer), narcotic, narcotic antagonist, or a mixed compound. Sedatives do not decrease pain. Their major use is during early labor, when they are given to decrease maternal anxiety and often produce sleep. However, sedatives may increase apprehension if they are given without analgesic agents. Use of sedatives should be limited to the early phase of the first stage of labor. These drugs may cause maternal central nervous system (CNS) depression, including respiratory and vasomotor depression and drowsiness. Hypotension, nausea, vomiting, vertigo, and lethargy also are often seen. Because of the risk of maternal hypotension, close monitoring of maternal and fetal status is essential. Interventions to promote uteroplacental circulation should be initiated.

Most often, barbiturates are the type of sedative used during labor. These can be divided into three groups: short-acting, such as secobarbital (Seconal); intermediate-acting, such as pentobarbital (Nembutal); and long-acting, such as phenobarbital (Luminal). Typically, the short- or intermediate-acting barbiturates are given because of their shorter duration. If the infant is born before the complete metabolism of these drugs, the infant often demonstrates respiratory depression, lethargy, and drowsiness for several hours.

Ataractics (tranquilizers) do not relieve pain during labor but do increase relaxation and may produce sleep in some women in addition to their antiemetic property. Frequently these drugs are given with a narcotic to potentiate their effectiveness. Most often, promethazine (Phenergan) and hydroxyzine (Vistaril) are used in labor. These drugs may be administered intramuscularly, with an onset of peak action within 30 to 60 minutes, or intravenously, with an onset within minutes.

The major side effect of ataractics is hypotension, which can impede the uteroplacental circulation. With administration of ataractics, the fetal status must be closely monitored, and methods to increase uteroplacental circulation should be employed as needed. If the infant is born shortly after drug administration, he or she is hypotonic, drowsy, and prone to hypothermia.

Narcotic analgesics produce a high level of pain relief without amnesic effects. The drugs rapidly cross into fetal circulation, where they are metabolized by the fetal liver and kidney. Some maternal breakdown of the drugs also occurs. Because the fetal and neonatal liver and kidney are less effective than the adult organ systems, the metabolism is much slower if the fetus is delivered before complete drug metabolism. Most commonly given narcotics include meperidine (Demerol), oxymorphone (Numorphan), and butorphanol (Stadol).

Meperidine is effective in decreasing pain but does not cause the respiratory depression that morphine does. This drug, when given intravenously, takes effect within minutes; when given intramuscularly, action peaks in about 45 minutes. The use of meperidine has not been reported to prolong labor.

Oxymorphone is a synthetic morphine and has many of the

properties of morphine. It has a peak action within 20 minutes after an intravenous injection or 2 hours after an intramuscular injection. There is often greater respiratory depression with this drug than with meperidine because the fetal brain is more responsive to its effects.

Mixed compounds combine a narcotic and a narcotic antagonist. These drugs give maximum relief of pain while counteracting the respiratory depression that occurs with the narcotic. Such mixed combinations include butorphanol (Stadol) and nalbuphine (Nubain).

Butorphanol (Stadol) is also a mixed agonist and antagonist agent. Butorphanol can provide a potent narcotic action while the antagonist portion is reversing the analgesic effects of the drug. This action-interaction causes drug withdrawal symptoms in narcotic-dependent mothers and fetuses. Butorphanol may be given intravenously, peaking in minutes, or intramuscularly, peaking in 30 minutes to 1 hour. This drug mixture rapidly crosses the placenta, but reports show that there is less respiratory depression in the neonate with butorphanol than with meperidine. Most women experience sedation as a side effect of butorphanol. Other side effects include clamminess of skin, nausea, and dizziness. Nalbuphine (Nubain), another combination drug, is similar to butorphanol in action except that respiratory depression is not increased with cumulative doses, as it is with butorphanol.

Narcotic antagonists reverse the effects of the narcotic-induced respiratory depression. The antagonist acts by displacing the narcotic at the receptor sites of the central nervous system. The antagonist is usually given intravenously for rapid results. This drug may be given up to 15 minutes before delivery. After delivery, the antagonist may be given directly to the neonate through the umbilical vein or through an endotracheal tube. Intramuscular or subcutaneous administration have a delayed onset of action. The action of the antagonist is rapid and the duration is short, and so repeat doses are often needed if respiratory depression recurs. The narcotic antagonist of choice is naloxone (Narcan). Naloxone is semisynthetic and does not function except in the presence of opiates. Therefore, even if maternal respiratory depression is of unknown cause, the drug can safely be administered without causing further respiratory depression. In addition, this drug may be used to reverse mild respiratory depression after small opiate dosages.

The analgesic methods of pain control for labor anesthesia may also be administered during active labor. Most often, a regional anesthetic is administered, and pain relief is provided by blocking the nerve impulses. The methods of administering a regional anesthetic agent are epidural block, spinal block, saddle block, subarachnoid block, caudal block, paracervical block, and pudendal block.

With an epidural block, analgesia is achieved within 10 to 30 minutes of administration. The medication is administered into the epidural space, where pain nervous intervention is blocked. The advantage is that the mother can remain awake and participate actively in the birth process. The disadvantage is that hypotension frequently develops, owing to the sympathetic involvement with this block. Hypotension can be prevented or minimized by hydrating the woman before beginning the anesthesia and by placing her on her side with a wedge under her to relieve the pressure on the vena cava. If the hypotension is moderate, the laboring woman may also be treated with O_2 by face mask. If this does not treat the problem, the woman's legs may be elevated to promote blood return, and ephedrine may be administered. In addition to hypotension, other side effects include nausea, vomiting, urinary retention, shivering, and headache. Medications used for an epidural block may be administered intermittently or continuously. The advantages of continuous infusion are consistency of the anesthesia level, lower blood concentrations, and reduced incidence of hypotension. The catheter may remain in place even after the delivery for pain control during the immediate postpartum period.

Spinal blocks, saddle blocks, and subarachnoid blocks are administered by injecting a local anesthetic into the spinal canal to provide anesthesia for delivery. If the delivery is to be vaginal, anesthesia is administered at the level of the T10 vertebra; for a cesarean delivery, at the level of T8. Saddle block is anesthesia injected into the spinal area that results in a blocking of nerve impulses through the perineal area and upper inner thighs (areas that touch a saddle). The major advantage of this type of anesthesia is the immediate onset and small dosage of medication needed. The major disadvantage is the hypotension that results from blocking of the sympathetic nerves.

Caudal block anesthesia is administered through the caudal area of the spine, providing anesthesia to the cervix, vagina, and perineum by blocking the sacral nerve. This method has been replaced in most areas by the epidural block.

A paracervical block results in interruption of the nerve impulses of the inferior hypogastric plexus and ganglia. This provides pain relief from cervical dilatation but not from uterine contractions and does not anesthetize the lower vagina or perineum. The major advantage is the speedy onset of the anesthesia. The disadvantages, which result from the high vascularity of the area, include possible hematoma formation resulting from trauma of labor or delivery or from the injection itself; rapid absorption of the medication; and fetal bradycardia resulting from the medication absorption.

The pudendal block provides anesthesia for the second and third stages of delivery and during repair of the episiotomy. The anesthetic agent is injected below the pudendal plexus, blocking the nerve impulse of the perineal muscles, urethral sphincter, perineal skin, and perianal muscles. It does not provide pain relief from uterine contractions. The major advantage is the lack of maternal hypotension, and effects on the fetus are rare unless there is injection into the vascular system.

All the regional anesthetics involve the use of a local anesthetic agent. Three types are currently available: ester-linked, amide-linked, and opiate. The ester-linked agents are short-acting and are quickly metabolized by plasma cholinesterase. They do not cross the placenta to the fetus. The longer acting ester-linked tetracaine (Pontocaine) lasts up to only 2 hours and provides an unreliable epidural block. The short-acting procaine (Novocain) is good for local infiltration but not for large areas, because it lasts approximately 1 hour. Chloroprocaine (Nesacaine) is used when fetal respiratory depression must be avoided. This drug lasts approximately 1 hour and has a rapid onset; however, injection into the spinal fluid should be avoided.

The amide-linked agents, which cross the placenta, are metabolized by liver enzymes. Because the fetal liver does not produce the same quantities of liver enzymes as those found in maternal circulation, the amide-linked agent is slowly metabolized by the fetus and neonate. Lidocaine (Xylocaine), mepivacaine (Carbocaine), and bupivacaine (Marcaine) all last at least 1 hour; bupivacaine may last as long as 3 hours. These drugs are good for prolonged relief of pain. However, they do affect the fetus, and effects include neurobehavioral changes, jaundice, and late decelerations.

Opiate use through the epidural catheter is relatively new in obstetrics. The advantages are the long-lasting pain relief and minimal effect on the fetus. Major disadvantages of epidural opiates include pruritus, nausea and vomiting, and occasionally respiratory depression. Morphine and meperidine are the drugs most often used.

Because the pain of labor is a complex response composed of physiologic and psychological aspects, many nurses encourage women to use a combination of pharmacologic agents as described earlier and cognitive management to decrease anxiety and tension (Lowe, 1996). Keeping the woman focused and participating in the process of pain control helps decrease the need for medication, thus decreasing the fetal/neonatal side effects of such therapies. Cultural aspects of childbearing pain should also be considered in the management plan. A Chinese woman may experience a great deal of pain but remain stoic according to her tradition (Weber, 1996). The nurse, in this case, must rely on the knowledge of the laboring process and subtle cues to assess the degree of pain being experienced.

INDICATIONS FOR TESTING FOR FETAL WELL-BEING

The effects of labor on the fetus are numerous and frequently unpredictable. The nurse must remain constantly alert for any subtle changes in maternal or fetal condition that signify fetal compromise or distress. These changes may occur suddenly and with very little warning. Often only a small amount of time is available for nursing intervention. Therefore, tests for fetal well-being are routinely performed on the mother with a high-risk pregnancy during the antenatal period. The mother is ideally observed closely during the antenatal period, and the information gained from this time can be useful for planning care during the crucial labor and delivery period. The nurse must be aware of situations in which antenatal testing is indicated. Antenatal testing for fetal well-being is indicated in certain maternal conditions that have the potential for causing decreased uteroplacental perfusion, such as chronic hypertension and PIH, renal disease, collagen vascular disease, cardiac disease, and diabetes mellitus. Testing is also indicated when maternal conditions have the potential to cause intrinsic placental disease that leads to placental insufficiency, as in the case of diabetes mellitus or postdate pregnancy. Other high-risk pregnancies that require close monitoring include multiple pregnancy and those in which there is intrauterine growth retardation or hemolytic disease. Situations that would entail higher than usual risk for fetal death would also include decreased perception of fetal movement and a history of previous unexplained stillbirth (Polin & Frangipane, 1986).

Tests for fetal well-being have been divided into biochemical and biophysical categories.

Biochemical Tests

Biochemical tests are appealing because they may be completed in a simple, quick manner at various intervals during the antenatal and labor period. There has been an ongoing search for serum and urine indicators of fetal distress. Human placental lactogen (HPL) and estriol levels have been researched in relation to their usefulness in managing high-risk pregnancies, but neither measurement has been found to ensure fetal well-being or to predict fetal distress. The trend in maternal-child testing has been away from the reliance on biochemical parameters and toward biophysical antenatal testing.

Biophysical Profile

The biophysical profile is a noninvasive assessment system that allows for evaluation of the fetal status on the basis of five or six parameters, whereby each area receives a score. This system is based on the premise that varying degrees of hypoxia affect different brain centers and the longer the hypoxia is present, the more systems are affected. The later in gestation that a fetal system develops, the more sensitive that system is to decreasing amounts of oxygen. Because the central nervous system develops late in gestation, it is most sensitive to oxygen deprivation. Development of the medulla is completed during the end of the second trimester or the beginning of the third trimester. It is therefore capable of responding to decreased oxygen concentration by losing heart rate variability. The ventral surface of the fourth ventricle completes development at 20 to 21 weeks and is responsible for fetal breathing movements, which cease after loss of heart rate variability. Fetal motor movement begins after development of the cortex nuclei at about 9 weeks' gestation, and fetal muscle begins to develop tone at about 7.5 to 8.5 weeks.

All the components of the biophysical profile except for the nonstress test are done with ultrasonographic visualization. The original areas evaluated include

1. Nonstress test (NST). This test evaluates the response of the FHR to fetal activity or stimulation. With activity, the fetus normally increases its heart rate by at least 15 beats for 15 seconds. This normally is done several times in a 10- to 20-minute time period.
2. Fetal breath movements (FBMs). This test is done under ultrasonographic visualization and involves assessing the fetal chest and abdomen for breathing movements.
3. Fetal movement (FM). Movement of the fetal trunk is assessed.
4. Fetal tone. The fetus is evaluated for extension and flexion of the fetal body or extremities.
5. Amniotic fluid volume (AFV). The amount of amniotic fluid present is measured. The amniotic sac is scanned for the presence of pockets of fluid that measure at least 2 mm in two different planes.

Vintzileos and associates (1983, 1985) later added placental grading. Placental grading entails examination of the basal and chorionic plates of the placenta. A grade 0 placenta is immature; a grade III placenta is significantly aged and may not be functioning optimally (Gaffney et al., 1990).

Each area is evaluated with specific criteria for a score of 2, 1, or 0 points. The scores from all areas are then totaled and evaluated. A total score of 8 or better indicates a normal infant, with low risk of chronic asphyxia. With a total score of 4 to 7, chronic asphyxia is suspected, and less than 4 is strongly suggestive of chronic asphyxia (Manning et al., 1985). Vintzileos and associates (1983, 1985) had defined an abnormal biophysical profile as a score less than 6.

PREPARATION FOR BIRTH

Each of the numerous delivery options has indications for fetal well-being. When spontaneous vaginal delivery is feasible, this is the option of choice. But there may be indications for the performance of a cesarean section, the use of forceps, or the use of vacuum extraction.

Although cesarean section has become a relatively safe procedure, this mode of delivery has been associated with a higher risk of morbidity and mortality than has vaginal delivery. Cesarean delivery has been associated with increases in neonatal respiratory morbidity at all gestational ages, in fetal asphyxia related to uteroplacental hypoperfusion secondary to anesthesia induction or maternal position, and in inadvertent scalpel lacerations (Creasy & Resnik, 1994). The neonatal nurse must be aware of the possible complications of cesarean section and perform an adequate and immediate assessment of the neonate for such complications.

Another alternative to spontaneous vaginal delivery is the use of low forceps or midforceps delivery to facilitate the birth of the infant's head. The use of forceps may serve to avoid maternal exhaustion from prolonged pushing and may be used to enable a vaginal birth in a mother who otherwise might have to undergo a cesarean section. Potential complications that the nurse must be alert to include vaginal, cervical, and perineal laceration; uterine rupture; uterine atony and bleeding; bladder trauma; infection;

and trauma to the fetal head. The nurse must emotionally support the mother during the procedure, monitor the fetus during the delivery, and assess carefully for any postpartum complications.

Vacuum extraction is another alternative mode of delivery. Indications for this delivery option are similar to those for the use of forceps: arrest of labor during the second stage and maternal need for shortening of the second stage (maternal exhaustion, cerebral or cardiovascular disease, or fetal distress). Contraindications to the use of the vacuum extractor may include unengaged fetal head; face, brow, or breech presentation; cephalopelvic disproportion; incomplete dilatation of the cervix; and prematurity. Fetal complications may include cephalhematoma, retinal hemorrhage, and, in rare instances, intracranial hemorrhage (Creasy & Resnik, 1994). The nurse must closely monitor the mother and the fetus for any possible complications. The nurse also must explain to the patient and family that the presence of a caput succedaneum at the suction site is normal and should resolve within approximately 24 hours after the procedure.

Regardless of the mode of delivery, the nurse should explain to the family the rationale for the delivery option and be present to provide support to the family during the actual birth process. The nurse also has a responsibility to be well aware of the advantages and potential complications of each type of delivery and to assess the mother and fetus accordingly.

CRITICAL CARE OBSTETRICS

The increase in acuity of many patients, coupled with an expansion of knowledge and technology, has provided the foundation for the growth of the notion of critical care obstetrics. Preterm and, consequently, high-risk infants are surviving for longer periods after birth at earlier gestations than ever before. Both the mothers and the infants are at high risk and in need of more complex care that is based on an expanded level of knowledge and skill. In addition to fetal electronic monitoring, nurses are now asked to monitor the mother with cardiac monitors, invasive hemodynamic monitoring catheters such as Swan-Ganz, central venous pressure catheters, and arterial lines. In complicated cases, mechanical ventilatory assistance is also introduced into the labor and delivery or recovery suite.

Nurses in all types of settings are now responsible for developing a plan of care to be executed in critical care situations. In some settings there is a merging of the roles of the traditional labor and delivery nurse and the traditional critical care nurse. Some nurses welcome the challenge of developing their expertise in both specialties. Nurses respond to the challenge by combining experience in high-risk labor and delivery settings with experience in critical care units. The development of obstetrical intensive or special care units is an emerging trend, and this development provides an opportunity for an increased expansion of clinical nursing collaboration, as well as an opportunity for the expansion of nursing knowledge through collaborative nursing research efforts.

CONCLUSION

Many neonatal nurses do not have the opportunity to work in an antenatal or intrapartal area; however, what happens during these periods directly affects the type of neonatal problems encountered. With a brief review of some of the principles of the effects of labor on the fetus, anticipatory care can be given either by the practitioner trying to stabilize the neonate in the delivery room or by the neonatal nurse trying to prevent complications in the NICU. This chapter, along with Chapter 11, The High-Risk Pregnancy, gives a good overview of the perinatal conditions that potentially compromise neonatal well-being.

REFERENCES

Adelsperger, D., Carr, J., Davis, D., Feinstein, N., & Schmidt, J. (1993). *AWHONN Fetal Heart Monitor Principles and Practices.* Washington, DC: Association of Women's Health, Obstetrical, and Neonatal Nurses.

Blair, R. G. (1973). Abruption of the placenta: A review of 189 cases occurring between 1965 and 1969. *Journal of Obstetrics and Gynaecology of the British Commonwealth, 80*(3), 242–245.

Bobak, I. M., & Jensen, M. D. (1993). *Maternity and gynecologic care: The nurse and the family* (5th ed.). St. Louis: C. V. Mosby.

Creasy, R. K., & Resnik, R. (1994). *Maternal-fetal medicine: Principles and practice* (3rd ed.). Philadelphia: W. B. Saunders.

Edelstone, D. I. (1984). Fetal compensatory responses to reduced oxygen delivery. *Seminars in Perinatology, 8*(3), 184–191.

Finnegan, L. P. (1986). Neonatal abstinence syndrome: Assessment and pharmacotherapy. In F. F. Rubaltelli & B. Granati (Eds.), *Neonatal therapy: An update* (pp. 122–145). New York: Elsevier Science Publishers B.V. (Biomedical Division).

Freeman, R. (1979). *Fetal monitoring: Policy, protocol, pitfalls* (#327). Paper presented for the Network for Continuing Medical Education, Columbus Circle, NY.

Gaffney, S. E., Salinger, L., & Vintzileos, A. M. (1990). The biophysical profile for fetal surveillance. *American Journal of Maternal Child Nursing, 15*(6), 356–360.

Gimovsky, M. L., & Caritis, S. N. (1982). Diagnosis and management of hypoxic fetal heart rate patterns. *Clinics in Perinatology,* 9(2), 313–324.

Kaunitz, A. M., Hughes, J. M., Grimes, D. A., et al. (1985). Causes of maternal mortality in the United States. *Obstetrics and Gynecology, 65*(5), 605–612.

Lin, C. C., Lindheimer, M. D., River, P., & Moawad, A. H. (1982). Fetal outcome in hypertensive disorders of pregnancy. *American Journal of Obstetrics and Gynecology, 142*(3), 255–260.

Lowe, N. K. (1996). The pain and discomfort of labor and birth. *Journal of Obstetric, Gynecologic, and Neonatal Nursing, 25*(1), 82–92.

Manning, F. A., Morrison, I., Lange, J. D., et al. (1985). Fetal assessment based on fetal biophysical profile scoring: Experience in 12,620 referred high risk pregnancies. *American Journal of Obstetrics and Gynecology, 151*(3), 343–380.

May, K. A., & Mahlmeister, L. R. (1994). *Maternal and neonatal nursing: Family-centered care* (3rd ed.). Philadelphia: J. B. Lippincott.

Moore, K. L. (1989). *Essentials of human embryology.* Toronto: B. C. Decker.

Moore, K. L., & Persaud, T. V. N. (1993). *Before we are born: Basic embryology and birth defects* (5th ed.). Philadelphia: W. B. Saunders.

Murphy, P. A. (1990). Assessment of fetal status. In K. Buckley & N. W. Kulb (Eds.), *High risk maternity nursing manual* (pp. 44–58). Baltimore: Williams & Wilkins.

Murray, M. (1988). *Essentials of electronic fetal monitoring: Antepartal and intrapartal fetal monitoring.* Washington, DC: Nurses Association of the American Association of Obstetrics and Gynecology (NAACOG).

Pedersen, H. (1990). Analgesia and anesthesia during pregnancy and labor. In K. Buckley & N. Kulb (Eds.), *High risk maternity nursing manual* (pp. 425–431). Baltimore: Williams & Wilkins.

Polin, J. I., & Frangipane, W. L. (1986). Current concepts in management of obstetric problems for pediatricians. *Pediatric Clinics of North America, 33*(3), 621–646.

Robertson, W. B., Brosens, I., & Dixon, H. G. (1967). The pathological response of the vessels of the placental bed to hypertensive pregnancy. *Journal of Pathology and Bacteriology, 93*(2), 581–592.

Tervila, L., Goecke, C., & Timonen, S. (1973). Estimation of gestosis of pregnancy (EPH in midline-gestosis). *Acta Obstetricia et Gynecologica Scandinavica, 52*(3), 235–243.

Tournaire, M., Sturbois, G., Zorn, J., et al. (1980). Clinical monitoring before and during labor. In S. Adadjern, A. K. Brown, & C. Sureau (Eds.), *Clinical perinatology* (pp. 331–361). St. Louis: C. V. Mosby.

Vintzileos, A. M., Campbell, W. A., Ingradia, C. J., & Nochimson, D. J. (1983). The biophysical profile and its predictive value. *Obstetrics and Gynecology, 62*(3), 271–278.

Vintzileos, A. M., Campbell, W. A., Nochimson, D. J., et al. (1985). The fetal biophysical profile in patients with premature rupture of membranes: An early predictor of fetal infection. *American Journal of Obstetrics and Gynecology, 153*(6), 624–633.

Weber, S. E. (1996). Cultural aspects of pain in childbearing women. *Journal of Obstetric, Gynecologic, and Neonatal Nursing, 25*(1), 67–72.

SUGGESTED READINGS

Finster, M., Ralston, D., & Pederson, H. (1993). Perinatal pharmacology. In S. Shnider & G. Levinson (Eds.), *Anesthesia for obstetrics* (3rd ed.). Baltimore: Williams & Wilkins.

Gin, T. (1993). Pharmacokinetic optimisation of general anaesthesia in pregnancy [Review]. *Clinical Pharmacokinetics, 25*(1), 59–70.

Neonatal Resuscitation Program. (1994). Textbook of neonatal resuscitation. Dallas: American Heart Association and American Academy of Pediatrics.

Taylor, T. (1993). Epidural anesthesia in the maternity patient [Review]. *American Journal of Maternal Child Nursing, 18*(2), 86–93.

Wright, R., Shnider, S., & Fong, C. (1993). Fetal and neonatal effects of maternally administered drugs. In S. Shnider & G. Levinson (Eds.), *Anesthesia for obstetrics* (3rd ed.). Baltimore: Williams & Wilkins.

CHAPTER 15

Resuscitation and Stabilization of the Neonate

LINDA L. McCOLLUM

RESEARCH AGENDA

What is the appropriate management of vigorous neonates born through meconium-stained amniotic fluid?

Is the use of a laryngeal mask airway a viable alternative to endotracheal intubation in terms of oxygenation and ventilation efficacy, complications, training time, and cost?

What rate and duty cycle provide the most effective myocardial and cerebral perfusion during chest compressions?

What is the optimal dose of epinephrine given by endotracheal route?

What is the risk:benefit ratio of sodium bicarbonate administration in neonatal resuscitation?

What is the comparative efficacy of naloxone hydrochloride when it is given by IV, ET, IM, and SQ routes?

VIGNETTE

It started out as a quiet 12-hour shift with a few patients in the NICU. The call came. A high-risk maternity patient was coming, admitted for decreased fetal movement and a biophysical profile of 2. I knew that this meant a compromised baby, probably with severe asphyxia. The neonatologist, Dr. B, had just finished rounds, and I informed him of the situation. Karen, a neonatal nurse practitioner, was on call and would be attending the delivery along with me and Sally, another nurse colleague.

We went to L & D to review Mrs. H's history and gather any additional data. She was a 32-year-old primigravida at 33 weeks' gestation. The only notable prenatal risk factor was gestational diabetes. Mrs. H had noticed decreased fetal movement overnight and had contacted her doctor this morning. Fetal monitoring was instituted and showed a widely varying rate. Late fetal heart decelerations with subsequent loss of beat-to-beat variability developed as labor progressed. Severe fetal bradycardia ensued, and an emergency C-section was performed.

Karen introduced herself and spoke briefly to Mr. H, who was nervously pacing in the corridor. I reviewed the steps of resuscitation in my mind and did another quick assessment of the equipment in the room. We checked everything to make sure it was functioning properly. The anticipation of an asphyxiated infant always elicits some anxiety. An established plan helps each person know his or her primary responsibility. Karen stated that she would assess the airway and provide ventilation. I would assess the heart rate and provide chest compressions if needed. Sally would draw up medications, check for venous access, and act as the "rover." One of the L & D nurses said that she would document the resuscitation efforts.

The baby was born at 10:15 A.M. She was pale and limp, and she had no respiratory effort. She was immediately placed under a preheated radiant warmer and dried, and wet linen was removed. Next she was positioned, and the mouth and nose were suctioned. There was still no respiratory effort despite tactile stimulation. Karen began ventilating with 100 percent oxygen 40 to 60 times per minute. I checked for a heart rate at 30 seconds. It was 40, so I began chest compressions. After about 30 seconds of positive-pressure ventilation and chest compressions, I checked the heart rate while Karen stopped ventilating. "Heart rate 50," I stated. I then continued chest compressions as Karen prepared to intubate the baby. "How big is this baby?" "Oh, about 1500 grams," I responded. Karen requested and administered 0.3 ml of epinephrine per the ET tube. Ventilation and chest compressions continued.

After 30 seconds, I checked the heart rate. "Pulse 90 and increasing," I said. I stopped compressions while Karen continued ventilation. At this point, I evaluated vital functions: the oximeter read 60 percent saturation, the arteriosound blood pressure was 34/15, and the baby continued with poor peripheral perfusion. Sally had set up the tray for umbilical line placement. I took over ventilation while Karen placed both arterial and venous umbilical lines. An ABG, glucose, and hematocrit were sent immediately to the lab; 15 ml of Plasmanate was then given during about 5 minutes, followed by 3 mEq of $NaHCO_3$. The baby's perfusion improved slightly, and the BP increased to 42/30. The NICU was notified that a very sick baby was on the way. They needed to prepare monitoring equipment, an IV of $D_{10}W$, and a ventilator with settings of 100 percent oxygen, rate of 60, PIP/PEEP of 22/3. Chest and abdominal radiographs were also ordered.

Everything happens so quickly in a resuscitation! I reminded myself to fill out the resuscitation evaluation form. It always helps me to review the events and critique the process and outcome. Karen, Sally, and I would also sit down to review it later that day.

The BP continued to be critically low, so dopamine (to relax the peripheral vessels) and dobutamine (to improve myocardial function) were started. The nursing care of an asphyxiated newborn should include these goals:

1. To provide a smooth transition from intrauterine to extrauterine life
2. To provide a patent airway
3. To provide adequate ventilation
4. To assess cardiac status and maintain cardiac output
5. To provide a neutral thermal environment
6. To maintain metabolic homeostasis and correct hypovolemia
7. To obtain appropriate lab tests, as ordered
8. To keep parents informed
9. To assess and reassess the effects of interventions essential to success of a resuscitation

Marianne McGraw

The transition from intrauterine to extrauterine life is perhaps the greatest challenge any human can face in the course of a lifetime. If the fetus is healthy and at term, the necessary adaptations are generally made with little difficulty. On the other hand, if the fetus is premature or compromised, some assistance may be needed. It is estimated that 1 of every 16 newborns requires such support. If the infant is premature or of low birth weight, the need rises dramatically (American Heart Association [AHA], 1992; Bloom & Cropley, 1994).

CARDIOPULMONARY EXTRAUTERINE ADAPTATION

For successful transition to be made to extrauterine life, spontaneous breathing, independent system functioning, and successive cardiopulmonary changes must occur. Before delivery, the fetus relies solely on the placenta for all gas exchange and the excretion of metabolic wastes. Oxygenated blood flows from the placenta to the fetus through the umbilical vein. Once the vein has penetrated the fetal abdominal wall, it divides into two branches. One branch, the ductus venosus, carries about half of the blood directly to the inferior vena cava just below the diaphragm. The other branch carries the remaining incoming blood to the hepatic microcirculation; after perfusing the liver, this blood is drained by the hepatic vein into the inferior vena cava where it joins blood returning from the lower body. Interestingly, flow studies have demonstrated that there is relatively little mixing of blood coming from different sites. The ductal blood that bypassed the liver tends to flow along the dorsal and left wall of the inferior vena cava, whereas the blood from the liver and lower body flows along the ventral and right wall. When the blood reaches the right atrium, a flap of tissue known as the eustachian valve directs the better oxygenated ductal blood across the foramen ovale into the left atrium (right-to-left shunting). The desaturated blood from the liver and lower body as well as the desaturated blood in the superior vena cava (from the head and upper body) and the coronary sinus (from the heart) is directed across the tricuspid valve into the right ventricle (Friedman & Fahey, 1993).

In the left atrium, the blood that flowed across the foramen ovale is mixed with the small amount of blood returning from the collapsed, dormant fetal lungs. This admixture flows across the mitral valve into the left ventricle, then across the aortic valve to be carried away from the heart by the ascending aorta. Therefore, as a result of the ductus venosus, the flap-like eustachian valve, and the foramen ovale, the majority of blood in the aorta comes directly from the umbilical vein and is relatively well oxygenated. As this blood moves to and through the aortic arch, the arterial branches carry the oxygenated blood to the heart, brain, head, and upper torso. The small amount of remaining blood continues into the descending aorta (Friedman & Fahey, 1993).

The desaturated blood in the right ventricle crosses the pulmonary valve to enter the pulmonary arteries. However, because the pulmonary vasculature is constricted and highly resistant to flow, only about 12 percent of this blood actually enters the pulmonary circulation. The remaining 88 percent of the blood follows the path of least resistance through the ductus arteriosus into the descending aorta (Friedman & Fahey, 1993).

There are two sources of blood to the descending aorta: the small amount of blood that was carried through the aortic arch from the left ventricle, and the large amount of blood that was carried through the ductus arteriosus from the right ventricle. About a third of this admixture is carried through the trunk, abdomen, and lower extremities; the remaining two thirds enters the umbilical artery and is returned to the placenta to be reoxygenated (Friedman & Fahey, 1993).

In summary, circulatory flow within the fetus is determined by the presence of anatomic ducts, which allow the most highly oxygenated blood to be directed toward the myocardium and brain while desaturated blood bypasses the highly resistant lung beds in favor of the low-resistance pathway back to the placenta. With the clamping of the cord and the infant's first breath, this flow pattern drastically changes. As the chest is squeezed during delivery, the bulk of pulmonary lung fluid is evacuated up and out through the mouth. When the chest recoils, air is drawn into the lungs. With this first breath, the PO_2 and pH begin to rise and the pulmonary vessels begin to dilate. This progressive vasodilation causes a steady drop in pulmonary resistance, and the pressure in the pulmonary artery and right side of the heart falls. At this same time, systemic resistance abruptly rises when the placenta is lost. This increase in systemic resistance causes the blood pressure in the aorta and the left side of the heart to increase. The peripheral vasoconstriction in response to skin cooling combined with the increased amount of blood flowing through the lungs and returning to the left atrium further accentuates the increase in left-sided heart pressures.

As the right atrial pressure falls and the left atrial pressure rises, the flap of the foramen ovale is pushed against the atrial septum and is effectively closed. The ductus venosus also closes as the result of simple mechanical forces, the vessel walls collapsing on themselves as umbilical venous return is terminated. Constriction and closure of the ductus arteriosus, however, are predominantly dependent on the net effects of increasing oxygen and falling levels of prostaglandin E_2 (PGE_2). The rise in oxygen tension is, of course, associated with the onset of spontaneous and regular respirations. The fall in PGE_2 (which held the ductus open in utero) is thought to be due to the removal of the placenta, which is a site of PGE_2 production, as well as to the increased blood flow to the lungs, where PGE_2 is metabolized (Friedman & Fahey, 1993; Heymann, 1987).

ASPHYXIA

Asphyxia occurs when the organ of gas exchange fails or in some way is prevented from carrying out its intended function. For the fetus, that organ is the placenta; for the neonate, it is the lungs. When infants become asphyxiated, either in utero or after delivery, the immediate consequence is progressive hypoxia and hypercarbia with mixed (metabolic and respiratory) acidosis. Under conditions of profound hypoxemia, the body shifts from aerobic to anaerobic metabolism. The final product of this alternative energy-producing pathway is lactic acid. As this strong acid accumulates, metabolic acidosis develops. Simultaneously, the carbon dioxide levels in the blood are steadily building. Excess carbon dioxide combines with water to form carbonic acid, which leads to the development of respiratory acidosis. As the mixed acidosis worsens, the myocardium fails. The heart rate falls, followed shortly thereafter by a fall in blood pressure. Blood flow to the tissues is reduced, and the hypoxia, hypercarbia, and acidosis worsen.

The closest model for human response to asphyxia has been provided by Dawes' (1968) study of the rhesus monkey fetus and asphyxia. The well-defined sequence of events that was observed is depicted in Figure 15–1. Shortly after the onset of asphyxia, rapid gasping begins and is often associated with thrashing movements of the arms and legs and brief elevation of heart rate. If the gasping does not relieve the asphyxia within about a minute, all respiratory activity ceases (primary apnea) and the heart rate begins to fall. This period of primary apnea lasts about 60 seconds and is then followed by a series of spontaneous deep gasps. If the asphyxia persists, the gasping respirations become progressively weaker, stopping altogether after about 4 to 5 minutes. Secondary apnea (or terminal apnea) follows the last gasp, beginning approximately 8 minutes after the anoxic event began. The heart rate continues to fall, and hypotension develops; if the asphyxia is not reversed within several minutes, extensive organ damage and ultimately death occur (Banagale & Donn, 1986).

In the early stages of asphyxia, adults and children at least initially attempt to maintain perfusion (and hence oxygen delivery) by increasing their cardiac output. This maintenance is accomplished by increasing both the heart rate and the stroke volume. However, the fetus and newborn, in comparison, have relatively fewer myofibrils and so the heart is unable to stretch sufficiently to hold an increased volume. Because of their inability to effectively increase stroke volume, they can increase cardiac output only by increasing their heart rate. Unfortunately, the heart rate of the normal fetus and newborn is already relatively high, 100 to 160 beats per minute, so there is little room for improvement. Instead, the fetus compensates for this liability by massive peripheral vasoconstriction, preferentially shunting and maintaining blood flow to the heart, brain, and adrenals at the expense of organs such as the gastrointestinal tract, kidney, skin, and skeletal muscle. This compensatory mechanism is something akin to the "diving reflex" of submerging mammals. The fetal brain and heart normally receive approximately 7 percent of the cardiac output, but as much as 26 percent of cardiac output may be shunted to these organs during fetal hypoxemia to ensure adequate tissue oxygenation. The placenta also receives a greater proportion of the cardiac output, as much as 16 percent in the presence of hypoxemia in conjunction with acidosis (Woods, 1983). However, with worsening fetal hypoxemia and hypercarbia, even this compensatory mechanism fails, and the familiar cascade of events (acidosis, bradycardia, and hypotension) is set into motion.

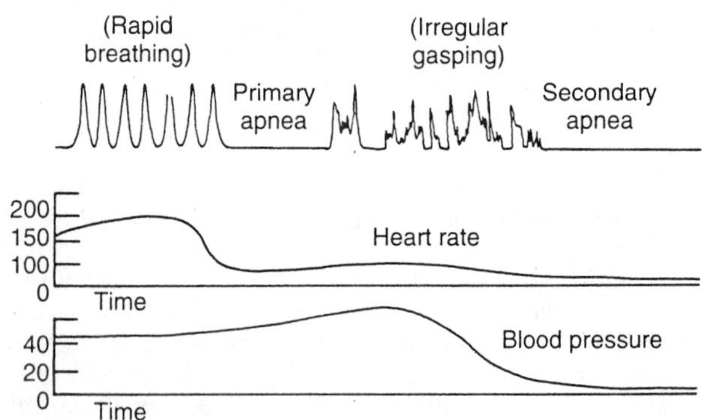

FIGURE 15–1. Effect of asphyxia on breathing, heart rate, and blood pressure. (From Bloom, R. S., & Cropley, C. [1994]. *Textbook of neonatal resuscitation* [pp. 1–5]. Elk Grove Village, IL: American Academy of Pediatrics and American Heart Association. Copyright American Heart Association, 1987, 1990, 1994.)

The passage of meconium in utero is estimated to occur in 10 to 15 percent of all fetuses and is considered a marker of antepartum or intrapartum asphyxia. Gasping by the fetus in utero can then cause aspiration. The pathophysiologic stimuli that trigger meconium passage are not clearly understood. It is generally thought to be due to some combination of vagal stimulation and hyperperistalsis after an episode of intestinal ischemia (Orlando, 1991; Wiswell & Bent, 1993). Meconium-stained amniotic fluid—and its potential sequela, meconium aspiration syndrome—may therefore be an unfortunate side effect of the diving reflex.

Ongoing monitoring of fetal status (by heart rate monitoring, scalp pH, or observation of meconium) allows early identification of the major clinical manifestations of fetal asphyxia. Once it is identified, every effort is made to expedite delivery so that the gas exchange functions can be transferred from the placenta to the lungs. Depending on how quickly this can be accomplished, the fetus may have already gone through primary apnea and be in secondary apnea at the time of birth. Practically speaking, it is difficult to differentiate primary from secondary apnea until after the event. Consequently, all newborns who are apneic or demonstrate evidence of cardiorespiratory depression should be treated as if they are in secondary apnea and provided urgent resuscitative care. Most infants who are in primary apnea resume breathing when they are stimulated and provided supplemental oxygen. On the other hand, infants who are in secondary apnea have been subjected to the asphyxiating event for a much longer time, long enough to exhibit signs of central nervous system involvement. They are hyporeflexive and hypotonic, and they are unresponsive to stimulation alone because the reflexes have been lost. These infants require ventilation and perhaps more aggressive therapy to maintain and improve their cardiorespiratory function.

The urgency of intervention cannot be overstressed. The closure of the foramen ovale and ductus arteriosus is at best tenuous until the sites become anatomically closed by fibrinous bands of tissue. Consequently, any event that causes delayed onset of respiration can potentially lead to hypoxia, hypercarbia, and acidosis. Under these circumstances, the pulmonary vasculature remains constricted and the pulmonary vascular resistance remains high, which in turn may cause a return to right-to-left shunting across the foramen ovale and ductus arteriosus as in perinatal circulation. If this occurs, blood will again largely bypass the lungs, but the placenta is no longer available for gas exchange. If this condition persists, the infant becomes progressively more hypoxic, hypercarbic, and acidotic, which produces a vicious circle of asphyxia from which the infant may not be able to escape.

CAUSES OF CARDIORESPIRATORY DEPRESSION IN THE NEWBORN

The condition of an infant at birth is determined by the combined effects of numerous maternal, fetal, and intrauterine factors. Some of these are listed in Table 15–1. It is at once obvious that although some of these factors arise only during the course of labor and delivery (cord prolapse, for instance), most come into being during gestation (e.g., placenta previa) or even before (e.g., maternal diabetes before conception). Regardless of the site or time of origin, the influence of each of these problems can become manifest as cardiorespiratory depression in the newborn.

To provide therapeutically effective care, the nurse must be able not only to recognize potential risk factors but to understand the ways in which they disrupt cardiorespiratory function. Although there are many potential risk factors, the underlying pathogenic processes can be divided into six major categories. The mnemonic TAMMSS can be used as a simple but effective way of remembering these etiologic groups:

T Trauma
A Asphyxia (intrauterine)
M Medication
M Malformation
S Sepsis
S Shock (hypovolemia)

Trauma

Traumatic injury to the central or peripheral nervous system is an infrequent occurrence that can result in either immediate or delayed respiratory depression. Because the skull is incompletely mineralized and has open sutures, it can undergo considerable distortion without fracture. However, the underlying membranes and vessels are much less resilient and are easily stretched or torn if they are overly compressed, particularly if the pressure is abruptly applied. Similarly, forced traction or torsion of the neck during delivery may damage the spinal cord or the phrenic nerve with consequent paralysis of the diaphragm. Unusually long and difficult labor, precipitous delivery, multiple gestation, abnormal presentation (especially breech), cephalopelvic disproportion (secondary to macrosomatia or a small or contracted pelvis), shoulder dystocia, or rapid extraction by forceps (as may be required for fetal distress) is frequently involved. Despite their generally low birth weight, premature infants may also be at risk because of the unusual compliance of their skulls.

Asphyxia (Intrauterine)

Of all the categories, the most common cause of cardiorespiratory depression at birth is fetal hypoxia and asphyxia. Any condition that reduces oxygen delivery to the fetus may be at fault. These factors include maternal hypoxia (due to hypoventilation or hyperventilation, respiratory or heart disease, anemia, postural hypotension, and so on), maternal vascular disease causing placental insufficiency (pre-existing or pregnancy-induced diabetes, primary or pregnancy-induced hypertension), and accidents involving the umbilical cord (compression, entanglement, or prolapse). Postterm pregnancies are also at risk, perhaps because of placental aging and progressive placental insufficiency. An asphyxial episode may occasionally trigger the passage and aspiration of meconium in utero.

TABLE 15–1 Conditions Associated With Asphyxiation of Newborns

Site or Source of Problem	Conditions
Maternal	Amnionitis Anemia Diabetes Pregnancy-induced hypertension Heart disease Hypotension Respiratory disease Maternal genetic Drugs Infection Maternal deformities
Uterine	Preterm labor Prolonged labor Multiple pregnancies Abnormal fetal presentations
Placental	Placenta previa Abruptio placentae Placental insufficiency Postterm pregnancy
Umbilical	Cord prolapse Cord entanglement Compression
Fetal	Cephalopelvic disproportion Congenital abnormalities Erythroblastosis fetalis Iatrogenic Mechanical Difficult forceps delivery Drugs Intrauterine infection

Medication

Pharmacologic agents given to the mother during labor and delivery may affect the fetus both directly and indirectly. Indirectly, these agents may cause maternal hypoventilation and hypotension or adversely affect placental perfusion. Hypnotic, analgesic, or anesthetic drugs may depress maternal respirations, resulting in reduced oxygen intake and delivery to the tissues and organs, including the uterus and placenta. Anesthetic agents, because of their effect on the sympathetic nervous system, may also cause peripheral vasodilation, decreased cardiac output, and hypotension with decreased placental perfusion. Oxytocin (Pitocin), on the other hand, may cause uterine hyperstimulation and reduced placental perfusion time. Each of these conditions, in turn, places the fetus at increased risk for fetal hypoxia and asphyxia. Furthermore, the narcotic analgesics, which rapidly cross the placenta, may directly depress neonatal respiratory drive.

Malformation

Infants may unfortunately exhibit a vast array of congenital anomalies, but the ones causing most concern during the first few minutes of life are those with associated facial or upper airway deformities and conditions leading to pulmonary hypoplasia. Whereas many of these conditions can be diagnosed by antenatal ultrasonography and other screening techniques, suspicion should also be raised if oligohydramnios or polyhydramnios is reported. Oligohydramnios is seen with prolonged rupture or leaking of membranes and in infants with renal agenesis or dysplasia or urethral obstruction. If fluid is lost or diminished, the developing fetal structures may be compressed, leading to characteristic Potter facies (including micrognathia) or pulmonary hypoplasia. Polyhydramnios is seen in infants who have impaired swallowing ability (those with anencephaly and neuromuscular disorders, for instance); in those with real or functional obstruction high in the gastrointestinal tract (e.g., esophageal atresia); and in those in whom large amounts of cerebrospinal fluid leaks, which contributes to the volume of amniotic fluid (as in neural tube defects). Polyhydramnios is also noted with diaphragmatic hernia and hydrops fetalis.

Sepsis

The fetus may acquire bacterial or viral agents from infected amniotic fluid, from maternal blood crossing the placenta, or by direct contact on passage through the birth canal. Premature infants (who are relatively immunocompromised), those with premature rupture of membranes, and those with a maternal history of infection or chorioamnionitis are especially susceptible. If infection is acquired in utero, the lungs tend to be heavily involved, and the alveoli may be filled with exudate. The infant may be apneic at birth, be slow to establish a spontaneous and regular breathing pattern, or exhibit frank signs of respiratory distress.

Shock (Hypovolemia)

Most of the blood lost during delivery is from the maternal side of the placenta and therefore is of no consequence to the newborn. However, blood loss from the fetal side of the placenta due to abruptio placentae or placenta previa can lead to acute hypovolemia and cardiovascular collapse. Whereas the normal umbilical cord is unusually strong, ruptures are possible if cord tension is suddenly increased (e.g., precipitous delivery) or if the vessels are superficially implanted into the placenta (velamentous insertions). Rarely, acute hypovolemia may occur without frank hemorrhage. With severe cord compression, for instance, blood flow to the fetus is impeded. The umbilical arteries, however, are much more resistant to compression and continue to pump blood back to the placenta. In this case, the effects of hypovolemia and asphyxia may be superimposed. Infants with chronic blood loss (e.g., from fetal-to-maternal hemorrhage or twin-to-twin transfusions) are generally asymptomatic immediately after delivery.

PREPARATION FOR DELIVERY

Success of resuscitation depends on three factors: (1) anticipation, (2) trained and available personnel, and (3) the necessary equipment and supplies. The most competent personnel and the finest equipment can be of no use if they are not present in the delivery room. Frantic calls for assistance or a scavenger hunt for equipment will needlessly delay intervention, can compromise the patient's outcome, and should not occur (Cropley, 1995).

Anticipation

The antepartum and intrapartum history of each pregnant woman must be carefully reviewed to identify those at risk for delivering a depressed infant. A fetus who clinically demonstrates the effects of asphyxia—nonreassuring fetal heart rate pattern (particularly bradycardia and loss of beat-to-beat variability), acidosis demonstrated by fetal scalp blood sampling, or meconium-stained amniotic fluid—is especially worrisome.

Personnel

Although most risk factors can be identified at some time during pregnancy, many may not become apparent until birth. Delivery through meconium-stained amniotic fluid and unexpected diaphragmatic hernia are just two cases in point. Consequently, at least one person competent in neonatal resuscitation should be present at every delivery. Obviously, additional personnel should be made available if a depressed newborn is expected (AHA, 1992; Bloom & Cropley, 1994).

When a team is required, the role each member is to play in the resuscitation should be predetermined. The "head" of the team is generally the person to establish and maintain the airway, the one responsible for ventilation and intubation. The second person is responsible for monitoring the heart rate and initiating chest compressions, if necessary. If intravenous (IV) medications are required, two additional persons will be needed—one to catheterize the umbilical cord and administer the drugs, the other to pass equipment and prepare the medications. The last individual may also be responsible for documenting the resuscitation process, but a fifth person is preferable because minute-to-minute notations must be made. The individual delivering the baby is not to be considered a part of the team.

Equipment and Supplies

The newly born infant is predisposed to heat loss (particularly evaporative and radiant losses) and, if unprotected, can quickly become cold stressed. The consequences of such stress include hypoxemia, metabolic acidosis, and rapid depletion of glycogen stores with hypoglycemia (see Chapter 16, Neonatal Thermoregulation). All are conditions that may exacerbate asphyxia and, in turn, make resuscitation more difficult. Clearly, measures to prevent hypothermia must be a part of any resuscitative effort. The delivery room should be kept warm, and the radiant bed should be preheated if possible. Prewarming of linens, towels, and caps (or other head coverings) is also helpful.

Possible exposure to blood and body fluids is of particular concern in the delivery room. Gloves, gowns, masks, and protective eyewear should be worn during procedures that are likely to generate droplets or splashes of blood or other body fluids (AHA, 1992).

The additional equipment and supplies needed to carry out a full resuscitation (Table 15–2) should be checked as a part of the daily routine. Small supplies should be organized according to their frequency of use and may be displayed on a wall board,

TABLE 15–2 Equipment and Supplies

Suction Equipment
Bulb syringe
Mechanical suction
Suction catheters: 5 French or 6 French, 8 French, 10 French
8 French feeding tube and 20-ml syringe
Meconium aspirator

Bag and Mask Equipment
Neonatal resuscitation bag with pressure-release valve or pressure gauge; the bag must be capable of delivering 90% to 100% oxygen
Face masks, newborn and premature sizes (cushioned rim masks preferred)
Oral airways, newborn and premature sizes
Oxygen with flowmeter and tubing

Intubation Equipment
Laryngoscope with straight blades, No. 0 (preterm) and No. 1 (term)
Extra bulbs and batteries for laryngoscope
Endotracheal tubes: 2.5-, 3.0-, 3.5-, 4.0-mm
Stylet
Scissors
Gloves

Medications
Epinephrine 1:10,000, 3-ml or 10-ml ampules
Naloxone hydrochloride: 0.4 mg/ml, 1-ml ampules; or 1.0 mg/ml, 2-ml ampules
Volume expander, one or more of these:
- 5% albumin–saline solution
- Normal saline
- Ringer's lactate

Sodium bicarbonate 4.2% (5 mEq/10 ml), 10-ml ampules
Dextrose 10%, 250 ml
Sterile water, 30 ml
Normal saline, 30 ml

Miscellaneous
Radiant warmer
Stethoscope
Cardiotachometer with electrocardiograph (oscilloscope desirable)
Adhesive tape, ½ or ¾ inch
Syringes: 1-, 3-, 5-, 10-, 20-, 50-ml
Needles: 25-, 21-, 18-gauge
Alcohol sponges
Umbilical artery catheterization tray
Umbilical tape
Umbilical catheters: 3.5 French, 5 French
Three-way stopcocks
Feeding tube, 5 French

From Bloom, R. S., & Cropley, C. (1994). *Textbook of neonatal resuscitation*. Elk Grove Village, IL: American Academy of Pediatrics and American Heart Association. Copyright American Heart Association, 1987, 1990, 1994.

kept in the radiant warmer (if there is sufficient drawer space), or stored in a cart or specially designed tackle box. Breakaway security clips may be used to safeguard materials when they are not in use, but foolproof or locking closures that require a key to open are not appropriate in delivery rooms, birthing rooms, or nurseries. A bedside table or flat surface (other than the bed) should be within reach to provide space for catheter trays and medication preparation. As the delivery nears, the team should double-check all supplies and make sure that the equipment is in working order. Hospital infection control policies dictate how far in advance packaged supplies can be opened, connected to tubing, and otherwise prepared. A back-up or duplicate set of materials should be maintained in case of equipment failure, contamination, or multiple births. Obviously, all items used should be restocked as soon as possible after a resuscitation (Cropley, 1995; Elliott, 1994).

GENERAL CONSIDERATIONS

The goals of resuscitation are (1) the removal or amelioration of the underlying cause of asphyxia and (2) the reversal or correction of the associated chain of events (hypoxia, hypercarbia, acidosis, bradycardia, and hypotension). To achieve these ends, resuscitation management should be centered on attempts to expand, ventilate, and oxygenate the lungs with cardiac assistance provided as necessary. However, intervention is infant specific in extent and form and must be determined by appropriate assessment.

Whereas the Apgar score provides a shorthand description of the infant's condition at specific intervals after birth and may be useful as a rough prognostic indicator of long-term outcome, it does have limitations. Although it is a quantitative tool, the scoring is often subjectively or retrospectively applied. It is often poorly correlated with other indicators of well-being, such as cord pH (Fields et al., 1983). Its usefulness is suspect with extremely preterm infants who may have poor respiratory drive and be relatively hyporeflexive and hypotonic because of immaturity rather than distress (Catlin et al., 1986). Finally, waiting until the first Apgar score is assigned at 1 minute of age causes unnecessary delay in care. For these reasons, the Apgar score should not be used to determine the need or course of resuscitation (AHA, 1992; Bloom & Cropley, 1994).

Instead, the initiation and conduct of resuscitation are based on three signs—the infant's respiratory effort, heart rate, and color. As soon as the infant is positioned under a radiant warmer, thoroughly dried, and suctioned, these signs are assessed at 30-second intervals with subsequent actions carried out accordingly. Figure 15–2 provides an overview describing the step-by-step approach currently recommended by the American Heart Association and the American Academy of Pediatrics.

AIRWAY CONTROL

Positioning

Airway control is a fundamental prerequisite for effective oxygenation and ventilation. To achieve this, the infant should first be placed in a flat supine position. The practice of placing the infant in a slight head-down tilt (Trendelenburg position) has been abandoned. This maneuver was historically used under the presumption that fluids from the lower extremities would be redistributed to the intrathoracic compartment. Studies with healthy adults in the Trendelenburg position have demonstrated improvement, albeit transient (<10 minutes), in the stroke volume of the heart but also indicated that as little as a 10-degree tilt may cause blood to pool in the dependent cerebrovascular

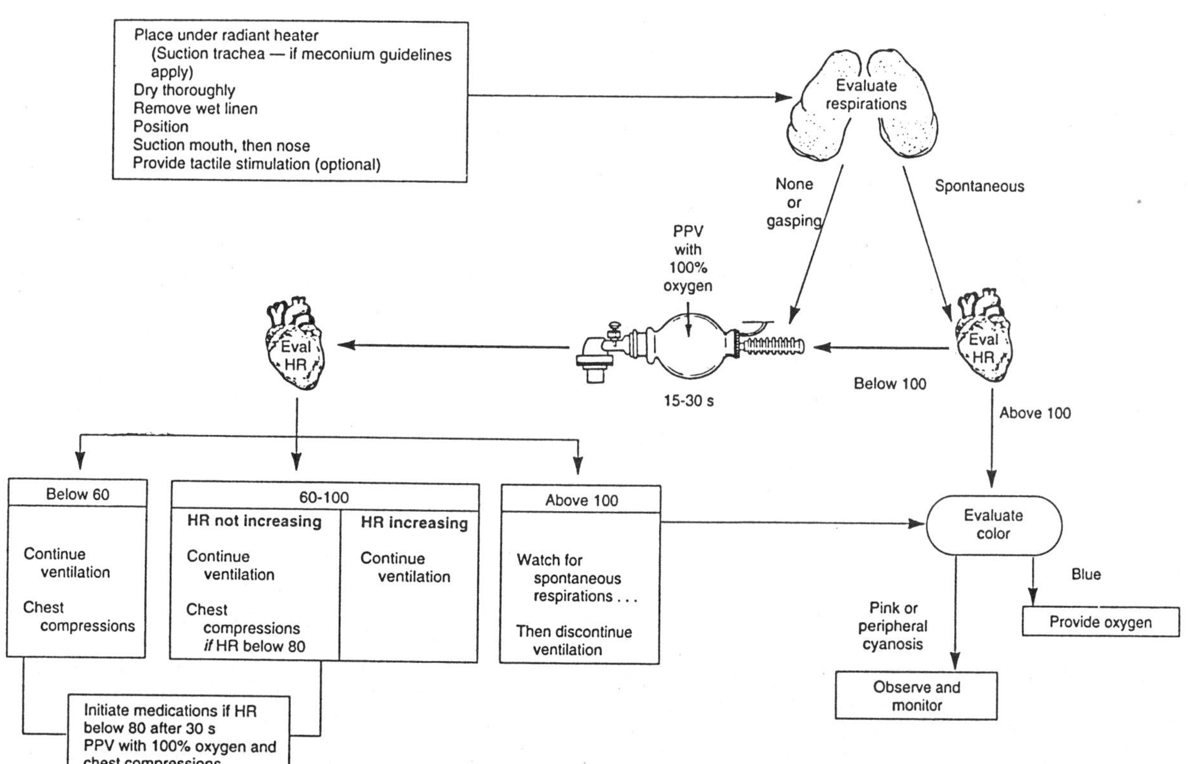

FIGURE 15–2. Overview of resuscitation in the delivery room. HR, heart rate; PPV, positive-pressure ventilation. (From Bloom, R. S., & Cropley, C. [1994]. *Textbook of neonatal resuscitation*. Elk Grove Village, IL: American Academy of Pediatrics and American Heart Association. Copyright American Heart Association, 1987, 1990, 1994.)

bed (Terai et al., 1995). Because infants are limited in their ability to increase stroke volume but are at increased risk for intraventricular hemorrhage secondary to rupture of the vulnerable microvessels of the germinal matrix, the potential benefit, if any, is not believed to be worth the risk.

Once the infant is in the supine position, the neck is placed in a neutral or slightly extended "sniff" position (AHA, 1992; Bloom & Cropley, 1994). Compared with the adult, the infant has a tongue that is relatively large in proportion to the mouth. This slight extension moves the tongue and epiglottis away from the posterior pharyngeal wall and opens the airway. Care must be taken to avoid full extension, however, because this causes narrowing of the airway caliber with increased airway resistance. The reasonably safe extension posture appears to be no more than 15 to 30 degrees from neutral (Reiterer et al., 1994; Todres, 1993). If the tongue is unusually large (e.g., Beckwith-Wiedemann syndrome) or the chin is unusually small causing posterior displacement of the tongue (e.g., Pierre Robin sequence or Potter's association), an oral airway should be placed. Because newborns also have a relatively large head in comparison with the chest and tend to naturally fall into a flexed position, a shoulder roll (¾ to 1 inch in thickness) may be used to raise the chest and align the cervical vertebrae. This roll may be particularly helpful if the occiput is exaggerated in size by molding or edema. If these procedures fail to provide an unobstructed airway, intubation is indicated (AHA, 1992; Bloom & Cropley, 1994; Todres, 1993).

Suctioning

If time permits, the mouth, nose, and posterior pharynx should be suctioned while the head is on the perineum before the thorax has been delivered. After delivery, the infant is placed on the bed, quickly dried, and positioned, and the airway is more thoroughly cleared with use of a bulb syringe. Because the process of suctioning may cause inadvertent stimulation and gasping, the mouth should always be suctioned before the nose. Mechanical suction is often mentioned as an alternative to the bulb syringe, but its use should generally be avoided immediately after delivery. A comparative study by Cordero and Hon (1971) demonstrated that 15 percent of infants suctioned with catheters during the first 5 minutes of life became apneic or developed significant arrhythmia (presumably due to vagal stimulation with reflex bradycardia), whereas none of the infants suctioned by bulb syringe was similarly affected. If mechanical suction is required (i.e., meconium removal), it should be applied for no more than 5 seconds at a time by use of an 8 or 10 French suction catheter and with the equipment set to produce no more than 100 mm Hg (136 cm H_2O) negative pressure (AHA, 1992; Bloom & Cropley, 1994).

If meconium is present in the amniotic fluid, endotracheal (ET) suctioning may be needed to achieve the most thorough clearing of the airway. This suction is performed *before* the infant is dried or otherwise stimulated and is conducted under laryngoscopy with suction directly applied to the trachea, using the ET tube as a suction catheter. Although there is some controversy regarding the benefit of ET suctioning if the infant is vigorous and the meconium is thin, it is generally recommended that suctioning be performed if the infant is depressed or the meconium is thick or particulate (Wiswell & Bent, 1993; Wiswell et al., 1990). The suction is applied as the ET tube is slowly withdrawn, and the procedure is repeated as needed until the meconium has been cleared. Techniques involving mouth suction should not be used because of the risk for exposure of personnel to blood and other body fluids. Also, passing a suction catheter through the ET tube or directly intubating the trachea with a suction catheter is an inadequate substitute for the ET tube. These catheters, with their small bore, are easily clogged with the thick, tenacious meconium (AHA, 1992; Bloom & Cropley, 1994).

TACTILE STIMULATION

Drying and suctioning generally produce enough stimulation to induce effective respirations in the mildly depressed infant. If the respiratory rate and depth are nevertheless diminished, the infant can be briefly stimulated by rubbing the spine or flicking or slapping the soles of the feet. If the infant's reflexes are intact, 10 to 15 seconds of stimulation should be sufficient to elicit a response. Longer and more vigorous methods of stimulation should be avoided (AHA, 1992; Bloom & Cropley, 1994).

OXYGENATION AND VENTILATION

Oxygenation and ventilation are the sine qua non of neonatal resuscitation. In fact, most infants who require resuscitation can be revived with oxygen and ventilation alone. Even when more aggressive therapies are required, they ultimately are undertaken to support oxygen delivery to the tissues—by optimizing the airway (i.e., intubation) or supporting the "pump" that "pushes" oxygen to the periphery (i.e., chest compressions, medications). Early administration of 100 percent oxygen is critical and may be delivered by multiple means. The potential risks associated with oxygen excess should not be a concern during the brief period required for resuscitation.

Free-Flow Administration

An infant who is breathing spontaneously but fails to become pink in room air needs supplemental oxygen. This supplemental oxygen can be provided directly from the end of the oxygen tube held in a cupped hand or by a funnel or face mask attached to the tubing or an anesthesia-type ventilation bag. The flow should be set to deliver at least 5 L/min, and the tubing, funnel, or mask should be held close to the infant's face to maximize the inhaled concentration (AHA, 1992; Bloom & Cropley, 1994).

Ventilation

If the infant still fails to become pink with free-flow oxygen or demonstrates other signs of cardiorespiratory decompensation (apnea or gasping respirations or heart rate less than 100 beats per minute), positive-pressure ventilation should be instituted. The initial breaths generally require pressures of 30 to 40 cm H_2O to inflate the lungs. Pressures for succeeding breaths vary with the condition of the infant. A ventilation rate of 40 to 60 breaths per minute should be used.

Ventilation Bags

Two types of ventilation bags are available for neonatal use—the self-inflating bag and the anesthesia bag. Self-inflating bags do not require gas flow for use but do require a reservoir to deliver high concentrations of oxygen. These bags are also traditionally fitted with a pressure-release "pop-off" valve that is preset at 30 to 40 cm H_2O pressure to prevent overinflation of the lungs and risk for pneumothorax. Most self-inflating bags must be squeezed to move gas through the circuit and may not be capable of passive, free-flow oxygen delivery.

Anesthesia bags, on the other hand, are closed systems and must therefore be connected to a compressed gas source before use. Whereas self-inflating bags have the advantage of being easy to operate and are gas flow independent, anesthesia bags provide more reliable oxygen concentrations (particularly at low flow rates), better control of inspiratory times, and greater range of peak inspiratory pressures and can be used to provide free-flow oxygen.

Both bags can be used to provide ventilation by either mask or

ET tube. Both can also be equipped with a manometer to monitor airway pressure, but visualization of the chest is equally if not more important. The degree of chest rise should simulate what one sees when the normal newborn takes an easy breath. Excessive chest rise reflects overzealous delivery of tidal volume; if there is no movement, delivery is inadequate. A bag with a maximal volume of 750 ml should be more than sufficient to deliver the normal tidal volume of 20 to 30 ml for the average newborn (AHA, 1992; Bloom & Cropley, 1994; Hermansen & Prior, 1993; Kain et al., 1993; Todres, 1993).

Methods of Ventilation

In mask ventilation, a face mask is used to provide an oxygen-enriched "microenvironment." An anatomically shaped mask with a cushioned rim is preferred. Because masks are available in a variety of sizes, care must be taken to select one that covers the tip of the chin, the mouth, and the nose but not the eyes. Mask ventilation is a simple, noninvasive method of oxygen delivery that can be initiated without delay, but use of a mask does have its disadvantages. First, it may be difficult to obtain and maintain a good seal between the mask and the infant's face, particularly around the nose. Any air leak will result in underventilation, which is further exaggerated when there is low lung compliance or high airway resistance (Todres, 1993). The seal should be "airtight" but without excessive application of pressure. Second, the mask itself has a considerable amount of dead space. Consequently, a sufficient tidal volume must be delivered to prevent accumulation and rebreathing of carbon dioxide. Masks used for neonatal resuscitation should ideally have a dead space of less than 5 ml. Finally, prolonged bag and mask ventilation may produce gastric distention from swallowed gas, which in turn impedes diaphragmatic excursions and places the infant at risk for regurgitation and aspiration. However, this final problem can be easily avoided by inserting an 8 French orogastric tube if mask ventilation continues beyond 2 minutes. The gastric contents should be suctioned and the tube left in place as a vent as long as mask ventilation is being provided (AHA, 1992; Bloom & Cropley, 1994).

Although mask ventilation suffices for most infants, if it has proved ineffective (as evidenced by poor chest rise or continuing bradycardia) or if prolonged ventilation is anticipated, an ET tube should be inserted. Premature infants (certainly those <1000 g) who have diminished lung compliance, immature respiratory musculature, and decreased respiratory drive may also benefit from early intubation (AHA, 1992; Bloom & Cropley, 1994). Indeed, research comparing outcomes for very low birth weight infants (≤1500 g) who were either selectively intubated at delivery or given a trial of spontaneous ventilation demonstrated that those who are immediately intubated have higher 5-minute Apgar scores, less acidosis, less hypoglycemia, and fewer pneumothoraces and require slower ventilatory rates (Drew, 1982). Infants with suspected diaphragmatic hernia, hydrops fetalis, or certain airway or gastrointestinal abnormalities also benefit from immediate intubation. Uncuffed tubes with a uniform internal diameter are to be used. The proper tube size (Table 15–3) and depth of insertion are determined by the infant's size by weight. Most neonatal ET tubes have a black line (vocal cord guide) near the tip of the tube that serves as a guide for insertion. When this guide is placed at the level of the vocal cords, the tube should be properly placed with its tip in the midtrachea. As an alternative, the distance from the midtrachea (tube tip) to the infant's upper lip may be calculated by use of the simple tip-to-lip formula:

$$\text{Weight (in kg)} + 6 = \text{tip-to-lip distance}$$

When the tube is properly situated, the centimeter marking on the side of the tube at the level of the upper lip should be at or near the tip-to-lip distance. That is, infants weighing 1 kg are intubated to a depth of 7 cm (1 + 6 = 7), those weighing 2 kg to a depth of 8 cm (2 + 6 = 8), and so on. Tubes with metallic markers or fiberoptic illumination at the tip may make it possible to transdermally determine the depth of the tube (by observing a circle of light on the skin or hearing an audible signal from a transcutaneous locator instrument), but these modifications do not allow one to differentiate between ET intubation and esophageal intubation and therefore offer no advantage in the emergency situation (Heller & Heller, 1994). Similarly, capnometers used during resuscitation to measure end-tidal carbon dioxide and thus confirm tube placement in the trachea may be inaccurate when pulmonary blood flow is poor or absent (Bhende & Thompson, 1995). Correct placement is best demonstrated by the "tried and true" methods—improved clinical signs (heart rate, color, and activity), symmetrical chest rise, bilateral and equal breath sounds (as auscultated in the axillae), and fogging of the tube on exhalation. Air should not be heard entering the stomach, and there should be no abdominal distention. If there are any doubts, tube placement can be checked by repeated laryngoscopy; the tube should be clearly seen passing through the glottic opening (AHA, 1992; Bloom & Cropley, 1994).

ET intubation is the definitive technique for airway management and ventilation. However, agility and accuracy in placement require ongoing practice. Also, many hospital personnel are restricted by policy or statute from learning or using the skill. The laryngeal mask airway (LMA), approved by the Food and Drug Administration in 1991, has been enthusiastically accepted in some settings as an alternative that offers most of the advantages of intubation but does not require laryngoscopy for placement. The LMA device (Figure 15–3) is a relatively long tube with a bag connector and inflation port at one end and an inflatable soft cuff at the other that is blindly passed into the hypopharynx so that the tip of the cuff lodges in the esophageal opening. Inflated, the cuff provides a seal around the larynx. The tube is then connected to a bag that delivers oxygen by ventilation through the central aperture of the laryngeal mask. Although little research has been conducted to compare LMA with ET tube use, particularly in the neonatal population, it appears that LMA under controlled circumstances can be as effective as but never more effective than intubation for ventilation. LMA placement is not necessarily easier than intubation. Studies have indicated wide variability in the successful placement of LMA on first attempt (68 to 100 percent by those with expertise in airway management), whereas reported success rates for intubation are generally always greater than 90 to 95 percent. Even when placement is initially successful, nearly a quarter of the infants with LMA subsequently develop airway obstruction, probably because of displacement during movement of the patient. The cuff provides only a low-pressure seal around the larynx, thereby placing a limit on the airway pressures that can be achieved during

TABLE 15–3 Endotracheal Tube Size and Placement

Weight (kg)	Tube Size (mm)	Insertion Depth (cm)
<1	2.5	<7
1–2	3.0	7–8
2–3	3.5	8–9
>3	3.5–4.0	>9

Data from American Heart Association Emergency Cardiac Care Committee and Subcommittees (1992). Guidelines for Cardiopulmonary Resuscitation and Emergency Cardiac Care (Part VII): Neonatal resuscitation. *Journal of the American Medical Association, 268* (16), 2276–2281; and Bloom, R. S., & Cropley, C. (1994). *Textbook of neonatal resuscitation.* Elk Grove Village, IL: American Academy of Pediatrics and American Heart Association. Copyright American Heart Association, 1987, 1990, 1994.

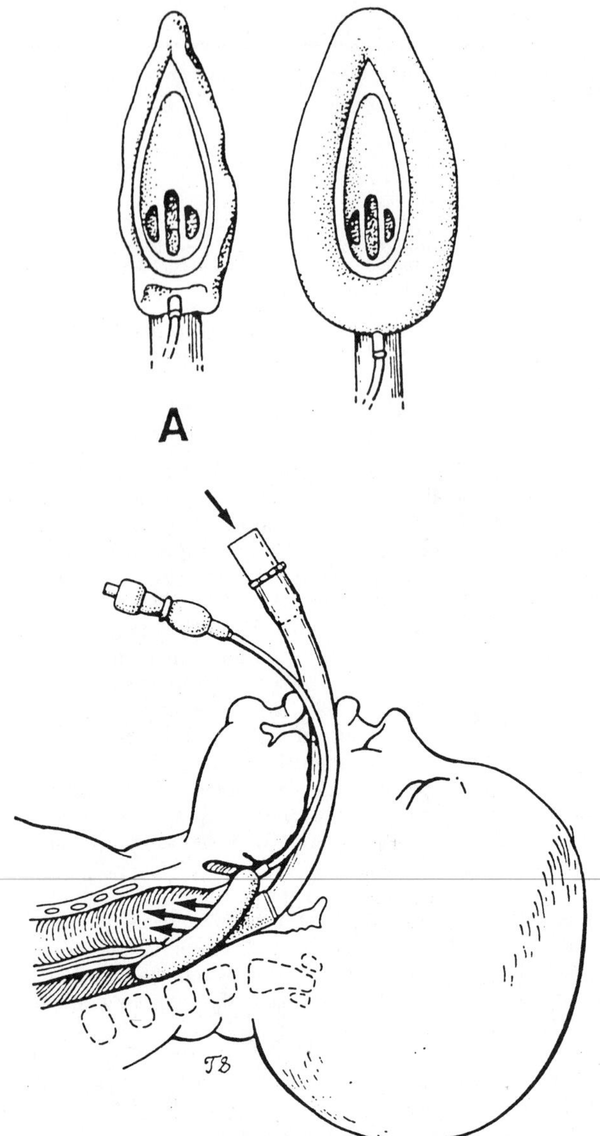

FIGURE 15–3. *A,* Laryngeal mask airway deflated for insertion *(left)* and with cuff inflated *(right)*. *B,* Laryngeal mask airway in position, with the cuff inflated around the laryngeal inlet. (From Efrat, R., Kadari, A., & Katz, S. [1994]. The laryngeal mask airway in pediatric anesthesia: Experience with 120 patients undergoing elective groin surgery. *Journal of Pediatric Surgery,* 29[2], 206–208.)

ventilation. Risk for gastric insufflation and regurgitation of gastric contents is reduced but not eliminated. Because of its size, current use is largely restricted to term infants, although successful use in very small infants (1.0 to 1.5 kg) has been anecdotally reported. The LMA does not provide access to the lower airway and is therefore not suitable for meconium removal or drug administration, nor does it preserve the airway during laryngospasm. Usefulness in neonates requiring chest compressions and in those with oropharyngeal disease or diaphragmatic hernia has yet to be assessed (Brimacombe, 1994, 1995; Brimacombe & Berry, 1995; Brimacombe & Gandini, 1995; Efrat et al., 1994; Lavies, 1993; Mizushima et al., 1992; Paterson et al., 1994; Pepe et al., 1993; Williams, 1995).

CHEST COMPRESSIONS

Chest compressions are rarely required as a component of resuscitation in the delivery room. They are performed in only 1 of every 1000 deliveries but are probably avoidable in the majority of these cases. According to one report, approximately one third of the infants who received compressions demonstrated biochemical evidence of asphyxia (acidemia), but the remaining two thirds were found to have a malpositioned ET tube or inadequate ventilatory support (i.e., insufficient rate or pressure). Clearly, the airway should be reassessed and respiratory support optimized before chest compressions are initiated (Perlman & Risser, 1995). Assuming these are satisfactory, chest compressions are begun if the heart rate is less than 60 or between 60 and 80 but not improving (AHA, 1992; Bloom & Cropley, 1994).

When used, chest compressions provide temporary support to circulation and oxygen delivery. Pressing on the sternum achieves two ends. First, the heart is compressed against the vertebral column. Second, the intrathoracic pressure is increased. Both effects cause blood to be pushed out of the heart into the arterial circulation. When the sternal pressure is released, the ventricles return to their original shape, intrathoracic pressure falls toward zero, and venous blood is pulled into the heart by a suction effect (Bloom & Cropley, 1994; Chandra, 1993; Elliott, 1994).

Either of two techniques may be used to perform chest compressions. The first is the thumb method. Both hands encircle the chest, the fingers support the back, and the thumbs (pointing cephalad either side-by-side or one on top of the other, depending on the size of the infant) are used to press the sternum downward. The second is the two-finger method. One hand supports the back from below while two fingers of the free hand are held perpendicular to the chest and the fingertips are used to apply downward pressure on the sternum. Comparative studies have demonstrated that higher systolic blood pressure, higher diastolic blood pressure, higher mean arterial pressure, and higher coronary perfusion pressure are generated with less external compression force when the thumb method is used. There are also fewer reports of trauma to the liver and other abdominal organs. Moreover, the thumb method is perhaps easier and certainly less tiring to perform (David, 1988; Menegazzi et al., 1993; Todres & Rogers, 1975). The thumb method is therefore preferred, but the two-finger method may be necessary if the hands are too small to properly encircle the chest or if access to the umbilicus is needed to facilitate placement of an umbilical venous catheter (UVC) for administration of emergency drugs (Bloom & Cropley, 1994; Elliott, 1994).

For both methods, the pressure is applied to the lower third of the sternum (just below the nipple line but above the xiphoid process) where the right ventricle lies closest to the sternum (Finholt et al., 1986). Just enough force is used to depress the sternum ½ to ¾ inches (AHA, 1992; Bloom & Cropley, 1994). Research indicates that myocardial and cerebral blood flow are optimal when the downward stroke and release phases of the compression are equal in time (Chandra, 1993). This equalization of the compression phases is best accomplished with a smooth, nonjerky rhythm.

Positive-pressure ventilation with 100 percent oxygen must be continued while chest compressions are performed. The most recent guidelines recommend interposing chest compressions with ventilations at a 3:1 ratio. Every fourth compression is dropped to allow delivery of a single, effective breath. During the course of a full minute, 90 compressions and 30 ventilations are given (AHA, 1992; Bloom & Cropley, 1994). Whereas faster rates have been recommended in the past, such rates only increase the chance of administering simultaneous compressions and ventilations (Bloom & Cropley, 1994; Trautman, 1995). Most research indicates that simultaneous delivery increases the intrathoracic pressure to such a level that ventilation is impeded and coronary perfusion is reduced. Whether there is any effect on cerebral blood flow is equivocal, but at least one research group has reported lower survival rates when simultaneous compression and ventilation was provided (Berkowitz et al., 1989; Burchfield et al., 1994; Krischer et al., 1989; Swenson et al., 1988).

Newer, experimental techniques—external circulatory assist devices (e.g., mechanical "thumpers," pneumatic vests, and abdominal binders), counterpoint abdominal compressions (e.g., cough cardiopulmonary resuscitation), and active decompression (e.g., plumber's plunger)—have shown promise in animal studies. However, few large-scale clinical trials have been conducted, and those that have been carried out have been limited to adults in selected settings (Babbs, 1993; Hoekstra et al., 1995; Niemann et al., 1985; Rudikoff et al., 1980; Ward et al., 1993; Wenzel et al., 1995). Consequently, use of these tools in neonatal resuscitation cannot be advocated at this time.

MEDICATIONS

Epinephrine

Epinephrine is a direct-acting catecholamine with both alpha-adrenergic and beta-adrenergic effects (Table 15–4). These lead to peripheral vasoconstriction, acceleration of the heart rate, and increase in the forcefulness of cardiac contractions. The net effect is a sharp rise in blood pressure (pressor effect) and increased cardiac output. Also, the marked pressor effect in combination with the increased aortic diastolic pressure in turn increases cerebral and myocardial perfusion pressure, thereby maintaining blood flow to these critical organs during resuscitation (Berkowitz et al., 1991; Zaritsky & Chernow, 1984). Epinephrine is therefore considered the drug of choice with asystole or persistent bradycardia (heart rate <80) despite adequate ventilation with 100 percent oxygen and chest compressions. For newborns, the recommended dose is 0.1 to 0.3 ml/kg of 1:10,000 solution (0.01 to 0.03 mg/kg) (AHA, 1992; Bloom & Cropley, 1994). The drug is rapidly inactivated by an enzymatically driven process known as sulfoconjugation wherein the active compound is bound to (conjugated with) sulfate (Schwab & von Stockhausen, 1994). The half-life of infused epinephrine is approximately 3 minutes (Fitzgerald et al., 1980). Consequently, the dose may be repeated every 3 to 5 minutes as clinically indicated.

Administration is by either ET or IV/UVC routes. Because IV/UVC placement may be difficult and time-consuming during resuscitation, initial doses tend to be given by ET tube. Unfortunately, absorption into the circulation from the pulmonary capillary bed may be highly variable because of the low blood flow state associated with resuscitation. In addition, much of the ET-instilled drug remains along the walls of the ET tube and in the conducting airways with a relatively small amount finding its way into the deep absorptive surfaces of the alveoli (Orlowski et al., 1990; Ralston et al., 1985). However, a number of steps can be taken to aid delivery when the ET route is necessary. First, to optimize blood flow to the lungs, every effort must be made to ensure that chest compressions are being effectively performed. Second, epinephrine may be dispersed more quickly to deeper pulmonary tissues by diluting the drug and following the instillation with a few forceful ventilations or a small amount of flush. When diluted, the medication should be mixed with a sufficient amount of normal saline to produce a final volume of 1 to 2 ml (AHA, 1992; Bloom & Cropley, 1994; Ralston et al., 1985; Zaritsky, 1993). Alternatively, some individuals prefer to administer the drug through a 5 French feeding tube positioned through the ET tube. Theoretically, the smaller lumen feeding tube would have less surface area for the drug to cling to, but the actual clinical significance, if any, is unknown. In view of the erratic absorption, subsequent doses should be given by the IV/UVC route as soon as access is achieved. In the rare situation when line placement is unattainable and the infant has failed to respond to standard doses given by the ET route, higher doses of 1 to 2 ml/kg (0.1 to 0.2 mg/kg) may be considered (AHA, 1992; Bloom & Cropley, 1994).

Although higher doses of epinephrine administered by the ET route may have a role in the exceptional situation, the routine IV/UVC administration of high-dose epinephrine is not recommended in the newborn. Although studies with adults and older children have demonstrated a dose–response relationship, with

TABLE 15–4 Effects of Stimulation of the Autonomic Nervous System*

Site	Adrenergic (Sympathetic) Effects: *Alpha-Receptors*	*Beta-Receptors*	*Dopaminergic Receptors*	Predominant Parasympathetic (Cholinergic) Effects
Heart				
SA node	—	↑ Heart rate	—	↓ Heart rate
AV node	—	↑ Conduction velocity	—	↓ Conduction velocity
Cardiac muscle	—	↑ Contractility	—	↓ Contractility
Lungs				
Bronchial muscle	Constrict	Relax	—	Constrict
Arteries				
Coronary	Constrict	Dilate	Dilate	Constrict
Pulmonary	Constrict	Dilate	?	—
Cerebral	Constrict	—	Dilate	Dilate
Renal	Constrict	Dilate	Dilate	—
Veins	Constrict	Dilate	Constrict	—

* The actions of the autonomic nervous system, which innervates cardiac muscle, smooth muscle, and the glands, depend on three factors: (1) the subdivision of the autonomic system (sympathetic versus parasympathetic) that is involved, (2) the chemical transmitter secreted at the nerve ending to carry the neural message across the synaptic gap, and (3) the type of receptor that is found within the cell membranes of the target organs. Parasympathetic nerve endings secrete acetylcholine and are therefore also known as cholinergic fibers. Receptors that are activated by acetylcholine are referred to as cholinergic receptors. Sympathetic nerve endings release both epinephrine (adrenaline) and the dopamine derivative norepinephrine (noradrenaline) and are therefore called adrenergic fibers. Receptors that are responsive to these substances are referred to as adrenergic receptors. Although an organ may contain more than one type of receptor, where two or more receptors coexist, one type generally occurs in greater density and thus its activity predominates. *Note*: In terms of molecular structure, the adrenergic transmitter substances are all dihydroxybenzenes (benzene with two OH groups) with an attached amine (nitrogen-containing group). The chemical name for a dihydroxybenzene is catechol. Therefore, these and structurally related substances are often referred to as catecholamines.

SA, sinoatrial; AV, atrioventricular.

Data from Zaritsky, A., & Chernow, B. (1984). Use of catecholamines in pediatrics. *Journal of Pediatrics, 105*(3), 341–350.

higher doses bringing about greater improvements in coronary and cerebral blood flow (Barton & Callaham, 1991; Goetting & Paradis, 1991; Gonzalez et al., 1989; Paradis et al., 1991), the efficacy and safety of high-dose IV/UVC epinephrine has not been adequately evaluated in the neonate. Most of these studies have been conducted with patients with a history of coronary artery disease presenting in ventricular fibrillation. Neonates, however, more commonly exhibit bradycardia due to hypoxia. These pathophysiologic differences prevent extrapolation of findings. Furthermore, administration of high doses has generally been followed by a prolonged period of hypertension. Because the newborn, particularly the prematurely born, has a vascular germinal matrix, the risk for intraventricular hemorrhage may be increased. In fact, this area of the brain is most susceptible to hemorrhage when hypertension is preceded by hypotension, which is the case with resuscitation (AHA, 1992; Burchfield, 1993). Consequently, at present, only the standard dose of epinephrine (0.1 to 0.3 ml/kg) should be given by the IV/UVC route.

Volume Expanders

Use of volume expanders is indicated when there is evidence or suspicion of acute blood loss with signs of hypovolemia. These signs include pallor in spite of oxygen therapy, hypotension with weak pulses despite a normal heart rate, and failure to respond to resuscitation (AHA, 1992; Bloom & Cropley, 1994). Low hematocrit and hemoglobin concentrations are diagnostic of blood loss, but the levels may be misleadingly normal immediately after acute loss. In general, it takes about 3 hours for a sufficient amount of fluid to shift from the interstitial to the intravascular space and produce the degree of compensatory hemodilution that would be reflected by a fall in laboratory values (Oski, 1993).

The basic requirement for any replacement solution is that its electrolyte and protein composition be roughly equivalent to that which was lost (Wayne & Fosburg, 1993). Otherwise, an osmotic pressure gradient is created and fluids are driven out of the capillaries into the interstitial tissue. The expansion of circulatory volume is only transient, and the infant is placed at risk for secondary problems, particularly pulmonary edema. Clearly, whole blood is the fluid of choice for volume replacement and offers the added benefit of oxygen-carrying capacity. Fresh O-negative blood crossmatched against the mother should be used. When blood is not readily available, 5 percent albumin-saline (or other plasma substitute) or isotonic fluids (normal saline or Ringer's lactate) may also be used (AHA, 1992; Bloom & Cropley, 1994). Glucose-containing fluids, such as D_5W or $D_{10}W$, should not be given by bolus because of the risk for profound hyperglycemia (Zaritsky, 1993). Hyperglycemia in the presence of untreated asphyxia may also aggravate metabolic acidosis (Jacobs & Phibbs, 1989; Williams et al., 1993).

For emergency treatment of hypovolemia, 10 ml/kg of volume expander is given slowly during 5 to 10 minutes by the IV/UVC route (AHA, 1992; Bloom & Cropley, 1994). Rapid infusion must be avoided because abrupt changes in vascular pressure in the vulnerable matrix capillaries place the infant, and especially the preterm infant, at increased risk for intraventricular hemorrhage (Volpe, 1989). The response is usually dramatic, with a prompt improvement in blood pressure, pulses, and color. If the signs of hypovolemia continue, however, a second volume replacement may be given. Persistent failure beyond this point probably indicates some degree of "pump failure," and further improvement is not likely to occur until cardiac function is improved. In fact, excessive volume administration may so engorge the heart and overstretch the cardiac muscle fibers that the strength of contractions is actually decreased. Use of sodium bicarbonate (to correct metabolic acidosis) or an inotropic agent (such as dopamine) should be considered (Bloom & Cropley, 1994).

Dopamine

When vascular volume has been restored but hypotension still exists because of myocardial decompensation (pump failure), dopamine may be used to increase cardiac output, increase blood pressure, and increase peripheral and organ perfusion. Dopamine, a precursor of norepinephrine, is a naturally occurring catecholamine with alpha-adrenergic, beta-adrenergic, and dopaminergic effects (see Table 15–4). The beta effects are elicited both directly (by direct interaction with the receptors) and indirectly (by releasing norepinephrine, which in turn interacts with receptors). The effects of dopamine are complex and dose related. In general, low doses (<2 μg/kg/min) primarily stimulate dopaminergic receptors. Moderate doses (2 to 10 μg/kg/min) activate dopaminergic receptors. High doses (>15 to 20 μg/kg/min) activate all three adrenergic receptors, but alpha stimulation negates the effect of beta stimulation (Crockett & Tappero, 1989; Driscoll, 1987; Keeley & Bohn, 1988; Young & Mangum, 1997; Zaritsky & Chernow, 1984).

Dopamine is metabolized rapidly with a serum half-life of 2 to 5 minutes. Duration of action is less than 10 minutes. Consequently, it must be given by continuous IV infusion. When used after a prolonged resuscitation, dopamine is infused at an initial dose of 5 μg/kg/min and titrated in increments of 3 to 5 μg/kg/min up to 20 μg/kg/min maximum until the blood pressure and perfusion improve. Heart rate and rhythm and blood pressure must be continuously monitored. Dopamine, like all catecholamines, is inactivated by alkaline solution and should therefore not be mixed with sodium bicarbonate (Bloom & Cropley, 1994; Crockett & Tappero, 1989; Young & Mangum, 1997).

Sodium Bicarbonate

Of the biochemical events that result from asphyxia, the most significant is the conversion from aerobic to anaerobic metabolism with the production of lactic acid. As this strong acid accumulates, metabolic acidosis develops and myocardial contractility is decreased, hypotension worsens, and the cardiac response to catecholamines is diminished (Burchfield, 1993; Leuthner et al., 1994; von Planta et al., 1993). The best treatment for acidosis in this circumstance is directed toward its cause—hypoxemia. Immediate therapy includes ventilation with 100 percent oxygen and cardiac compressions to restore blood flow and tissue oxygenation. However, if the resuscitation is prolonged and the infant remains unresponsive, alkali therapy may be helpful (AHA, 1992; Bloom & Cropley, 1994). Sodium bicarbonate is the most frequently used alkalinizing agent.

Sodium bicarbonate ($NaHCO_3$) is a physiologic buffer. When it is added to a solution of strong acid, such as hydrochloric acid (HCl), the bicarbonate anion (HCO_3^-) combines with the hydrogen ion (H^+) from the acid to form the weaker carbonic acid (H_2CO_3) and a neutral salt, such as sodium chloride (NaCl):

$$HCl + NaHCO_3 \rightarrow H_2CO_3 + NaCl$$

The carbonic acid rapidly dissociates into water (H_2O) and carbon dioxide (CO_2). The dissolved carbon dioxide is then transported by the blood to the lungs, where it is eliminated:

$$H_2CO_3 \rightarrow H_2O + CO_2$$

Although it was historically considered a pharmacologic mainstay in neonatal resuscitation, a growing body of research suggests that sodium bicarbonate administration may actually be counterproductive and possibly injurious (Hein, 1993; Howell, 1987). First and foremost, effective removal of carbon dioxide by the lungs is dependent on both ventilation and pulmonary blood flow. If either is inadequate (which is frequently the case during resuscitation), carbon dioxide accumulates with a shift from metabolic to respiratory acidosis without any real resolution of acid–base balance (Burchfield, 1993; Leuthner et al., 1994; Ostrea & Odell, 1972). Second, carbon dioxide diffuses across cell membranes much more rapidly and easily than does bicarbonate. That is, carbon dioxide quickly moves out of the capillaries into cells while bicarbonate lags behind in the intravascular space. Blood pH rises, but intracellular pH transiently falls. Thus, when the cells of the heart are involved, intramyocardial acidosis worsens and cardiac performance is further diminished (Burchfield, 1993; Graf et al., 1985; Kette et al., 1990; Leuthner et al., 1994). Other potential consequences of sodium bicarbonate administration include intraventricular hemorrhage (due to rapid infusion of hypertonic solution) and hypernatremia (Papile et al., 1978; Simmons et al., 1974).

Clearly, administration of sodium bicarbonate should not be undertaken lightly and is, in fact, discouraged for brief resuscitation or episodes of bradycardia (AHA, 1992). Its use is reserved for prolonged arrest unresponsive to other therapy, and then only after effective ventilation and compressions have been established. The dose currently recommended is 4 ml/kg of 4.2 percent solution (2 mEq/kg) by the IV/UVC route. This hypertonic solution contains 0.5 mEq/ml and should therefore be given slowly during at least 2 minutes (1 mEq/kg/min) (Bloom & Cropley, 1994). At the first opportunity, samples for blood gas analysis should be drawn from whatever site is available to confirm metabolic acidosis.

Naloxone

Narcotic analgesics administered to mothers provide an effective means of pain control during labor. Unfortunately, these lipid-soluble drugs rapidly cross the placenta and can therefore cause neonatal respiratory depression. Peak fetal narcotic levels occur 30 minutes to 2 hours after administration to the mother. The degree and duration of depression exhibited by the newborn depend on the dose, route, and length of time before delivery that the drug is given. Affected infants present with decreased respiratory effort and muscle tone but typically have a good heart rate and perfusion. If these signs are demonstrated and the mother has received a narcotic within 4 hours of delivery, a narcotic antagonist should be given (AHA, 1992; Bloom & Cropley, 1994; Wimmer, 1994).

Naloxone hydrochloride is a synthetic narcotic antagonist designed to reverse narcotic-induced respiratory depression. It acts by competing with narcotics for their receptor sites in the central nervous system. As a pure competitive antagonist, it binds with but does not activate receptors. Consequently, in the absence of narcotics, naloxone exhibits essentially no pharmacologic activity (Evans et al., 1976; Handal et al., 1983; Young & Mangum, 1997).

Naloxone is available in ampules at a variety of concentrations; however, the American Academy of Pediatrics Committee on Drugs currently recommends use of either the 0.4 mg/ml or 1.0 mg/ml preparation. Neonatal naloxone (0.02 mg/ml) should not be used because of the fluid volume that would be given. The dose is 0.1 mg/kg and may be repeated every 2 to 3 minutes as needed. Administration by the IV/UVC or ET routes is preferred, but it can also be given intramuscularly (IM) or subcutaneously (SQ) because affected newborns generally have good perfusion. The most rapid onset of action is obtained by the IV/UVC route (generally apparent within 2 minutes), but IM injection produces a more prolonged effect. Adequate ventilatory assistance must be provided until reversal is complete. Close monitoring should continue for 4 to 6 hours after administration. Because naloxone is rapidly metabolized by the liver, the duration of its effect may be shorter than that of some narcotics and respiratory depression may recur. If signs reappear, additional doses of naloxone should be given (American Academy of Pediatrics Committee on Drugs, 1989, 1990; AHA, 1992; Bloom & Cropley, 1994; Wimmer, 1994). Although naloxone has no known short-term toxic effects, it is contraindicated in infants born to narcotic-dependent mothers. Because abrupt and complete reversal of narcotic effect may precipitate seizures (withdrawal reaction), assisted ventilation is provided in this circumstance until the respiratory drive is adequate (AHA, 1992; Bloom & Cropley, 1994; Young & Mangum, 1997).

Because several studies have suggested that hypoxia and acidosis stimulate the release of endogenous opiates (endorphins), it has been theorized that these endorphins might accentuate the depressing effect of hypoxemia on the cardiorespiratory system. However, clinical trials of naloxone administration to infants with 1-minute Apgar scores of 6 or less have demonstrated no effect on either spontaneous respiratory frequency or heart rate (Chernick & Craig, 1982; Chernick et al., 1988; Wardlaw et al., 1979).

Other Drugs

Calcium ions play a critical role in the depolarization of cardiac pacemaker cells in the sinoatrial and atrioventricular nodes, and the movement of calcium into and within the cells of the cardiac and vascular smooth muscle accelerates and maintains the chemical reactions necessary for muscle contraction. As a result, administration of calcium salt (e.g., calcium gluconate, calcium chloride) has been widely recommended in the past to increase heart rate, improve myocardial contractility, and raise blood pressure during resuscitation (Proano et al., 1995). Although it is theoretically plausible, several studies have failed to demonstrate the anticipated improvement in cardiovascular function (Dembo, 1981; Stueven et al., 1984). On the other hand, adverse side effects have been reported even at standard doses (Kuhn, 1991). Although preterm and sick newborns may develop hypocalcemia in the first week of life from a variety of causes, low calcium levels are rarely if ever exhibited at birth because calcium is actively transported across the placenta from mother to fetus. Administration of calcium in the first few minutes of life may therefore produce dangerously high serum calcium levels. Pacemaker blockade, bradycardia, and even arrest may result from fatigue after excessive and sustained stimulation. Moreover, high intracellular free calcium levels have been implicated in the activation of aberrant enzyme systems, intracellular release of free fatty acids, generation of oxidative free radicals, and cerebral arterial spasm, which may trigger many of the undesirable consequences of asphyxia (Clark, 1989; Palmer & Vannucci, 1993; White et al., 1983). In summary, no data are currently available to support the use of calcium, but a considerable amount of evidence indicates that it may actually be deleterious. Whereas administration may be appropriate in other circumstances as therapy for documented hypocalcemia or to antagonize the adverse effects of hyperkalemia or hypermagnesemia, calcium should not be used for neonatal resuscitation in the delivery room (AHA, 1992; Bloom & Cropley, 1994; Keenan, 1994).

Another drug that has fallen out of use in neonatal resuscitation is atropine. It is an anticholinergic drug that blocks the action of acetylcholine at cholinergic receptor sites. Parasympathetic (vagal) stimulation of the heart normally inhibits and decelerates cardiac function (see Table 15–4). If this stimulation is blocked, cardiac tone and activity are returned to normal. Whereas atropine may be useful in reversing bradycardia of vagal origin (e.g., airway manipulation during intubation), infants requiring resuscitation in the delivery room are typically bradycardic because of hypoxia. Administration of atropine in this situation has a transient effect at best, and bradycardia will return if the hypoxia persists (Burchfield, 1994; Gonzalez, 1993; Mendez-Bauer et al., 1963; Zaritsky, 1993).

SPECIAL SITUATIONS

Certain situations necessitate alterations in or variations of the usual resuscitative measures needed by most newborns. Table 15–5 lists several of these problem conditions, key features for differential diagnosis, and the immediate therapy required in the delivery room. They are discussed in greater detail in the appropriate systems chapters in this text.

TERMINATION OF RESUSCITATION

The law and its underlying ethical principles mandate that treatment be provided and continued as long as it is judged to be effective in ameliorating or correcting an underlying pathophysiologic process. Unfortunately, there are insufficient data to support a general recommendation for how long resuscitation should be performed before continuation can be deemed futile and efforts are terminated (Jain & Vidyasagar, 1993; Landwirth, 1993). There is evidence that neonates with birth weights of less than 750 g who require cardiac compressions in the delivery room do not survive to discharge (Davis, 1993). Survival is also unlikely at any birth weight if the Apgar score remains zero after 10 minutes of aggressive resuscitation (Jain et al., 1991).

Whereas many hospitals have guidelines for withholding full resuscitation for extremely low birth weight infants and those with lethal anomalies, early and well-documented discussion with parents is recommended when such events are anticipated prenatally. When the event was unanticipated, great attention should be given to postmortem evaluation. Blood for chromosome examination and other pertinent laboratory work, radiographs, and autopsy are important for both family counseling and evaluation of the resuscitation process (Edwards, 1988; Landwirth, 1993).

POSTRESUSCITATION STABILIZATION

The successfully resuscitated neonate requires special consideration during stabilization. The goal of care after resuscitation is to reverse the causes of cell death and tissue injury (hypoxia, ischemia, acidosis) and avoid any exacerbating conditions (hypothermia, hypoglycemia). The mnemonic STABLE can aid in re-

TABLE 15–5 Special Situations in the Delivery Room

Condition	Perinatal Associations	Clinical Features	Immediate Therapy
Abdominal wall defects Omphalocele Gastroschisis	Abnormal prenatal ultrasound findings	Immediately apparent	Supine or side-lying position without tension to bowel, cover defect with warm sterile saline soaks and wrap with sterile plastic wrap, orogastric tube for decompression
Choanal atresia	None	Cyanosis at rest, pink when crying; inability to pass catheter through nares, noisy upper airway sounds	Placement of oral airway
Diaphragmatic hernia	Polyhydramnios	Severe respiratory distress usually soon after birth, dyspnea, cyanosis, scaphoid abdomen, shift in cardiac impulse, bowel sounds heard over thorax	*Immediate* intubation, assisted ventilation with low inspiratory pressures, orogastric tube for decompression, sedation
Esophageal atresia	Polyhydramnios	Abundant oral secretions, swallowing difficulties, respiratory distress, inability to pass catheter into stomach	Elevate head, suction upper esophageal pouch, humidified oxygen
Hydrops fetalis	Rh isoimmunization, cardiac arrhythmias, structural heart disease, polyhydramnios, toxemia	Edema, respiratory distress, or apnea; distant breath sounds, ascites	Intubation, assisted ventilation, needle aspiration of pleural or peritoneal fluid
Laryngeal lesions, webs, or partial atresia	None	Inspiratory stridor, direct visualization most helpful	Percutaneous placement of large-bore catheter into trachea, distal to obstruction; assisted ventilation
Neural tube defects	Abnormal prenatal ultrasound findings, elevated alpha-fetoprotein levels, polyhydramnios	Immediately apparent	Prone or side-lying position without tension to sac, cover defect with warm sterile saline soaks and wrap with sterile plastic wrap
Pneumothorax	Meconium-stained amniotic fluid, respiratory distress syndrome, requirement for assisted ventilation	Acute onset of retractions, tachypnea, cyanosis, chest asymmetry, or shift in position of cardiac impulse; positive findings on transillumination	Needle aspiration, oxygen

Adapted from Ringer, S. A., & Stark, A. R. (1989). Management of neonatal emergencies in the delivery room. *Clinics in Perinatology, 16*(1), 23–41.

membering the basic components of the stabilization process (Karlsen, 1994):

S Sugar
T Temperature
A Artificial breathing
B Blood pressure
L Laboratory work
E Emotional support for the family

Sugar

Hypoglycemia can occur rapidly in newborns recovering from asphyxia, particularly in those with diminished glycogen stores due to prematurity or growth retardation. Serial screening of blood glucose levels must be instituted, with the first test done as soon as possible after emergency measures have been de-escalated. Hypoglycemia can be effectively managed and perhaps prevented by supplying a continuous dextrose infusion (4 to 6 mg/kg/min). Bolus administration is not advised because it may precipitate rebound hypoglycemia and transient hyperosmolarity, which in turn may injure the cerebral circulation (Jacobs & Phibbs, 1989).

Temperature

Hypothermia and the resultant sequelae of cold stress (see Chapter 16, Neonatal Thermoregulation) are best avoided by providing rapid and thorough drying of the newborn during resuscitation, but maintaining warmth after resuscitation is equally important. Temperature should be monitored and the radiant warmer or incubator regulated by servocontrol through a skin probe to maintain the infant's temperature between 35.5°C and 36.5°C. If additional heat sources are required, they must be judiciously applied to avoid skin damage. Infants with open defects, such as meningomyelocele, omphalocele, and gastroschisis, require special attention for prevention of excessive heat and fluid losses. These anomalies and their care are discussed in the appropriate systems chapters in this text.

Artificial Breathing

Many infants respond immediately to the respiratory support provided them during resuscitation, wean quickly, and have little or no need for continued therapy. Others may suffer postasphyxial respiratory distress (probably due to ischemic lung injury), meconium pneumonitis, or confounding hyaline membrane disease and need to have their ventilations artificially supported for days or weeks thereafter. Response must be diligently observed, and assisted ventilation and oxygen therapy must be adjusted to changing pulmonary function (Jacobs & Phibbs, 1989). Determination of the changes in pulmonary function is best accomplished by ongoing transcutaneous oxygen monitoring or pulse oximetry with trends confirmed by blood gas determinations. Arterial blood gas is the best indicator of ventilation, but a venous gas can be used to provide an approximation if arterial access is difficult or delayed. A chest radiograph should also be obtained to verify ET tube placement, to confirm underlying pathophysiologic changes, and to rule out potential air leaks.

Blood Pressure

One of the main causes of circulatory insufficiency and hypotension in the postresuscitation period is overzealous ventilation. Pulmonary function may change rapidly in the first hours after birth, leading to extreme changes in P_{CO_2}, which if undetected and allowed to continue can lead to acute hypocarbia. The hypocarbia, in turn, produces marked systemic hypotension. Administration of volume expanders is not appropriate in this situation. Rather, ventilation should be adjusted so that the P_{CO_2} returns to normal (Jacobs & Phibbs, 1989).

If the infant has survived severe asphyxia, postasphyxial myocardiopathy may occur secondary to ischemic injury. The heart becomes enlarged, myocardial contractility is diminished, and pulmonary edema may develop. True myocardiopathy is vigorously treated, usually with assisted ventilation, correction of any residual acidosis, and, if necessary, administration of dopamine (Jacobs & Phibbs, 1989).

Continuous monitoring of the infant's status with a cardiorespiratory monitor is recommended. Normal blood pressure is proportional to birth weight, and this must be kept in mind when the measurements are studied. In addition to heart rate and blood pressure, the electrocardiogram should be checked for wave changes (Jacobs & Phibbs, 1989).

Laboratory Work

Renal injury with oliguria (<1 ml/kg/h of urine), azotemia (elevated blood urea nitrogen), and elevated serum creatinine levels frequently occur, probably as a consequence of the redistribution of blood flow during asphyxia (Perlman, 1989). Sodium levels may be either decreased or increased. Hyponatremia is most frequently the result of inappropriate antidiuretic hormone secretion; hypernatremia is usually iatrogenic in infants who received large quantities of sodium bicarbonate during resuscitation. Hypocalcemia may be due to anoxic stimulation of calcitonin. This thyroid hormone lowers blood calcium levels by inhibiting calcium resorption from the bone and increasing calcium excretion by the kidneys. Hypomagnesemia, in association with hypocalcemia, may also be noted (Banagale & Donn, 1986). Finally, release of potassium by lysed cells, transcellular shifts of potassium, and decreased renal excretion of potassium can lead to hyperkalemia.

In light of the many fluid and electrolyte problems that can occur, urine output and specific gravity must be carefully measured. The serum and urine electrolytes and osmolality are closely monitored. Overall hydration is evaluated by skin turgor and weight changes. Infants are given nothing by mouth, and IV fluids are initially infused at a rate to provide 60 to 80 ml/kg/day, depending on the infant's gestational age. If renal damage becomes apparent, fluids may be restricted to 40 to 60 ml/kg/day to avoid overload and the attendant risks of cerebral edema and worsening hyponatremia.

Emotional Support for the Family

Parents confronted with the situation of having a sick newborn may have considerable emotional needs—feelings of guilt, anxiety, and fear are compounded by loss of control. Time must be taken to answer questions honestly and to listen to their concerns. If at all possible, speak to the parents and family in a group so that information is shared simultaneously. This group approach allows either parent or both parents to avoid the added responsibility of communicating information that may not be fully understood. Once the newborn is stabilized, the parents should be encouraged to see and touch their infant (Paxton, 1990).

DOCUMENTATION

No resuscitative event can go unrecorded. Unfortunately, the circumstances surrounding resuscitation are fraught with medicolegal hazards. Assessment of the infant is generally limited to the most basic of measurements (respiratory rate, heart rate, and color). Immediate response may be affected by many factors that are unrelated to professional competence. Furthermore, the ultimate outcome may not become apparent for years after the event. Even the best, most appropriate care can look "bad" in retrospect if documentation is incomplete or inaccurate. Yet no area of the hospital is perhaps less conducive to quality documentation than the delivery room, where a variety of professionals (nurses, physicians, and respiratory therapists) from different clinical areas (obstetrics, neonatology, anesthesiology), each with a unique perspective on the situation, are brought together in an emergency. Notes are jotted on bed linen, scrub clothes, paper towels, or anything at hand. More often than not, these brief notes are so hastily written that they are little more than a list of the medications given. When transcribed, the events may be documented in two totally separate charts, one for the mother, another for the infant. Great care must be taken so that events and actions can be accurately reconstructed many years in the future (Holzman, 1993; McCulloch & Vidyasagar, 1993; Thigpen, 1995).

Descriptive charting is most appropriate to this situation. The record should include the pertinent perinatal factors, the physical findings, the activities performed, and the infant's response, but definitive diagnoses should not be offered. It is particularly important that information concerning the pregnancy, labor, and delivery be based on fact and not hearsay. Terms such as "fetal distress" and "asphyxia" tend to take on a life of their own once they have been committed to paper, even if they are not supported by clinical evidence. It is best to record factual data, such as vital signs and blood gas determinations, without adding an interpretation. Ventilation, chest compressions, and administration of medications are essential items for documentation, but the basics should not be dismissed. It is just as important to note that attempts were made to keep the infant dry and warm (Holzman, 1993, 1994).

Accurate timing of notes can be critical because actions will be judged by the minute-to-minute changes noted in the chart. Use of a preprinted recording tool not only is helpful in this regard but can also provide a structure for evaluation and making decisions. It is recommended that any form used be printed in triplicate. One copy (the original) is retained for the medical record, the second is sent to the pharmacy so that medications can be quickly restocked, and the third is used for quality assessment purposes (McCulloch & Vidyasagar, 1993; Thigpen, 1995).

CONCLUSION

Although most depressed infants will respond to drying, warming, positioning, suctioning, and tactile stimulation, every obstetrical and neonatal unit should be adequately equipped and well prepared to handle neonatal emergencies when they arise. Effective management requires an understanding of cardiorespiratory transition; the identification of factors that may interfere with successful transition; an appreciation of the principles of resuscitation; and intervention based on assessment of respirations, heart rate, and color.

REFERENCES

American Academy of Pediatrics Committee on Drugs (1989). Emergency drug doses for infants and children and naloxone use in newborns: Clarification. *Pediatrics, 83*(5), 803.

American Academy of Pediatrics Committee on Drugs (1990). Naloxone dosage and route of administration for infants and children: Addendum to emergency drug doses for infants and children. *Pediatrics, 86*(3), 484–485.

American Heart Association Emergency Cardiac Care Committee and Subcommittees (1992). Guidelines for cardiopulmonary resuscitation and emergency cardiac care (Part VII): Neonatal resuscitation. *Journal of the American Medical Association, 268*(16), 2276–2281.

Babbs, C. F. (1993). Interposed abdominal compression–CPR: A case study in cardiac arrest research. *Annals of Emergency Medicine, 22*(1), 24–32.

Banagale, R. C., & Donn, S. M. (1986). Asphyxia neonatorum. *Journal of Family Practice, 22*(6), 539–545.

Barton, C., & Callaham, M. (1991). High-dose epinephrine improves the return of spontaneous circulation rates in human victims of cardiac arrest. *Annals of Emergency Medicine, 20*(7), 722–725.

Berkowitz, I. D., Chantarojanasiri, T., Koehler, R. C., et al. (1989). Blood flow during cardiopulmonary resuscitation with simultaneous compression and ventilation in infant pigs. *Pediatric Research, 26*(6), 558–564.

Berkowitz, I. D., Gervais, H., Schleien, C. L., et al. (1991). Epinephrine dosage effects on cerebral and myocardial blood flow in an infant swine model of cardiopulmonary resuscitation. *Anesthesiology, 75*(6), 1041–1050.

Bhende, M. S., & Thompson, A. E. (1995). Evaluation of an end-tidal CO_2 detector during pediatric cardiopulmonary resuscitation. *Pediatrics, 95*(3), 395–399.

Bloom, R. S., & Cropley, C. (1994). *Textbook of neonatal resuscitation.* Elk Grove Village, IL: American Academy of Pediatrics and American Heart Association.

Brimacombe, J. (1994). The laryngeal mask airway for neonatal resuscitation [Letter]. *Pediatrics, 93*(5), 874.

Brimacombe, J. (1995). Laryngeal mask airway for emergency medicine. *American Journal of Emergency Medicine, 13*(1), 111–112.

Brimacombe, J., & Berry, A. (1995). The laryngeal mask airway—A consideration for the Neonatal Resuscitation Programme guidelines? *Canadian Journal of Anaesthesia, 42*(1), 88–89.

Brimacombe, J., & Gandini, D. (1995). Resuscitation of neonates with the laryngeal mask airway—A caution. *Pediatrics, 95*(3), 453–454.

Burchfield, D. J. (1993). Medication use in neonatal resuscitation: Epinephrine and sodium bicarbonate. *Neonatal Pharmacology Quarterly, 2*(2), 25–30.

Burchfield, D. J. (1994). Why *not* use atropine in neonatal resuscitation. *NRP News Intermountain West, 1*(4), 1.

Burchfield, D., Erenberg, A., Mullett, M. D., et al. (1994). Why change the compression and ventilation rates during CPR in neonates? *Pediatrics, 93*(6), 1026–1027.

Catlin, E. A., Carpenter, M. W., Brann, B. S., et al. (1986). The Apgar score revisited: Influences of gestational age. *Journal of Pediatrics, 109*(5), 865–868.

Chandra, N. C. (1993). Mechanisms of blood flow during CPR. *Annals of Emergency Medicine, 22*(2, Part 2), 281–288.

Chernick, V., & Craig, R. J. (1982). Naloxone reverses neonatal depression caused by fetal asphyxia. *Science, 216*(4551), 1252–1253.

Chernick, V., Manfreda, J., De Booy, V., et al. (1988). Clinical trial of naloxone in birth asphyxia. *Journal of Pediatrics, 113*(3), 519–525.

Clark, G. D. (1989). Role of excitatory amino acids in brain injury caused by hypoxia-ischemia, status epilepticus, and hypoglycemia. *Clinics in Perinatology, 16*(2), 459–474.

Cordero, L., & Hon, E. H. (1971). Neonatal bradycardia following nasopharyngeal stimulation. *Journal of Pediatrics, 78*(3), 441–447.

Crockett, M., & Tappero, E. (1989). Dopamine and dobutamine: Neonatal indications and implications. *Neonatal Network, 7*(5), 13–20.

Cropley, C. (1995). How to make sure you can find what you are looking for when you need it. *NRP News Intermountain West, 2*(4), 1.

David, R. (1988). Closed chest cardiac massage in the newborn infant. *Pediatrics, 81*(4), 552–554.

Davis, D. J. (1993). How aggressive should delivery room cardiopulmonary resuscitation be for extremely low birth weight neonates? *Pediatrics, 92*(3), 447–450.

Dawes, G. S. (1968). *Fetal and neonatal physiology.* Chicago: Year Book Medical Publishers.

Dembo, D. H. (1981). Calcium in advanced life support. *Critical Care Medicine, 9*(5), 358–359.

Drew, J. H. (1982). Immediate intubation at birth of the very-low-birth-weight infant. *American Journal of Diseases of Children, 136*(3), 207–210.

Driscoll, D. J. (1987). Use of inotropic and chronotropic agents in neonates. *Clinics in Perinatology, 14*(4), 931–949.

Edwards, M. C. (1988). Delivery room resuscitation of the neonate. *Pediatric Annals, 17*(7), 458–466.

Efrat, R., Kadari, A., & Katz, S. (1994). The laryngeal mask airway in pediatric anesthesia: Experience with 120 patients undergoing elective groin surgery. *Journal of Pediatric Surgery, 29*(2), 206–208.

Elliott, R. D. (1994). Neonatal resuscitation: The NRP guidelines. *Canadian Journal of Anaesthesia, 41*(8), 742–753.

Evans, J. M., Hogg, M. I. J., & Rosen, M. (1976). Reversal of narcotic depression in the neonate by naloxone. *British Medical Journal, 2*(19), 1098–1100.

Fields, L. M., Entman, S. S., & Boehm, F. H. (1983). Correlation of the one-minute Apgar score and the pH value of umbilical arterial blood. *Southern Medical Journal, 76*(12), 1477–1479.

Finholt, D. A., Kettrick, R. G., Wagner, H. R., & Swedlow, D. B. (1986). The heart is under the lower third of the sternum. *American Journal of Diseases of Children, 140*(7), 646–649.

Fitzgerald, G. A., Barnes, P., Hamilton, C. A., & Dollery, C. T. (1980). Circulating adrenaline and blood pressure: The metabolic effects and kinetics of infused adrenaline in man. *European Journal of Clinical Investigation, 10*(5), 401–406.

Friedman, A. H., & Fahey, J. T. (1993). The transition from fetal to neonatal circulation: Normal response and implications for infants with heart disease. *Seminars in Perinatology, 17*(2), 106–121.

Goetting, M. G., & Paradis, N. A. (1991). High-dose epinephrine improves outcome from pediatric cardiac arrest. *Annals of Emergency Medicine, 20*(1), 22–26.

Gonzalez, E. R. (1993). Pharmacologic controversies in CPR. *Annals of Emergency Medicine, 22*(2, Part 2), 317–323.

Gonzalez, E. R., Ornato, J. P., Garnett, A. R., et al. (1989). Dose-dependent vasopressor response to epinephrine during CPR in human beings. *Annals of Emergency Medicine, 18*(9), 920–926.

Graf, H., Leach, W., & Arieff, A. I. (1985). Evidence for a detrimental effect of bicarbonate therapy in hypoxic lactic acidosis. *Science,* 227(4688), 754–756.

Handal, K. A., Schauben, J. L., & Salamone, F. R. (1983). Naloxone. *Annals of Emergency Medicine, 12*(7), 438–445.

Hein, H. A. (1993). The use of sodium bicarbonate in neonatal resuscitation: Help or harm? *Pediatrics, 91*(2), 496–497.

Heller, R. M., & Heller, T. W. (1994). Experience with the illuminated endotracheal tube in the prevention of unsafe intubations in the premature and full-term newborn. *Pediatrics, 93*(3), 389–391.

Hermansen, M. C., & Prior, M. M. (1993). Oxygen concentrations from self-inflating resuscitation bags. *American Journal of Perinatology, 10*(1), 79–80.

Heymann, M. A. (1987). Prostaglandins and leukotrienes in the perinatal period. *Clinics in Perinatology, 14*(4), 857–880.

Hoekstra, O. S., van Lambalgen, A. A., Groeneveld, A. B. J., et al. (1995). Abdominal compressions increase vital organ perfusion during CPR in dogs: Relation with efficacy of thoracic compressions. *Annals of Emergency Medicine, 25*(3), 375–385.

Holzman, I. (1993). Delivery room scenario may prompt legal tangles. *AAP News,* 9(8), 3, 13.

Holzman, I. (1994). Legal defense requires precise medical records. *AAP News, 10*(9), 4.

Howell, J. H. (1987). Sodium bicarbonate in the perinatal setting—Revisited. *Clinics in Perinatology, 14*(4), 807–816.

Jacobs, M. M., & Phibbs, R. H. (1989). Prevention, recognition, and treatment of perinatal asphyxia. *Clinics in Perinatology, 16*(4), 785–807.

Jain, L., & Vidyasagar, D. (1993). Cardiopulmonary resuscitation of newborns: Its application to transport medicine. *Pediatric Clinics of North America, 40*(2), 287–302.

Jain, L., Ferre, C., Vidyasagar, E., et al. (1991). Cardiopulmonary resuscitation of apparently stillborn infants: Survival and long-term outcome. *Journal of Pediatrics, 118,* 778–782.

Kain, Z. N., Berde, C. B., Benjamin, P. K., & Thompson, J. E. (1993). Performance of pediatric resuscitation bags assessed with an infant lung simulator. *Anesthesia and Analgesia, 77*(2), 261–264.

Karlsen, K. A. (1994). *A mnemonic approach to neonatal stabilization: "Transporting newborns the S.T.A.B.L.E. way." Development of an outreach educational program* [Abstract]. Presented at the 6th National Outreach Conference, Telluride, CO, September, 1994.

Keeley, S. R., & Bohn, D. J. (1988). The use of inotropic and afterload-reducing agents in neonates. *Clinics in Perinatology, 15*(3), 467–489.

Keenan, B. (1994). Calcium use for neonatal resuscitation. *NRP News Intermountain West, 1*(5), 1–2.

Kette, F., Weil, M. H., von Planta, M., et al. (1990). Buffer agents do not reverse intramyocardial acidosis during cardiac resuscitation. *Circulation, 81,* 1660–1666.

Krischer, J. P., Fine, E. G., Weisfeldt, M. L., et al. (1989). Comparison of prehospital conventional and simultaneous compression-ventilation cardiopulmonary resuscitation. *Critical Care Medicine, 17*(12), 1263–1269.

Kuhn, M. (1991). Severe bradyarrhythmias following calcium pretreatment. *American Heart Journal, 6*(1), 1812–1813.

Landwirth, J. (1993). Ethical issues in pediatric and neonatal resuscitation. *Annals of Emergency Medicine, 22*(2, Part 2), 502–507.

Lavies, N. G. (1993). Use of the laryngeal mask airway in neonatal resuscitation [Letter; comment]. *Anaesthesia, 48*(4), 352.

Leuthner, S. R., Jansen, R. D., & Hageman, J. R. (1994). Cardiopulmonary resuscitation of the newborn: An update. *Pediatric Clinics of North America, 41*(5), 893–907.

McCulloch, K. M., & Vidyasagar, D. (1993). Assessing adherence to standards for neonatal resuscitation taught throughout the perinatal referral area. *Pediatric Clinics of North America, 40*(2), 431–438.

Mendez-Bauer, C., Poseiro, J. J., Arellano-Hernandez, G., et al. (1963). Effects of atropine on the heart rate of the human fetus during labor. *American Journal of Obstetrics and Gynecology, 85*(8), 1033–1053.

Menegazzi, J. J., Auble, T. E., Nicklas, K. A., et al. (1993). Two-thumb versus two-finger chest compression during CPR in a swine infant model of cardiac arrest. *Annals of Emergency Medicine, 22*(2), 240–243.

Mizushima, A., Wardall, G. J., & Simpson, D. L. (1992). The laryngeal mask airway in infants. *Anaesthesia, 47*(10), 849–851.

Niemann, J. T., Rosborough, J. P., Niskanen, R. A., et al. (1985). Mechanical "cough" cardiopulmonary resuscitation during cardiac arrest in dogs. *American Journal of Cardiology, 55*(1), 199–204.

Orlando, S. (1991). Pathophysiology of acute respiratory distress. In J. Nugent (Ed.), *Acute respiratory care of the neonate* (pp. 27–46). Petaluma, CA: NICU Ink.

Orlowski, J. P., Gallagher, J. M., & Porembka, D. T. (1990). Endotracheal epinephrine is unreliable. *Resuscitation, 19*(2), 103–113.

Oski, F. A. (1993). The erythrocyte and its disorders. In D. G. Nathan & F. A. Oski (Eds.), *Hematology of infancy and childhood* (Vol. 1, pp. 18–43). Philadelphia: W. B. Saunders.

Ostrea, E. M., & Odell, G. B. (1972). The influence of bicarbonate administration on blood pH in a "closed system": Clinical implications. *Journal of Pediatrics, 80*(4), 671–680.

Palmer, C., & Vannucci, R. C. (1993). Potential new therapies for perinatal cerebral hypoxia-ischemia. *Clinics in Perinatology, 20*(2), 411–432.

Papile, L., Burstein, J., Burstein, R., et al. (1978). Relationship of intravenous sodium bicarbonate infusions and cerebral intraventricular hemorrhage. *Journal of Pediatrics, 93*(5), 834–836.

Paradis, N. A., Martin, G. B., Rosenberg, J., et al. (1991). The effect of standard- and high-dose epinephrine on coronary perfusion pressure during prolonged cardiopulmonary resuscitation. *Journal of the American Medical Association, 265*(9), 1139–1144.

Paterson, S. J., Byrne, P. J., Molesky, M. G., et al. (1994). Neonatal resuscitation using the laryngeal mask airway. *Anesthesiology, 80*(6), 1248–1253.

Paxton, J. M. (1990). Transport of the surgical neonate. *Journal of Perinatal and Neonatal Nursing, 3*(3), 43–49.

Pepe, P. E., Zachariah, B. S., & Chandra, N. C. (1993). Invasive airway techniques in resuscitation. *Annals of Emergency Medicine, 22* (2, Part 2), 393–403.

Perlman, J. M. (1989). Systemic abnormalities in term infants following perinatal asphyxia: Relevance to long-term neurologic outcome. *Clinics in Perinatology, 16*(2), 475–484.

Perlman, J. M., & Risser, R. (1995). Cardiopulmonary resuscitation in the delivery room: Associated clinical events. *Archives of Pediatric and Adolescent Medicine, 149*(1), 20–25.

Proano, L., Chiang, W. K., & Wang, R. Y. (1995). Calcium channel blocker overdose. *American Journal of Emergency Medicine, 13*(4), 444–450.

Ralston, S. H., Tacker, W. A., Showen, L., et al. (1985). Endotracheal versus intravenous epinephrine during electromechanical dissociation with CPR in dogs. *Annals of Emergency Medicine, 14*(11), 1044–1048.

Reiterer, F., Abbasi, S., & Bhutani, V. K. (1994). Influence of head-neck posture on airflow and pulmonary mechanics in preterm neonates. *Pediatric Pulmonology, 17*(3), 149–154.

Rudikoff, M. T., Maughan, W. L., Effron, M., et al. (1980). Mechanisms of blood flow during cardiopulmonary resuscitation. *Circulation, 61*(2), 345–352.

Schwab, K. O., & von Stockhausen, H. B. (1994). Plasma catecholamines after endotracheal administration of adrenaline during postnatal resuscitation. *Archives of Disease in Childhood, 70*(3), F213–F217.

Simmons, M. A., Adcock, E. W., Bard, H., & Battaglia, F. C. (1974). Hypernatremia and intracranial hemorrhage in neonates. *New England Journal of Medicine, 291*(1), 6–10.

Stueven, H. A., Thompson, B. M., Aprahamian, C., & Tonsfeldt, D. J. (1984). Calcium chloride: Reassessment of use in asystole. *Annals of Emergency Medicine, 13*(9, Part 2), 820–822.

Swenson, R. D., Weaver, W. D., Niskanen, R. A., et al. (1988). Hemodynamics in humans during conventional and experimental methods of cardiopulmonary resuscitation. *Circulation, 78*(3), 630–639.

Terai, C., Anada, H., Matsushima, S., et al. (1995). Effects of mild Trendelenburg on central hemodynamics and internal jugular vein velocity, cross-sectional area, and flow. *American Journal of Emergency Medicine, 13*(3), 255–258.

Thigpen, J. (1995). Neonatal resuscitation record. *Neonatal Network, 14*(1), 57–58.

Todres, I. D. (1993). Pediatric airway control and ventilation. *Annals of Emergency Medicine, 22*(2, Part 2), 440–444.

Todres, I. D., & Rogers, M. C. (1975). Methods of external cardiac massage in the newborn infant. *Journal of Pediatrics, 86*(5), 781–782.

Trautman, M. S. (1995). Neonatal resuscitation: Be prepared. *Contemporary Pediatrics, 12*(3), 101–110, 113.

Volpe, J. J. (1989). Intraventricular hemorrhage and brain injury in the premature infant. *Clinics in Perinatology, 16*(2), 361–386.

von Planta, M., Bar-Joseph, G., Wiklund, L., et al. (1993). Pathophysiologic and therapeutic implications of acid-base changes during CPR. *Annals of Emergency Medicine, 22*(2, Part 2), 404–410.

Ward, K. R., Menegazzi, J. J., Zelenak, R. R., et al. (1993). A comparison of chest compressions between mechanical and manual CPR by monitoring end-tidal PCO_2 during human cardiac arrest. *Annals of Emergency Medicine, 22*(4), 669–674.

Wardlaw, S. L., Stark, R. I., Baxi, L., & Frantz, A. G. (1979). Plasma ß-endorphin and ß-lipotropin in the human fetus at delivery: Correlation with arterial pH and pO_2. *Journal of Clinical Endocrinology and Metabolism, 49*, 888–891.

Wayne, A. S., & Fosburg, M. T. (1993). Therapeutic plasma exchange and cataphoresiscytapheresis. In D. G. Nathan & F. A. Oski (Eds.), *Hematology of infancy and childhood* (Vol. 2, pp. 1819–1831). Philadelphia: W. B. Saunders.

Wenzel, V., Fuerst, R. S., Idris, A. H., et al. (1995). Automatic mechanical device to standardize active compression-decompression CPR. *Annals of Emergency Medicine, 25*(3), 386–389.

White, B. C., Winegar, C. D., Wilson, R. F., et al. (1983). Possible role of calcium blockers in cerebral resuscitation: A review of the literature and synthesis for future studies. *Critical Care Medicine, 11*(3), 202–207.

Williams, C. E., Mallard, C., Tan, W., & Gluckman, P. D. (1993). Pathophysiology of perinatal asphyxia. *Clinics in Perinatology, 20*(2), 305–325.

Williams, R. K. (1995). Resuscitation of neonates with the laryngeal mask airway: A caution [In reply]. *Pediatrics, 95*(3), 454.

Wimmer, J. E. (1994). Neonatal resuscitation. *Pediatrics in Review, 15*(7), 255–265.

Wiswell, T. E., & Bent, R. C. (1993). Meconium staining and the meconium aspiration syndrome: Unresolved issues. *Pediatric Clinics of North America, 40*(5), 955–981.

Wiswell, T. E., Tuggle, J. M., & Turner, B. S. (1990). Meconium aspiration syndromes: Have we made a difference? *Pediatrics, 85*(5), 715–721.

Woods, J. (1983). Birth asphyxia: Pathophysiologic events and fetal adaptive changes. *Clinics in Perinatology, 10*(2), 473.

Young, T. E., & Mangum, O. B. (1997). *Neofax '97: A manual of drugs used in neonatal care* (8th ed.). Columbus, OH: Ross Products Division, Abbott Laboratories.

Zaritsky, A. (1993). Pediatric resuscitation pharmacology. *Annals of Emergency Medicine, 22*(2, Part 2), 445–455.

Zaritsky, A., & Chernow, B. (1984). Use of catecholamines in pediatrics. *Journal of Pediatrics, 105*(3), 341–350.

CHAPTER 16

Neonatal Thermoregulation

STEPHANIE ROCKWERN AMLUNG

RESEARCH AGENDA

Is there a positive correlation among tympanic, axillary, and rectal temperatures measured in the first 24 hours after birth?

What is the effect of skin-to-skin contact and thermal regulation in the very low birth weight neonate?

What is the normal temperature range for a neonate weighing 1000 g or more?

What is the effect of high humidity on overall temperature regulation in the very low birth weight neonate?

What is the impact of environmental temperature on neonatal temperatures, especially during the weaning process from isolette to open crib?

VIGNETTE

It was a cold November night, and I was getting ready to give report to the next shift when our new admission arrived: Baby Eric, a 31-week neonate, born 2 hours ago at an outlying community hospital. Eric's mother had developed gestational diabetes. As we were taking Eric from the transporter, I realized his skin was cool and pale. The transport nurse was giving report. "We monitored his glucose levels, with his last Dextrostix reading 60. He's receiving D5W at 8 ml/hr through a 24-G angiocath in his right arm. His respiratory status has been stable, color pale pink, respirations 60 to 70 with mild retractions in 45% O_2." "What was his temperature?" I asked. "Well, when we arrived at the hospital, Eric's temperature was 97°F rectally, but on the trip back his skin temperature was registering at 95.8°F."

Even though Eric had good Apgar scores and was demonstrating signs of only mild respiratory distress, I knew temperature regulation was a priority. Instead of putting him on a cool scale, I warmed a blanket, weighed it, and put it over the scale so Eric would not lose heat through conduction. After weighing Eric, I put him in a heated incubator. His vital signs were stable except for a rectal temperature of 95.8°F and skin temperature of 95°F. Being LGA, Eric had a greater surface area from which to lose heat. His ability to produce heat was limited. His posture was relaxed, and he was unable to shiver to produce more heat. The transport note stated the delivery room had been cold and the radiant warmer was not functioning at the time of his birth, all factors adding to his thermal problems. Eric had been dried immediately and placed on his mother's chest to provide skin-to-skin warmth. He was covered with a blanket, and a hat was put on him. His color and respiratory status were monitored to ensure his condition did not worsen before transport.

Now that the transport was over, Eric would need prewarmed items. The stethoscope, diapers, and even hands are things that we do not always think of as playing a part in thermoregulation. The oxygen he was receiving via an Oxy-Hood was warmed and humidified, as was the incubator's air. I maintained the temperature in the incubator at about 2°F higher than his core temperature to prevent warming him too rapidly. Eric was already experiencing occasional apneic spells, and these would only increase if I warmed him too quickly.

As I completed my assessment, I sat down to set care priorities. A neutral thermal environment was top on the list. There were several key components in accomplishing this goal. Because Eric was LGA, he probably had enough subcutaneous fat to help him maintain his temperature but most likely had limited brown fat stores to assist in thermogenesis. As an IDM, Eric's glucose levels would have to be closely monitored. If he became hypoglycemic, that would complicate his ability to generate heat through metabolic means. Also, his being designated as NPO would have implications in his ability to produce heat. If his respiratory status worsened, that would also affect his ability to maintain warmth. Evaporative losses would be affected. Hypoglycemia and increased respiratory effort would decrease the amount of energy available to produce heat.

Eric was carefully monitored throughout the next 24 hours. He gradually warmed to a core temperature of 98.4°F. His color improved; respirations stabilized with minimal apneic episodes; head hood O_2 was weaned to 30%. Feedings were begun. Eric's metabolic rate increased, thus fostering his ability to produce heat. As feedings were tolerated, the IV was converted to a heparin well. Initially he lost some weight, but it remained within 5% of his birth weight. I knew that Eric had stabilized, but I still felt it important to continue basic thermoregulatory interventions. Keeping a hat on was one way to prevent heat loss. Once out of the incubator, keeping him from drafty rooms or outside windows would be important. Also, not allowing him to be exposed for long periods of time during examination would be important to Eric's continued thermal stability.

Stephanie Rockwern Amlung

Since the 1960s, temperature control of the newborn has played a significant role in altering the rate of infant morbidity and mortality. Currently, temperature control continues to play a major role in neonatal health care, as technologic advancements make it possible for smaller infants to survive. These small infants have limited energy and fat stores that can be called upon to support thermal needs. The infants must be supported in an environment that provides for these needs.

Newborns' thermoregulation must be carefully managed. This management cannot be addressed by a single protocol for maintaining thermoneutrality, inasmuch as each infant's needs are different. These differences are the result of gestational age and feeding methods. Access to warming devices is also a factor that impacts the nurse's ability to manage thermoneutrality. Within each institution, variables such as humidity, air flow, and infant temperature are important factors affecting temperature management.

Although the infant is capable of heat production at the time of birth, maintenance of the thermal needs plays an important part in the collaborative neonatal management. Full-term infants are capable of limited heat production by use of brown fat stores, which are sufficient to meet normal heat energy needs. Such infants, however, must also be monitored for thermal balance, because environmental and neonatal factors may make thermal self-regulation difficult without proactive nursing intervention.

Providing for the needs of an unstable or premature infant often requires special techniques for assisting the infant to maintain adequate body temperature. Infants who have been stressed in utero have depleted reserves of brown fat stores. Neonates who are premature, small for gestational age (SGA), or growth retarded have insufficient brown fat stores. They are less able to produce sufficient heat for thermal self-regulation. The last trimester is the period in which the greatest transfer of nutrients across the placenta to the fetus occurs for energy use. The infant born before this time has fewer nutrient stores to produce heat.

Once stabilized after delivery, the infant's ability to generate heat improves. The metabolic rate increases to provide energy for growth. This metabolic increase also affects the neonate's ability to self-regulate or maintain thermocontrol and to yield heat energy (Sauer et al., 1984). As the neonate matures, thermal support needs change. The full-term infant may require only light clothing to assist in maintenance of temperature stability. The premature infant requires gradually lower ambient temperatures and fewer interventive techniques to conserve body heat than were required at the time of birth.

Although thermoregulation is a basic requirement for good neonatal management, it is probably one of the most complex aspects of the care. This chapter outlines the basic principles of thermoregulation. Neonatal assessment and thermal management are explained, as are the complications of thermal stress.

THERMOREGULATION AT BIRTH

Before birth, the infant's core temperature is slightly higher than the maternal core temperature. If the mother experiences hypothermia, depending on the degree of severity, the fetus may also be cold (Dunn, 1994). The physiologic mechanism that dictates higher fetal than maternal temperatures has not been established. After birth, the neonate is exposed to the relatively cold environment of the delivery room. The infant experiences a sudden increase in demand to produce heat to maintain a stable body temperature. Although delivery rooms employ methods to prevent heat loss postnatally, the infant's temperature can fall as much as 2.6°C (Besch et al., 1971). During the course of a normal delivery, the wet infant can lose as much as 200 calories of heat for every 1 kg of body weight during each minute that the heat loss is allowed to continue (Nalepka, 1976). Thus, one of the most important points of neonatal stabilization in the delivery room is rapid drying to decrease the chance of iatrogenic hypothermia (Ringer & Stark, 1990).

Neonatal peripheral cooling stimulates heat production even before a fall in core temperature is detected. Facial cooling alone is sufficient to initiate this response. The response results from stimulation of the skin receptors, especially in the area of the facial trigeminal nerve. These receptors transmit the stimuli to the pituitary to begin heat production. The same stimuli are also transmitted to the respiratory center at the time of birth. Contraction of the diaphragm, in turn, is initiated to trigger respiration. (This mechanism has implications for neonatal resuscitation, because the blowing of cold air across the face can produce respirations; however, it can also result in significant heat loss. This heat loss can, as explained later in the chapter, compromise the neonate.)

Heat Loss

Heat can be lost via four processes: conduction, convection, evaporation, and radiation. Heat loss resulting from conductive losses at the time of birth occurs in two stages. In the first stage, interior body heat is lost to the skin's surface by conduction via the tissues and body organs. The second stage involves the release of heat from the skin's surface to environmental surfaces, such as a cold infant scale (Swyer, 1978). Minimal heat losses may also occur through the urine and feces.

Convective losses are due to air flowing across body surfaces; evaporative losses are related to heat rising from the skin to the air. These are usually related to differences in water concentrations between the skin and the air. Convective and evaporative losses occur in three ways. First, heat is lost from the interior body to the skin through the blood's circulation. Second, there is further heat loss as air moves over the neonate's wet skin. Third, inspired air is heated and moistened in the pulmonary capillary bed and then exhaled. Radiant losses result as the neonate is placed near objects that are cooler than the skin's surface.

The majority of heat loss in the neonate is through radiative and convective losses. Prevention of heat loss is the first goal in neonatal thermoregulation. The secondary goal is to minimize the energy necessary for the infant to produce heat.

Heat Production

The neonate is capable of heat production through three ways: voluntary muscle activity, shivering, and nonshivering or chemical thermogenesis. Of these three, shivering is the most inefficient method of heat production. Although it is the primary method of heat production in the adult, the full-term infant has limited ability to produce heat in this manner. The preterm infant has virtually no ability to generate heat through shivering.

Voluntary muscle activity is used by full-term neonates to some extent to generate heat. This activity is generally related to positioning in an effort to conserve heat losses. Full-term infants are capable of assuming a flexed position, unless impeded, to conserve heat loss from exposed surfaces. The preterm infant, however, has a limited ability to assume a flexed position. It is more common for the preterm infant to assume a relaxed posture, leaving the skin's surface exposed. Thus heat loss is inevitable unless steps are taken to protect such a vulnerable infant. Another group of vulnerable infants is the critically ill or sick neonates. In these infants, the flaccid, outstretched position may be observed.

The main source of heat production for the infant, therefore, is chemical thermogenesis. Stimulated by norepinephrine, brown fat metabolism occurs. The availability of glucose initiates glycolysis. Digestion may also play a limited role in heat production. Thus, without adequate sources of brown fat and glucose or in the absence of enteral feeding, the neonate is at risk for thermal instability secondary to the inability to carry out effective thermogenesis.

Once the heat generation response is initiated, oxygen consumption rises as the infant metabolizes brown fat, resulting in heat energy. The infant who requires resuscitation or who is unable to meet the demands of increased oxygen intake is at greatest risk for decreased ability to achieve early thermoregulation (Schubring, 1986).

Thermoneutrality

The goal of maintaining a stable body temperature is to ensure normal growth and maintenance of energy needs. This thermoneutral state is one in which body temperature is maintained within a normal range and calorie expenditure and oxygen consumption are minimal. What defines a normal range is not clear, and further research in this area is needed. The thermoneutral body temperature of a full-term infant may be within the range of 36.6°C to 37°C but may be as low as 35°C for a preterm infant. The broad range of what constitutes normal body temperature is related more to gestational age than to birth weight, inasmuch as infants who are SGA may have a better ability to self-regulate than their size indicates (Sauer & Visser, 1984).

Determination of what constitutes a thermally neutral temperature may be complicated in very premature infants. In such neonates, oxygen uptake may not increase sufficiently to meet heat production needs, especially in the first few weeks of life.

Thermoneutrality may be difficult to achieve in the very low birth weight (VLBW) infant and in the extremely low birth weight (ELBW) infant in the first few days after delivery. Despite an inability to sweat, premature infants (<37 weeks' gestational age) have high evaporative heat losses as the result of increased permeability of their skin. The very thin, gelatinous epidermis, typical of gestationally immature neonates, affords very little protection against heat losses. The thermoneutral ambient temperature range that best meets the metabolic needs of the infant may be narrow and fluctuate less than 0.5°C (Wheldon & Hull, 1983). In some cases, the environmental temperatures tolerated by the premature infant may have a range of less than 3°C, depending on the source of heat and amount of humidity. The addition of humidity in the range of 40 to 60 percent may lower environmental temperature needs of the premature infant by 1°C or more.

Determination of appropriate environmental temperatures is related to the infant's ability to maintain a satisfactory body temperature by using the least amount of energy. Maintenance of a thermoneutral environment can be achieved for the full-term infant in an incubator with an air temperature between 32°C and 35°C. The premature infant often needs air temperatures between 35°C and 37°C (Dodman, 1987). If the infant is clothed, the air temperature can often be reduced by 2°C to 4°C. As the infant matures, air temperature needed to maintain thermoneutrality declines (Table 16–1).

TABLE 16–1 Environmental Assessment

Macroenvironment

What is the temperature within the room in general?
What is the actual temperature at specific infant care areas?
What is the method of delivery of heat and air conditioning (i.e., baseboard units, wall units, ceiling units)?
Where do air currents and drafts occur?
What is the actual percentage of humidity within the room?
What electrical equipment in the unit contributes to the temperature and humidity within the unit?

Microenvironment

What type of bed is being used for the infant (e.g., open crib, incubator)?
What type of heating source is being used (i.e., convection, conduction, radiation)?
What amount of humidity is being delivered?
What other therapies have been instituted that impact on temperature regulation (e.g., phototherapy, oxygen and ventilator therapy)?
Where is the location of the bed in relation to air currents?
What is the temperature of incubator walls?

Mechanisms of Neonatal Heat Regulation

The infant has a much greater potential for losing heat than does the adult, because of a greater body surface area in comparison to weight. A decrease in neonatal fat stores prevents insulation from heat losses resulting from external environmental changes. Heat production by the neonate and environmental control by the health care team serve to provide for the thermoregulatory needs.

Healthy full-term babies (appropriate for gestational age [AGA]), when clothed and fed, are able to produce heat in order to self-thermoregulate. In the presence of a cold environment, these infants are able to increase basal heat production by two to three times the normal rate within a day or two of birth (Laburn & Laburn, 1985).

Neonates who are large in comparison with the normal weight and size for their gestational age (large for gestational age [LGA]) may be expected to be able to generate sufficient heat to maintain self-thermoregulation. In reality, they may lack sufficient brown fat stores. These infants may also be poor feeders and lack sufficient oral intake to generate heat.

Several other factors may limit the infant's ability to thermally self-regulate. The presence of hypoxia or hypoglycemia may prevent the infant from generating sufficient heat through metabolism. Infants are also at risk after episodes of stress or prolonged periods of increased metabolic demands. These infants may have depleted stores of brown fat and glucose and are unable to generate heat.

Central nervous system (CNS) defects or infection may alter the temperature-regulating ability of the brain. In the infant with CNS alterations, hypothalamic control may be absent. Anencephalic infants and infants with intracranial defects and/or hemorrhage may be unable to produce heat. Use of maternal analgesia may inhibit the infant's ability to generate heat in the first few days of life, because metabolism is slowed by these drugs (Schwartz et al., 1978). Anesthetic or muscle relaxant use in infants may also alter thermal response through neural inhibition of temperature response.

Heat production in the newborn gradually improves during the first few days of life with the institution of feedings (Hull & Smales, 1978). Oral feedings have been shown to cause an increase in neonatal heat production that is not present when protein hydrolysate is administered parenterally (Mestyán, 1978). It is not clear as to why heat is produced with oral feedings, but it may result from increased metabolism during digestion or heat gain that can be generated when sufficient energy is provided via ingestion.

Infants who are SGA are a group for whom it seems to be especially difficult to provide care. Many nurseries use infant weight to determine when care should be provided in an incubator or under a radiant warmer. The SGA infant may be better served by providing for thermoregulatory needs on the basis of the individual needs of the infant. If the size of the infant dictates the use of only a diaper in the confines of an incubator, the SGA infant may use more energy trying to "be comfortable" than if lightly clothed in the incubator with the air temperature set slightly lower. Physical contact, even with clothing, may serve as a source of comfort to such an infant.

Preterm infants are at risk for difficulties in generating heat and energy because of large body surface area in relation to weight, limited brown fat stores, and delayed or absent mediating responses to initiate heat production. In addition to limited stores of fat, glucose, liver enzymes, and hormones, norepinephrine may not be released in sufficient amounts for the preterm infant to initiate metabolic thermogenesis (Williams & Lancaster, 1976).

Growth and energy needs as well as heat production in the VLBW infant are dependent on the source of metabolic energy. Energy needs can be met through absorption of nutrients via the gastrointestinal tract or by direct intravenous infusion. Ingestion of human milk has been found to increase metabolism in the VLBW infant, leading to production of heat (Rubecz & Mestyán, 1986).

Despite the seemingly small size of the premature infant, the body surface area is proportionately larger than that of the normal full-term infant. Fat stores, necessary for heat production, are minimal. The layer of fat and brown fat stores is generally not complete until the last few weeks of gestation. Brown fat begins to develop around 26 to 30 weeks' gestation and continues to develop until after the birth of the full-term infant. The thin layer of subcutaneous fat increases the internal convective loss of heat in the small infant because of the lack of insulation.

Although sweat glands are almost nonexistent in the preterm infant, the infant loses enormous amounts of water through the skin's surface. These losses rise dramatically when radiant heating sources are used or when the infant is placed under phototherapy lights. Under these circumstances, premature infants can lose as much as 120 ml of water per kilogram per day (Swyer, 1978). Humidification of the environment in the range of 40 to 60 percent may protect the premature infant from heat loss resulting from evaporative losses.

Heat conservation is limited in most infants 24 to 25 weeks' gestational age because of their flaccid posture. Thus, limited heat sources coupled with the inability to conserve heat place these infants at risk for cold stress. Therefore, they are very sensitive to even the slightest alterations in environmental temperature (Brueggemeyer, 1995).

Gluconeogenesis

Although glycogenolysis is the main source of energy for the infant after birth, gluconeogenesis plays a role in energy stabilization for the infant. The process of gluconeogenesis converts proteins and lipids into glucose for use in the body. The anterior pituitary is responsible for releasing corticotropin. The release of corticotropin then stimulates the release of glucocorticoid hormone from the adrenal cortex. Cortisol, the glucocorticoid hormone, mobilizes proteins within the cells for metabolism into glucose.

In the preterm or SGA infant, glycogen stores are limited. A decreased rate of gluconeogenesis in these infants may also influence glucose and energy stabilization. The delay in the ability for the preterm infant to initiate gluconeogenesis may be related to insufficient hepatic maturity. Liver substrates necessary for gluconeogenesis to occur include glycerol, lactate, and amino acids.

Hormonal levels may also be inadequate in preterm infants to initiate gluconeogenesis. Thyroid-stimulating hormone (TSH) and adrenocorticotropic hormone (ACTH) influence thyroxine and the adrenal cortex necessary in the regulation of gluconeogenesis. Protein levels that are insufficient and the presence of little or no muscle mass make gluconeogenesis difficult if not impossible. Gluconeogenesis may be inhibited in some infants who have high levels of insulin (Maniscaleo & Warshaw, 1978).

Glycolysis

The infant derives most of his or her heat production from the metabolism of brown fat. The term *brown fat* refers to the reddish-brown coloring of the fat, which is caused by the high vascularization of the tissue. Brown fat is stored in pockets throughout the neonate's body. The majority of brown fat is located around the neck, along the line of the spinal column between the scapulae, across the clavicle line, and down the sternal line. It also surrounds the major thoracic vessels and pads the kidneys. The full-term infant has sufficient brown fat to meet minimum heat needs for 2 to 4 days after birth (Holdcroft, 1980). Use of fat stores can be delayed by the infusion of glucose.

Heat production is activated in the presence of a cold stimulus, which is then transmitted to the hypothalamus. Both the anterior and posterior portions of the hypothalamus play a role in regulating temperature. Heat loss mechanisms related to maintenance of the body's set point temperature are controlled by the anterior hypothalamus. The posterior hypothalamus responds to cold stimuli and initiates brown fat thermogenesis. The stimulation of the release of norepinephrine and catecholamines triggers the production of glucose needed for thermogenesis in brown fat. More research on the role of catecholamines in adaptation and thermogenesis is needed (Copper & Goldenberg, 1990).

The purpose of brown fat is heat energy production. It is well suited for this function because of the presence of multiple fat vacuoles within the cytoplasm. The brown fat cell also contains a round central nucleus, glycogen, and a number of mitochondria, the cell's powerhouse, which are used for energy production. The fat vacuoles rapidly convert into heat energy because they are small and yet numerous and are readily available within the cell. The high number of mitochondria makes it easy to provide the energy (adenosine triphosphate [ATP]) for metabolic conversion and heat energy. Glycogen is available for ready use within the cell to mediate the ATP response.

Thermogenesis through brown fat stores cannot occur independently of other factors. Cell energy is also directly dependent on thyroxine, norepinephrine, triglycerides, glucose, and oxygen to metabolize fat and produce heat energy (Davis, 1980). The absence of any of these components makes thermogenesis impossible.

Mechanisms of Heat Transfer

Hypothermia is the most common concern for neonatal nurses. Hyperthermia, although a serious concern, occurs less frequently. Fluctuations in temperature cannot always be predicted or controlled. Sepsis and reactions to medication may cause a previously stable temperature to change suddenly and drastically. Monitoring the infant's temperature as well as the environmental temperature (including ambient air and incubator surface temperatures) helps identify potential temperature regulation needs of the infant (Thomas, 1994).

Heat is transferred through four basic mechanisms: radiation, convection, conduction, and evaporation. Heat can be gained through the mechanisms of radiation, conduction, and convection.

Radiation

Radiant energy is transferred between two objects in the environment that are not in direct contact with each other. The infant can readily gain heat from a warm object in the immediate environment, such as a radiant heater. The unprotected infant can also lose heat to objects in the immediate surroundings. Incubator walls, crib walls, and unwarmed objects placed near the infant all may serve as avenues for heat loss for the infant.

The ambient air temperature of the incubator is only one part of the assessment of the environmental status of the infant, inasmuch as large radiant heat losses may occur even with seemingly normal ambient air temperatures. Radiative heat loss is the most common type of loss for infants of less than 28 weeks' gestation after the first week after birth, as well as the main source of heat loss for all infants throughout the neonatal period (Hammarlund et al., 1986).

Radiant heat is commonly used to warm the infant because it is fast and efficient. Radiant heat is especially useful in the period immediately after birth, when easy access to the infant must be maintained. Radiant heat sources can also be used in tandem with other sources of heat for the infant.

Convection

Convection occurs when heat is exchanged between the environment and an object within the environment. In an open crib, the infant loses heat into the atmosphere. The amount of exposed skin determines the amount of heat lost through convection. To maintain a normal body temperature, a clothed infant who is exposed to air currents or cool air temperatures may be required to use a great deal of energy that is needed for growth.

In a radiant warming bed, a cool room or high air currents may counterbalance the effect of high heat output from the radiant warmer, thus cooling the infant. Inside the incubator, the infant gains heat from the warm internal environment. Clothed or unclothed, the infant is prevented from losing heat within this warmed setting.

Conduction

Conduction involves the transfer of heat from one object to another when they are in contact with each other. Conductive losses occur when the infant is placed on a cool surface. In the delivery room, the infant should be placed on a prewarmed surface. Linens should be prewarmed as well. Once stabilization has occurred, conductive heat losses must be continually avoided. Radiographic plates and infant weight scales, although used briefly, may cause a decrease in temperature stability in the infant who is premature or clinically unstable.

Evaporation

Evaporation is the loss of heat through water lost through the skin to the environment. Heat loss due to evaporation is the chief form of heat loss in the premature infant during the first week of life (Hammarlund et al., 1986). High evaporative loss is counterbalanced by a decrease in radiative and convective losses.

Evaporation cannot be used to provide heat for the infant, but there exist techniques for preventing loss of heat through excessive evaporation. Evaporative losses can be minimized by protecting body surfaces from the cooling effects of the environment. Protective clothing, skin barrier creams, and the use of high humidity in the infant's environment serve to decrease the evaporative heat losses of the infant. Evaporative losses occur most commonly after delivery and after bathing. During these times, the cool room air is most likely to cause heat losses through moist, uncovered skin surfaces.

Environmental Effects

The immediate environment of the infant can play a major role in thermoregulation. The room temperature is often kept slightly warmer than would be expected in the home. Air currents must be monitored. Drafts from air conditioners or blowers could easily effect conductive heat losses in the infant even when room air temperature is stable. External windows, especially during cool weather, may serve as sources of radiant heat loss for an infant in a warm room.

Thermal environment also plays a role in insensible water loss. As the ambient temperature rises to the maximum level for thermoneutrality or even surpasses it, the amount of insensible water loss of the infant rises (Bell et al., 1980). The preterm infant has greater insensible water loss than the full-term infant.

Concerns over the impact of environmental temperatures have played a role in the process of self-weaning from an isolette to an open crib. Proponents of this self-weaning method believe that an infant that is weaned in this manner will do better than one that is regulated only by waiting until a certain weight is reached and by mechanically controlling the isolette's temperature and moving back and forth between the isolette and open crib if there is a temperature problem. One study conducted to address environmental temperatures and their impact on neonatal temperatures was sponsored by the Association of Women's Health, Obstetric, and Neonatal Nurses (AWHONN) (Gelhar et al., 1994). This project's purpose was to determine the effects of temperatures in the neonatal intensive care unit (NICU) on neonatal temperatures during weaning from an isolette to an open crib. The research question was "Was there a relationship between the infant's temperature and the environmental temperature during the weaning period with infants wrapped in layers according to protocol?" (Gelhar et al., 1994, p. 342). This procedure is a common neonatal nursing care task that certainly has implications for length of stay and patient outcomes.

Six project sites were used, and 151 infants participated. The mean gestational age was 34.2 weeks; weights ranged from 1500 to 1800 g, with a mean of 1566 g (Gelhar et al., 1994). Weaning was initiated at 1500 g. The protocol for thermoregulation consisted of a double-thickness cap, cotton shirt, and diaper. Infants were covered by hospital-supplied blankets (one layer of insulation) and quilts (each quilt being heavier than a blanket and counted as two layers of insulation). These layers of insulation were added or subtracted as necessary to keep the infant's temperature in the range of 36°C to 37°C. Eight sets of temperatures were measured on each infant for 3 days, hence a total of 24 measurements per infant. A calibrated thermistor was used for these measurements. The findings did not support any significant effect of the environmental temperature on the infant's temperature. The researchers suggest this may be a result of the effectiveness of the insulating layers at keeping the infant in a neurally thermal environment. Swaddling practices in developing countries have been used for years to keep newborns warm. It has been in the high-technology environments of the NICU where thermoregulation has been a problem.

To critical consumers of research, what do these findings mean? Statistically they are not important, but clinically they suggest that nursing care can stabilize a neonatal temperature even in a 1500-g infant when attention is paid to insulating layers, swaddling practices, and frequent temperature measurements. It is an area of neonatal care that is in need of further research, because the move is on to decrease vital sign measurements and move infants home faster. To consumers of research, availability of personnel for measurements, institutional policies on weaning practices, and what problems a particular unit has had with temperature regulation should all be examined before the practice described is embraced as a new acceptable method of thermoregulation.

These findings supported an earlier AWHONN Research Utilization Project conducted by Meier and associates in 1993. Theirs was a similar study with 10 clinical sites, the purpose of which was "to develop and test a research-based weaning protocol that would be easy and practical to use" (p. 9). They included 270 infants whose birth weights were under 1550 g. The mean gestational age was 29.3 weeks at birth. This protocol was based, not

TABLE 16–2 Protocols Used in the AWHONN Research Utilization Project: Transition to an Open Crib for the Very Low Birth Weight Infant

Insulating the Infant

Clothe infants as soon as they are considered medically stable.

The clothing of the infant may occur several days or weeks before the infant is ready to be weaned to an open crib.

Clothing consists of double thickness cap, cotton shirt, and diaper.

Decreasing Incubator Temperature

Establish that infant is eligible to begin weaning process:

- approximately 1500 g
- 5 days of consistent weight gain
- stabilization of apnea and bradycardia episodes
- enteral nutrition
- medically stable
- not requiring assisted ventilation

Once the above requirements are met, the second step of the transition process can begin.

1. Add two layers of blankets and place the incubator on manual control. (During the Research Utilization project, a Yellow Springs probe was placed on the abdomen. While such a probe may be used to document temperature, it is not considered to be necessary during clinical use.)
2. The starting point of the incubator temperature should be the average temperature of the last 5 days minus 5% of the average temperature.
3. Record the temperature from the continuous monitor every 15 minutes for first hour after the incubator temperature has been decreased. Optimal infant abdominal skin temperature is between 36 and 37°C.
4. If the infant's temperature is greater than 37°C, lower the incubator temperature another 0.5°.
5. If the infant's temperature is less than 36°C, increase 0.5°C.
6. The goal is to have four stable temperature readings over a 1-hour time period. (Temperature monitoring every 15 minutes should be maintained until four stable temperature readings are obtained).
7. After the infant's temperature is stable, temperature should be recorded q3–4h.

After 24 Hours, Each Day

1. Lower incubator 1.5°. (There may be smaller decreases for the smaller infants and larger decreases for the bigger infants.)
2. Continually monitor temperature, with q3–4h recording of values.

Once the Infant Has Reached a 28°C Incubator

1. Keep the incubator at 28°C for 8 to 24 hours.
2. If weight gain has remained stable over the entire weaning course, remove infant to open crib.

Open Crib: First Day

1. Place open crib in draft-free environment.
2. If temperature in nursery is greater than 3° different from the incubator temperature, add additional blanket on infant.
3. Recheck infant's temperature. If infant's temperature is less than 36°C, then add another blanket, for a total of two more layers from the incubator.
4. Record infant temperature every 15 minutes for first hour, then during routine vital signs (q3–4h).
5. Do not bathe the infant on the first day of the open crib.
6. Record daily weight.

Second and Third Day in an Open Crib

1. Record every 3- to 4-hour temperature.
2. Record daily weight.
3. If an infant's temperature drops below 36°C, record temperature more frequently and take action to increase the temperature.

Transition Failure

1. If temperature is less than 36°C for more than 1 hour after a second blanket is added, return the infant to the incubator until temperature is stable. Record any identified problems. Try weaning again 72 hours later.
2. If there is a failure due to any other problems, document.

From Meier, P., Bliss-Holtz, J., Lund, C., et al. (1993). Transition of the preterm infant to an open crib. *AWHONN Voice, 1*(10), 10.

on weight alone, but rather on a steady weight gain over a 1-week period before the "thermal challenge." When the protocol listed in Table 16–2 was used, the average time of the "thermal challenge" was 3 days; 90 percent were weaned in 2 days or less. The incubator temperature at the beginning of the challenge was 28°C. Twenty percent required an extra blanket during the first day or so in an open crib. Only eight infants failed the weaning process. Therefore, they found that the environmental temperature could be controlled with insulated layers of blankets and standardized temperature monitoring (Meier et al., 1993).

INFANT ASSESSMENT

The first step in managing the thermal needs of the infant is to conduct a thorough assessment in order to identify normal and extraordinary thermal needs. Once risk factors are identified, appropriate action can be taken to provide for the needs of the infant. The following may be used as an assessment guide for factors that may influence the ability of the infant to generate heat or maintain thermoregulation:

I. Gestational age
   A. Comparison to size (AGA, SGA, LGA)
   B. Degree of prematurity (influencing skin's permeability and infant's ability to flex or extend)
II. Neurologic status
   A. Presence of CNS defects
      1. Anencephaly or absence of hypothalamus
      2. Myelomeningocele or encephalocele
   B. Neurologic insult
      1. Intracranial bleeding
      2. Prolonged hypoxia or asphyxia
III. Use of drugs that inhibit thermoregulatory response
   A. Maternal use during late pregnancy or labor
      1. Diazepam
      2. Meperidine
      3. Reserpine
      4. CNS depressants
   B. Infant drug intake
      1. CNS depressants
      2. Prostaglandins E_1 and E_2 (can cause increase in temperature)
      3. Atropine (may increase infant temperature)
IV. Cardiorespiratory response
   A. Cardiac insufficiency
      1. Cardiac failure
      2. Congenital heart disease
   B. Respiratory insufficiency
      1. Respiratory distress syndrome
      2. Persistent pulmonary hypertension
      3. Artificial ventilation
   C. Hypoxemia
   D. Exchange transfusion
V. Endocrine response
   A. Maternal use of thiourea compounds, leading to transient infant hypothyroidism
   B. Infant hypothyroidism
VI. Nutritional response
   A. Sufficient intake of calories

B. Use of oral feedings (may improve heat production)
C. Excess energy in the ingestion of nutrients
D. Balance of electrolytes, especially sodium and potassium

VII. Infection (Tappero & Honeyfield, 1996).

Assessment of temperature in the infant is easily accomplished in a variety of ways. No single method has been found to be universally superior. Temperature measurement instruments range from single-use paper thermometers to glass and mercury thermometers to a variety of electronic thermometers. Each method is satisfactory for accurate temperature measurement when used correctly.

The length of time that the thermometer is left in place influences the accuracy of the reading. Studies indicate that a temperature can be optimally measured in 5 to 10 minutes (Haddock et al., 1986, 1988). Although thermometer readings do not always stabilize during a period of 10 minutes, these minor variations may be insignificant (Haddock et al., 1988).

Rectal temperature historically has been considered the most accurate measurement of core body temperature. Although it may identify internal organ temperature, it may not truly reflect the stability of the infant's body temperature, because skin surfaces may cool before a drop in internal body temperature. The core temperature does not decline until the infant has lost the ability to produce heat (Dodman, 1987). The use of rectal temperature assessment has also been used to determine patency of the anal canal. Once this has been documented, the rectal route of temperature evaluation may not be necessary. Possible adverse effects of the use of rectal thermometers include rectal perforation and bradycardia secondary to neurologic response.

Axillary or skin surface temperatures may be lower than rectal temperature by as much as 1°C, but the difference is generally less than 0.4°C (Haddock et al., 1986). Skin temperature readings taken over the site of large brown fat stores may yield a falsely high reading, because these skin areas tend to remain warmer (Dawes, 1968). High evaporative losses may produce falsely high readings in abdominal skin temperature measurements (Hey, 1994). Inguinal site temperature may be more closely aligned to rectal temperature, and the measurement of core temperature at the inguinal site is less traumatic (Bliss-Holtz, 1989).

Since the mid-1980s, infrared tympanic thermometers have been available. Some institutions use these for all age groups. The rationale for using the ear canal is that it is a highly vascular region in which the amount of blood perfusion is the same as that in the hypothalamic region, the area responsible for temperature control. The temperature readings that are obtained by placing a small probe into the ear canal should approximate the core temperature. Newbold (1991) conducted a study in which three brands of infrared tympanic thermometers were compared. Results showed that when the tympanic thermometer was used correctly, there was only about a 0.3°F to 0.5°F difference between the three tympanic temperatures and an axillary temperature on the same child, the axillary temperature being lower. Tympanic thermometers are gaining acceptance and may be used in many more NICUs in the near future.

The timing of the temperature assessment of the infant on the basis of behavioral state is not significant. Although core body temperature declines in the active sleep states in adults, infants maintain active thermoregulation during sleep (Darnall & Ariagno, 1982).

Physiologic Response

A change in measured temperature may not occur until the infant has lost the ability to generate heat. The infant may display subtle signs of distress. Heart rate may rise. Tachypnea may manifest in an infant with temperature instability. In the cold stressed infant, tachypnea results from an increased need for oxygen as the result of an increase in metabolism. The heat-stressed infant becomes tachypneic in order to increase expiratory heat losses.

In the short-term response, the infant may exhibit changes in behavior and response. Long-term responses may include poor growth patterns and behavioral changes.

Temperature Stability

The variance of temperature readings in relation to the method used is less significant than the variability of the temperature of the infant over a period of time. After temperature fluctuations over a period of time, use of the same method of assessment is more important in evaluating thermoregulation than is the actual temperature value at one point in time. Assessing the infant for other factors, such as growth, oxygen needs, and feeding tolerance, also contributes to the determination of appropriate thermal control. Record review of growth charts, fractional inspired oxygen (FiO_2) needs, and notation of feedings and emesis provides ready access to these data.

Growth

Changes in normal growth patterns are frequently overlooked as an indicator of temperature instability. Energy demands for temperature control take precedence over the demands for growth. The infant who is exhibiting slow weight gain or erratic growth patterns may be experiencing poor thermal control. Infants who follow a normal growth curve are usually receiving sufficient intake of nutrients for both thermal control and weight gain. Infants who fail to gain weight despite adequate calorie intake may indicate poor temperature regulation or other environmental stress. After the ingestion of feedings, especially in the preterm infant, there is a rise in metabolic rate as well as in heat production. The increase in metabolism after the ingestion of human milk in the preterm infant may result from the metabolic demands of ingestion, digestion, and absorption (Rubecz & Mestyán, 1986). Infant thermal response may also be related to the temperature of the ingested milk. It is unclear whether these changes contribute to or inhibit growth.

Oxygen Requirements

Each infant has an individual rate of oxygen consumption in a neutral thermal environment. There is more of an increase in metabolic rate and oxygen consumption in a cool environment. This increase in metabolic rate is even greater in smaller infants (Dawes, 1968).

Using energy to produce heat also requires an increase in oxygen consumption. The infant who has increased demands for oxygen or has decreased ability to maintain basic oxygen needs through normal respiration is also at risk for impaired heat generation. As tissue oxygen levels decline, anaerobic metabolism of glucose yields relatively few heat energy molecules. The hypoxic tissues continue to metabolize greater stores of glucose and glycogen to meet energy demands, depleting already limited supplies. The anaerobic glucose response in the cold stressed infant is amplified (Maniscaleo & Warshaw, 1978).

The infant responds to thermal stress and energy demands by hyperventilation. In the healthy infant who is cold stressed, the consumption of oxygen may double or triple (James, 1973). In an infant with an elevated temperature, metabolic response may rise 10 percent for every degree of temperature elevation. The healthy infant may be able to compensate for increased oxygen demands, but the infant with respiratory or CNS compromise is unable to do so.

The VLBW infant, as the result of immaturity of the respiratory tract, may be unable to meet the metabolic demands. Without sufficient oxygenation, asphyxiated or hypoxic infants have a decreased ability to generate heat. Preterm infants are at risk for decreased oxygen intake even if distress is not apparent, because such infants may not be able to hyperventilate on the basis of metabolic needs. Thermogenesis is directly dependent on tissue oxygenation in order to use heat energy.

Behavioral Instability

The infant may exhibit behavioral signs that indicate poor temperature control. These signs may be subtle at first, but as the infant's temperature continues to change, the signs may become more recognizable.

Body positioning is one of the first signs that the infant is attempting to respond to internal or environmental temperature changes. The full-term infant is able to assume a flexed body position in order to generate and retain body heat. The premature infant has a very limited ability to assume a flexed position and may indeed be incapable of changing position.

In the infant who is overheated, the body tends to achieve a more open or flaccid position to allow for a greater surface area for heat loss. Premature infants, unless assisted in achieving a flexed position, may remain in a heat-losing flaccid position even in a cool or neutral thermal environment.

Skin changes may occur in infants when thermoregulation has been disturbed. In the infant who is cool, skin color may range from pale to cyanotic. Mottling in peripheral areas may also occur as a response to cooling attempts to retain core body temperature. The overheated infant may become slightly plethoric. Although the sweating mechanism is poorly developed in infants, diaphoresis may occur.

The infant with disturbances in temperature control may exhibit feeding difficulties. If energy is being used to generate heat, sufficient energy for sucking may not be available. The infant who is gavage-fed may vomit feedings if he or she is too cool or overheated.

THERMAL MANAGEMENT

There is no single normal temperature for the infant. A normal range for an individual infant must be broad enough to allow for temperature variations that can occur during sleep or feedings. Premature infants are often stabilized at temperatures slightly lower than what is considered acceptable for full-term infants.

The healthy full-term infant is able to initiate heat production within a few hours after birth. The infant usually requires assistance in maintenance of body temperature during this time. After delivery, infants are often cared for in a warming bed until temperature stabilization has occurred. Once the infant has stabilized, a shirt and diaper may be put on and the infant wrapped in one or two cotton blankets. If the ambient temperature is cool or if drafts occur in the immediate area, the head of the infant may be covered with a cotton stocking-knit cap.

The thermal management of the low birth weight or premature infant requires special attention. There is no set temperature for which an infant is considered to be in a neutral thermal environment. For some low birth weight infants, a skin temperature of 36°C to 36.5°C may be acceptable. For others, a lower temperature range may be more appropriate as long as adequate calorie needs are being met, especially in the form of gastric feedings (Hey, 1994).

Environmental temperature is not the only factor in determining temperature stability. Use of humidity alters the need to increase the ambient temperature by as much as 1.5°C (Hey, 1994). Conversely, when humidity is lowered, the ambient temperature must be raised to provide for temperature stability in the infant.

Interventions

Thermal management can be controlled in a variety of ways. No single way works best for every infant under all conditions. Use of incubators to control environmental changes and effects is generally believed to be a safe and efficient method of providing for the heat needs of the infant. The ambient temperature of the incubator can be controlled manually, through air temperature control, or through skin control. Each method, when monitored appropriately, can provide a mechanism for thermocontrol (Bell & Rios, 1983a) (Table 16–3).

Radiant Warmer Beds

The radiant warmer bed has the advantage of being a powerful and efficient means of providing heat for the newborn. It does, however, allow for a great deal of convective heat loss in the infant (Baumgart, 1985). Through the use of the radiant warmer bed in the delivery room, the infant can be assessed properly, inasmuch as clothing would obstruct careful head-to-toe analysis. Once the infant has been dried and wrapped, the heat from a radiant warmer may serve as adjunct warmth for the infant attempting to achieve self-regulation.

In the nursery, radiant warmers are a useful way to provide for heat needs of the infant who requires treatment or resuscitation and stabilization. The radiant warmer may also be used for infants who are too large for standard incubators but require assistance in thermoregulation.

Stabilized infants in radiant heaters have shown a significantly higher insensible water loss and higher oxygen intake than have infants who are cared for in incubators (LeBlanc, 1982; Marks et al., 1980). Evaporative heat losses can be decreased through the use of plastic blankets, which also play a role in convective losses (Baumgart et al., 1981). Many NICUs use radiant warmers for all infants, regardless of size. These units prefer compensating for the insensible water losses that are encountered even in the smallest of infants. Liberalization of fluids requires meticulous monitoring of intake and output to avoid fluid overload. Other units would rather have VLBW infants in incubators to reduce the difficulty in maintaining fluid balance.

Incubator

The incubator is the ideal environment for the infant who is unable to thermoregulate. Radiant and convective heat losses are kept to a minimum in the infant who is cared for in an incubator,

TABLE 16–3 Assessment Factors to Consider in Determining Appropriate Method of Temperature Control for Selected Neonates

Gestational age at the time of birth
Current age of the infant
Infant weight
Established baseline temperature for infant if other than unit standard
Amount of clothing or coverings being used for the infant
Need for frequent handling of infant
Need for full visibility of infant at all times
High fluid loss potential (e.g., poor skin integrity or open wounds or lesions)
Use of equipment that may alter temperature or fluid loss (e.g., phototherapy lights)
Method of heater regulation available (i.e., skin, rectal, or air servocontrol)

because ambient temperature is high, warming the incubator walls. Appropriate nursing care and assessment can be performed whether the infant is naked or is dressed and wrapped. The air temperature of the incubator is adjusted according to the infant's needs.

Portholes and doors must be kept closed unless a specific intervention is being carried out. Incubator temperature may drop several degrees if the portholes are left open for several minutes. The temperature drops dramatically if the door is left open for any period of time. It may take from 10 to 20 minutes for the incubator temperature to reach the previous level and stabilize.

Use of computer-assisted temperature control in incubators was shown to be effective in decreasing the mortality rates for infants whose temperatures were closely monitored (Perlstein et al., 1976). Computer regulation of servocontrolled incubators decreases the amount of ambient temperature variations, thus decreasing physiologic responses to cold stress (Endo, 1981). These systems are quite costly and have not been widely adopted.

Premature infants who are having difficulty in thermoregulating inside an incubator may achieve better results in a double-walled incubator. The double wall serves as a barrier to radiative heat losses to the cool walls, because the inside wall is warmed by the ambient air temperature of the incubator (Marks et al., 1981). Double-walled incubators may lead to high convective heat losses in some infants, even though radiative heat losses may be lowered (Bell & Rios, 1983b). Infant temperature stabilization must be monitored to determine the effectiveness of the incubator. A double-walled transport incubator may be more effective in maintaining infant temperature than is a single-walled incubator (LeBlanc, 1984a). Incubators can be heated by using either conduction or radiation sources. Oxygen consumption is not significantly different between infants who are in radiative heated incubators and those in conductive heated incubators (LeBlanc, 1984b).

The nurse often is the one who reminds other health professionals to cluster the times when the incubator is opened. Collaboration is necessary if heat is to be preserved and the neonate is to be protected from temperature fluctuations. Signs by the bed to remind personnel to keep the time in the incubator to a minimum are sometimes helpful in providing thermal stability to the infant. Regulation of the incubator's environmental temperature is also dependent on the amount of humidity that is maintained.

Humidity

Humidity lowers the evaporative losses in the infant. The infant who is cared for in an environment of at least 50 percent humidity requires lower ambient temperature than if humidity is not provided. Use of humidity remains controversial, in that the moisture or water reservoir serves as a potential source of infection for the infant. Use of humidity above 50 percent supports the growth of gram-negative microorganisms, which compromise the sick or premature infant (Nalepka, 1976). In incubator in which water is used in the reservoirs, the addition of silver nitrate has been effective in controlling the growth of these organisms. If no treatment is used to prevent colonization, the water should be drained every few days and prewarmed water should be added.

Because heat is lost through the respiratory tract, humidity is always provided for the infant receiving oxygen therapy or assisted ventilation. Humidified air delivered to the infant via an endotracheal tube decreases the insensible water loss in the infant, although this humidification does not contribute to thermal equilibrium in the infant (Sosulski et al., 1983).

Heat Shields

Heat shields have been shown to be effective in some cases when thermoregulation could not be achieved through the use of radiant or convective heat sources alone. Plexiglas tents have been used as a method of shielding the infant within the incubator. Infants in radiant warmers have been shielded with plastic sheeting placed over the area of the infant. It must also be remembered that effective heat loss shields may block the warming equipment from providing heat to the infant. In the cold stressed infant, heat shields may be inappropriate.

Warming Pads

Heated water pads have been shown to be effective in decreasing the heater output when used on infants who are cared for under radiant warmers (Topper & Stewart, 1984). A decrease in heater output may decrease the ill effects of radiant heat on infants who must be cared for under radiant warmers. Heated mattress pads are also effective in maintaining incubator heat in transport incubators before and during transport of the infant (Nielsen et al., 1976).

A major concern with the use of heated pads is the occurrence of thermal burns on the skin of the infant. The infant who is most likely to require assistance with heat gain is the preterm infant. The skin of the preterm infant is extremely fragile and may suffer from thermal injury at lower temperatures than expected. Warming pads may best be used only if no other source of heat is available.

Head Coverings

It is well recognized that the infant's head is the largest heat-losing body surface. Traditionally, the head was left uncovered, providing a vehicle for heat loss. Current thermoregulatory care needs incorporate the use of head coverings in most newborn care settings. In the delivery room, the infant is dried and wrapped in a prewarmed blanket. The infant's head is also covered at this time. The most common head covering used is a cotton stocking-knit cap (D'Apolito, 1994).

Once the infant is stabilized, the hat may continue to be used to prevent heat loss in drafty rooms or during periods of exposure for nursing care or examination. The premature infant may benefit from the addition of a plastic lining in the cap, which further insulates the head from evaporative and conductive heat losses (Greer, 1988; Rowe et al., 1983). If the infant has become cool, however, the use of a lined cap may prevent the infant from gaining heat through radiation or conduction (Templeman & Bell, 1986). In this case, the insulated cap should be removed; a plain cotton cap may be used. Some institutions prefer the use of woolen caps, but their use should be discontinued if skin irritation occurs.

Plastic Wraps and Coverings

Plastic wraps have been used on infants to decrease the amount of evaporative losses in the early postdelivery stage of life. Bubble plastic has also been shown to be an effective insulator, while allowing visualization of the infant (Besch et al., 1971). In infants under radiant warmers, loosely fitting plastic wraps have been effective in decreasing insensible water loss and oxygen consumption as well as decreasing the heater output (Baumgart, 1984).

In the premature infant, the use of plastic wraps decreases insensible water and heat loss. Use of plastic wraps also assists in achieving thermal control in incubators at a lower ambient air temperature than for infants who are not wrapped (Darnall & Ariagno, 1979).

Skin Protectors

Paraffin has been used with some success as a skin barrier in preventing evaporative heat losses (Brice et al., 1981). Although helpful in some infants, its use must be balanced with other methods of thermoregulation. Skin irritation is possible and necessitates termination of treatment with this method.

Barrier creams have also been used as a method for decreasing evaporative losses. However, there may be much absorption of the chemicals within the cream, as a result of the thin layer of skin of the preterm infant.

Skin protector treatments may necessitate repeated applications, which disturb the infant. The skin of the infant must be assessed regularly for irritation. The contents of the products used must be analyzed to prevent complications in the infant.

Skin-to-Skin Care

Skin-to-skin care of the infant has been reintroduced as a method of caring for infants, especially stable low birth weight infants (Ludington-Hoe et al., 1991, 1994). This method of care involves the placement of the infant against the mother's skin in an upright position between her breasts. The infant is clothed only in a diaper and perhaps a hat.

Although not widely accepted as a means of thermal control, the skin-to-skin control method, or "kangaroo" care, is a means of providing warmth to low birth weight infants who are stable when other methods of thermal control are unavailable or limited. Ludington-Hoe and colleagues (1991) reported that in a study of stable premature infants with an average gestational age of 34.5 weeks, significant increases in heart rate as well as skin and rectal temperatures were demonstrated during skin-to-skin contact. These increases were all within the normal ranges for these vital signs.

A secondary use of skin-to-skin care has been to facilitate early parent–infant contact to promote attachment. This method of care has been shown to improve the length of lactation in mothers of these infants (Vaughans, 1990; Whitelaw et al., 1981).

Low birth weight infants who have been cared for in this manner for at least brief daily periods sometimes show a slight decline in temperature readings of 0.2°C; conversely, there may be a slight increase in maternal as well as infant temperature (Anderson, 1989; Bosque et al., 1988; Whitelaw et al., 1981). Although this type of care may not be used widely as a method for providing heat stabilization for infants, it can be safely used in stable infants to assist in improving lactation and parent–infant attachment (Sloan et al., 1994). Ludington (1990) studied preterm infants, 34 to 36 weeks' gestation, who participated in skin-to-skin contact and found that these infants exhibited less purposeless activity and state-related energy consumption.

THERMAL STRESS

Despite attempts at maintaining thermoneutrality, the infant may experience changes in temperature that may cause physiologic stress. Changes that lead to both increased and decreased temperature produce changes in the infant that may be difficult to regulate. Brief episodes of cold stress in the first few days of life, however, may assist the infant in thermoregulation when cold stress occurs after the third day of life (Perlstein et al., 1974). Even a full-term infant experiences cold stress and must be assessed for it by simultaneous temperature site comparisons (Bliss-Holtz, 1991, 1993). The preterm infant may not display a similar response. Decreased stress and conservation of calories places the infant at less risk for temperature instability—at least for instability resulting from depleted energy stores.

Cold Stress

The infant is placed at risk for cold stress when in transport from one warmed environment to another. Cold stress can occur in a premature infant who is being transferred from one incubator to another. When infants must be transported from one hospital to another, cold stress is a common problem because environmental temperature changes cannot easily be controlled. Infants who require surgery are at risk for cold stress from the time they are transported to the operating room until the time they are returned to the unit. Anesthetic agents may inhibit the infant's ability to generate heat or maintain thermoneutrality.

Three mechanisms are involved in cold stress. The first mechanism involves the sympathetic nervous system. Peripherally, vasoconstriction occurs to limit the loss of heat. The heart rate increases to compensate for the increased demand of metabolism to maintain heat. The second mechanism involves shivering and posturing. Although infants have limited ability to shiver, some heat may be generated in this manner. Posture changes, chiefly toward a more flexed position, also help the infant retain body heat. The preterm infant has no ability to shiver and extremely limited ability to change position. The third mechanism involves the stimulation of the pituitary and the release of chemicals to initiate chemical responses to achieve heat energy output.

The effects of cold stress can be detected in all aspects of body functioning. Each system that is affected may then have a feedback mechanism that affects another body system. Before temperature changes are recorded, oxygen consumption has already increased. The prevention of cold stress is essential in protecting the infant from multisystem stress.

The cardiorespiratory system manifests the most obvious symptoms when the infant is cold stressed. As the temperature declines, peripheral vasoconstriction occurs in order to conserve heat. As central blood volume increases, pulse and blood pressure increase. Once central cooling has occurred, diuresis may result, with a decline in pulse and blood pressure, leading to decreased cardiac output. Arrhythmias may occur secondary to acidosis as fatty acids break down in an attempt to generate heat.

The CNS can be affected by cold stress secondary to cardiovascular changes. As peripheral vasoconstriction occurs, cerebral blood flow diminishes. Decreased blood flow to the brain compromises metabolic activity. Electroencephalographic activity may decline. In order to obtain an accurate electroencephalogram, body temperature must be in the normal range. Peripheral nerve conduction may also be delayed. Pupils may become dilated and fixed.

Metabolic response to cold stress encompasses fluid, electrolyte, and glucose aberrations. In the early stages, diuresis occurs. If cold stress continues, further changes take place. With decreased perfusion to the kidneys, glomerular filtration declines, along with the reabsorption of sodium, water, and glucose. Hypoglycemia results as the consumption of glucose rises with the rise in metabolic rate. Unstable glucose levels can lead to further acidosis and neurologic damage. As the release of nonesterified fatty acid increases, the liver slows metabolism of glucose, inhibiting thermogenesis. As liver function declines, drugs are metabolized and excreted more slowly.

Acidosis occurs as the result of a variety of contributing factors. As tissue perfusion declines, lactic, pyruvic, and organic acids build. The kidneys and liver are unable to metabolize and secrete these products. The enzymatic action within the kidneys is blocked, preventing acid–base regulation through a diminished excretion of hydrogen ions (Holdcroft, 1980). Fluid balance is further complicated by poor gastrointestinal absorption and decreased peristalsis.

As acidosis continues, there is an increase in dissociation of the indirect bilirubin from albumin-binding sites. The increase in nonesterified fatty acids is caused by their high affinity for the albumin-binding sites. In the presence of high levels of nonesterified fatty acids, kernicterus can occur in the cold stressed infant with relatively low bilirubin levels (Williams & Lancaster, 1976).

The cold stressed infant may be at risk for bleeding, because clotting factors may be altered. Besides thrombocytopenia, there is an increase in hematocrit and in viscosity of the blood. This may be secondary to fluid shifts that occur with cold stress.

Clinically, the infant becomes lethargic and refuses to eat when cold stressed. The respirations of the infant become slow and shallow. If stimulated, the infant has a weak cry. There is a decreased response to painful stimuli. A ruddy coloring, secondary to the failure of dissociation of oxyhemoglobin, belies the seriousness of the infant's condition (Klaus et al., 1993). As the condition continues, the infant becomes edematous or scleremic.

Methods of Rewarming

To keep oxygen consumption to a minimum during rewarming, the incubator temperature should be adjusted to 1° to 1.5° higher than the infant's temperature (Dodman, 1987). Hourly, the incubator temperature may be adjusted upwardly by 1° until the infant's temperature has been stabilized (Brueggemeyer, 1995). If the infant has been severely cold stressed, his or her temperature may continue to decline during the early stages of rewarming (Laburn & Laburn, 1985). Caps, plastic wrap, and heat shields should be removed to prevent them from interfering with heat gain.

Ingested fluids can be warmed before their introduction to the infant. Feedings should always be warmed before being given to a premature or cold stressed infant. In most cases, feedings should be withheld from a cold stressed infant in order to prevent problems caused by a decrease in gastrointestinal motility. Intravenous fluids may also be warmed by using blood-warming devices or by placing an extra length of tubing inside the incubator to allow the warmed environment to warm the fluids.

High levels of serum sodium are associated with increased temperatures, whereas high levels of calcium indicate decreased temperatures. The exact mechanism for this is unknown but may be related to the ratio of sodium to calcium and not isolated elevations of either electrolyte (Abels, 1986). Normal saline may be given intravenously during the rewarming process to assist the infant in raising the body temperature (Klaus et al., 1993).

Heat Stress

Heat stress, excluding the febrile state, should never be allowed to occur in the neonate. When it does occur, it is generally caused by improper use or monitoring of equipment to warm infants. Occasionally, the neutral thermal temperature for the infant may be overestimated, causing heat stress when the infant's temperature is raised to a level that is too high for the infant.

Overheating can often be differentiated from febrile episodes by determining the differences in core or rectal temperature from the skin temperatures of the central body and distal extremities. When core temperatures are elevated in febrile conditions, the skin temperature of the distal extremities remains cool in comparison to the skin temperature of the trunk (Harpin et al., 1983). This difference may also be evident in VLBW infants if thermoregulation has not been satisfactorily achieved.

Overheating can lead to a variety of responses in the infant. All infants tend to be less active as the environmental temperature increases. Heat stress may be evident in a preterm infant below 36°C. Mature infants may become more restless or irritable. Both preterm and full-term infants generally attempt to achieve an extended posture and become more flaccid. Cardiovascular changes may be subtle. Elevations in heart rate and respiratory rate may be negligible.

Color changes may be more evident in the infant and more indicative of heat stress. Color change in the overheated infant often occurs first in the soles of the feet, which become more pink to red (Harpin et al., 1983). Overall increase in redness may not occur until the infant is heat stressed. The febrile infant often becomes more pale with cool extremities.

The heat-stressed infant should be assisted in keeping metabolic heat production to a minimum. The infant who assumes an extended position should be left in this position in order to encourage heat loss. Skin surfaces can be left exposed to enhance evaporative loss. Active temperature reduction methods should be kept at a minimum to prevent a dramatic loss of heat, potentially leading to cold stress and shock.

Apnea

Apnea is a problem associated with temperature changes, especially in the premature infant. Sudden or dramatic infant temperature changes can lead to apnea (Fanaroff & Martin, 1997). Overheating can cause an increase in apneic spells in premature infants (Harpin et al., 1983).

Special attention must be paid to the infant during rewarming to prevent complications from rapid temperature changes. Sudden increases in ambient temperature may also lead to an increase in apneic spells as well as overly rapid rewarming of the cold stressed infant (Perlstein et al., 1970; Perlstein, 1987).

CONCLUSION

Temperature is an integral part of the environment of the infant. Although there are a variety of ways to assist the infant in achieving thermoregulation, each must be used appropriately to achieve its goal and to prevent complications. The nurse is in the pivotal role of protecting the infant from thermal stress and assisting the infant in achieving thermoregulation.

REFERENCES

Abels, L. (1986). *Critical care nursing: A physiologic approach* (pp. 548–587). St. Louis: C. V. Mosby.

Anderson, G. C. (1989). Skin-to-skin: Kangaroo care in Western Europe. *American Journal of Nursing, 89*(5), 662–666.

Baumgart, S. (1984). Reduction of oxygen consumption, insensible water loss, and radiant heat demand with use of a plastic blanket for low-birth-weight infants under radiant warmers. *Pediatrics, 74*(6), 1022–1028.

Baumgart, S. (1985). Partitioning of heat losses and gains in premature infants under radiant warmers. *Pediatrics, 75*(1), 89–99.

Baumgart, S., Engle, W. D., Fox, W. W., & Polin, R. A. (1981). Effect of heat shielding on convective and evaporative heat losses and on radiant heat transfer in the premature infant. *Journal of Pediatrics, 99*(6), 948–956.

Bell, E. F., Gray, J. C., Weinstein, M. R., & Oh, W. (1980). The effects of thermal environment on heat balance and insensible water loss in low-birth-weight infants. *Journal of Pediatrics, 96*(3), 452–459.

Bell, E. F., & Rios, G. R. (1983a). Air versus skin temperature servocontrol of infant incubators. *Journal of Pediatrics, 103*(6), 954–959.

Bell, E. F., & Rios, G. R. (1983b). A double-walled incubator alters the partition of body heat loss of premature infants. *Pediatric Research, 17,* 135–140.

Besch, N. J., Perlstein, P. H., Edwards, N. K., et al. (1971). The transparent baby bag. *New England Journal of Medicine, 284*(3), 121–124.

Bliss-Holtz, J. (1989). Comparison of rectal, axillary, and inguinal temperatures in full-term newborn infants. *Nursing Research, 38*(2), 85–87.

Bliss-Holtz, J. (1991). Determining cold stress in full term newborns through temperature site comparisons. *Scholarly Inquiry for Nursing Practice, 5*(2), 113–123.

Bliss-Holtz, J. (1993). Determination of thermoregulatory state in full-term infants. *Nursing Research, 42*(4), 204–207.

Bosque, E. M., Brady, J. P., Affonso, D. D., & Wahlberg, V. (1988). Continuous physiological measures of kangaroo versus incubator care in a tertiary level nursery [Abstract #1204]. *Pediatric Research, 23*(4, part 2), 402A.

Brice, J. E. H., Rutter, N., & Hull, D. (1981). Reduction of skin water loss in the newborn: Clinical trial of two methods in very low birthweight babies. *Archives of Disease in Childhood, 56*(9), 673–675.

Brueggemeyer, A. (1995). Thermoregulation. In L. P. Gunderson & C. Kenner (Eds.), *Care of the 24–25 week gestational age infant: Small baby protocol* (2nd ed., pp. 27–42). Petaluma, CA: Neonatal Network.

Copper, R. L., & Goldenberg, R. L. (1990). Catecholamine secretion in fetal adaptation to stress. *Journal of Obstetric, Gynecologic, and Neonatal Nursing, 19*(3), 223–226.

D'Apolito, K. (1994). Hats used to maintain body temperature. *Neonatal Network, 13*(5), 93–94.

Darnall, R. A., & Ariagno, R. L. (1979). Resting oxygen consumption of premature infants covered with a plastic thermal blanket. *Pediatrics, 63*(4), 547–551.

Darnall, R. A., & Ariagno, R. L. (1982). The effect of sleep state on active thermoregulation in the premature infant. *Pediatric Research, 16*, 512–514.

Davis, V. (1980). The structure and function of brown adipose tissue in the neonate. *Journal of Obstetric, Gynecologic, and Neonatal Nursing, 9*(1), 368–372.

Dawes, G. (1968). *Foetal and neonatal physiology* (pp. 191–209). Chicago: Year Book Medical Publishers.

Dodman, N. (1987). Newborn temperature control. *Neonatal Network, 5*(6), 19–23.

Dunn, P. (1994). Maternal hypothermia: Implications for obstetric nurses. *Journal of Obstetric, Gynecologic, and Neonatal Nursing, 23*(3), 238–242.

Endo, A. S. (1981). Using computers in newborn intensive care settings. *American Journal of Nursing, 81*(7), 1336–1337.

Fanaroff, A. A., & Martin, R. J. (1997). *Neonatal-perinatal medicine: Diseases of the fetus and newborn* (6th ed.). St. Louis: C. V. Mosby.

Gelhar, D. K., Miserendino, C. A. K., O'Sullivan, P. L., & Vessey, J. A. (1994). Research from the research utilization project: Environmental temperatures. *Journal of Obstetric, Gynecologic, and Neonatal Nursing, 23*(4), 341–344.

Greer, P. S. (1988). Head coverings for newborns under radiant warmers. *Journal of Obstetric, Gynecologic, and Neonatal Nursing, 17*(4), 265–271.

Haddock, B. J., Merrow, D. L., & Vincent, P. A. (1988). Comparisons of axillary and rectal temperatures in the preterm infant. *Neonatal Network, 6*(5), 67–71.

Haddock, B., Vincent, P., & Merrow, D. (1986). Axillary and rectal temperatures of full-term neonates: Are they different? *Neonatal Network, 5*(1), 36–40.

Hammarlund, K., Strömberg, B., & Sedin, G. (1986). Heat loss from the skin of preterm and fullterm newborn infants during the first weeks after birth. *Biology of the Neonate, 50*(1), 1–10.

Harpin, V. A., Chellappah, G., & Rutter, N. (1983). Responses of the newborn infant to overheating. *Biology of the Neonate, 44*(2), 65–75.

Hey, E. (1994). Thermoregulation. In G. B. Avery, M. A. Fletcher, & M. G. MacDonald (Eds.), *Neonatology: Pathophysiology and management in the newborn* (4th ed., pp. 357–365). Philadelphia: J. B. Lippincott.

Holdcroft, A. (1980). *Body temperature control in anesthesia, surgery & intensive care*. London: Baillière Tindall.

Hull, D., & Smales, O. R. C. (1978). Heat production in the newborn. In J. C. Sinclair (Ed.), *Temperature regulation and energy metabolism in the newborn* (pp. 129–156). New York: Grune & Stratton.

James, L. S. (1973). Acid-base changes in the perinatal period. In R. W. Winters (Ed.), *The body fluids in pediatrics* (pp. 185–206). Boston: Little, Brown.

Klaus, M. H., Martin, R. J., & Fanaroff, A. A. (1993). The physical environment. In M. H. Klaus & A. A. Fanaroff (Eds.), *Care of the high-risk neonate* (4th ed., pp. 114–129). Philadelphia: W. B. Saunders.

Laburn, D. M., & Laburn, H. P. (1985). Pathophysiology of temperature regulation. *Physiologist, 28*(6), 507–517.

LeBlanc, M. H. (1982). Relative efficacy of an incubator and an open warmer in producing thermoneutrality for the small premature infant. *Pediatrics, 69*(4), 439–445.

LeBlanc, M. H. (1984a). Evaluation of two devices for improving thermal control of premature infants in transport. *Critical Care Medicine, 12*(7), 593–595.

LeBlanc, M. H. (1984b). Relative efficacy of radiant and convective heat in incubators in producing thermoneutrality for the premature. *Pediatric Research, 18*(5), 425–428.

Ludington, S. M. (1990). Energy conservation during skin-to-skin contact between premature infants and their mothers. *Heart and Lung, 19*(5, Part 1), 445–451.

Ludington-Hoe, S. M., Hadeed, A. J., & Anderson, G. C. (1991). Physiologic responses to skin-to-skin contact in hospitalized premature infants. *Journal of Perinatology, 11*(1), 19–29.

Ludington-Hoe, S. M., Thompson, C., Swinth, J., et al. (1994). Kangaroo care: Research results, and practice implications and guidelines. *Neonatal Network, 13*(1), 19–37.

Maniscaleo, W. M., & Warshaw, J. B. (1978). Cellular energy metabolism during fetal and perinatal development. In J. Sinclair (Ed.), *Temperature regulation and energy metabolism in the newborn* (pp. 1–37). New York: Grune & Stratton.

Marks, K. H., Gunther, R. C., Rossi, J. A., & Maisels, M. J. (1980). Oxygen consumption and insensible water loss in premature infants under radiant heaters. *Pediatrics, 66*(2), 228–232.

Marks, K. H., Lee, C. A., Bolan, C. D., & Maisels, M. J. (1981). Oxygen consumption and temperature control of premature infants in a double-wall incubator. *Pediatrics, 68*(1), 93–98.

Meier, P., Bliss-Holtz, J., Lund, C., et al. (1993). Transition of the preterm infant to an open crib. *AWHONN Voice, 1*(10), 9–10.

Mestyán, J. (1978). Energy metabolism and substrate utilization in the newborn. In J. Sinclair (Ed.), *Temperature regulation and energy metabolism in the newborn* (pp. 39–74). New York: Grune & Stratton.

Nalepka, C. D. (1976). Understanding thermoregulation in newborns. *Journal of Obstetric, Gynecologic, and Neonatal Nursing, 5*(6), 17–19.

Newbold, M. S. (1991). Evaluation of a new infrared tympanic thermometer: Comparison of three brands. *Journal of Pediatric Nursing, 6*(4), 281–283.

Nielsen, H. C., Jung, A. L., & Atherton, S. O. (1976). Evaluation of the Porta-warm mattress as a source of heat for neonatal transport. *Pediatrics, 58*(4), 500–504.

Perlstein, P. H. (1987). Routine and special care: Physical environment. In A. A. Fanaroff & R. J. Martin (Eds.), *Neonatal-perinatal medicine: Diseases of the fetus and infant* (pp. 398–415). St. Louis: C. V. Mosby.

Perlstein, P. H., Edwards, N. K., Atherton, H. D., & Sutherland, J. M. (1976). Computer-assisted newborn intensive care. *Pediatrics, 57*(4), 494–501.

Perlstein, P. H., Edwards, N. K., & Sutherland, J. M. (1970). Apnea in premature infants and incubator-air-temperature changes. *New England Journal of Medicine, 282*(9), 461–466.

Perlstein, P. H., Hersh, C., Glueck, C. J., & Sutherland, J. M. (1974). Adaptation to cold in the first days of life. *Pediatrics, 54*(4), 411–415.

Ringer, S. A., & Stark, A. R. (1990). Management of neonatal emergencies in the delivery room. *Clinics in Perinatology, 16*(1), 23–41.

Rowe, M. I., Weinberg, G., & Andrews, W. (1983). Reduction of neonatal heat loss by an insulated head cover. *Journal of Pediatric Surgery, 18*(6), 909–913.

Rubecz, I., & Mestyán, J. (1986). Postprandial thermogenesis in human milk–fed very low birth weight infants. *Biology of the Neonate, 49*(6), 301–306.

Sauer, P. J. J., Dane, H. J., & Visser, H. K. A. (1984). Longitudinal studies on metabolic rate, heat loss, and energy cost of growth in low birth weight infants. *Pediatric Research, 18*(3), 254–259.

Sauer, P. J. J., & Visser, H. K. A. (1984). The neutral temperature of very low-birth-weight infants. *Pediatrics, 74*(2), 288–289.

Schubring, C. (1986). Temperature regulation in healthy and resuscitated newborns immediately after birth. *Journal of Perinatal Medicine, 14*, 27–33.

Schwartz, R., Hay, E., & Baum, J. (1978). Management of newborn thermal environment. In J. Sinclair (Ed.), *Temperature regulation and energy metabolism in the newborn* (pp. 129–156). New York: Grune & Stratton.

Sosulski, R., Polin, R. A., & Baumgart, S. (1983). Respiratory water loss and heat balance in intubated infants receiving humidified air. *Journal of Pediatrics, 103*(2), 307–310.

Sloan, N. L., Camacho, L. W. L., Rojas, E. P., et al. (1994). Kangaroo mother method: Randomised controlled trial of an alternative method of care for stabilised low-birthweight infants. *Lancet, 344*(8925), 782–785.

Swyer, P. (1978). Heat loss after birth. In J. Sinclair (Ed.), *Temperature regulation and energy metabolism in the newborn* (pp. 91–128). New York: Grune & Stratton.

Tappero, E., & Honeyfield, M. (1996). *Physical assessment of the newborn: A comprehensive approach to the art of physical examination.* Petaluma, CA: NICU Ink.

Templeman, M. C., & Bell, E. F. (1986). Head insulation for premature infants in servocontrolled incubators and radiant warmers. *American Journal of Diseases of Children, 140*, 940–942.

Thomas, K. (1994). Thermoregulation in neonates. *Neonatal Network, 13*(2), 15–25.

Topper, W. H., & Stewart, T. P. (1984). Thermal support for the very-low-birth-weight infant: Role of supplemental conductive heat. *Journal of Pediatrics, 105*(5), 810–814.

Vaughans, B. (1990). Early maternal infant contact and neonatal thermoregulation. *Neonatal Network, 8*(5), 19–21.

Wheldon, A. E., & Hull, D. (1983). Incubation of very immature infants. *Archives of Disease in Childhood, 58*(7), 504–508.

Whitelaw, A., Heisterkamp, G., Sleath, K., et al. (1981). Skin to skin contact for very low birthweight infants and their mothers. *Archives of Disease in Childhood, 63*, 1377–1381.

Williams, J. K., & Lancaster, J. (1976). Thermoregulation of the newborn. *Maternal Child Nursing, 1*(6), 355–360.

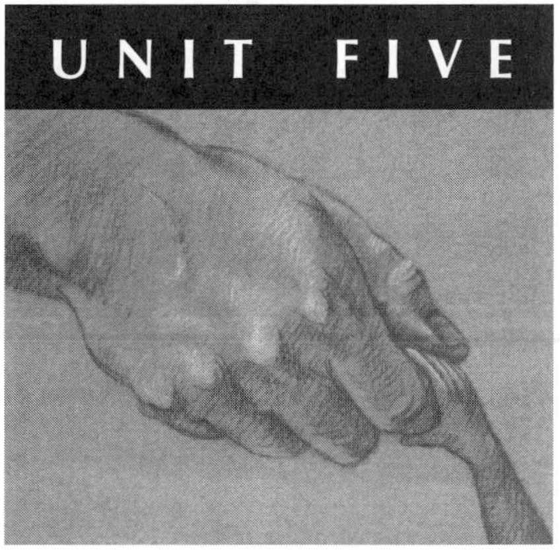

Physiologic Adaptation of the Neonate

It seemed that all the K9 nurses knew that today was Emily's day for surgery. Many stopped by to give us little pep talks, or simply to smile at Emily and wish her luck. The sense of community among this disparate collection of humanity had never felt stronger.

As luck would have it, Leslie was not scheduled to work today. This was as disappointing for her as it was for Fox and me, because at this point, she seemed as close to Emily as we were. I knew Leslie was skilled at avoiding excessive emotional involvement in her work. If not, how could she have survived more than a decade of K9's joys and heartaches? But I was also certain that she had meant it when she had said she came to love these babies as if they were her own. I had heard that theme from too many of the NICU nurses not to believe it was true—and I had seen it in action myself, over and over.

ELIZABETH MEHREN
Born Too Soon

CHAPTER 17

Neonatal Assessment

KAREN KATZ ELAINE NISHIOKA

RESEARCH AGENDA

What factors affect the reliability of the gestational assessment instruments?

What is the relationship between neonatal behavioral states and the accuracy of the gestational assessment?

Is the neurologic portion of the Ballard gestational examination valid before 24 hours of age?

Do the periods of reactivity have an effect on the neonatal assessment findings?

Is there a relationship between conducting a newborn assessment with the parents present and their understanding of the competency of their infant?

VIGNETTE

The sound of new life filled the nursery, each with a different pitch and tone of its own. The buzzer rang, and in came a new member of the chorus. The L & D nurse gave a concise report of the delivery. Michael, the 38-week product of a diabetic mother, weighed in at 10 lb, 15 oz. Quite a big baby for a vaginal delivery, even when forceps are used to assist with delivery. His Apgar scores were 7 (1 minute) and 9 (5 minutes).

I noticed a man standing at the nursery window and found out that he was Michael's father. I introduced myself and explained that I was going to do a physical assessment of his son. A smile of excitement appeared, and as I walked back to Michael, the father's video camera rolled.

Michael was lying in a bassinet under a radiant warmer. This way he could be more visible for assessment, yet warm. His temperature registered at 98.4°F; apical pulse was 158 bpm; respirations were 48 and easy; and arteriosound blood pressure was 56/40. I touched his scalp. He had thick black hair like his father's. His fontanelles were soft, yet level. His head was molded, with caput present. His face was symmetrical; eyes were clear and bright. Michael's ears were in normal position with instant recoil. I placed a gloved finger into his mouth. His palate was intact; no teeth were present. His suck was present but sporadic. His neck was normal. I was careful with his clavicles because of his large size. I wanted to make sure that there was no crepitus, indicative of a fracture. The skin was smooth with rare veins and cracking. Lips were pink. No rashes or marks of any kind were present. Capillary refill was brisk. Chest was symmetrical, with breast buds measuring 3 to 4 mm in size. Michael's heart rate was regular, with no murmur on auscultation. His femoral pulses were equal and strong bilaterally. I next listened to his breath sounds, which were clear and equal bilaterally. There were no signs of respiratory distress, such as retractions, grunting, or flaring.

Michael's father tapped at the window to get my attention. When I went to the door he asked if anything was wrong. I assured him that so far in my exam Michael was fine, but that I had a few more things to check before I would be finished.

I continued the assessment. All fingers and toes were present. There were no unusual hand creases; plantar creases covered half of his feet. I picked Michael up to examine his spine, which was intact and straight. I placed him back into his bassinet. I checked for hip clicks; none present. There were three umbilical vessels. Bowel sounds were audible on auscultation, and his abdomen was soft and symmetrical. His anus was patent, with no fissures present. Both testes were descended, with deep rugae covering the scrotal sac. Michael appeared to be a normal male infant.

Neurologically, he was alert with normal muscle tone. Reflexes were present; his cry was normal. Yet he was "jittery." I started thinking about the connection between jitteriness and being an infant of a diabetic mother. I obtained a blood glucose from his heel, along with a hematocrit specimen. The glucose read at 30, the hematocrit at 56 to 58 percent. According to the institution's standing policy, I offered formula to Michael. He gagged and spit for a few seconds. Then, as if he had been given instructions, he latched on to the bottle and drank his fill, about 1 oz. Thirty minutes later I obtained a postprandial glucose. The result was 46. His physician ordered preprandial glucose determinations for the next three feedings.

Later I discussed with Michael's parents the normal physical exam and low blood glucose level. I told them that the pediatrician was aware of this and that we would monitor his blood glucose before the next three feedings. I pointed out that low blood glucose is a common and correctable finding in infants of diabetic mothers. I also pointed out how alert Michael was and how well he took his bottle. I answered the parents' questions and reassured them.

I documented my exam findings and interactions with the parents. I drafted a plan of care using nursing diagnosis, outcome goals, and dependent and independent nursing orders to address his low glucose.

I followed Michael throughout his hospital stay. He continued to feed well and experienced only one more preprandial low blood glucose, which responded quickly to feeding.

Vicky Merritt

Assessment of the neonate serves to evaluate the adaptation to extrauterine life, to identify any deviations from expected growth and development, and to facilitate mutual attachment between parents and their unique newborn. Assessment is a complex activity that in practice occurs continually during the giving of care. That is, assessment may be seen not as a static event but as a result of constant evaluation of the neonate's condition and response to intervention. Being the person most consistently present at the bedside, the nurse is in an ideal position to observe neonatal behavior, to identify any changes from the individual neonate's baseline, and to evaluate the progress of bonding within the family.

From another perspective, however, it is clear that more standardized, comprehensive assessments are needed periodically to compare various aspects of the individual neonate with those of the usual neonatal population and thus to ensure timely, accurate identification of present or potential problems. For this purpose, a number of instruments with specific objectives have been developed; when administered by knowledgeable and proficient staff, they provide a useful picture of the neonate at the time the assessment was conducted. These results form a data base that can be readily shared with other members of the health team.

For reasons of comprehensiveness and clarity, this chapter focuses on the "formal" assessments (i.e., physical and gestational assessments). One should constantly bear in mind, however, that many of the considerations and techniques described are applicable and at times essential to the ongoing assessments made by the professional nurse during daily neonatal care. This chapter is meant to serve only as a brief overview of the general principles of assessment and gestational examination. Comprehensive reviews are discussed in the individual systems chapters.

GENERAL CONSIDERATIONS

In any assessment activity, one must avoid compromising the infant through any procedure. The neonate exhibits physiologic, hormonal, metabolic, and behavioral responses to stressors that often are more intense than those of an adult despite immature brain dendrite and axonal branching and incomplete myelinization (Blackburn & Loper, 1992; Gardner, 1994). The physiologic system responses include autonomic functions initiating and controlling respiration, oxygen saturation, cardiac activity, temperature, fluid balance, enzyme and hormone production, and processes involved with digestion and elimination. The behavioral system involves motor activities and states of consciousness. Organized behavior describes the ability of the infant to react to the environment without disrupting these systems to self-regulate. Disorganized behavior occurs when there is a disturbance between these systems evidenced by the inability to self-regulate (D'Apolito, 1991). The Neonatal Individualized Developmental Care and Assessment Program, for example, focuses on identifying communication signals sent forth by the infant and individualizing care to the infant and family (Koszarek, 1992). These programs are an outgrowth of observations by many individual nurse care providers searching to improve quality of neonatal care (see Chapter 49, Assessment and Management of Neonatal Neurobehavioral Development).

It is imperative that any measures possible be used to alleviate stressors and conserve the newborn's limited energy stores. The transition period after delivery is a precarious time when a newborn is stressed because of adaptation to the extrauterine environment. A vigorous, strong newborn manifests almost excess energy and aggressively demands to breastfeed and quiets with bundling and cuddling. On the other end of the continuum is a newborn who is more fragile by virtue of either events related to birth or prematurity.

The admission process in itself may influence that adaptation in a negative way to an extent that a marginal transition newborn may require aggressive cardiorespiratory intervention. Energy conservation can be considered from many aspects, including cardiorespiratory support, thermal regulation, maintenance of fluids and nutrition, attention to aseptic technique, and decrease of environmental stressors. The degree to which a particular infant can cope and remain organized will be seen by observing the infant and assessing autonomic parameters (Koszarek, 1992).

Cardiorespiratory function is the sum of all of the processes that ultimately supply energy to all the cells of the body. A number of factors affect availability of oxygen to the cells: (1) reduced alveolar oxygen tension (PaO_2), resulting in partially saturated hemoglobin; (2) anemia; (3) inadequate blood flow; and (4) reduced oxygen uptake by the cells (Blackburn & Loper, 1992, p. 310). Maintaining an open airway for optimal air exchange and providing a necessary oxygen supply can be challenging during the admission procedure. Signs of increased work of breathing are retractions of the chest wall, tachypnea, and nasal flaring. An accurate assessment requires a pulse oximeter (set at lowest interval time response) or a transcutaneous oxygen monitor followed by a correlating blood gas analysis. Positioning on the abdomen supports the chest wall and allows greater lung excursion. However, according to the American Academy of Pediatrics (AAP), the prone position should not be used for most newborns because of the possible link to sudden infant death syndrome. If the prone position is used, the head should be turned to one side with the neck straight for maximal airway alignment. The infant's autonomic responses provide clues to the optimal position: increase or decrease in heart rate; color changes; changes in quality and rate of respirations; jitteriness; body, face, and limb twitching; gagging or spitting.

Maintenance of an optimal thermal environment is necessary to minimize energy consumption for all neonates; cold stress may be devastating to the small or ill individual. A hypoxic infant undergoes a greater than normal drop in core temperature because hypoxia blunts the normal response to cold (Fanaroff et al., 1994). The infant with a large surface:mass ratio is extremely susceptible to cold stress from a cold delivery room. The delivery room should be draft free, and the dried newborn should immediately be placed in a preheated radiant warmer or prewarmed incubator for assessment and care. During subsequent examinations in the nursery, continued vigilance is necessary to prevent heat loss by radiation, conduction, evaporation, or convection (see Chapter 16, Neonatal Thermoregulation). Modern double-walled incubators improve insulation, and much information can be obtained through observation and porthole access. Simply standing and looking at the infant—observing body position, quality and rate of breathing, and state—yields a great deal of information before the actual laying on of hands. For the larger, stable infant who may be assessed in an examination room, a warm draft-free environment, warm examination table, and warmed equipment not only help prevent heat loss but also avoid upsetting an otherwise quiet and cooperative infant. Suggestions for supportive care include warming hands and stethoscope, weighing the infant on a prewarmed scale or under an overhead heater, warming fluids, cleansing skin with water for attaching monitor leads, placing the infant in a flexed position with blanket rolls, and decreasing sensory input from bright lights and environmental noise.

Maintenance of an optimal glucose level and hydration supports homeostasis. Individual nurseries vary in protocols, but a generally acceptable level of serum glucose is equal to or greater than 40 mg/dl. The nurse should obtain a Chemstrip or Dextrostix to assess glucose level, using careful technique to prevent pain and bruising (bundle and comfort when possible); assess hydration and nutrition; and examine the skin for turgor and the anterior fontanelle for fullness (a sunken fontanelle can be indicative of dehydration). Nutritional status can be evaluated by such indicators as thin hair, narrow flat face, thin neck with wrinkles, accordion folding of the lower arm skin, skin loose and easily lifted from the scapular area, lack of gluteal fat and skin on the buttocks, prominent ribs, and loose skin that is easily lifted on the abdomen (Metcoff, 1994). Starting an intravenous infusion without stressing an infant is an art. The nurse should plan to have all the necessary "tools" at hand, and bundle the infant even under a radiant warmer; it is comforting to have boundaries such as blanket rolls for nesting. A soft humming voice or music and a finger or pacifier is soothing. The nurse should observe for subtle clues and provide a break for a minute or two if it is needed to help the infant reorganize.

Attention must also be given to aseptic technique to avoid introducing infection to the neonate and possibly cross-infecting the nursery group. Handwashing remains one simple, effective, proven method of preventing infection in the nursery (Davenport, 1992; Kelly, 1994; Larson, 1987). In one study, the hands of hospital personnel were shown to be not only a means of transmission of microorganisms but also a significant reservoir of bacteria (Klein & Remmington, 1995). Gowning, which has evolved from operating room practices, has been shown to be ineffective in reducing risk for infection of the infant (Larson, 1987). Current recommendations of the AAP and American College of Obstetricians and Gynecologists (1992) state that the benefit of gowning to prevent infection is not supported by research. The examiner's hands must be scrupulously clean, and all equipment must be cleaned appropriately between use with successive infants. Should any laboratory specimens be obtained, each must without fail be taken and handled according to institutional infection control procedures and the universal precautions guidelines of the Occupational Safety and Health Administration (1991) to avoid infecting the neonate, the nursery cohort, or the nursery or laboratory personnel.

Environmental stressors such as lighting and noise affect not only infants but also staff and families. Several studies have demonstrated that intense ambient, white fluorescent lighting can cause chromosome damage, interfere with endocrine gland and gonadal function, disrupt diurnal rhythms, and interfere with vitamin D synthesis (Gunderson & Kenner, 1995). Of further concern is the possible damage to the retina of preterm infants. The noise in different nurseries varies, depending on acoustics, equipment (number and type), physical layout, and staffing patterns. In one study (Vandenberg, 1995), the highest noise level in one nursery occurred during admissions, at change of shift, and during medical rounds at the bedside. The AAP (1988) reported that hospital noise, including incubator noise, must be considered a possible cause of childhood deafness. Noise also interferes with sleep–wake cycles, and changes in heart rate and peripheral vasoconstriction occur with levels as low as 70 dB. Above 55 dB, the mother's voice is obliterated (Graven, 1996). At all times, we must be cognizant of ways to protect infants from these environmental factors by reducing light, sound, and activity in the nursery.

Tribotti (1990) has developed an admission care plan that prioritizes the admission process to conserve the infant's energy while providing necessary support for survival and optimal outcome. Principles of thermoregulation and infection control should be included in a comprehensive orientation and in-service program for all nursery staff. Consideration should be given to all iatrogenic factors, such as use of invasive procedures, hospitalization, and nosocomial transmission while the newborn is hospitalized (Lott & Kenner, 1994a, 1994b). Infections remain a leading cause of neonatal mortality and morbidity. Nurses need to be especially careful in caring for the infant and the family. Nurses must also be sure to teach infection control measures to the family (Lott & Kenner, 1994a, 1994b).

Periodic review of techniques and patient care outcomes helps ensure compliance with the highest standards of care. Personnel specifically concerned with gestational or physical assessment will, of course, need additional preparation for these activities. Assessment tools for specific objectives are selected or prepared by each institution for reliability, ease of comprehension, and efficiency of use. The current trend in mother–newborn nursing is case management through use of the critical pathway, a tool to track the progress of the infant by defining interventions appropriate for the infant's position on the pathway (Rogers et al., 1993). The critical pathway is a multidisciplinary tool that outlines expected patient outcomes from the time of admission, including consultations, tests, activities, treatments, medications, nutrition, discharge planning, and parent teaching, in an organized format (Elizondo, 1995; McGregor, 1994). Critics of the critical pathway method question its usefulness in the neonatal intensive care unit because assessment and care of a complex infant do not readily lend themselves to a systematized cookbook approach (Lynam, 1994). (For a sample critical pathway, see the Appendix.)

The examiner proceeds in an organized manner to obtain complete, accurate results. To avoid tiring or otherwise stressing the infant, assessments should be done as quickly as is compatible with completeness and accuracy and from the least to the most disturbing activities. If the infant becomes tired or irritable, portions of an assessment may be postponed to a more appropriate time. New staff will initially be guided by a skilled mentor, improving in speed and dexterity through guided experiences. The physical examination remains one of the most professionally challenging procedures embraced by nurses. Each infant is a unique individual. The art and challenge of discovery is always enticing, especially at the first examination. The communication with the patient is nonverbal, but the language of the infant is guiding each step of palpation, auscultation, touch, and observation.

Assessments are also an excellent opportunity for interaction with the newborn's family. Some parents may have little knowledge of normal characteristics and behaviors of an infant, particularly with a first child. They may worry unnecessarily ("What are those funny spots?") or be anxious about handling their new infant. Excoriated skin, not uncommon to premature infants on monitors, often represents pain, discomfort, abnormality, and imperfection to a new parent (Kuller, 1995). Many parents today are more aware of the capabilities of their infant even in utero, through preparation in parenting classes and reading popular magazines. Then again, popular misconceptions, such as "Babies can't see when they're first born," may inhibit a parent's efforts to establish eye contact, interact, and bond. This time is an ideal opportunity to assess parents' needs, to teach focal distance, and to point out changes in infant state that allow greater attentiveness. Research has provided increasing evidence that an infant, including the preterm neonate, has a more mature central nervous system and memory function than was previously recognized (AAP, 1987; Anand & Hickey, 1987). While explaining normal newborn characteristics, the nurse may also point out an individual infant's coping skills and clues to temperament, such as being vigorously active or readily consoled (Brazelton, 1994). A modification of the Brazelton Neonatal Behavioral Assessment Scale is often helpful in acquainting parents with the uniqueness of their infant's patterns of behavior, temperament, and states (Brazelton, 1984). Another behavioral assessment instrument is the Barnard Infant State Chart, which gives detailed explanations of behaviors that are exhibited in a particular state (Blackburn & Kang, 1995).

All families need support at the time of birth as they adjust to the new member and their new roles (Prudhoe & Peters, 1995). The family of today is part of a diverse cultural, ethnic, and religious background that affects the assimilation of the newborn into the family. The nurse's care, role modeling, and teaching are received by the parents to a great extent on the basis of their cultural customs. Nonverbal communication is often the strongest communicator. Nurses caring for families of a culture different from their own should become knowledgeable about different customs and recognize cultural coping patterns (Callister, 1995). Characteristics of selected cultures and religions are outlined in current nursing textbooks (Betz et al., 1994; Pillitteri, 1995; Wong, 1995).

Facilitating bonding between a preterm or ill infant and the parents clearly presents a greater challenge. Even the healthy, 32-week-gestation infant who is "fine" (or even "big") to the nursery staff can be alarming to parents ("She's so small! She just lies there!"). The nurse can explain differences in the normal posture of the premature versus the term infant and point out "normal baby" behaviors, such as the sucking reflex. With an ill neonate, the assessor explains the rationale for procedures and offers reassurances as appropriate while recognizing the family's concerns. These parents are also encouraged to touch and talk to their infant and to make eye contact.

The examiner thus uses assessment occasions to build rapport and trust with parents, listening to parental concerns and offering understandable explanations. The assessor considers aspects of assessment beyond the physical and gestational and evaluates the presence of financial, social, cultural, or other difficulties in the family. The nurse functions in many ways as a "consultant to the family throughout the neonatal period" (Kiernan & Scoloveno, 1986). The neonatal nurse, as part of the caregiving team, can be instrumental in helping parents recognize their own support network that helps them cope with their specific set of circumstances (Prudhoe & Peters, 1995).

MAJOR ASSESSMENTS IN THE NEONATAL PERIOD

The total neonatal assessment includes evaluating risk status based on review of pregnancy and delivery history, gestational age, physical parameters, laboratory reports (i.e., hematocrit, blood type, blood glucose level, acid–base status), behavioral components, and parent–child interaction (Kenner, 1990; Volpe, 1995; Wong, 1995). Assessment begins at birth and is continued at every contact with the infant.

The assessment at birth is primarily a physical assessment, with the objective being the evaluation of adaptation to extrauterine life. The generally accepted instrument for this assessment is the Apgar score (Apgar, 1953), which measures heart rate, respiratory effort, color, muscle tone, and reflex response at 1 and 5 minutes. Scores range from 0 (cyanotic, bradycardic, unresponsive, little if any respiratory effort) to a "perfect 10." Scores that remain low on repeated scoring at 10 to 15 minutes after birth have traditionally been thought to be predictive of a poor outcome (Fanaroff et al., 1994). Initial low Apgar scores may not be predictive of fetal asphyxia. Multiple factors other than a hypoxic-ischemic insult influence a low Apgar score. Examples include varying quantitation by different observers, assigning of equal numerical values to each of the five factors evaluated, transient airway problems (such as vagal stimulation and maternal drugs), and prematurity (Volpe, 1995). (See Chapter 29, Assessment and Management of Neurologic Dysfunction.)

It is imperative that every effort be made to anticipate (if not prevent) the birth of a depressed infant. Apgar scores are an assessment, in a sense, of prenatal and intrapartal care, with the score at 5 minutes or later reflecting the success of resuscitation. The Neonatal Resuscitation Program (1994) now used in most delivery units has overshadowed the initial reliance on the 1-minute Apgar assessment for the decision to intervene. The infant who remains unstable or in need of significant assistance requires admission to a tertiary care nursery.

The second major assessment is performed in the nursery, generally 1 to 4 hours after birth. For the well neonate, this consists of both a short physical examination to confirm a stable condition and a gestational assessment. The ill neonate receives a physical examination as required for full clinical evaluation and a gestational assessment as early as possible, deferring to the infant's organization and coping.

The primary purpose of the gestational assessment is to anticipate problems related to development. In the past, a birth weight of 2500 g divided premature from term infants. It gradually became evident, however, that a given infant's clinical course could not be predicted from weight alone; many premature neonates progressed better than some term infants. Further research has demonstrated that gestational age and whether the individual's development is appropriate for that age have considerable influence on outcome (Battaglia & Lubchenco, 1967).

Battaglia and Lubchenco (1967) found that 80 percent of births occur in a range within 40 ± 2 weeks of gestation. Because they further found that infants born before 38 weeks have a higher frequency of morbidity and mortality, they accepted 38 weeks as the dividing line between preterm and term births. Graphs show the distribution of birth weights at various gestational ages and define large for gestational age (LGA; weight greater than the 90th percentile) and small for gestational age (SGA; weight less than the 10th percentile) (Fig. 17–1). Infants who are average for gestational age (AGA) and born at term are at least risk for neonatal difficulties.

Other infants (preterm or postterm, SGA or LGA) are at greater risk, and the nature of probable neonatal morbidities has been identified as a function of birth weight and gestational age (Fig. 17–2). It is thus possible through the gestational age assessment to identify the newborn at increased risk and to anticipate to some degree the problems that may develop (Fig. 17–3). It also provides a basis for research to improve care. In 1948, Dancis and colleagues attempted to predict growth for infants with birth weights of 750 g because few very low birth

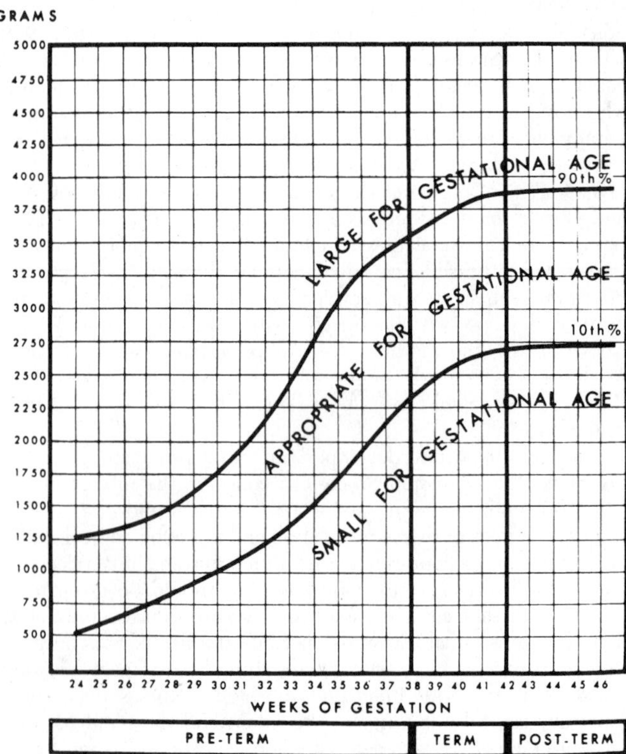

FIGURE 17–1. University of Colorado Medical Center classification of newborns by birth weight and gestational age. (From Battaglia, F. C., & Lubchenco, L. O. [1967]. A practical classification of newborn infants by weight and gestational age. *Journal of Pediatrics, 71*[2], 159–163.)

weight infants at that time survived. The rate of hyperalimentation and overall better supportive care have been reflected in a report by Adamkin and coworkers (1994) in which 750-g birth weight infants did not lose as much weight as predicted by Dancis and gained weight at a faster rate.

Various tools have been developed to facilitate estimation of gestational age. In most widespread use are those of Lubchenco, Dubowitz (Fig. 17–4 and Table 17–1), and Ballard (Fig. 17–5). These assessments consist of an observation of external physical characteristics, such as skin condition and ear development, and an evaluation of neuromuscular development. The physical findings remain relatively unchanged in the immediate newborn period. By contrast, the neurologic system of the newborn is unstable. If results obtained in this portion of the gestational examination are grossly inconsistent with other findings, the examination may be repeated in 24 hours or, in the case of the Lubchenco evaluation, supplemented by a more detailed confirmatory examination on the second postnatal day.

A complete physical assessment performed by a physician or nurse practitioner is on record for legal reasons before discharge. Various guides are in use to ensure completeness and accuracy of this evaluation, which provides baseline data for well-child care and any other follow-up required.

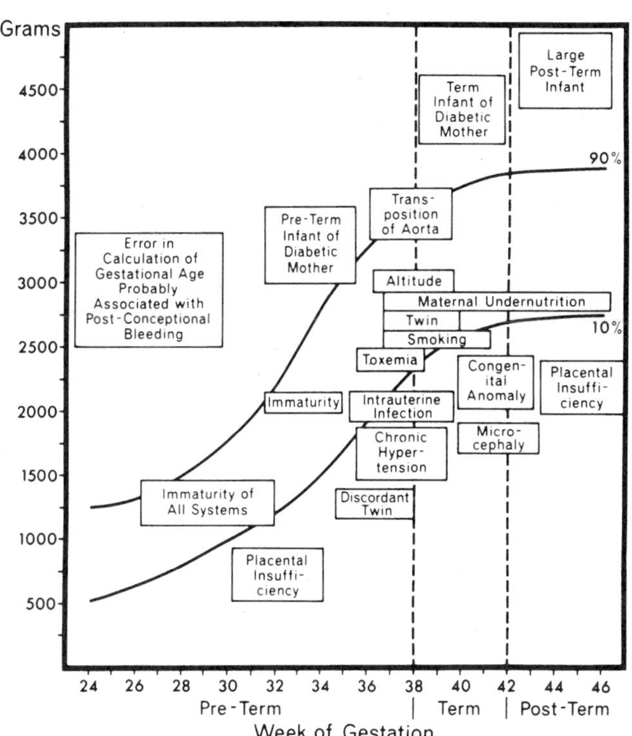

FIGURE 17–3. Deviations of intrauterine growth: neonatal morbidity by birth weight and gestational age. (From Lubchenco, L. O. [1967]. *The high risk infant* [p. 6]. Philadelphia: W. B. Saunders; as adapted from Lubchenco, L. O., Hansman, C., & Backstrom, L. [1968]. In J. H. P. Jonxis, H. K. A. Visser, & J. A. Troelstra [Eds.], *Aspects of prematurity and dysmaturity*. Springfield, IL: Charles C Thomas.)

GESTATIONAL ASSESSMENT

The gestational assessment is a determination of the approximate duration of fetal development, and a comparison against standardized norms of neonatal growth versus weeks of gestation, to identify those infants unusually large or small for gestational age. In clinical practice, the gestational assessment tools in common use are generally considered accurate within a range of ±2 weeks (see Figs. 17–4 and 17–5 and Table 17–1). Furthermore, a study has shown that the widely used fetal growth curve developed in Denver (see Fig. 17–1) is not completely applicable to a neonatal population at sea level (Lugo & Tominey, 1989). Specifically, use of a growth curve appropriate for high altitudes may cause one to overlook some truly SGA infants born at lower altitude (high altitudes shift growth distributions to the left or smaller end of the scale). Thus, along with other factors, the limitations of various instruments, possibly including the "normal" growth curves in some settings, leave some uncertainty in the process of gestational assessment. Nevertheless, it seems clear that the majority of SGA, LGA, and premature and postmature neonates may be identified as infants at risk and given closer observation in the nursery.

There are several approaches to estimating gestational age before birth. First, a careful menstrual history is obtained as early as possible. Naegele's rule is applied to the date of onset of the last menstrual period (LMP) to determine the estimated date of confinement, which is calculated by counting backward 3 calendar months from the first day of the LMP and adding 7 days (Pillitteri, 1995). Less than 5 percent of pregnancies end exactly 280 days from the LMP, and less than half end within 1 week of the 280th day. Recall of the date of the onset of the LMP is accurate in 75 to 85 percent of women (Korones, 1981). Miscalculation is possible, however, for reasons other than an inadequate history (e.g., irregular menses, postconceptual bleeding). Two studies by a group of researchers investigating the accuracy of the Ballard instrument found that it sometimes overestimated the gestational age of preterm infants, which resulted in an underestimation of the very preterm infant, and that there may be ethnic variations in fetal growth that make the use of the LMP criteria invalid (Alexander et al., 1992a, 1992b).

Various obstetrical milestones are also used to estimate progres-

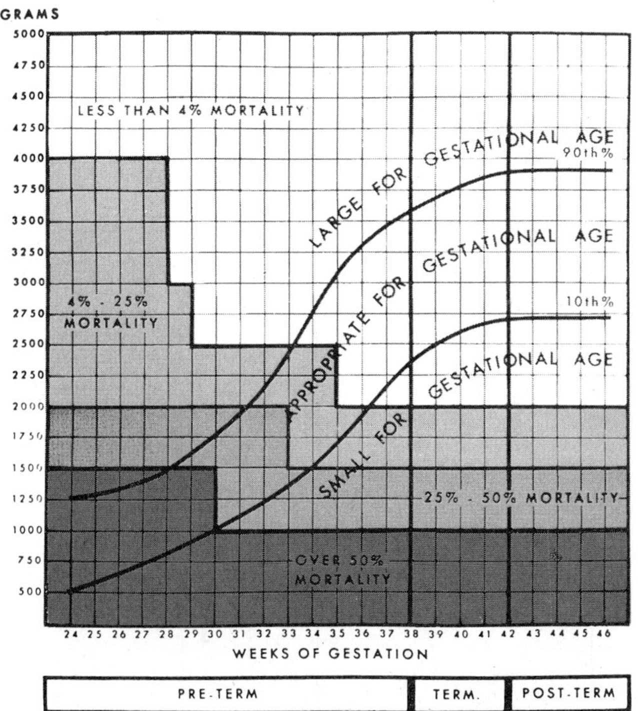

FIGURE 17–2. University of Colorado Medical Center classification of newborns by birth weight and gestational age and by neonatal mortality risk. (From Battaglia, F. C., & Lubchenco, L. O. [1967]. A practical classification of newborn infants by weight and gestational age. *Journal of Pediatrics, 71*[2], 159–163.)

sive gestational age. These include the first auscultation of fetal heart tones by fetoscope (approximately 20 weeks), the measurement of fundal height (directly related to weight of fetus and duration of pregnancy), and the mother's report of quickening (about 18 weeks in primigravidas and slightly earlier in multigravidas). Ultrasonography may be used to monitor fetal growth as well as to identify certain abnormalities of development. Gestational age can be ascertained by ultrasound examination within a range of ±1 week in early pregnancy (6 to 18 weeks), decreasing in certainty to ±3 weeks from 29 weeks to term (Petrucha, 1989). Measurements of fetal biparietal diameter may identify the growth retarded fetus: in early pregnancy, the head grows appropriately but the body is disproportionately small; later, the rate of increase of biparietal diameter also slows, and the fetus or neonate is more in proportion but SGA (Leppink, 1986). Smith and Bottoms (1993) found that biparietal diameter reflected fetal maturity more accurately than did estimated fetal weight. Huang and Yeh (1991) found that a simplified ultrasonographic system based on cerebral sulcal development correlated better with gestational age by dates than with the Dubowitz scoring system.

NEUROLOGICAL SIGN	SCORE					
	0	1	2	3	4	5
POSTURE						
SQUARE WINDOW	90°	60°	45°	30°	0°	
ANKLE DORSIFLEXION	90°	75°	45°	20°	0°	
ARM RECOIL	180°	90–180°	<90°			
LEG RECOIL	180°	90–180°	<90°			
POPLITEAL ANGLE	180	160°	130°	110°	90°	<90°
HEEL TO EAR						
SCARF SIGN						
HEAD LAG						
VENTRAL SUSPENSION						

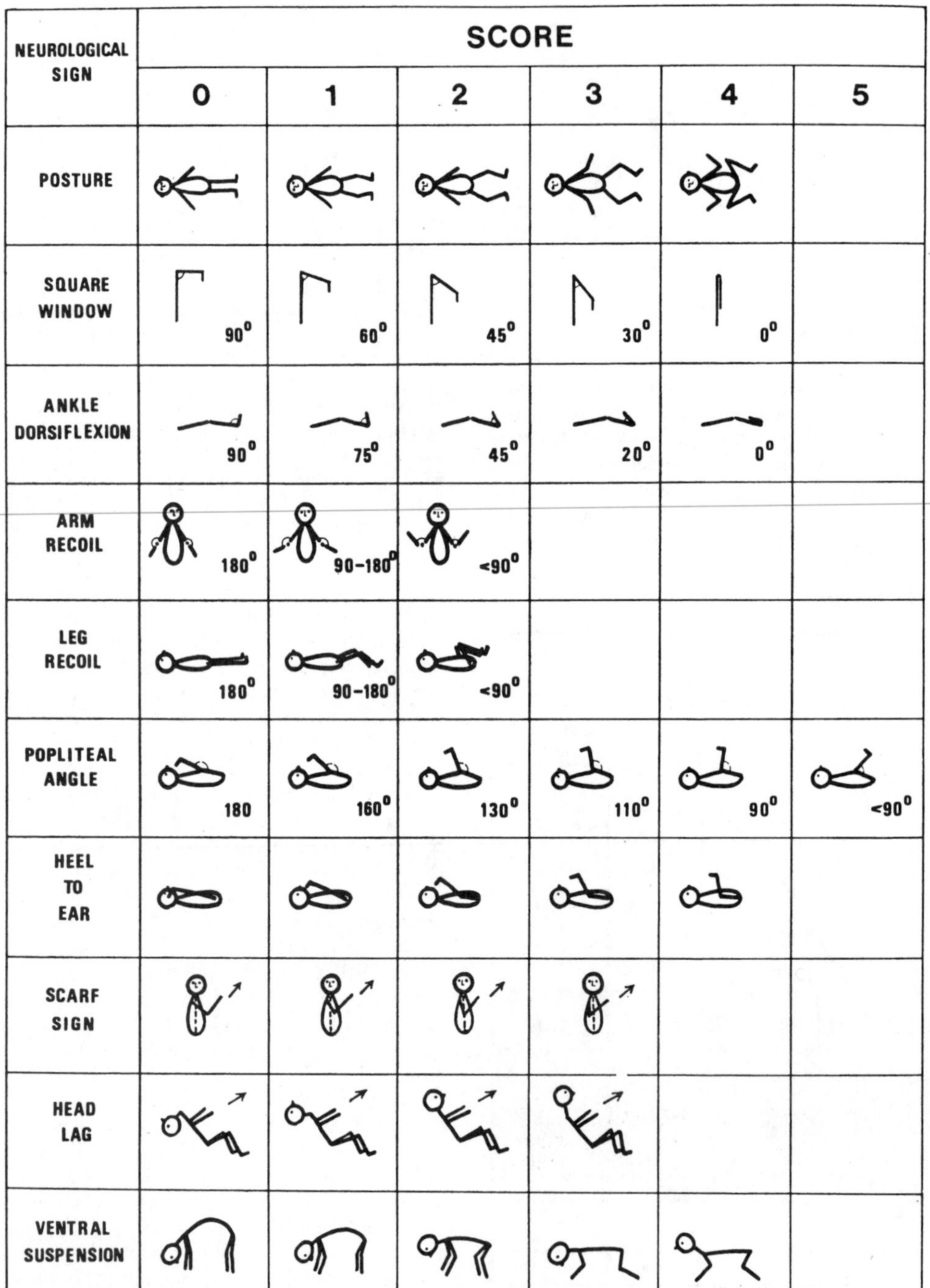

FIGURE 17–4. Dubowitz scoring system for neurologic criteria. (From Dubowitz, L. M.., Dubowitz, V., & Goldberg, C. [1970]. Clinical assessment of gestational age in the newborn infant. *Journal of Pediatrics, 77*[1], 1–10.)

Legend continued on opposite page

Amato and associates (1991) found that use of biometric parameters (i.e., anterior vascular capsule of the lens, internipple distance, and foot length) early in the postnatal period could improve assessment of gestational age in very low birth weight infants. Another group of researches found that the fetal sacral length could predict gestational age (Sherer et al., 1993).

Laboratory tests, particularly on amniotic fluid obtained by amniocentesis, are increasingly accurate in estimating fetal development, but availability, cost, and risk factors generally limit their use to high-risk pregnancies. Elliott and Cassano (1991) used an objective laboratory test, the flow cytometric analysis of erythroid differentiation antigens, to predict gestational age. This test would be useful whenever fetal blood sampling is performed for other diagnostic studies (see Chapter 11, The High-Risk Pregnancy).

Instruments for Gestational Assessment

After delivery, the neonate's gestational age is estimated by assessing physical, neurologic, and neuromuscular development. Although electroencephalographic patterns and motor nerve conduction times correlate well with gestational age (Leppink, 1986), to date there seems to be no rationale for using them as routine screening tools. Instead, one of several checklist-type screening tools is generally used (see Figs. 17–4 and 17–5 and Table 17–1). These instruments provide acceptably high accuracy in a short time, at low cost, and with little risk to the neonate. All are based on the observations that fetal development normally proceeds in an organized, predictable manner and that a fetus or neonate at a given gestational age ordinarily has many common characteristics. For example, the resting supine posture of a newborn less than about 28 to 30 weeks' gestation is hypotonic extension of all extremities. By 34 weeks, the legs are flexed ("frog-like") while the arms remain extended; by 38 weeks, a neonate normally shows hypertonic flexion of all extremities. Increased muscle tone with progressive gestational age is also demonstrated by the arm recoil test (flexion of the arm after brief passive extension by the examiner; strong "recoil" flexion by term) and the scarf sign (drawing arm of supine neonate across chest toward opposite shoulder; no resistance until about 32 weeks, resistance just before midline at 40 weeks). Joint mobility increases with gestational age, as demonstrated by the square window sign (wrist flexion; the wrist can be bent to a 90-degree angle with the forearm until about 31 weeks but to progressively smaller angles decreasing to zero at term) or the ankle dorsiflexion sign (parallels change in wrist flexion).

Similarly, physical characteristics are seen to vary consistently. Vernix is assessed immediately after delivery. The 36-week neonate is heavily covered with vernix. After 36 weeks, the amount of vernix decreases until it is found only in skin creases by 40 to 41 weeks. Ear cartilage is soft until about 32 to 33 weeks, and the pinnae, if folded, remain folded. By 36 weeks, the pinnae recoil after folding unless they are glued down by excess vernix. At term, the ear is firm with well-defined incurving. Lanugo (fine hair over the entire body) decreases in amount from 20 weeks to term. By 40 weeks, it may be found only on a portion of the back or shoulders. See the physical assessment section for a more complete discussion.

FIGURE 17–4 *Continued.* Some notes on techniques of assessment of neurologic criteria.

POSTURE: Observed with infant quiet and in supine position. Score 0: arms and legs extended; 1: beginning of flexion of hips and knees, arms extended; 2: stronger flexion of legs, arms extended; 3: arms slightly flexed and abducted; 4: full flexion of arms and legs.

SQUARE WINDOW: The hand is flexed on the forearm between the thumb and index finger of the examiner. Enough pressure is applied to get as full flexion as possible, and the angle between the hypothenar eminence and the ventral aspect of the forearm is measured and graded according to diagram. (Care is taken not to rotate the infant's wrist while doing this maneuver.)

ANKLE DORSIFLEXION: The foot is dorsiflexed onto the anterior aspect of the leg, with the examiner's thumb on the sole of the foot and other fingers behind the leg. Enough pressure is applied to get as full flexion as possible, and the angle between the dorsum of the foot and the anterior aspect of the leg is measured.

ARM RECOIL: With the infant in the supine position, the forearms are first flexed for 5 seconds, then fully extended by pulling on the hands, and then released. The sign is fully positive if the arms return briskly to full flexion (score 2). If the arms return to incomplete flexion or the response is sluggish, it is graded as score 1. If they remain extended or are only followed by random movements, the score is 0.

LEG RECOIL: With the infant supine, the hips and knees are fully flexed for 5 seconds, then extended by traction on the feet, and released. A maximal response is one of full flexion of the hips and knees (score 2). A partial flexion scores 1, and minimal or no movement scores 0.

POPLITEAL ANGLE: With the infant supine and the pelvis flat on the examining couch, the thigh is held in the knee–chest position by the examiner's left index finger and thumb supporting the knee. The leg is then extended by gentle pressure from the examiner's right index finger behind the ankle, and the popliteal angle is measured.

HEEL-TO-EAR MANEUVER: With the infant supine, draw the infant's foot as near to the head as it will go without forcing it. Observe the distance between the foot and the head as well as the degree of extension at the knee. Grade according to diagram. Note that the knee is left free and may draw down alongside the abdomen.

SCARF SIGN: With the infant supine, take the infant's hand and try to put it around the neck and as far posteriorly as possible around the opposite shoulder. Assist this maneuver by lifting the elbow across the body. See how far the elbow will go across and grade according to illustrations. Score 0: elbow reaches opposite axillary line; 1: elbow between midline and opposite axillary line; 2: elbow reaches midline; 3: elbow will not reach midline.

HEAD LAG: With the infant lying supine, grasp the hands (or the arms if a very small infant) and pull infant slowly toward the sitting position. Observe the position of the head in relation to the trunk and grade accordingly. In a small infant, the head may initially be supported by one hand. Score 0: complete lag; 1: partial head control; 2: able to maintain head in line with body; 3: brings head anterior to body.

VENTRAL SUSPENSION: The infant is suspended in the prone position, with examiner's hand under the infant's chest (one hand in a small infant, two in a large infant). Observe the degree of extension of the back and the amount of flexion of the arms and legs. Also note the relation of the head to the trunk. Grade according to diagrams.
If the score differs on the two sides, take the mean.

TABLE 17–1 Dubowitz Scoring System for External Criteria

External Sign	Score*				
	0	*1*	*2*	*3*	*4*
Edema	Obvious edema of hands and feet; pitting over tibia	No obvious edema of hands and feet; pitting over tibia	No edema		
Skin texture	Very thin, gelatinous	Thin and smooth	Smooth; medium thickness; rash; superficial peeling	Slight thickening; superficial cracking and peeling, especially of hands and feet	Thick and parchment-like; superficial or deep cracking
Skin color	Dark red	Uniformly pink	Pale pink; variable over body	Pale; only pink over ears, lips, palms, or soles	
Skin opacity	Numerous veins and venules clearly seen, especially over abdomen	Veins and tributaries seen	A few large vessels clearly seen over abdomen	A few large vessels seen indistinctly over abdomen	No blood vessels
Lanugo	No lanugo	Abundant; long and thick over whole back	Hair thinning, especially over lower back	Small amount of lanugo and bald areas	At least half of back devoid of lanugo
Plantar creases	No skin creases	Faint red marks over anterior half of sole	Definite red marks over > anterior half; indentations over < anterior third	Indentations over > anterior third	Definite deep indentations over > anterior third
Nipple formation	Nipple barely visible, no areola	Nipple well defined; areola smooth and flat, diameter <0.75 cm	Areola stippled, edge not raised, diameter <0.75 cm	Areola stippled, edge raised, diameter >0.75 cm	
Breast size	No breast tissue palpable	Breast tissue on one or both sides, <0.5 cm diameter	Breast tissue both sides; one or both 0.5–1.0 cm	Breast tissue both sides; one or both >1 cm	
Ear form	Pinna flat and shapeless, little or no incurving of edge	Incurving of part of edge of pinna	Partial incurving whole of upper pinna	Well-defined incurving whole of upper pinna	
Ear firmness	Pinna soft, easily folded, no recoil	Pinna soft, easily folded, slow recoil	Cartilage to edge of pinna but soft in places, ready recoil	Pinna firm, cartilage to edge, instant recoil	
Genital, male	Neither testis in scrotum	At least one testis high in scrotum	At least one testis right down		
Genital, female (with hips half abducted)	Labia majora widely separated, labia minora protruding	Labia majora almost cover labia minora	Labia majora completely cover labia minora		

* If the score differs on the two sides, take the mean.

From Dubowitz, V., Dubowitz, I., & Goldberg, C. (1970). Clinical assessment of gestational age in the newborn infant. *Journal of Pediatrics, 77*(1), 1–10. As adapted from Farr, V., Mitchell, R. G., Neligan, G. A., et al. (1966). The definition of some external characteristics used in the assessment of gestational age in the newborn infant. *Developmental Medicine and Child Neurology, 8,* 507–511.

Neuromuscular Maturity

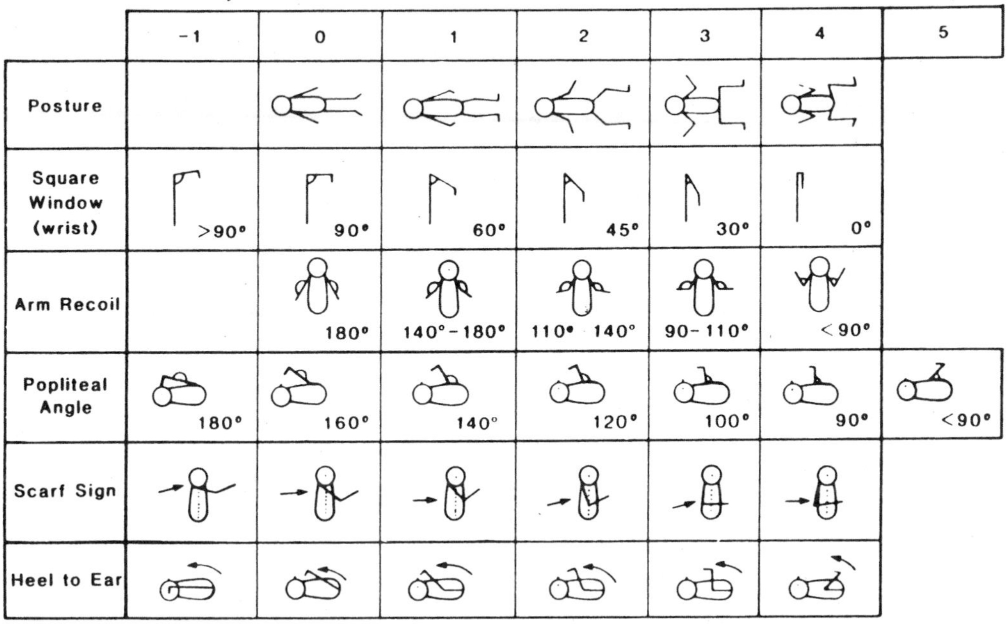

	-1	0	1	2	3	4	5
Posture							
Square Window (wrist)	>90°	90°	60°	45°	30°	0°	
Arm Recoil		180°	140°-180°	110° 140°	90-110°	<90°	
Popliteal Angle	180°	160°	140°	120°	100°	90°	<90°
Scarf Sign							
Heel to Ear							

Physical Maturity

Skin	sticky friable transparent	gelatinous red, translucent	smooth pink, visible veins	superficial peeling &/or rash. few veins	cracking pale areas rare veins	parchment deep cracking no vessels	leathery cracked wrinkled
Lanugo	none	sparse	abundant	thinning	bald areas	mostly bald	
Plantar Surface	heel-toe 40-50 mm: -1 <40 mm: -2	>50mm no crease	faint red marks	anterior transverse crease only	creases ant. 2/3	creases over entire sole	
Breast	imperceptible	barely perceptible	flat areola no bud	stippled areola 1-2mm bud	raised areola 3-4mm bud	full areola 5-10mm bud	
Eye/Ear	lids fused loosely:-1 tightly:-2	lids open pinna flat stays folded	sl. curved pinna; soft; slow recoil	well-curved pinna; soft but ready recoil	formed &firm instant recoil	thick cartilage ear stiff	
Genitals male	scrotum flat, smooth	scrotum empty faint rugae	testes in upper canal rare rugae	testes descending few rugae	testes down good rugae	testes pendulous deep rugae	
Genitals female	clitoris prominent labia flat	prominent clitoris small labia minora	prominent clitoris enlarging minora	majora & minora equally prominent	majora large minora small	majora cover clitoris & minora	

Maturity Rating

score	weeks
-10	20
-5	22
0	24
5	26
10	28
15	30
20	32
25	34
30	36
35	38
40	40
45	42
50	44

FIGURE 17–5. Maturational assessment of gestational age: Ballard score. (From Ballard, J. L., Khoury, J. C., Wedig, K., et al. [1991]. New Ballard Score, expanded to include extremely premature infants. *Journal of Pediatrics*, *119*[3], 417–423.)

Clinical Estimation of Gestational Age (Lubchenco)

The Clinical Estimation of Gestational Age scale, developed by Lubchenco (1970) and colleagues at the University of Colorado, was designed for use in the first hours of life and requires little handling or exposure of the newborn. Completion of all items on this assessment form yields a profile of the neonate's development and an estimation of gestational age. If there is a significant discrepancy between this finding and gestational age based on the mother's menstrual history, a confirmatory neurologic examination may be done after 24 hours, when the infant is more stable and may be less stressed by handling during the more extensive examination. Lubchenco suggested that the *pattern* of results in the initial examination may provide information beyond a simple gestational age, such as evidence of intrauterine growth retardation.

Clinical Assessment of Gestational Age (Dubowitz)

Dubowitz and colleagues (1970) developed the Clinical Assessment of Gestational Age scale, which assigns a score of 0 to 5 to each of 10 neurologic signs and a score of 0 to 4 to each of 11 external (physical) signs. The totals are added to yield a composite score, which is correlated with weeks of gestation. This composite has a higher degree of correlation than does either the neurologic or the external portion considered separately (±2 weeks with 95 percent confidence). Furthermore, although SGA infants tend to underscore on external signs and overscore on neurologic signs, the composite is again reliable (Taylor, 1982).

Dubowitz and colleagues (1977) published *Gestational Age of the Newborn: A Clinical Manual*, which explains their testing and scoring procedure in detail. The examination should be conducted within the first 5 days of life because physical characteristics begin to change thereafter (see Fig. 17–4 and Table 17–1).

Newborn Maturity Rating (Ballard)

Ballard and coworkers (1979) developed the Newborn Maturity Rating, a simplified version of the Dubowitz tool. This version was later modified by Ballard (1988) to assess neonates from 20 to 44 weeks (see Fig. 17–5). As with the Dubowitz tool, the Ballard tool may be used from birth through the first 5 days and involves assigning a score of 0 to 5 to each of six neurologic and six physical criteria. However, it requires less time (3 to 4 minutes versus 10 to 15 minutes) and eliminates neurologic assessment signs requiring active muscle tone, which might be difficult if not impossible to assess in severely ill newborns. The Ballard instrument in its older form has been found reliable when it was tested against the Dubowitz tool as a standard as well as on comparison of the composite score against known dates of a group of infants (Ballard et al., 1979). The newest Ballard tool, as shown in Figure 17–5, which can be used as early as 20 weeks of gestation, has also proved to be reliable and valid (Ballard et al., 1991).

Clinical Assessment of Nutritional Status at Birth (CANSCORE)

Metcoff (1994) has looked at the Clinical Assessment of Nutritional Status at Birth (CANSCORE) as an assessment tool to further differentiate infants who may be classified SGA, intrauterine growth retarded, or even AGA but have clinical characteristics indicative of fetal malnutrition. Fetal malnutrition affects body composition and impairs brain development. If maternal malnutrition is appropriately evaluated to predict the birth of small infants 20 weeks later and appropriate nutritional therapy is instituted, fetal malnutrition could be potentially corrected before birth. This treatment could, perhaps, have an impact on 3 million infants worldwide.

Interpretation of Results

The examiner should attempt to perform the gestational assessment under the optimal conditions previously described. The examination should be done as soon as is feasible after birth, when the infant is alert and not too hungry, so that an infant at risk may be promptly identified and given closer observation and prompt intervention as needed. When practical, the examiner may wish to assess the infant before reviewing maternal history to avoid biasing the examination by knowing the calculated estimated date of confinement. Many of these currently used instruments were developed and tested on white, middle-class infants. Cultural differences in birth weight are not reflected; therefore, use of these charts with minorities, such as African-American or Latino infants, whose average birth weights are slightly less than that of the average white infant, should take cultural differences into account (Kenner, 1990).

Test procedures should be followed exactly. Stick figures accompanying tools should be used as guides. Staff members not yet adept at gestational assessment should be given ample instruction and guidance by more experienced colleagues. Dubowitz found, however, that there is good interexaminer reliability between more and less experienced medical and nursing staff when the instructions on the assessment form are carefully followed (Taylor, 1982.) Gestational age is compared with infant weight, length, and head circumference to identify deviations from expected intrauterine growth.

If a significant discrepancy is found between maternal dates and the neonatal gestational assessment, several possibilities exist. The neonate should certainly be re-evaluated after 24 hours, possibly with use of a more elaborate tool such as the Lubchenco Confirmatory Neurological Examination. One should also bear in mind that the examination may be affected by neonatal or maternal conditions. For example, infants with respiratory distress may be relatively flaccid, and infants of diabetic mothers may have accelerated physical growth with retarded neurologic development. (The nursery is of course particularly observant of such infants at known risk, even in the absence of SGA or LGA classification.) If the infant is premature or postmature or has experienced intrauterine growth retardation, efforts should be made to identify the probable cause. This information may be useful in counseling the mother about future pregnancies, although great care must be taken not to add the burden of guilt to that of anxiety about her infant.

In any event, the gestational assessment is only one means of identifying the neonate who may develop problems early in life. Dubowitz and associates (1984) found a positive correlation between the neurologic portion of the gestational examination performed at 40 weeks' gestational age and the neurologic status of the child at the end of the first year of life. Classification as AGA and term does not guarantee an uneventful clinical course. If the institution has an early discharge policy for mothers and well infants, the nurse should instruct the parents in normal appearance and behavior so that an infant developing a problem at home (jaundice, digestive disorders, respiratory distress) will receive prompt care. Accuracy of gestational instruments depends on the assessor's expertise at conducting the examination (Kenner, 1990).

PHYSICAL ASSESSMENT

The first physical assessment is done immediately at birth. The skilled practitioner will readily apprehend much about the infant's condition from color, general vigor, responsiveness, and other factors well in advance of the 1-minute Apgar score. Resuscitation of the distressed neonate begins immediately (see Chapter 15, Resuscitation and Stabilization of the Neonate); staff certainly does not wait for a low Apgar score to give the go-ahead. Apgar scores are calculated and recorded, along with notes of obvious deviations from expected maturity, congenital anomalies, or evidence of disease. Resuscitative efforts and the neonate's response are recorded in full. Results of this initial assessment determine whether the newborn is admitted to the primary care nursery or to a secondary or tertiary care nursery (possibly requiring transport to another facility).

A more complete physical examination is generally not performed until the infant is stable in the nursery. The attending nurse must be particularly alert during this transition period for deterioration of the well infant. The physician or neonatal nurse practitioner should be notified immediately. Nursing interventions are consistent with the agency's policy, the physician's or practitioner's orders, and the nurse's clinical judgment and may include nasopharyngeal suction, estimating blood sugar by Dextrostix or Chemstrip, and initiating oxygen support by head hood or blowing oxygen to the face. The neonatal clinical specialist or nurse practitioner may carry out more vigorous resuscitation as permitted by law and agency policy.

Before the formal physical assessment, the practitioner should be familiar with the maternal and paternal medical histories; course of pregnancy; birth history, including type of delivery, medications received during labor and delivery, condition of the infant at birth, Apgar scores, and any resuscitative measures; any laboratory values available; and treatments, if any, in progress. The nurse may thus identify, in advance, many potential problems of a particular infant and plan the examination for efficiency and thoroughness.

The practitioner obtains much valuable information by hands-off observation of the quiet infant. Many aspects of neonatal assessment come from indirect or observational methods as discussed previously (Bruno, 1995; Kenner, 1990). The term, healthy infant displays a flexed posture, indicating good muscle tone. Preterm infants often have a relaxed posture with less or little flexion. Besides prematurity, a lack of flexion may indicate hypotonicity resulting from severe nervous system trauma or an overstressed system. Excessive flexion (hypertonicity) may be evidence of a complicated delivery or, in some cases, prematurity. Normal spontaneous activity should be symmetrical, with alternate flexion and extension of arms and legs. Fine tremors of the extremities are seen in the jitteriness of hypoglycemia or hypocalcemia as well as in the vigorous crying of normal term infants.

A head-to-toe approach is generally taken, but the areas of most concern are evaluated first. Similarly, baseline measurements of body length and head circumference may be deferred to the end because they are not affected by infant state. The following sections provide an overview of the elements of the physical assessment. The reader is referred to Chapters 18 through 34 for a detailed evaluation of each system.

Color and Skin

Color is best evaluated in the quiet infant. Crying may cause cyanosis, resulting from generalized poor oxygenation or possibly a temporary reopening of the ductus arteriosus. Acrocyanosis (blue hands and feet) is common and generally insignificant in the transition period immediately after birth and reflects poor peripheral perfusion. However, it is also seen with cold stress (see Chapter 16, Neonatal Thermoregulation) and may improve as the infant is warmed. Generalized cyanosis may be present with serious cardiac or respiratory dysfunction. Evaluation of hypoxia without blood gas analysis can be difficult. Many infants with cyanotic mucous membranes are not hypoxic, and some hypoxic infants have pink lips (Korones, 1981). Color is best interpreted in the context of the overall clinical assessment.

The neonate's skin indicates maturity. A full-term neonate has layers of subcutaneous fat, which provide for temperature regulation. The preterm infant lacks subcutaneous fat, and blood vessels are evident over the chest and abdomen.

The skin of white infants should be pink. The presence of pallor or plethora should be noted. They may reflect low or high hematocrit or vasoconstriction (shock, infection, and so on) versus vasodilation and should be investigated for cause. Dark-skinned or Asian infants may be somewhat more difficult to assess, but the mucous membranes should be pink. These infants often have a mongolian spot over the buttocks—a dark, hyperpigmented area resembling a large bruise. Parents may need to be informed that this is a normal finding and will disappear with time. Mottling of the skin in response to chilling or stress is referred to as cutis marmorata. The harlequin sign is deep pink coloring of one side of the body on the dependent side while the other side is pale. This sign has no pathologic significance. It is believed to be indicative of the immaturity of the neurologic system.

The skin should also be observed for petechiae, plethora, and jaundice. Petechiae, pinpoint hemorrhagic spots on the skin that do not blanch with pressure, if present, are usually related to birth trauma and generally disappear in a few days. Persistent petechiae warrant further evaluation because they may be indicative of platelet disorders. Similarly, ecchymoses of the presenting part are frequently noted as purplish blue irregular areas caused by blood outside the vessel. Milia (small white shiny nodules caused by sebaceous gland secretion) are often found on the nose and chin and disappear with treatment in a few days. Telangiectatic nevi ("stork bites") are localized areas of redness caused by capillary dilation and can be seen on the eyelids as well as the back of the neck and head and across the bridge of the nose. They generally disappear by 2 weeks of age. Excellent color plates of skin lesions can be found in *Physical Assessment of the Newborn: A Comprehensive Approach to the Art of Physical Examination* (Tappero & Honeyfield, 1996).

Jaundice is considered physiologic if it occurs after day 2 and is resolving by days 5 to 7. In the premature infant, this jaundice may peak slightly later, usually around day 5. Breast milk jaundice normally appears just as the physiologic jaundice is beginning to subside. It normally peaks around days 10 to 15 of life. Jaundice may be difficult to evaluate in a plethoric or dusky newborn. Application of pressure to the skin reveals jaundice, if it is present, in the blanched area.

Cheesy vernix caseosa develops in the third trimester and is present to term. Lanugo first appears at 20 weeks, is most abundant at 28 to 30 weeks, and decreases as the infant matures; it is best evaluated on the upper back. Both, if present, contribute to the gestational assessment.

Cardiopulmonary Status

The chest should be observed for overall symmetry. It is generally round and 1 to 2 cm smaller in circumference than the head. Chest excursion should be observed during quiet respiration. Movement should be unlabored and equal bilaterally. The ribs are compliant, and therefore subcostal and intercostal retractions can be common even in healthy newborns. Infants breathe diaphragmatically in a paradoxical pattern: on inspiration, the lower thorax draws in and the abdomen protrudes; on expiration, the reverse occurs. With respiratory distress, a variety of signs are present. Flaring of the nostrils with mild retractions is seen in early or mild conditions. Severe retractions (substernal, supracostal, intracostal), respiratory grunt, and stridor indicate serious distress. Suprasternal retractions are never normal.

Respirations should be counted for a full minute. The normal range for the quiet infant is 40 to 60 breaths per minute. There can be considerable variability in rate and breathing pattern in the premature infant. Transient tachypnea may be present for the first few hours after birth, particularly for cesarean section births, because some lung fluid may be retained. Most infants with transient tachypnea of the newborn (TTN) develop difficulty within the first 30 minutes of life and are cyanotic. Rales and rhonchi are usually heard, and breath sounds are diminished bilaterally. Hyperexpansion of the lungs occurs, and there is a "barrel chest" appearance. Persistent or developing tachypnea may also indicate respiratory distress or sepsis. A work-up for sepsis including white blood cell count and chest radiograph along with an antenatal history may assist in the diagnosis of pneumonia. Periodic respiration (intermittent cessation of respiration for up to 10 seconds) is a normal finding, especially among premature infants. Apneic episodes, in contrast, are of longer duration (more than 20 seconds) and are accompanied by duskiness or cyanosis. These infants clearly require further respiratory assessment and intervention.

Spontaneous pneumothoraces occur within the first 48 hours of life in 2 to 10 percent of full-term and postterm newborns (Merenstein & Gardner, 1993). Predisposing factors are intrapartum stressors or asphyxia and aspiration of meconium or amniotic fluid (Wyatt, 1995). Many may be asymptomatic and resolve without ever being noticed. Cardinal signs and symptoms include cyanosis, dyspnea, decreased breath sounds on the affected side, and a shift in the point of maximal impulse (PMI). Breath sounds may be diminished bilaterally as both lungs are compressed (Wyatt, 1995). A chest radiograph is needed for a definitive diagnosis, but transillumination with a high-intensity fiberoptic light affords rapid diagnosis and emergency evaluation.

Auscultation of the chest should always be done with a warm neonatal stethoscope with a diaphragm no larger than 2.5 cm in diameter (Bruno, 1995). Assessment of neonatal breath sounds is difficult for the novice because sounds are readily transmitted in the small chest, which makes it difficult to localize their source. There may be considerable interference from heart sounds and gastric noises. Breath sounds should be clear anteriorly and posteriorly, with the possible exception of a few fine rales soon after birth in the otherwise asymptomatic neonate. Stridor, a high-pitched hoarse breath sound heard on inspiration or expiration, indicates partial obstruction of the airway and must be evaluated immediately (Simon, 1991). During the first period of reactivity (2 to 4 hours after birth), rates and rhythms may be irregular. Increased heart rate (up to 180 beats per minute) and respiratory rate (up to 80 breaths per minute) are usual (Kenner, 1990). Diagnosis of pathologic conditions such as atelectasis, effusion, and pneumothorax is made on the basis of diminished or congested breath sounds or radiographic studies (see Chapter 36, Diagnostic Imaging). Rhonchi and rales can often be heard together. Respirations are counted by looking at the upper abdomen for a full minute. As soon as the infant is touched, the rate and depth of breathing change with the infant's arousal.

In assessment of the heart, the chest should first be observed for pulsation. Chest pulsations are readily seen in preterm infants owing to thin skin and relative absence of subcutaneous tissue. The PMI is usually found at the fourth or fifth intercostal space. The PMI can shift if the baby has a pneumothorax or another pulmonary pathologic process (Bruno, 1995). The heart rate is counted for a full minute by auscultation. Normal range is 100 to 160 beats per minute. Newborns are more likely to have abnormalities in rate and rhythm than are older children. Premature infants frequently have marked sinus rhythms, sinus arrests, and premature ventricular contractions (Leppink, 1986). Murmurs are common in neonates. A slight murmur may be heard before complete closure of the ductus arteriosus. Bradycardia, tachycardia, and strong or persistent murmurs are abnormal findings requiring evaluation. Differential diagnoses include congenital heart defects, sepsis, prematurity (e.g., patent ductus arteriosus), and precipitating respiratory dysfunction.

Neonatal blood pressure must be assessed with an appropriately sized cuff (50 to 60 percent of upper arm length). Blood pressure should be approximately equal in all four extremities. Significant differences, particularly between upper and lower extremities, may indicate a cardiac defect. Normally, blood pressure increases with an increase in gestational age. Blood pressure can be measured either directly or indirectly (Kenner, 1990). The average systolic pressure at 28 to 32 weeks is 52 mm Hg; at 32 to 36 weeks, 56 mm Hg, and at term, 63 mm Hg (Cantu et al., 1991; Kenner et al., 1988). Infants less than 1000 g have a range of 22 to 42 mm Hg, with the systolic range 30 to 60 mm Hg and the diastolic range 20 to 38 mm Hg (Gunderson, 1995). Infants whose mothers are hypertensive have higher blood pressures (Hegyi et al., 1994).

Head

The head of the infant should be observed for shape and symmetry. A vaginal delivery in the vertex presentation may cause the sutures to override, resulting in an irregularly shaped head "molding." This condition disappears spontaneously in the term infant within a few days but may persist for several weeks in the premature infant. Infants delivered by cesarean section generally have a well-rounded head.

Caput succedaneum, or hemorrhage with edema external to the periosteum, manifests with subcutaneous edema of the soft tissues of the scalp extending across suture lines; it is caused by pressure on the head during labor and delivery in the vertex presentation. Caput is evident at birth and is gradually reabsorbed and disappears within a few days. Rarely is it a problem to the newborn.

Cephalhematoma, a collection of blood from ruptured blood vessels that forms between the skull and the periosteum, may also be caused by trauma to the head during the birth process. The hematoma does not cross suture lines. It may not become apparent for several hours and is not obvious in the delivery room. The cephalhematoma increases in size within 24 to 48 hours. Reabsorption may take 2 to 3 weeks or longer. Cephalhematoma is associated with an underlying fracture in 10 percent of cases.

A subgaleal hemorrhage is rarely seen but is potentially serious. It is most commonly associated with vacuum extraction. Pallor and hypotonicity may be the first early clues followed by increased heart rate and respiratory rate (Cavlovich, 1995). The scalp may present with features similar to caput succedaneum. Large volumes of fluid become redistributed and deplete total body volumes, leading to hypovolemic shock. The subgaleal hemorrhage may involve the entire scalp bilaterally and extend into the soft tissues of the neck and face, producing marked swelling of the forehead and eyelid closure. The hematocrit needs to be closely monitored along with signs and symptoms of anemia.

Further inspection may reveal bruising from forceps or bleeding or irritation from placement of an internal monitor electrode. The hair of a term newborn has identifiable strands and is predominantly over the top of the head. More generally dispersed "fuzz" indicates prematurity (Kenner et al., 1988). Extreme hair unruliness with microcephaly, SGA, or unusual facies may indicate poor early fetal brain growth, typically seen with Cornelia de Lange and Down syndromes (Avery et al., 1994).

The skull is gently palpated to assess the fontanelles, the soft membranous spaces where the skull bones join. The anterior fontanelle is diamond shaped and lies between the sagittal and coronal sutures. It is usually about 2 to 3 cm wide and 3 to 4 cm long and normally closes at about 12 to 18 months of age.

The posterior fontanelle is triangle shaped and lies between the lambdoid and sagittal sutures. It measures 1 to 2 cm and usually closes by 2 months. Either or both of the fontanelles may be difficult to palpate immediately after birth because of molding. The fontanelles should be assessed for fullness when the infant is quiet. Fullness is most readily assessed in the larger anterior fontanelle. Although some enlargement may be seen in the normal crying infant, a bulging fontanelle when the infant is at rest can indicate increased intracranial pressure. A depressed or sunken fontanelle is a sign of dehydration.

Head circumference is measured and plotted on a normal growth curve to determine whether head size is appropriate for age and body length (normocephalic). The presence of edema or molding may account for the head's seeming large or small for age; therefore, the measurement should be repeated when these conditions have subsided. An unusually small head (microcephaly) is seen in a number of congenital syndromes and underdevelopment of the brain. A large head is seen with hydrocephalus, in which either the circulation of cerebrospinal fluid (CSF) is blocked or the CSF is produced in excess. In intrauterine growth retardation, the head may appear large owing to the relative thinness of the body, although it is actually within normal range on the growth curve.

Eyes

Because the ophthalmic examination is frequently upsetting to the infant, it may be reserved until the latter part of the physical assessment. Assessment of the eyes in the initial head-to-toe examination may be confined to readily observed aspects.

The eyes should be clear with no redness, jaundice, or discharge. Swelling of the eyelids may occur from pressure during the delivery process or after instillation of silver nitrate to prevent gonorrheal conjunctivitis. The current trend is to apply erythromycin ointment, which prevents gonorrheal conjunctivitis as well as chlamydial ophthalmia with no evidence of chemical conjunctivitis (Bryant, 1984). Subconjunctival hemorrhages, which result from pressure during delivery and are not pathologic, can frequently be seen in the sclera. They disappear spontaneously in 1 to 3 weeks. Lagophthalmos describes the inability to close the eyes and results from facial nerve pressure from forceps (Fanaroff et al., 1994). It usually resolves within a week but necessitates covering the exposed corneas and use of moisturizing eye drops.

The iris should be evenly colored. The color appears bluish in the white infant, although color may not be permanently established for several months. Dark-skinned or Asian infants usually have dark eyes at birth. The presence of small spots in the iris may be a sign of congenital abnormality (Brushfield's spots).

The corneas should be bright and shiny. The *p*upils should be *e*qual, *r*ound, and *r*eactive to *l*ight *a*ccommodation (PERRLA). Pupil reaction occurs consistently after 32 weeks' gestation but may be present as early as 28 weeks (Avery et al., 1994). The lens should be observed for whiteness or opacity that could indicate congenital cataracts. Opacities are sometimes best visualized by cross-illumination rather than by a light shined directly toward the eye. An opacity of the lens in early infancy is referred to as a cataract, and 1 in 250 infants has some form of congenital cataract (Symanski et al., 1994). The white pupillary reflex seen instead of a red reflex is called leukokoria. Cataracts of infancy and childhood may be hereditary, infectious, traumatic, or metabolic; about one third have no clear cause. Before surgery, no special care is needed (Symanski et al., 1994).

Ears

The development of the ears (cartilage formation; recoil) is an indication of maturity. It is also important to assess the position of the ears. The pinna of the ear should align with the inner canthus of the eye. Use of an otoscope to visualize ear canals is generally deferred unless it is indicated by the condition of the infant. Hearing can be assessed by observing the infant's turning the head to sound or blinking the eyes after sound. Hematomas of the external ear, usually caused by delivery trauma, liquefy slowly and may develop into a cauliflower ear and therefore need to be treated by evacuation (Fanaroff et al., 1994).

Nose

The nose of the newborn is generally slightly flattened. It should be midline, with both nares present and patent. A malpositioned or malformed nose may be seen with a variety of congenital syndromes. Because newborns are nose breathers, patency of the nares should be confirmed by passing a suction catheter into each nostril or by observing the infant breathe with the mouth shut and each nostril occluded one at a time. The nurse should take care to prevent nasal obstruction from developing (from mucous plugs and edema from frequent irritation or suctioning). An infant who has experienced nasal trauma during delivery may demonstrate stridor and cyanosis. A nasal septal dislocation may be identified by finger pressure on the tip of the nose. Where the septum is dislocated, the nostrils collapse and the septal deviation is more obvious. Early identification and surgical consultation are essential along with airway support as indicated.

Mouth

Complete assessment of the mouth may be done toward the end of the examination because it may upset the infant. Although crying may greatly facilitate the oral examination, it hinders assessment of other areas, such as the abdomen.

The mouth should be midline and symmetrical in structure and movement. The lips should be fully formed, with mouth, chin, and tongue in proportion. Micrognathia or small lower jaw may be seen in some trisomies. Macroglossia, or large tongue, may be associated with Beckwith-Wiedemann syndrome, hypothyroidism, or mucopolysaccharidosis (Tappero & Honeyfield, 1996). The mucous membranes should be pink and moist, indicating good hydration and oxygenation. Thrush, a candidal infection transmitted during the birth process, may be identified by white patches that are difficult to remove. Hard and soft palates are examined for cleft. Excessive salivation indicates possible tracheoesophageal fistula or esophageal atresia. Natal teeth are usually malformed and loose and are therefore usually removed.

Several reflexes may be demonstrated at this time. The term infant with normal neurologic function has a gag reflex, a sucking reflex (sucking on a nipple or examiner's finger), and a rooting reflex (turning toward the cheek that is stroked). If a reflex is absent, an explanation is sought; prematurity and dysfunction of the nervous system are the most common causes.

If the infant is intubated with either an oral or a nasal endotracheal tube, the tube should be comfortably secured and marked such that displacement may be readily recognized. Breath sounds should be auscultated frequently. Presence of bilateral breath sounds helps confirm correct tube placement, whereas sounds unilaterally diminished or absent indicate poor ventilation on that side (possibly secondary to tube displacement).

Neck

The neck should be symmetrical and the head able to turn in full range of motion bilaterally. No lymph nodes or masses should be palpable. The clavicles should be symmetrical and even in appearance. Asymmetrical or "bumpy" clavicles indicate fracture secondary to birth trauma. Crepitus, if present, is easily palpable.

Trunk

Much of this area is described under cardiopulmonary status. The examiner further assesses the breast, abdomen, and back.

Breast

Two nipples should be present, in normal alignment. The size of the areola depends on the gestational age. The term infant has a raised areola and breast tissue approximately 1 cm in diameter. A slight discharge ("witch's milk") may be present owing to the influence of maternal hormones.

Abdomen

The neonate's abdomen is soft, rounded, and slightly protuberant. Asymmetry, distention, weak musculature, visible peristaltic waves, masses, or herniations are clearly abnormal findings requiring prompt evaluation and possible intervention. Distention may be secondary to factors such as resuscitative measures, mechanical ventilation, enlargement of organs, or obstruction of the bowel.

The umbilical cord stump should be bluish, shiny, and moist, with no oozing or bleeding. Three vessels should be present (two arteries and one vein); a single artery is associated with congenital anomalies, most often renal. Meconium staining indicates stress before birth. Redness, discharge, and a foul odor are signs of infection. An arterial or venous line, if present, should be securely taped to prevent displacement and possible hemorrhage.

The bowel sounds are auscultated before palpation. The abdomen is palpated gently to locate vital organs as well as any abnormal masses.

Flexing the knees and legs toward the hips allows the abdominal muscles to relax. This position is similar to the fetal position and calms the infant. The liver margin is palpated inferior to the right costal margin, and the spleen tip can frequently be felt at the left costal margin. Both kidneys as well as the descending colon in the left lower quadrant may be palpated.

Back

The spinal column should be straight and flexible. There should be no visible defects. A meningocele presents as a soft rounded mass on the back, usually skin covered. A meningomyelocele presents as a herniated sac containing meninges as well as neural tissue. It is usually flat at birth with spinal cord tissue lying exposed on the surface and surrounded by a bluish pink membrane. A spina bifida occulta is located in the lower lumbar and lumbosacral area and is a result of absence of one or more posterior arches of the spine. The meninges and spinal cord are normal. The defect is covered with skin although there may be a dimple on the skin surface. The vertebrae should be palpable without pain.

Anogenital Area

The anus should be inspected for patency to rule out imperforate anus. Patency is indicated by the passage of meconium. A closed anus can be diagnosed when it is impossible to insert a rectal thermometer; this practice may be disappearing, however, because there is increasing controversy surrounding rectal temperatures in the neonate. An area of current research is the validity of temperatures in the axillary and inguinal areas as reflective of core temperature (Bliss-Holtz, 1989). This is an effort to avoid rectal perforations. Tympanic thermometers are acceptable for rapid screening in the neonate, but accuracy variation is believed by some to be too extreme to be reliable (Weiss et al., 1993).

In both male and female preterm infants, the genitalia are useful in determining gestational age. The female genitals consist of the labia majora, labia minora, and clitoris. In a full-term infant, the labia majora usually cover the labia minora; but in preterm infants, the labia minora and clitoris may be more prominent. A hymenal tag may be present and may protrude from the vagina. The labia may be engorged as a result of circulating maternal hormones. These hormones are also responsible for a milky vaginal discharge tinged with mucus or blood (pseudomenstruation).

The male genitals consist of scrotum, testes, and penis. The external urinary meatus is usually covered by the prepuce. The foreskin should never be forced. The placement of the external meatus on the glans penis should be evaluated to rule out hypospadias (meatal opening on the ventral portion of the penile shaft) or epispadias (meatal opening on the dorsal portion of the penile shaft). The scrotum should be inspected for size, amount of rugae, and presence of testicles. In preterm infants, inguinal hernias are common. A chordee, ventral bowing of the penis, is often seen with hypospadias, and a malformed prepuce may represent a malformed urethra.

Extremities

The extremities are first observed in the resting state for symmetry, degree of flexion, and movement. Asymmetrical limbs are associated with trauma, maternal diabetes, drug use, and congenital syndromes.

There should be full range of joint motion in all extremities. Birth trauma resulting in damage to the fifth or sixth cervical nerves results in a paralysis of the upper portion of the arm called Erb-Duchenne paralysis. The grasp reflex is normal, but the Moro reflex is absent. Klumpke's palsy involves C8 to T1, and the hand and lower arm are paralyzed; it has a poor prognosis. Brachial plexus palsy is a stretch injury and is serious from a functional standpoint. Neurologic function returns in a few days, and hemorrhage and edema resolve.

Flexion is related to the gestational age of the infant. Flexion begins in the lower portion of the body and moves upward to the arms. The hands and feet should be observed for extra digits, clubbing, or webbing. The hands and feet are observed for presence of creases. The most common one found is the simian crease, a palmar crease associated with trisomy 21, or Down syndrome. Because this crease is found in the general population as well, its presence alone is not diagnostic.

The lower extremities are evaluated for congenital hip dislocation. Ortolani's maneuver is performed by placing the fingers on both trochanters while the thumbs grip the medial aspects of the femur. Both legs are flexed and abducted so that they nearly touch the examining table. If dislocation is present, a click may be felt or heard as the femoral head is reduced into the acetabulum. Conversely, Barlow's maneuver tests for ready dislocation of the femoral head from the acetabulum. With the examiner's hands placed as for Ortolani's maneuver, the infant's legs are adducted and pressed down gently. Dislocation, if present, is palpable. Both Ortolani's and Barlow's tests should be performed to confirm presence or absence of abnormality.

The feet are examined for presence of clubfoot or rocker-bottom feet. Either of these conditions should be referred to an orthopedist or geneticist, or both, because both conditions require further assessment and intervention. The presence of rocker-bottom feet is often related to a chromosomally induced congenital syndrome such as trisomy 13 or 18.

Newborn physical and gestational assessment is reviewed in Table 17–2.

Text continued on page 249

TABLE 17–2 Newborn Physical and Gestational Assessment

System	Normal	Significance	Abnormal	Significance
Color—good indicator of overall status of infant, especially cardiopulmonary system				
Inspection	Pink; in dark-skinned infants, mucous membranes should be pink	No cardiopulmonary compromise	Duskiness or cyanosis (other than acrocyanosis)	Poor circulation or respiratory difficulty or distress
	Acrocyanosis of hands and feet during first 24 hours of life	Sluggish peripheral circulation caused by transition to the cool extrauterine life	Acrocyanosis lasting longer than first 24 hours	Poor peripheral circulation, may have cardiac compromise
	Reddish hue (especially noted immediately after birth)	Adjustment in oxygen levels in extrauterine environment	Plethora	Elevated hematocrit or hemoglobin levels, polycythemia, or hyperviscosity of blood
			Pale	Cardiopulmonary compromise or failure
	Ecchymosis over presenting part (to differentiate between cyanosis and ecchymosis, apply pressure to darkened area; cyanotic area blanches, whereas ecchymotic area remains dark)	Pressure over presenting part, causing bruising and trapping of blood in external tissue layers		
	Mongolian spots over buttocks, may extend to sacral region (usually in dark-skinned infants)	Hyperpigmentation		
	Jaundice after first 48 hours of age, receding by days 4–5 (peak occurs later in premature infant, may be after day 4)	Physiologic jaundice; transition of blood supply to liver, increased red blood cell count with decreased life span of cells, decreased plasma protein level, and decreased glucuronosyl transferase that aids in bilirubin conjugation	Jaundice on day 1 or after day 4	Isoimmunity such as Rh or ABO incompatibility, polycythemia, enzyme deficiencies, excessive bruising or bleeding, Hirschsprung's disease, pyloric stenosis, other intestinal obstructions that increase blood supply or shunt blood to the liver; maternal diabetes, SGA
General appearance—indicative of nutritional status, infant maturity, and general well-being				
Inspection	Well-formed and rounded, with presence of subcutaneous tissue; no obvious anomalies	Good nutritional status; generally healthy	Little or no subcutaneous tissue, wasting muscle, loose skin, thin extremities, anomalies	Malnourished or with a variety of congenital defects, such as cleft lip and/or palate, omphalocele, gastroschisis, meningomyelocele; infant stressed in utero
	Vernix	Increases with gestational age		
	Lanugo	Decreases with gestational age		
Posture				
Inspection	Fetal position: fists clenched; arms adducted, flexed; hip abducted; knees flexed (extension of extremities may be normal in prematurity but abnormal in full term, because extension of legs and then flexion occurs as development progresses); flexion moves upward to arms; spinal column straight	Full term	Opisthotonos (neck in extension)	Brain damage, birth asphyxia; neurologic abnormality
			"Frog position" of legs	Prematurity
			Bulge or curvature of the spinal column	Spina bifida or meningomyelocele

Table continued on following page

TABLE 17–2 Newborn Physical and Gestational Assessment *(Continued)*

System	Normal	Significance	Abnormal	Significance
	Spontaneous, symmetrical movement, may be slightly tremulous (flexion and extension should be equal bilaterally)	Full-term newborn activity	No movement; or asymmetrical, irregular, tremulous (jerky motions, unequal movement)	Birth asphyxia; neurologic dysfunction; prematurity; drug-induced birth injury
Muscle strength and tone				
Inspection	Strength and tone strong	May be full term	Strength and tone weak, hypotonic, or flaccid	Birth asphyxia or prematurity
	Palmar grasp strong	Good overall strength; may be full term	Palmar grasp weak	Prematurity
Alertness and cry				
Inspection	Mood ranges from quiet to alert; consolable when upset	Normal newborn activity	Not easily aroused, not alert	Prematurity; stressed; septic; states of wakefulness from neurologic problem
	Cry strong	No increased intracranial pressure	Weak, high-pitched, or absent cry	Brain damage or increased intracranial pressure
			Raspy	Upper airway problem
			Expiratory grunt	Respiratory distress
			Unilateral drooping of mouth when crying	Nerve damage
Cardiopulmonary				
Inspection				
Respiratory effort	Easy, unlabored rhythm; may be irregular, but periods of apnea >15 seconds are abnormal; abdominal breathing	No respiratory distress or difficulty	Dyspnea: accessory muscle retraction (substernal, supracostal, intercostal, supraclavicular); flared nostrils, stridor, or grunting	Respiratory distress or difficulty
Respiratory rate	40–60 breaths per minute	Normal rate	Apnea lasting >15 seconds and accompanied by duskiness, cyanosis, or respiratory rate >60 breaths per minute	Prematurity; respiratory difficulty; sepsis; tachypnea in C-section or in full-term infants may be transient (from retention of lung fluid)
Thorax	Symmetrical excursion	Normal respiratory pattern	Asymmetry or unequal excursion	Diaphragmatic hernia; pneumothorax; phrenic nerve damage
Anteroposterior diameter	Normal	Normal respiratory pattern	Exaggerated: ratio greater than 1:1, barrel chest; hyperinflation equal without exaggeration	Respiratory distress
Auscultation				
Breath sounds	Clear; equal bilaterally, anteriorly, and posteriorly; a few rales may be present the first few hours after birth because of residual fetal lung fluid: no color changes or cyanosis should accompany this finding	Clear lung fields	Rales after first day; rhonchi; expiratory grunting; wheezing	Lung congestion; respiratory distress; pulmonary edema; pneumonia
			Unequal breath sounds	Pneumothorax or diaphragmatic hernia
Heart rate	100–160 beats per minute; regular, without murmurs (initially may hear slight murmur until ductus arteriosus closes)	Normal cardiac rhythm without significant abnormalities	Bradycardia <100 beats per minute or tachycardia >160 beats per minute; murmur (usually heard at left sternal border or above apical pulse)	May be secondary to respiratory difficulty; increased workload of the heart; prematurity sepsis; congenital heart defect with or without cyanosis
Bruit	No bruit in cranium or abdomen	No arteriovenous malformation	Bruit either in abdomen or cranium	Arteriovenous malformation

TABLE 17–2 Newborn Physical and Gestational Assessment *(Continued)*

System	Normal	Significance	Abnormal	Significance
Palpation				
Apical pulse	At fourth or fifth intercostal space, midclavicular line, left anterior chest (point of maximal impulse at fourth intercostal space just right of midclavicular line, may be shifted to the right during the first few hours of life)	Normal position of cardiac pulse; no shifting; without cardiomegaly	Displaced apical pulse	May have cardiac defect or cardiomegaly
Thrill	No thrill	No increased cardiac activity	Thrill after first few hours of life	Increased cardiac activity
Blood pressure	Average systolic rate 28–32 weeks: 52; 32–36 weeks: 56; full term: 63; equal in all four extremities	Normal cardiac output; good circulation; possibly no cardiac defect	Decreased blood pressure	Shock or hypovolemia
			Unequal blood pressure in the extremities, especially between upper and lower extremities	Cardiac defect: coarctation of the aorta
Percussion	No increased tympany over lung fields	Normal lung field borders	Increased tympany over lung fields	Hyperinflation of the lungs
Skin				
Inspection	Moist, warm to touch, without peeling	Normal, well hydrated	Dry, peeling, cracked	Postmature infant
			Wrinkled	Intrauterine growth retardation
			Gelatinous with visible veins (transparent skin and visible veins disappear with increasing gestational age)	Prematurity
	Vernix (thick, white cheesy material)	Increases with gestational age	No vernix	Prematurity
	Scant lanugo (fine hair over body)	Full term; decreases with gestational age	Abundant lanugo	Prematurity
	Milia	Blocked sebaceous glands (common in newborns)		
	Erythema toxicum	Newborn rash over body, usually on days 1–3	Nevus flammeus	Hyperpigmentation
			Meconium staining	Fetal distress
			Petechiae	Hematopoietic disorder
			Edematous, shiny, taut skin	Kidney dysfunction, cardiac failure, and/or renal failure
			Skin tags	Extra folds of skin, overgrowth of tissue; sometimes associated with anomalies
	Mottling	May be normal reaction to immaturity of organ systems	Mottling	May be abnormal if associated with cold stress, color changes, bradycardia
Palpation	Warm (axillary temperature 35.5°C–36.5°C)	Normal range	Cool (<35.5°C)	Poor peripheral perfusion; prematurity
			Warm (>37°C)	Hyperthermia or fever
Head				
Inspection	Normocephalic in proportion to body (head circumference for average full-term newborn is 32–38 cm)	Normal	Microcephalic	Congenital syndromes or decreased brain growth as with substance abuse
			Hydrocephalic	Blockage of the passage of CSF such as in meningomyelocele; or excessive production of CSF

Table continued on following page

TABLE 17–2 Newborn Physical and Gestational Assessment *(Continued)*

System	Normal	Significance	Abnormal	Significance
			Anencephaly	Absent cerebral tissue and/ or scant or absent skull
			Encephalocele	Brain and spinal cord that have herniated
			Bradycephalic	Premature closure of coronal suture line; AP diameter shortened and lateral growth increased
			Craniosynostosis	Premature closure of suture lines
			Molding: cranial distortion lasting 5–7 days	Excessive pressure on cranium during vaginal delivery
			Overriding sutures	Excessive pressure on cranium during vaginal delivery
			Caput succedaneum	Edematous region of scalp extending over suture lines, resulting from pressure on presenting part during vaginal delivery
			Cephalhematoma	Trapping of blood in tissues not crossing the suture lines and lasting up to 8 weeks
			Forceps marks; edematous or reddened areas	Forceps delivery
Head lag (pull newborn up, supporting the arms, from supine to sitting position; grade degree of head lag by position of head in relationship to trunk part of gestational examination)	Not greater than 10 degrees in full term	Decreases with maturity	Greater than 10 degrees; little or no support of head	Hypotonia or prematurity
Hair distribution	Over top of head, with single strands identifiable	Full term	Fine, fuzzy, may be over entire head	Prematurity
Palpation	Without masses or soft areas over skull bones	Normal	Masses or soft areas such as craniotabes over parietal bones	May be normal variation if no abnormality present
Auscultation	No bruit	Normal	Bruit	Cerebral arteriovenous malformation
Fontanelles				
Inspection and palpation				
Anterior fontanelle (open until 12–18 months)	Diamond shaped, 5 × 4 cm along the coronal and sagittal sutures	Normal	Craniosynostosis	Premature closure of suture lines may result from brain growth retardation
Posterior fontanelle	Triangle shaped, small, 1 × 1 cm along sagittal and lambdoid suture lines; or closed at birth	Normal	Bulging fontanelle (usually anterior fontanelle)	Increased intracranial pressure
			Sunken fontanelle	Dehydration
Facies				
Inspection	Eyes on line with ears; nose midline	Normal	Low-set ear; asymmetry of features	Congenital syndromes such as Down syndrome, or genetic defect
			Wide-eyed, worried	Postmature; SGA; or intrauterine growth retardation
			Hypertelorism >2.5 cm	Congenital syndrome: genetic disorders
			Hypotelorism <2.5 cm	Trisomy 13

TABLE 17–2 Newborn Physical and Gestational Assessment *(Continued)*

System	Normal	Significance	Abnormal	Significance
Oral cavity				
Inspection				
Mouth	Midline of face, symmetrical	Normal	Drooping or slanting unilaterally with crying; movement of mouth	Seventh cranial nerve damage; facial nerve damage
	Shape and size in proportion with face	Normal	Bird-like mouth: shortened vermilion border	Fetal alcohol syndrome
			Wide mouth (macrostomia)	Metabolic disorder
			Small mouth (microstomia)	Down syndrome
Mucous membranes	Moist, pink	Well hydrated and oxygenated	Dry, dusky	Dehydrated or poorly oxygenated
Chin	Shape and size in proportion with face	Normal	Micrognathia	Pierre Robin sequence
Lips	Completely formed, pink, moist	Normal	Cleft lip	Congenital anomaly: failure of midline fusion during first trimester
Palate	Without arching; intact (determine by palpating)	Normal	High-arched palate	Turner's syndrome
			Cleft palate	Failure of midline fusion during first trimester
Tongue	Size in proportion with mouth	Normal	Macroglossia	Hypothyroidism
			Microglossia	Hypothyroidism
	Midline	Normal: no neurologic dysfunction	Deviation from midline	Cranial nerve damage
Uvula	Midline, rises with crying	Normal function of glossopharyngeal and vagus nerves	Not midline or does not rise with crying	Neurologic dysfunction
Gag reflex	Present (reflexes generally develop from head to toe during gestation)	Normal neurologic function of glossopharyngeal and vagus nerves	Absent	Neurologic dysfunction
Sucking reflex	Present and strong when nipple or finger offered	Normal maturity and intact hypoglossal nerve	Absent	Prematurity or brain dysfunction
Rooting reflex	Present when cheek is stroked, infant turns toward stroking	Normal maturity and intact trigeminal nerve	Absent	Prematurity or brain dysfunction
Salivation	Without excess	Normal	Excessive	Tracheoesophageal fistula; esophageal atresia
Nose				
Inspection				
Position	Midline	Normal	Off midline	Congenital malformation or syndrome
			Flattened nasal bridge	Congenital syndromes
			Beaked	Treacher Collins syndrome
			Enlarged or bulbous	Trisomy 13
Nares	Bilaterally present	Intact	Not present bilaterally	Congenital malformation or syndrome
	Patent (occlude neonate's nostrils one at a time while holding mouth closed; infant should be able to breathe through one side at a time; passing a catheter into newborn's nares, one at a time, also demonstrates patency)	Normal	Not patent	Nasal obstruction; choanal atresia
Response to strong odors passed under nose	Grimace or cry	Normal; intact olfactory nerve	No response	Olfactory nerve damage
Auscultation				
Nares (with a stethoscope, auscultate for breathing, one side at a time)	Breathing detected bilaterally	Patent	Breathing not detected bilaterally	Not patent; nasal obstruction

Table continued on following page

TABLE 17–2 Newborn Physical and Gestational Assessment *(Continued)*

System	Normal	Significance	Abnormal	Significance
Eyes—indicate many systemic problems				
Inspection				
Sclera	Clear	Normal	Yellow	Jaundice
			Hemorrhage	Birth trauma
			Blue	Osteogenesis imperfecta
Conjunctiva	Clear	Normal	Hemorrhage	Birth trauma
			Pink	Conjunctivitis, may be chemical, caused by silver nitrate
Iris	Colored evenly, bilaterally	Normal	Brushfield's spots (these gold flecks may be normal if not found with other anomalies)	Down syndrome or congenital syndrome
			Coloboma (opening of pupil that extends into iris on one side)	May be associated with congenital malformation (internal)
Pupils (examination done in darkened room with penlight or flashlight; if done with newborn in incubator or in nursery, shield infant's eyes as much as possible)	Equal bilaterally and reactive to light	Normal: intact oculomotor nerve	Unequal bilaterally; nonreactive	Brain damage or increased intracranial pressure
Cornea	Clear	Normal: intact	Hazy	Prematurity
			Milky	Congenital cataracts possibly due to congenital rubella
Retina	Transparent	Normal: intact	Areas of pigmentation	Damaged retina
			Blood vessels without clear demarcation, or tortuous	Retinal hemorrhage
Lacrimal duct	Patent	Normal	Blocked or absent	Congenital obstruction
Blink reflex	Reactive (responds to bright light)	Intact optic nerve	Nonreactive or absent	Facial nerve paralysis or optic nerve damage
Red reflex	Present	Lens intact	Absent	Congenital cataracts
Eyelids	Without ptosis or edema	Normal; intact oculomotor nerve	Edema	Birth trauma
			Ptosis	Oculomotor nerve damage
			Epicanthal folds	Down syndrome or cri du chat syndrome
Doll-eye response (with infant in supine position, turn head from one side to the other: eyes move to opposite side from which head is turned)	Present	Normal: intact trochlear, abducens, and oculomotor nerves	Absent	Damage to trochlear, abducens, and oculomotor nerves
Eye position	Without slant	Normal	Slant upward	Down syndrome
			Slant downward	Treacher Collins syndrome
			Sunset eyes (downward slope of pupils below lids)	Hydrocephalus
Ears				
Inspection				
Position	Ears in straight line with eyes; vertical angle that is greater than straight vertical line; without slant	Normal	Set below eyes; ears slant, internally or externally rotated	Down syndrome
Skin tags	Absent	Normal	Present	Congenital renal anomaly
Cartilage formation	Well-curved pinna, sturdy, stiff cartilage, instant recoil	Normal	Flattened or folded, slow recoil	Prematurity

TABLE 17–2 Newborn Physical and Gestational Assessment *(Continued)*

System	Normal	Significance	Abnormal	Significance
Reaction to loud noise or snapping fingers	Neonate startles or cries	Hearing intact: auditory nerve intact	Absent or little response (further testing can be done with hearing tests done in the crib or other hearing tests)	Deaf or decreased hearing
Otoscopic examination (this examination is often omitted because it is difficult to perform and may be potentially harmful if the examiner is not skilled; ear should be pulled down and back for examination)	Umbo (cone) of light present, pearl-gray tympanic membrane may have vernix; membrane is movable without bulging	Normal: intact ear without infection	Umbo of light dull or absent; dull or immobile tympanic membrane, may be	Congenital malformation or infection
			Red	Infection
			Blue	Hemorrhage
			Bulging	Infected: otitis media
Neck				
Inspection	Shape: symmetrical	Normal	Shape: asymmetrical	Fetal position
	Head: turns from side to side equally, full range of joint motion	Normal	Shape: asymmetrical	Fetal position
	Short without excessive skin	Normal	Short and webbed	Down syndrome
Tonic neck reflex (place infant in supine position; turn one side with body restrained; extremities toward side that head is turned are extended, but other extremities are flexed: attempt by newborn to right head when turned to side in position tests accessory nerve)	Asymmetrical and present but decreases	Normal	Asymmetrical and strongly present	Prematurity
			Symmetrical	Neurologic dysfunction
Palpation				
Thyroid	Midline	Normal	Enlarged	Goiter (rare)
Lymph nodes	Not palpable	Normal	Palpable	Congenital infection
Mass	No masses	Normal	Mass in neck	Cystic hygroma
			Sternocleidomastoid enlarged	Torticollis: birth or in utero injury resulting in hematoma of sternocleidomastoid muscle
Carotid	Pulse rate strong and regular (do not massage carotid artery or neck: can result in reflex bradycardia)	Normal cardiac and circulatory function	Pulse rate weak or absent	Cardiac defect or circulatory problem
Clavicles	Even and without "lumps" along bones; symmetrical	No fractures	Fracture or lump felt; uneven; asymmetrical	Birth injury
Abdomen and thorax				
Inspection				
Chest circumference	30–36 cm	Average for full-term neonate	<30 cm	Prematurity; or SGA
			Chest circumference >36 cm	Barrel chest: respiratory difficulty; or LGA
Excursion of diaphragm	Equal	Normal	Unequal	Phrenic nerve damage
Ribs	Symmetrical	Normal	Asymmetrical	Birth injury or congenital syndrome

Table continued on following page

TABLE 17–2 Newborn Physical and Gestational Assessment *(Continued)*

System	Normal	Significance	Abnormal	Significance
Breast	Nipple spacing on line without extra nipples	Normal	Nipple spacing not on line, or extra nipples	Congenital syndrome
Areola	Raised and without discharge	Full term	Flat and/or discharge	Prematurity or discharge from hormonal influence
			Hypertrophy	Maternal hormonal influence
Abdomen	Rounded, contoured, symmetrical	Normal	Scaphoid	Diaphragmatic hernia
			Distended (if suspected, measure the abdominal girth every 4 hours to detect changes)	Intestinal obstruction, renal problem; ascites: edema caused by a variety of problems, including congenital kidney or cardiac defects, prematurity, fetal hydrops
			Distention in left upper quadrant	Pyloric stenosis or duodenal or jejunal obstruction
			Asymmetrical	Abdominal mass
Umbilical cord	3 vessels (2 arteries, 1 vein)	Normal	2 vessels (1 artery, 1 vein)	Internal congenital anomalies possible
	Bluish white	Normal	Meconium-stained	Distress in utero
			Reddened with discharge	Infection
			Thick cord	LGA
			Small cord	SGA or malnourished
			Mass	Hernia
			Hernia of the cord through which abdominal viscera, intestines, sometimes other organs enter	Omphalocele
			Hernia (lateral to the cord may contain abdominal content)	Gastroschisis
Abdominal musculature	Strong	Normal	Weak	Prune-belly syndrome, may have associated renal problems, including hypoplastic kidneys
			Visible abdominal wall defect over bladder areas	Exstrophy of the bladder
	No visible peristaltic waves	Normal bowel activity	Visible peristaltic waves	Intestinal obstruction, usually not present immediately after birth
Auscultation				
Bowel sounds	Present	Normal	Absent	Obstruction
			Hyperactive (unless just after feeding)	Hypermotility
Abdomen	No bruit	Normal	Bruit	Arteriovenous malformation
Renal	No bruit	Normal	Bruit	Renal artery stenosis
Palpation				
Xiphoid process	Present	Normal: intact	Absent or depressed	Fracture (sometimes due to resuscitation)
Ribs	Without masses or crepitus	Intact, without defects or "air leaks"	Masses or crepitus	Fractures or mass; subcutaneous air due to air leaks from pulmonary dysfunction
Breast tissue	1 cm	Normal: full term	<1 cm, may be ≤5 mm	Prematurity
Abdomen	Soft and not tender; without masses	Normal	Tense, rigid, tender, masses	Intestinal deformity or obstruction; renal or urinary tract deformity
			Separation of rectus muscles of abdominal wall (diastasis recti)	Common in newborns, especially premature

TABLE 17–2 Newborn Physical and Gestational Assessment *(Continued)*

System	Normal	Significance	Abnormal	Significance
Kidneys	4–5 cm in length; right kidney lower than left, found in abdomen and posteriorly in lumbar or flank area (palpate with newborn's legs flexed in fetal position to relax infant)	Normal	Enlarged Absent	Polycystic Potter's association
Liver	Sharp edge just above right costal margin; firm	Normal	Below right costal margin	Respiratory distress or congestive heart failure
			Hard	Liver damage or cardiopulmonary problems
Spleen	1 cm below left costal margin	Normal	Absent or not palpable	Congenital heart defects
Bladder	Not distended (unless just before void)	Normal kidney and urinary tract system	Distended; may be visible above pubic bone	Urinary tract obstruction
Groin	Femoral pulse rate strong and regular bilaterally	Normal	Femoral pulse rate weak or absent bilaterally	Coarctation of the aorta
			Bounding femoral pulses	Patent ductus arteriosus
	No hernias or groin masses	Normal	Groin masses	Inguinal hernia
Percussion				
Gastric bubble	Just below left costal margin and toward midline; tympanic	Normal	No tympany	Esophageal atresia or gastric deformity
Abdomen	Tympanic except dull over liver, spleen, and bladder	Normal liver, spleen, bladder, no masses (indicated by dullness)	Increased tympany	Increased presence of fluid or air
			Increased areas of dullness (if liver or spleen is enlarged, dullness extends below the costal margins; if bladder is enlarged, dullness extends toward umbilicus: be sure to re-examine after void)	Masses or enlarged abdominal organs, located where the dullness is increased
Genitourinary tract				
Inspection of female newborn				
Labia majora	Present and extend beyond labia minora	Full term	Smaller than labia minora	Prematurity
Labia minora	Present and well-formed	Full term	Larger than labia majora	Prematurity
Clitoris	Present, may be enlarged	Full term or prematurity		
Urethral meatus	Present in front of vaginal orifice	Normal	Displaced	Urinary malformation
Vagina	Patent with or without white discharge	Normal	Not patent, with or without slight bleeding	Hormonal influence
Genitalia	Distinguishable as female or male	Normal	Not clearly distinguishable as to sex, may have organs of both sexes	Ambiguous genitalia; endocrine problems
Perineum	Smooth	Normal	Dimpling or extra opening	Urinary or genital malformation, or urinary fistula
Anus	Midline, patent (test by inserting small finger)	Normal	Shifted anteriorly or posteriorly	Anal defect
			Nonpatent or dimpling	Imperforate anus
Anal wink	Present (light stroking of anal area produces constriction of sphincter)	Normal sphincter	Absent	Poor muscle strength of sphincter
Inspection of male newborn				
Penis	Straight; proportionate to body (length: 2.8–4.3 cm)	Normal	Curved Enlarged	Chordee Renal problems

Table continued on following page

TABLE 17–2 Newborn Physical and Gestational Assessment *(Continued)*

System	Normal	Significance	Abnormal	Significance
Urinary meatus (if neonate is uncircumcised, gently retract the foreskin; if circumcised, also check for edema or bleeding)	Midline and at tip of glans	Normal	Displaced to ventral surface	Hypospadias
			Displaced to dorsal surface	Epispadias
Urinary stream (first void should occur no later than 24 hours postnatally)	Straight from penis	Normal urinary pattern	Not straight	Urinary obstruction or malformation
			From opening in abdomen or perineum	Urinary fistula
			Failure to void within first 24 hours of life	Renal or urinary obstruction or malformation
Testes and scrotum	Full, numerous rugae	Full term	Flaccid, smooth, or few rugae	Prematurity
	Darkly pigmented	Normal	Bluish testes or scrotal sac	Torsion of the testicles
			Enlarged or edematous	Hydrocele or breech delivery
			Dimpling	Torsion of the testicles
Perineum	Smooth	Normal	Dimpling or extra opening	Urinary or genital malformation, or urinary fistula
Anus	Midline, patent (test by inserting small finger)	Normal	Shifted anteriorly or posteriorly	Anal defect
			Nonpatent or dimpling	Imperforate anus
Anal wink	Present (light stroking of anal area produces constriction of sphincter)	Normal sphincter	Absent	Poor muscle strength or sphincter
Palpation of male newborn	Testes descended on at least one side	Full term	Testes not palpable (may be found high in the inguinal canal)	Prematurity or undescended testes
Upper extremities				
Inspection				
Length	In proportion to each other; lower extremities and body symmetrical	Normal	Shortened extremities or asymmetrical	Diabetic mother; congenital syndrome; maternal drug use
Range of motion	Full range of joint motion: includes abduction, adduction, internal and external rotation, flexion, extension as applicable to joint (full flexion of upper extremities comes with maturity)	Normal	Limited range of joint motion	Birth injury or trauma
			Limited range of flexion	Prematurity
Shoulder	Full range of motion	Normal	Limited range of motion or flexion of shoulder	Dystocia; brachial plexus damage
Clavicles	Full range of motion	Normal	Limited range of motion of clavicles	Clavicle injury; osteogenesis imperfecta
Elbow	Full range of motion	Normal	Limited range of motion or flexion of elbow	Birth injury or fetal position
Wrist	Full range of motion	Normal	Limited range of motion or flexion of wrist	Birth injury or fetal position
Square window (test by flexing infant's wrist on forearm, then measure angle according to gestational examination chart)	0-degree angle for term	Maturity	Angle greater than 0 degree	Prematurity
Hand: grasp reflex	Present, strong, equal bilaterally	Normal; maturity	Weak or absent, or unequal bilaterally	Hand injury or fetal position; prematurity or birth injury

TABLE 17–2 Newborn Physical and Gestational Assessment *(Continued)*

System	Normal	Significance	Abnormal	Significance
Scarf sign (grasp infant's hand and gently pull hand around neck toward the opposite shoulder; observe position of elbow to chest; grade position according to gestational chart)	Elbow short of midline	Maturity	Elbow beyond midline	Prematurity
Arm recoil (quickly flex neonate's forearms for 5 seconds, next pull them to full extension, then release; recoil time is graded)	Instant	Maturity	Slow	Prematurity
Palm	No simian creases	Normal	Simian creases	Down syndrome
Fingers	10 digits and without webbing; equal spacing	Normal	More than 10 digits (polydactyly)	May be part of syndrome
			Webbed, digital tags (syndactyly), or unequal spacing	Congenital syndrome
Carpals and metacarpals	Present and equal bilaterally	No fractures; bone formation normal	Absent or unequal bilaterally	Fractures or absence of bone, may be associated with congenital syndromes
Nails	Extend beyond nail beds	Normal; full term	Short; spoon-shaped	Congenital syndromes, fetal alcohol syndrome
			Absent	May have absent radius
			Meconium-stained	Fetal distress
Nail beds	Pink, brisk capillary refill (≤3 seconds), equal bilaterally	Normal peripheral perfusion, normal oxygenation	Dusky, or slow capillary refill (>3 seconds), bilaterally	Poor peripheral perfusion or oxygenation
Palpation (in the presence of a fracture may produce crying or facial grimace; observe infant's response)				
Clavicles	Without fractures or pain; symmetrical	Normal	Asymmetrical or pain on palpation	Fractures, shoulder dystocia, brachial plexus damage, or palsy
Humerus, radius, and ulna	Present; symmetrical and without fractures	Normal bone formation	Absent or asymmetrical	Absence of any of these bones may be associated with syndromes
			Painful fractures	Birth injury
Pulses	Brachial and radial strong and equal bilaterally; in comparison with femoral pulses: equal	Good peripheral perfusion, without obvious cardiac defects	Brachial and/or radial weak, absent, or unequal bilaterally	Poor peripheral perfusion, possible cardiac defects
Lower extremities				
Inspection				
Length	In proportion to body and equal bilaterally; limbs straight	Normal extremity length	Not in proportion to body; short or unequal; limbs not straight, leg internally rotated or bowed	Congenital syndrome; diabetic mother
Toes	10 toes and without webbing; equal spacing	Normal	More than 10 digits or with webbing or unequal spacing	May be associated with congenital syndromes
Feet	Straight	Normal	Turned valgus	Absent fibula or fetal position
			Turned varus	Absent tibia or fetal position
Ankle dorsiflexion (foot is flexed back on ankle, then angle between foot and ankle is measured)	0-degree angle	Maturity	Angle >0 degrees, may be up to 90 degrees in very premature infant	Prematurity

Table continued on following page

TABLE 17–2 Newborn Physical and Gestational Assessment *(Continued)*

System	Normal	Significance	Abnormal	Significance
Popliteal angle (flex newborn's leg, then flex thigh; next release and extend leg; measure angle of knee)	≤90 degrees	Maturity	>90 degrees and ≤180 degrees in very immature infant	Prematurity
Heel-to-ear maneuver (gently pull leg to ear without forcing)	Heel will not reach ear but only near shoulder area in full-term infant	Maturity	Heel reaches ear, or just short of the ear	Prematurity
Nails	Extend to end of nail bed	Normal; maturity	Do not extend to end of nail bed	Prematurity
Nail beds	Pink; brisk capillary refill (≤3 seconds)	Good peripheral perfusion	Dusky, or slow capillary refill (>3 seconds)	Poor peripheral perfusion
			Pedal edema	Pressure due to fetal position, can also be associated with poor peripheral perfusion, syndromes such as Turner's syndrome
Plantar creases	Cover the sole of foot	Maturity	Few or only anterior third of sole of foot	Prematurity
Buttocks	Creases symmetrical	Normal hips	Creases asymmetrical	Congenital hip dysplasia
Palpation (in the presence of a fracture may produce crying or facial grimacing; observe infant's response)				
Fibula, tibia, trochanter, and femur	Present and equal bilaterally	No fractures; bone formation normal	Absent or unequal bilaterally	Fractures or absence of bone, may be associated with congenital syndromes
Tarsals and metatarsals	Present and equal bilaterally	No fractures; bone formation normal	Absent or unequal bilaterally	Fractures or absence of bone, may be associated with congenital syndromes
Range of motion	Full range of joint motion: includes abduction, adduction, internal and external rotation, flexion and extension as applicable to respective joints of legs, knees, ankles, feet, toes	Normal; maturity	Limited range of joint motion	Birth injury or trauma
			Flexion of legs, knees, ankles, feet, toes is limited	Prematurity
Hips (Ortolani's maneuver: flex newborn's hips and knees, then abduct and adduct hip to detect a slipping of the hip out of the acetabulum or an uneven motion unilaterally; Barlow's maneuver: flex newborn's hips and knees, then place finger on the femur and trochanter, put hip through full range of joint motion and listen for audible click)	Without clicks and full range of joint motion	Normal range of joint motion and no clicks	Limited range of motion or positive result of Ortolani's or Barlow's maneuvers	Congenital hip dysplasia
Knee jerk or patellar reflex	Present, symmetrical	Normal; mature	Absent, weak, or asymmetrical	Neurologic deficit or prematurity
Plantar reflex	Present, symmetrical	Normal; mature	Absent, weak, or asymmetrical	Neurologic deficit or prematurity

TABLE 17–2 Newborn Physical and Gestational Assessment *(Continued)*

System	Normal	Significance	Abnormal	Significance
Back				
Inspection				
Spinal column	Straight	Normal alignment	Curved	Altered alignment that should gradually resolve if resulting from fetal positioning
	No visible deviations or defects	Intact	Visible defects: mass, dimple, or bulge with or without a tuft of hair	Spina bifida
			Open spinal defect or may be covered with tissues, involving the meninges and spinal cord or just spinal cord	Meningomyelocele
			Sinus tracts present	Pilonidal cysts
Palpation				
Vertebrae	Present, without enlargement or pain	Normal spinal column	With bulge, enlarged area, or pain	Mass, bulge, or cyst; fracture of a vertebra; spina bifida; occult meningomyelocele or pilonidal cyst
Anus	See genitourinary tract			
Buttocks	See lower extremities			

AP, anteroposterior; CSF, cerebrospinal fluid; LGA, large for gestational age; SGA, small for gestational age.
Adapted from Kenner, C., Harjo, J., & Brueggemeyer, A. (1988). *Neonatal surgery: A nursing perspective* (pp. 12–42). Orlando, FL: Grune & Stratton.

Interpretation of Results and Intervention

The physical assessment findings are recorded in a clear, complete, concise, and systematic manner. The health team may wish to collaborate on the development of a standardized form for this purpose if one is not already in use. Standardization facilitates both communication among team members and comparison of infants (or comparison of a given infant with normal findings). The examiner should list problems identified and recommendations for follow-up (e.g., request for a chest radiograph or consultation with an orthopedist). Problems requiring immediate attention, such as respiratory distress, are appropriately communicated.

The family is ideally present during the physical examination. If so, the examiner should explain each step simply and reassure the family of normal findings. In the case of suspected or apparent abnormality, great tact is clearly needed. The nurse must be honest but must avoid causing undue anxiety. A calm statement of what will be done next to evaluate the infant's condition may be sufficient, along with positive comments about the infant's vigor or attractive features.

PREDICTIVE VALUE OF NEWBORN ASSESSMENTS

The various elements of newborn assessment are designed not only to identify problems present at birth or at the moment of the assessment but also to anticipate, insofar as possible, those problems likely to develop hours, days, months, or possibly years later. With what confidence can one use neonatal assessments to predict the future development of the child? In the case of some congenital anomalies, the treatment, if any, and probable clinical course are fairly well defined. For example, congenital hip dislocation, if detected by the presence of Ortolani's sign during the early neonatal assessment, is frequently correctable by double-diapering for a time. It is far more difficult to detect or to predict the outcome of many other conditions.

Many attempts have been made to correlate Apgar scores with neurologic outcomes (Schifrin, 1989). Although Apgar scores remain a clinically useful indicator of problems at birth, they apparently have no predictive value for a particular infant.

The prognosis for an SGA infant depends on the timing, duration, and cause of the intrauterine growth retardation, such as infection, congenital anomalies, poor maternal nutrition, or asphyxia (Fanaroff et al., 1994). Particular effort must be made to nourish and nurture the SGA infant during the first year of life, because such infants seldom catch up in weight after that time. It is therefore imperative that the family's socioeconomic situation be assessed and support provided as indicated.

Infants with abnormal neurologic assessments should also be closely observed because the outcomes are variable. It is essential that infants at risk for neurodevelopmental sequelae be identified as early as possible so that programs may begin without delay to enhance the functional potential of these children and provide feedback as to the efficacy of rehabilitation efforts (Majnemer et al., 1994; Oehler et al., 1993). Dubowitz and colleagues (1984) found that infants assessed as neurologically normal at 40 weeks' postmenstrual age have a 91 percent chance of being normal at 1 year, regardless of earlier deficits or insults. Whereas multiple abnormal signs at 40 weeks indicate possible later abnormality, the nature of the signs does not predict the type of deficit observed at 1 year (Dubowitz et al., 1984). Most at risk for cognitive deficits are very small premature infants (less than 1250 g) and those with a complicated neonatal clinical course (Leonard et al., 1990).

In general, it can be said that most high-risk newborns develop normally and that most children with developmental disabilities were not high-risk infants. It cannot be overemphasized that each newborn must be assessed as a unique individual in the context of the family and the environment. The infant's ability to interact with the family and the surrounding environment is an important consideration as well.

CONCLUSION

Neonatal assessment is an essential part of nursing management. It provides the data base from which problems are identified, from which interventions are planned and implemented, and with which later developments of the infant can be compared. It is an ongoing process, beginning at the moment of birth and continuing in all caregiving activities, so that subtle changes may be noted. Frequently, problems may be anticipated and prevented or minimized through early intervention.

Because the nurse is most consistently at the infant's bedside, it is critical that both gestational and physical assessments be recognized as nursing functions and not be restricted to physicians. Optimal care of the neonate demands a team effort to ensure the best possible outcome for the patient.

REFERENCES

Adamkin, D., Klingbeil, R., & Radmacher, P., (1994). Forty years after Dancis: The very-very low birthweight infant grids. *Journal of Perinatology, 14*(3), 187–189.

Alexander, G. R., de Caunes, F., Hulsey, T. C., et al. (1992a). Validity of postnatal assessments of gestational age: A comparison of the method of Ballard et al. and early ultrasonography. *American Journal of Obstetrics and Gynecology, 166*(3), 891–895.

Alexander, G. R., de Caunes, F., Hulsey, T. C., et al. (1992b). Ethnic variation in postnatal assessments of gestational age: A reappraisal. *Paediatric Perinatal Epidemiology 6*(4), 423–433.

Amato, M., Huppi, P., & Claus, R. (1991). Rapid biometric assessment of gestational age in very low birth weight infants. *Journal of Perinatology, 19*(5), 367–371.

American Academy of Pediatrics. (1987). Neonatal anesthesia. *Pediatrics, 80*(3), 446.

American Academy of Pediatrics and American College of Obstetricians and Gynecologists. (1988). *Guidelines for perinatal care* (2nd ed.). Elk Grove Village, IL: Authors.

American Academy of Pediatrics and American College of Obstetricians and Gynecologists. (1992). *Guidelines for perinatal care* (3rd ed.). Elk Grove Village, IL: Authors.

Anand, K. J., & Hickey, P. R. (1987). Pain and its effect in human neonate and fetus. *New England Journal of Medicine, 317*(21), 1321–1329.

Apgar, V. (1953). A proposal for a new method of evaluation of the newborn infant. *Current Researches in Anesthesia and Analgesia, 32*, 260–267.

Avery, G., Fletcher, M., & MacDonald, M. (1994). *Neonatology: Pathophysiology and management of the newborn* (4th ed.). Philadelphia: J. B. Lippincott.

Ballard, J. (1988). *Maturational assessment of gestational age: Ballard score.* Cincinnati, OH: University of Cincinnati.

Ballard, J. L., Khoury, J. C., Wedig, K., et al. (1991). New Ballard Score, expanded to include extremely premature infants. *Journal of Pediatrics, 119*(3), 417–423.

Ballard, J. L., Novak, K. K., & Driver, M. (1979). A simplified score for assessment of fetal maturation of newly born infants. *Journal of Pediatrics, 95*(5, Part 1), 769–774.

Battaglia, F. C., & Lubchenco, L. O. (1967). A practical classification of newborn infants by weight and gestational age. *Journal of Pediatrics, 71*(2), 159–163.

Betz, C., Hunsberger, M., & Wright, S. (1994). *Family-centered nursing care of children* (2nd ed.). Philadelphia: W. B. Saunders.

Blackburn, S., & Kang, R. (1995). *Early parent-infant relationships. The first six hours of life series, module 3* (2nd ed.). White Plains, NY: National Foundation/March of Dimes.

Blackburn, S., & Loper, D. (1992). *Maternal, fetal, and neonatal physiology: A clinical perspective.* Philadelphia: W. B. Saunders.

Bliss-Holtz, J. (1989). Comparison of rectal, axillary, and inguinal temperatures in full-term newborn infants. *Nursing Research, 38*(2), 85–87.

Brazelton, T. (1984). *Neonatal behavioral assessment scale in planning care for parents and newborns* (2nd ed.). St. Louis: J. B. Lippincott/Spastics International Medical Publishers.

Brazelton, T. (1994). Behavioral competence. In G. Avery, M. Fletcher, & M. MacDonald (Eds.), *Neonatology: Pathophysiology and management of the newborn* (4th ed., pp. 289–300). Philadelphia: J. B. Lippincott.

Bruno, J. (1995). Systematic neonatal assessment and intervention. *MCN; American Journal of Maternal Child Nursing, 20*(1), 21–24.

Bryant, B. G. (1984). Unit dose erythromycin ophthalmic ointment for neonatal ocular prophylaxis. *Journal of Obstetric, Gynecologic, and Neonatal Nursing, 13*(2), 83–87.

Callister, L. (1995). Cultural meanings of childbirth. *Journal of Obstetric, Gynecologic, and Neonatal Nursing, 24*(4), 327–331.

Cantu, D., Vaello, L., & Kenner, C. (1991). Neonatal assessment. In S. M. Cohen, C. A. Kenner, & A. O. Hollingsworth (Eds.), *Maternal, neonatal, and women's health nursing* (pp. 832–870). Philadelphia: Springhouse.

Cavlovich, F. (1995). Subgaleal hemorrhage in the neonate. *Journal of Obstetric, Gynecologic, and Neonatal Nursing, 24*(5), 397–404.

Dancis, J., O'Connell, J., & Holte, L. (1948). A grid for recording the weight of premature infants. *Journal of Pediatrics, 33*, 570–572.

D'Apolito, K. (1991). What is an organized infant? *Neonatal Network, 10*(1), 23–29.

Davenport, S. (1992). Frequency of handwashing by registered nurses caring for infants on radiant warmers and in incubators. *Neonatal Network, 11*(1), 21–25.

Dubowitz, L. M., Dubowitz, V., & Goldberg, C. (1970). Clinical assessment of gestational age in the newborn infant. *Journal of Pediatrics, 77*(1), 1–10.

Dubowitz, V., Dubowitz, L., & Goldberg, C. (1977). *Gestational age of the newborn: A clinical manual.* London: Addison-Wesley.

Dubowitz, L. M., Dubowitz, V., Palmer, P. C., et al. (1984). Correlation of neurologic assessment in the preterm newborn infant with outcome at 1 year. *Journal of Pediatrics, 105*(3), 452–456.

Elizondo, A. (1995). Nursing case management in the neonatal intensive care unit, part 2: Developing critical pathways. *Neonatal Network, 14*(1), 11–19.

Elliott, M., & Cassano, W. (1991). Alternative method of gestational age assessment by the measurement of human erythrocyte differentiation antigen expression. *Journal of Perinatology, 11*(3), 268–272.

Fanaroff, A., Martin, R., & Miller, M. (1994). Identification and management of high risk problems in the neonate. In R. Creasy & R. Resnick (Eds.), *Maternal-fetal medicine: Principles and practice* (3rd ed., pp. 1135–1172.) Philadelphia: W. B. Saunders.

Gardner, S. (1994). Pain and pain relief in the neonate. *MCN: American Journal of Maternal Child Nursing, 19*(2), 85–90.

Graven, S. (1996). *The physical and developmental environment of the high risk neonate.* Presentation at the Sheraton Sand Key, Clearwater Beach, FL, January 30, 1996.

Gunderson, L. (1995). Embryology and development of the infant born at 24–25 weeks of gestation. In L. P. Gunderson & C. Kenner (Eds.), *Care of the 24–25 week gestational age infant (small baby protocol* (2nd ed., pp. 1–26). Petaluma, CA: NICU Ink.

Gunderson, L., & Kenner, C. (Eds.). (1995). *Care of the 24–25 week gestational age infant (small baby protocol)* (2nd ed.). Petaluma, CA: NICU Ink.

Hegyi, T., Carbone, M. T., Anwar, M., et al. (1994). Blood pressure ranges in premature infants. I. The first hours of life. *Journal of Pediatrics, 124*(4), 627–633.

Huang C., & Yeh, T. (1991). Assessment of gestational age in newborns by neurosonography. *Early Human Development, 25*(3), 209–220.

Kelly, J. (1994). General care. In G. Avery, M. Fletcher, & M. MacDonald (1994). *Neonatology: Pathophysiology and management of the newborn* (4th ed., pp. 301–304). Philadelphia: J. B. Lippincott.

Kenner, C. (1990). Measuring neonatal assessment. *Neonatal Network, 9*(4), 17–22.

Kenner, C., Harjo, J., & Brueggemeyer, A. (1988). *Neonatal surgery: A nursing perspective.* Orlando, FL: Grune & Stratton.

Kiernan, B. S., & Scoloveno, M. A. (1986). Assessment of the neonate. *Clinical Nursing, 8*(1), 1–10.

Klein, J., & Remmington, J. (1995). Current concepts of infections of the fetus and newborn infant. In J. Remmington & J. Klein (Eds.), *Infectious diseases of the fetus and newborn infant* (pp. 1–19). Philadelphia: W. B. Saunders.

Korones, S. B. (1981). *High-risk newborn infants: The basis for intensive care* (3rd ed.). St. Louis: C. V. Mosby.

Koszarek, K. (1992). It's common sense. *Neonatal Network, 11*(6), 7–9.

Kuller, J. (1995). Skin care management of the low birth weight infant. In L. Gunderson & C. Kenner (Eds.), *Care of the 24–25 week gestational infant (small baby protocol)* (2nd ed., pp. 107–144). Petaluma, CA: NICU Ink.

Larson, E. (1987). Rituals in infection control: What works in the newborn nursery? Handwashing and gowning. *Journal of Obstetric, Gynecologic, and Neonatal Nursing, 16*(6), 411–416.

Leonard, C. H., Clyman, R. I., Piecuch, R. E., et al. (1990). Effect of medical and social risk factors on outcome of prematurity and very low birth weight. *Journal of Pediatrics, 116*(4), 620–626.

Leppink, M. A. (1986). Assessment of the newborn. In N. Streeter (Ed.), *High-risk neonatal care* (pp. 57–60). Rockville, MD: Aspen.

Lott, J., & Kenner, C. (1994a). Keeping up with neonatal infections: Designer bugs, part 1. *MCN; American Journal of Maternal Child Nursing, 19*(4), 207–213.

Lott, J., & Kenner, C. (1994b). Keeping up with neonatal infections: Designer bugs, part 2. *MCN; American Journal of Maternal Child Nursing, 19*(5), 264–271.

Lubchenco, L. O. (1970). Assessment of gestational age and development at birth. *Pediatric Clinics of North America, 17*(1), 125–145.

Lugo, E. J., & Tominey, T. M. (1989). The adverse effects of utilizing altitude-inappropriate fetal growth curves. *Journal of Perinatology,* 9(2), 147–149.

Lynam, L. (1994). Case management and critical pathways: Friend or foe? *Neonatal Network, 13*(8), 48–51.

Majnemer, A., Rosenblatt, B., & Riley, P. (1994). Predicting outcome in high-risk newborns with a neonatal neurobehavioral assessment. *American Journal of Occupational Therapy, 48*(8), 723–732.

McGregor, L. (1994). Short, shorter, shortest: Improving the hospital stay for mothers and newborns. *MCN; American Journal of Maternal Child Nursing, 19*(2), 91–96.

Merenstein, G., & Gardner, S. (1993). *Handbook of neonatal intensive care* (3rd ed.). St. Louis: C. V. Mosby.

Metcoff, J. (1994). Clinical assessment of nutritional status at birth: Fetal malnutrition and SGA are not synonymous. *Pediatric Clinics of North America, 41*(5), 875–891.

Neonatal Resuscitation Program. (1994). *Textbook of neonatal resuscitation.* Dallas, TX: American Heart Association and American Academy of Pediatrics.

Occupational Safety and Health Administration. (1991). *Occupational exposure to bloodborne pathogens; final rule 29 CRF part 1910, 1030.* Washington, DC: Department of Labor.

Oehler, J., Goldstein, R., Catlett, A., et al. (1993). How to target infants at highest risk for developmental delay. *MCN; American Journal of Maternal Child Nursing, 18*(1), 20–23.

Petrucha, R. (1989). Fetal maturity/gestational age evaluation. *Journal of Perinatology, 9*(1), 100–101.

Pillitteri, A. (1995). *Maternal and child health nursing: Care of the childbearing and childrearing family* (2nd ed.). Philadelphia: J. B. Lippincott.

Prudhoe, C., & Peters, D. (1995). Social support of parents and grandparents in the neonatal intensive care unit. *Pediatric Nursing, 21*(2), 140–146.

Rogers, A., Batterson, J., & Shurak, E. (1993). User friendly forms for mother-baby nursing. *MCN; American Journal of Maternal Child Nursing, 19*(2), 297–301.

Schifrin, B. S. (1989). Polemics in perinatology: The Apgar score—What shall we call it? *Journal of Perinatology, 9*(3), 331–332.

Sherer, D., Abramowicz, J., Plessinger, M., & Woods, J.(1993). Fetal sacral length in the ultrasonographic assessment of gestational age. *American Journal of Obstetrics and Gynecology, 168*(2), 626–633.

Simon, N. (1991). Evaluation and management of stridor in the newborn. *Clinical Pediatrics, 30*(4), 211–216.

Smith, R., & Bottoms, S. (1993). Ultrasonographic prediction of neonatal survival in extremely low birth weight infants. *American Journal of Obstetrics and Gynecology, 169*(3), 490–493.

Symanski, M., Newman, C., & Bachynski, B. (1994). Treating congenital cataracts. *MCN; American Journal of Maternal Child Nursing, 19*(6), 335–338.

Tappero, E., & Honeyfield, M. (1996). *Physical assessment of the newborn: A comprehensive approach to the art of physical examination* (2nd ed.). Petaluma, CA: NICU Ink.

Taylor, K. M. (1982). Gestational age assessment. In S. Humenick (Ed.), *Analysis of current assessment strategies in the health care of young children and childbearing families* (pp. 129–145). Norwalk, CT: Appleton-Century-Crofts.

Tribotti, S. (1990). Admission to the neonatal intensive care unit: Reducing the risks. *Neonatal Network, 8*(4), 17–22.

Vandenberg, M. (1995). Behaviorally supportive care for the extremely premature infant. In L. P. Gunderson & C. Kenner (Eds.), *Care of the 24–25 week gestational age infant (small baby protocol)* (2nd ed., pp. 145–170). Petaluma, CA: NICU Ink.

Volpe, J. (1995). *Neurology of the newborn* (3rd ed.). Philadelphia: W. B. Saunders.

Weiss, M., Poeltler, D., & Gocka, I. (1993). Infrared tympanic thermometry for neonatal temperature assessment. *Journal of Obstetric, Gynecologic, and Neonatal Nursing,* 23(9), 798–804.

Wong, D. (1995). *Whaley & Wong's nursing care of infants and children* (5th ed.). St. Louis: C. V. Mosby.

Wyatt, T. (1995). Pneumothorax in the neonate. *Journal of Obstetric, Gynecologic, and Neonatal Nursing, 24*(3), 211–216.

CHAPTER 18

Assessment and Management of Respiratory Dysfunction

JAVIER CIFUENTES JAMES L. HAYWOOD MADELINE ROSS
WALDEMAR A. CARLO

RESEARCH AGENDA

What should the temperature of humidified air be for a premature infant?

How often should a neonate with respiratory distress syndrome (RDS) undergo suctioning?

Should solution be used with endotracheal suctioning?

Does chest physiotherapy or vibration have any beneficial effects in the early stages of RDS?

How should an endotracheal tube be secured to prevent accidental extubation?

VIGNETTE

I first met Denise S. during a nursing consultation on our antepartum unit when she was 26 weeks pregnant and experiencing signs of premature labor. Denise had previously lost a baby at 20 weeks. She had been diagnosed as having an incompetent cervix, and a cerclage procedure had been performed in an attempt to prolong the pregnancy.

Denise had many questions about the potential outcome of a premature baby. I provided her with information on, and pictures of, premature infants. I showed her NICU scenes. I discussed the major difficulties experienced by premature babies, such as immaturity of respiratory and other organ systems and the accompanying problems. We discussed IV therapy, nutrition, and breastfeeding. "Premature babies face many problems in the extrauterine environment; however, we have improved our knowledge about the needs of premature neonates, and there are many new treatments available to help the babies overcome the problems of prematurity," I told her. "We have specially trained physicians, nurses, respiratory therapists, nutritionists, pharmacologists, and many other health care workers available to provide the best possible care for your baby." I told Denise to call me if she had further questions, and I promised to keep in touch.

Three weeks later, Denise began premature labor that did not respond to tocolysis. Labor was progressing so rapidly that only one dose of betamethasone could be administered before delivery. Abby was born at 2:00 A.M., weighing 1000 g. Both I and the neonatologist attended the delivery. Bag and mask ventilation was immediately required for Abby's poor color and inadequate respiratory effort. Abby responded to the positive pressure ventilation rapidly with improved color, tone, heart rate, and activity. She was transported to the NICU in an incubator with free-flow O_2.

Upon admission to the NICU, Abby was initially placed in a head hood with 50 percent O_2. She was pink, with expiratory grunting, nasal flaring, and intercostal and substernal retractions. Bilateral breath sounds were equal with crackles present. Her respiratory rate was 88 per minute. Initial laboratory data revealed a glucose of 43, hematocrit of 45%, and a normal CBC. The chest x-ray was consistent with RDS. Arterial blood gas was as follows: pH, 7.18; $Pa{O_2}$, 40 mm Hg; $Pa{CO_2}$, 55 mm Hg; HCO_3^-, 18 mEq/L; B.E., −4 mEq/L. Because of the immaturity of the infant, the respiratory acidosis, and the degree of respiratory distress present, Abby was intubated, begun on mechanical ventilation, and given exogenous surfactant therapy.

Primary goals for Abby's care were the following:

1. To maintain adequate oxygenation and ventilation
2. To maintain a neutral thermal environment
3. To provide fluids and nutrition sufficient to meet metabolic requirement and growth needs
4. To maintain intact skin without breakdown
5. To provide an environment free of noxious stimulation
6. To foster positive parent–infant interaction

The respiratory distress continued to progress, requiring high ventilator support for several days. After the first week, however, the ventilatory requirement decreased, and by day 14 of life, Abby was extubated and placed in an Oxy-Hood. Episodes of apnea developed but were successfully treated with aminophylline.

Like most other preterm infants, Abby experienced many small successes and setbacks during her hospitalization, including nutritional management problems, sepsis, and a grade I intraventricular hemorrhage. She overcame these difficulties, however, and was discharged home after a 9-week NICU stay. Abby's parents had difficulty in handling the anxiety and fear that having a premature infant involved. However, through the combined efforts of the hospital staff, family, and friends, these parents were able to cope with the challenges and maintain their involvement with their infant. At discharge, the parents were prepared to take their baby home.

Marianne McGraw

Respiratory illness, especially pulmonary immaturity, is the most common cause for admission to the neonatal intensive care unit

(NICU). Perhaps nothing is more frightening to the parents, separated from their infant by barriers of wires, plastic tubing, and thermal wrap, than the realization that their baby is not breathing well. At delivery (if modern technology has not answered this question prenatally), there is the time-honored, invariable question, "Is it a boy or a girl?" The next question is, "Is she breathing; is she pink?" Or perhaps, "Why is my baby blue?" The care of the infant with cyanosis and respiratory distress so visibly apparent to the apprehensive parent represents a unique challenge to the neonatal nurse.

To develop a systematic and intellectually reliable method of assessing infants with respiratory distress, the mechanisms that bring about normal pulmonary function must be understood. Well founded on the physiologic basis for newborn respiratory illness, the nurse, as part of the collaborative team, can then direct care through diagnostic evaluation and carry that forward to treatment, culminating in the best possible outcome.

EMBRYOLOGIC DEVELOPMENT OF THE LUNG

During gestation, gas exchange is carried out by the placenta. Throughout this period, pulmonary development of the embryo proceeds along a predetermined sequence. It begins with formation of an outpouching of the embryonic foregut during the fourth week of gestation and continues on to form sufficient alveoli to maintain gas exchange in most infants by 32 to 36 weeks of estimated gestational age. Additional alveoli continue to develop in the newborn infant and well into childhood, perhaps as late as the seventh year of life (Thibeault & Gregory, 1986) (Table 18–1).

The *embryonic phase* of lung development is marked by sequential branching of the lung bud, which appears at about 4 weeks and is complete by the sixth week. The following 10 weeks are marked by the formation of conducting airways by branching of the aforementioned lung buds. This phase, the *pseudoglandular phase*, continues through week 16 and ends with completion of the conducting airways. The *canalicular phase* follows through week 28, when gas exchange units, known as acini, develop. Type II alveolar cells, the surfactant-producing cells, begin to form during the latter part of this phase. Mature, vascularized gas-exchange sites form during the *saccular phase*, which spans the 29th through 35th weeks. During this phase, the interstitial space between alveoli thins, so respiratory epithelial cells tightly contact developing capillaries. The *alveolar development phase*, marked by expansion of gas-exchange surface area, begins at 36 weeks and extends into the postnatal period. The alveolar wall and interstitial spaces become very thin, and the single capillary network comes into close proximity to the alveolar membrane.

There are no firm boundaries separating these phases, and gas exchange, albeit inefficient, is possible relatively early in gestation, even before mature, vascularized gas-exchange sites form. Lung development is a continuum marked by rapid structural change.

TABLE 18–1 Stages of Normal Lung Growth

Phase	Timing	Major Event
Embryonic	Weeks 4–6	Formation of proximal airway
Pseudoglandular	Weeks 7–16	Formation of conducting airways
Canalicular	Weeks 17–28	Formation of acini
Saccular	Weeks 29–35	Development of gas exchange sites
Alveolar	Weeks 36 through postnatal life	Expansion of surface area

Interference at any time by premature birth or by disease introduces the possibility of inducing iatrogenic disease through intervention.

NEWBORN PULMONARY PHYSIOLOGY AND THE ONSET OF BREATHING

The fetal lung is fluid filled, underperfused, and dormant with regard to gas exchange. It receives only approximately 10 percent of the cardiac output. Because the placenta is the gas-exchange organ in fetal life, a high blood flow is directed toward it rather than to the lungs (Fig. 18–1). Consequently, most of the right ventricular output is shunted from the pulmonary artery across the ductus arteriosus into the aorta, bypassing the pulmonary circulation.

Within moments after the umbilical cord is clamped, the newborn undergoes an amazing transformation from a fetus floating in amniotic fluid to an air-breathing neonate. When the normal onset of breathing occurs, the ensuing chain of events converts the fetal circulation to the circulation pattern of an adult. The lung fluid is absorbed and replaced with air, thus establishing lung volume and allowing for normal neonatal pulmonary function (Nelson, 1994; Ross Laboratories, 1978). The process of fetal lung fluid absorption begins before birth, when the rate of alveolar fluid secretion declines. Reabsorption speeds up during labor. Animal data suggest that as much as two thirds of the total clearance of lung fluid occurs during labor (Bland et al., 1982). This clearance probably results from the cessation of active chloride secretion into the alveolar space. Oncotic pressure favors the movement of water from the air space back into the interstitium and into the vascular space. With the onset of breathing and lung expansion, water moves rapidly from the air spaces into the interstitium and is removed from the lung by lymphatic and pulmonary blood vessels (Bland, 1988). Because a large portion of the clearance of lung fluid occurs during labor, neonates born without labor after cesarean section are at particularly high risk for delayed absorption of fetal lung fluid and thus for transient tachypnea of the newborn.

With the onset of breathing, highly negative intrathoracic pressures are generated with inspiratory efforts, filling the alveoli with air. Replacing alveolar fluid with air causes a precipitous decrease in hydrostatic pressure in the lung; therefore, pulmonary artery pressure decreases, lowering pressure in the right atrium and causing an increase in pulmonary blood flow. These changes result in an increase in alveolar oxygen tension (PaO_2), causing constriction of the ductus arteriosus, which normally shunts right ventricular blood away from the lungs. By clamping of the cord, the large, low-resistance, placental surface area is removed from the circulation. This change in resistance causes an abrupt increase in systemic arterial pressure, reflected all the way back to the left atrium. As left atrial pressure rises, the opening between the atria, known as the foramen ovale, is closed by its flap valve. This closure prevents blood from bypassing the lungs by eliminating the shunt across the foramen ovale from the right atrium to the left atrium. As a result of closure of fetal pathways and decreased pulmonary artery pressure, systemic pressure is greater than pulmonary artery pressure. The infant successfully converts from the pattern of fetal circulation to neonatal circulation when blood coming from the right ventricle flows in its new path of least resistance (lower pressure) to the lungs, instead of shunting across the foramen ovale to the left atrium or across the ductus arteriosus from the pulmonary artery to the aorta.

An understanding of ventilation enables the clinician to assess the infant in respiratory distress and devise strategies for management. The respiratory system is composed of (1) the pumping system (the chest wall muscles, diaphragm, and accessory muscles of respiration), which moves free gas into the lungs; (2) the bony

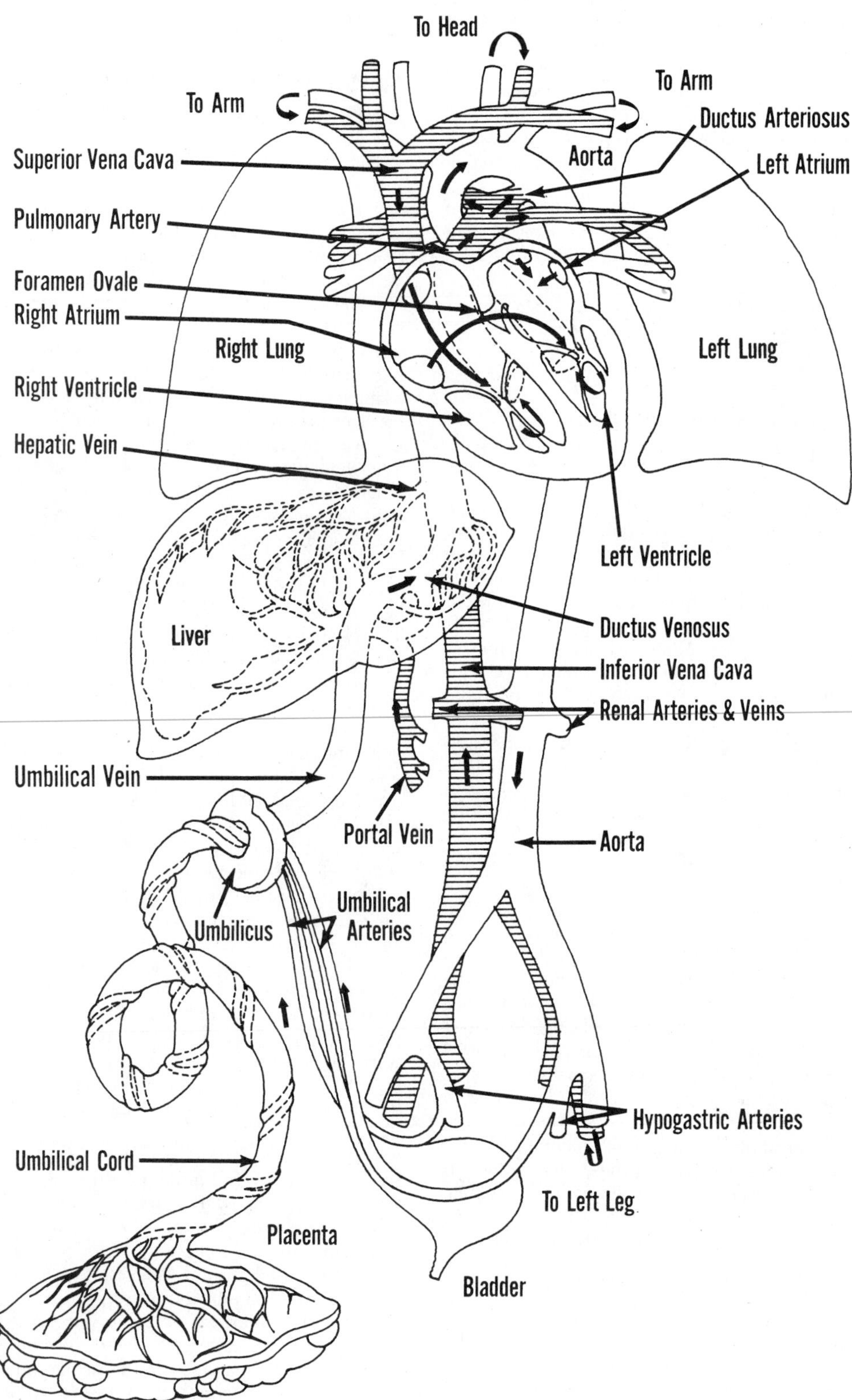

FIGURE 18–1. Fetal circulation. (Reprinted with permission of Ross Laboratories, Columbus, OH 43216, from Clinical Education Aid, Copyright 1985, Ross Laboratories.)

rib cage, which provides structural support for the respiratory muscles and limits lung deflation; (3) the conducting airways, which connect gas-exchanging units with the outside but offer resistance to gas flow; (4) an elastic element, which offers some resistance to gas flow but provides pumping force for moving stale air out of the system; (5) air–liquid interfaces, which generate surface tension that opposes lung expansion on inspiration but supports lung deflation on expiration; and (6) the abdominal muscles, which aid exhalation by active contraction (Harris, 1988).

The respiratory system of the newborn is limited, making it susceptible to respiratory difficulty. The circular, poorly ossified rib cage, with a flat instead of angular insertion of the diaphragm, is less efficient at generating negative intrathoracic pressure to move air into the system. The strength and endurance of respiratory muscles are hindered by small muscles and a relative paucity of type I muscle fibers. The newborn has a relatively low functional residual capacity (lung volume at the end of exhalation) because its comparatively floppy chest wall offers little resistance to collapse, even when there is a normal amount of functional surfactant present.

Surface tension is dependent upon alveolar diameter. According to Laplace's law, increasingly higher pressures are required to inflate the alveolus as its diameter decreases. The inflating pressure is also related to the surface tension, as shown in the following equation:

$$P = 2\frac{ST}{r}$$

where *P* is pressure, *ST* is surface tension, and *r* is radius of the alveolus. It is difficult to inflate a small or collapsed alveolus because it has a very small diameter. As its volume increases, the pressure needed to continue inflation becomes progressively less; that is, compliance of the alveolus, and thus compliance of the lung, has improved. Coating the alveoli with an agent that decreases surface tension reduces the effort required to inflate the lungs from a low volume. Pulmonary surfactant is a surface tension–reducing mixture of phospholipids and proteins found in mature alveoli. Surfactant is produced by an alveolar cell known as the type II pneumocyte. Surfactant coats alveoli, preventing alveolar collapse and loss of lung volume during expiration; that is, as expiration ensues and elasticity of the lung deflates it, the alveolar diameter becomes smaller. Surfactant coating the alveolus reduces surface tension so that collapse is prevented and less pressure is required to reinflate it with the next inspiration. Neonates with respiratory distress syndrome (RDS) have surfactant deficiency. In the absence of surfactant, surface tension is high, and the tendency is toward collapse of alveoli at end expiration.

Compliance is the elasticity, or distensibility, of the lung. It is expressed as the change in volume caused by a change in pressure as follows:

$$C_L = \frac{\Delta V}{\Delta P}$$

where C_L is compliance of the lung, *V* is volume, and *P* is pressure. The higher the compliance, the larger the volume delivered to the alveoli per unit of applied inspiratory pressure.

Surface tension and compliance are particularly important in the preterm infant with RDS. Surface tension is a force that opposes lung expansion. Surfactant deficiency leads to increased surface tension in the alveoli. Lungs with higher surface tension are more difficult to inflate. During expiration, some alveoli collapse, so lung volume at the end of expiration is decreased (low functional residual capacity). Clinically, the effects of this increased surface tension are manifested by the presence of retractions. Respiratory muscles contract to inflate the lungs against surface tension that acts in the opposite direction. The floppy thoracic wall of the preterm infant is easily deformed by the negative pleural pressure. When a preterm infant with RDS is intubated, a high peak inspiratory pressure (PIP) is required to expand the thorax (i.e., tidal volume is obtained only with a high change in pressure). After surfactant is administered, the chest rise increases without changes in PIP. This PIP stability is due to a decrease in surface tension (i.e., a smaller force opposing lung distention). Thus tidal volume obtained with the same PIP is increased. Before surfactant is administered, it is very difficult to inflate the lung because compliance is low. After surfactant is administered, surface tension decreases, and it becomes easier to inflate the lung (i.e., compliance is improved).

Resistance is a term used to describe characteristics of gas flow through the airways and pulmonary tissues. Resistance can be thought of as the capacity of the lung to resist air flow. The principal component of resistance is determined by the small airway. Pressure is required to force gas through the airways (airway resistance) and to overcome the elasticity of the lung and chest wall, which work to deflate the respiratory system (tissue resistance). At a specific flow rate, resistance is described by the following equation:

$$R = \frac{P_1 - P_2}{\dot{V}}$$

where P_1 and P_2 are pressures at opposite ends of the airway and $\dot{V}$ *is the flow rate of gas (volume per unit of time)*. Resistance increases as airway diameter decreases. Because the infant has airways of relatively small radius, the resistance to gas flow through those airways is high.

The *time constant* is the time necessary for airway pressure to equilibrate throughout the respiratory system and equals the mathematic product of compliance and resistance. In other words, the time constant is a measure of how quickly the lungs can inhale or exhale. The time constant (*Kt*) is directly related to both compliance (*C*) and resistance (*R*). This relationship is described by the equation $Kt = C \times R$. An infant with RDS has decreased compliance, so the time constant of the respiratory system is relatively short. In such an infant, little time is required for pressure to equilibrate between the proximal airway and alveoli, so short inspiratory and expiratory times may be appropriate during mechanical ventilation. When compliance improves (increases), however, the time constant becomes longer. If sufficient time is not allowed for expiration, alveoli may become overdistended and an air leak may result (Carlo et al., 1994).

Blood Gas Analysis and Acid–Base Balance

Oxygen diffuses across the alveolar-capillary membrane, moved by the difference in oxygen pressure between the alveolus and the blood. In the blood, oxygen dissolves in the plasma and binds to hemoglobin. Thus arterial oxygen content (Cao_2) is the sum of dissolved and hemoglobin-bound oxygen, as shown by the following equation:

$$Cao_2 = (1.37 \times Hb \times Sao_2) + (0.003 \times Pao_2)$$

where Cao_2 = arterial oxygen content (ml/100 m of blood); 1.37 = milliliters of oxygen bound to 1 g of hemoglobin at 100 percent saturation; Hb = hemoglobin concentration (g/100 ml); Sao_2 = percentage of hemoglobin bound to oxygen (%); 0.003 = solubility factor of oxygen in plasma (ml/mm Hg); and Pao_2 = oxygen partial pressure in arterial blood (mm Hg).

In the equation for arterial oxygen content, the first term—($1.37 \times Hb \times Sao_2$)—is the amount of oxygen bound to hemoglobin. The second term—($0.003 \times Pao_2$)—is the amount of oxygen dissolved in plasma. Most of the oxygen in the blood is carried by hemoglobin. For example, if a premature infant has a PaO_2 of 60 mm Hg, an SaO_2 of 92 percent, and a hemoglobin concentration of 14 g/100 ml, then CaO_2 is the sum of oxygen bound to hemoglobin ($1.37 \times 14 \times 92/100$) = 17.6 ml, plus the oxygen dissolved in plasma (0.003×60) = 0.1 ml. In this example, only 1 percent of oxygen in blood is dissolved in plasma; 99 percent is carried by hemoglobin. If the infant has an intraventricular hemorrhage and the hemoglobin concentration decreases to 10.5 g/dl but PaO_2 and SaO_2 remain the same, then CaO_2 ($1.37 \times 10.5 \times 92/100$) + ($0.003 \times 600$) equals 13.4 ml/100 ml of blood. Thus, without any change in PaO_2 or SaO_2, a 25 percent decrease in hemoglobin concentration (from 14 to 10.5 g/dl) reduces the amount of oxygen in arterial blood by 24 percent (from 17.6 to 13.4 ml/100 ml of blood). This is an important concept for persons caring for patients with respiratory disease. PaO_2, SaO_2, and hemoglobin should be monitored and, if low, corrected to keep an adequate level of tissue oxygenation.

The force that loads hemoglobin with oxygen in the lungs and unloads it in the tissues is the difference in partial pressure of oxygen. In the lungs, alveolar oxygen partial pressure is higher than capillary oxygen partial pressure, so that oxygen moves to the capillaries and binds to the hemoglobin. Tissue partial pressure of oxygen is lower than that of the blood, so oxygen moves from hemoglobin to the tissues. The relationship between partial pressure of oxygen and hemoglobin is better understood with the oxyhemoglobin dissociation curve (Fig. 18–2). Several factors can affect the affinity of hemoglobin for oxygen. Alkalosis, hypothermia, hypocapnia, and decreased levels of 2,3-diphosphoglycerate (2,3-DPG) increase the affinity of hemoglobin for oxygen (as shown in Fig. 18–2 by a left shift of the curve). Acidosis, hyperthermia, hypercapnia, and increased 2,3-DPG have the opposite effect, decreasing the affinity of hemoglobin for oxygen, so that the hemoglobin dissociation curve shifts to the right. This characteristic of hemoglobin facilitates oxygen loading in the lung and unloading in the tissue where the pH is lower and alveolar carbon dioxide tension ($PaCO_2$) is higher. Fetal hemoglobin, which has a higher affinity for oxygen than adult hemoglobin, is more fully oxygen saturated at lower PaO_2 values. This is represented by a left shift on the curve of dissociation of hemoglobin.

Once loaded with oxygen, the blood should reach the tissues to transfer oxygen to the cells. Oxygen delivery to the tissue depends on cardiac output (CO) and CaO_2, as described in the following equation:

$$\text{Oxygen delivery} = CO \times CaO_2$$

In the case of the infant discussed previously, the decrease in CaO_2 resulting from anemia is compensated for by increased CO. The key concept is that when a patient's oxygenation is assessed, more information than just PaO_2 and SaO_2 should be considered. PaO_2 and SaO_2 may be normal but, if hemoglobin concentration is low or CO is decreased, oxygen delivery to the tissues is decreased. With this approach, the clinician should be able to better plan the interventions needed to improve oxygenation.

As in the adult, the acid–base balance in the neonate is maintained within narrow limits by complex interactions between the pulmonary system, which eliminates carbon dioxide, and the kidneys, which conserve carbon dioxide and eliminate metabolic acids. Carbon dioxide elimination, which is more efficient than oxygenation across the alveolar capillary membrane, is usually not as problematic as oxygenation. Carbon dioxide has a high solubility coefficient, so cellular diffusion is very efficient and no measurable partial pressure gradient exists between venous blood and the tissues. Therefore, elevated carbon dioxide tension (PCO_2) values in arterial blood samples nearly always indicate ventilatory dysfunction. Dissolved carbon dioxide moves rapidly across cell membranes of peripheral chemoreceptors, thus making them sensitive to changes in ventilation. Increased intracellular PCO_2 elevates the cellular hydrogen ion concentration as carbon dioxide combines with water to form carbonic acid. This stimulates neural impulses to the medulla, stimulating respiration. However, excessively high PCO_2 levels can depress ventilation.

Acid–base balance is controlled by homeostatic mechanisms and is expressed as follows as pH (the negative logarithm of the hydrogen ion concentration):

$$pH = 6.1 + \log \frac{HCO_3^-}{0.03 \times PCO_2}$$

It can be seen from this mathematical relationship that acid–base balance depends on the interplay of bicarbonate ion (HCO_3^-) and carbon dioxide. Serum pH is tightly regulated in the normal range. Low pH (acidosis) can contribute to vasoconstriction, resulting in worsening hypoxemia caused by extrapulmonary shunt across the ductus or foramen ovale. A pH of less than 7.0 is not well tolerated and is associated with a poor survival rate.

If $PaCO_2$ rises above normal, as in hypoventilation, pH declines and the patient suffers from respiratory acidosis. The patient with a chronic respiratory acidosis may retain bicarbonate, self-inducing a compensatory metabolic alkalosis. A patient who is hyperventilated with a low $PaCO_2$ has respiratory alkalosis. Depressed bicarbonate ion concentration (less than approximately 20 mmol/L in plasma) is called *metabolic acidosis* and can be associated with any cause of anaerobic metabolism, such as poor CO from congenital heart disease, such as hypoplastic left heart syndrome or severe aortic coarctation, or from myocardial ischemia, myocardiopathy, myocarditis, or septic shock. Metabolic acidosis resulting from renal bicarbonate wasting may develop in extremely immature infants. Less common causes for prolonged and severe metabolic acidosis are the inborn errors of metabolisms, including urea cycle defects and amino acidopathies.

The clinician should become proficient at interpreting blood gas data. With a knowledge of the accepted normal values and definitions of the simple blood gas disorders and their compensatory mechanisms, the clinician can examine data in light of the disease process and interpret blood gas values in a fairly straightforward manner. Normally, the body does not overcompensate for a pH above or below the normal range. Therefore, when presented with an abnormal pH, the clinician rapidly determines whether acidosis (Fig. 18–3*A*) or alkalosis exists (see Fig. 18–3*B*).

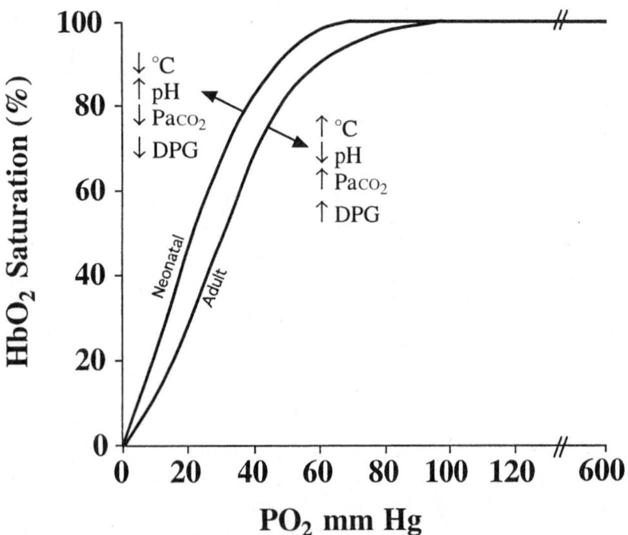

FIGURE 18–2. Oxyhemoglobin equilibrium curves of blood from term infants at birth and from adults (at pH 7.40).

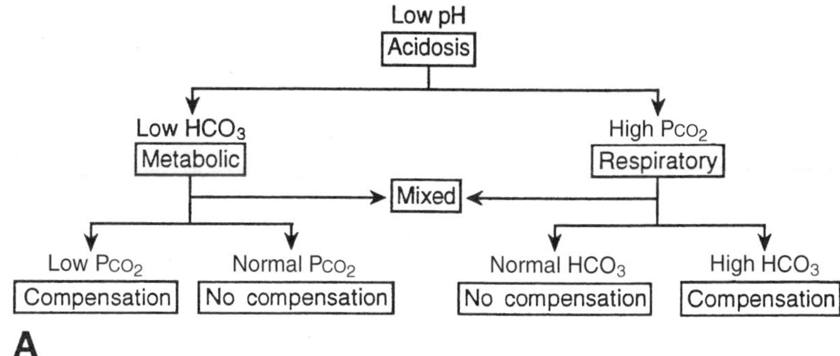

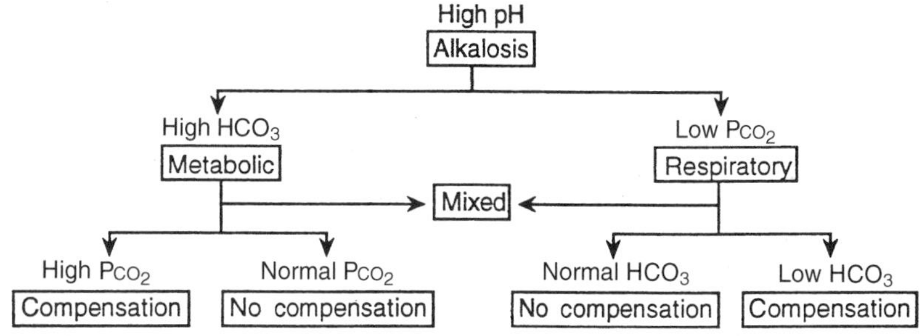

FIGURE 18–3. Acid–base balance: diagnostic approach.

An examination of $Paco_2$ and HCO_3^- determines whether the process is respiratory, metabolic, or mixed. The clinician should determine which derangement occurred first. For example, an acidotic, acutely ill hypoxemic infant with a high $Paco_2$ and depressed HCO_3^- is usually hypoventilating and suffering metabolic acidosis secondary to anaerobic metabolism. The infant with a low $Paco_2$ is hyperventilating, either spontaneously or secondary to overzealous mechanical ventilation. A concomitantly low pH and low HCO_3^- indicate that the infant is compensating for metabolic acidosis with hyperventilation in an effort to normalize the pH. A pure metabolic alkalosis with high pH is nearly always caused by bicarbonate administration. The infant with chronic lung disease has a compensated respiratory acidosis, with an elevated $Paco_2$ and concomitantly elevated HCO_3^-. The pH may be in the normal range or slightly acidotic. A severely depressed pH indicates acute decompensation.

ASSESSMENT OF THE NEONATE WITH RESPIRATORY DISTRESS

The assessment of a neonate with respiratory distress should always begin with the compilation of a detailed perinatal history. In many cases, the history is difficult to obtain, especially when the infant has been transferred from one center to another, often with inadequate records. Even so, every effort should be made to obtain as much information as possible. The nurse is often able to gain important supplemental information from the father or visiting relatives at the bedside. A review of the maternal-perinatal history and a complete physical examination, combined with a limited laboratory and radiologic evaluation, lead to a timely diagnosis in most circumstances. Many neonatal diseases, including many with nonpulmonary origins, may manifest with signs of respiratory distress. Therefore, a comprehensive differential diagnosis must be considered (Fig. 18–4).

History

Data from a patient's history direct the clinician to the correct diagnosis in most situations, and neonatal respiratory distress is no exception. The mother's prenatal record should be reviewed carefully for clues to the cause of her infant's difficulties. The mother's age, gravidity, parity, blood type, and Rh status should be recorded. The duration of rupture of membranes before delivery, the presence of maternal fever, and the presence of amnionitis are important pieces of information that may help in the differential diagnosis of a newborn with respiratory distress. Administration of steroids to the mother reduces the likelihood that RDS will develop in the infant; administration of narcotics to the mother close to delivery may result in poor respiratory effort by an otherwise normal infant.

A history of prior preterm births is associated with increased risk of premature delivery in subsequent pregnancies. The obstetrician's best estimate of gestational age should be recorded, and it should be documented whether early ultrasonography contributed to dating of the pregnancy. In addition, anomalies are often diagnosed prenatally through ultrasound examination.

Maternal weight gain should be adequate; an excess weight gain may be indicative of diabetes, multiple gestation, or polyhydramnios. Abnormal glucose tolerance screening results alert the clinician to the possibility of gestational diabetes.

PHYSICAL EXAMINATION OF THE RESPIRATORY SYSTEM

One or more of the major signs of respiratory difficulty (e.g., cyanosis, tachypnea, grunting, retractions, and nasal flaring) are

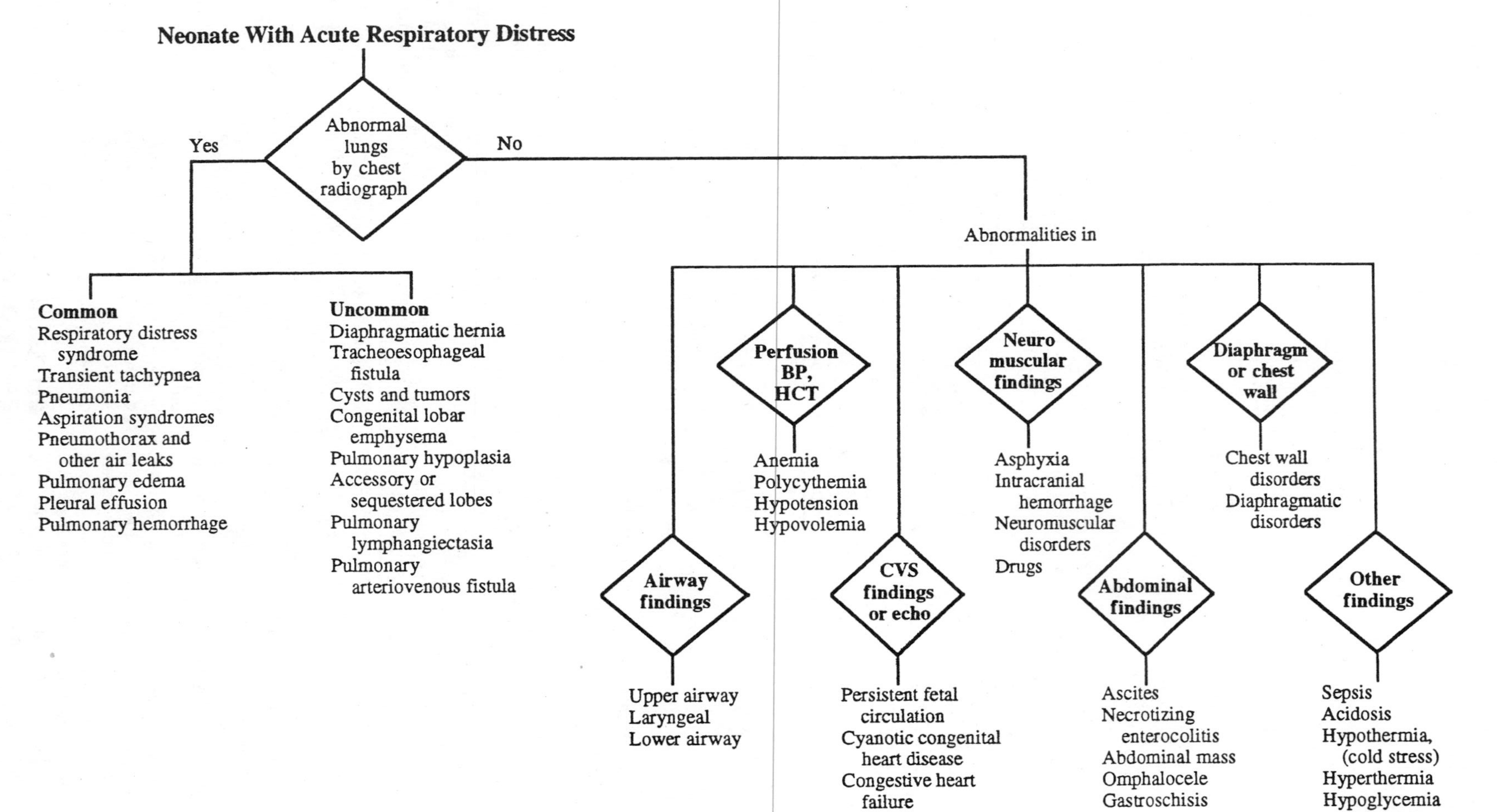

FIGURE 18–4. Neonate with acute respiratory distress.

usually present in neonates with both pulmonary and nonpulmonary causes of respiratory distress. Observation of the distressed infant with the unaided eye and ear is the clinician's first step in the physical assessment. Cyanosis may be central, as caused by pulmonary disease and cyanotic heart disease, or peripheral, as occurs in conditions with impaired CO. Tachypnea typically manifests in patients with decreased lung compliance such as RDS, whereas patients with high airway resistance (e.g., airway obstruction) usually have deep but slow breathing. Grunting, which helps maintain lung volume, is more typical of infants with decreased functional residual capacity. Chest wall retractions occur more frequently in the very premature infants because of the highly compliant chest wall (Avery, 1994; Bueuvalas & Balisteri, 1995). When the infant is intubated, careful observation of the chest gives important information. Close observation of chest wall excursions produced by the ventilator allows the clinician to adjust the magnitude of the ventilator pressure so that better gas exchange is achieved while risk of barotrauma is minimized. An overinflated thorax is a sign of gas trapping. In the intubated infant, this observation should prompt the clinician to adjust the positive end-expiratory pressure (PEEP) or expiratory time so that gas trapping and air leakage are prevented. The observation of an anguished intubated infant, with cyanosis and gasping efforts, may be diagnostic of endotracheal tube obstruction.

Careful attention should be given to the various sounds emanating from the respiratory tract, because their quality often aids in localization of the source of respiratory distress. Stridor is common in neonates with upper airway and laryngeal lesions. Inspiratory stridor occurs most frequently with upper airway and laryngeal lesions, whereas wheezing commonly accompanies lower airway disorders. Hoarseness is a common sign of laryngeal disorders. Forced inspiratory efforts may indicate upper airway or laryngeal involvement, whereas expiratory wheezes suggest a lower airway disease. Congenital airway disorders that may cause respiratory distress in the neonate are included in Figure 18–4.

Auscultation of the chest further aids the examiner. Because they have low lung volumes, infants with RDS have faint breath sounds, usually without rales. In contradistinction, the infant with pneumonia may have rales indicative of alveolar filling. Auscultation allows the clinician to detect the presence of secretion in the airway and to evaluate the response to physiotherapy and suctioning. Rhonchi may be heard in neonates with airway disease, such as meconium aspiration syndrome (MAS). Unequal breath sounds may be due to a pneumothorax or to one of the many causes of diminished ventilation to a lung lobe (e.g., atelectasis, mainstream bronchial intubation, and pleural effusion). A shift of the apex of the heart can occur with a pneumothorax, diaphragmatic hernia, unilateral pulmonary interstitial emphysema, pleural effusion, or atelectasis. Transillumination of the chest may help to differentiate the conditions. Dullness to percussion may be due to a pleural effusion or solid mass. Muffled heart tones suggest a pneumopericardium.

Respiratory distress may occur in many chest wall disorders that restrict rib cage movements. Increased oral secretions and choking with feedings are common in neonates with a tracheoesophageal fistula. Because newborns are obligate nasal breathers, those with choanal atresia typically improve with crying and have worsening respiratory distress with rest and feeding. Characteristic Potter facies and other compression deformities and contractures may be present in neonates with hypoplastic lungs secondary to oligohydramnios.

Examination of the cardiovascular system and assessment of peripheral perfusion yield many clues toward arriving at a diagnosis. Pallor and poor perfusion may indicate anemia, hypotension, or hypovolemia. Polycythemia with plethora may also cause respiratory distress. Cardiovascular signs of congestive failure (e.g., hyperactive precordium, tachycardia, and hepatomegaly), poor CO, pathologic murmurs, decreased femoral pulses, and nonsinus rhythm suggest a primary cardiac cause for the respiratory distress.

TABLE 18–2 Neuromuscular Disorders That May Cause Respiratory Distress in the Neonate

Myopathies	Spinal cord disorder
Myasthenia gravis	Poliomyelitis
Werdnig-Hoffmann disease	Others

Adapted from Battista, M. A., & Carlo, W. A. (1992). Differential diagnosis of acute respiratory distress in the neonate. *Tufts University School of Medicine and Floating Hospital for Children Reports on Neonatal Respiratory Diseases*, 2(3), 1–4, 9–11.

When hypotonia, muscle weakness, or areflexia accompanies respiratory distress, a neuromuscular cause should be considered (Table 18–2). In such cases, there is often an accompanying history of less frequent fetal movement. Sometimes there is a history of muscular disease in the family. Brachial plexus injury or fracture of a clavicle may accompany phrenic nerve injury and diaphragm paralysis.

Abnormalities found on abdominal examination enlighten the examiner to other causes of respiratory difficulty. Abdominal distention resulting from causes such as ascites, necrotizing enterocolitis, abdominal mass, ileus, or tracheoesophageal fistula can cause respiratory distress, whereas a scaphoid configuration of the abdomen suggests a diaphragmatic hernia.

Other nonpulmonary disorders such as sepsis, metabolic acidosis, hypothermia, hyperthermia, hypoglycemia, and methemoglobinemia may also cause respiratory distress in the neonate.

RADIOGRAPHIC AND LABORATORY INVESTIGATION

Radiographic examination is often the most useful part of the laboratory evaluation and may serve to narrow the differential diagnosis. An anteroposterior view is usually sufficient, but lateral chest radiograph may be useful if fluid, masses, or free air is suspected. Other diagnostic imaging techniques (ultrasonography, fluoroscopy, computed tomography, or magnetic resonance imaging) may be helpful in selected patients. Bronchoscopy allows direct visualization of the upper airway. This technique, albeit invasive and technically difficult, may in selected cases be a great aid in differential diagnosis and treatment of obstructive lesions.

Much can be learned from a relatively small battery of laboratory tests. In the NICU setting, the nurse is often called upon not only to interpret results of physiologic testing but also to collect the specimens. Considerable skill is required in sampling both venous and arterial blood from small patients who are at substantial risk for iatrogenic anemia and vascular damage. Ideally, the hospital laboratory is equipped to do most routine tests on microliter quantities of blood. The nurse must monitor total quantities of blood sampled from the infant and be alert to the development of anemia.

Analysis of arterial blood for pH and gas tensions is perhaps one of the most common tasks of the nurse in caring for the infant with respiratory illness. Noninvasive methods to assess gas exchange, such as transcutaneous blood gas measurements or oxygen saturation, may also be used. Because oxygen delivery to the tissues is so intimately dependent on circulating red blood cell volume, a hematocrit should be performed on a central sample.

COMMON DISORDERS OF THE RESPIRATORY SYSTEM

A large variety of disorders afflict neonates. The most common disorders are discussed here. See Figure 18–4 for a listing of both

TABLE 18–3 Causes of Late Respiratory Distress in the Neonate

Bronchopulmonary dysplasia
Pneumonia (bacterial, viral, or fungal)
Congestive heart failure
Recurrent pneumonitis or aspiration
Upper airway obstruction
Wilson-Mikity syndrome
Idiopathic pulmonary fibrosis (Hamman-Rich syndrome)
Pulmonary lymphangiectasia
Cystic fibrosis
Immature lungs

pulmonary and nonpulmonary congenital anomalies that cause respiratory symptoms in the newborn infant. Several diseases may start later in the neonatal period and extend into infancy (Table 18–3). The most common is bronchopulmonary dysplasia (BPD), a chronic lung disease that affects newborns, mainly premature infants exposed to mechanical ventilation and oxygen for RDS or other respiratory problems (see Chapter 20, Complications of Respiratory Management).

Respiratory Distress Syndrome

RDS, or hyaline membrane disease, is the most common cause of respiratory distress in premature neonates (Bueuvalas & Balisteri, 1995). It is estimated that there are more than 40,000 cases of RDS per year in the United States (Farrell & Wood, 1976). Sixty percent of infants born before 29 weeks' gestation have the disorder (Usher et al., 1971), accounting for thousands of patient days in the NICUs and millions of dollars in health care expenditures. In rare cases, RDS develops in full-term infants born to diabetic mothers or full-term infants who have experienced asphyxia. The radiograph displays a characteristic ground-glass, reticulogranular appearance with air bronchograms. Lung inflation is poor. Arterial blood gas analysis reveals respiratory acidemia as well as hypoxemia.

RDS is progressively more common the lower the infant's gestational age. The lung is deficient in pulmonary surfactant, a surface tension–reducing agent that prevents alveolar collapse at end expiration and loss of lung volume. Progressive atelectasis leads to intrapulmonary shunting, owing to perfusion of unventilated lung, and subsequent hypoxemia.

Therapy is directed toward improving oxygenation as well as maintaining optimal lung volume. Continuous positive airway pressure (CPAP) or PEEP is applied to prevent volume loss during expiration. In severe cases, mechanical ventilation via tracheal tube is required. Exogenous surfactants (artificial and natural), which are available for intratracheal instillation, improve survival and reduce some of the associated morbidity of RDS, such as air leaks. High-frequency ventilation for treatment of RDS has met with mixed results and should be considered experimental except in specific circumstances, such as in infants with air leaks and severe hypercapnia. Near-term infants with RDS and respiratory failure unresponsive to ventilatory management have been salvaged with extracorporeal membrane oxygenation (ECMO). See Chapter 19, New Technologies Applied to the Management of Respiratory Dysfunction, for detailed discussions of surfactant therapy and of high-frequency ventilation and ECMO.

Nursing care for infants with RDS is demanding; infants who are the most ill require intensive nursing care, often by a dedicated nurse with no other patient care responsibilities. The nurse must monitor the quality of respirations, observing their depth and the degree of difficulty that the baby is experiencing. Worsening retractions may signal progressive volume loss and impending respiratory failure. Arterial blood gas tensions and pH should be measured frequently and continuous noninvasive monitoring of oxygenation may help early identification of gas exchange problems. The risk of pneumothorax is high, and the symmetry of breath sounds must be verified regularly. The patient receiving nasal CPAP must be kept calm, because a crying baby loses airway pressure when the mouth is open. The intubated infant must be monitored for appropriate endotracheal tube position and patency. Suctioning of the airway should be done carefully. The suction catheter should be passed only as far as the end of the endotracheal tube, because overzealous suctioning can denude the tracheal epithelium (Bailey et al., 1988). Lung volume can be lost during prolonged disconnection from the ventilator. This disconnection time is particularly important when high-frequency ventilation is being used, because rapid loss of lung volume can precipitate hypoxemia in these patients. Any sudden decompensation should alert the nurse to investigate for ventilator failure, pneumothorax, or tracheal tube plugging (Fig. 18–5). These infants often have invasive catheters and the nurse should be adept at caring for them.

A frequent complication of RDS in the tiny premature infant is BPD. BPD generally refers to a chronic obstructive pulmonary disorder characterized by pulmonary fibrosis, bronchiolar metaplasia, emphysema, and interstitial edema. It is most commonly seen in survivors of extreme prematurity who had RDS and, often, air leaks as well. Infants with BPD generally include those who continue to require oxygen supplementation at 28 days of age or 36 weeks of postconceptional age. The incidence of BPD is estimated at 1300 cases per year in the United States (Bancalari, 1985). The incidence of BPD increases as gestational age decreases. Approximately 10 percent of premature infants with birth weight less than 1500 g have BPD, and BPD develops in more than one third of infants with birth weight less than 751 g (Hack et al., 1995).

Air Leak

Pneumothorax is a frequent complication of RDS and other neonatal respiratory disorders. Pneumothorax is just one of a number of entities that compose the air leak syndromes, which are characterized by air in an ectopic location (Table 18–4). Many air leak syndromes begin with at least some degree of pulmonary interstitial emphysema, which is the result of alveolar rupture from overdistention, usually concomitant with mechanical ventilation or continuous distending airway pressure. It occurs most commonly in preterm infants but may be seen in infants of any gestational age. Lung compliance is nonuniform, and there are areas of poor aeration and alveolar collapse. Interspersed are alveoli of normal or near-normal compliance, which become overdistended. The more normal lung units (those with better compliance) become overdistended and eventually rupture. Air is forced from the alveolus into the loose tissue of the interstitial space and dissects toward the hilum of the lung, where it may track into the mediastinum, causing a pneumomediastinum, or into the

TABLE 18–4 Types of Air Leaks Associated With Respiratory Distress in the Neonate

Pneumothorax	Pneumoperitoneum
Pulmonary interstitial emphysema	Pulmonary venous air embolism
Pneumomediastinum	Subcutaneous emphysema
Pneumopericardium	Pseudocyst

Adapted from Battista, M. A., & Carlo, W. A. (1992). Differential diagnosis of acute respiratory distress in the neonate. *Tufts University School of Medicine and Floating Hospital for Children Reports on Neonatal Respiratory Diseases*, 2(3), 1–4, 9–11.

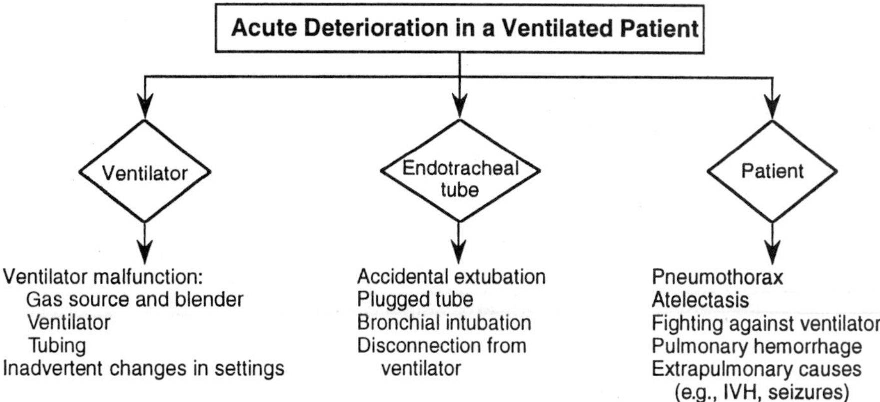

FIGURE 18–5. Acute deterioration in a ventilated patient.

pericardium, causing a pneumopericardium. The astute nurse may notice that an infant's chest becomes barrel-shaped with overdistention and that breath sounds become distant on the affected side. Typically, the infant who suffers a pneumothorax becomes unstable, with development of cyanosis, oxygen desaturation, and carbon dioxide retention. The infant may become hypotensive and bradycardic because high intrathoracic pressure impedes CO. A tension pneumothorax, in which free pleural air compresses the lung, is a medical emergency, and prompt relief by thoracentesis or tube thoracostomy is indicated.

Transient tachypnea of the newborn occurs typically in infants born by cesarean section, particularly in the absence of labor. The cause of the disorder is thought to be a transient pulmonary edema, resulting from the infant's "missed" chance during labor to absorb pulmonary alveolar fluid (Avery et al., 1966). The chest radiograph may show increased perihilar interstitial markings and small pleural fluid collections, especially in the minor fissure. In contrast to the infant with RDS, the infant with transient tachypnea has relative normocarbia or hypocarbia as shown by arterial blood gas analysis. Hypocapnia decreases the amount of carbon dioxide in the blood; pH remains normal. Oxygenation can usually be maintained by supplementing oxygen with a hood, although some infants benefit from a short course of positive pressure support. The infant usually recovers in 24 to 48 hours.

Pneumonia

Pneumonia may be of bacterial, viral, or of other infectious origin (Table 18–5). Pneumonia may be transmitted transplacentally, as has been shown with group B streptococcus, or via an ascending bacterial invasion associated with maternal amnionitis and prolonged rupture of the membranes. The usual organisms of active postamnionitis pneumonia are group B streptococcus, *Escherichia coli, Haemophilus influenzae,* and, less commonly, *Streptococcus viridans, Listeria,* monocytogenes, and anaerobes.

There is a strong association of bacterial pneumonias with premature birth, which may be due to a developmental deficiency of bacteriostatic factors in the amniotic fluid (Schlievert et al., 1975), or the infection may be a precipitating factor in preterm labor. Amnionitis can occur even in the presence of intact membranes (Naeye & Peters, 1978). Blood cultures and other diagnostic tests are necessary to help direct specific antimicrobial therapy. The nurse should be attuned to the labor history. Were membranes ruptured for more than 12 to 24 hours? Did the mother have a fever before delivery? The full-term infant who remains tachypneic, has prolonged grunting, or has retractions or in whom temperature instability develops should be evaluated carefully. Blood counts may be helpful, and the neutropenic infant in particular should be carefully monitored. Careful consideration of infection should be given to any newborn with respiratory distress and more than transient oxygen requirements. Tracheal aspirates obtained within 8 hours of birth that show both bacteria and white blood cells on Wright's stain are highly predictive of pneumonia (Brook et al., 1980).

Treatment is usually begun with broad-spectrum antibiotics, such as ampicillin, and an aminoglycoside, pending culture results. Lumbar puncture may be undertaken or may be postponed until results of blood culture are obtained. When cultures result in the identification of the organism, the study of antibiotic sensitivity allows the clinician to choose the most effective antibi-

TABLE 18–5 Organisms That May Cause Pneumonia in the Neonate

Bacterial	Viral	Other
Group B streptococcus	Cytomegalovirus	*Candida* (and other fungi)
Escherichia coli	Adenovirus	*Ureaplasma*
Klebsiella	Rhinovirus	*Chlamydia*
Staphylococcus aureus	Respiratory syncytial virus	Syphilis
Listeria monocytogenes	Parainfluenza	*Pneumocystis carinii*
Enterobacter	Enterovirus	Tuberculosis
Haemophilus influenzae	Rubella	
Pneumococcus		
Pseudomonas		
Bacteroides		
Others		

Adapted from Battista, M. A., & Carlo, W. A. (1992). Differential diagnosis of acute respiratory distress in the neonate. *Tufts University School of Medicine and Floating Hospital for Children Reports on Neonatal Respiratory Diseases*, 2(3), 1–4, 9–11.

otic or combination of antibiotics for the causative agent. Antibiotic treatment for up to 10 to 14 days may be necessary.

Persistent Pulmonary Hypertension of the Newborn

Persistent pulmonary hypertension of the newborn (PPHN), or persistent fetal circulation, is a term applied to the combination of pulmonary hypertension (high pressure in the pulmonary artery), subsequent right-to-left shunting through fetal channels (the foramen ovale or ductus arteriosus) away from the pulmonary vascular bed, and a structurally normal heart. The syndrome may be idiopathic, or, more commonly, it is secondary to another disorder such as MAS, congenital diaphragmatic hernia, RDS, asphyxia, sepsis, hyperviscosity of the blood, or hypoglycemia.

The neonatal pulmonary vasculature is sensitive to changes in PaO_2 and pH, and, during stress, it can become even hyperreactive, constricting to cause increased pressure against which the neonatal heart cannot force blood flow to the lungs. If the pulmonary artery pressure is higher than systemic pressure, blood flows through the path of least resistance, away from the lungs through the foramen ovale and the ductus arteriosus. The infant becomes progressively hypoxemic and acidemic, and the cycle perpetuates.

Collaborative management of infants with PPHN demands the greatest diligence that the health care professional can summon. Because the pulmonary vasculature is unstable, almost any event can precipitate severe hypoxemia.

Sedation and induced muscle paralysis are often necessary to prevent episodes of hypoxemia associated with nursing procedures (e.g., suctioning and position changes) or with asynchrony of patient and ventilator breaths. Alkalosis, either with bicarbonate infusion or by hyperventilation, often relaxes the pulmonary vascular bed and allows better pulmonary perfusion and thus oxygenation. The approach to therapy should be directed toward preventing hypoxemia and acidosis, because the infant may be stable with a PaO_2 around 100 mm Hg and a high pH (usually more than 7.55) (Drummond et al., 1981). The critical pH necessary for overcoming pulmonary vasoconstriction seems to be unique to the individual and may be referred to as a "set point." High applied ventilator pressures predispose the lung to air leak syndromes, further increasing the risk of sudden destabilization. Vasopressor therapy with dopamine and dobutamine is often used in conjunction with hyperventilation. Presumably, they act both to improve contractility of the stressed myocardium, improving CO, and to raise systemic arterial pressure above pulmonary artery pressure so that right-to-left shunting is reduced.

When conventional therapies fail, high-frequency ventilation may be attempted. Approximately 30 to 60 percent of patients who fail conventional mechanical ventilation respond to high-frequency ventilation (Carlo et al., 1989; Carter et al., 1990; Clark et al., 1994). However, the exact role of high-frequency ventilation on mortality or in preventing ECMO needs further evaluation. Since the early 1990s, inhalation of nitric oxide has been shown to be a promising new therapy for PPHN (Kinsella et al., 1992; Kinsella et al., 1993; Roberts et al., 1992), but further studies are needed to determine which patients benefit from this therapy. When oxygenation cannot be accomplished despite the use of conventional mechanical ventilation, high-frequency ventilation, or even a trial with nitric oxide, ECMO has been shown to salvage approximately 80 percent of patients with reversible causes of lung disease. There is disagreement among neonatologists regarding the exact indications for ECMO, and some centers report impressive survival statistics without the use of ECMO. However, ECMO is frequently the only treatment that improves some infants who fail less invasive therapies. A detailed discussion of ECMO is presented in Chapter 19, New Technologies Applied to the Management of Respiratory Dysfunction.

Meconium Aspiration Syndrome

MAS is the most common aspiration syndrome that causes respiratory distress in neonates. The role of meconium in the pathophysiology of aspiration pneumonia has become controversial. It is unclear whether the material itself causes severe enough pneumonia to lead to hypoxemia, acidosis, and pulmonary hypertension, or whether the presence of meconium in the amniotic fluid is merely a marker for other events that may have predisposed the fetus to severe pulmonary disease. The severely ill infant with meconium aspiration pneumonia typically comes from a stressed labor and has depressed cord pH resulting from metabolic acidosis. Frequently, these infants are postmature and exhibit classic signs of weight loss, skin peeling, and deep staining of the nails and umbilical cord.

Pulmonary disease arises both from chemical pneumonitis, interstitial edema, and small airway obstruction and from concomitant persistent pulmonary hypertension. The infant may have uneven pulmonary ventilation with hyperinflation of some areas and atelectasis of others, leading to ventilation–perfusion mismatching and subsequent hypoxemia. The hypoxemia may then exacerbate pulmonary vasoconstriction, leading to deeper hypoxemia and acidosis. Infants with MAS may have evidence of lung overinflation with a barrel-chested appearance. Auscultation reveals rales and rhonchi. The radiograph shows patchy or streaky areas of atelectasis and other areas of overinflation.

There is debate among neonatologists as to whether infants born through thinly meconium-stained fluid should be intubated at delivery for suctioning, but most agree that the stressed infant with thick or particulate meconium may benefit from airway suctioning. Ideally, the nose, mouth, and pharynx are emptied before delivery of the shoulders; then the infant is rapidly intubated under direct laryngoscopy for suctioning of the airway. An endotracheal tube of adequate caliber to remove particulate matter should be used.

As with other cases of pulmonary hypertension, nursing care of infants with MAS centers on maintenance of adequate oxygenation and acid–base balance and on avoidance of cold stress, which contributes to acidosis. There is a high incidence of air leaks in these infants, and positive pressure ventilation is best avoided if the patient can be adequately oxygenated, even at very high inspired oxygen concentrations. Use of antibiotics for these infants is also controversial. No studies have shown that infection is causal, but meconium itself may enhance bacterial growth as a culture medium. Antibiotics are often used, however, particularly in desperately ill infants, at least until a bacterial infection is ruled out. The infant is often exquisitely sensitive to environmental stimuli and should be nursed in as quiet an environment as possible (Langer, 1990). Interventions should be preplanned to maximize efficiency of handling the infant.

Less common than aspiration of meconium, aspiration of blood, amniotic fluid, or gastrointestinal contents may make a neonate symptomatic. The history is important in the differential diagnosis because radiographs are nondiagnostic.

Pulmonary Hemorrhage

Pulmonary hemorrhage is rarely an isolated condition and usually occurs in an otherwise sick infant. RDS, asphyxia, congenital heart disease, aspiration of gastric content or maternal blood, and disseminated intravascular coagulation and other bleeding disorders may play a role in the cause of pulmonary hemorrhage. Pulmonary hemorrhage affects approximately 10 percent of infants who receive either natural or artificial surfactant (Horbar et al., 1993). Massive bleeding may also occur as a complication of airway suction secondary to direct trauma of the respiratory epithelium.

Pulmonary hemorrhage is manifested by the presence of

bloody fluid from the trachea. When massive, it may be heralded by a sudden deterioration with pallor, shock, cyanosis, or bradycardia. Attention must be given to maintenance of a patent airway because the tracheal tube may become obstructed and require emergency replacement. Suctioning must be done with great care to avoid precipitation of further bleeding. Clotting factors can be consumed rapidly, and the nurse should be alert to signs of generalized bleeding.

Pleural Effusions

Pleural effusions may be caused by accumulation of fluid between the parietal pleura of the chest wall and the visceral pleura enveloping the lung. A pleural effusion may also be due to chylothorax (lymphatic fluid) or hemothorax (blood). Lymphatics drain fluid that filters into the pleural space. Fluid accumulates in the pleural space as a result of either increased filtration or decreased absorption. An increase in filtration pressure, as seen with increased venous pressure in hydrops fetalis or congestive heart failure, leads to pleural effusion. The rate of filtration into the pleural space also increases if the pleural membrane becomes more permeable to water and protein, as occurs with infection.

Pleural effusion with high glucose content in an infant receiving parenteral nutrition via a central venous catheter should raise the suspicion of catheter perforation into the pleural space. If the infant is also receiving lipid infusion, the fluid may appear milky and be confused with chylothorax.

Chylothorax may be congenital or acquired and is associated with obstruction or perforation of the thoracic duct. It may also be a surgical complication of repair of diaphragmatic hernia, tracheoesophageal fistula, and congenital heart defects. Congenital chylothorax may be suspected in the infant who cannot be ventilated in the delivery room. Breath sounds are difficult to hear, and chest movement with ventilation is minimal. Bilateral thoracenteses may be lifesaving. The typical pleural fluid in a chylothorax—opalescent and rich in fat—is present only if the infant has been fed.

Pleural effusions that embarrass respiratory function typically require drainage, by either thoracentesis or tube thoracostomy. It may be necessary for chest tubes placed for chylothorax and thoracic duct injury to remain in place for extended periods while the infant is given total parenteral nutrition, receiving nothing by mouth, minimizing thoracic duct flow.

Apnea

Apnea is the common end product of a myriad of neonatal physiologic events. Apnea can be caused by hypoxemia, infection, anemia, thermal instability, gastroesophageal reflux, metabolic derangement, drugs, and intracranial disease (Kattwinkel, 1977). An infant with visible respiratory excursions but absent air entry should be examined for obstructive causes of apnea. The presence of a cardiac murmur with bounding pulses should alert the nurse to patent ductus arteriosus as a possible contributor to worsening apnea in the small preterm infant. These causes should be ruled out before idiopathic apnea of prematurity is diagnosed.

Apnea is observed in more than half of surviving premature infants weighing less than 1.5 kg at birth. The respiratory control mechanism and central responsiveness to carbon dioxide is progressively less mature the lower the gestational age. In contrast to adults, infants respond to hypoxemia with only a brief hyperpneic response, followed by hypoventilation or apnea. In any infant who has apnea, hypoxemia should always be ruled out before the clinician embarks on any other workup or institutes therapy.

Care of the infant with apnea requires constant attentiveness. Obstructive apnea cannot be detected with the impedance respiratory monitor, because there are normal or pronounced respiratory excursions of the chest wall. Prompt tactile stimulation for mild "spells" is often sufficient to abort the episode of apnea, obviating the need for further therapy. Infants with apneic episodes accompanied by cyanosis and profound bradycardia need prompt attention to their immediate needs as well as more aggressive diagnostic and therapeutic intervention.

Sensory stimulation with water beds or other means can sometimes be used to manage these infants, particularly those with mild apnea. Many apneic neonates respond to nasal CPAP at low pressures, because the apnea may be due to airway obstruction or intermittent hypoxemia (Speidel & Dunn, 1976). Pressure support may also stimulate pulmonary stretch receptors, thus stimulating respiration. Excellent nursing care directed toward maintenance of the neutral thermal environment, normoxia, good pulmonary toilet, and prevention of aspiration is essential in the care of neonates at risk for apnea.

Use of methylxanthines, such as aminophylline, has markedly simplified the treatment of apnea in some premature infants. Xanthines appear to exert a central stimulatory effect on brain stem respiratory neurons and often markedly decrease the frequency and severity of apneic episodes. The nurse must be attuned to the toxicities of aminophylline, including tachycardia, excessive diuresis, and vomiting, which may precede neurologic toxicity at inadvertently high blood drug levels.

CONGENITAL ANOMALIES AFFECTING RESPIRATORY FUNCTION

Diaphragmatic Hernia

Congenital diaphragmatic hernia occurs at a frequency of 1 in 2500 live births, and it may be unsuspected until birth. Herniation of abdominal contents into the chest cavity early in gestation is accompanied by ipsilateral pulmonary hypoplasia. By mechanisms that are not well understood, there is often some degree of pulmonary hypoplasia on the contralateral side. Most infants are symptomatic at birth, with severe respiratory distress in the delivery room. The affected newborn's abdomen is usually scaphoid, and breath sounds are absent on the side of the defect (a left-sided defect occurs in 90 percent of cases). Bowel sounds may be heard in the chest, and heart sounds may be heard on the right side because the herniated abdominal contents push the mediastinum to the right (Chernick & Kendig, 1990; Langston & Thurlbeck, 1986).

As soon as the diagnosis is suspected, bag and mask ventilation should be avoided because it fills the hernia contents with air and can compress the lungs and worsen ventilation. An orogastric tube should be placed to aid in decompression of the herniated abdominal viscera. The trachea should be intubated promptly and mechanical ventilation begun. Ventilation should be attempted with a rapid rate and low inflation pressure. Symptomatic neonates often have pulmonary hypertension and progressive right-to-left shunting. Hypotension is common, and, when adequate intravascular volume is established, dopamine infusion may be helpful. Pulmonary vasodilators have been advocated by some clinicians and have met with variable success, but they should not be used unless adequate systemic blood pressure can be maintained.

Survival rate is poor in infants who are symptomatic at birth, but their condition may be improved by ECMO. Even with ECMO, rate of survival is poor in infants whose Pa_{CO_2} cannot be decreased to less than 60 mm Hg before cardiopulmonary bypass. Surgery to repair the defect is indicated. There is controversy among pediatric surgeons regarding the urgency of the procedure, and some prefer to stabilize the patient with mechanical ventilation, vasopressors, and correction of acidosis before undertaking surgical intervention (Sakai et al., 1987); others perform surgical repair while the patient is maintained on ECMO (Breaux et al., 1991). (See Chapter 19, New Technologies Applied to the Management of Respiratory Dysfunction.)

Congenital Heart Disease

Congenital heart disease frequently manifests with signs of respiratory distress. Neonates with congenital heart disease demonstrating right-to-left shunting and decreased pulmonary blood flow (e.g., tetralogy of Fallot, pulmonary valve atresia, and tricuspid valve atresia or stenosis) usually present with profound cyanosis unresponsive to oxygen supplementation. Neonates with congenital heart disease demonstrating increased pulmonary blood flow or obstruction to the left outflow tract (e.g., transposition of the great vessels, total anomalous pulmonary venous return, atrioventricular canal, hypoplastic left heart syndrome, and critical coarctation of the aorta) may transiently improve with oxygen supplementation. Neonates with noncyanotic lesions such as patent ductus arteriosus and ventricular septal defect may present with signs of congestive heart failure. (See Chapter 21, Assessment and Management of Cardiovascular Dysfunction, for a complete description.)

Choanal Atresia

Choanal atresia causes upper airway obstruction in the neonate. The choanae, or nasal passages, are separated from the nasopharynx by a structure known as the bucconasal membrane, which normally perforates during gestation. Failure of this developmental event results in an obstructed airway, occurring bilaterally in 50 percent of cases. Most affected infants are female and half of affected infants have associated anomalies. Because newborns are obligate nasal breathers, they have chest retractions and severe cyanosis (particularly during feeding), and they paradoxically turn pink when crying. Emergency treatment consists of tracheal intubation or placement of an oral airway. Surgical correction is indicated (Hall, 1979).

Cystic Hygroma

A variety of space-occupying lesions can impose on the airway of the newborn (Table 18–6). Most are derived from embryonic tissues. Cystic hygroma, derived from lymphatic tissue, is the most common lateral neck mass in the newborn. It is multilobular, is multicystic, and, when large, obstructs the airway. Surgery is curative, although it is sometimes technically difficult. The nurse must always be mindful of the airway and its patency. Many of these lesions are of great cosmetic concern and cause great distress in the parents. A care plan should address these parental concerns. It is sometimes helpful to facilitate contact with parents of other children with similar problems who can share their experiences.

TABLE 18–6 Thoracic Cysts and Tumors That May Cause Respiratory Distress in the Neonate

Teratoma	Gastrogenic cyst
Cystic hygroma	Hemangioma
Neurogenic tumor	Angiosarcoma
Neuroblastoma	Mediastinal goiter
Ganglioneuroma	Thymoma
Neurofibroma	Mesenchymoma
Bronchial or bronchogenic cyst	Lipoma
Intrapulmonary cyst	Cystic adenomatous malformation

Adapted from Battista, M. A., & Carlo, W. A. (1992). Differential diagnosis of acute respiratory distress in the neonate. *Tufts University School of Medicine and Floating Hospital for Children Reports on Neonatal Respiratory Diseases*, 2(3), 1–4, 9–11.

Pierre Robin Syndrome or Sequence

The major feature of Pierre Robin syndrome or sequence is micrognathia (a small mandible). The tongue is posteriorly displaced into the oropharynx, obstructing the airway. Sixty percent of affected patients also have a cleft palate. Obstructive respiratory distress and cyanosis are common and may be severe. In an emergency, as with all airway obstructions (obstructive apnea), tracheal intubation should be undertaken. Infants with Pierre Robin syndrome or sequence are nursed in the prone position to prevent the tongue from falling backward. Nasogastric tube feedings are usually required in the neonatal period. With good care, the infant has a good prognosis for survival; the mandible usually grows and the problem resolves by 6 to 12 months of age.

The newer term for this condition, in many cases, is *sequence*, but *syndrome* can also be used because there are many ways that the clusters of symptoms can occur. *Sequence* refers to a pattern that is a result of a single problem in morphogenesis that leads to this variety of problems. *Syndrome* is usually used when no one determinant can be identified. For example, it may result from multifactorial inheritance, may be part of other conditions, or may be genetic (whereby one or more genes are responsible). Thus this condition is more than just an explainable, describable syndrome or a sequence of visible defects (Prows, 1997).

COLLABORATIVE MANAGEMENT OF INFANTS WITH RESPIRATORY DISORDERS

Supportive Care

Supportive care of the infant in respiratory distress requires attention to detail. The health care professional's primary goals are to minimize oxygen consumption and carbon dioxide production. These goals are accomplished by maintaining a neutral thermal environment and ensuring normoxia. The nurse must be skilled in physical assessment to interpret signs and symptoms, such as cyanosis, gasping, tachypnea, grunting, nasal flaring, and retractions. By understanding the pathophysiology of breathing, the nurse knows that the infant with retractions has decreased lung compliance and that the cyanotic infant has poor tissue oxygenation (Polin & Burg, 1983).

The neonatal nurse and the rest of the neonatal team need excellent communication skills. Acutely ill neonates with respiratory disease are often unstable and their condition can deteriorate rapidly, so astute observation skills are necessary. Assessment is a continuous process and effective communication among nurses, respiratory therapists, physicians, and supportive staff is necessary for proper delivery of intensive care. The nurse, who is the primary bedside caregiver, is the gatekeeper for all interactions between the patient and the environment. The nurse caring for an unstable patient should be the patient's advocate, whether such a role involves the timing of a physical examination by the physician or venipuncture for laboratory investigation.

Technical competence is an important facet of the nurse's repertoire. The nurse is responsible for maintaining intravenous lines and tracheal tube patency, accurately measuring volumes of intravenous intake as well as urinary output, and operating advanced electronic machinery. Moreover, the nurse must also be adept at interpreting arterial blood gas and laboratory data in order to communicate these to the rest of the care team and to develop a cogent management plan.

Many functions are shared to some degree with respiratory

therapists. Whether ventilator changes are made by nurses or respiratory therapists, the nurse should become familiar with the effects of ventilator setting changes on blood gases. Briefly, $Paco_2$ is affected by changes in ventilator rate and tidal volume. Tidal volume depends on the difference between PIP and PEEP. Thus, to decrease $Paco_2$, rate or inspiratory pressure should be increased. Pao_2 is dependent on the fraction of inspirated oxygen concentration (Fio_2) and mean airway pressure (MAP). MAP depends on gas flow, PIP, PEEP, and inspiratory to expiratory time ratio. To improve Pao_2, the most effective changes are to increase MAP by increasing PIP or PEEP or to increase Fio_2. Table 18–7 shows the effect of ventilator setting changes on blood gases. The nurse should also be generally familiar with ventilator functioning so that malfunctions can be detected promptly. The nurse should always be prepared to bag-ventilate an intubated neonate in case decompensation occurs while the status of the ventilatory apparatus is checked. Nurses and therapists often share such functions as airway suctioning, monitoring and recording of inspired oxygen concentration, and delivery of chest physical therapy.

The delivery of oxygen therapy should always be carefully monitored. Desired oxygenation parameters should be recorded in the nurses' notes and followed up with measurement of arterial blood gases or by noninvasive means. The acutely ill infant should have Fio_2 measured continuously and recorded frequently.

Care of the infant receiving CPAP can be particularly challenging. These infants should be kept calm and swaddled if necessary. Crying releases pressure through the mouth, and lung volume is lost. Nasal CPAP can be effective, but, at the same time, particular attention must be given to maintaining patency of the nose, the nasal prongs, and the pharynx. The infant's nares and nasal septum should be guarded from pressure necrosis from inappropriately applied prongs.

The infant requiring mechanical ventilation must be constantly assessed for airway patency. If the infant is unable to grunt against a closed glottis and to maintain positive airway pressure, the condition may worsen if airway pressure is not maintained properly. Suctioning of the airway should be done only as often as necessary to remove pulmonary secretions that could occlude the airway. The suction catheter should be passed only to the end of the tracheal tube because epithelium is easily damaged. Vibration and percussion should be used judiciously in the infant with pulmonary secretions to loosen them and allow removal via suction. There is perhaps little need to suction the intubated baby with RDS vigorously in the first 24 hours because secretions are minimal and lung volume is lost with every disconnection of the ventilator circuit (Cassani, 1984). The sudden decompensation of a ventilated infant should alert the nurse to look for disconnection of the ventilator, pulmonary air leak, ventilator failure, or obstructed tracheal tube (see Fig. 18–5). The very small infant who suddenly decompensates may have had a severe intracranial hemorrhage.

TABLE 18–7 Effects of Ventilator Setting Changes on Blood Gases

Ventilator Setting Changes	Effects on Blood Gases	
	$Paco_2$	*Pao_2*
≠ PIP	Ø	≠
≠ PEEP	≠	≠
≠ Frequency	Ø	± ≠
≠ I:E ratio	æ	≠
≠ Fio_2	æ	≠
≠ Flow	± Ø	± ≠

≠, increase; Ø, decrease; ±, minimal effect; æ, no consistent effect; Fio_2, fraction of O_2 in dry inspired air; PEEP, positive end-expiratory pressure; PIP, peak inspiratory pressure.

Modified from Carlo, W. A., Greenough, A., & Chatburn, R. L. (1994). Advances in conventional mechanical ventilation. In B. R. Boynton, W. A. Carlo, & A. H. Jobe (Eds.), *New therapies for neonatal respiratory failure* (p. 144). New York: Cambridge University Press.

ASSESSMENT AND MONITORING

The most important aspect in monitoring patients with respiratory disease is the close and continuous observation of signs and symptoms. The color of the patient gives important clues: An infant with pink lips and oral mucosa has good oxygenation and perfusion; a cyanotic patient has poor tissue oxygenation. If the hemoglobin concentration is too low, the patient can be hypoxemic, but because the concentration of deoxyhemoglobin is low, there may be no cyanosis. An infant with tachypnea and retraction usually has decreased lung compliance. A patient with barrel-shaped thorax, taking deep breaths and with a normal or low respiratory rate, probably has an increased airway resistance and gas trapping. Observation of the intubated patient is especially important. An anguished infant, who is cyanotic and breathing deeply, may have an obstructed endotracheal tube. An infant with RDS and increased chest expansion over time, despite no change in ventilatory pressure, is experiencing improvement in lung compliance. The same infant with later asymmetry in chest and sudden deterioration of oxygenation may have a pneumothorax. Cardiac beats easily seen through the thoracic wall may be caused by the presence of a symptomatic patent ductus arteriosus. A recently extubated infant in whom increased retractions and inspiratory stridor develop has upper airway obstruction. Auscultation helps in the diagnosis of increased airway resistance or the presence of secretions. It also allows the clinician to assess the response to different treatment maneuvers, such as suctioning, chest physiotherapy, and bronchodilation. Asymmetries in auscultation suggest mainstream bronchial intubation, atelectasis, pneumothorax, or pleural effusion.

Great progress has been made in noninvasive monitoring of blood gas tensions, but blood sampling is still necessary for pH determination. Arterial samples are preferable. Capillary specimens are undependable, especially for Po_2. If peripheral perfusion is adequate, capillary blood approximates arterial values of pH and Pco_2. However, capillary blood Pao_2 values do not reliably reflect arterial oxygenation.

Neonatal care has changed dramatically with the advent and widespread use of transcutaneous monitoring of Pao_2, $Paco_2$, and Sao_2. The neonatal intensive care team should become familiar with the devices used in noninvasive gas monitoring. It is especially important to know the basis for their functioning and how to interpret the information they provide, and to be aware of clinical situations in which the information provided is not reliable or needs to be complemented before any management decisions are made. Transcutaneous Po_2 ($TcPo_2$) is measured with an electrode applied over the skin and heated to 42°C to 44°C. The electrode measures skin Po_2, not arterial Po_2. Skin Po_2 measurement depends on skin perfusion and on oxygen diffusion across the epidermis. Warming the skin to 42°C to 44°C under the electrode increases skin perfusion so that $TcPo_2$ correlates better with arterial Po_2. When initiating $TcPo_2$ monitoring, 10 to 15 minutes are needed to obtain a stable reading. After that, $TcPo_2$ reflects changes on Fio_2 with a 10- to 20-second delay. After 4 to 6 hours, the method becomes unreliable because of changes in skin secondary to hyperthermia (Pollitzer et al., 1980), so the electrode position should be changed. In premature infants with more labile skin, the electrode placement should be changed even more frequently to avoid skin burns.

The nurse should be aware of situations that make $TcPo_2$ lose its reliability. Overestimation of oxygenation occurs when there is an air bubble or leak between the electrode and the skin or when the calibration is improper. Underestimation occurs with skin hypoperfusion, in older infants (increased thickness of the skin), with insufficient heating of the electrodes, or with improper calibration.

$TcPo_2$ is being supplanted by continuous pulse oximetry. Arterial oxygen saturation is computed from absorption of emitted low-intensity red or infrared light. The probe is attached to a finger or toe in large infants or to a hand or foot in small premature infants. Pulse oximetry offers several advantages over transcutaneous oxygen monitoring: (1) avoidance of heating of the skin and risk of burns, (2) elimination of a delay period for transducer equilibration, (3) accurate measurement regardless of presence of edema or patient age, (4) no requirement of in vitro calibration, and (5) no requirement for frequent position changes. However, the nurse should be aware that Sao_2 higher than 97 percent may be associated with Pao_2 higher than 100 mm Hg. This is important in premature infants who are at risk for retinopathy of prematurity. Sao_2 between 92 and 97 percent is associated with a safe range of Pao_2, that is, 45 to 100 mm Hg (Hay et al., 1989). With Sao_2 over 97 percent and especially when it is 100 percent, the clinician cannot predict a patient's Pao_2. When the saturation is 100 percent, the Pao_2 can be 100 mm Hg or even higher (see Fig. 18–2). This situation is particularly important in infants with PPHN because the decision whether to wean ventilator settings depends on Pao_2. In these patients, the simultaneous use of $TcPo_2$ and pulse oximetry is a useful alternative.

A common problem of pulse oximetry is the presence of motion artifacts, an altered signal caused by movement of the part of the body where the sensor is applied. This movement is recognized by the loss of correlation between the oximeter pulse rate and the electrical monitor heart rate, because the pulse wave form is not detected. Peripheral pulse oximetry may not detect pulse signals in patients with hypotension and poor perfusion. $TcPo_2$ may also give false readings in this situation. The clinician should be aware that pressure of the probe over the skin can produce skin pressure necrosis. This consideration is particularly important in the premature infant. Phototherapy may interfere with accuracy of Sao_2 monitoring, but this problem can be avoided by covering the sensor with an opaque material (e.g., a diaper).

$TcPo_2$ monitoring and pulse oximetry are useful in several clinical situations. They may be used in neonates with mild respiratory distress, such as transient tachypnea, to assess the oxygen requirement, and to allow weaning without placement of an arterial catheter. In infants receiving mechanical ventilation, $TcPo_2$ or pulse oximetry helps to assess the effects of ventilator setting changes, reducing the need for arterial blood sampling. Continuous oxygenation monitoring reduces the risk of hyperoxemia or hypoxemia during interventions such as airway suctioning, position change, lumbar puncture, or venous cannulation. This monitoring is particularly helpful in the care of infants who are intolerant of excessive stimulation, such as those with PPHN.

$TcPo_2$ and pulse oximetry monitoring are also useful in caring for patients with PPHN because simultaneous monitoring of preductal (head, right arm, right upper chest) and postductal (left arm, abdomen, legs) $TcPo_2$ or Sao_2 allows assessment of the magnitude of ductal shunting or the response to therapies such as vasodilation or alkalinization.

Transcutaneously measured Pco_2 is accomplished with a glass electrode that is pH sensitive. Transcutaneous Pco_2 response is slower than that of $TcPo_2$, and the value measured must be corrected for skin production of carbon dioxide. Thus, transcutaneously measured values are 1.37 times higher than arterial Pco_2 values (Herrell et al., 1980). Most modern monitors display an electronically corrected value to $TcPo_2$. This modality is especially useful for monitoring chronically ventilated patients without indwelling catheters. Blood gas values during arterial puncture or vigorous crying during the procedure are often affected by breath holding and shunt, and may be misleading.

ENVIRONMENTAL CONSIDERATIONS

Maintenance of the therapeutic environment is an important nursing function. Much attention has been given recently to the effects of sensory stimulation on the infant with respiratory distress. The sick newborn often has unstable pulmonary vasculature and may be particularly prone to hypoxic vasoconstriction. This phenomenon may be triggered in some individuals by excess stimulation, such as loud noise, handling, or venipuncture. It has been shown that the agitated neonate has more difficulty with oxygenation and that a quiet, minimally stimulating environment allows for more stable oxygenation (Als, 1996; Catlett & Holditch-Davis, 1991). The bedside nurse should develop a care plan that allows the baby long periods of undisturbed rest, clustering interventions into short periods whenever possible. Positioning the infant in the flexed, or fetal, position or "nesting" may help in calming some infants.

FAMILY CARE

Neonates with respiratory distress frequently require multiple instrumentation. They may have endotracheal tubes, umbilical catheters, oximeter probes, chest leads, and other paraphernalia attached or applied to their skin. All of these interventions can give parents a feeling of unnaturalness or separation from their infant. The nurse should explain the function of all equipment surrounding the bedside as well as the function of invasive catheters, monitoring leads, and tracheal tubes. Terminology appropriate to the parents' level of understanding should be used. Even the most astute parents may be bewildered, and repetition is necessary. Staff should maintain consistent terminology so that the parents do not become confused between "respirators" and "ventilators." Whenever possible, the use of frightening or inaccurate terms should be avoided. Imagine the fear engendered by the phrase, "We paralyzed your baby last night."

Parents should be brought into the care of their baby as much as possible. The mother who plans to breastfeed can be assisted in pumping her breasts and freezing the milk, even if enteral feedings are delayed for some time. This pumping may be the only thing that she alone can do for her baby.

Often lost in the bustle of critical care is the need for privacy. The perceptive nurse senses this need and backs away from the bedside when appropriate, allowing the parent some time with the infant.

CONCLUSION

Most infants admitted to the NICU have respiratory illness. Nursing care of these infants requires a broad knowledge of newborn physiology and practical skills in the application of therapies directed toward solving the many problems that sick infants can have. The nurse often must anticipate problems. The neonatal nurse works with two or three patients; he or she must care for a sick infant who desperately needs attention, and he or she must give support to the infant's parents, who are in shock and often are physically and emotionally drained. The rewards for meeting the needs of these individuals are not always immediately evident, but they are great nonetheless.

REFERENCES

Als, H. (1996). The very immature infant enviromental and care issues (pp. 97–107). Presentation at The Physical and Developmental Environment of the High Risk Neonate. Graven Conference, Graven Study Groups of the Physical and Developmental Environment of the High Risk Neonate, Clearwater Beach, FL.

Avery, G. B. (1994). *Neonatology: Pathophysiology and management of the newborn* (4th ed.). Philadelphia: J. B. Lippincott.

Avery, M. E., Gatewood, O. B., & Brumley, G. (1966). Transient tachypnea of the newborn: Possible delayed resorption of fluid at birth. *American Journal of Diseases in Childhood, 111*(4), 380–385.

Bailey, C., Kattwinkel, J., Teja, K., & Buckley, T. (1988). Shallow versus deep endotracheal suctioning in young rabbits: Pathologic effects on the tracheobronchial wall. *Pediatrics, 82*(5), 746–751.

Bancalari, E. (1985). Bronchopulmonary dysplasia. In A. D. Milder & R. J. Martin (Eds.), *Neonatal and pediatric respiratory medicine*. London: Butterworths.

Bland, R. D. (1988). Lung liquid clearance before and after birth. [Review]. *Seminars in Perinatology, 12*(2), 124–133.

Bland, R. D., Hansen, T. N., Haberkern, C. M., Bressack, M. A., Hazinski, T. A., Raju, J. U., & Goldberg, R. B. (1982). Lung fluid balance in lambs before and after birth. *Journal of Applied Physiology, 53*(4), 992–1004.

Breaux, C. W., Jr., Rouse, T. M., Cain, W. S., & Georgeson, K. E. (1991). Improvement in survival of patients with congenital diaphragmatic hernia utilizing a strategy of delayed repair after medical and/or extracorporeal membrane oxygenation stabilization. *Journal of Pediatric Surgery, 26*(3), 333–338.

Brook, I., Martin, W. J., & Finegold, S. M. (1980). Bacteriology of tracheal aspirates in intubated newborn. *Chest 78*(6), 785–877.

Bueuvalas, J. C., & Balisteri, W. F. (1995). The neonatal gastrointestinal tract: Development. In A. A. Fanaroff & R. Martin (Eds.), *Neonatal-perinatal medicine: diseases of the fetus and infant* (15th ed., pp. 1019–1023). St. Louis: C. V. Mosby.

Carlo, W. A., Beoglos, A., Chatburn, R. L., et al. (1989). High frequency jet ventilation in neonatal pulmonary hypertension. *American Journal of Diseases in Childhood, 143*(2), 233–238.

Carlo, W. A., Greenough, A., & Chatburn, R. L. (1994). Advances in conventional mechanical ventilation. In B. R. Boynton, W. A. Carlo, & A. H. Jobe (Eds.), *New therapies for neonatal respiratory failure*. New York: Cambridge University Press.

Carter, J. M., Gerstmann, D. R., Clark, R. H., et al. (1990). High-frequency oscillatory ventilation and extracorporeal membrane oxygenation for the treatment of acute neonatal respiratory failure. *Pediatrics, 85*(2), 159–164.

Cassani, V. L., III (1984). Hypoxemia secondary to suctioning in the neonate. *Neonatal Network, 2*(6), 8–16.

Catlett, A. T., & Holditch-Davis, D. (1991). Environmental stimulation of the acutely ill premature infant: Physiologic effects and nursing implications. *Neonatal Network, 8*(6), 19–26.

Chernick, V. (1990). *Kendig's disorders of the respiratory tract in children* (5th ed.). Philadelphia: W. B. Saunders.

Clark, R. H., Yoder, B. A., & Sell, M. S. (1994). Prospective, randomized comparison of high frequency oscillation and conventional ventilation in candidates for extracorporeal membrane oxygenation. *Journal of Pediatrics, 124*(3), 447–454.

Drummond, W. H., Gregory, G. A., Heymann, M. A., & Phibbs, R. A. (1981). The independent effects of hyperventilation, tolazoline and dopamine on infants with persistent pulmonary hypertension. *Journal of Pediatrics, 98*(4), 603–611.

Farrell, P. M., & Wood, R. E. (1976). Epidemiology of hyaline membrane disease in the United States: Analysis of national mortality statistics. *Pediatrics, 58*(2), 167–176.

Hack, M., Wright, L. L., Shankaran, S., et al. (1995). Very-low-birth weight outcomes of the National Institute of Child Health and Human Development Neonatal Network, November 1989 to October 1990. *American Journal of Obstetrics and Gynecology, 172*(2, Part 1), 457–464.

Hall, B. D. (1979). Choanal atresia and associated multiple anomalies. *Journal of Pediatrics, 95*(3), 395–398.

Harris, T. R. (1988). *Physiologic principles*. In J. P. Goldsmith & E. H. Karotkin (Eds.), *Assisted ventilation of the neonate* (2nd ed.). Philadelphia: W. B. Saunders.

Hay, W. W., Jr., Brockway, J. M., & Eyzaguirre, M. (1989). Neonatal pulse oximetry: Accuracy and reliability. *Pediatrics, 83*(5), 717–722.

Herrell, N., Martin, R. J., Pultusker, M., Lough, M., & Fanaroff, A. (1980). Optimal temperature for the measurement of transcutaneous carbon dioxide tension in the neonate. *Journal of Pediatrics, 97*(1), 114–117.

Horbar, J. D., Wright, L. L., Soll, R. F., et al. (1993). A multicenter randomized trial comparing two surfactants for the treatment of neonatal respiratory distress syndrome. *Journal of Pediatrics, 123*(5), 757–766.

Kattwinkel, J. (1977). Neonatal apnea: Pathogenesis and therapy. *Journal of Pediatrics, 90*(3), 342–347.

Kinsella, J. P., Neish, S. R., Ivy, D. D., et al. (1993). Clinical responses to prolonged treatment of persistent pulmonary hypertension of the newborn with low doses of inhaled nitric oxide. *Journal of Pediatrics, 123*(1), 103–108.

Kinsella, J. P., Neish, S. R., Shaffer, E., & Abman, S. H. (1992). Low-dose inhalation nitric oxide in persistent pulmonary hypertension of the newborn. *Lancet, 340*(8823), 819–820.

Langer, V. S. (1990). Minimal handling protocol for the intensive care nursery. *Neonatal Network, 9*(3), 23–27.

Langston, C. J., & Thurlbeck, W. (1986). Conditions altering normal lung growth & development. In D. Thibeault & G. Gregory (Eds.), *Neonatal pulmonary care* (2nd ed.). Norwalk, CT: Appleton-Century-Crofts.

Naeye, R. L., & Peters, E. C. (1978). Amniotic fluid infections with intact membranes leading to perinatal death: A prospective study. *Pediatrics, 61*(2), 171–177.

Nelson, N. (1994). Physiology of transition. In G. B. Avery, M. A. Fletcher, & M. G. MacDonald (Eds.), *Neonatology, pathophysiology and management of the newborn* (4th ed., pp. 223–247). Philadelphia: J. B. Lippincott.

Polin, R. A., & Burg, F. D. (1983). *Workbook in practical neonatology*. Philadelphia: W. B. Saunders.

Pollitzer, M. J., Whitehead, M. D., Reynolds, E. O., & Delpy, D. (1980). Effect of electrode temperature and in vivo calibration on accuracy of transcutaneous estimation of arterial oxygen tension in infants. *Pediatrics, 65*(3), 515–522.

Prows, C. (1997). Craniofacial defects. Presentation at the University of Cincinnati College of Nursing and Health, Genetics and Fetal Development Class.

Roberts, J. D., Jr., Polaner, D. M., Lang, P., & Zapol, W. M. (1992). Inhaled nitric oxide (NO) in persistent pulmonary hypertension of the newborn. *Lancet, 340*(8823), 818–819.

Ross Laboratories. (1978). *Clinical educations aid #1: Fetal Circulation*. Columbus, OH: Ross Laboratories.

Sakai, H., Tamura, M., Hosokawa, Y., et al. (1987). Effect of surgical repair on respiratory mechanics in congenital diaphragmatic hernia. *Journal of Pediatrics, 111*(3), 432–438.

Schlievert, P., Larsen, B., Johnson, W., & Galask, R. P. (1975). Bacterial growth inhibition by amniotic fluid. Studies on the nature of bacterial inhibition with the use of plate-count determinations. *American Journal of Obstetrics and Gynecology, 122*(7), 814–819.

Speidel, B. D., & Dunn, P. M. (1976). Use of nasal continuous positive airway pressure to treat severe recurrent apnea in very preterm infants. *Lancet, 2*(7987), 658–660.

Thibeault, D. W., & Gregory, G. A. (1986). *Neonatal pulmonary care* (2nd ed.). Norwalk, CT: Appleton-Century-Crofts.

Usher, R. H., Allen, A. C., & McLean, F. H. (1971). Risk of respiratory distress syndrome related to gestational age, route of delivery and maternal diabetes. *American Journal of Obstetrics and Gynecology, 111*(6), 826–832.

CHAPTER 19

New Technologies Applied to the Management of Respiratory Dysfunction

EDWARD F. DONOVAN JONATHAN E. SCHWARTZ LISA M. MOLES

RESEARCH AGENDA

Determine whether neurodevelopmental outcome is improved by methods of ECMO that spare the carotid artery.

Does nitric oxide improve survival of infants with persistent pulmonary hypertension?

Does nitric oxide decrease the necessity of ECMO in infants with persistent pulmonary hypertension?

What types of neonatal respiratory dysfunction are benefited by high-frequency ventilation?

Does one type of high-frequency ventilation have advantages over another for specific types of neonatal lung disease processes?

Is liquid ventilation effective and practical for use in the NICU for infants with surfactant-deficient respiratory distress syndrome?

VIGNETTE

Shawn was born at 28 weeks' gestation and weighed 1.2 kg. He was born at an outlying hospital, where he was managed for approximately 6 hours with head hood O_2. When he needed more ventilatory support, he was intubated and transferred to the regional center for newborn intensive care (RCNIC). At the time of his birth, the RCNIC had just begun to use surfactant therapy for neonatal respiratory distress syndrome (RDS). Shawn was evaluated when he arrived in our unit, and it was determined that he should be given "rescue" surfactant treatment. Within the first hour, Shawn became pink. Pa_{O_2} went from 40 to 80, pH from 7.3 to 7.4, and Pa_{CO_2} from 50 to 35. His ventilator settings were gradually decreased from a peak inspiratory pressure of 30 to 24, rate of 40 to 20, and the end-expiratory pressure was decreased from 4 to 2. During the next 6 hours, Shawn's RDS seemed to worsen. He again required increased ventilatory support. He received a second dose of surfactant. His blood gases improved dramatically. Again his ventilator settings were weaned.

During the next few weeks, Shawn could not be effectively weaned from the ventilator. He had developed pneumonia. In spite of surfactant therapy, he developed mild bronchopulmonary dysplasia (BPD). His parents watched as smaller and less mature infants went home.

Shawn's parents were upset and angry over their son's illness, but they never took their anger out on the staff. As Shawn became a chronic BPD infant, his parents wondered if it might have helped him to receive a dose of surfactant earlier. When I spoke with Shawn's parents several weeks after his birth, they wondered why the "miracle" drug had not worked. I explained that it helped some babies dramatically. With Shawn, the benefit was limited. I talked with them about how Shawn might have been much worse without the drug but that there was no way of knowing for sure. They nodded and stated their hope that they would soon see some progress and that Shawn would be able to go home.

Lisa Spangler-Torok
Lisa Moles

This chapter focuses on innovative technologies and strategies for the management of intractable hypoxemia in the newborn. These include exogenous surfactant administration, extracorporeal membrane oxygenation, high-frequency ventilation, inhaled nitric oxide, and liquid ventilation. To understand the context in which these new techniques were developed, it is important to briefly review the pathophysiology of neonatal hypoxemia as well as the standard modes of therapy for hypoxemia in the newborn.

The prevention of cell injury caused by lack of oxygen is a major focus of newborn intensive care. For appropriate management strategies to be developed for care of the sick neonate, caretakers must have a thorough knowledge of the biochemistry and physiology of the transfer of oxygen from the external environment to the mitochondria, where oxygen-dependent energy supplies (e.g., adenosine triphosphate) are generated. Lack of oxygen availability and therefore decreased cellular energy production lead, in a matter of minutes, to permanent cell injury or cell death.

OVERVIEW OF NORMAL NEONATAL CARDIORESPIRATORY PHYSIOLOGY

For the newborn, the transition from complete dependence on the maternal-placental unit for adequate oxygen delivery to complete respiratory self-reliance must occur rapidly after birth. For oxygen delivery to occur appropriately after separation from the maternal-placental unit, a cascade of newborn responses must

TABLE 19–1 The Neonatal Respiratory System

Components	Functions
Central and peripheral nervous system	Control of breathing
Chest wall (ribs and respiratory muscles)	Pump
Pulmonary circulation	Oxygen uptake from alveoli
Hemoglobin	Oxygen transport
Systemic cardiac output	Oxygen delivery
Mitochondria	Oxygen-dependent energy production

occur immediately (Table 19–1). The newborn's central nervous system must respond to changes in oxygen and carbon dioxide tensions and to other stimuli by generating the necessary efferent signals to establish a regular respiratory pattern with a rate and tidal volume that deliver enough oxygen to the alveoli to meet tissue needs. The newborn chest wall, including its respiratory muscles, must be of sufficient stiffness and strength to respond to the signals received from the central nervous system. The newborn's pulmonary blood flow, both amount and distribution, must be adequate for the task of removing oxygen from the alveolus at a rate that meets the body's needs. Shunting through the ductus arteriosus and foramen ovale must be minimal so that oxygenated blood is delivered systemically and not recirculated to the lungs. The oxygen-carrying capacity of the blood must be appropriate to the limits of cardiac output. The newborn's systemic cardiac output, that is, blood flow to organs other than the lungs, must provide oxygen to the tissues at a rate equivalent to oxygen use. The affinity of hemoglobin for oxygen must be such that oxygen, once delivered, can be appropriately released to the tissues. The distances between the newborn's capillaries and mitochondria must be sufficiently small so that oxygen tension is greater than the minimum needed for normal mitochondrial function. Finally, there must be sufficient activity of the enzymes necessary for oxygen-dependent energy production (Carlo & Chatburn, 1988).

Many neonatal systems must be fully operational within minutes of birth for adequate tissue oxygenation to be achieved. It is not surprising, therefore, that a large proportion of the problems that are dealt with in neonatal intensive care units (NICUs) relate to tissue oxygenation.

PATHOGENESIS OF NEONATAL HYPOXEMIA

Preterm Newborns

The preterm newborn is at risk for multiorgan system dysfunction related to inadequate oxygenation. In the preterm infant, the brain's respiratory control centers sometimes lack sufficient maturity to sustain regular respiration, as manifested by the frequent occurrence of periodic breathing and apnea (Martin et al., 1986). The preterm infant's chest wall has a high compliance, which leads to inefficient breathing. Inward or expiratory movement of the rib cage (retractions) during the inspiratory phase of breathing is seen particularly when the inspiratory effort is increased (Avery et al., 1981). The preterm newborn's respiratory muscles have exercised less in utero compared with those of the full-term newborn; and preterm muscle fiber type distribution suggests that these muscles may be more susceptible to fatigue (Keens & Ianuzzo, 1979).

In the preterm infant, a floppy chest wall (high compliance) is often confronted with a stiff lung (low compliance) owing to surfactant deficiency (Scarpelli et al., 1978). Low compliance means increased work for the respiratory muscles and increased retractions because of the requirement for low intrapleural pressures. In addition, surfactant deficiency leads to airway collapse and intrapulmonary shunting, which severely limit systemic arterial oxygen tension (Boyle & Oh, 1978). The preterm ductus arteriosus tends to remain patent, thus shunting blood away from the systemic organs (Long, 1990).

The preterm newborn's blood hemoglobin concentration is lower than that of the full-term newborn, thereby limiting oxygen-carrying capacity (Strang, 1977). Finally, there may be limits to how much the preterm infant can increase cardiac output to respond to increased oxygen demand or to compensate for other deficits in oxygen delivery (Long, 1990).

Near-Term and Full-Term Newborns

Near-term and full-term newborns frequently experience problems that challenge the neonate's ability to establish adequate tissue oxygenation at birth. Aspiration of meconium, infectious pneumonia, and air leak syndromes occur frequently in these newborns (Miller et al., 1992). Each of these demands increases the work of breathing, and each may be associated with intrapulmonary shunting and hypoxemia. In addition, pulmonary vascular smooth muscle is well developed and normally constricted in the late-gestation fetus (Haworth & Reid, 1976). In the face of lung disease or peripartum asphyxia, pulmonary arterioles may not dilate normally, resulting in a compensatory effort to push blood through the constricted arterioles. It takes higher pressure to attempt to provide adequate oxygenation, with the resultant condition being persistent pulmonary hypertension of the newborn (PPHN). PPHN may result in large right-to-left shunts through the foramen ovale and ductus arteriosus and is therefore associated with severe and sometimes protracted neonatal hypoxemia (Fox & Duara, 1983).

Two additional threats to normal tissue oxygenation at birth are anemia and polycythemia (Ramamurthy & Brans, 1981; Shurin, 1987). Fetal blood is partitioned between the fetus and the placenta, which become separated at birth. It is evident that a variety of events may lead to neonatal anemia secondary to blood loss, including abruption, placenta previa, fetal-maternal hemorrhage, trauma to the cord or fetal placental vessels, nuchal cord, position of the newborn relative to the placenta when the umbilical cord blood flow ceases, and timing of cord clamping. Anemia by any of these mechanisms means decreased blood oxygen-carrying capacity and thus an increased risk for inadequate tissue oxygenation. Polycythemia, often defined as a venous hematocrit greater than 65 percent, may be caused by intrauterine events such as chronic hypoxia and twin-to-twin transfusion or extrauterine events such as delayed cord clamping. Paradoxically, polycythemia increases blood oxygen-carrying capacity but may decrease tissue oxygen delivery by causing poor tissue blood flow or right-to-left ductal shunting.

Neonatal Pulmonary Hypertension

Potentially reversible hypoxemia in newborns that does not respond to increased inspired oxygen concentrations or mechanical ventilation often occurs as a consequence of increased pulmonary vascular resistance. Termed PPHN or persistent fetal circulation, increased pulmonary vascular resistance in newborns with patent fetal circulatory pathways (foramen ovale and ductus arteriosus) leads to a vicious circle of right-to-left (pulmonary-to-systemic) shunting, arterial hypoxemia, and maintenance of pulmonary vasoconstriction.

The fetal pulmonary circulation is characterized by arterial vasoconstriction that produces shunting of umbilical venous blood away from the fetal lung, which, of course, does not serve a respiratory function in utero. Pulmonary vasoconstriction is maintained by relative hypertrophy of the medial smooth muscle of pulmonary arterioles (especially in the third trimester) and fetal hypoxemia. At birth, a variety of events associated with the first breath produce a rapid although incomplete decrease in pulmonary vascular resistance. The most important of these events is an increase in the alveolar and arterial oxygen tension. Other factors leading to pulmonary vasodilation at birth include the mechanical effects of lung expansion and an increase in pH associated with a decrease in PCO_2. Muscularized pulmonary arterioles become remodeled during a period of weeks in the newborn and young infant. This remodeling is associated with a decrease in resting pulmonary vascular resistance.

PPHN is associated with a variety of pathologic perinatal events. After birth, any event associated with alveolar hypoxia may produce a return to the fetal condition of intense pulmonary vasoconstriction. Thus, pneumonia, meconium aspiration syndrome, pneumothorax, and surfactant deficiency may be complicated by pulmonary hypertension because of the associated hypoxia. Perinatal asphyxia complicated by hypoxia and acidosis may also be associated with pulmonary hypertension. Pulmonary hypoplasia as a primary event or secondary to thoracic space-occupying masses such as diaphragmatic hernia is often complicated by increased pulmonary vascular resistance as a consequence of decreased pulmonary vascular cross-sectional area. In addition, pulmonary hypertension may be seen in newborns whose mothers have ingested prostaglandin synthesis inhibitors such as aspirin or indomethacin in the third trimester.

Whatever its cause, PPHN is difficult to treat. Once established, especially when there is a delay in recognition, pulmonary vasoconstriction may not respond as it does with the first breath at birth. Increasing alveolar oxygen tension by giving supplemental oxygen, expanding the lungs with positive-pressure ventilation, and increasing pH by hyperventilation or administration of alkali may have negligible or only transient effects on constricted pulmonary arterioles.

A variety of newborn problems may adversely affect tissue oxygenation. Some of the more common ones have been mentioned. The common denominator for the caretaker in the NICU is the knowledge that inadequate tissue oxygenation for even a brief period may result in permanent cell injury or cell death. The perinatal caretaker's knowledge and skills must include (1) strategies for prevention of the diseases associated with poor tissue oxygenation, (2) an ability to recognize the pathologic event, (3) a detailed understanding of the pathophysiology and treatment of the particular disease entity, and (4) a strategy for rapidly correcting inadequate tissue oxygenation as soon as it is recognized regardless of whether one has made a specific diagnosis.

CONVENTIONAL MANAGEMENT OF NEONATAL HYPOXEMIA

The perinatal caregiver's first line of defense for the prevention or treatment of hypoxemia is to provide an increased inspired oxygen concentration. Although fetal hypoxemia does not respond dramatically to an increase of maternal inspired oxygen concentrations, providing oxygen by mask or nasal cannula to mothers whose fetuses show signs of hypoxia is an accepted mode of therapy in most obstetrical units. Although fetal arterial oxygen tension (PaO_2) increases only a few millimeters of mercury even when maternal PaO_2 increases dramatically, the fact that fetal PaO_2 is usually on the steep portion of the oxygen-hemoglobin dissociation curve means that small changes in fetal PaO_2 are associated with relatively large increases in fetal blood oxygen content (Meschia, 1989).

For the hypoxemic newborn, the response to an increased inspired oxygen concentration depends on the cause of the hypoxemia. When hypoxemia is caused by hypoventilation, PaO_2 increases in an approximately one-to-one relationship with alveolar oxygen tension. Thus, the PaO_2 increases by approximately 60 mm Hg in the hypoventilating newborn placed in 30 percent oxygen. On the other hand, when hypoxemia is caused by an intrapulmonary or extrapulmonary right-to-left shunt (pulmonary-to-systemic shunt), the neonatal PaO_2 increases minimally in response to an increased inspired oxygen concentration. For example, a newborn with a 50 percent right-to-left shunt (i.e., 50 percent of right ventricular output does not pass through the lungs) has a PaO_2 of approximately 50 to 55 mm Hg in room air. Placing the newborn in a head hood containing 100 percent oxygen may raise the PaO_2 to only 60 to 65 mm Hg. Although little is gained in terms of PaO_2, blood oxygen content may increase significantly because of the position and shape of the oxygen-hemoglobin dissociation curve (Strang, 1977). Although increasing the inspired oxygen concentration in the hypoxemic newborn may be essential to prevent permanent cell injury or cell death, this benefit must be weighed against the risk for chronic lung disease due to the toxic effects of pulmonary oxygen.

A second mainstay of current management of the newborn at risk for hypoxemia is the maintenance of an adequate oxygen-carrying capacity by intermittent blood transfusion. Although few scientific studies have been published, it is empirically accepted that prevention and treatment of anemia in the newborn with cardiorespiratory disease are important aspects of management. For example, transfusion of infants with bronchopulmonary dysplasia results in decreased use of oxygen (Alverson et al., 1988). Early studies of human erythropoietin administration to sick newborns suggested that caregivers may be able, in the future, to manage some newborns at risk for anemia without the associated risks of repeated blood transfusions. In one study, six of seven anemic preterm infants receiving human recombinant erythropoietin had an increased or stabilized hematocrit (Halpérin et al., 1990).

A third strategy that may be used to reduce the risk for cell injury secondary to tissue hypoxia is to minimize oxygen demand by minimizing the newborn's metabolic rate. Depending on the specific thermal environment, the neonatal energy (and oxygen) expenditure necessary to keep warm may be great or small (Adamsons et al., 1965). This relationship has been recognized for more than 40 years and has resulted in many studies attempting to define the thermal environment at which the energy expended to keep warm is minimal (neutral thermal environment). Attempts to create a near-neutral thermal environment have been associated with improved survival of sick premature newborns, presumably by favorably affecting the balance between oxygen demand and oxygen supply (Perlstein, 1987).

Another critical factor that affects the delivery of oxygen to the tissues is the adequacy of organ blood flow. Organ blood flow may be globally decreased owing to decreased cardiac output, thus increasing the risk for tissue hypoxia. Methods commonly employed for maintenance of adequate cardiac output include volume expansion of the hypovolemic newborn and inotropic drugs to stimulate the poorly contractile myocardium (Long, 1990). Clinical evaluation is often used to estimate cardiac output, including determination of the rate of capillary refill; determination of the presence or absence of acrocyanosis, skin mottling, or relative coolness of the extremities; and determination of pulse strength and blood pressure. Laboratory aids, including serial hematocrit determinations to diagnose acute blood loss and echocardiography to evaluate cardiac contractility, are at times helpful. Bedside evaluation of neonatal cardiac output remains an inexact science. Techniques for more precise estimation of cardiac output in larger patients, such as indwelling cardiac catheters for measuring mixed venous oxygen, cardiac output, pulmonary vascular resistance, and pulmonary capillary wedge pressure, are not widely available for use in the newborn with evidence of low cardiac output. Research continues in the use of pulsed Doppler and thoracic impedance techniques for the measurement of cardiac output (Belik & Pelech, 1988; Walther et al., 1985).

If determination of the neonatal cardiac output is difficult, determination of the distribution of organ blood flow is almost impossible. Cardiac output may be normal or nearly normal, but some organs may suffer hypoxic insults because of low blood flow. If, for example, necrotizing enterocolitis results in part from decreased intestinal blood flow and thus decreased intestinal oxygenation, it would be useful to be able to estimate that flow. Similarly, decreased urine output may indicate decreased renal blood flow; however, waiting for changes in blood and urine chemistries, such as elevated creatinine, which could be used, for example, in the determination of fractional excretion of sodium, may mean that an irreversible renal hypoxic injury has already occurred. Rapid determination of the distribution of neonatal organ blood flow awaits the development of new methods.

A discussion of strategies now available in NICUs for the management of hypoxemia and hypoxia would not be complete without at least mentioning the widespread use of techniques for measuring or estimating blood oxygen tension or blood oxygen saturation. The direct measurement of PaO_2 and oxygen saturation in small samples of blood (0.1 to 0.2 ml) has been available for several years. Although not in widespread use, indwelling vascular catheters for the continuous measurement of blood PaO_2 or oxygen saturations are available (Harris & Nugent, 1973; Sperinde & Senelly, 1985). Perhaps the most significant technologic development aiding the management of potentially hypoxic sick newborns has been that of noninvasive methods of measuring transcutaneous PaO_2 and transcutaneous oxygen saturation nearly continuously to provide fairly reliable estimations of blood oxygen levels. These critically important new tools for management of sick newborns are discussed in more detail in Chapter 35, Monitoring Neonatal Biophysical Parameters.

TREATMENT OF NEONATAL LUNG DISEASE WITH EXOGENOUS SURFACTANT

It has generally been accepted for more than 30 years that respiratory distress syndrome (RDS), or hyaline membrane disease, is associated with an abnormal gas–liquid interface in the lung (Avery et al., 1981). Normal airways contain a surface-active substance, now called surfactant, that reduces airway and alveolar surface tension and therefore increases lung compliance. In the late 1950s, it was determined that the liquid found in the airways of premature infants and infants of diabetic mothers who died with RDS had a diminished ability to decrease surface tension in vitro (Avery & Mead, 1959; Pattle, 1958). Thus, the hypothesis was developed that decreased lung compliance in infants with RDS was due to lack of surfactant.

RDS is characterized by diffuse pulmonary microatelectasis (Stern, 1984). Manifestations of this atelectasis include tachypnea, low tidal volume breathing, increased inspiratory work with retractions as a consequence of decreased lung compliance, expiratory grunting with increased expiratory airway pressure presumably to prevent further atelectasis, and hypoxemia secondary to intrapulmonary shunting. RDS, as a clinical syndrome, is therefore defined as the immediate onset after birth of tachypnea, retractions, grunting, and cyanosis in a premature infant or infant of a diabetic mother. The chest radiograph in these patients usually confirms the presence of diffuse microatelectasis with uniform increased opacity of the alveolar portions of the lung and widespread air bronchograms (Johnson & Dean, 1982). The arterial carbon dioxide tension ($PaCO_2$) reflects the infant's ability to compensate for decreased lung compliance. Therefore, $PaCO_2$ may be either increased or normal. The PaO_2 on breathing room air is always decreased owing to intrapulmonary shunting. The arterial hydrogen ion concentration (pH) reflects the presence or absence of an elevated $PaCO_2$ and the adequacy of tissue oxygenation. Infants with RDS often have both a metabolic and a respiratory acidosis.

Surfactant Biochemistry and Physiology

Surfactant is generally defined as the noncellular liquid found in the more distal airways and alveoli of normal lungs. Although surfactant contains a mixture of various phospholipids, proteins, and neutral lipids, the extent to which each of these components contributes to the surface tension–decreasing properties of surfactant is not certain.

Surfactant is produced and secreted by cuboid type II pneumocytes that line the distal airways (Stevens et al., 1989). Phospholipids and surfactant-specific proteins are packaged within intracellular lamellar bodies. These are secreted by exocytosis into the liquid lining layer of the airway. Within the hypophase of this liquid interface between the pneumocytes and lung gas, surfactant forms a regular microscopic latticework called tubular myelin. It is thought that surfactant exerts its surface tension–decreasing activity by the movement of certain surfactant components from the hypophase to the gas–liquid interface. Surface tension is decreased by molecular interactions occurring as the gas–liquid interface is compressed during expiration. There is probably an intrapulmonary conservation of surfactant in which "used surfactant" is reabsorbed by the type II pneumocyte, repackaged, and resecreted (Glatz et al., 1982).

Surfactant Replacement

Exogenous surfactant was first given to premature infants with RDS in the mid-1960s. In these studies, dipalmitoylphosphatidylcholine (DPPC) was administered by nebulized aerosol (Chu et al., 1967; Robillard et al., 1964). Clear benefits were not seen in these studies or in similar human trials in the mid-1970s (Enhorning et al., 1973). Studies of tracheal instillation of exogenous surfactants in surfactant-deficient premature rabbits and lambs, also performed in the 1970s, showed more promise than the early human studies of aerosolized surfactant. Survival was improved, and decreased ventilator pressures were required after instillation of surfactant (Enhorning & Robertson, 1972; Nilsson et al., 1978).

The first convincing human study pointing to the possible benefits of exogenous surfactant administration to premature humans with RDS was that of Fujiwara and associates (1980). Fujiwara added extra DPPC and phosphatidylglycerol to an acetone extract of minced bovine lung. Ten premature infants with RDS were given 10 ml of this mixture into the endotracheal tube. These infants were given surfactant on the first day of life. All 10 showed a decreased oxygen requirement and a decreased ventilator positive-pressure requirement.

Since Fujiwara's pioneering work, several different exogenous surfactants have been developed and tested in infants with RDS. These exogenous surfactants can be broadly classified into two types: (1) natural surfactants derived from animal lungs or human amniotic fluid and (2) artificial surfactants composed of "off-the-shelf" chemical mixtures (Table 19–2).

Natural Surfactants

The natural surfactants that have been developed and tested in premature infants include those of bovine, porcine, and human origin. At least three different bovine surfactant preparations have

TABLE 19–2 Exogenous Surfactants

Name	Source	Key Reference
Calf lung surfactant extract	Bovine	Enhorning et al., 1985
Human	Amniotic fluid	Merritt et al., 1986
Curosurf	Porcine	Collaborative European Multicenter Study Group, 1988
Survanta	Bovine	Liechty et al., 1991
Infasurf	Bovine	Kendig et al., 1991
Exosurf	Artificial	Long et al., 1991

been evaluated in premature newborns by use of randomized controlled clinical trials.

An organic solvent extract of fluid obtained by lavage of recently slaughtered calves was developed by Enhorning and coworkers and first reported in 1985. This procedure resulted in a surfactant that contained approximately 97 percent phospholipid, mostly phosphatidylcholine, and a small amount of protein. The solvent extract procedure reduced the proportion of protein in the surfactant from approximately 10 percent to approximately 1 percent. Several controlled trials using this particular surfactant, now referred to as calf lung surfactant extract (CLSE), have been published.

Given intratracheally in the delivery room to 39 newborns of less than 30 weeks' gestation, CLSE resulted in improved oxygenation, decreased respiratory support during the first 72 hours of life, shorter duration of total oxygen therapy, and fewer infants with pulmonary interstitial emphysema (Enhorning et al., 1985). In newborns between 30 and 36 weeks' gestation with RDS, both single and multiple doses of CLSE resulted in improved oxygenation. Improved oxygenation could be maintained by giving up to three additional doses of surfactant. No differences in overall mortality were seen in either of these studies (Dunn et al., 1990).

A similar organic solvent extract of calf lung lavage fluid was used by Egan and associates (1983). This natural surfactant has been extensively studied in premature newborn infants. As with most other surfactants evaluated in recent years, CLSE has been studied as a method of preventing RDS and as a method of improving outcome in newborns who have already developed RDS. As a preventive therapy, surfactant is given intratracheally in the delivery room in the first minutes of life to premature newborns at risk for developing RDS. A double-blind randomized controlled trial of this CLSE given in the delivery room to very premature infants between 24 and 28 weeks' gestation showed that oxygenation was improved and ventilator pressures were decreased in the 14 CLSE-treated infants compared with 13 control infants. The overall death rate and the frequency of bronchopulmonary dysplasia were not different in this study (Kwong et al., 1985).

In another study, a single dose of CLSE given in the delivery room to infants of less than 30 weeks' gestation resulted in improved oxygenation and decreased respiratory support during the first 24 to 72 hours of life, reduced duration of oxygen therapy, and decreased occurrence of pulmonary interstitial emphysema. CLSE in this study was not associated with decreased overall mortality or decreased frequency of bronchopulmonary dysplasia (Shapiro et al., 1985).

Administering surfactant in the delivery room to infants at risk for developing RDS inevitably means that some infants who may not have surfactant deficiency will be subjected to the adverse effects of intratracheal surfactant administration. In a large randomized controlled trial, use of CLSE in a prevention mode (delivery room administration) was compared with use of CLSE in a rescue mode (given only to infants with established RDS). More infants less than 30 weeks' gestation survived in the prevention group: 88 percent versus 80 percent (Kendig et al., 1991).

Although these results are encouraging, the adverse effects of delivery room intubation of infants who do not otherwise require intubation are poorly understood. One study of long-term outcome demonstrated some advantages of rescue therapy compared with prevention (Vaucher et al., 1990). Avery and Merritt (1991) suggested that early identification of those infants with documented surfactant deficiency may allow us to maximize the benefits of early surfactant therapy. In addition, strategies for assisted ventilation could be improved to minimize lung injury in the hours before surfactant administration.

The other bovine surfactant subjected to controlled clinical trial was developed by Fujiwara in Japan and adopted by Abbott Laboratories for testing in the United States. This natural surfactant has also been tested in both the prevention and the rescue modes. Given as a single preventive dose in the first 15 minutes of life to infants between 750 and 1250 g birth weight, this bovine surfactant (Survanta) was associated with a decreased average fraction of inspired oxygen (FiO_2). No differences in alveolar to arterial oxygen ratio, mean airway pressure, or severity of respiratory disease at age 28 days were noted (Soll et al. & Ross Collaborative Surfactant Prevention Study Group, 1990).

In a multicenter placebo-controlled rescue study of single-dose Survanta given before 8 hours of age, infants with birth weights between 750 and 1750 g showed no differences in survival or respiratory outcome at age 28 days. Oxygenation was improved and mean airway pressure was decreased during the first 72 hours of life (Horbar et al., 1989). Similar results were observed in two smaller trials of single-dose Survanta used in the rescue mode (Gitlin et al., 1987; Raju et al., 1987).

Several controlled clinical trials of multiple doses of Survanta given either as rescue or as prevention demonstrated significantly decreased mortality in Survanta-treated infants. Unfortunately, the frequency of bronchopulmonary dysplasia is not reduced (Hoekstra et al., 1991; Liechty et al., 1991) (Fig. 19–1).

A protein-depleted organic solvent extract of minced porcine lung (Curosurf) has been evaluated in Europe. In the rescue mode, Curosurf was administered to infants with RDS with birth weights between 700 and 2000 g between 2 and 15 hours of age. Infants randomized to receive Curosurf showed improved oxygenation, decreased occurrence of air leaks, decreased frequency of bronchopulmonary dysplasia, and improved survival (51 percent versus 31 percent). The relatively high mortality in the control group in this study suggests significant unknown differences between this population and those studied with use of other surfactants (Collaborative European Multicenter Study Group, 1988).

A small multicenter randomized study of infants weighing 700 to 1500 g compared Curosurf with Survanta (Speer et al., 1995). This study found that both drugs rapidly reduced oxygen and ventilatory requirements. Curosurf-treated infants had significantly higher arterial to alveolar oxygen ratios and significantly lower mean airway pressures. Trends that did not reach statistical significance showed a lower frequency of pneumothorax (6 percent versus 12.5 percent), intracranial hemorrhage (3 percent versus 12.5 percent), and mortality (3 percent versus 12.5 percent) in the Curosurf group.

The only other natural surfactant to have been subjected to controlled clinical trial was extracted from human amniotic fluid collected at the time of cesarean section delivery. Sterilely collected amniotic fluid was centrifuged to produce a surfactant-containing pellet. Purified human surfactant was obtained by passing the pellet over a discontinuous buffered sucrose density gradient (Hallman et al., 1983). Appropriate surface activity was ensured before use. This preparation of human surfactant contains larger amounts of protein than do the other natural surfac-

Store Refrigerated

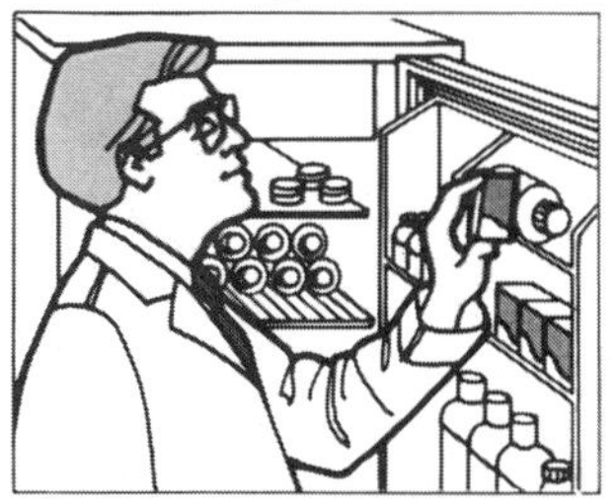

Store unopened SURVANTA vials at refrigeration temperature (2 to 8 C). Protect from light. Store vials in carton until ready for use. Some settling may occur during storage. If this occurs, swirl the vial gently (DO NOT SHAKE) to redisperse.

Do NOT Shake

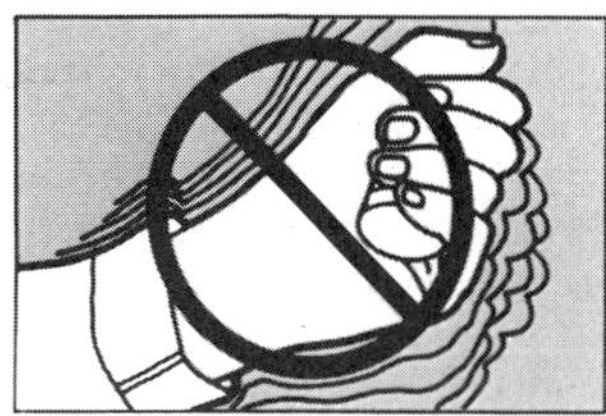

SURVANTA does not require reconstitution or sonication. If settling occurs during storage, swirl the vial gently to redisperse. Single-dose SURVANTA vials are for SINGLE USE ONLY. Discard used SURVANTA vials.

Warm at Room Temperature or With the Hand

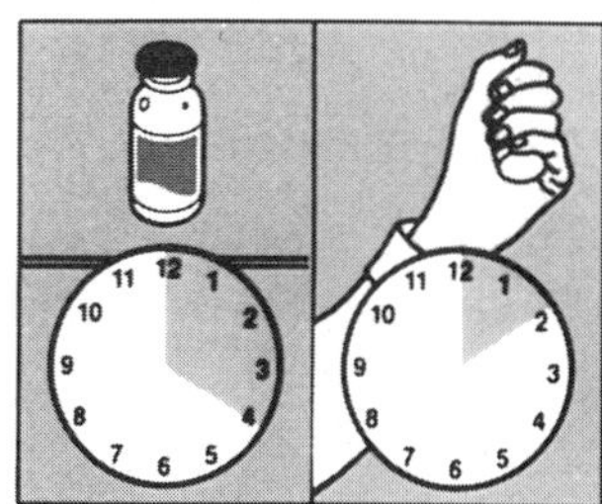

SURVANTA does not require reconstitution or sonication. Do not use artificial warming methods. Before use, warm by standing the vial at room temperature for 20 minutes or holding in the hand for 8 minutes.
DO NOT SHAKE.

Administration Requirements

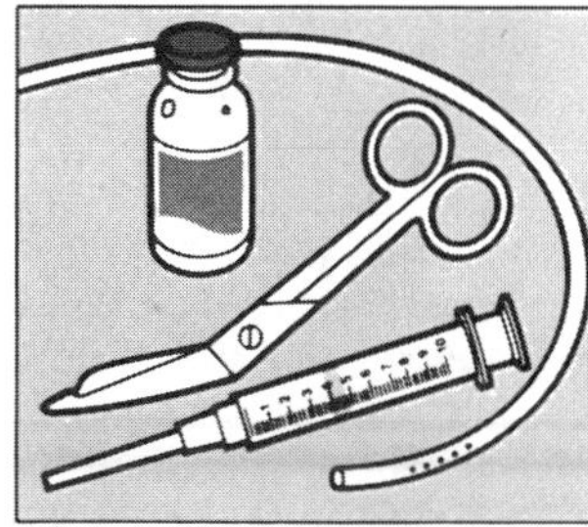

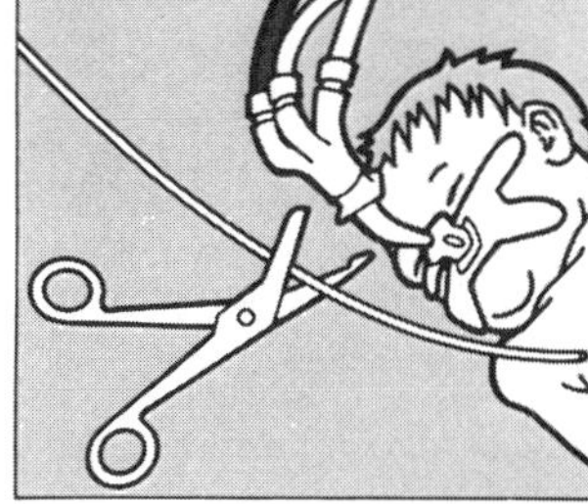

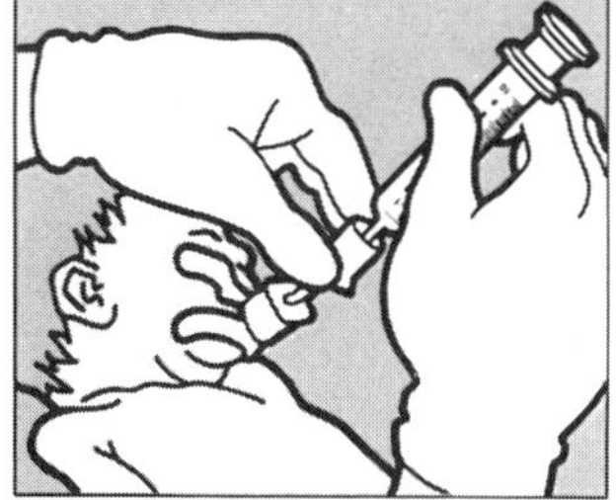

SURVANTA is administered intratracheally by instillation through a 5 French end-hole catheter inserted into the infant's endotracheal tube. Before inserting the catheter through the endotracheal tube, the length of the catheter should be shortened sufficiently so that when passed through the endotracheal tube, the tip of the catheter will protrude just beyond the end of the endotracheal tube in the infant's trachea. The end of the endotracheal tube should be positioned above the infant's carina. SURVANTA should not be instilled into a main-stem bronchus. SURVANTA is withdrawn from the vial into the syringe through a large (16 gauge) needle. DO NOT FILTER SURVANTA.

Dosing

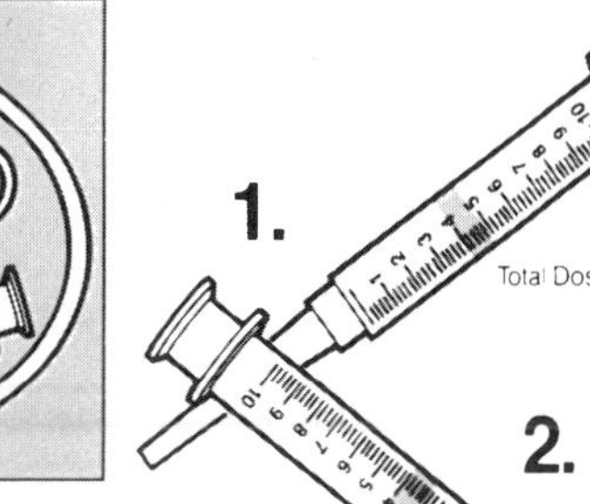

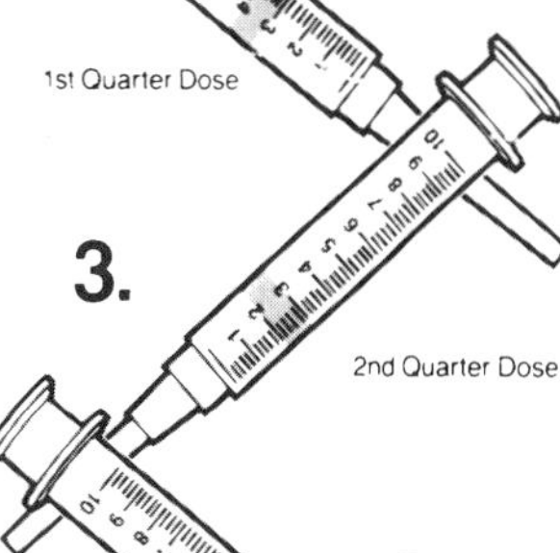

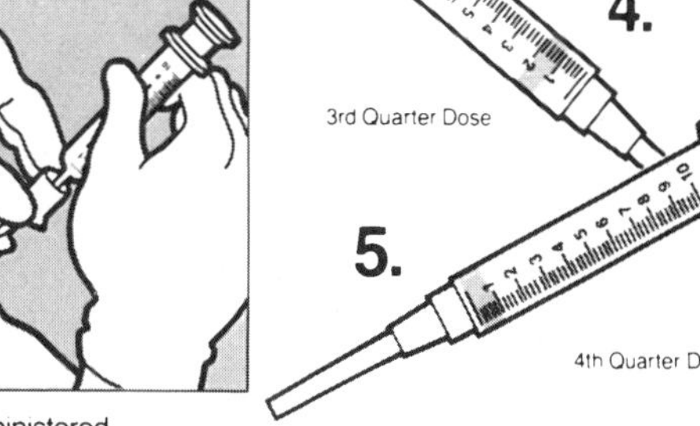

Each dose of SURVANTA is 100 mg phospholipids kg birth weight (4 mL kg). This total dose is administered to the infant in four separate quarter doses. The volume of each quarter dose is approximately one fourth the total dose (approximately 1 mL kg per quarter dose). The dose pictured is for an infant 951 to 1000 g birth weight only.

Gently inject each quarter dose through the catheter over 2 to 3 seconds.

Administration

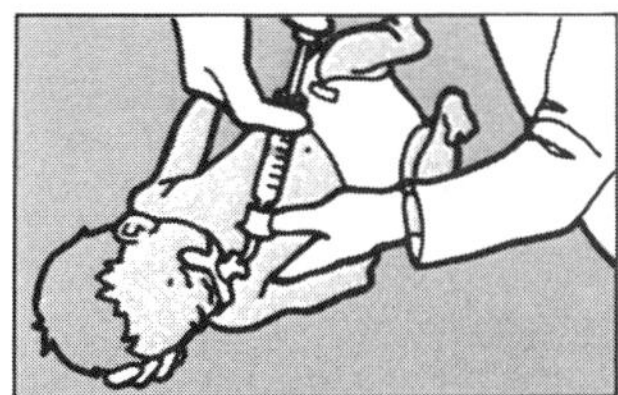

1. Infant's head and body inclined slightly down, head turned to the right.

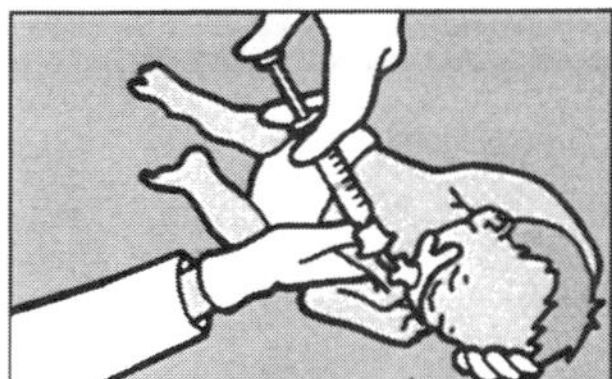

2. Head and body inclined slightly down, head turned to the left.

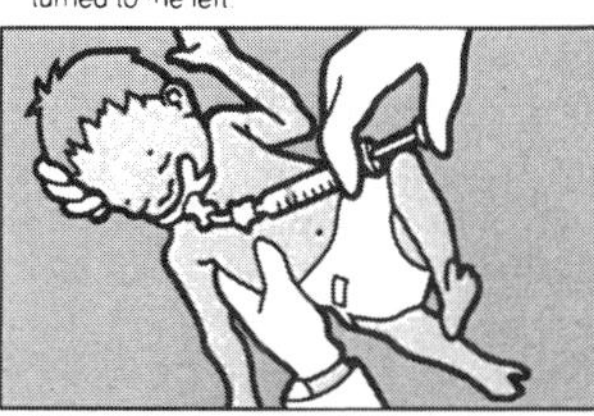

3. Head and body inclined slightly up, head turned to the right.

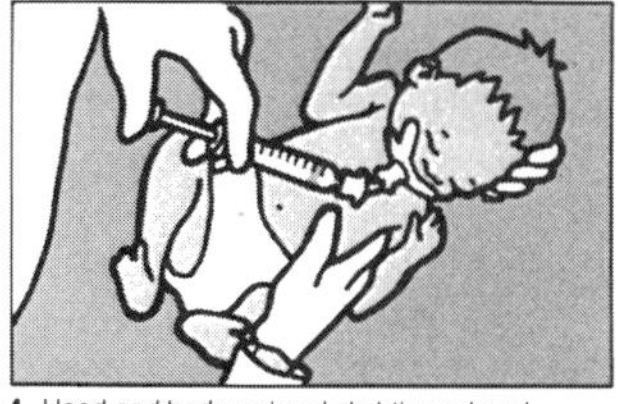

4. Head and body inclined slightly up, head turned to the left.

The total dose of SURVANTA is administered in four separate quarter doses. To ensure uniform distribution of SURVANTA throughout the lungs, each quarter dose should be administered with the infant in a different position. A recommended sequence is pictured above. The dosing procedure is facilitated if one person administers the dose while another person positions and monitors the infant.

Please see package enclosure for full prescribing information.

FIGURE 19–1. Survanta product preparation and administration guide. (Reprinted with permission of Ross Laboratories, Columbus, OH 43216.)

tants that have been evaluated. There is accumulating evidence that the specific proteins found as components of surfactant in the airways are integral to surfactant turnover and function (Robertson et al., 1988). Administered as a single dose intratracheally in the delivery room to newborns between 24 and 29 weeks' gestation, human surfactant was associated with reduced mortality (from 84 percent to 48 percent), decreased frequency of bronchopulmonary dysplasia, and fewer air leaks (Merritt et al., 1986). In the rescue mode, one or two doses of human surfactant resulted in improved oxygenation, decreased ventilator pressures, and decreased frequency of air leaks. In this study of infants less than 30 weeks' gestation with RDS, fewer surfactant-treated infants died or developed bronchopulmonary dysplasia before age 28 days (Hallman et al., 1985). In another study using a similar rescue study design, neither mortality nor frequency of bronchopulmonary dysplasia was improved in infants between 24 and 32 weeks' gestation receiving one or two doses of human surfactant. Although early surfactant therapy was statistically associated with improved survival, this was apparently a retrospective observation (Lang et al., 1990).

One study has been designed to determine whether up to four doses of human surfactant given as preventive therapy at birth is of greater net benefit than human surfactant given after the onset of severe RDS in infants of 24 to 29 weeks' gestation. Compared with infants who received placebo, human surfactant–treated infants had improved oxygenation and decreased frequency of pulmonary interstitial emphysema. Overall mortality was not reduced, and no benefit of treatment at birth compared with treatment at a mean age of 220 minutes was seen (Merritt et al., 1991).

Artificial Surfactants

Two different artificial surfactants have been tested in newborn infants with RDS. Artificial surfactants may be distinguished from natural surfactants by the absence of the surfactant-associated proteins.

A mixture of DPPC and phosphatidylglycerol has been evaluated by several investigators in England. Two controlled clinical trials have been published: a preventive trial and a rescue or treatment trial. This particular surfactant is administered as a dry powder that is forced down an endotracheal tube by positive-pressure bag breathing. Use of this dry surfactant resulted in no improvement in oxygenation, no reduction in ventilator pressures, and no reduction in mortality (Wilkinson et al., 1985). In a multicenter trial, 100 mg of a similar phospholipid mixture was suspended by shaking it in 1 ml of saline and administering it into the pharynx at birth in newborn infants between 25 and 29 weeks' gestation. If they were endotracheally intubated, infants received up to three additional doses of this artificial surfactant. Control infants received saline. In this large study, artificial surfactant significantly reduced mortality from 27 percent to 14 percent (Ten Centre Study Group, 1987).

Exosurf Neonatal, an artificial surfactant manufactured by Burroughs Wellcome Company (1990), is composed of DPPC, cetyl alcohol, and tyloxapol. Several studies have evaluated the safety and efficacy of this product. A multicenter placebo-controlled trial of a single delivery room dose of Exosurf given to infants between 700 and 1350 g birth weight revealed that Exosurf administration resulted in a decreased fraction of inspired oxygen to maintain adequate oxygenation. Neither neonatal death nor bronchopulmonary dysplasia was significantly decreased by Exosurf administration (Phibbs et al., 1991).

A much larger trial of a single prophylactic dose of Exosurf demonstrated more promising results. A total of 446 newborns between 700 and 1100 g were randomly assigned to receive either 5 ml of Exosurf or 5 ml of air endotracheally. Mortality at both age 28 days and age 1 year was significantly reduced. Air leaks, oxygen requirements, and ventilator pressures were also reduced (Corbet et al. & the American Exosurf Pediatric Study Group, 1991).

Two doses of Exosurf were given as rescue therapy to infants with RDS weighing 700 to 1350 g in a multicenter double-blind placebo-controlled trial. The first dose was given between 2 and 24 hours of age. The second dose was given 12 hours after the first dose. Pulmonary function improved with Exosurf, as evidenced by an improvement in the arterial to alveolar oxygen pressure ratio and decreased ventilator pressure requirement. The neonatal mortality rates were decreased from 23 percent to 11 percent. The frequency of bronchopulmonary dysplasia was not decreased (Long et al. & the American Exosurf Neonatal Study Group, 1991).

A large multicenter randomized study comparing Exosurf and Survanta in neonates 501 to 1500 g reported by the National Institutes of Child Health and Human Development Neonatal Research Network suggested that both surfactants are reasonable choices for use in infants with RDS (Horbar et al., 1993). There were no significant differences between the two surfactants in frequency of death, bronchopulmonary dysplasia, intracranial hemorrhage, pulmonary hemorrhage, or patent ductus arteriosus. There was, however, a difference in response to treatment in the first 72 hours as evidenced by significantly lower FiO_2 and mean airway pressures in the Survanta-treated group.

Although a variety of different surfactants have been evaluated and are currently in use, we do not yet have an optimal method of surfactant administration. Because surfactant is expected to reach noncolonized portions of the lung, sterile technique must be used during dosing. Surfactant exerts its effect in the distal airways, yet it must be delivered to the upper airway and find its way distally. Surfactant has been given as a dry or wet aerosol and as a liquid bolus into the pharynx or trachea. As a detergent-type substance, surfactant spreads rapidly on the gas–liquid interface of the lung to reach its primary site of action. Because surfactant must be delivered into the upper airway, administration is associated with transient interruption of ventilation. Some surfactants are given by bolus during disconnection of the endotracheal tube from the ventilator tubing. Exosurf is given through a side port on specially designed endotracheal tube adapters. All surfactants produce transient gas-exchange abnormalities during administration of the dose, usually hypoxemia and hypercarbia. Transcutaneous PO_2, PCO_2, and oxygen saturation should be monitored continuously during the dosing procedure. Physiologic instability should be expected during dosing. The studies previously described suggest that respiratory compliance will often increase after a dose of surfactant is given. The time course of this change in compliance has not been studied but probably varies with the type of patient and the type of surfactant used. Thus, close monitoring of blood gases and ventilator settings is warranted for a period of 8 to 12 hours after each dose. Under all but emergency circumstances, the American Academy of Pediatrics recommends that surfactant be administered only in nurseries able to sustain long-term mechanical ventilation (Merenstein et al., 1991).

Although exogenous surfactant is used in most tertiary NICUs in the United States, many questions about surfactant administration remain unanswered. The importance of the surfactant-associated proteins to neonatal outcome is unknown. Determination of the appropriate timing, dose, and method of surfactant administration awaits additional clinical trials. There is general agreement that exogenous surfactant administration provides a net benefit to sick newborns with RDS. However, the mortality rates and frequency of chronic lung disease remain high in surfactant-treated infants. Moreover, well-designed research studies to address the questions surrounding the use of surfactant in infants with respiratory compromise need to be done.

Nursing Care: Surfactant Therapy

Nurses play an important role in caring for infants receiving surfactant replacement therapy in the NICU. The nursing care of the infants before, during, and after surfactant administration is unique to this treatment modality. It is important for nurses to have a working knowledge of the specific care needs of infants treated with surfactant.

Before administration of surfactant, nurses should consider several factors. Accurate weights of the infants must be determined to ensure the proper doses of surfactant to be given. Confirmation of proper placement of the infants' endotracheal tubes by chest radiographs must be documented. These infants should have continuous cardiac and respiratory monitoring. Cardiac monitoring may include electrocardiograms as well as arterial catheters. Respiratory monitoring may include transcutaneous measurement of PO_2 or PCO_2 and pulse oximetry. Nurses may also suggest sedation or increases in ventilator settings before dosing for infants who do not tolerate handling or who become hypoxic quickly. Another essential component of nursing care of infants before surfactant therapy is administered is endotracheal suctioning. These infants should be suctioned approximately 15 minutes before surfactant dosing to rid the infants of secretions that may inhibit the administration of the surfactant.

The nursing care of infants during surfactant dosing is also unique to this treatment modality. Of utmost importance during dosing is the ongoing nursing assessment and monitoring of the infants. Because dosing with surfactant may be stressful for the infants, nurses must be alert for signs that indicate the need to slow or stop the dosing momentarily to allow the infants to recover. Some signs that the infants may be stressed by dosing include bradycardia, duskiness, and decrease in transcutaneous Po_2 or oxygen saturation. During administration of surfactant, assessment and monitoring of the infants need not be minimized.

Optimal positioning of infants during surfactant administration is another critical facet of nursing care. Infants receive some surfactants, such as Survanta, in four aliquots, each in a different body position (see Fig. 19–1).

The infants are positioned head down, head turned to the right; head down, head turned to the left; head up, head turned to the right; and head up, head turned to the left (Horbar et al., 1989). The infants are held in each position for 30 seconds after the dose is administered into the endotracheal tube. Administration of Exosurf requires only turning the head from midline to the right, then midline to the left.

Last, nurses have specific responsibilities after surfactant is administered to infants. Again, nursing assessment and monitoring are important, just as during dosing. Immediately after dosing, the nurse should assess the infant's skin color, respirations, oxygen saturation, and transcutaneous monitoring. Arterial blood gas should be sampled and the ventilator weaned appropriately. Surfactant produces changes in pulmonary compliance that may require rapid weaning of ventilator settings. However, infants may also experience respiratory distress immediately after dosing. Therefore, astute assessment skills are necessary in caring for infants after they have received surfactant therapy. Endotracheal suctioning is delayed after dosing of surfactant for at least 1 to 2 hours to prevent removal of the instilled surfactant (Miller & Armstrong, 1990).

These infants require continuous monitoring of oxygen saturations. The surfactant may suddenly raise a saturation from the 40s to well above 100 to 200. The side effects of this effective therapy are sudden changes in cerebral blood flow, which makes intraventricular hemorrhage a real possibility, and changes in retinal blood flow increase chances for retinopathy of prematurity. Just as rapidly as the arterial oxygen saturation improved after administration, it may fall back to presurfactant levels. The nurse must monitor the situation and often adjust the ventilator settings or oxygen percentage. This situation is a catch-22 in the sense that the side effects of the therapy are also natural adverse reactions to RDS as well.

CONVENTIONAL VENTILATORY SUPPORTS AND RESPIRATORY CONSIDERATIONS

Although this chapter focuses on new technologies, it is important that standard ventilation therapies be mentioned. Conventional techniques include time-cycled ventilation; pressure-limited ventilation; continuous or intermittent ventilation; continuous positive airway pressure (CPAP) ventilation; and intermittent mandatory ventilation (IMV), which may or may not be synchronized with neonatal spontaneous breathing. A brief description of each is given.

Time-cycled ventilators are based on lung compliance. Positive inspiratory pressure (PIP) is directly related to the lung's compliance or ability to distend and the gas flow through the ventilator's circuit. Changes in pressure relate to the neonate's oxygen saturation level (Hargett, 1995). The caregiver sets the cycle of time in which breaths are delivered. Pressure, rates, flow, PIP, and positive end-expiratory pressure (PEEP) are adjusted on the basis of the pulmonary assessment of the infant. This form of ventilation is standard therapy in many NICUs today.

Volume-dependent ventilators are sometimes used but with caution. The concern is that these can lead to barotrauma by delivering more pressure than is necessary. The settings on this machine are regulated according to value changes and the pressure changes in response. The pressure changes reflect the lung compliance and pulmonary resistance. Tidal volumes of 6 to 15 ml/kg are necessary for this type of ventilation (Hargett, 1995). Hargett set volume of 2 to 3 ml/cm H_2O, depending on circuit and humidifier being used (p. 298). This is due to compression of some of the volume within the circuit itself. Difficulties arise when there are any air leaks in the system (i.e., around an endotracheal tube) because these translate into loss of volume delivered to the neonatal lung.

CPAP is on the way back into favor in NICUs. It was a method in the past for weaning a neonate from conventional mechanical ventilation (CMV). However, with the initiation of use of maternal steroids and surfactant in the very low birth weight infant, many neonates go most immediately to CPAP. This allows spontaneous breathing while a continuous gas volume is being delivered to the pulmonary circuit. This continuous pressure inflates the lung, makes breathing easier, and facilitates alveolar gas exchange. This type of support is often all that is needed if compliance is not the underlying problem. CPAP is still used for weaning purposes too because it provides pulmonary support but no set breaths per minute. It is often maintained by an endotracheal tube that allows quick return to CMV if necessary. It may also be done by nasal prong or orally. A complication of CPAP is barotrauma from overdistention of the lungs. A neonate may also tire out from the work of breathing, and it may result too in carbon dioxide build-up. Capillary blood flow at the pulmonary level can also be impeded, especially if there is an overdistention of the entire lung or areas of blebs that become overinflated (Bateman et al., 1995).

IMV provides a continuous flow of oxygen/air through the ventilatory circuit; however, the neonate can breathe spontaneously. The term mandatory refers to the number of mandatory breaths per minute that are set by the caregiver. The settings allow PIP, rates, inspiratory time, and flow to be adjusted to individual ventilation. This type of ventilation has been used as a method of weaning (Hargett, 1995).

An alternative form of IMV is referred to as synchronized IMV. This system encourages the neonate to breathe in synchrony with the ventilator. It is patient triggered. Hargett (1995) identified the neonatal benefits of this ventilation to be generally centered on improved oxygenation through better tidal volume at the same PIP (p. 200), reduced need for long-term ventilation or for sedation, and reduced complications such as barotrauma and intracranial bleeds.

Ventilatory adjustments must be based on thorough assessments of the pulmonary system. This includes physical assessment and laboratory tests. It must be done with full consideration of the total clinical case situation of the neonate. PIP is based on the lowest level that will maintain an acceptable tidal volume. Tidal volumes are gauged at 6 to 15 ml/kg (Hargett, 1995). When adjustments are made of 1 to 2 cm H_2O, the expected change is in the arterial oxygen. It should always be started at a low level and increased on the basis of the clinical picture.

PEEP is used to distend the alveolar tissue, which has a tendency in the neonate to collapse with each breath. If PEEP is not maintained, the neonate is always taking the first breath and expending a tremendous amount of energy. Levels, like PIP, should be started low at 2 to 6 cm H_2O and adjusted in relationship to the PIP so that the tidal volume is affected. It is the difference between these two values that determines the tidal volume.

Oxygen levels are aimed at keeping arterial blood gases within normal ranges of 80 to 100 mm Hg. The lowest level that maintains normal ranges should be sought. A Fio_2 of 0.4 to 0.6

is usually considered an acceptable safe level (Hargett, 1995, p. 303).

Rate is set on the basis of the neonate's alveolar ventilation needs. A conservative approach is to set a low rate of about half the expected respiratory rate (i.e., 30 breaths per minute). The PIP in this case would generally be set slightly higher than normal to maintain a normal tidal volume. If a higher rate in the range of 40 to 60 breaths per minute is used, less PIP will generally be needed to maintain the tidal volume.

Inspiratory time is generally set in relationship to the expiratory time. The less compliant the lungs, the shorter the inspiratory time, because lungs are not expanding easily. Long inspiratory times have been associated with barotrauma caused by overdistention of the lungs (Hargett, 1995). However, longer inspiratory times are needed when there are mechanical obstructions to gas flow, such as in meconium aspiration.

Adjustments of inspiratory time result in changes in arterial oxygen levels. An inspiratory time of 0.25 to 0.4 second is acceptable in most cases (Hargett, 1995). Inspiratory time to expiratory time ratios are normally maintained at 1:2 or 1:3.

Flow rate of the ventilatory circuit is calculated as twice the minute volume of the infant (Hargett, 1995, p. 305). This is usually between 3 and 10 ml/min.

These are just a few of the conventional respiratory supports that are commonly used in neonatal care. They give a framework for understanding the new technologies, such as high-frequency ventilation (HFV).

HIGH-FREQUENCY VENTILATION

In contrast to HFV, CMV uses ventilator rates and tidal volumes that correspond to the spontaneous ventilation patterns of newborns. High mean and peak airway pressures may be required during CMV to adequately ventilate noncompliant lungs (Carlo & Chatburn, 1988). Exposure to high inflating pressures may lead to lung and airway injury, including pulmonary interstitial emphysema, pneumothoraces, bronchopleural fistulas, and bronchopulmonary dysplasia. HFV attempts to avoid these complications by delivering low tidal volumes at high frequencies. HFV may be used as a "rescue" technique to prevent further damage in infants who have developed complications secondary to CMV. HFV allows severely ill infants to be adequately ventilated at lower volumes than with CMV while improving gas exchange (Merenstein & Gardner, 1989). HFV may be used perioperatively and postoperatively to reduce movement of the airway and thoracic cavity (Carlo & Chatburn, 1988). HFV may be beneficial to infants who have pre-existing pneumothoraces or bronchopleural fistulas. One study showed that when these infants were treated with HFV, there was a decrease in air flow through the pneumothorax and the fistula. They were also able to wean the peak and mean airway pressures of these infants while maintaining adequate gas exchange (Gonzalez et al., 1987).

There is no generally accepted ventilator rate at which one may use the term high frequency. Respiratory disease in the newborn is commonly associated with tachypnea. Thus, respiratory rates in the spontaneously breathing newborn with surfactant deficiency, pneumonia, or meconium aspiration often reach 80 to 100 breaths per minute. Under the assumption that tachypnea represents an efficient, spontaneous breathing strategy that minimizes respiratory work, CMV frequencies often mimic this tachypnea. Another common rationale for selecting a rapid ventilator rate is so that the newborn may breathe in synchrony with the ventilator. The tachypneic newborn who breathes spontaneously during CMV often makes spontaneous inspiratory efforts at frequencies that exactly match the selected mechanical ventilation rate as long as this rate is sufficiently great. Thus, a newborn who tends to breathe "against the ventilator" when the ventilator rate is set at so-called normal frequencies (40 to 50 breaths per minute) may breathe in synchrony with the ventilator if the ventilator rate is increased to 60 to 80 breaths per minute.

A definition of high frequency based on the physical characteristics of gas transport has been suggested (Venegas et al., 1986). At low frequencies, gas transport may be accounted for entirely by convective or bulk flow in which the gas volume transported is proportional to the product of velocity and cross-sectional area. At these frequencies, carbon dioxide excretion by the lung, for example, can be attributed entirely to the bulk flow of gas from the alveolus to the airway opening. At very high frequencies, carbon dioxide elimination cannot be explained by bulk flow calculations. The respiratory rate or frequency at which gas transport begins to occur by mechanisms other than bulk flow has been called the transitional frequency. For the adult human, the transitional frequency has been calculated to be approximately 170 breaths per minute. Thus, adult ventilators that operate at frequencies greater than 170 breaths per minute might be called high-frequency ventilators. Because the transitional frequency may be greater for the respiratory system of the newborn than for that of the adult, neonatal high-frequency ventilators, by this definition, are likely to operate at frèquencies greater than 200 to 300 breaths per minute.

High-frequency ventilators, however one defines them, may be characterized by their expiratory phase as either passive or active (Fredberg et al., 1987) (Table 19–3). With some high-frequency ventilators, such as the jet and flow interrupter, expiration occurs by passive recoil of the distended respiratory system (lung and chest wall). With passive HFV, the expired volume is limited by both the flow rates generated during passive recoil and the small expiratory time. Because these factors may act in concert to decrease expired volume, hyperinflation is more common with passive HFV. Hyperinflation during passive HFV is likely to result in the same complications as those of hyperinflation due to other causes, namely, air leak, increased carbon dioxide levels, and decreased cardiac output. Hyperinflation is made worse when the expiratory time is decreased, when tidal volume is increased, and when the infant's respiratory time constant is increased by either increased compliance or increased resistance.

The oscillator-type high-frequency ventilators are characterized by active expiration, during which gas is sucked out of the lung. These high-frequency ventilators function by a reciprocating pump analogous to a syringe's being alternately pushed and pulled. A bias flow flushes the system and maintains constant inspired gas concentrations. Because expired volume equals inspired volume with active high-frequency ventilators, the risk for hyperinflation is decreased compared with that associated with the use of passive high-frequency ventilators. Gas trapping or hyperinflation may still occur, however, when patients are mechanically ventilated with active high-frequency ventilators. Because pressure within the airway is subatmospheric during the active expiratory phase, portions of the airway may close during expiration, thus trapping gas distally.

Passive and active high-frequency ventilators differ in the manner in which airway pressure is monitored. During passive HFV, airway pressure is monitored distally in specially designed endotracheal tubes. Despite these special techniques, the measured

TABLE 19–3 Classification of High-Frequency Neonatal Ventilators

Type	Maximal Rate (breaths/min)	Expiration
Pressure limited, time cycled	150	Passive
Jet	250–300	Passive
Oscillator	1800	Active

airway pressure may not accurately reflect the actual pulmonary distending pressure. By use of appropriate ventilator circuits and ventilators, airway pressure during active HFV may be monitored more accurately even when conventional endotracheal tubes are used (Bancalari et al., 1987).

Passive and active high-frequency ventilators differ in two additional important ways. First, the very high driving pressure required during the inspiratory phase of passive HFV creates very high, although brief, inspiratory flow rates. Maintaining adequate humidification at these flow rates requires specially designed humidification systems. In contrast, active HFV requires conventional gas flows, and therefore humidification may be achieved with the same humidifiers as are used in CMV. Another difference between passive and active HFV is that very high rates (greater than 300 breaths per minute) cannot be used with passive HFV because of hyperinflation. Active HFV, on the other hand, allows the use of ventilator rates as high as 1800 breaths per minute.

Although important functional differences between passive and active high-frequency ventilators exist, experience with neonatal HFV is limited and controlled clinical trials are few. It is generally accepted that HFV has been useful in the management of newborns with severe pulmonary interstitial emphysema. The primary benefit of HFV in the management of pulmonary interstitial emphysema is that airway pressures may be significantly reduced, thus theoretically decreasing the risk for further air leak, other pressure-related airway injury, and decreased cardiac output (Gaylord et al., 1987). At this time, no controlled trials have been performed to evaluate the safety and efficacy of HFV, either active or passive, in the treatment of pulmonary interstitial emphysema.

Uncontrolled trials of HFV in the management of neonatal pulmonary hypertension have been published (Carlo et al., 1989). These experiences suggest that HFV may be helpful in the management of newborns with meconium aspiration syndrome, congenital diaphragmatic hernia, and neonatal pulmonary hypertension without primary lung disease. Although difficult to perform, randomized clinical trials are necessary to demonstrate that HFV does indeed carry a net benefit in newborns with these diseases. In the absence of such trials, the clinician must rely on determining whether conventional therapy has failed in a given patient and whether a new, unproven therapy should be attempted.

The first randomized trial of HFV used in the management of premature newborns with RDS has been published (HIFI Study Group, 1989). In this multicenter trial, 673 newborns with RDS were randomly assigned to either CMV or HFV with active expiration. No differences in mortality or frequency of bronchopulmonary dysplasia were seen. A greater occurrence of intraventricular hemorrhage was seen in newborns assigned to the high-frequency ventilator with active expiration. Although these findings are disappointing, animal studies suggest that the ventilator strategy used in this trial may have been as important as the type of ventilator used in determining the outcome. This study was carried out at a time when the chief benefit of HFV was thought to be that it allowed a lower mean airway pressure. Thus, the ventilator strategies used may have emphasized higher frequency at low pressures, thus producing alveolar collapse.

A randomized trial compared modes of ventilation in 83 infants less than 1.75 kg with acute respiratory failure (Clark et al., 1992). Infants were randomized to receive CMV alone, high-frequency oscillatory ventilation (HFOV) alone, or HFOV for 72 hours followed by CMV. No differences were seen between any groups with respect to death, pulmonary air leak syndromes, or intracranial hemorrhage. There was a significantly lower frequency of bronchopulmonary dysplasia at 30 days of age and 36 weeks of postconceptional age in infants managed with HFOV alone. This finding was not seen in infants who received HFOV for 72 hours and were then switched to CMV.

When surfactant-deficient rabbits were managed with active HFV at either a low or a high mean lung volume, there were marked differences in the degree of lung injury seen. Rabbits ventilated at low lung volumes had physiologic and histologic evidence of significantly greater lung injury compared with rabbits ventilated at high volumes (Froese et al., 1988). Thus, the degree of alveolar recruitment may be an important determinant of pulmonary outcome in surfactant-deficient animals treated with HFV. Another trial in premature monkeys examined pathologic lung changes in animals after 6 hours of management with one of four strategies: CMV alone, HFOV alone, CMV plus surfactant, and HFOV plus surfactant (Jackson et al., 1994). The group treated with HFOV and surfactant had significantly less proteinaceous edema than with any other management strategy, allowing speculation that this treatment strategy might reduce the risk for bronchopulmonary dysplasia.

The appropriate role of HFV in the management of sick newborns with severe hypoxemia is not yet well understood. Gas exchange is improved in newborns with pulmonary interstitial emphysema. In near-term newborns with meconium aspiration syndrome or persistent pulmonary hypertension, few studies have been performed to evaluate the efficacy of HFV. The use of HFV may not be appropriate in the premature infant with RDS, in which outcome was not improved in a randomized controlled trial. We should continue to evaluate HFV as a possibly beneficial therapeutic modality for future newborns. Perhaps ventilator strategies that maximize alveolar recruitment while avoiding hyperinflation will lead to as yet unseen benefits. Those who wish to employ HFV in the NICU must have a detailed understanding of the underlying pathophysiologic mechanisms of neonatal respiratory disease and recognize that different types of high-frequency ventilators and different ventilator strategies are likely to have vastly different physiologic and pathologic effects. There are four modes of HFV; each is discussed separately.

Modes of High-Frequency Ventilation

High-Frequency Positive-Pressure Ventilation

High-frequency positive-pressure ventilation (HFPPV) may be referred to as CMV with increased frequencies of 60 to 150 breaths per minute. In HFPPV, the tidal volume is greater than anatomic dead space but less than that commonly used during CMV, and it is delivered with short inspiratory times (Carlo & Chatburn, 1988). HFPPV comes from the Sjostrand technique and employs passive expiration. HFPPV may be used for airway surgeries because of its open system design (Gordin, 1989).

High-Frequency Flow Interruption

High-frequency flow interruption (HFFI) ventilation delivers tidal volumes that may be less than or greater than anatomic dead space at frequencies of 300 to 900 breaths per minute. HFFI works by interrupting the flow of gas with a motor-driven valve. The gas flows through the humidifier, flows through the interrupting valve, and is propelled down the endotracheal tube (Carlo & Chatburn, 1988). There is an expiratory limb through which passive expiration occurs. Clinical experience, research, and literature on HFFI are limited. It is sometimes classified as a type of HFOV.

High-Frequency Oscillatory Ventilation

HFOV delivers low tidal volumes, less than anatomic dead space, at high frequencies of 300 to 3000 breaths per minute. Expiration is active and is achieved by a piston pump or acoustic speaker. Active expiration decreases the risk for air trapping and may explain the minimal air trapping with HFOV (HIFI Study

Group, 1989). HFOV consists of a fresh gas source to provide oxygen and remove carbon dioxide, an exit port, an oscillator to direct the pressurized gas down the airway, and an airway adapter. The oscillator, which may be a vibrating loudspeaker or a piston and flywheel combination, generates air movement toward the patient (Wetzel & Gioia, 1987). HFOV may also be delivered by pressure to the external chest wall. This delivery method can be achieved with "a thoracoabdominal chamber connected to a vacuum source that maintains lung volume by controlling the negative pressure" (Carlo & Chatburn, 1988, p. 372).

High-Frequency Jet Ventilation

High-frequency jet ventilation (HFJV) delivers tidal volumes that may be less than or greater then anatomic dead space at frequencies of 60 to 600 breaths per minute. HFJV operates similarly to constant flow time-cycled ventilation with passive expiration (Carlo & Chatburn, 1988). Adequate humidification is needed with HFJV to prevent tracheal injury. In HFJV, a high-pressure gas source is connected to a small airway cannula with use of a high-frequency flow interrupter valve. This valve opens and closes rapidly, propelling the pressurized gas into the airway. As much as 50 percent of the tidal volume gases are entrained from a continuous gas flow circuit (Gordin, 1989; Wetzel & Gioia, 1987). Gas entrainment is the addition of gas from areas surrounding the airway cannula to the gas flow being delivered by the jet ventilator (Carlo & Chatburn, 1988). This important aspect of jet ventilation is needed to force the nonmoving gas into the moving stream of gases. HFJV requires a specific endotracheal tube with a lumen for the jet gas flow and a lumen for the fresh gas flow. The fresh gas flow allows entrainment of gases and addition of PEEP. There is a port, near the jet gas flow lumen, for the instillation of nebulized saline to prevent tracheal erosion (Wetzel & Gioia, 1987). A conventional ventilator may be used with a jet ventilator to provide "background" ventilation or sighs at a low rate. Background ventilation may decrease the risk for microatelectasis that may occur with long-term HFJV (Gordin, 1989).

Complications Associated With High-Frequency Ventilation

Whereas HFV can provide adequate ventilation to infants, it is not without the possibility of complications. The gases used during HFV need to be heated to avoid the delivery of cold gas into the airway. Cold air can lead to fluid overload, hypothermia, and necrotizing tracheobronchitis (NTB) (Carlo & Chatburn, 1988). NTB is a lesion of the airway, commonly found near the distal end of the endotracheal tube. This lesion may be caused by epithelial erosion and loss of cells in the airway, which can lead to the formation of granulation tissue. Granulation tissue may lead to impaired gas exchange, airway obstruction, or atelectasis (Carlo & Chatburn, 1988). One study of infants treated with HFJV showed that 44 percent of the survivors and 83 percent of the nonsurvivors had NTB (Boros et al., 1985). Although NTB is most often associated with HFJV, it has been reported in studies of HFOV and CMV.

Humidification of gas during HFV is needed to prevent tracheal inflammation and copious secretions. Use of nebulized saline in the stream of gases appears to prevent tracheal inflammation (Wetzel & Gioia, 1987). Some studies conflict in reports of the effects of HFV on mucous flow but agree that HFOV applied to the external chest wall enhances the clearance of tracheal secretions (Wetzel & Gioia, 1987). Regardless of the type of ventilation, decreased humidification leads to the presence of thick secretions that can impair gas exchange and plug an endotracheal tube. This plugging will require frequent reintubations and thus cause further trauma to the airway.

With high ventilatory frequencies, the inspiratory and expiratory times are decreased, which may increase the risk for gas trapping in the lungs. Gas trapping occurs less frequently during HFOV because it is the only form of HFV in which expiration is active. Gas trapping can lead to decreased lung compliance and retention of carbon dioxide. Microatelectasis may occur with HFV but can be combated by use of a low-rate conventional mechanical ventilator for background breaths to provide PEEP and extra gas flow for entrainment (Gordin, 1989).

Nursing Care—High-Frequency Ventilation

Caring for infants receiving HFV presents many challenges to NICU nurses. These nurses must adopt new skills and alter those used in caring for infants who are conventionally ventilated. Specific care need areas unique to infants receiving HFV include physical assessment, airway management, and positioning and comfort (Tables 19–4 and 19–5).

One of the most challenging yet critical aspects of caring for these infants is the physical assessment. Heightened physical assessment skills are critical because of the importance of recognizing subtle changes in assessment parameters that may signify changes in the infants' conditions. One necessary assessment parameter is astute observation of the degree of chest wall vibration, an indicator of tidal volume. Even small changes in the vibrations may indicate a change in the neonate's condition. Decreased chest vibration may indicate pneumothorax, endotracheal secretions, and mechanical malfunction (Avila et al., 1994).

The noise of the ventilator and the constant vibration of the infants make auscultation of breath sounds, heart tones, and bowel sounds difficult. If oscillating ventilators are used, this evaluation is best done when the infants are momentarily removed from the ventilator (for routine circuit changes) or when the ventilator is in standby (interruption of oscillation but not from ventilator mean airway pressure). Disconnection from HFV is discouraged because of possible alveolar collapse. Therefore, when necessary, disconnection from HFV should be limited to short periods. If the infants are receiving HFOV, it is also important to auscultate breath sounds while they are being oscillated to assess the symmetry of oscillatory intensity (Avila et al., 1994).

TABLE 19–4 Nursing Responsibilities and Interventions for Oscillated Infants Before High-Frequency Ventilation

Responsibility	Intervention
Obtain and record baseline physiologic data	Record temperature, heart rate, respiratory rate, systolic and diastolic blood pressures, transcutaneous Po_2, and Pco_2
Obtain and record baseline biochemical data	Draw blood samples for arterial gases
Maintain current ventilation	Record ventilator parameters: rate, PIP, PEEP, MAP, inspiratory:expiratory ratio, Fio_2
Assemble and prepare equipment	Ensure that infant is attached to monitoring devices for heart rate, intra-arterial blood pressure, transcutaneous oxygen and carbon dioxide Check alarms on all monitors Assist with arterial line insertion

PIP, peak inspiratory pressure; PEEP, positive end-expiratory pressure; MAP, mean airway pressure.

From Inwood, M. S. (1991). High-frequency oscillation. In J. Nugent (Ed.), *Acute respiratory care of the neonate* (p. 180). Petaluma, CA: NICU Ink.

TABLE 19–5 Nursing Responsibilities and Interventions for Oscillated Infants During Oscillation

Responsibility	Intervention
Monitor and document physiologic parameters	Record hourly temperature, heart rate, spontaneous respirations, systolic and diastolic blood pressure
	Measure and record accurate intake and output of fluids every 8 hours
Monitor and document biochemical parameters	Draw arterial blood gas samples as ordered
Maintain patent airway	Monitor for continuous vibration of chest
	Assess transcutaneous Po_2 and Pco_2 hourly
	Perform endotracheal suctioning every 2 hours and prn
	Record amount, color, and consistency of secretions
	Assess bilateral air entry while hand bagging at sigh pressures, before and after suctioning
	Ensure adequate humidification of gas flow
Prevent pneumothorax	Maintain ordered MAP
	Observe for decreased vibrations of the chest
	Assess infant for signs of respiratory difficulty: increase spontaneous respirations, increased chest retraction, diminished air entry, increased Fio_2 requirements, increased transcutaneous Pco_2 readings
	Obtain chest radiograph as required, ensuring that oscillator is stopped during filming
Provide pulmonary support	Monitor and record MAP, amplitude, frequency, and Fio_2 hourly
	Perform a sustained inflation after endotracheal suctioning and disconnection at ordered pressure and duration
	Record infant's response to sigh
Provide physical care	Reposition infant from side to side, or prone to supine, every 2 hours
Provide emotional support to family	Provide accurate, consistent information
	Promote bonding by encouraging nurse specialist or social worker for assistance with coping skills
	Encourage parents to attend parents' support group

MAP, mean airway pressure.
From Inwood, M. S. (1991). High-frequency oscillation. In J. Nugent (Ed.), *Acute respiratory care of the neonate* (p. 181). Petaluma, CA: NICU Ink.

The second specific area of care unique to infants receiving HFV is airway management. Suctioning of infants receiving HFV requires two people: one person to suction and the other person to either manually ventilate or return the infants to HFV. Remember that disconnection from HFV may lead to alveolar collapse, so the infants may need to be manually ventilated or the mean airway pressure increased after suctioning. The need for manual ventilation or increase in mean airway pressure is individually based. It is generally accepted practice to suction infants while they are disconnected from HFOV and HFJV. With HFOV, there is a possibility of air trapping during rapid rate ventilation (Avila et al., 1994). With HFJV, a possible shearing force on the airway results from the simultaneous occurrence of negative-pressure suction and high-frequency positive pressure (Gordin, 1989). Therefore, the use of closed tracheal suction systems with HFV is discouraged.

Positioning and comfort of infants receiving HFV are also important facets of care. Because of the physical restraints of the delivery devices and the importance of disconnecting the infant from the ventilator for only short durations, positioning and repositioning become challenging. Two caregivers should be used for repositioning: one to turn the infant and stabilize the endotracheal tube, and one to reposition the circuit and ventilator (Avila et al., 1994). Although water mattresses are not recommended, sheepskins, lamb's wool, and egg-crate mattresses may be used to provide comfort and prevent skin breakdown.

Sedatives, paralytics, and analgesics may be necessary to facilitate comfort for infants while they are receiving HFV. However, the necessity of pharmacologic agents is influenced by the infants' conditions rather than by the mode of ventilation. Interventions such as bundling and soothing music may decrease the need for pharmacologic agents. Whereas some believe that the noise and the constant vibration may be disturbing to the infants, others believe them to have a calming effect.

TREATMENT OF NEONATAL HYPOXEMIA WITH EXTRACORPOREAL MEMBRANE OXYGENATION

The first heart–lung machines, designed to serve the function of cardiopulmonary bypass during pediatric cardiac surgery, were developed in the 1950s. Blood was removed from the patient and pumped through an oxygenator before return to the systemic circulation. At the end of the surgical procedure, the patient was disconnected from the machine and pulmonary and systemic flows were restored with the patient's own heart as the pump. In the mid-1970s, the first attempts at prolonged cardiopulmonary bypass in infants with potentially reversible hypoxemia were made (Bartlett et al., 1977). The differences between these efforts and those employed during cardiac surgery were that the duration of bypass was measured in days rather than hours and the underlying disease leading to hypoxemia was potentially reversible lung disease rather than primary cardiac disease.

In the last 20 years, prolonged cardiopulmonary bypass, also known as extracorporeal membrane oxygenation (ECMO) or extracorporeal life support, has been used in thousands of newborn infants with hypoxemia that appears to be intractable to aggressive nonsurgical management. Few controlled clinical trials of ECMO have been performed (Bartlett et al., 1985; O'Rourke et al., 1989). In the absence of such trials, much controversy still exists about the uses of ECMO. Despite its efficacy in improving oxygen delivery in sick newborns, the mortality and morbidity associated with its use remain in the range of 13 to 33 percent, depending on the underlying disease process (Hofkosh et al., 1991; Schumacher et al., 1991). The long-term morbidities associated with ECMO use thus far are primarily adverse neurodevelopmental outcomes. The proponents of ECMO use argue that mortality and morbidity would actually be greater in these patients if ECMO were not available. The opponents of ECMO use argue that without additional trials, we will be unable to distinguish ECMO-related complications from disease-related complications.

A 1995 study examined neurodevelopmental status at age 5 years in ECMO-treated infants compared with a cohort of normal 5-year-olds (Glass et al., 1995). In the group treated with ECMO, 17 percent of children had major developmental disabilities, similar to rates seen in infants born weighing less than 750 g. The average IQ was lower for ECMO-treated infants (115 ± 16 for control children versus 96 ± 20 for those treated with ECMO). ECMO patients were at significantly higher risk for school failure and behavioral problems. Differences between the two groups may be related to initial severity of illness or to the ECMO process itself or both.

Despite these controversies, ECMO is widely used in NICUs in the United States as well as in several other industrialized nations. Neonatal ECMO is used in the management of intractable hypoxemia in near-term newborns with meconium aspiration syndrome, RDS, pneumonia/sepsis, and congenital diaphragmatic hernia. A variety of criteria are used to determine the point at which the risk for persistent hypoxemia is greater than the risk of ECMO. At Children's Hospital Medical Center in Cincinnati, for example, an alveolar-arterial oxygen partial pressure difference of greater than 620 torr for more than 12 hours is considered an indication for ECMO use. Other centers take into account the degree of ventilation support to determine whether a maximal medical effort is being made and to evaluate the risks associated with persisting in the use of increased ventilator pressures and increased inspired oxygen concentrations (Bartlett et al., 1977). Most ECMO centers probably use a combination of oxygenation criteria, ventilation criteria, and clinical judgment.

There are a variety of contraindications to the use of ECMO. The most important contraindication is prematurity. Early reports of ECMO use in premature infants revealed alarmingly high rates of intracranial hemorrhage (Cilley et al., 1986). Whether intracranial hemorrhage in these patients is related to the systemic anticoagulation required with ECMO or to the abnormal cerebrovascular pressures and flows associated with ECMO use is unknown. Other contraindications to ECMO use include preexisting intracranial hemorrhage and hypoxemia that is not potentially reversible, such as that seen in patients with cyanotic congenital heart disease.

ECMO is most commonly applied by use of a venoarterial approach. Blood is removed from the patient by gravity with use of a large-bore, jugular-venous, multiholed catheter advanced into the right atrium. Oxygenated blood is returned to the infant's aortic arch through a large-bore, multiholed catheter advanced through the carotid artery from a point of introduction in the neck.

The apparatus used for prolonged neonatal cardiopulmonary bypass (ECMO) begins with the right atrial catheter, which drains deoxygenated venous blood into a small pressure-sensitive reservoir placed below the level of the right atrium to take advantage of the effect of gravity (Fig. 19–2). The pressure-sensitive reservoir (bladder box) is connected in a servocontrol mode to the ECMO pump. If venous drainage from the infant is inadequate, a pressure decrease in the bladder box automatically shuts off the pump. Thus, venous outflow is matched to arterial inflow, resulting in a constant blood volume in the infant. After exiting the bladder box, tubing that contains the infant's venous blood passes through a pump that maintains constant, nonpulsatile flow in the ECMO circuit. Venous blood is pumped through a multilamellar, Teflon-coated membrane oxygenator. The membrane oxygenator provides a large surface area that separates the blood in the ECMO circuit from controlled concentrations of oxygen and carbon dioxide gas on the opposite side of the membrane. The postmembrane blood gases may be adjusted by altering gas concentrations in the oxygenator, thus ensuring that appropriately arterialized blood is returned to the newborn's aorta. The final step in the ECMO circuit, before blood is returned to the arch of the aorta, is the reheating of the blood, which cools as it passes through the large surface area of the membrane oxygenator. The blood is warmed by passage through a countercurrent heat exchanger, which is servocontrolled to increase the blood temperature to the desired body temperature of the infant.

Before the jugular venous and carotid artery catheters are placed, the ECMO circuit is primed with heparinized adult donor blood. Heparinization prevents clotting as the blood is exposed to surfaces of foreign substances that compose the ECMO circuit. Because platelets are trapped in the membrane oxygenator and because platelets are decreased in banked donor blood, fresh platelets are added to the circuit before bypass is begun.

Jugular venous and carotid arterial catheters are placed after a skin incision is made over these vessels in the neck. Before opening of the jugular vein, the infant is paralyzed by an appropriate neuromuscular blocking agent such as pancuronium bromide. This paralysis is necessary to avoid air embolization in the spontaneously breathing child. If possible, the positions of both catheters are verified radiographically before bypass is begun. After both catheters are connected to the bypass circuit, bypass flow is gradually increased to ensure adequate venous return to the circuit and to ensure the integrity of the bypass circuit. To maintain adequate gas exchange and normal acid–base balance, bypass flow rates of 100 to 150 ml/kg/min are usually required in the first hours after bypass is begun.

To avoid further pulmonary injury, ventilator pressures and the inspired oxygen concentration are decreased to minimal levels during ECMO. Because a large fraction of systemic venous return is drained from the right atrium, it is assumed that pulmonary blood flow is minimal during the first hours of bypass. If this is true, tissue oxygen delivery is provided almost entirely by the ECMO circuit. The activated clotting time is measured frequently while the infant is receiving ECMO. The heparin dosage is adjusted as necessary to maintain adequate anticoagulation. Fluids, nutrients, transfusions, volume expanders, and medications are delivered directly into the ECMO circuit. Blood gases and pH are measured frequently while the patient is on bypass. The bypass flow rate and membrane oxygenator oxygen and carbon dioxide concentrations are adjusted to maintain blood gas and acid–base homeostasis.

Weaning from ECMO is accomplished by periodic reductions in the bypass flow rate. As lung function improves, gas exchange may be gradually returned to the mechanically ventilated lungs. Periodic chest radiographs and estimates of pulmonary function can be used to determine the appropriate time for decreasing the bypass flow rate. Typically, ECMO may be required for 4 to 7 days. In general, the more severe the lung disease, the slower the rate of improvement in lung function and the greater the duration of the ECMO procedure. The infant is often weaned from the ventilator within a few days of discontinuation of bypass.

ECMO is an expensive and labor-intensive procedure. Two caretakers are required 24 hours per day: one to provide nursing care directly to the patient and one to monitor the functional integrity of the circuit and its various components. A variety of technical malfunctions have been reported, including rupture or disconnection of the circuit tubing, pump failure, oxygenator rupture, and heat exchanger malfunction. Heat exchangers have been reported to disintegrate partially, leading to aluminum particulate embolization in the patient (Vogler et al., 1988). The most frequently reported ECMO complication is hemorrhage

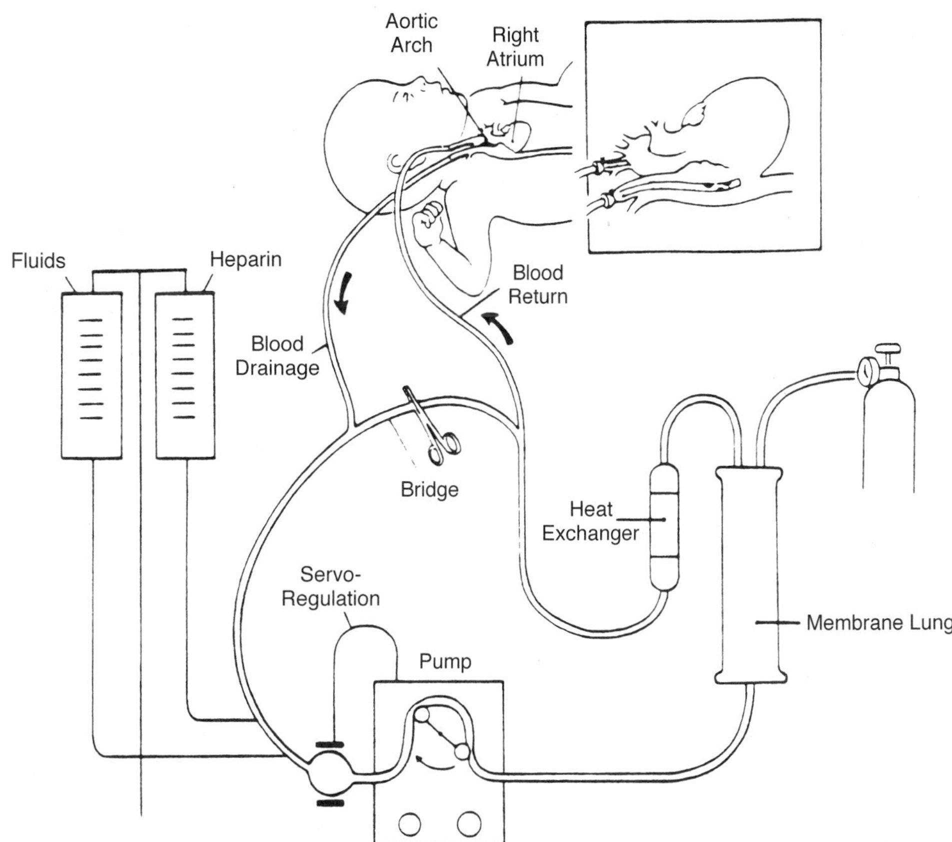

FIGURE 19–2. Extracorporeal membrane oxygenation setup. (From *Extracorporeal membrane oxygenation: Technical specialist manual* [7th ed.]. [1984]. Ann Arbor, MI: University of Michigan Department of Surgery, University of Michigan Hospitals.)

secondary to continuous systemic anticoagulation. Hemorrhage may lead to acute asphyxia or death due to blood loss or, as has been documented more frequently, to long-term neurologic sequelae as a consequence of intracranial hemorrhage. Efforts to avoid potentially preventable morbidity and mortality include attempts to avoid permanent carotid artery ligation and the evaluation of methods for avoiding systemic anticoagulation.

In an effort to avoid permanent carotid artery ligation, two new approaches are currently being evaluated. Several ECMO centers are now reanastomosing the proximal and distal carotid artery segments after removal of the carotid artery catheter. This was not performed in early ECMO patients because of concern about thrombus formation at the repair site with subsequent cerebral embolization. Another approach that avoids carotid artery ligation is the venovenous bypass (Andrews et al., 1983). With this technique, blood is both removed from and returned to the systemic venous circulation. A double-lumen catheter is inserted through the external jugular vein. With this specially designed catheter, one lumen opens distally in the right atrium while the more proximal lumen sits in the superior vena cava. Blood is removed by gravity from the proximal lumen, and oxygenated blood, which has passed through the ECMO circuit, is pumped back into the distal lumen. The most important functional limitation of venovenous bypass using this particular technique is the sufficiency of circuit flow. Because blood is both withdrawn from and returned to the same vessel, flow may be inadequate to meet the patient's oxygen use rate. Therefore, only infants whose pulmonary function is such that less than maximal bypass flow rates are required may be candidates for venovenous bypass. However, sicker infants may still require venoarterial bypass. For a list of common complications of ECMO, see Table 19–6.

Efforts to avoid the need for systemic anticoagulation are in their rudimentary stages. The most promising of these involve the use of ECMO circuit materials to which heparin has been bonded. Although these materials are being evaluated, such a circuit is not yet commercially available.

ECMO, although widely used, is likely to be replaced by less invasive and less risky preventive and therapeutic procedures. Prevention of PPHN is obviously a primary goal. Appropriate assessment of fetal lung maturity before elective cesarean section, fetal monitoring to avoid intrapartum asphyxia, early and aggressive resuscitation in the event of neonatal asphyxia (including tracheal suction for meconium), and early recognition of hypoxia are all necessary and effective means of preventing PPHN. In those instances in which prevention is ineffective, basic science research and clinical studies are necessary to minimize the risk and maximize the benefit of therapeutic interventions. For a summary of nursing responsibilities before and during cannulation and during the ECMO run, see Table 19–7.

INHALED NITRIC OXIDE

In the past 20 years, it has become apparent that vascular endothelium has an important role in the regulation of blood vessel smooth muscle tone as well as other important physiologic functions. Relaxation of vascular smooth muscle in response to acetylcholine requires an intact endothelium (Furchgott & Zawadski, 1980). Nitric oxide (NO) is thought to be the molecule released from the endothelium that is responsible for vascular smooth muscle relaxation (Ignarro et al., 1987). These findings were the catalyst for additional investigations of the biologic effects of NO.

NO has an unpaired electron and therefore rapidly combines with other free radicals. The biologic half-life of the molecule is estimated to be 110 to 130 msec (Lunn, 1995). In vivo, biologic activity of NO is limited because it is rapidly inactivated within

TABLE 19–6 Complications of Extracorporeal Membrane Oxygenation

Complication	Rationale and Treatment
Physiologic	
Electrolyte/glucose/fluid imbalance	Sodium requirements decrease to 1–2 mEq/kg/day; potassium requirements increase to 4 mEq/kg/day secondary to action of aldosterone Calcium replacement may be required if citrate is a component of prime blood anticoagulant Hyperglycemia may occur if citrate–phosphate–dextrose anticoagulated blood is used; reduce dextrose concentration of maintenance and heparin infusions Maintain total fluid intake of 100–150 ml/kg/day Fluid intake should balance output; furosemide may be required if positive fluid balance occurs
Central nervous system deterioration: cerebral edema, intracranial hemorrhage, seizures	This significant complication of ECMO can be related to pre-ECMO hypoxia, acidosis, hypercapnia, or vessel ligation Drug of choice for seizures is phenobarbital Serial electroencephalograms and cranial ultrasound examinations may be required
Generalized edema	Extracellular space is enlarged by distribution of crystalloid solution from the prime fluid and action of aldosterone and antidiuretic hormone Furosemide or hemofiltration may be indicated if edema causes brain or lung dysfunction
Renal failure	Acute tubular necrosis results from pre-ECMO hypotension and hypoxia Monitor output and indicators of renal failure: blood urea nitrogen, creatinine Increase renal perfusion by increasing pump flow and use of dopamine (5 μg/kg/min) Hemodialysis may be added to the circuit if necessary
Bleeding/thrombocytopenia	Most frequent cause of death Large foreign surface of ECMO circuit lowers platelet function and count Most common in infants requiring surgery or chest tubes Minimize with good control of ACT (180–200 seconds) and judicious use of platelets and frozen plasma All surgical procedures must be done with electrocautery
Decreased venous return/hypovolemia	Infant must have adequate circulating volume to obtain adequate flow rates Manifested by collapsing silicone bladder triggering bladder box alarm and decrease in extracorporeal flow rate, arterial pressure, and arterial pulse amplitude Blood sampling, wound drainage, or peripheral dilatation may account for hypovolemia Check for pneumothorax, partial venous catheter occlusion, or malposition, which may decrease venous drainage and return Replace volume with packed cells, fresh frozen plasma Treat pneumothorax with chest tube placement Raise level of bed to enhance gravity drainage of venous blood
Hypervolemia	Caused by overinfusion of blood products, which causes a larger percentage of blood to flow through malfunctioning lungs Can also be caused by renal ischemia and excretion of renin/angiotensin Manifested by widening pulse amplitude and decreasing systemic oxygenation at an extracorporeal flow rate Treat overinfusion by removing blood from the circuit; renal hypertension may dictate use of captopril or labetalol
Patent ductus arteriosus	Left-to-right shunting may occur, causing increased blood flow to the lungs, necessitating high pump flows without expected increase in PaO_2 Ligation may be indicated because weaning will not be successful
Mechanical	
Tubing rupture, air in oxygenator	Increase ventilator to pre-ECMO parameters; take patient off bypass (repair circuit, aspirate air, replace malfunctioning oxygenator); be prepared to resuscitate infant
Power failure	Always plug pump into hospital's emergency power supply; hand crank until emergency power is available
Decannulation	Apply firm pressure; come off bypass; increase ventilator parameters; repair vessel; replace blood volume; be prepared to resuscitate infant

ACT, activated coagulation time; ECMO, extracorporeal membrane oxygenation.

From Nugent, J. (1991). *Acute respiratory care of the neonate* (p. 210). Petaluma, CA: NICU Ink. Adapted from Nugent, J. (1986). Extracorporeal membrane oxygenation in the neonate. *Neonatal Network*, 4(5), 33.

TABLE 19–7 Nursing Responsibilities and Interventions for Extracorporeal Membrane Oxygenation

Responsibility	Intervention
Before Cannulation	
Obtain and document baseline physiologic data	Record weight, length, head circumference Draw blood samples for CBC, electrolytes, calcium, glucose, BUN, creatinine, PT, PTT, platelets, arterial blood gases Record vital signs: heart rate; respiratory rate; systolic, diastolic, mean blood pressure; temperature
Ensure adequate supply of blood products for replacement	Draw type and crossmatch samples for 2 units of packed red cells and fresh frozen plasma Keep 1 unit of packed cells and fresh frozen plasma always available in blood bank
Maintain prescribed pulmonary support	Maintain ventilator parameters Administer muscle relaxants if indicated
Assemble and prepare equipment	Prepare infusion pumps to maintain arterial lines and infusion of parenteral fluids and medications into the ECMO circuit Place the infant on a radiant warmer with the head positioned at the foot of the bed to provide thermoregulation and access for cannulation Attach infant to physiologic monitoring devices for heart rate, intra-arterial blood pressure, transcutaneous oxygen, and other parameters Insert urinary catheter and nasogastric tube; place to gravity drainage Remove intravenous lines just before heparinization (optional) Prepare loading dose of heparin (100 U/kg) Prepare heparin solution of continuous infusion (100 U/ml/D_5W) Prepare paralyzing drug (pancuronium bromide, 0.1 mg/kg, or succinylcholine, 1–4 mg/kg) Assist in insertion of arterial line (umbilical or peripheral) Administer prophylactic antibiotics
During Cannulation	
Monitor cardiopulmonary status during procedure	Monitor heart rate and intra-arterial blood pressure continuously Obtain samples for blood gas analysis after paralysis and during cannulation as indicated by infant's response to procedure
Be prepared to administer cardiopulmonary support	Have available medications and blood products to correct hypovolemia, bradycardia, acidosis, cardiac arrest
Administer medications	Give loading dose of heparin systemically when vessels are dissected free and are ready to be cannulated Give paralyzing drug systemically just before cannulation of internal jugular vein if infant has not been previously paralyzed
Reduce ventilator parameters	Once adequate bypass is achieved, reduce PIP to 16–20 cm H_2O, PEEP to 4 cm H_2O, ventilator rate to 10–20 breaths per minute, and FiO_2 to 21%–30%
During ECMO Run	
Monitor and document physiologic parameters	Record hourly heart rate, blood pressure (systolic, diastolic, mean), respiration, temperature, transcutaneous PO_2, carbon dioxide, oxygen saturation, ACT, ECMO flow Measure hourly accurate intake and output of all body fluids (urine, gastric contents, blood); measure every 4 hours: urine pH, protein, glucose, specific gravity; test all stools for blood (Hematest) Assess hourly: color, breath sounds, heart tones, murmurs, cardiac rhythm, arterial pressure wave form, peripheral perfusion Perform hourly neurologic check, including fontanelle tension, pupil size and reaction, level of consciousness, reflexes, tone, and movement of extremities Record ventilator parameters hourly Assess weight and head circumference daily
Monitor and document biochemical parameters	Draw samples for arterial blood gas analysis from umbilical or peripheral line hourly All other blood specimens are drawn from the ECMO circuit by the ECMO specialist: electrolytes, calcium, platelets, Chemstrip, hematocrit every 4–8 hours, CBC, PT, PTT, BUN, creatinine, total and direct bilirubin, plasma hemoglobin, fibrinogen, fibrin split products, and daily blood culture as indicated
Administer medications	Remove air bubbles and double-check dosages before infusion
Administer no medications intramuscularly or by venipuncture	Place all medications and fluids into the venous side of the ECMO circuit Prepare and administer the arterial line (umbilical or peripheral) infusion Administer parenteral alimentation
Provide pulmonary support	Perform endotracheal suctioning on the basis of individual assessment and need Maintain patent airway; be alert to extubation or plugging Obtain daily chest films and tracheal aspirant cultures as indicated Maintain ventilator parameters
Prevent bleeding	Avoid all of the following: rectal probes, injections, venipunctures, heel sticks, cuff blood pressures, chest tube stripping, restraints, chest percussion Avoid invasive procedures: do not change nasogastric tube, urinary catheters, or endotracheal tube unless absolutely necessary; use premeasured endotracheal tube suction technique Observe for blood in the urine, stools, endotracheal tubes, or nasogastric tubes

Table continued on following page

TABLE 19–7 Nursing Responsibilities and Interventions for Extracorporeal Membrane Oxygenation *(Continued)*

Responsibility	Intervention
Maintain excellent infection control	Change all fluids and tubing daily Change dressings daily and prn Clean urinary catheter site daily Maintain strict aseptic and handwashing technique Use universal barrier precautions
Provide physical care	Keep skin dry, clean, and free from pressure points Give mouth care prn Provide range of motion as indicated Turn side to side every 1–2 hours
Provide pain management, sedation, stress management	Minimize noise level Cluster patient care to maximize sleep period Administer analgesia: fentanyl 9–18 μg/kg/h (increased dosage due to binding of fentanyl to membrane oxygenator) Manage iatrogenic physical dependency by following a dose reduction regimen (reduce dose 10% every 4 hours)
Be alert to complications and emergencies	

ACT, activated coagulation time; BUN, blood urea nitrogen; CBC, complete blood count; ECMO, extracorporeal membrane oxygenation; PEEP, positive end-expiratory pressure; PIP, peak inspiratory pressure; PT, prothrombin time; PTT, partial thromboplastin time.

From Nugent, J. (1991). *Acute respiratory care of the neonate* (pp. 212–213). Petaluma, CA: NICU Ink. Adapted from Nugent, J. (1986). Extracorporeal membrane oxygenation in the neonate. *Neonatal Network*, 4(5), 34–35.

the vessel lumen. Inactivation occurs because NO has a high affinity for hemoglobin and avidly binds to the iron of heme proteins to form a biologically inactive compound, nitrosyl-hemoglobin. Nitrosyl-hemoglobin is then oxidized to form methemoglobin and nitrate.

The NO molecule is synthesized from the amino acid L-arginine in a reaction catalyzed by a group of enzymes called the nitric oxide synthases (NOS). The by-product of this reaction is L-citrulline:

$$\text{L-arginine} + \text{molecular } O_2 > NO + \text{L-citrulline}$$

There are three major types or isoforms of NOS. The first isoform is the endothelial or constitutive type, which is located in vascular endothelial cell wall, endocardium, myocardium, and platelets. Neuronal NOS is the isoform located in both the peripheral and central nervous systems. The third isoform, called inducible NOS, is not present under normal physiologic conditions but is produced in response to various inflammatory stimuli. Excitation of the inducible NOS causes production of much greater quantities of NO than activation of other isoforms. Activation of inducible NOS during sepsis plays a major part in producing vasodilation and consequent hypotension.

The biologic actions of NO are mediated through the guanylate cyclase–cyclic guanosine monophosphate (cGMP) system. After formation from L-arginine in the endothelial cell, NO readily diffuses into the cytosol of smooth muscle because it is a small, lipophilic molecule. Once inside the smooth muscle cell, NO binds soluble guanylate cyclase, which in turn catalyzes the formation of cGMP from guanosine triphosphate. Increases in cGMP lead to activation of cGMP-dependent protein kinase, which triggers a reduction in intracellular calcium concentration through extrusion and sequestration. The decreased calcium concentration causes smooth muscle relaxation.

NO is a biologic mediator of a variety of physiologic responses in numerous systems in the body. In the healthy state, the arterial circulation is partially dilated by basal production of NO in the endothelium. At birth, production of endogenous NO in response to rhythmic distention of the lung, shear stress, and acetylcholine release plays a major role in mediating a decrease in pulmonary vascular resistance (Cornfield et al., 1992). In addition to being an important determinant of basal tone in small arteries and arterioles, NO inhibits platelet aggregation and adherence and may alter vascular permeability (Moncada & Higgs, 1993). In the nervous system, NO may have a role in memory formation, pain perception, and electrocortical activation. In the gastrointestinal and genitourinary tracts, NO participates in control of signals regulating smooth muscle relaxation. NO is produced in large quantities in response to various immunologic stimuli. It may also have a role in nonspecific immunity because it is generated when macrophages are activated.

A particularly frustrating problem for caregivers in the NICU is the treatment of acute hypoxic respiratory failure due to pulmonary arterial vasoconstriction. Successful adaptation for extrauterine life depends on the ability of the fetus to make a transition from fetal to postnatal circulation. A variety of factors, probably related to adverse intrauterine events, may alter the ability of the newborn to decrease pulmonary vascular resistance at birth and make this adaptation. When pulmonary vascular resistance remains elevated postnatally, blood is shunted right to left across the ductus arteriosus and foramen ovale and away from the lungs, causing hypoxemia. This condition, PPHN, is seen either in isolation or in conjunction with various diseases such as meconium aspiration syndrome, severe birth asphyxia, sepsis, congenital diaphragmatic hernia, and RDS. In the past, pharmacologic interventions, such as tolazoline, an alpha-adrenergic blocker with histamine-like properties, have been used to decrease pulmonary vascular resistance. However, the effects of these drugs are unpredictable and inconsistent; and because they are not selective for the pulmonary bed, nearly 50 percent of patients develop systemic hypotension. Sodium nitroprusside is another drug that causes vasodilation through activation or release of NO, but it is not selective for the pulmonary arterial bed and decreases systemic vascular resistance as well. Other intravenous vasodilators, such as prostaglandin I_2 and adenosine triphosphate–magnesium chloride, may selectively decrease pulmonary vascular resistance and are currently being investigated (Roberts & Shaul, 1993). The ideal agent for the treatment of pulmonary hypertension would be one that causes pulmonary vasodilation without decreasing systemic vascular resistance.

Beginning in the early 1990s, it was theorized that inhaled NO would diffuse from the alveolar space across the epithelium to directly mediate vascular smooth muscle relaxation. Ultimately, NO would diffuse into the lumen of the pulmonary blood vessels and be inactivated on binding hemoglobin, thus avoiding effects on the systemic circulation. Theoretically, inhaled NO could increase systemic oxygenation by two mechanisms: global pulmonary arterial vasodilation with increased pulmonary blood flow and cardiac output, and improved matching of ventilation and perfusion in the lung.

There is concern, however, with potential toxic effects that might be associated with the use of inhaled NO. One potential problem is the formation of excess amounts of methemoglobin, causing the clinical condition known as methemoglobinemia. This condition is serious and associated with hypoxemia because of the inability of methemoglobin to carry oxygen. The body's defense mechanism against the formation of methemoglobin is the enzyme methemoglobin reductase, which readily converts methemoglobin back to hemoglobin. If the rate of accumulation of methemoglobin is slow, this enzyme will limit increases in methemoglobin. To date, significant methemoglobin levels have not been reported when low concentrations of inhaled NO are used in neonates.

Another possible problem is the production of nitrogen dioxide and higher oxides of nitrogen such as peroxynitrite when NO is used with high concentrations of oxygen. Nitrogen dioxide and peroxynitrite in high concentration have been shown to directly damage the lung (Haddad et al., 1993). By using low concentrations of NO and limiting the time of mixing of NO and oxygen, the formation of these toxic molecules is minimized.

Animal studies suggest that inhaled nitric oxide (INO) might indeed be a selective pulmonary vasodilator. When pulmonary hypertension was induced in newborn lambs with a thromboxane analogue or hypoxia, pulmonary hypertension was rapidly reversed with the addition of 40 to 80 parts per million (ppm) of INO. In this study, the use of INO was not associated with a decrease in systemic blood pressure (Frostell et al., 1991).

In fetal lambs, hypoxia-induced pulmonary hypertension is reversed with INO. Administration of INO caused a decrease in pulmonary vascular resistance but no change in systemic vascular resistance. Echocardiography performed during administration of NO demonstrated increased left-to-right shunt across the ductus (Roberts et al., 1992).

In the first use of INO in humans, decreased pulmonary vascular resistance was observed in adult patients with pulmonary hypertension with no change in systemic vascular resistance (Higenbottam et al., 1988). These findings were subsequently confirmed (Pepke-Zaba et al., 1991). In adults with adult respiratory distress syndrome (ARDS), decreased intrapulmonary shunting resulting from improved ventilation–perfusion matching and pulmonary vasodilation occurred shortly after administration of INO (Rossaint et al., 1993).

In infants, studies of small sample size have been reported by three groups of investigators. In a 1992 study, seven full-term infants with PPHN received INO at 80 ppm for 30 minutes. All infants had a rapid improvement in preductal oxygen saturation, and six of the seven had a postductal increase (Roberts et al., 1992). In Denver, nine patients with echocardiographic evidence of PPHN who were candidates for ECMO (oxygen index >40, PaO_2 <40 despite maximal therapy) were given 10 to 20 ppm of INO for approximately 4 to 24 hours. These nine infants demonstrated a 66 percent decrease in mean oxygen index during the first 30 minutes of treatment without a decrease in mean arterial pressure. Six infants who were treated for longer periods (up to 24 hours) had sustained improvement in systemic oxygenation. None of these six infants subsequently needed ECMO or developed methemoglobinemia (Kinsella et al., 1992). In a Canadian study, 23 near-term infants referred for ECMO who had an oxygen index greater than 20 were given randomized doses of 5 to 80 ppm of INO. If there was less than a 10 torr increase in PaO_2 or 10 percent increase in saturation after two doses of INO given in a randomized fashion, then ECMO was instituted. Thirteen infants in this study had PPHN documented by echocardiography. Eleven of these infants had improvement in PaO_2 and saturation after receiving INO and were not placed on ECMO. Ten had hypoxic respiratory failure without documented PPHN, and only three of these infants improved after INO. The other seven were placed on ECMO. There was no significant benefit in PaO_2 response with increasing doses of INO. No toxic effects from methemoglobin or dangerously increased levels of nitrogen dioxide were seen in this study (Finer et al., 1994).

At present, INO is not approved by the Food and Drug Administration. Several multicenter, double-masked, randomized, placebo-controlled studies are currently being conducted to further delineate the benefits and toxic effects of INO.

NO gas is supplied in aluminum tanks containing high concentrations of gaseous NO in equilibrium with inert nitrogen. This gas is added to the inspiratory limb of the ventilator circuit by flowmeters and blenders. By use of high flow rates, NO mixing time with oxygen is limited and the formation of nitrogen dioxide is decreased. Scavenging equipment at the expiratory limb of the ventilator eliminates potentially toxic exhaust gases. In-line monitoring of NO and nitrogen dioxide is performed by a chemoluminescence analyzer. Samples of gas in the ventilator circuit are aspirated, and the concentrations of these two molecules are determined. Blood is periodically monitored for methemoglobin levels in patients receiving INO.

INO holds promise as a selective pulmonary vasodilator that may soon be added to the clinician's armamentarium. Several small pilot studies suggest that INO may be effective in decreasing pulmonary vascular resistance and improving oxygenation without reducing systemic blood pressure or cardiac output. Extreme care must be taken to monitor blood levels of methemoglobin and the formation of higher oxides of nitrogen when NO is used. Until larger controlled trials are completed, the benefit:risk ratio of INO as a possible treatment for neonatal pulmonary hypertension is unknown.

Nursing Care: Nitric Oxide

Multicenter trials are currently under way to determine the efficacy and safety of NO use in the management of newborns with respiratory dysfunction. If this treatment modality does prove to be effective and safe, the nursing care of these infants as we know it today will change. Like liquid ventilation, NO therapy would bring with it many new challenges to NICU nurses.

LIQUID VENTILATION

A historical review of management of the premature infant provides insight into the logic behind the search for new treatment methods. With the advent of technology to manage temperature control and metabolic requirements, premature infants began to survive. Because of the increased survival of premature infants, it became necessary to understand and treat the difficulties of immature lung function. Thirty years ago, it became possible to mechanically ventilate premature infants, and more immature infants became candidates for intensive care and potential survival. Ten years ago, surfactant replacement became a standard of care, again improving survival of preterm infants. The skills, technologies, and resources for managing respiratory compromise of infants have continued to improve. Despite these advancements, prematurity and respiratory distress are still associated with significant morbidity and mortality. Modern therapies cause lung injury that often results in a chronic, incapacitating lung disease—bronchopulmonary dysplasia.

To decrease lung injury, efforts have concentrated on decreasing inspired oxygen concentration and decreasing inspiratory pressure. New ventilatory techniques such as HFV, early and repeated surfactant administration, and ECMO are used to decrease iatrogenic lung injury. Surface tension in the alveoli must be uniformly decreased to decrease inspiratory pressure and work of breathing and to improve ventilation. This surface tension arises because of the air–liquid interface at the lining of the alveolar membrane. Even optimal surfactant therapy does not distribute homogeneously and uniformly decrease surface tension. The concept of uniformly and maximally reducing surface tension has been explored with use of liquid ventilation techniques.

Background

As early as the 1920s, Neergaard demonstrated that oxygenated saline could be used to inflate the lung and improve ventilation (Shaffer, 1987). However, saline proved to be inadequate owing to its low gas-carrying ability and its high viscosity. In 1966, Clark and Gollan demonstrated that perfluorochemical liquids could support the respiration of animals. Perfluorochemical liquids are inert, have high solubility for respiratory gases, and minimize surface tension. They appear to be only minimally absorbed through the mature epithelium. Limited clinical experience and extensive work in animals suggest that these compounds are relatively nontoxic, even when given intravenously.

Rationale for Liquid Breathing

The alveolus is lined by a liquid gel, surfactant, that acts to decrease surface tension, enhance alveolar stability, and protect the respiratory epithelium. The surface tension forces within the alveolus are the result of the air–fluid interface and are dramatically increased by the absence of surfactant. Surfactant production and function are usually deficient in preterm infants. This deficiency results in noncompliant alveoli that tend to collapse spontaneously. Because surfactant deficiency tends to be nonhomogeneous, alveolar surface tension varies from one portion of the lung to another. Respiratory function in preterm infants is characterized by stiff lungs, increased work of breathing, uneven ventilation, and ventilation–perfusion mismatch. One way to decrease alveolar surface tension is to eliminate the air–liquid interface in the alveolus by filling it with liquid. This elimination of the air–liquid interface could improve alveolar compliance, reverse ventilation–perfusion abnormalities, and—if the liquid contains oxygen—increase oxygen uptake.

Strategies of Liquid Ventilation

Tidal Liquid Ventilation

Efforts were initially made to entirely replace gas breathing with liquid respiration. In tidal liquid ventilation (TLV), a liquid is used to transport dissolved oxygen and carbon dioxide; inhaled liquid brings dissolved oxygen to the lungs, and exhaled liquid carries off carbon dioxide. During TLV, both functional residual capacity and tidal volume are replaced by perfluorocarbon liquid. The advantages of this technique were substantiated in liquid-ventilated preterm lambs with surfactant deficiency (Wolfson et al., 1988) and during short-term liquid ventilation of human preterm infants (Greenspan et al., 1990). Technically, TLV is difficult. Clinically, provisions need to be made to mechanically deliver and withdraw liquid from the lung, and there needs to be equipment for eliminating carbon dioxide from the liquid and equilibrating it with oxygen. TLV requires new equipment and procedures. Moreover, the high viscosity of the perfluorocarbon liquid limits the number of breaths per minute that can be delivered.

Perfluorocarbon-Associated Gas Exchange

Perfluorocarbon-associated gas exchange (PAGE) is a hybrid method that attempts to overcome some of the limitations of TLV while retaining the advantages of liquid ventilation. During PAGE, functional residual capacity is replaced by liquid, but tidal ventilation is conventional, using oxygen-enriched gas and standard ventilator equipment. The lung is filled with perfluorocarbon liquid to a volume equivalent to the normal pulmonary functional residual capacity (about 30 ml/kg). This volume of liquid is left in the lung, and gas ventilation is resumed with use of conventional gas ventilators. On inspiration, oxygen is pushed down the airway into the liquid-filled alveoli where it forms bubbles. By a process similar to the bubble oxygenation during ECMO, oxygen and carbon dioxide are exchanged from bubble to liquid. This process oxygenates the alveolar perfluorocarbon reservoir and purges it of carbon dioxide. On exhalation, the gas is expelled from the lung. Breaths can be delivered at a frequency appropriate for the size and needs of the patient because respiratory rate is not limited by the viscosity of the liquid. PAGE has been shown to be effective in surfactant-deficient premature lambs. PAGE improved oxygenation and carbon dioxide elimination and improved lung compliance. It has also been shown to work in two models of ARDS, oleic acid lung injury (Papo et al., 1992) and saline lavage (Tutuncu et al., 1993).

Experimental experience with oxygenated perfluorocarbon liquid ventilation suggests that this technology will eventually provide a strong addition to the available strategies for managing preterm infants. Liquid ventilation offers the ability to effectively manage respiratory function and decrease barotrauma. Several fluids meet the physiologic requirements, and high-purity, medical-grade perfluorocarbons are now available. Realistically, PAGE or TLV can be envisioned to benefit premature infants with surfactant deficiency. Liquid ventilation may also prove beneficial in other conditions of respiratory insufficiency. Careful clinical trials remain to be done, but in the absence of unforeseen problems of toxicity or adverse effects, it is likely that liquid ventilation techniques will assume an important role in care of neonates with lung disease.

Nursing Care: Liquid Ventilation

The nursing care of infants with respiratory compromise may be greatly affected if future advances prove liquid ventilation to be safe and effective. Because of the complexity of the delivery systems, a specialized team, similar to an ECMO team, will be required to care for these infants. A two-person team will manage these infants. One team member would care for the infant while a second team member would be responsible for the breathing device. These specialists will need to be trained in fluid mechanics and liquid breathing techniques. In summary, if found beneficial to infants with respiratory compromise, liquid ventilation will bring with it many new and exciting nursing challenges.

Conclusion

Hypoxemia continues to contribute significantly to both morbidity and mortality in NICUs. As our understanding of the pathophysiology of neonatal hypoxemia improves, new approaches to prevention and treatment are suggested. The development of new therapeutic techniques, such as surfactant replacement, ECMO, HFV, NO, and liquid ventilation, holds the promise of improved neonatal outcome. As demonstrated by these examples, however, the development phase may be prolonged. We are tempted to employ these techniques at the bedside perhaps before the risks and benefits are well understood. The discovery of new safe and effective methods of prevention and treatment of neonatal hypoxemia requires the collaborative efforts of basic science research to describe the underlying pathophysiologic process and randomized clinical trials to evaluate appropriate new interventions.

REFERENCES

Adamsons, K., Jr., Gandy, G. M., & James, L. S. (1965). The influence of thermal factors upon oxygen consumption of newborn human infants. *Journal of Pediatrics, 66,* 495–508.

Alverson, D. C., Isken, V. H., & Cohen, R. S. (1988). Effect of booster blood transfusions on oxygen utilization in infants with bronchopulmonary dysplasia. *Journal of Pediatrics, 113*(4), 722–726.

Andrews, A. F., Klein, M. D., Toomasian, J. M., et al. (1983). Venovenous extracorporeal membrane oxygenation in neonates with respiratory failure. *Journal of Pediatric Surgery, 18*(4), 339–346.

Avery, M. E., & Mead, J. (1959). Surface properties in relation to atelectasis and hyaline membrane disease. *American Journal of Diseases of Children, 97,* 517–523.

Avery, M. E., & Merritt, T. A. (1991). Surfactant replacement therapy [Editorial]. *New England Journal of Medicine, 324*(13), 910–912.

Avery, M. E., Fletcher, B. D., & Williams, R. G. (1981). *The lung and its disorders in the newborn infant* (4th ed.). Philadelphia: W. B. Saunders.

Avila, K., Mazza, L., & Morgan-Trujillo, L. (1994). High-frequency oscillatory ventilation: A nursing approach to bedside care. *Neonatal Network, 13*(5), 23–30.

Bancalari, A., Gerhardt, T., Bancalari, E., et al. (1987). Gas trapping with high-frequency ventilation: Jet versus oscillatory ventilation. *Journal of Pediatrics, 110*(4), 617–622.

Bartlett, R. H., Gazzaniga, A. B., Huxtable, R. F., et al. (1977). Extracorporeal circulation (ECMO) in neonatal respiratory failure. *Journal of Thoracic and Cardiovascular Surgery, 74*(6), 826–833.

Bartlett, R. H., Roloff, D. W., Cornell, R. G., et al. (1985). Extracorporeal circulation in neonatal respiratory failure: A prospective randomized trial. *Pediatrics, 76*(4), 479–487.

Bateman, L., Hooper, R., Losh, T., & Miller, L. (1995). Continuous positive airway pressure. In S. L. Barnhart & M. P. Czervinske (Eds.), *Perinatal and pediatric respiratory care* (pp. 335–353). Philadelphia: W. B. Saunders.

Belik, J., & Pelech, A. (1988). Thoracic electric bioimpedance measurement of cardiac output in the newborn infant. *Journal of Pediatrics, 113*(5), 890–895.

Boros, S. J., Mammel, M. C., Coleman, J. M., et al. (1985). Neonatal high-frequency jet ventilation: Four years' experience. *Pediatrics, 75*(4), 657–663.

Boyle, R. J., & Oh, W. (1978). Respiratory distress syndrome. *Clinics in Perinatology, 5*(2), 283–297.

Burroughs Wellcome Company. (1990). *Synthetic lung surfactant for the treatment of neonatal respiratory distress syndrome* (Product Monograph). Research Triangle Park, NC: Author.

Carlo, W. A., & Chatburn, R. L. (1988). *Neonatal respiratory care.* Chicago: Year Book Medical Publishers.

Carlo, W. A., Beoglos, A., Chatburn, R. L., et al. (1989). High-frequency jet ventilation in neonatal pulmonary hypertension. *American Journal of Diseases of Children, 143*(2), 233–238.

Chu, J., Clements, J. A., Cotton, E. K., et al. (1967). Neonatal pulmonary ischemia. I. Clinical and physiological studies. *Pediatrics, 40*(4, Suppl.), 709–782.

Cilley, R. E., Zwischenberger, J. B., Andrews, A. F., et al. (1986). Intracranial hemorrhage during extracorporeal membrane oxygenation in neonates. *Pediatrics, 78*(4), 699–704.

Clark, L. C., Jr., & Gollan, F. (1966). Survival of mammals breathing organic liquid equilibrated with oxygen at atmospheric pressure. *Science, 152*(730), 1755–1756.

Clark, R. H., Gerstmann, D. R., Null, D. M., Jr., & deLemos, R. A. (1992). Prospective randomized comparison of high-frequency oscillatory and conventional ventilation in respiratory distress syndrome. *Pediatrics, 89*(1), 5–12.

Collaborative European Multicenter Study Group. (1988). Surfactant replacement therapy for severe neonatal respiratory distress syndrome: An international randomized clinical trial. *Pediatrics, 82*(5), 683–691.

Corbet, A., Bucciarelli, R., Goldman, S., et al., & The American Exosurf Pediatric Study Group 1. (1991). Decreased mortality rate among small premature infants treated at birth with a single dose of synthetic surfactant: A multicenter controlled trial. *Journal of Pediatrics, 118*(2), 277–284.

Cornfield, D. N., Chatfield, B. A., McQueston, J. A., et al. (1992). Effects of birth-related stimuli on L-arginine–dependent pulmonary vasodilation in ovine fetus. *American Journal of Physiology, 262*(5, Part 2), H1474–H1481.

Dunn, M. S., Shennan, A. T., & Possmayer, F. (1990). Single- versus multiple-dose surfactant replacement therapy in neonates of 30 to 36 weeks gestation with respiratory distress syndrome. *Pediatrics, 86*(4), 564–571.

Egan, E. A., Notter, R. H., Kwong, M. S., & Shapiro, D. L. (1983). Natural and artificial surfactant replacement in premature lambs. *Journal of Applied Physiology: Respiratory, Environmental, and Exercise Physiology, 55*(3), 875–883.

Enhorning, G., & Robertson, B. (1972). Lung expansion in the premature rabbit fetus after tracheal deposition of surfactant. *Pediatrics, 50*(1), 58–66.

Enhorning, G., Grossman, G., & Robertson, B. (1973). Tracheal deposition of surfactant before the first breath. *American Review of Respiratory Disease, 107*(6), 921–927.

Enhorning, G., Shennan, A., Possmayer, F., et al. (1985). Prevention of neonatal respiratory distress syndrome by tracheal instillation of surfactant: A randomized clinical trial. *Pediatrics, 76*(2), 145–153.

Finer, N. N., Etches, P. C., Kamstra, B., et al. (1994). Inhaled nitric oxide in infants referred for extracorporeal membrane oxygenation: Dose-responses. *Journal of Pediatrics, 124*(2), 302–308.

Fox, W. W., & Duara, S. (1983). Persistent pulmonary hypertension in the neonate: Diagnosis and management [Review]. *Journal of Pediatrics, 103*(4), 505–514.

Fredberg, J. J., Glass, G. M., Boynton, B. R., & Frantz, I. D., III. (1987). Factors influencing mechanical performance of neonatal high-frequency ventilators. *Journal of Applied Physiology, 62*(6), 2485–2490.

Froese, A. B., Hill, P. E., Bond, D. M., & Moller, F. (1988). Maintaining alveolar expansion facilitates surfactant repletion in ventilated atelectasis-prone rabbits. *Journal of the Federation of American Societies of Experimental Biology, 2,* A1183.

Frostell, C., Fratacci, M. D., Wain, J. C., et al. (1991). Inhaled nitric oxide. A selective pulmonary vasodilator reversing hypoxic pulmonary vasoconstriction. *Circulation, 83*(6), 2038–2047.

Fujiwara, T., Maeta, H., Chida, S., et al. (1980). Artificial surfactant therapy in hyaline membrane disease. *Lancet, 1*(8159), 55–59.

Furchgott, R. F., & Zawadski, J. W. (1980). The obligatory role of endothelial cells in the relaxation of arterial smooth muscle by acetylcholine. *Nature, 288*(5789), 373–376.

Gaylord, M. S., Quissell, B. J., & Lair, M. E. (1987). High-frequency ventilation in the treatment of infants weighing less than 1500 grams with pulmonary interstitial emphysema: A pilot study. *Pediatrics, 79*(6), 915–921.

Gitlin, J. D., Soll, R. F., Parad, R. B., et al. (1987). Randomized controlled trial of exogenous surfactant for the treatment of hyaline membrane disease. *Pediatrics, 79*(1), 31–37.

Glass, P., Wagner, A. E., Papero, P. H., et al. (1995). Neurodevelopmental status at age five years of neonates treated with extracorporeal membrane oxygenation. *Journal of Pediatrics, 127*(3), 447–457.

Glatz, T., Ikegami, M., & Jobe, A. (1982). Metabolism of exogenously administered natural surfactant in the newborn lamb. *Pediatric Research, 16*(9), 711–715.

Gonzalez, F., Harris, T., Black, P., & Richardson, P. (1987). Decreased gas flow through pneumothoraces in neonates receiving high-frequency jet versus conventional ventilation. *Journal of Pediatrics, 110*(3), 464–466.

Gordin, P. (1989). High-frequency jet ventilation for severe respiratory failure. *Pediatric Nursing, 15*(6), 625–629.

Greenspan, J. S., Wolfson, M. R., Rubenstein, S. D., & Shaffer, T. H. (1990). Liquid ventilation of human preterm neonates. *Journal of Pediatrics, 117*(1, Part 1), 106–111.

Haddad, I. Y., Ischiropoulus, H., Holm, B. A., et al. (1993). Mechanisms of peroxynitrite-induced injury to pulmonary surfactants. *American Journal of Physiology, 265*(6, Part 1), L555–L564.

Hallman, M., Merritt, T. A., Jarvenpaa, A. L., et al. (1985). Exogenous human surfactant for treatment of severe respiratory distress syndrome: A randomized prospective clinical trial. *Journal of Pediatrics, 106*(6), 963–969.

Hallman, M., Merritt, T. A., Schneider, H., et al. (1983). Isolation of human surfactant from amniotic fluid and a pilot study of its efficacy in respiratory distress syndrome. *Pediatrics, 71*(4), 473–482.

Halpérin, D. S., Wacker, P., Lacourt, G., et al. (1990). Effects of recombinant human erythropoietin in infants with the anemia of prematurity: A pilot study. *Journal of Pediatrics, 116*(5), 779–786.

Hargett, K. D. (1995). Mechanical ventilation of the neonate. In S. L. Barnhart & M. P. Czervinske (Eds.), *Perinatal and pediatric respiratory care* (pp. 294–312). Philadelphia: W. B. Saunders.

Harris, T. R., & Nugent, M. (1973). Continuous arterial oxygen tension monitoring in the newborn infant. *Journal of Pediatrics, 82*(6), 929–939.

Haworth, S. G., & Reid, L. (1976). Persistent fetal circulation: Newly recognized structural features. *Journal of Pediatrics, 88*(4), 614–620.

HIFI Study Group. (1989). High-frequency oscillatory ventilation compared with conventional mechanical ventilation in the treatment of respiratory failure in preterm infants. *New England Journal of Medicine, 320*(2), 88–93.

Higenbottam, T. W., Pepke-Zaba, J., Scott, J., et al. (1988). Inhaled "endothelial-derived relaxing factor" (EDRF) in primary hypertension. *American Review of Respiratory Disease, 137,* A107.

Hoekstra, R. E., Jackson, J. C., Myers, T. F., et al. (1991). Improved neonatal survival following multiple doses of bovine surfactant in very premature neonates at risk for respiratory distress syndrome. *Pediatrics, 88*(1), 10–18.

Hofkosh, D., Thompson, A. E., Nozza, R. J., et al. (1991). Ten years of extracorporeal membrane oxygenation: Neurodevelopmental outcome. *Pediatrics, 87*(4), 549–555.

Horbar, J. D., Soll, R. F., Sutherland, J. M., et al. (1989). A multicenter randomized, placebo-controlled trial of surfactant therapy for respiratory distress syndrome. *New England Journal of Medicine, 320*(15), 959–965.

Horbar, J. D., Wright, L. L., Soll, R. F., et al., for the National Institutes of Child Health and Human Development Neonatal Research Network. (1993). A multicenter randomized trial comparing two surfactants for the treatment of neonatal respiratory distress syndrome. *Journal of Pediatrics, 123*(5), 757–761.

Ignarro, L. J., Buga, G. M., Wood, K. S., et al. (1987). Endothelium derived relaxing factor produced and released from artery and vein is nitric oxide. *Proceedings of the National Academy of Sciences of the United States of America, 84*(24), 9265–9269.

Jackson, J. C., Truog, W. E., Standaert, T. A., et al. (1994). Reduction in lung injury after combined surfactant and high-frequency ventilation. *American Journal of Respiratory and Critical Care Medicine, 150*(2), 534–539.

Johnson, J. F., & Dean, B. L. (1982). The expiratory film in hyaline membrane disease: Preliminary observations. *American Journal of Roentgenology, 139*(1), 31–34.

Keens, T. G., & Ianuzzo, C. D. (1979). Development of fatigue-resistant muscle fibers in human ventilatory muscles. *American Review of Respiratory Disease, 119*(2, Part 2), 139–141.

Kendig, J. W., Notter, R. H., Cox, C., et al. (1991). A comparison of surfactant as immediate prophylaxis and as rescue therapy in newborns of less than 30 weeks gestation. *New England Journal of Medicine, 324*(13), 865–871.

Kinsella, J. P., & Abman, S. H. (1995). Recent developments in the pathophysiology and treatment of persistent pulmonary hypertension of the newborn. *Journal of Pediatrics, 126*(6), 853–863.

Kwong, M. S., Egan, E. A., Notter, R. H., & Shapiro, D. L. (1985). Double-blind clinical trial of calf lung surfactant extract for the prevention of hyaline membrane disease in extremely premature infants. *Pediatrics, 76*(4), 585–592.

Lang, M. J., Hall, R. T., Reddy, N. S., et al. (1990). A controlled trial of human surfactant replacement therapy for severe respiratory distress syndrome in very low birth weight infants. *Journal of Pediatrics, 116*(2), 295–300.

Liechty, E. A., Donovan, E., Purohit, D., et al. (1991). Reduction of neonatal mortality after multiple doses of bovine surfactant in low birth weight neonates with respiratory distress syndrome. *Pediatrics, 88*(1), 19–28.

Long, W. A. (1990). *Fetal and neonatal cardiology.* Philadelphia: W. B. Saunders.

Long, W., Thompson, T., Sundell, H., et al., & the American Exosurf Neonatal Study Group 1. (1991). Effects of two rescue doses of a synthetic surfactant on mortality rate and survival without bronchopulmonary dysplasia in 700- to 1350-gram infants with respiratory distress syndrome. *Journal of Pediatrics, 118*(4, Part 1), 595–605.

Lunn, R. J. (1995). Inhaled nitric oxide therapy. *Mayo Clinic Proceedings, 70,* 247–255.

Martin, R. J., Miller, M. J., & Carlo, W. A. (1986). Neonatal apnea: Pathogenesis of apnea in preterm infants [Review]. *Journal of Pediatrics, 109*(5), 733–741.

Merenstein, G. B., & Gardner, S. L. (1989). *Handbook of neonatal intensive care.* St. Louis: C. V. Mosby.

Merenstein, G. B., Cassady, G., Erenberg, A., et al., Committee on Fetus and Newborn, American Academy of Pediatrics. (1991). Surfactant replacement therapy for respiratory distress syndrome. *Pediatrics, 87*(16), 946–947.

Merritt, T. A., Hallman, M., Berry, C., et al. (1991). Randomized, placebo-controlled trial of human surfactant given at birth versus rescue administration in very low birth weight infants with lung immaturity. *Journal of Pediatrics, 118*(4, Part 1), 581–594.

Merritt, T. A., Hallman, M., Bloom, B. T., et al. (1986). Prophylactic treatment of very premature infants with human surfactant. *New England Journal of Medicine, 315*(12), 785–790.

Meschia, G. (1989). Placental respiratory gas exchange and fetal oxygenation. In R. K. Creasy & R. Resnik (Eds.), *Maternal-fetal medicine: Principles and practice* (pp. 303–313). Philadelphia: W. B. Saunders.

Miller, E. D., & Armstrong, C. L. (1990). Surfactant replacement therapy: Innovative care for the premature infant. *Journal of Obstetric, Gynecologic, and Neonatal Nursing, 19*(1), 14–17.

Miller, M. J., Fanaroff, A. A., & Martin, R. J. (1992). Respiratory disorders in preterm and term infants. In A. A. Fanaroff & R. J. Martin (Eds.), *Neonatal-perinatal medicine: Diseases of the fetus and infant* (6th ed., pp. 1040–1064). St. Louis: C. V. Mosby.

Moncada, S., & Higgs, A. (1993). The L-arginine–nitric oxide pathway [Review]. *New England Journal of Medicine, 329*(27), 2002–2011.

Nilsson, R., Grossman, N. G., & Robertson, B. (1978). Lung surfactant and the pathogenesis of neonatal bronchiolar lesions induced by artificial ventilation. *Pediatric Research, 12*(4, Part 1), 249–255.

O'Rourke, P. P., Crone, R. K., Vacanti, J. P., et al. (1989). Extracorporeal membrane oxygenation (ECMO) and conventional medical therapy in neonates with persistent pulmonary hypertension of the newborn: A prospective randomized study. *Pediatrics, 84*(6), 957–963.

Papo, M., Paczan, P., & Fuhrman, B. (1992). Improved oxygenation and lung compliance using perfluorocarbon-assisted gas exchange (PAGE) in a pediatric animal model with oleic acid induced lung injury. *Pediatric Colloquium Proceedings,* 1992.

Pattle, R. E. (1958). Properties, function and origin of alveolar lining layer. *Proceeding of the Royal Society of London, B148,* 217–240.

Pepke-Zaba, J., Higenbottam, T. W., Dinh-Xuan, A. T., et al. (1991). Inhaled nitric oxide as a selective pulmonary vasodilator in pulmonary hypertension. *Lancet, 338*(8776), 1173–1174.

Perlstein, P. (1987). Physical environment. In A. A. Fanaroff & R. J. Martin (Eds.), *Neonatal-perinatal medicine: Diseases of the fetus and infant* (5th ed., pp. 401–419). St. Louis: C. V. Mosby.

Phibbs, R. H., Ballard, R. A., Clements, J. A., et al. (1991). Initial clinical trial of Exosurf, a protein-free synthetic surfactant, for the prophylaxis and early treatment of hyaline membrane disease. *Pediatrics, 88*(1), 1–9.

Raju, T. N., Vidyasagar, D., Bhat, R., et al. (1987). Double-blind controlled trial of single-dose treatment with bovine surfactant in severe hyaline membrane disease. *Lancet, 1*(8434), 651–656.

Ramamurthy, R. S., & Brans, Y. W. (1981). Neonatal polycythemia: I. Criteria for diagnosis and treatment. *Pediatrics, 68*(2), 168–174.

Roberts, J. D., Jr., & Shaul, P. W. (1993). Advances in the treatment of persistent pulmonary hypertension of the newborn [Review]. *Pediatric Clinics of North America, 40*(5), 983–1004.

Roberts, J. D., Polander, D. M., Lang, P., & Zapol, W. M. (1992). Inhaled nitric oxide in persistent pulmonary hypertension of the newborn. *Lancet, 340*(8823), 818–819.

Robertson, B., Curstedt, T., Grossman, G., et al. (1988). Prolonged ventilation of the premature newborn rabbit after treatment with natural or apoprotein-based artificial surfactant. *European Journal of Pediatrics, 147*(2), 168–173.

Robillard, E., Alarie, Y., Dagenais-Perusse, P., et al. (1964). Microaerosol administration of synthetic B-Y-dipalmitoyl-D-lecithin in the respiratory distress syndrome: A preliminary report. *Canadian Medical Association Journal, 90,* 55–57.

Rossaint, R., Falke, K. J., Lopez, F., et al. (1993). Inhaled nitric oxide for adult respiratory distress syndrome. *New England Journal of Medicine, 328*(6), 399–405.

Scarpelli, E. M., Auld, P. A .M., & Golman, H. S. (1978). *Pulmonary disease of the fetus, newborn and child.* Philadelphia: Lea & Febiger.

Schumacher, R. E., Palmer, T. W., Roloff, D. W., et al. (1991). Follow-up of infants treated with extracorporeal membrane oxygenation for newborn respiratory failure. *Pediatrics*, 87(4), 451–457.

Shaffer, T. H. (1987). A brief review: Liquid ventilation. *Undersea Biomedical Research, 14,* 169-179.

Shapiro, D. L., Notter, R. H., Morin, F. C., III, et al. (1985). Double-blind, randomized trial of a calf lung surfactant extract administered at birth to very premature infants for prevention of respiratory distress syndrome. *Pediatrics, 76*(4), 593–599.

Shurin, S. B. (1987). Hematologic problems in the fetus and neonate. In A. A. Fanaroff & R. J. Martin (Eds.), *Neonatal-perinatal medicine: Diseases of the fetus and infant* (5th ed., pp. 941–988). St. Louis: C. V. Mosby.

Soll, R. F., Hoekstra, R. E., Fangman, J. J., et al., & Ross Collaborative Surfactant Prevention Study Group (1990). Multicenter trial of single-dose modified bovine surfactant extract (Survanta) for prevention of respiratory distress syndrome. *Pediatrics, 85*(6), 1092–1102.

Speer, C. P., Gefeller, O., Groneck, P., et al. (1995). Randomized clinical trial of two treatment regimens of natural surfactant preparations in neonatal respiratory distress syndrome. *Archives of Disease in Childhood, Fetal and Neonatal Edition,* 72(1), F8–F13.

Sperinde, J. M., & Senelly, K. M. (1985). The Oximetrix Opticath oximetry system: Theory and development. In P. J. Fabey (Ed.), *Continuous measurement of blood oxygen saturation in the high risk patient. Theory and practice in monitoring mixed venous oxygen saturation* (Vol. 2, pp. 59–80). San Diego: Beach International.

Stern, L. (Ed.). (1984). *Hyaline membrane disease: Pathogenesis and pathophysiology.* New York: Grune & Stratton.

Stevens, P. A., Wright, J. R., & Clements, J. A. (1989). Surfactant secretion and clearance in the newborn. *Journal of Applied Physiology, 67*(4), 1597–1605.

Strang, L. B. (1977). *Neonatal respiration: Physiological and clinical studies.* Oxford: Blackwell Scientific Publications.

Ten Centre Study Group. (1987). Ten centre trial of artificial surfactant (artificial lung expanding compound) in very premature babies. *British Medical Journal, Clinical Research Edition, 294*(6578), 991–1000.

Tutuncu, A., Faithfull, N., & Lachmann, B. (1993). Intratracheal perfluorocarbon administration combined with mechanical ventilation in experimental respiratory distress syndrome: Dose-dependent improvement of gas exchange. *Critical Care Medicine, 21*(7), 962–969.

Vaucher, Y. E., Merritt, T. A., Hallman, M., et al. (1990). Improved outcome following rescue versus prophylactic surfactant treatment in RDS. *Pediatric Research, 27,* 260A.

Venegas, J. G., Hales, C. A., & Strieder, D. J. (1986). A general dimensionless equation of gas transport by high-frequency ventilation. *Journal of Applied Physiology, 60*(3), 1025–1030.

Vogler, C., Sotelo-Avila, C., Lagunoff, D., et al. (1988). Aluminum-containing emboli in infants treated with extracorporeal membrane oxygenation. *New England Journal of Medicine, 319*(2), 75–79.

Walther, F. J., Siassi, B., Ramadan, N. A., et al. (1985). Pulsed Doppler determinations of cardiac output in neonates: Normal standards for clinical use. *Pediatrics, 76*(5), 829–833.

Wetzel, R. C., & Gioia, F. R. (1987). Extracorporeal membrane oxygenation: Its use in neonatal respiratory failure. *AORN Journal, 45*(3), 725–739.

Wilkinson, A., Jenkins, P. A., & Jeffrey, J. A. (1985). Two controlled trials of dry artificial surfactant: Early effects and later outcome in babies with surfactant deficiency. *Lancet,* 2(8450), 287–291.

Wolfson, M. R., Tran, N., & Bhutani, V. K. (1988). A new experimental approach for the study of cardiopulmonary physiology during early development. *Journal of Applied Physiology,* 65, 1436–1443.

CHAPTER 20

Complications of Respiratory Management

CAROLE KENNER

RESEARCH AGENDA

What factors influence the development of bronchopulmonary dysplasia (BPD)?

What is the effect of the diagnosis of BPD on the family?

What is the effect of surfactant therapy on the incidence of BPD?

What is the effect of maternal steroids and surfactant therapy on the incidence of BPD?

In the 25 years of modern neonatal intensive care, great advances have been made in respiratory treatments. Many newborns suffer from life-threatening respiratory compromise—from premature infants with respiratory distress syndrome (RDS) to full-term infants with congenital heart disease or pneumonia. Advances in respiratory technology, together with clinical expertise honed by long practice, have enabled survival of many infants who previously would not have even been treated. These technologies have their cost, however, and, even though many acute respiratory problems are treatable, the long-term consequences of that treatment must also be addressed. Chronic respiratory disease has become a fact of life for many neonatal intensive care unit (NICU) survivors and has resulted in increased health care costs and quality-of-life concerns.

This chapter discusses the pathogenesis of respiratory complications, focusing primarily on BPD, treatment of complications, and infant outcomes.

BRONCHOPULMONARY DYSPLASIA

Definition

Many sources agree that BPD has become more of a problem with the increase in survival of very low birth weight (VLBW) infants, but no consensus exists about any other aspect of the disease. According to Sinkin and Phelps (1987), for comparisons to be made across study sites and at different points in time, first a concise definition of the disease process or condition is needed. The condition must be described according to severity and risk factors for its development. Subjects who are at greatest risk must also be identified. None of these criteria exist for BPD.

For BPD, there is neither a precise definition nor standardized diagnostic criteria (Monin & Vert, 1987; Sinkin & Phelps, 1987). Both are necessary to identify risk groups, pinpoint affected infants for study and treatment, track incidence and prevalence, and provide guidance for the study of causes and treatment options.

The current definitions agree that BPD is a chronic neonatal respiratory problem that is caused by a complex interaction of iatrogenic factors and characteristics of the at-risk group. Significant variability in incidence exists from center to center, even within regions (Avery et al., 1987; Boynton, 1988), and may be due to any or all of the following (Boynton, 1988):

1. Variability in diagnostic criteria
2. Variability in criteria for identification of the at-risk population
3. Differences in composition of patient population
4. Temporal changes in survival rates of VLBW neonates
5. Differences in clinical management of neonates with respiratory disease

The classical classification of Northway (Northway et al., 1967), shown in Table 20–1, is no longer useful because of changes in the natural history of the disease, the nature of the neonatal population, and NICU practices over the years (Boynton, 1988).

A 1987 definition in a national comparative study of incidence, prevalence, and causal factors used as its criteria for BPD a requirement for oxygen therapy at 30 days of age accompanied by an abnormal chest radiograph (Avery et al., 1987). This definition lacks specificity, however, and may include infants who do not have BPD.

Toce and colleagues (1984) have proposed a classification system to be used at 21 days of age that includes measures of gas exchange, respiratory distress, and growth, together with a chest radiograph scoring assessment (Tables 20–2 and 20–3). This system identifies infants with BPD by chart review, quantifies severity at specific ages, and determines disease resolution. However, it does not include infants with chronic BPD-like changes on their chest radiographs who do not require oxygen therapy or who have clinical respiratory distress. The criteria also lack the predictive ability to identify, at early ages, infants at risk who might benefit from preventive therapies.

Bancalari and associates (1979) have developed widely used criteria (Table 20–4) that contain some measurable historic, clini-

TABLE 20–1 Northway's Stages of Bronchopulmonary Dysplasia

Stage I (2 to 3 days): period of acute respiratory distress syndrome
Stage II (4 to 10 days): period of regeneration
Stage III (10 to 20 days): period of transition to chronic disease
Stage IV (beyond 1 month): period of chronic disease

TABLE 20–2 Bronchopulmonary Dysplasia Clinical Scoring Chart*

Variable	Score			
	0 (Normal)	*1 (Mild)*	*2 (Moderate)*	*3 (Severe)*
Respiratory rate† No./min	<40	40–60	61–80	>80
Dyspnea (retractions)	0	Mild	Moderate	Severe
FIO_2‡ requirement (for PaO_2 of 50–70 mm Hg) (%)	21	21–30	31–50	>50
PCO_2 (mm Hg)	<45	46–55	56–70	>70
Growth rate (g/day)	>25	15–24	5–14	<5

*Modified from the National Institutes of Health Workshop on Bronchopulmonary Dysplasia.

†Average per minute value over one nursing shift. If patient is receiving mechanical ventilation for respiratory failure, a total score of 15 points is assigned. Total score is the summation of values for the live categories, the maximum being 15 points.

‡FIO_2 indicates forced inspiratory oxygen.

From Toce, S. S., Farrell, P. M., Leavitt, L. A., et al. (1984). Clinical and roentgenographic scoring systems for assessing bronchopulmonary dysplasia. *American Journal of Diseases of Children, 138,* 581–585. Copyright 1984, American Medical Association. Reprinted with permission.

cal, and radiographic aspects. This system has advantages and disadvantages similar to those of the Toce criteria.

The natural history of the disease is not well understood. Not all infants who meet some of the BPD criteria have had RDS at birth requiring oxygen therapy and mechanical ventilation, the two factors thought to trigger BPD. Nor do all infants with BPD require supplemental oxygen therapy after discharge, even though they continue to have abnormalities in lung function and chest radiographs for years. Some therapies are effective for some infants, but not for others.

However, these infants do have some outcomes in common (Boynton, 1988). First, they have an excessively high postnatal mortality rate within the first year of life. Second, they have recurrent lower respiratory tract infections in the first few years of life, often requiring hospitalization. Third, they have delays in growth and development, despite what may appear to be adequate or even excessive nutritional support. Fourth, although pulmonary dysfunction does decrease with time, measurable abnormalities persist in pulmonary mechanics, even in the absence of an oxygen requirement or other clinical symptoms.

ETIOLOGY OF BRONCHOPULMONARY DYSPLASIA

BPD does not appear to have one discrete cause; it is brought on by a combination of iatrogenic factors and patient characteristics (Boynton, 1988) (Table 20–5). The classic BPD formula of Philip (1975) could be altered to include the following interaction:

$$\text{Oxygen} + \text{pressure} + \text{time} + \text{susceptible host} = \text{BPD}$$

Two commonly used respiratory treatments, oxygen therapy and mechanical ventilation, have been strongly implicated in initiating a cascade of events that lead to the development of BPD (Boynton, 1988) (Fig. 20–1).

Oxygen Toxicity: Mechanisms

In humans breathing 0.21 FIO_2 (room air), energy is derived from an electron transport system based on the controlled reduction of molecular oxygen to water (Wispe & Roberts, 1987). Also

TABLE 20–3 A System for Scoring Roentgenographic Severity of Bronchopulmonary Dysplasia

Variable	Score		
	0	*1*	*2*
Cardiovascular abnormalities	None	Cardiomegaly	Gross cardiomegaly, or right ventricular hypertrophy, or enlarged
Hyperexpansion	Anterior plus posterior rib count* of 14 or less	Anterior plus posterior rib count of 14½ to 16	Anterior plus posterior rib count of 16½ or more, or hemidiaphragms flat or concave on lateral view
Emphysema	No focal areas seen	Scattered small abnormal lucencies	One or more large blebs or bullae
Fibrosis/ interstitial abnormalities	None seen	Few streaks of abnormal density interstitial prominence†	Many abnormal strands; dense fibrotic bands
Subjective‡	Appears mildly diseased	Appears moderately diseased	Appears severely diseased

*Counts of anterior and posterior ribs intersecting the level of the dome of the right hemidiaphragm. If the level of the right hemidiaphragm is at the sixth anterior rib and the eighth posterior intercostal space, the total rib count is 14½.

†Enlarged lymphatics and areas of atelectasis cannot usually be distinguished from fibrosis.

‡"Subjective" factor is based on overall roentgenographic judgment of the severity of disease.

From Toce, S. S., Farrell, P. M., Leavitt, L. A., et al. (1984). Clinical and roentgenographic scoring systems for assessing bronchopulmonary dysplasia. *American Journal of Diseases of Children, 138,* 581–585. Copyright 1984, American Medical Association. As modified from Edwards, D. K. (1982). Radiology of hyaline membrane disease: Transient tachypnea of the newborn and bronchopulmonary dysplasia. In P. M. Farrell (Ed.), *Lung development: Biological and clinical perspectives* (Vol. 2, pp. 47–89). New York: Academic Press.

TABLE 20–4 Bancalari's Criteria for Bronchopulmonary Dysplasia

1. Required intermittent positive pressure ventilation during the first week of life and for a minimum of 3 days.
2. Developed clinical signs of chronic respiratory disease characterized by tachypnea, intercostal and subcostal retraction, and rales on auscultation, all persisting for longer than 28 days.
3. Required supplemental oxygen for more than 28 days to maintain a PaO_2 over 50 mm Hg.
4. Chest radiograph showed persistent strands of densities in both lungs, alternating with areas of normal or increased lucency.

From Bancalari, E., Abdenour, G. E., Feller, R., & Gannon, J. (1979). Bronchopulmonary dysplasia: Clinical presentation. *Journal of Pediatrics*, *95*, 819–823. Reprinted with permission.

TABLE 20–5 Risk Factors for Bronchopulmonary Dysplasia

Immaturity of the pulmonary parenchyma
Surfactant deficiency
Exposure to elevated concentrations of inspired oxygen
Barotrauma from postive-pressure ventilation
Systemic-to-pulmonary shunt through a patent ductus arteriosus
Pulmonary edema
Pulmonary air leak
Protease–antiprotease imbalance
Family history of reactive airway disease
Tissue type HLA-A2
Vitamin A deficiency

From Boynton, B. R. (1988). Epidemiology of bronchopulmonary dysplasia. In T. A. Merritt, W. H. Northway, Jr., & B. R. Boynton (Eds.), *Bronchopulmonary dysplasia* (p. 26). Boston: Blackwell Scientific Publications. By permission of Blackwell Scientific Publications.

generated during this process are a series of free radicals, which are toxic, partially reduced oxygen intermediates that have the capacity to damage and kill tissue. In the normal human, enzyme and nonenzyme systems operate to scavenge and neutralize these radicals as soon as they are produced. Under hypoxic conditions requiring oxygen therapy in the premature infant, however, not only can the rate of production of these radicals exceed the capacity of these protective systems but also the systems themselves are immature and functioning at a lower level than those of the adult (Wispe & Roberts, 1987). Unscavenged radicals have a direct toxic effect on pulmonary epithelial cells, causing cell membrane injury, enzyme inactivation, and structural protein damage (Shannon & Epstein, 1986). Depending on the overall importance of the altered proteins to cellular function and on the ability of the cell to repair or replace the protein, the damage has different effects. Reaction of the free radicals with proteins may also generate by-products that amplify the initial damage (Wispe & Roberts, 1987).

Damage to the alveolar-capillary membrane causes the loss of the membrane's integrity as a barrier, resulting in a leak of fluids and proteins into the lung (Shannon & Epstein, 1986; Sinkin & Phelps, 1987). This phenomenon is referred to as *capillary leak syndrome*. One of the factors believed to be related to this development is fibronectin. Fibronectin is a glycoprotein whose action is not completely understood. It acts as an opsonin by coating bacteria and enhancing phagocytosis. Located within the neutrophils and their storage pools, fibronectin is carried by the polymorphonuclear leukocytes to the site of invasion by a foreign substance (Polin, 1990). Fibronectin sometimes complicates the neonate's physical well-being by changing the vascular permeability of the surrounding tissue. It appears to have a role in the regulation of vascular permeability. The implication is that microvascular integrity and permeability are also regulated by its presence. It may also be responsible for the build-up of fibrinous

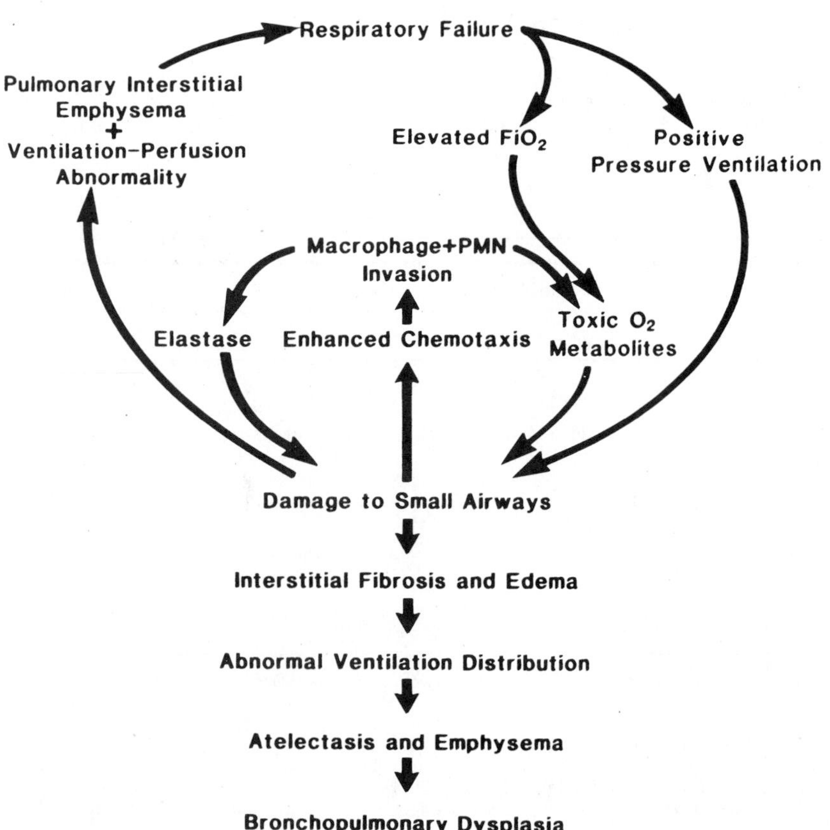

FIGURE 20–1. Interaction of factors involved in the pathogenesis of bronchopulmonary dysplasia. (From Boynton, C. A. [1988]. Epidemiology of bronchopulmonary dysplasia. In T. A. Merritt, W. H. Northway, Jr., & B. R. Boynton [Eds.], *Bronchopulmonary dysplasia* [p. 27]. Boston: Blackwell Scientific Publications. By permission of Blackwell Scientific Publications. As adapted from Bancalari, E. (1985). In A. D. Milner & R. Martin, [Eds.], *Neonatal and pediatric respiratory medicine*. London: Butterworths. Reprinted with permission.)

tissue in the pulmonary tree, which is often associated with chronic lung changes in the neonate. Thus, alveolar macrophages most likely produce fibronectin (Polin, 1990).

An inflammatory response, together with an influx of polymorphonuclear cells and macrophages that release proteolytic enzymes, further aggravates the damage. The influx of fluid, proteins, and enzymes causes an inactivation of any surfactant that is present, worsening the initial lung disease (Merritt & Hallman, 1988b). This influx also causes the release of more oxygen radicals, adding to the initial damage. The proteases released during this inflammatory response are ineffectively opposed by endogenous proteinase inhibitors, which are at low levels in premature infants (Merritt & Hallman, 1988b; Sinkin & Phelps, 1987), and cause damage to lung elastin, proteoglycan, basement membranes, and collagen.

Destruction of elastin causes disruption of alveolar septal development in the developing lung and may have long-term effects on the ability of the lung to grow and develop normally in infancy and childhood (Monin & Vert, 1987). All this damage, together with resulting alveolar and bronchiolar necrosis, causes regenerative efforts by the lung, that is, the growth of new alveolar lining cells with a fibroproliferative response. This cycle of lung injury and necrosis followed by fibrotic repair mechanisms is typical of BPD and is also associated with the other iatrogenic trigger, barotrauma.

Barotrauma: Mechanisms

Barotrauma, the damage done to lung structures (primarily small airways and alveoli) by mechanical stress, has been implicated as a major contributor to the incidence of BPD. Barotrauma occurs when lung volume exceeds physiologic limits, especially when tissue structures are "stiff" or noncompliant. Overdistention of the airways and alveoli in the premature infant is most often caused by the large and frequently oscillating pressure differences associated with mechanical ventilation (Thibeault, 1986). Premature infants are especially susceptible to barotrauma, not only because they are likely to need assisted ventilation but also because their lungs are noncompliant owing to increased surface tension from surfactant deficiency and increased interstitial fluid (Thibeault & Lang, 1988). Mechanical stresses occur in all planes of the alveolar wall, but the strain is especially significant at the junction of the alveolus and the related bronchioles, where large excursions in diameter occur during ventilation (Monin & Vert, 1987; Thibeault, 1986). Tissue breakdown, epithelial necrosis, and alveolar rupture occur as a consequence of these large, unbalanced stresses (Thibeault, 1986). In the bronchi and bronchioles, these stresses produce desquamation of epithelium and ciliary apparatus, an increase in goblet cells and smooth muscle, and necrotizing bronchiolitis that heals with fibrosis. The pathologic process of BPD is summarized in Figure 20–2 (Merritt & Hallman, 1988b).

Oxygen Toxicity and Barotrauma: Consequences

BPD is a disease characterized by two stages: (1) an exudative and early reparative stage followed by (2) a chronic fibroproliferative stage. The chronic phase consists of obliterative airway disease, widespread parenchymal fibrosis, alternating areas of atelectasis and emphysema, and capillary damage. These processes have both short- and long-term consequences for the infant with BPD.

PATHOGENESIS OF BRONCHOPULMONARY DYSPLASIA

Alterations in Lung Mechanics

BPD infants have both short- and long-term alterations in lung mechanics that may persist even after clinical symptoms disappear (Boynton, 1988). These alterations are a result of the lung pathology of BPD (Agiagno, 1988) (Table 20–6). Protein leakage inhibits surfactant production and function, leading to increased surface tension, decreased dynamic compliance, and increased atelectasis (Obladen, 1988) (Fig. 20–3). Some reports indicate that surfactant synthesis in BPD survivors does not return to normal even with recovery (Obladen, 1988). These infants also have an increase in pulmonary resistance because of increased mucus production, decreased mucus transport caused by damaged cilia, low lung volume, and airway occlusion. Hypoxia and hypercapnia cause an elevation in minute ventilation, respiratory rate, work of breathing, and oxygen consumption (Monin & Vert, 1987). Functional residual capacity may be increased or decreased, but is usually not normal. These infants also have recurrent lower respiratory tract infections.

Postnatal Mortality

Infants with BPD have an excessive postnatal mortality rate in the first year of life. The incidence of sudden infant death in these infants is reported to be as much as seven times the normal rate (Boynton, 1988).

Bronchial Reactivity

Bronchial reactivity is a significant clinical problem (Monin & Vert, 1987). Reactivity appears to be a response to different factors that induce bronchoconstriction and smooth muscle hypertrophy. Reactivity can develop both at the onset of clinical and radiologic signs of BPD and as a late sign of severe disease.

TABLE 20–6 Pathology of the Lung in Bronchopulmonary Dysplasia

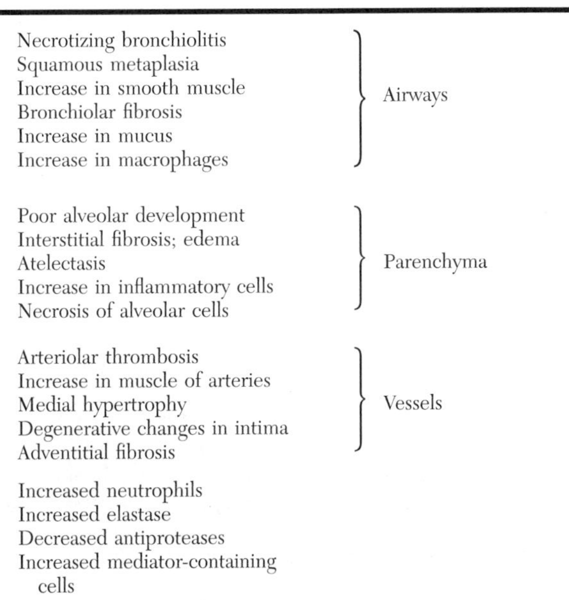

Finding	Site
Necrotizing bronchiolitis Squamous metaplasia Increase in smooth muscle Bronchiolar fibrosis Increase in mucus Increase in macrophages	Airways
Poor alveolar development Interstitial fibrosis; edema Atelectasis Increase in inflammatory cells Necrosis of alveolar cells	Parenchyma
Arteriolar thrombosis Increase in muscle of arteries Medial hypertrophy Degenerative changes in intima Adventitial fibrosis	Vessels
Increased neutrophils Increased elastase Decreased antiproteases Increased mediator-containing cells	

Reprinted with permission of Ross Laboratories, Columbus, OH 43216, from 90th Ross Conference on Pediatric Research, p. 127. Copyright 1986, Ross Laboratories.

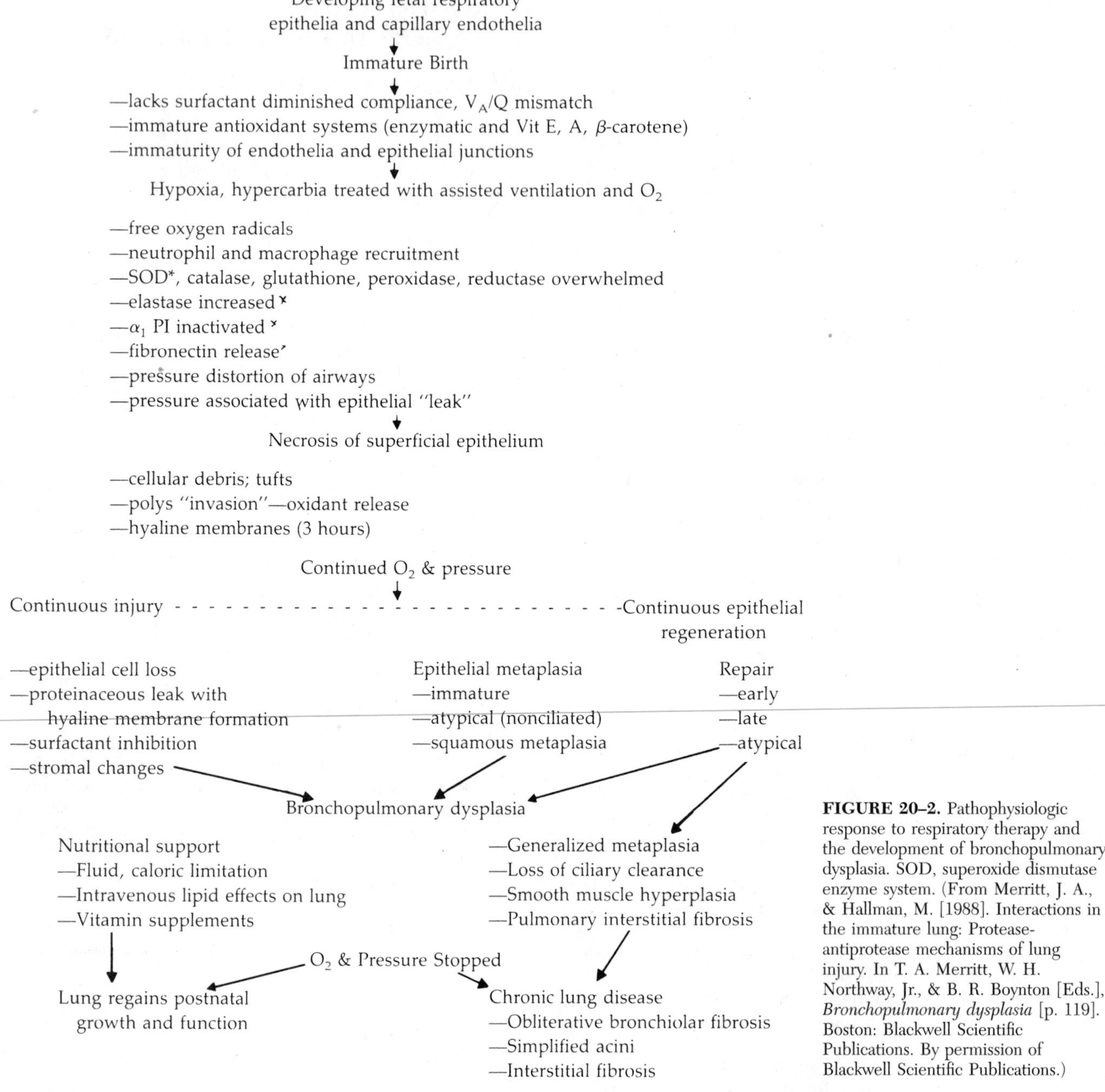

FIGURE 20–2. Pathophysiologic response to respiratory therapy and the development of bronchopulmonary dysplasia. SOD, superoxide dismutase enzyme system. (From Merritt, J. A., & Hallman, M. [1988]. Interactions in the immature lung: Protease-antiprotease mechanisms of lung injury. In T. A. Merritt, W. H. Northway, Jr., & B. R. Boynton [Eds.], *Bronchopulmonary dysplasia* [p. 119]. Boston: Blackwell Scientific Publications. By permission of Blackwell Scientific Publications.)

Pulmonary Hypertension and Cardiac Failure

Infants with BPD are often acidemic and hypoxemic because of the alterations in lung mechanics. These conditions induce pulmonary arteriolar vasoconstriction, vascular muscular hypertrophy, and hypertension. Pulmonary blood flow may be significantly decreased, resulting in further hypoxemia and acidemia. In severe cases of BPD, a cyclic process of pulmonary hypertension and cardiac dysfunction is present (Perkin & Anas, 1984) (Figs. 20–4 through 20–6), complicating the treatment for respiratory compromise with cardiac failure and for cor pulmonale (Sherman, 1988).

Changes in cardiac function and their effects are not easily evaluated in the individual patient, however, because echocardiographic data and direct cardiac catheterization measurements do not always correlate (Goodman et al., 1988; Sherman, 1988). In some infants with severe pulmonary hypertension, large collateral pulmonary vessels develop. These patients often do not respond to conventional treatment (e.g., oxygen, antihypertensive drugs) and have a high mortality rate (Goodman et al., 1988).

Alterations in Lung Growth and Development

A large portion of lung growth and development occurs after birth, with full adult size and numbers of respiratory units and arteriolar networks being developed by 8 years of age (Moore & Persaud, 1993). This future growth was once thought to be an advantage for infants with BPD because large amounts of new, unscarred, functional lung would eventually make the amount of damaged lung insignificant. However, the process of BPD appears

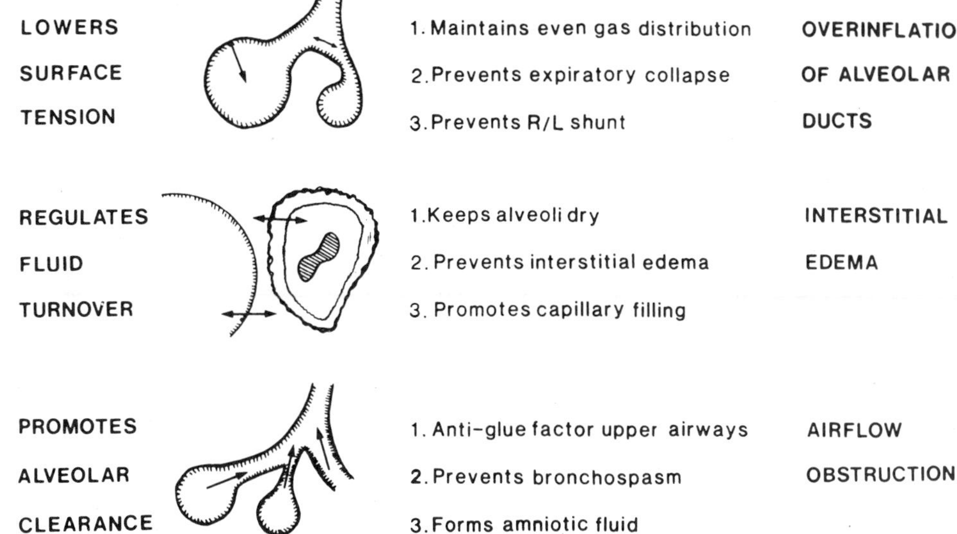

FIGURE 20–3. Basic surfactant functions and possible contribution of persisting surfactant inadequacy to specific features of bronchopulmonary dysplasia. (Adapted from Obladen, M. [1988]. Alterations in surfactant composition. In T. A. Merritt, W. H. Northway, Jr., & B. R. Boynton [Eds.], *Bronchopulmonary dysplasia* [p. 138]. Boston: Blackwell Scientific Publications. By permission of Blackwell Scientific Publications.)

to have inhibitory effects on future lung growth and development, preventing some of these infants from ever reaching fully normal capacity and function (Bonikos & Bensch, 1988). The proposed mechanisms for these inhibitory effects are injury-caused alterations in nucleic acid formation and function (Wispe & Roberts, 1987) and a mechanical interruption and alteration of the normal development sequences of vascular and alveolar formation (Bonikos & Bensch, 1988). The pulmonary capillary bed is further directly damaged by hyperoxia in the fibroproliferative repair process of BPD. The result of all these processes is a smaller lung with decreased alveolarization and diminished alveolar and vascular surface area for diffusion.

Alteration of Total Growth and Development

Delays and retardation of total growth and development are common but not universal in the infant with BPD (Kurzner et al., 1988a, 1988b). The reason why some infants grow and develop normally and some do not, even those with similar morbidity, is not clear. However, studies have suggested that increased oxygen consumption, increased resting metabolic expenditure, and inefficient substrate utilization may combine to create a state of relative protein–calorie malnutrition, even with nutritional supplementation calculated to be more than adequate for growth needs (Kurzner et al., 1988a, 1988b).

Tracheobronchial Injury

Many of the same factors that contribute to the development of BPD also cause tracheobronchial abnormalities, often in the same patient. Reported complications include partial to near-total airway occlusion by abnormal growth of granulation tissue, subglottic stenosis, tracheobronchiomalacia, tracheomegaly, necrotizing tracheobronchitis, vocal cord injuries, and inspissated secretions (Miller et al., 1987). All of these lesions are thought to be acquired as a consequence of respiratory treatments because they are not present before therapy is initiated and appear only after prolonged therapy (Miller et al., 1987). Several risk factors for these lesions are listed in Table 20–7.

Destruction of epithelium from oxygen toxicity, barotrauma, and suctioning creates necrotic areas that later heal with granulation tissue and thickening of the respiratory mucosa, leading to airway occlusion. Prolonged intubation, repeated reintubation, and large endotracheal tubes cause mechanical trauma to the

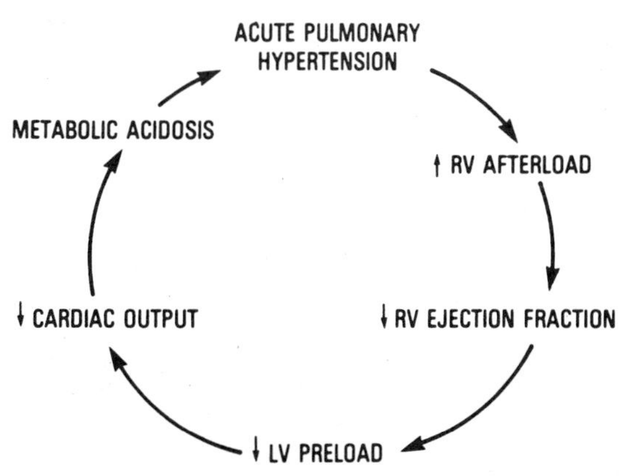

FIGURE 20–4. Effect of pulmonary hypertension on cardiac output. RV, right ventricle; LV, left ventricle. (From Perkin, R. M., & Anas, N. G. [1984]. Pulmonary hypertension in pediatric patients. *Journal of Pediatrics, 105*(4), 516–517. Reprinted with permission.)

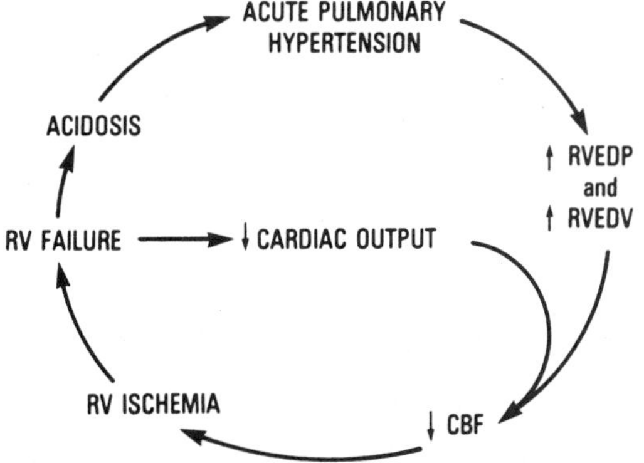

FIGURE 20–5. Effect of pulmonary hypertension on right ventricular function. RV, right ventricle; RVEDP, right ventricular end diastolic pressure; RVEDV, right ventricular end diastolic volume; CBF, coronary blood flow. (From Perkin, R. M., & Anas, N. G. [1984]. Pulmonary hypertension in pediatric patients. *Journal of Pediatrics, 105*(4), 516–517. Reprinted with permission.)

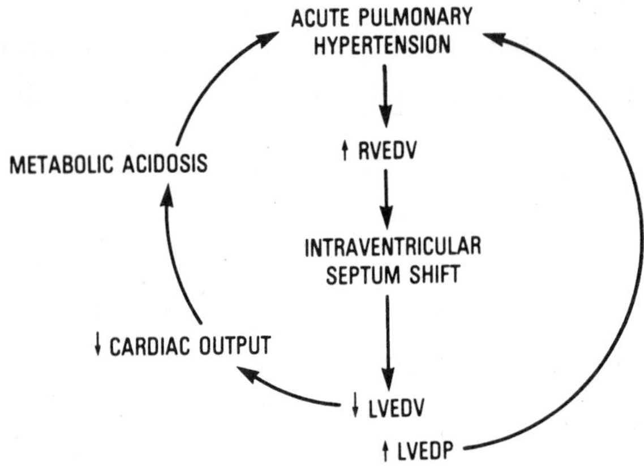

FIGURE 20–6. Effect of pulmonary hypertension on left ventricular function. RVEDV, right ventricular end diastolic volume; LVEDV, left ventricular end diastolic volume; LVEDP, left ventricular end diastolic pressure. (From Perkin, R. M., & Anas, N. G. [1984]. Pulmonary hypertension in pediatric patients. *Journal of Pediatrics, 105*(4), 516–517. Reprinted with permission.)

trachea and vocal cords, resulting in stenosis, necrotizing tracheobronchitis, and vocal cord injuries that can cause permanent interference with airway patency and normal vocalization. Intubation and barotrauma can also cause tracheomegaly and tracheobronchiomalacia. At best, these lesions interfere with the process of recovery from RDS and BPD; at worst, they cause permanent disabilities or even death.

Pulmonary Air Leaks

Pulmonary air leaks are primarily caused by rupture of the alveoli when the lung is overdistended by the oscillating pressures of mechanical ventilation (Thibeault, 1986). They are rarely seen in neonates who have not been intubated and ventilated. Air leaks can be acute or chronic and can vary in severity from benign to acutely life-threatening, depending on the location, amount, and dissection of air. Most pulmonary air leaks are preceded by intrapulmonary interstitial emphysema (IIE).

Intrapulmonary Interstitial Emphysema

IIE is a common air leak in ventilated VLBW neonates. Table 20–8 lists predisposing factors for IIE (or pulmonary interstitial emphysema [PIE] as it is often referred) (Thibeault, 1986). Mechanical ventilation at high pressures causes stress and rupture of the alveoli, probably at the bases or ducts. The air then dissects perivascularly and peribronchially, probably along lymphatic channels (Thibeault, 1986). The lungs on chest radiograph have a "bubbly" appearance either unilaterally or bilaterally, and the affected lung is usually hyperventilated. The effects of IIE are summarized in Table 20–9 (Thibeault, 1986). Preterm neonates with widespread IIE, especially those with diffuse IIE and flattened diaphragms, have a high mortality rate. Significant BPD usually develops in those who survive (Thibeault, 1986).

TABLE 20–7 Risk Factors for Tracheobronchial Injury

- Prolonged intubation
- Lack of air leak around endotracheal tube
- Repeated reintubation
- Mechanical trauma secondary to suctioning
- Amount and duration of positive-pressure ventilation
- Hyperoxia
- Unbalanced lung expansion pattern
- Respiratory infection
- Excessive movement of endotracheal tube

TABLE 20–8 Predisposing Factors for Intrapulmonary Interstitial Emphysema

- Lung immaturity
  - Increased connective tissue and interstitial fluid
  - Atelectasis
- RDS
- Aspiration syndromes
- Lung infection
- Pulmonary anomalies
  - Hypoplastic lung and diaphragmatic hernia
- Overzealous resuscitation at birth
- Intubation of a bronchus followed by positive-pressure ventilation
- Iatrogenic needle puncture of a lung
- Transient tachypnea of the newborn
- Inhomogeneity of alveolar ventilation
- Assisted ventilation

RDS, respiratory distress syndrome.
From Thibeault, D. W. (1986). Pulmonary barotrauma: Interstitial emphysema, pneumomediastinum, and pneumothorax. In D. W. Thibeault & G. A. Gregory (Eds.), *Neonatal pulmonary care* (2nd ed., pp. 504–505). Norwalk, CT: Appleton-Century-Crofts, Reprinted with permission.

Congenital Lobar Emphysema

Congenital lobar emphysema is not as common as IIE, but the side effects are similar, except that congenital lobar emphysema is really an overdistention of lung tissue, a lobe that occurs in utero (Lazar & Stolar, 1995). The cause is not exactly known. Congenital lobar emphysema is sometimes diagnosed in the newborn period when RDS seems to worsen. Ideally, it is identified in the delivery room if the lesion is large and causes immediate distress or cardiac compromise. Otherwise, attempts to compensate for respiratory distress follow the normal course of mechanical ventilation, with higher and higher pressures until adequate oxygenation is achieved, while the lobe continues to distend,

TABLE 20–9 Intrapulmonary Interstitial Emphysema and Physiologic Derangements

Effect of Interstitial Gas Collection	Physiologic Abnormality
Trapped interstitial air splints	Decreased compliance
Lung and thorax in inflated position	Decreased tidal volume Decreased negative interstitial pressure Pulmonary hypertension Right-sided heart failure Right-to-left extrapulmonary shunts
Alveoli compressed	Venous admixture
Lymphatics, capillaries, and arterioles compressed	Lung edema and hypoperfusion
Airway compression	Gas trapping or atelectasis

From Thibeault, D. W. (1986). Pulmonary barotrauma: Interstitial emphysema, pneumomediastinum, and pneumothorax. In D. W. Thibeault & G. A. Gregory (Eds.), *Neonatal pulmonary care* (2nd ed., p. 509). Norwalk, CT: Appleton-Century-Crofts. Reprinted with permission.

leading to circulatory collapse (Lazar & Stolar, 1995). If there is a chest tube inserted without recognition of the problem, damage from the tube eventually necessitates resection of the lobe. A normal chest radiograph can usually confirm the presence of lobar emphysema. If lobar emphysema is allowed to progress, increased respiratory distress, cardiac collapse, and chronic lung changes occur. The only treatment is removal of the cyst (Lazar & Stolar, 1995).

Pneumomediastinum

A pneumomediastinum is almost always preceded by IIE. The air usually collects anterior to the heart, and pneumomediastinum is often benign. A pneumomediastinum that does not cause clinical symptoms of cardiac or respiratory embarrassment does not need treatment (Thibeault, 1986).

Pneumothorax

A pneumothorax is preceded by rupture of the alveoli, with interstitial air traveling via fascial planes to the mediastinum, where it breaks through the mediastinal pleura to form collections of air outside the lung (Thibeault, 1986). Pneumothoraces are usually caused by one or more of the following:

1. High-pressure gradients from mechanical ventilation or continuous positive airway pressure (CPAP) across poorly compliant alveoli
2. Obstructive pulmonary pathology such as ball-valve air trapping associated with meconium aspiration syndrome
3. Rupture of subpleural blebs from IIE or BPD

Occasionally, a pneumothorax is benign and asymptomatic. More serious leaks needing treatment are usually larger, occur in neonates with pre-existing serious lung disease, are under tension, and compress the heart and lungs, compromising their function. Serious pneumothoraces are accompanied by acute, profound respiratory and cardiac decompensation and often require cardiopulmonary resuscitation along with evacuation of the air by needle aspiration and chest tube placement.

Pneumopericardium

A pneumopericardium is a very rare complication of mechanical ventilation caused by lung overdistention with high peak inspiratory and positive end-expiratory pressures. A pneumopericardium is usually preceded by either IIE or a pneumomediastinum, or both. The exact mechanism of air dissection into the pericardial space is unknown.

A pneumopericardium can be benign and the neonate asymptomatic (Thibeault, 1986). If the air pocket is sufficiently large or under tension, however, a cardiac tamponade results, dramatically reducing cardiac output and producing a life-threatening situation. Immediate evacuation of the air is often needed.

TREATMENT OF BRONCHOPULMONARY DYSPLASIA

Early Treatment Strategies

New treatment strategies for BPD are aimed at preventing or inhibiting the events that trigger the cascade of underlying pathogenic mechanisms in the development of the disease (Goetzman, 1986) (Table 20–10). Whereas previous strategies treated the symptoms of the disease once it occurred, current understanding of the interaction of host susceptibility and iatrogenic factors allows caretakers to intervene earlier in the process and save other strategies for the treatment of the fixed disease (Sinkin & Phelps, 1987). This discussion is directed toward BPD, but the principles also apply to airway injury and air leaks.

Prevention of Risk Group

Ideally, prevention of BPD at various levels is the goal of treatment (Boynton, 1988) (Table 20–11). The first defense is to identify and prevent the creation of susceptible hosts. Although more work needs to be done in prospectively identifying risk groups, BPD is more likely to develop in VLBW neonates with RDS who are exposed to intubation, mechanical ventilation, and supplemental oxygen than in more mature neonates. Decreasing the numbers of these neonates, first by prevention of prematurity and second by prevention of RDS, is a primary intervention. Tocolysis for control of preterm labor and delay of delivery is a widespread practice. This practice can delay delivery either until the point of natural lung maturity or until artificial induction of surfactant synthesis can take place. For the preterm infant weighing less than 1000 g at birth, delay of delivery with tocolysis

TABLE 20–10 Proposed Pathogenesis of, Factors Involved in, and Therapies for Bronchopulmonary Dysplasia

Proposed Pathogenesis		Factors Involved		Potential Therapies
Susceptible host	◆	Premature birth Genetic predisposition Fetal asphyxia Fetal infection	◆	Prenatal care Antenatal care Intrapartum care
+				
Acute lung injury	◆	Surfactant deficiency Barotrauma Infection	◆	Surfactant replacement Decrease inflation pressure Decrease bacterial damage
+				
Secondary lung injury	◆	Oxidants Proteolytic enzymes	◆	Antioxidants Antiproteases
+				
Abnormal healing	◆	Hyperoxia/hypoxia Vitamin A deficiency Interstitial fibrosis	◆	Monitoring oxygenation Vitamin A Anti-inflammatory and antifibrotic agents
↓				
Bronchopulmonary dysplasia			◆	Supportive care

From Goetzman, B. W. (1986). Understanding bronchopulmonary dysplasia. *American Journal of Diseases of Children*, *140*, 332–334.

TABLE 20–11 Bronchopulmonary Dysplasia: Levels of Prevention

Primary prevention
- Prevention of preterm birth
- Prevention of respiratory distress

Secondary prevention
- Use of less toxic therapies
- Exogenous surfactants
- High-frequency ventilation
- More insightful use of conventional ventilation
- Antidotes for toxic therapies
  - Antioxidants
    - Vitamins A and E
    - Superoxide dismutase
- Corticosteroids

Tertiary prevention
- Optimal treatment of bronchopulmonary dysplasia
- Screening for complications
- Early detection of neurodevelopmental delay

From Boynton, B. R. (1988). Epidemiology of bronchopulmonary dysplasia. In T. A. Merritt, W. H. Northway, Jr., & B. R. Boynton (Eds.), *Bronchopulmonary dysplasia* (p. 26). Boston: Blackwell Scientific Publications. By permission of Blackwell Scientific Publications.

for at least 24 hours and enhancement of surfactant synthesis by betamethasone reduces not only the incidence of RDS but also subsequent mortality and morbidity (Papageorgiou et al., 1989). In 1994, the National Institutes of Health (NIH) published the *NIH Consensus Statement: Effect of Corticosteroids for Fetal Maturation on Perinatal Outcomes*. The findings indicated that, if women at risk for delivering an infant of 24 to 34 weeks' gestation received antenatal corticosteroids (betamethasone or dexamethasone), then the incidence of BPD would be significantly decreased. If these same infants then received surfactant therapy postnatally, there would be another decrease in the BPD incidence (National Institutes of Health, 1994). With the changes in health care, however, many at-risk women do not receive adequate prenatal care in a timely fashion, thus contributing to the incidence of BPD (Maloni et al., 1996). Optimal timing of the therapy is at least 24 hours before or less than 7 days before delivery. Additionally, positive effects have been documented when delivery occurs before or after this time period (National Institutes of Health, 1994).

Another preventive therapy is the use of antenatal steroids concomitantly with thyrotropin-releasing hormone. The latter does not cross the placental barrier; however, when given with maternal steroids, the incidence of BPD is decreased more than if steroids alone were used (National Institutes of Health, 1994).

Postnatally, surfactant replacement therapy is very effective against RDS; however, it does not prevent all chronic lung problems, including BPD. Treated infants have decreased incidence and severity of RDS and therefore a decreased need for respiratory support (Merritt & Hallman, 1988a; Sinkin & Phelps, 1987). It is the respiratory support in many instances that leads to chronic lung changes or barotrauma and eventually the development of BPD.

When preterm delivery cannot be prevented, identification of the subgroup prone to BPD would be helpful so that early treatment could be directed toward them. It may be possible to pinpoint susceptible neonates as early as the end of the first week of life by the presence of proteolytic enzymes and polymorphonuclear cells in their lung fluid and by abnormal pulmonary function tests (PFTs) (Sinkin & Phelps, 1987).

Neonates with RDS in whom BPD does not later develop have a predominance of antiproteolytic enzymes, macrophages, and early regenerative processes detectable in their lung fluid by the end of the first week of life. Neonates in whom BPD will later develop have a predominance of proteolytic enzymes, polymorphonuclear cells, and fibrotic processes, indicating that the BPD cycle of tissue destruction and fibrosis is already present.

Although the significance of PFTs is not well known enough for their use as predictors, early alterations in these tests have been noted in neonates in whom BPD later develops (Tepper, 1988). The PFTs could be used to define pathophysiology and dysfunction, to monitor the natural history of BPD, to evaluate interventions, and to predict the specific groups at risk for BPD (Tepper, 1988). If a reliable predictive early scoring system using PFTs and other indicators could be developed that has specificity, then preventive and direct therapies could be used.

Limitation of Injury

In the first few weeks of life of the premature infant with RDS requiring respiratory support, the strategy is to limit the iatrogenic tissue injury that leads to the development of chronic BPD. This strategy includes the prevention of oxygen toxicity injury by (1) limiting intubation and mechanical ventilation, (2) applying extracorporeal membrane oxygenation (ECMO) and alternative ventilation techniques, and (3) applying developmental enhancement techniques.

Oxygen therapy in the premature newborn is a balancing act between providing adequate oxygenation to prevent hypoxic damage and limiting complications related to hyperoxia. There is a lack of agreement as to what levels of oxygen are appropriate to reach this balance (Avery et al., 1987; Davis & Rosenfeld, 1994; Rhodes et al., 1983; Sinkin & Phelps, 1987; Usher, 1987). Based on experience with increased rates of retinopathy of prematurity associated with liberal oxygen use in the 1940s and with increased rates of cerebral palsy associated with restricted oxygen use in the 1950s and 1960s, many current protocols maintain PaO_2 in a midrange (50 to 70 mm Hg). Guidelines are complicated by other factors: the prevention of pulmonary hypertension, natural or stress-induced fluctuations in oxygenation, and unknowns in the interpretation of noninvasive readings.

For many premature infants, a PaO_2 of approximately 25 mm Hg would have been their normal environment for many more weeks if they had remained in utero. Even allowing for the need for increased blood oxygen levels to compensate for the increased oxygen demands of respiratory disease, metabolism, and cost of interaction with the extrauterine environment, no minimally acceptable levels have been established. Present guidelines are based on experience with much larger infants, and whether such levels are appropriate or toxic to VLBW infants is unknown. Are the tissues of VLBW infants more susceptible to injury from oxygen toxicity? Would any level be too high? How much oxygenation do their developing tissues need? Many authors advocate minimizing oxygenation (PaO_2, 35 to 40 mm Hg) as long as perfusion, hematocrit, blood pressure, and other parameters of tissue oxygenation are normal (Avery et al., 1987; Rhodes et al., 1983; Usher, 1987). Further controlled investigations are needed to determine minimum safe levels for oxygenation in various gestational ages.

A promising trend is the use of antioxidant therapy to neutralize and clear free oxygen radicals (Rosenfeld & Concepcion, 1988). Both premature infants and infants with BPD have immature or poorly functioning enzymatic and nonenzymatic antioxidant systems and low serum antioxidant levels. In one double-blind study (Rosenfeld et al., 1984), infants experimentally treated with superoxide dismutase (SOD) had decreased radiologic and clinical signs of BPD and required fewer days on CPAP than did control infants, but they had no difference in survival or amount of oxygen or mechanical ventilation needed. The activity of natural protease inhibitors may also be increased in SOD-treated infants, thereby providing another protection from tissue damage in the cycle of BPD. Further studies are needed to establish whether SOD therapy is safe and efficacious in the newborn.

The prevention of barotrauma injury also requires rethinking of standard practices of intubation and mechanical ventilation (Avery et al., 1987; Rhodes et al., 1983; Southwell, 1995; Usher, 1987). Which infants are susceptible? What pattern of rate, pressure, inspiratory time, and mean airway pressure produces adequate oxygenation with minimal damage? Are alternative therapies to endotracheal intubation and conventional mechanical ventilation as useful in maintaining homeostasis and preventing injury? These questions need to be answered by controlled clinical investigations before practices can be standardized and individualized appropriately. Until then, various guidelines for the use of intubation and ventilation have been suggested and are summarized in Table 20–12 in increasing order of invasiveness and risk of barotrauma (Monin & Vert, 1987; Sinkin & Phelps, 1987).

High-frequency ventilation (HFV), both jet and oscillation, decreases barotrauma by (1) decreasing airway pressures (Karp et al., 1986), (2) changing the mechanics of airflow (Inwood et al., 1986; Karp et al., 1986; Karp, 1991), and (3) decreasing the development of hyaline membranes (Sinkin & Phelps, 1987). Study results with HFV have been difficult to interpret owing to selection of subjects (Sinkin & Phelps, 1987). Most infants put on HFV already have evidence of early BPD, have been on high rates of pressure on conventional ventilation for varying lengths of time, or are "rescue" subjects for whom all other therapy has failed. In the evaluation of outcomes, the contribution of these factors versus the contribution of HFV is difficult to interpret. HFV needs to be used in studies of a preventive nature in an at-risk population before its impact on mortality and morbidity can be known (Boyle et al., 1995). Since the use of HFV involves complications (Karp et al., 1986; Karp, 1991), it should be used with caution. (See Chapter 19, New Technologies Applied to the Management of Respiratory Dysfunction, for a complete discussion of high-frequency ventilation.)

ECMO appears to be of some use in preventing mortality and morbidity in larger infants with respiration disease (Bartlett et al., 1985). ECMO decreases barotrauma and oxygen toxicity by controlling oxygenation outside the lungs, thereby decreasing the need for mechanical ventilation and oxygen (Nugent, 1986). Chronic lung changes often develop in such infants when treated with conventional ventilation because of the high pressures, rates, and oxygen levels that are a part of the treatment. Although ECMO has complications and its use is currently limited to larger infants, future improvements may make ECMO an option for preterm infants (Nugent, 1986; Boyle et al., 1995). (See Chapter 19, New Technologies Applied to the Management of Respiratory Dysfunction, for a complete discussion of ECMO.)

Another experimental therapy is nitric oxide (NO). Although most of the research with NO has been for term or close to term infants with persistent pulmonary hypertension, it has been used with some premature infants. The inhalation of NO activates vasorelaxation, thus diminishing pulmonary vascular resistance (Southwell, 1995). The result is an increase in effective oxygenation and perfusion at lower mechanical ventilation pressures. The downside is the side effects. Methemoglobinemia is a breakdown product of NO that does not effectively carry oxygen, and there is increased susceptibility to lung injury owing to increased permeability of the tissue. This change in permeability can cause bleeding tendencies to increase (Southwell, 1995). More clinical research needs to be done with this population before the therapy can be widely used.

Developmental enhancement techniques also offer hope in decreasing barotrauma and oxygen toxicity by preventing or handling adverse patient reactions to environmental stress that might otherwise result in the need for increased ventilatory support. The influence of the techniques on respiratory problems is discussed here.

Premature infants have difficulty in interacting appropriately with the extrauterine environment, that is, the stress of light, noise, and handling. They have greater difficulty than larger infants in organization and regulatory control, often not being able to keep the primitive functions of heart and respiratory rates stable when exposed to increasing environmental stress (Lawhon, 1986; Linton, 1986). Infants with BPD have similar difficulty in self-regulation, organization, and integration of the developmental systems (Boynton & Jones, 1988). A controlled study of a small group of infants in a preventive developmental program has indicated that such programs can improve both respiratory and motor development outcomes (Als et al., 1986). Further studies with such techniques are needed to clarify the contribution of developmental programs to the prevention and treatment of respiratory complications.

TABLE 20–12 Guidelines for Use of Intubation and Mechanical Ventilation

Tolerance of increased $Pa{CO_2}$ and decreased pH and $Pa{O_2}$ levels if evidence of adequate tissue oxygenation and normoacidemia is present.
Increased use of nasal CPAP rather than routine intubation.
If mechanical ventilation is needed:
- The lowest pressures and MAP possible should be used to establish adequate oxygenation and ventilation.
- The option of high rates with lower pressures may be used.
- Mechanical ventilation should be weaned as soon and as quickly as possible.

Suctioning, reintubation, and manipulation of the tube should be kept to a minimum.
Ventilatory adjustments should be made by the same practitioner for consistency.
The use of high-frequency ventilators should be considered for those infants needing mechanical ventilation who are at high risk for air leaks and BPD and those with early signs of chronic lung changes.
The use of ECMO should be considered in those larger infants who meet treatment criteria.

BPD, bronchopulmonary dysplasia; CPAP, continuous positive airway pressure; ECMO, extracorporeal membrane oxygenation; MAP, mean airway pressure.

Medical Treatment of Fixed Bronchopulmonary Dysplasia

Once BPD is present, treatment of the disease is focused on the twin goals of enhancing the natural healing process to restore whatever normal function is possible and controlling complications caused by the damaged lung tissue and abnormal lung mechanics of BPD. Generally used treatments are still in the evolutionary phase, are still largely empirical, and have little experimental clinical data to support any one standard procedure. Such treatments include oxygen therapy, diuretics, bronchodilators, steroids, and nutritional support.

Oxygen Therapy

Although oxygen is part of the cause of BPD, it is also a large part of the supportive treatment of fixed BPD. Supplemental oxygen is often needed to ensure adequate and stable oxygenation for growth and healing and to prevent recurrent hypoxemia during the fluctuating oxygen demands of exercise and stress (Blanchard et al., 1987; Monin & Vert, 1987). Chronic hypoxemia can cause abnormal muscularization of the pulmonary arterioles, pulmonary hypertension, cor pulmonale, reduction in weight gain, and increase in oxygen consumption. No exact parameters exist for adequate oxygen levels, but some authors suggest maintenance of $Pa{O_2}$ at 55 mm Hg or greater, or oxygen saturation at

95 percent or greater, or both (Blanchard et al., 1987; Goodman et al., 1988).

The need of infants with BPD to have oxygen therapy varies in amount and duration. Frequent noninvasive oxygenation monitoring, especially during periods of exercise and stress, is important to assess any increased need for oxygen. BPD infants are often discharged on low-flow nasal cannula oxygen, with regular outpatient oxygenation assessment by clinic or home care professionals (Dorkin, 1988).

Diuretics

Because increased interstitial fluid and pulmonary edema play a role both in the origin and the ongoing complications of BPD, the elimination or control of this extra fluid is thought to improve outcomes (Blanchard, 1987; Yeh, 1988). The absence of an expected early diuresis in the neonate with RDS has been correlated with a higher incidence of BPD; therefore, inducing diuresis in these neonates has been advocated as a means of preventing BPD (Blanchard et al., 1987). However, although the restriction of fluid and prevention of fluid overload in these infants has been helpful, induced diuresis has not been found to be effective (Blanchard et al., 1987; Monin & Vert, 1987). In the infant with fixed BPD, regular diuretic therapy has been found to be helpful both in preventing fluid overload and in decreasing pulmonary resistance and increasing compliance (Boyle et al., 1995; Monin & Vert, 1987; Martin et al., 1993). Occasional extra doses may be necessary to correct intermittent fluid overload or retention. The commonly used diuretics, their doses, and their complications are listed in Table 20–13 (Roberts, 1984a).

Bronchodilators

Hypoxemia caused by reactive airway disease (because of muscular hypertrophy and peribronchial edema) and peripheral airway closure (because of hypoventilation) is common in infants with BPD. Treatment with bronchodilators is thought to modify or overcome some of these effects (Blanchard et al., 1987; Katz & Murphy, 1988; Monin & Vert, 1987). Bronchodilators, both oral and inhalation, decrease pulmonary resistance, increase compliance, increase minute ventilation, decrease diaphragmatic fatigue by increasing contractility without increasing oxygen consumption, decrease pulmonary edema, and prevent dyspneic attacks (Blanchard et al., 1987; Katz & Murphy, 1988; Monin & Vert, 1987). However, there is no evidence that they alter the evolution of the disease. The commonly used bronchodilators are listed in Table 20–14 (Roberts, 1984b).

Steroids

Steroids have been used both in the early stages of BPD to promote weaning from ventilatory support and in the later stages of BPD to decrease inflammatory responses and promote improvement in PFTs. Which actions of steroids have an effect on BPD is uncertain, but short-term improvement in lung function has been documented (Avery et al., 1985). Table 20–15 indicates the mechanisms of action of steroids that might affect BPD (Agiagno, 1988). Although steroids apparently have helpful effects in the treatment of BPD, steroid therapy has a large potential for side effects and must be used with caution (Boyle et al., 1995; Rimsza, 1978) (Table 20–16). Dexamethasone can be used as soon as 24 to 48 hours before weaning (Boyle et al., 1995). Some health professionals do not use steroids to prevent or treat BPD but only use them for weaning. Dexamethasone can be administered even in VLBW infants to help wean them from a ventilator to CPAP and then to extubation, or when extubation is going to be done with no intermediate CPAP. Nebulized epinephrine immediately following the extubation helps keep the airway open. Some centers use long-term steroids for weaning, sometimes over several weeks. The concern is that there may be an increased risk of infections, especially fungal infections, but this has not been well documented. Clinical trials of long-term steroid use are ongoing.

Nutrition

Adequate nutrition is needed in infants with BPD to restore a balance between lung injury and lung repair, to promote normal lung growth and development, and to compensate for increased oxygen and caloric consumption. Providing adequate nutrition is complicated by intolerance of increased fluid intake, inefficient substrate utilization, relative protein–calorie malnutrition, gastro-

TABLE 20–13 Dosage Recommendations and Signs of Toxicity for Diuretic Agents in Neonates

Drug	Recommended Dosage	Signs of Toxicity
Acetazolamide	5 mg/kg q 6–8 hours PO; increase as required to 25 mg/kg/dose	Metabolic acidosis, hypokalemia, drowsiness, paresthesias, rare allergic reaction
Ethacrynic acid (Edecrin)	Same as furosemide	Dehydration and electrolyte (Na, Cl, K) imbalances, gastrointestinal bleeding, ototoxicity
Furosemide	Initial dose: 1 mg/kg IV, IM, or PO; increase as required to maximum of 2 mg/kg IV or IM and 6 mg/kg PO; repeat as required, but no more often than q 12 hours (full term) or 24 hours (premature); >1 month old may tolerate dosing as often as q 6 hours	Dehydration and electrolyte (Na, Cl, K) imbalances, ototoxicity, metabolic alkalosis
Spironolactone	1–3 mg/kg q 24 hours PO	Hyperkalemia, drowsiness, gastrointestinal upset, rash
Chlorothiazide (Diuril)	10–20 mg/kg q 12 hours PO	Dehydration and electrolyte (Na, Cl, K) imbalances, hyperglycemia, hypercalcemia, liver and renal disease, metabolic alkalosis, hyperuricemia
Hydrochlorothiazide (Esidrix, HydroDIURIL, Oretic)	1–2 mg/kg q 12 hours PO	Same as chlorothiazide

Cl, chlorine; K, potassium; Na, sodium; PO, by mouth; IV, intravenously; IM, intramuscularly; q, every.
From Roberts, R. J. (1984). Diuretics. In R. J. Roberts (Ed.), *Drug therapy in infants* (p. 229). Philadelphia: W. B. Saunders. Reprinted with permission.

TABLE 20–14 Dosage Recommendations for Caffeine and Theophylline in Neonates

	Recommended Dosage		Serum Concentration (μg/ml)	
	Loading	*Maintenance*	*Therapeutic*	*Toxic*
Caffeine	10 mg/kg IV or PO	2.5 mg/kg IV or PO q 24 hours (first dose given 24 hours after loading dose)	5–25	>40–50
Theophylline	5 mg/kg IV	2 mg/kg IV q 12 hours (first dose given 12 hours after loading dose)	2–15	>15–20

IV, intravenously; PO, by mouth; q, every.
From Roberts, R. J. (1984). Methylxanthine therapy: Caffeine and theophylline. In R. J. Roberts. *Drug therapy in infants* (p. 125). Philadelphia: W. B. Saunders. Reprinted with permission.

esophageal reflux, and disturbed feeding mechanics such as uncoordinated suck and increased vomiting (Boyle et al., 1995; Boynton & Jones, 1988; Kurzner et al., 1988a, 1988b).

Nursing Care

Because BPD is partially caused by medical therapy and because the nurse carries out that therapy, the nurse is in a unique position to influence the outcome of these patients, both in preventing the disease and in treatment of the fixed disease. Nurses need to have a knowledge of disease processes, indications for and consequences of therapy, and developmental theory. Their focus should be on prevention, early intervention, and individualization of care rather than merely on the implementation of medical therapies.

The various levels of nursing intervention in patients with BPD are listed in Table 20–17.

Consistency of Caretakers and Early Problem Detection

Consistency of care in the small premature neonate at risk for BPD or in the infant with fixed BPD is important for accurate assessment of the patient. The primary or associate nurse who is familiar with a particular infant's behavior and responses to care is more likely to assess the impact of both medical treatment and nursing care quickly and accurately. This advantage is important for early detection of and intervention in problems, for designing a helpful developmental enhancement program, and for individualizing care in general to maximize benefits and minimize costs. A system of primary nursing in an NICU is a good way to provide consistency. Case management is another good approach, but it is not often implemented in NICUs.

TABLE 20–15 Potential Beneficial Effects of Steroids on Lung Function

- Gross
  - Reduction in pulmonary edema
  - Reduction of bronchial edema and bronchospasm
  - Decrease in collagen deposition in tissues
- Cellular
  - Polymorphonuclear effects
    - Decrease in polymorphonuclear recruitment to lung
    - Decreased breakdown of granulocyte aggregation with improvement in pulmonary microcirculation
  - Stabilization of cell and lysosomal membranes
- Biochemical
  - Increased surfactant synthesis
  - Enhancement of β-adrenergic activity
  - Prostaglandin effects
    - Inhibition of prostaglandin and leukotriene synthesis
  - Enhancement of prostaglandin F_2 degradation
  - Increased prostaglandin I_2 levels

From Agiagno, R. L. (1988). Use of steroids. In T. A. Merritt, W. H. Northway, Jr., & B. R. Boynton (Eds.), *Bronchopulmonary dysplasia* (p. 396). Boston: Blackwell Scientific Publications. By permission of Blackwell Scientific Publications.

Developmental Enhancement

The results of early studies (Als et al., 1986) indicate that planning and implementing a developmental enhancement pro-

TABLE 20–16 Complications of Steroid Therapy

- Ophthalmologic
  - Posterior subcapsular cataracts
  - Glaucoma
  - Reactivation of herpes keratitis
- Central nervous system
  - Pseudotumor cerebri
  - Psychiatric disturbances and dependency
- Hematopoietic system
  - Leukocytosis, neutrophilia, monocytopenia, lymphopenia, eosinopenia
  - Purpura
- Gastrointestinal system
  - Pancreatitis
  - Peptic ulcer (?)
  - Fatty infiltration of the liver
- Renal system
  - Nephrocalcinosis
  - Nephrolithiasis
  - Uricosuria
- Musculoskeletal system
  - Mycopathy
  - Osteoporosis and fractures
  - Aseptic necrosis of bone
- Endocrine and metabolic
  - Diabetes
  - Adrenal insufficiency
  - Growth failure
  - Hyperlipidemia
  - Lipomatosis
  - Hypocalcemia
  - Hypokalemic alkalosis
  - Sodium retention and hypertension

From Rimsza, M. E. (1978). Complications of corticosteroid therapy. *American Journal of Diseases of Children, 132*, 806. Copyright 1978, American Medical Association. Reprinted with permission.

TABLE 20–17 Levels of Nursing Intervention in Infants With Bronchopulmonary Dysplasia

1. Consistency of caretakers
2. Developmental enhancement
3. Early detection of problems
4. Assessment of need for and response to treatment
5. Assessment of respiratory function
6. Detection of complications of oxygen and mechanical ventilation
7. Evaluation of need for suctioning
8. Suctioning techniques
9. Control and evaluation of weaning from respiratory support
10. Feeding evaluation and techniques
11. Parent teaching
12. Discharge evaluation
13. Home care

gram based on individualized assessment may be helpful in decreasing morbidity in the VLBW neonate. In infants with fixed BPD who have decreased exercise and stress tolerance, feeding difficulties, and delayed growth and development, an individualized program of appropriate stimulation regulation can aid in maximizing their potential and minimizing the effects of stress on weight gain, respiratory function, and development (Boynton & Jones, 1988). Suggested interventions are listed in Table 20–18.

Collaborative Management of Respiratory Complications

The nurse not only implements ordered medical therapy but also assesses the need for and response to treatment. The nurse provides the physician with criteria by which to evaluate and change therapy in individual patients. The nurse is the only caretaker who is consistent enough to provide ongoing comparative assessment of the individual infant's ever-changing status and response to treatment. This information can be of great assistance to physicians both in response to acute situations such as pneumothoraces and in planning medical care that is most beneficial and least harmful to the patient.

Evaluation of Suctioning Needs and Techniques

Suctioning the endotracheal tube has been correlated with significant morbidity, including tracheal injury and hypoxemia (Miller et al., 1987). The nurse can decrease adverse reactions associated with suctioning by various means: suctioning only when assessment shows a clear patient need, implementing noninvasive oxygenation monitoring during the procedure, measuring suction catheters so as to reach only the end of the endotracheal tube, and increasing FiO_2 and using two-person technique for hypoxemic infants (Boynton & Jones, 1988). The primary goals are that suctioning be done only when it benefits the patient, that homeostasis be maintained during the procedure as much as possible, and that the stress of the procedure be minimized.

Weaning From Respiratory Support

Weaning from respiratory support, whether for the preterm neonate with RDS or the infant with fixed BPD, is a balancing of the benefits of removing treatments that may cause morbidity and the costs of exceeding the infant's physiologic limits by re-

TABLE 20–18 Stimulus Reduction for Stress-Intolerant Infants

Environmental
1. Place sign on incubator indicating extreme stress intolerance.
2. Place incubator in quiet area, away from traffic, telephones, and noisy machinery.
3. Make a personalized developmental care plan for the infant.
4. Provide signs that encourage staff and visitors to speak quietly.

Auditory
1. Eliminate radios, loud laughter, and loud conversations.
2. Place felt strips on portholes, waste cans, and drawers.
3. Provide appropriate stimulation such as quiet rattles, soft music, or tapes of parents' voices when the infant is alert.
4. Provide auditory stimulation alone without visual and vestibular stimulation to assess tolerance.
5. Alter voice to observe the effect of changes in tone and frequency on the infant. Watch for symmetrical reactions, hearing better on one side than the other, and require appropriate modification of auditory stimuli.

Visual
1. Place blanket over incubator to shield infant from bright light or make a canopy for an open crib.
2. Limit visual input by presenting a simple face on incubator or some stable visual pattern.
3. Avoid massive visual overload such as colorful sheets and blankets with complicated designs or multiple, brightly colored stuffed animals.
4. Observe infant for signs of sensory overload such as a hyperalert state, hypervigilant stare, or withdrawal.
5. Visual stimulation should be given at an appropriate distance (8 to 12 inches from face) and timed to coincide with the infant's natural rhythms. It is not appropriate to awaken a sleeping infant to provide stimulation.

Tactile
1. Provide maximal postural support with blanket rolls and provide physical boundaries by encasing the limbs in a flexed position on the body. The trunk should be held in flexion without airway compromise.
2. Change the infant's position. The trunk should be turned slowly with gentle unwrapping and undressing. During bathing, expose only the area being washed.
3. Use heat lamps to prevent cold stress. Take care to avoid overheating.
4. Use a pacifier and bundle the infant during any painful procedure.
5. Position the infant properly to help prevent gastroesophageal reflux.
6. Remain with the infant after a procedure until his motor activity returns to the baseline level.
7. Allow the infant to grip your finger or a small roll of gauze.
8. Awaken the infant slowly; first speak quietly to him, then touch him, and finally unwrap him.
9. If infant is able to suck on his fingers, position hand near face to allow him to do so.
10. Use fabrics with different textures (silk, satin, velvet) for stimulation.

Olfactory
1. Use sterile gauze to protect the mouth and eyes from alcohol and tincture of benzoin during reintubation. Uncap bottles of adhesive remover away from the bedside.
2. Place mild, pleasant-smelling substances such as mother's lotion, perfume, or breast milk on gauze pad in the incubator. Scratch-and-smell books and stickers can also be placed in the incubator.
3. Check the incubator and linen for unpleasant smells. Remove soiled diapers immediately after changing.

From Boynton, C. A., & Jones, B. (1988). Nursing care of the infant with bronchopulmonary dysplasia. In T. A. Merritt, W. H. Northway, Jr., and B. R. Boynton (Eds.), *Bronchopulmonary dysplasia* (pp. 322–323). Boston: Blackwell Scientific Publications. By permission of Blackwell Scientific Publications.

TABLE 20–19 Discharge Teaching Goals and Plan for Parents of Infants With Bronchopulmonary Dysplasia

Teaching Goals

1. Understanding of bronchopulmonary dysplasia (BPD) pathophysiology.
2. Assessment of respiratory rate and effort. Detection of cyanosis. Ability to suction the airway, perform chest physiotherapy, and use oxygen equipment.
3. Assessment of weight changes and fluid overload.
4. Role of bronchodilators, diuretics, and electrolyte supplements.
5. Recognition of emergency situations.
6. Ability to prepare formula and feed infant with respiratory compromise.
7. Understanding of infant behavioral responses. Ability to provide environmental and behavioral support.
8. Understanding of basic infant care.

Teaching Plan

Upon discharge from the hospital the parent(s) will

1. Be able to verbalize their understanding of BPD, its chronic nature, the course of the illness, and the need for follow-up.
2. Demonstrate their ability to evaluate their infant's respiratory status:
   a. Count respirations.
   b. Identify retractions.
   c. Identify color changes.
   d. Identify fluid overload (puffiness, irritability, refusal of feeds).
3. Describe the key aspects of feeding their infant:
   a. Importance of high caloric intake and the need for rest periods during feeding.
   b. Importance of positioning in "head up" posture.
   c. How to obtain formula supplements.
   d. How to fix formula.
   e. Technique of spoon feeding and plan for introduction of solids when instructed by pediatrician.
   f. Understanding the need for fluid restriction.
   g. Awareness of possible need for increased FiO_2 during feeding.
4. Explain the purpose, dose, schedule, and method of administration for each medication as well as precautions and side effects.
   a. Demonstrate how to draw up medications in a syringe accurately.
   b. Demonstrate how each type of medication (e.g., oral, inhaled) is to be administered to the infant.
5. Demonstrate and describe care and use of oxygen equipment.
   a. Demonstrate how to change and secure catheter or cannula.
   b. Describe how to adjust oxygen flow rate and know appropriate levels for infant.
   c. Describe precautions for use of home oxygen.
   d. Understand how oxygen flow and rate will be decreased for weaning.
   e. Know what to do if oxygen supply runs out.
6. Describe the special care needs of infant.
   a. Obtain handicapped parking sticker for motor vehicle.
   b. Understand the need for rest periods and protection from infection.
   c. Understand the need to avoid smoking in the home.
   d. Understand the need for developmental evaluation.
   e. Have a means of transportation (public or private) to medical appointments.
7. Describe indications for emergency action and the steps that need to be taken.
   a. Know signs and symptoms of respiratory distress and which problems should be referred to the pediatrician and which to the pulmonologist.
   b. Have phone numbers of pediatrician, pulmonologist, paramedics, oxygen supply company, monitor company, fire department, and police department.
   c. Know cardiopulmonary resuscitation.
   d. Understand the operation and use of the home monitor.
   e. Know the location of the nearest emergency room.

From Boynton, C. A., & Jones, B. (1988). Nursing care of the infant with bronchopulmonary dysplasia. In T. A. Merritt, W. H. Northway, Jr., & B. R. Boynton (Eds.), *Bronchopulmonary dysplasia* (pp. 327–328). Boston: Blackwell Scientific Publications. By permission of Blackwell Scientific Publications.

moving needed supports. Clear parameters for respiratory function should be established for each patient, and continued assessment of compensatory abilities should occur with each decrease in support. Ideally, those elements highly associated with increased morbidity—positive inspiratory pressure and oxygen—should be decreased first (Boynton & Jones, 1988), but individual patient response may indicate other weaning techniques. Decreasing one parameter at a time and evaluating its effects before changing another aids in assessment of weaning tolerance. The infant with fixed BPD often requires very slow weaning with small increments of change followed by long periods of equilibrium. This weaning process can be enhanced by use of dexamethasone as previously discussed (Boyle et al., 1995). If there is no improvement in the oxygenation and weaning process after 4 to 5 days of steroid therapy, it should be stopped (Davis & Rosenfeld, 1994).

Feeding Evaluation and Techniques

The infant with BPD has high caloric requirements, low fluid and stress tolerances, and maladaptive feeding behaviors. Individualized interventions such as increasing FiO_2, promoting nonnutritive sucking, reducing extraneous stimulation during feeding, swaddling, fortifying feedings, and individualizing a feeding schedule within overall caloric and fluid goals can promote maximum growth and development with fewer complications (Boynton & Jones, 1988). Usually, 120 to 150 kcal/kg/day is adequate for growth, but some infants may need more (Kurzner et al., 1988a, 1988b). These infants are prone to gastroesophageal reflux and feeding intolerances so there is an increased risk for aspiration (Boyle et al., 1995). Metoclopramide may be necessary to decrease the reflux (Boyle et al., 1995).

Parent Teaching, Discharge Planning, and Home Care

After discharge, infants with BPD often need specialized care at home by parents or health care practitioners, so clear and complete discharge instructions are necessary to ensure continuity of care. Table 20–19 lists suggestions for common parental teaching needs and interventions.

CONCLUSION

It is much easier to write on a disease than a remedy. The former is in the hands of nature, and a faithful observer with an eye to tolerable judgment cannot fail to delineate a likeness; the latter will ever be subject to the whim, the inaccuracy, and the blunder of man (William Withering, 1758).

With improvement in ventilation techniques, the treatment of neonatal respiratory disease has become possible, but significant morbidity has been the price. Now that we have the ability to help the smallest of infants, we need to learn how not to harm them at the same time. The next challenge of neonatology is to find ways to reduce morbidity and to improve the quality of life for these infants.

Because BPD is a complex problem in origin, we should not expect the remedy to be easy. Correcting the problems that we have caused may mean major changes in our philosophy and practice, that is, giving up things that we have used in the past to increase survival. We will need to find new ways to achieve the same ends.

REFERENCES

Agiagno, R. L. (1988). Use of steroids. In T. A. Merritt, W. H. Northway, Jr., & B. R. Boynton (Eds.), *Bronchopulmonary dysplasia* (pp. 375–402). Boston: Blackwell Scientific Publications.

Als, H., Lawhon, G., Brown, E., et al. (1986). Individualized behavioral and environmental care for the very low birth weight preterm infant at high risk for bronchopulmonary dysplasia: Neonatal intensive care unit and developmental outcome. *Pediatrics, 78*(16), 1123–1132.

Avery, G. B., Fletcher, A. B., Kaplan, M., & Brudno, D. S. (1985). Controlled trial of dexamethasone in respirator-dependent infants with bronchopulmonary dysplasia. *Pediatrics, 75*(1), 106–111.

Avery, M. E., Tooley, W. A., Keller, J. B., et al. (1987). Is chronic lung disease in low birth weight infants preventable? A survey of eight centers. *Pediatrics, 79*(1), 26–30.

Bancalari, E., Abdenour, G. E., Feller, R., & Gannon, J. (1979). Bronchopulmonary dysplasia: Clinical presentation. *Journal of Pediatrics, 95*(5, Part 2), 819–823.

Bartlett, R. H., Roloff, D. W., Cornell, R. G., et al. (1985). Extracorporeal circulation in neonatal respiratory failure: A prospective randomized study. *Pediatrics, 76*(4), 479–487.

Blanchard, P. W., Brown, T. M., & Coates, A. L. (1987). Pharmacotherapy in bronchopulmonary dysplasia. *Clinics in Perinatology, 14*(4), 881–910.

Bonikos, D. S., & Bensch, K. G. (1988). Pathogenesis of bronchopulmonary dysplasia. In T. A. Merritt, W. H. Northway, Jr., & B. R. Boynton (Eds.), *Bronchopulmonary dysplasia* (pp. 33–58). Boston: Blackwell Scientific Publications.

Boyle, K. M., Baker, V. L., & Cassaday, C. J. (1995). Neonatal pulmonary disorders. In S. L. Barnhart & M.P. Czervinske (Eds.), *Perinatal and pediatric respiratory care* (pp. 445–479). Philadelphia: W. B. Saunders.

Boynton, B. R. (1988). Epidemiology of BPD. In T. A. Merritt, W. H. Northway, Jr., & B. R. Boynton (Eds.), *Bronchopulmonary dysplasia* (pp. 19–32). Boston: Blackwell Scientific Publications.

Boynton, C. A., & Jones, B. (1988). Nursing care of the infant with bronchopulmonary dysplasia. In T. A. Merritt, W. H. Northway, Jr., & B. R. Boynton (Eds.), *Bronchopulmonary dysplasia* (pp. 313–330). Boston: Blackwell Scientific Publications.

Davis, J. M., & Rosenfeld, W. N. (1994). Chronic lung disease. In G. B. Avery, M. A. Fletcher, & M. G. MacDonald (Eds.), *Neonatalogy: Pathophysiology and management of the newborn* (4th ed., pp. 453–477). Philadelphia: J. B. Lippincott.

Dorkin, H. I. (1988). Home respiratory care. In T. A. Merritt, W. H. Northway, Jr., & B. R. Boynton (Eds.), *Bronchopulmonary dysplasia* (pp. 331–342). Boston: Blackwell Scientific Publications.

Goetzman, B. W. (1986). Understanding bronchopulmonary dysplasia [Review]. *American Journal of Diseases of Children, 140*(4), 332–334.

Goodman, G., Perkin, R. M., Anas, N. G., et al. (1988). Pulmonary hypertension in infants with bronchopulmonary dysplasia. *Journal of Pediatrics, 112*(1), 67–72.

Inwood, S., Finley, G. A., & Fitzhardinge, P. M. (1986). High-frequency oscillation: A new mode of ventilation for the neonate. *Neonatal Network, 4*(5), 53–58.

Karp, T. B. (1991). High-frequency jet ventilation: Impact on neonatal nursing. In J. Nugent (Ed.), *Acute respiratory care of the neonate* (pp. 147–170). Petaluma, CA: NICU Ink.

Karp, T. B., Solon, J. F., Olson, D. L., et al. (1986). High frequency jet ventilation: A neonatal nursing perspective. *Neonatal Network, 4*(5), 42–50.

Katz, R., & Murphy, S. (1988). Bronchodilators and anti-inflammatory agents. In T. A. Merritt, W. H. Northway, Jr., & B. R. Boynton (Eds.), *Bronchopulmonary dysplasia* (pp. 293–312). Boston: Blackwell Scientific Publications.

Kurzner, S. J., Garg, M., Bautista, D. B., et al. (1988a). Growth failure in infants with bronchopulmonary dysplasia: Nutrition and elevated resting metabolic expenditure. *Journal of Pediatrics, 81*(3), 379–384.

Kurzner, S. J., Garg, M., Bautista, D. B., et al. (1988b). Growth failure in bronchopulmonary dysplasia: Elevated metabolic rates and pulmonary mechanics. *Journal of Pediatrics, 112*(1), 73–80.

Lawhon, G. (1986). Management of stress in premature infants. In D. J. Angelini, C. M. Whelan Knapp, & R. M. Gibbs (Eds.), *Perinatal/neonatal nursing: A clinical handbook* (pp. 319–328). Boston: Blackwell Scientific Publications.

Lazar, E. L., & Stolar, C. J. H. (1995). Congenital pulmonary and chest wall malformations. In S. L. Barnhart & M. P. Czervinske (Eds.), *Perinatal and pediatric respiratory care* (pp. 526–536). Philadelphia: W. B. Saunders.

Linton, P. T. (1986). Behavioral development of the premature infant. *Perinatology/Neonatology, 10*(4), 27–33.

Maloni, J. A., Cheng, C.-Y., Liebl, C. P., & Maier, J. S. (1996). Transforming prenatal care: Reflections of the past and present with implications for the future. *Journal of Obstetric, Gynecologic, and Neonatal Nursing, 25*(1), 17–23.

Martin, R. J., Fanaroff, A. A., & Klaus, M. H. (1993). Respiratory problems. In M. H. Klaus & A. A. Fanaroff (Eds.), *Care of the high-risk neonate* (4th ed., pp. 228–259). Philadelphia: W. B. Saunders.

Merritt, J. A., & Hallman, M. (1988a). Impact of surfactant therapy for respiratory distress in preventing or reducing bronchopulmonary dysplasia. In T. A. Merritt, W. H. Northway, Jr., & B. R. Boynton (Eds.), *Bronchopulmonary dysplasia* (pp. 343–350). Boston: Blackwell Scientific Publications.

Merritt, J. A., & Hallman, M. (1988b). Interactions in the immature lung: Protease-antiprotease mechanisms of lung injury. In T. A. Merritt, W. H. Northway, Jr., & B. R. Boynton (Eds.), *Bronchopulmonary dysplasia* (pp. 117–130). Boston: Blackwell Scientific Publications.

Miller, R. W., Woo, P., Kellman, R. K., & Slagle, T. S. (1987). Tracheobronchial abnormalities in infants with bronchopulmonary dysplasia. *Journal of Pediatrics, 111*(5), 779–782.

Monin, P., & Vert, P. (1987). The management of bronchopulmonary dysplasia [Review]. *Clinics in Perinatology, 14*(3), 531–549.

Moore, K. L., & Persaud, T. V. N. (1993). *The developing human: Clinically oriented embryology* (5th ed.). Philadelphia: W. B. Saunders.

National Institutes of Health (NIH). (1994). *NIH consensus statement: Effect of corticosteroids for fetal maturation on perinatal outcomes.* Rockville, MD: National Institutes of Health.

Northway, W. H., Jr., Rosan, R. C., & Porter, D. Y. (1967). Pulmonary disease following respirator therapy of hyaline membrane disease. Bronchopulmonary dysplasia. *New England Journal of Medicine, 276*(7), 357–368.

Nugent, J. (1986). Extracorporeal membrane oxygenation in the neonate. *Neonatal Network, 4*(5), 27–38.

Obladen, M. (1988). Alterations in surfactant composition. In T. A. Merritt, W. H. Northway, Jr., & B. R. Boynton (Eds.), *Bronchopulmonary dysplasia* (pp. 131–142). Boston: Blackwell Scientific Publications.

Papageorgiou, A. N., Doray, J. L., Ardila, R., & Kunos, I. (1989). Reduction of mortality, morbidity, and respiratory distress syndrome in infants weighing less than 1000 grams by treatment with betamethasone and ritodrine. *Pediatrics, 83*(4), 493–497.

Perkin, R. M., & Anas, N. G. (1984). Pulmonary hypertension in pediatric patients [Review]. *Journal of Pediatrics, 105*(4), 511–522.

Philip, A. G. S. (1975). Oxygen plus pressure plus time: The etiology of bronchopulmonary dysplasia. *Pediatrics, 55*(1), 44–50.

Polin, R.A. (1990). Role of fibronectin in disease of newborn infants and children. *Reviews of Infectious Diseases, 12*(Suppl. 4), S428–S438.

Rhodes, P. G., Graves, G. R., Patel, D. M., et al. (1983). Minimizing pneumothorax and bronchopulmonary dysplasia in ventilated infants with hyaline membrane disease. *Journal of Pediatrics, 103*(4), 634–637.

Rimsza, M. E. (1978). Complications of corticosteroid therapy [Review]. *American Journal of Diseases of Children, 132*(8), 806–810.

Roberts, R. J. (1984a). Diuretics. In R. J. Roberts, *Drug therapy in infants* (p. 229). Philadelphia: W. B. Saunders.

Roberts, R. J. (1984b). Methylxanthine therapy: Caffeine and theophylline. In R. J. Roberts, *Drug therapy in infants* (pp. 119–137). Philadelphia: W. B. Saunders.

Rosenfeld, W., & Concepcion, L. (1988). Pharmacologic intervention: Use of the antioxidant superoxide dismutase. In T. A. Merritt, W. H. Northway, Jr., & B. R. Boynton (Eds.), *Bronchopulmonary dysplasia* (pp. 365–374). Boston: Blackwell Scientific Publications.

Rosenfeld, W., Evans, H., Concepcion, L., et al. (1984). Prevention of bronchopulmonary dysplasia by administration of bovine superoxide dismutase in preterm infants with respiratory distress syndrome. *Journal of Pediatrics, 105*(5), 781–785.

Shannon, D. C., & Epstein, M. (1986). Bronchopulmonary dysplasia. In D. W. Thibeault & G. A. Gregory (Eds.), *Neonatal pulmonary care* (2nd ed., pp. 697–707). Norwalk, CT: Appleton-Century-Crofts.

Sherman, F.S. (1988). Cor pulmonale. In T. A. Merritt, W. H. Northway,

Jr., & B. R. Boynton (Eds.), *Bronchopulmonary dysplasia* (pp. 251–262). Boston: Blackwell Scientific Publications.

Sinkin, R. A., & Phelps, D. L. (1987). New strategies for the prevention of bronchopulmonary dysplasia [Review]. *Clinics in Perinatology, 14*(3), 599–620.

Southwell, S. M. (1995). Respiratory management. In L. P. Gunderson & C. Kenner (Eds.), *Care of the 24–25 week gestational age infant: A small baby protocol* (2nd ed., pp. 43–68). Petaluma, CA: NICU Ink.

Tepper, R. S. (1988). Assessment of pulmonary function in the post neonatal period. In T. A. Merritt, W. H. Northway, Jr., & B. R. Boynton (Eds.), *Bronchopulmonary dysplasia* (pp. 263–276). Boston: Blackwell Scientific Publications.

Thibeault, D. W. (1986). Pulmonary barotrauma: Interstitial emphysema, pneumomediastinum, and pneumothorax. In D. W. Thibeault & G. A. Gregory (Eds.), *Neonatal pulmonary care* (2nd ed., pp. 499–517). Norwalk, CT: Appleton-Century-Crofts.

Thibeault, D. W., & Lang, M. J. (1988). Mechanisms and pathobiologic effects of barotrauma. In T. A. Merritt, W. H. Northway, Jr., & B. R. Boynton (Eds.), *Bronchopulmonary dysplasia* (pp. 79–101). Boston: Blackwell Scientific Publications.

Toce, S. S., Farrell, P. M., Leavitt, L. A., et al. (1984). Clinical and roentgenographic scoring systems for assessing bronchopulmonary dysplasia. *American Journal of Diseases of Children, 138*(6), 581–585.

Usher, R. (1987). Extreme prematurity. In G. B. Avery (Ed.), *Neonatology: Pathophysiology management of the newborn* (pp. 264–298). Philadelphia: J. B. Lippincott.

Wispe, J. R., & Roberts, R. J. (1987). Molecular basis of pulmonary oxygen toxicity [Review]. *Clinics in Perinatology, 14*(3), 651–666.

Yeh, T. F. (1988). Diuretic therapy in bronchopulmonary dysplasia. In T. A. Merritt, W. H. Northway, Jr., & B. R. Boynton (Eds.), *Bronchopulmonary dysplasia* (pp. 277–292). Boston: Blackwell Scientific Publications.

CHAPTER 21

Assessment and Management of Cardiovascular Dysfunction

JUDY WRIGHT LOTT

RESEARCH AGENDA

What nursing interventions can be initiated to help families cope with the implications of the diagnosis of a congenital heart defect in their newborn or infant?

Are there methods to reduce environmental influences on the development of cardiac defects?

Is there a relationship between early surgical intervention in severe congenital heart defect (CHD) and long-term infant development?

What is the relationship between morbidity and mortality during the surgical correction of a defect and time of the initial diagnosis?

What nursing interventions can be used to improve oxygenation of neonates with cardiac defects?

VIGNETTE

Matthew, a 3-day-old infant, was referred for evaluation of a CHD from a small community hospital. Matthew's parents accompanied him to the tertiary center.

Matthew had been delivered by normal spontaneous vaginal route with a low forceps assist, after a term, uncomplicated pregnancy. At delivery, the amniotic fluid was meconium stained, but there was no meconium below the cords. The Apgar scores were 8 and 9, and the baby was taken to the regular nursery. Birth weight was 3980 g and length was 53 cm. There were no obvious physical defects on initial assessment. Matthew was described as a poor nipple feeder when first offered a feeding. Later, when the nursery nurse examined Matthew, he was tachypneic and slightly mottled. A review of the nursing notes revealed that tachypnea had been observed since delivery. No murmur was heard on auscultation. The nurse contacted the pediatrician, who ordered an x-ray and CBC. The CBC was unremarkable, but the x-ray showed moderate cardiomegaly and a slight streaky pattern in the lung fields. At 50 hours of age, Matthew was transported to our unit for cardiac evaluation.

Matthew cried and moved about normally during admission procedures. An ABG was obtained, and the cardiology department was contacted. I performed a quick head-to-toe assessment and documented the following abnormal information:

General: tachypneic and ashen in 40% O_2; facies normal and no gross anomalies.
Heart: rate rapid at 172, regular but with a strong S_2 and a gallop quality. No murmur. PMI at left sternal border with increased precordial activity. Pulses were diminished, especially in the legs. Four extremity blood pressures: 79/38 and 72/43 in the arms and 63/35 and 68/38 in the legs.
Resp: rapid with breath sounds equal and clear; no grunting, flaring, or retractions. Oxygen saturation 95% to 100%, Tco_2, 58; $TcCo_2$, 36.
Skin: pale/gray with delayed capillary refill at 4 seconds.

The working diagnosis was left obstructive congenital heart disease with a differential diagnosis of sepsis. The neonatologist ordered PGE by continuous infusion.

The cardiologist examined Matthew, evaluated his medical history, and obtained an echocardiogram. The blood gas at this time was pH, 7.36; Pco_2, 27; Po_2, 137; base deficit, −12.1. I prepared the PGE_1 infusion and readied the bag and mask should apnea occur. The parents listened intently as the doctors explained. I listened too, knowing they might need repeated explanations and clarification of terminology. The echocardiogram revealed a small left ventricle, small aortic root, coarctation of the aorta, and small mitral valve. We weaned the oxygen and began the PGE continuous infusion at 0.05 μg/kg/minute. Also, I added no stopcock to this line and clearly marked the IV tubing as a PGE_1 infusion. A note was hung on the O_2 blender to alert personnel to the diagnosis. Within 20 minutes, Matthew's color was better and a ductal murmur was heard. His follow-up blood gas was pH, 7.37; Pco_2, 37; Po_2, 68; base deficit, −3.6.

The nursing care would be directed toward (1) maintaining the PGE infusion, (2) decreasing Matthew's oxygen demand, (3) frequent monitoring and assessment, and (4) supporting Matthew's parents. Umbilical artery and venous catheters were inserted. Matthew fussed as he was positioned for his line placement. His O_2 saturation read 82%, and his tachypnea worsened. Decreasing Matthew's oxygen demand and managing his activity intolerance would mean keeping him happy. Sedation was an option, but his mother and a pacifier worked well, so we kept both of them close. The lines were placed, and the PGE infusion was switched to the umbilical venous line. Matthew was sleeping quietly.

The cardiologists returned to discuss treatment options with the parents. The parents looked dazed when the discussion was complete. After the conference, Matthew was scheduled for a coarctotomy–arch repair. The changes that had taken place and the seriousness of the diagnosis were overwhelming. I took the parents to our "quiet room." They actually had a good grasp of everything that was said and needed some time alone.

I sat with Matthew and his parents for another 15 minutes to provide support and to make sure all their questions had been answered. I also initiated a social services referral for family support. The family would receive continual assessment and support throughout Matthew's hospitalization.

Rita Kunk

This chapter presents the physiology of normal cardiac function, including fetal circulatory patterns and the changes that occur during transition to extrauterine life. The most common cyanotic and acyanotic CHDs are discussed. Information about incidence, hemodynamics, manifestations, diagnosis, and medical and surgical management is included. Because some CHDs are not identified during the neonatal period, information about presentation in infants is also included. The chapter concludes with a discussion about the support of the family of an infant with a CHD.

CARDIOVASCULAR ADAPTATION AT BIRTH

Fetal Circulation

Knowledge of the normal route of fetal blood flow is essential for understanding the circulatory changes that occur in the newborn at delivery. The pattern of fetal circulation is illustrated in Figure 21–1. Fetal circulation involves four unique anatomic features:

1. The placenta is the exchange organ for oxygen and carbon dioxide and for nutrients and wastes.
2. The ductus venosus permits the majority of blood from the placenta to bypass the liver and enter the inferior vena cava.
3. The foramen ovale is the opening in the interatrial septum, which permits a portion of the blood to flow from the right atrium directly to the left atrium.
4. The patent ductus arteriosus (PDA) is a tubular communication between the pulmonary artery and the descending aorta, which allows blood to flow from the pulmonary artery to the aorta, bypassing the fetal lungs (Moller, 1987).

Oxygen diffuses into the fetal circulation from the maternal uterine arteries in the placenta. From the placenta, the oxygenated blood flows through the umbilical vein to the fetus. The fetal circulation divides at the liver, with about half of the blood entering the liver and the remainder bypassing the liver through the ductus venosus. Blood from the ductus venosus enters the inferior vena cava. Blood of lower oxygen content coming from the gastrointestinal tract, legs, and liver mixes with the blood of higher oxygen content in the inferior vena cava. The mixed blood then enters the right atrium (Hazinski, 1984; Moller, 1987; Sacksteder, 1978).

From this point, the blood from the right atrium flows directly to the left atrium through the foramen ovale. From the left atrium, the blood goes to the left ventricle and then to the head and neck through the ascending aorta. This circulatory pattern ensures that the fetal brain constantly receives well-oxygenated blood.

The blood returns from the head and neck through the superior vena cava to the right atrium. This blood then flows into the right ventricle. From the right ventricle, the blood enters the pulmonary arteries. Only a small portion of this blood enters the pulmonary circuit to perfuse the lungs; most of the blood is shunted through the ductus arteriosus into the aorta to supply oxygen and nutrients to the trunk and lower extremities (Moller, 1987).

Most of the blood flow from the lower extremities rejoins the fetal circulation through the internal iliac arteries via the umbilical cord to the placenta, where it is reoxygenated and recirculated. A small amount of the blood from the lower extremities passes back into the ascending vena cava, where it is mixed with fresh blood from the umbilical vein and recirculated without reoxygenation. Thus, fetal circulation can be described as two parallel circuits rather than as the serial circuit present in extrauterine life (Avery et al., 1994).

Neonatal Circulation

The cardiac and pulmonary systems undergo drastic changes at birth. These changes usually occur functionally, immediately upon onset of respirations. The most significant change is that the primary oxygenation organ becomes the lungs rather than the placenta. Clamping of the umbilical cord and subsequent removal of the placenta cause immediate circulatory changes in the neonate. With the first breath and occlusion of the umbilical cord, systemic resistance is elevated, which reduces blood flow through the ductus arteriosus (Brook & Heymann, 1995). Cord occlusion causes a prompt increase in blood pressure and a corresponding stimulation of the aortic baroreceptors and the sympathetic nervous system. The onset of respirations and lung expansion causes a decrease in pulmonary vascular resistance secondary to the direct effect of oxygen and carbon dioxide on the blood vessels. Resistance decreases as arterial oxygen increases and arterial carbon dioxide decreases (Sacksteder, 1978).

Most of the right ventricular output flows through the lungs and increases the pulmonary venous return to the left atrium. The increased amount of blood in the lungs and the heart causes increased pressure in the left atrium. The increased pressure in the left atrium, combined with the increased systemic resistance, functionally closes the foramen ovale.

The ductus arteriosus normally closes within 15 to 24 hours of birth in response to increased arterial oxygen content caused by the initiation of pulmonary respiratory effort of the newborn and the effects of sympathomimetic amines and prostaglandins. The ductus arteriosus is anatomically obliterated by constriction by 3 to 4 weeks of age.

Blood flow through the ductus venosus ceases when the umbilical cord is clamped, functionally closing the ductus venosus. The ductus venosus is anatomically obliterated by approximately 1 to 2 weeks of life. After birth, the umbilical vein and arteries no longer transport blood and are obliterated. *Functional closure* refers to the cessation of flow through the structure caused by changes in pressure. *Anatomic closure* refers to obliteration of the structure by constriction or growth of tissue (Moller, 1987).

Because anatomic closure of the fetal pathways lags behind functional closure, the shunts may open and close intermittently before complete closure, resulting in functional murmurs. Pulmonary artery pressure remains high for several hours. As the pulmonary vascular resistance declines, the direction of blood flow through the ductus arteriosus reverses. Initially bidirectional, the flow becomes entirely left to right and then becomes functionally insignificant by approximately 15 hours of life (Brook & Heymann, 1995; Sacksteder, 1978). Intermittent or functional murmurs do not cause any clinical compromise for the newborn and are not significant. Conditions that cause transient opening of fetal shunts, allowing unoxygenated blood to shunt from the right side of the heart to the left and bypassing the pulmonary circuit, produce transient cyanosis. Any murmur or cyanosis in the new-

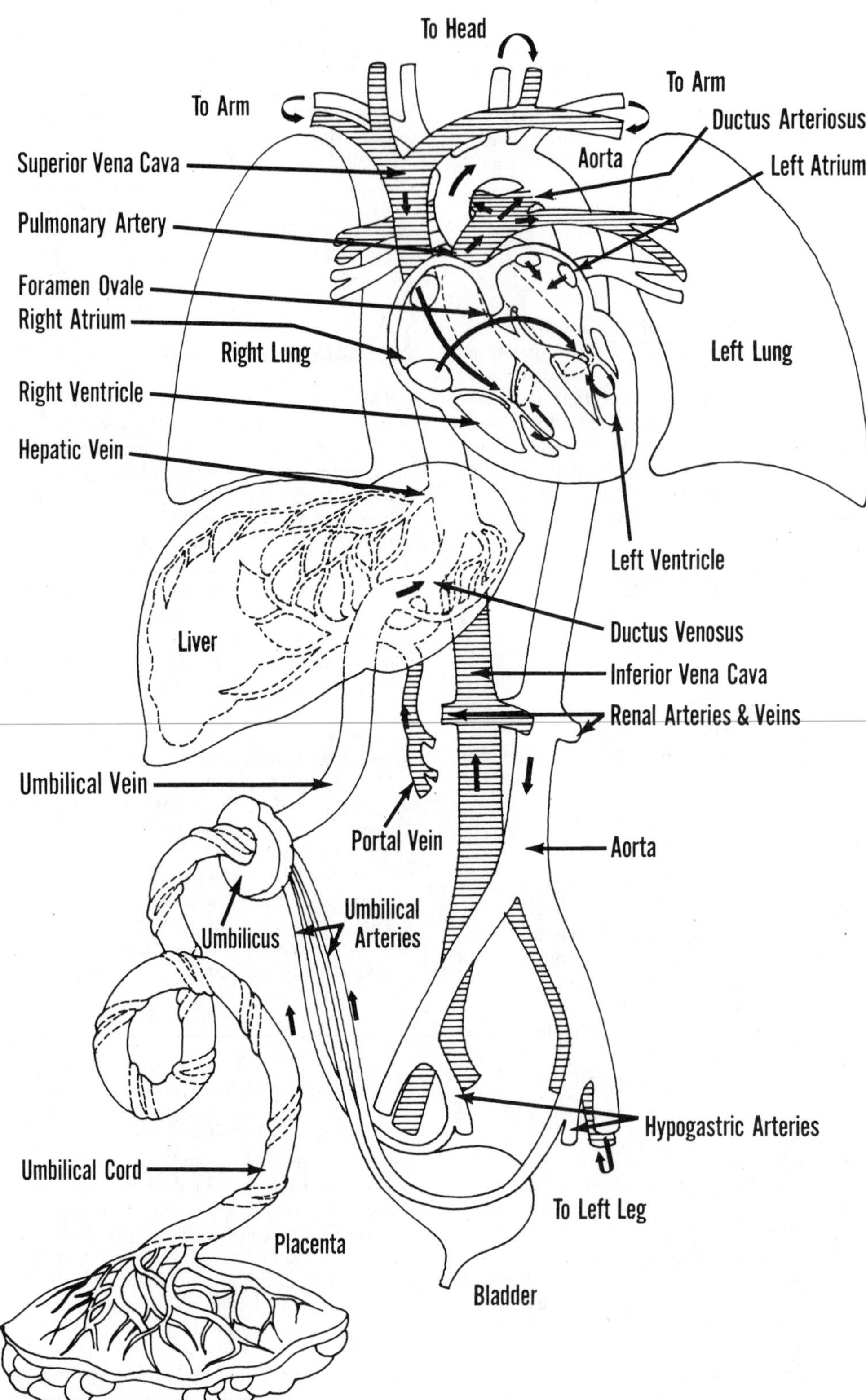

FIGURE 21–1. Fetal circulation. (Reprinted with permission of Ross Laboratories, Columbus, OH 43216, Clinical Education Aid, © 1985, Ross Laboratories.)

born should be carefully monitored and evaluated to detect abnormalities.

Hypoxemia can cause a constricted ductus to reopen and may reestablish increased pulmonary vascular resistance, leading to persistent pulmonary hypertension of the newborn. The ductus arteriosus responds to hypoxemia by opening, whereas the pulmonary arterioles respond by constricting.

NORMAL CARDIAC FUNCTION

The normal anatomy of the heart is shown in Figure 21–2.

Heart Valves

Blood flow through the heart is directed through two sets of one-way valves. The semilunar valves consist of the pulmonary valve and the aortic valve. The pulmonary valve connects the right ventricle and the pulmonary artery. The aortic valve connects the left ventricle and the aorta. The atrioventricular (AV) valves consist of the tricuspid valve and the mitral valve. The tricuspid valve connects the right atrium and the right ventricle. The mitral valve connects the left atrium and the left ventricle.

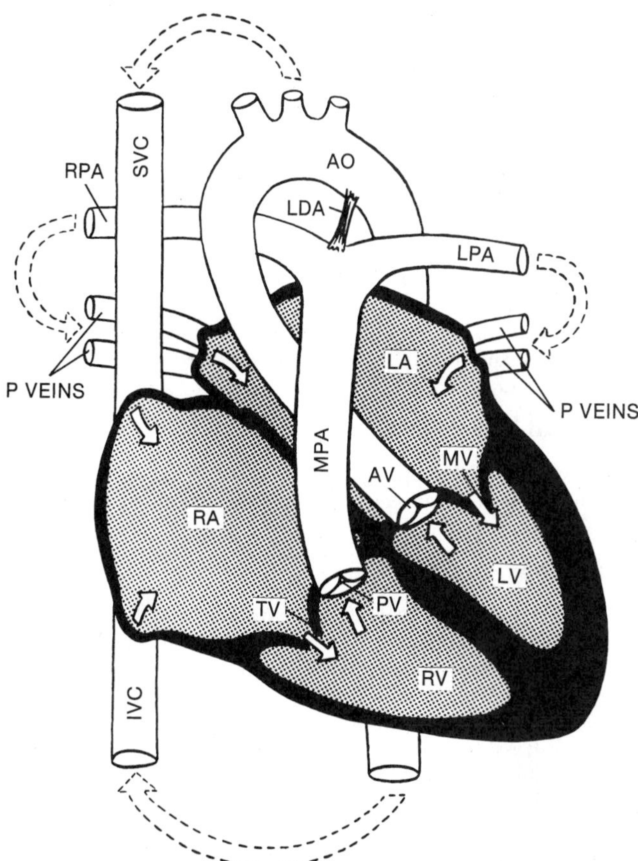

FIGURE 21–2. Normal cardiac anatomy and circulation. AO, aorta; AV, aortic valve; IVC, inferior vena cava; LA, left atrium; LDA, ligamentum ductus arteriosus; LPA, left pulmonary artery; LV, left ventricle; MPA, main pulmonary artery; MV, mitral valve; PV, pulmonary valve; P VEINS, pulmonary veins; RA, right atrium; RPA, right pulmonary artery; RV, right ventricle; SVC, superior vena cava; TV, tricuspid valve. (Reprinted with permission of Ross Laboratories, Columbus, OH 43216, Clinical Education Aid, © 1985, Ross Laboratories.)

Cardiac Cycle

Normal cardiac function involves two stages: systole and diastole. During systole, contraction of the ventricle causes the pressure inside the ventricle to increase to approximately 70 mm Hg in neonates (approximately 120 mm Hg in adults). When sufficient pressure is generated, the aortic and pulmonary valves open and blood is ejected from the ventricles. As the blood flows from the ventricles, the pressure decreases, causing the aortic and pulmonary valves to close (Conover, 1988).

During diastole, the mitral and tricuspid valves open and 70 percent of the blood in the atria flows into the ventricles. A small portion of the blood flows back into the aorta and enters the coronary arteries for perfusion of the heart. At the end of diastole, a small atrial contraction occurs (4 to 6 mm Hg on the right side; 7 to 8 mm Hg on the left side), and the mitral and tricuspid valves close. Metabolism of the heart is decreased during diastole. The average neonate's cardiac cycle is approximately 0.4 second, with 0.2 second for diastole and 0.2 second for systole (based on a heart rate of approximately 150 beats per minute) (Conover, 1988).

Cardiac Output

Cardiac output is the amount of blood pumped by the left ventricle in 1 minute. Cardiac output is equal to the stroke volume times the heart rate (CO = SV × HR). The stroke volume is the volume of blood pumped per beat from each ventricle. The greater the stroke volume, the larger the amount of blood in the systemic circulation. An increase in cardiac output increases systole and decreases diastole. Cardiac output is influenced by changes in heart rate, pulmonary vascular resistance, and systemic resistance to flow.

Cardiac output is influenced by the amount of blood returned to the heart, as explained by the Frank-Starling law. This law states that, within physiologic limits, the heart pumps all the blood that enters it without allowing excessive accumulation of blood in the veins. Venous return is determined by the passive movement of blood through the veins, the thoracic pump, and the venous muscle pump. Normally, when increased volume enters the heart, contractility is increased as a response to stimulation of stretch receptors in the heart muscle. The newborn's heart has fewer fibers and is unable to stretch sufficiently to accommodate increased volume; therefore, increased heart rate is the only effective mechanism by which the newborn can respond to increased volume (Braunwald et al., 1988; Talner, 1995).

When the volume exceeds the ability of the heart to pump, cardiac failure results. Local factors that affect venous return to the heart include hypoxia, acidosis, hypercarbia, hyperthermia, increased metabolic demand, and increased metabolites (potassium, adenosine triphosphate, and lactic acid) (Conover, 1988).

Other factors that influence cardiac output include pressure and resistance. Pressure and resistance are inversely related: if pressure in the arterial bed is increased, resistance is decreased and flow is improved. The size (radius) of vessels influences resistance: the greater the radius of a vessel, the lower the resistance. Vessels obstructed by thromboses or constriction have greater resistance to vascular flow (Heymann, 1995).

Autonomic Cardiac Control

Cardiovascular function is modulated by the autonomic nervous system. Baroreceptors and chemoreceptors in the aorta and carotid sinus provide feedback to the autonomic nervous system. Feedback from these receptors stimulates the parasympathetic or sympathetic nervous system (Hazinski, 1984).

The parasympathetic nervous system is less powerful than the sympathetic system. Stimulation of the parasympathetic and sympathetic nervous systems results in vagal nerve stimulation and a decrease in heart rate. Most parasympathetic and sympathetic nervous system effects are on the atria, but decreased ventricular contractility may also occur. Right vagal stimulation affects the sinoatrial (SA) node, and left vagal stimulation affects the AV node. Acetylcholine is the active neurotransmitter for the parasympathetic and sympathetic nervous systems (Braunwald et al., 1988; Talner, 1995).

Stimulation of the sympathetic nervous system through the ganglionic chain releases norepinephrine and epinephrine, which act on the SA node, the AV node, the atria, and the ventricles. Maximal stimulation of the sympathetic nervous system can increase heart rate to 250 to 300 beats per minute. Contractility can be improved by approximately 100 percent. Alpha- and beta-adrenergic receptors are stimulated. Alpha receptors cause increased contractility (inotropic) and increased rate (chronotropic); β_2 receptors cause vasodilation, bronchodilatation, and smooth muscle relaxation.

Term newborns have a decreased number of receptors but are capable of normal cardiovascular system function. The preterm infant is not able to smoothly maintain autonomic function, and energy expenditure is increased. Hence, the cardiovascular signs such as color changes and bradycardia may occur as a result of an excessive demand for autonomic nervous system function.

CARDIAC ASSESSMENT

Cardiac assessment includes history taking, physical assessment, and diagnostic tests. Review of the maternal, fetal, and neonatal history is helpful in cardiac evaluation of the newborn. Associated with CHDs are (1) maternal infections, especially viral and protozoal infections early in pregnancy, (2) maternal use of tobacco, alcohol, or drugs, and (3) maternal diseases. Table 21–1 lists heart defects commonly associated with maternal history. Birth weight may also aid in the identification of a CHD. Macrosomia is associated with maternal diabetes and transposition of the great arteries (TGA), whereas infants of mothers with viral diseases are frequently small for gestational age (Park, 1988).

TABLE 21–1 Maternal Condition and Associated Congenital Heart Defects

Condition	Defect
Maternal Disease	
Diabetes mellitus	Cardiomyopathy, TGA, VSD, PDA
Lupus erythematosus	Congenital heart block
Collagen disease	Congenital heart block
Congenital heart defect	Increased risk for congenital heart defect (3%–4%)
Viral Disease	
Rubella	
First trimester	PDA, pulmonary artery branch stenosis
Later	Various cardiac and other defects
Cytomegalovirus	Various cardiac and other defects
Herpesvirus	Various cardiac and other defects
Coxsackievirus B	Cardiomyopathy
Drugs	
Amphetamines	VSD, PDA, ASD, TGA
Phenytoin	PS, AS, COA, PDA
Trimethadione	TGA, TOF, HLHS
Progesterone/estrogen	VSD, TOF, TGA
Alcohol	VSD, PDA, ASD, TOF

AS, aortic stenosis; ASD, atrial septal defect; COA, coarctation of the aorta; HLHS, hypoplastic left heart syndrome; PDA, patent ductus arteriosus; PS, pulmonary stenosis; TGA, transposition of the great arteries; TOF, tetralogy of Fallot; VSD, ventricular septal defect.

Data from Hazinski, M. F. (1984). Cardiovascular disorders. In M. F. Hazinski (Ed.), *Nursing care of the critically ill child* (pp. 63–252). St. Louis: C. V. Mosby; Park, M. K. (1988). *Pediatric cardiology for practitioners*. Chicago: Mosby–Year Book.

TABLE 21–2 Congenital Heart Defects Associated With Specific Genetic or Chromosomal Abnormalities

Disease or Syndrome	Defect
Trisomy 13, 18	PDA, VSD
Trisomy 21	ECD, VSD, PDA
Turner's syndrome	COA
Marfan syndrome	AS, MVS, aortic aneurysms, TAPVR
Williams syndrome or elfin facies	AS, PPAS
DiGeorge syndrome	Interrupted aortic arch
Neurofibromatosis	PVS

AS, aortic stenosis; COA, coarctation of the aorta; ECD, endocardial cushion defect; MVS, mitral valve stenosis; PDA, patent ductus arteriosus; PPAS, peripheral pulmonic arterial stenosis; PVS, pulmonic valvular stenosis; TAPVR, total anomalous pulmonary venous return; VSD, ventricular septal defect.

Data from Park, M. F. (1988). *Pediatric cardiology for practitioners*. Chicago: Mosby–Year Book.

Family history of hereditary disease, congenital heart disease, or rheumatic fever is significant. Certain hereditary diseases have a CHD as part of the expression (Clark, 1995) (Table 21–2). (Chapter 10, Fetal Development: Environmental Influences and Critical Periods, discusses hereditary conditions.) The overall incidence of CHDs is approximately 1 percent, or 8 per 1000 live births, excluding persistent PDA in preterm infants. If the mother had a CHD, however, the incidence increases in the offspring to approximately 3 to 4 percent (Hazinski, 1984; Heymann, 1995; Park, 1988).

A neonatal history of cyanosis, tachypnea without pulmonary disease, sweating, poor feeding, edema, or, in older infants, failure to gain weight is suggestive of congenital heart disease. Careful evaluation of the maternal, fetal, and neonatal history in conjunction with a thorough physical assessment identifies infants for whom further diagnostic testing is indicated.

Physical Assessment

Assessment of the newborn with a suspected cardiovascular dysfunction includes inspection, palpation, and auscultation.

Inspection

Valuable information about the cardiovascular system of the newborn can be obtained by observation of the infant's general appearance before examination. The following states of the neonate should be observed: sleeping or awake, alert or lethargic, anxious or relaxed. Respiratory effort, including signs of respiratory distress such as nasal flaring, expiratory grunting, stridor, retractions, or paradoxical respirations, should be observed. Tachypnea and tachycardia are early signs of left ventricular failure. Severe left ventricular failure also causes dyspnea and retractions (Park, 1988).

The color of the neonate should be observed. Cyanosis is the bluish color of the skin, mucous membranes, and nailbeds that occurs when there is at least 5 g/100 ml of deoxygenated hemoglobin in the circulation. If cyanosis is present, the nurse should differentiate between peripheral and central cyanosis and whether it improves with crying, does not change, or becomes worse with crying. Cyanosis can result from pulmonary, hematologic, central nervous system, or metabolic diseases, as well as from cardiac defects (Driscoll, 1990). Pulmonary and cardiac defects are the two most common causes of central cyanosis in the newborn (Avery et al., 1994; Friedman, 1988).

Pallor may indicate vasoconstriction resulting from congestive heart failure (CHF) or circulatory shock caused by severe anemia. Prolonged physiologic jaundice may occur in infants with CHF or congenital hypothyroidism, which is associated with PDA and pulmonary stenosis. A ruddy or plethoric appearance is often seen in polycythemia. These infants may appear cyanotic without significant arterial desaturation.

The presence of sweating is very suggestive of a CHD in the newborn. The cause of sweating is sympathetic overactivity as a compensatory mechanism for decreased cardiac output (Driscoll, 1990).

The presence of precordial bulging is suggestive of a chronic cardiac enlargement. The presence of precordial activity without bulging may be associated with more acute onset of cardiac dysfunction. Precordial activity is a reliable parameter of cardiac dysfunction. Pectus excavatum may cause a pulmonary systolic ejection murmur or a large cardiac silhouette on an anteroposterior chest radiograph because of the decreased anteroposterior chest diameter. Pectus excavatum does not cause cardiac dysfunction (Park, 1988).

Palpation

Palpation includes the palpation of the precordium and peripheral pulses. Palpation of the precordium detects hyperactivity, thrill, and the point of maximal impulse (PMI). By counting the peripheral pulse rate, any irregularities or inequalities of rate or volume can be observed. Evaluation of the carotid, brachial, femoral, and pedal pulses detects differences between sides and upper and lower extremities. If pulses are unequal, four extremity blood pressures should be measured. Weak leg pulses and strong arm pulses suggest coarctation of the aorta (COA). If the right brachial pulse is stronger than the left, supravalvular aortic stenosis or coarctation proximal to or near the origin of the left subclavian artery may be present (Hazinski, 1984).

Heart defects that lead to "aortic runoff," such as PDA, aortic insufficiency, large arteriovenous fistula, or persistent truncus arteriosus, cause bounding pulses. However, preterm newborns frequently have a bounding pulse secondary to relatively decreased subcutaneous tissue. Also, preterm infants frequently have PDA secondary to their prematurity. Cardiac failure or circulatory shock causes weak or thready pulses (Park, 1988).

The hyperactive precordium indicates a heart defect with increased volume, such as CHDs with large left-to-right shunts (e.g., PDA, ventricular septal defect [VSD]) or heart disease with valvular regurgitation (e.g., aortic regurgitation or mitral regurgitation). The location of the PMI depends on whether the right or left ventricle is dominant. With right ventricular dominance, the PMI is at the lower left sternal border. Left ventricular dominance places the PMI at the apex. A diffuse, slow-rising PMI is called a *heave*. Heaves are associated with volume overload. A sharp, fast-rising PMI is called a *tap* and is associated with pressure overload. The normal newborn has a right ventricular dominance (Park, 1988).

The apical impulse of the newborn is normally felt in the fourth intercostal space to the left of the midclavicular line. Displacement of the apical impulse downward or laterally may indicate cardiac enlargement (Park, 1988).

The presence and location of a thrill provide important diagnostic information. The palms of the hands rather than the fingertips should be used to feel for a thrill, except in the suprasternal notch and carotid arteries. The examiner should palpate for the presence of thrills in the upper left, upper right, and lower left sternal border, in the suprasternal notch, and over the carotid arteries. A thrill in the upper left sternal border is derived from the pulmonary valve or pulmonary artery. Thrills in the lower left sternal border suggest pulmonary stenosis, pulmonary artery atresia, or, occasionally, PDA. A thrill felt in the upper right sternal border signifies aortic origin, usually aortic stenosis or, less frequently, pulmonary stenosis, PDA, or COA. A thrill over the carotid arteries along with a thrill in the suprasternal notch suggests COA or aortic stenosis, or other defects of the aorta or aortic valve (Park, 1988).

Palpation of the abdomen determines the size, consistency, and location of the liver and spleen. Increased liver size is a frequent finding with CHF.

Auscultation

Careful auscultation by a skilled evaluator is an essential component of any cardiovascular assessment. Auscultation includes heart rate and regularity, heart sounds, systolic and diastolic sounds, and heart murmurs. The skillful evaluation of cardiac sounds requires systematic auscultation and much practice.

Identification of Heart Sounds

Individual heart sounds should be identified and evaluated before evaluation of cardiac murmurs is attempted. There are four individual heart sounds: S_1, S_2, S_3, and S_4. However, S_3 and S_4 are rarely heard in the newborn. S_1 is the sound resulting from closure of the mitral and tricuspid valves following atrial systole. S_1 is best heard at the apex or lower left sternal border. S_1 is the beginning of ventricular systole. Splitting of S_1 is infrequently heard in newborns. Wide splitting of S_1 is heard in right bundle branch block or Ebstein's anomaly (McNamara, 1990; Park, 1988).

S_2 is the sound created by closure of the aortic and pulmonary valves, which marks the end of systole and the beginning of ventricular diastole. S_2 is best heard in the upper left sternal border or pulmonic area. Evaluation of the splitting of S_2 is important diagnostically. The timing of the closure of the aortic and pulmonary valves is determined by the volume of blood ejected from the aorta and pulmonary artery and the resistance against which the ventricles must pump (McNamara, 1990).

In the immediate newborn period, there may be no appreciable splitting of S_2. Because the right and left ventricles pump similar quantities of blood and the pulmonary pressure is close to the aortic pressure, these valves close almost simultaneously. Thus, S_2 is heard as a single sound. As the pulmonary vascular resistance decreases, the pulmonary resistance decreases and becomes lower than the aortic pressure, causing a splitting of S_2 as the valve leaflets on the left side of the heart (aortic valve) close before those on the right (pulmonary valve).

By 72 hours of life, S_2 should be split. The absence of a split S_2 or the presence of a widely split S_2 usually indicates an abnormality. A fixed, widely split S_2 occurs in conditions that prolong right ventricular ejection time or shorten left ventricular ejection time. It occurs in (1) atrial septal defect (ASD) and partial anomalous pulmonary venous return (amount of blood ejected by right ventricle is increased, resulting in volume overload), (2) pulmonary stenosis (stenosis delays right ventricular ejection time, resulting in pressure overload), (3) right bundle branch block (delayed electrical activation of right ventricle), (4) mitral regurgitation (decreased forward output, decreased left ventricular ejection time), and (5) idiopathic dilated main pulmonary artery (increased capacity of main pulmonary artery produces less recoil to close the valves, delaying closure) (Park, 1988).

A narrowly split S_2 occurs when there is early closure of the pulmonary valve (pulmonary hypertension) or a delay in aortic closure. A single S_2 is significant because it could represent the presence of only one semilunar valve (e.g., aortic or pulmonary atresia and truncus arteriosus). A single S_2 may also occur with a critical pulmonary stenosis, TGA, or tetralogy of Fallot (TOF), in which the pulmonary closure is not audible. Severe aortic stenosis may also cause a single S_2 because aortic closure is delayed. Severe pulmonary hypertension may cause early closure of the pulmonary valve, thus causing a single S_2.

The relative intensity of the aortic and pulmonary components of S_2 must be assessed. In the pulmonary area (upper left sternal border), the aortic component is usually louder than the pulmonary component. Increased intensity of the pulmonary component, compared with the aortic component, occurs with pulmonary hypertension. Conditions that cause decreased diastolic pressure of the pulmonary artery (e.g., critical pulmonary stenosis, TOF, tricuspid atresia) may cause decreased intensity of the pulmonary component. Evaluation of intensity is difficult, requiring frequent practice listening to heart sounds (McNamara, 1990; Park, 1988).

As discussed, S_3 and S_4 are rarely heard in the neonatal period; their presence denotes pathologic origin. Likewise, a gallop rhythm, the result of a loud S_3 and S_4, and tachycardia are abnormal.

After evaluation of individual heart sounds, the systolic and diastolic sounds are evaluated. The ejection sound, or click, occurs after S_1 and may sound like splitting of S_1. The ejection click is best heard at the upper left or right sternal border or base. The pulmonary click can best be heard at the second or third left intercostal space and is louder with expiration. The aortic click, best heard at the second right intercostal space, does not change in intensity with change in respiration. Ejection clicks are associated with pulmonary or aortic stenosis or with the dilated great arteries seen in systemic or pulmonary hypertension, idiopathic dilation of the main pulmonary artery, TOF, or truncus arteriosus (Park, 1988).

CARDIAC MURMURS

Cardiac murmurs should be evaluated for intensity (grades 1 to 6), timing (systolic or diastolic), location, transmission, and quality (musical, vibratory, or blowing).

The grade scale for murmurs is as follows:

Grade 1: barely audible
Grade 2: soft but easily audible
Grade 3: moderately loud; no thrill
Grade 4: loud; thrill present
Grade 5: loud; audible with stethoscope barely on chest
Grade 6: loud; audible with stethoscope near chest

The murmur grade is recorded as 1/6, 2/6, and so on. Again, practice in auscultation improves the listener's evaluation skills. The intensity of the murmur is affected by cardiac output; anything that increases cardiac output (e.g., anemia, fever, exercise) increases the intensity of the murmur (Park, 1988).

The next step in evaluating a murmur is its classification in relation to S_1 and S_2. There are three types of murmurs: systolic, diastolic, and continuous.

Systolic Murmurs

Most heart murmurs are systolic, occurring between S_1 and S_2. Systolic murmurs are either ejection or regurgitation murmurs. Ejection murmurs occur after S_1 and end before S_2. Ejection murmurs are caused by flow of blood through stenotic or deformed semilunar valves or increased flow through normal semilunar valves (Talner, 1995). Systolic ejection murmurs are best heard at the second left or right intercostal space. Regurgitant systolic murmurs begin with S_1, with no interval between S_1 and the beginning of the murmur. Regurgitation murmurs generally continue throughout systole (pansystolic or holosystolic). Regurgitation systolic murmurs are caused by flow of blood from a chamber at a higher pressure throughout systole than the receiving chamber. Regurgitation systolic murmurs are associated with only three conditions: (1) VSD, (2) mitral regurgitation, and (3) tricuspid regurgitation (Park, 1988).

Location

The location of the maximal intensity of the murmur is helpful in evaluation of the cardiac murmur. Figure 21–3 shows the locations at which various systolic murmurs can be heard.

Related to the location is the transmission of the murmur. Knowledge of transmission can assist in determining the origin of the murmur. A systolic ejection murmur that transmits well to the neck is usually aortic in origin, whereas one that transmits to the back is usually pulmonary in origin. An apical systolic murmur that transmits well to the left axilla and lower back is characteristic of mitral regurgitation, but one that transmits to the upper right sternal border and neck is likely to be aortic in nature (McNamara, 1990).

Quality

Murmurs are described as musical, vibratory, or blowing (Park, 1988). VSDs or mitral regurgitation murmurs have a high-pitched, blowing quality. Aortic stenosis and pulmonary valve stenosis murmurs have a rough, grating quality. Establishing the quality of the murmur is subjective, and expertise is gained only after extensive practice.

Diastolic Murmurs

Diastolic murmurs occur between S_1 and S_2. Diastolic murmurs are classified according to their timing in relation to heart sounds as early diastolic, middiastolic, or presystolic.

Early diastolic (protodiastolic) murmurs occur early in diastole, right after S_2, owing to incompetence of the aortic or pulmonary valve. Aortic regurgitation murmurs are high pitched and are best heard with the diaphragm at the third left intercostal space. This murmur radiates to the apex. Bounding pulses are present with significant regurgitation. Aortic regurgitation murmurs occur with bicuspid aortic valve, subaortic stenosis, and subarterial infundibular VSD. Pulmonary regurgitation murmurs are medium pitched unless pulmonary hypertension is present, in which case they are high pitched. Diastolic regurgitation murmurs are heard best at the second left intercostal space, radiating along the left sternal border. Pulmonary regurgitation murmurs occur with postoperative TOF, pulmonary hypertension, postoperative pulmonary valvotomy for pulmonary stenosis, or other deformity of the pulmonary valve (Park, 1988).

Middiastolic murmurs result from abnormal ventricular filling. These murmurs are low pitched and can best be heard with the bell of the stethoscope placed lightly on the chest wall. The murmur results from turbulent flow through the tricuspid or mitral valve that is caused by stenosis. Mitral middiastolic murmurs are best heard at the apex and are referred to as *apical rumbles*. They are associated with mitral stenosis or large left-to-right shunt VSD or PDA, producing relative mitral stenosis secondary to increased flow across the normal-sized mitral valve. Tricuspid middiastolic murmurs can best be heard along the lower left sternal border and are associated with ASD, total or partial anomalous pulmonary venous return, endocardial cushion defects, or abnormal stenosis of the tricuspid valve.

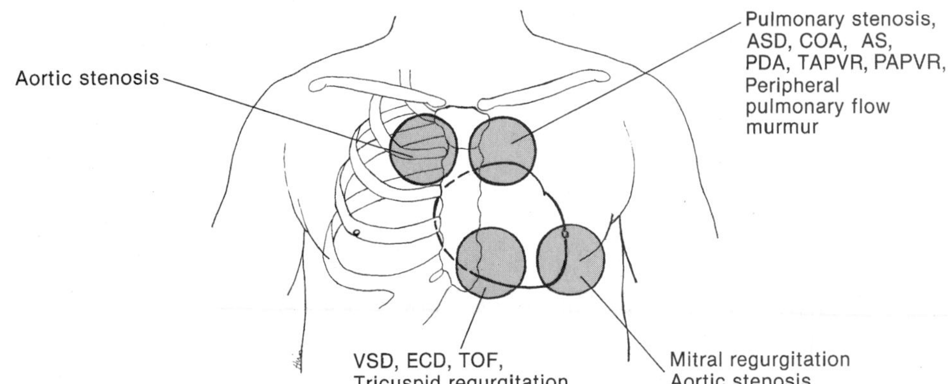

FIGURE 21–3. Location of systolic murmurs. AS, aortic stenosis; ASD, atrial septal defect; COA, coarctation of the aorta; ECD, endocardial cushion defect; PAPVR, partial anomalous pulmonary venous return; PDA, patent ductus arteriosus; TAPVR, total anomalous pulmonary venous return; TOF, tetralogy of Fallot; VSD, ventricular septal defect.

Presystolic or late diastolic murmurs result from flow through AV valves during ventricular diastole as a result of active atrial contraction ejecting blood into the ventricle. These are low-frequency murmurs found with true mitral or tricuspid valve stenosis.

Continuous Murmurs

Continuous murmurs begin in systole and continue throughout S_2 into all or part of diastole. Continuous murmurs are caused by (1) aorticopulmonary or AV connection (e.g., PDA, AV fistula, or persistent truncus), (2) disturbances of flow in veins (e.g., venous hum), and (3) disturbances of flow in arteries (e.g., COA or pulmonary artery stenosis) (Park, 1988).

PDA is the most commonly heard continuous murmur in the newborn. The PDA murmur is described as a machinery murmur, louder during systole, peaking at S_2, and decreased in diastole. PDA murmurs are loudest in the left infraclavicular area or the upper left sternal border (Avery et al., 1994).

Other Murmurs

Functional or innocent cardiac murmurs are common in children and can occur in newborns. These murmurs occur in the absence of abnormal cardiac structures. Functional murmurs are asymptomatic. The presence of any unusual or abnormal finding warrants consultation. Findings such as cyanosis, enlarged heart size on examination or enlarged cardiac silhouette on radiograph, abnormal electrocardiogram (ECG), diastolic murmur, grade 3/6 systolic murmur or a less intense murmur with a thrill, weak or bounding pulses, or other abnormal heart sounds have pathologic origins and must be investigated.

Commonly found in low birth weight infants is the pulmonary flow murmur. These infants have relative hypoplastic right and left pulmonary arteries at birth, which are a result of the small amount of blood flow during fetal life. The increased flow after birth creates turbulence in the small vessels, which is transmitted along the smaller branches of the pulmonary arteries. This murmur is best heard at the upper left sternal border. The pulmonary flow murmur has a grade of 1/6 to 2/6 intensity, but is transmitted to the right and left chest, both axillae, and back. There are no other significant cardiac findings. It usually disappears by 3 to 6 months of age. Persistence beyond this period should lead to further evaluation for anatomic pulmonary artery stenosis (Park, 1988).

CONGENITAL HEART DEFECTS

Etiology

Cardiac development occurs during the first 7 weeks of gestation. Major structural defects can occur if there is an interference with the maternal-placental-fetal unit during this critical period. Causes of CHDs are classified as chromosomal (10 to 12 percent), genetic (1 to 2 percent), maternal or environmental (1 to 2 percent), or multifactorial (85 percent) (Moller, 1987).

Many chromosomal abnormalities are associated with structural heart defects. Thirty to 50 percent of infants with trisomy 21 (Down syndrome) have a structural heart defect. The most common CHDs with trisomy 21 are endocardial cushion defects and VSD. Specific genetic abnormalities account for only a small percentage of CHDs. Marfan syndrome is associated with defects of the aorta, such as aortic insufficiency or an aortic aneurysm (Baraitser & Winter, 1996; Hoffman, 1990; Park, 1988).

Maternal or environmental factors include maternal illness and drug ingestion. Maternal rubella during the first 7 weeks of pregnancy carries a 50 percent risk of congenital rubella with major defects of multiple organ systems. Heart defects include PDA and pulmonary artery branch stenosis. Other viral diseases, such as cytomegalovirus, or protozoal diseases, such as toxoplasmosis, are also associated with CHDs. The diagnosis of a CHD calls for a careful maternal history to identify viral-like illnesses that may have been unrecognized or unreported at the time of occurrence (Park, 1988).

Maternal drug use may also cause cardiac malformations. Fifty percent of newborns with fetal alcohol syndrome have a CHD. Only a few drugs are proven teratogens (e.g., thalidomide); however, *no* drugs are known to be completely safe. The threat of environmental hazards to fetal development have only recently been recognized.

Metabolic disease of the mother increases the risk for CHDs. Infants of diabetic mothers have a 10 percent risk of having a CHD. TGA, VSD, or generalized hypertrophic cardiomyopathy are the most common types of defects found in infants of diabetic mothers (Hazinski, 1984; Heymann, 1995; Park, 1988).

Most CHDs are considered to be of multifactorial origin. These defects are probably the result of an interaction effect of the other causes. Research into genetic causes of cardiac defects may identify specific genetic causes for some heart defects that are currently thought to have multifactorial origin. Infants with other congenital defects often have associated CHDs. Multiple defects affect the development of structures that are forming at the time of the interference with normal development.

Incidence

Estimates of incidence of CHD vary from 4.05 to 10.2 per 1000 live births (Hoffman, 1990). The overall incidence of CHD is slightly less than 1 percent, or 8 per 1000 live births, excluding PDA in the preterm infant (Hoffman, 1990; Park, 1988). Because the overall incidence of CHD is approximately 1 percent of all live births and because the incidence of individual defects is less than 1 percent, the incidence of individual defects is usually given as a percent of all CHDs. The incidence of a specific defect within the overall incidence of CHDs is included in the discussion of that defect.

Some CHDs are not detected in the neonatal period. Others are detected but are initially managed medically. Thus, the following discussion of CHDs extends beyond the neonatal period. Table 21–3 is an overview of the diagnosis of CHDs.

The discussion of defects is based on the common pathophysiologic features. CHDs can be classified in numerous ways. The simplest classification is based on whether the defect produces cyanosis. Cyanosis is the bluish discoloration of the skin that occurs when there is approximately 5 g/100 ml of desaturated hemoglobin in the circulating volume. Thus, the appearance of cyanosis depends on the hemoglobin concentration. An infant with low hemoglobin may be hypoxic but may not appear cyanotic, thus low hemoglobin cannot be the sole criterion for determining pathologic origin. Cyanosis in the extremities, or acrocyanosis, is frequently seen in newborns because of reduced blood flow through the small capillaries. Oxygen is extracted from the hemoglobin in the capillaries, giving the skin a blue appearance. This blue appearance is a normal phenomenon in the newborn. Differentiation of central cyanosis from peripheral or acrocyanosis is essential (Driscoll, 1990).

Acyanotic Heart Defects

Acyanotic heart defects are those that produce a left-to-right shunt. Typically, these defects do not produce cyanosis because there is sufficient oxygenated blood in the circulation. The left-to-right shunts produce increased pulmonary blood flow and increased workload on the heart. The acyanotic heart defects discussed here are PDA, VSD, ASD, endocardial cushion defects, and aortic stenosis.

Patent Ductus Arteriosus

The ductus arteriosus is a wide muscular connection between the pulmonary artery and the aorta. The ductus arteriosus originates from the left pulmonary artery and enters the aorta below the subclavian artery. The ductus arteriosus allows oxygenated blood from the placenta to bypass the lungs and enter the circulation (Friedman, 1988; Hazinski, 1984; Moller, 1987).

The ductus arteriosus closes functionally by about 15 hours of life. During the first 24 hours of life, there may be some shunting of blood, but the ductal opening must be greater than 2 mm for significant shunting to occur.

Closure of the ductus arteriosus occurs in response to increased arterial oxygen concentration after the initiation of pulmonary function. Other factors that contribute to closure of the ductus arteriosus include a decrease in prostaglandin E (PGE) and an increase in acetylcholine and bradykinin (Park, 1988). The persistence of the ductus arteriosus beyond 24 hours of life is considered a PDA in the term newborn. PDA in the preterm neonate presents a different clinical problem and is discussed separately from PDA in the term newborn.

Patent Ductus Arteriosus in the Term Newborn

Incidence

PDA accounts for approximately 5 to 10 percent of all CHDs, excluding preterm neonates. There is a higher ratio of PDA in females (about 3:1) (Park, 1988).

Hemodynamics

In extrauterine life, the flow of blood through the ductus arteriosus is reversed. The PDA allows blood to flow from left-to-right, thereby reentering the pulmonary circuit and increasing pulmonary blood flow.

The amount of blood flow through the PDA and the effects of the ductal flow depend on (1) the difference between systemic and pulmonary vascular resistance, (2) the diameter of the ductus, and (3) the length of the ductus. High pulmonary blood flow causes increased pulmonary vascular resistance, pulmonary hypertension, and right ventricular hypertrophy. Figure 21–4 shows the hemodynamics of PDA.

Manifestations

A small PDA may be asymptomatic. A large PDA with significant shunting may cause signs of CHF with tachypnea, dyspnea, hoarse cry, frequent lower respiratory tract infections, and coughing. Poor weight gain is common.

Diagnosis

The diagnosis of PDA is based on history and physical examination, radiograph, ECG, and echocardiogram. On physical examination, there may be bounding peripheral pulses, widened pulse pressure, and a hyperactive precordium. A systolic thrill may be felt at the upper left sternal border. A grade 1/6 to 4/6 continuous "machinery" murmur is audible at the upper left sternal border or left infraclavicular area. The murmur is heard throughout the entire cardiac cycle because of the pressure gradient between the aorta and the pulmonary artery in both systole and diastole. In severe PDA with large shunt, the S_2 is accentuated because of pulmonary hypertension (Brook & Heymann, 1995; Park, 1988).

A small PDA may not be distinguishable on radiograph. With more severe shunting, there may be cardiomegaly and increased pulmonary vascularity. ECG may show left atrial and ventricular enlargement and an abnormal QRS axis for age. The definitive diagnosis is made with an echocardiogram. With two-dimensional echocardiogram, PDA can be directly visualized. A ductus is considered to be hemodynamically significant if the left atrium to aortic root ratio (LA:AO) is greater than 1:3 in term newborns or greater than 1:0 in preterm newborns (Friedman, 1988; Brook & Heymann, 1995; Park, 1988).

Management

Medical management includes prophylactic antibiotics against bacterial endocarditis. There are no exercise restrictions in the absence of pulmonary hypertension. Definitive treatment is surgical ligation through a posterolateral thoracotomy. The surgery is performed in patients between 1 and 2 years of age, unless there is CHF, recurrent pneumonia, or pulmonary hypertension. The mortality rate is less than 1 percent (excluding preterm newborns). The prognosis is excellent, and complications are rare (Brook & Heymann, 1995; Park, 1988).

Patent Ductus Arteriosus in the Preterm Newborn

PDA in preterm newborns is a common complicating factor in their care. As the newborn recovers from respiratory distress, pulmonary vascular resistance decreases as oxygenation improves. The ductus in the preterm newborn is not as responsive to increased oxygen content and does not close. The decreased pulmonary vascular resistance causes blood to shunt from left to right and reenter the pulmonary circuit. This shunting causes increased pulmonary venous congestion, which decreases lung compliance, making the lungs stiff. Large shunts result in symptoms of CHF and an inability to wean ventilatory support or an increased oxygen requirement (Avery et al., 1994).

TABLE 21–3 Diagnosis of Congenital Heart Defects

Defect	Chest Radiograph	ECG	Echocardiogram	Catheterization	Lab Tests
PDA	Increased pulmonary vascularity; cardiac enlargement; left aortic arch	Left atrial and ventricular enlargement; abnormal QRS axis for age	LA:AO ratio >1.3 (term), 1.0 (preterm); increased left atrium and ventricle (2-D)	Increased O_2 saturation in pulmonary artery; increased right ventricular and pulmonary artery pressure (with pulmonary hypertension)	NA
ASD	Mild heart enlargement; prominent main pulmonary artery; increased pulmonary vascularity	Right axis deviation; incomplete right bundle branch block; right ventricular hypertrophy	Dilated right ventricle; paradoxical movement of ventricular septum	Increased O_2 in right atrium; normal right side atrium; normal right side pressure; 10%: PAPVR	NA
AS	Normal heart size; slight prominence of left ventricle and aorta	Normal or mild left ventricular hypertrophy; inverted T waves	Prominent septal thickening; abnormal mitral valve motions	Anatomic and physiologic alterations in cardiac function	NA
VSD	Enlarged heart; increased pulmonary markings	Left and right ventricular hypertrophy	Large left atrium (M-mode); presence or absence of other defects (2-D)	Increased O_2 in right ventricle; increased systolic pressure in right ventricle and pulmonary artery	NA
ECD	Cardiomegaly; increased pulmonary vascularity	Left axis deviation; prolonged P-R interval; right and left atrial enlargement; right ventricular hypertrophy; incomplete right bundle branch block	Ventricular dilation; abnormal mitral and tricuspid valves	Increased O_2 in right atrium; increased right ventricular and/or pulmonary artery pressure; with angiography, a "goose neck" deformity of ventricular outflow area	NA
TOF	Normal heart size; boot-shaped contour; decreased pulmonary markings; prominent aorta; right aortic arch in ⅓ cases	Right axis deviation; right ventricular hypertrophy	Large VSD, aortic dextroposition, and PS; size of main, right, and left pulmonary arteries (2-D)	Demonstrates anatomy of right ventricular outflow region; microcytic anemia	Increased Hgb and HCT clotting time
PS	Normal heart size; normal pulmonary vascularity; enlarged pulmonary artery; right ventricle filling (lateral)	Right axis deviation; right atrial enlargement; right ventricular hypertrophy	Decreased valve leaflet motion; small changes in right ventricular wall thickness	Elevated right ventricular pressure; normal or slightly lowered pulmonary artery pressure	NA
TA	Cardiomegaly; absence of main pulmonary artery segment; large aorta; increased pulmonary vascularity	Right and/or left ventricular hypertrophy	Absence of two semilunar valves	Left-to-right shunt at level of ventricle; pressure equal in ventricles, truncus, and pulmonary arteries	Increased Hgb and HCT
TGA	Enlarged heart with narrow base; enlarged ventricles; increased pulmonary vascularity	Right axis deviation; right ventricular hypertrophy	Abnormal origin of great vessels	Increased right ventricular pressure; catheter can enter aorta from right ventricle; pulmonary artery can be entered only through PDA or ASD	Increased Hgb and HCT; polycythemia
COA	Cardiomegaly; postcoarctation dilation (by age 5 years); notching of ribs from collateral vessels	Left ventricular hypertrophy; inverted T waves in left precordial leads; right ventricular hypertrophy (severe)	Visualization of narrowed aorta and location of associated defects; allows evaluation of aortic valve movement, structure, and function and left ventricular size and function	Performed to determine exact location and evaluation	NA
HLHS	Cardiomegaly; increased pulmonary vascularity; interstitial emphysema	Prominent right ventricular forces; decreased left ventricular forces	Small left ventricle	Performed for evaluation for surgical intervention or if echocardiogram is inconclusive	NA
TAPVR	Cardiac enlargement; large pulmonary artery; increased pulmonary flow	Right ventricular hypertrophy; right axis deviation; right atrial hypertrophy (after 1 month)	Presence of right atrial enlargement; patent foramen ovale; inability to demonstrate continuity between the pulmonary veins and left atrium (2-D)	Higher O_2 saturation in right atrium; angiography reveals opacification of pulmonary arterial circulation, pulmonary venous circulation, and abnormal circulation	NA

AS, aortic stenosis; ASD, atrial septal defect; COA, coarctation of the aorta; ECG, electrocardiogram; HCT, hematocrit; Hgb, hemoglobin; HLHS, hypoplastic left heart syndrome; LA:AO, left atrium to aortic root; Lab, laboratory; NA, not applicable; PAPVR, partial anomalous pulmonary venous return; PDA, patent ductus arteriosus; PS, pulmonary stenosis; TA, truncus arteriosus; TAPVR, total anomalous pulmonary venous return; TGA, transposition of the great arteries; TOF, tetralogy of Fallot; VSD, ventricular septal defect.

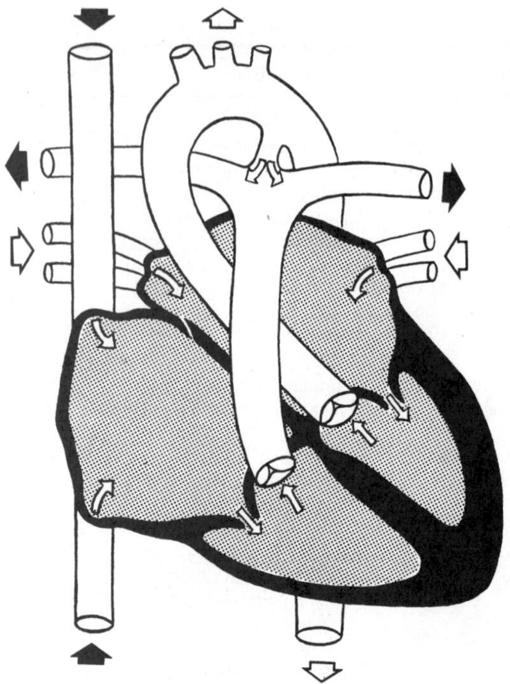

FIGURE 21–4. Patent ductus arteriosus is a communication between the pulmonary artery and the aorta. (Reprinted with permission of Ross Laboratories, Columbus, OH 43216, Clinical Education Aid, © 1985, Ross Laboratories.)

Clinical findings indicative of PDA include bounding peripheral pulses, hyperactive precordium, widened pulse pressures (greater than 25), and a continuous murmur, best heard at the upper left and middle sternal border. Radiographic findings include increased pulmonary vascularity and cardiomegaly. PDA can be directly visualized by two-dimensional echocardiogram and Doppler flow studies (Avery et al., 1994; Park, 1988).

Management of PDA depends on the severity of the symptoms. Conservative management consists of fluid restriction and diuretic therapy. Use of cardiac glycosides is controversial in the preterm newborn. The preterm newborn's myocardium has a higher amount of connective tissue and water, which may decrease the left ventricular distensibility; thus, digitalis would have no effect. Digitalis toxicity may occur because of poor elimination of the drug. If digitalis is used, the dose should be decreased and monitored carefully (Park, 1988).

Indomethacin, a prostaglandin synthetase inhibitor, may be used to close the ductus. PGE_2 is produced in the walls of the ductus arteriosus to prevent closure during fetal life. Indomethacin inhibits the production of PGE_2 and promotes ductal closure. Smaller babies may require a higher dose to obtain effective plasma levels. Indomethacin works best if used in newborns younger than 13 days of life; it is not effective after 4 to 6 weeks of life. The dosage for indomethacin is 0.2 mg/kg intravenously every 12 hours for three doses. Indomethacin is highly nephrotoxic, so the blood urea nitrogen (BUN) and creatinine levels must be monitored. Contraindications to using indomethacin include renal failure, low platelet count, bleeding disorders, necrotizing enterocolitis, and hyperbilirubinemia (Avery et al., 1994; Park, 1988).

Surgical ligation is reserved for cases in which indomethacin failed or was contraindicated. The mortality rate for ligation is slightly less than 2 percent. Mortality rate is highest in the more preterm, sicker infants, especially if pulmonary hypertension has developed.

Ventricular Septal Defect

A VSD is a defect or opening in the ventricular septum that results from imperfect ventricular division during early fetal development. The defect can occur anywhere in the muscular or membranous ventricular septum. The size of the defect and the degree of pulmonary vascular resistance are more important in determining the severity than the location. With a small defect, there is a large resistance to the left-to-right shunt at the defect and the shunt is not dependent on the pulmonary vascular resistance. With a large VSD, there is little resistance at the defect and the amount of left-to-right shunt is dependent on the level of pulmonary vascular resistance (Graham & Gutgesell, 1995).

Incidence

VSD is the most common CHD. It accounts for approximately 20 to 25 percent of all CHDs.

Hemodynamics

The hemodynamic consequences of a VSD depend on its size: small, moderate, and large defects.

Small VSD. Small VSDs produce minimal shunting and may not be symptomatic. Chest radiograph and ECG are also normal. There is usually a loud, harsh pansystolic heart murmur, best heard in the third and fourth left intercostal space at the sternal border. Figure 21–5 shows a VSD (Moller, 1987; Park, 1988).

Moderate VSD. With moderate-sized VSDs, the blood is shunted from the left to right ventricle because of higher pressure in the left ventricle and higher systemic vascular resistance. The shunt of VSD occurs during systole, when the right ventricle contracts, so that the blood enters the pulmonary artery rather

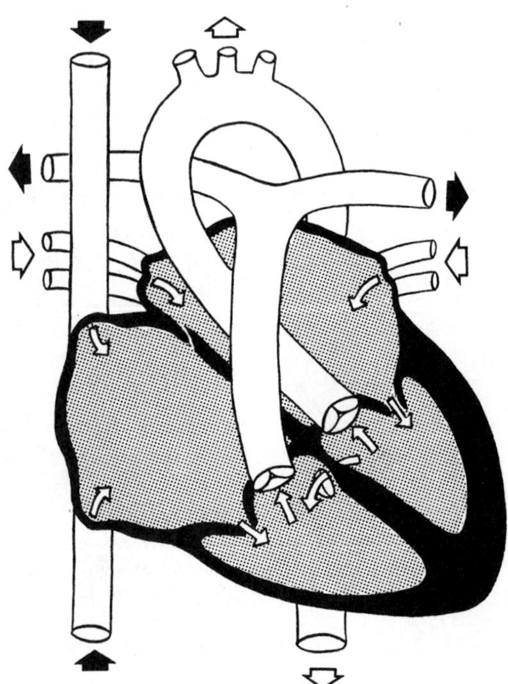

FIGURE 21–5. Ventricular septal defect is a communication between the right and left ventricles. (Reprinted with permission of Ross Laboratories, Columbus, OH 43216, Clinical Education Aid, © 1985, Ross Laboratories.)

than remaining in the right ventricle. This prevents the development of right ventricular hypertrophy.

Large VSD. With large VSDs, blood is shunted from the left to right ventricle. The larger the VSD, the greater the shunt and the higher the pressure in the right ventricle and pulmonary artery. If pulmonary artery pressure is increased, thickening of the walls of the pulmonary arterioles may develop and the increased resistance may decrease the left-to-right shunt. Pulmonary vascular disease can lead to right-to-left shunting and cyanosis (Graham & Gutgesell, 1995).

Manifestations

Manifestations of VSD depend on the degree of shunting. Small VSDs may produce no hemodynamic compromise and be asymptomatic. Larger defects are associated with decreased exertional tolerance, recurrent pulmonary infections, poor growth, and symptoms of CHF. With severe VSD, there may be pulmonary hypertension and cyanosis.

Diagnosis

In VSD, a systolic thrill may be palpated at the lower left sternal border. There may be a precordial bulge with very large VSDs. A grade 2/6 to 5/6 regurgitant systolic murmur is heard at the lower left sternal border. There may also be an apical diastolic rumble. The pulmonary heart sound may be loud.

Radiographs show cardiomegaly involving the left atrium, left ventricle, and possibly the right ventricle. There is also increased pulmonary vascularity. ECG may reveal left ventricular hypertrophy. Right ventricular hypertrophy may also be present in severe cases. Echocardiogram (M-mode) shows a large left atrium. Two-dimensional echocardiogram shows other defects and the size and location of the VSD (Avery et al., 1994; Park, 1988).

Physical examination of infants with a large VSD not detected in the neonatal period may reveal inadequate weight gain, cyanosis, and clubbing of the digits.

Management

Initial management of the hemodynamically significant VSD includes monitoring for signs of CHF and prompt initiation of therapy. CHF is treated with diuretics and digitalis. Unless there is pulmonary hypertension, there is no need to restrict activities. Prophylaxis against bacterial endocarditis is indicated.

Surgical management involves direct closure of the VSD. Cardiopulmonary bypass is required for the surgical correction. The timing of the surgery depends on the severity of the circulatory and pulmonary compromise. Infants with significant left-to-right shunting with evidence of severe compromise require surgery. Signs of CHF that do not respond to conservative medical management or increasing pulmonary vascular resistance are indications for surgical correction. Asymptomatic children with a moderate VSD usually have surgical correction between 2 and 4 years of age.

The mortality rate for VSD correction is approximately 5 percent. The mortality rate is higher among smaller infants, those with other defects, and those with multiple VSDs (Graham & Gutgesell, 1995).

Atrial Septal Defect

An ASD is a defect or opening in the atrial septum that develops as a result of improper septal formation early in fetal cardiac development.

There are three types of ASDs (Park, 1988):

1. Ostium secundum, commonly associated with mitral valve
2. Ostium primum, an endocardial cushion defect associated with anomalies of one or both AV valves
3. Sinus venosus, often associated with partial anomalous pulmonary venous connection

Incidence

ASDs account for 5 to 10 percent of all CHDs.

Hemodynamics

An ASD usually does not produce symptoms until pulmonary vascular resistance begins to decrease and right ventricular end-diastolic and right atrial pressures decline. All types of ASDs produce some blood flow alterations (Porter et al., 1995; Feldt et al., 1995).

With an ASD, blood shunts from left to right across the defect because the right ventricle, being more compliant than the left, offers less resistance to filling. Any factors that decrease right ventricular distensibility or obstruct flow into the right ventricle (e.g., pulmonary stenosis or tricuspid stenosis) can reduce or reverse the shunt direction. The left-to-right shunt increases right ventricular volume, but pulmonary vascular resistance decreases, so pulmonary artery pressure is almost normal. The large pulmonary blood flow eventually leads to increased pulmonary artery pressures. These changes are gradual. Figure 21–6 shows an ASD (Feldt et al., 1995).

Manifestations

Neonates with ASDs are usually asymptomatic or there may be a grade 2/6 to 3/6 systolic ejection murmur, which can best be heard at the upper left sternal border.

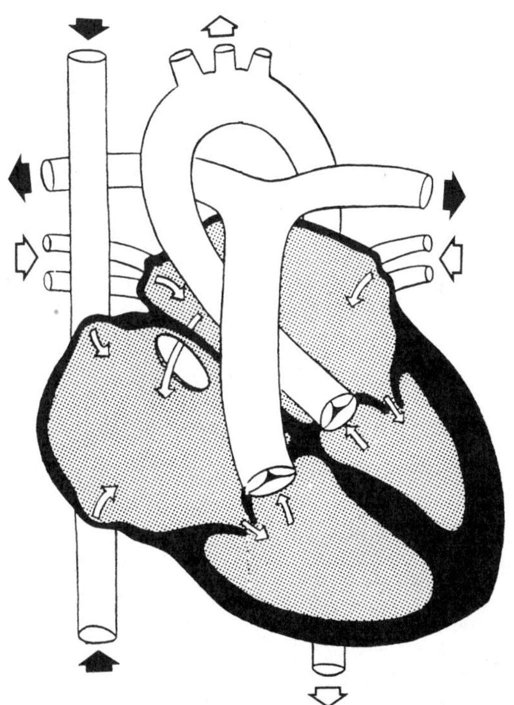

FIGURE 21–6. Atrial septal defect is a communication between the right and left atria. (Reprinted with permission of Ross Laboratories, Columbus, OH 43216, Clinical Education Aid, © 1985, Ross Laboratories.)

S_2 may be widely split and fixed. With a large ASD, there may be a middiastolic rumble caused by the relative tricuspid stenosis audible at the lower left sternal border (Park, 1988). On chest radiograph, the heart is enlarged, with a prominent main pulmonary artery segment and increased pulmonary vascularity. ECG shows right axis deviation and mild right ventricular hypertrophy. There may be incomplete right bundle branch block.

Echocardiogram by M-mode shows increased right ventricular dimension and paradoxical movement of the ventricular septum. Diagnosis can be made by two-dimensional echocardiogram, which shows the location and size of the defect. Children with ASDs are usually thin and may be easily fatigued. By late infancy, there may be a precordial bulge caused by enlargement of the right side of the heart.

Management

Untreated ASD can lead to CHF, pulmonary hypertension, and atrial arrhythmias in adults. Spontaneous closure of ASDs occurs in the first 5 years of age in up to 40 percent of children (Park, 1988). Medical management of ASD consists of prevention or treatment of CHF. There is no need to limit activity. Surgical correction is accomplished by a simple patch or with direct closure during open heart surgery using cardiopulmonary bypass. Timing of surgery depends on the severity of the defect. The presence of a significant left-to-right shunt is an indication for surgical correction. Surgery is performed when the patient is between 2 and 5 years of age. The surgery is not performed in infants unless there is CHF that is unresponsive to medical management. The mortality rate of the surgery is less than 1 percent. The highest risk is for small infants with CHF or increased pulmonary vascular resistance.

Endocardial Cushion Defects

Endocardial cushion defects result from inappropriate fusion of the endocardial cushions during fetal development. Endocardial cushion defects produce abnormalities of the atrial septum (ostium primum), ventricular septum, and AV valves. Endocardial cushion defects take many forms and are characterized by downward displacement of the AV valves as a result of deficiency in ventricular septal tissue and an elongation of the left ventricular outflow tract. The term *complete AV canal* describes the large opening in the center of the heart between the atria and the ventricles. The following defects can occur in the AV canal: (1) an ostium primum ASD, (2) a VSD in the inlet portion of the ventricular septum, (3) a cleft in the anterior mitral valve leaflet, and (4) a cleft in the septal leaflet of the tricuspid valve, which results in common anterior and posterior cusps of the AV valve (Feldt et al., 1995; Park, 1988).

Incidence

Endocardial cushion defects account for 2 percent of all CHDs. Thirty percent of the endocardial cushion defects present in infants with Down syndrome. Ten percent of infants with endocardial cushion defects also have PDA, and 10 percent have TOF (Feldt et al., 1995; Park, 1988).

Hemodynamics

The hemodynamic consequences of endocardial cushion defects depend on their type and severity. There may be interatrial and interventricular shunts, left ventricle to right atrium shunts, or AV valve regurgitation (Hazinski, 1984). Figure 21–7 shows an endocardial cushion defect.

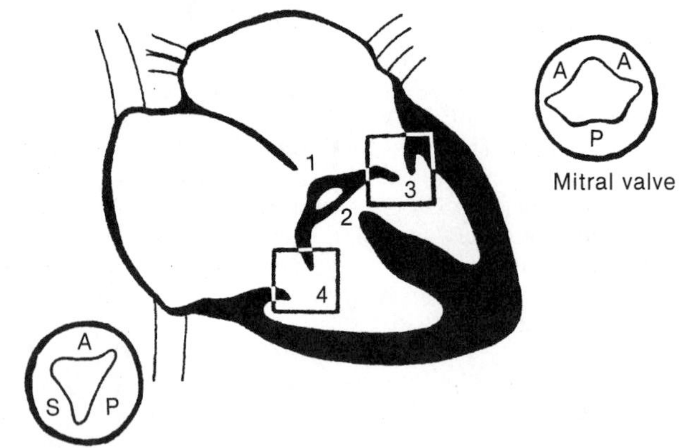

FIGURE 21–7. Endocardial cushion defect. *1*, ostium primum atrial septal defect; *2*, a ventricular septal defect in the inlet portion of ventricular septum; *3*, cleft in anterior mitral valve leaflet; *4*, cleft in septal leaflet of the tricuspid valve, resulting in common anterior and posterior cusps of the atrioventricular valve. A, anterior; S, septal; P, posterior.

Manifestations

The manifestations of endocardial cushion defects result from the increased pulmonary blood flow caused by the abnormal connection between both ventricles and the atria and by absent or malformed AV valves. The neonate may have respiratory distress, signs of CHF, tachycardia, and a cardiac murmur. The mitral regurgitation may be heard as a grade 3/6 to 4/6 holosystolic regurgitant murmur audible at the lower left sternal border, which transmits to the left back and may be audible at the apex. There is also a middiastolic rumble at the lower left sternal border or at the apex caused by the relative stenosis of tricuspid and mitral valves. S_1 is accentuated, and S_2 is narrowly split. The sound of the pulmonary closure is increased in intensity (Feldt et al., 1995; Hazinski, 1984; Park, 1988).

Chest radiograph reveals generalized cardiomegaly with increased pulmonary vascularity and a prominent main pulmonary artery segment. ECG shows left axis deviation with a prolonged P-R interval, right and left atrial enlargement, right ventricular hypertrophy, and incomplete right bundle branch block.

An infant with an endocardial cushion defect may demonstrate signs of CHF, recurrent respiratory infections, and failure to thrive. Physical examination reveals a poorly nourished infant with signs of respiratory distress and tachycardia.

Management

Initial medical management is aimed at preventing or treating CHF with diuretics and digitalis. Prophylaxis against bacterial endocarditis is required before and after surgical correction. Definitive management consists of surgical closure of the ASD and VSD, with reconstruction of AV valves under cardiopulmonary bypass, deep hypothermia, or both. In some cases, pulmonary artery banding may be performed as a palliative procedure if there is not significant mitral regurgitation. This procedure carries a slightly higher mortality risk than when primary surgical repair is performed.

Surgery is indicated when there is CHF that is unresponsive to medical therapy, recurrent pneumonia, failure to thrive, or a large shunt with development of pulmonary hypertension and increasing pulmonary vascular resistance. The repair is performed in patients aged approximately 6 months to 2 years. The mortality rate has declined in recent years to approximately 5 to 10 percent.

The mortality rate for patients who undergo pulmonary banding is approximately 15 percent. Factors that increase the risks of this procedure include (1) very young age, (2) severe AV valve incompetence, (3) hypoplastic left ventricle, and (4) severe symptoms before surgery (Feldt et al., 1995; Park, 1988).

Aortic Stenosis

Aortic stenosis is one of a group of defects that produce obstruction to ventricular outflow. Aortic stenosis may be valvular, subvalvular, or supravalvular. Valvular stenosis is the most common, and supravalvular is the least common (Park, 1988).

In valvular stenosis, there is usually a bicuspid valve. Subvalvular stenosis can involve either a simple diaphragm or a long tunnel-like ventricular outflow tract. Idiopathic hypertrophic subaortic stenosis is a form of subvalvular stenosis that presents as a cardiomyopathy. Supravalvular stenosis is associated with Williams' syndrome, or elfin facies, characterized by mental retardation, short palpebral fissures, and thick lips (Baraitser & Winter, 1996; Park, 1988).

Incidence

Aortic stenosis accounts for 5 percent of all CHDs. It is four times more common in males.

Hemodynamics

Aortic stenosis causes increased pressure load on the left ventricle, leading to left ventricular hypertrophy. The resistance to blood flow through the stenosis gradually causes a pressure gradient between the ventricle and the aorta. Eventually, coronary blood flow decreases. Aortic stenosis is illustrated in Figure 21–8.

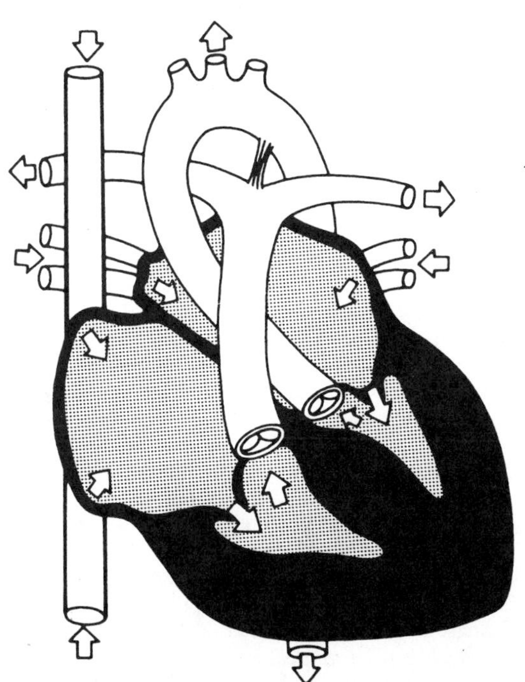

FIGURE 21–8. Aortic stenosis is a narrowing or thickening of the aortic valvular region. (Reprinted with permission of Ross Laboratories, Columbus, OH 43216, Clinical Education Aid, © 1985, Ross Laboratories.)

Manifestations

Symptoms depend on the severity of the defect. Mild aortic stenosis may not cause symptoms. With more severe defects, there is activity intolerance, chest pain, or syncope. With severe defects, CHF develops (Friedman, 1988).

Diagnosis

Physical examination reveals normal development without cyanosis. There may be a narrow pulse pressure and a higher systolic pressure in the right arm with severe supravalvular aortic stenosis. There is a systolic murmur of approximately grade 2/6 to 4/6, best heard at the second right or left intercostal space with transmission to the neck. With valvular aortic stenosis, there may be an ejection click. With severe aortic stenosis, there may be paradoxical splitting of S_2. Aortic insufficiency may cause a high-pitched, early diastolic decrescendo murmur if there is bicuspid aortic valve or subvalvular stenosis (Friedman, 1995; Hazinski, 1984; Park, 1988).

Chest radiographs may be normal or may show a dilated ascending aorta or, in the case of valvular stenosis, a prominent aortic "knob" caused by poststenotic dilation (Park, 1988). Cardiomegaly is present if there is CHF or severe aortic regurgitation. ECG may be normal or may show mild left ventricular hypertrophy and inverted T waves. Echocardiogram shows prominent thickening of the septum and abnormal mitral valve motions. Two-dimensional echocardiogram shows the anatomy of the aortic valve (bicuspid, tricuspid, or unicuspid) and that of subvalvular and supravalvular aortic stenosis.

Cardiac catheterization may be performed. Its purpose is to identify the exact anatomy and to analyze pressure gradients.

Management

Management is aimed at preventing or treating the CHF with fluid restriction, diuretics, and digitalis. In children with moderate to severe aortic stenosis, activity is restricted to prevent increased demand on the heart. Balloon valvuloplasty is sometimes performed at the time of cardiac catheterization to improve circulation. In critical aortic stenosis, maintenance of the patency of the ductus arteriosus with PGE_1 is necessary to prevent hypoxia (Avery et al., 1994).

The type of surgical correction depends on the exact location and severity of the defect. The procedure may consist of aortic valve commissurotomy or valve replacement with a prosthetic valve or a graft. The placement of prosthetic valves is usually deferred until adult-sized prosthetic valves can be inserted. The timing of the surgery depends on the severity of the defect. Infants with critical aortic stenosis with CHF must have corrective surgery. Surgery is performed on children when there is a peak systolic pressure gradient greater than 80 mm Hg or when there are symptoms of chest pain (Friedman, 1988).

The mortality risk for infants and small children is 15 to 20 percent. As in all cases, the sicker, smaller infants have the highest mortality rate. The mortality rate in older children is approximately 1 to 2 percent (Park, 1988).

Cyanotic Heart Defects

Cyanotic heart defects are those defects with a right-to-left shunt with either reduced or increased pulmonary blood flow. The cyanotic heart defects discussed here include TOF, pulmonary valve atresia or stenosis, truncus arteriosus, TGA, COA, hypoplastic left heart syndrome (HLHS), and total anomalous pulmonary venous return (TAPVR).

Tetralogy of Fallot

TOF was first described in 1888. Tetralogy of Fallot develops as a result of lack of development of the subpulmonary conus during fetal life. TOF consists of a large VSD, pulmonary stenosis or other right ventricular outflow tract obstruction, overriding aorta, and hypertrophied right ventricle. The right ventricle may not be hypertrophied initially. In the most severe form, there is pulmonary valve atresia (Zuberbuhler, 1995).

Incidence

TOF accounts for 10 percent of all CHDs. Because repair is generally not carried out in the first year of life, TOF is the most common cyanotic heart defect beyond infancy.

Hemodynamics

In TOF, the VSD causes equalization of pressure in the ventricles. Unsaturated blood flows through the VSD into the aorta because of the obstruction to blood flow from the right ventricle into the pulmonary artery. TOF is illustrated in Figure 21–9.

Manifestations

Cyanosis, hypoxia, and dyspnea are the cardinal signs of TOF. Newborns can present with just a loud murmur or they may be cyanotic. Severe decompensation or "tet" spells are common in infants or children but can also occur in neonates. Children instinctively assume a squatting position, which traps venous blood in the legs and decreases systemic venous return to the heart. Chronic arterial desaturation stimulates erythropoiesis, causing polycythemia. Increased viscosity of the blood caused by the increased red blood cells and microcytic anemia may lead to cerebrovascular accident (stroke). Brain abscesses may also occur as a result of bacteremia and compromised cerebral flow in the microcirculation. The chronic hypoxemia and polycythemia cause (1) an increased risk of hemorrhagic diathesis because decreased platelet survival time and reduced platelet aggregation cause thrombocytopenia and (2) impaired synthesis of vitamin K–dependent clotting factors (Hazinski, 1984; Park, 1988; Pinsky & Arciniegas, 1990; Zuberbuhler, 1995).

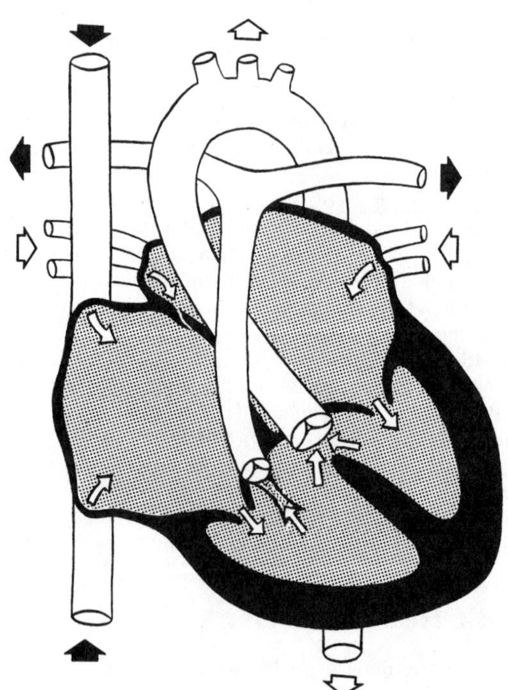

FIGURE 21–9. Tetralogy of Fallot consists of pulmonary stenosis, ventricular septal defect, overriding aorta, and hypertrophy of the right ventricle. (Reprinted with permission of Ross Laboratories, Columbus, OH 43216, Clinical Education Aid, © 1985, Ross Laboratories.)

Diagnosis

Neonates with TOF exhibit varying degrees of cyanosis, depending on the severity of the obstruction of blood flow through the right ventricular outflow tract. A long, loud, grade 3/6 to 5/6 systolic ejection murmur is heard at the middle and upper left sternal border. There may also be a ventricular tap along the lower left sternal border and a systolic thrill at the lower and middle left sternal border. A PDA murmur may also be heard in severe TOF (Park, 1988).

Chest radiograph demonstrates decreased or normal heart size with decreased pulmonary vascularity. The contour of the heart may be a typical boot shape caused by the concave main pulmonary artery segment with upturned apex. There may also be right atrial enlargement and a right aortic arch.

Echocardiography shows a large VSD and overriding aorta. The anatomy of the right ventricular outflow tract and pulmonary valve can be identified by two-dimensional echocardiogram (Moller, 1987).

In addition to the manifestations present in the neonate, clubbing of the fingers may be present in the infant or child with TOF.

Management

The definitive therapy for TOF is surgical repair under cardiopulmonary bypass. The surgical correction can sometimes be delayed with careful medical management. Neonates with only mild cyanosis improve when the pulmonary vascular resistance decreases. Medical management is aimed at prevention or treatment of hypoxemia, polycythemia, infection, and microcytic hypochromic anemia. Careful follow-up is essential to detect signs of clinical deterioration. Parents need adequate education and support for home management (Moller, 1987; Park, 1988; Zuberbuhler, 1995).

Dehydration must be avoided to prevent increased risk of cerebral infarcts caused by hemoconcentration. Polycythemia develops as a compensatory mechanism to increase the oxygen-carrying capacity of the blood. In the presence of decreased volume, however, the increased viscosity of the blood may further impede cerebral circulation (Hazinski, 1984).

Parents must be taught how to recognize the early signs and symptoms of decompensation. They must also be taught to recognize and treat hypercyanotic or tet spells (Table 21–4). Tet spells are precipitated by events that lower the systemic vascular resistance, producing a large right-to-left ventricular shunt. Increased activity, crying, nursing, or defecation may trigger a hypoxemic episode. The right-to-left shunt causes a decreased P_{O_2}, increased P_{CO_2}, and decreased pH, which stimulates the respiratory center, causing increased rate and depth of respirations (hyperpnea). The hyperpnea causes increased systemic venous return by increasing the efficiency of the thoracic pump. The right ventricular outflow tract obstruction prevents the increased blood flow from entering the pulmonary artery, so the increased flow is shunted through the aorta, which further decreases the arterial P_{O_2}. Severe, uninterrupted tet spells lead to loss of consciousness, hypoxemia, seizures, and death (Zuberbuhler, 1995).

Surgical treatment is indicated in the presence of tet spells that result in increased hypoxemia, metabolic acidosis, inadequate systemic perfusion, increased cyanosis, or polycythemia. Systemic

TABLE 21–4 Recognition and Treatment of Tet Spells

Manifestations	
Irritability, crying	
Hyperpnea	
Cyanosis	
Diaphoresis	
Loss of consciousness	
Seizures	
Decreased murmur	
Metabolic acidosis	
Treatment	***Rationale***
Knee–chest or squatting position	Traps blood in lower extremities to decrease systemic venous return; increases pulmonary blood flow
Oxygen administration	Improves arterial oxygen saturation
Morphine sulfate (0.1–0.2 mg/kg/dose)	Suppresses respiratory center to decrease hyperpnea
Bicarbonate	Corrects acidosis and eliminates stimulation of respiratory center
Propranolol (Inderal) (0.15–0.25 mg/kg/dose)	May decrease spasm of right ventricular outflow tract or may act peripherally to stabilize

perfusion can be evaluated by observing peripheral pulse intensity, urine output, capillary filling time, blood pressure, or peripheral vasoconstriction.

Surgical management can be either palliative or corrective. Palliative procedures are undertaken to improve pulmonary blood flow by creating a pathway between the systemic and pulmonary circulation. In addition, these procedures allow time for the right and left pulmonary arteries to grow. Palliative procedures are indicated for newborns with TOF and pulmonary atresia, severely cyanotic infants younger than 6 months old, infants with medically unmanageable tet spells, or children with a hypoplastic pulmonary artery, in whom corrective surgery is difficult (Park, 1988; Zuberbuhler, 1995). Common surgical procedures are listed in Table 21–5.

Surgical correction is performed under cardiopulmonary bypass after the infant is 6 months old. Surgery may be delayed until age 2 to 4 years in asymptomatic children or in children who undergo palliative procedures. The defect is repaired by patch closure of the VSD and resection and widening of the right ventricular outflow tract (Pinsky & Arciniegas, 1990). Complications of cardiac surgery are listed in Tables 21–6 and 21–7. The mortality rate for TOF varies with the severity of the circulatory compromise caused by the defect. The postoperative mortality rate is 5 to 10 percent in the first 2 years for uncomplicated TOF. More severe cases have a higher mortality rate, exhibit residual pulmonary outflow tract obstruction, and may require further surgery (Hazinski, 1984). Because myocardial damage may occur from the restriction of the right ventricular blood flow during the surgery, cardiac support is needed to ensure adequate myocardial perfusion. Extracorporeal membrane oxygenation (ECMO) is being used by some centers to support the cardiovascular perfusion (Suddaby & O'Brien, 1993). ECMO is also being attempted after surgical procedures for TGA and TAPVR, but infants with TOF make up the largest group of patients who benefit from its use (Suddaby & O'Brien, 1993). Many of these infants experience pulmonary hypertension secondary to the cardiac problem or the surgical correction. With ECMO, management of cases can focus

TABLE 21–5 Common Cardiac Surgical Procedures

Procedure	Type	Defect	Description
Blalock-Hanlon	Palliative	TGA	Surgical creation of an ASD: rarely used; still useful for complex TGA or mitral atresia and single ventricle
Blalock-Taussig	Palliative	TOF, PA, PS, VSD	Anastomosis of the subclavian artery and pulmonary artery to improve pulmonary blood flow
Brock	Corrective	PVA	Blind pulmonary valvotomy incision of PV
Fontan	Corrective	HLHS (stage 2), tricuspid atresia, tricuspid stenosis	Bypass of the right ventricle by connection of the right atrium to pulmonary artery
Gore-Tex shunt	Palliative	TOF	Interposition of Gore-Tex between subclavian artery and ipsilateral pulmonary artery
Jatene	Corrective	TGA	Switching of transposed great arteries to their anatomically correct position
Mustard	Corrective	TGA	Use of a pericardial or synthetic baffle in the atria so that venous blood is shunted across the right atrium to the left ventricle and into the pulmonary artery. Systemic blood is shunted across the left atrium to the right ventricle, which delivers blood to the aorta.
Norwood	Palliative	HLHS (stage 1)	1. Main pulmnary artery is divided, and the proximal stump is anastomosed to the descending aorta; distal main pulmonary artery is closed. 2. Right-sided Gore-Tex shunt is performed to increase pulmonary blood flow. 3. Excision of atrial septum to allow interatrial mixing.
Potts	Palliative	TOF	Surgical creation of a window between descending aorta and left pulmonary artery; difficult to take down; rarely used
Pulmonary artery banding	Palliative	VSD, single ventricle	Placement of a band around the pulmonary artery to decrease the blood flow to the lungs
Rashkind	Corrective	PA, TGA	Atrial septostomy created at cardiac catheterization by passing a balloon-tipped catheter through the patent foramen ovale, inflating the balloon, and snapping it back through the patent foramen
Rastelli	Corrective	TGA, TOF, PA, TA	Commonly applied to all valved conduits from the right ventricle to pulmonary artery
Senning	Corrective	TGA	Creation of an intra-atrial baffle, using atrial tissue, to shunt blood from the vena cava to the left ventricle and from the pulmonary veins to the right ventricle
Waterston	Palliative	TOF	Window created between the ascending aorta and the pulmonary artery, improving oxygenation of systemic blood; rarely used because of the distortion and/or obstruction of pulmonary artery

ASD, atrial septal defect; HLHS, hypoplastic left heart syndrome; PA, pulmonary artery; PS, pulmonary stenosis; PV, pulmonary valve; PVA, pulmonic valve atresia; TA, truncus arteriosus; TGA, transposition of the great arteries; TOF, tetralogy of Fallot; VSD, ventricular septal defect.

TABLE 21–6 Complications of Cardiac Surgery

- Low cardiac output
  - Hypovolemia
    - Hemorrhage
    - Diuresis
    - Inadequate fluid volume
  - Tamponade
    - Mediastinal bleeding
    - Inadequate mediastinal drainage
  - Decreased cardiac contractility
    - Hypervolemia
    - Electrolyte imbalance
    - Cardiac dysfunction
  - Increased systemic vascular resistance
  - Increased pulmonary vascular resistance
  - Arrhythmias
  - Hypothermia
- Congestive heart failure
  - Uncorrected CHD (after palliative procedure)
  - Corrected CHD, causing alterations in ventricular preload, contractility, and afterload
  - Hypervolemia
  - Electrolyte imbalance
  - Arrhythmias
- Respiratory distress
  - Atelectasis
  - Pneumothorax
  - Hemothorax
  - Pleural effusion
  - Chylothorax
- Respiratory distress *(Continued)*
  - Congestive heart failure
  - Low cardiac output
  - Pulmonary hypertension
  - Inadequate ventilatory support
  - Ineffective pleural drainage
  - Hypoventilation secondary to pain
- Renal dysfunction or failure
  - Poor systemic and renal perfusion
  - Intravascular hemolysis
  - Thromboembolus
  - Nephrotoxic drugs
- Electrolyte imbalance
  - Effects of cardiopulmonary bypass
  - Diuretics
  - Stress response
  - Fluid administration
  - Blood administration
  - Renal failure
- Neurologic abnormalities
  - Hypoxia
  - Acidosis
  - Poor systemic perfusion
  - Thromboembolism
  - Electrolyte imbalance
- Infection
  - Surgery
  - Prosthetic material
  - Invasive monitoring and/or procedures
  - Inadequate nutrition

CHD, congenital heart defect.

TABLE 21–7 Complications of Cardiac Surgery: Postoperative Syndromes

- Postcoarctectomy syndrome
  - Results from changes in pressure and flow
  - Symptoms: severe intermittent abdominal pain, fever, and leukocytosis; abdominal distention, melena, and ascites with gangrenous bowel; rebound systemic hypertension
  - Management: monitor blood pressure; prevent hypertension; delay postoperative feeding
- Postpericardiotomy syndrome
  - Causes: immunologic syndrome in response to blood in the pericardial sac
  - Manifestations: fever, chest pain, pericardial and pleural effusions, hepatomegaly, leukocytosis, left shift, increased ESR, persistent ST and T wave changes on ECG
  - Rare in children younger than 2 years of age
  - Treatment: rest, aspirin for pain, corticosteroids in severe cases, pericardiocentesis if tamponade develops, diuretics
- Postperfusion syndrome
  - Cause: cytomegalovirus
  - Manifestations: onset 3 to 6 weeks after surgery; fever, splenomegaly, atypical lymphocytosis
  - Treatment: supportive care; self-limiting disease process
- Hemolytic anemia syndrome
  - Cause: trauma of RBCs or autoimmune action
  - Manifestations: onset 1 to 2 weeks postoperatively; fever, jaundice, hepatomegaly, reticulocytosis
  - Treatment: iron supplementation or blood transfusions, correction of turbulent flow

ESR, erythrocyte sedimentation rate; RBC, red blood cell.

on decreasing pulmonary vascular resistance and diminishing right-to-left shunting during the immediate postoperative period (Suddaby & O'Brien, 1993).

Pulmonary Atresia

Pulmonary atresia results in the absence of communication between the right ventricle and the pulmonary artery. The atresia can be at the level of the main pulmonary artery or the pulmonary valve. Atresia of the pulmonary valve, with a diaphragm-like membrane, is the most common type. The right ventricle is usually hypoplastic, with thick ventricular walls. Less frequently, the right ventricle is of normal size with tricuspid regurgitation. The presence of a PDA, ASD, or patent foramen ovale to allow mixing of blood is crucial for survival (Mair et al., 1995a).

Incidence

Pulmonary atresia accounts for less than 1 percent of all CHDs (Park, 1988).

Hemodynamics

Pulmonary atresia with ASD results in a small, hypoplastic right heart. The absence of a right ventricular outflow tract results in high right ventricular end-diastolic pressures. Tricuspid insufficiency occurs and right atrial pressures increase, causing systemic venous blood to shunt from the right to the left atrium through the patent foramen ovale or ASD. Mixed venous blood flows into the left ventricle and aorta. The PDA produces the only pulmonary blood flow. Closure of the PDA causes severe cyanosis, hypoxemia, and acidosis.

In the presence of a VSD, right ventricular size is usually adequate. Systemic venous blood shunts from the right ventricle through the VSD to the left ventricle and enters the aorta. The PDA still provides the only pulmonary blood flow. Pulmonary atresia is shown in Figure 21–10.

Manifestations

Pulmonary atresia usually is seen with cyanosis at birth. Tachypnea is present, but there is no obvious respiratory distress. S_2 is single and a soft systolic PDA murmur can be heard in the upper left sternal border. Tricuspid insufficiency may produce a harsh

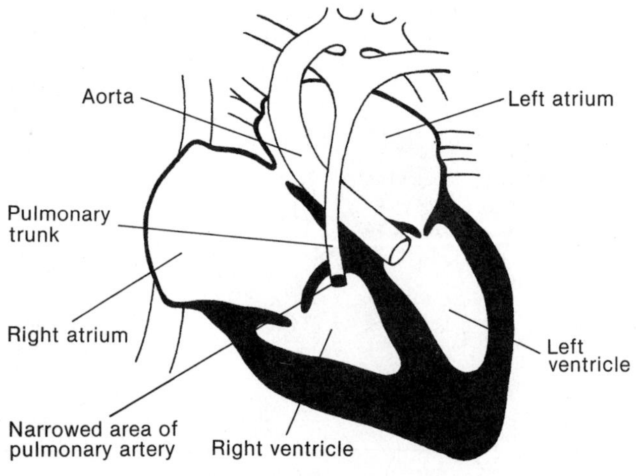

FIGURE 21–10. Pulmonary atresia.

systolic murmur along the lower right and left sternal border (Hazinski, 1984; Mair et al., 1995a; Park, 1988).

Heart size may be normal or enlarged on radiograph. The main pulmonary artery segment is concave and similar to the radiographic appearance of tricuspid atresia. Pulmonary vascular markings are decreased and continue to decrease as the PDA closes.

ECG may reveal a normal QRS axis, left ventricular hypertrophy (type I), or, less frequently, right ventricular hypertrophy (type II). Right atrial hypertrophy is seen in approximately 70 percent of cases (Park, 1988). Two-dimensional echocardiogram reveals the atretic pulmonary valve and the hypoplastic right ventricular cavity and tricuspid valve. The location and size of the atrial communication are estimated by echocardiogram.

Management

Immediate management of pulmonary atresia is administration of prostaglandin to maintain ductal patency. PGE_1 (Prostin) is given as a continuous intravenous infusion. The initial dose is started at 0.1 μg/kg/minute. When the desired effect is achieved, the dose is incrementally decreased to a maintenance of 0.01 μg/kg/minute. Careful attention to the site of the infusion is important.

A balloon atrial septostomy is performed at cardiac catheterization to promote better mixing of systemic and pulmonary venous blood in the atria. As soon as the newborn is stabilized, surgical correction is performed. Initially, a systemic-pulmonary artery shunt using Gore-Tex between the left subclavian artery and the left pulmonary artery (Blalock-Taussig procedure) is performed. If pulmonary valve atresia is present, a closed heart pulmonary valvotomy (Brock's procedure) may be performed. The mortality rate for these procedures is 10 to 25 percent.

If the initial systemic-pulmonary shunt is not effective, a second shunt is attempted in another location. Right ventricular outflow tract reconstruction can be attempted if the right ventricle size is adequate. This procedure has a mortality rate of 25 percent. The Fontan procedure is attempted in the presence of a hypoplastic right ventricle in late childhood. The mortality rate for this procedure can be as high as 40 percent.

The prognosis for pulmonary atresia depends on the size of the pulmonary outflow tract established through surgery and the degree of fibrosis of the right ventricle. If there is severe fibrosis and significant outflow tract obstruction, there is an increased risk of development of dysrhythmias and right ventricular dysfunction (Hazinski, 1984; Mair, 1995a; Park, 1988).

Pulmonary Stenosis

Pulmonary stenosis is caused by abnormal formation of the pulmonary valve leaflets during fetal cardiac development. Pulmonary stenosis can be valvular, subvalvular (infundibular), or supravalvular. Valvular pulmonary stenosis is the most common, accounting for 90 percent of cases. Pulmonary stenosis is frequently seen in Noonan's syndrome. It is one of the four defects found in TOF. Isolated infundibular pulmonary stenosis is uncommon.

Incidence

Pulmonary stenosis makes up 5 to 8 percent of all CHDs. It is often associated with other defects.

Hemodynamics

Pulmonary stenosis results in obstruction to blood flow from the right ventricle to the pulmonary artery. The right ventricle hypertrophies in response to the increased pressure caused by the obstruction to outflow. Pulmonary blood flow volume is normal in the absence of intracardiac shunting (Rocchini & Emmanouilides, 1995). Pulmonary stenosis is shown in Figure 21–11.

Manifestations

Pulmonary stenosis may be asymptomatic if it is mild. Moderate pulmonary stenosis may cause easy tiring. Severe or critical pulmonary stenosis causes CHF.

Diagnosis

The findings of pulmonary stenosis depend on the severity of the defect. A pulmonary systolic ejection click can be heard at the upper left sternal border. S_2 may be widely split, and the pulmonary component may be soft and delayed. A systolic ejection murmur (grade 2/6 to 5/6) is audible at the upper left sternal border and transmits across the back. The severity of the pulmonary stenosis is directly related to the loudness and duration of the murmur. A systolic thrill can sometimes be felt at the upper left sternal border. Hepatosplenomegaly may be present along with CHF.

The ECG is normal in mild pulmonary stenosis. There may be right axis deviation and right ventricular hypertrophy with moderate stenosis. Right atrial hypertrophy and right ventricular strain occur with severe pulmonary stenosis.

Radiographically, the heart size is normal, with a prominent main pulmonary artery segment. In mild to moderate pulmonary stenosis, pulmonary markings are normal. The critical type of pulmonary stenosis causes decreased pulmonary markings. CHF results in increased heart size. Echocardiogram demonstrates decreased motion of the pulmonary valve leaflets and poststenotic dilation of the main pulmonary artery segment (Park, 1988; Rocchini & Emmanouilides, 1995).

Management

Management of pulmonary stenosis is determined by the severity of the obstruction to flow. The mild type generally requires

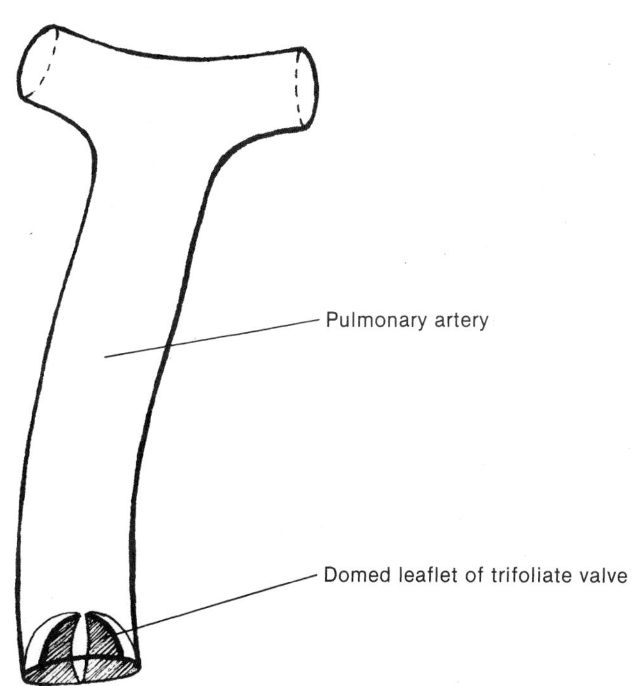

FIGURE 21–11. Pulmonary stenosis.

no therapy except antimicrobial prophylaxis against subacute infective endocarditis (SAIE). Moderate pulmonary stenosis is treated through balloon valvuloplasty during cardiac catheterization. Surgical correction is performed in children when the right ventricular pressure measures 80 to 100 mm Hg and balloon valvuloplasty is not successful or when the pulmonary stenosis is infundibular in origin. Infants with critical pulmonary stenosis and CHF require PGE_1 infusion to maintain ductal patency until surgery is performed (Park, 1988; Rocchini & Emmanouilides, 1995).

The overall prognosis for pulmonary stenosis is excellent. The mortality rate is less than 1 percent in older infants. The mortality rate is higher in newborns with critical pulmonary stenosis and CHF (Park, 1988).

Truncus Arteriosus

The truncus arteriosus is a large vessel located in front of the developing fetal heart. The truncus arteriosus gives rise to the coronary and pulmonary arteries and the aorta. The persistence of the truncus arteriosus results from inadequate division of the common great vessel into a separate aorta and pulmonary artery during fetal cardiac development. A single, large great vessel arises from the ventricles and gives rise to the systemic, pulmonary, and coronary circulations. Inadequate closure of the conal ventricular septum results in a VSD. Four types of this defect have been described; see Table 21–8 for the classifications (Park, 1988).

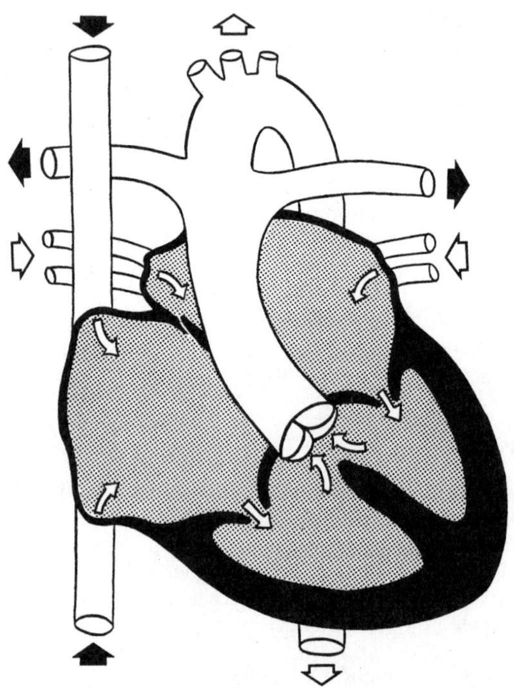

FIGURE 21–12. Persistent truncus arteriosus is a single arterial vessel that gives rise to the coronary arteries, pulmonary arteries, and aorta. (Reprinted with permission of Ross Laboratories, Columbus, OH 43216, Clinical Education Aid, © 1985, Ross Laboratories.)

Incidence

Persistent truncus arteriosus accounts for less than 1 percent of all CHDs.

Hemodynamics

Desaturated blood from the right ventricle and oxygenated blood from the left ventricle are received in the truncus arteriosus. The pressures of both ventricles are equal. The truncus arteriosus supplies blood to the systemic and pulmonary circuits. The amount of flow depends on the resistance of the two circulations. Pulmonary vascular resistance is high at birth, so pulmonary and systemic flow is relatively equal initially. Pulmonary resistance gradually decreases, causing increased pulmonary blood flow. CHF may develop as a result of increased pulmonary blood flow. If not corrected, pulmonary vascular disease develops in response to high pressure and increased pulmonary blood flow; this decreases pulmonary blood flow. These changes, although compensatory initially, complicate the hemodynamics after surgical correction. Frequently, the volume overload is compounded by incompetent truncal valves, allowing regurgitation of blood into the ventricles (Mair et al., 1995b). Truncus arteriosus is illustrated in Figure 21–12.

TABLE 21–8 Four Major Types of Truncus Arteriosus

Type	Incidence (%)	Description
I	60	Main pulmonary artery arises from truncus and divides into left and right pulmonary artery; results in increased pulmonary blood flow
II	20	Pulmonary artery arises from posterior portion of truncus arteriosus; pulmonary blood flow is normal
III	10	Pulmonary artery arises from sides of truncus arteriosus; pulmonary blood flow is normal
IV	10	Bronchial arteries arise from descending aorta to supply lungs; pulmonary blood flow is decreased

Manifestations

The presence of cyanosis depends on the amount of pulmonary blood flow. Signs of CHF may be the first indication of persistent truncus arteriosus. On auscultation, there may be a systolic click at the apex and upper left sternal border. The VSD may produce a harsh, grade 2/6 to 4/6 systolic murmur along the lower sternal border. Increased pulmonary blood flow may produce an atrial rumble. Truncal valve insufficiency produces a high-pitched, early diastolic decrescendo murmur. There may be bounding arterial pulses and a widened pulse pressure. S_2 is single. If truncus arteriosus is not detected in the newborn period, symptoms of poor feeding, failure to thrive, frequent respiratory infections, and signs of CHF appear.

Diagnosis

On radiographic study of truncus arteriosus, the heart size is increased and pulmonary blood flow may be increased. Fifty percent of cases have a right aortic arch (Park, 1988). ECG reveals a normal QRS axis and ventricular hypertrophy. Echocardiography demonstrates the presence of the truncus arteriosus overriding a VSD and the absence of the pulmonary valve (Mair et al., 1995a; Park, 1988).

Management

Medical management consists primarily of treatment of CHF and prophylaxis with antimicrobials. Pulmonary artery banding, instituted as a palliative measure, may be performed in small infants with increased pulmonary blood flow and CHF unresponsive to medical management. The mortality rate for this group of infants is close to 30 percent (Park, 1988).

The definitive surgical correction is Rastelli's procedure. (See Table 21–5 for a description of common surgical procedures.) Surgery is performed in infants because there is a high mortality rate for uncorrected truncus arteriosus. The mortality rate associated with surgery is also high, ranging from 20 to 60 percent. Reoperation may be required to enlarge the conduit as growth occurs (Moller, 1987; Park, 1988).

Complete Transposition of the Great Arteries or Vessels

TGA is the result of inappropriate septation and migration of the truncus arteriosus during fetal cardiac development. TGA may be dextrotransposition of the great arteries (D-TGA) or levotransposition of the great arteries (L-TGA). In D-TGA, the aorta arises from the right ventricle and the pulmonary artery arises from the left ventricle. The aorta receives unoxygenated systemic venous blood and returns it to the systemic arterial circuit. The pulmonary artery receives oxygenated pulmonary venous blood and returns it to the pulmonary circulation.

In L-TGA, the great vessels are transposed, with the aorta arising from the right ventricle and the pulmonary artery arising from the left ventricle. The aorta is to the left and anterior to the pulmonary artery. This type of transposition is called *corrected* because functionally the hemodynamics are normal. The oxygenated blood comes into the left atrium, enters the right ventricle, and goes through the aorta to the systemic circulation. However, frequently there are other associated cardiac defects (Park, 1988; Paul, 1995).

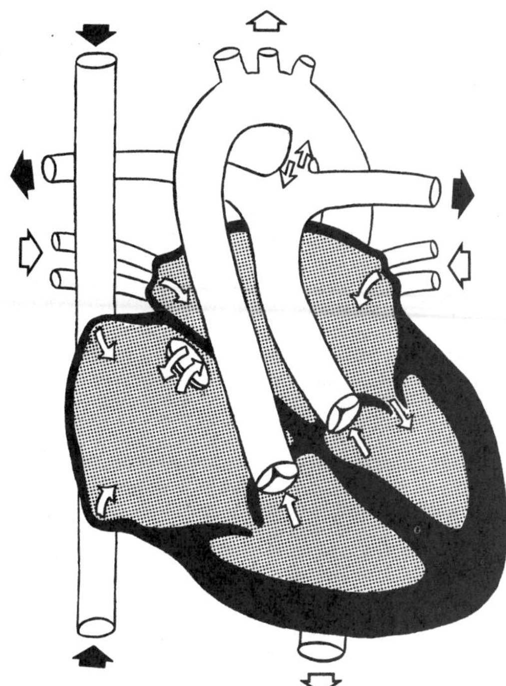

FIGURE 21–13. Transposition of the great arteries or vessels is a condition in which the aorta arises from the right ventricle and the pulmonary artery arises from the left ventricle. The result is two distinct circulatory (parallel) pathways. (Reprinted with permission of Ross Laboratories, Columbus, OH 43216, Clinical Education Aid, © 1985, Ross Laboratories.)

Incidence

TGA accounts for 5 percent of all CHDs. It is more common in males (3:1). D-TGA is the most common cyanotic heart defect in newborns.

Hemodynamics

Hemodynamically, two separate parallel circulations result from complete D-TGA. Oxygenated blood from the lungs is returned to the left atrium, enters the left ventricle, and goes through the pulmonary artery to the lungs again. Desaturated blood from the systemic circulation enters the right atrium, goes to the right ventricle, enters the aorta, and is directed back into the systemic circulation. The end result is that the heart and brain and other vital tissues are perfused with desaturated blood. This defect is incompatible with life. A communication between the two circulations must exist to allow mixing of the oxygenated and desaturated blood. This communication can be at the ductal, atrial, or ventricular level. The best mixing occurs with a large VSD. Figure 21–13 shows TGA (Park, 1988; Paul, 1995).

Manifestations

Marked cyanosis is the prominent sign of TGA. The degree of cyanosis varies with the amount of communication between the two circulations. Signs of CHF are present. S_2 is loud and single. If a VSD is present, there is a loud, harsh systolic murmur of variable intensity. Hypoglycemia, hypocalcemia, and metabolic acidosis are frequently present.

Diagnosis

On radiographic study of TGA, the heart is enlarged and has a narrow base because the aorta is over the pulmonary artery. The heart is described as egg shaped (Park, 1988). Pulmonary blood flow is increased. On ECG, there is right axis deviation of the QRS and right ventricular hypertrophy. Echocardiography reveals the abnormal origin of the great arteries from the ventricles. Associated defects can also be visualized by echocardiography.

Management

TGA is a cardiac emergency. Immediate medical management includes correction of acidosis, hypoglycemia, hypocalcemia, administration of oxygen and infusion of PGE_1, and treatment of CHF. A cardiac catheterization is performed and a balloon atrial septostomy is carried out to promote mixing of oxygenated and desaturated blood in the atria. If the septostomy and PGE_1 infusion do not sufficiently improve oxygenation, surgical excision of the posterior aspect of the atrial septum (Blalock-Hanlon procedure) is performed without cardiopulmonary bypass as a palliative measure. This procedure has a 10 to 25 percent mortality rate (Park, 1988).

Definitive surgical correction involves switching the right- and left-sided structures at the ventricular level (Rastelli's procedure), the artery level (Jatene's procedure), or the atrial level (Senning's or Mustard's procedure). See Table 21–5 for a description of these procedures.

The prognosis for TGA without surgical intervention is poor; 90 percent of patients die within the first year of life. The surgical procedures have high mortality rates and a high rate of postoperative complications (e.g., dysrhythmias, obstruction to systemic or pulmonary venous return, and right ventricular dysfunction). Jatene's procedure is newer but seems to minimize many complications associated with the intra-atrial repair operations. Long-term results of this procedure must be evaluated. The type and timing of surgical correction depend on the condition of the patient and the anatomic defect, so each case must be decided individually (Kirklin et al., 1990). A typical management approach is presented in the flow diagram in Figure 21–14.

Coarctation of the Aorta

Coarctation is a narrowing or constriction of the aorta in the aortic arch segment. The most common location is below the origin of the left subclavian artery. Coarctation may occur as a single lesion due to improper development of the aorta or may occur secondary to constriction of the ductus arteriosus. The severity of the circulatory compromise depends on the location of the constriction and the degree of constriction. Coarctation proximal to the ductus arteriosus (preductal COA) has associated defects in 40 percent of cases. Associated defects include VSD, TGA, and PDA. Collateral circulation is poorly developed with preductal COA. Postductal COA is usually not associated with other defects, and collateral circulation is more effective. Infants with postductal COA may not be symptomatic. More than half of infants with COA have a bicuspid aortic valve (Beekman, 1995; Park, 1988).

Incidence

COA accounts for 8 percent of all CHDs. Coarctation occurs twice as often in males. It is found in 30 percent of infants with Turner's syndrome (Park, 1988).

Hemodynamics

Coarctation causes obstruction to flow, which leads to varying pressure across the aortic segment. The portion of aorta proximal to the constriction has an elevated pressure, which leads to increased left ventricular pressure. The increased left ventricular pressure results in left ventricular hypertrophy and dilation. Collateral circulation develops from the proximal to distal arteries, bypassing the constricted segment of the aorta. This is a compensatory mechanism to increase flow to the lower extremities and abdomen, producing lower pulses in the lower extremities. COA is shown in Figure 21–15 (Beekman, 1995; Park, 1988).

Manifestations

The severity and time of appearance of symptoms of coarctation depend on the location and degree of constriction, as well as the presence of associated cardiac defects. Symptoms of coarctation include signs of CHF and absent, weak, or delayed pulses in the lower extremities with bounding pulses in the upper extremities. In the presence of CHF, however, all pulses may be weak. With severe COA, S_2 is loud and single. A systolic thrill may be felt in the suprasternal notch. An ejection click may be audible at the apex if there is a bicuspid aortic valve or if systemic hypertension is present. A systolic ejection murmur of grade 2/6 to 3/6 can be heard at the upper right and middle or lower left sternal border, and at the left interscapular area in the infant's back; however, no murmur is heard in more than half of infants with COA. Correction of CHF may produce the murmur (Beekman, 1995; Hazinski, 1984; Park, 1988).

Diagnosis

Diagnosis of COA is based on history, physical findings, radiograph, ECG, and echocardiographic data. In asymptomatic infants and children, radiographs may show a normal or slightly enlarged heart. Dilation of the ascending aorta may be evident. The "E" sign on barium swallow is characteristic, but is usually not evident until at least 4 months of age. The "E" appearance is due to the large proximal aortic segment or prominent subclavian artery above and the poststenotic dilation of the descending aorta below the constricted segment (Park, 1988). In symptomatic infants and children, radiographs show cardiomegaly and increased pulmonary venous congestion.

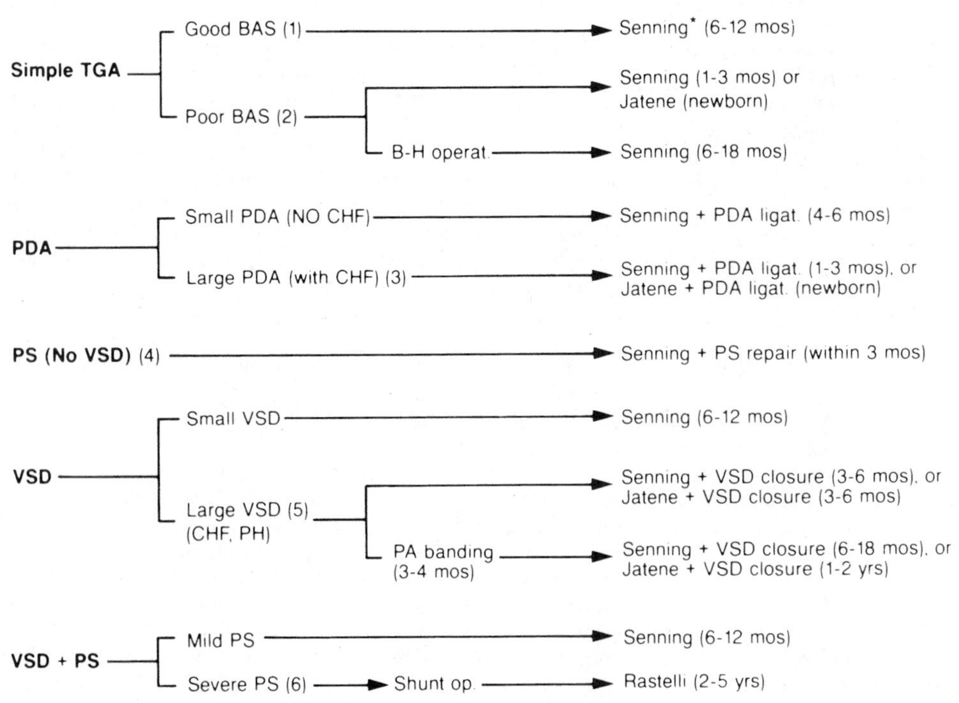

FIGURE 21–14. Management of transposition of the great arteries: flow diagram. (*Senning is used to represent an intra-atrial repair, either the Senning operation or the Mustard operation.) (From Park, M. K. [1988]. *Pediatric cardiology for practitioners* [p. 164]. Chicago: Mosby–Year Book. Reprinted with permission.)

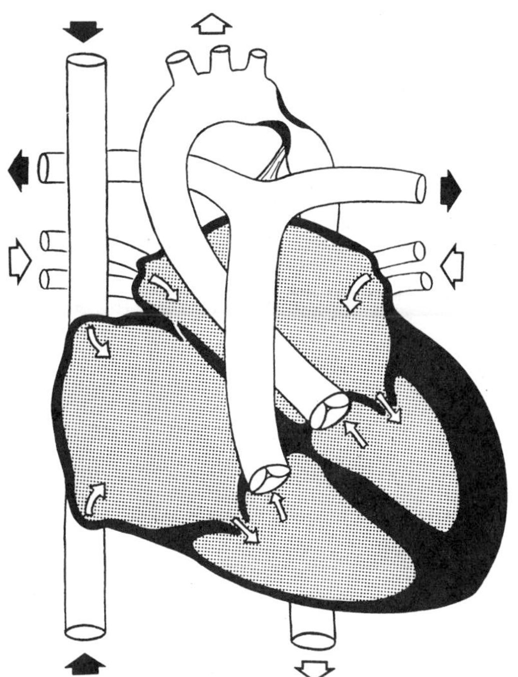

FIGURE 21–15. Coarctation of the aorta is a narrowing or constriction of the aorta near the ductus arteriosus. (Reprinted with permission of Ross Laboratories, Columbus, OH 43216, Clinical Education Aid, © 1985, Ross Laboratories.)

The ECG of asymptomatic children may show left axis deviation of the QRS and left ventricular hypertrophy. In symptomatic children, the ECG reveals normal or right axis deviation of the QRS. Right ventricular hypertrophy or right bundle branch block is present in infants, whereas left ventricular hypertrophy is present in older children (Park, 1988). Two-dimensional echocardiogram demonstrates the location and degree of the constriction and the presence of associated defects (Beekman, 1995).

Management

Surgical correction of COA is the definitive treatment. Surgery is performed in patients aged 3 to 5 years if signs and symptoms can be medically controlled. Earlier surgery is indicated if medical management is not successful.

Medical management is aimed at providing adequate oxygenation, preventing or treating CHF, and preventing SAIE. PGE_1 may be needed to maintain ductal patency if the constricted segment is at the level of the ductus arteriosus (Park, 1988).

Surgical intervention of COA involves the excision of the constricted segment of the aorta with end-to-end anastomosis, patch graft, bypass tube graft, or Dacron graft (Park, 1988). Alternatively, a subclavian flap aortoplasty may be performed. Surgery is indicated in the presence of CHF with or without circulatory shock. In the presence of a large VSD, pulmonary artery banding may be performed at surgery to reduce pulmonary blood flow in an attempt to prevent pulmonary hypertension. The pulmonary artery banding is removed and the VSD is repaired at 6 months to 2 years of age. The mortality rate for surgical corrections is less than 5 percent. Postoperative complications include renal failure and recoarctation (Beekman, 1995).

Hypoplastic Left Heart Syndrome

HLHS consists of a group of cardiac defects, including a small aorta, aortic and mitral valve stenosis or atresia, and a small left atrium and ventricle. The great vessels are usually normally related.

Incidence

HLHS accounts for 1 to 2 percent of all CHDs, but it accounts for 7 to 8 percent of heart defects producing symptoms in the first year of life (Bailey & Gundry, 1990). It is the leading cause of death from CHDs in the first month of life (Norwood et al., 1983). HLHS is not associated with abnormalities in other organ systems.

Hemodynamics

Left ventricular output is greatly reduced or eliminated secondary to the valvular obstruction and small size of the left ventricle. Left atrial and pulmonary venous pressures are elevated, and there is pulmonary edema and pulmonary hypertension. With a PDA, blood shunts from the pulmonary artery into the aorta. The PDA provides the only cardiac output because there is little or no flow across the aortic valve. Retrograde flow through the aortic arch supplies the head, upper extremities, and coronary arteries (Freedom & Benson, 1995).

Although circulation is abnormal in utero, the high pulmonary vascular resistance and the low systemic vascular resistance make survival possible. The right ventricle maintains normal perfusion pressure in the descending aorta by a right-to-left ductal shunt. At birth, the onset of pulmonary ventilation causes the pulmonary vascular resistance to decrease. The systemic vascular resistance increases because the placenta is eliminated. Closure of the ductus arteriosus further decreases systemic cardiac output and aortic pressure, leading to metabolic acidosis and circulatory shock. Increased pulmonary blood flow causes increased left atrial pressure and pulmonary edema. Figure 21–16 shows HLHS.

Manifestations

Progressive cyanosis, pallor, and mottling are presenting symptoms of HLHS. Tachycardia, tachypnea, dyspnea, and pulmonary rales are present. The S_2 is loud and single. Poor peripheral pulses and vasoconstriction of the extremities is noted on examination. A cardiac murmur may be absent or there may be a grade 1/6 to 3/6 nonspecific systolic murmur (Park, 1988).

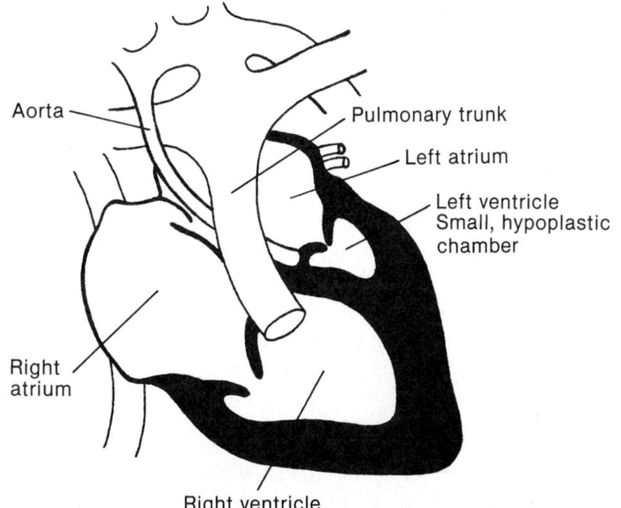

FIGURE 21–16. Hypoplastic left heart syndrome.

Diagnosis

On radiographic study of HLHS, there is mild to moderate heart enlargement and pulmonary venous congestion or pulmonary edema. Metabolic acidosis found on arterial blood gas study is a result of decreased cardiac output. Right ventricular hypertrophy is the characteristic finding on ECG. Echocardiography is usually diagnostic. Findings demonstrate the components of the small left-sided heart structures and the dilated or hypertrophied right-sided heart structures. Findings include a small left ventricle, small ascending aorta and aortic root, absent or abnormal mitral valve, and enlarged right ventricle. An abnormal left ventricle to right ventricle end-diastolic ratio is present (Freedom & Benson, 1995; Park, 1988).

Management

Medical management of HLHS is aimed at prevention of hypoxemia and correction of metabolic acidosis. PGE_1 is administered through continuous infusion to maintain ductal patency. Balloon atrial septostomy may be performed to decompress the left atrium.

Surgical correction of the HLHS is experimental and has a high mortality rate. However, this defect was once considered 100 percent fatal. Surgical correction is performed in stages. The first stage, the modified procedure, is performed in the neonatal period to maintain pulmonary blood flow and create interatrial mixing of blood. The second stage, a modified Fontan procedure, is performed in patients at 6 months to 2 years of age. This procedure closes the Gore-Tex shunt, closes the atrial communication, and forms a direct anastomosis of the right atrium and pulmonary artery. See Table 21–5 for a description of these procedures (Bailey & Gundry, 1990; Park, 1988).

The mortality rate for HLHS remains high. The first-stage surgical repair has a mortality rate of nearly 75 percent. For the survivors, there is a 50 percent mortality rate with the second-stage operation (Freedom & Benson, 1995; Park, 1988). Nursing care is critical after the first-stage repair. Callow (1992) outlines this management as twofold: (1) assessing changes in homeostasis and pulmonary blood flow and (2) assessing changes in nutritional status. These changes require close monitoring of the following:

1. Vital signs for symptoms of blood loss
2. Chest tube output greater than 10 percent of the total blood volume per hour, lasting over a period of several hours
3. Platelet counts that may require treatment with fresh-frozen plasma, platelets, or cryoprecipitate at 10 ml/kg until the patient is stable
4. Daily liver function studies that may indicate vitamin K treatment
5. Guaiac testing of bodily fluids such as stool and gastric drainage
6. Ventilatory status, with maintenance of mean airway pressure of less than 10 cm H_2O or peak inspiratory pressure of less than 25 cm H_2O
7. Blood gases for persistent acidosis or systemic hypotension as evidenced by arterial oxygen pressures greater than 45 mm Hg or saturations greater than 85 percent

Use of dopamine at 5 to 10 μg/kg/minute may be necessary to decrease pulmonary vasoconstriction (Callow, 1992). Use of dobutamine or isoproterenol may only dilate the pulmonary arterioles, making the situation worse. Fentanyl may be used to balance pulmonary vascular resistance (Callow, 1992). Diuretic or peritoneal dialysis may be necessary to maintain a fluid balance. High-frequency jet ventilation is sometimes used to support pulmonary function when there is acidosis and stiffening lungs. ECMO has also been used in these infants.

Initially, nutritional support for homeostasis is provided through parenteral nutrition. Monitoring of daily weights, of urine for ketones, glucose, and protein, and of serum levels of electrolytes and trace minerals is necessary to adjust the parenteral fluids (Callow, 1992). Enteral feedings may be started in the first 2 weeks postoperatively if the infant is stable and when the greatest danger of necrotizing enterocolitis is past.

Pericardial effusion may not occur until several days or weeks after the Fontan procedure. Alterations in tissue perfusion and changes in system blood flow return are indicative of this effusion (Smith & Vernon-Levett, 1993).

Cardiac transplantation, although experimental, may provide improved prognosis for infants with HLHS (Chiavarelli et al., 1993). It is essential that parents be informed of all available treatments, including risks and prognosis if surgical intervention is an option.

Total Anomalous Pulmonary Venous Return

With TAPVR, the pulmonary veins drain into the right atrium (rather than the left atrium) directly or through connection with the systemic veins. There is no direct connection between the pulmonary veins and the left atrium. Four types of TAPVR have been identified (Park, 1988).

Incidence

TAPVR accounts for 1 percent of all CHDs. There is a 1:1 male to female ratio of occurrence.

Hemodynamics

If there is an ASD or patent foramen ovale in TAPVR, a portion of the mixed blood from the right atrium can cross into the left atrium, into the left ventricle, and on into the systemic circulation. The direction of the blood flow and the amount that crosses the atrial communication into the left atrium or that enters the left ventricle are determined by the compliance of the ventricles.

Two clinical hemodynamic states exist with TAPVR. If there is no obstruction to pulmonary blood flow, this flow is greatly increased. The result is highly saturated blood in the right atrium and mild cyanosis. If there is obstruction to pulmonary blood flow, the volume of flow is decreased and cyanosis is severe. Pulmonary edema often occurs secondary to elevated pulmonary venous pressure. Obstruction to pulmonary blood flow is a common occurrence when the TAPVR is below the diaphragm (Park, 1988). TAPVR is shown in Figure 21–17.

Manifestations

The manifestations of TAPVR depend on the presence of pulmonary venous obstruction (PVO). TAPVR without PVO includes a history of mild cyanosis, frequent pulmonary infections, poor growth, and CHF. TAPVR with PVO involves severe cyanosis and respiratory distress in the neonatal period, with progressive growth failure. Feeding is associated with increased cyanosis secondary to the compression of the common pulmonary vein by the filled esophagus (Park, 1988). Signs and symptoms of CHF are also present.

Diagnosis

TAPVR without PVO produces a precordial bulge with hyperactive right ventricular impulse. The PMI is at the xiphoid process or lower left sternal border. S_2 is widely split and fixed; the pulmonic sound may be pronounced. A grade 2/6 to 3/6 systolic

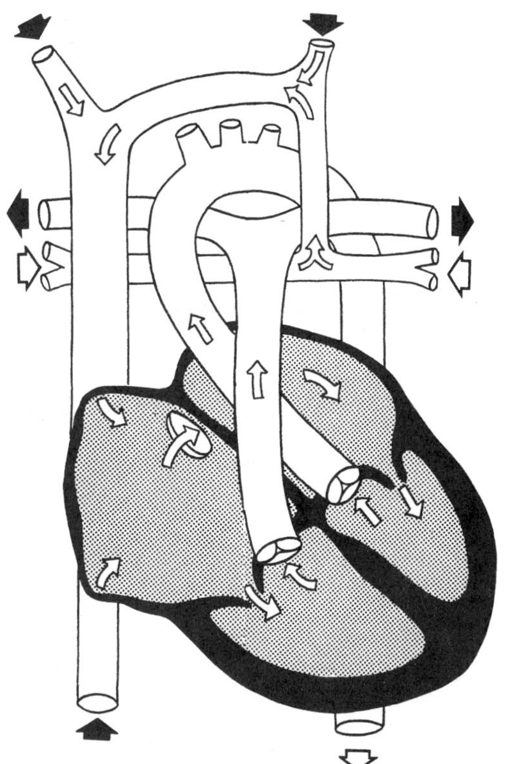

FIGURE 21–17. Total anomalous pulmonary venous return is a condition in which all the pulmonary veins empty into the right atrium. (Reprinted with permission of Ross Laboratories, Columbus, OH 43216, Clinical Education Aid, © 1985, Ross Laboratories.)

ejection murmur can be heard at the upper left sternal border, and there is always a middiastolic rumble at the lower left sternal border. The rhythm is a quadruple or quintuple gallop (Park, 1988).

TAPVR with PVO may produce minimal cardiac findings. S_2 is loud and single and there is a gallop rhythm. There may be a faint systolic ejection murmur at the upper left sternal border. Pulmonary rales may be audible.

Radiographic findings of TAPVR without PVO include mild to moderate cardiomegaly and increased pulmonary markings. The characteristic "snowman" sign occurs because of the anatomic appearance of the left superior vena cava, the left innominate vein, and the right superior vena cava. This sign is seldom visible before the patient is 4 months of age. With TAPVR with PVO, the heart size is normal on radiograph and there are signs of pulmonary edema (Park, 1988).

On ECG, TAPVR without PVO has right axis deviation of the QRS and sometimes right atrial hypertrophy. TAPVR with PVO has right axis deviation for age and right ventricular hypertrophy in the form of tall R waves in the right precordial leads.

Echocardiography of TAPVR without PVO reveals the pulmonary veins draining into a common chamber posterior to the left atrium. The ASD and small left atrium and left ventricle are visualized. A dilated coronary sinus protruding into the left atrium or a dilated innominate vein and superior vena cava can be visualized, if present. Two-dimensional echocardiography of TAPVR with PVO shows the small left atrium and left ventricle. Anomalous pulmonary venous return below the diaphragm can be directly visualized. Doppler echocardiography can be used to detect the venous flow pattern (Park, 1988).

Management

Management of TAPVR is surgical, and surgery is emergent when PVO is below the diaphragm. Medical management is aimed at preventing or treating CHF and preventing hypoxemia. Diuretics may be required to manage pulmonary edema. Balloon atrial septostomy at cardiac catheterization is performed to enlarge the interatrial communication and promote better mixing of blood. Surgery may be delayed when response to medical management is good, but it is usually performed when the patients are infants (Park, 1988).

The surgical procedure depends on the site of the anomalous drainage. Cardiopulmonary bypass is required. Surgery involves the anastomosis of the pulmonary veins to the left atrium, closure of the ASD, and division of the anomalous connection. The surgical mortality rate is high, 10 to 25 percent, but it is lower than with medical management alone. The highest mortality rate is with the infracardiac type.

Experimental Treatments in the Postoperative Period

As discussed, morbidity and mortality rates remain high after surgery in many of the cardiac defects. Treatments that are aimed at decreasing pulmonary vascular resistance, decreasing persistent pulmonary hypertension, and improving cardiac output are being tried at many centers. These include ECMO, especially in infants with TOF, and high-frequency jet ventilation in infants who have undergone stage-one repair of the Norwood procedure for stage 1 HLHS. Other newer treatments include nitric oxide (NO) and ultrafiltration.

Inhaled NO acts as a pulmonary dilator. It directly impacts on pulmonary and systemic vascular resistance. Its use is being researched in infants who have undergone procedures that require cardiac bypass, such as bidirection Glenn or Fontan procedures (Frostell et al., 1993; Roberts et al., 1992).

Ultrafiltration is an experimental procedure undertaken after open heart surgery (Journois et al., 1994). This process is similar to peritoneal dialysis in that it removes water and solutes to increase the hematocrit and blood pressure and to decrease cardiac workload and pulmonary vascular resistance. The action is probably due to a change in the pressure gradient between the blood and the dialysing solution. The result is restoration or maintenance of blood volume, which reduces the need for transfusions. The better perfusion lessens the edema. As contractility of the heart improves, cardiac workload decreases, possibly because cardiodepressant proteins that are present after cardiac surgery are removed. The exact action of this procedure is being researched. It does appear to be a potential treatment for capillary leak syndrome that is prevalent after cardiac surgery (Journois et al., 1994).

Complications of Congenital Heart Defects

Congestive Heart Failure

CHF is a condition in which the blood supply to the body is insufficient to meet the metabolic requirements of the organs. CHF is a manifestation of an underlying disease or defect, rather than a disease itself. Before development of CHF, compensatory mechanisms are activated to maintain adequate cardiac output (Hazinski, 1984; Park, 1988). Normal mechanisms for regulation of cardiac output are listed in Table 21–9. CHF is classified according to the cause. Table 21–10 shows common causes of CHF in newborns.

Increased volume may be caused from fluid overload or fluid retention. In the normally functioning myocardium, fluid retention does not cause CHF; however, fluid retention complicates CHF from other causes. In neonates, the most common cause of increased volume is CHD or altered hemodynamics, as in PDA.

TABLE 21–9 Regulation of Cardiac Output

Sympathetic nervous system activated by
Vasomotor center through peripheral sympathetic fibers
Secretion of norepinephrine from adrenal medulla—"fight or flight" response
Characterized by tachycardia, increased contractility, peripheral vasoconstriction, pupil dilation
Parasympathetic nervous system activated by vagal fibers
Atria—stimulation causes decreased heart rate
Ventricles—stimulation causes decreased contractility
Baroreceptor reflexes
Located in walls of carotid sinuses and in aortic arch
Pressure receptors stimulated by blood pressure
Stimulation causes inhibition of the sympathetic portion of the vasomotor center and stimulation of the parasympathetic (vagal) center; decreased arterial blood pressure

CHF caused by obstruction to outflow occurs when the normal myocardium pumps against increased resistance. This increased resistance may be caused by structural defects, such as valvular stenosis or COA, or by pulmonary disease or pulmonary hypertension. CHF caused by pulmonary disease is called *cor pulmonale*. Severe systemic hypertension can also cause increased resistance.

CHF in the neonate usually results from abnormal stresses placed on the heart rather than from an ineffective myocardium. However, electrolyte imbalances, acidosis, and myocardial ischemia affect the ability of the heart to function effectively. Conditions such as rheumatic fever, infectious myocarditis, Kawasaki disease, and anomalous origin of the left coronary artery reduce the effectiveness of the heart.

Dysrhythmias that may produce CHF include complete AV block or sustained primary tachycardia. AV block results in a severe bradycardia that prohibits adequate circulation of blood. Tachycardia causes insufficient time for ventricular filling, decreasing cardiac output.

Severe anemia can cause CHF because of excessive demand for cardiac output. Because the oxygen-carrying capacity of the blood is diminished, the heart must pump more blood per minute to meet the tissue oxygenation requirements. If the heart cannot meet the excessive demand, CHF develops (Hazinski, 1984; Park, 1988).

Compensatory mechanisms function to meet the body's increased demand for cardiac output. These mechanisms are regulated by the sympathetic nervous system and mechanical factors. The compensatory mechanisms can sustain adequate cardiac output for only a short period of time. If the underlying condition is not corrected, CHF develops.

TABLE 21–10 Causes of Congestive Heart Failure in the Newborn

Causes of Congestive Heart Failure
Increased volume
Obstruction to flow
Ineffective myocardial function
Arrhythmias
Excessive demand for cardiac output
Congenital Heart Defects
Hypoplastic left heart syndrome
Interrupted aortic arch
Coarctation of the aorta
Total anomalous pulmonary venous return with obstruction
Arteriovenous malformation (cranial or hepatic)
Transposition of the great arteries
Patent ductus arteriosus (in preterm infants)
Acquired Heart Defects
Myocardial dysfunction
Anemia
Polycythemia or hyperviscosity
Tachyarrhythmias
Myocarditis

Sympathetic Nervous System Compensatory Mechanisms

Decreased blood pressure stimulates vascular stretch receptors and baroreceptors in the aorta and carotid arteries, which trigger the sympathetic nervous system. Decreased systemic blood pressure inactivates baroreceptors, causing (1) increased sympathetic stimulation, (2) increased heart rate, (3) increased cardiac contractility, and (4) increased arterial blood pressure. Catecholamine release and beta-receptor stimulation increase the rate and force of myocardial contraction. Catecholamines also increase venous tone, so that blood is returned to the heart more effectively. Circulation to the skin, kidneys, extremities, and splanchnic bed is decreased, allowing better circulation to the brain, heart, and lungs. Decreased renal blood flow stimulates the release of renin, angiotensin, and aldosterone. This release causes retention of sodium and fluid, resulting in increased circulating volume. The increased volume puts additional work on the heart (Hazinski, 1984).

Mechanical Compensatory Mechanisms

The heart muscle thickens to increase myocardial pressure. The hypertrophy is effective in the early stages, but as soon as the muscle mass increases, compliance decreases. This change in compliance requires greater filling pressure for adequate cardiac output. The hypertrophied heart eventually becomes ischemic because it does not receive adequate circulation to meet its metabolic needs. Ventricular dilation occurs as myocardial fibers stretch to accommodate heart volume. Initially, this increases the force of the contraction, but it, too, fails after a point.

Effects of Congestive Heart Failure

When the right ventricle is unable to pump blood into the pulmonary artery, less blood is oxygenated by the lungs, there is increased pressure in the right atrium and systemic venous circulation, and edema occurs in the extremities and viscera. When the left ventricle is unable to pump blood into the systemic circulation, there is increased pressure in the left atrium and pulmonary veins. The lungs become congested with blood, causing elevated pulmonary pressures and pulmonary edema (Talner, 1995).

The end effects of CHF are the following:

1. Decreased cardiac output. This stimulates the sympathetic nervous system, causing tachycardia, increased contractility, increased vasomotor tone, peripheral vasoconstriction, and diaphoresis.
2. Decreased renal perfusion. This stimulates the renin–angiotensin–aldosterone mechanism, causing sodium and water retention.
3. Systemic venous engorgement. This results in hepatomegaly, jugular venous distention, periorbital and facial edema, and, occasionally, ascites and dependent edema.
4. Pulmonary venous engorgement. This results in tachypnea, decreased tidal volume, decreased lung compliance, increased airway resistance, early closure of the small airways with air trapping, increased work of breathing, and increased respiratory effort, grunting, and rales. Stimulation of the

j-receptors in the lung causes the infant to become apprehensive (Talner, 1995).

Diagnosis

The diagnosis of CHF is based on clinical signs and symptoms, laboratory data, and chest radiography. In contrast to infants with cyanotic heart disease, infants with CHF usually have significant respiratory distress with tachypnea, grunting, and retractions. They exhibit peripheral pallor, appearing to be ashen or gray in color. The precordium is active, and there are usually loud murmurs heard throughout systole and diastole. Pulses are usually full, but there may be a difference between the upper and the lower extremities. Hepatomegaly is common. The infants are irritable.

In addition to demonstrating hypoxemia, arterial blood gas may reveal a metabolic acidosis resulting from the decreased systemic blood flow. If acidosis is severe, there may be concurrent respiratory acidosis because of the pulmonary edema caused by left-sided heart failure. Pulmonary ventilation–perfusion mismatch may cause hypoxemia. Hypocalcemia is often present in infants with CHF because they have an inappropriate response to stress. In addition, infants with DiGeorge syndrome may have hypocalcemia because of absent parathyroids. Aortic arch abnormalities (e.g., interrupted aortic arch, hypoplastic left heart, and COA) are commonly associated with DiGeorge syndrome (Park, 1988; Talner, 1995).

Hypoglycemia may be present in infants with severe CHF. The myocardium is dependent on glucose; decreased glucose levels diminish the ability of the heart to compensate for CHF. On chest radiograph, the heart is enlarged and there is increased pulmonary congestion. ECG is not generally diagnostic, unless the CHF is caused by an arrhythmia. There may be nonspecific changes in the T waves, changes in the ST segment, and an increase in the height of the P wave (Talner, 1995).

Electrolyte imbalances usually include relative hyponatremia, which is due to the increase in free water. Hypochloremia and increased bicarbonate may result from respiratory acidemia and the use of loop diuretics. Hyperkalemia results from the release of intracellular cations, which is related to poor tissue perfusion. Elevated lactic acid levels are also indicative of tissue hypoxia (Talner, 1995). Atrial natriuretic factor (ANF), a peptide hormone, may be important in the regulation of volume and blood pressure. ANF is released from the atria when they are distended. ANF release causes natriuresis, diuresis, and vasodilation. ANF acts with other volume regulators, such as renin, aldosterone, and vasopressin. An increased ANF level may be found when there is increased pulmonary blood flow, increased left atrial pressure, or pulmonary hypertension (Talner, 1995).

Treatment

The goal of management of CHF is to improve cardiac function while identifying and correcting the underlying cause. General measures that decrease the demand on the heart are helpful; however, pharmacologic intervention is the most efficacious therapy.

General Measures. General measures to manage CHF include the administration of oxygen to improve ventilation and perfusion at the alveolar level. Ventilation with positive end-expiratory pressure at 6 to 10 cm H_2O may relieve the effects of CHF by reducing pulmonary edema (Talner, 1995).

Fluid restriction may decrease the circulating volume. Careful monitoring of serum electrolytes, intake and output, and weight is essential. It is imperative that *all* fluid be counted in the total daily fluid volume. Infants with CHF do not usually feed well and may require caloric supplementation with hyperalimentation or gavage feedings (Park, 1988).

Infants with CHF are irritable and agitated, which further complicates their status. Sedation with continuous infusions of morphine sulfate or fentanyl may improve the infant's comfort and oxygenation. Other measures that reduce cardiac demand include maintenance of a normal hematocrit, maintenance of the thermoneutral environment, and minimal stimulation. Cautious use of sedation may reduce anxiety and agitation, increasing comfort and decreasing the demand for oxygen.

Pharmacologic Interventions. Table 21–11 lists the medications most commonly used in the management of cardiac conditions. The mainstay of management of CHF beyond the neonatal period is digitalis (digoxin). Digoxin slows conduction through the AV node, prolongs the refractory period, and slows the heart rate through vagal effects on the SA node.

The use of digoxin in preterm or term neonates is controversial. The preterm newborn is at risk for digitalis toxicity because of the narrow range between therapeutic and toxic drug levels. The preterm infant requires a lower maintenance dose because of limited renal excretion of the drug (Table 21–12). If digoxin is used, the neonate must be carefully monitored for signs and symptoms of digitalis toxicity. Lead II ECGs should be obtained before each dose for the first 3 days; the dose should be withheld if the P-R interval is greater than 0.16 second or if there is an arrhythmia present. Digoxin levels should be monitored and should be less than 2.0 ng/ml (Avery et al., 1994; Beckman & Brent, 1994; Park, 1988; Talner, 1995). Blood samples for digoxin levels should be drawn after the drug has achieved equilibrium in the body, approximately 6 to 8 hours after administration (Yeh, 1985).

Other inotropic agents can be used to improve cardiac output. Dopamine, a norepinephrine precursor, has direct and indirect beta-adrenergic effects that are dose dependent. At low doses (2 to 5 μg/kg/minute), there is increased renal blood flow with minimal effect on heart rate, blood pressure, or contractility. Medium doses (5 to 10 μg/kg/minute) increase renal blood flow, heart rate, blood pressure, and contractility. Pulmonary artery pressure may be increased; peripheral resistance is not affected. High doses (10 to 20 μg/kg/minute) cause alpha effects, resulting in peripheral vasoconstriction, increased cardiac rate, and increased contractility (Park, 1988).

Dobutamine is a synthetic catecholamine that acts on beta- and alpha-adrenergic receptors. Dobutamine (2 to 10 μg/kg/minute) has decreased effects on the heart rate and rhythm and causes less peripheral vasoconstriction.

Isoproterenol (Isuprel), a synthetic epinephrine-like substance, has $beta_1$- and $beta_2$-adrenergic effects. The usefulness of Isuprel in the neonate is limited because it produces increased heart rate, arrhythmias, and decreased systemic vascular resistance, which may worsen the hypotension (Park, 1988; Talner, 1995).

DIURETICS. Diuretics are useful in the treatment of CHF to decrease sodium and water retention. The primary goal is to increase renal perfusion (with inotropic agents or vasodilators) and to increase sodium delivery to distal diluting sites of the renal tubules. Diuretic agents increase the renal excretion of sodium and other anions by inhibition of tubular reabsorption of sodium (Park, 1988).

Furosemide (Lasix), a loop diuretic, blocks sodium and chloride reabsorption in the ascending limb of the loop of Henle. Loop diuretics interfere with the formation of free water and free water reabsorption by preventing the transport of sodium, potassium, and chloride into the medullary interstitium. Loop diuretics cause increased excretion of potassium by delivering increased quantities of sodium to sites in the distal nephron where potassium can be excreted. Furosemide also increases excretion of calcium, but

TABLE 21–11 Drugs Used in the Management of Congenital Heart Defects

Drug	Dosage	Action	Onset	Comments
Diuretics				
Furosemide (Lasix)	1 mg/kg/dose IV 1–3 mg/kg/dose	Loop diuretic; inhibits sodium and chloride reabsorption in proximal tubule	15–30 minutes 30–60 minutes	Associated with increased PDA; calcium loss
Spironolactone (Aldactone)	1.5–3.0 mg/kg/day PO	Competitive antagonist of aldosterone	3–5 days	Potassium sparing
Chlorothiazide	20–40 mg/kg/day PO	Inhibits sodium and chloride reabsorption along the distal tubules	1–2 hours	
Inotropic Agents				
Dopamine	Low: 2–5 μg/kg/minute	Increased renal blood flow; beta-adrenergic effects		Monitor ECG; BP
	Mod: 5–10 μg/kg/minute	Increased renal blood flow; heart rate, BP, and contractility		
	High: 10–20 μg/kg/minute	Peripheral vasoconstriction, increased heart rate, and contractility		
Dobutamine	2–10 μg/kg/minute	Increased renal blood flow; increased contractility	Rapid	Decreased systemic vascular resistance; increased pulmonary wedge pressure
Isoproterenol	0.05–0.5 mg/kg/minute	Increased venous return to heart and decreased pulmonary vascular resistance		Tachycardia, dysrhythmias, decreased renal perfusion
Vasodilators				
Sodium nitroprusside (Nipride)	0.5–6 μg/kg/minute	Directly relaxes smooth muscles in arteriolar and venous walls; increases cardiac output if the decrease is secondary to myocardial dysfunction	Seconds	Monitor BP and thiocyanate levels; light sensitive; monitor heart rate
Prostaglandins				
PGE_1	0.05–0.1 mg/kg/minute	Produces vasodilation and smooth muscle relaxation of ductus arteriosus and pulmonary and systemic circulations; increased arterial saturation by 25%–100%	Rapid	Monitor BP; vasopressors may be required; apnea, flush, fever, seizure-like activity; decreased heart rate
Prostaglandin Synthetase Inhibitors				
Indomethacin	0.2 mg/kg IV (1st) q 24 hours 0.1 mg/kg IV (2nd and 3rd) >48 hours and <14 days: 0.3 mg/kg IV and 3 doses q 24 hours >14 days and <6 weeks: 0.2–0.3 mg/kg q 12 hours	Promotes ductal closure by inhibition of PGE_2 in the walls of the ductus	12–24 hours	Monitor renal function, bilirubin, electrolytes, glucose, platelets, bleeding

BP, blood pressure; ECG, electrocardiogram; IV, intravenously; PDA, patent ductus arteriosus; PO, by mouth; q, every.

does not affect the ability of the kidney to regulate acid–base balance (Oh, 1985).

An aldosterone antagonist such as spironolactone (Aldactone) may be useful because it is a potassium-sparing diuretic. Spironolactone works by binding to the cytoplasmic receptor sites and blocking aldosterone action, thus impairing the reabsorption of sodium and the secretion of potassium and hydrogen ion. Spironolactone has no effect on free water production and absorption. Thiazide diuretics (chlorothiazide and hydrochlorothiazide) inhibit sodium and chloride reabsorption along the distal tubules. They are not as effective as the loop diuretics and are infrequently used (Park, 1988).

COMPLICATIONS OF DIURETIC THERAPY. Diuretic therapy can provide severe electrolyte imbalances if not monitored carefully. The complications of diuretic therapy include (1) volume contraction, (2) hyponatremia, (3) metabolic alkalemia or acidemia, and (4) hypokalemia or hyperkalemia (Hazinski, 1984; Talner, 1995). When using diuretics, fluid and electrolyte balance must be maintained by administration of water and electrolytes. The adequacy of the volume can be determined by monitoring serum electrolytes, BUN, creatinine, urinary output, weight, specific gravity, and skin turgor.

The increased renal losses of sodium can lead to hyponatremia, because adequate amounts of sodium are not supplied. There may also be increased antidiuretic hormone release secondary to changes in the osmoreceptors or inhibition of antidiuretic hormone action. This can best be managed by decreasing the amount of total water and improving the cardiac output, thus increasing renal perfusion.

Metabolic alkalosis can result from administration of loop diuretics that interfere with sodium- and potassium-dependent chloride reabsorption. Hypochloremia results in a greater aldosterone production and an increase in bicarbonate concentration.

TABLE 21–12 Digoxin Prescription Information

Total Digitalizing Dose (TDD)	Maintenance Dose
Preterm	
0.025–0.05 mg/kg	0.008–0.012 mg/kg/day
Term	
0.04–0.08 mg/kg	0.01–0.02 mg/kg/day (⅛ TDD)

To digitalize:

1. Give ½ TDD.
2. Six to 8 hours later, give ¼ TDD.
3. Six to 8 hours later, get a rhythm strip; if normal, give ¼ TDD.
4. Give maintenance dose (⅛ TDD) 12 hours after last digitalizing dose and then every 12 hours.

Slow digitalization, with decreased risk of toxicity, can be achieved by starting with the maintenance dose.

Hypokalemia is a frequent complication of loop diuretic therapy. An increased ratio of intracellular to extracellular potassium results in the clinical signs and symptoms of hypokalemia. Hypokalemia increases the risk for digoxin toxicity. In contrast, hyperkalemia may result when the cardiac output is low and tissue perfusion is severely compromised. Other complications of diuretic therapy include increased calcium excretion, hyperuricemia, and glucose intolerance (Talner, 1995).

Vasodilators may be used in severe CHF to reduce the right and left ventricular preload and afterload to improve cardiac function (Hazinski, 1983). Vasodilators cause arterial and venous dilation, resulting in decreased systemic and pulmonary vascular resistance. Sodium nitroprusside (Nipride) is a smooth muscle relaxant that decreases ventricular afterload by decreasing pulmonary and systemic vascular resistance and decreases venous return and ventricular preload. This leads to decreased ventricular end-diastolic volume, increased ejection fraction, increased heart rate and cardiac index, and decreased pulmonary and systemic resistance. Sodium nitroprusside is sensitive to light and must be stored in dark containers. Side effects are cyanide toxicity and decreased platelet function (Hazinski, 1984; Park, 1988).

The prognosis for CHF depends on the severity of the underlying condition and on the degree of CHF.

Subacute Infective Endocarditis

SAIE can be a complication of CHD. Two factors are important in the development of SAIE: (1) structural abnormalities that create turbulent flow or pressure gradients and (2) bacteremia. All cardiac defects that produce turbulent flow or have a significant pressure gradient predispose the patient to bacterial invasion of the cardiac endothelium. The turbulent flow damages the endothelial lining and platelet–fibrin thrombus formation. Prevention of bacterial SAIE requires scrupulous daily oral care as well as prophylactic antimicrobials for dental procedures (Park, 1988). All CHDs, except secundum-type ASDs, predispose the patient to SAIE. VSDs, TOF, and aortic stenosis are the CHDs most commonly associated with SAIE (Park, 1988).

Vegetation of SAIE is usually on the low pressure side of the defect, where endothelial damage is established by the jet effect of the defect. More than 90 percent of SAIE cases are caused by *Streptococcus viridans, Streptococcus faecalis* (enterococcus), and *Staphylococcus aureus.* Other organisms include *Haemophilus influenzae, Pseudomonas, Escherichia coli, Proteus, Aerobacter,* and *Listeria. Candida* may infect infants who have been on long-term antimicrobial or steroid therapy (Dajani & Taubert, 1995).

Prevention

Procedures for which SAIE prophylaxis is indicated include (1) all dental procedures, (2) tonsillectomy or adenoidectomy, (3) surgical procedures involving the respiratory mucosa, (4) bronchoscopy, (5) incision and drainage of infected tissue, and (6) gastrointestinal or genitourinary procedures.

For complete prescribing and dosing information, refer to the Committee on Rheumatic Fever and Infective Endocarditis of the Council on Cardiovascular Diseases in the Young (Schulman et al., 1984). The recommendations for children are listed in Table 21–13.

SUPPORT OF THE FAMILY OF THE INFANT WITH A CONGENITAL HEART DEFECT

Families with infants with CHDs feel confusion, guilt, anger, and fear. The family needs support to cope with the short- and long-term consequences of the CHD. The severity of the CHD, the availability of treatment, and the prognosis influence the amount and kind of support required. Parents need frequent contact with members of the health care team. Caretakers should

TABLE 21–13 Antimicrobial Prophylaxis to Prevent Subacute Infective Endocarditis in Children With Cardiac Defects

I. Dental procedures and oral respiratory tract surgery
   A. Standard regimen
      1. Amoxicillin 50 mg/kg 1 hour before procedure, followed by 25 mg/kg 6 hours after procedure.
   B. Alternative regimens
      1. Allergic to penicillin and/or amoxicillin: erythromycin ethylsuccinate or erythromycin stearate 20 mg/kg orally 2 hours before procedure, followed by erythromycin 10 mg/kg 6 hours after initial dose.
      2. Children unable to take oral medications: ampicillin 50 mg/kg IV or IM 30 minutes before procedure, followed by ampicillin 25 mg/kg IV or IM 6 hours after initial dose.
      3. Allergic to penicillin and/or amoxicillin and unable to take oral medications: clindamycin 10 mg/kg IV 30 minutes before procedure, followed by clindamycin 5 mg/kg IV 6 hours after initial dose.
      4. High-risk children not candidates for standard regimen: ampicillin 50 mg/kg IV or IM plus gentamicin 2.0 mg/kg IV or IM 30 minutes before procedure, followed by amoxicillin 25 mg/kg orally 6 hours after initial dose or a repeat of the ampicillin plus gentamicin regimen.
      5. High-risk children allergic to ampicillin, amoxicillin, or penicillin: vancomycin 20 mg/kg IV over 1 hour, starting 1 hour before procedure. No repeat dose necessary.

II. Gastrointestinal or genitourinary procedure
   A. Standard regimen
      1. Ampicillin 50 mg/kg plus gentamicin 2.0 mg/kg IV or IM 30 minutes before procedure, followed by amoxicillin 25 mg/kg 6 hours after initial dose; or repeat ampicillin plus gentamicin regimen 8 hours after initial dose.
   B. Alternative regimens
      1. Ampicillin/amoxicillin/penicillin-allergic children: vancomycin 20 mg/kg IV over 1 hour plus gentamicin 2.0 mg/kg IV or IM 1 hour before procedure; repeat the vancomycin plus gentamicin regimen 8 hours after initial dose.
      2. Low-risk patient alternative regimen: amoxicillin 50 mg/kg orally 1 hour before procedure, followed by amoxicillin 25 mg/kg 6 hours after initial dose.

From Dajani, A. S., Bisno, A. L., Chung, K. J., et al. (1990). Prevention of bacterial endocarditis: Recommendations by the American Heart Association. *Journal of the American Medical Association*, 264:2919–2922.

speak with the parents routinely, not just when there are major changes in the infant's condition.

Family members should be given an accurate description of the defect; diagrams and models illustrating the defect should be used. Parents need frequent reassurance and repetition of information. Parents of infants who do not require immediate surgery but who will eventually require surgery, must be educated about all aspects of the infant's care, including signs and symptoms of deterioration, medication administration, activity limitations, and normal development. Careful follow-up is important to prevent complications.

Identification of support persons for the family is extremely valuable. Parents may be encouraged to talk to other parents of newborns with the same or similar defects. Many neonatal intensive care units have active support groups consisting of parents of patients. Care should be taken in selection of supporters. Parents with a term newborn with a CHD may not be able to relate to parents of a preterm neonate. Other family members or friends should not be overlooked; they can become valuable support persons if they are provided appropriate guidance and education. The needs of siblings should also be assessed. Siblings need support, education, and guidance appropriate for their age and comprehension of the situation. Parents may not recognize their needs because of the overwhelming situation. Health care providers can facilitate the parent–child relationship during the initial period and throughout the course of the management.

Financial resources should be addressed because preoperative, operative, and postoperative care is expensive. Many parents need assistance in obtaining aid to which they are entitled. Even the most knowledgeable of parents may not be aware of resources available to them. If experimental surgery is contemplated, parents may need assistance in speaking with private insurance companies regarding coverage. Referrals to appropriate local, state, federal, or private organizations that pertain to the CHD should be made for the parents. These include the Department of Family and Children Services, the March of Dimes, and Children's Medical Services. The family may qualify for the Special Supplemental Nutrition Program for Women, Infants, and Children.

Discharge planning must be comprehensive for the neonate who will receive medical management for a CHD before corrective surgery. A thorough assessment of the home should be obtained before discharge. Contact with the primary care provider who will perform the routine management of the infant is imperative. Initial contact by telephone should be followed up with a copy of the complete medical record and discharge summary. If the infant requires any special equipment for home care, the equipment should be obtained before discharge so that the parents can be taught how to use it. Also, practical details such as whether there are enough electrical outlets in the infant's room must be determined. Notification of local emergency medical services, power companies, and other relevant companies should be completed before discharge.

REFERENCES

Avery, G. B., Fletcher, M. A., & MacDonald, M. G. (Eds.). (1994). *Neonatology: Pathophysiology and management of the newborn* (4th ed.). Philadelphia: J. B. Lippincott.

Bailey, L. L., & Gundry, S. R. (1990). Hypoplastic left heart syndrome [Review]. *Pediatric Clinics of North America, 37*(1), 137–151.

Baraitser, M., & Winter, R. M. (1996). *Color atlas of congenital malformation syndromes.* St. Louis: Mosby-Wolfe.

Beckman, D. A., & Brent, R. L. (1994). Effects of prescribed and self-administered drugs during the second and third trimesters. In G. B. Avery, M. A. Fletcher, & M. G. MacDonald (Eds.), *Neonatology: Pathophysiology and management of the newborn* (4th ed., pp. 197–206). Philadelphia: J. B. Lippincott.

Beekman, R. H. (1995). Coarctation of the aorta. In G. C. Emmanouilides, H. Allen, T. Riemenschneider, & H. Gutgesell (Eds.), *Moss and Adams heart disease in infants, children, and adolescents including the fetus and young adult* (5th ed., pp. 1111–1132). Baltimore: Williams & Wilkins.

Braunwald, E., Sonnenblick, E. H., & Ross, J. (1988). Mechanisms of cardiac contraction and relaxation. In E. Braunwald (Ed.), *Heart disease: A textbook of cardiovascular medicine* (pp. 383–425). Philadelphia: W. B. Saunders.

Brook, M. M., & Heymann, M. A. (1995). Patent ductus arteriosus. In G. C. Emmanouilides, H. Allen, T. Riemenschneider, & H. Gutgesell (Eds.), *Moss and Adams heart disease in infants, children, and adolescents including the fetus and young adult* (5th ed., pp. 746–763). Baltimore: Williams & Wilkins.

Callow, L. B. (1992). Current strategies in the nursing care of infants with hypoplastic left-heart syndrome undergoing first-stage palliation with the Norwood operation. *Heart & Lung, 21*(5), 463–470.

Chiavarelli, M., Gundry, S. R., Razzouk, A. J., & Bailey, L. L. (1993). Cardiac transplantation for infants with hypoplastic left-heart syndrome. *Journal of the American Medical Association, 270*(24), 2944–2947.

Clark, E. B. (1995). Epidemiology of congenital cardiovascular malformations. In G. C. Emmanouilides, H. Allen, T. Riemenschneider, & H. Gutgesell (Eds.), *Moss and Adams heart disease in infants, children, and adolescents including the fetus and young adult* (5th ed., pp 60–69). Baltimore: Williams & Wilkins.

Conover, M. B. (1988). Anatomy and physiology of the heart. In M. B. Conover (Ed.), *Understanding electrocardiography: Arrhythmias and the 12-lead KG* (pp. 1–14). St. Louis: C. V. Mosby.

Dajani, A. S., & Taubert, K. A. (1995). Infective endocarditis. In G. C. Emmanouilides, H. Allen, T. Riemenschneider, & H. Gutgesell (Eds.), *Moss and Adams heart disease in infants, children, and adolescents including the fetus and young adult* (5th ed., 1541–1554). Baltimore: Williams & Wilkins.

Driscoll, D. J. (1990). Evaluation of the cyanotic newborn. Congenital heart disease [Review]. *Pediatric Clinics of North America, 37*(1), 1–23.

Feldt, R. H., Porter, C. J., Edwards, W. D., et al. (1995). Atrioventricular septal defects. In G. C. Emmanouilides, H. Allen, T. Riemenschneider, & H. Gutgesell (Eds.), *Moss and Adams heart disease in infants, children, and adolescents including the fetus and young adult* (5th ed., pp. 704–723). Baltimore: Williams & Wilkins.

Freedom, R. M., & Benson, L. (1995). Hypoplastic left heart syndrome. In G. C. Emmanouilides, H. Allen, T. Riemenschneider, & H. Gutgesell (Eds.), *Moss and Adams heart disease in infants, children, and adolescents including the fetus and young adult* (5th ed., pp. 1133–1153). Baltimore: Williams & Wilkins.

Friedman, W. F. (1988). Congenital heart disease in infancy and childhood. In E. Braunwald (Ed.), *Heart disease: A textbook of cardiovascular medicine* (pp. 896–975). Philadelphia: W. B. Saunders.

Friedman, W. F. (1995). Aortic stenosis. In G. C. Emmanouilides, H. Allen, T. Riemenschneider, & H. Gutgesell (Eds.), *Moss and Adams heart disease in infants, children, and adolescents including the fetus and young adult* (5th ed., pp. 1087–1110). Baltimore: Williams & Wilkins.

Frostell, C. G., Blomquist, H., Hedenstierna, G., et al. (1993). Inhaled nitric oxide selectively reverses human hypoxic pulmonary vasoconstriction without causing systemic vasodilation. *Anesthesiology, 78*(3), 427–435.

Graham, T. P., & Gutgesell, H. P. (1995). Ventricular septal defects. In G. C. Emmanouilides, H. Allen, T. Riemenschneider, & H. Gutgesell (Eds.), *Moss and Adams heart disease in infants, children, and adolescents including the fetus and young adult* (5th ed., pp. 724–745). Baltimore: Williams & Wilkins.

Hazinski, M. F. (1983). Congenital heart disease in the neonate (part III): Congestive heart failure. *Neonatal Network, 1*(6), 8–17.

Hazinski, M. F. (1984). Cardiovascular disorders. In M. F. Hazinski (Ed.), *Nursing care of the critically ill child* (pp. 63–252). St. Louis: C. V. Mosby.

Heymann, M. A. (1995). Fetal and postnatal circulations: Pulmonary circulation. In G. C. Emmanouilides, H. Allen, T. Riemenschneider, & H. Gutgesell (Eds.), *Moss and Adams heart disease in infants, children, and adolescents including the fetus and young adult* (5th ed., pp. 41–46). Baltimore: Williams & Wilkins.

Hoffman, J. I. (1990). Congenital heart defects: Incidence and inheritance [Review]. *Pediatric Clinics of North America, 37*(1), 25–43.

Journois, D., Pouard, P., Greel W. J., et al. (1994). Hemofiltration during cardiopulmonary bypass in pediatric cardiac surgery: Effects on hemostasis, cytokines and complement components. *Anesthesiology, 81*(5), 1181–1189.

Kirklin, J. W., Colvin, E. V., McConnell, M. E., & Bargeron, L. M. (1990). Complete transposition of the great arteries: Treatment in the current era. *Pediatric Clinics of North America, 37*(1), 171–177.

Mair, D. D., Edwards, W. D., Julsrud, P. R., et al. (1995a). Pulmonary artresia and ventricular septal defect. In G. C. Emmanouilides, H. Allen, T. Riemenschneider, & H. Gutgesell (Eds.), *Moss and Adams heart disease in infants, children, and adolescents including the fetus and young adult* (5th ed., pp. 983–997). Baltimore: Williams & Wilkins.

Mair, D. D., Edwards, W. D., Julsrud, P. R., et al. (1995b). Truncus arteriosus. In G. C. Emmanouilides, H. Allen, T. Riemenschneider, & H. Gutgesell (Eds.), *Moss and Adams heart disease in infants, children, and adolescents including the fetus and young adult* (5th ed., pp. 1026–1041). Baltimore: Williams & Wilkins.

McNamara, D. G. (1990). Value and limitations of auscultation in the management of congenital heart disease. *Pediatric Clinics of North America, 37*(1), 93–113.

Moller, J. H. (1987). Clinical education aid: Congenital heart anomalies. Columbus, OH: Ross Laboratories.

Norwood, W. I., Lang, P., & Hansen, D. D. (1983). Physiologic repair of aortic atresia—Hypoplastic left heart syndrome. *New England Journal of Medicine, 308*(1), 23–26.

Oh, W. (1985). Diuretic therapy. In T. F. Yeh (Ed.), *Drug therapy in the neonate and small infant* (pp. 299–304). Chicago: Year Book Medical Publishers.

Park, M. K. (1988). *Pediatric cardiology for practitioners.* Chicago: Mosby–Year Book.

Paul, M. H. (1995). Transposition of the great arteries. In G. C. Emmanouilides, H. Allen, T. Riemenschneider, & H. Gutgesell (Eds.), *Moss and Adams heart disease in infants, children, and adolescents including the fetus and young adult* (5th ed., pp. 1154–1224). Baltimore: Williams & Wilkins.

Pinsky, W. W., & Arciniegas, E. (1990). Tetralogy of Fallot [Review]. *Pediatric Clinics of North America, 37*(1), 179–192.

Porter, C. J., Feldt, R. H., Edwards, W. D., et al. (1995). Atrial septal defects. In G. C. Emmanouilides, H. Allen, T. Riemenschneider, & H. Gutgesell (Eds.), *Moss and Adams heart disease in infants, children, and adolescents including the fetus and young adult* (5th ed., pp. 687–703). Baltimore: Williams & Wilkins.

Roberts, J. D., Polaner, D. M., Lang, P., & Zapol, W. M. (1992). Inhaled nitric oxide in persistent pulmonary hypertension of the newborn. *Lancet, 340*, 818–819.

Rocchini, A. P., & Emmanouilides, G. C. (1995). Pulmonary stenosis. In G. C. Emmanouilides, H. Allen, T. Riemenschneider, & H. Gutgesell (Eds.), *Moss and Adams heart disease in infants, children, and adolescents including the fetus and young adult* (5th ed., pp. 930–961). Baltimore: Williams & Wilkins.

Sacksteder, S. (1978). Congenital cardiac defects: Embryology and fetal circulation. *American Journal of Nursing, 78*(2), 262–264.

Schulman, S. T., Ameren, D. P., Bisno, A. L., et al. (1984). Committee on Rheumatic Fever and Infective Endocarditis: A statement for professionals by the Council on Cardiovascular Disease in the Young. *Circulation,* 70(6), 1123A–1128A.

Smith, J. B., & Vernon-Levett, P. (1993). Care of infants with hypoplastic left heart syndrome. *AACN Clinical Issues, 4*(2), 329–339.

Suddaby, E. C., & O'Brien, A. M. (1993). ECMO for cardiac support in children. *Heart & Lung, 22*(5), 401–407.

Talner, N. S. (1995). Heart failure. In G. C. Emmanouilides, H. Allen, T. Riemenschneider, & H. Gutgesell (Eds.), *Moss and Adams heart disease in infants, children, and adolescents including the fetus and young adult* (5th ed., pp. 1746–1772). Baltimore: Williams & Wilkins.

Yeh, T. F. (1985). Congestive heart failure. In T. F. Yeh (Ed.), *Drug therapy in the neonate and small infant* (pp. 139–160). Chicago: Year Book Medical Publishers.

Zuberbuhler, J. R. (1995). Tetralogy of Fallot. In G. C. Emmanouilides, H. Allen, T. Riemenschneider, & H. Gutgesell (Eds.), *Moss and Adams heart disease in infants, children, and adolescents including the fetus and young adult* (5th ed., pp. 998–1017). Baltimore: Williams & Wilkins.

CHAPTER 22

Fluids, Electrolytes, Vitamins, and Trace Minerals: Basis of Ingestion, Digestion, Elimination, and Metabolism

REGINALD C. TSANG SERGIO DEMARINI LINDA L. RATH

■ RESEARCH AGENDA

Which infants are at greatest risk for fluid and electrolyte problems?

What are the risk factors associated with fluid and electrolyte problems?

What is the relationship between early hyponatremia and perinatal asphyxia?

Is there a relationship between vitamin E and cerebral hemorrhages?

Is there a relationship between phototherapy and neonatal hypocalcemia?

Water and electrolytes are vital components of the body at any age. The laws that regulate fluid and electrolyte balance in the newborn are the same as in children and adults. However, the newborn's body water distribution is both quantitatively and qualitatively different. Furthermore, rapid changes take place at the time of birth, and so special care is necessary to maintain an appropriate fluid and electrolyte balance, especially in very low birth weight (VLBW) infants.

In this chapter, whenever possible, the recommendations of the American Academy of Pediatrics (AAP) have been followed. In all other instances, the conclusions have been based on the current standard medical practice in the field.

WATER AND ELECTROLYTES

Water

Physiology

Water is the main component of the human body. It is distributed both inside and outside the cells; therefore, a practical simplification is to classify total body water (TBW) into intracellular water (ICW) and extracellular water (ECW). ICW is the total amount of water in all the body cells. ECW is the total amount of water outside the cells; it comprises the water in the interstitial space and in the intravascular space (plasma).

The distribution of TBW between intracellular and extracellular spaces depends on the water's relative content of solutes (electrolytes, proteins): that is, on its relative osmolality. The osmolality of a solution is determined by the total number of solute particles in solution. Osmolality values are expressed in osmoles or milliosmoles per kilogram of water (Osm/kg or mOsm/kg). Because cell membranes are completely permeable to water but not to most solutes, water shifts from one compartment to the other until equilibrium between osmolalities on both sides of the membrane is achieved. The osmolality of intracellular and extracellular spaces is therefore equal, although the composition of ICW is different from that of ECW: sodium (Na) is the main extracellular ion, whereas potassium (K) is the main intracellular ion. The size of a compartment therefore depends on the amount of osmoles within it, which in turn determines the water content.

In each compartment, there is a main solute that acts to keep water within the compartment: (1) The volume of the intracellular compartment is mainly maintained by K salts and regulated by the Na-K cellular pump; (2) the volume of the extracellular compartment is mainly maintained by Na salts and regulated by the kidneys; (3) within the extracellular space, the volume of the intravascular compartment is maintained mainly by the colloidal osmotic pressure of plasma proteins.

Changes in Water Distribution

TBW decreases over age (Fig. 22–1): it constitutes more than 90 percent of the total body weight in the first trimester of gestation, about 80 percent at 32 weeks' gestation, about 78 percent at 40 weeks' gestation, and approximately 60 to 65 percent at the end of the first year of life. The ratio of ECW to ICW also changes with growth. ECW decreases from approximately 60 percent of body weight in the second trimester to about 45 percent at term. Correspondingly, ICW increases from about 25 percent of body weight in the second trimester to approximately 33 percent at term (Friis-Hansen, 1957, 1961).

At birth, an acute expansion of ECW is superimposed upon the gradual changes that took place during fetal life. Through an unknown mechanism, water and electrolytes shift from the intracellular to the extracellular space (Cassady, 1971; Costarino & Baumgart, 1986; Coulter & Avery, 1980; MacLaurin, 1966). Therefore, the newborn at birth is in a state of excess extracellular fluid, and this is particularly prominent in the preterm infant (TBW and ECW are larger at lower gestational ages). The excess ECW is lost through diuresis; thus some weight loss (5 to 10

Much of the content of this chapter is based on studies funded in part by the National Institutes of Health (NIH) with the following grants: HD 11725, Diabetes in Pregnancy Program Project; NIHL-T32-HD07200, Research Training in Perinatology; and NIH-HD20748, Perinatal Emphasis Research Center.

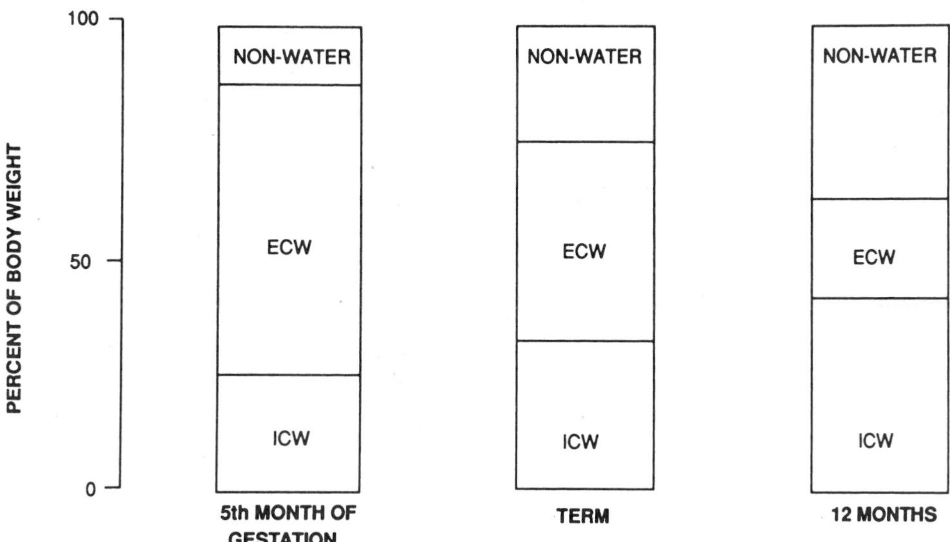

FIGURE 22–1. Changes in body water distribution.

percent) usually takes place as a consequence of these physiologic changes in body water distribution (Aperia et al., 1981; Hanna, 1963; Kagan et al., 1972). Postnatal weight loss and regaining reflect changes in the interstitial water component of ECW, whereas plasma volume remains essentially unchanged (Bauer et al., 1991). In preterm infants, a postnatal weight loss of more than 10 percent occurs more frequently in clinically unstable infants with inadequate caloric intake. If energy intake is adequate, the decrease in extracellular volume is compensated by an increase in intracellular volume, and weight loss is minimal (Heimler et al., 1993). On the basis of these characteristics, it may be inappropriate both to administer large amounts of fluids and to replace all fluid losses during the first days of life.

Water Balance and Body Metabolism

The human body loses a variable amount of water and electrolytes daily. To maintain body fluid balance, fluid losses must be replaced periodically. Maintenance fluid requirements are calculated to replace water and electrolytes normally lost through urine, stools, skin, and the respiratory tract. Water turnover is part of cellular metabolism and is usually related precisely to basal metabolic rate. Basal metabolic rate is the amount of energy that the body must produce to maintain homeostasis at rest and in a thermally neutral environment (see Chapter 16, Neonatal Thermoregulation).

Carbohydrates, lipids, and proteins are the substances used to produce energy. Waste products are heat, nitrogen, carbon dioxide, and water. To excrete waste products, water is normally lost through kidneys (to eliminate nitrogen), skin (to eliminate excess heat), and the respiratory tract (to eliminate carbon dioxide). Therefore, a high body energy expenditure means a large amount of waste products and, consequently, large water losses.

Some water is generated by the cells as a by-product of cell metabolism (water of oxidation). This amount of water, which must be subtracted from fluid requirements, is approximately equal to water losses in stools. Thus the latter can be omitted from the usual calculations of required water intake (Bell & Oh, 1979; Winters, 1973).

Water Requirements

To maintain the overall body water and salt composition, renal water and electrolyte losses and insensible water losses from respiratory tract and skin evaporation should ordinarily be replaced. According to the classical definition of maintenance fluids, 100 ml of water is needed for each 100 kcal of energy expended (Winters, 1973).

Although this relationship between metabolic rate and water loss holds true in full-term infants, it is not valid in preterm infants. Immature renal function, very high insensible water losses caused by skin immaturity and higher body surface area:body mass ratio, and neonatal illnesses have significant influences on fluid balance (Costarino & Baumgart, 1988). Although values for fluid requirements are available (Table 22–1), these values provide only an approximate guideline for the individual infant.

Accuracy for fluid requirements may be improved by taking into account factors that influence insensible water losses (Table 22–2). For example, radiant warmers and phototherapy increase insensible water losses, whereas a plastic blanket under a radiant warmer or adequate humidification in an incubator decreases insensible water losses. Appropriate administration of fluid is

TABLE 22–1 Approximate Water Requirements (ml/kg/day) in Newborns in the First Week of Life

Time	Birth Weight Category			
	<1000 g	*1000–1500 g*	*1501–2000 g*	*Full Term*
First 48 hours	110–140	90–120	80–110	65
End of first week	150–200	120–150	110–150	100–150

TABLE 22–2 Factors Affecting Water Losses

Increase	Decrease
Water Losses From the Skin	
Low gestational age	High humidity in incubator
Forced convection in incubator	Double-walled incubator
Radiant warmer	Plastic heat shield
Hyperthermia	Plastic blanket
Activity	Patches applied to the infant's skin
Phototherapy	
Water Losses From the Respiratory Tract	
Tachypnea	Continuous distending pressure with humidified gas
Inadequate humidification	Artificial ventilation with humidification
Renal Water Losses	
Diuretics	Renal failure
Osmotic diuresis (hyperglycemia, mannitol)	Inappropriate secretion of antidiuretic hormone
Congenital adrenal hyperplasia	Congestive heart failure

important because both excessive fluid restriction and overload lead to clinical consequences (Fig. 22–2). Excessive fluid restriction may lead to dehydration, hyperosmolality, hypoglycemia, and hyperbilirubinemia (Beard et al., 1963; Smallpiece & Davies, 1964; Wu et al., 1967). In preterm infants, high volumes of parenteral fluids have been associated with increased incidence of bronchopulmonary dysplasia (BPD), patent ductus arteriosus, and intraventricular hemorrhage (Bell et al., 1980; Palta et al., 1991; Papile et al., 1978). Close monitoring of clinical hydration, weight, urine output, and serum Na concentration should enable the best possible decisions on fluid administration.

Sodium

Na is the main extracellular ion, constituting with its salts more than 90 percent of the total amount of solutes in the extracellular space. Na is absorbed in both the small intestine and the colon, the largest amount being absorbed in the jejunum. Na absorption involves several mechanisms: (1) passive absorption, after glucose absorption, secondary to the flow of water; (2) active absorption, stimulated by glucose and amino acids; (3) active absorption, uncoupled with glucose, involving the Na-K pump; and (4) active absorption in exchange with hydrogen ions (H^+) (Fordtran, 1975). The overall process is very efficient: Adults normally absorb 98 percent of ingested Na.

Na is excreted by the kidney; it is filtered by glomeruli and reabsorbed throughout the tubules and the collecting ducts. Most of the Na is absorbed with chloride (Cl), but small amounts are absorbed in exchange with K^+ or H^+. Under normal circumstances, 96 to 99 percent of filtered Na is reabsorbed (Ganong, 1993; Spitzer, 1982). The main factors involved in the regulation of Na reabsorption are the oncotic and hydrostatic pressure in the peritubular capillaries and the action of the hormone aldosterone, which increases the absorption of Na in exchange with K^+ or H^+. Although antidiuretic hormone does not affect Na excretion directly, it can influence serum Na concentration indirectly, inasmuch as it regulates the excretion or the reabsorption of free water.

The Na concentration in human milk is 12 to 20 mEq/L (12 to 20 mmol/L) (Aperia et al., 1979). The current recommendation for standard formulas is 6 to 17 mEq/L (6 to 17 mmol/L), whereas preterm formulas provide about 2.5 to 3.5 mEq/kg/day (2.5 to 3.5 mmol/kg/day). Because of high urinary loss of Na, VLBW infants (<1500 g) may temporarily require up to 4 to 8 mEq/kg/day (4 to 8 mmol/kg/day) in the first week of life (American Academy of Pediatrics, Committee on Nutrition, 1985). Thereafter, the urinary losses are markedly reduced. Normal serum concentrations range between 130 and 150 mEq/L (130 and 150 mmol/L). Disorders of Na balance are summarized in Table 22–3.

Hyponatremia

Hyponatremia (serum Na < 130 mEq/L, or < 130 mmol/L) is caused by retention of water relative to Na. When serum Na concentration and, therefore, serum osmolality decrease, water moves into cells. The increased water content in the brain causes the symptoms and signs of hyponatremia. Vomiting, lethargy, and apnea may occur with various degrees of hyponatremia, but seizures and coma do not usually occur unless serum Na concentration is less than 115 mEq/L (<115 mmol/L) (Arieff & Guisado, 1976). Neonatal hyponatremia is usually classified by the timing of the occurrence into early and late hyponatremia.

Early Hyponatremia

Early hyponatremia often occurs in the first 2 days of life and results from extrinsic perinatal factors. It is not influenced by parenteral administration of additional Na and water.

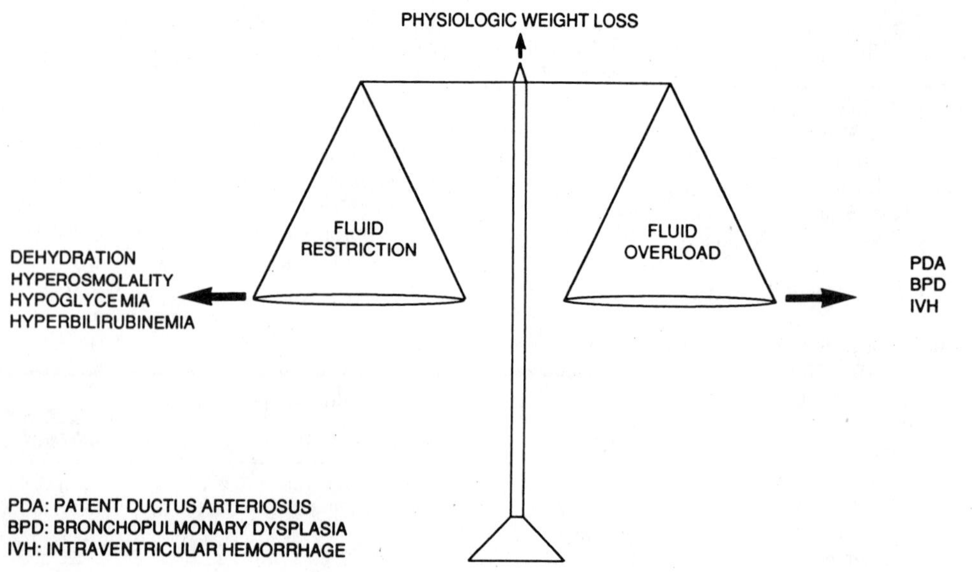

FIGURE 22–2. Risks of fluid administration.

TABLE 22–3 Disorders of Sodium Balance

Hyponatremia
Early
Perinatal asphyxia
Respiratory distress syndrome
Diuretics
Nebulization associated with nasal continuous positive airway pressure
Hypotonic fluid to mother during labor
Late
Very low birth weight infants fed human milk/standard formula
With overhydration: congestive heart failure, renal failure
With dehydration: adrenal insufficiency, vomiting, diarrhea, peritonitis
Hypernatremia
With dehydration
Vomiting, diarrhea with inadequate fluid replacement
Osmotic diuresis (hyperglycemia, mannitol)
Radiant warmers
"Hyperosmolar state" in infants <800 g
With overhydration
Excessive administration of $NaHCO_3$
Errors in administration of NaCl

The most common cause is perinatal asphyxia. The mechanism is a decreased excretion of free water, which is apparently caused by an increased secretion of antidiuretic hormone (syndrome of inappropriate antidiuretic hormone [SIADH]) and to an impairment of renal function by hypoxia (Weinberg et al., 1977). Severe respiratory distress syndrome (RDS) also predisposes newborns to hyponatremia, probably for the same reasons (Guignard et al., 1976), and diuresis precedes the resolution of the acute phase of RDS.

Iatrogenic causes of early hyponatremia include administration of large volumes of hypotonic fluid to the mother during labor; nebulization with nasal continuous positive airway pressure, resulting in water intoxication (Rosenfeld et al., 1976); and use of diuretics with excessive free water replacement (Savage et al., 1975). Infants with early hyponatremia are usually in a state of excess water, and fluid restriction is the appropriate treatment.

Late Hyponatremia

The most common form of late hyponatremia is typically seen after the first week of life in growing VLBW infants fed either human milk or standard proprietary formulas (Day et al., 1976; Engelke et al., 1978). These infants have a negative Na balance in the first weeks of life owing to a combination of factors, including an inadequate Na intake, a small surface of reabsorption in renal tubules, and a temporary unresponsiveness of renal tubules to aldosterone (Aperia et al., 1985). Whereas preterm infants heavier than 1500 g usually require 2 to 3 mEq/kg/day (2 to 3 mmol/kg/day) of Na, the daily requirements of VLBW infants to obtain a positive Na balance may initially be as high as 4 to 8 mEq/kg/day (4 to 8 mmol/kg/day). Spontaneous improvement in Na balance in several weeks is the rule. At any time, neonatal hyponatremia may occur in association with overhydration (dilutional hyponatremia) or dehydration (true hyponatremia).

Hyponatremia with overhydration may occur in newborns with congestive heart failure (congenital heart disease, patent ductus arteriosus), renal failure, or SIADH. Because total body Na is increased but TBW is even more increased, the administration of Na would only cause an additional expansion of the extracellular space, which can aggravate the infant's condition.

Hyponatremia with dehydration can be caused by either renal or extrarenal Na and water losses. Renal losses usually result from adrenal insufficiency (salt-losing type of congenital adrenal hyperplasia, adrenal hemorrhage), although infants with urinary tract obstruction may have similar electrolyte disorders. Extrarenal losses may result from disorders such as vomiting, diarrhea, and peritonitis. Treatment is directed both at the underlying disorder and at volume replacement with NaCl-containing solutions. The amount of Na needed to correct low serum Na level can be calculated according to the following formula:

$$\text{Na to be given (mEq/mmol)} = 0.6 \times \text{weight (kg)} \times (\text{desired serum Na} - \text{actual serum Na})$$

Usually, the correction is given over several hours, and the target is a serum Na concentration of about 135 mEq/L (135 mmol/L). However, there are two important exceptions to this general rule: (1) If shock is present or impending, normal saline should be given rapidly at 10 to 20 ml/kg intravenously over 20 to 30 minutes and repeated until arterial blood pressure is normalized; and (2) in symptomatic hyponatremia (which almost always occurs only when serum Na < 115 mEq/L, or < 115 mmol/L), hypertonic saline should be infused. However, because an abrupt or large increase in osmolality carries the risk of intracranial hemorrhage and congestive heart failure (CHF), the aim of the initial correction in this case should be a serum Na concentration of 120 to 125 mEq/L (120 to 125 mmol/L) (Perkin & Levin, 1980).

Hypernatremia

Hypernatremia (serum Na > 150 mEq/L, or > 150 mmol/L) is an increase in Na serum concentration. It may be accompanied by dehydration or, rarely, overhydration. Hypernatremia with dehydration is caused by an insufficient intake of water, by increased renal or extrarenal water losses, or by a combination of both. Hypernatremia with overhydration is usually of iatrogenic origin.

When hypernatremia and, therefore, hyperosmolality develop, water moves out of the cells into the extracellular space to achieve an osmotic equilibrium between intracellular and extracellular fluid. This attempt to equilibrate results in volume depletion of intracellular space. Brain cells can protect themselves, maintaining their intracellular volume by generating new solutes or idiogenic osmoles (Feig & McCurdy, 1977). Idiogenic osmoles are amino acids, polyols, and trimethylamines synthesized by the brain as a protective response to serum hyperosmolality. Idiogenic osmoles are neither produced nor catabolized rapidly. Therefore, this mechanism is effective within certain limits and only if hyperosmolality does not develop too rapidly. Similarly, corrections of hypernatremia with hypotonic solutions should not be performed rapidly, because idiogenic osmoles probably cannot be metabolized quickly and cerebral edema can occur because of movement of water into brain cells.

In VLBW infants, Na restriction during the first 3 to 5 days of life (no Na other than with transfusions) may prevent the occurrence of hypernatremia and decrease the need for parenteral fluid (Costarino et al., 1992).

Hypernatremia With Dehydration

Hypernatremia with dehydration results from water losses with inadequate replacement fluids. Water losses may occur from the gastrointestinal tract (vomiting, diarrhea). Inadequate replacement of fluids may include failure of appropriate water intake, especially when compounded by administration of high-solute fluids. Renal water losses may occur when an increased amount of solute, such as glucose or mannitol, must be excreted (osmotic diuresis). Significant insensible water losses through the skin occur when infants are placed under radiant warmers; the magnitude of these losses is inversely related to gestational age.

The correction of hypernatremia with dehydration must be carried out slowly, since cerebral edema can easily develop. Intravascular volume should be restored quickly with isotonic fluids, whereas water deficits should be corrected slowly and with great caution by administration of hypotonic fluids (Finberg, 1973).

Baumgart and colleagues (1982) and Gruskay and associates (1988) described a hyperosmolar state that occurs in the first days of life in infants of less than 800 g and less than 26 weeks' gestation. The immature skin and the large surface area cause massive evaporative losses of free water. This loss of free water results in a significant dehydration (weight loss ≥ 20 percent in the first 48 hours) accompanied by hypernatremia, hyperkalemia, and hyperglycemia, without oliguria. The correction of this hyperosmolar state, once fully established, involves the risk of volume overload. The suggested strategy to prevent this syndrome includes: (1) reduction of insensible water losses through the skin (using an incubator instead of an overhead warmer, with or without a plastic shield or a Saran wrap blanket); (2) frequent monitoring of weight, urine output, serum Na, and glucose concentrations; and (3) Na restriction and the administration of the least volume of fluids to maintain serum Na concentration within normal limits (initial rate 80 to 100 ml/kg/day with subsequent increases, usually without exceeding 150 ml/kg/day) (Costarino & Baumgart, 1986).

Hypernatremia With Overhydration

Hypernatremia with overhydration is almost always iatrogenic. It may occur after administration of sodium bicarbonate during cardiopulmonary resuscitation, acidosis, or RDS or because of accidental errors in the administration of NaCl with fluids. Because Na administration increases serum osmolality, it results in a shift of water into the intravascular space. An acute expansion of plasma volume may result in intracranial bleeding and heart failure with pulmonary edema. Treatment includes restriction of Na intake and diuretic therapy.

Potassium

Potassium (K) is the main intracellular cation. Its concentration within cells is maintained by the membrane Na^+,K^+-ATPase pump. Since potassium is involved in the regulation of cell membrane potential, variations in serum potassium concentrations have important effects. Although every cell is susceptible to fluctuations in serum potassium concentrations, the effects on myocardial cells are the most prominent and severe.

Dietary potassium is mainly absorbed in the jejunum by passive absorption, and it is actively secreted in the colon (Turnberg, 1971b). Potassium is excreted by the kidney. Probably all filtered potassium is reabsorbed in the proximal tubule. Potassium is then secreted by the distal tubules in exchange with Na in a process regulated by aldosterone. The amount of secreted potassium is normally proportional to the intake so that balance is maintained (Ganong, 1993).

The potassium requirement for both preterm and full-term infants is 2 to 3 mEq/kg/day (2 to 3 mmol/kg/day). The current recommendation for infant formulas is 14 to 34 mEq/L (14 to 34 mmol/L) (American Academy of Pediatrics, Committee on Nutrition, 1985). Normal serum concentrations are 3.5 to 5.0 mEq/L (3.5 to 5.0 mmol/L). Disorders of potassium balance are summarized in Table 22–4.

TABLE 22–4 Disorders of Potassium Balance

Hypokalemia
Inadequate intake
Gastrointestinal losses: vomiting, diarrhea, continuous gastric aspiration
Renal losses: diuretics, steroids, renal tubular acidosis
Hyperkalemia
Excessive intake
Impaired excretion: renal failure, congenital adrenal hyperplasia
Movement of potassium out of cells: catabolic states, acidosis

Hypokalemia

Hypokalemia (serum potassium < 3.5 mEq/L, or < 3.5 mmol/L) can result from inadequate intake, gastrointestinal losses (diarrhea, vomiting, continuous aspiration, and removal of gastrointestinal contents), and renal losses (diuretics, steroid therapy, renal tubular acidosis, Bartter's syndrome).

The consequences of hypokalemia are related to the effects on muscle cells. Although abdominal distention and decreased bowel motility may occur, cardiac effects are of much more concern, and an electrocardiogram (ECG) may be a better measure of serious toxicity than is serum potassium concentration. ECG changes include depression of the ST segment, flattening of the T wave, and increased height of the U wave. Prolongation of the P-R interval, widening of the QRS complex, and various arrhythmias may follow, particularly in newborns treated with digoxin (Surawicz, 1967).

Treatment is potassium replacement: potassium chloride should be given very slowly (<0.3 mEq/kg/hour, or <0.3 mmol/kg/hour), and serum potassium concentration or ECG, or both, should be checked frequently (Rose, 1977). Rapid intravenous potassium administration may cause fatal arrhythmias.

Hyperkalemia

Hyperkalemia (usually defined as serum potassium > 6.5 mEq/L, or > 6.5 mmol/L) can be caused by excessive intake, impaired excretion (renal failure, salt-losing congenital adrenal hyperplasia), and increased movement of potassium from intracellular to extracellular space (catabolic states, acidosis of any origin). Spurious hyperkalemia, caused by venipuncture (injury to red blood cells), must be ruled out. Hyperkalemia occurs in approximately 50 percent of infants with birth weight less than 1000 grams and especially in infants with low urine output in the first hours of life (Shaffer et al., 1992). The proposed mechanism is an increased potassium flow from the intracellular to the extracellular compartment, resulting from a decreased activity of Na^+,K^+-ATPase (Stefano et al., 1993), whereas increased catabolism does not seem to play a role (Stefano & Norman, 1993). Cardiac toxicity is the main issue and is better reflected by ECG changes than by serum potassium concentrations. The typical sequence is as follows: peaked T waves, disappearance of P waves, and widening of QRS complex and its fusion with the T wave to form a sine wave. Ventricular fibrillation may follow.

While treatment is being directed at the underlying disorder, several temporary measures can be taken: (1) 10 percent calcium gluconate, 1 ml/kg intravenously (to antagonize the effect of hyperkalemia on cell membranes); (2) sodium bicarbonate, 1 to 2 mEq/kg intravenously (to increase potassium influx into cells); (3) infusion of glucose and insulin at a ratio of 4 g of glucose to 1 unit of insulin (to increase cellular uptake of potassium); (4) intravenous furosemide, 1 mg/kg (to increase renal excretion); and (5) potassium-binding resin, Kayexalate, 1 g/kg per rectum or per os (to increase intestinal excretion) (Perkin & Levin, 1980). All these measures are temporary; if serum potassium concentration continues to increase and exceeds 8 mEq/L (8 mmol/L), peritoneal dialysis or exchange blood transfusions using fresh blood or a mixture of washed red blood cells and fresh-frozen plasma (to avoid high blood potassium) should be instituted.

Chloride

Chloride (Cl) is the main inorganic anion in the extracellular fluid and, together with Na, is essential for maintenance of plasma volume. Cl is administered as NaCl in the diet. Intestinal absorption is passive in the jejunum and secondary to Na absorption. In the ileum and colon, Cl is actively absorbed in exchange with bicarbonate. Normally, only minimal amounts of Cl are lost in the feces (Turnberg et al., 1970). Cl is excreted by the kidneys. Like Na, Cl is filtered by the glomeruli and reabsorbed throughout the tubules and collecting ducts. Three mechanisms of reabsorption have been described: passive diffusion, cotransport with Na, and exchange with OH^-. Normally, 99 percent of the filtered Cl is reabsorbed (Ganong, 1993).

Cl reabsorption is inversely related to bicarbonate reabsorption. Serum concentrations of Cl and bicarbonate are also inversely correlated, keeping the total anion concentration ($Cl^- + HCO_3^-$) constant. For this reason, although Cl has no buffer effect, it plays an important part in acid–base regulation. When Cl is retained in the body, serum bicarbonate decreases and metabolic acidosis follows. When Cl is lost from the body, serum bicarbonate increases and metabolic alkalosis ensues. Current recommendations for infant formulas are 11 to 29 mEq/100 kcal (11 to 29 mmol/100 kcal). Normal serum concentrations are 90 to 112 mEq/L (90 to 112 mmol/L) in full-term infants and 100 to 115 mEq/L (100 to 115 mmol/L) in preterm infants. Disorders of Cl balance are summarized in Table 22–5.

Hypochloremia

Hypochloremia (serum Cl < 90 mEq/L, or < 90 mmol/L) may be caused by decreased intake or by increased losses of Cl (gastrointestinal or renal). Clinical manifestations include metabolic alkalosis, hypokalemia, and, in the case of a chronic disturbance, failure to thrive.

Decreased intake has occurred with soy formulas with Cl contents that were very low (Anderson et al., 1982). The diagnosis is based on the dietary history and on the absence of urinary Cl, indicating a normal ability to retain Cl to compensate for the low intake. Increased gastrointestinal losses of Cl, as HCl, may be caused by prolonged vomiting (pyloric stenosis) or continuous aspiration and removal of gastric content (necrotizing enterocolitis, abdominal surgery).

Congenital chloridorrhea is a rare disorder of severe diarrhea, beginning at birth, caused by an impairment of the active Cl transport system in the ileum and colon. Analysis of feces demonstrates an acid pH and a greatly increased Cl concentration. Diarrhea is caused by the osmotic purgative effect of excess Cl, and hypokalemia ensues as a secondary consequence of diarrhea. Treatment includes a diet low in NaCl, with potassium supplement (Turnberg, 1971a). The most common cause of increased renal losses of Cl is diuretic therapy. Frequent indications for this treatment in infancy are congestive heart failure and, especially, BPD.

TABLE 22–5 Disorders of Chloride Balance

Hypochloremia
Decreased intake: some soy formulas
Increased gastrointestinal losses: vomiting (pyloric stenosis), continuous gastric aspiration, congenital chloridorrhea
Increased renal losses: diuretics, Bartter's syndrome

Hyperchloremia
Increased bicarbonate losses: renal tubular acidosis
Excessive administration of NaCl: absolute, relative (renal failure)
Hypertonic dehydration (apparent hyperchloremia)

Chronic administration of furosemide is often necessary in BPD and may cause Cl deficiency with secondary metabolic alkalosis. Alkalosis, in turn, causes hypoventilation and increased arterial carbon dioxide pressure ($Paco_2$). This clinical picture can simulate pulmonary edema, but in this case the treatment should include not additional diuretic therapy (as in pulmonary edema), but rather correction of the hypochloremia (Blanchard et al., 1987).

Increased renal loss of Cl is the characteristic feature of Bartter's syndrome, whose underlying mechanism is a defect in tubular reabsorption of Cl. Increased urinary Cl and prostaglandin concentrations are diagnostic, and therapy with indomethacin (a prostaglandin antagonist) is usually effective (Bartter, 1980).

Hyperchloremia

Hyperchloremia (serum Cl > 115 mEq/L, or > 115 mmol/L) is usually associated with metabolic acidosis and can be caused by either bicarbonate depletion or excessive Cl intake. Diarrhea is the most common cause of hyperchloremic metabolic acidosis, because in the intestine Cl is absorbed together with Na, and bicarbonate is excreted with potassium. Increased losses of bicarbonate occur with renal tubular acidosis. The proximal type is usually diagnosed in the neonatal period and occurs mainly in male infants (Spitzer et al., 1992). A decreased renal threshold for bicarbonate and a failure to decrease the acid level of the urine occur in this condition and result in a hyperchloremic metabolic acidosis. This condition is self-limited, and the diagnosis is based on the demonstration that (1) the renal bicarbonate threshold is lower than normal and (2) when serum bicarbonate concentrations are lower than the threshold, bicarbonate is retained and acid urine is produced.

Hyperchloremia may follow an excessive administration of NaCl. Overtreatment with NaCl may be absolute, as in accidental errors in administration, or relative, as in renal failure. In the latter case, excretion is impaired and can be exceeded by an otherwise "normal" intake; NaCl administration must therefore be reduced accordingly. Finally, apparent hyperchloremia together with increased serum concentration of other electrolytes can occur with dehydration when there is a water deficit in relation to solute.

Calcium and Phosphorus

Calcium (Ca) is the most abundant mineral in the human body. It is an essential component of the skeleton and plays an important role in muscle contraction, neural transmission, and blood coagulation. Phosphorus (P) is essential for bone mineralization, erythrocyte function, cell metabolism, and the generation and storage of energy.

In human milk, the Ca content is about 39 mg/100 kcal (0.97 mmol/100 kcal), and the P content is about 19 mg/100 kcal (0.61 mmol/100 kcal). Current recommendations for standard formulas are 50 mg (1.25 mmol) of Ca per 100 kcal and 25 mg (0.80 mmol) of P per 100 kcal. In preterm formulas, Ca concentrations range between 75 and 144 mg/dl (18.7 and 35.9 mmol/L) and P concentrations range between 40 and 72 mg/dl (12.9 and 23.2 mmol/L) (American Academy of Pediatrics, Committee on Nutrition, 1985).

Calcium

Ca transport in the intestine occurs by both passive and active processes (Greer & Tsang, 1985; Kalser, 1985b; Kimberg, 1969). An important prerequisite for intestinal absorption is the ionization of Ca compounds, such as Ca caseinate and phosphate; ionization requires an acid pH and takes place in the stomach.

Active intestinal transport involves carriers named Ca-binding proteins. Vitamin D in its active form, 1,25-dihydroxyvitamin D, is essential for the active process. Parathyroid hormone is involved only through stimulation of production of 1,25-dihydroxyvitamin D. Vitamin D deficiency and almost any form of intestinal malabsorption can impair Ca transport. Corticosteroids decrease Ca absorption by inhibiting its transfer in the intestinal mucosa. Anticonvulsants can directly inhibit intestinal transfer of Ca (phenytoin) or can interfere with vitamin D metabolism (phenobarbital and phenytoin) (Hahn, 1980).

Serum Ca concentration is maintained within narrow limits by the action of parathyroid hormone and 1,25-dihydroxyvitamin D, which increase serum Ca, and of calcitonin, which decreases serum Ca.

Ca is excreted by the kidneys; filtered Ca is reabsorbed in most segments of the tubules. Parathyroid hormone increases tubular reabsorption of Ca, whereas calcitonin is thought to increase Ca excretion. The current recommendation for enteral feedings is a daily intake of 120 to 230 mg/kg (3.0 to 5.75 mmol/kg). With regard to parenteral nutrition, a Ca intake of 60 to 90 mg/kg/day (1.5 to 2.25 mmol/kg/day) is currently recommended (Tsang et al., 1993). Ca concentration in the parenteral solution should be maintained between 500 to 600 mg/L (12.5 to 15.0 mmol/L) to avoid precipitation. Disorders of Ca balance are summarized in Table 22–6.

Hypocalcemia

Neonatal hypocalcemia is defined as an ionized serum Ca concentration of less than 4.4 mg/dl (1.10 mmol/L) in full-term infants. For preterm infants, in view of insufficient normative data on ionized Ca, a total serum Ca concentration of less than 7.0 mg/dL (1.75 mmol/L) continues to be a reasonable definition. Hypocalcemia is conventionally divided into early hypocalcemia, which occurs in the first 2 days of life, and late hypocalcemia, which occurs after the first 2 days, usually at about 1 week of age. Neonatal hypocalcemia may be asymptomatic or can cause symptoms such as irritability, tremors, poor feeding, muscle twitching, and seizures.

Early hypocalcemia is a relatively frequent event and is deemed to be caused by perinatal factors. Thirty percent of preterm infants (37 weeks' gestation) (Tsang & Oh, 1970), 35 percent of birth-asphyxiated infants (Tsang et al., 1974), 17 to 32 percent of infants of insulin-dependent diabetic mothers (Demarini et al., 1994), and 90 percent of VLBW infants (<1500 g) (Venkataramaran et al., 1986) develop hypocalcemia in the first days of life. Several factors appear to be involved: abrupt termination of maternal Ca supply, temporary functional hypoparathyroidism (in infants of diabetic mothers), increased calcitonin concentrations (in asphyxiated and preterm infants), and 1,25-dihydroxyvitamin D resistance (in VLBW infants).

TABLE 22–6 Disorders of Calcium Balance

Hypocalcemia
Early
Preterm infants
Infants of diabetic mothers
Perinatal asphyxia
Late
Cow's milk–based formulas
Hypomagnesemia
Hypoparathyroidism
Phototherapy
Maternal vitamin D deficiency
Hypercalcemia
Excessive administration of calcium and/or vitamin D
Subcutaneous fat necrosis
Williams syndrome
Idiopathic hypercalcemia

Late hypocalcemia typically occurs by the end of the first week of life and is caused by increased dietary phosphate load. It was relatively common with the use of evaporated cow's milk formulas, in which the phosphate content greatly exceeds that of human milk. With modern "adapted" formulas, whose P content is closer to that of human milk, late neonatal hypocalcemia has become much less common but has not disappeared (Venkataramaran et al., 1985). Maternal vitamin D deficiency may represent a predisposing factor (Roberts et al., 1973). Phototherapy appears to be an additional factor associated with neonatal hypocalcemia, especially in preterm infants (Mimouni & Tsang, 1992). The mechanism is incompletely understood.

Rarely, late hypocalcemia can also occur as a consequence of subclinical maternal hyperparathyroidism: maternal hypercalcemia leads to fetal hypercalcemia, which suppresses fetal parathyroid glands. After birth, when the maternal source of Ca is no longer available, the suppressed parathyroid glands are unable to maintain a normal serum Ca concentration. Because the maternal hyperparathyroidism is often asymptomatic, neonatal hypocalcemia may provide the initial clue to the maternal disease (Wilson et al., 1983). Another infrequent but serious condition that can cause symptomatic hypocalcemia is severe hypomagnesemia (see the section on magnesium).

The choice of treatment of neonatal hypocalcemia is complicated by several factors: (1) It may coexist with other perinatal complications, such as asphyxia and hypoglycemia, which can cause similar clinical signs (Brann & Schwartz, 1992); (2) it may be associated with seizures without being the cause of the seizures (Volpe, 1977); and (3) in most cases, it is an asymptomatic and self-limited condition (Scott et al., 1984).

If hypocalcemia is asymptomatic, 10 percent calcium gluconate (9.4 mg of elemental Ca/ml) may be given orally at a rate of 75 mg/kg/day divided into six equal doses per day. If hypocalcemia is symptomatic, 10 percent calcium gluconate must be given intravenously at a rate of 2 ml/kg over 10 minutes; the heart rate should be closely monitored and the infusion stopped immediately at the first sign of bradycardia.

Hypercalcemia

Hypercalcemic disorders (serum Ca > 11 mg/dl, or > 2.75 mmol/L) such as subcutaneous fat necrosis, Williams syndrome, congenital hyperparathyroidism, hyperprostaglandin E syndrome, and familial hypocalciuric hypercalcemia are exceedingly rare among newborns. Usually, hypercalcemia is of iatrogenic origin and results from excessive administration of Ca or vitamin D.

Signs and symptoms are nonspecific and include constipation, polyuria, and bradycardia. Nephrocalcinosis and nephrolithiasis caused by hypercalcemia can be worsened by dehydration and diuretics (DeCristofaro & Tsang, 1986). Treatment consists of suspension of Ca and vitamin D administration, promotion of urinary Ca excretion by fluid administration, and, in the case of vitamin D intoxication, glucocorticoids to decrease intestinal absorption and bone resorption of Ca.

Phosphorus

P is absorbed mainly in the jejunum by both active and passive diffusion. Absorption depends mainly on the absolute amount of P in the diet, on the relative concentrations of Ca and P (an excessive amount of either one can reduce the absorption of the other), and on the presence of substances that bind to P and

TABLE 22–7 Disorders of Phosphorus Balance

Hypophosphatemia
Rickets/osteopenia of prematurity
Inadequate parenteral phosphorus administration
Familial hypophosphatemias: vitamin D–resistant rickets, X-linked hypophosphatemia, Fanconi's syndrome

Hyperphosphatemia
Impaired excretion of phosphorus (renal failure)
Hypoparathyroidism
Excessive parenteral/enteral administration of phosphorus

make it unavailable for absorption (phytates in soy-based formulas) (Greer & Tsang, 1985; Koo & Tsang, 1988).

P is excreted by the kidneys; 10 to 15 percent of the filtered P is normally excreted. Parathyroid hormone directly influences P excretion through its phosphaturic effect. The current recommendation for enteral feedings is a daily intake of 60 to 140 mg/kg (1.9 to 4.5 mmol/kg). With regard to parenteral nutrition, a P intake of 47 to 70 mg/kg/day (1.5 to 2.25 mmol/kg/day) is currently recommended (Tsang et al., 1993). P concentration in the parenteral solution should be maintained between 390 and 470 mg/L (12.5 to 15.0 mmol/L) to avoid precipitation. Disorders of phosphorus balance are summarized in Table 22–7.

Hypophosphatemia

Hypophosphatemia (serum P $<$ 4 mg/dl, or $<$ 1.29 mmol/L) is a common feature in preterm infants with rickets of prematurity (Koo et al., 1984). Rickets is caused by insufficient intake of Ca and P (Steichen et al., 1980). Rickets of prematurity is frequent in VLBW infants fed regular formulas, especially human milk with low P content. Preterm formulas provide a higher intake of Ca and P and can result in bone mineralization similar to intrauterine bone mineralization (Greer & McCormick, 1988; Steichen et al., 1980). In very rare cases, hypophosphatemia is caused by neonatal hyperparathyroidism.

In infancy, hypophosphatemia can be caused by diseases of vitamin D metabolism (vitamin D–dependent rickets) or by disorders of renal P transport (familial hypophosphatemic rickets).

Severe hypophosphatemia (serum P $<$ 1.0 mg/dl, or $<$ 0.32 mmol/L) is uncommon and may occur only in newborns receiving parenteral alimentation with inadequate P administration. Respiratory failure, decreased myocardial performance, and neurologic abnormalities have been described as possible consequences of severe hypophosphatemia in adults (Lentz et al., 1978).

Hyperphosphatemia

Neonatal hyperphosphatemia (serum P $<$ 7.0 mg/dl, or 2.26 mmol/L) can be caused by ingestion of milk formulas containing high amounts of P, by excessive parenteral P administration, by impaired P excretion (renal failure), or by defects in hormonal regulation (hypoparathyroidism). Severe hyperphosphatemia may cause metastatic calcifications and hypocalcemia. Management includes alimentation with a low-P formula, such as Similac PM 60/40, and Ca supplementation to increase binding to P and its fecal excretion. Reduction of parenteral P intake usually resolves parenteral hyperphosphatemia. In renal failure, 1,25-dihydroxyvitamin D or dihydrotachysterol, whose actions are independent of functioning renal tissue, can be given to counteract hypocalcemia secondary to hyperphosphatemia.

Hypoparathyroidism from maternal hyperparathyroidism (transient hypoparathyroidism) and from DiGeorge's syndrome (permanent hypoparathyroidism, which includes aplasia of the thymus and parathyroid glands, T cell immunodeficiency, defects of the aortic arch, and peculiar facies) may be treated by 1,25-dihydroxyvitamin D and Ca supplementation.

Magnesium

Magnesium (Mg) is distributed primarily in the skeleton and the intracellular space. It is involved in energy production, cell membrane function, mitochondrial function, and protein synthesis.

Mg is absorbed by passive diffusion throughout the small intestine. Absorption is related to intake, and approximately 50 to 70 percent of the dietary Mg is absorbed (Moya & Domenech, 1982; Okamoto et al., 1982). Regulation of serum Mg concentration is performed mainly by the kidney; under normal circumstances, 3 to 5 percent of the filtered Mg is excreted. Parathyroid hormone increases serum Mg concentration, possibly through mobilization from bone. Whereas an acute decrease in serum Mg concentration increases parathyroid hormone secretion, a chronic Mg deficiency decreases secretion and therefore may cause hypocalcemia (Shaul et al., 1987). The Mg content of human milk is about 5 mg/100 kcal (0.21 mmol/100 kcal). The current recommendation for formulas is 6 mg/100 kcal (0.25 mmol/100 kcal) (American Academy of Pediatrics, Committee on Nutrition, 1985). A parenteral intake of 4.3 to 7.2 mg/kg/day (0.18 to 0.30 mmol/kg/day) is currently recommended (Tsang et al., 1993). Mg concentration in the parenteral solution should be maintained between 36 and 48 mg/L (1.5 to 2.0 mmol/L) to avoid precipitation. Disorders of Mg balance are summarized in Table 22–8.

Hypomagnesemia

Mg transfer from mother to fetus theoretically might be impaired in the presence of placental malfunction, and placental insufficiency appears to predispose the infant to neonatal hypomagnesemia (serum Mg $<$ 1.6 mg/dl, or $<$ 0.66 mmol/L). In infants of diabetic mothers, hypomagnesemia appears to be a consequence of maternal Mg depletion (Tsang et al., 1975). Any severe malabsorption syndrome can cause Mg deficiency (Kalser, 1985b), and an isolated defect in intestinal absorption of Mg has been described (Paunier et al., 1968).

Hypomagnesemia in the neonatal period is usually transient (except for the cases of malabsorption) and asymptomatic but can cause hyperexcitability (Nelson et al., 1987) and, occasionally, severe intractable hypocalcemic seizures that are unresponsive to Ca infusion and anticonvulsants (Turner et al., 1977). The mechanism for resultant hypocalcemia is a decreased secretion of parathyroid hormone caused by Mg depletion (Shaul et al., 1987). The treatment is 0.2 ml/kg of 50 percent magnesium sulfate given intramuscularly. This dose can be repeated, with monitoring of serum Mg concentration every 12 hours, until normomagnesemia is achieved.

TABLE 22–8 Disorders of Magnesium Balance

Hypomagnesemia
Infants of diabetic mothers
Infants small for gestational age
Malabsorption syndromes
Isolated intestinal magnesium malabsorption

Hypermagnesemia
Maternal treatment with magnesium sulfate for preeclampsia
Excessive magnesium administration with parenteral nutrition

Hypermagnesemia

Neonatal hypermagnesemia (serum Mg >2.8 mg/dl, or 1.15 mmol/L) is an iatrogenic event caused either by parenteral nutrition or, more commonly, by maternal treatment of preeclampsia with magnesium sulfate ($MgSO_4$). Other causes are administration of Mg-containing antacid for treatment of stress ulcers (Brand & Greer, 1990) and treatment of persistent pulmonary hypertension of the newborn with $MgSO_4$ (Abu-Osba et al., 1992). Reported symptoms and signs include hyporeflexia, lethargy, and respiratory depression (Lipsitz & English, 1967). However, with current treatment of preeclampsia, neonatal serum Mg concentrations generally do not rise to potentially dangerous levels and gradually return to normal after several days (Donovan et al., 1980; McGuinness et al., 1980). Hypermagnesemia does not cause hypocalcemia in the neonatal period and appears to be associated only with hypotonia. No treatment is usually necessary. In severe cases, exchange blood transfusion has been used to lower the elevated serum concentrations.

WATER-SOLUBLE VITAMINS

Thiamine (Vitamin B_1)

Thiamine is a necessary coenzyme in carbohydrate and amino acid metabolism. Intestinal absorption is both active and passive: The transport is active at physiologic concentrations and passive at pharmacologic concentrations. Thiamine is absorbed throughout the small intestine, but active transport is greatest in the duodenum (Kalser, 1985a). The vitamin is excreted by the kidneys, and urinary excretion varies according to dietary intake.

Thiamine content is about 30 μg/100 kcal (0.09 μmol/100 kcal) in human milk, about 100 μg/100 kcal (0.29 μmol/100 kcal) in regular formulas, and between 100 and 250 μg/100 kcal (0.29 to 0.74 μmol/100 kcal) in preterm formulas (Schanler, 1988). The American Academy of Pediatrics (1976) recommended a minimum content of 40 μg/100 kcal (0.12 μmol/419 kJ), whereas 150 to 200 μg/100 kcal (0.45 to 0.59 μmol/419 kJ) are currently recommended for preterm infants (Tsang et al., 1993).

Deficiency. Thiamine deficiency results in beriberi. Infantile beriberi occurs only in breastfed infants of thiamine-deficient mothers. Clinical signs become apparent after 1 to 4 months and include aphonia, cardiac signs (dyspnea and cyanosis), and neurologic signs (bulging fontanelle and seizures). Thiamine deficiency can be determined from reduced activity of the erythrocyte enzyme transketolase or by measurement of whole blood thiamine concentration.

Toxicity. Thiamine toxicity has not been reported for oral administration and is very rare in parenteral administration; very large intravenous doses of thiamine have caused anaphylaxis and respiratory depression (Goodhart & Shils, 1980).

Riboflavin (Vitamin B_2)

As part of the coenzymes flavin adenine dinucleotide (FAD) and flavin mononucleotide (FMN), riboflavin is involved in electron transport and is essential in glucose, amino acid, and lipid metabolism. Riboflavin is absorbed in the proximal part of the small intestine, and amounts in excess of needs are excreted unchanged in the urine (Schanler, 1988). The average content of riboflavin (vitamin B_2) in human milk is approximately 50 to 60 μg/100 kcal (0.13 to 0.16 μmol/100 kcal) and about 150 μg/100 kcal (0.40 μmol/100 kcal) in milk formulas. The American Academy of Pediatrics, Committee on Nutrition (1976), recommends 60 μg/100 kcal (0.16 μmol/419 kJ), whereas 200 to 300 μg/100 kcal (0.53 to 0.80 μmol/419 kJ) are currently recommended for preterm infants (Tsang et al., 1993). Riboflavin 5-phosphate (FMN) is more resistant to light and is the form used for parenteral nutrition.

Deficiency. Riboflavin deficiency results in epithelial abnormalities (stomatitis, cheilosis, glossitis, seborrheic dermatitis), normocytic anemia, and vascularization of the cornea. Transient biochemical deficiency, without clinical signs, has been reported in full-term infants fed human milk (Hovi et al., 1979); riboflavin supplementation, however, is not recommended in full-term, human milk–fed infants. Riboflavin intake does not seem to be sufficient in preterm infants fed human milk (Ronnholm, 1986). Although the clinical significance of this deficiency is unclear, at present a supplementation of 0.9 μmol/100 kcal (or 1.1 to 1.3 μmol/day) may be reasonable.

In spite of riboflavin's inactivation by light, clinical riboflavin deficiency during phototherapy has not been reported. If riboflavin supplementation is to be given, it should probably not be administered during phototherapy, but rather after its completion; mutational changes in cellular DNA structure induced by photodynamic alteration of riboflavin have been demonstrated in vitro (Pascale et al., 1976).

Toxicity. Toxic effects have not been reported. Some concern remains for preterm infants, since renal clearance of the vitamin may be inadequate and deposition of riboflavin crystals in kidneys has been observed in animals (Christensen, 1971).

Vitamin B_6

Vitamin B_6 is the generic term used to describe three substances: pyridoxine, pyridoxal, and pyridoxamine. The metabolic functions of these vitamins include the synthesis of neurotransmitters, heme, and prostaglandins and the interconversion of amino acids (Schanler, 1988). Absorption occurs in the proximal small intestine by passive diffusion.

The vitamin content in human milk depends on the maternal nutritional status: the concentration of vitamin B_6 in human milk ranges between 9 and 79 μg/100 kcal (0.05 and 0.47 μmol/100 kcal), according to the maternal intake of the vitamin (Styslinger & Kirksey, 1985; West & Kirksey, 1976). The American Academy of Pediatrics, Committee on Nutrition (1976, 1985), recommends 60 μg/100 kcal (0.35 μmol/419 kJ) for standard formulas, whereas 125 to 175 μg/100 kcal (0.61 to 0.85 μmol/419 kJ) are currently recommended for preterm infants (Tsang et al., 1993). Vitamin B_6 is inactivated by light. Pyridoxal and pyridoxamine are heat labile, whereas pyridoxine is heat stable.

Deficiency. Vitamin B_6 deficiency can result from severe malabsorption and dietary deprivation (human milk with low vitamin B_6 content, goat's milk). Signs and symptoms include microcytic anemia, failure to thrive, irritability, and seizures (Schanler, 1988).

Isoniazid binds to and inactivates vitamin B_6; therefore, infants receiving this drug may need vitamin B_6 supplementation (Moran & Greene, 1979). Neonatal pyridoxine-dependent seizures are caused by a congenital abnormality of vitamin B_6 metabolism, and pharmacologic doses of vitamin B_6 are needed.

Toxicity. A sensory neuropathy has been described in adults taking extremely large doses (Schaumburg et al., 1983).

Cyanocobalamin (Vitamin B_{12})

Vitamin B_{12} is essential in the synthesis of DNA nucleotides and in carbohydrate and lipid metabolism. It can be synthesized only by microorganisms and is absent in plants. Absorption of vitamin B_{12} takes place in the distal third of the ileum and requires the presence of intrinsic factor, a glycoprotein secreted by the stomach. In plasma, the vitamin is transported by a specific protein (transcobalamin II); vitamin B_{12} is stored in the liver. Human milk provides approximately 0.3 μg/day (0.22 nmol/day) (Ek, 1985), and 0.15 μg/100 kcal (0.11 nmol/100 kcal) is the current recommendation for formulas (American Academy of Pediatrics, Committee on Nutrition, 1976, 1985).

Deficiency. Vitamin B_{12} deficiency causes hematologic changes (megaloblastic anemia, thrombocytopenia, leukopenia) and neurologic changes (demyelination) of the spinal cord and mental retardation). Neurologic manifestations may precede anemia. At birth, liver stores are very large and usually sufficient for most of the first year of life (Ek, 1985). Therefore, vitamin B_{12} deficiency rarely develops in infancy.

Nutritional deficiency occurs exclusively in infants fed breast milk from strictly vegetarian mothers and has been described as early as 4 months of age (Lampkin et al., 1966). Deficiency can develop in infants with short bowel syndrome, if terminal ileum (the site of absorption) is resected. The onset of vitamin B_{12} deficiency from intrinsic factor deficiency occurs at about 6 months of age. Congenital transcobalamin II deficiency is a rare but important cause of vitamin B_{12} deficiency, inasmuch as signs can occur after only 6 weeks of life and mental retardation is invariably present (Kalser, 1985a). Because both folic acid and vitamin B_{12} deficiency can cause megaloblastic anemia, and because folic acid can interfere with vitamin B_{12} metabolism, the differential diagnosis becomes important. A large folate intake may mask vitamin B_{12} deficiency and can aggravate the neurologic damage (Dallman, 1988). vitamin B_{12} and folate supplementation may reduce the severity of anemia of prematurity (Worthington-White et al., 1994).

Toxicity. Toxicity from vitamin B_{12} has not been reported.

Folic Acid

Folic acid is essential for the synthesis of nucleic acids and for the metabolism of some amino acids. Maximum absorption of folic acid takes place in the proximal jejunum. Absorption is active with physiologic doses of folic acid and mainly passive with pharmacologic doses. Folic acid is stored in the liver in small amounts, so deficiency can develop within weeks (Dallman, 1988; Ek, 1985; Kalser, 1985a).

Folic acid concentration is approximately 50 to 60 μg/L (113 to 135 nmol/L) in human milk (Ek, 1983) and about 160 μg/L (362 nmol/L) in formulas. Heat treatment decreases the folic acid concentration in milk. The current recommendation for standard formulas is 4 μg/100 kcal (9 nmol/100 kcal). For preterm infants, 21 to 42 μg/100 kcal (48 to 95 nmol/419 kJ) are recommended at present (Tsang et al., 1993).

Deficiency. Signs of deficiency include hypersegmentation of neutrophils, megaloblastic anemia, poor growth, irritability, and hypotonia. Neurologic disorders such as seizures and mental retardation are seen only in the congenital isolated defect of folic acid absorption (Poncz et al., 1981). Folic acid deficiency may be associated with prematurity (rapid growth and decreased hepatic stores), hemolytic disease of the newborn (increased erythropoiesis), anticonvulsant therapy (interference with absorption), prolonged antibiotic therapy (decreased production from intestinal bacterial flora), and any malabsorption syndrome. Folic acid and vitamin B_{12} supplementation may ameliorate anemia or prematurity (Worthington-White et al., 1994).

Toxicity. There are no reports on toxic effects of folic acid in infancy. However, at least theoretically, extremely large oral doses of folic acid may partially reverse the effects of anticonvulsants (Reynolds, 1968).

Ascorbic Acid (Vitamin C)

Vitamin C is required for collagen synthesis, for normal function of osteoblasts and fibroblasts, and for metabolism of some amino acids. Ascorbic acid is actively absorbed in the small intestine. A feedback mechanism apparently regulates the absorption of vitamin C, according to studies measuring serum vitamin C concentration. Very large doses of the vitamin appear to result in decreased efficiency of intestinal absorption of vitamin C and render affected persons prone to rebound deficiency once intake decreases. Vitamin C is excreted by the kidney either unchanged or as oxalic acid. Vitamin C concentration is about 8 mg/100 kcal (45 μmol/100 kcal) in both human milk (Byerley & Kirksey, 1985) and standard formulas, whereas in preterm formulas it ranges between 8.6 and 37 mg/100 kcal (49 and 210 μmol/100 kcal). The American Academy of Pediatrics, Committee on Nutrition (1976, 1985), currently recommends a minimum intake of 8 mg/100 kcal or 35 mg/day (45 μmol/100 kcal or 199 μmol/419 kJ) (Tsang et al., 1993). Heat treatment of milk significantly decreases vitamin C content. Pasteurization of banked human milk decreases its content of vitamin C (Ford, 1977).

Deficiency. Vitamin C deficiency is very rare but can occur in infants fed pasteurized, unsupplemented cow's milk or vitamin C–deficient breast milk. Vitamin C deficiency is associated with transient tyrosinemia and neonatal scurvy.

Transient tyrosinemia results from a partial enzymatic deficiency, which causes an elevation in serum concentration of the amino acid tyrosine. The enzymatic activity increases and tyrosine concentration decreases with vitamin C administration. Transient tyrosinemia is a common event, occurring in as many as 10 percent of full-term infants and 30 percent of preterm infants during the first week of life (Pereira & Zucker, 1986). The amount of dietary tyrosine also plays a role, inasmuch as both a high intake of protein and the use of casein-predominant formulas can increase serum tyrosine concentrations. In view of their frequency, it seems unlikely that these transiently elevated concentrations could be regarded as abnormal. However, in preterm infants, this transient disorder has been associated with mild mental impairment later in life (Menkes et al., 1972). Neonatal scurvy is very rare and is characterized by hemorrhages in the skin, subperiosteal spaces, and costochondral cartilage; by anemia resulting from decreased iron absorption; and by failure to thrive.

Toxicity. Large doses of vitamin C may decrease vitamin B_{12} absorption, increase iron absorption, and increase the incidence of nephrolithiasis in congenital disorders such as oxalosis and cystinuria (Schanler, 1988). In spite of regular intake, discontinuation of extremely large doses of vitamin C can lead rapidly to deficiency, caused apparently by a continuous "conditioned" need for high doses of the vitamin (Levine, 1986).

Niacin (Vitamin B_3)

Niacin includes both nicotinic acid and its amide, nicotinamide. As components of the coenzymes nicotinamide adenine dinucleotide (NAD) and nicotinamide adenine dinucleotide phosphate (NADP), niacin is involved in mitochondrial electron transport, lipid synthesis, and glycolysis.

Because niacin can also derive from the amino acid tryptophan, dietary intake of both niacin and tryptophan is evaluated to calculate niacin requirements. Therefore, it is customary to use niacin equivalents (1 mg of niacin = 1 niacin equivalent = 60 mg of tryptophan) (Goldsmith, 1975).

The concentration of niacin in human milk is 0.8 niacin equivalents/100 kcal, and this is the recommendation of the American Academy of Pediatrics, Committee on Nutrition (1985). For preterm infants, 3 to 4 mg/100 kcal (25 to 33 μmol/419 kJ) are currently recommended (Tsang et al., 1993). Heating and storage do not significantly affect niacin content in milk.

Deficiency. Pellagra (rough skin) is the consequence of niacin deficiency. Signs include dermatitis and inflammation of the mucous membranes, diarrhea, and dementia.

Toxicity. Toxicity is related to the portion of a component of niacin (nicotinic acid) and may include cutaneous vasodilatation, arrhythmias, and increased intestinal motility and acid gastric secretion.

FAT-SOLUBLE VITAMINS

Vitamin A

Vitamin A exists in many isomeric forms: the basic and most active component is all-*trans* retinol. Vitamin A can be administered in different forms (retinol itself, palmitate esters of retinol, provitamins) and in different units (micrograms, international units [IU]). Vitamin A activity is usually defined as the equivalent weight of retinol (retinol equivalent [RE]). One RE is equal to 1 μg or 3.33 IU of retinol and to 6 μg or 10 IU of the provitamin beta carotene. Placental transfer of the vitamin appears to be limited, and hepatic retinol stores are low at birth. Dietary retinol is absorbed in the proximal intestine; under normal circumstances, about 50 percent is absorbed. Retinol is incorporated into chylomicrons and transported to the liver, where it is stored. From the liver, retinol is released into the circulation according to the needs and is transported in plasma bound to retinol-binding protein and delivered to tissues. Retinol facilitates the visual process in rod cells of the retina and plays a role in regulation and differentiation of epithelial cells (Zachman, 1988).

During parenteral nutrition, a considerable amount of retinol is lost in the delivery set. Loss during infusion can be corrected by (1) adding vitamin A to intravenous lipids (Werkman et al., 1994) or (2) infusing the daily dose of multivitamin preparation over 6 hours, as opposed to 24 hours (Inder et al., 1995).

Retinol concentration in human milk is approximately 50 μg/dl (1.74 μmol/L). The American Academy of Pediatrics, Committee on Nutrition (1985), recommends 75 RE/100 kcal for formulas. For preterm infants the current recommendation is 583 to 1250 IU/100 kcal. An intake of 1250 to 2333 IU/100 kcal is recommended in infants with chronic lung disease (Tsang et al., 1993).

Deficiency. The classic signs of vitamin A deficiency (night blindness, dryness of the cornea progressing to ulceration, perifollicular dermatitis) are of no value in the neonatal period. In practice, serum retinol concentration of less than 10 μg/dl (<0.35 μmol/L) is currently accepted as indicative of vitamin A deficiency (Pitt, 1983).

Vitamin A deficiency may occur with any form of fat malabsorption (decreased absorption), in preterm infants (low hepatic stores and decreased intake), in infants on parenteral nutrition (adherence of retinol to plastic tubing), and in infants with BPD. Lower serum retinol concentrations have been reported in infants with BPD than in controls without BPD (Shenai et al., 1985). In infants with BPD, vitamin A deficiency is not absolute but relative, possibly owing to increased vitamin A requirements. It has been speculated that vitamin A deficiency might result from increased requirements during the healing process of the bronchiolar epithelium. It is still unclear whether morbidity associated with BPD can be reduced by vitamin A supplementation (Pearson et al., 1992).

Toxicity. Vitamin A toxicity occurs from significant overdosage. Clinical signs include bulging anterior fontanelle, vomiting, and other neurologic symptoms.

Vitamin D

Vitamin D is essential for normal metabolism of Ca and P. Through the effects of its active form, 1,25-dihydroxyvitamin D, it is necessary for parathyroid hormone action in mobilizing Ca and P from bone; for intestinal absorption of Ca and P; and, indirectly, for bone formation (Tsang, 1983).

Vitamin D can be obtained through the diet or can be synthesized by the skin after exposure to sunlight. Regardless of its origin, vitamin D is transported to the liver, where it is converted into 25-hydroxyvitamin D (25 OHD) and subsequently to the kidney where it is converted into the final, active metabolite, 1,25-dihydroxyvitamin D. 25-Hydroxyvitamin D is the major circulating vitamin D metabolite, and it is regarded as an indicator of vitamin D status. It is transferred from mother to fetus, and maternal vitamin D deficiency may be a predisposing factor for late neonatal hypocalcemia (Roberts et al., 1973).

The serum concentration of 1,25-dihydroxyvitamin D appears to be tightly regulated. The synthesis of 1,25-dihydroxyvitamin D is facilitated by parathyroid hormone, hypocalcemia, and hypophosphatemia. Under normal circumstances, placental transfer of 1,25-dihydroxyvitamin D does not appear to occur, at least in significant amounts (Marx et al., 1980).

The current recommendation is a daily intake of 400 IU for both full-term and preterm infants (American Academy of Pediatrics, Committee on Nutrition, 1985), or 125 to 333 IU/100 kcal (Tsang et al., 1993). Breastfed full-term infants receiving adequate exposure to sunlight (0.5 to 2 hours per week average with face and hands exposed) do not appear to require vitamin D supplementation (Specker et al., 1985).

Deficiency. Vitamin D deficiency results in bone demineralization or rickets. Clinical signs are craniotabes, frontal bossing, widened ribs with enlargement of costochondral junctions, and muscle weakness.

Laboratory findings include low serum 25-hydroxyvitamin D concentration (resulting from decreased intake), increased serum parathyroid hormone stimulated by transiently low blood Ca (to maintain normal serum Ca), normal or increased 1,25-dihydroxyvitamin D (resulting from parathyroid hormone stimulation), and normal serum Ca and low serum P concentrations (resulting from the effects of parathyroid hormone).

Rickets can be caused by inadequate vitamin D intake, by inadequate exposure to sunlight, and by any form of fat malabsorption. Rickets can also be caused by abnormalities of vitamin D metabolism, such as occurs in renal failure or in vitamin D–dependent rickets (Type 1: deficient activity of renal 1α-hydroxylase, which converts 25-hydroxyvitamin D to 1,25-dihydroxyvitamin D; Type 2: defective hormone receptor with end-organ resistance to 1,25-dihydroxyvitamin D).

Rickets or osteopenia of prematurity, a common disorder in VLBW infants, is believed to be generally caused not by dietary deficiency or abnormality of metabolism of vitamin D but by insufficient intake of Ca and P.

Toxicity. Excessive doses of vitamin D can cause restlessness, diarrhea, polyuria, and growth retardation. Calcinosis occurs mainly in kidneys and in the cardiovascular system but may also occur in lungs and intestine (Specker et al., 1988).

Vitamin E

Vitamin E comprises several compounds, named tocopherols, which are important biologic antioxidants; among these, α-tocopherol is believed to be most active. Vitamin E protects the polyunsaturated fatty acid of biologic membranes from peroxidation.

Oral administration of both forms of tocopherols, α-tocopherol and α-tocopherol acetate, results in satisfactory absorption, even in very small preterm infants (Bell et al., 1979). However, absorption may be decreased in sick infants (Zipursky et al., 1987). Tocopherols are absorbed in the jejunum and transported by either chylomicrons or low-density lipoproteins to body tissues. Fixed oral or intramuscular daily doses of vitamin E can produce variable serum concentrations (Zipursky et al., 1987). Serum tocopherol concentrations may not reflect tissue concentrations, because tocopherol is carried by plasma lipoproteins, which are decreased in the newborn.

Vitamin E is excreted mainly in feces. Biliary excretion is small, and urine excretion is almost negligible. The half-life of tocopherol is approximately 2 days. Because excretion is minimal, vitamin E is cleared from serum by tissue uptake or metabolic degradation or both. Administration of α-tocopherol acetate (α-tocopherol ester) results in lower serum tocopherol concentrations and faster clearance in comparison with tocopherol itself (Knight & Roberts, 1986).

Vitamin E concentration in human milk is 0.5 to 2.2 IU/100 kcal. The recommendations of the American Academy of Pediatrics, Committee on Nutrition (1985), for formulas are based on both caloric intake and on dietary content of polyunsaturated fatty acids: 0.3 IU (full-term) and 0.7 IU (preterm) of vitamin E per 100 kcal; or 0.7 IU (full-term) and 1.0 IU (preterm) of vitamin E per gram of linoleic acid. During the first 2 to 3 weeks of life of enterally fed preterm infants, intake is usually too low to achieve vitamin E sufficiency, and therefore a supplement of 5 to 25 IU/day should be given.

No benefits have been demonstrated for pharmacologic doses of vitamin E with regard to physiologic anemia of prematurity (Chadd & Fraser, 1970) and BPD (Ehrenkranz et al., 1979). The effects on retinopathy of prematurity (ROP) are controversial (Finer et al., 1983; Hittner et al., 1981; Phelps et al., 1987). Vitamin E supplementation may decrease both incidence and severity of intraventricular hemorrhage (Chiswick et al., 1983; Phelps, 1988; Speer et al., 1984).

If pharmacologic doses of vitamin E must be given, a dosage exceeding 25 IU/kg/day may result in tissue concentrations greater than needed for maximum antioxidant effect. Furthermore, in view of its long half-life, vitamin E could probably be administered every other day (Roberts & Knight, 1987).

Deficiency. Vitamin E deficiency can occur in two categories of patients. Infants with severe forms of fat malabsorption can develop vitamin E deficiency and neurologic and myopathic abnormalities over several years. Preterm infants fed milk formulas both low in vitamin E and high in polyunsaturated fatty acids may develop, at about 2 months of age, a syndrome consisting of anemia, thrombocytosis, and peripheral edema (Oski & Barness, 1967). This syndrome does not seem to occur with current preterm formulas.

Toxicity. Very large doses of vitamin E can cause calcifications at injection sites, creatinuria, inhibition of wound healing, and fibrinolysis. An increased incidence of necrotizing enterocolitis has been associated with high oral doses of hyperosmolar preparation (Finer et al., 1984). An intravenous preparation, E-Ferol (tocopherol acetate in polysorbate), is no longer available because it was associated with a fatal syndrome consisting of renal failure, thrombocytopenia, hepatomegaly, cholestasis, and ascites (Balistreri et al., 1986).

Vitamin K

Two forms of vitamin K are naturally available: vitamin K_1, or phylloquinone, which is synthesized by plants, and vitamin K_2, or menaquinone, which is synthesized by animals.

Vitamin K is required for the synthesis of coagulation factors II, VII, IX, and X and for the conversion of inactive precursors into active clotting factors. Dietary vitamin K is absorbed in the small intestine and transported with chylomicrons through the lymphatic system. Approximately 29 percent of orally administered vitamin K is absorbed in the newborn. Vitamin K synthesized by intestinal bacteria is believed to be absorbed in the colon. It has been estimated that in adults, about 50 percent of the total amount of vitamin K manufactured in the body comes from intestinal bacteria. Vitamin K is stored in the liver, but storage capacity appears to be limited. Excretion mainly occurs with bile in the feces, whereas urinary excretion is quantitatively less important.

The concentration of phylloquinone is about 2.1 μg/ml (4.6 μmol/L) in human milk, 4.9 μg/ml (10.9 μmol/L) in cow's milk, and 55 to 58 μg/ml (122 to 129 μmol/L) in milk formulas (Greer & Suttie, 1988). Therefore, dietary intake of vitamin K depends on both quality and quantity of ingested milk. A deficiency state (plasma vitamin K concentration < 0.2 ng/mL) occurs in breastfed infants who do not receive vitamin K (Hathaway et al., 1993). Current recommendations for vitamin K include (1) administration of 0.5 to 1.0 mg (1.1 to 2.2 μmol) intramuscularly or 1.0 to 2.0 mg (2.2 to 4.4 μmol) orally, at birth; (2) weekly intramuscular administration of 0.5 to 1.0 mg (1.1 to 2.2 μmol) to infants on total parenteral nutrition; and (3) a minimum concentration of 4 μg/100 kcal (0.009 μmol/100 kcal) in milk formulas (American Academy of Pediatrics, Committee on Nutrition, 1985). For preterm infants an intake of 6.66 to 8.33 μg/100 kcal (15 to 18.5 nmol/410 kj) is currently recommended (Tsang et al., 1993).

Deficiency. Vitamin K deficiency may result in hemorrhagic disease of the newborn. Bleeding may occur from the umbilical stump or after minor procedures, such as circumcision or blood sampling, but serious events such as gastrointestinal and cerebral hemorrhages are also possible.

Three clinical forms of this disease have been described by Lane and Hathaway (1985): (1) the early type, which occurs on the first day of life in infants born to mothers receiving anticonvulsant therapy (phenytoin, phenobarbital); (2) the classic type, which occurs between 2 and 10 days of life in breastfed infants unsupplemented with vitamin K at birth; and (3) the late type, which occurs after 2 to 4 weeks of age in infants with severe forms of fat malabsorption; this type is now the most common, is frequently complicated by intracranial bleeding, and carries a high mortality rate. To prevent the disease, doses as small as 100 μg (0.22 μmol) intramuscularly have been demonstrated to be effective. With regard to oral administration, although as little as 15 μg (0.03 μmol) appears to be effective in the majority of infants (Motohara et al., 1989), the occasional finding of infants with vitamin K malabsorption supports the recommendation of 1.0 to 2.0 mg (2.2 to 4.4 μmol) as a safe dose for all newborns.

Infants born to mothers receiving anticonvulsant therapy should receive vitamin K intramuscularly immediately after birth, because they are at risk for the early form of the disease. This form can be prevented by antepartum maternal vitamin K supplementation.

Toxicity. There is no evidence of vitamin K toxicity, except for red blood cell hemolysis and hyperbilirubinemia after the administration of large doses of the synthetic vitamin K_3 (menadione).

TRACE MINERALS

Zinc

Zinc, as a cofactor, is necessary for the synthesis of nucleic acids and for the metabolism of proteins, lipids, and carbohydrates; therefore, it is essential for normal growth and development.

Zinc accumulation in the fetus mainly occurs during the third trimester. Consequently, preterm infants have lower body stores than do full-term infants. However, stores are limited in both full-term and preterm infants, and dietary intake is essential for maintaining optimal zinc status in the newborn (Shaw, 1979).

Zinc is absorbed in the duodenum and proximal jejunum; zinc absorption from cow's milk formula is 32 percent, whereas zinc added to preterm human milk has 52 percent absorption (Ehrenkranz et al., 1989). Absorption can be significantly improved by increased amounts of medium-chain triglycerides in the diet (Voyer et al., 1982).

Although there have been cases of zinc deficiency in breastfed infants, zinc absorption is greater from human milk than from formulas. Excretion occurs mainly through feces, whereas urinary excretion is far less important.

Zinc concentration in human milk ranges between 825 μg/dl (126 μmol/L) in the first days of life and 340 μg/dl (52 μmol/L) at the end of the first month (Pereira & Zucker, 1986). Maternal zinc supplementation has no effect on serum zinc concentration in infants (Salmenpera et al., 1994). Zinc intake in breastfed infants is adequate through 5 months of age but subsequently becomes marginal without introduction of solid food (Krebs et al., 1994).

The current recommendation for enteral feedings is a daily intake of 500 to 800 μg/kg (7.6 to 12.2 μmol/kg) during the transitional period, when infants are still unstable, and 1000 μg/kg (15 μmol/kg) in stable, growing preterm infants. With regard to parenteral nutrition, a zinc intake of 150 μg/kg/day (2.29 μmol/kg/day) is currently recommended during the transitional phase and 400 μg/kg (6.1 μmol/kg/day) in stable, growing preterm infants (Tsang et al., 1993).

Deficiency. Zinc deficiency can be caused by inadequate intake, decreased absorption (preterm infant), and increased losses (malabsorption syndromes, ostomies). Serum zinc concentrations of less than 40 μg/dl (<6.1 mmol/L) are generally accepted as indications of deficiency.

Zinc deficiency is not uncommon in breastfed preterm infants, owing to the large variations in breast milk zinc concentration. Signs include reduced growth velocity, acro-orificial rash, hypoproteinemia, and generalized edema (Kumar & Anday, 1984). Acrodermatitis enteropathica is an autosomal recessive disease in which there is a defect in the intestinal absorption of zinc. It is characterized by a dermatitis affecting extremities and perioral/perigenital areas, diarrhea, and failure to thrive, which progresses to thymic atrophy and immunodeficiency (Moynahan, 1974).

Toxicity. Zinc overdosage may result in copper deficiency and increased serum cholesterol concentrations.

Copper

Copper is necessary for normal functions of oxidative enzymes and for the synthesis of collagen, melanin, and catecholamines. Both full-term and preterm infants are born with significant liver stores (Casey & Walravens, 1988). Active absorption takes place mainly in the duodenum. Copper absorption appears to be greater with human milk than with formulas (Mendelson et al., 1983). In plasma, approximately two thirds of copper is bound to ceruloplasmin. In newborns, limited ceruloplasmin synthesis results in low plasma ceruloplasmin and, consequently, low serum copper concentrations. Neither serum copper nor ceruloplasmin concentrations are therefore adequate indices of copper status in the first 6 to 12 weeks of life. Copper excretion occurs almost exclusively through the bile.

Human milk, in spite of wide variation in copper content, appears adequate for both full-term and preterm infants. Current recommendations for milk formulas are a daily intake of 120 μg/100 kcal (1.9 μmol/kg) during the transitional period, when infants are still unstable, and 120 to 150 μg/kg (1.9 to 2.4 μmol/kg) in stable growing preterm infants. With parenteral nutrition, a copper intake of 20 μg/kg/day (0.31 μmol/kg/day) is currently recommended in stable growing preterm infants (Tsang et al., 1993).

Deficiency. Copper deficiency can result from inadequate intake (cow's milk, total parenteral nutrition) or increased losses (malabsorption syndromes, ostomies).

Clinical signs include pallor, hypotonia, psychomotor retardation, hypochromic anemia unresponsive to iron therapy, neutropenia, osteoporosis, and failure to thrive (Al-Rashid & Spangler, 1971).

Toxicity. Acute overdosage can cause vomiting, abdominal pain, and diarrhea. Chronic overdosage or intravenous administration of normal amounts to infants with cholestasis results in liver damage, because excess copper cannot be excreted.

NURSING MANAGEMENT

Obtaining vascular access on a sick newborn has become as routine a part of the admission procedure as obtaining a weight and vital signs. Nurses are responsible for the correct and safe delivery of intravenous fluids, recognizing signs and symptoms of disorders in hydration, and preventing complications associated with fluid administration (Donler, 1990).

Assessment and Evaluation of Fluid and Electrolyte Therapy

Estimating fluid needs depends on the infant's age, weight, and disease process. The fluid and electrolyte needs of a 4-kg infant with perinatal asphyxia and seizures are different from those of a 32-week, 1750-g infant with RDS or a 23-week, 460-g infant with multiple, complex needs. Each of these infants represents varying points on the continuum of fetal growth and development and represents a different disease process, and yet each requires careful management of fluid and electrolytes to maintain homeostasis.

Fluid needs can be calculated by using body weight, body surface area, or caloric expenditure (Behrman et al., 1995). An easy method is that of caloric expenditure, whereby caloric needs are calculated and fluid and electrolyte requirements are related to it. To begin these calculations, it must be remembered that 1 kcal is the amount of heat needed to raise 1 L of water 1°C. "Caloric expenditures up to 10 kilograms = 100 calories/kilogram/24 hours" (Donler, 1990). For example, a 1700-g infant would expend 170 calories in 24 hours, whereas a 460-g infant would expend 46 calories in 24 hours. Caloric expenditures can be modified by an increase or decrease in body temperature as well as by specific disease states. Caloric expenditure can be used to determine water needs, because for every 100 calories metabolized, 100 ml of fluid are needed (Behrman et al., 1995; Donler, 1990). Water needs are determined on the basis of calculated insensible losses from the skin and pulmonary system and actual losses from the urine, stool, and sweat (Table 22–9).

Insensible water loss can be affected by a variety of factors, including skin integrity and the degree of that integrity. An example of this is the newborn infant with a large gastroschisis. This midline abdominal wall defect predisposes to large amounts of insensible water loss because of the exposed abdominal organs with an absent omentum or peritoneum. Another example is the 23-week, 400-g infant with the typical "translucent" skin that has not yet formed a protective keratin layer, thus predisposing the infant to dehydration secondary to large insensible water losses. Also affecting insensible water loss are environmental factors, including the presence or absence of humidity and increased or decreased ambient temperature. The use of radiant warmers has long been understood to affect the infant's fluid status by increasing insensible losses in a relatively open, unprotected environment. Phototherapy has similar effects, with the additional problems of thermoregulation. Other factors include increased metabolic rate, body temperature, and activity, all of which must be accounted for in calculating fluid needs.

Fluids are usually calculated on a daily basis, taking into consideration past losses, projected losses, and maintenance requirements. However, depending on the disease process, fluids may need to be calculated more often, even as often as every 4 hours, to keep up with ongoing losses and to make appropriate adjustments in fluid therapy. A general estimate of fluid requirements can be calculated on the basis of the following guidelines (for normal, full-term newborns):

Day 1: 80 ml/kg/day
Day 2: 100 ml/kg/day
Day 3: 120 ml/kg/day
Day 4: 135 ml/kg/day
Day 5: 150 ml/kg/day

Again, these are just guidelines, and requirements may be different on the basis of the gestational age and disease process. A premature, low birth weight infant may require as much as 150 to 200 ml/kg/day during the first 24 hours of life, whereas a full-term, asphyxiated infant may be restricted to no more than 40 to 50 ml/kg/day for the first 72 hours of life.

Electrolyte requirements are usually calculated on the basis of 100 calories metabolized:

Na: 2 to 3 mEq/100 cal/24 hours (or 2 to 3 mEq/kg/day)

K: 1 to 2 mEq/100 cal/24 hours (or 1 to 2 mEq/kg/day)

TABLE 22–9 Fluid Intake and Output

	Range (ml/100 cal/24 hours)	Average (ml/100 cal/24 hours)
Output		
Insensible water losses:		
Pulmonary	10–20	15
Skin	25–35	30
Urine	50–70	60
Stool	5–10	7
Sweat	0–20	0
Intake		112
Water of oxidation		−12
		100 ml/100 cal/day average maintenance requirements

TABLE 22–10 Electrolyte Components of Intravenous Fluids

Solution	mEq Na/1000 ml	mEq Na/100 ml
D_5W ½ NS	77	7.7
D_5W ¼ NS	38.5	3.8

Standard intravenous solutions containing a predetermined quantity of sodium are routinely used in neonatal intensive care units (for example, 5 percent dextrose in 0.45 percent NaCl) with potassium chloride added as indicated (Table 22–10).

Caloric requirements cannot be met solely by the intravenous solutions commonly used in neonatal intensive care units (i.e., 5 or 10 percent dextrose). These solutions are relatively low in calories; there are only 4 calories per gram of glucose (carbohydrate), and the number of calories in intravenous solutions is calculated on a percent solution and based on grams per 100 ml. Therefore, 5 percent dextrose in water (D_5W) contains 5 g/100 ml of fluid, and a 10 percent dextrose in water ($D_{10}W$) solution contains 10 g/100 ml. To carry this calculation further, D_5W and $D_{10}W$ intravenous solutions contain 20 and 40 calories, respectively (for example, D_5W = 5 g/100 ml at 4 cal/g = 20 cal).

The dextrose concentration administered to the infant also depends on the infant's gestational age and renal function. Glucose excretion may be altered by the premature kidney's inability to concentrate urine and conserve electrolytes and glucose, thus "spilling sugar" into the urine. An essential test of the infant's response to intravenous glucose therapy can easily be done at the bedside with the urine dipstick. This test requires only a few drops of urine on a dipstick to determine the presence of glucose, protein, ketones, and blood and to determine the pH level, an important indicator of acid–base balance. Another essential bedside test requiring only a few drops of urine is specific gravity. Specific gravity is normally between 1.008 and 1.012 and is an early indicator of hydration status (Korones, 1986). Urine dipstick and specific gravity tests should be performed at least every shift and more often as the infant's condition warrants. Along with these two parameters, fluid intake and output should be strictly monitored to ensure adequate hydration status. Urine output (UOP) is monitored and calculated on an hourly basis over a 24-hour period. UOP should be no less than 1 ml/kg/hour/day. For example, for a 2-kg infant,

$$\text{UOP} = 240 \text{ ml/24 hr} = 10 \text{ ml/2 kg} = 5 \text{ ml/kg/hr}$$

To promote improved nutritional status for infants requiring long-term intravenous therapy, total parenteral nutrition (TPN) is used and may be started within the first 24 to 72 hours of life. TPN spares protein, increases calories, and, when used in conjunction with intralipids, further increases caloric intake. When infused through a peripheral vein, glucose concentration is limited to no more than 12.5 percent because of the risks of tissue irritation and sloughing with infiltration; however, when it is infused through central lines, higher concentrations may be used. In addition to the increased glucose concentrations (thus increasing calories), higher concentrations of protein, fat,* and other essential minerals and trace elements may be infused. Caloric supplementation with TPN is calculated as follows:

Protein (4 cal/g): 1 to 2.5 g/kg/day; 4 to 10 cal/kg/day

Fat (9 cal/g): up to 4 g/kg/day; 10 percent emulsion = 1.1 cal/ml; 20 percent emulsion = 2.0 cal/ml

The nurse is responsible for monitoring hourly fluid intake and

*Fat calories should not exceed 50 percent of the total caloric intake.

should always double-check fluid orders to ensure that the ordered rate and solution are appropriate for that infant.

Weight is an important indicator of overall fluid status. Infants are usually weighed on a daily basis; extremely low birth weight infants and infants with excessive fluid losses and needs may be weighed more often, on an every-12-hour schedule or even on an every-6-hour schedule, with ongoing fluid needs recalculated on the basis of weight changes. It is important to use care when weighing infants, for inaccuracies that show extreme weight fluctuations can have a detrimental impact on therapy. For example, an inaccurate weight measurement showing an increase of 100 g in a 12-hour period for an infant with severe RDS may result in an unnecessary dose of furosemide. The infant should be weighed nude, with as much equipment removed as possible (ECG leads, probes, etc.), at the same time each day, and on the same scale. Newer, in-bed scales that give a constant weight read-out, simplifying the weighing process, are now available (Kavanaugh et al., 1990).

The physical examination can reveal changes in the infant's fluid status and should be used in conjunction with laboratory data to plan interventions in fluid and electrolyte therapy. A general assessment includes the infant's color, skin turgor, activity, mucous membranes, fontanelles, and vital signs:

Color: pink and well-perfused versus pale and mottled
Activity: active with good tone versus lethargic and hypotonic
Mucous membranes: pink and moist versus dry and gray
Fontanelles: soft and flat versus depressed or full and tense
Vital signs: bradycardia/tachycardia, slowed respirations/tachypnea, normotensive versus hypotensive or hypertensive, hypothermia versus hyperthermia, or temperature instability
Urine output: normal versus excessive, decreased, or absent

CONCLUSION

The care of infants with alterations in fluid and electrolyte balance presents a management challenge for both physicians and nurses. By having a thorough understanding of the underlying pathophysiology and rationale for therapy, the health care team is able to provide more informed care for these infants and able to anticipate and prevent problems.

REFERENCES

Abu-Osba, Y. K., Galal, O., Manasra, K., & Rejjal, A. (1992). Treatment of severe persistent pulmonary hypertension of the newborn with magnesium sulfate. *Archives of Disease in Children, 67*(1, special issue), 31–35.

Al-Rashid, R. A., & Spangler, J. (1971). Neonatal copper deficiency. *New England Journal of Medicine, 285*(15), 841–843.

American Academy of Pediatrics, Committee on Nutrition. (1976). Commentary on breast-feeding and infant formula, including proposed standards for formulas. *Pediatrics, 57*(2), 278–285.

American Academy of Pediatrics, Committee on Nutrition. (1985). Nutritional needs of low-birth-weight infants [Review]. *Pediatrics, 75*(5), 976–986.

Anderson, S. A., Chinn, H. I., & Fisher, K. D. (1982). History and current status of infant formulas [Review]. *American Journal of Clinical Nutrition, 35*(2), 381–397.

Aperia, A., Broberger, O., Elinder, G., et al. (1981). Postnatal development of renal function in preterm and full-term infants. *Acta Paediatrica Scandinavica, 70*(2), 183–187.

Aperia, A., Broberger, O., Herin, P., & Zetterstrom, R. (1979). Salt content in human breast milk during the first three weeks after delivery. *Acta Paediatrica Scandinavica, 68*(3), 441–442.

Aperia, A., Herin, P., & Zetterstom, R. (1985). Sodium, chloride and potassium in very low birthweight infants. In R. C. Tsang (Ed.), *Vitamin and mineral requirements in preterm infants* (pp. 137–151). New York: Marcel Dekker.

Arieff, A., & Guisado, R. (1976). Effects on the central nervous system of hypernatremic and hyponatremic states. *Kidney International, 10*(1), 104–116.

Balistreri, W. F., Farrell, M. K., & Bove, K. E. (1986). Lessons from the E-Ferol tragedy. *Pediatrics, 78*(3), 503–506.

Bartter, F. C. (1980). On the pathogenesis of Bartter's syndrome. *Mineral and Electrolyte Metabolism, 3*, 61–65.

Bauer K., Bovermann, G., Roithmeier, A., et al. (1991). Body composition, nutrition, and fluid balance during the first two weeks of life in preterm neonates weighing <1500 grams. *Journal of Pediatrics, 118*(4, Part 1), 615–620.

Baumgart, S., Langman, C. B., Sosuski, R., et al. (1982). Fluid, electrolyte and glucose maintenance in the very low birthweight infant. *Clinical Pediatrics, 21*(4), 199–206.

Beard, A. G., Panos, T. C., Burroughs, J. C., et al. (1963). Perinatal stress and the premature neonate: I. Effect of fluid and calorie deprivation. *Journal of Pediatrics, 63*, 361–385.

Behrman, R. E., Kliegman, R. M., & Arvin, A. M. (Eds.). (1995). *Nelson textbook of pediatrics* (15th ed.). Philadelphia: W. B. Saunders.

Bell, E. F., Brown, E. J., Milner, R., et al. (1979). Vitamin E absorption in small premature infants. *Pediatrics, 63*(6), 830–832.

Bell, E. F., & Oh, W. (1979). Fluid and electrolyte balance in very low birth weight infants [Review]. *Clinics in Perinatology, 6*(1), 139–150.

Bell, E. F., Warburton, D., Stonestreet, B. S., & Oh, W. (1980). Effect of fluid administration on the development of symptomatic patent ductus arteriosus and congestive heart failure in premature infants. *New England Journal of Medicine, 302*(11), 598–604.

Blanchard, P. W., Brown, T. M., & Coates, A. L. (1987). Pharmacotherapy in bronchopulmonary dysplasia. *Clinics in Perinatology, 14*(4), 881–910.

Brand, J. M., & Greer, F. A. (1990). Hypermagnesemia and intestinal perforation following antacid administration in a premature infant. *Pediatrics 85*(1), 121–124.

Brann, A. W., & Schwartz, J. F., Jr. (1992). Seizures. In A. A. Fanaroff & R. J. Martin (Eds.), *Neonatal-perinatal medicine* (5th ed., pp. 729–733). St. Louis: C. V. Mosby.

Byerley, L. O., & Kirksey, A. (1985). Effects of different levels of vitamin C intake on the vitamin C concentration in human milk and the vitamin C intakes of breastfed infants. *American Journal of Clinical Nutrition, 41*(4), 665–671.

Casey, C. E., & Walravens, P. A. (1988). Trace elements. In R. C. Tsang & B. L. Nichols (Eds.), *Nutrition during infancy* (pp. 190–215). St. Louis: C. V. Mosby.

Cassady, G. (1971). Effect of cesarean section on neonatal body water spaces. *New England Journal of Medicine, 285*(16), 887–891.

Chadd, M. A., & Fraser, A. J. (1970). A controlled trial of vitamin E therapy in infancy. *International Journal of Vitamin Research, 40*(5), 610–616.

Chiswick, M. L., Johnson, M., Woodhall, C., et al. (1983). Protective effect of vitamin E (DL-alpha-tocopherol) against intraventricular hemorrhage in premature babies. *British Medical Journal Clinical Research Education, 287*(6385), 81–84.

Christensen, S. (1971). Renal excretion of riboflavin in the rat. *Acta Pharmacologica et Toxicologica, 29*(5), 428–440.

Costarino, A., & Baumgart, S. (1986). Modern fluid and electrolyte management of the critically ill premature infant [Review]. *Pediatric Clinics of North America, 33*(1), 153–178.

Costarino, A. T., & Baumgart, S. (1988). Controversies in fluid and electrolyte therapy for the premature infant [Review]. *Clinics in Perinatology, 15*(4), 863–878.

Costarino, A. T., Gruskay, J. A., Corcoran, L., et al. (1992). Sodium restriction versus daily maintenance replacement in very low birth weight premature neonates: A randomized blind therapeutic trial. *Journal of Pediatrics 120*(1), 99–106.

Coulter, D. M., & Avery, M. E. (1980). Paradoxical reduction in tissue hydration with weight gain in neonatal rabbit pups. *Pediatric Research, 14*(10), 1122–1126.

Dallman, P. R. (1988). Nutritional anemia of infancy: Iron, folic acid and vitamin B_{12}. In R. C. Tsang & B. L. Nichols (Eds.), *Nutrition during infancy* (pp. 175–189). St. Louis: C. V. Mosby.

Day, G. M., Radde, I. C., Balfe, J. W., & Chance, G. W. (1976). Electrolyte abnormalities in very low birthweight infants. *Pediatric Research, 10*(5), 522–526.

DeCristofaro, J. D., & Tsang, R. C. (1986). Calcium [Review]. *Emergency Medicine Clinics of North America, 4*(2), 207–221.

Demarini S., Mimouni F., Tsang, R. C., et al. (1994). Impact of metabolic control of diabetes during pregnancy on neonatal hypocalcemia: A randomized study. *Obstetrics and Gynecology, 83*(6), 918–922.

Donler, J. (1990). Fluid and electrolyte balance. In P. Beachy & J. Deacon (Eds.), *Neonatal intensive care nursing review* (p. 137). Washington, DC: Nurses Association of the American Association of Obstetrics and Gynecology (NAACOG).

Donovan, E. F., Tsang, R. C., Steichen, J. J., et al. (1980). Neonatal hypermagnesemia: Effect on parathyroid hormone and calcium homeostasis. *Journal of Pediatrics, 96*(2), 305–310.

Ehrenkranz, R. A., Ablow, R. C., & Warshaw, J. B. (1979). Prevention of bronchopulmonary dysplasia with vitamin E administration during the acute stages of respiratory distress syndrome. *Journal of Pediatrics,* 95(5, Part 2), 873–878.

Ehrenkranz, R. A., Gettner, P. A., Nelli, C. M., et al. (1989). Zinc and copper nutritional studies in very low birth weight infants: Comparison of stable isotopic extrinsic tag and chemical balance methods. *Pediatric Research,* 26(4), 298–307.

Ek, J. (1983). Plasma, red cell and breast milk folacin concentrations in lactating women. *American Journal of Clinical Nutrition, 38*(6), 929–935.

Ek, J. (1985). Folic acid and vitamin B_{12} requirement in premature infants. In R. C. Tsang (Ed.), *Vitamin and mineral requirements in preterm infants* (pp. 23–38). New York: Marcel Dekker.

Engelke, S. C., Shah, B. L., Vasan, U., & Raye, J. R. (1978). Sodium balance in very low birthweight infants. *Journal of Pediatrics, 93*(5), 837–841.

Feig, P. A., & McCurdy, D. K. (1977). The hypertonic state [Review]. *New England Journal of Medicine, 297*(26), 1444–1454.

Finberg, L. (1973). Hypernatremic (hypertonic) dehydration in infants [Review]. *New England Journal of Medicine, 289*(4), 196–198.

Finer, N. N., Peters, K. L., Hayek, Z., & Merkel, C. L. (1984). Vitamin E and necrotizing enterocolitis. *Pediatrics, 73*(3), 387–393.

Finer, N. N., Schindler, R. F., Peters, K. L., & Grant, G. D. (1983). Vitamin E and retrolental fibroplasia. Improved visual outcome with early vitamin E. *Ophthalmology, 90*(5), 428–435.

Ford, R. F. (1977). Morbidity in breast fed and artificially fed infants. *Journal of Pediatrics, 91*(6), 1033–1034.

Fordtran, J. S. (1975). Stimulation of active and passive sodium absorption by sugars in the human jejunum. *Journal of Clinical Investigation, 55*(4), 728–737.

Friis-Hansen, B. (1957). Changes in body water compartments during growth. *Acta Paediatrica Scandinavica, 43*(Suppl. 110), 1–12.

Friis-Hansen, B. (1961). Body water compartments in children: Changes during growth and related changes in body composition. *Pediatrics, 28,* 169–181.

Ganong, W. F. (1993). *Review of medical physiology* (16th ed.). Norwalk, CT: Appleton-Lange.

Goodhart, R. S., & Shils, M. E. (1980). *Modern nutrition in health and diseases* (6th ed.). Philadelphia: Lea & Febiger.

Goldsmith, G. A. (1975). Vitamin B complex. Thiamine, riboflavin, niacin, folic acid (folacin), vitamin B_{12}, biotin [Review]. *Progress in Food and Nutrition Science, 1*(9), 559–609.

Greer, F. R., & McCormick, A. (1988). Improved bone mineralization and growth in premature infants fed fortified own mother's milk. *Journal of Pediatrics, 112*(6), 961–969.

Greer, F. R., & Suttie, J. W. (1988). Vitamin K and the newborn. In R. C. Tsang & B. L. Nichols (Eds.), *Nutrition during infancy* (pp. 289–297). St. Louis: C. V. Mosby.

Greer, F. R., & Tsang, R. C. (1985). Calcium, phosphorus, magnesium and vitamin D requirements for the preterm infant. In R. C. Tsang (Ed.), *Vitamin and mineral requirements in preterm infants* (pp. 99–136). New York: Marcel Dekker.

Gruskay, J. A., Costarino, A. T., Polin, R. A., & Baumgart, S. (1988). Non-oliguric hyperkalemia in the premature infant less than 1000 grams. *Journal of Pediatrics, 113*(2), 381–386.

Guignard, J., Torrado, A., Mazouni, S. M., & Gautier, E. (1976). Renal function in respiratory distress syndrome. *Journal of Pediatrics, 88*(5), 845–850.

Hahn, T. J. (1980). Drug induced disorders of vitamin D and mineral metabolism. *Clinics in Endocrinology and Metabolism, 9*(1), 107–129.

Hanna, F. M. (1963). Changes in body composition of normal infants in relation to diet. *Annals of New York Academy of Science, 110,* 840–848.

Hathaway, W. E., Isarangkura, P. B., Mahasandana, C., et al. (1993). Comparison of oral and parenteral vitamin K prophylaxis for prevention of late hemorrhagic disease of the newborn. *Journal of Pediatrics, 119*(3), 461–463.

Heimler, R., Doumas, B. T., Jendrzjaczak, B. M., et al. (1993). Relationship between nutrition, weight change, and fluid compartments in preterm infants during the first week of life. *Journal of Pediatrics 122*(1), 110–114.

Hittner, H. M., Godio, L. B., Rudolph, A. J., et al. (1981). Retrolental fibroplasia: Efficacy of vitamin E in a double-blind clinical study of preterm infants. *New England Journal of Medicine, 305*(23), 1365–1371.

Hovi, L., Hekali, R., & Slimes, M. A. (1979). Evidence of riboflavin depletion in breast-fed newborns and its further acceleration during treatment of hyperbilirubinemia by phototherapy. *Acta Paediatrica Scandinavica, 68*(4), 567–570.

Inder, T. E., Carr, A. C., Winterbourn, C. C., et al. (1995). Vitamin A and E status in very low birth weight infants: Development of an improved parenteral delivery system. *Journal of Pediatrics, 126,* 128–131.

Kagan, B. M., Stanincova, V., Felix, N. S., et al. (1972). Body composition of premature infants: Relation to nutrition. *American Journal of Clinical Nutrition, 25*(11), 1153–1164.

Kalser, M. H. (1985a). Absorption of cobalamin (vitamin B_{12}), folate and other water-soluble vitamins. In J. E. Berk (Ed.), *Gastroenterology* (4th ed., pp. 1553–1566). Philadelphia: W. B. Saunders.

Kalser, M. H. (1985b). Water and mineral transport. In J. E. Berk (Ed.), *Gastroenterology* (4th ed., pp. 1538–1552). Philadelphia: W. B. Saunders.

Kavanaugh, K., Engstrom, J. L., Meier, P. P., & Lysakowski, T. Y. (1990). How reliable are scales for weighing preterm infants? *Neonatal Network, 9*(3), 29–32.

Kimberg, D. V. (1969). Effects of vitamin D and steroid hormones on intestinal calcium transport [Review]. *New England Journal of Medicine, 280*(25), 1396–1405.

Knight, M. E., & Roberts, R. J. (1986). Disposition of intravenously administered pharmacologic doses of vitamin E in newborn rabbits. *Journal of Pediatrics, 108*(10), 145–150.

Koo, W. W., Antony, G., & Stevens, L. H. (1984). Continuous nasogastric phosphorus infusion in hypophosphatemic rickets of prematurity. *American Journal of Diseases in Children,* 138(2), 172–175.

Koo, W. W., & Tsang, R. C. (1988). Calcium, magnesium and phosphorus. In R. C. Tsang & B. L. Nichols (Eds.), *Nutrition during infancy* (pp. 175–189). St. Louis: C. V. Mosby.

Korones, S. (1986). *High-risk newborn infants: The basis for intensive nursing care* (4th ed., p. 199). St. Louis: C. V. Mosby

Krebs, N. F., Reidinger, C. J., Robertson, A. D., & Hambidge, K. M. (1994). Growth and intakes of energy and zinc in infants fed human milk. *Journal of Pediatrics, 124*(1), 32–39.

Kumar, S. P., & Anday, E. K. (1984). Edema, hypoproteinemia and zinc deficiency in low birthweight infants. *Pediatrics, 73*(3), 327–329.

Lampkin, B. C., Shore, N. A., & Chadwick, D. (1966). Megaloblastic anemia of infancy secondary to maternal pernicious anemia. *New England Journal of Medicine, 274*(21), 1168–1171.

Lane, P. A., & Hathaway, W. E. (1985). Vitamin K in infancy. *Journal of Pediatrics, 106*(3), 351–359.

Lentz, R. D., Brown, D. M., & Kjellstrand, C. M. (1978). Treatment of severe hypophosphatemia. *Annals of Internal Medicine, 89*(6), 941–944.

Levine, M. (1986). New concepts in the biology and biochemistry of ascorbic acid. *New England Journal of Medicine, 314*(14), 892–902.

Lipsitz, P. J., & English, I. C. (1967). Hypermagnesemia in the newborn infant. *Pediatrics, 40*(5), 856–862.

MacLaurin, J. C. (1966). Changes in body water distribution during the first two weeks of life. *Archives of Disease in Childhood, 41*(217), 286–291.

Marx, S. J., Swart, E. G., Hamstra, A. J., & Deluca, H. F. (1980). Normal intrauterine development of a fetus of a woman receiving extraordinarily high doses of 1,25-dihydroxyvitamin D_3. *Journal of Clinical Endocrinology and Metabolism, 51*(5), 1138–1142.

McGuinness, G. A., Weinstein, M. M., Cruikshank, D. P., & Pitkin, R. M. (1980). Effects of magnesium sulfate treatment of perinatal calcium metabolism: II. Neonatal responses. *Obstetrics and Gynecology, 56*(5), 595–600.

Mendelson, R. A., Bryan, M. H., & Anderson, G. H. (1983). Trace mineral balances in preterm infants fed their own mother's milk. *Journal of Pediatric Gastroenterology and Nutrition, 2*(2), 256–261.

Menkes, J. H., Welcher, D. W., Levi, S. H., et al. (1972). Relationship of elevated blood tyrosine to the ultimate intellectual performance of premature infants. *Pediatrics, 49*(2), 218–224.

Mimouni, F., & Tsang, R. C. (1992). Pathophysiology of neonatal hypocalcemia. In R. A. Polin & W. W. Fox (Eds.), *Fetal and neonatal physiology* (pp. 1761–1767). Philadelphia: W. B. Saunders.

Moran, J. R., & Greene, H. L. (1979). The B vitamins and vitamin C in human nutrition: I. General considerations and "obligatory" B vitamins. *American Journal of Diseases of Childhood, 133*(2), 192–199.

Motohara, K., Matsukane, I., Endo, F., et al. (1989). Relationship of milk intake and vitamin K supplementation to vitamin K status in newborns. *Pediatrics, 84*(1), 90–93.

Moya, M., & Domenech, E. (1982). Role of calcium phosphate ratio of milk formulae on calcium balance in low birth weight infants during the first three days of life. *Pediatric Research, 16*(8), 675–681.

Moynahan, E. J. (1974). Acrodermatitis enteropathica: A lethal, inherited human zinc deficiency disorder [Letter]. *Lancet, 2*(7877), 399–400.

Nelson, N., Finnstrom, O., & Larson, L. (1987). Neonatal hyperexcitability in relation to plasma ionized calcium, magnesium, phosphate and glucose. *Acta Paediatrica Scandinavica, 76*(4), 579–584.

Okamoto, E., Muttart, C., Zucker, C., & Heird, W. (1982). Use of medium-chain triglycerides in feeding the low birthweight infant. *American Journal of Diseases of Children, 136*(5), 428–431.

Oski, F. A., & Barness, L. A. (1967). Vitamin E deficiency: A previously unrecognized cause of hemolytic anemia in the premature infant. *Journal of Pediatrics, 70*(2), 211–220.

Palta, M., Gabbert, D., Weinstein, M. R., & Peters, M. E. (1991). Multivariate assessment of traditional risk factors for chronic lung disease in very low birth weight infants. *Journal of Pediatrics, 119*(2), 285–292.

Papile, L. A., Burstein, J., Burstein, R., et al. (1978). Relationship of intravenous sodium bicarbonate infusions and cerebral intraventricular hemorrhage. *Journal of Pediatrics, 93*(5), 834–836.

Pascale, J. A., Mims, L. C., Greenberg, M. H., et al. (1976). Riboflavin and bilirubin response during phototherapy. *Pediatric Research, 10*(10), 854–856.

Paunier, L., Ingeborg, C. R., Kooh, S. Y., et al. (1968). Primary hypomagnesemia with secondary hypocalcemia in an infant. *Pediatrics, 41*(2), 385–402.

Pearson, E., Bose, C., Snidow, T., et al. (1992). Trial of vitamin A supplementation in very low birth weight infants at risk for bronchopulmonary dysplasia. *Journal of Pediatrics, 121*(3), 420–427.

Pereira, G. R., & Zucker, A. H. (1986). Nutritional deficiencies in the neonate [Review]. *Clinics in Perinatology, 13*(1), 175–189.

Perkin, R. M., & Levin, D. L. (1980). Common fluid and electrolyte problems in the pediatric intensive care unit. *Pediatric Clinics of North America, 27*(3), 558–567.

Phelps, D. L. (1988). The role of vitamin E therapy in high-risk neonates [Review]. *Clinics in Perinatology, 15*(4), 955–963.

Phelps, D. L., Rosenbaum, A. L., Isenberg, S. J., et al. (1987). Tocopherol efficacy and safety for preventing retinopathy of prematurity: A randomized controlled, double-masked trial. *Pediatrics, 79*(4), 489–500.

Pitt, G. A. (1983). The assessment of vitamin A status [Review]. *Proceedings of the Nutritional Society, 40*(2), 173–178.

Poncz, M., Colman, N., Herbert, V., et al. (1981). Therapy of congenital folate malabsorption. *Journal of Pediatrics, 98*(1), 76–79.

Reynolds, E. H. (1968). Mental effects of anticonvulsants and folic acid metabolism. *Brain, 91*(2), 197–214.

Roberts, R. A., Cohen, M. D., & Forfar, J. O. (1973). Antenatal factors associated with neonatal hypocalcemic convulsions. *Lancet, 2*(833), 809–811.

Roberts, R. J., & Knight, M. E. (1987). Pharmacology of vitamin E in the newborn [Review]. *Clinics in Perinatology, 14*(4), 843–855.

Ronnholm, K. A. R. (1986). Need for riboflavin supplementation in small prematures fed with human milk. *American Journal of Clinical Nutrition, 43*(1), 1–6.

Rose, B. D. (1977). *Clinical physiology of acid-base and electrolyte disorders.* New York: McGraw-Hill.

Rosenfeld, W. N., Linshaw, M., & Fox, H. A. (1976). Water intoxication: A complication of nebulization with nasal CPAP. *Journal of Pediatrics, 89*(1), 113–114.

Salmenpera, L., Perheentupa, J., Nato, V., & Siimes, N. (1994). Low zinc intake during exclusive breast-feeding does not impair growth. *Journal of Parenteral and Enteral Nutrition, 18*(3), 361–370.

Savage, M. D., Wilkinson, A. R., Baum, J. D., & Roberton, N. R. (1975). Furosemide in respiratory distress syndrome. *Archives of Disease in Childhood, 50*(9), 709–713.

Schanler, R. J. (1988). Water-soluble vitamins: C, B_1, B_2, B_6, niacin, biotin and pantothenic acid. In R. C. Tsang & B. L. Nichols (Eds.), *Nutrition during infancy* (pp. 236–252). St. Louis: C. V. Mosby.

Schaumburg, H., Kaplan, J., Widebank, A., et al. (1983). Sensory neuropathy from pyridoxine abuse. A new megavitamin syndrome. *New England Journal of Medicine, 309*(8), 445–448.

Scott, S. M., Ladenson, J. H., Aguanna, J. J., et al. (1984). Effect of calcium therapy in the sick premature infant with early neonatal hypocalcemia. *Journal of Pediatrics, 104*(5), 747–751.

Shaffer, S. G., Kilbride, H. W., Hayen, L. K., et al. (1992). Hyperkalemia in very low birth weight infants. *Journal of Pediatrics, 121*(2), 275–279.

Shaul, P. W., Mimouni, F., Tsang, R. C., & Specker, B. L. (1987). The role of magnesium in neonatal calcium homeostasis: Effects of magnesium infusion on calcitropic hormones and calcium. *Pediatric Research, 22*(3), 319–323.

Shaw, J. C. L. (1979). Trace elements in the fetus and young infant: I. Zinc [Review]. *American Journal of Diseases of Children, 133*(12), 1260–1268.

Shenai, J. P., Chityl, F., & Stahlman, M. T. (1985). Vitamin A status of neonates with bronchopulmonary dysplasia. *Pediatric Research, 19*(2), 185–188.

Smallpiece, V., & Davies, P. A. (1964). Immediate feeding of premature infants with undiluted breast milk. *Lancet, 2*, 1349–1352.

Specker, B. L., Greer, F., & Tsang, R. C. (1988). Vitamin D. In R. C. Tsang & B. L. Nichols (Eds.), *Nutrition during infancy* (pp. 264–276). St. Louis: C. V. Mosby.

Specker, B. L., Valanis, B., Hertzberg, V., et al. (1985). Sunshine exposure and serum 25-hydroxyvitamin D concentrations in exclusively breast-fed infants. *Journal of Pediatrics, 107*(3), 372–376.

Speer, M. E., Blifeld, C., Rudolph, A. J., et al. (1984). Intraventricular hemorrhage and vitamin E in the very low birthweight infant: Evidence for efficacy of early intramuscular vitamin E administration. *Pediatrics, 74*(6), 1107–1112.

Spitzer, A. (1982). The role of the kidney in sodium homeostasis during maturation. *Kidney International, 21*(4), 539–545.

Spitzer, A., Berstein, J., Boichis, H., & Edelmann, C. M., Jr. (1992). The kidney and urinary tract. In A. A. Fanaroff & R. J. Martin (Eds.), *Neonatal-perinatal medicine* (5th ed., pp. 1293–1327). St. Louis: C. V. Mosby.

Stefano, J. L., & Norman, M. E. (1993). Nitrogen balance in extremely low birth weight infants with non-oliguric hyperkalemia. *Journal of Pediatrics, 123*(4), 632–635.

Stefano, J. L., Norman, M. E., Morales, M. C., et al. (1993). Decreased erythrocyte Na^+,$K(^+)$-ATPase activity associated with cellular potassium loss in extremely low birth weight infants with non-oliguric hyperkalemia. *Journal of Pediatrics, 122*(2), 276–284.

Steichen, J. J., Gratton, T. L., & Tsang, R. C. (1980). Osteopenia of prematurity: The cause and possible treatment. *Journal of Pediatrics, 96*(3, Part 2), 528–534.

Styslinger, L., & Kirksey, A. (1985). Effects of different levels of vitamin B_6 supplementation on vitamin B_6 intakes of breastfed infants. *American Journal of Clinical Nutrition, 41*(1), 21–31.

Surawicz, B. (1967). Relationship between electrocardiogram and electrolytes. *American Heart Journal, 73*(6), 814–834.

Tsang, R. C. (1983). The quandary of vitamin D in the newborn infant. *Lancet, 1*(8338), 1370–1372.

Tsang, R. C., Chen, I. W., Friedman, M. A., et al. (1975). Parathyroid function in infants of diabetic mothers. *Journal of Pediatrics, 86*(3), 399–404.

Tsang, R. C., Chen, I., Hayes, W., et al. (1974). Neonatal hypocalcemia in infants with birth asphyxia. *Journal of Pediatrics, 84*(3), 428–433.

Tsang, R. C., Lucas, A., Uauy R., & Zlotkin, S. (1993). *Nutritional needs of the preterm infant. Scientific basis and practical guidelines.* Baltimore: Williams & Wilkins.

Tsang, R. C., & Oh, W. (1970). Neonatal hypocalcemia in low birthweight infants. *Pediatrics, 45*(5), 773–781.

Turnberg, L. A. (1971a). Abnormalities in intestinal electrolyte transport in congenital chloridorrhea. *Gut, 12*(7), 544–551.

Turnberg, L. A. (1971b). Potassium transport in the human small bowel. *Gut, 12*(10), 811–818.

Turnberg, L. A., Bieberdort, F. A., Mordowsky, S. G., & Fordtran, J. S. (1970). Interrelations of chloride, bicarbonate, sodium and hydrogen transport in human ileum. *Journal of Clinical Investigation, 49*(3), 557–567.

Turner, T. L., Cockburn, F., & Forfar, J. O. (1977). Magnesium therapy in neonatal tetany. *Lancet, 1*(8006), 283–284.

Venkataramaran, P. S., Tsang, R. C., Greer, F. R., et al. (1985). Late infantile tetany and secondary hyperparathyroidism in infants fed humanized cow milk formula. *American Journal of Diseases of Children, 139*(7), 664–668.

Venkataramaran, P. S., Tsang, R. C., Steichen, J. J., et al. (1986). Early neonatal hypocalcemia in extremely preterm infants. *American Journal of Diseases of Children, 140*(10), 1004–1008.

Volpe, J. J. (1977). Management of neonatal seizures. *Critical Care Medicine, 5*(1), 43–49.

Voyer, M., Davakis, M., Antener, I., & Valleur, D. (1982). Zinc balances in preterm infants. *Biology of the Neonate, 42*(1–2), 87–92.

Weinberg, J. A., Weitzman, R. E., Zakauddin, S., & Leake, R. D. (1977). Inappropriate secretion of antidiuretic hormone in a premature infant. *Journal of Pediatrics, 90*(1), 111–114.

Werkman, S. H., Peeples, J. M., Cooke, R. J., et al. (1994). Effect of vitamin A supplementation of intravenous lipids on early vitamin A intake and status of premature infants. *American Journal of Clinical Nutrition, 59*(3), 586–592.

West, K. D., & Kirksey, A. (1976). Influence of vitamin B_6 intake on the content of the vitamin in milk. *American Journal of Clinical Nutrition, 29*(9), 961–969.

Wilson, R. D., Martin, T., Christensen, R., et al. (1983). Hyperparathyroidism in pregnancy: Case report and review of the literature. *Canadian Medical Association Journal, 129*(9), 986–989.

Winters, R. W. (1973). Maintenance fluid therapy. In R. W. Winters (Ed.), *The body fluids in pediatrics* (pp. 113–133). Boston: Little, Brown.

Worthington-White, D. A., Behnke, M., & Gross, S. (1994). Premature infants require additional folate and vitamin B_{12} to reduce the severity of the anemia of prematurity. *American Journal of Clinical Nutrition, 60*(6), 930–935.

Wu, P. Y., Teilman, P., Gabler, M., et al. (1967). "Early" versus "late" feeding of low birthweight neonates: Effect on serum bilirubin, blood sugar and responses to glucagon and epinephrine tests. *Pediatrics, 39*(5), 733–739.

Zachman, R. D. (1988). Vitamin A. In R. C. Tsang & B. L. Nichols (Eds.), *Nutrition during infancy* (pp. 253–263). St. Louis: C. V. Mosby.

Zipursky, A., Brown, E. J., Watts, J., et al. (1987). Oral vitamin E supplementation for the prevention of anemia in premature infants: A controlled trial. *Pediatrics, 79*(1), 61–68.

CHAPTER 23

Nutrition: Physiologic Basis of Metabolism and Management of Enteral and Parenteral Nutrition

LINDA LEFRAK DONNA A. DOWLING

RESEARCH AGENDA

What effect does nasal versus oral gavage have on an infant's tolerance of enteral feedings?

How often should an indwelling gavage tube be changed?

What amount of aspirate obtained prior to gavage feedings indicates feeding intolerance?

What is the ideal rate of bolus feedings?

What is the relationship between infant birth weight and responses to enteral feedings?

What is the effect of milk temperature, infusion rates, infant position, and use of nonnutritive sucking on feeding tolerance and weight gain?

What is the effect of infant position during gavage feedings on feeding tolerance and oxygenation?

What is the relationship between suck–swallow coordination and weight and maturational age?

What is the difference between preterm and term infants' early hunger cues?

Meeting the nutritional needs of premature and sick infants is essential to their intact recovery and survival. This subject, however, receives only token discussion in many neonatal intensive care units (NICUs). As pointed out by Adamkin (1986), the very low birth weight premature infant's body contains approximately 1 percent fat and 8.5 percent protein owing to its high body water content. Under conditions of total starvation, these infants have reserves for only 4½ days, and daily provision of intravenous (IV) glucose prolongs survival to only about 7 days. Therefore, the mandate is to meet the basic nutrient requirements of these infants and to understand their metabolic limitations to avoid physiologic stress and morbidity related to the delivery of enteral and parenteral nutrition.

This chapter briefly reviews the metabolism of nutrients, minerals, and vitamins in the neonate. It then discusses the developmental and physiologic disabilities that are unique to the premature and sick infant. Finally, it includes a discussion regarding practical issues that affect nursing practice in the delivery and monitoring of enteral and parenteral nutrition.

NUTRIENTS

Protein

Protein digestion and absorption can be divided into three phases: gastric, pancreatic, and intestinal. All mechanisms occur to some extent in the developing fetus and have been documented to occur at some level as early as 12 weeks' gestation. The role of protein absorption in the fetus is still unclear (Lebenthal, 1989). In the stomach, protein is broken down into polypeptides and amino acids. This occurs through the activity of pepsin and hydrochloric acid. Although these substances are found as early as 16 weeks in the fetus, at term they have reached only about 10 percent of adult levels (Lebenthal et al., 1983). The second mechanism of protein absorption is the pancreatic or intraluminal phase, during which the polypeptides are broken down into smaller peptides and amino acids. The enzymes responsible for this process are also found early in gestation, but at term they have reached only 20 percent of adult levels. The last phase of protein absorption, intestinal absorption, is a two-step process, during which the small polypeptides continue to break down into amino acids and these substances are subsequently absorbed. This second mechanism is the direct absorption of macromolecules. It is most likely the mechanism that leads to some allergies later in life. In the NICU, the second mechanism is of concern. When feeding a neonate with a damaged bowel, the absorption of macromolecules may be responsible for the antibody response to cow's milk protein (Walker, 1985). Protein absorption in the preterm and term infant is inefficient when compared with that in the adult, but it allows adequate utilization of enteral protein, even in the very small premature infant. As long as the intake is adjusted slightly higher to account for the relative inefficiency of absorption, nitrogen balance is achieved (Kerner, 1983).

Fat

Fat absorption can also be divided into three phases: intraluminal, mucosal, and transport or delivery (Lebenthal, 1989). In the intraluminal phase, triglycerides are converted into free fatty acids and monoglycerides, which are absorbed into mucosal cells. Long-chain fatty acids require bile acids for absorption and, owing to the slow rate of bile acid synthesis and the increased rate of turnover, this process is extremely inefficient in preterm infants

(Lebenthal, 1989). This fat source is avoided when possible. In the mucosal phase of absorption, the free fatty acids are taken through a number of steps, forming phospholipids, cholesterol esters, cholesterol, chylomicrons, and very low density lipoproteins. Chylomicrons are transported through the lymphatic system to the thoracic duct and eventually into the superior vena cava (SVC). Damage to the thoracic duct, which can occur in chest surgery, can then lead to the collection of chyle in the chest and require that dietary fat be modified or totally avoided until the leak resolves. This entire process of fat absorption, although found to occur as early as 22 to 26 weeks' gestation, remains inefficient in preterm infants. Only about 65 to 75 percent of dietary fat is absorbed in the 32-week premature infant, as compared with 95 percent absorption in the adult (Lebenthal, 1989). This translates into the need to adjust dietary fat in quantity and quality when feeding the premature or sick infant. Fat contributes 35 to 55 percent of the dietary calories and is therefore an essential nutrient to adequate growth.

Carbohydrates

Carbohydrate absorption is a three-phase mechanism. During the pancreatic or intraluminal phase, the polysaccharides are broken down into mono- and disaccharides. Amylase is the primary enzyme responsible for this process, and it is secreted by the pancreas into the small intestine. At term, amylase is only at 10 percent of adult levels. The brush border of the neonate's intestines contains the enzymes that break down the disaccharides. Although maltase, isomaltase, invertase, sucrase, and palatinase are all found at functional levels in the fetus as early as 23 weeks, lactase levels remain low even in a full-term birth when compared with those of the adult (Lebenthal, 1989). This fact accounts for the presence of sugars other than lactose in most premature formulas. Lastly, there is active mucosal transport of monosaccharides or simple sugars such as glucose. This mechanism is found even in the fetus and continues to provide a simple mechanism for carbohydrate absorption when other mechanisms fail. Infants with intestinal damage following necrotizing enterocolitis or prolonged ileus with atrophy may be disaccharide intolerant and yet absorb glucose or glucose polymers such as Polycose. The absorption of carbohydrates is therefore somewhat inefficient in the premature infant. The provision of corn syrup solids in premature formulas is meant to reduce carbohydrate malabsorption due to the relative lactase deficiency. The transient nature of lactose malabsorption when the infant's own mother's milk is used confirms the infant's ability to adapt rapidly once fed an exclusive disaccharide-containing enteral diet.

In summary, the absorption of the three major nutrients is relatively inefficient in the preterm as well as in the term infant. For nurses, a basic understanding of these mechanisms of digestion and absorption is essential so that the rationale for various dietary adjustments can be understood. It is also essential for the understanding of risk factors of dietary intolerance and screening for intolerance in individual neonates. For a complete discussion of nutrient absorption and current research, the reader should refer to one of many texts devoted to the subject.

VITAMINS, MACROMINERALS, AND TRACE MINERALS

Little is known about fat-soluble vitamin absorption in the infant at term (Tsang, 1985). Even less is known about these mechanisms in the premature infant. Although the function of vitamins A, D, E, and K is better understood, a great deal is still hypothesized, and additional study in infants is needed. For a review of fat-soluble vitamin function, the reader is referred to Tsang (1985).

Water-soluble vitamins, the B and C group, are less likely to create deficiency states owing to their relative availability and method of absorption in infants. An explanation of their absorption, function, and metabolism can be found in Tsang (1985). Little is known about the needs of premature infants and how to evaluate for deficiency states. References for current recommended intakes can be found in Kerner (1991).

The absorption of sodium, potassium, chloride, and bicarbonate across the intestinal mucosa in the infant appears to differ from that in the adult as inferred by fetal rat studies (Lebenthal, 1989). Under normal circumstances, this difference appears to be of no consequence. In unusual circumstances, such as when hypertonic feedings are used or when diarrhea occurs, the increased intestinal permeability leads to large intestinal losses of these electrolytes as well as of water. This causes the infant to experience dehydration and electrolyte imbalance more rapidly than does the adult. Basic requirements also vary in the infant because renal absorption and excretion of these minerals are not well regulated owing to organ immaturity, which is accentuated in the premature infant.

Calcium absorption occurs through a carrier-mediated mechanism and passive diffusion (Lebenthal, 1989). The carrier-mediated mechanism is dependent on a vitamin D_3 metabolite. Passive diffusion occurs across the intestinal mucosa against a concentration gradient. If bulk water flow through the intestinal tract occurs, as with diarrhea, calcium losses will be exaggerated owing to the diffusion mechanism (Lebenthal, 1989).

Ingested zinc is absorbed in the proximal small bowel. Absorption varies based on the bioavailability of the source and the presence of other minerals in the diet such as iron and copper, which are known to interfere with absorption (Tsang & Nichols, 1988). Much remains to be investigated about the specific absorption of the other trace minerals, such as chromium and selenium.

The reader is encouraged to seek in-depth information about the current recommended intake and utilization of these trace minerals in Tsang (1985) (see Chapter 22, Fluids, Electrolytes, Vitamins, and Trace Minerals: Basis of Ingestion, Digestion, Elimination, and Metabolism).

GASTROINTESTINAL FUNCTION OF THE PREMATURE INFANT

Research on the developing fetus has determined that much of the gastrointestinal tract begins to function at some level early in fetal life. Anatomically, the foregut and hindgut are present at 3½ weeks' gestation, and intestinal villi begin to develop at 8 weeks (Lebenthal et al., 1983). It is clear, however, that even in the full-term infant, the gastrointestinal tract is inefficient in its ability to propel, absorb, and utilize nutrients and maintain homeostasis during stress.

Developmentally, the disabilities of the premature infant begin with the inability to suck, swallow, and breathe in a coordinated fashion. This disability places a heavy burden on the caregiver to provide adequate nutrient intake via all artificial methods. Suck, swallow, and breath coordination develops as early as 32 weeks' gestation (Lebenthal et al., 1983; Meier & Pugh, 1985). There are many reasons why this coordination can be delayed. For example, it is common to observe late coordination in infants who have cardiorespiratory disease and who are physiologically unstable. Another large group of infants who cannot regulate their own intake are those who remain on assisted ventilation. The sequence of the infant suck, swallow, and breathe pattern has been described as a suck once every 2 seconds, a swallow every five to six sucks, and a breath every 2 seconds. This sequence not only presumes maturity of the infant but also depends on physiologic stability. Several studies have made an association between the initial sucking bursts in hypoxemia with or without bradycardia in premature infants and in more mature infants with lung disease (Guilleminault & Coons, 1984; Mathew, 1988b; Rosen et al., 1984). Nonnutritive sucking has some obvious differences from nutritive sucking that make it only one of several indicators of readiness for oral feedings in a premature infant.

The second physiologic disability of the premature infant is the absence or weakness of the gag and cough reflexes. This disability increases the risks to premature infants when gastric enteral feedings are used. The risk of aspiration must be considered when the stomach is filled with food. The assessment for the presence of the gag reflex is easy to perform by direct observation while passing a feeding tube. It is difficult if not impossible to assess the adequacy of the gag reflex for the prevention of aspiration if vomiting or reflux occurs. The risk of aspiration should be considered in all premature infants who are beginning enteral feeding.

The third disability is the relative incompetence of the cardiac sphincter. The purpose of the cardiac sphincter is to close after swallowing and prevent reflux of stomach contents into the esophagus. Even in term infants, sphincter maturation is not complete until about 5 to 7 weeks postnatally. Inadequate sphincter function adds an additional risk factor to all premature infants who are fed orally. In addition, if the infant actually vomits owing to this disability, chronic loss of nutrients becomes a problem. Reflux can also lead to a vagal stimulus, which can precipitate an apneic event (Plaxico & Loughlin, 1981).

Delayed gastric emptying is the fourth physiologic disability in premature infants. Gastric emptying appears to be relatively delayed in all infants. Term and preterm infants improve their emptying times within the first 24 to 48 hours of life. Gastric emptying is delayed in disease states, and nurses find that milk feedings do not predictably empty in preterm infants or sick term infants. This disability may be the single limiting factor when the premature infant is given enteral feedings in that there is little that can be done toward progression until stomach emptying occurs. If gastric emptying remains a limiting factor, transpyloric feedings can be implemented.

Intestinal motility is the fifth major disability in the premature infant. Although this disability is obvious to most clinicians, studies have described the phenomenon and identified the postconceptional age at which motility dramatically improves (Berseth, 1990; Morriss et al., 1986). The investigators looked at the frequency of duodenal contractions in newborns, the number of contractions per burst, and the intraluminal peak pressure per burst. The frequency and strength of the bursts increased after delivery regardless of the gestational age at the time of delivery. There was considerable improvement at 32 weeks' gestation, and infants whose mothers had received prenatal steroids showed a more mature pattern than that of infants of comparable gestations. Other studies of infants with known central nervous system abnormalities or insult had bursts at half the rate expected for their gestational age. Motility is thus a function of gestation, postnatal maturation, and disease state, with a definite link to the central nervous system. If intestinal motility is the limiting factor in the progression of enteral feedings, it should be identified as such before multiple formula changes are tried. It is essential to identify the specific source of the enteral feeding baseline so that a plan can be devised to eliminate the causative factor.

Incompetence of the ileocecal valve, the sixth disability, is not plainly assessed by the clinician. This valve acts as a barrier between small and large bowel contents, thus separating bacterial flora as well as regulating the time needed for the small bowel to absorb nutrients before its contents are delivered to the colon for water absorption. When reflux through this valve occurs, the small bowel is colonized with bacteria. With the presence of undigested nutrients in the small bowel, bacteria proliferate and can produce hydrogen gas. This mechanism is part of the sequence of events hypothesized in the process that leads to necrotizing enterocolitis.

The seventh and last disability is the premature infant's impaired rectosphincteric reflex, which creates a delay in stool evacuation, sometimes to the point of a functional obstruction. Many premature infants require rectal stimulation with a thermometer or a glycerin suppository to evacuate the rectum. Although the passage of the first stool in a premature infant is slightly delayed when compared with term infants, failure to pass meconium by 72 hours of life should alert the nurse that a suppository may be necessary (Jhaveri & Kumar, 1987). Thereafter, rectal evacuation should be looked at in relation to oral feeding volumes and symptoms of obstruction. Isolated intestinal perforations without the histologic findings of necrotizing enterocolitis may in part be due to the distention of the premature bowel to the point of perforation. Although described in association with IV indomethacin, it has also been described in very low birth weight infants who have had no indomethacin, and therefore the mechanism of immature gastrointestinal function most likely plays a role (Buchheit & Stewart, 1994).

In summary, the premature infant has many developmental and mechanical disabilities that make use of the gastrointestinal tract difficult or impossible. The digestive tract matures with postnatal age and physiologic stability and needs to be reassessed regularly so that its use is not delayed. Increasing evidence exists suggesting that small amounts of enteral nutrient delivery enhance maturation of the gastrointestinal tract (Berseth, 1990; Lucas et al., 1986; Slagle & Gross, 1988). With the use of manometrics (a tool to evaluate intestinal motor activity in response to various feeding techniques), there may be clearer recommendations in the future on the methods of feeding best suited for the premature infant (Koenig et al., 1995).

PARENTERAL NUTRITION

Based on the knowledge that the premature or sick infant has a gastrointestinal system that may not allow the safe or feasible delivery of enteral feeding, the clinician must consider the alternate route, total parenteral nutrition (TPN). Until the early 1970s, infants who could not be fed orally could receive only IV glucose with electrolytes and crude IV vitamin preparations. The mortality and morbidity associated with many neonatal conditions were directly related to how long the infant could survive on inadequate nutrient delivery. Over almost three decades, there has been continued refinement of the clinician's ability to provide adequate and safe IV nutrition, not only to improve survival but also to promote normal growth and avoid the morbidity of nutritional deficiencies, many of which we have yet to appreciate fully.

Basic Needs

There are many controversies about what infants need nutritionally. This chapter provides the current range of recommendations for parenteral nutrients and refers the reader to references in which the controversies are discussed in depth.

It is generally accepted that infants require at least 50 kcal/kg/day to meet the basic metabolic requirement (BMR). Two recent studies that calculated BMR in premature infants receiving assisted ventilation and in premature infants with chronic lung disease with growth failure found resting energy expenditure or BMR was 67 kcal/kg/day and 72 kcal/kg/day, respectively (Billeaud et al., 1992; Kurzner et al., 1988). This caloric need assumes that infants do not break down any of their own tissue to sustain body functions. Since IV calories are utilized most efficiently, providing 50 kcal/kg/day to an infant solely by the IV route will almost assuredly meet BMR only in the most stable infants. If these calories are provided enterally, the loss of calories via inefficient absorption must be considered. Meeting the BMR translates into an infant receiving 125 ml/kg/day of $D_{10}W$ to obtain 50 kcal/kg/day, using the value of 0.4 kcal/ml of $D_{10}W$. When D_5W is used, the amount is prohibitive (250 ml/kg/day). Once the BMR is met, calories and protein are increased to allow positive nitrogen balance, protein sparing and, ultimately, growth requirements. The recommendations for target calories vary from 70 to 100 kcal/kg/day intravenously. Providing this intake using peripheral IV access is impractical and risky (Pereira, 1995). Technical considerations are discussed further on.

Enteral fluid and nutrient needs will not be discussed here, but in most cases the total fluid volume that the infant can safely receive, based on organ maturity and disease state, dictates the concentration of all other nutrients to be delivered. The basic principles governing the calculation of fluid to be delivered are no different for total IV nutrition than for IV glucose or volume. Fluid issues focus on providing that which is balanced and adequate in a volume that can be safely handled by the infant (see Chapter 22 for a complete discussion of fluids and electrolytes).

As mentioned, infants' nutrient needs—protein, carbohydrate, and fat—are still somewhat controversial. It is now possible to deliver adequate, balanced IV nutrition to even the smallest premature neonate. It is essential that nurses understand the makeup and rationale of the IV nutrient bottles that they hang. As with any IV medication, these solutions have the potential to create short- and long-term complications, and the nurse must have a clear understanding of these complications and how to monitor for them. Recently, there have been reports of severe hyperglycemia as a result of human error in hanging bags for automixer, the most common error being the transposing of the water bag and the bag of 50 to 70 percent dextrose. The result is a bag containing a very high concentration of glucose. To prevent this type of error, pharmacists can implement the use of a refractive index measurement (Meyer et al., 1987). The instrument measures what essentially is the specific gravity of the solution from a known value based on the percent of glucose and amino acid. Solutions once mixed are tested rapidly and mixing errors are determined before the bags are sent to the nursery. All pediatric pharmacies should consider the use of this device because it is inexpensive and may prevent mixing errors that lead to severe central nervous system bleeding, neurologic devastation, and death. The $300 cost for the instrument is offset, potentially averting the dramatic adverse effects of only one error.

IV nutrient delivery must be balanced and must provide maintenance as well as growth needs. IV protein intake most likely should be 3 g/kg/day. Some preliminary observations have led to recommendations of 3.5 g/kg/day for preterm infants (Kerner, 1991; Pereira, 1995; Shulman et al., 1985). Although third-trimester accretion is approximately 2 to 3 g/kg/day, certain postnatal events such as surgery, respiratory disease, or necrotizing enterocolitis increase the protein needs and deplete the protein stores rapidly. Fat needs are minimal to prevent a deficiency state, but fats should make up 40 to 50 percent of total caloric intake and therefore are a large contributor to total required calories. If IV fats in the range of 3 to 4 g/kg/day are used, there is a risk of excess owing to the complications of fat overload syndrome, the potential for a harmful effect on oxygen diffusion, and additional concerns if triglyceride and cholesterol levels are elevated (Kerner, 1991). IV fat intake should not exceed 3 to 4 g/kg/day for all infants and should be monitored at least weekly with triglyceride and cholesterol levels (Kerner, 1983, 1991). Several authors have shown that the 20 percent lipid solutions are better tolerated because of the efficiency of triglyceride clearance in the 20 percent solutions. Carbohydrate intake should also represent 40 to 50 percent of the total caloric intake. Excesses should be avoided even if the blood glucose level is normal, owing to the potential development of cholestasis and its contribution to carbon dioxide production and oxygen consumption. If no more than 20 g/kg/day is delivered, these risks are considered reduced. More commonly, the technical problems related to delivering adequate glucose arise when peripheral access is used or when the infant is very hyperglycemic in the face of low glucose intake. These issues are discussed in the following section.

To summarize, the balance and absolute amount of nutrients needed for TPN are

Protein:	8 to 12 percent of total caloric intake; 2.5 to 3.5 g/kg/day
Fat:	40 to 50 percent of total caloric intake; 3 to 4 g/kg/day
Carbohydrate:	40 to 50 percent of total caloric intake; as tolerated to 20 g/kg/day

Methods of Delivery and Technical Problems

Parenteral nutrients can be delivered in many ways in today's NICU. Table 23–1 lists the methods and the risks and benefits of each. The clinician must then decide how best to deliver IV nutrients in the face of immaturity and disease. Premature infants of less than 32 weeks' gestation rarely have a gastrointestinal tract that will function fully within 2 weeks. In premature infants of all gestations, disease affects the gastrointestinal tract, rendering it immobile for days to weeks. Gastrointestinal dysfunction also occurs in many term infants in the NICU who come to the setting with asphyxia, severe lung disease, or congenital anomalies. For this reason, 2 to 3 weeks of some form of IV nutrition is common.

There are two major constraints to peripheral IV nutrient delivery: the amount of glucose and the amount of protein that can be administered. The maximal carbohydrate (glucose) concentration that can be delivered is 10 to 12.5 percent, and the amount of protein is 2 g/dl. These values are based on the subsequent osmolality of the solution that is tolerated by peripheral veins. The higher the osmolality, the more likely that infiltration and tissue damage will occur. Although it is possible to infuse 15 percent glucose solutions into a peripheral vein, the risk of infiltration and tissue damage is not only high but also likely (Kerner, 1983). Considering that most sick infants require fluid limitations, it is almost impossible to administer 80 kcal/kg/day and 3 g of protein/kg/day by this method. Other major issues of peripheral administration are the adequacy of peripheral veins, pain of intermittent "restarts," hypoxia from crying, cost of personnel time, and poor subsequent growth if nutrient delivery is low or frequently interrupted.

It is for these reasons that the use of percutaneous central venous catheters (PCVCs) has become so widespread in this population of sick infants. Several authors describe the procedure and the risks, feasibility, and care of these lines (Dolcourt & Bose, 1982; Durand et al., 1986; Leick-Rude, 1990; Mactier et al., 1986; Nakamura et al., 1990; Oellrich et al., 1991; Riordan, 1979; Stringer et al., 1992). There are currently five devices on the market that can be used for this procedure. All PCVCs are made of polymeric silicone (Silastic), silicone, or polyurethane, and all go through needles that break away or are threaded out of the system. There are now double-lumen devices and devices small enough to thread a 24-gauge breakaway needle. The vein of choice for cannulation is the cephalic or basilic vein of the arm. These veins can be cannulated at the hand or the antecubital fossa; they flow in a direct way to become the auxiliary vein, then the innominate vein, and finally the SVC. The saphenous veins at the ankle or knee are also safe sites for insertion and thread to the femoral vein, the iliac vein, and eventually the inferior vena cava (IVC). In our practice, this site has the same low risk for insertion as do the upper extremity veins. The tips of PCVCs are usually threaded to the SVC or IVC–right atrial junction to pro-

TABLE 23–1 Methods of Intravenous Access Techniques and the Risks and Benefits of Each

Pros–Benefits	Cons–Risks
Peripheral	
Reduced risk of systemic infection Multiple team members have insertion skills No central venous access risks Low cost per device	Limited percent glucose and percent protein High fluid volumes required to meet energy and protein needs of sick infants (150–200 ml/kg) Intermittent pain, hypoxia, cold stress, and hypoglycemia with restarts Possible tissue damage with infiltration Restriction of positioning and motion when extremities used Limited veins in very small infants and infants with long-term IV needs
Central	
Nutrient needs met with limited fluids (high caloric density possible) Staff time minimal once inserted (no need for restarts) No positional restraints Percutaneous access can be attained with no vein loss, no surgical incision; small size reduces thrombus, embolus, and effusion risks of central access No intermittent loss of therapy (glucose and fluids) due to infiltration	Central access risks effusion, thrombus, and infection If surgical access used, vein loss, cost increased for device and surgeon fee Need for radiograph to determine tip and follow-over time Increased nursing skill required for patient monitoring and troubleshooting device

IV, intravenous.

vide the highest flow area, which minimizes the risk of infiltration and extravasation and reduces the possibility of arrhythmia. Concentrations of glucose and protein intake can be increased to meet the infant's needs even in the circumstance of conservative fluid restriction. In our practice, we use glucose concentrations of 20 to 25 percent and protein concentrations as high as 4 percent when clinically indicated to achieve adequate nutrient intake.

The position of the PCVC tip should be confirmed by radiography, using contrast injection. Although the device is radiopaque, the densities within the chest and abdomen of a neonate make tip placement impossible to determine accurately without additional contrast injection. The clinician should document that there is good blood return and that flushing meets no resistance. Both of these factors help ensure a high-flow area that allows rapid dilution of these hypertonic solutions. Broviac catheters, which are placed surgically, are reserved for infants who need months of parenteral nutrition, such as those with short bowel syndrome or the rare infant who cannot have a peripheral vein successfully cannulated for a PCVC. The success of this technique (PCVC insertion) requires skill and knowledge; most important, however, is staff education about the maintenance and troubleshooting of the lines and the commitment to early insertion before peripheral sites are used for other venous punctures. A comprehensive review of maintenance and troubleshooting can be found in an article by Chathas, who has contributed greatly to this technology and has supported it as a nursing procedure under standardized protocol (Chathas, 1986).

If peripheral access is chosen, the device for delivery should be one of the Intracath-Jelco types because their mean life is at least twice that of the stainless steel needle (Batton et al., 1982). There is also a device on the market that expands 2 gauges after insertion into the vein and is made of a new soft plastic that provides a longer dwelling time in adults and may do the same in neonates (Hickey et al., 1989; Sheehan et al., 1992). Peripheral access, no matter what the device, involves nutritional limitations in all premature and sick infants and is realistic for only a few days.

The other issue related to peripheral access is the care of the site if the solution infiltrates. All NICUs that use peripheral alimentation must have a procedure or protocol for initial treatment of the site. Hyaluronidase (Wydase) has been used for this purpose for several years and has been found to reduce the extent of tissue necrosis dramatically by breaking down the cell membrane and dissipating the chemical irritant (TPN) (Pettit & Hughes, 1993; Zenk et al., 1981). A dose of 15 units given in three to four subcutaneous injections around the perimeter of the edema within an hour will give best results. Another factor that contributes to tissue necrosis is the vascular supply to the site of infiltration. If arterial flow is adequate and venous return is unrestricted, damage is reduced. For these reasons, the site for peripheral TPN must be selected carefully. For example, a foot vein should not be used if 2 days before that foot showed vascular compromise from an umbilical artery line. Although the color of the foot may be normal and the pulse palpable, there may be unexpected tissue damage, probably owing to a clinically undetected decreased arterial flow.

The technical risks of central access are many (Carey, 1989; Dhande et al., 1983; Grisoni et al., 1986; MacDonald & Chou, 1986; Opitz & Toyama, 1982). The most common risks are infiltration, infection, and loss of the device resulting from technical difficulties such as occlusion. Infiltration risks can all but be eliminated when the tips of the catheters are left at the SVC or IVC–right atrial junction. When this is not feasible, or when the infant grows and the catheter tip begins to migrate, staff must begin to monitor closely for signs that the TPN fluid is collecting in the subcutaneous space. For catheter tips in the innominate, subclavian, auxiliary, or jugular vein, swelling can usually be detected with regular inspection of the neck or chest wall. When the patient has generalized edema, detection becomes more difficult, and an asymmetrical swelling that does not disappear with position change may be detected first. Careful review for the presence of differential edema on a radiograph may be helpful. Infiltration, although possible, is actually rare. To minimize risk, lower glucose solutions can be used in very low birth weight infants when it is not feasible to thread the catheter tip to the SVC. For instance, if the first catheter tip can be threaded only to the subclavian vein in an 800-g infant, the glucose limit may need to remain at 15 percent until the time a second catheter can be threaded to the SVC. However, most very low birth weight infants cannot tolerate 15 percent glucose at the maintenance fluid rates until they are about 2 weeks old, so this limit is usually not a factor in the delivery of adequate calories.

The infectious risks of the PCVC are also reported to be low (Chathas, 1986; Chathas et al., 1990; Ramanathan & Durand, 1987; Shulman et al., 1986). All invasive devices increase the risk of infection in sick infants. The PCVC is no exception but should not be implicated immediately as the focus of infection in all infants who have positive cultures. It is well known that certain resistant bacterial strains and fungi are present on the skin of these infants within a few days after admission to a NICU (Evans et al., 1988). Any loss of skin integrity, tracheal trauma, or skin puncture—such as with a chest tube insertion or arterial puncture—can introduce the flora into the blood stream. If PCVC insertion is performed under sterile conditions, if a sterile occlusive dressing is placed and not disturbed, and if all breaks into the system are carried out under sterile technique, the risk of infection is reduced. Fungal infection remains a problem because the presence of IV fat in the system provides an ideal culture medium for *Candida albicans* and all yeasts, including *Malassezia furfur*. This fungus can cause infection and will also occlude the line (Aschner et al., 1987; Azimi et al., 1988; Powell et al., 1984). An occlusion with fungus, such as *M. furfur*, requires that the line be pulled because at this time there is no pharmacologic treatment for this fungus. If fungal infections are suspected, the contents of the catheters must be antiseptically flushed into a container and sent to the laboratory for identification, with specific instructions to examine the specimen for fungus. Fungal growth requires that fat be added to the traditional agar plates; recovery of the organism from catheter tips and blood cultures is low (Azimi et al., 1988).

The technical difficulties of maintaining PCVCs can be minimized with staff education and systematic, ongoing monitoring. Clinicians should maintain a record of insertion complications, which should be followed up systematically, and the nursing quality assurance or quality improvement committee ideally should monitor for maintenance problems. Through this process, staff can be informed and educated about how to handle technical problems. Through two prospective, descriptive studies to quantify technical problems in our practice, we have been able to extend the mean catheter life so that elective removal now occurs 70 to 80 percent of the time compared with a rate of only 40 percent in 1982 (Lefrak-Okikawa, unpublished data).

Finally, there are complications related to patient intolerance of the solution components themselves. These complications include metabolic imbalances, such as hyperglycemia or hyponatremia, and clinically significant deficiency states if essential nutrients, minerals, or vitamins are omitted. All NICUs should have system checks in place to aid in the comprehensive ordering of these solutions. Systems include standardized order sheets, computer programs that calculate solution additives based on target orders per kilogram per day, or manual pharmacist checks to determine safety and completeness (Ball et al., 1985; Yamamoto et al., 1986). It is no longer acceptable to leave to chance that the ordering of these solutions is complete and accurate. It is also essential that ongoing quality assurance–improvement monitoring occurs to determine whether the systems are adequate. TPN has now been in use for 20 years; although there is still controversy on the ideal amino acid mix and the exact amount of trace minerals and vitamins needed, the basic nutrient mineral needs are known.

It should be possible to avoid metabolic problems by systematically advancing fluid constituents and regularly monitoring with weekly laboratory tests, growth graphs, and daily screens such as bedside serum glucose testing or reagent strip tests (Chemstrip). Hyperglycemia and hypoglycemia are probably the most common ongoing problems associated with the use of TPN. One way to reduce these problems is through a system that requires a calculation of grams of glucose per kilogram per day or milligrams per kilogram per minute when the TPN rate is ordered. Traditionally, the percent glucose is ordered incrementally; thus, as IV rate changes are made, the glucose load either exceeds that which is tolerated or is inadequate. For example, a 1-kg infant may be receiving a 7.5 percent glucose solution on day 3 of life and the blood glucose or reagent strip result remains stable. The order for day 4 is for 10 percent glucose, which is incremental, but at the same time the fluids are liberalized and the ultimate glucose received jumps from 8 to 12 g/kg/day. Most preterm infants cannot adequately metabolize this increased glucose load and experience hyperglycemia, which may require a work-up for sepsis, since hyperglycemia is a symptom of many other complications, including infection. Hyperglycemia sometimes occurs under the best circumstances in very low birth weight infants. With the mandate of providing calories to meet the BMR as soon as possible, it is sometimes necessary to use insulin additives in the TPN solution. It has been shown that this practice is feasible and can improve the glucose tolerance in very low birth weight infants, providing better caloric intake early on in hospitalization (Binder et al., 1989; Ostertag et al., 1986; Simeon et al., 1994; Vaucher et al., 1982).

It is no longer acceptable for the NICU nurse to hang a TPN bottle that is checked only for patient name, rate, and glucose concentration. The bottle must be checked for all contents, and the potential risks of all constituents must be understood if safe patient care is to be delivered. This therapy is collaborative: it is ordered by the physician, checked and mixed by the pharmacist, and monitored by the nurse. Nurses will most likely be the first to observe technical or metabolic complications, and they must know what these complications are. In our own unit we have asked nurses to screen the label for accuracy of patient weight (as additives are based on a per kilogram calculation), milliequivalent of sodium and potassium per deciliter, and clarity and color of the solution. If an infant exhibits a dramatic change in serum glucose or electrolyte levels, part of the differential diagnosis includes the possibility of a TPN solution mixing error. A sample from the TPN bag is sent to the laboratory for analysis of the additive in question. The laboratory must be informed what the concentration is thought to be so that appropriate dilutions can be performed before the sample is analyzed.

An article on Y-site compatibility by Zenk (1992) provides current compatibility information for medications that can be administered with TPN including IV fat. Of particular importance is the information about the compatibility of dopamine with TPN and fat and the compatibility of vancomycin with TPN. This information assists nurses in the administration of these common medications using only one line for IV access.

For more discussion of the rare metabolic complications, the reader is referred to the references at the end of this chapter (see Chapter 25, Assessment and Management of Metabolic Dysfunction).

ENTERAL NUTRITION

From the 1920s until the 1950s, the management of enteral feeding was the responsibility of the "premature nursery" nurse (Lundeen, 1939). Preparing and administering feedings and assisting mothers in acquiring feeding skills were major components of the nursing role. Techniques of feeding (gavage, medicine dropper, bottle, and breast) for preterm infants and approaches to parent education about feeding have been detailed in the historical nursing literature (Lundeen, 1939, 1954, 1959). However, as premature nurseries were replaced by NICUs during the 1960s and 1970s, physicians began to assume increasing control of enteral feeding decisions for preterm infants. These decisions include (1) the timing of the initiation of enteral feedings; (2) the route of feeding, for example, oral, nasogastric, or transpyloric; (3) the volume of the feeding; (4) the periodicity of the feeding, for example, intermittent or continuous; and (5) the constituents and concentration of the feeding.

The enteral caloric needs of premature and sick infants vary widely based on size, age, disease state, and genetic factors. However, there are target numbers that should be committed to memory as a safe starting place; with daily monitoring this number can be modified appropriately. Preterm infants require approximately 120 kcal/kg/day for tissue repair and growth. Term infants who have a disease state may require as many calories but usually will grow while receiving 100 to 110 kcal/kg/day owing to more efficient digestion and absorption. Many authors have broken down the intake based on BMR, specific dynamic action, stool losses, and so on. It is, however, hard to find any data on specific genetic considerations, and it is essential that all units have growth charts that can assist in the assessment of an individual infant's growth pattern.

Growth charts allow clinicians to plot weight, length, and head circumference of infants as immature as 24 weeks; compare individual infants with standardized norms of infants of similar gestation; and establish the infant's baseline. Whether an infant's relative size at birth is due to his or her intrauterine environment or genetic potential is never clear, but a fall below that baseline should alarm physicians and nurses. The graphs that should be used are those that show intrauterine growth curves, which demonstrate what would have happened had the gestation been carried to full term. Postnatal growth is almost never ideal in this population owing to disease states and technical constraints of nutrient delivery. The specific growth chart should be evaluated before we ascertain if it is appropriate to use for the specific population, for example, the Dancis growth charts provide a poor comparison because they show postnatal curves and were established at a time when nutrient delivery was minimal and crude at best (Dancis et al., 1948). The Babson growth charts are probably most amenable to generalization in that they show intrauterine growth curves, allowing an infant to be plotted from 24 weeks to 1 year adjusted age (Babson & Benda, 1976). NICUs located high above sea level should consider other curves, since data for the Babson graph were taken from infants born at sea level. Neonatal specialists in Denver and Arizona have developed modified growth curves for infants born at high altitudes. Once the infants' measurements have been plotted on the birth parameters, caloric adjustments should be made to keep them on this curve. Daily gains should aim for about 15 to 20 g/kg/day. Two studies have shown that when gain is looked at as a per kilogram number, all infants are comparable (Fenton et al., 1990; Shaffer et al., 1987). For example, although the 600-g infant may gain only 9 g/day, this is equivalent to 14 g/kg/day. Published data on average percent of weight loss by birth weight also exist (Brosius et al., 1984; Fenton et al., 1990; Shaffer et al., 1987). Although this information comes from descriptive data, it has been observed in other units that have similar nutritional goals. If weight losses in premature infants are high and time to regain birth weight exceeds 3 weeks, there may be a need for some change in therapy, even in very immature infants.

Although it is clear that the caloric intake should be higher when enteral nutrition is started, it should be gradually increased as parenteral nutrition is gradually reduced. The ultimate target intake may take many weeks to achieve. Therefore, IV nutrient supplementation is essential until full enteral feedings are tolerated. This transition must be monitored closely for adequacy and balance of nutrients. IV calories should not be withdrawn until infants are receiving target calories of 100 to 120 kcal/kg/day for at least a day or two. Since this is when a great deal of intolerance to enteral nutrients tends to develop, including necrotizing enterocolitis, it is sometimes helpful to use a heparin lock on the IV device for several days in case enteral feedings need to be reduced (Barnard et al., 1985).

Fluid intake should not be less than 100 ml/kg/day to provide basic hydration, and the upper limits need to be determined based on each infant's assessment. Infants with lung disease may need moderate restriction of 140 to 150 ml/kg/day or conservative restriction of 120 ml/kg/day. If there are no fluid constraints due to disease or an inability of intake, premature infants have been observed to take in as much as 250 ml/kg/day of formula during the recovery phase of illness with no ill effects. If fluid restraints are ongoing, the caloric density of the formula needs to be adjusted to allow the target caloric intake.

Nutrient needs should not be a major issue if fortified human milk or premature formulas are used. These diets provide the premature infant with the additional protein, vitamins, and minerals needed when target caloric intake is achieved. Standard infant formulas should not be used in this population because they are too low in protein and have an inadequate vitamin and mineral content for the growing preterm infant (Anderson, 1987). There are also good data showing that pooled mature human milk is also inadequate in protein and minerals and that growth rate and quality are poor when it is used in premature infants (Gross, 1983; Modanlou et al., 1986; Putet et al., 1984). It may also be a source of the human immunodeficiency virus. When an elemental diet is needed, such as with infants who have had bowel resection for necrotizing enterocolitis, the most commonly prepared diet currently available is protein hydrosylate formula (Pregestimil). It contains protein in an enzymatically hydrolyzed casein mixed with three amino acids. The carbohydrate consists of glucose polymers, which are easily digestible. The fat content is 60 percent medium chain triglycerides, 20 percent oleic safflower oil, and 20 percent corn oil. It is almost isotonic. A soy protein formula (Alimentum) is being used by some practitioners. Its protein is casein hydrolysate, with amino acids cystine, tyrosine, and tryptophan. The carbohydrate is sucrose and modified tapioca starch, with the fat being medium chain triglycerides and safflower and soy oils with linoleic acid. Its osmolarity is 330 mOsm/L per 100 kcal. If either is used, there may be a need for some adjustments when possible in calcium, phosphorus, and protein content. Table 23–2 presents a comparison of standard formulas.

Methods of Enteral Feeding

Historically, nurses have based enteral feeding protocols for preterm infants on experience and tradition rather than on a scientific foundation, primarily because little research has been conducted on this topic. Consequently, considerable variability exists in the management of gavage feeding, bottle feeding, and breastfeeding for preterm infants. In a survey of directors of NICUs (Churella et al., 1985), investigators found that neonatologists make decisions about feeding methods for low birth weight infants based primarily on infant weight at birth. Although making feeding decisions based on infant weight provides for standardization of practice in a busy NICU, it does not incorporate individual infant differences with respect to enteral feeding. Although no previously published research has demonstrated an association between infant birth weight and responses to enteral feeding, research has been described that supports the use of early, small-volume enteral feeding to promote maturation of intestinal motor function in preterm infants (Berseth & Nordyke, 1993; Meetze et al., 1992). Additionally, a recent research report described the effect of different volumes and concentrations of gastric and transpyloric feedings on the intestinal motor response to feeding in preterm infants (Koenig et al., 1995). Research in this arena will provide a scientific basis for decisions concerning the initiation of enteral feeding for preterm infants (Lebenthal, 1995).

Issues Common to All Methods of Enteral Feeding

Numerous published reports have demonstrated that enteral feeding is accompanied by physiologic and biochemical changes for term and preterm infants. In general for gavage and bottle

TABLE 23–2 Comparison of Human Milk, Soy Protein Formulas, and Cow's Milk

	Mother's Milk	SMA*	Similac with Iron	Gerber with Iron*	Enfamil with Iron*	Good Start	Whole Cow's Milk
Protein (%) (weight/volume)	1.1	1.5	1.5	1.5	1.5	—	3.6
Casein (%)	40	40	82	82	40	—	82
Whey protein (%)	60	60	18	18	60	100†	18
Fat (%) (weight/volume)	3.9	3.6	3.6	3.7	3.8	3.5	3.7
Monounsaturated (%)	41.6	41.3	17.6	17.6	16.0	25.6	30.4
Polyunsaturated (%)	14.2	14.5	37.3	37.3	29.0	31.9	3.8
Saturated (%)	44.2	44.2	45.1	45.1	55.0	42.5	65.8
Oils							
Soy (%)	—	15	60	60	45	—	—
Coconut (%)	—	27	40	40	55	18	—
High oleic safflower–sunflower (%)	—	25	—	—	—	22	—
Palmolein (%)	—	—	—	—	—	60	—
Oleo (%)	—	33	—	—	—	—	—
Minerals (milligrams/liter)							
Total (ash)	2000	2500	3300	NA	3000	NA	7200
Sodium	150	150	190	225	180	162	520
Potassium	550	560	730	730	720	662	1480
Calcium	340	420	510	510	460	433	1220
Phosphorus	140	280	390	390	320	243	960
Chloride	360–480	375	450	475	420	400	960
Iron	0.5	12‡	12‡	12‡	13‡	10	0.6
Zinc	3	5	5	5	5	5	5
Selected Vitamins (per liter)							
Vitamin A (IU)	2000	2000	2030	2030	2100	2030	1400
Contains beta-carotene	Yes	Yes	No§	No§	No§	No§	Yes
Vitamin C (mg)	40	55	60	60	54	54	10
Vitamin D (IU)	22	400	410	406	420	406	20
Carbohydrate (%) (weight–volume)	7.2 lactose	7.2 lactose	7.2 lactose	7.2 lactose	6.9 lactose	7.4 lactose, maltodextrin	4.8 lactose
Nucleotides	Yes	Yes	No§	No§	No§	No§	No§

NOTE: All data for competitive products are derived from product labels, *Physicians' Desk Reference*, or analyses.
*Concentrated liquid with iron (standard dilution).
†Partially hydrolyzed whey protein.
‡SMA Lo-iron and Similac contain 1.5 mg of iron per liter. Enfamil low-iron and Gerber low-iron contain 1.1 mg of iron per liter. Infants fed these formulas should receive supplemental dietary iron from an outside source to meet daily requirements.
§Trace amounts only.
NA, not available.
Courtesy of Wyeth-Ayerst Laboratories, Philadelphia, Pa.

feeding, these changes include hypoxemia, hypercarbia, ventilatory disruption, circulatory alterations, thermal changes, apnea, bradycardia, and cyanosis (Bodefeld et al., 1979; Eckburg et al., 1987; Guilleminault & Coons, 1984; Herrell et al., 1980; Mathew et al., 1985a, 1985b; Mukhtar & Strothers, 1982; Patel et al., 1977; Shivpuri et al., 1983; Wilkinson & Yu, 1974; Yu, 1976; Yu & Rolfe, 1976). The extent to which these changes have been identified as clinically significant varies with the individual studies, sample characteristics, and specifics of the feeding techniques.

In general, the few studies that have been conducted during breastfeeding for preterm infants suggest that only minor physiologic and biochemical changes occur. Specifically, oxygenation is unaltered during and after breastfeeding, and body temperature increases during breastfeeding (Meier, 1988; Meier & Anderson, 1987). However, these studies had a small sample size, and additional research is necessary prior to widespread generalization of results.

Gavage Feedings

Gavage feedings, either by the orogastric or the nasogastric route, are indicated for preterm infants who are unable to feed orally. Generally, infants are transferred gradually from parenteral nutrition to gavage feedings, receiving them until sucking and swallowing reflexes are coordinated sufficiently to prevent aspiration of milk during oral feedings. A major controversy in the administration of gavage feedings for preterm infants is whether continuous or intermittent feedings, or some combination of these routes, should be used. A secondary consideration is whether selected nursing interventions might minimize the physiologic and biochemical alterations that have been noted during and after intermittent gavage or bolus feedings.

Continuous Versus Intermittent Gavage or Bolus Feedings

Prior to the 1970s, preterm infants received gavage or bolus feedings intermittently, at 1- to 4-hour intervals. Clinical distress and regurgitation during and after feedings were managed by administering milk in smaller volumes, at slower rates, and at more frequent intervals. In the 1970s, an alternative to intermittent gavage or bolus feedings was introduced and was referred to as transpyloric continuous nasojejunal (CNJ) alimentation

(Cheek & Staub, 1973; Rhea & Kilby, 1970). This technique became widely used, especially for small, ill preterm infants. CNJ feedings involved insertion of a small feeding tube through the nose into the stomach; gastrointestinal peristalsis moved the tube into the jejunum within a 24-hour period. Once correct tube placement was documented, milk feedings were connected to an infusion pump and allowed to flow continuously at a prescribed rate (milliliters per hour). Theoretically, preterm infants could receive larger daily volumes of milk with minimal physiologic and biochemical alterations. The continuous milk flow minimized gastric distention and consequent circulatory and respiratory changes. Additionally, the milk was delivered into the jejunum, bypassing both the cardiac and the pyloric sphincters, so the probability of regurgitation and aspiration was reduced.

CNJ feedings were gradually replaced with continuous nasogastric (CNG) feedings (Landwirth, 1974). CNG feedings were administered by slow infusion rates into the stomach so that rapid distention of the stomach was avoided. By employing the CNG route, clinicians hoped to avoid the adverse physiologic and biochemical responses—tachycardia, tachypnea, bradycardia, apnea, cyanosis, and hypoxemia—associated with intermittent gavage or bolus feedings (Heldt, 1988; Herrell et al., 1980; Mukhtar & Strothers, 1982; Patel et al., 1977; Wilkinson & Yu, 1974; Yu, 1976; Yu & Rolfe, 1976).

CURRENT CLINICAL PRACTICES

There is no consensus in the literature or among clinicians about whether gavage feedings for small preterm infants should be administered continuously by infusion pump (CNG) or intermittently by gavage or bolus into the infant stomach. Proponents of CNG feedings cite the previously mentioned adverse physiologic and biochemical responses to intermittent feedings, emphasizing that these responses do not occur with CNG feedings. Proponents of intermittent gavage or bolus feedings have expressed concern that CNG feedings permit bacterial growth and that infusion pumps and disposable infusion tubing, which must be used with CNG feedings, represent an additional, perhaps unnecessary, patient expense.

Controlled clinical trials are needed in which infant outcomes are compared for intermittent and CNG feedings. One published study compared weight gain and the incidence of complications in infants fed by continuous and gavage methods with those in infants fed by bolus methods (Toce et al., 1987). Although this study demonstrated minor differences in mean infant weight gain for the two feeding methods, numerous methodologic limitations compromise the study results. In a separate study, patterns of enteroinsular hormone secretion were noted to differ for preterm infants, depending on whether feedings were administered by the intermittent or CNG route. Interestingly, in this research no differences in weight gain were noted for the two groups of infants (Aynsley-Green et al., 1982). A recent study reported adverse effects on pulmonary function for preterm infants after intermittent gavage feedings when compared with infants who received continuous feedings (Blondheim et al., 1993). After intermittent feeding administered over a 15- to 20-minute period, infants demonstrated significant decreases in tidal volume, minute ventilation, and dynamic compliance and a significant increase in pulmonary resistance. Infants who were studied after receiving the same volume per body weight by continuous feedings given over a 3-hour period demonstrated no significant changes in pulmonary function data.

Gavage Feedings of Expressed Mother's Milk

Milk expressed by mothers of preterm infants can be fed to the infants by gavage until the infant is able to suckle at the breast provided that certain safeguards are observed. Two outcomes preclude administration of expressed mother's milk by the CNG route when traditional infusion tubing is used: (1) nutrient loss (Brennan-Behm et al., 1994; Brooke & Barley, 1978; Greer et al., 1984; Lemons et al., 1983; Narayanan et al., 1984; Stocks et al., 1985) and (2) bacterial growth in expressed mother's milk that has been colonized previously (Botsford et al., 1986; Lemons et al., 1983; Meier & Wilks, 1987; Wilks & Meier, 1988).

Six separate studies have documented that milk lipid losses during CNG infusion are significant (Brennan-Behm et al., 1994; Brooke & Barley, 1978; Greer et al., 1984; Lemons et al., 1983; Narayanan et al., 1984; Stocks et al., 1985). Investigators from one study reported large protein losses during CNG infusion (Stocks et al., 1985). These nutrient losses are especially significant for very low birth weight preterm infants, and it is this population that usually receives CNG feedings. In one study, investigators compared lipid losses for two types of infusion tubing: one with a lumen capacity of 5 ml and the other with a lumen capacity of 0.6 ml (Brennan-Behm et al., 1994). The CNG feedings were simulated, and expressed mother's milk was infused at a rate of 2 ml/hour. The findings revealed that statistically and clinically significant lipid losses occurred for both types of tubing; however, the mean difference between lipid values before and after feeding was greatest for the larger lumen tubing.

In one study, investigators proposed that lipid losses during CNG feedings could be reduced by elevating the tip of the infusion syringe to an angle between 25 and 40 degrees (Narayanan et al., 1984). However, pre- and postfeeding lipid concentrations were measured from milk remaining in the infusion syringe rather than from the distal end of the infusion tubing. Thus, it is unclear whether the infant actually received a greater concentration of lipids. In combination, these data suggest that nutrient loss, especially milk lipids, may be unavoidable when expressed mother's milk is administered by the CNG route.

The potential for bacterial growth in already colonized expressed mother's milk has been widely recognized in recent years. Contrary to widespread opinion, expressed mother's milk is seldom sterile (Eidelman & Szilagyi, 1979; Meier & Wilks, 1987) and may contain a variety of potentially pathogenic organisms (Meier & Wilks, 1987). The particular concern with respect to CNG feedings is that expressed mother's milk is allowed to remain at room temperature, often for several hours, before reaching the infant's stomach. The warm temperature permits further bacterial growth, so the infant may receive a sizable inoculate of bacteria. Although term infants can apparently consume a variety of bacteria during breastfeeding without adverse effects (Eidelman & Szilagyi, 1979), this principle cannot be generalized to small preterm infants, who have immature immune systems and do not receive milk directly from the breast (Meier & Wilks, 1987).

Continuous infusion of expressed mother's milk by syringe pump may circumvent problems with bacterial growth (McCoy et al., 1988) in that the syringe pump and infusion tubing can be changed frequently (e.g., every 2 hours), with minimal wasting of expressed mother's milk. There is also theoretical support, but no empirical evidence, for feeding infants fresh rather than frozen expressed mother's milk. The anti-infective properties of expressed mother's milk are optimally preserved if the expressed mother's milk is not frozen or heat processed (American Academy of Pediatrics, 1980a, 1980b; Liebhaber et al., 1977). Thus, the preterm infant would receive maximal protection from expressed mother's milk contaminants if (1) the expressed mother's milk has only small concentrations of skin flora ($\leq 10^3$), (2) the expressed mother's milk is administered within 24 hours of expression, and (3) the tubings are changed every 2 to 3 hours. However, there is no indication that these management strategies minimize the nutrient losses that occur with CNG feeding.

Orogastric and Nasogastric Routes for Intermittent Gavage or Bolus Feedings

A clinical dilemma concerning intermittent gavage or bolus feedings is whether orogastric or nasogastric intubation should be used for milk administration. Clinically, nasogastric tubes are simpler to insert and maintain in position than are orogastric tubes; determining the correct insertion length is essential for both methods (Gallaher et al., 1993). However, three reports have suggested that the use of indwelling nasogastric tubes may compromise respiration for smaller preterm infants (Greenspan et al., 1990; Stocks, 1980; van Someren et al., 1984). In one study (Greenspan et al., 1990), pulmonary function was studied in preterm infants with nasogastric and orogastric tubes in place, but not during infusion of milk. Infants weighing less than 2 kg demonstrated diminished minute ventilation and respiratory rate, increased pulmonary resistance and work of breathing, and peak transpulmonary pressure change with nasogastric but not orogastric intubation. The investigators proposed that the nasogastric tube partially occluded the nares, especially in smaller infants, causing acute pulmonary compromise, for which smaller, less mature infants may be unable to compensate.

In another study, investigators reported significantly less periodic breathing and apnea and higher transcutaneous partial pressure of oxygen ($tcPO_2$) values when preterm infants had orogastric rather than nasogastric tubes in place (van Someren et al., 1984). Through a study design that incorporated two related projects, these investigators proposed that these adverse outcomes become manifested over several days rather than immediately after nasogastric tube placement. They suggested that initially the infant compensates for the increased work of breathing induced by the indwelling tube, but that the infant's ability to do this diminishes over time. In this study, the authors proposed that orogastric tubes represent a safe and convenient alternative to nasogastric tubes if the former are stabilized with a palatal appliance.

Type of Gavage Tube

Two decisions with respect to selection of a tube for gavage feedings are tube size and tube material. Ideally, the tube used for gavage feedings should have the smallest bore to deliver the feeding, especially for nasogastric intubation in which the nare will be partially occluded. For nasally placed tubes, a 5 French size is desirable. However, the 5 French has a very small end hole and may become occluded during feeding. An 8 French may be used for orogastric intubation because occlusion of the nare is not a consideration.

Available materials for gavage tubes are polyvinyl chloride and polyurethane. The majority of gavage tubes are constructed of polyvinyl chloride, a stiff plastic that hardens over time, with potential for perforating the gastrointestinal tract during or after insertion. Tubes made of polyvinyl chloride should be used for a single feeding or left in place for no more than 1 day. Thus, if these tubes are used routinely, nurses need to develop a mechanism whereby the tubes are changed on a daily basis. For gavage tubes that will remain in place for longer than 1 day, a tube made of a softer, more biocompatible plastic, such as polymeric silicone or polyurethane, should be used. Several types of polyurethane feeding tubes are available commercially in sizes 5, 6, and 8 French. Small-bore polyurethane feeding tubes with weighted tips are also available and should be considered for infants with reflux.

Selected Nursing Interventions During Intermittent Gavage or Bolus Feedings

Selected nursing interventions have been proposed to ameliorate the adverse physiologic and biochemical responses during intermittent gavage or bolus feedings. These interventions can be categorized as follows: (1) controlling the rate of milk flow, (2) warming the milk to body temperature, (3) optimizing infant position, (4) using intermittently placed gavage tubes rather than indwelling gavage tubes, and (5) providing nonnutritive sucking opportunities. At present, well-controlled clinical trials in which these interventions have been tested, either singly or in combination, have not been conducted. Additionally, these interventions, because of their potential to influence a variety of other outcome measures, should be controlled when other feeding-related interventions are under investigation. For example, a study that focuses on the effect of milk temperatures should include controls for infusion rate, infant position, and nonnutritive sucking. However, these variables have not been well controlled in previous published research, so conclusions from this body of literature are not optimal.

Administration Rate. As previously mentioned, a major controversy exists as to whether gavage or bolus feedings should be administered continuously or intermittently owing to concerns about distending the infant stomach with rapid infusion rates. However, *continuous* usually refers to milliliters per hour, whereas *intermittent* usually refers to numbers of minutes to complete the infusion, regardless of volume to be administered. Thus, allowing 10 minutes for infusion of a gavage or bolus feeding may be a relatively rapid or slow rate, depending on the volume to be infused. Thus, clinical protocols for intermittent gavage or bolus feedings should reflect an infusion rate (in milliliters per kilogram of body weight per minute) rather than an infusion time.

Milk Temperature. Although early feeding techniques for preterm infants included warming milk to approximately body temperature prior to feeding, this procedure was abandoned with the advent of commercially prepared "ready-to-feed" formula. Thus, in clinical practice, preterm infants receive formula that may be as much as –3.88°C to – 1.11°C (25°F to 30°F) lower than body temperature. Although a single study (Gibson, 1958) reported that term infants "accepted" cold formula, a decrease in body temperature was noted for preterm infants following the feeding of unwarmed formula in one early report (Holt et al., 1962). Studies in the late 1980s suggested that milk temperature may influence the body temperature response of preterm infants; one study was conducted with gavage feedings (Eckburg et al., 1987), whereas other studies were conducted with oral feedings (Meier, 1988; Meier & Anderson, 1987). A recent study found significant improvement in feeding tolerance, as measured by volume of gastric residual, for preterm infants gavage-fed milk warmed to body temperature when compared with infants receiving milk warmed to room temperature (24°C) or cool milk (10°C) (Gonzales et al., 1995). Additionally, there were no significant differences in body temperature for infants in any of the three milk temperature groups in this study. However, it is important to generalize this finding cautiously, as the infants in this study were maintained in a neutral thermal environment, with heating equipment keeping the body temperature within set parameters during data collection. A study in which infants are allowed to self-regulate body temperature in an incubator or open crib may produce different findings regarding the effect of milk temperature on infant body temperature.

Infant Position. Two reports have described the effect of infant position on oxygenation: one report included gavage feeding for which two positions were compared (Herrell et al., 1980), whereas the other compared infant position (prone versus supine) in the absence of feeding (Martin et al., 1979). No studies could be located in which other infant positions were studied during gavage infusion. For example, gavage infusions are frequently administered while the mother or nurse holds the infant or while the infant remains in the incubator in a "contained" position (Als, 1986). In the absence of definitive data concerning an optimal infant position, the nurse should recognize that infant position may influence oxygenation during gavage feeding. For infants who demonstrate hypoxemia, modification of position may promote improved oxygenation.

Intermittent Versus Indwelling Tube Placement. Gavage tube placement may result in adverse effects for the infant. These effects may include bradycardia as a result of vagal stimulation, reflux, and aspiration. To minimize these effects, some nurseries prefer to secure gavage tubes in place between feedings, decreasing the frequency with which infants are subjected to the procedure. In contrast, other clinicians feel that because nasogastric tubes compromise breathing, and orogastric tubes are prone to accidental removal, gavage tubes should be placed for every feeding and removed when the feeding is completed. One research report was found that measured the incidence of apneic and bradycardic episodes and the amount of weight gain for preterm infants with indwelling versus intermittently placed gavage tubes (Symington et al., 1995). Although no significant differences were found in the incidence of apneic and bradycardic episodes between the two groups, the percentage of infants exhibiting such episodes was smaller for the indwelling group than for the intermittent group, despite the fact that all indwelling tubes were placed via the nasogastric route and all intermittent tubes were placed via the orogastric route. This study suggests that indwelling tubes could be used safely for this population, resulting in an economic advantage. Although this study has clinical merit, a study controlling for the feeding route while comparing infant response to indwelling and intermittent feeding tubes would help further understanding in this controversy.

Nonnutritive Sucking. The beneficial long-term effects of providing nonnutritive sucking with a pacifier during intermittent gavage feeding have been described for preterm infants (Bernbaum et al., 1983; Field et al., 1982; Measel & Anderson, 1979; Szabo et al., 1985) and include fewer gavage feedings; accelerated maturation of the sucking reflex, with earlier initiation of bottle feedings; greater daily weight gain; shorter hospital stay; and hospital cost savings. However, in a well-controlled prospective study, nonnutritive sucking was not associated with improved growth outcome for very low birth weight preterm infants (Ernst et al., 1989). Thus, the data on long-term outcome measures with respect to offering nonnutritive sucking during gavage feeding are inconclusive, and further study is needed. However, no published studies have reported adverse outcomes associated with nonnutritive sucking provided that safe pacifiers are used.

Although studies have demonstrated that nonnutritive sucking in preterm infants is accompanied by the more immediate benefit of increased oxygenation, as measured by $tcPo_2$ (Anderson et al., 1983; Burroughs et al., 1978), these infants were studied while at rest, not during gavage feeding.

Oral Feedings

In clinical practice, preterm infants are seldom allowed to feed orally, by bottle or breast, until they weigh at least 1500 g and have reached a postconceptional age of 34 to 35 weeks (Batton et al., 1982; Churella et al., 1985; Lefrak-Okikawa, 1988). These practices are based on the untested assumption that suck–swallow coordination coincides with weight and maturity and does not reflect individual characteristics such as clinical stability and presence of complications affecting feeding. Once oral feedings are established, infants are usually placed on a 3- or 4-hour feeding schedule until discharge.

Issues Common to the Management of Both Methods of Oral Feeding. Clinically, two major issues are important to the management of both bottle feeding and breastfeeding. The first issue concerns the transition of preterm infants from gavage to oral feedings, and the second issue concerns whether preterm infants should be fed according to a 3- or 4-hour schedule, or whether feedings should be cue based.

Transition From Gavage to Oral Feedings. Although all preterm infants who require gavage feedings undergo a "transition" period in which gavage feedings are discontinued and oral feedings are initiated, few research-based guidelines have been developed for managing this process. However, most NICUs have written policies concerning when oral feedings can be introduced to preterm infants; criteria usually include a minimal weight and postconceptional age. Kinneer and Beachy (1994) reported factors that nurses ranked as the most important indicators of an infant's readiness to initiate oral feeding. These factors included nonnutritive sucking, a strong gag reflex, demanding feedings, and a gestational age greater than or equal to 34 weeks of gestation. The authors suggested that further research was needed to determine the predictive validity of nonnutritive sucking and other infant behaviors for nutritive sucking ability.

Feeding orally requires the integration of three functions: sucking, swallowing, and breathing. According to the classic study by Gryboski (1969), sucking movements precede swallowing, which, in turn, inhibits respiration. Initially, preterm infants demonstrate an "immature sucking pattern," which is characterized by short sucking bursts, which, in turn, are preceded or followed by swallows. As preterm infants mature, sucking bursts become more prolonged, with multiple swallows occurring during these bursts (Gryboski, 1969). The integration of sucking, swallowing, and breathing is apparently related to both the maturity and the general health status of the preterm infant.

The problem with most NICU feeding protocols is that they do not incorporate individual infant differences with respect to oral feeding. Some preterm infants may be able to feed orally as early as 32 weeks' postconceptional age, whereas other infants may demonstrate difficulty in the coordination of sucking, swallowing, and breathing until near term or even beyond. At present, there are no universally accepted clinical tools for assessing readiness to feed orally or for quantitatively measuring an infant's ability to feed. A tool developed for either purpose should include noninvasive measures of oxygenation, because a primary goal of early oral feeding is the avoidance of hypoxemia. Thus, oximetry or $tcPo_2$ measures should be a part of management protocols for the transition of preterm infants from gavage to oral feedings.

Scheduled Versus Cue-Based Feedings. Two separate investigations (Collinge et al., 1982; Horton et al., 1952) have supported the practice of cue-based, or self-regulatory, feedings for clinically stable preterm infants. Self-regulatory feedings involve feeding the infant based on caregiver interpretation of infant hunger versus feeding the infant every 3 or 4 hours independent of the presence or absence of behaviors that suggest hunger. Demand feedings generally refer to an infant's being fed when crying commences, whereas cue-based feedings refer to an infant's being fed based on demonstrated hunger cues, that is, alert state, hand-to-mouth movement, and rooting reflex, which precede the onset of crying (Gill et al., 1984). Previous research has documented the presence of these early hunger cues for term infants (Gill et al., 1984). One brief research report was found that described a cluster pattern of state or activity changes (orally directed behaviors, such as mouthing, sucking, and rooting, and clinical indices, such as cough, yawn, or sneeze) that occurred prior to feeding for preterm infants at 32 to 33 weeks of gestation (Cagan, 1995). This study suggests that cue-based feeding would be feasible for young preterm infants.

In the study by Collinge and associates (1982), preterm infants were randomly assigned to either a scheduled or a demand feeding group; the scheduled group was fed at intervals of 3 to 4 hours. Although no differences were reported between groups for 24-hour volume of intake or calories consumed, infants fed on demand required fewer gavage feedings and fewer feedings per day and were discharged a mean of 6.2 days earlier than infants in the scheduled group. Although these data support the practice of establishing self-regulatory feeding protocols for clinically stable preterm infants and suggest potential advantages for infants, parents, nurses, and third-party payers, this study should be replicated with a larger sample of preterm infants.

Clinicians, although supportive of self-regulatory feedings in theory, have raised legitimate questions about how to institute such a policy in the NICU. One major unanswered question is whether preterm infants demonstrate the same early hunger cues as term infants and, if so, will the busy NICU nurse be able to identify those cues prior to the onset of crying. An additional concern evolves from the reality that each NICU nurse may be caring for three to four clinically stable preterm infants, all of whom may awake to feed at the same time. Clearly, self-regulatory feedings would be implemented most successfully in a NICU in which parents were present to recognize and respond to their infant's hunger cues.

Bottle Feeding

The process of feeding by bottle results in significant physiologic and biochemical alterations for many term infants (Bodefeld et al., 1979; Durand et al., 1981; Mathew & Bhatia, 1989; Mathew et al., 1985a, 1985b; Rosen et al., 1984) and preterm infants (Guilleminault & Coons, 1984; Meier, 1988; Meier & Anderson, 1987; Rosen et al., 1984; Shivpuri et al., 1983). The general consensus of these studies is that hypoxemia, hypercarbia, decreased minute ventilation, and more extreme manifestations of distress (apnea, bradycardia, and cyanosis) occur owing to immaturity in the integration of sucking, swallowing, and breathing. One study suggests that these responses are more severe when a nasogastric tube is in place during bottle feedings (Shiao et al., 1995).

In general, as the infant begins to suck with the bottle, minute ventilation falls owing to a combination of decreases in respiratory frequency and tidal volume. Consequently, oxygenation declines and carbon dioxide levels increase. A more exaggerated response includes apnea, bradycardia, and cyanosis. Research in which infants were fed during polygraphic studies suggests that clinically significant hypoxemia during bottle feeding may go undetected during routine nursery care for both term and preterm infants (Guilleminault & Coons, 1984; Mathew et al., 1985a, 1985b; Rosen et al., 1984). In one report (Rosen et al., 1984), investigators noted that one fifth of all neonates referred for polygraphic studies demonstrated profound hypoxemia and cardiorespiratory disturbances during bottle feeding. These same investigators suggested that mild feeding disturbances may even be more common than suspected because of nursery practices of disconnecting monitoring equipment from "well" infants during feeding or removing the bottle frequently during feedings for preterm infants.

In combination, these data suggest that considerably more attention should be directed toward evaluation of physiologic and biochemical changes during feeding, especially for preterm infants. Although more research must be conducted in this area, selected nursing measures to minimize these changes can be instituted.

Nursing Interventions

Traditionally, nurses have not identified bottle feeding as an intervention that requires professional attention. Consequently, convalescing preterm infants have been referred to as "feeders" or "growers," suggesting that staff other than professional nurses can provide their care. Given the documented frequency of hypoxemia during bottle feeding, nurses should refocus professional care on the assessment and management of feeding-related hypoxemia.

The assessment of hypoxemia should include routine noninvasive monitoring of small preterm infants as bottle feedings are initiated. Numerous studies have emphasized that clinical indices alone are inadequate in the identification of hypoxemia. For initial bottle feedings, a preterm infant should be fed while attached to a cardiorespiratory monitor and either an oximeter or a $tcPo_2$ monitor, preferably with a trend recorder to document the oxygenation pattern throughout the feeding. Parameters on the oxygenation tracing that should be evaluated include: (1) percentage of decline from baseline during sucking, (2) extent of recovery of oxygenation during rest periods and in the period after feeding, and (3) which phases of the tracing, if any, were accompanied by tachycardia, bradycardia, or apnea. Noninvasive monitoring of oxygenation can be discontinued for an individual infant based on the nurse's decision that the infant does not demonstrate significant hypoxemia.

A second intervention is to select the appropriate nipple for the infant. In a simulated study of sucking, a variety of nipple units routinely recommended for term and preterm infants were compared (Mathew, 1988a). Results of this study revealed marked variation in rates of flow for different nipple units; variations were noted not only for different types of nipples but also for different nipple units of the same type. In particular, the Nuk-type nipple, often recommended for use with breastfed infants, was characterized by higher flow than comparable standard nipple units. The investigator raised the consideration that feeding-related apnea and bradycardia in preterm infants might be related, in part, to nipple units that permit high flow (Mathew, 1988a).

Milk that flows rapidly from the nipple necessitates more frequent swallowing on the part of the infant. Because swallowing interrupts respiration, more frequent swallowing might compromise ventilatory function for the preterm infant. However, Dowling (1995) reported that selected preterm infants were able to maintain regular breathing patterns, and consequently oxygenation, during bottle feeding with Nuk-type nipples. Therefore, each infant should be evaluated individually to determine the infant's ability to regulate milk flow from a particular nipple unit.

A third nursing intervention, related to controlling the rate of milk flow, is to allow the infant to set the pace of the feeding. In a well-controlled study of nine term and nine preterm infants (Jain et al., 1987), investigators found that preterm infants generated lower sucking pressures and expended less energy than did term infants to obtain the same total volume of milk. Additionally, preterm infants sucked at a slower rate than did term infants and consumed less volume per suck. These data suggest that preterm infants may require more time to complete a feeding than do term infants and that the ability to pace the bottle feeding may be a protective mechanism, allowing the infant to expend less energy while feeding.

A related intervention is the avoidance of force feeding for preterm infants. In the nonresearch literature, a frequent recommendation for feeding preterm infants is to stimulate the infant in order to complete a bottle feeding. Consequently, in the clinical setting it is not unusual to see nurses manipulating infants' faces, mouths, and the bottle, forcing an already fatigued infant to complete the remainder of a feeding. One research report described apnea, documented on a polygraph tracing, associated with nurse-induced sucks (Dowling, 1995). Thus, stimulating an infant to suck has the potential for interfering with the infant's self-regulation of sucking and breathing, which, especially for a fatigued infant, may precipitate hypoxemia.

The preceding is an example of a situation in which noninvasive monitoring would alert the nurse to an infant who is hypoxemic and fatigued and who should be allowed to rest while the remainder of a feeding is infused by gavage. In one study in which $tcPo_2$ was compared during bottle feedings and breastfeedings for preterm infants, the investigator noted that clinical indices of fatigue during bottle feeding were manifested when $tcPo_2$ values were between 40 and 50 mm Hg (Meier, 1988), a finding that is clearly suggestive of hypoxemia.

Breastfeeding

Preterm infants are seldom allowed to breastfeed until bottle feedings have been well established and an arbitrary weight criterion is achieved. However, delay in initial breastfeedings is associated with undesirable outcomes for mothers and preterm infants (Ehrenkranz et al., 1985; McCoy et al., 1988; Measel et al., 1987; Meberg et al., 1982; Meier & Anderson, 1987; Meier & Pugh, 1985; Pereira et al., 1984; Verronen, 1985). The most important of these is breastfeeding failure, defined as the cessation of breastfeeding during the infant's hospitalization or in the early period after discharge, prior to the mother's intended weaning. The breastfeeding failure rate for mothers of preterm infants may exceed 50 percent of those mothers who try to breastfeed by the time infants are discharged from the hospital nursery (Pereira et al., 1984).

Significance of Breastfeeding for Preterm Infants and Mothers

Successful breastfeeding has numerous advantages for preterm infants and their mothers. Infants receive the unique immunologic and nutritional properties of human milk, which cannot be reproduced in commercial formulas (American Academy of Pediatrics, 1980a; World Health Organization, 1981). Breastfeeding is associated with lower rates of postneonatal morbidity than is formula feeding in the United States (Kovar et al., 1984) and with lower rates of postneonatal mortality and morbidity in developing countries (Jason et al., 1984). Also, preterm infants, subjected to painful procedures and separation from their mothers after birth, experience the pleasurable sensations and closeness of breastfeeding (Meberg et al., 1982). Physiologically, pilot research has demonstrated that contrary to popular assumption, breastfeeding is less stressful than bottle feeding, especially when infants are smallest and least mature (Meier, 1988; Meier & Anderson, 1987). For mothers, breastfeeding may facilitate mother–infant attachment (Alberts et al., 1983; Newton & Newton, 1967) and provide a sense that they are contributing something to the care of their infant that no one else can (Ehrenkranz & Ackerman, 1986; Measel et al., 1987).

Model for Providing Breastfeeding Support in the Neonatal Intensive Care Unit

In one study, investigators reported that 72 percent of mothers of high-risk infants who began milk expression were still breastfeeding at the time of the infant's discharge from the NICU (Meier & Mangurten, 1993). These investigators proposed a five-phase temporal model for supporting lactation in the NICU: (1) assisting the mother in the collection and storage of milk, (2) gavage feeding of expressed mother's milk, (3) managing in-hospital breastfeeding sessions, (4) breastfeeding support after discharge, and (5) consultation with the family or nursery personnel or both. Investigators proposed two additional recommendations based on the data generated by this study. First, the amount of time required to provide breastfeeding interventions for mothers of infants in the NICU probably necessitates retaining a full-time nurse to coordinate support if more than 100 mothers per year elect to breastfeed. Second, the nurse who coordinates such a program should have experience not only in lactation management but also in the clinical care of high-risk infants.

Assisting With Milk Collection and Storage. Within the proposed model of lactation support, each mother who expresses an interest in breastfeeding should be contacted by the nurse, and a suitable breast pump should be obtained prior to the mother's discharge from the hospital. Mothers should be encouraged to rent an electric breast pump, and if milk expression is anticipated to last more than 2 weeks, a double-pump collecting device should be recommended. Initial studies indicate that prolactin levels are higher when double-pump collecting devices, rather than single-pump ones, are used for milk expression (Neifert & Seacat, 1985). Mothers should be instructed to initiate milk expression as soon as possible after delivery and to express their milk 8 to 12 times in a 24-hour period, a schedule that corresponds to breastfeeding patterns of low-risk term infants.

Management of In-Hospital Breastfeeding Sessions. Previously published research has suggested that contrary to popular opinion, breastfeeding may be less stressful than bottle feeding for small preterm infants (Meier, 1988; Meier & Anderson, 1987; Meier & Pugh, 1985). In a study in which preterm infants served as their own controls for 32 bottle feedings and 39 breastfeedings, the $tcPo_2$ declined during bottle feedings but not during breastfeedings (Fig. 23–1). Additionally, at young gestational ages, infants demonstrated different suck–breathe patterns during breast- and bottle feedings. During breastfeeding, infants breathed within sucking bursts. However, during bottle feeding, bouts of breathing were alternated with sucking bursts, rather than being integrated into the sucking bursts (deMonterice, 1993). These different patterns of suck–swallow–breathe coordination for small preterm infants result in less ventilatory disruption during breastfeeding.

In a study by Meier and Mangurten (1993), preterm infants as small as 1200 g and as immature as 32 weeks' gestation were permitted to breastfeed. Most infants had not attempted bottle feeding at the time of initial breastfeeding. During initial breastfeedings, these infants organized sucking into bursts of three to five sucks, with audible swallowing. These data support the results of previously published research suggesting that preterm infants can breastfeed earlier in the hospital stay than currently thought.

For clinical purposes, breastfeeding should be initiated for preterm infants when bottle feedings would ordinarily have been started. A preterm infant does not need to demonstrate the ability to feed by bottle prior to the initiation of breastfeeding. Other components of breastfeeding protocols should include (1) noninvasive monitoring of cardiorespiratory and oxygenation responses to feeding, as recommended previously for bottle feeding; (2) test weighing with electronic scales to estimate volume of intake during breastfeeding (Meier et al., 1990); and (3) observation and recording characteristics of infant sucking and maternal milk flow. According to the model of lactation support described previously (Meier & Mangurten, 1993), the mean amount of time spent in assisting mothers with in-hospital breastfeeding sessions was 1 hour per feeding session. This phase of lactation support is extremely time-consuming and should be managed by a nurse who is knowledgeable about lactation and high-risk preterm infants.

Breastfeeding Consultation After Discharge. Anecdotal responses of mothers who participated in the model of lactation support study suggest that a different set of concerns originates during the period after discharge with respect to breastfeeding a preterm infant. A recent report indicates that paramount among these concerns is the mother's fear that the infant will not con-

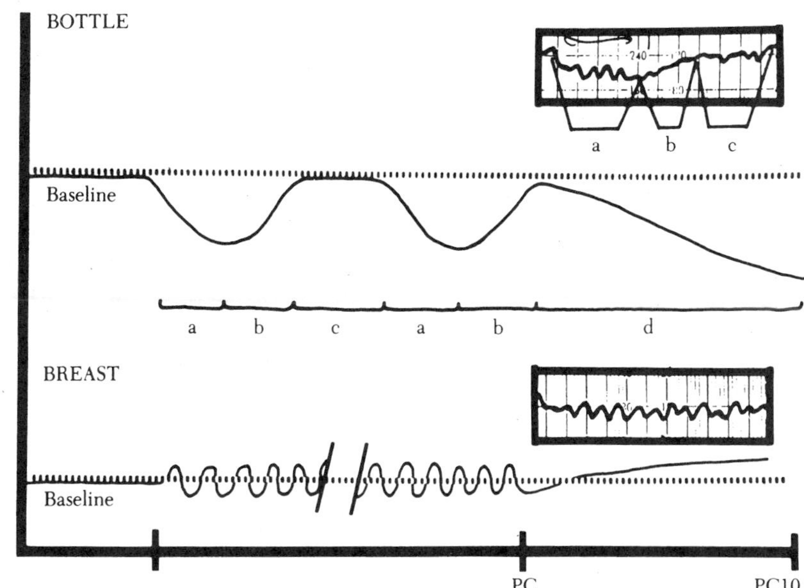

FIGURE 23–1. Schematic of typical $tcPO_2$ patterns during bottle feeding and breastfeeding. Note in bottle feeding (a) decline, (b) recovery, (c) plateau, and (d) decline between end of feeding (PC) and 10 minutes postfeeding (PC10). Both schematics have been magnified somewhat for clarity. Also, note interruption in the breastfeeding line to show that breastfeedings were generally longer than bottle feedings. Insets are from actual $tcPO_2$ recordings. (Copyright 1988 American Journal of Nursing Company. Reprinted from *Nursing Research*, Jan./Feb., 1988, Vol. 37, No. 1. Used with permission. All rights reserved.)

sume enough milk during breastfeeding (Kavanaugh et al., 1995). This concern is not the same as the concern of mothers of full-term infants that their milk supply is inadequate; mothers of these preterm infants were able to observe the adequacy of their milk supply with milk expression for complementary or supplemental feedings. Their concern, instead, was related to the adequacy of milk transfer, which involves the synchrony of maternal milk ejection and infant sucking. Mothers managed this concern with the use of complementary or supplemental bottles until they felt infant intake was adequate, approximately 2 weeks after discharge. Another appropriate method for mothers breastfeeding preterm infants in the early period after discharge is test weighing, using a scale designed for this purpose (Meier et al., 1994). The BabyWeigh (Medela, Inc., McHenry, Illinois) was found to give an accurate estimate of intake when used by mothers and investigators, whereas evaluation of infant cues, such as infant latching onto the breast and infant sucking, were not accurate for estimating the volume of intake.

Previously, most consumer-oriented information has focused on generalizing recommendations for term, healthy infants to smaller, less stable preterm infants. For example, mothers of preterm infants were frequently told just to "trust" lactation and to feed their infants on demand or to wake their infants frequently (i.e., every 1 to 2 hours) so that they can feed small volumes from the breast. These recommendations are not research based and can be potentially dangerous for preterm infants.

Until the knowledge base has been developed in this area, neonatal nurses need to use in-hospital breastfeeding information to help mothers prepare for discharge. For example, an evaluation of serial test weighings during breastfeedings will provide the nurse with information about an individual infant's pattern of milk intake, and interventions can be planned to meet the breastfeeding needs of a particular mother–infant pair. An additional helpful intervention is to prepare the mother for the types of advice that she is likely to receive from family members, friends, and even primary care providers. This will help the mother identify information that is erroneous so that she will know to question it and to contact the nurse concerning appropriate management strategies.

As a component of the lactation model, the nurse coordinator should telephone the mother within 48 hours after infant discharge and again 48 hours after the first telephone call. Mothers should be encouraged to telephone the nurse following the visit to the pediatrician at 1 week after discharge to share information and recommendations from the pediatrician. Even though mothers have access to the nurse coordinator in the period after discharge, they often hesitate to call, thinking that the call will be a disturbance. Thus, when the nurse initiates the call, the mother is likely to have at least one major question concerning breastfeeding management strategies.

CONCLUSION

This chapter has reviewed the principles of digestion, absorption, and metabolic processes involved. It included developmental and physiologic considerations of the premature or sick neonate. Practical issues were addressed regarding neonatal nutrition.

REFERENCES

Adamkin, D. H. (1986). Nutrition in very very low birth weight infants. *Clinics in Perinatology, 13*(2), 419–443.

Alberts, E., Kalverboer, A. F., & Hopkins, B. (1983). Mother-infant dialogue in the first days of life: An observational study during breastfeeding. *Journal of Child Psychology and Psychiatry and Applied Disciplines, 24*(1), 145–161.

Als, H. (1986). A synactive model of neonatal behavioral organization: Framework for the assessment of neurobehavioral development in the premature infant and for support of infants and parents in the neonatal intensive care environment. *Physical and Occupational Therapy in Pediatrics, 6*(3/4), 3–55.

American Academy of Pediatrics. (1980a). Encouraging breast-feeding. *Pediatrics, 65*(3), 657–658.

American Academy of Pediatrics, Committee on Nutrition. (1980b). Human milk banking. *Pediatrics, 65*(4), 854–857.

Anderson, D. M. (1987). Nutrition care for the premature infant. *Topics in Clinical Nutrition, 2*, 1–9.

Anderson, G. C., Burroughs, A. K., & Measel, C. P. (1983). Nonnutritive sucking opportunities: A safe and effective treatment for preterm neonates. In T. M. Field & A. K. Sostek (Eds.), *Infants born at risk: Physiological, perceptual, and cognitive processes* (pp. 129–146). New York: Grune & Stratton.

Aschner, J. L., Punsalang, A., Jr., Maniscalco, W. M., & Menegus, M. A. (1987). Percutaneous central venous catheter colonization with *Malassezia furfur*: Incidence and clinical significance. *Pediatrics, 80*(4), 535–539.

Aynsley-Green, A., Adrian, T. E., & Bloom, S. R. (1982). Feeding and the development of enteroinsular hormone secretion in the preterm infant: Effects of continuous gastric infusions of human milk compared with intermittent boluses. *Acta Pediatrica Scandinavica, 71*, 379–383.

Azimi, P. H., Levernier, K., Lefrak, L. M., et al. (1988). *Malassezia furfur:* A cause of occlusion of percutaneous central venous catheters in infants in the intensive care nursery. *Pediatric Infectious Disease Journal, 7*(2), 100–103.

Babson, S. G., & Benda, G. I. (1976). Growth graphs for the clinical assessment of infants of varying gestational age. *Journal of Pediatrics, 89*(5), 814–820.

Ball, P. A., Candy, D. C. A., Puntis, J. W. L., & McNeish, A. S. (1985). Portable bedside microcomputer system for management of parenteral nutrition in all age groups. *Archives of Disease in Childhood, 60*(5), 435–439.

Barnard, J. A., Cotton, R. B., & Lutin, W. (1985). Necrotizing enterocolitis: Variables associated with the severity of disease. *American Journal of Diseases of Children, 139*(4), 375–377.

Batton, D. G., Maisels, M. J., & Appelbaum, P. (1982). Use of peripheral intravenous cannulas in premature infants: A controlled study. *Pediatrics, 70*(3), 487–490.

Bernbaum, J. C., Pereira, G. R., Watkins, J. B., & Peckham, G. J. (1983). Nonnutritive sucking during gavage feeding enhances growth and maturation in premature infants. *Pediatrics, 71*(1), 41–45.

Berseth, C. L. (1990). Neonatal small intestinal motility: Motor responses to feeding in term and preterm infants. *Journal of Pediatrics, 117*(4), 777–782.

Berseth, C. L., & Nordyke, C. (1993). Enteral nutrients promote postnatal maturation of intestinal motor activity in preterm infants. *American Journal of Physiology, 264*(6, Part 1), G1046–G1051.

Billeaud, C., Piedboeuf, B., & Chessex, P. (1992). Energy expediture and severity of respiratory disease in very low birth weight infants receiving long-term ventilatory support. *Journal of Pediatrics, 120*(3), 461–464.

Binder, N. D., Raschko, P. K., Benda, G. I., & Reynolds, J. W. (1989). Insulin infusion with parenteral nutrition in extremely low birth weight infants with hyperglycemia. *Journal of Pediatrics, 114*(2), 273–280.

Blondheim, O., Abbasi, S., Fox, W. W., & Bhutani, V. K. (1993). Effect of enteral gavage feeding rate on pulmonary functions of very low birth weight infants. *Journal of Pediatrics, 122*(5, Part 1), 751–755.

Bodefeld, E., Schachinger, H., Huch, A., et al. (1979). Continuous $tcPo_2$ monitoring in healthy and sick newborn infants during and after feeding. In A. Huch, R. Huch, & J. F. Lucey (Eds.), *Continuous transcutaneous blood gas monitoring* (pp. 503–508). New York: Alan R. Liss.

Botsford, K. B., Weinstein, R. A., Boyer, K. M., et al. (1986). Gram-negative bacilli in human milk feedings: Quantitation and clinical consequences for premature infants. *Journal of Pediatrics, 109*(4), 707–710.

Brennan-Behm, M., Carlson, E., Meier, P., & Engstrom, J. (1994). Caloric loss from expressed mother's milk during continuous gavage infusion. *Neonatal Network, 13*(2), 27–32.

Brooke, O. G., & Barley, J. (1978). Loss of energy during continuous infusions of breast milk. *Archives of Disease in Childhood, 53*(4), 344–345.

Brosius, K. K., Ritter, D. A., & Kenny, J. D. (1984). Postnatal growth curve of the infant with extremely low birth weight who was fed enterally. *Pediatrics, 74*(5), 778–782.

Buchheit, J. Q., & Stewart, D. L. (1994). Clinical comparison of localized intestinal perforation and necrotizing enterocolitis in neonates. *Pediatrics, 93*(1), 32–36.

Burroughs, A., Asonye, U. O., Anderson-Shanklin, G. C., & Vidyasagar, D. (1978). The effect of nonnutritive sucking on transcutaneous oxygen tension in noncrying, preterm neonates. *Research in Nursing and Health, 1*(2), 69–75.

Cagan, J. (1995). Feeding readiness behavior in preterm infants. *Neonatal Network, 14*(2), 82.

Carey, B. E. (1989). Major complications of central lines in neonates [Review]. *Neonatal Network, 7*(6), 17–28.

Chathas, M. K. (1986). Percutaneous central venous catheters in neonates. *Journal of Obstetric, Gynecologic and Neonatal Nursing, 15*(4), 324–332.

Chathas, M. K., Paton, J. B., & Fisher, D. E. (1990). Percutaneous central venous catheterization: Three years' experience in a neonatal intensive care unit. *Archives of Diseases of Childhood, 144*(11), 1246–1250.

Cheek, J. A., Jr., & Staub, G. F. (1973). Nasojejunal alimentation for premature and full-term newborn infants. *Journal of Pediatrics, 82*(6), 955–962.

Churella, H. R., Bachhuber, W. L., & MacLean, W. C. (1985). Survey: Methods of feeding low-birth-weight infants. *Pediatrics, 76*(2), 243–249.

Collinge, J. M., Bradley, K., Perks, C., et al. (1982). Demand vs. scheduled feedings for premature infants. *Journal of Obstetric, Gynecologic, and Neonatal Nursing, 11*(6), 362–367.

Dancis, J., O'Connell, J. R., & Holt, L. E. (1948). A grid for recording the weight of premature infants. *Journal of Pediatrics, 33*, 570–572.

deMonterice, D. (1993). *Differences in coordination of sucking and breathing during breast and bottle feeding.* Paper presented at the Perinatal Nursing Research Forum, January 1993. Santa Fe, NM: Mead Johnson Nutritionals.

Dhande, V., Kattwinkel, J., & Alford, B. (1983). Recurrent bilateral pleural effusions secondary to superior vena cava obstruction as a complication of central venous catheterization. *Pediatrics, 72*(1), 109–113.

Dolcourt, J. L., & Bose, C. L. (1982). Percutaneous insertion of Silastic central venous catheters in newborn infants. *Pediatrics, 70*(3), 484–486.

Dowling, D. A. (1995). *Responses of preterm infants to enteral feeding.* Unpublished doctoral dissertation. Chicago: University of Illinois.

Durand, M., Leahy, F. N., MacCallum, M., et al. (1981). Effect of feeding on the chemical control of breathing in the newborn infant. *Pediatric Research, 15*(12), 1509–1512.

Durand, M., Ramanathan, R., Martinelli, B., & Tolentino, M. (1986). Prospective evaluation of percutaneous central venous Silastic catheters in newborn infants with birth weight of 510–3920 grams. *Pediatrics, 78*(2), 245–250.

Eckburg, J. J., Bell, E. F., Rios, G. R., & Wilmoth, P. K. (1987). Effects of formula temperature on postprandial thermogenesis and body temperature of premature infants. *Journal of Pediatrics, 111*(4), 588–592.

Ehrenkranz, R. A., & Ackerman, B. A. (1986). Metoclopramide effect on faltering milk production by mothers of premature infants. *Pediatrics, 78*(4), 614–620.

Ehrenkranz, R. A., Ackerman, B. A., Mezger, J., & Bracken, M. B. (1985). Breastfeeding and premature infant: Incidence and success. *Pediatric Research, 19*, 99A (Abstract 530).

Eidelman, A. L., & Szilagyi, G. (1979). Patterns of bacterial colonization of human milk. *Obstetrics and Gynecology, 53*(5), 550–552.

Ernst, J. A., Rickard, K. A., Neal, P. R., et al. (1989). Lack of improved growth outcome related to nonnutritive sucking in very low birth weight premature infants fed a controlled nutrient intake: A randomized prospective study. *Pediatrics, 83*(5), 706–716.

Evans, M. E., Schaffner, W., Federspiel, C. F., et al. (1988). Sensitivity, specificity, and predictive value of body surface cultures in a neonatal intensive care unit. *Journal of the American Medical Association, 259*(2), 248–252.

Fenton, T. R., McMillan, D. D., & Sauve, R. S. (1990). Nutrition and growth analysis of very low birth weight infants. *Pediatrics, 86*(3), 378–383.

Field, T., Ignatoff, E., Stringer, S., et al. (1982). Nonnutritive sucking during tube feedings: Effects on preterm neonates in an intensive care unit. *Pediatrics, 70*(3), 381–384.

Gallaher, K. J., Cashwell, S., Hall, V., et al. (1993). Orogastric tube insertion length in very low birth weight infants. *Journal of Perinatology, 13*(2), 128–131.

Gibson, J. P. (1958). Reaction of 150 infants to cold formulas. *Journal of Pediatrics, 52*, 404–406.

Gill, N. E., White, M. A., & Anderson, G. C. (1984). Transitional newborn infants in a hospital nursery: From first oral cue to first sustained cry. *Nursing Research, 33*(4), 213–217.

Gonzales, I., Duryea, E., Vasquez, E., & Geraghty, N. (1995). Effect of enteral feeding temperature on feeding tolerance in preterm infants. *Neonatal Network, 14*(3), 39–43.

Greenspan, J. S., Wolfson, M. R., Holt, W. J., & Shaffer, T. H. (1990). Neonatal gastric intubation: Differential respiratory effects between nasogastric and orogastric tubes. *Pediatric Pulmonology, 8*(4), 254–258.

Greer, F. R., McCormick, A., & Loker, J. (1984). Changes in fat concentration of human milk during delivery by intermittent bolus and continuous mechanical pump infusion. *Journal of Pediatrics, 105*(5), 745–749.

Grisoni, E. R., Mehta, S. K., & Connors, A. F. (1986). Thrombosis and infection complicating central venous catheterization in neonates. *Journal of Pediatric Surgery, 21*(9), 772–776.

Gross, S. J. (1983). Growth and biochemical response of preterm infants fed human milk or modified infant formula. *New England Journal of Medicine, 308*(5), 237–241.

Gryboski, J. D. (1969). Suck and swallow in the premature infant. *Pediatrics, 43*(1), 96–102.

Guilleminault, C., & Coons, S. (1984). Apnea and bradycardia during feeding in infants weighing >2000 grams. *Journal of Pediatrics, 104*(6), 932–935.

Heldt, G. P. (1988). The effect of gavage feeding on the mechanics of the lung, chest wall, and diaphragm of preterm infants. *Pediatric Research, 24*(1), 55–58.

Herrell, N., Martin, R. J., & Fanaroff, A. (1980). Arterial oxygen tension during nasogastric feeding in the preterm infant. *Journal of Pediatrics, 96*(5), 914–916.

Hickey, R. F., Cason, B. A., & Charles, R. (1989). Lower incidence of intravenous catheter complications with an elastomeric hydrogel catheter. *Anesthesia and Analgesia, 68*, S1-S321.

Holt, L. E., Davies, E. A., Hasselmeyer, E. G., & Adams, A. O. (1962). A study of premature infants fed cold formulas. *Journal of Pediatrics, 61*, 556–561.

Horton, F. H., Lubchenco, L. O., & Gordon, H. H. (1952). Self-regulation feeding in a premature nursery. *Yale Journal of Biological Medicine, 24*, 263–272.

Jain, L., Sivieri, E., Abbasi, S., & Bhutani, V. K. (1987). Energetics and mechanics of nutritive sucking in the preterm and term neonate. *Journal of Pediatrics, 111*(6, Part 1), 894–898.

Jason, J. M., Nieburg, P., & Marks, J. S. (1984). Mortality and infectious disease associated with infant-feeding practices in developing countries [Review]. *Pediatrics, 74*(4, Part 2), 702–727.

Jhaveri, M. K., & Kumar, S. P. (1987). Passage of the first stool in very low birth weight infants. *Pediatrics, 79*(6), 1005–1007.

Kavanaugh, K., Mead, L., Meier, P., & Mangurten, H. H. (1995). Getting enough: Mothers' concerns about breastfeeding a preterm infant after discharge. *Journal of Obstetric, Gynecologic, and Neonatal Nursing, 24*(1), 23–32.

Kerner, J. A. (1983). *Manual of pediatric parenteral nutrition* (pp. 63–68, 117–217). New York: John Wiley & Sons.

Kerner, J. A. (1991). Parenteral nutrition. In W. A. Walker, P. Durie, R. Hamilton, et al. (Eds.), *Pediatric gastrointestinal diseases* (Vol. 2). Philadelphia: B. C. Decker.

Kinneer, M. D., & Beachy, P. (1994). Nipple feeding premature infants in the neonatal intensive-care unit: Factors and decisions. *Journal of Obstetric, Gynecologic, and Neonatal Nursing, 23*(2), 105–112.

Klaus, M. H., & Kennell, J. H. (1982). *Parent-infant bonding*. St. Louis: C. V. Mosby.

Koenig, W. J., Amarnath, R. P., Hench, V., & Berseth, C. L. (1995). Manometrics for preterm and term infants: A new tool for old questions. *Pediatrics, 95*(2), 203–206.

Kovar, M. G., Serdula, M. K., Marks, J. S., & Fraser, D. W. (1984). Review of the epidemiologic evidence for an association between infant feeding and infant health. *Pediatrics, 74*(4, Part 2), 615–638.

Kurzner, S. I., Garg, M., Bautista, D. B., et al. (1988). Growth failure in infants with bronchopulmonary dysplasia: Nutrition and elevated resting metabolic expenditure. *Pediatrics, 81*(3), 379–384.

Landwirth, J. (1974). Continuous nasogastric infusion feedings of infants of low birth weight. *Clinical Pediatrics, 13*(7), 603–608.

Lebenthal, E. (Ed.). (1989). *Textbook of gastroenterology and nutrition in infancy.* New York: Raven Press.

Lebenthal, E. (1995). Gastrointestinal maturation and motility patterns as indicators for feeding the premature infant. *Pediatrics, 95*(2), 207–209.

Lebenthal, E., Lee, P. C., & Heitlinger, L. A. (1983). Impact of development of the gastrointestinal tract on infant feeding. *Journal of Pediatrics, 102*(1), 1–9.

Lefrak-Okikawa, L. (1988). Nutritional management of the very low birth weight infant. *Journal of Perinatal and Neonatal Nursing, 2*(1), 66–77.

Lefrak-Okikawa, L. (1988). Unpublished data, University of California, San Francisco.

Leick-Rude, M. K. (1990). Use of percutaneous Silastic intravascular catheters in high-risk neonates. *Neonatal Network, 9*(1), 17–25.

Lemons, P. M., Miller, K., Eitzen, H., et al. (1983). Bacterial growth in human milk during continuous feeding. *American Journal of Perinatology, 1*(1), 76–80.

Liebhaber, M., Lewiston, N. J., Asquith, M. T., et al. (1977). Alterations of lymphocytes and of antibody content of human milk after processing. *Journal of Pediatrics, 91*(6), 887–900.

Lucas, A., Bloom, S. R., & Aynsley-Green, A. (1986). Gut hormones and "minimal enteral feeding." *Acta Paediatrica Scandinavica, 75*(5), 719–723.

Lucey, J. F. (1981). Clinical uses of transcutaneous oxygen monitoring [Review]. *Advances in Pediatrics, 28*, 27–56.

Lundeen, E. C. (1939). Feeding the premature baby. *American Journal of Nursing, 39*, 3–11.

Lundeen, E. C. (1954). Prematures present special problems: Basic factors in nursing care. *Modern Hospital, 82*(4), 60–65.

Lundeen, E. C. (1959). Newer trends in the care of premature infants. *Nursing World, 133*(5), 133–137.

MacDonald, M. G., & Chou, M. M. (1986). Preventing complications from lines and tubes [Review]. *Seminars in Perinatology, 10*(3), 224–233.

Mactier, H., Alroomi, L. G., Young D. G., & Raine, P. A. (1986). Central venous catheterization in very low birth weight infants. *Archives of Disease in Childhood, 61*(5), 449–453.

Martin, R. J., Herrell, N., Rubin, D., & Fanaroff, A. (1979). Effect of supine and prone positions on arterial oxygen tension in the preterm infant. *Pediatrics, 63*(4), 528–531.

Mathew, O. P. (1988a). Nipple units for newborn infants: A functional comparison. *Pediatrics, 81*(5), 688–691.

Mathew, O. P. (1988b). Respiratory control during nipple feeding in preterm infants. *Pediatric Pulmonology, 5*(4), 220–224.

Mathew, O.P., & Bhatia, J. (1989). Sucking and breathing patterns during breast- and bottle-feeding in term neonates. Effects of nutrient delivery and composition. *American Journal of Diseases of Children, 143*(5), 588–592.

Mathew, O. P., Clark, M. L., & Pronske, M. H. (1985). Apnea, bradycardia, and cyanosis during oral feeding in term neonates [Letter]. *Journal of Pediatrics, 10*(5), 857.

Mathew, O. P., Clark, M. L., Pronske, M. L., et al. (1985). Breathing pattern and ventilation during oral feeding in term newborn infants. *Journal of Pediatrics, 106*(5), 810–813.

McCoy, R., Kadowaki, C., Wilks, S., et al. (1988). Nursing management of breastfeeding for preterm infants. *Journal of Perinatal and Neonatal Nursing, 2*(1), 42–55.

Measel, C. P., & Anderson, G. C. (1979). Nonnutritive sucking during tube feedings: Effect on clinical course in premature infants. *Journal of Obstetric, Gynecologic, and Neonatal Nursing, 8*(5), 265–272.

Measel, C. P., Neu, J., & Anderson, G. C. (1987). *Establishing and maintaining lactation: Experiences of mothers of very low birth weight infants.* Unpublished manuscript.

Meberg, A., Willgraff, S., & Sande, H. A. (1982). High potential for breastfeeding among mothers giving birth to pre-term infants. *Acta Paediatrica Scandinavica, 71*(4), 661–662.

Meetze, W. H., Valentine, C., McGuigan, J. E., et al. (1992). Gastrointestinal priming prior to full enteral nutrition in very low birth weight infants. *Journal of Pediatric Gastroenterology and Nutrition, 15*(2), 163–170.

Meier, P., & Anderson, G. C. (1987). Responses of preterm infants to bottle and breast-feeding. *MCN: American Journal of Maternal Child Nursing, 12*(2), 97–105.

Meier, P. P. (1988). Bottle and breastfeeding: Effects on transcutaneous oxygen pressure and temperature in preterm infants. *Nursing Research, 37*(1), 36–41.

Meier, P. P., & Mangurten, H. H. (1993). Breastfeeding the preterm infant. In J. Riordan & K. Auerbach (Eds.), *Breastfeeding and human lactation* (pp. 253–278). Boston: Jones & Bartlett.

Meier, P. P., & Pugh, E. J. (1985). Breast-feeding behavior of small preterm infants. *MCN: American Journal of Maternal Child Nursing, 10*(6), 396–401.

Meier, P. P., & Wilks, S. O. (1987). The bacteria in expressed mothers' milk. *MCN: American Journal of Maternal Child Nursing, 12*(6), 420–423.

Meier, P. P., Engstrom, J. L., Crichton, C. L., et al. (1994). A new scale for in-home test-weighing for mothers of preterm and high risk infants. *Journal of Human Lactation, 10*(3), 163–168.

Meier, P. P., Engstrom, J. L., Mangurten, H., et al. (1993). Breastfeeding support services in the neonatal intensive care unit. *Journal of Obstetric, Gynecologic and Neonatal Nursing, 22*(4), 338–347.

Meier, P. P., Lysakowski, T. Y., Engstrom, J. L., et al. (1990). The accuracy of test-weighing for preterm infants. *Journal of Pediatric Gastroenterology and Nutrition, 10*(1), 62–65.

Meyer, G. E., Novielli, K. A., & Smith, J. E. (1987). Use of refractive index measurement for quality assurance of pediatric parenteral nutrient solutions. *American Journal of Hospital Pharmacy, 44*(7), 1617–1620.

Modanlou, H. D., Lim, M. O., Hansen, J. W., & Sickles, V. (1986). Growth, biochemical status, and mineral metabolism in very-low-birthweight infants receiving fortified preterm human milk. *Journal of Pediatric Gastroenterology and Nutrition, 5*(5), 762–767.

Morriss, F. H., Jr., Moore, M., Weisbrodt, N. W., & West, M. S. (1986). Ontogenic development of gastrointestinal motility: IV. Duodenal contractions in preterm infants. *Pediatrics, 78*(6), 1106–1113.

Mukhtar, A. I., & Stothers, J. K. (1982). Cardiovascular effects of nasogastric tube feeding in the healthy preterm infant. *Early Human Development, 6*(1), 25–30.

Nakamura, K. T., Sato, Y., & Erennberg, A. (1990). Evaluation of a percutaneously placed 27-gauge central venous catheter in neonates weighing <1200 grams. *Journal of Parenteral and Enteral Nutrition, 14*(3), 295–299.

Narayanan, I., Singh, B., & Harvey, D. (1984). Fat loss during feeding of human milk. *Archives of Disease in Childhood, 59*(5), 475–477.

Neifert, M. A., & Seacat, J. (1985). *Milk yield and prolactin rise with simultaneous breast pumping.* Paper presented at the Ambulatory Pediatric Association Meeting, Washington, DC, May 7–10.

Newton, N., & Newton, M. (1967). Psychologic aspects of lactation [Review]. *New England Journal of Medicine, 277*(22), 1179–1188.

Oellrich, R. G., Murphy, M. R., Goldberg, L. A., & Aggarwal, R. (1991). The percutaneous central venous catheter for small or ill infants. *MCN: American Journal of Maternal Child Nursing, 16*(2), 92–96.

Opitz, J. C., & Toyama, W. (1982). Cardiac tamponade from central venous catheterization: Two cases in premature infants with survival. *Pediatrics, 70*(1), 139–140.

Ostertag, S. G., Jovanovic, L., Lewis, B., & Auld, P. A. (1986). Insulin pump therapy in the very low birth weight infant. *Pediatrics, 78*(4), 625–630.

Patel, B. D., Dinwiddie, R., Kumar, S. P., & Fos, W. W. (1977). The effects of feeding on arterial blood gas and lung mechanics in newborn infants recovering from respiratory disease. *Journal of Pediatrics, 90*(3), 435–438.

Pereira, G. R. (1995). Nutritional care of the extremely premature infant [Review]. *Clinics in Perinatology, 22*(1), 61–75.

Pereira, G. R., Schwartz, D., Gould, P., & Grim, N. (1984). Breastfeeding in neonatal intensive care: Beneficial effects of maternal counseling. *Perinatology/Neonatology, 8*(2), 35–42.

Pettit, J. D., & Hughes, K. (1993). Intravenous extravasation: Mechanisms, management and prevention. *Journal of Perinatal and Neonatal Nursing, 6*(4), 74–85.

Plaxico, D. T., & Loughlin, G. M. (1981). Nasopharyngeal reflux and neonatal apnea. *American Journal of Diseases of Children, 135*(9), 793–794.

Powell, D. A., Aungst, J., Snedden, S., et al. (1984). Broviac catheter–related *Malassezia furfur* sepsis in five infants receiving intravenous fat emulsions. *Journal of Pediatrics, 105*(6), 987–990.

Putet, G., Senterre, J., Rigo, J., & Salle, B. (1984). Nutrient balance, energy utilization, and composition of weight gain in very-low-birth-weight infants fed pooled human milk or a preterm formula. *Journal of Pediatrics, 105*(1), 79–85.

Ramanathan, R., & Durand, M. (1987). Blood cultures in neonates with percutaneous central venous catheters. *Archives of Disease in Childhood, 62*(6), 621–623.

Rhea, J. W., & Kilby, J. O. (1970). A nasojejunal tube for infant feeding. *Pediatrics, 46*(1), 36–40.

Riordan, T. P. (1979). Placement of central venous lines in the premature infant. *Journal of Parenteral and Enteral Nutrition, 3*(5), 381–382.

Rosen, C. L., Glaze, D. G., & Frost, J. D., Jr. (1984). Hypoxemia associated with feeding in the preterm and full-term neonate. *American Journal of Diseases of Children, 138*(7), 623–628.

Shaffer, S. G., Quimiro, C. L., Anderson, J. V., & Hall, R. T. (1987). Postnatal weight changes in low birth weight infants. *Pediatrics, 79*(5), 702–705.

Sheehan, A. M., Palange, K., Rasor, J. S., & Moran, M. A. (1992). Significantly improved peripheral intravenous catheter performance in neonates: Insertion ease, dwell time, complication rate and costs. *Journal of Perinatology, 12*(4), 369–376.

Shiao, S. Y., Youngblut, J. M., Anderson, G. C., et al. (1995). Nasogastric tube placement: Effects on breathing and sucking in low-birth-weight infants. *Nursing Research, 44*(2), 82–88.

Shivpuri, C. R., Martin, R. J., Carlo, W. A., & Fanaroff, A. A. (1983). Decreased ventilation in preterm infants during oral feeding. *Journal of Pediatrics, 103*(2), 285–289.

Shulman, R. J., Buffone, G., & Wise, L. (1985). Enteric protein loss in necrotizing enterocolitis as measured by fecal 1-anti-trypsin excretion. *Journal of Pediatrics, 107*(2), 287–289.

Shulman, R. J., Pokorny, W. J., Martin, C. G., et al. (1986). Comparison of percutaneous and surgical placement of central venous catheters in neonates. *Journal of Pediatric Surgery, 21*(4), 348–350.

Simeon, P. S., Geffner, M. E., Levin, S. R., & Lindsey, A. M. (1994). Continuous insulin infusions in neonates: Pharmacologic availability of insulin in intravenous solutions. *Journal of Pediatrics 124*(5, Part 1), 818–820.

Slagle, T. A., & Gross, S. J. (1988). Effect of early low-volume enteral substrate on subsequent feeding tolerance in very low birth weight infants. *Journal of Pediatrics, 113*(3), 526–531.

Stocks, J. (1980). Effect of nasogastric tubes on nasal resistance during infancy. *Archives of Disease in Childhood, 55*(1), 17–21.

Stocks, R. J., Davies, D. P., Allen, F., & Sewell, D. (1985). Loss of breast milk nutrients during tube feeding. *Archives of Disease in Childhood, 60*(2), 164–166.

Stringer, M. D., Brereton, R. J., & Wright, V. M. (1992). Performance of percutaneous Silastic central venous feeding catheters in surgical neonates. *Pediatric Surgery International, 7*, 79–81.

Symington, A., Ballantyne, M., Pinelli, J., & Stevens, B. (1995). Indwelling versus intermittent feeding tubes in premature neonates. *Journal of Obstetric, Gynecologic, and Neonatal Nursing, 24*(4), 321–326.

Szabo, J. S., Hillemeier, C., & Oh, W. (1985). Effect on non-nutritive and nutritive suck on gastric emptying in premature infants. *Journal of Pediatric Gastroenterology and Nutrition, 4*(3), 348–351.

Toce, S. S., Keenan, W. J., & Homan, S. M. (1987). Enteral feeding in very-low-birth-weight infants: A comparison of two nasogastric methods. *American Journal of Diseases of Children, 141*(4), 439–444.

Tsang, R. (Ed.). (1985). *Vitamin and mineral requirements in preterm infants.* New York: Marcel Dekker.

Tsang, R. E., & Nichols, B. L. (Eds.). (1988). *Nutrition during infancy.* Philadelphia: Hanley & Belfus.

van Someren, V., Linnett, S. J., Stothers, J. K., & Sullivan, P. G. (1984). An investigation into the benefits of resiting nasoenteric feed tubes. *Pediatrics, 74*(3), 379–383.

Vaucher, Y. E., Walson, P. D., & Morrow, G., III. (1982). Continuous insulin infusion in hyperglycemic, very low birth weight infants. *Journal of Pediatric Gastroenterology and Nutrition, 1*(2), 211–217.

Verronen, P. (1985). Breastfeeding of low birthweight infants. *Acta Paediatrica Scandinavica, 74*(4), 495–499.

Walker, W. A. (1985). Absorption of protein and protein fragments in the developing intestine: Role in immunologic allergic reactions. *Pediatrics 75*(Suppl. 1, Part 2), 167–171.

Wilkinson, A., & Yu, V. Y. H. (1974). Immediate effects of feeding on blood-gases and some cardiorespiratory functions in ill newborn infants. *Lancet, 1*(866), 1083–1085.

Wilks, S., & Meier, P. (1988). Helping mothers express milk suitable for preterm and high-risk infant feeding. *MCN: American Journal of Maternal Child Nursing, 13*(2), 121–123.

World Health Organization. (1981). *Contemporary patterns of breastfeeding: Report on the WHO collaborative study of breast-feeding.* Geneva: Author.

Yamamoto, L. G., Gainsley, G. J., & Witek, J. E. (1986). Pediatric parenteral nutrition management using a comprehensive user-friendly computer program designed for personal computers. *Journal of Parenteral and Enteral Nutrition, 10*(5), 535–539.

Yu, V. Y. (1976). Cardiorespiratory response to feeding in newborn infants. *Archives of Disease in Childhood, 51*(4), 305–309.

Yu, V. Y. H., & Rolfe, P. (1976). Effect of feeding on ventilation and respiratory mechanics in newborn infants. *Archives of Disease in Childhood, 51*(4), 310–313.

Zenk, K. E. (1992). Y-site compatibility of drugs commonly used in the NICU. *Neonatal Pharmacology Quarterly, 1*(2), 13–22.

Zenk, K. E., Dungy, C. I., & Greene, G. R. (1981). Nafcillin extravasation injury. Use of hyaluronidase as an antidote. *American Journal of Diseases of Children, 135*(12), 1113–1114.

CHAPTER 24

Assessment and Management of Gastrointestinal Dysfunction

LINDA L. McCOLLUM JANET L. THIGPEN

RESEARCH AGENDA

What is the relationship between gastric tube placement (for feeding or decompression) and respiratory compromise?

What feeding practices are most beneficial in stimulating early gut maturation (priming) in preterm infants?

What is the relationship between ischemia, bacteria, and feeding and the development of necrotizing enterocolitis (NEC)?

What factors regulate the establishment and composition of intestinal microflora and how might these factors be regulated to prevent the development of NEC?

How can the postoperative reestablishment of feedings best be accomplished?

How does the presence of an obvious external defect affect the development of the parent–child relationship?

How can the nurse best help the family develop realistic expectations concerning outcome?

VIGNETTE

Ashley was born 8 weeks prematurely. After her initial assessment and stabilization, I bundled her in a warm, dry blanket and handed her to her parents' eagerly waiting arms.

On her arrival in the special care nursery, I weighed Ashley and placed her in a warm incubator to maintain a neutral thermal environment. I then continued to assess and plan her care. She required minimal ventilatory assistance with low oxygen setting. Her bilateral breath sounds were equal and clear, with symmetrical chest movements. The abdomen was soft without distention. Active bowel sounds were present. The remainder of my assessment was within normal limits.

Her parents visited later that evening. At first they were hesitant to hold such a tiny baby. I acknowledged their feelings and encouraged them to just touch her at first. When they were ready, I placed her in their arms. I pointed out her competencies and personified her by calling her by her name, Ashley. These interventions allow the parents to begin to integrate the baby into their family unit.

When I returned the next day, I began to develop a feeding plan in collaboration with Ashley's physician. Throughout the shift, I closely monitored her nutritional status and began gavage feedings of formula. The plan was to increase the feedings gradually over the next several days, while decreasing her IV fluid. She continued to tolerate her feedings with minimal aspirates, and on the fourth day we discontinued her IV. She was taking 24 ml every 3 hours without problems.

Later, as I passed by the nursery window, my heart sank when I saw Ashley with a gastric tube attached to low suction and an IV. X-ray was waiting by the door. I quickly changed into scrubs and went to see what had happened. During the last 16 hours she had presented several symptoms: spitting, increased gastric aspirates, temperature instability, and apnea. A bloody stool and abdominal distention happened as I arrived. The physician had ordered several diagnostic studies: abdominal films, CBC with differential, blood gas, blood cultures, and stool Hematest. In the meantime, I maintained the basic NEC protocol: NPO, NG tube to suction, work-up, and lab monitoring. The lab results had come back, revealing an elevated white blood cell count with a left shift. The blood gas revealed a slight metabolic acidosis.

With NEC, early assessment and intervention are vital. We had begun the initial management. I then reviewed in my mind the nursing goals, that is, maintenance of a neutral thermal environment, GI decompression, maintenance of fluid and electrolyte balance, prevention of infection, proper positioning and nutrition, and assessment of abdominal girth.

The physician informed the parents about Ashley's condition. They both came close to the bedside. I said, "Go on and touch her. She needs to know that you are here." At this point, the x-ray results had come back, showing pneumatosis intestinalis and portal venous gas consistent with NEC. Ashley would need to be transferred to a level III neonatal unit.

I asked a nursing colleague to notify the transport team and prepare the paperwork so that I could spend some time with the parents. Fear of the unknown and fear for survival are very common with parents of any sick infant. I acknowledged their fears and reassured them that Ashley would receive the best possible care.

The transport was uneventful. The goals of care at the tertiary center were to

1. Maintain NPO status.
2. Provide total parenteral nutrition.

3. Monitor intake and output.
4. Maintain a neutral thermal environment.
5. Maintain gastric decompression.
6. Test stool for occult blood.
7. Monitor cardiopulmonary status.
8. Provide skin care, especially over the abdominal wall.
9. Monitor abdominal status, including girths, during the disease process and during realimentation.
10. Minimize parental anxiety and provide support.

I called the center several days later to get an update on Ashley's condition. My colleague informed me that Ashley was doing fairly well. She would be kept on NPO status for the next 2 weeks and receive antibiotic therapy. If Ashley was doing well at that point, gavage feedings would gradually be resumed.

Marianne McGraw

The intake and digestion of foodstuffs and the elimination of waste products are critical to long-term survival. Although many complex metabolic processes are involved, the ability to maintain adequate nutrition ultimately requires that the gastrointestinal (GI) tract be patent and structurally intact. With only a few exceptions, the vast majority of conditions causing GI dysfunction are the result of congenital anatomic malformations. The discovery and management of GI dysfunction thus require a knowledge of both embryogenesis and normal anatomy. Although some anomalies involve external defects and are immediately apparent, most causes of dysfunction are hidden from view and may initially cause few symptoms unless allowed to progress to the point at which serious pathophysiologic changes present a major threat to life. The input and support of a variety of nursing, medical, and other specialists are required for optimal outcomes, that is, the infant's physiologic well-being and the parents' psychosocial stability. The emotional needs of parents and their work through the process of grief over the loss of the expected "perfect" child cannot be underestimated. Visible defects, especially those involving the face, appear to be particularly difficult for parents to accept (Roberts, 1977). The frequent GI malformations are associated with other congenital anomalies and prematurity, and the possible need for transport to a distant center where corrective surgery can be accomplished places additional demands on parental coping.

The GI tract is the site of the many complex transport and enzymatic mechanisms required for the biologic absorption and digestion of nutrients. The successful intake and assimilation of these nutrients, however, rests on the capability of the gut to act as a conduit for ingestion, digestion, and elimination. Congenital malformations, particularly those involving anatomic or functional obstruction, clearly hinder this process. Even when structurally intact, however, the supporting gastric and intestinal musculature of the newborn is relatively deficient, making peristaltic movements more infrequent and irregular when compared with those of adults, thus increasing the tendency toward distention (Smith, 1976). Transport of materials through the tract is further diminished in premature infants, who are characterized by poor sucking and swallowing abilities, small gastric capacity, and incompetent cardioesophageal sphincter (Fletcher, 1994). Debilitated, hypotonic infants may similarly exhibit poor sucking and swallowing and decreased motility. In addition, the bowel seems particularly susceptible to ischemic conditions in which blood flow is preferentially directed away from the GI tract (as well as the kidneys and peripheral vascular bed) toward the brain and heart. Untoward effects of drugs commonly used in the nursery may further compromise intestinal function or integrity. For example, morphine, in addition to its desired analgesic effect, also slows gastric emptying and reduces propulsive peristalsis. Conversely, the antibiotic erythromycin has been shown to accelerate gastric emptying. Ulceration of the GI tract with possible bleeding and perforation are reported side effects of tolazoline, dexamethasone, and indomethacin (Giacoia et al., 1993; Kubota et al., 1994; Young & Mangum, 1997).

The basics of ingestion, digestion, elimination, and metabolism are discussed in Chapter 22, Fluids, Electrolytes, Vitamins, and Trace Minerals: Basis of Ingestion, Digestion, Elimination, and Metabolism and in Chapter 23, Nutrition: Physiologic Basis of Metabolism and Management of Enteral and Parenteral Nutrition. The major purposes of this chapter are to discuss the embryologic development of the GI tract and resultant normal anatomic structure and to describe common causes of neonatal dysfunction with their implications for care.

EMBRYOLOGIC DEVELOPMENT OF THE GASTROINTESTINAL TRACT

The formation of the GI tract is largely dependent on the folding that the embryo undergoes at the end of the first month of development. Initially, the embryo is shaped like a flat, circular plate. However, in the third week, with the beginning development of the nervous system, the area that becomes the cranial region expands, and the neural plate elongates so that the flat disk assumes a shape more closely resembling a pear, with a broad cephalic and more narrow caudal end. The continued longitudinal growth of the primitive central nervous system causes the embryonic disk to bend so that the cranial and caudal portions fold ventrally toward one another. Simultaneously, the rapid proliferation of cells alongside the primitive neural tube causes the disk to fold laterally so that the sides also move ventrally toward each other. By 4 weeks' gestation, the head-to-toe and side-to-side folding is complete, and the embryo more closely resembles a horseshoe-shaped cylinder. The hollow internal cavity, lined by what once was the dorsal portion of the yolk sac that was invaginated during the folding process, forms the basis of the primitive GI tract. The ventral flexure partitions the tube-like cavity into three regions: (1) the foregut, (2) the midgut, and (3) the hindgut. The cephalic area is called the *foregut* and gives rise to the esophagus, stomach, proximal duodenum (above the bile duct), liver, pancreas, and biliary apparatus as well as the lower respiratory system. The mouth develops from a surface depression in the ectoderm called the *stomodeum*, or primitive mouth, and involves the most cranial part of the foregut, which is referred to by some as the *pharyngeal gut*. The middle region is the *midgut*, from which the distal duodenum, the remainder of the small intestine, the ascending colon, and most of the transverse colon are formed. The *hindgut*, the most distal portion of the cavity, gives rise to the rest of the colon, rectum, and upper anal canal as well as the genitourinary structures. The anus originates from an ectodermal depression called the *proctodeum*, or anal pit, and involves the most caudal part of the hindgut, which is referred to as the *cloaca* (Moore & Persaud, 1993; Sadler, 1985). For the purposes of discussion, further review of embryogenesis correlates with these major regions.

Pharyngeal Gut

Early in the fourth week of fetal life, a depression appears on the ventral surface of the head called the *stomodeum*. Oval thickenings, the nasal placodes, develop above and on either side of this primitive mouth. Subsequently, C-shaped elevations, called simply the *nasal elevations*, develop at the margins of the nasal placodes. As this development continues, the nasal placodes deepen and sink to form the nasal pits that become the nostrils. The medial nasal elevations and the area above the stomodeum continue to grow and eventually merge with each other to form the future philtrum, the vertical groove in the middle of the upper lip. Maxillary processes on either side of the stomodeum grow forward and fuse first with the lower edge of the lateral nasal elevations and then extend below the nasal pits to reach and merge with the primitive philtrum to form a continuous ridge above the stomodeum during the eighth embryonic week. It is from this ridge that the upper lip develops. Similarly, two mandibular processes below the stomodeum meet and fuse to form the lower lip and jaw (Habib, 1978a, 1978b; Krogman, 1979; Moore & Persaud, 1993).

The palate is formed between the 5th and 12th weeks of embryonic development. A wedge-shaped extension of the maxillary processes grows beneath the olfactory pits, separating the future nostrils from the upper lip to form the median palatine process or primary palate. The maxillary process also gives rise to a shelf-like projection called the *lateral palatine process.* Initially, the palatine process projects downward on each side of the tongue, but as the tongue descends, the processes gradually grow toward each other in a horizontal plane. The free edges of these lateral processes fuse first with the posterior portion of the primary palate and then with each other in the midline, starting from the front and progressing posteriorly until the fusion is complete. The palate formed by the fusion of these two lateral palatine processes is called the *secondary palate;* this palate subsequently merges with the free edge of the nasal septum (Habib, 1978a, 1978b; Krogman, 1979; Moore & Persaud, 1993).

Foregut

Between 4 and 5 weeks' gestation, a small diverticulum or outpouching appears on the ventral wall of the newly established foregut. As this diverticulum grows, folds develop along its length and eventually grow together in a zipper-like fashion to form an esophagotracheal septum. When completed, this septum divides what was once the proximal foregut into a ventral portion, the primitive respiratory system with its set of lung buds, and a dorsal portion, the esophagus. Initially very short, the esophagus rapidly lengthens over the next 2 to 3 weeks to accommodate the development of the lungs, heart, and neck. During this same interval, at about 4 weeks, a more distal area along the foregut begins to dilate and gradually develops into the stomach. At first this primitive stomach is located in the neck, but it gradually descends during the next 8 weeks to its final abdominal position as the esophagus lengthens, whereas descending, differential growth rates along the sides of the primitive stomach result in the formation of the greater and lesser curvatures. Around 11 weeks, differentiated glandular epithelial cells (primitive parietal cells) begin to appear and have the potential to produce hydrochloric acid as early as 13 weeks' gestation. However, actual acid secretion is not significant until after 33 weeks' gestation (Kelly & Newell, 1994; Kelly et al., 1992, 1993; Loper, 1983; Moore & Persaud, 1993; Sadler, 1985).

The most terminal portion of the foregut, the part that eventually becomes the duodenum, undergoes both external and internal changes during the remainder of the first trimester. Internally, the duodenum begins to generate villi between 5 and 6 weeks' gestation. Interestingly, these villi grow so profusely that the lumen of the duodenum is filled and becomes temporarily occluded by these prolific cells. Not until about 1 month later, between 9 and 10 weeks' gestation, does the duodenum recanalize, thus opening the lumen. Externally, by the beginning of the fourth week, the primitive liver appears as a small bud formed from the lining of the foregut. Shortly thereafter, another outgrowth begins along the stalk connecting the liver to the duodenum, giving rise to the gallbladder and bile ducts. Although initially a hollow organ, the gallbladder and its ducts also experience temporary occlusion as a result of the proliferation of its lining, subsequently recanalizing to allow formation and secretion of bile by the 12th week of gestation. The pancreas also begins with the protrusion of two buds at about 5 weeks' gestation. These buds fuse 1 week later to form a single, definitive pancreas (Moore & Persaud, 1993; Sadler, 1985).

Midgut

Initially, the tube-like gut lengthens in tandem with the overall elongation of the embryo. However, by the sixth week of gestation, the rate of growth of the intestinal tube outpaces the elongation of the body, causing the tube to bend ventrally. With the simultaneously rapid growth of the liver, the space within the abdominal cavity quickly becomes limited. Consequently, at about 7 weeks' gestation, loops of intestine begin to protrude into the umbilical cord. As the midgut literally herniates, it rotates in a counterclockwise fashion (approximately 90 degrees) around an axis formed by the superior mesenteric artery. At around 10 weeks, when the abdominal cavity has expanded sufficiently and the growth of the liver has slowed, the loops of intestine are retracted into the abdomen (undergoing counterclockwise rotation an additional 180 degrees). Thus, during the processes of herniation and return, the intestine has rotated a full 270 degrees. This counterclockwise rotation allows the transverse colon to pass in front of the duodenum and places the cecum and appendix in the right lower quadrant of the abdomen (Loper, 1983; Moore & Persaud, 1993; Sadler, 1985).

Hindgut

The major embryologic process occurring in this third region of the gut involves the formation of the anus. This process takes place in the most terminal part of the hindgut, the cloaca, which is separated from the caudal ectoderm by only a thin barrier called the *cloacal membrane.* When the embryo is 4 weeks old, a ridge of tissue referred to as the urorectal septum develops in the area that becomes the umbilicus. As this septum grows caudally, the cloaca is divided into a ventral portion, the primitive urogenital sinus, and a dorsal portion, the anorectal canal. By the end of the sixth week of gestation, the septum has reached the cloacal membrane, dividing it into smaller membranes as well: the urogenital membrane, which bounds the ventral urogenital sinus, and the anal membrane, which bounds the dorsal anorectal canal. In the meantime, the tissues around the anal membrane swell so that by the eighth week of gestation this anal membrane is found at the bottom of a depression known as the *proctodeum* or anal pit. In the ninth week, the anal membrane ruptures and an open pathway is established between the rectum and the outside (Moore & Persaud, 1993; Sadler, 1985).

Relationship to Nervous System

Before concluding the discussion of GI embryogenesis, it is necessary to review briefly the concurrent development of the nervous system. The primitive neural tube and the neural crest cells proliferating along its side, which were responsible for the initial folding of the embryo (transforming it from a flat disk into a hollow cylinder) continue their own growth and differentiation while the gut is undergoing its transformation. The primitive neural tube ultimately gives rise to the brain, spinal cord, and central nervous system; the neural crest cells give rise to the peripheral nervous system. The relationship between the peripheral nervous system and the GI system begins immediately on completion of the folding process, at about 5 weeks' gestation, when primitive nerve cells begin migrating along the intestinal tube in a cephalocaudal direction. By 12 weeks, the muscular layers of the intestine have appeared, and the primitive nerve cells, or neuroblasts, have completed their head-to-toe migration so that the entire length of the GI tract is innervated (Moore & Persaud, 1993; Sadler, 1985). Thus, by the end of the first trimester, the main structures of the intestinal system have all been established. The last two trimesters are characterized by maturation of the tissues and organs and the rapid growth of the body.

PHYSIOLOGY OF THE GASTROINTESTINAL TRACT

The major function of the GI tract is to transfer food and water from the external to the internal environment, where they can be digested, absorbed, and distributed to the cells of the body by the circulatory system. While these processes are occurring, contractions of the smooth muscle lining the walls of the intestine move the contents through the lumen, releasing any material not digested and absorbed during transit back into the external environment. Technically speaking, this released material is composed of very few "waste products." Although some end products, such as the breakdown products of hemoglobin, are contained in the stool, most metabolic end products are actually eliminated from the body by the kidneys and lungs (Vander et al., 1975).

Structure

The GI tract consists of a tube of variable diameter with the same general structure throughout most of its length. Moving from the outside inward toward the lumen, six concentric layers in the wall of the intestine can be identified (Fig. 24–1). The first, outermost layer is composed of connective tissue. In the esophagus, where the connective layer is continuous with the deep fascia, it is called the *adventitia;* in all other portions of the gut, the connective tissue layer is covered with peritoneal epithelial cells and is called the *serosa.* The next two layers are both made up of smooth muscle, but with each exhibiting a different orientation of its muscle fibers. The outer layer of muscle has its fibers running longitudinally along the gut; the fibers in the inner muscle layer circle the gut. The fourth layer, the submucosa, is composed primarily of connective tissue as well as a few exocrine gland cells, blood vessels, and lymphatics. The fifth layer is again composed of smooth muscle but is of mixed orientation with both longitudinal and circular fibers. The last layer, which actually lines the lumen of the gut, is known as the *mucosa* and contains most of the exocrine gland cells as well as epithelial cells. The mucosal surface is highly convoluted in the small intestine, with many ridges and valleys giving it a larger surface area for absorption. Elsewhere, the mucosa has a smoother surface (Guyton, 1996; Landau, 1980; Moog, 1981; Vander et al., 1975).

In addition to these six structural layers, two major nerve plexuses are found in the gut wall; they regulate the contraction of the smooth muscles. The myenteric plexus lies between the longitudinal and circular layers of muscle and is largely motor in function. The submucosal plexus, as its name implies, is located in the submucosa and is mainly sensory. Synaptic connections between the two nerve networks allow one plexus to stimulate activity in the other and vice versa, leading to activity that is conducted both up and down the length of the gut (Guyton, 1996; Vander et al., 1975).

Motility

Once food enters the esophagus, it is moved along by peristaltic waves initiated by impulses from autonomic nerves and coordinated by the swallowing center in the medulla. As the wave of contraction begins, the gastroesophageal sphincter temporarily relaxes to allow the bolus to enter the stomach. Although this sphincter is anatomically indistinct from the remainder of the esophagus, it normally remains tonically contracted so that the contents of the stomach, which are under relatively higher internal pressure in relation to that experienced in the esophagus, do not reflux (Guyton, 1996; Vander et al., 1975).

When filled with food, the peristaltic waves spread across the stomach toward the small intestine. However, the contractions are no longer mediated by the medulla but rather by the nerve plexuses and the effect of smooth muscle stretching. Because the muscle layers are thicker in the distal portion of the stomach (antrum) in comparison with the relatively thin layer surrounding the upper portion of the stomach (fundus), the contractions are most powerful and intense in the antrum. These strong antral contractions fulfill two functions. First, they are the primary force acting to break up the gastric contents and mix them with enzymes to form a semifluid mixture called *chyme.* Second, they force the chyme past the pyloric sphincter into the duodenum. Normally the rate of gastric emptying is controlled by the chemical composition and amount of chyme, but when the stomach is distended or subjected to increased calorific density or high loads of carbohydrate, fat, or acid, the gastric motility may actually decrease so that more time can be devoted to digestion and absorption in the small intestine. In general, formula empties more slowly than breast milk. The effect of infant positioning and

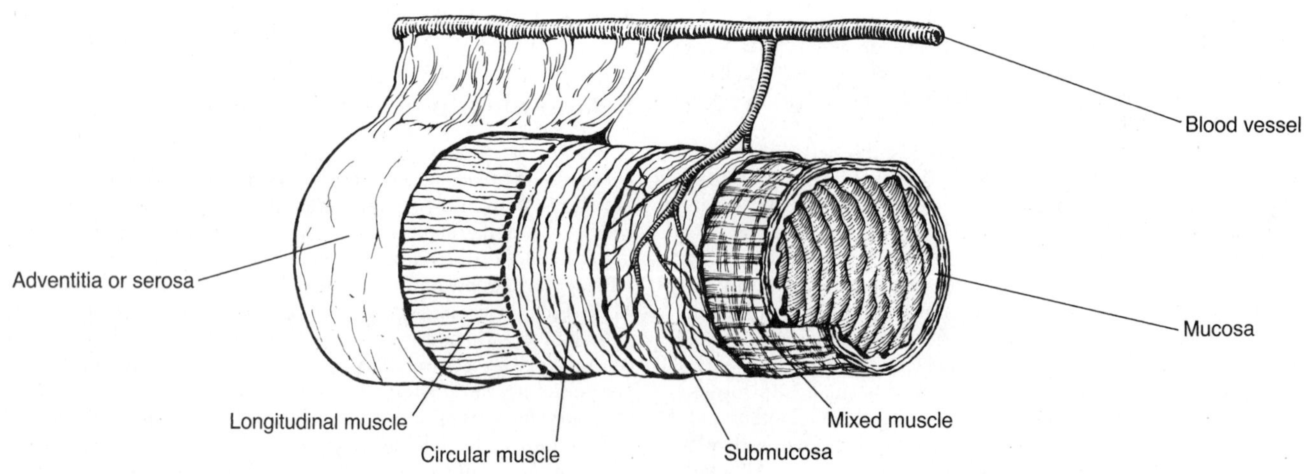

FIGURE 24–1. Anatomy of the intestinal wall.

the temperature of the feed on gastric emptying are less clear (Cavell, 1979; Ewer et al., 1994; Guyton, 1996; Vander et al., 1975).

The contractions that sweep strongly over the stomach become more oscillatory in nature in the small intestine, promoting the digestive and absorptive processes that occur there. Assisting in the process are pancreatic secretions and bile secreted by the liver into the duodenum just below the stomach. Although contractions become progressively slower in the small intestine as chyme passes from the duodenum to the jejunum to the ileum, the muscular activity is sufficient to move the contents slowly downward toward the colon. However, distention and luminal injury may bring muscular activity to a halt (Vander et al., 1975).

The colon functions primarily as a storage area. Consequently its structure differs from that of the small intestine in several major ways. Because only a minuscule amount (approximately 4 percent) of the total intestinal contents is absorbed here, no digestive enzymes are secreted, the lumen is no longer convoluted, and it lacks villi. In addition, the longitudinal smooth muscle layer is incomplete. The contractions of the remaining circular smooth muscle layer therefore produce only segmental, not propulsive, movement. Consequently, when the luminal contents enter the colon through the ileocecal sphincter, they are merely concentrated (through the reabsorption of water) until distention of the rectum initiates the defecation reflex and the fecal matter is expelled (Vander et al., 1975).

MATURATION OF GASTROINTESTINAL FUNCTION

The gross anatomy of the supporting musculature and the functional development of GI motility have not been as well studied as has the development of the secretory and absorptive capabilities of the bowel. In general, however, it appears that these supporting structures are relatively thinner in the newborn, especially in the premature newborn, than in the adult. The muscular layers of the stomach are somewhat deficient, with the longitudinal muscle layer being especially thin over the greater curvature. Similarly, the musculature of the intestine is also relatively thin, constituting approximately 53 percent of the bowel wall in the newborn as compared with approximately 60 percent in the adult (Smith, 1976).

The presence of lanugo and squamous cells in meconium in the newborn bowel indicates that there is at least some movement of materials from swallowed amniotic fluid. Under normal circumstances, however, there appears to be little propulsive peristaltic muscle activity until late in gestation, and even at term such activity is somewhat irregular and slowed in comparison with that occurring in the adult (Smith, 1976). Measurable duodenal contractions have been demonstrated by indwelling intraluminal manometry to be present in the infant born as early as the 26th week of gestation, although they occur infrequently (mean of 1.9 contractions per minute) and are relatively weak (mean of 6.3 mm Hg at peak pressure). Between 29 and 32 weeks of gestation, motility spontaneously and significantly improves, with contractions occurring at an average rate of 6.5 per minute and with an average force of 17.1 mm Hg (Morriss et al., 1986). Neither postnatal age nor type of enteral feed given (breast milk versus formula) nor mode of feeding (instillation by orogastric versus transpyloric tube) appears to affect the timing of this narrow maturational window. Evidence does point to a somewhat enhanced maturation in infants who receive early enteral feedings with volumes as small as 4 ml/g/hour. Use of diluted formula for these early feedings is, however, controversial because the onset, strength, and duration of motor activity appears to be inversely related to the concentration formula. Manometric studies, in fact, indicate that the routine use of diluted formula (even one-third strength) may not provide an optimal stimulus for gut motility (Koenig et al., 1995). Antenatal corticosteroid treatment to initiate production of pulmonary surfactant does appear to promote gut maturation, but maturation appears to be delayed in infants affected with significant central nervous system insult or abnormality such as asphyxia and hydrocephalus. After 32 weeks' gestation, duodenal function steadily improves and by term reaches a contraction frequency of approximately 10 per minute. Thus, the duodenal contraction rate at term approaches but is less than that found in fasting adults of roughly 11 per minute. Furthermore, the number of contractions occurring in a burst or rapid sequence is often fewer than that measured in adults (Morriss et al., 1986).

The motor mechanism of the colon also appears to be affected by maturation and illness. Although virtually all healthy, full-term newborns (99.8 percent) pass meconium within 48 hours of delivery (Sherry & Kramer, 1955), the first passage of stool is frequently delayed in premature infants. Only 94 percent of infants with birth weight less than 2500 g (Kramer & Sherry, 1957), 80 percent of infants weighing less than 1500 g at birth (Jhaveri & Kumar, 1987), and 43 percent of infants with birth weight less than 1000 g (Verma & Dhanireddy, 1993) have passed their first stool by the end of 48 hours. Further delay may be experienced by low birth weight infants who are ill, especially those with severe respiratory distress syndrome, in whom enteral feedings are consequently delayed. Data for such infants with birth weights less than 1500 g reveal a mean time of passage of the first stool at 91 hours for those receiving early feedings versus an average of 168 hours for those receiving delayed feedings. Thus, even in the absence of congenital GI problems, very low birth weight infants might not be expected to pass their first stool until as late as 7 to 12 days of age.

In summary, even when structurally intact, the relatively deficient supporting musculature and immature motor mechanisms of the newborn, particularly the premature newborn, at best allow only irregular peristaltic activity that occurs in somewhat disorganized patterns. This infrequent and irregular activity increases the tendency toward distention in the infant and in the ill or premature infant, increasing the likelihood of delayed transit and stooling. Complete and thorough assessment of the GI tract therefore becomes essential if the expected physiologic deficiencies of the newborn are to be distinguished from pathologic causes of dysfunction.

ASSESSMENT OF THE GASTROINTESTINAL TRACT

History

Assessment of the newborn infant ideally begins during the prenatal period. Although newly born, each infant has a history dating to the time of conception. Consequently, historical antecedents to birth may serve as an indicator of increased likelihood of dysfunction of a specific organ system such as the GI tract (Scanlon et al., 1979; Tappero & Honeyfield, 1996). Although most cases of isolated abdominal and GI defects occur sporadically, some (such as cleft lip or palate, or both, and pyloric stenosis) may exhibit familial recurrence patterns, suggesting at least some degree of genetic influence mediated by environmental factors (McCormack, 1979). Thus, any initial history taking should include a screen to identify parents who have had a previous child with related genetic or congenital anomaly or other positive family history. Major syndromes that have frequently associated GI anomalies are listed in Table 24–1.

Although a certain degree of risk may be established through genetic screening, the best evidence of fetal GI anomalies is obtained through prenatal ultrasonography. The fetal abdomen can be identified as early as 10 weeks from the last menstrual

TABLE 24–1 Major Syndromes Associated With Gastrointestinal Dysfunction

Syndrome	Gastrointestinal Component
Apert's syndrome	Narrow palate with or without cleft palate or bifid uvula Pyloric stenosis Ectopic anus
Beckwith-Wiedemann syndrome	Omphalocele
Fetal hydantoin syndrome	Cleft lip and palate Pyloric stenosis Duodenal atresia Anal atresia
Meckel-Gruber syndrome	Cleft palate with or without cleft lip Bile duct proliferation fibrosis, cysts Omphalocele Malrotation Imperforate anus
Sirenomelia (mermaid syndrome)	Imperforate anus Esophageal atresia with tracheoesophageal fistula
Trisomy 13	Cleft lip with or without cleft palate Omphalocele Incomplete rotation of colon
Trisomy 18	Cleft lip with or without cleft palate Pyloric stenosis Biliary atresia Omphalocele Incomplete rotation of colon Imperforate anus
Trisomy 21	Short palate Tracheoesophageal fistula Duodenal atresia
VATER association	Imperforate anus with or without fistula Esophageal atresia with tracheoesophageal fistula

Data from Jones, K. L. (1988). *Smith's recognizable patterns of human malformation: Genetic, embryologic and clinical aspects* (4th ed.). Philadelphia: W. B. Saunders.

period, and the stomach can be visualized at 13 weeks' gestation. The transient herniation of the intestine into the umbilical cord has even been documented by ultrasonography. However, since embryogenesis is still under way at this time, first-trimester diagnosis of defects, particularly small ones, is exceptionally difficult. It is generally not until the second and third trimesters, when the GI structures are established, that reliable visualization becomes possible. Scanning at that point would include a survey of the abdominal wall and insertion of the umbilical cord, visualization of the fluid-filled stomach, and a search for bowel dilation or abnormal echolucencies resembling cysts that might indicate collection of fluid within the bowel owing to obstruction (Hirata et al., 1990). Abnormal facial features such as clefting may even be identified if fetal position allows and examination is targeted for that area (Graham & Otto, 1990). The presence of polyhydramnios may provide an additional clue to defects high in the GI tract. Normally, in utero the fetus swallows, absorbs, and metabolizes amniotic fluid. However, if the fetus is unable to swallow effectively owing to a GI obstruction, polyhydramnios results.

Postnatally, three cardinal signs point to the possibility of GI obstruction, whether structural or functional: (1) persistent vomiting, especially if it is bile stained; (2) abdominal distention; and (3) failure to pass meconium within the first 48 hours of birth (Chang, 1980b; Ghory & Sheldon, 1985).

Vomiting, as differentiated from reflux, indicates an attempt by an irritated or overdistended bowel to rid itself of its contents. Although vomiting may be initiated by distention or irritative stimuli at any point along the length of the gut, the stomach and duodenum appear to be the most sensitive to these stimuli (Guyton, 1996). Consequently, vomiting is most often considered an indicator of defects high in the GI tract. The presence of bile further indicates that the point of obstruction is distal to the ampulla of Vater, where bile is emptied from the common bile duct into the duodenum. Conversely, nonbilious vomiting would be noted if obstruction were proximal to the ampulla (Ricketts, 1984). Because the mechanism for vomiting requires expulsion of the offending contents up through the esophagus, a patent esophagus is required for true vomiting to occur.

Abdominal distention occurs when large amounts of swallowed air and fluid collect in the bowel and because of obstruction can pass through the gut no further. The situation is compounded as digestive fluids and electrolytes continue to be secreted and proteins are lost from the circulation into the lumen of bowel that becomes progressively edematous as the result of distention (Guyton, 1996). Because the stomach is shielded by the rib cage, such distention is generally observed when obstruction occurs in the lower small intestine or colon (Chang, 1980b).

Most normal full-term infants pass their first stool by 48 hours of age. Failure to pass meconium within the first 2 days of life therefore generally indicates obstruction of the large intestine, unless such delay can be attributed to the case of an oversedated, debilitated, or premature infant.

Physical Assessment

A systematic approach to assessment of the newborn GI tract includes inspection, auscultation, and palpation. Percussion, although useful in the examination of adults, is unreliable and difficult to perform in the infant because the internal abdominal organs are so small and close together. Consequently, the examiner tends to rely on radiography and other diagnostic procedures instead of percussion.

Inspection

Since many of the GI defects are grossly apparent even to the untrained eye, inspection is a fundamental part of assessment. The mouth is observed for its position, shape, size, and symmetry, and the lips, palate, and uvula are evaluated for clefts. Although complete separation of the lip extending up into the nasal area is obvious, close attention must also be paid for any niche in the lip that might easily be overlooked. Abundant oral secretions or saliva provides an early clue to esophageal atresia, particularly when a history of polyhydramnios has been reported (Johnson, 1993; Scanlon et al., 1979).

The abdomen is next inspected for contour, symmetry, and integrity. Distention of the abdomen, which is normally slightly rounded, serves as a hallmark of obstruction. Although the decreased muscle tone in a premature infant may allow visualization of peristalsis, such movement is not normally observed, and when noted in the presence of vomiting or distention, it again suggests the possibility of obstruction. The character of the umbilical cord and site of insertion are checked. Although most cases of omphalocele are obvious, an abnormal thickness to the stump or cord itself should raise suspicion of a single herniated loop of intestine. Any such enlargement must be differentiated from a Wharton's jelly cyst or umbilical hernia through the lax rectus muscles. The anus is examined for position, and the perineal area is inspected for fistulas. The muscle tone of the anal sphincter can be determined by stroking the anal area with a gloved finger and observing for the contraction "wink" that normally occurs around the anal opening. If clinically indicated, the examiner can assess for anal patency by digital examination using the gloved little finger (Conner, 1993; Gluck, 1979; Kiernan & Scoloveno,

1986; Scanlon et al., 1979). Insertion of a rectal thermometer presents the risk of perforating the rectum and should not be performed for assessment purposes (Merenstein, 1970).

Auscultation

Although initially absent, bowel sounds generally become audible within the first 15 to 30 minutes of life, as the bowel fills with swallowed air and peristaltic activity is activated by the parasympathetic nervous system (Desmond & Rudolph, 1965; Lepley, 1980). Normally these sounds should be of a metallic tinkling quality, occurring approximately two to five times per minute (Roberts, 1977). Although often helpful in the assessment of the adult, in the case of neonatal obstruction, sounds may be hyperactive, absent, or even normal (Sunshine et al., 1983). Therefore, the presence and intensity of bowel sounds must be interpreted in relation to other pertinent historical and clinical findings. Hyperdynamic sounds in a recently fed infant with a benign history and otherwise insignificant examination should be considered normal; however, marked concern should be raised if hyperdynamic sounds are found in an infant with concurrent findings of distention and vomiting (Conner, 1993; Scanlon et al., 1979). More often than not, however, the abdomen is misleadingly silent (Flake & Ryckman, 1997).

Palpation

Abdominal palpation is performed with the infant in a supine position and is best carried out when the infant is quiet and preferably during the first 24 hours of life, when the abdominal musculature is lax. Holding the infant's knees and hips in a flexed position also helps to relax the abdominal musculature. Using the pads of the fingers, the liver, spleen, and kidneys should be felt with a warm hand using slow, gentle pressure. Care to perform abdominal palpation in as gentle a manner as possible cannot be overemphasized. The multiple maneuvers involved are often distressing to the newborn and the pressure applied even during a routine examination may result in significant, although transient, elevations in both systolic and diastolic blood pressures (Conner, 1993; Sinkin et al., 1985).

The liver is found by placing the index finger just above and to the right of the groin and slowly advancing upward until the edge of the liver can be felt to slip beneath the pad of the finger. Normally the organ is firm (but not hard) with a sharp edge that extends 1 to 2 cm below the right costal margin and can be followed across the abdomen into the left upper quadrant. The spleen is found on the left side in a similar manner, but generally only the tip of the organ is felt at the left costal margin, or it may be entirely unpalpable. The kidneys are located in the flank areas above the level of the umbilicus and are normally 4.5 to 5 cm in length in the term infant. Palpation may be performed bimanually (with one hand supporting and stabilizing the flanks posteriorly while the thumb or a finger of the free hand is moved anteriorly over the same area), or a single hand may be used (with the fingers of the hand supporting the flank posteriorly while the free thumb of the same hand explores the flank anteriorly). Although the upper position of the right kidney may be obscured by the overlying liver, the entire left kidney should be felt easily. The remainder of the abdominal examination consists of a gentle search for pathologic masses. Although most masses found are of renal origin, it may be possible to detect stool-filled bowel, particularly in the case of meconium ileus (Conner, 1993; Gluck, 1979; Scanlon et al., 1979).

Related Findings

Prenatal ultrasonography and direct postnatal visualization of external defects are diagnostic of GI anomalies. In the absence of these obvious signs, a history of maternal polyhydramnios, vomiting, distention, and failure to pass stool are most indicative of GI dysfunction. Other relatively subtle, and oftentimes nonspecific, signs may also be noted (Ghory & Sheldon, 1985).

Respiratory difficulty may arise as the result of an inability to handle the abundant oral secretions commonly found in esophageal atresia or may develop as a result of aspiration of gastric contents by way of an associated tracheoesophageal fistula. Abdominal distention may impede diaphragmatic excursions and therefore decrease ventilation. Frank airway obstruction may even occur in the case of cleft palate, if the negative inspiratory pressure pulls the tongue into the hypopharynx (Avery et al., 1981).

Jaundice may occur if the removal of bilirubin is hampered. In the case of biliary atresia, the conjugated bilirubin, which is a normal component of bile, is unable to pass into the duodenum for excretion in the stool. In the case of intestinal atresias, meconium ileus, and Hirschsprung's disease, the enterohepatic circulation becomes exaggerated as stasis of the luminal contents promotes intestinal reabsorption of the bilirubin that is present (Poland & Ostrea, 1993).

Systemic hypertension may be an additional, although rarely noted, subtle sign. This increase in blood pressure may be appreciated in situations in which masses or distention significantly increase intra-abdominal pressure (Sinkin et al., 1985).

Risk Factors

Maternal, neonatal, and other risk factors associated with GI dysfunction may be found in Table 24–2. These factors are discussed in the sections outlining the management of specific problems.

Diagnostic Procedures

Radiologic Examination

Air in the GI tract serves as a naturally occurring contrast medium that makes radiologic evaluation of the abdomen a useful tool in the diagnosis of obstruction. At birth, the gut is fluid-filled, but as air is swallowed by the infant after delivery, the radiolucent gas may be followed radiographically as it passes through the bowel. Within the first 30 minutes of life, air should be present in the stomach. By 3 to 4 hours, gas should be seen in the small bowel. After 6 to 8 hours, the entire gut including the colon and rectum should be filled with air (Heller & Kirchner, 1979; Morrison et al., 1992; Singleton, 1963). However, this normal progression of gas through the GI tract cannot occur if obstruction is present. No air is able to pass beyond the point of obstruction, so the portion of the intestine distal to the obstruction is generally airless. Nevertheless, air continues to be swallowed so that the part of the alimentary tract that lies above the obstruction can become quite distended and is demonstrated on radiography by often dramatic radiolucent (black) bubbles. Flat and upright radiographic studies of the chest and abdomen may suffice for identifying esophageal or intestinal atresias. Cross-table lateral radiographs may be helpful by identifying air in the rectum in infants suspected of having intestinal obstruction. A left lateral decubitus film may determine the presence of free air in the intestinal wall or the peritoneal cavity.

Barium swallow is often used to demonstrate GE reflux, pyloric stenosis, and malrotation. Contrast material is swallowed or administered by nasogastric tube and observed by fluoroscopy as it passes through the digestive tract. The procedure may last 30 minutes to 4 hours, depending on the rate of small intestine motility. The patient need not be placed on a nothing by mouth status prior to the examination and may continue feedings after the examination (Kenner et al., 1988).

TABLE 24–2 Risk Factors Associated With Gastrointestinal Dysfunction

Risk Factor	Gastrointestinal Dysfunction
Maternal	
Cigarette smoking	Cleft lip with or without cleft palate
Diabetes	Small left colon syndrome
Hypovitaminosis	Cleft lip with or without cleft palate
Influenza with fever	Cleft lip with or without cleft palate
Ionizing radiation exposure	Biliary atresia
Polyhydraminos	Esophageal atresia with or without TE fistula, duodenal atresia, meconium ileus
Stress and anxiety	Pyloric stenosis
Medications:	
Doxylamine succinate–pyridoxine hydrochloride	Pyloric stenosis
Benzodiazepines	Cleft lip with or without cleft palate
Cortisone	Cleft lip with or without cleft palate
Phenytoin	Cleft lip with or without cleft palate
Magnesium sulfate	Meconium plug syndrome
Opiates	Cleft lip with or without cleft palate
Penicillin	Cleft lip with or without cleft palate
Salicylates	Cleft lip with or without cleft palate
Positive family history:	
"Apple peel" type of jejunoileal atresia	Similar anomaly
Cleft lip with or without cleft palate	Similar anomaly
Cystic fibrosis	Meconium ileus
Hirschsprung's disease	Similar anomaly
Neonatal	
Apnea	Necrotizing enterocolitis
Aseptic environment	Necrotizing enterocolitis
Asphyxia or ischemic episodes	Biliary atresia, necrotizing enterocolitis
Cyanotic spells	Necrotizing enterocolitis
Exchange transfusion	Necrotizing enterocolitis
Feeding practices	Pyloric stenosis, necrotizing enterocolitis
Hyperbilirubinemia	Duodenal atresia, jejunoileal atresia
Polycythemia	Necrotizing enterocolitis
Respiratory distress	Necrotizing enterocolitis
Vascular catheterization	Necrotizing enterocolitis
Infections:	
Cytomegalovirus	Biliary atresia
Gastroenteritis	Intussusception
Hepatitis A and B	Biliary atresia
Reovirus type 3	Biliary atresia
Respiratory infection	Intussusception
Rubella	Biliary atresia
Viral infection	Pyloric stenosis
Medications:	
Hyperosmolar medications	Necrotizing enterocolitis
Xanthines	Gastroesophageal reflux
Other	
Congenital deafness	Hirschsprung's disease
Congenital heart disease	Esophageal atresia with or without TE fistula, duodenal atresia, biliary atresia, omphalocele, anorectal atresia
Diaphragmatic hernia	Malrotation
Genitourinary anomalies	Esophageal atresia with or without TE fistula, duodenal atresia, biliary atresia, omphalocele, Hirschsprung's disease, malrotation, anorectal atresia
Imperforate anus	Esophageal atresia with or without TE fistula, duodenal atresia
Intestinal atresia or obstruction	Gastroesophageal reflux, esophageal atresia with or without TE fistula, biliary atresia, omphalocele gastroschisis, malrotation
Malrotation	Duodenal atresia, jejunoileal atresia
Meckel's diverticulum	Malrotation, intussusception
Meconium ileus	Jejunoileal atresia
Neurologic abnormalities	Hirschsprung's disease, meconium plug syndrome
Ocular neurocristopathies	Hirschsprung's disease
Pancreatic defects	Meconium ileus
Tracheoesophageal anomalies	Duodenal atresia, anorectal atresia
Vertebral malformations	Esophageal atresia with or without TE fistula

TE, tracheoesophageal.

Barium enema is used for examination of the large intestine after contrast solution is instilled through the rectum. It may be diagnostic in cases of malrotation, suspected Hirschsprung's disease, meconium ileus, and meconium plug syndrome. The procedure should be performed prior to any planned upper GI examination. The rationale for this is that barium from the upper GI tract may take several days to clear and may interfere with the lower GI study. No special preparation is made other than placing the infant on a nothing by mouth status 4 to 6 hours prior to the study (Kenner et al., 1988). Gentle saline enemas may be helpful in clearing barium and trapped air after the contrast procedure. If barium is allowed to harden and form concretions that can become impacted, more aggressive procedures may be required for evacuation (Gilger et al., 1995).

Ultrasonography

Ultrasonography may be diagnostic in cases of pyloric stenosis, enteric duplication, GE reflux, or biliary atresia if the intrahepatic or proximal extrahepatic tracts are dilated. Conducting gel is placed on the abdomen and the transducer is placed against the gel on the abdomen. Reflected sound waves from tissues are transformed by a computer into scans, graphs, or audible sound (Kee, 1995).

Gastric Aspirate

A gastric aspirate may be obtained to measure the pH of the gastric contents. A premeasured feeding tube is passed into the stomach. At least 1 ml of gastric contents is gently aspirated into a syringe, and the feeding tube is withdrawn. The syringe is capped, labeled, and sent for testing.

Apt Testing

The Apt test may be used to determine the origin of blood in vomitus or stool by differentiating neonatal GI blood loss from swallowed maternal blood. Bloody aspirate or bloody stool is centrifuged in 5 ml water. One part 0.25 sodium hydroxide is added to five parts supernatant. The fluid remains pink in the presence of fetal blood but turns brown in the presence of maternal blood (Cloherty & Stark, 1985).

Stool Culture

A stool culture may differentiate between an intestinal lining insult and an infection as the cause of bloody diarrhea. A stool sample is taken from a diaper, placed in a specimen container, labeled, and sent for testing.

Stool Hematest

A stool Hematest is a rapid and convenient method for detection of fecal occult blood, possibly indicating GI disease. The test is based on the oxidation of guaiac by hydrogen peroxide, resulting in a blue compound. A thin smear of stool is placed on guaiac paper. Developer is applied over the smear. Results are read in 60 seconds. Any blue colorization on or at the edge of the smear indicates a positive occult blood result. Fecal samples need not be tested if there is hematuria present or obvious rectal bleeding. Drugs influencing positive results include iron preparations, indomethacin, potassium preparations, salicylates, and steroids. Large amounts of ascorbic acid may cause a false-negative result (Kee, 1995).

Stool-Reducing Substances

Carbohydrate intolerance is detected by the presence of reducing substances in the stool. To perform this test, the liquid portion of stool, which can be collected in a diaper, is aspirated into a syringe. A 1:2 ratio of stool to water is obtained. Fifteen drops of this supernatant are placed in a clean test tube, and a Clinitest (test for urinary glucose) tablet is added. After 15 seconds, the test tube is shaken gently and the color of the liquid is compared with the color chart provided with the Clinitest tablets. More than 0.5 percent glucose in the stool indicates an abnormal amount of sugar (Krom & Frank, 1989).

pH Probe Test

A 24-hour esophageal pH study detects nighttime and intermittent GE reflux. A pH microelectrode is placed in the distal third of the esophagus. Reflux episodes are recorded by computer when the esophageal pH is less than 4. Scoring for abnormal results is based on frequency of reflux, number of episodes greater than 4 minutes' duration, time of the longest episode, and the percentage of time in reflux (Meyers et al., 1985). Nursing responsibilities include recording the time of feedings and describing the activity level of the infant throughout the test.

GENETIC CONSULTATION

Some GI disorders are related to chromosomal and single-gene defects. Omphalocele, duodenal atresia, and stenosis have a high association with trisomy disorders. At least 95 percent of cases of meconium ileus occur in infants with cystic fibrosis (Merenstein & Gardner, 1989). Since cystic fibrosis is inherited as an autosomal recessive disease, there may be a family history of the disease. There is a familiar association with pyloric stenosis. Five percent of infants of affected men have pyloric stenosis, and approximately 20 percent of infants of affected women are also affected by the disease. Genetic consultation is suggested for infants with these disorders to provide additional counseling to parents on the risk of recurrence (Lincoln-Boyea & Cefalo, 1996). Chromosomal studies should be performed if there are additional physical findings associated with GI anomaly.

NURSING MANAGEMENT

General Principles

Early recognition accompanied by medical or surgical intervention for infants with GI obstructions or alterations is necessary to decrease the likelihood of a poor outcome. The general considerations that guide nursing care in alterations of the GI system include GI decompression, fluid and electrolyte balance, thermoregulation, positioning, prevention of infection, and nutrition.

Gastric Decompression

Gastric decompression is extremely important to prevent aspiration, respiratory compromise, or gastric perforation. If the intestinal obstruction is not relieved, abdominal distention may become severe and the upward pressure on the diaphragm may compromise respirations. Connection of an orogastric tube to low intermittent suction minimizes the risk of aspiration and prevents distention from swallowed air. Tube patency is essential if gastric decompression is to be maintained. A 10 French soft vinyl, double-lumen gastric sump tube provides sufficient decompression for most infants. Irrigating the tube every 2 hours with 2 ml air ensures that the tube remains open and functioning.

Fluid and Electrolyte Balance

Large amounts of extracellular fluid pass into and out of the GI tract as part of the normal digestive process. In intestinal obstruction, the fluids that are normally reabsorbed by the intestine become trapped. Additionally, infants with obstruction frequently experience "third-spacing," with a shift of fluid from the vascular into the interstitial compartment. This third-spacing is also referred to as capillary leak syndrome. If severe, this loss of intravascular volume can result in relative hypovolemia and hypoperfusion with all their attendant risks. Furthermore, vomiting, diarrhea, and gastric suction can cause excessive volume depletion and electrolyte abnormalities, especially losses of sodium, potassium, and chloride.

The goal of nursing management is to maintain fluid and electrolyte balance. Guidelines for maintenance fluids are usually 60 to 80 ml/kg for the first 24 hours of life and then 120 to 160 ml/kg/day (Kenner et al., 1988). A rate should be maintained at which urine output is at least 1 ml/kg/hour and maintains a specific gravity of 1.005 to 1.012. Sodium is provided at a rate 2 to 3 mEq/kg/day and potassium at 2 mEq/kg/day, as serum electrolytes indicate.

For the infant receiving gastric suction, the amount of gastric loss is determined by measuring drainage every 4 to 8 hours. The amount of gastric output should be replaced milliliter for milliliter every 4 to 8 hours with 5 percent dextrose in 0.9 percent sodium chloride with 10 mEq potassium chloride per liter (Kenner et al., 1988). This amount of fluid is given in addition to maintenance fluids. Fluid volume deficit and electrolyte imbalances may occur if replacement therapy is inadequate. The adequacy for fluid replacement is assessed by changes in vital signs, amount of urinary output, urine specific gravity, levels of electrolytes and blood urea nitrogen, and hematocrit readings.

Metabolic alkalosis may occur with pyloric stenosis or high jejunal obstruction because of loss of acidic gastric juice. In obstructions in the distal segment of the small intestine, larger quantities of alkaline fluids than acidic fluids may be lost, resulting in metabolic acidosis. If the obstruction is below the proximal colon, acid–base balance may be maintained because most of the GI fluids are absorbed before reaching the obstruction. Respiratory acidosis may develop in patients with abdominal distention owing to carbon dioxide retention from hypoventilation (Methany, 1987). Correction of acid–base imbalances would be made in the instance of a pH less than 7.35 or greater than 7.45 or for base excess below -4 or above $+4$ (Merenstein & Gardner, 1989).

Thermoregulation

Thermoregulation is vital in the care of all newborns and becomes more critical for the stressed neonate. Cold stress dramatically increases oxygen requirements and predisposes the infant to hypoglycemia and metabolic acidosis. An appropriate heat source and monitoring must be ensured for any infant with GI dysfunction. Gastroschisis and omphalocele in particular cause profound heat loss from exposed bowel. Nursing intervention includes provision of an external heat source and head covering, hourly monitoring of temperature and, in the case of exposed bowel, use of a bowel bag from the feet to the axillae. The use of the plastic wrap also helps decrease evaporative losses.

Positioning

Head-up positioning accomplishes two management goals in the infant with GI dysfunction. It minimizes pressure that a distended bowel places on the diaphragm, and it minimizes gastric reflux. A 30-degree prone position has been shown to be the most effective position to decrease reflux (Meyers & Herbst, 1982).

Prevention of Infection

Newborn infants are uniquely at risk for infections acquired prenatally, intrapartally, and postnatally. Infants requiring specialized care as the result of medical or surgical problems have an increased susceptibility for infection. Broad-spectrum antibiotics are administered immediately in presumed neonatal infections. Many institutions administer antibiotics preoperatively to prevent infection.

Nutrition

Meeting the caloric and metabolic needs postoperatively in the infant with GI dysfunction is challenging. Enteral feeding is delayed owing to surgery of the alimentary tract. Hyperalimentation is indicated to supply these needs. When the infant is ready to begin enteral feedings, clear liquids are begun, progressing to elemental feedings such as Pregestimil (protein hydosylate formula), gradually increasing from one-quarter to one-half to full strength. Bowel loss or severity of the defect influences the infant's tolerance to feedings. Initial feedings are small, frequent or continuous drip, supplemented with intravenous hyperalimentation, and are gradually advanced. Advancement of feeding should be stopped if there are signs of intolerance, such as diarrhea, vomiting, abdominal distention, or presence of reducing substances in stool (Kenner et al., 1988).

General Preoperative Management

Although the infant is already afflicted by GI dysfunction, surgery presents an additional stress that the child is often ill equipped to tolerate. Therefore, all the principles of preoperative management revolve around the prevention or minimization of identified stressors by replacing all fluid losses, decompressing the distended bowel, and supporting failing organ systems by means of assisted ventilation, radiant heating, parenteral nutrition, and so on. Constant monitoring for potential derangements is essential (Leape, 1987). The specifics of both pre- and postoperative care of the surgical neonate are discussed in Chapter 39, The Surgical Neonate.

General Postoperative Management

Hydration, maintenance of electrolyte balance, and gastric decompression are continued postoperatively, along with respiratory and other therapy that the individual case warrants. If enteral feedings are expected to be delayed beyond 3 to 5 days, total parenteral nutrition should be instituted to prevent excessive catabolism. Otherwise, feedings may generally start when bowel sounds are present, stools are being passed normally, and the gastric drainage clears and lessens in amount (Pereira & Ziegler, 1989).

Infants with ostomies require special management. Skin care is a major concern, owing to frequent problems associated with excoriation and fungal and other infections. To prevent skin breakdown, great care must be given to the construction of appliances so that the skin is maximally protected from contact with effluent, and the stomal appliance should be changed if the seal is broken. Allergic reaction to the products used for stomal appliances is rare (<1 percent). Assessment of hydration and monitoring of urine and stool output, gastric drainage, and stomal drainage should be carried out (Harrell-Bean & Klell, 1983). The normal stoma should be dark pink to red, with a smooth, moist surface that protrudes slightly. Any deviation or change in appearance should be reported immediately.

The short bowel (short gut) syndrome is an unfortunate complication of many neonatal surgeries involving extensive resection of the GI tract. The loss of considerable absorptive surface results in a complex malabsorptive problem with episodic diarrhea, steatorrhea, and dehydration, which if allowed to progress may cause metabolic derangements and ultimately poor growth and development. In the presence of short bowel syndrome, a 1- to 2-year hospitalization may not be unusual (Leape, 1987). The duration of initial hospitalization and length of dependence on parenteral nutrition are both inversely related to the length of remaining bowel (Chaet et al., 1994). Most infants eventually experience progressive small bowel adaptation, and the surgically shortened intestine grows, the mucosal wall hypertrophies, and the villi become hyperplastic so that the absorptive area is increased. Blood flow to the residual intestine and the proportion of the villus that is enzymatically active are both initially increased but gradually decline as the surface area and length continue to increase with time (Swaniker et al., 1995). However, completely normal absorption may never be achieved in cases of extensive resection in which less than 75 cm of the bowel remains (the approximate length of the small intestine in the normal newborn is 200 cm), particularly when the ileocecal valve has also been removed. General survival is considered possible with as little as 11 cm of residual jejunoileum if the ileocecal valve is intact, and with as little as 25 cm when the valve is removed (Dorney et al., 1985). Perhaps owing to improved techniques and advances in enteral nutrition to stimulate the adaptation response, one case has recently been reported of a survivor with 12 cm of jejunum without an ileocecal valve (Surana et al., 1994). Infants with massive resection and those demonstrating no spontaneous adaptation after 6 to 12 months (refractory short bowel syndrome) may require radical surgery to slow intestinal transit (e.g., intestinal valves, reversed segment, colon interposition, intestinal pacing) or increase mucosal surface area (e.g., intestinal lengthening, tapering enteroplasty, neomucosa, small bowel transplantation) and thus increase absorption (Warner & Ziegler, 1993). Whatever the means, until the intestine adapts and full oral feedings have been achieved, the nurse should work collaboratively with others to monitor fluid and electrolyte status and the calories and nutrients taken in. Prevention of skin breakdown (due to diarrhea) and infection are critical. Parents must be involved in their infant's care and every effort made to stimulate normal growth and development (Gantt & Thompson, 1985).

Support of Parents

The birth of an infant with a congenital anomaly or the birth of an infant who is acutely ill elicits feelings of loss, guilt, and confusion for parents. Nurses must expect grief reactions and help the family cope with the crisis. Strategies to help parents cope include support for early contact between parents and infant and explanation with factual information of the infant's condition and plan of care. The lines of communication must be kept open to reinforce information that the family has not been able to process and to assist the family in responding to their grief. Understanding of the disease process is essential for parents to deal later with the prognosis and ongoing health care needs.

CONSIDERATION OF ETHICAL ISSUES

Congenital malformations rarely occur in isolation. When another defect or organ system dysfunction places a major threat on life, decisions regarding the timing of surgical intervention must be made. For example, repair of a serious heart lesion may necessarily precede repair of esophageal atresia, but the resection of necrotic bowel must precede both conditions. Such scheduling decisions are made difficult when it is recognized that some conditions may be improved only at the expense of others. Even when surgical correction of GI dysfunction can be achieved successfully, in the face of multiple malformations (which may not be equally amenable to operative treatment or may result in early demise), the appropriateness of intervention must be reevaluated. Each affected newborn deserves individual consideration. The wishes of the parents and the opinion of each member of the management team must be considered (Leape, 1987).

MANAGEMENT OF PROBLEMS WITH INGESTION

Cleft Palate and Cleft Lip

Pathophysiology

Although cleft lip and cleft palate are often associated, these defects are embryologically distinct disorders. Cleft lip occurs when the maxillary process fails to merge with the medial nasal elevation on one or both sides. Cleft palate occurs when the lateral palatine processes fail to meet and fuse with each other, the primary palate, or the nasal septum (Moore & Persaud, 1993). When both cleft lip and cleft palate occur together, studies indicate that the failure of the secondary palate to close may be a developmental consequence of the abnormalities in the primary palate associated with the cleft lip, rather than an intrinsic defect in the secondary palate. It is possible, therefore, that isolated cleft lip and cleft lip with an associated cleft palate represent varying degrees of the same embryologic defect (Fraser, 1970; Habib, 1978a).

Risk Factors

Cleft lip with or without an associated cleft palate affects 14 of every 10,000 newborns, with rates higher in males than in females and in Asians than in whites. In contrast, isolated cleft palate has a lower incidence rate of 4 in 10,000 infants, occurs more frequently in females, and has no clear racial variation (Habib, 1978a, 1978b; Oka, 1979). Although rates of recurrence risks indicate that genetic factors are often involved, environmental factors also appear to contribute in some way, indicating a multifactorial mode of inheritance.

Maternal medication during the first trimester—especially benzodiazepines, phenytoin, opiates, penicillin, salicylates, and cortisone—has been associated with clefting. Occurrence of fever and influenza during the first trimester has also been demonstrated as a possible factor; however, it is questionable as to whether the viral agent or the therapeutic drugs are the causative factors. Threatened abortion in the first and second trimesters and premature delivery of neonates with clefts have also been reported, but it is uncertain whether this indicates an unfavorable intrauterine environment or simply a symptom of an already malformed fetus (e.g., Pierre Robin syndrome or sequence). An association between clefting and variables such as maternal smoking, hypovitaminosis, and hypervitaminosis, especially of vitamin A, has also been supported. Maternal age, however, does not appear to be a factor, although there may be a small but nonsignificant increase in the incidence of clefting with increasing paternal age (Briggs, 1976; Fraser, 1970; Habib, 1978a, 1978b; Khoury et al., 1989; Oka, 1979; Saxen, 1975; Walantas, 1986).

Clearly, cleft lip or cleft palate, or both, can have multiple causes and consequently may represent a malformation, a disruption, or a deformation. When the defect is the result of an inherently abnormal developmental process, as in the case of genetic derangement, it is appropriately called a *malformation*. When the developmental process is originally normal but goes awry because of extrinsic factors, as in the case of teratogenic exposure, it is called a *disruption*. Lastly, when mechanical forces interfere with normal development, as in the case of Pierre Robin syndrome in which mandibular hypoplasia causes the tongue to be posteriorly displaced thus interfering with the fusion of the lateral palatine shelves, the result is called a *deformation* (Saal & Rosenbaum, 1988).

Clinical Manifestations

Generally defined, *cleft lip* is the term that signifies a congenital fissure in the upper lip, whereas cleft palate indicates a congenital fissure in either the soft palate alone or in both the hard and soft palates. The two conditions may occur in isolation or together. Isolated cleft lip may be either unilateral or bilateral and may range in severity from a slight notch in the lip to a complete cleft into the nostril. Isolated cleft palate may also be unilateral or bilateral and may be as mild as a submucous cleft characterized by a notch at the posterior edge of the hard palate, an imperfect muscle union across the palate, a thin mucosal surface, and a bifid uvula. In this mild form, the diagnosis may never be made. Combined clefts of the lip and palate are the most severe form of the defect, particularly if they are bilateral (Shah & Wong, 1980).

Differential Diagnosis

The major condition requiring differential diagnosis is van der Woude's syndrome, which is inherited as an autosomal dominant trait. This syndrome ranges in appearance from a single, barely visible lower lip depression to frank pits or fistulas usually occurring in pairs on the vermilion of the lower lips, with clefting of the lip with or without palate involvement (Bowers, 1970; Jones, 1988; Schneider, 1973).

Prognosis

Although an excellent prognosis for survival can be expected, an individual born with a cleft defect is faced with more than just a cosmetic problem. Language and speech tend to be retarded in affected individuals. This retardation is further compounded by the fact that hearing impairment is more frequent in these individuals (Bergstrom, 1978; Krogman, 1979; Shah & Wong, 1980). Olfactory defects have also been demonstrated in males with cleft palate; however, females appear to be affected less frequently (Richman et al., 1988). Dental problems, such as malocclusion, irregularity of the teeth, and increased frequency of caries, may also be encountered in affected individuals (Shah & Wong, 1980). Although the majority of cases of cleft lip or palate, or both, are not associated with any recognizable syndrome, there are more than 154 syndromes that include cleft lip or palate, or both, as a feature (Cohen, 1978). Obviously, the prognosis in such cases varies with the associated anomalies involved.

Collaborative Management

The management of an individual born with a cleft defect is beyond the capabilities of any one professional. Rather, effective care requires the services of a team of individuals: pediatrician, plastic surgeon, audiologist, speech pathologist, dental specialist, geneticist, social worker, and nursing personnel at various levels.

Surgical repair is a priority, not only to achieve closure of the defect but also to minimize maxillary growth retardation, to limit dental deformity, and to allow normal speech development. If the infant is healthy and no complications are expected, a cleft lip can be repaired at about 3 months of age. Repair of an associated cleft palate is generally postponed until a later time to allow medial movement of the palatal shelves, which appears to be initiated by lip closure. Depending on the involvement, palate closure may occur as a two-step process, with the hard palate being corrected at 14 to 16 months of age, followed by soft palate repair at 18 to 20 months of age. If additional repair of the lip or nose is required for aesthetic purposes, it is postponed until sufficient structural growth has been achieved, generally after 12 years of age (Krogman, 1979; Shah & Wong, 1980).

Emotional preparation of the parents is frequently the most immediate and demanding nursing problem encountered. The birth of a defective child comes as both a shock and a disappointment to the parents. Information and reassurance are desperately needed at this critical time. Nurses can also provide a role model to influence the parents' attitude toward the child positively and to provide guidance and support as the family copes with the reactions of others (MacDonald, 1979; Pate, 1987; Shah & Wong, 1980).

Feeding is another important aspect in the care of an infant with cleft lip or palate and is one that requires a great deal of patience and attention to technique. In the presence of cleft lip, the infant may have difficulty not only in holding the nipple in the mouth but also in creating the vacuum necessary for adequate sucking. The bottle should be held securely and the cheeks grasped so that the cleft is pushed closed. Even then, large amounts of air may be swallowed, so frequent burping should be performed. The infant with cleft palate should be held in an upright or semiupright position to avoid choking, and the flow of milk should be directed to the side of the mouth. Use of a "preemie" nipple or a special cleft palate nipple may also be helpful. Frequent, small feedings help in preventing fatigue and frustration. Breastfeeding is certainly possible, although considerable creativity may be required. A pillow placed between the infant's back and the mother's arm can maintain the infant in an upright position. Because the clefted areas easily become encrusted with milk and are therefore prone to excoriation and infection, a small amount of sterile water should be offered after each feeding (Pate, 1987; Styer & Freeh, 1981).

Esophageal Atresia and Tracheoesophageal Fistula

Pathophysiology

Esophageal atresia and tracheoesophageal (TE) fistula occur when the trachea fails to differentiate and separate from the esophagus. The atresia appears most likely to be the result of either a spontaneous posterior deviation of the esophagotracheal septum or some mechanical force that pushes the dorsal wall of the foregut in an anterior direction. A fistula occurs when the lateral ridges of the septum fail to close completely in their normal zipper-like fashion so that a communication is left between the foregut and the primitive respiratory tree (Moore & Persaud, 1993; Sadler, 1985).

Risk Factors

Esophageal atresia with or without TE fistula occurs approximately once in every 3000 live births. Although rare cases of familial occurrence have been reported, most cases represent an accident of embryology. A history of maternal polyhydramnios is reported in 14 to 90 percent of cases (Sunshine et al., 1983). The higher rates are found with an isolated esophageal atresia; the lower rates are found when a fistula allows passage of swallowed amniotic fluid around the obstruction. Associated malformations are present in 30 to 70 percent of infants. Congenital heart disease is reported most frequently (25 to 40 percent), with ventricular and atrial septal defects being the most common lesions. Other associated anomalies include vertebral malformations (25 to 30 percent), atresias of the small intestine (5 percent), imperforate anus (10 to 20 percent), and genitourinary anomalies (10 to 21 percent). Approximately 15 percent present as part of the VATER association, the acronym representing a complex of vertebral and ventricular septal defects, anal atresia, TE fistula with esophageal atresia, and radial and renal anomalies. VACTERL association is used by some experts to describe the same cluster of symptoms. The C stands for congenital heart defects, and the L is for limb deformities. Overall, 20 to 30 percent of these infants are premature or small for gestational age, but in the case of isolated esophageal atresia, the incidence of prematurity approaches 50 percent (Chang, 1979; Desjardins, 1987; Dienno, 1987; Ein & Shandling, 1994; Holder & Ashcraft, 1981; Jones, 1988; Martin & Alexander, 1985).

Clinical Manifestations

Although the infant may appear well at birth, oral secretions and saliva collect in the upper esophageal pouch and appear in the mouth and around the lips because effective swallowing is not possible. The typical description of "excessive" secretions, however, is a misnomer. The body does not produce greater amounts of secretions; they simply cannot be handled properly and thus become more visible. Respiratory difficulty may be encountered if the secretions and mucus fill the esophageal pouch and overflow into the upper airway or find their way into the trachea through a proximal fistula. Any attempts at feeding are generally accompanied by coughing, choking, and cyanosis. If a distal fistula is present, crying may force air into the stomach, where it collects and causes progressive distention. This gastric distention may impede diaphragmatic excursions, leading to worsening respiratory status or a reflux of gastric contents back up through the fistula into the trachea. If there is no distal fistula, the abdomen is more likely to appear scaphoid owing to the lack of swallowed air. True vomiting is not possible (except in the case of an isolated TE fistula) because the esophagus and stomach are not connected. This triad of "excessive" secretions, reflux, and respiratory distress, particularly in association with a maternal history of polyhydramnios, indicates esophageal atresia until proved otherwise (Chang, 1979; Gryboski & Walker, 1983; Holder & Ashcraft, 1981). However, the clinical presentation may vary slightly, depending on the specific type of anomaly found (Fig. 24–2). Although there are five major pathologic types of esophageal atresia with or without TE fistula, approximately 100 subtypes have been described (Kluth, 1976; Lambrecht & Kluth, 1994).

Differential Diagnosis

Diagnosis of esophageal atresia is confirmed by attempting to pass a radiopaque catheter from the nares through the esophagus into the stomach. If the esophagus is atretic, the catheter cannot be advanced further than a depth of approximately 9 to 12 cm

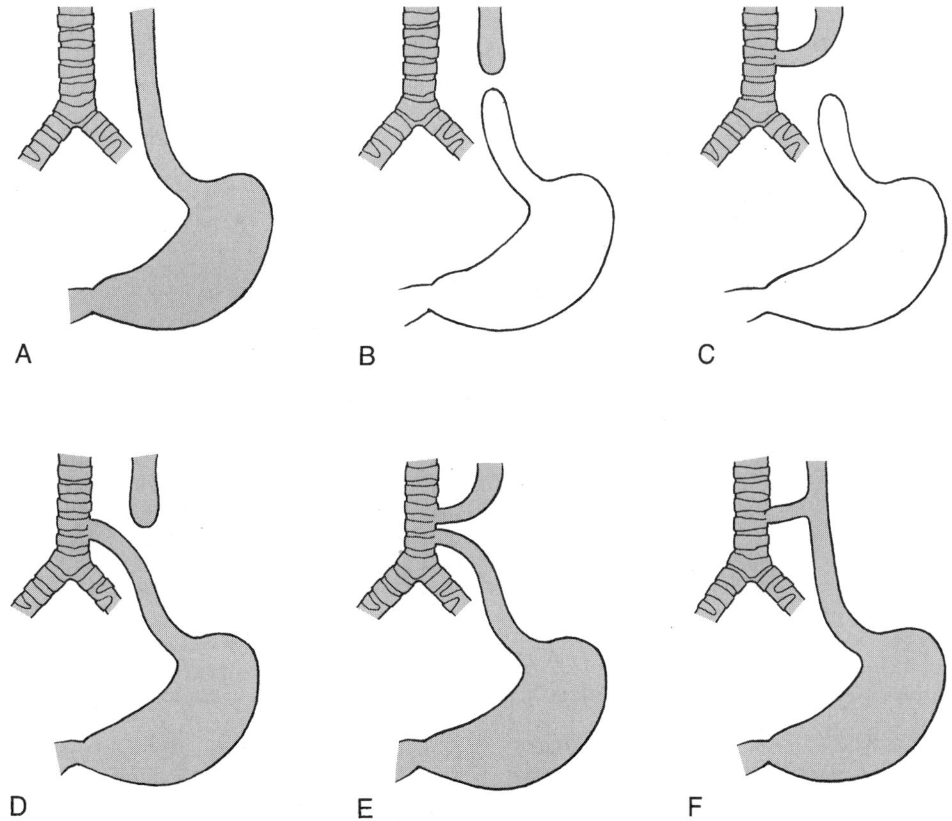

FIGURE 24–2. Esophageal atresia and transesophageal (TE) fistula. Shading represents areas of lucency typically found on radiographs. Percentages reflect relative occurrence. *A*, Normal. *B*, Isolated esophageal atresia (8 percent), characterized by excessive salivation. *C*, Esophageal atresia with proximal TE fistula (1 percent), characterized by respiratory distress, especially with feeding. *D*, Esophageal atresia with distal TE fistula (86 percent), characterized by excessive salivation, respiratory distress, and reflux. *E*, Esophageal atresia with both proximal and distal TE fistulas (1 percent), characterized by respiratory distress, especially with feeding, and reflux. *F*, Isolated (H-type) TE fistula (4 percent), characterized by respiratory distress, especially with feeding, and reflux. (Data from Cassani, V. L. [1984]. Tracheoesophageal anomalies. *Neonatal Network*, 3[2], 20–27; Desjardins, J. G. [1987]. Esophageal atresia. In L. Stern & P. Vert [Eds.], *Neonatal medicine* [pp. 1036–1042]. New York: Masson Publishing; Sunshine, P., Sinatra, F. R., Mitchell, C. H., & Santulli, T. V. [1983]. The gastrointestinal system. In A. A. Fanaroff & R. J. Martin [Eds.], *Behrman's neonatal-perinatal medicine: Diseases of the fetus and infant* [3rd ed., pp. 477–535]. St. Louis: C. V. Mosby.)

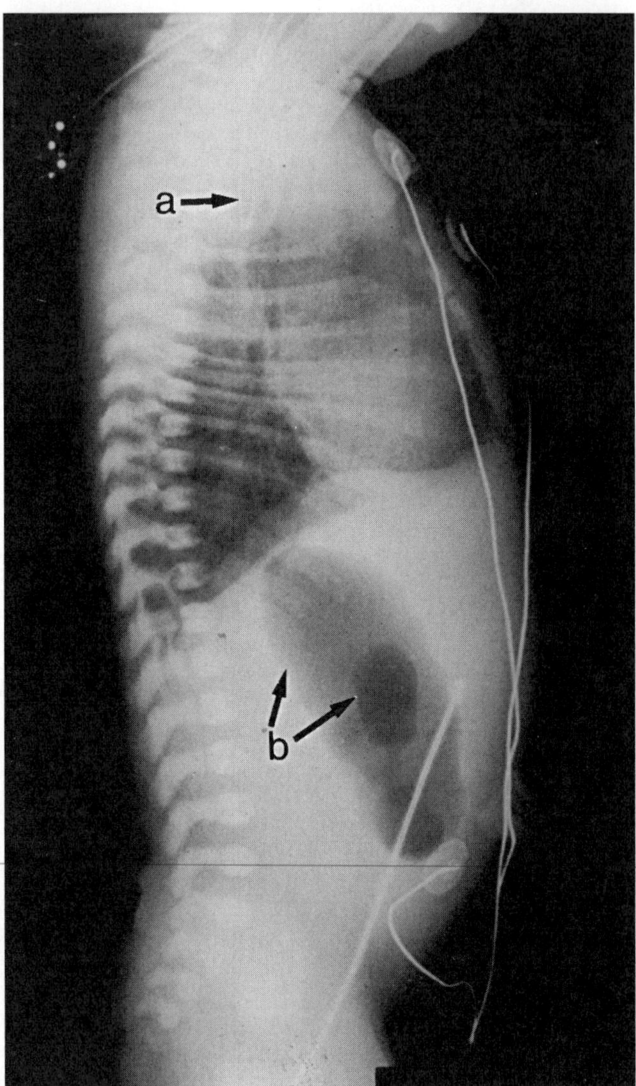

FIGURE 24–3. Coexisting atresia with TE fistula and duodenal atresia. Catheter (a) is seen curled in the upper esophageal pouch. Air in abdomen indicates presence of a distal TE fistula. The "double bubbles" (b) characteristic of duodenal atresia appear to overlie one another on this lateral film. This infant survived surgical repair but later died as a result of multiple congenital anomalies.

before meeting resistance, and any contents that are aspirated are alkaline rather than acidic. A chest radiograph shows the tube ending or coiling in the upper esophageal pouch (Fig. 24–3). Air in the bowel indicates the presence of a distal TE fistula. If the abdomen is airless, no such fistula is present. Contrast studies are generally contraindicated owing to the danger of aspiration but may become necessary in the diagnosis of an isolated or H-type TE fistula. In these cases, which are more difficult to diagnose, bronchoscopy or endoscopy may be required to allow direct visualization of the fistulous site (Chang, 1979; Chang & Saing, 1995; Holder & Ashcraft, 1981; Martin & Alexander, 1985; Ryckman et al., 1992).

Prognosis

With early diagnosis and efforts to prevent aspiration pneumonia, most full-term infants do well, with a survival rate of 97 percent. However, mortality dramatically increases in the presence of prematurity or associated major anomalies, particularly cardiac disease. When birth weight is less than 1500 g or major cardiac disease is present, survival is approximately 60 percent. When both conditions are present, survival falls to 22 percent (Holder & Ashcraft, 1981; Spitz et al., 1994).

Collaborative Management

Surgical correction involves esophageal anastomosis (esophagoesophagostomy) and obliteration of any fistula that is present. The exact technique varies with the type of defect present, but if a great distance separates the two ends of the esophagus, the repair is made more difficult and must often be staged. In this case, the ends may be brought into closer approximation either preoperatively by stretching the upper esophageal pouch daily with a bougie to produce progressive elongation or intraoperatively by performing multiple circular myotomies so that the upper esophageal segment can be lengthened in a telescoping fashion. Alternatively, a combination of the two methods may be used. If these procedures are not effective, or if the gap is particularly large, a segment of the small or large intestine or an inverted tube of gastric tissue may be used for esophageal replacement (Cusick et al., 1993). Such a dramatic procedure is generally delayed until 1 year of age. When the gap makes primary repair impossible, the upper esophageal pouch can be brought to the surface as a cervical esophagostomy ("spit fistula") to allow the drainage of saliva, with gastrostomy performed for feeding. In these protracted cases, sham feeding may be attempted in which orally fed milk is collected with saliva in the ostomy bag attached to the esophagostomy stoma and refed through the gastrostomy tube into the stomach (Chang, 1979; Holder & Ashcraft, 1981; Kimura & Soper, 1994; Martin & Alexander, 1985).

Generally, repair is performed through an incision at the base of the neck, but if the lesion is exceptionally low within the chest, a thoracic approach may be used, necessitating chest tube placement. A gastrostomy may also be performed to allow feeding during healing (Ashcraft & Holder, 1981; Holder & Ashcraft, 1981; Kemmotsu et al., 1995).

Preoperative care is focused primarily on the reduction of symptoms. To prevent overflow of secretions, a sump catheter (Replogle's tube) is placed in the upper esophageal pouch and connected to low intermittent suction. The tube lumen becomes easily occluded by tenacious secretions and should therefore be changed daily. Catheter irrigation is potentially dangerous and is not recommended. If the secretions are particularly thick, humidified air may assist in liquefying them for easier removal. Elevating the head 30 to 40 degrees helps avoid reflux of gastric secretions into the trachea via a distal fistula. Comfort measures to prevent crying reduce the amount of air swallowed through the fistula, thus limiting gastric distention and further reducing the risk of reflux. If no TE fistula is present, a flat or head-down position may be preferable to avoid gravity drainage of saliva from an overflowing esophageal pouch. Fluids and electrolytes should be given by the intravenous route. Supplemental oxygen and intubation may be needed if respiratory distress occurs. However, use of positive-pressure ventilation increases the propensity for gastric distention and may even necessitate preoperative gastrostomy for decompression (Cassani, 1984; Chang, 1979; Dienno, 1987; Martin & Alexander, 1985).

Postoperatively, vital signs are monitored closely and frequent assessment is made looking for potential leaking at the anastomotic site. If a chest tube has been placed, such leakage presents as persistent or increased drainage. The endotracheal tube is generally left in place for at least 24 hours to allow full recovery from anesthesia and relaxants. When suctioning the airway, the catheter should be well marked and inserted to a predetermined depth above the site to avoid disruption or trauma. The quantity and appearance of secretions and any respiratory difficulties are reported. Feeding by gastrostomy may be started within 48 hours, with oral feedings generally withheld for 5 to 10 days to ensure healing. Gastroesophageal reflux is a common complication because of the upward pull on the lower esophageal pouch and stomach and generally poor peristalsis, occurring in 50 to 75 percent of infants, and should be managed as described in the next section. Postoperative complications frequently seen arising over time include stricture of the anastomosis (40 to 50 percent) and recurrence of the fistula (5 to 12 percent). Support and communication are the cornerstones of parental care throughout hospitalization (Cassani, 1984; Chang, 1979; Dienno, 1987; Ein & Shandling, 1994; Gutierrez et al., 1994; Martin & Alexander, 1985; Ravelli et al., 1994).

Gastroesophageal Reflux

Pathophysiology

Gastroesophageal reflux is the spontaneous passage of acidic gastric contents from the stomach into the esophagus. Berenberg and Neuhauser (1950) described the classic and radiologic findings of GE reflux in infants. They suggested the term *chalasia*, referring to an abnormal relaxation of the gastroesophageal junction.

The distal esophagus possesses a physiologic sphincter, approximately 0.5 cm long in the infant, called the *esophageal vestibule*. The upper portion of the esophagus lies in the thorax, the middle section at the diaphragm, and the lower segment in the abdomen. This segment of terminal esophagus has a higher pressure than that of the stomach below or the esophagus above and helps prevent retrograde flow of gastric contents into the esophagus. Any condition delaying or altering the maturation of this valve may cause reflux of stomach contents in the infant.

Adult lower esophageal segment pressure is usually 5.6 ± 3 mm Hg. In the newborn, it remains low during the first 2 weeks of life, increases markedly between 2 and 4 weeks of age, and reaches adult pressure measurements by 1 to 2 months of age.

Risk Factors

Premature infants are at risk for reflux owing to immaturity of the esophagogastric junction. In otherwise normal term infants, this junction may not mature normally, and reflux into the esophagus may continue. Infants with high bowel obstructions have delayed maturation of the valve mechanism and are at risk for chalasia resulting from structural weakness. Nearly 12 percent of infants with congenital diaphragmatic hernia experience reflux after repair, most likely due to deviation of the esophagus to the affected side, malposition of the stomach, increased intra-abdominal pressure, gastric dysmotility, or a combination of these factors (Nagaya et al., 1994; Sigalet et al., 1994). A high percentage of infants with neurologic damage exhibit GE reflux, possibly due to reduced swallowing frequency and weaker esophageal sphincter control (Hlusko & McMurray, 1991).

Clinical Manifestations

The primary symptoms of GE reflux in infants are vomiting, growth retardation, aspiration pneumonia, apneic spells, and esophagitis (Guzzetta et al., 1994). Persistent vomiting due to GE reflux often leads to failure to thrive. Such infants tend to be pale, thin, hypoactive, listless, and underweight and are often misdiagnosed as having a nutritional deficiency. Infants with growth retardation due to reflux usually improve promptly and dramatically following corrective surgery.

The most commonly recognized pulmonary symptom associated with GE reflux is recurrent aspiration pneumonia. It is characterized by fever, cough, poor appetite, and typical findings on radiography.

Apneic spells, most commonly seen in the early weeks of life, may be caused by reflux. Gastroesophageal reflux is capable of causing laryngospasm, with cardiac slowing or arrest, apnea, and death if this sequence is not halted (Avery & Taeusch, 1984). Well-documented recurrent apneic spells have been completely eliminated in many cases after antireflux surgery. Asthma or asthma-like symptoms related to reflux are rare during the first year of life but have been seen occasionally in infants.

Esophagitis is generally not seen in the early months of life. Infants suffering from esophagitis caused by GE reflux are usually fussy, irritable, and colicky. Frank bleeding is rare but may be present with anemia and guaiac-positive stools.

Differential Diagnosis

Differential diagnosis includes other causes of vomiting (distal outlet obstruction as in pyloric stenosis or neurologic or metabolic disease). Cystic fibrosis and bronchitis may present with a similar clinical picture.

Prognosis

Most infants can be safely treated medically for 3 months before it may be judged that conservative therapy has failed. Seventy-five percent recover when treated medically, 10 to 15 percent require prolonged medical management, and 10 to 15 percent require surgery. When symptoms are controlled by medical means, reflux ceases by 15 months of age and therapy can be discontinued. Surgical long-term results are good, with reported 95 percent total clinical cures assessed at check-ups after 10 years or more (Bettex & Oesch, 1983; Herbst, 1983). Adverse side effects, including mild gas bloating, slow eating, an inability to burp, or vomiting, are seen in approximately one third of surgically treated patients.

Collaborative Management

Nursing and medical collaboration is necessary to assess the effectiveness of conservative treatment modalities. These methods include positioning, thickening of feedings, monitoring for apnea, antacids in the presence of esophagitis, and use of bethanechol, metoclopramide, or cisapride. Physical and occupational therapy input may be helpful for issues of positioning and techniques of feeding.

If medical management fails to control life-threatening complications, surgical intervention is indicated. Although many procedures have been devised, the Nissen fundoplication is most widely used in the neonate. In this procedure, the proximal stomach is wrapped around the distal esophagus, creating a junction that is effective in preventing reflux. Most infants have a temporary gastrostomy placed postoperatively to vent swallowed air and decrease bloating. The tube is usually removed after 3 to 6 weeks. Associated problems usually improve promptly with corrective surgery.

Nursing assessment of the infant with GE reflux and its related problems is important in the diagnostic process. The history, physical examination, and test results of upper GI series or pH probe testing confirm or deny the diagnosis. Conservative therapy generally falls under the direct supervision of the primary nurse.

A 30-degree prone position after feedings is better than the upright and supine positions, when the infant is both awake and asleep (Lynn, 1986; Meyers & Herbst, 1982; Orenstein, 1992). Contrary to popular thinking, infants placed in infant seats had 50 percent more reflux episodes that lasted twice as long as when they were in the prone position (Orenstein, 1992). Sitting in an infant seat places the gastroesophageal junction in an embedded or dependent position.

Thickening of formula with rice cereal (at a ratio of 15 ml cereal to 30 ml formula), which is then fed by nipple with an enlarged hole, has been found to decrease vomiting, decrease crying time, and increase sleep in the postprandial period (Orenstein, 1992; Orenstein et al., 1987). The possible tendency of thickened feedings to increase coughing mandates caution in using this form of therapy in infants with pulmonary symptoms and reflux (Orenstein et al., 1992). Unless coupled with a 30-degree prone position after feeding, the full efficacy of thickened feeding to decrease vomiting may not be appreciated (Bailey et al., 1987).

Apneic episodes and recurrent aspiration pneumonia have been associated with GE reflux. Infants suspected of and documented as having clinically significant reflux should therefore undergo continuous respiratory monitoring. This monitoring is particularly important when xanthines are used to treat the apnea. Although xanthines are used to improve respiratory function and reduce apnea, they also increase gastric acid secretion and decrease lower esophageal sphincter pressure, which may further increase GE reflux (Young & Mangum, 1997).

Antacids and H_2 antagonists (cimetidine, famotidine, or ranitidine) are used, not to prevent reflux but to treat esophagitis. Bethanechol increases lower esophageal sphincter pressure, decreases vomiting, and increases weight gain in reflux patients with failure to thrive. Because of its cholinergic effect, it must be used with care in infants with chronic lung disease (Herbst, 1983; Orenstein, 1992). Metoclopramide increases the tone and amplitude of gastric contractions, relaxes the pyloric sphincter and duodenal bulb, increases peristalsis of the duodenum and jejunum, and increases the resisting tone of the lower esophageal sphincter. Once medication is begun, the infant must still be monitored carefully for apnea and regurgitation. Cisapride acts by selectively stimulating release of acetylcholine from neurons within the myenteric plexus. Clinical studies have shown that cisapride increases esophageal sphincter pressure, gastric emptying, and propulsive activity in the small and large intestine. Unlike metoclopramide, cisapride possesses no antagonism at the dopamine receptor; therefore, it is not associated with dystonic reactions. As a new prokinetic drug approved in the use of GE reflux, studies are needed to assess its role in pediatric GE reflux. Until such studies are completed, cisapride should be reserved for patients in whom other pharmacologic agents fail (Arura & Spino, 1991; McCallum, 1991).

Pyloric Stenosis

Pathophysiology

Although many cases of pyloric stenosis are believed to be acquired postnatally, this disorder is properly referred to as *congenital hypertrophic pyloric stenosis.* The pathologic picture consists of marked hypertrophy of the pylorus with spasm of the muscular coat, creating a tumor-like nodule constricting the lumen of the pyloric canal. The cause is poorly understood but probably has a genetic basis with a polygenic mode of inheritance, modified by gender (Jedd et al., 1988). The prevalence rate typically ranges from 1.5 to 4 per 1000, with higher rates in whites than in blacks (Mitchell & Risch, 1993). More males, specifically first-born males, have the disease than do females, and approximately 5 percent of affected infants are born to women who themselves have the disease (Merenstein & Gardner, 1989).

Risk Factors

Associated factors include maternal stress and anxiety, feeding practices, and antenatal exposure to doxylamine succinate–pyridoxine hydrochloride (Bendectin). Seasonal factors such as infection have also been reported (Jedd et al., 1988).

Clinical Manifestations

The infant typically appears healthy for the first 2 weeks of life and then begins vomiting (nonbilious), which worsens to frequent projectile vomiting. The infant may be anxious, irritable, and excessively hungry; have decreased frequency of stool; and lose weight. Vomiting may cause dehydration, metabolic alkalosis, hypochloremia, and hypokalemia. The level of indirect bilirubin is significantly elevated in 5 percent of affected infants but resolves when stenosis is corrected.

Differential Diagnosis

Most cases (89 percent) of pyloric stenosis may be clinically diagnosed by palpation of a small, olive-sized mass below the liver. However, if the mass cannot be felt, a barium swallow or ultrasound examination is indicated (Breaux et al., 1988). The differential diagnosis of nonbilious vomiting includes sepsis, withdrawal syndromes, GE reflux, and metabolic diseases such as organic acidemias, hyperammonemia, galactosemias, and adrenogenital syndrome.

Prognosis

Once diagnosed and surgically treated, the prognosis is excellent, with complete relief of symptoms. The mortality rate is less than 1 percent provided that the infant has not become too dehydrated and malnourished (Mitchell & Risch, 1993).

Collaborative Management

Medical and nursing assessment and management of the infant are critical throughout the process of management. On diagnosis of pyloric stenosis, which is reached in consultation with the radiologist, surgical correction should be performed. There is no effective medical treatment. The repair is by pyloromyotomy. A simple incision is made in the hypertrophied longitudinal and circular muscles of the pylorus, thus releasing the obstruction (Leape, 1987).

As with any vomiting infant, fluid and electrolyte management is paramount. A nasogastric tube connected to low continuous suction is maintained to prevent distention and vomiting and to decrease the risk of aspiration. Vital signs are monitored every 2 to 4 hours. Thermoregulation is maintained to prevent exacerbation of symptoms.

Postoperatively, intravenous hydration and electrolyte balance must be maintained. Nasogastric suction is continued for 4 to 24 hours. The tube may be disconnected when the infant is fully awake and bowel sounds are present. Assessment of the suture line is made for signs of infection or skin breakdown. Feedings are begun 6 to 24 hours postoperatively, beginning with clear liquids and progressing slowly with formula administration. Full feedings should be reached in 3 to 5 days (Kenner et al., 1988).

MANAGEMENT OF PROBLEMS WITH DIGESTION

Biliary Atresia

Pathophysiology

Biliary atresia is the complete obstruction of bile flow due to fibrosis of the extrahepatic ducts. It is the most common form of ductal cholestasis, occurring in approximately 1 in every 10,000 births, with a female predominance. The cause remains unclear. Some clinicians theorize that the obstruction is due to injured bile ducts leading to atresia, others describe the disease as an inflammatory process, whereas still others propose an intrauterine insult from environmental factors or failure of ducts to recanalize. Pathologically, the obstruction of the common bile duct prevents bile from entering the duodenum. Consequently, digestion and absorption of fat are impaired, leading to deficiencies in fat-soluble vitamins and vitamin K, which have an impact on bleeding tendencies. Owing to the obstruction, bile accumulates in the ducts and gallbladder and causes distention of these structures. The atresia appears to progress to the intrahepatic ducts, leading to biliary cirrhosis and ultimately death if the bile flow is not established.

Risk Factors

Associated congenital defects, found in 15 percent of reported cases, include congenital heart disease, polysplenic syndrome, small bowel atresia, bronchobiliary atresia, and trisomies 17 and 18. Teratogenic factors include ionizing radiation, drugs, ischemic episode, and viruses such as reovirus type 3, cytomegalovirus, rubella, and hepatitis A and B (Oellrich & Cusumano, 1987).

Clinical Manifestations

Infants appear normal at birth and pass stools with appropriate pigmentation. Clinical signs are subtle, with jaundice persisting after the first week of life. The direct bilirubin level slowly increases, resulting in a greenish bronze appearance of the skin. Gradually stools become clay-colored to pale to yellowish tan, and the urine becomes dark as the result of bile excretion.

Over a 2- to 3-month period, the liver becomes cirrhotic. Portal hypertension is a major complication. The reverse blood flow results in enlargement of esophageal, umbilical, and rectal veins, which is manifested as splenomegaly, hemorrhoids, enlarged abdominal veins, ascites, and blood in the stools. Additional complications include decreased clotting ability, anemia, and ineffective metabolism of nutrients. End-stage liver disease may lead to rupture of veins in the esophagus and stomach or hepatic coma with eventual death from liver failure (Oellrich & Cusumano, 1987).

Differential Diagnosis

There are multiple causes of cholestasis in the infant. All causes must be considered in the presence of conjugated hyperbilirubinemia, other causes excluded, and proper therapy instituted. The differential diagnosis includes neonatal hepatitis, choledochal cyst, inborn errors of metabolism, trisomies 18 and 21, α_1-antitrypsin deficiency, neonatal hypopituitarism, cystic fibrosis, TORCH infectious agents (the acronym representing toxoplasma, rubella, cytomegalovirus, and herpes virus, with the O standing for other agents such as syphilis) or bacterial sepsis, drug-induced cholestasis, and cholestasis associated with parenteral nutrition (Vanderhoof et al., 1994).

Prognosis

Survival in untreated cases of biliary atresia is less than 2 years. Success rates for surgical intervention range from 45 to 85 percent with satisfactory bile drainage. The complication of cholangitis is high.

Many children grow naturally and lead normal lives. Prognosis is best when the original surgery takes place before 2 months of age, when there is minimal hepatocellular damage, when there are ducts in the porta hepatis, and when postoperative complications are minimal (Zink, 1985).

When portoenterostomy is unsuccessful, liver transplantation is an acceptable alternative therapy, with 1-year survival rates ranging from 57 to 70 percent and 4-year survival rates ranging from 28 to 69 percent (Oellrich & Cusumano, 1987; Zink, 1985).

Collaborative Management

Medical, surgical, and nursing staff must strive diligently in the diagnostic work-up and ultimate treatment. Consultation and follow-up care by a gastroenterologist provides guidance for feeding and drug therapy modalities. Parents of these infants can profit from ongoing support from social services, chaplains, or support counseling sources.

Surgical intervention involves a hepatic portoenterostomy, called the *Kasai procedure,* which consists of dissection and resection of the extrahepatic bile duct. The porta hepatis, where the ducts normally occur, is cut, and a loop of bowel is brought up to permit bile drainage from the liver surface to the GI tract. If the Kasai procedure is unsuccessful, the only alternative for treatment is transplantation (see Chapter 43, Hepatic and Renal Transplantation in Infants and Children).

Nurses take an active role in the complex task of diagnosis and treatment of the infant with biliary atresia. Because of the portal hypertension and bleeding tendencies, there should be careful monitoring of vital signs and blood pressure. Efficient collection of multiple blood samples is required for tests, including bilirubin, aspartate transaminase (AST), alanine transaminase (ALT), alkaline phosphatase, albumin, protein, and cholesterol determinations; prothrombin time; complete blood count; reticulocyte count; Coombs' test; measurement of platelets and red blood cell morphologic features, thyroxine, thyroid-stimulating hormone, and glucose determinations; cultures; and TORCH titers. Urine is collected for urinalysis, culture, and metabolic screens. Radiography, ultrasonography, and liver biopsy may be performed.

Meeting nutritional requirements is difficult because the infant needs one and one-half to two times the normal caloric requirements owing to affected metabolism, yet ascites and pressure on the stomach make it difficult for the child to eat. Formulas must contain medium-chain triglycerides for easier absorption. Supplementation with fat-soluble vitamins is required because of impaired absorption. Parenteral nutrition is given to provide adequate calories. Phenobarbital may be an ongoing therapy to stimulate bile flow (Haber & Lake, 1990).

The whole family requires comprehensive psychosocial support. Family and work life are disrupted by lengthy, repeated hospitalizations. The emotional and physical toll is high because of complex care demands, and dealing with the suffering of the child places further stress on the parents. Social support systems need to be explored to assist families in dealing with the long-term health crisis of an infant with biliary atresia.

Duodenal Atresia

Pathophysiology

Duodenal atresia occurs as the result of incomplete recanalization of the lumen. The mechanism by which recanalization is prevented is not known but most likely occurs when the proliferative villi adhere abnormally to one another. The result is the formation of a transverse diaphragm of tissue that completely obstructs the lumen (Davis, 1985; Gryboski & Walker, 1983; Moore & Persaud, 1993; Sadler, 1985). Overall occurrence is approximately 1 in every 6000 to 10,000 live births (Avery & Taeusch, 1984; Chang, 1980b; Davis, 1985).

Risk Factors

Polyhydramnios has been identified as a significant risk factor, occurring in one quarter to one half of women who deliver affected infants. Associated anomalies, present in 60 to 70 percent of patients, are numerous and include trisomy 21, malrotation, TE anomalies, imperforate anus, congenital heart disease, VATER or VACTERL association, and renal anomalies. An annular pancreas—resulting from the failure of the two pancreatic buds to fuse normally, allowing the deformed pancreas to encircle the duodenum—is found in approximately 20 percent of patients. Nearly half of all infants are premature or of low birth weight, and 40 percent acquire hyperbilirubinemia (Davis, 1985; Ducharme & Ghosn, 1987a; Flake & Ryckman, 1997; Bucuvalas & Balistreri, 1997; Gryboski & Walker, 1983; Leape, 1987).

Clinical Manifestations

The significance of polyhydramnios has been noted previously, but in its absence a large amount of gastric aspirate may be obtained on routine delivery room screening. Normally, only small amounts of aspirate are expected (4 to 7 ml), but if more than 10 to 15 ml is obtained, atresia should be suspected (Bloom, 1997; Gryboski & Walker, 1983; Pickering & Adcock, 1980).

Although atresia may be located at any point along the duodenum, most obstructions (80 to 90 percent) are situated below the ampulla of Vater. Consequently, bilious vomiting is a common presenting sign. Failure to pass meconium is noted in approximately 70 percent of patients. Both the onset of vomiting and the ability to pass stool are related to the site of obstruction. Proximal duodenal obstructions tend to present with vomiting within a few hours of birth, although stool may be passed normally. Distal obstructions tend to present with a later onset of vomiting and failure to pass stool. Abdominal distention is generally not noted, but when present, it is confined to the upper abdomen, giving the lower abdomen an almost scaphoid appearance in contrast (Avery & Taeusch, 1984; Davis, 1985; Leape, 1987; Ricketts, 1984; Touloukian, 1978).

Differential Diagnosis

Radiographic examination provides confirmation of duodenal atresia with the classic finding of a "double bubble" (see Fig. 24–3). These bubbles reflect the localization of swallowed air in the stomach and in the distended portion of the duodenum lying above the obstruction; the remainder of the bowel is totally airless. If gas is present elsewhere, other anomalies causing partial obstruction must be presumed. An upper GI series may be helpful in identifying incomplete obstructions such as duodenal stenosis, duodenal web, or annular pancreas, or in ruling out associated malrotation (Davis, 1985; Gryboski & Walker, 1983; Ricketts, 1984).

Prognosis

A 65 to 84 percent survival rate is reported, with deaths attributed to associated cardiac or renal anomalies or to infectious or respiratory complications (Chang, 1980b; Davis, 1985; Ghory & Sheldon, 1985).

Collaborative Management

Surgical treatment involves excision of the atretic site (unless the area so closely approximates the pancreatic and bile ducts that injury to these structures is risked) and side-to-side anastomosis of the free ends. The level of the obstruction determines whether a duodenoduodenostomy or a duodenojejunostomy is carried out. A gastrostomy also is performed for decompression to avoid trauma to the anastomotic site (Chang, 1980b; Davis, 1985; Ghory & Sheldon, 1985; Gryboski & Walker, 1983; Touloukian, 1978). A combined nursing and medical approach facilitates both preoperative stabilization and postoperative recuperation.

Preoperative care is directed toward decompression and hydration. Intermittent gastric suction by use of a sump tube reduces the risk of aspiration or perforation due to overdistention. Vital signs, fluid intake and output, urine specific gravity, and serum electrolytes must be closely monitored, with fluids, electrolytes, and crystalloid provided as needed. Antibiotics may be instituted for preoperative prophylaxis or when perforation or sepsis is suspected (Chang, 1980b; Davis, 1985; Touloukian, 1978).

Continued decompression and nutrition are the major postoperative concerns. Total parenteral nutrition is given initially. Oral feedings are generally begun at 10 to 14 days with an oral electrolyte solution, advancing to low-osmolality formulas such as Nutramigen or Pregestimil (protein hydrosylate formulas) before moving to regular formula (Chang, 1980b; Davis, 1985; Touloukian, 1978).

Jejunoileal Atresia

Pathophysiology

Atresias of the jejunum and ileum are thought to be the result of mesenteric vascular compromise with necrosis and eventual resorption of the involved area. The presence of bile, meconium, epithelial cells, and lanugo distal to the atresia indicates that this ischemic injury occurs relatively late in utero, possibly as late as 3 to 6 months' gestation (Bishop, 1976; Chang, 1980b; Flake & Ryckman, 1997; Touloukian, 1978). The occurrence rate is 1 in 20,000 live births, with an apparently equal distribution of atresias between the jejunum and the ileum (Gryboski & Walker, 1983).

Risk Factors

Owing to the surface area available for absorption proximal to the obstruction, maternal polyhydramnios does not generally present as a risk factor, as it does in the higher atresias of the esophagus and duodenum (Chang, 1980b). Polyhydramnios is reported in only one third of those with jejunal atresia; ileal atresias rarely present with polyhydramnios (Flake & Ryckman, 1992). Because this group of defects arises after embryogenesis is complete, associated anomalies are rare and when they do occur, they are primarily restricted to the GI tract, with malrotation and meconium ileus being most common (Sunshine et al., 1983; Touloukian, 1978). Between 25 and 30 percent of patients experience hyperbilirubinemia, and 25 to 38 percent are born prematurely. Of the four types of jejunoileal atresia that have been identified (Fig. 24–4), only the "apple peel" or "Christmas tree" type is typically familial, indicating that this one form alone may involve some autosomal recessive or multifactorial type of inheritance (Gryboski & Walker, 1983). Although it is the rarest form of jejunoileal atresia, it carries the highest mortality rate (54 percent) and higher rates of prematurity and malrotation in comparison with the more conventional types (Seashore et al., 1987).

Clinical Manifestations

Signs and symptoms generally present at 1 or 2 days of age and are virtually the same for all four types of jejunoileal atresia. Presentation includes bilious vomiting, failure to pass stool, and generalized abdominal distention (Avery & Taeusch, 1984; Gryboski & Walker, 1983; Ricketts, 1984; Touloukian, 1978).

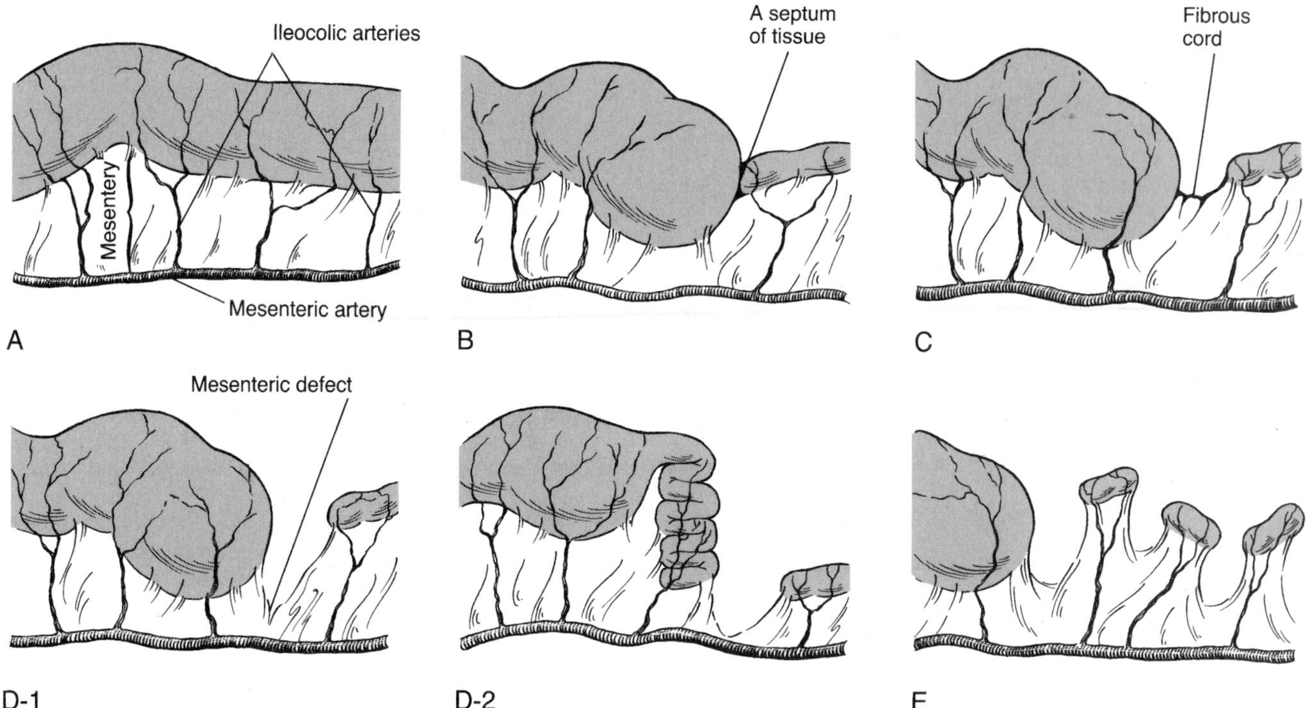

FIGURE 24–4. Jejunoileal obstruction. Percentages reflect relative occurrence. *A*, Normal anatomy. *B*, Type I or diaphragmatic form (20 percent): single atresia in which the integrity of the bowel wall is preserved, but its lumen is obstructed by a septum of tissue; the mesentery is intact. *C*, Type II or cord anomaly (30 to 35 percent): single but discontinuous atresia with opposing ends connected by a long, fibrous cord; the mesentery is intact. *D-1*, Type IIIa or mesenteric defect (35 to 45 percent): single but discontinuous atresia with a V-shaped defect in the intervening mesentery. *D-2*, Type IIIb or "apple peel" (<1 percent): single but discontinuous atresia with a V-shaped defect in the intervening mesentery; the intestine coils around a single ileocolic artery, which is its sole source of circulation. *E*, Type IV or multiple atresias (5 to 10 percent): multiple discontinuous atresias with intervening V-shaped mesenteric defects, giving it the appearance of sausage links. (Data from Gryboski & Walker, 1983; Leape, 1987; Touloukian, 1978.)

Differential Diagnosis

Abdominal radiographs show multiple bubbles, reflecting dilation and collection of swallowed air proximal to the obstruction. Intraperitoneal calcifications are present in 10 percent of patients, which indicates antenatal intestinal perforation with resultant meconium peritonitis. The peritonitis in this case is due to chemical irritation (there is no infection because the bowel and meconium are sterile before birth), causing fibrosis, granuloma formation, and ultimately calcifications. The perforated site usually heals spontaneously before delivery, leaving no evidence of what occurred other than the residual calcifications. The airless, unused distal portion of the gut is generally contracted and of a much smaller caliber than normal. Visualization of this distal "microcolon" by barium or meglumine diatrizoate (Gastrografin) enema may be necessary to rule out malrotation and meconium ileus (Avery & Taeusch, 1984; Bucuvalas & Balistreri, 1997; Chang, 1980b; Ghory & Sheldon, 1985; Ricketts, 1984; Touloukian, 1978).

Prognosis

With the availability of parenteral alimentation, survival rates have risen to as high as 84 to 96 percent. Deaths are generally the result of prematurity, postoperative short gut or bowel syndrome, or infectious complications (Avery & Taeusch, 1984; Ghory & Sheldon, 1985; Touloukian, 1978).

Collaborative Management

Surgical management begins with resection of the dilated proximal gut and atretic, bulbous ending and a search for multiple distal atresias. Primary closure by end-to-end or side-to-end anastomosis generally follows, but preliminary tapering of the distended distal segment may be required; as a third alternative, an end-to-oblique closure may be performed. However, if there is considerable discrepancy (more than 2:1) between the dilated proximal portion and the distal microcolon, an ostomy (either double-barrel or single) is created (Bishop, 1976; Chang, 1980b; Ghory & Sheldon, 1985). Once surgical correction is complete, collaboration with the nutritional support team and enterostomal therapist is essential.

The principles of preoperative care involve bowel decompression and intravenous hydration with the correction of any electrolyte imbalance that may occur as the result of vomiting or third-spacing. Antibiotics may be given prophylactically but certainly should be used in the case of peritonitis (Touloukian, 1978).

Recovery of bowel peristalsis and enzymatic integrity may be delayed, necessitating parenteral nutrition. When started, initial feedings are of a clear electrolyte solution, progressing serially to elemental formulas such as Nutramigen or Pregestimil (protein hydrosylate formulas) until standard formula can be tolerated. The nurses should assess diligently for evidence of short bowel syndrome, commonly seen with atresias that are multiple or of the "apple peel" variety, necessitating excision of an extensive length of bowel (Chang, 1980b; Leape, 1987; Touloukian, 1978).

Omphalocele

Pathophysiology

Omphalocele results from the failure of the intestines to return from the umbilical cord into the abdominal cavity. Because some defects can be sufficiently large that they also contain the liver and other organs that do not normally participate in the migratory process, it has been further proposed that their passage can be accommodated only when there is incomplete folding of the embryonic disk so that the future abdominal wall cannot close completely, resulting in an unusually large umbilical ring (Avery & Taeusch, 1984; Frentner, 1987; Meller et al., 1989; Moore & Persaud, 1993; Sadler, 1985; Seashore, 1978).

Risk Factors

Omphalocele occurs in roughly 1 of every 5000 to 6000 live births, with a male predominance. Multiple and often life-threatening syndromes and anomalies occur with an unusually high frequency (50 to 77 percent) and include trisomy 13, trisomy 18, Beckwith-Wiedemann syndrome, pentalogy syndrome, congenital heart defects, diaphragmatic and upper midline defects, malrotation, intestinal atresia, and genitourinary anomalies. Additionally, 30 to 33 percent of affected infants are premature, and approximately 19 percent are small for gestational age (Avery & Taeusch, 1984; Frentner, 1987; Leape, 1987; Meller et al., 1989; Seashore, 1978).

Clinical Manifestations

Omphalocele is generally an immediately apparent anomaly, ranging between 2 and 15 cm in size. However, the small defects involving perhaps a single loop of intestine may be easily overlooked unless the physical examination is carried out in an unhurried fashion and the umbilical ring is clearly absent on palpation. The larger defects generally contain the intestine and possibly the liver, spleen, stomach, bladder, ovaries and tubes, or testicles. These two extremes most likely reflect the difference in the time at which normal embryogenesis is interrupted. If the interruption is early, around the 3- to 4-week window when infolding is in its last stages, the defect is large. If the interruption occurs later, at about 9 to 10 weeks when migration is generally completed, the defect is smaller. However, in both cases, the intestine, and possibly other abdominal organs, herniate into the umbilical cord. The viscera are covered by a thin, transparent membrane composed of peritoneum and amnion, and the visible bowel has a normal appearance. The abdominal cavity is often relatively small and underdeveloped, having never held the growing intestine (Avery & Taeusch, 1984; Frentner, 1987; Gryboski & Walker, 1983; Kim, 1976; Richey, 1990).

Differential Diagnosis

Although omphaloceles are generally covered by a membrane, intrauterine rupture of that membrane occurs in 11 to 23 percent of patients (Seashore, 1978; Yazbeck & Bensoussan, 1987). As a consequence of prolonged exposure to the amniotic fluid, the bowel becomes matted and edematous in appearance and difficult to differentiate from gastroschisis. Closer examination may reveal the sac remnants, but if none are noted, one need only look to the base of the cord. In gastroschisis, the umbilical cord is intact, inserted normally at the abdominal wall, and separated from the defect by a small amount of skin (Frentner, 1987).

Prognosis

The overall mortality rate is 30 percent and is primarily dependent on the size of the defect, associated chromosomal and other anomalies, and coincidental prematurity or low birth weight (Frentner, 1987; Gryboski & Walker, 1983; Richey, 1990). Malrotation with the resultant danger of volvulus, ischemia, and necrosis is common. Antenatal membrane rupture may also add the dimension of potential sepsis.

Collaborative Management

If surgery is contraindicated because of coexisting chromosomal or other syndromes, the defect may be treated medically by repeatedly painting the sac with silver nitrate solution, merbromin (Mercurochrome), or alcohol. These topical agents promote eschar formation and epithelization with complete coverage by skin within 6 to 8 weeks. Should the patient survive, a later repair of the muscle wall becomes necessary. Biologic dressings have also been used to provide temporary protection (Avery & Taeusch, 1984; Frentner, 1987; Kim, 1976; Leape, 1987; Seashore, 1978).

The definitive surgical treatment is return of the viscera into the abdominal cavity and closure of the defect. However, the procedure employed varies with the size of the defect. Primary closure is preferred, but larger defects (>5 cm) may require a staged repair with a polymeric silicone (Silastic) pouch or chimney (silo) used to suspend the viscera above the patient. Reduction maneuvers are carried out daily to return the suspended organs into the relatively small abdominal cavity. A forceful return and closure under pressure would risk compression of the inferior vena cava, with reduced filling of the heart and decreased cardiac output and impedance of the diaphragmatic excursions, resulting in respiratory compromise. A gastrostomy to provide decompression and an appendectomy to avoid atypically presenting appendicitis in later life may be carried out with both primary and staged procedures, depending on the preferences of the surgical team (Leape, 1987; Yazbeck & Bensoussan, 1987). If a staged repair is performed, complete return of the organs into the abdominal cavity is generally achieved over a period of 7 to 10 days. At that time, the infant is returned to surgery for final closure of the abdominal wall (Frentner, 1987; Kim, 1976; Meller et al., 1989).

These children often require aggressive postoperative respiratory management followed by prolonged total parenteral nutrition. Early psychosocial support of parents must be provided to promote their involvement in what is commonly an extended hospital stay. Genetic counseling may also be required.

The cornerstones of preoperative management include protection of the eviscerated organs, decompression of the gut, and hydration. Thermoregulation is a particular concern, since massive evaporative and radiant heat losses may occur through the exposed defect. One researcher has reported that 44 percent of infants in one patient survey experienced temperatures of less than 35°C (95°F) (Seashore, 1978). Care directed in these four areas may overlap, but all are necessary. The first step is to loosely apply sterile, warmed, saline-soaked gauze in a turban style around the defect, wrapping the ends around the body. Great care must be taken to prevent tight application, which might create pressure; two fingers should fit easily between the trunk and the encircling gauze. Some clinicians suggest that an outer, dry sterile dressing also be applied. The dressing is then covered with plastic wrap. As an alternative, sterile bowel bags may be used. Both wrapping and bag techniques provide protection to the defect from trauma and infection and help limit the loss of fluids and body heat. Clearly, sterile gloves must be worn during the necessary manipulation of the bowel. If the defect is small, the infant may be positioned on the back, but if the defect is large, it may be best to place the infant on the side. In the side-lying position, a small blanket or diaper may be slipped between the covered viscera and the bed surface so that no traction is placed on the bowel, which might cause physical injury to the gut or impede circulation. A gastric tube should be passed and set to low intermittent suction for decompression. Appropriate comfort measures to reduce or prevent crying with concomitant air swallowing should also be employed. Intravenous fluids should be started immediately to counteract direct fluid losses from exposure and the loss of fluids from the circulation caused by inflammation and third-spacing. Poor venous return from the lower extremities is also a concern owing to the ever-present potential for vena cava compression. Hydration status, fluid intake and output, and vital signs should be monitored closely for any evidence of hypovolemia, such as tachycardia, thready pulses, hypotension, poor perfusion, and decreased output of urine with increased specific gravity. Umbilical catheterization for venous access is contraindicated because of the nature and site of the defect. Prophylactic antibiotic administration should also be started (Frentner, 1987; Richey, 1990).

Postoperative support varies slightly according to the repair procedure used, but both methods should generally include measures of hydration, decompression, and a search for evidence of increased intra-abdominal pressure. Third-spacing, or capillary leak syndrome, may continue to be a problem and may actually be exacerbated by the trauma of surgical manipulation of the bowel. Assessment for signs of hypovolemia should be documented. Serum electrolytes, albumin, and total serum protein values should also be followed, with fluid and other replacements as necessary. Decompression by gastric tube or gastrostomy is generally required for a considerable time until peristaltic activity returns. Ileus and cholestasis are common following repair, so enteral feedings may be considerably delayed and parenteral alimentation is provided during the interval. When feedings are begun, an elemental formula is used initially. Respiratory support with increased pressures may be required to achieve adequate ventilation if diaphragmatic movements are hampered. Inspection of the lower extremities and palpation of pedal pulses are helpful in assessing for impaired circulation. Elevating the extremities may promote venous return to the heart. In addition to these measures, if a staged repair is undertaken, particular attention must be paid to the infant's tolerance of daily reduction attempts. Furthermore, the silo provides an open port for bacterial invasion. Povidone–iodine or silver sulfadiazine (Silvadene) ointment may be applied with dressing changes, and most certainly antibiotic therapy is continued postoperatively (Frentner, 1987).

Gastroschisis

Pathophysiology

Gastroschisis is a full-thickness defect in the abdominal wall through which the uncovered intestines protrude. The defect is generally thought to arise as the result of incomplete lateral infolding of the embryonic disk. As a result of this primary failure, the abdominal wall is incompletely formed, allowing herniation of the gut (Frentner, 1987; Meller et al., 1989; Richey, 1990; Seashore, 1978). Three other accepted theories have also been offered. The first suggests that the umbilical coelom (cavity) fails to form, so normal herniation of the midgut into the cord cannot occur. Consequently, during its rapid growth phase the intestine ruptures through the embryonic body wall. Another view considers that a vascular accident occurring in utero leads to occlusion of the omphalomesenteric artery. With its circulation removed, the base of the cord becomes necrotic, leaving an opening through which the intestine can eviscerate. The last theory proposes that gastroschisis may simply be a variant of omphalocele, with early intrauterine rupture of its membranous covering. The membrane remnants are subsequently reabsorbed, and the umbilical cord is re-formed around the offset umbilical vessels. For the last two theories, the gap between the evisceration and cord base is presumably filled in by skin (Frentner, 1987; Meller et al., 1989; Richey, 1990; Seashore, 1978).

Risk Factors

Prematurity (58 percent) and low birth weight (92 percent) are extremely common. Malrotation is found in all affected infants, and a few may exhibit intestinal atresia, but anomalies of systems other than the GI tract are infrequent and relatively minor (Seashore, 1978). The overall incidence is approximately 1 per 30,000 to 50,000 live births (Frentner, 1987).

Clinical Manifestations

Gastroschisis is an immediately apparent defect in the abdominal wall through which the intestine and possibly portions of the colon protrude. The liver and other solid organs generally remain in the abdominal cavity, although evisceration is possible. The defect is usually small (2 to 5 cm) and located to the right of the umbilicus, from which it is separated by a narrow margin of skin. The bowel is uncovered and, as a consequence of chemical peritonitis caused by long exposure to the amniotic fluid, appears as an edematous and matted mass with no identifiable loops. The abdominal cavity is small and underdeveloped (Frentner, 1987; Meller et al., 1989; Richey, 1990).

Differential Diagnosis

Although it is often confused with a ruptured omphalocele, in gastroschisis the umbilical cord is inserted normally. The defect is next to, rather than in, the umbilical cord and there is no protective sac or remnants thereof (Leape, 1987; Richey, 1990).

Prognosis

A 13 to 28 percent mortality rate is reported for gastroschisis, with all deaths directly related to the defect. Early deaths are largely attributable to a combination of shock, sepsis (associated with perforation or contamination of the exposed bowel), and hypothermia. Profound hypothermia (temperature lower than 35°C [95°F]) is reported to occur in 67 percent of affected infants. Late deaths come as a result of sepsis, respiratory failure, and the inability of the bowel to sustain nutrition (Seashore, 1978; Yazbeck & Bensoussan, 1987).

Collaborative Management

Although a primary closure may be possible in gastroschisis, the majority of defects are closed by staged repair using the polymeric silicone pouch as described for omphalocele. Although gastroschisis is a smaller defect than omphalocele, the distortion of the viscera with typical thickening and edema of the bowel make primary closure more difficult. Often the defect must be surgically enlarged to allow thorough inspection of the entire length of the GI tract and to avoid restricting the passage of the eviscerated intestine back into the abdominal cavity. All display some degree of malrotation, predisposing them to both intestinal atresias and infarction. Bowel resection and anastomosis are frequently necessary; however, primary anastomosis is contraindicated in the face of peritonitis or inflammation. In such situations, an enterostomy is performed away from the defect, with anastomosis delayed until final closure of the abdominal wall. The visceral mass is returned to the abdominal cavity as a whole. Because of the potential for bowel injury and blood loss, no attempt is made to unravel the adherent loops of bowel (Meller et al., 1989; Seashore, 1978).

Postoperative nutritional and respiratory support is essential. Consultation with social services is helpful in providing parental support and the establishment of healthy parent–child relationships.

The care of patients with gastroschisis is much like that for omphalocele. The intestines should be covered to protect them from injury and to reduce the loss of fluids and heat. Gastric decompression, fluid resuscitation, and antibiotic prophylaxis round out preoperative care (Frentner, 1987).

Following surgery, the major concerns are venous stasis, respiratory compromise, infection, and nutrition. Edema and cyanosis of the lower extremities and evidence of decreased cardiac output should be reported immediately. Intensive respiratory support is provided and oxygenation and ventilation are monitored closely. Infection is prevented by careful aseptic dressing changes, daily applications of bacteriostatic solutions or ointments, and systemic administration of antibiotics. Total parenteral nutrition is generally continued for several weeks until intestinal function returns. Feedings are begun with elemental formula, eventually progressing to standard formula, with diligent assessment for evidence of intestinal obstruction during the process (Frentner, 1987; Leape, 1987).

MANAGEMENT OF PROBLEMS WITH ELIMINATION

Hirschsprung's Disease

Pathophysiology

Hirschsprung's disease (also known as congenital megacolon or aganglionic megacolon) is an abnormality of the colon marked by the congenital absence of ganglion cells (aganglionosis). Failure of the neural crest cells to migrate in their usual craniocaudal fashion results in aberrant bowel innervation and interrupted neuromuscular conduction of the messages promoting peristalsis of the anal sphincters. This local failure of relaxation results in functional intestinal obstruction. Fecal matter accumulates in the normally innervated proximal bowel, producing dilation (megacolon) and hypertrophy of the muscular wall as normal peristaltic activity works against the obstruction. The distal, aganglionic segment is unused and may appear narrowed in relation to the proximal dilation, but it is in fact of normal caliber. Between the ganglionic proximal section and the distal aganglionic section lies a "transition zone" of tapered bowel (Boley et al., 1978; Flake & Ryckman, 1997; Kenner & Brueggemeyer, 1984; Martin & Torres, 1985; Ricketts, 1984; Sadler, 1985).

The rectum is always involved, and most cases (85 percent) involve the sigmoid colon as well. Rarely, aganglionosis may also be found in the upper portion of the colon or throughout the entire intestine (Chang, 1980b; Stringer et al., 1994). Atypical forms of Hirschsprung's disease have also been described, in which areas of normal innervation are found between aganglionic areas, but the presence of such "skip areas" is extremely rare (Martin & Torres, 1985).

The cause of the interrupted migration of ganglion cells is not known, but anoxia is frequently cited. The theory is that local anoxemia due to an interference with the source of oxygen to the site may lead to ischemia, atrophy, and regression of the cells (Kenner & Brueggemeyer, 1984).

Risk Factors

The incidence of Hirschsprung's disease is 1 in 2000 to 5000 live births, with males predominating. Associated anomalies are relatively infrequent but include trisomy 21 and asymptomatic urologic anomalies. The ganglionic plexuses of the bowel are derived from the same craniocervical neural crest as are the oral, facial, and cranial ganglia. Consequently, a limited number of infants may also exhibit congenital deafness and ocular neurocristopathies, most commonly in association with Waardenburg's syndrome (Meire et al., 1987). Approximately 5 percent have associated neurologic abnormalities ranging from developmental delay to mental retardation or cerebral palsy. Overall, a positive family history is found in 17 to 30 percent of cases, rising to 50 percent when total colonic aganglionosis is present (Boley et al., 1978; Kenner & Brueggemeyer, 1984; Marty et al., 1995). The fact that more males than females are affected has caused some to theorize that a form of X-linked recessive transmission is occurring (Reyna, 1994). More recently, however, a gene has been identified on chromosome 10 that may be involved in the differentiation or proliferation, or both, of neural crest cells (Martucciello et al., 1995).

Clinical Manifestations

The signs and symptoms of Hirschsprung's disease in the newborn are primarily those of intestinal obstruction, including bilious vomiting, distention, and failure to pass meconium. The rectum is empty of stool unless the aganglionic segment is very short, in which case rectal examination with the gloved little finger may cause explosive release of gas and evacuation of meconium. If the disease goes undiagnosed, fecal stagnation may lead to increased intraluminal pressures, reduced colonic blood flow, and bacterial overgrowth with resultant enterocolitis. This severe bowel irritation and inflammation may cause "overflow" diarrhea, with complicating dehydration, hypoproteinemia, electrolyte imbalance, and sometimes perforation and shock (Boley et al., 1978; Jones, 1978; Kenner & Brueggemeyer, 1984; Ricketts, 1984).

Differential Diagnosis

Hirschsprung's disease may be clinically indistinguishable from jejunoileal atresia, meconium ileus, meconium plug syndrome, and small left colon syndrome (Ricketts, 1984; Stringer et al., 1994). Plain radiographic examination offers little or no help in differentiation. All conditions show large gas-filled loops of bowel consistent with intestinal obstruction. The rectum may or may not contain air, but when air is present, it generally is of a reduced amount consistent with partial or functional obstruction (Chang, 1980b).

Barium contrast studies are therefore indicated to determine the caliber of the distal colon. Microcolon is typically found with jejunoileal atresia and meconium ileus, but if the colon is of normal size or somewhat enlarged, the obstruction may be the result of Hirschsprung's disease, meconium plug syndrome, or small left colon syndrome. Occasionally, barium enema demonstrates the "pigtail" or "funnel" sign characteristic of Hirschsprung's disease. This sign is simply a demonstration of the tapering transition zone lying between the dilated, innervated proximal segment and the normal-caliber, aganglionic distal bowel. Unfortunately in most newborns (75 percent) the dilation of the proximal colon may not yet be sufficiently dramatic for visualization. When the sign is present, usually in infants older than 2 months of age, it is highly suggestive of Hirschsprung's disease, but it may also be found in small left colon syndrome; in its absence, no judgment can be made. However, the margins of the distal colon generally have a saw-toothed appearance in Hirschsprung's disease, whereas smooth margins are typically described with small left colon syndrome. Retention of barium noted by follow-up film 24 hours later is suggestive of Hirschsprung's disease but may also be noted in its absence (Boley et al., 1978; Chang, 1980b; Davis & Campbell, 1975; Davis et al., 1974; Kenner & Brueggemeyer, 1984).

Anorectal manometry is frequently discussed in the literature as an alternative diagnostic tool. The test is performed to determine the ability of the internal sphincter to relax, but results are generally unreliable in the neonate (Boley et al., 1978; Youssef, 1987).

Final diagnosis can be made only by suction or punch rectal biopsy through the anus and histologic examination of the specimen obtained. No anesthesia is required, and the procedure can easily be performed in the nursery. If ganglionic bowel is obtained, either meconium plug syndrome or small left colon syndrome is possible. However, the absence of ganglionic cells in the submucosal plexus firmly establishes the diagnosis of Hirschsprung's disease (Boley et al., 1978; Chang, 1980b; Ricketts, 1984). Should questions regarding diagnosis persist, a full-thickness operative biopsy under general anesthesia may be performed to collect deeper nerve plexuses, but this is rarely needed (Boley et al., 1978).

Prognosis

The mortality rate for Hirschsprung's disease is generally less than 5 percent but may be as high as 15 to 20 percent in the neonatal period, when diagnosis is often delayed and enterocolitis develops (Kenner & Brueggemeyer, 1984; Youssef, 1987). Good surgical results can be expected in the vast majority of patients (90 percent), but diarrhea, constipation with distention, and intermittent colitis may occur in 2 to 34 percent of patients as the result of residual aganglionosis, postoperative stricture formation, overactivity of the sphincter, or motility disorders. Delayed toilet training is frequently reported, and 14 to 44 percent of patients experience problems with soiling, with the actual rate varying in direct proportion to the length of the aganglionic segment (Boley et al., 1978; Elhalaby et al., 1995; Heij et al., 1995; Marty et al., 1995; Moore et al., 1994).

Collaborative Management

Although older children with mild symptoms of Hirschsprung's disease may be managed medically with a daily colonic lavage of normal saline to evacuate the bowel (Jones, 1978), such conservative therapy is inappropriate in the neonatal period owing to the risk of fatal enterocolitis with perforation, peritonitis, and septicemia. In the newborn, the immediate treatment is a temporary colostomy, placed proximal to the aganglionic segment, to decompress the bowel and divert the fecal contents. The definitive repair is carried out between 6 and 12 months of age and involves resection of the affected, aganglionic bowel and anastomosis of the normal bowel to the anus (Boley et al., 1978; Leape, 1987). The enterostomal therapist is clearly an important member of the patient care team.

Initial nursing care is directed toward abdominal decompression, return of fluid and electrolyte balance, and the treatment of sepsis (Sugar, 1981). A gastric tube is set to low intermittent suction, and all drainage is measured. Fluids with appropriate electrolytes for the maintenance and replacement of gastric losses should be provided. Actions to combat the fluid shifts that are common following contrast studies with hyperosmolar media may also be necessary. Prophylactic antibiotic therapy is initiated because of the high risk of enterocolitis (Kenner & Brueggemeyer, 1984). If enterocolitis is present, aggressive therapy with fluids, blood, or plasma may be required (Leape, 1987). The infant should be monitored closely after rectal biopsy. Any bleeding can be controlled with digital pressure (Chang, 1980b).

Colostomy is possible when the diagnosis of Hirschsprung's disease is confirmed by rectal biopsy. A preoperative colonic lavage or enema is given to evacuate and prepare the bowel for surgery. Only isotonic solutions such as normal saline should be used to avoid water intoxication and resultant hyponatremia (Kenner & Brueggemeyer, 1984; Leape, 1987). Following colostomy, the infant must be assessed frequently for respiratory compromise, abdominal distention, hemorrhage, wound dehiscence, and infection. The stomal perfusion and appearance should also be noted and appropriate skin care provided. Intravenous fluids are continued until oral feedings can be started (Sugar, 1981). Routine rectal irrigations with normal saline may reduce the incidence of postoperative enterocolitis (Marty et al., 1995).

As the infant becomes ready for discharge, the focus of nursing care shifts to readying the parents for home management of the colostomy. Family teaching should include skin care, normal stomal appearance and stool output, and the construction or application of appliances. Because the definitive repair is generally delayed until the end of the first year, the neonatal nurse most likely is not involved in patient care at that time.

Small Left Colon Syndrome

Pathophysiology

Neonatal small left colon syndrome is a condition of functional immaturity of the large bowel in which the left colon is uniformly narrowed from the anus to the splenic flexure. The proximal colon above the flexure is dilated and distended with meconium. A cone-shaped transition zone lies between the dilated and narrowed distal segments (Davis & Campbell, 1975; Woodhurst & Kliman, 1976). The cause is unclear but is generally thought to involve the myenteric plexuses that innervate the GI tract in a cephalocaudal direction between 5 and 12 weeks' gestation. Once the plexuses are in position, their maturation and function are largely determined by gestational age. The impression that this condition results from intramural immaturity is supported by histologic findings of increased numbers of small, immature neuronal elements in contrast to the larger, multipolar ganglion cells that normally predominate at term. The neuronal plexuses are present but immature; morphologically they resemble the structure expected at approximately 32 weeks' gestation. The syndrome might therefore be best described as a disease of decreased intestinal motility (Davis et al., 1974; Philippart et al., 1975).

Risk Factors

Approximately 40 percent of those with small left colon syndrome are the infants of diabetic mothers (Davis et al., 1974; Philippart et al., 1975). Furthermore, a survey of asymptomatic infants of diabetic mothers has shown that 50 percent have a demonstrable narrowed colonic configuration in the absence of frank symptoms (Davis & Campbell, 1975). Variable degrees of hypoglycemia, hypocalcemia, and hyperbilirubinemia have also been reported (Philippart et al., 1975), but these findings may simply reflect the predisposition for hyperinsulinemia and polycythemia in the general population of infants of diabetic mothers. The overall incidence of small left colon syndrome is believed to be 1 of every 855 deliveries (Davis et al., 1974).

Clinical Manifestations

Presenting signs and symptoms are those associated with low intestinal obstruction. These manifestations include bile-stained vomitus, abdominal distention, and failure to pass meconium spontaneously. However, rectal examination may be followed by the passage of very small amounts of meconium in approximately a third of patients (Philippart et al., 1975).

Differential Diagnosis

On clinical presentation and with plain radiographic studies, this condition is indistinguishable from Hirschsprung's disease and meconium plug syndrome. Multiple gas-filled loops of bowel are seen proximally, with decreased air noted distally (Davis & Campbell, 1975).

Barium enema shows the uniformly small left colon with a zone of transition at the splenic flexure. Although a zone of transition may also be noted with Hirschsprung's disease, the margins of the distal colon generally appear smooth with small left colon syndrome rather than jagged or serrated as described in Hirschsprung's disease (Davis & Campbell, 1975; Davis et al., 1974). Perhaps more distinguishing from Hirschsprung's disease is the incidental finding that following contrast studies, the majority (71 percent) of infants with small left colon syndrome promptly evacuate the barium and begin passing stools spontaneously. As a consequence, the signs and symptoms of low intestinal obstruction disappear. The meconium rarely (5 percent) contains a significant rubbery plug (Davis et al., 1974; Philippart et al., 1975).

Rectal biopsy for the presence of ganglion cells, although they may appear atypically immature in small left colon syndrome, may ultimately be required to differentiate this syndrome from Hirschsprung's disease (Ricketts, 1984). If the possibility of meconium plug persists, a follow-up contrast examination should be performed. Despite the passage of meconium, the transition zone persists in infants suffering from small left colon syndrome (Philippart et al., 1975).

Prognosis

Although the initial presentation may be dramatic, many cases are apparently asymptomatic and go undiagnosed. In either case, the condition spontaneously resolves within the neonatal period with no subsequent stooling problems encountered (Cowett & Schwartz, 1987; Davis & Campbell, 1975; Davis et al., 1974). Late intermittent obstruction with or without cecal perforation is reported rarely (Philippart et al., 1975).

Collaborative Management

Management is of a conservative nature. The diagnostic barium enema is generally curative. Only in the rare case of significant intermittent obstruction or cecal perforation is a colostomy required. If the diagnosis of small left colon syndrome is made in the face of a negative maternal history, the suggestion of maternal diabetes may be made to the obstetric team (Davis et al., 1974; Philippart et al., 1975).

As with all intestinal obstructions, initial management involves decompression, intravenous fluids for hydration, and the treatment of electrolyte imbalance. Symptoms generally resolve following barium enema, and oral feeding may be instituted gradually. The nurse must be diligent, however, for evidence of persistent or recurrent obstruction and report abnormal findings accordingly (Philippart et al., 1975).

Meconium Ileus

Pathophysiology

Meconium ileus is an obstruction of the distal ileum due to an accumulation of abnormally thick, tarry meconium. The condition is a result of pancreatic insufficiency. Pancreatic hydrolytic enzymes are normally responsible for the metabolism of fat and protein. Consequently, if these enzymes are absent, the meconium has an unusually high protein content and abnormal mucous glycoprotein, making it more viscid than usual. The resultant thick, tenacious material literally becomes impacted within the ileal lumen, producing a functional obstruction (Avery & Taeusch, 1984; Chang, 1980b; Cohn & Roth, 1983; Leape, 1987).

Risk Factors

Virtually all children (95 percent) with meconium ileus have cystic fibrosis, although only a small proportion (10 to 15 percent) of infants with cystic fibrosis present with meconium ileus. Cystic fibrosis, also known as mucoviscidosis, is a genetic disorder with an autosomal recessive inheritance pattern that occurs in 1 of every 2000 live births. All exocrine glands are affected, producing tenacious mucus that causes not only GI dysfunction but also ultimate respiratory malfunction (AAP Committee on Genetics, 1989; Chawls et al., 1988; Leape, 1987; Wells & Meghdadpour, 1988).

Rarely (5 percent) meconium ileus occurs in the absence of cystic fibrosis, but generally pancreatic duct stenosis or partial pancreatic aplasia can be demonstrated. The cause of these isolated findings is not known (Leape, 1987; Lebenthal et al., 1983).

Additional findings associated with meconium ileus include maternal polyhydramnios (5 to 10 percent) and prematurity (10 to 33 percent) (Chawls et al., 1988; Leape, 1987).

Clinical Manifestations

Meconium ileus generally presents first with progressive abdominal distention (within 12 to 24 hours of birth), followed by bilious vomiting and a failure to pass meconium. On physical examination the meconium mass may be palpated as a movable, doughy or putty-like ball; smaller pellet-like concretions of inspissated meconium may be felt distally. Rectal examination should produce no meconium, but normal sphincter tone should be felt (Avery & Taeusch, 1984; Chang, 1980b; Chawls et al., 1988; Ghory & Sheldon, 1985; Leape, 1987).

Differential Diagnosis

Plain abdominal films show distended loops proximal to the point of obstruction, but unlike the uniformly lucent areas seen in jejunoileal atresia, the dilated areas typical of meconium ileus are of varying sizes and have a "soap-bubble" or "ground-glass" appearance. This appearance reflects the mixture of trapped air and meconium. Calcifications that are the result of antenatal intestinal perforation and consequent meconium peritonitis may also be noted. Barium enema demonstrates a distally unused microcolon, thus differentiating this condition from Hirschsprung's disease. The smaller pellet-like masses of meconium may also be noted in the distal segment (Chang, 1980b; Chawls et al., 1988; Dirkes et al., 1995; Ghory & Sheldon, 1985; Leape, 1987; Ricketts, 1984). A history of cystic fibrosis in siblings virtually ensures the diagnosis of meconium ileus. An immunoreactive trypsin test using a dry blood spot provides a screen for cystic fibrosis, with confirmation by sweat test (AAP Committee on Genetics, 1989).

Prognosis

Cystic fibrosis is a condition of delayed mortality, with a mean survival of 22 years. At this age, death comes as a result of obstructive pulmonary disease and infection. The intervening period is marked by poor growth and chronic respiratory and GI dysfunction. The infant mortality rate in cystic fibrosis is 13 percent, with these early deaths attributed to malabsorption and malnutrition (AAP Committee on Genetics, 1989). For a complete discussion of cystic fibrosis, see Chapter 26, Assessment and Management of Endocrine Dysfunction.

Collaborative Management

In the case of uncomplicated meconium ileus, the bowel can generally be evacuated using a hyperosmolar contrast enema such as meglumine diatrizoate. Because of its hyperosmolarity, fluid is drawn from the interstitial and intravascular spaces into the intestinal lumen, softening the impacted meconium and allowing it to pull away from the intestinal wall. The mass can then be evacuated by normal peristalsis. This nonoperative treatment is generally successful in 15 to 20 percent of patients (Chang, 1980b; Chawls et al., 1988; Leape, 1987).

If repeated enemas are not productive, or if meconium ileus is complicated by bowel ischemia, sepsis, or hypovolemic shock, the obstructing meconium may be surgically removed. A temporary ileostomy may be established. Such an ileostomy is irrigated daily with dilute acetylcysteine until any residual meconium is softened and evacuated. Chest physiotherapy, acetylcysteine sodium aerosols (Mucomyst), and extra humidity may be helpful in preventing postoperative pulmonary complications (such as atelectasis and pneumonia), to which infants with cystic fibrosis are particularly prone (Avery & Taeusch, 1984; Bishop, 1976; Chang, 1980b; Ghory & Sheldon, 1985; Leape, 1987).

Genetic counseling should be provided to parents of affected children, with appropriate referral to a geneticist or genetic counselor. A social worker or other mental health professional may help parents explore their feelings concerning their child's prognosis and their future reproductive plans (Wells & Meghdadpour, 1988). Extensive parent teaching of pulmonary toilet and enzyme supplementation is needed. Respiratory therapy personnel and the nutritional support team should consequently be included in parent teaching. Many larger communities have special follow-up clinics for cystic fibrosis patients that may be used to ensure continuity and coordination of care after discharge.

Immediate stabilization of the child with meconium ileus requires decompression with gastric suction and the correction of fluid and electrolyte imbalances. Hydration is particularly important in patients being treated medically with hyperosmolar enemas. Fluids drawn into the intestinal lumen to allow softening and evacuation of the meconium are by default removed from the effective circulation, placing the infant at risk for severe hypovolemia and vascular collapse. The extracted fluids should be replaced accordingly. Generally 4 ml of one-half normal saline solution is given for every 1 ml of retained enema. Fluids and suction are continued until the meconium is evacuated and the clinical manifestations of obstruction resolve. When intestinal function is deemed adequate, protein hydrosylate formula feedings may be started, together with the pancreatic enzyme supplement pancrilipase (Viokase) (Chawls et al., 1988; Leape, 1987).

If the obstruction is not relieved, decompression, fluids, and electrolytes are continued until surgical treatment can be carried out. Postoperatively, ostomy care becomes a part of nursing management, along with assistance in providing pulmonary toilet. The infant's respiratory status should be monitored closely. If there are adhesions secondary to meconium peritonitis or surgical manipulation, or if the meconium is incompletely removed, signs of obstruction may recur. These signs of persistent or recurrent obstruction must be reported immediately to allow early intervention and reoperation as needed. Feedings are delayed until the obstruction is relieved, the ileostomy is functioning, and bowel activity has returned. Protein hydrosylate formula with added pancrilipase is given initially. Many of these infants feed quite poorly, however, and total parenteral nutrition may be required for these special patients (Chang, 1980b; Leape, 1987).

Meconium Plug Syndrome

Pathophysiology

Meconium plug syndrome is a condition in which intestinal obstruction (generally of the lower colon and rectum) occurs as the result of unusually thick meconium in the absence of demonstrable enzymatic deficiency. The syndrome is most likely the result of abnormal gut motility associated with immaturity or hypotonia; ganglion deficiency is not found. The plug is formed primarily from mucus and secretions and therefore appears yellowish white and is gelatinous in consistency, lacking the usual flow properties of normal meconium (Gryboski & Walker, 1983).

Risk Factors

Premature infants are especially prone to meconium plug syndrome; however, the condition may also be found in hypotonic infants with central nervous system damage, and some infants of diabetic mothers are also affected. In the latter case, meconium plug syndrome is considered to be a variant of small left colon syndrome. Treatment of the mother with magnesium sulfate is an additional risk factor that has been noted by some clinicians (Avery & Taeusch, 1984; Bucuvalas & Balistreri, 1997). Meconium plugs are found in about 1 of every 100 newborns, but only a quarter of these infants are unable to evacuate the plug spontaneously and thus experience intestinal obstruction (Gryboski & Walker, 1983).

Clinical Manifestations

The signs are those of low intestinal obstruction with failure to stool, followed by abdominal distention and bilious vomiting. Hyperactive bowel sounds are often noted on auscultation, and normal sphincter tone is generally felt on rectal examination. The meconium plug and flatus are often passed after digital examination (Bucuvalas & Balistreri, 1997; Gryboski & Walker, 1983).

Differential Diagnosis

Plain radiographs indicate a low intestinal obstruction with multiply distended loops of proximal bowel, thus bringing to mind a number of possible conditions, including jejunoileal atresia, meconium ileus, Hirschsprung's disease, small left colon syndrome, or meconium plug syndrome. On barium enema the colon is generally described as being of normal caliber with no evidence of microcolon, thus eliminating the diagnosis of jejunoileal atresia or meconium ileus. The presence of normal ganglion cells on rectal biopsy removes Hirschsprung's disease from the differential diagnosis. In the absence of a history of maternal diabetes, meconium plug syndrome becomes the most logical cause for the symptoms presented (Bucuvalas & Balistreri, 1997; Ricketts, 1984).

Prognosis

Once the meconium plug is expelled, complete recovery should follow (Gryboski & Walker, 1983).

Collaborative Management

Small enemas of warm saline, meglumine diatrizoate, or acetylcysteine are usually all that are needed to dislodge the obstructing meconium plug if it has not already been expelled following rectal examination. Normal stooling patterns should follow. Surgical intervention is rarely needed (Avery & Taeusch, 1984; Bucuvalas & Balistreri, 1997; Gryboski & Walker, 1983).

Decompression, hydration, and electrolyte balance are the immediate concerns. The special care required following meglumine diatrizoate enema and rectal biopsy has already been discussed. Once the plug is evacuated, symptoms have resolved, and normal intestinal function has returned, feedings can be started.

Anorectal Agenesis

Pathophysiology

Anorectal agenesis (imperforate anus) refers to a group of congenital malformations involving the anus or rectum or the junction between the two structures. If the urorectal septum deviates during its growth, the cloaca is abnormally or incompletely partitioned, resulting in rectal stenosis or atresia. Rectourethral and rectovaginal fistulas frequently occur in association with these defects. If the anal membrane fails to rupture, the result is a membranous anal atresia (Boles, 1978; Moore & Persaud, 1993; Sadler, 1985).

A whole spectrum of defects is possible, but they are generally classified into four major types (Fig. 24–5). The cause of deviated or arrested anorectal development is not known.

Risk Factors

Anorectal agenesis occurs in 1 of every 1500 to 5000 live births. Between 20 and 75 percent of all affected infants have an associated anomaly. Considering its common origin from the cloaca, it is not surprising that genitourinary tract abnormalities are found most frequently (25 to 50 percent); approximately 4 percent of affected infants have the lethal defects of bilateral renal agenesis or dysplasia. Cryptorchidism is noted in 3 to 19 percent of affected males. Congenital heart disease and esophageal atresia are also reported occasionally, and when the latter is found, the VATER and VACTERL associations should be considered. Approximately half of affected patients have spinal dysraphism, ranging from occult spina bifida (2.2 percent) to myelomeningocele (2 to 4.4 percent), including scoliosis (13.3 percent), hemivertebra (6.7 percent), extra segments (8.9 percent), tethered cord (4 to 13.3 percent), and fibrolipoma of the cord (8.9 to 38 percent) (Adkins & Kiesewetter, 1976; Boles, 1978; Chang, 1980b; Cortes et al., 1995; Flake & Ryckman, 1997; Rivosecchi et al., 1995; Tsakayannis & Shamberger, 1995).

Clinical Manifestations

Presenting signs and symptoms vary slightly with the particular type of defect present. For the majority (those with type III agenesis), the anus is clearly imperforate. Owing to the high incidence of fistulas, meconium may be passed in the urine (in males) or its presence may be noted at the vaginal outlet (in females). With anal stenosis (type I), the anus and rectal vaults are patent but narrowed so that the pasty stools of the newborn may be passed. The stenosis is generally suspected by the microscopic appearance of the anus and is confirmed on rectal examination. With the remaining two types, the anus may appear misleadingly normal on first inspection. In the membranous type (type II), the anal membrane may become visible within 24 to 48 hours as meconium bulges from beneath the thin epithelial covering, but by then the signs of low intestinal obstruction (distention, bilious vomiting, and failure to pass stool) are also becoming apparent. The atretic type (type IV), which is fortunately rare, generally first presents with the full-blown manifestations of obstruction (Avery & Taeusch, 1984; Boles, 1978; Chang, 1980b).

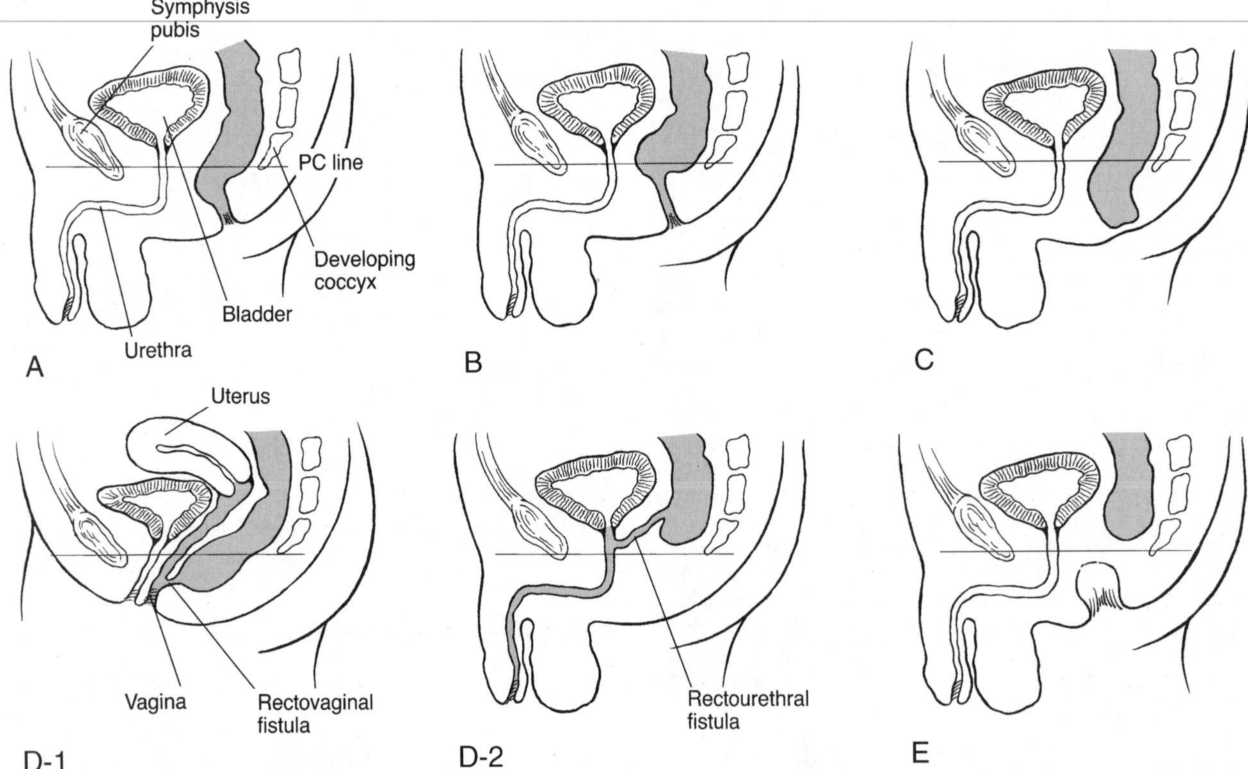

FIGURE 24–5. Anorectal agenesis. Shading represents areas of lucency typically found on radiograph. Percentages reflect relative occurrence. *A*, Normal anatomy. *B*, Type I or anal stenosis (5 to 6 percent): anus or lower rectum is narrowed but patent. *C*, Type II or anal membrane (5 to 7 percent): anal opening covered by a membranous diaphragm. *D*, Type III or anal agenesis (85 percent): anus is clearly imperforate; fistulas are present in three quarters of cases. *D-1*, Type IIIA or low agenesis: bowel ends as a blind pouch below the pubococcygeal (PC) line; most common in females. *D-2*, Type IIIB or high agenesis: bowel ends as a blind pouch above the pubococcygeal line; most common in males. *E*, Type IV or anal atresia (3 percent): rectum and anus are present as blind pouches but are separated by a variable distance. (Data from Avery & Taeusch, 1984; Chang, 1980b; deVries & Cox, 1985; Gryboski & Walker, 1983; Moore & Persaud, 1993; Sadler, 1985.)

Differential Diagnosis

Visual and digital rectal examinations are generally diagnostic. In the presence of a fistula, the urine may also be examined for meconium epithelial cells (Gryboski & Walker, 1983; Leape, 1987).

An inverted lateral radiograph (upside-down Wangensteen-Rice technique) may demonstrate air collected in the blind-ending upper rectal pouch but is generally unreliable for determining the level of obstruction, owing to the considerable time required for swallowed air to reach this portion of the gut. Even when sufficient time is given, air may be prevented by meconium from reaching the end of the pouch. Nevertheless, if a fistula is present, air may be seen in the bladder or vagina on the plain film (Boles, 1978; Gryboski & Walker, 1983; Leape, 1987).

Contrast studies with barium injected into the blind rectum confirm obstruction but provide no indication of the distance that separates the distal and proximal pouches. Barium injected through the urethra or vagina confirms the presence of a fistula and through retrograde filling indicates the level of the rectal pouch (Boles, 1978; Flake & Ryckman, 1992; Leape, 1987). In those rare situations in which a fistula is not present and the level of the obstruction has still not been determined, a perineal puncture contrast rectogram or needle aspiration may be required. For the rectogram, a needle is inserted through the perineum and guided (by sonography) into the rectal pouch to inject the barium. The needle aspiration is a more conservative alternative and involves advancement of the needle while attempting to aspirate. If the needle has been advanced to a depth of 1.5 cm and no meconium has been obtained, the defect is assumed to be of a high type (Adkins & Kiesewetter, 1976; deVries & Cox, 1985; Leape, 1987).

Prognosis

The outcome for infants with anorectal anomalies is largely dependent on the type of defect and the level of the upper rectal pouch in relation to the puborectal muscle, which is the main muscle of sphincter function and continence. This muscle is a central component of the levator ani muscle, which spans the pelvis much like a sling to support the lower end of the rectum. On radiography, the position of this muscle can be estimated by drawing an imaginary line between the symphysis pubis and the developing coccyx (see Fig. 24–5). Based on the relation of the pouch to this pubococcygeal line, anorectal anomalies can be classified into three groups indicating a low, high, or intermediate level defect. In low (translevator) types, the rectum descends through and is surrounded by the puborectalis and levator ani muscles so that the sensorimotor mechanisms are generally intact. With high (supralevator) defects, the rectal pouch ends above the puborectalis and levator ani muscles so that the neurologic and muscular mechanisms of continence may be impaired. In intermediate types (supralevator), the rectum again ends above the puborectalis, but the pouch is cradled in the muscular hammock formed by the levator ani so that neuromuscular function is variable and repair more complicated (Adkins & Kiesewetter, 1976; Chang, 1980b; deVries & Cox, 1985; Leape, 1987).

The overall mortality rate is approximately 20 percent, with death largely a reflection of the nature of the defect and the presence of associated anomalies. In general, the supralevator types of defects carry the highest mortality (31 percent), with intermediate supralevator lesions having the highest death rate of all (45 percent), followed by high supralevator lesions (29 percent) and low translevator defects (7 percent). As a group, the cause of death for most defects is due to the presence of associated anomalies (Adkins & Kiesewetter, 1976).

For survivors, the main criterion for outcome is fecal continence. When anorectal anomalies are reviewed as a whole, 74 percent of patients can be expected to have good results, with normal anal function and control of defecation; 14 percent have fair results, with only occasional soiling or straining; and 12 percent have poor results, being nearly or completely incontinent or requiring permanent colostomy. Here again, however, outcome is determined largely by the level of the defect. Most low translevator (92 percent) and intermediate supralevator (83 percent) types have a good outcome. Far fewer (51 percent) of the high supralevator defects have good postoperative results, and a large proportion (23 percent) have frankly poor results (Adkins & Kiesewetter, 1976).

Collaborative Management

As might be expected, the treatment of anorectal anomalies varies with the nature of the defect. The higher the lesion, the more technically complicated its repair becomes.

The treatment of anal stenosis (type I defect) consists of repeated dilation using Hegar dilators. When the anus is sufficiently enlarged, and if the infant is otherwise stable, the patient is discharged, with daily digital dilation (using the little finger) to be performed by the parents (Adkins & Kiesewetter, 1976; Chang, 1980b; Leape, 1987).

Membranous defects (type II) require minimal surgical therapy. The membrane is simply punctured with a hemostat or excised using a scalpel. Repeated dilation is performed as needed (Adkins & Kiesewetter, 1976; Chang, 1980b).

Low agenesis (translevator, type III lesion) is corrected by perineal anoplasty. After locating the position of the superficial external sphincter using a nerve stimulator, the rectal pouch is brought down through the sphincter to the opening on the anal skin. The fistulous connection, if present, is removed. Gentle irrigations help facilitate stooling and keep the anastomotic site clean until daily dilations can be started, generally between 10 and 14 days postoperatively (Adkins & Kiesewetter, 1976; Chang, 1980b; Hendren & Kim, 1974; Leape, 1987).

High agenesis (intermediate or high supralevator, type III lesions) and atresia (supralevator, type IV lesions) generally are treated in two phases. The first step is immediate placement of a colostomy for decompression and diversion of fecal contents. If present, the urethrorectal fistula is generally closed or excised to avoid "spill-over" fecal contamination with resultant urinary tract infection. The definitive repair is generally delayed 3 to 12 months to allow growth and pelvic enlargement. At that time, an abdominal-perineal pull-through procedure is performed in which the rectal pouch is literally pulled through the levator sling and anchored to the skin. The colostomy is left intact until healing is complete (Boles, 1978; Chang, 1980b; deVries & Cox, 1985; Leape, 1987).

Nonemergent cases (typically stenosis) usually require little in the way of stabilization, other than replacement and correction of fluid and electrolyte imbalance. If a fistula is present, these infants are at risk for the development of hyperchloremic acidosis owing to the absorption of urine from the colon (Leape, 1987). Gastric suction for decompression is instituted prophylactically (in the case of agenesis when the defect is obvious on inspection) or therapeutically (when membranous and atretic types begin to display symptoms of obstruction).

Postoperatively, wound care and monitoring for postoperative complications are added to the regimen. If anoplasty is performed, the site should be inspected (as allowed by the surgical team) for mucosal prolapse, which may occur if there is inadequate sphincter preservation. A colostomy placed for higher defects should receive the standard care and monitoring. Dilatory procedures are initially carried out by the surgeon, but when digital dilation becomes possible, the nurse may assume this task, making sure to provide bedside parent teaching. Throughout recuperation, the urine (or vaginal outlet) should be closely observed for the presence of meconium, which would indicate a recurrent fistula. If such a fistula is suspected, electrolyte and acid–base status should also be monitored for hyperchloremic acidosis. Otherwise, feeding may begin when the colostomy or anoplasty is sufficiently healed and intestinal function resumes. Stool-softening agents may be required (Leape, 1987).

As children age, psychosocial counseling should become an integral part of continuing care. Longitudinal data indicate that 29 percent of affected children experience some behavioral problem, ranging from mild (10 percent) to levels severe enough to influence their daily lives (19 percent). These maladjustments generally involve social withdrawal, depression, anxiety, and other internalizing behavior and are most apparent in those who achieve continence late or who suffer frequent accidents (Ludman & Spitz, 1995). Adults similarly report social problems related to fecal continence (83 percent) in addition to problems with sexual function (30 percent) (Rintala et al., 1994).

Malrotation With Volvulus

Pathophysiology

Malrotation is an anomaly of intestinal rotation and fixation. Although alternative theories have been offered (Kluth et al., 1995), the abnormality most likely arises as the intestine rotates around the axis of the superior mesenteric artery during its entry into and movement from the umbilical cord. Once returned to the abdominal cavity, the intestinal mesentery lies along and eventually adheres to the posterior abdominal wall, thus fixing the intestine in place (Chang, 1980a; Moore & Persaud, 1993; Sadler, 1985). The normal 270-degree counterclockwise rotation can be interrupted or deviated at any time, and consequently a variety of rotation and fixation anomalies is possible (Fig. 24–6).

The major danger with malrotation is that the intestinal loops may become kinked, knotted, or otherwise obstructed. This knotting and twisting of the bowel is called a *volvulus*. The resultant occlusion of the intestinal tract or its blood supply can lead to widespread ischemia and necrosis. Nearly two thirds of all cases of malrotation are complicated by volvulus, with the incidence varying with age at the onset of symptoms. Eighty-five percent of patients less than 1 month of age have volvulus compared with 43 percent of older children (Gryboski & Walker, 1983; Messineo et al., 1992; Seashore & Touloukian, 1994).

Risk Factors

Owing to the rarity of rotational anomalies, their incidence is not known. However, the busiest surgical referral services typically see only two to four cases a year (Ducharme & Ghosn, 1987b; Messineo et al., 1992; Reyes et al., 1989; Seashore & Touloukian, 1994). The anomaly does appear to predominate in males; however, no specific cause has been identified (Chang, 1980a).

Because of the nature of these defects, almost all cases of omphalocele, gastroschisis, and diaphragmatic hernia entail some component of malrotation. The frequency is in fact so high that many clinicians do not consider malrotation an anomaly associated with these conditions but rather an expected component of them. In addition to these defects, associated anomalies such as intestinal atresias, annular pancreas, Meckel's diverticulum, and urinary tract malformation as well as congenital heart disease are found in 8 to 24 percent of patients (Chang, 1980a; Messineo et al., 1992; Reyes et al., 1989; Seashore & Touloukian, 1994).

Clinical Manifestations

Only about half of all affected infants present with symptoms in the first week of life. In those who do, the symptoms are generally intermittent or recurrent, indicating that most of these obstructions are partial rather than complete. Most infants demonstrate progressive bilious vomiting and little else (Chang, 1980a). However, when a previously well infant presents with sudden bilious vomiting, a malrotation with volvulus should be the first thought of the clinician. In the case of volvulus, the abdomen may become distended and the stools may be bloody. Bleeding occurs when twisting is severe enough to interfere with venous return from the bowel, causing the vessels to become engorged and leak blood into the gut (Hendren & Kim, 1974).

Differential Diagnosis

The differential diagnosis generally includes pyloric stenosis, duodenal atresia, and jejunoileal atresia. The possibility of pyloric stenosis is generally considered, owing to vomiting in the absence of any other typical signs of GI obstruction. However, the emesis of pyloric stenosis is seldom bile-stained, and this condition is quickly dropped from further consideration (Chang, 1980a).

On plain radiograph, the stomach and upper small intestine are generally distended with air and may mimic the characteristic "double-bubble" of duodenal atresia. However, the presence of small amounts of gas in the distal positions of the gut is more reflective of a partial obstruction by malrotation than of an atresia in the jejunum or ileum. In adults, the gas-filled loops may appear to converge to a point ("convergency sign"). A "spoke wheel" sign of mucosal folds radiating from the center has also been described. However, these radiographic signs have not been reported in neonates (Lee et al., 1995). If doubt persists, a barium enema can be given to locate the position of the cecum under fluoroscopy. If a misplaced colon is seen, the diagnosis of malrotation is confirmed. However, some malrotations (notably reverse rotation) may not be demonstrated. An upper GI series is diagnostic in all cases, allowing the exact position of the duodenum to be seen. When volvulus is present, the barium column is noted to end with a peculiar "beaking" effect. This beaking appearance is pathognomonic of a volvulus and is caused by the twisting of the bowel into a sharp point resembling the beak of a bird (Chang, 1980a; Leape, 1987). Suspected malrotation is the only situation that warrants an upper GI series; otherwise the procedure should not be carried out in infants (Ricketts, 1984).

Prognosis

When the condition is uncomplicated by infarction or associated anomalies, the survival rate is excellent and may be as high as 99 percent. However, in the presence of necrosis, survival falls to 35 percent. An increased risk of dying is also noted with younger age (<3 months) at the time of surgery (Chang, 1980a; Ducharme & Ghosn, 1987b; Messineo et al., 1992).

Collaborative Management

The goals for surgical management are the release of obstruction and counterclockwise rotational reduction of the bowel (Chang, 1980a). If a volvulus is present, it is immediately apparent on opening the abdomen. Normally, the transverse colon is the first structure that is seen. In the case of volvulus, however, the small bowel typically lies anterior to the colon, making it the first structure that is encountered. The volvulus is relieved by counterclockwise rotation, and the viability of the bowel is determined with necrotic sections removed. If the necrosis is extensive, rather than perform massive bowel resection, the abdomen is closed. A return "second look" surgery is performed in 24 to 48 hours, at which time it becomes mandatory to remove any unrecovered, infarcted bowel. If the bowel appears viable, the Ladd bands (if present) are divided and the entrapped duodenum

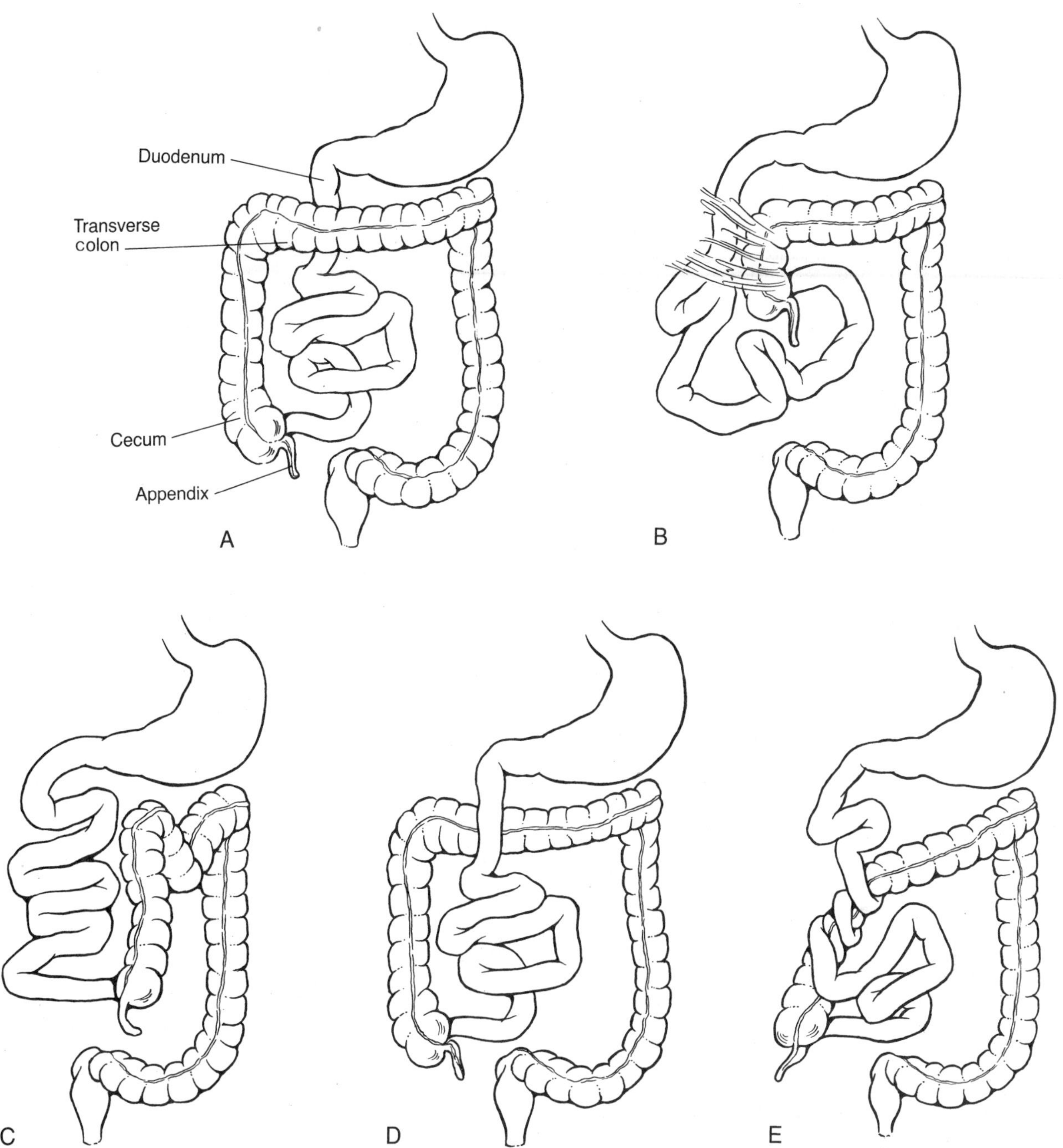

FIGURE 24–6. Anomalies of rotation and fixation. *A*, Normal anatomy: cecum lies in right lower quadrant; transverse colon overlies duodenum. *B*, Incomplete rotation (Ladd bands): cecum lies just below and anterior to the duodenum, where it becomes fixed to the posterior wall by abnormal peritoneal bands; the bands cross over, compress, and obstruct the duodenum. *C*, Nonrotation ("left-sided colon"): entire small intestine lies in the right side of the abdominal cavity, whereas all of the large intestine lies on the left; volvulus may occur, but the condition is more frequently asymptomatic. *D*, Reverse (clockwise) rotation: duodenum overlies and may obstruct the transverse colon. *E*, Nonfixation ("midgut volvulus"): mesentery fails to adhere to the posterior abdominal wall so that the small intestine hangs loosely from the superior mesenteric artery and is free to twist around it or on itself to create a volvulus, typically involving the duodenum. (Data from Chang, 1980a; Leape, 1987, Moore & Persaud, 1993; Sadler, 1985.)

is freed. The entire length of the bowel is then inspected for patency and associated defects and returned to the abdominal cavity; the small intestine is placed on the right and the colon is placed on the left side of the abdominal cavity. Suture fixation of the replaced bowel generally is not necessary. Appendectomy and gastrostomy are generally performed as well (Bucuvalas & Balistreri, 1997; Ducharme & Ghosn, 1987b; Ghory & Sheldon, 1985; Leape, 1987).

The major postoperative complication is short bowel syndrome, resulting from the excision of major portions of the gut (Leape, 1987). The complex malabsorption problems and prolonged hospitalization with total parenteral nutrition call for consultation and close collaboration with members of the nutritional support team and social services. Wound problems and prolonged ileus may also be noted (Seashore & Touloukian, 1994).

The principles of preoperative stabilization include gastric decompression and correction of fluid and electrolyte deficits. The presence of volvulus places the infant at particular risk for both hypovolemia and metabolic acidosis. Hypovolemia occurs as a result of fluid accumulation in the bowel wall, which effectively reduces the circulating blood volume (Leape, 1987). Clinically, as the infant worsens, the abdomen becomes distended, erythematous, and tender, and blood is passed into the stool. The heart rate quickens in an attempt to maintain cardiac output, and the infant's color may become ashen. This state constitutes a true surgical emergency (Ducharme & Ghosn, 1987b).

The same principles of decompression and fluid and electrolyte resuscitation apply postoperatively. Total parenteral nutrition is instituted and continued, often for months in the case of short bowel syndrome, until the intestine has had an opportunity to recover and grow. When feedings are begun, very dilute formula (one-quarter strength protein hydrosylate formula) is given initially; the volume and then the concentration are gradually increased until a normal amount of full-strength formula can be tolerated. This feeding progression is often a tedious process fraught with many setbacks that are frustrating to both the nurse and the parents (Leape, 1987).

Intussusception

Pathophysiology

Intussusception is an acquired obstruction in which a part of the intestine prolapses into the lumen of an adjoining distal intestinal segment (Fig. 24–7). This luminal prolapse may occur at any site in the GI tract, but typically there are four varieties: (1) enteric intussusception, in which the small intestine prolapses into itself; (2) colic intussusception, in which the large intestine prolapses into itself; (3) ileocecal intussusception, in which the ileocecal valve is inverted and pushed into the cecum, pulling a segment of ileum with it; and (4) ileocolic intussusception, in which the ileocecal valve remains in place but the ileum prolapses through it into the colon (Taylor, 1988). Rarely, a retrograde intussusception may occur in which a distal intestinal segment prolapses upward into a proximal part. In the neonate, the majority of cases are of the enteric (most often involving the terminal ileum) or ileocecal type (Avery & Taeusch, 1984).

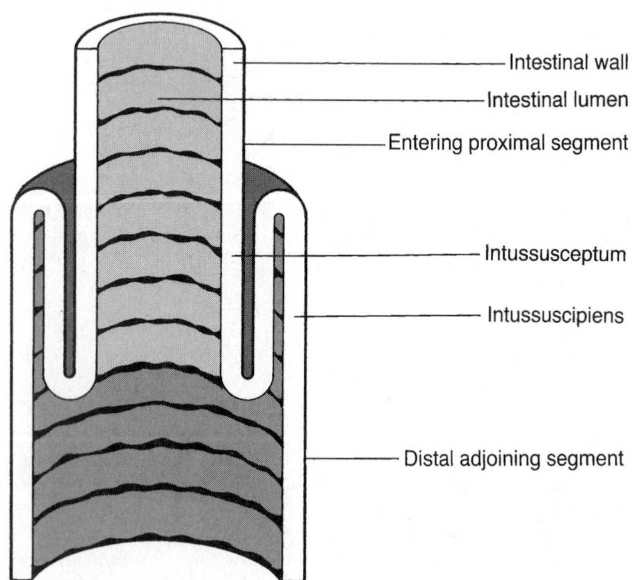

FIGURE 24–7. Schematic representation of intussusception. The proximal intestinal segment has prolapsed into the lumen of an adjacent distal intestinal segment.

Risk Factors

Intussusception is an acquired condition and therefore not easily explained by any one causative factor. A small proportion of cases (5 to 13 percent) appear to have a "lead point," a demonstrable anatomic lesion or defect that may have been the cause of intussusception. Such lead points may include Meckel's diverticula, duplication defects, polyps, hematomas, and lymphomas. The viscid stool common in cystic fibrosis may even be a potential cause. In most situations, the cause is not known (idiopathic intussusception). However, there is often a history of preceding upper respiratory infection or gastroenteritis. Nearly half of all patients demonstrate infection with adenovirus on stool culture. The role played by infection in the phenomenon of intussusception has not yet been determined. The inflammatory response of the intestine to infection may possibly cause an abnormal hyperplasia of lymphoid tissue. The hyperplastic site might then serve as a lead point for intussusception (Avery & Taeusch, 1984; Leape, 1987; Lipschitz et al., 1995).

Intussusception is extremely rare in the newborn period; consequently, an overall incidence rate is not known. Even if one could be involved in the care of each affected newborn, one might expect to encounter only one case every 5 years (Rachelson et al., 1955). The usual age for intussusception is between 3 and 24 months, with males predominating (Gryboski & Walker, 1983; Hendren & Kim, 1974; Leape, 1987).

Clinical Manifestations

Regardless of the site, the intussusception gives rise to two problems. First, it causes a simple mechanical obstruction as the result of the blockage of the distal intestinal lumen by the prolapsed proximal segment. Second, as the intestinal walls are telescoped into one another, the mucosal blood vessels become compressed, congested, and prone to ischemia or infarction (Avery & Taeusch, 1984). Thus, the symptoms of intussusception typically include vomiting, colicky pain, and bloody stools or red "currant jelly" stools (Gryboski & Walker, 1983; Shanbhogue et al., 1994).

Differential Diagnosis

Plain radiographs may not be helpful in the diagnosis, with 20 to 30 percent showing only a general picture of intestinal obstruction with dilated proximal loops and an airless distal bowel. On ultrasonography, the affected area often appears as a "doughnut sign" on cross-section. Definitive diagnosis is by barium enema with the contrast media outlining the gut and end proximally in a characteristic "coiled spring" pattern. This pattern is caused by barium trickling into the transverse folds of the luminal mucosa between the intussusceptum and the intussuscipiens (Avery & Taeusch, 1984; Gryboski & Walker, 1983; Hendren & Kim, 1974; Leape, 1987; Shanbhogue et al., 1994).

Prognosis

The prognosis for intussusception in newborns is not good, basically because they present with so few of the signs that classically appear in infants and older children. Consequently, intussusception is rarely considered in the differential diagnosis of intestinal obstruction. When diagnosed, the mortality rate is approximately 41 percent (Avery & Taeusch, 1984).

Collaborative Management

Intussusception is so rare that little medical research has been undertaken to determine the best approach for treatment. In older children and adults, an attempt is first made to reduce the intussusception using the hydrostatic pressure produced by a barium enema. Barium is injected into the rectum and allowed to flow distally until the "coiled-spring" pattern appears. A balloon-tipped catheter is then inserted into the rectum. The balloon is inflated with air, and gentle traction is applied until the balloon is pulled back against the muscular sling of the levatores, thus preventing any outflow of barium. The administration of barium is restarted, causing the intraluminal pressure to rise slowly as more and more contrast medium is added without an avenue for escape. The pressure is maintained until the intussusception is pushed distally and freed. The procedure can be likened to taking a surgical glove in which one fingertip has been pulled inward, closing the cuff around the mouth, and slowly exhaling until the fingertip of the glove is blown outward. If the intussusception is fully reduced, the barium is seen suddenly to flow freely into the proximal bowel, and the clinical status of the patient should immediately improve. Unfortunately, in infants, full reduction is generally not accomplished and surgical reduction is required (Avery & Taeusch, 1984; Gryboski & Walker, 1983; Leape, 1987). Recently, an alternate approach of rectal insufflation of air has been reported. Pneumatic reduction, however, generally is not performed in infants less than 3 months of age because of the risk of bowel perforation and rapid tension pneumoperitoneum (Lipschitz et al., 1995; Shiels, 1995; Zheng et al., 1994).

Surgical intervention involves a manual reduction of the intussusception using a "milking" motion on the proximal bowel. The pressure and squeezing are continued until the loop is freed; traction and pulling should never be applied. The bowel is carefully inspected, any necrotic tissue is removed, and lead points are resected (Avery & Taeusch, 1984; Leape, 1987).

The major concerns prior to reduction are sepsis and shock. In light of the strong association with adenovirus and the frequent history of gastroenteritis or respiratory infection, sepsis should be expected and the appropriate blood work carried out. Antibiotic therapy is initiated pending culture results. Fluid lost into the wall of the trapped intestine or blood lost from congested vessels into the lumen of the intestine, or a combination of both, predisposes to shock and should be appropriately managed with fluid resuscitation and volume expansion. Decompression by gastric suction is also recommended (Leape, 1987).

Postoperative care is fairly routine, with fluids, electrolytes, and decompression provided as needed. However, the nurse must be aware that intussusception may recur. The recurrence risk is 2 to 20 percent, being more common following hydrostatic reduction (8 to 13 percent) than after surgical reduction (0 to 4 percent). Consequently, even though the intussusception has presumably been resolved, the nurse must be alert for the return of associated signs and symptoms. Increasing gastric drainage may be a particularly helpful clue (Champous et al., 1994; Leape, 1987).

Necrotizing Enterocolitis

Pathophysiology

Necrotizing enterocolitis (NEC) is an acquired disorder characterized by necrosis of the mucosal and submucosal layers of the GI tract. Any portion of the bowel can be affected, but the ileocecal area predominates (66 percent), with the antimesenteric side most typically being involved (Lemelle et al., 1994). To the naked eye, the affected intestine appears irregularly dilated with patchy areas of discoloration ranging from pale to dark purple. The pale color indicates areas of ischemic necrosis where the tissues have been deprived of their blood supply; the purple color indicates areas of hemorrhagic necrosis where blood has leaked into the tissues from capillary hemorrhage. Gas-containing cysts (pneumatosis) may be seen in the wall of the intestine as the result of gas dissecting beneath the serosa or submucosa (Fig. 24–8). If perforation has occurred, it is usually found in the ileocecal area.

On microscopic examination, the mucosa appears edematous, and the necrotic areas may extend beyond the mucosa and submucosa into the muscular layers. Microthrombi may also be noted in the tiny arterioles and venules of the mesentery, but frank thrombosis of the larger arteries or veins rarely occurs. Contrary to what the name NEC implies, there is really little inflammation in the acute stages of the disease (Kosloske & Musemeche, 1989).

The etiology and pathogenesis of NEC have been the focus of extensive debate and research for the past 30 years. Many theories have been offered concerning the factors that cause the disease and their method of introduction to the neonate, but few absolute answers have been found. At present the sum of knowledge indicates that there are three major pathologic mechanisms occurring in combination that lead to the development of NEC. These three mechanisms involve selective ischemia of the bowel, establishment of bacterial flora, and the effect of feeding (Kosloske & Musemeche, 1989; Santulli et al., 1975).

The selective bowel ischemia is really an asphyxial defense mechanism, serving to protect the brain and heart from hypoxia by shunting blood away from the mesenteric, renal, and peripheral vascular bed. This redistribution of blood flow is similar to the "diving reflex" typical of aquatic birds and mammals. Unfortunately, in human infants this relative circulatory insufficiency to the bowel may result in intestinal ischemia. Asphyxiated infants and those suffering respiratory distress syndrome, apneic episodes, or cyanosis are most commonly affected. Although these conditions undoubtedly affect intestinal perfusion, such compromise may be intermittent in nature and of insufficient magnitude alone to induce necrosis without some additional factor. Any condition or procedure that holds potential for causing hemodynamic change may also be at fault. Polycythemia, umbilical artery catheterization, and exchange transfusion as well as maternal cocaine abuse have been implicated in bowel ischemia (Buyukunal et al., 1994; Kosloske, 1994a; Kosloske & Musemeche, 1989; Lloyd, 1969; Nowicki & Nankervis, 1994; Santulli et al., 1975; Topalian & Ziegler, 1984).

Colonization of the intestine with bacteria that normally reside within its lumen is a postnatal process. In utero the intestines are sterile, but during the process of delivery and subsequent contact with the surrounding environment, the gut becomes seeded with a wide variety of aerobic and anaerobic bacteria, which then

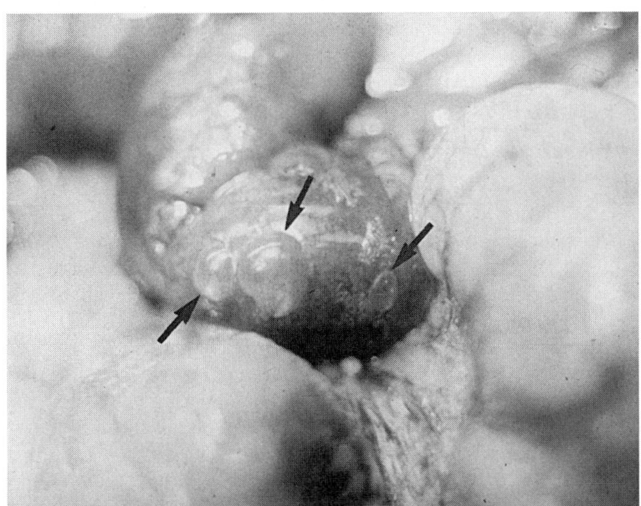

FIGURE 24–8. Gross operative findings in necrotizing enterocolitis. The gas-filled intramural cysts *(arrows)* are typical of pneumatosis intestinalis. (Courtesy of Drs. David A. Clark and Jeffery E. Thompson and Wyeth-Ayerst Laboratories, Philadelphia, PA.)

multiply and spread with enteral feedings. In healthy newborn infants, the intestinal flora is established by about 10 days of age; however, in premature and sick infants, the colonization may be delayed, with fewer species of bacteria than are normally present. Attempts at controlling infectious disease within the special care nursery and skill at employing aseptic technique may in large part be responsible. Nevertheless, the result is a newborn with a GI tract that is both structurally and immunologically immature and susceptible to injury from bacterial toxins, that is, the passage of bacteria or bacterial products (such as endotoxins) across the mucosal wall (Deitch, 1994; Israel, 1994; Kosloske & Musemeche, 1989). This decreased immunity and lack of resistance may explain the fact that most of the bacteria cultured from affected infants are of species that are otherwise considered a part of the normal intestinal flora (Roy, 1987). The organisms that are typically isolated include *Escherichia coli* and *Enterobacter, Klebsiella,* and *Clostridium* species. These enteric bacilli do not usually invade normal tissue but are opportunistic pathogens (Blakey et al., 1985; Chan et al., 1994; Kosloske, 1994a; Kosloske & Musemeche, 1989; Santulli et al., 1975). Based on these observations, several research groups are currently working to develop a means of prophylaxis. Although the administration of oral antibiotics to modify intestinal flora has provided mixed results, oral administration of an immunoglobulin preparation (IgA or IgG, or both) appears promising (Fast & Rosegger, 1994; Maxson et al., 1995; Rubaltelli et al., 1991; Wolf & Eibl, 1994). The administration of glucocorticoids to accelerate maturation of the GI system may also be potentially beneficial (Faix & Adams, 1994; Halac et al., 1990; Vasan & Gotoff, 1994).

Formula feedings have also been cited as an important factor in making the gut susceptible to NEC. In fact, virtually all infants in whom the disease develops (98 percent) have previously been fed either formula or dextrose solution (Kliegman & Fanaroff, 1981; Santulli et al., 1975). It is believed that such intake may simply provide a substance on which bacteria can feed and flourish. In comparison, infants who receive fresh breast milk are rarely affected with NEC, presumably being protected by the secretory immunoglobulin (IgA) and anti-inflammatory components it provides (Barlow et al., 1974; Buescher, 1994; Kosloske, 1994a; Kosloske & Musemeche, 1989).

Hyperosmolar loads of formula or medications may further compound the situation. In response to the osmotic gradient and in a futile attempt to reduce the osmolarity, intestinal secretions are increased and fluid moves into the lumen of the GI tract. As a result of this fluid shift, blood volume is decreased, GI blood flow is reduced, and the intestinal mucosa becomes relatively ischemic, increasing the risk of NEC (Finer et al., 1984; Santulli et al., 1975; Sunshine et al., 1983). Furthermore, in vitro studies have demonstrated that the tissue fluid content of the bowel wall itself is also decreased as fluid moves into the lumen. This dehydration of the epithelium causes both morphologic and functional alterations in the mucosal lining of the intestine. The height and width of the villi decrease, the intercellular spaces close, and as a result the overall absorptive capacity of the bowel is decreased (Norris, 1973). Malabsorption with varying degrees of stasis and ileus in turn allows the development of abnormal flora, which further increases the risk of NEC (Johnson et al., 1985). The complex mechanism of vascular and cellular changes occurring in response to hyperosmolar loads is believed to be responsible for the increased incidence of NEC reported for low birth weight infants historically receiving hyperosmolar feedings and certain oral medications, particularly high-dose vitamin E (100 to 200 mg/kg/day, producing tocopherol levels in excess of 3.5 mg/dl), which was given to impede the development of retinopathy of prematurity (Bell, 1989; Book et al., 1975; Finer et al., 1984; Johnson et al., 1985). Although vitamin E is no longer given at such high doses, other medications frequently used in neonatal therapy also possess high osmolality and must be considered potentially damaging to the gut. Even when diluted in formula, a medication such as phenobarbital elixir can increase the osmolality of a feeding by more than twofold. In many cases it may be preferable to give the intravenous preparation of the drug by the oral route to avoid such hypertonic feedings (White & Harkavy, 1982).

The development of NEC apparently occurs as a result of the three pathologic mechanisms—ischemia, bacteria, and feeding (particularly hyperosmolar feeding)—operating in concert. Injured by ischemia, the mucosal cells lining the gut stop secreting protective enzymes. The unprotected luminal cells are destroyed by the digestive enzymes present (autodigestion). Enteric bacteria proliferate in the substrate-rich but immunologically deficient environment and invade the intestinal wall, where they release toxins and produce hydrogen gas. The gas is formed as a result of the catalytic activity of bacterial enzymes acting on formula as a substrate (Engel et al., 1973). The gas initially dissects beneath the serosal and submucosal layers of the intestine (pneumatosis intestinalis), but if this gas ruptures into the mesenteric vascular bed, it can be distributed through the systemic vessels into the venous system of the liver (portal venous gas). The bacterial toxins together with ischemia result in necrosis. If the full thickness of the intestinal wall is damaged, perforation can result, with the release of free air into the peritoneal cavity (pneumoperitoneum), producing a true surgical emergency (Avery & Taeusch, 1984; Leape, 1987; Santulli et al., 1975).

Risk Factors

NEC is the most common GI disorder seen in the intensive care nursery, affecting approximately 5 percent of all admissions, although wide differences are reported from center to center (from a low of 1 percent to a high of 8 percent). Any condition or situation leading to ischemia and bacterial overgrowth in the presence of formula feedings can logically be considered a risk factor. However, prematurity is probably the greatest risk factor of all. Although cases in term infants are noted (Wiswell et al., 1988), NEC is almost exclusively a disease of the prematurely born. Of all infants affected, 62 to 94 percent are premature, with the highest rates in those with lowest birth weight and gestational age. No consistent associations between NEC and sex, race, socioeconomic status, or season of the year have been found (Kliegman & Fanaroff, 1981; Kosloske, 1994a; Kosloske & Musemeche, 1989; Stoll, 1994).

Clinical Manifestations

Symptoms generally present on an overall average (mean) at 12 days of age, although the most common age at onset (mode) is 3 days. However, cases have been reported to occur in infants as old as 90 days (Kliegman & Fanaroff, 1981). Covert and associates (1989) have suggested that this wide range in age at onset may actually reflect the presence of two distinct patient subgroups. Patients with early-onset NEC (those 21 days of age or younger) typically have less severe respiratory disease and require shorter periods of mechanical ventilation and oxygen supplementation than do patients with late-onset NEC (those older than 21 days). As a consequence, those with early-onset NEC are generally fed early (beginning at an average of 4 days of life) and advanced quickly to full feedings (over a 9-day period on average). Patients with late-onset NEC typically are not fed until 9 days of age and advance to full feedings more slowly over a 22-day period. When these subgroups are reviewed separately, the early cases typically present with symptoms at 12 days of age; the late cases typically present at 35 days. Regardless of age at onset, there does not appear to be any significant difference between the groups in terms of symptoms, severity, or sequelae of NEC.

Early signs are highly variable but generally include nonspecific signs of GI compromise (abdominal distention, gastric residuals, vomiting that may or may not be bilious, and bloody stools) or nonspecific signs of infection (lethargy, temperature instability, apnea, and bradycardia), or both. Laboratory findings include abnormal blood gases caused by apnea and acidosis, abnormal blood counts resulting from sepsis, thrombocytopenia resulting from consumption by the necrotic process and infection, and reducing substances in the stool caused by carbohydrate malabsorption. As the disease progresses, hypovolemia occurs as the result of the third-spacing of fluids in the interstitial compartments of the damaged intestine, blood pressure falls, urinary output decreases, and the poorly perfused, often septic infant appears gray, pale, or mottled. Peritonitis is evident by erythema, edema, and tenderness of the abdominal wall. If clotting factors continue to be consumed, disseminated intravascular coagulation may even occur (Gupta et al., 1994; Kanto et al., 1994; Kliegman & Fanaroff, 1981; Kosloske & Musemeche, 1989; Leape, 1987; Santulli et al., 1975; Schober & Nassiri, 1994).

Differential Diagnosis

Radiographic findings change as the disease progresses (Fig. 24–9). Radiographs taken early in the course of the disease generally exhibit little more than fixed, dilated bowel loops with thickened walls, all due to local edema. The invasion of gas-forming bacteria into the intestinal wall produces the diagnostic picture of pneumatosis intestinalis. This intraluminal air, found in 85 percent of affected infants, generally appears as tiny, lucent bubbles that may come so close together in some places that they coalesce to form curvilinear or crescent-shaped streaks. If extensive disease is present, air may enter the venous system and outline the hepatic veins. Portal venous gas, found in 15 to 30 percent of patients, is also diagnostic of NEC. Ultimately, perforation may occur, presenting the characteristic appearance of pneumoperitoneum with a layer of free air lying immediately inferior to the abdominal wall. This free air is best seen by a lateral view, but on anteroposterior view it may be noted by the characteristic "football sign" due to air outlining the falciform ligament (Fotter & Sorantin, 1994; Kosloske & Musemeche, 1989; Leape, 1987; Morrison & Jacobson, 1994; Rabinowitz & Siegle, 1976; Santulli et al., 1975).

Other diagnostic studies are used sporadically but may be of diagnostic benefit, particularly in the early stages of NEC. These studies include assays of hydrogen in expired breath (which may be increased owing to the fermentative activity of bacteria), hepatic vein ultrasonography (which may detect microbubbles in the portal vein before air can be identified on the plain radiograph), and metrizamide upper GI series (to detect pneumatosis unappreciated radiographically) (Cheu et al., 1989; Fotter & Sorantin, 1994; Keller & Chawla, 1985; Lindley et al., 1986).

Prognosis

Mortality rates have dramatically decreased over time with improved medical-surgical care and the use of total parenteral nutrition, falling from a rate of 24 to 65 percent in the 1960s and 1970s to a rate of 9 to 28 percent in the 1990s. Within groups, mortality varies with treatment, with lower rates in those who are managed medically compared with those requiring surgical intervention. Persistent acidosis, severe pneumatosis, and the presence of portal venous air are poor prognostic indicators (Buras et al., 1986; Kosloske, 1994b; Stoll, 1994).

Of those who survive, approximately 31 percent experience strictures (mostly colonic) as the result of structural changes in nonperforated, healed ischemic sites. Somewhat fewer patients suffer from short bowel syndrome (9 to 23 percent) and sepsis (9 percent). More than 80 percent of infants with NEC demonstrate evidence of failure of organ systems other than the GI tract. Respiratory failure (91 percent), renal failure (85 percent), cardiovascular failure (33 percent), and hepatic failure (15 percent) are reported most frequently. The number of systems involved increases with the severity of disease and is highest in nonsurvivors. Neurologic, psychomotor, and psychosocial impairment of a moderate to severe nature may be exhibited, but the rate is not significantly different from the rate appearing in the general premature and very low birth weight population (Horwitz et al., 1995; Kosloske & Musemeche, 1989; Mayr et al., 1994; Morecroft et al., 1994).

Recurrent NEC has been reported in 4 to 6 percent of patients, with an average onset of symptoms approximately 5 weeks after the original episode. Neither the type nor timing of enteral

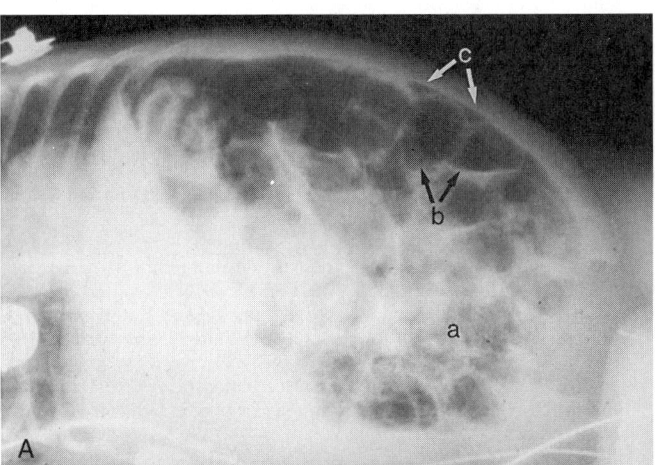

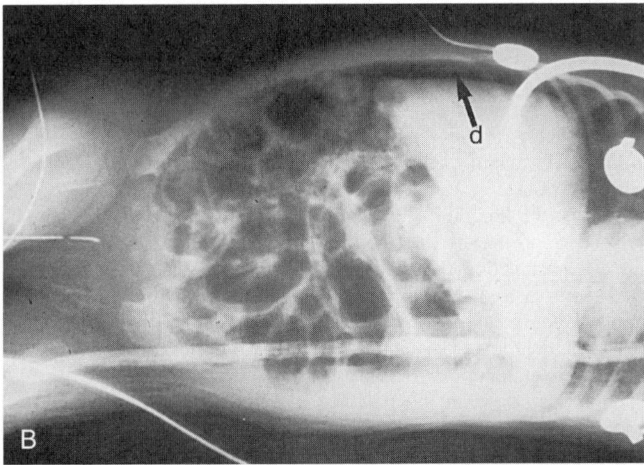

FIGURE 24–9. Extensive necrotizing enterocolitis in a premature infant. The infant died following a "second look" operation. *A*, Right lateral decubitus view of the abdomen demonstrates the widespread bubbly lucencies of pneumatosis intestinalis (a), particularly in the right lower quadrant. In comparison, note the few uniformly dark air-filled loops of normal appearing bowel (b). The small triangular lucencies (c) inferior to the left abdominal wall are formed by free air filling in the spaces between bowel loops and are seen only in the very early stages of pneumoperitoneum immediately following perforation. *B*, Left lateral decubitus view of the abdomen taken 20 minutes later. The lucency overlying the liver (d) demonstrates continued collection of free air in the peritoneal cavity and worsening pneumoperitoneum.

feedings nor the anatomic site or method of management of the initial episode appears to be an influencing factor. Those affected tend to be recovering premature infants (63 percent), although recurrence is also seen in mature infants with major congenital anomalies (31 percent), primarily cyanotic congenital heart disease. The mortality rate is similar to that seen with primary NEC (Ricketts, 1994; Ricketts & Jerles, 1990; Stringer et al., 1993).

Collaborative Management

Aggressive medical management may be successful in approximately half of all affected neonates (Ricketts, 1994). Such management is based on three traditional principles: (1) bowel rest, (2) prevention of progressive injury, and (3) normalization of systemic responses. Enteral nutrition is discontinued, the stomach is decompressed by low intermittent suction through a large-bore orogastric tube, and fluids and electrolytes are closely monitored and adjusted. Antibiotic therapy (after blood for cultures is drawn), early intubation and ventilation, management of acid–base derangements, and efforts to support blood pressure and blood flow to the gut are undertaken both to prevent continuing injury and to correct systemic responses. Serial abdominal films are made at 6- to 8-hour intervals during acute illness to monitor progression of the disease and to detect perforation (Kanto et al., 1994; Kosloske & Musemeche, 1989; Leape, 1987).

Criteria for surgery are somewhat controversial and may vary slightly from institution to institution. However, expedient laparotomy is ideally performed after the advent of intestinal gangrene but prior to perforation. Absolute indications are pneumoperitoneum or confirmation of intestinal gangrene by positive paracentesis (peritoneal tap producing ≥0.5 ml of fluid that is yellowish brown or brown or contains bacteria that is demonstrated on Gram stain, or both). Nonspecific but supportive findings include clinical deterioration in spite of vigorous clinical management (metabolic acidosis, ventilatory failure, thrombocytopenia, leukopenia or leukocytosis with shift to the left, oliguria, and so on), portal venous air, erythema of the abdominal wall, or persistently dilated and fixed bowel loop (Kosloske, 1994b; Kosloske & Musemeche, 1989; Parigi et al., 1994; Ricketts, 1994).

The principles of surgical management include careful examination of the bowel, with resection of all grossly necrotic intestine or perforated sites. If the viability of extensive portions of the gut is in question, resection is deferred, with a follow-up second look operation carried out in 24 to 48 hours. Otherwise the bowel ends are brought to the surface to create an ostomy (Kosloske & Musemeche, 1989; Ricketts, 1994).

Extensive respiratory therapy may be required throughout hospitalization, especially when marked abdominal distention may interfere with ventilation. Long-term parenteral nutrition can be anticipated, making collaboration with the nutritional support team essential.

Because of the high incidence of NEC in the intensive care nursery, a premature infant who experiences any of the early signs of obstruction (vomiting, distention, increased gastric aspirates), one who demonstrates increased episodes of apnea and bradycardia, or one who passes bloody stools should be regarded with a high index of suspicion. Should two or more of the early signs appear together, one should presume NEC until other diagnostic studies can be performed. Feedings are immediately stopped and venous access obtained. A gastric tube is set to intermittent suction for decompression. Vigorous hydration and antibiotic therapy are provided, and total parenteral nutrition is initiated as soon as possible. Circulatory status must be evaluated frequently by monitoring perfusion, vital signs including blood pressure, and urinary output. All stools are routinely checked for blood. Hematologic studies are performed to look for anemia, thrombocytopenia, and disordered coagulation, and blood, platelets, or fresh frozen plasma is given as needed. Oxygenation and acid–base status are also monitored, with respiratory support provided accordingly. Careful, gentle re-examination of the abdomen should be carried out every 8 hours (Kosloske & Musemeche, 1989; Leape, 1987).

Ventilatory and circulatory support are maintained in the postoperative period, and antibiotic therapy is continued for 10 to 14 days past resolution of pneumatosis. Ostomy care is performed as previously described. When stabilized GI function has resumed (generally in 7 to 14 days), feedings are cautiously and slowly begun with small amounts of dilute elemental formula. The amount and concentration of feedings are advanced as tolerated, but these attempts are frequently frustrated by malabsorption associated with short bowel syndrome or the development of strictures. Recurrent distention, residuals, vomiting, intractable constipation, or bloody stools may be noted with partial or complete obstruction due to such strictures (Rushton, 1990).

CONCLUSION

The present management of infants with GI disorders aims for early recognition with relief of symptoms and eventual resumption of normal function to support nutritional needs. Diligent nursing assessment allows early intervention, and appropriate research-based care ensures the best possible long-term results.

REFERENCES

AAP Committee on Genetics. (1989). Newborn screening fact sheets. *Pediatrics, 83*(3), 449–464.

Adkins, J. C., & Kiesewetter, W. B. (1976). Imperforate anus. *Surgical Clinics of North America, 56*(2), 379–394.

Arura, V., & Spino, M. (1991). Cisapride: A novel gastroprokinetic drug. *Canadian Journal of Hospital Pharmacy, 44*(4), 175–181.

Ashcraft, K. W., & Holder, T. M. (1981). Esophageal atresia and tracheo-esophageal fistula malformations. *Continuing Education, 15*(4), 51–60.

Avery, M. E., & Taeusch, H. W. (1984). *Schaffer's diseases of the newborn* (5th ed.). Philadelphia: W. B. Saunders.

Avery, M. E., Fletcher, B. D., & Williams, R. G. (1981). *The lung and its disorders in the newborn infant* (4th ed.). Philadelphia: W. B. Saunders.

Bailey, D. J., Andres, J. M., Danek, G. D., & Pineiro-Carrero, V. M. (1987). Lack of efficacy of thickened feeding as treatment for gastroesophageal reflux. *Journal of Pediatrics, 110*(2), 187–189.

Barlow, B., Santulli, T. V., Heird, W. C., et al. (1974). An experimental study of acute necrotizing enterocolitis: The importance of breast milk. *Journal of Pediatric Surgery, 9*(5), 587–595.

Bell, E. F. (1989). Upper limit of vitamin E in infant formulas. *Journal of Nutrition, 119*(12S), 1829–1831.

Berenberg, W., & Neuhauser, E. B. D. (1950). Cardio-esophageal relaxation (chalasia) as a cause of vomiting in infants. *Pediatrics, 5,* 414–419.

Bergstrom, L. V. (1978). Congenital and acquired deafness in clefting and craniofacial syndromes. *Cleft Palate Journal, 15*(3), 254–261.

Bettex, M., & Oesch, I. (1983). The hiatus hernia saga. Ups and downs in gastroesophageal reflux: Past, present, and future perspectives. *Journal of Pediatric Surgery, 18*(6), 670–680.

Bishop, H. C. (1976). Small bowel obstructions in the newborn. *Surgical Clinics of North America, 56*(2), 329–348.

Blakey, J. L., Lubitz, L., Campbell, N. T., et al. (1985). Enteric colonization in sporadic neonatal necrotizing enterocolitis. *Journal of Pediatric Gastroenterology and Nutrition, 4*(4), 591–595.

Bloom, R. S. (1997). Delivery room resuscitation of newborn. In A. A. Fanaroff & R. J. Martin (Eds.), *Neonatal-perinatal Medicine: Diseases of the fetus and infant* (6th ed., pp. 376–402). St. Louis: Mosby–Year Book.

Boles, E. T. (1978). Imperforate anus. *Clinics in Perinatology, 5*(1), 149–161.

Boley, S. J., Dinari, G., & Cohen, M. I. (1978). Hirschsprung's disease in the newborn. *Clinics in Perinatology, 5*(1), 45–60.

Book, L. S., Herbst, J. J., Atherton, S. O., & Jung, A. L. (1975). Necrotizing enterocolitis in low-birth-weight infants fed an elemental formula. *Journal of Pediatrics, 87*(4), 602–605.

Bowers, D. G. (1970). Congenital lower lip sinuses with cleft palate. *Plastic and Reconstructive Surgery, 45*(2), 151–154.

Breaux, C. W., Georgeson, K. E., Royal, S. A., & Curnow, A. J. (1988). Changing patterns in the diagnosis of hypertrophic pyloric stenosis. *Pediatrics, 81*(2), 213–217.

Briggs, R. M. (1976). Vitamin supplementation as a possible factor in the incidence of cleft lip/palate deformities in humans. *Clinics in Plastic Surgery, 3*(4), 647–652.

Bucuvalas, J. C., & Balistreri, W. F. (1997). The neonatal gastrointestinal tract. In A. A. Fanaroff & R. J. Martin (Eds.), *Neonatal-perinatal medicine: Diseases of the fetus and infant* (6th ed., pp. 1288–1293). St. Louis: Mosby–Year Book.

Buescher, E. S. (1994). Host defense mechanisms of human milk and their relations to enteric infections and necrotizing enterocolitis. *Clinics in Perinatology, 21*(2), 247–262.

Buras, R., Guzzetta, P., Avery, G., & Naulty, C. (1986). Acidosis and hepatic portal venous gas: Indications for surgery in necrotizing enterocolitis. *Pediatrics, 78*(2), 273–277.

Buyukunal, C., Kilic, N., Dervisoglu, S., & Altug, T. (1994). Maternal cocaine abuse resulting in necrotizing enterocolitis: An experimental study in a rat model. *Acta Paediatrica, 83*(Suppl. 396), 91–93.

Cassani, V. L. (1984). Tracheoesophageal anomalies. *Neonatal Network, 3*(2), 20–27.

Cavell, B. (1979). Gastric emptying in preterm infants. *Acta Paediatrica Scandinavia, 68*(5), 725–730.

Chaet, M. S., Farrell, M. K., Ziegler, M. M., & Warner, B. W. (1994). Intensive nutritional support and remedial surgical intervention for extreme short bowel syndrome. *Journal of Pediatric Gastroenterology and Nutrition, 19*(3), 295–298.

Champous, A. N., DelBeccaro, M. A., & Nazar-Stewart, V. (1994). Recurrent intussusception. *Archives of Pediatric and Adolescent Medicine, 148*(5), 474–478.

Chan, K. L., & Saing, H. (1995). Combined flexible endoscopy and fluoroscopy in the assessment of the gap between the two esophageal pouches in esophageal atresia without fistula. *Journal of Pediatric Surgery, 30*(5), 668-670.

Chan, K. L., Saing, H., Yung, R. W. H., et al. (1994). A study of pre-antibiotic bacteriology in 125 patients with necrotizing enterocolitis. *Acta Paediatrica, 83*(Suppl. 396), 45–48.

Chang, J. H. T. (1979). Neonatal surgical emergencies: Part II. Esophageal atresia and tracheoesophageal fistula. *Perinatology/Neonatology, 3*(5), 26–27, 78.

Chang, J. H. T. (1980a). Neonatal surgical emergencies: Part IV. Malrotation of the intestine. *Perinatology/Neonatology, 4*(1), 50–52.

Chang, J. H. T. (1980b). Neonatal surgical emergencies: Part V. Intestinal obstruction. *Perinatology/Neonatology, 4*(2), 34–40.

Chawls, W. J., Lally, K. P., & Mahour, G. H. (1988). Neonatal surgical casebook: Meconium ileus in premature twins. *Journal of Perinatology, 8*(1), 62–64.

Cheu, H. W., Brown, D. R., & Rowe, M. I. (1989). Breath hydrogen excretion as a screening test for the early diagnosis of necrotizing enterocolitis. *American Journal of Diseases of Children, 143*(2), 156–159.

Cloherty, J. P., & Stark, A. R. (1985). *Manual of neonatal care* (2nd ed.). Boston: Little, Brown.

Cohen, M. M. (1978). Syndromes with cleft lip and cleft palate. *Cleft Palate Journal, 15*(4), 306–328.

Cohn, R. M., & Roth, K. S. (1983). *Metabolic disease: A guide to early recognition.* Philadelphia: W. B. Saunders.

Conner, G. K. (1993). Abdomen assessment. In E. P. Tappero & M. E. Honeyfield (Eds.), *Physical assessment of the newborn: A comprehensive approach to the art of physical examination* (pp. 81–89). Petaluma, CA: NICU Ink.

Cortes, D., Thorup, J. M., Nielsen, O. H., & Beck, B. L. (1995). Cryptorchidism in boys with imperforate anus. *Journal of Pediatric Surgery, 30*(4), 631–635.

Covert, R. F., Neu, J., Elliott, M. J., et al. (1989). Factors associated with age of onset of necrotizing enterocolitis. *American Journal of Perinatology, 6*(4), 455–460.

Cowett, R. M., & Schwartz, R. (1987). Glucose metabolism and homeostasis. In L. Stern & P. Vert (Eds.), *Neonatal medicine* (pp. 809–830). New York: Masson Publishing.

Cusick, E. L., Batchelor, A. A. G., & Spicer, R. D. (1993). Development of a technique for jejunal interposition in long-gap esophageal atresia. *Journal of Pediatric Surgery, 28*(8), 990–994.

Davis, D. W. (1985). Congenital duodenal obstruction. *Neonatal Network, 3*(6), 9–13.

Davis, W. S., & Campbell, J. B. (1975). Neonatal small left colon syndrome. *American Journal of Diseases of Children, 129*(9), 1024–1027.

Davis, W. S., Allen, R. P., Favara, B. E., & Slovis, T. L. (1974). Neonatal small left colon syndrome. *American Journal of Roentgenology, 120*(2), 322–329.

Deitch, E. A. (1994). Role of bacterial translocation in necrotizing enterocolitis. *Acta Paediatrica, 83*(Suppl. 296), 33–36.

Desjardins, J. G. (1987). Esophageal atresia. In L. Stern & P. Vert (Eds.), *Neonatal medicine* (pp. 1036–1042). New York: Masson Publishing.

Desmond, M. M., & Rudolph, A. J. (1965). Progressive evaluation of the newborn infant. *Postgraduate Medicine, 37*(2), 207–212.

deVries, P. A., & Cox, K. L. (1985). Surgery of anorectal anomalies. *Surgical Clinics of North America, 65*(5), 1139–1169.

Dienno, M. E. (1987). Esophageal atresia: Corrective procedures and nursing care. *AORN Journal, 45*(6), 1356–1367.

Dirkes, K., Crombleholme, T. M., Craigo, S. D., et al. (1995). The natural history of meconium peritonitis diagnosed in utero. *Journal of Pediatric Surgery, 30*(7), 979–982.

Dorney, S. F. A., Ament, M. E., Berquist, W. E., et al. (1985). Improved survival in very short small bowel of infancy with use of long-term parenteral nutrition. *Journal of Pediatrics, 107*(4), 521–525.

Ducharme, J. C., & Ghosn, P. B. (1987a). Congenital duodenal obstruction. In L. Stern & P. Vert (Eds.), *Neonatal medicine* (pp. 1050–1052). New York: Masson Publishing.

Ducharme, J. C., & Ghosn, P. B. (1987b). Intestinal malrotation. In L. Stern & P. Vert (Eds.), *Neonatal medicine* (pp. 1065–1068). New York: Masson Publishing.

Ein, S. H., & Shandling, B. (1994). Pure esophageal atresia: A 50-year review. *Journal of Pediatric Surgery, 29*(9), 1208–1211.

Elhalaby, E. A., Coran, A. G., Blane, C. E., et al. (1995). Enterocolitis associated with Hirschsprung's disease: A clinical-radiological characterization based on 168 patients. *Journal of Pediatric Surgery, 30*(1), 76–83.

Engel, R. R., Virnig, N. L., Hunt, C. E., & Levitt, M. D. (1973). Origin of mural gas in necrotizing enterocolitis. *Pediatric Research, 7,* 292.

Ewer, A. K., Durbin, G. M., Morgan, M. E. I., & Booth, I. W. (1994). Gastric emptying in preterm infants. *Archives of Disease in Childhood, 71*(1), F24–F27.

Faix, R. G., & Adams, J. T. (1994). Neonatal necrotizing enterocolitis: Current concepts and controversies. [Review]. *Advances in Pediatric Infectious Disease, 9,* 1–36.

Fast, C., & Rosegger, H. (1994). Necrotizing enterocolitis prophylaxis: Oral antibiotics and lyophilized enterobacteria vs. oral immunoglobulins. *Acta Paediatrica, 83*(Suppl. 396), 86–90.

Finer, N. N., Peters, K. L., Hayek, Z., & Merkel, C. L. (1984). Vitamin E and necrotizing enterocolitis. *Pediatrics, 73*(3), 387–393.

Flake, A. W., & Ryckman, F. C. (1997). Selected anomalies and intestinal obstruction. In A. A. Fanaroff & R. J. Martin (Eds.), *Neonatal-perinatal medicine: Diseases of the fetus and infant* (6th ed., pp. 1307–1330). St. Louis: C. V. Mosby.

Fletcher, M. A. (1994). Nutrition. In G. B. Avery, M. S. Fletcher, & M. D. MacDonald (Eds.), *Neonatology: Pathophysiology and management of the newborn* (4th ed., pp. 330–356). Philadelphia: J. B. Lippincott.

Fotter, R., & Sorantin, E. (1994). Diagnostic imaging in necrotizing enterocolitis. [Review]. *Acta Paediatrica, 83*(Suppl. 396), 41–44.

Fraser, F. C. (1970). The genetics of cleft lip and cleft palate. *American Journal of Human Genetics, 22*(3), 336–352.

Frentner, S. (1987). Abdominal wall defects: Omphalocele and gastroschisis. *Neonatal Network, 6*(3), 29–41.

Gantt, L., & Thompson, C. (1985). Short gut syndrome in the infant. *American Journal of Nursing, 85*(11), 1263–1266.

Ghory, M. J., & Sheldon, C. A. (1985). Newborn surgical emergencies of the gastrointestinal tract. *Surgical Clinics of North America, 65*(5), 1083–1098.

Giacoia, G. P., Azubuike, D., & Taylor, J. R. (1993). Indomethacin and recurrent ileal perforations in a preterm infant. *Journal of Perinatology, 13*(4), 297–299.

Gilger, M. A., Wagner, M. L., & Kelley, G. T. (1995). Dissolution of a barium impaction ileus in a child using the PIEE procedure. *Journal of Pediatric Gastroenterology and Nutrition, 21*(1), 119.

Gluck, L. (1979). Examining the newborn. *Family Practice Annual, 1,* 65–79.

Graham, J. M., & Otto, C. (1990). Clinical approach to prenatal detection of human structural defects. *Clinics in Perinatology, 17*(3), 513–546.

Gryboski, J., & Walker, W. A. (1983). *Gastrointestinal problems in the infant* (2nd ed.). Philadelphia: W. B. Saunders.

Gupta, S. K., Burke, G., & Herson, V. C. (1994). Necrotizing enterocolitis: Laboratory indicators of surgical disease. *Journal of Pediatric Surgery, 29*(110), 1472–1475.

Gutierrez, C., Barrios, J. E., Lluna, J., et al. (1994). Recurrent tracheoesophageal fistula treated with fibrin glue. *Journal of Pediatric Surgery, 29*(120), 1567–1569.

Guyton, A. C. (1996). *Textbook of medical physiology* (9th ed.). Philadelphia: W. B. Saunders.

Guzzetta, P. C., Anderson, K. D., Eichelberger, M. R., et al. (1994). General surgery. In G. B. Avery, M. A. Fletcher, & M. D. MacDonald (Eds.), *Neonatology: Pathophysiology and management of the newborn* (4th ed., pp. 914–951). Philadelphia: J. B. Lippincott.

Haber, B. A., & Lake, A. M. (1990). Cholestatic jaundice in the newborn. *Clinics in Perinatology, 17*(2), 483–506.

Habib, Z. (1978a). Factors determining occurrence of cleft lip and cleft palate. *Surgery, Gynecology and Obstetrics, 146*(1), 105–110.

Habib, Z. (1978b). Genetic counseling and genetics of cleft lip and cleft palate. *Obstetrical and Gynecological Survey, 33*(7), 441–447.

Halac, E., Halac, J., Begue, E. F., et al. (1990). Prenatal and postnatal corticosteroid therapy to prevent neonatal necrotizing enterocolitis; A controlled trial. *Journal of Pediatrics, 117*(1, Part 1), 132–138.

Harrell-Bean, H. A., & Klell, C. A. (1983). Neonatal ostomies. *Journal of Obstetric, Gynecologic, and Neonatal Nursing, 12*(Suppl. 3), 69s–73s.

Heij, H. A., deVries, X., Bremer, I., et al. (1995). Long-term anorectal function after Duhamel operation for Hirschsprung's disease. *Journal of Pediatric Surgery, 30*(3), 430–432.

Heller, R. M., & Kirchner, S. G. (1979). *Advanced exercises in diagnostic radiology: The newborn* (Vol. 12). Philadelphia: W. B. Saunders.

Hendren, W. H., & Kim, S. H. (1974). Abdominal surgical emergencies of the newborn. *Surgical Clinics of North America, 54*(3), 489–527.

Herbst, J. J. (1983). Diagnosis and treatment of gastroesophageal reflux in children. *Pediatrics in Review, 5*(3) 75–79.

Hirata, G. I., Medearis, A. L., & Platt, L. D. (1990). Fetal abdominal abnormalities associated with genetic syndromes. *Clinics in Perinatology, 17*(3), 675–702.

Hlusko, D. L., & McMurray, J. (1991). Gastroesophageal reflux: Treatment and nursing care. *Neonatal Network, 9*(5), 33–35.

Holder, T. M., & Ashcraft, K. W. (1981). Developments in the care of patients with esophageal atresia and tracheoesophageal fistula. *Surgical Clinics of North America, 61*(5), 1051–1061.

Horwitz, J. R., Lally, K. P., Cheu, H. W., et al. (1995). Complications after surgical interventions for necrotizing enterocolitis: A multicenter review. *Journal of Pediatric Surgery, 30*(7), 994–999.

Israel, E. J. (1994). Neonatal necrotizing enterocolitis, a disease of the immature intestinal mucosal barrier. *Acta Paediatrica, 83*(Suppl. 396), 27–32.

Jedd, M. B., Melton, L. J., Griffin, M. R., et al. (1988). Factors associated with infantile hypertrophic pyloric stenosis. *American Journal of Diseases of Children, 142*(3), 334–337.

Jhaveri, M. K., & Kumar, S. P. (1987). Passage of the first stool in very low birth weight infants. *Pediatrics, 79*(6), 1005–1007.

Johnson, C. B. (1993). Head, eyes, ears, nose, throat (HEENT) assessment. In E. P. Tappero & M. E. Honeyfield (Eds.), *Physical assessment of the newborn; A comprehensive approach to the art of physical examination* (pp. 41–54). Petaluma, CA: NICU Ink.

Johnson, L., Bowen, F. W., Abbasi, S., et al. (1985). Relationship of prolonged pharmacologic serum levels of vitamin E to incidence of sepsis and necrotizing enterocolitis in infants with birth weight 1,500 grams or less. *Pediatrics, 75*(4), 619–638.

Jones, K. L. (1988). *Smith's recognizable patterns of human malformation: Genetic, embryologic and clinical aspects* (4th ed.). Philadelphia: W. B. Saunders.

Jones, K. M. (1978). Love and lavage: The urgent needs of children with Hirschsprung's disease. *Nursing '78, 8*(7), 33–39.

Kanto, W. P., Hunter, J. E., & Stoll, B. J. (1994). Recognition and medical management of necrotizing enterocolitis. *Clinics in Perinatology, 21*(2), 335–346.

Kee, J. L. (1995). *Laboratory and diagnostic tests with nursing implications* (4th ed.). Norwalk, CT: Appleton & Lange.

Keller, M. S., & Chawla, H. S. (1985). Neonatal metrizamide gastrointestinal series in suspected necrotizing enterocolitis. *American Journal of Diseases of Children, 139*(7), 713–716.

Kelly, E. J., & Newell, S. J. (1994). Gastric ontogeny: Clinical implications. *Archives of Disease in Childhood, 71*(2), F136–F141.

Kelly, E. J., Brownlee, K. G., & Newell, S. J. (1992). Gastric secretory function in the developing human stomach. *Early Human Development, 31*(2), 163–166.

Kelly, E. J., Newell, S. J., Brownlee, K. G., et al. (1993). Gastric acid secretion in preterm infants. *Early Human Development, 35*(3), 215–220.

Kemmotsu, H., Joe, K., Nakamura, H., & Yamashita, M. (1995). Cervical approach for the repair of esophageal atresia. *Journal of Pediatric Surgery, 30*(4), 549–552.

Kenner, C., & Brueggemeyer, A. (1984). Hirschsprung's disease: Current trends and practices. *Neonatal Network, 3*(1), 7–16.

Kenner, C., Harjo, J., & Brueggemeyer, A. (Eds.). (1988). *Neonatal surgery: A nursing perspective.* Orlando, FL: Grune & Stratton.

Khoury, M. J., Gomez-Farias, M., & Mulinare, J. (1989). Does maternal cigarette smoking during pregnancy cause cleft lip and palate in offspring? *American Journal of Diseases of Children, 143*(3), 333–337.

Kiernan, B. S., & Scoloveno, M. A. (1986). Assessment of the neonate. *Topics in Clinical Nursing, 8*(1), 1–10.

Kim, S. H. (1976). Omphalocele. *Surgical Clinics of North America, 56*(2), 361–371.

Kimura, K., & Soper, R. T. (1994). Multistaged extrathoracic esophageal elongation for long gap esophageal atresia. *Journal of Pediatric Surgery, 29*(4), 566-568.

Kliegman, R. M., & Fanaroff, A. A. (1981). Neonatal necrotizing enterocolitis: A nine-year experience. I. Epidemiology and uncommon observations. *American Journal of Diseases of Children, 135*(7), 603–607.

Kluth, D. (1976). Atlas of esophageal atresia. *Journal of Pediatric Surgery, 11*(6), 901–919.

Kluth, D., Kaestner, M., Tibboel, D., & Lambrecht, W. (1995). Rotation of the gut: Fact or fantasy? *Journal of Pediatric Surgery 30*(3), 448–453.

Koenig, W. J., Amarnath, R. P., Hench, V., & Berseth, C. L. (1995). Manometrics for preterm and term infants: A new tool for old questions. *Pediatrics, 95*(2), 203–206.

Kosloske, A. M. (1994a). Epidemiology of necrotizing enterocolitis. *Acta Paediatrica, 83*(Suppl. 396), 2–7.

Kosloske, A. M. (1994b). Indications for operation in necrotizing enterocolitis revisited. *Journal of Pediatric Surgery, 29*(5), 663–666.

Kosloske, A. M., & Musemeche, C. A. (1989). Necrotizing enterocolitis of the neonate. *Clinics in Perinatology, 16*(1), 97–111.

Kramer, I., & Sherry, S. N. (1957). The time of passage of the first stool and urine by the premature infant. *Journal of Pediatrics, 51*(4), 373–376.

Krogman, W. M. (1979). Craniofacial growth: Prenatal and postnatal. In H. K. Cooper, R. L. Harding, W. M. Krogman, et al. (Eds.), *Cleft palate and cleft lip: A team approach to clinical management and rehabilitation of the patient.* (pp. 22–107). Philadelphia: W. B. Saunders.

Krom, F. A., & Frank, C. G. (1989). Clinitesting neonatal stools. *Neonatal Network, 8*(2), 37–40.

Kubota, M., Nakamura, T., Motokura, T., et al. (1994). Erythromycin improves gastrointestinal motility in extremely low birthweight infants. *Acta Paediatrica Japonica, 36*(4), 564–465.

Lambrecht, W., & Kluth, D. (1994). Esophageal atresia: A new anatomic variant with gasless abdomen. *Journal of Pediatric Surgery, 29*(4), 564–565.

Landau, B. R. (1980). *Essential human anatomy and physiology* (2nd ed.). Glenview, IL: Scott, Foresman.

Leape, L. L. (1987). *Patient care in pediatric surgery.* Boston: Little, Brown.

Lebenthal, E., Wynn, R., & Lebenthal, H. (1983). Digestive disorders in neonates: Part 2. Congenital and acquired disease. *Perinatology/Neonatology, 7*(4), 53–59.

Lee, T. Y., Ko, S. F., Wan, Y. L., et al. (1995). "Spoke wheel" sign of small intestinal volvulus. *American Journal of Emergency Medicine, 13*(4), 477-478.

Lemelle, J. L., Schmitt, M., deMiscault, G., et al. (1994). Neonatal necrotizing enterocolitis: A retrospective and multicenter review of 331 cases. *Acta Paediatrica, 83*(Suppl. 396), 70–73.

Lepley, C. J. (1980). *Assessment of risk in the newborn: Evaluation during the transitional period.* White Plains, NY: March of Dimes Birth Defects Foundation.

Lincoln-Boyea, B., & Cefalo, R. C. (1996). Principles of Genetic Counseling. (pp. 16–22). In J. A. Kuller, N. C. Chescheir, & R. C. Cefalo (Eds.). *Prenatal diagnosis & reproductive genetics.* St. Louis: C. V. Mosby.

Lindley, S., Mollitt, D. L., Seibert, J. J., & Golladay, E. S. (1986). Portal vein ultrasonography in the early diagnosis of necrotizing enterocolitis. *Journal of Pediatric Surgery, 21*(6), 530–532.

Lipschitz, B., Patel, Y. T., & Kazlow, P. (1995). Endoscopic pneumatic reduction of an intussusception with simultaneous polypectomy in a child. *Journal of Pediatric Gastroenterology and Nutrition, 21*(1), 91–94.

Lloyd, J. R. (1969). The etiology of gastrointestinal perforations in the newborn. *Journal of Pediatric Surgery, 4*(1), 77–84.

Loper, D. L. (1983). Gastrointestinal development: Embryology, congenital anomalies, and impact on feedings. *Neonatal Network, 2*(1), 27–36.

Ludman, L., & Spitz, L. (1995). Psychosocial adjustment of children treated for anorectal anomalies. *Journal of Pediatric Surgery, 30*(3), 495–499.

Lynn, M. R. (1986). Use of infant seats for gastroesophageal reflux. *Journal of Pediatric Nursing, 1*(2), 127–129.

MacDonald, S. K. (1979). Parental needs and professional responses: A parental perspective. *Cleft Palate Journal, 16*(2), 188–192.

Martin, L. W., & Alexander, F. (1985). Esophageal atresia. *Surgical Clinics of North America, 65*(5), 1099–1113.

Martin, L. W., & Torres, A. M. (1985). Hirschsprung's disease. *Surgical Clinics of North America, 65*(5), 1171–1180.

Martucciello, G., Favre, A., Takahashi, M., & Jasonni, V. (1995). Immunohistochemical localization of RET protein in Hirschsprung's disease. *Journal of Pediatric Surgery, 309*(3), 433–436.

Marty, T. L., Seo, T., Matlak, M. E., et al. (1995). Gastrointestinal function after surgical correction of Hirschsprung's disease: Long-term follow-up in 135 patients. *Journal of Pediatric Surgery, 30*(5), 655-658.

Marty, T. L., Seo, T., Sullivan, J. J., et al. (1995). Rectal irrigations for the prevention of postoperative enterocolitis in Hirschsprung's disease. *Journal of Pediatric Surgery, 30*(5), 652–654.

Maxson, R. T., Jackson, R. J., & Smith, S. D. (1995). The protective role of enteral IgA supplementation in neonatal gut origin sepsis. *Journal of Pediatric Surgery, 30*(2), 231–234.

Mayr, J., Fasching, G., & Hollwarth, M. E. (1994). Psychosocial and psychomotoric development of very low birthweight infants with necrotizing enterocolitis. *Acta Paediatrica, 83*(Suppl. 396), 96–100.

McCallum, R. W. (1991). Cisapride: A new class of prokinetic agent. *American Journal of Gastroenterology, 86*(2), 135–149.

McCormack, M. K. (1979). Medical genetics and family practice. *American Family Physician, 20*(3), 142–154.

Meire, F., Standaert, L., deLaey, J. J., & Zeng, L. H. (1987). Waardenburg syndrome, Hirschsprung megacolon, and Marcus Gunn ptosis. *American Journal of Medical Genetics, 27*(3), 683–686.

Meller, J. L., Reyes, H. M., & Loeff, D. S. (1989). Gastroschisis and omphalocele. *Clinics in Perinatology, 16*(1), 113–122.

Merenstein, G. B. (1970). Rectal perforation by thermometer. *Lancet, 1*(7654), 1007.

Merenstein, G. B., & Gardner, S. L. (1989). *Handbook of neonatal intensive care.* St. Louis: C. V. Mosby.

Messineo, A., MacMillan, J. H., Palder, S. B., & Filler, R. M. (1992). Clinical factors affecting mortality in children with malrotation of the intestine. *Journal of Pediatric Surgery, 27*(10), 1343–1345.

Methany, N. M. (1987). *Fluid and electrolyte balance: Nursing considerations.* Philadelphia: J. B. Lippincott.

Meyers, W. F., & Herbst, J. J. (1982). Effectiveness of positioning therapy for gastroesophageal reflux. *Pediatrics, 69*(6), 768–772.

Meyers, W. F., Roberts, C. C., Johnson, D. G., & Herbst, J. J. (1985). Value of tests for evaluation of gastroesophageal reflux in children. *Journal of Pediatric Surgery, 20*(5), 515–520.

Mitchell, L. E., & Risch, N. (1993). The genetics of infantile hypertrophic pyloric stenosis: A reanalysis. *American Journal of Diseases of Children, 147*(11), 1203–1211.

Moog, F. (1981). The lining of the small intestine. *Scientific American, 245*(5), 154–176.

Moore, K. L., & Persaud, T. V. N. (1993). *Before we are born: Basic embryology and birth defects* (4th ed.). Philadelphia: W. B. Saunders.

Moore, S. W., Millar, A. J. W., & Cywes, S. (1994). Long-term clinical, manometric, and histological evaluation of obstructive symptoms in the postoperative Hirschsprung's patient. *Journal of Pediatric Surgery, 29*(1), 106–111.

Morecroft, J. A., Spitz, L., Hamilton, P. A., & Holmes, S. J. K. (1994). Necrotizing enterocolitis—multisystem organ failure of the newborn? *Acta Paediatrica, 83*(Suppl. 296), 21–23.

Morrison, S. C., & Jacobson, J. M. (1994). The radiology of necrotizing enterocolitis. *Clinics in Perinatology, 21*(2), 347–363.

Morrison, S. C., Fletcher, B. D., & Yulish, B. S (1992). Diagnostic imaging. In A. A. Fanaroff & R. J. Martin (Eds.), *Neonatal-perinatal medicine: Diseases of the fetus and infant* (5th ed., pp. 543–563). St. Louis: C. V. Mosby.

Morriss, F. H., Moore M., Weisbrodt, N. W., & West, M. S. (1986). Ontogenic development of gastrointestinal motility: IV. Duodenal contractions in preterm infants. *Pediatrics, 78*(6), 1106–1113.

Musemeche, C. A., Kosloske, A. M., Bartow, S. A., & Umland, E. T. (1986). Comparative effects of ischemia, bacteria, and substrate on the pathogenesis of intestinal necrosis. *Journal of Pediatric Surgery, 21*(6), 536–538.

Nagaya, M., Akatsuka, H., & Kato, J. (1994). Gastroesophageal reflux occurring after repair of congenital diaphragmatic hernia. *Journal of Pediatric Surgery, 29*(11), 1447–1451.

Norris, H. T. (1973). Response of the small intestine to the application of a hypertonic solution. *American Journal of Pathology, 73*(3), 747–759.

Nowicki, P. T., & Nankervis, C. A. (1994). The role of the circulation in the pathogenesis of necrotizing enterocolitis. *Clinics in Perinatology, 21*(2), 219–234.

Oellrich, R. G., & Cusumano, M. M. (1987). Biliary atresia. *Neonatal Network, 5*(5), 25–32.

Oka, S. W. (1979). Epidemiology and genetics of clefting: With implications for etiology. In H. K. Cooper, R. L. Harding, W. M. Krogman, et al. (Eds.), *Cleft palate and cleft lip: A team approach to clinical management and rehabilitation of the patient* (pp. 108–143). Philadelphia: W. B. Saunders.

Orenstein, S. R. (1992). Controversies in pediatric gastroesophageal reflux. *Journal of Pediatric Gastroenterology and Nutrition, 14*(3), 338–348.

Orenstein, S. R., Magill, H. L., & Brooks, P. (1987). Thickening of infant feedings for therapy of gastroesophageal reflux. *Journal of Pediatrics, 110*(2), 181–186.

Orenstein, S. R., Shalaby, T. M., & Putnam, P. E. (1992). Thickened feedings as a cause of increased coughing when used as therapy for gastroesophageal reflux in infants. *Journal of Pediatrics 121*(6), 913–915.

Parigi, G. B., Bragheri, R., Minniti, S., & Verga, G. (1994). Surgical treatment of necrotizing enterocolitis: When? How? *Acta Paediatrica, 83*(Suppl. 296), 58–61.

Pate, C. M. H. (1987). Care of the family following the birth of a child with a cleft lip and/or palate. *Neonatal Network, 5*(6), 30–37.

Pereira, G. R., & Ziegler, M. M. (1989). Nutritional care of the surgical neonate. *Clinics in Perinatology, 16*(1), 233–253.

Philippart, A. I., Reed, J. O., & Georgeson, K. E. (1975). Neonatal small left colon syndrome: Intramural not intraluminal obstruction. *Journal of Pediatric Surgery, 10*(5), 733–740.

Pickering, L. K., & Adcock, E. W. (1980). Gastrointestinal disorders in infants. *Family Practice Annual, 2*, 57–76.

Poland, R. L., & Ostrea, E. M. (1993). Neonatal hyperbilirubinemia. In M. H. Klaus & A. A. Fanaroff (Eds.), *Care of the high-risk neonate* (4th ed., pp. 302–322). Philadelphia: W. B. Saunders.

Rabinowitz, J. G., & Siegle, R. L. (1976). Changing clinical and roentgenographic patterns of necrotizing enterocolitis. *American Journal of Roentgenology, 126*(3), 560–566.

Rachelson, M. H., Jernigan, J. P., & Jackson, W. F. (1955). Intussusception in the newborn infant with spontaneous expulsion of the intussusception. *Journal of Pediatrics, 47*(1), 87–94.

Ravelli, A. M., Spitz, L., & Milla, P. J. (1994). Gastric emptying in children with gastric transposition. *Journal of Pediatric Gastroenterology and Nutrition, 19*(4), 403–409.

Reyes, H. M., Meller, J. L., & Loeff, D. (1989). Neonatal intestinal obstruction. *Clinics in Perinatology, 16*(1), 85–96.

Reyna, T. M. (1994). Familial Hirschsprung's disease: Study of a Texas cohort. *Pediatrics, 94*(3), 347–349.

Richey, D. A. (1990). Transporting the infant with an abdominal wall defect. *Neonatal Network, 9*(2), 53–56.

Richman, R. A., Sheehe, P. R., McCanty, T., et al. (1988). Olfactory deficits in boys with cleft palate. *Pediatrics, 82*(6), 840–844.

Ricketts, R. R. (1984). Workup of neonatal intestinal obstruction. *American Surgeon, 50*(10), 517–521.

Ricketts, R. R. (1994). Surgical treatment of necrotizing enterocolitis and the short bowel syndrome. *Clinics in Perinatology, 21*(2), 365–387.

Ricketts, R. R., & Jerles, M. L. (1990). Neonatal necrotizing enterocolitis: Experience with 100 consecutive surgical patients. *World Journal of Surgery, 14*(5), 600–605.

Rintala, R., Mildh, L., & Lindahl, H. (1994)). Fecal continence and quality of life for adult patients with an operated high or intermediate anorectal malformation. *Journal of Pediatric Surgery, 29*(6), 777–780.

Rivosecchi, M., Lucchetti, M. C., Zaccara, A., et al. (1995). Spinal dysraphism detected by magnetic resonance imaging in patients with anorectal anomalies: Incidence and clinical significance. *Journal of Pediatric Surgery, 30*(3), 488–490.

Roberts, F. B. (1977). *Perinatal nursing: Care of newborns and their families.* New York: McGraw-Hill.

Roy, C. C. (1987). Intestinal adaptation, maturation and related disorders. In L. Stern & P. Vert (Eds.), *Neonatal medicine* (pp. 987–1011). New York: Masson Publishing.

Rubaltelli, F. F., Benini, F., & Sala, M. (1991). Prevention of necrotizing enterocolitis in neonates at risk by oral administration of monomeric IgG1. *Developmental Pharmacology Therapeutics, 17*(3–4), 138–143.

Rushton, C. H. (1990). Necrotizing enterocolitis: Part II. Treatment and nursing care. *MCN, American Journal of Maternal Child Nursing, 15*(5), 309–313.

Ryckman, F. C., Flake, A. W., & Balistreri, W. F. (1992). Upper gastrointestinal disorders. In A. A. Fanaroff & R. J. Martin (Eds.), *Neonatal-perinatal medicine: Diseases of the fetus and infant* (5th ed., pp. 1024–1029). St. Louis: C. V. Mosby.

Saal, H. M., & Rosenbaum, K. N. (1988). Screening the newborn for anatomic and metabolic defects. *Pediatric Annals, 17*(7), 467–476.

Sadler, T. W. (1985). *Langman's medical embryology* (5th ed.). Baltimore: Williams & Wilkins.

Santulli, T. V., Schullinger, J. N., Heird, W. C., et al. (1975). Acute necrotizing enterocolitis in infancy: A review of 64 cases. *Pediatrics, 55*(3), 376–387.

Saxen, I. (1975). Epidemiology of cleft lip and palate. *British Journal of Preventive and Social Medicine, 29*(2), 103–110.

Scanlon, J. W., Nelson, T., Grylack, L. J., & Smith, Y. F. (1979). *A system of newborn physical examination.* Baltimore: University Park Press.

Schneider, E. L. (1973). Lip pits and congenital absence of second premolars: Varied expression of the lip pits syndrome. *Journal of Medical Genetics, 10*(4), 346–349.

Schober, P. H., & Nassiri, J. (1994). Risk factors and severity indices in necrotizing enterocolitis. *Acta Paediatrica, 83*(Suppl. 396), 49–52.

Seashore, J. H. (1978). Congenital abdominal wall defects. *Clinics in Perinatology, 5*(1), 61–77.

Seashore, J. H., & Touloukian, R. J. (1994). Midgut volvulus: An ever-present threat. *Archives of Pediatrics and Adolescent Medicine, 148*(1), 43–46.

Seashore, J. H., Collins, F. S., Markowitz, R. I., & Seashore, M. R. (1987). Familial apple peel jejunal atresia: Surgical, genetic, and radiographic aspects. *Pediatrics, 80*(4), 540–544.

Shah, C. P., & Wong D. (1980). Management of children with cleft lip and palate. *Canadian Medical Association Journal, 122*(1), 19–24.

Shanbhogue, R. L. K., Hussain, S. M., Meradji, M., et al. (1994). Ultrasonography is accurate enough for the diagnosis of intussusception. *Journal of Pediatric Surgery, 29*(2), 324–328.

Sherry, S. N., & Kramer, I. (1955). The time of passage of the first stool and first urine by the newborn infant. *Journal of Pediatrics, 46*(2), 158–159.

Shiels, W. E. (1995). Childhood intussusception: Management perspectives in 1995. *Journal of Pediatric Gastroenterology and Nutrition, 21*(1), 15–17.

Sigalet, D. L., Nguyen, L. T., Adolph, V., et al. (1994). Gastroesophageal reflux associated with large diaphragmatic hernias. *Journal of Pediatric Surgery, 29*(9), 1262–1265.

Singleton, E. B. (1963). Radiologic evaluation of intestinal obstruction in the newborn. *Radiologic Clinics of North America, 1*(3), 571–581.

Sinkin, R. A., Phillips, B. L., & Adelman, R. D. (1985). Elevation in systemic blood pressure in the neonate during abdominal examination. *Pediatrics, 76*(6), 970–972.

Smith, C. A. (1976). Physiology of the digestive tract. In C. A. Smith & N. M. Nelson (Eds.), *The physiology of the newborn infant* (4th ed., pp. 459–479). Springfield, IL: Charles C Thomas.

Spitz, L., Kiely, E. M., Morecroft, J. A., & Drake, D. P. (1994). Oesophageal atresia: At-risk groups for the 1990s. *Journal of Pediatric Surgery, 29*(6), 723–725.

Stoll, B. J. (1994). Epidemiology of necrotizing enterocolitis. *Clinics in Perinatology, 21*(2), 205–218.

Stringer, M. D., Brereton, R. J., Drake, D. P., et al. (1994). Meconium ileus due to extensive intestinal aganglionosis. *Journal of Pediatric Surgery, 29*(4), 501–503.

Stringer, M. D., Brereton, R. J., Drake, D. P., et al. (1993). Recurrent necrotizing enterocolitis. *Journal of Pediatric Surgery, 28*(8), 979–981.

Styer, G. W., & Freeh, K. (1981). Feeding infants with cleft lip and/or palate. *Journal of Obstetric, Gynecologic, and Neonatal Nursing, 10*(5), 329–332.

Sugar, E. C. (1981). Hirschsprung's disease. *American Journal of Nursing, 81*(11), 2065–2067.

Surana, R., Quinn, F. M. J., & Puri, P. (1994). Short-gut syndrome: Intestinal adaptation in a patient with 12 cm of jejunum. *Journal of Pediatric Gastroenterology and Nutrition, 19*(2), 246–249.

Swaniker, F., Guo, W., Fonkalsrud, E. W., et al. (1995). Adaptation of rabbit small intestinal brush-border membrane enzymes after extensive bowel resection. *Journal of Pediatric Surgery, 30*(7), 1000–1003.

Tappero, E. P., & Honeyfield, M. E. (1996). *Physical assessment of the newborn: A comprehensive approach to the art of physical examination* (2nd ed.). Petaluma, CA: NICU Ink.

Taylor, E. J. (Ed.). (1988). *Dorland's illustrated medical dictionary* (27th ed.). Philadelphia: W. B. Saunders.

Topalian, S. L., & Ziegler, M. M. (1984). Necrotizing enterocolitis: A review of animal models. *Journal of Surgical Research, 37*(4), 320–336.

Touloukian, R. J. (1978). Intestinal atresia. *Clinics in Perinatology, 5*(1), 3–18.

Tsakayannis, D. E., & Shamberger, R. C. (1995). Association of imperforate anus with occult spinal dysraphism. *Journal of Pediatric Surgery, 30*(7), 1010–1012.

Vander, A. J., Sherman, J. H., & Luciano, D. S. (1975). *Human physiology: The mechanisms of body function* (2nd ed.). New York: McGraw-Hill.

Vanderhoof, J. A., Zach, T. L, & Adrian, T. E. (1994). Gastrointestinal Disease. In G. B. Avery, M. A. Fletcher, & M. G. MacDonald (Eds.), *Neonatalology: Pathophysiology and management of the newborn* (4th ed., pp. 605–629). Philadelphia: J. B. Lippincott.

Vasan, U., & Gotoff, S. P. (1994). Prevention of neonatal necrotizing enterocolitis. *Clinics in Perinatology, 21*(2), 425–435.

Verma, A., & Dhanireddy, R. (1993). Time of first stool in extremely low birth weight (≤1000 grams) infants. *Journal of Pediatrics, 122*(4), 626–629.

Walantas, R. J. (1986). Discordant microform cleft lip in a dizygotic female twin. *Journal of Obstetric, Gynecologic, and Neonatal Nursing, 15*(6), 467–470.

Warner, B. W., & Ziegler, M. M. (1993). Management of the short bowel syndrome in the pediatric population. *Pediatric Clinics of North America, 40*(6), 1335–1350.

Wells, P. W., & Meghdadpour, S. (1988). Research yields new clues to cystic fibrosis. *MCN, American Journal of Maternal Child Nursing, 13*(3), 187–190.

White, K. C., & Harkavy, K. L. (1982). Hypertonic formula resulting from added oral medications. *American Journal of Diseases of Children, 136*(10), 931–933.

Wiswell, T. E., Robertson, C. F., Jones, T. A., & Tuttle, D. J. (1988). Necrotizing enterocolitis in full-term infants: A case-control study. *American Journal of Diseases of Children, 142*(5), 532–535.

Wolf, H. M., & Eibl, M. M. (1994). The anti-inflammatory effect of an oral immunoglobulin (IgA-IgG) preparation and its possible relevance for the prevention of necrotizing enterocolitis. *Acta Paediatrica, 83*(Suppl. 396), 37–40.

Woodhurst, W. B., & Kliman, M. R. (1976). Neonatal small left colon syndrome: Report of two cases. *American Surgeon, 42*(7), 479–481.

Yazbeck, S., & Bensoussan, A. L. (1987). Omphalocele and gastroschisis. In L. Stern & P. Vert (Eds.), *Neonatal medicine* (pp. 1078–1081). New York: Masson Publishing.

Young, T. E., & Mangum, O. B. (1997). *Neofax '97: A manual of drugs used in neonatal care* (10th ed.). Columbus, OH: Ross Products Division, Abbott Laboratories.

Youssef, S. (1987). Congenital megacolon. In L. Stern & P. Vert (Eds.), *Neonatal medicine* (pp. 1073–1075). New York: Masson Publishing.

Zheng, J. Y., Frush, D. P., & Guo, J. Z. (1994). Review of pneumatic reduction of intussusception: Evolution, not revolution. *Journal of Pediatric Surgery, 29*(1), 93–97.

Zink, M. (1985). Biliary atresia: Nursing diagnoses and management. *Journal of Enterostomal Therapy, 12*(4), 128–139.

CHAPTER 25

Assessment and Management of Metabolic Dysfunction

CATHERINE JURSICH THEORELL MARGUERITE DEGENHARDT

RESEARCH AGENDA

What are the risk factors that predispose a neonate to inborn errors of metabolism?

What are the fetal and neonatal effects of adherence to a normal diet during the pregnancy of a mother with PKU?

What is the impact on parent–infant interaction when there is a diagnosis of a metabolic disease?

What is the effect of social support on a family coping with a metabolic disease?

Should all infants be tested for several metabolic diseases even though some of the diseases have no cure?

VIGNETTE

John and Sarah were thrilled the day they brought their new baby, a first-born child, home from the hospital. Sarah's pregnancy had been uncomplicated. She spontaneously went into labor at term. Labor proceeded as expected with an unmedicated vaginal delivery. Anthony weighed 8 lb, 1 oz, and was 21 inches. His Apgar scores were 8 and 10. Discharge was planned for 48 hours post delivery, just after completion of the required PKU test.

Things were going well for Sarah and Anthony. Sarah had chosen to breastfeed. Both she and the baby found this to be a very satisfying experience. Then a shocking call came from the pediatrician 2 weeks later. Anthony had an abnormal result of the test for PKU. It was only a screening test, but Sarah was instructed to take the baby immediately to the hospital for another blood test. Sarah remembered a pamphlet from the hospital, something about PKU and mental retardation. What a horrible mistake; anyone could see that Anthony was perfect!

The team at the Metabolic Disease Center was notified of the possibility of a new baby with PKU. They responded to the anxious parents and doctor by offering to repeat the test the same day if the parents and baby could get to the hospital by noon.

The second test result was positive, with a serum phenylalanine level of 60 mg/dl. A normal value is less than 2 mg/dl. A family meeting was arranged for the same day. Our immediate goal was to begin a diet designed to lower the blood phenylalanine level and thereby protect the infant's developing brain.

As we arrived in the clinic area, we saw Sarah cuddling her baby. John was pale with downcast eyes. I introduced myself as the team nurse. Sarah, almost in tears, told me angrily that the nurse who drew the baby's blood had stuck him twice and she was not sure that people knew what they were doing. I agreed that it was upsetting to be summoned for a blood test for some obscure unpronounceable disease.

Sarah was in tremendous shock and pain on hearing that her little Anthony had a rare genetic disease called PKU. Sarah and John's responses were typical. Denial and anger are common defenses. Initially the parents need time to vent their feelings. After I acknowledged how frightening the situation was, Sarah was able to express how upsetting and confusing it seemed. She again pointed out how normal and healthy Anthony was.

For a child with PKU, our job is to work with the family to prevent brain damage and permit the child to develop as a normal and healthy person. However, the nurse is aware that denial of the disease on the part of the parents can jeopardize the success of the diet. Teaching the parents about the disease and the underlying biochemical defect is an essential part of helping the family cope with the treatment.

I asked Sarah if she had ever heard of PKU before our meeting. She said that she knew it had something to do with mental retardation and burst into tears. Over the years, I came to realize that the words "mental retardation" frightened parents to such a degree that they often were unable to hear the subsequent discussion.

Asking the parents to repeat their understanding of PKU and the reason for the diet often uncovers or elucidates areas that need more explanation. I provided John and Sarah with some simple written information so that once they were home they could again go over the facts about the disease.

The successful treatment of PKU, although familiar to experts in the field of metabolic diseases, is still not well understood by the community. PKU is rare; it occurs in 1 in 15,000 births. The average pediatrician does not see a single patient with PKU in a lifetime of practice. The stigma and fears associated with mental retardation may loom so large that the fact that there is a successful treatment is lost. Therefore, the nurse listens carefully to learn what the family fears the most and then proceeds to clarify and reassure as indicated. Sarah began to relax as I reassured her that the majority of children did very well. I thought of my peer counselors who had spent hours explaining to anxious parents like Sarah and John how bringing their special formula to school was a "pain" but could be done.

Both parents began asking questions about the diet. As my

colleague, the team's nutritionist, started to outline the treatment, the mysteries of the diet unfolded. The baby would be fed a special formula supplemented with small amounts of milk. At this the mother again broke into tears, exclaiming she would have to stop breastfeeding. No, she did not have to stop breastfeeding entirely. Yes, it would take extra effort to continue, but it was possible. The baby's protein requirements would be met with the special formula, one in which the phenylalanine had been reduced. Since phenylalanine was essential to normal growth, the baby would need a certain amount of phenylalanine from natural foods. Breast milk could certainly be used, but in small amounts. Anthony's tolerance for phenylalanine in mother's milk would be determined by frequently measuring his blood phenylalanine concentrations. The mother again relaxed at the thought that she might be able to continue partial breastfeeding.

The family left with a new feeding plan, telephone numbers for questions, and clearly written instructions. The months ahead were trying for the family. The nurse would not only review information about PKU with the immediate family as well as with grandmothers and grandfathers, aunts and uncles, and other caretakers, but also point out the baby's healthy development and praise and encourage the family for their good efforts. Questions about everything from birthday parties to athletics to future pregnancies would be explored.

The diet would be the mainstay of the treatment for Anthony. There is new research into improvements not only with the diet, such as VIL, but also in the molecular area. Prenatal diagnosis is already available, and there is the possibility of an eventual treatment in the form of a genetic cure. However, for a nurse watching families cope with the needs of children with genetic diseases, nothing holds more hope than watching one of our young patients with PKU blossom into a fine adult.

Pamela White

Metabolic dysfunction in the neonate is a relatively rare occurrence that is not always identified until after discharge from the neonatal intensive care unit (NICU). Most dysfunctions of this system result from inborn errors of metabolism that are linked to genetic disturbances in DNA synthesis. It is essential for these problems to be detected as early as possible if long-term complications such as developmental delays and mental retardation are to be avoided. This chapter describes prenatal and postnatal detection, biochemical defects and clinical manifestations of some of the more common metabolic disorders, and their collaborative management.

ROUTINE NEONATAL SCREENING TESTS

The purpose of routine neonatal screening for metabolic disease is to search for the population of individuals with a certain genotype, or change of the gene structure, that either is already associated with the disease or predisposes the carrier to the disease. It involves the nonselective testing of large numbers of newborns with the aim of identifying individuals with disorders caused by mutant genes. Implicit in the concept of neonatal screening is the availability of specific treatment, the hope of improved medical management, and the availability of informative genetic counseling (Ampola, 1982; Benson, 1983; Duran et al., 1994; Fost, 1992; Hammersen & Bickel, 1982; Holtzman, 1992; Irons, 1993; Natowicz & Alper, 1991; Paul et al., 1980; Wu, 1991).

Routine neonatal screening occurred after Bickel's demonstration of the effectiveness of phenylalanine-restricted diets in phenylketonuria (PKU) (Bickel et al., 1954). Before this time, no treatment existed for newborns with PKU, and survivors had severe neurologic and mental impairment. In addition, at that time, the method for screening urine for phenylpyruvic acid was unsuccessful in detecting this disorder in newborns, because the urinary levels of phenylpyruvic acid may not become elevated for weeks despite markedly high plasma levels of phenylalanine (Paul et al., 1980). By the time that PKU could be detected by this test, severe neurologic impairment had occurred. Early identification of affected newborns was then needed to ensure maximum effectiveness of phenylalanine restriction on neurologic outcome.

It was not until 1962 that Guthrie's development of a bacterial inhibition assay of whole blood for phenylalanine made available a reliable, specific screening measure to identify newborns with PKU (Bickel et al., 1980). Guthrie's test is based on the inhibition of bacterial growth of certain species by biochemical compounds normally present in whole blood disk specimens. The elevated blood phenylalanine levels in newborns with PKU resulted in more vigorous bacterial growth around the blood specimen in direct proportion to the elevation of phenylalanine (Bickel et al., 1980). Thus elevations in blood phenylalanine levels could be identified and quantified. The ingenuity of this test was not the microbiologic test per se but the method of using a capillary whole blood specimen impregnated on filter paper. In addition to PKU, Guthrie adapted his bacteriologic test to other disorders, including defects in the metabolism of leucine, methionine, histidine, lysine, tyrosine, and galactose, by using different inhibitors and different bacterial strains (Bickel et al., 1980; Crawford et al., 1982; LeGrys, 1984; Nyhan, 1984).

The Guthrie bacterial inhibition assay is considered the most significant contribution to screening populations for metabolic diseases (Ampola, 1982; Hammersen & Bickel, 1982; Wapnir, 1985). Thus the research conducted on PKU demonstrated that neonatal screening programs were feasible and practical and that defects with a fixed genotype do respond to therapeutic interventions (Ampola, 1982; Benson, 1983; Bickel, 1980; Cockburn & Gitzelmann, 1980; Crawford et al., 1982; Dhondt et al., 1991; Durand-Zaleski et al., 1992; Galjaard, 1980; Komrower, 1980; Scriver et al., 1995a, 1995b; Wu, 1991).

Since the discoveries related to PKU, research on inherited metabolic disorders has intensified. The explosion of knowledge has helped identify affected individuals as early as the first trimester of pregnancy, define the biochemical complexities of metabolic disease, and propose and evaluate new treatment modalities. Despite these rapid advances, the understanding of metabolism and metabolic disorders is not yet complete.

The success of widespread screening for PKU in newborns led to the belief that all metabolic disorders could be identified in a similar manner. Although theoretically possible in numerous cases, mass screening for all metabolic disorders is not justifiable. A screening test to detect a metabolic disorder is readily justifiable when it can be used for the same blood sample used for PKU and when the corresponding disorder is relatively frequent in the population tested and effectively treatable (Benson, 1983; Bickel et al., 1980; Crawford et al., 1982; Fanaroff & Martin, 1997; Fost, 1992; Hammersen & Bickel, 1982; Levy & Hammersen, 1978; Holtzman, 1992; Irons, 1993; Paul et al., 1980; Stern & Vert, 1987). For example, screening for congenital hypothyroidism by thyroid-stimulating hormone (TSH) analysis is justifiable, because the disorder occurs in 1 in 3500 births, a sensitive, specific measure is available, and early initiation of treatment limits the severity of the resulting mental disorders (Benson, 1983; Bickel et al., 1980; Dhondt et al., 1991; Durand-Zaleski et al., 1992; Hammersen & Bickel, 1982; Missiou-Tsagaraki, 1992).

In 1978, the International Symposium on Newborn Screening for Inborn Errors of Metabolism was held in Heidelberg, and the National Academy of Sciences defined criteria for the selection of diseases amenable to neonatal screening. These criteria are the following: (1) The disease presents a significant problem when the diagnosis is delayed (i.e., high rates of mortality and morbidity); (2) the condition occurs in a population with a high frequency; (3) the condition is amenable to treatment; (4) a simple, inexpensive screening method is available; (5) the test is sensitive and specific, and quality control is maintained; (6) there exists a mechanism for collecting samples and delivering them to the laboratory; (7) a reliable means of reporting results exists; (8) resources for treatment or counseling are available; and (9) the cost of screening, diagnosis, and treatment during the asymptomatic phase is outweighed by savings in human misery and fiscal expenditure (Benson, 1983; Bickel et al., 1980; Crawford et al., 1982; Dhondt et al., 1991; Hammersen & Bickel, 1982; Holtzman, 1992; Levy & Hammersen, 1978; Paul et al., 1980).

Using these criteria, the symposium members identified four diseases for which there are reliable tests for large-scale screening of infants and that should receive priority in detection: (1) PKU; (2) congenital hypothyroidism; (3) galactosemia; and (4) maple syrup urine disease (MSUD) (Benson, 1983; Bickel et al., 1980; Crawford et al., 1982; Hammersen & Bickel, 1982; Irons, 1993; Scriver et al., 1995a; Wu, 1991). The symposium also identified three other diseases—tyrosinemia, homocystinuria, and histidinemia—that cannot be considered for priority screening because they have important clinical variants that escape detection on testing (homocystinuria, tyrosinemia) or because treatment has not proved effective (histidinemia) (Benson, 1983; Bickel et al., 1980; Crawford et al., 1982; Hammersen & Bickel, 1982; Irons, 1993; Scriver et al., 1995a; Wu, 1991). Today some states (e.g., Ohio) do, however, require the test for homocystinuria. Four years after the Heidelberg symposium, the priority diseases amenable to routine neonatal screening were expanded to include a fifth test to detect congenital adrenal hyperplasia (Benson, 1983; Bickel et al., 1980; Hammersen & Bickel, 1982; Irons, 1993; Scriver et al., 1995a, 1995b; Wu, 1991).

Other amino acid disorders, the organic acidurias, the transport disorders, and cystic fibrosis are not routinely screened. Tests for hemoglobin disorders and hemolytic anemias resulting from erythrocyte abnormalities can be proposed only for high-risk groups. However, in 1989 Ohio mandated routine neonatal screening for hemoglobinopathies sickle cell anemia and beta-thalassemia (Scriver et al., 1995a, 1995b). Screening for hyperlipidemias should be performed only in high-risk families (Benson, 1983; Bickel et al., 1980; Crawford et al., 1982; Hammersen & Bickel, 1982; Irons, 1993; Scriver et al., 1995a, 1995b).

Neonatal screening, the purpose of which is to diagnose shortly after birth the infants with genetic diseases for which early treatment will prevent or minimize serious, irreversible complications or even death, is not mandated by the federal government. The first mandatory screening law to detect PKU was passed in 1963 in Massachusetts (Bickel et al., 1980; Hammersen & Bickel, 1982); since then, each state has defined which tests are to be included in the routine newborn screen. As the genetic complexities of more metabolic disorders are understood, the neonatal screening tests may change over time and from state to state. The United States Department of Health Resources and Services Administration, in the Department of Health and Human Services (DHHS), has developed a manual entitled "Newborn Screening: An Overview of Newborn Screening Programs in the United States and Canada." Originally published in the 1980s, the manual is updated every 3 years to provide the current state-by-state parameters for their neonatal screening programs, testing methods, and follow-up for affected families. To obtain a copy of the manual, readers are referred to their medical center libraries or their states' Departments of Public Health.

PRENATAL AND NEONATAL DIAGNOSIS OF INHERITED METABOLIC DISORDERS

The prenatal diagnosis of inherited metabolic disorders developed concurrently with the advances in chromosomal analysis, molecular genetics, and fetal cell culture. Successful growth of fetal cells in culture soon had researchers interested in investigating the enzymatic machinery of these tissues and resulted in the prenatal diagnosis of a substantial number of inherited metabolic disorders. Each year additional information that facilitates the prenatal diagnosis of increasing numbers of metabolic disorders is discovered.

The prenatal diagnosis of inherited metabolic disorders is not often indicated (Bickel, 1980; Bickel et al., 1980; Crawford et al., 1982; Durand-Zaleski et al., 1992; Fost, 1992; Hammersen & Bickel, 1982; Natowicz & Alper, 1991; Scriver et al., 1995a, 1995b). Because most inherited metabolic disorders are rare, and some extremely so, prenatal diagnosis involves a delicate balance that demands a thorough understanding of the technical, biochemical, ethical, and psychological difficulties experienced by those involved.

Prenatal screening via amniocentesis, chorionic villus sampling, or cordocentesis can be carried out in a considerable number of metabolic disorders (Gregory, 1992; Rossiter & Johnson, 1992; Scriver et al., 1995a, 1995b). These procedures require sophisticated techniques and should be performed only by laboratories experienced in these procedures. However, certain metabolic conditions are not amenable to prenatal investigation (Evans & Shulman, 1991) and necessitate postnatal screening at the earliest opportunity. In addition, prenatal screening is not justifiable when satisfactory treatment is available after early postnatal diagnosis (Bickel et al., 1980; Hammersen & Bickel, 1982; Dhondt et al., 1991; Durand-Zaleski et al., 1992; Fost, 1992; Holtzman, 1992; Natowicz & Alper, 1991; Scriver et al., 1995a, 1995b).

Newborns are not screened for all inherited metabolic disorders. Only newborns suspected of having an inherited metabolic disorder should undergo the rigorous investigation of metabolism. If a neonatal screening test is positive for an inherited metabolic disorder (e.g., PKU), the investigation is not complete. It is important not to make a diagnosis of an inherited metabolic disorder too quickly. Ancillary tests are often needed to confirm the diagnosis and avoid errors in management. For example, galactosuria can be observed in newborns without galactosemia or galactokinase deficiency (Levy & Hammersen, 1978; Scriver et al., 1995a, 1995b). Also, an increase in serum phenylalanine, tyrosine, and methionine levels may be observed in various hepatic disorders or in immature newborns receiving excessive protein intake (Benson, 1983; Blaskovics et al., 1974; Fanaroff & Martin, 1997; Nyhan, 1984; Scriver et al., 1995a, 1995b). Severe hyperammonemia is not always caused by a specific enzyme deficiency but may be due to hepatic dysfunction from other causes (Ballard et al., 1978). If there is severe hypoglycemia, hyperinsulinemia should first be ruled out, especially if there is no ketosis present (Cornblath et al., 1963; Cornblath & Schwartz, 1966; Ogata, 1986; Scriver et al., 1995a, 1995b; Wallach, 1983).

In the analysis and investigation of metabolic disorders, a positive screening test result must be followed up with complementary determinations of compounds. For example, a positive result of the screening test for PKU must be followed up by determining the levels of phenylalanine, tyrosine, orthohydroxyphenylacetic acid, phenylpyruvic acid, and urinary biopterins to confirm the diagnosis and specify the exact type of hyperphenylalaninemia (Blaskovics et al., 1974; Qu et al., 1991; Scriver et al., 1995a, 1995b). This confirmational stage is critical because moderate transient hyperphenylalaninemias and immaturity tyrosinemias are frequent and do not necessitate treatment, whereas biopterin deficiency as a cause for hyperphenylalaninemia does not respond to dietary restrictions and necessitates different treatment; thus moderate increases in phenylalanine should not be falsely reassuring (Ampola, 1982; Benson, 1983; Bickel et al., 1980; Bickel et al., 1954; Blaskovics et al., 1974; Cockburn & Gitzelmann, 1980; Crawford et al., 1982; Lloyd & Scriver, 1985; Nyhan, 1984;

Scriver et al., 1995a, 1995b; Winick, 1979). For more information, see the section on hyperphenylalaninemias later in this chapter.

Clinical manifestations of inherited metabolic disorders may be general or specific (Schmidt, 1989). The nurse has the first opportunity to take a detailed history from the parents. Often, there is a history of recurrent spontaneous abortions (Shaw et al., 1991), unexplained neonatal deaths, or psychomotor deficiencies in the family, and a precise study of genealogy is warranted (Clark & Cockburn, 1991; Rossiter & Johnson, 1992). Specific investigation of consanguinity should be performed to analyze for the presence of an autosomal recessive disorder. An X-linked disorder might be suspected if male siblings, cousins, and uncles are affected. The medical histories of siblings should be analyzed for the occurrence of neonatal deaths or abnormalities, even if they were supposedly caused by acquired disorders such as septicemia, anoxia, or subarachnoid hemorrhages. Previous children with a history of hypoglycemia, acute encephalopathy, ataxia, metabolic acidosis, hepatomegaly, or acute episodes of "intoxication" or vomiting should increase suspicion that an inherited metabolic disorder may exist (Clark & Cockburn, 1991; Irons, 1993; Schmidt, 1989; Scriver et al., 1995a, 1995b).

Circumstances leading to the onset of symptoms are very important in the investigation of inherited metabolic disorders. An important negative finding is the absence of fetal or perinatal distress that may explain the abnormalities. Metabolic disorders are often characterized by an interval of variable duration during which the newborn is apparently normal. For example, in Tay-Sachs disease, the clinical manifestations may take months to appear; in MSUD, the symptoms appear after 5 to 6 days; and in pyruvate carboxylase deficiency, symptoms begin several hours after birth (Ampola, 1982; Benson, 1983; Bickel et al., 1980; Cockburn & Gitzelmann, 1980; Crawford et al., 1982; Fanaroff & Martin, 1997; Galjaard, 1980; Irons, 1993; Komrower, 1980; Levy & Hammersen, 1978; Lloyd & Scriver, 1985; Natowicz & Alper, 1991; Schmidt, 1989; Scriver et al., 1995a, 1995b; Wapnir, 1985). Clinical manifestations may also take on an intermittent or cyclic character brought about by increases in protein intake or tissue catabolism (Ampola, 1982; Benson, 1983; Bickel et al., 1980; Cockburn & Gitzelmann, 1980; Cohn & Roth, 1983; Crawford et al., 1982; Dixon & Leonard, 1992; Komrower, 1980; Lloyd & Scriver, 1985; Scriver et al., 1995a, 1995b; Thomas, 1992).

Often, the neonate with an inherited metabolic disorder exhibits neurologic manifestations such as hypotonia, hypertonia, lethargy, alternating hyperexcitability and somnolence, myoclonia, abnormal eye movements, alteration in levels of consciousness, coma, and seizures (Ampola, 1982; Benson, 1983; Cockburn & Gitzelmann, 1980; Cohn & Roth, 1983; Durand-Zaleski et al., 1992; Fanaroff & Martin, 1992; Galjaard, 1980; Komrower, 1980; Lloyd & Scriver, 1985; Natowicz & Alper, 1991; Scriver et al., 1995a, 1995b; Wapnir, 1985). Additional clinical manifestations that would lead to the suspicion of an inherited metabolic disorder include vomiting, diarrhea, poor feeding, weight loss, dehydration, and failure to thrive. There may be hepatomegaly with hyperbilirubinemia (Missiou-Tsagaraki, 1992). The infant may appear to have a hemorrhagic syndrome and splenomegaly (Ampola, 1982; Benson, 1983; Cockburn & Gitzelmann, 1980; Cohn & Roth, 1983; Fanaroff & Martin, 1997; Irons, 1993; Schmidt, 1989; Scriver et al., 1995a, 1995b; Wapnir, 1985; Wu, 1991). There may be an unusual odor of the infant's breath or sweat or an unusual odor or color of the urine.

The clinical manifestations in an infant with an undiagnosed inherited metabolic disorder usually occur in the absence of infection, central nervous system hemorrhage, or congenital defects (Ampola, 1982; Durand-Zaleski et al., 1992; Fanaroff & Martin, 1997; Irons, 1993; Natowicz & Alper, 1991; Stern & Vert, 1987; Wapnir, 1985). Despite the institution of conventional therapy, there is no relief of these symptoms. There may be some transient improvement in clinical manifestations after an exchange transfusion, venovenous hemofiltration, or peritoneal dialysis (Ampola, 1982; Cohn & Roth, 1983; Crawford et al., 1982; Falk et al., 1994; Komrower, 1980; Lloyd & Scriver, 1985; Thompson et al., 1991).

The initial laboratory investigation of an infant with a suspected metabolic disorder should include blood determinations for glucose level, acid–base equilibrium, and ammonia levels. In addition, a complete blood count, coagulation studies, and electrolyte, calcium, magnesium, blood urea nitrogen, and creatinine measurements should be performed to rule out other potential causes of the symptoms (Ampola, 1982; Benson, 1983; Cockburn & Gitzelmann, 1980; Durand-Zaleski et al., 1992; Fanaroff & Martin, 1997; LeGrys, 1984; Natowicz & Alper, 1991; Qu et al., 1991; Schmidt, 1989; Wallach, 1983; Wapnir, 1985; Wu, 1991). The urine should be tested for ketones (Acetest), reducing sugars (Clinitest), glucose (Clinistix), phenylpyruvic acid (Phenistix), and toxic substances (Fanaroff & Martin, 1997; LeGrys, 1984; Schmidt, 1989; Wallach, 1983). Of importance, when an inherited metabolic disorder is suspected, a sample or a series of samples of blood and urine should be set aside for later testing (Duran et al., 1994; Fanaroff & Martin, 1997; Irons, 1993; LeGrys, 1984; Schmidt, 1989; Stern & Vert, 1987; Wu, 1991), preferably before the administration of any blood products.

Certain clinical manifestations may be found in isolation or in association with abnormal laboratory findings. For example, neurologic symptoms may occur in isolation or in association with metabolic acidosis or alkalosis, ketosis, hypoglycemia, or hyperammonemia; hypoglycemia may be associated with ketosis; and severe acidosis may be associated with hematologic symptoms, pancytopenia, or hepatic insufficiency (Ampola, 1982; Benson, 1983; Durand-Zaleski et al., 1992; Galjaard, 1980; Lloyd & Scriver, 1985; Scriver et al., 1995a, 1995b; Wu, 1991). Depending on the suspected etiology, more sophisticated testing can be undertaken, such as ion exchange or gas chromatography of blood and urine for amino acid quantification, gas chromatography of urinary organic acids coupled with mass spectrometry, and determinations of pyruvemia, erythrocyte galactose-1-phosphate, and urinary oligosaccharides and mucopolysaccharides (Duran et al., 1994; Holtzman, 1992; LeGrys, 1984; Qu et al., 1991; Schmidt, 1989; Wu, 1991). Enzyme and complex DNA analysis can also be done on blood cells, hepatocytes, or cultured skin fibroblasts to assist in the diagnosis of the metabolic disorder (Ampola, 1982; LeGrys, 1984; Scriver et al., 1995a, 1995b; Wapnir, 1985). In addition, a positive response to treatment provides an additional diagnostic finding: For example, the symptoms associated with galactosemia rapidly improve when galactose is removed from the diet (Ampola, 1982; Benson, 1983; Crawford et al., 1982; Irons, 1993; Komrower, 1980; Levy & Hammersen, 1978; Lloyd & Scriver, 1985; Scriver et al., 1995a, 1995b; Wapnir, 1985).

Because metabolic disorders may be inherited, it is necessary to make an accurate diagnosis even if the infant has died. After death, skin samples should be obtained for fibroblast cultures and enzyme analysis in all infants suspected of having a metabolic disorder. If possible, blood and urine samples should be obtained for biochemical analysis and needle biopsy specimens of the liver, kidneys, brain, and muscle should be obtained as soon as possible after death for ultrastructural studies. Delay in obtaining these tissue specimens makes ultrastructural studies difficult and enzyme analysis impossible (Ampola, 1982; Benson, 1983; Duran et al., 1994; Fanaroff & Martin, 1997; LeGrys, 1984; Lloyd & Scriver, 1985; Qu et al., 1991; Scriver et al., 1995a, 1995b; Wapnir, 1985; Wu, 1991).

To understand how disorders of metabolism affect the neonate, a brief description of normal metabolism is presented, followed by a description of the metabolic disturbances encountered in clinical practice.

CARBOHYDRATE METABOLISM

Circulating glucose plays an essential role in providing fuel for many tissues. Glucose occupies a unique position in intermediary metabolism for two reasons: (1) It is the substrate of glycolysis that is the sole pathway that produces adenosine triphosphate (ATP) in anaerobic life; although humans as a whole do not exist in an anaerobic condition, erythrocytes, which are devoid of mitochondria, are completely dependent on glycolysis for their supply of ATP. (2) Glucose is the major substrate of brain metabolism. Ketone bodies are easily utilized by brain tissue, but the normal concentrations of these substances are low and increase only during fasting. Fatty acids are bound to albumin in the blood and cannot penetrate the blood–brain barrier. Thus, a decrease in the level of blood glucose may result in neurologic injury. This is, in itself, a justification for the development of rather elaborate mechanisms of hepatic control over blood glucose (Benson, 1983; Bier et al., 1977; Cornblath et al., 1963; Cornblath & Schwartz, 1966; Ogata, 1986; Stave, 1978).

Figure 25–1 presents a brief summary of carbohydrate metabolism. The main dietary carbohydrates are starch, sucrose, and lactose, which are hydrolytically degraded into the free sugars, glucose, fructose, and galactose. Hydrolysis of the oligosaccharides occurs through the action of oligosaccharidases located in the wall of the intestine (Burman et al., 1978; Fanaroff & Martin, 1997; Stave, 1978; Stern & Vert, 1987).

Fructose is very rapidly used by the liver and converted to glucose and lactate. Intravenous administration of fructose results in the development of lactic acidemia from the intense usage of that sugar. In addition, fructose-1-phosphate accumulates in the liver, causing depletion of inorganic phosphate and ATP, followed by the conversion of adenine nucleotides to uric acid, resulting in hyperuricemia (Burman et al., 1978; Cornblath et al., 1963; Cornblath & Schwartz, 1966; Stern & Vert, 1987).

Galactose is also rapidly used by the liver, and its metabolism normally causes no problem (Burman et al., 1978; Levy & Hammersen, 1978). It is only in congenital galactosemia that galactose concentration in the blood increases. Galactosemia is discussed in greater detail later in this chapter. The metabolism of fructose and galactose is not subject to the tight regulation of control as is that of glucose.

Glucose is used by all tissues of the body, and its penetration into muscle and adipose tissue is controlled by insulin. As the primary regulator of blood glucose, the liver takes up glucose during times of abundance after meals and converts it mostly to glycogen. The liver uses very little of this glucose for its own energy needs but instead consumes mostly fatty acids. By the breakdown of glycogen and gluconeogenesis during times of fasting, the liver delivers a large amount of glucose to the blood for use by the brain, erythrocytes, and other tissues. The concentration of glucose in the blood is the primary stimulus that elicits glucose uptake or glucose output by the liver. The hepatic threshold of glucose is the glucose concentration at which the liver is converted from an organ of glucose output to an organ of glucose uptake (Burman et al., 1978; Cornblath et al., 1963; Cornblath & Schwartz, 1966).

Glucose transport across the hepatic membrane is an efficient carrier-mediated process that is not influenced by insulin. The primary effect of glucose in the hepatocyte is to bind to phosphorylase *a*, an active hepatic enzyme. The activity of phosphorylase *a* is inhibited by glucose, and the glucose-bound phosphorylase *a* is rapidly converted to phosphorylase *b* by phosphorylase phos-

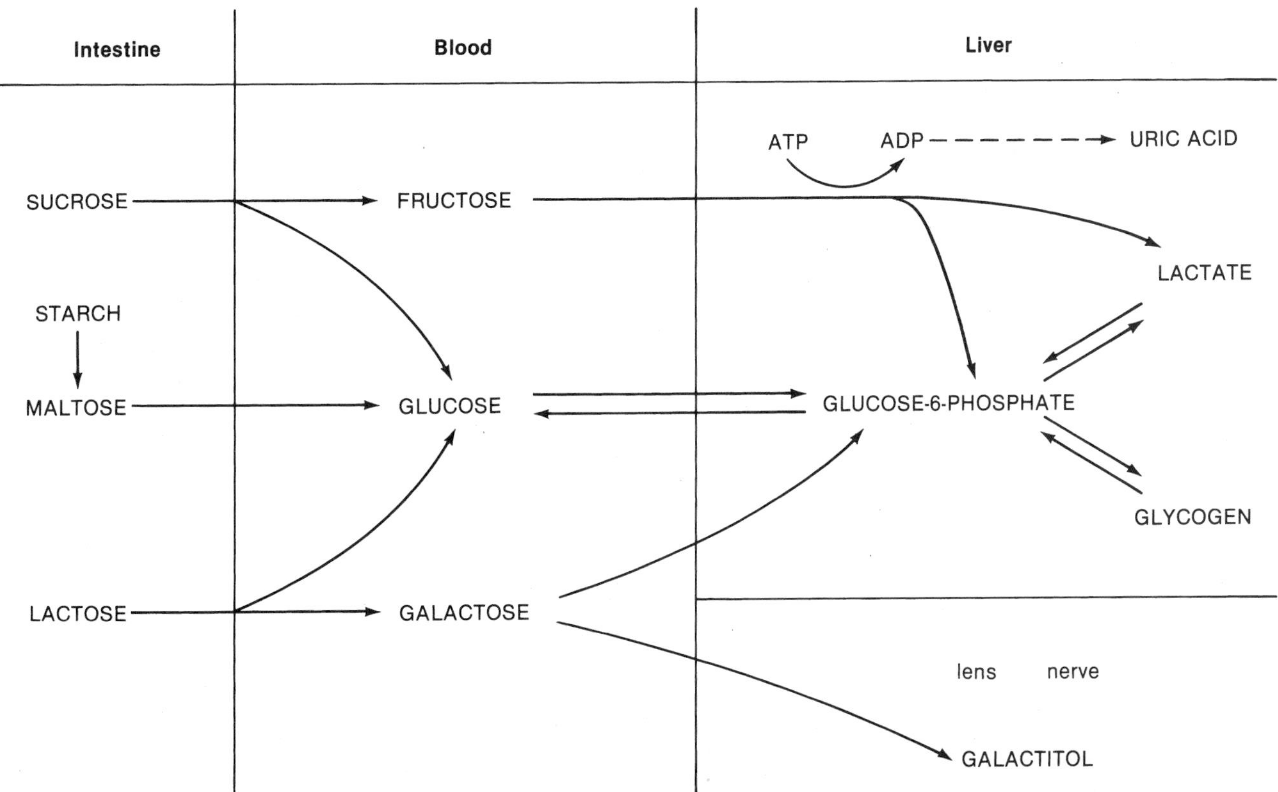

FIGURE 25–1. A summary of carbohydrate metabolism. The primary dietary carbohydrates are starch, sucrose, and lactose, which are hydrolytically degraded into the free sugars glucose, fructose, and galactose. Hydrolysis of the oligosaccharides occurs through the action of oligosaccharidases located in the intestinal wall. This specific location of the enzymes prevents the accumulation of free sugars in the intestine and their utilization by microorganisms. ADP, adenosine diphosphate; ATP, adenosine triphosphate.

phatase. Thus, the first effect of an elevated blood glucose level is to decrease and eventually arrest glycogen degradation in the liver (Burman et al., 1978; Cornblath et al., 1963; Cornblath & Schwartz, 1966).

An elevated blood glucose level also stimulates glycogen synthesis by allowing the activation of glycogen synthetase. The enzyme responsible for glycogen synthesis, synthetase phosphatase, is strongly inhibited by phosphorylase *a*. This mechanism thus prevents glycogen synthesis when blood glucose levels are low (Burman et al., 1978; Cornblath et al., 1963).

Gluconeogenesis is the mechanism by which lactate and amino acids are converted to glucose. It occurs in the liver and the kidney and has a major role in the control of the level of glucose under fasting conditions. It also allows the removal of a large amount of lactic acid from the blood. Gluconeogenesis seems to operate continuously in the liver even in fed states. The rate of gluconeogenesis is increased by glucagon and also in fasting states (Burman et al., 1978; Cornblath et al., 1963; Fanaroff & Martin, 1997; Stave, 1978; Stern & Vert, 1987).

Most of the enzymes in gluconeogenesis are freely reversible and are common to glycolysis (Fig. 25–2). There are, however, three exceptions: (1) at the level of interconversion of pyruvate and phosphoenolpyruvate, at which the glycolytic enzyme pyruvate kinase is reversed by a two-step conversion involving pyruvate carboxylase and pyruvate carboxykinase; (2) at the level of the interconversion between fructose diphosphate and fructose-6-phosphate, at which phosphofructokinase is reversed by hexose diphosphatase; and (3) at the level of interconversion of glucose and glucose-6-phosphate, at which glucokinase is reversed by glucose-6-phosphate (Burman et al., 1978; Cornblath et al., 1963; Stern & Vert, 1987).

The main advantage of the interconversion recycling system is that it allows very large changes in glucose uptake and output to be controlled only by substrate concentration. An increase in glucose concentration influences the phosphorylase synthetase system, and the recycling of glucose and glucose-6-phosphate allows the second system to keep pace with the first (Burman et al., 1978; Cornblath et al., 1963).

Disorders of Carbohydrate Metabolism

Carbohydrates are important components of diets throughout the world and, after intestinal hydrolysis and absorption, provide a critical source of metabolic energy. Defects in hydrolysis or absorption result in retention of residues in the intestinal tract and GI symptoms. Carbohydrate intolerance is a common clinical problem and may have serious consequences, particularly when it occurs early in life.

The predominant symptoms of an infant with carbohydrate intolerance are intestinal. They are the result of the osmotic effects of unabsorbed carbohydrate in the lumen of the small intestine and of the products of bacterial fermentation in the large intestine. The osmotic pressure of the unabsorbed carbohydrate in the small intestine leads to a secretion of water and electrolytes into the lumen until osmotic equilibrium is reached.

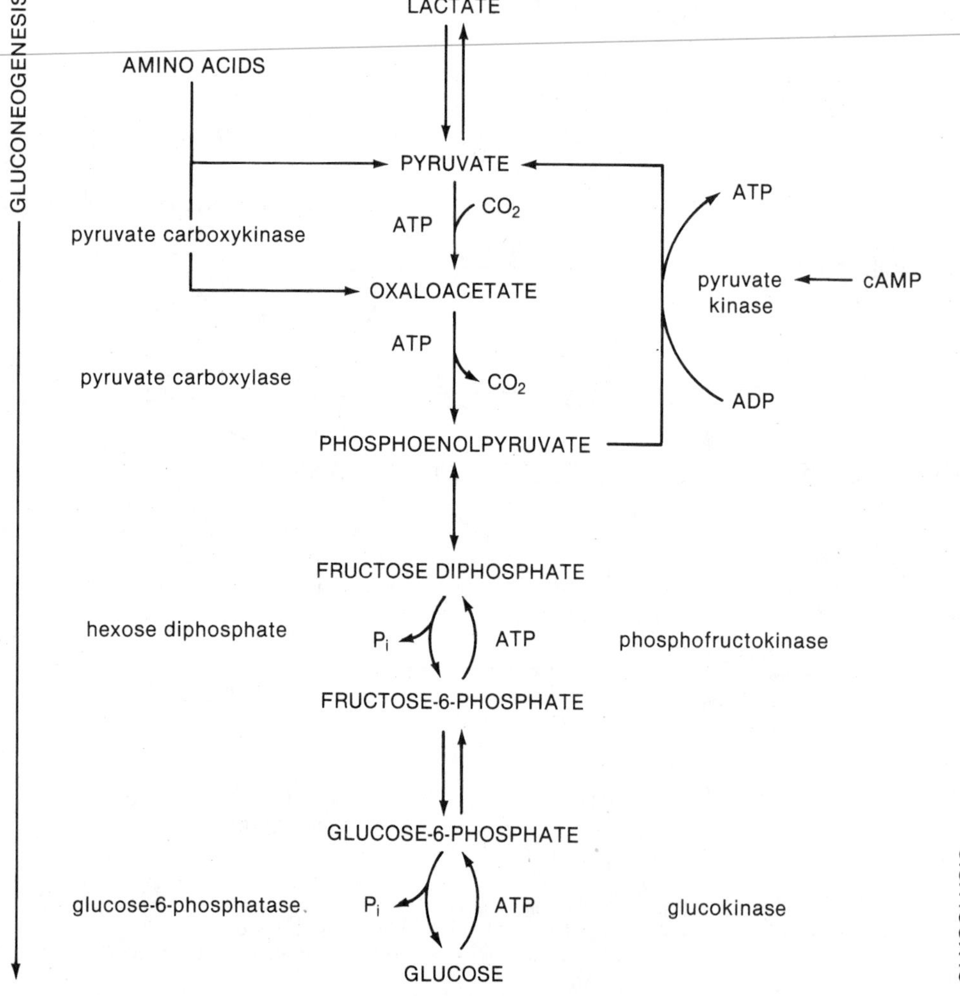

FIGURE 25–2. The pathway of glycolysis and gluconeogenesis. Most of the enzymes responsible for gluconeogenesis are freely reversible and are common to glycolysis. The three exceptions are at the level of interconversion of pyruvate to phosphoenolpyruvate, the interconversion between fructose diphosphate and fructose-6-phosphate, and the interconversion of glucose and glucose-6-phosphate. ADP, adenosine diphosphate; ATP, adenosine triphosphate; cAMP, cyclic adenosine monophosphate; P_i, inorganic phosphate.

A proportion of the carbohydrate may be excreted unchanged in the stool, but the majority is hydrolyzed (reduced) by ideal and colonic bacteria to small carbohydrate molecules, short-chain organic acids, hydrogen, carbon dioxide, and other fermentative products. The organic acids lower the stool pH, inhibit water absorption from the colon, and contribute to the increased mobility (Burman et al., 1978; Wapnir, 1985; Winick, 1979). The severity of the symptoms varies with age, the extent of the enzyme deficiency, the load of the offending carbohydrate, and the colon's ability to reabsorb the excessive fluid delivered to it by the small intestine (Winick, 1979).

Watery acid diarrhea with excoriated buttocks is the hallmark of carbohydrate intolerance in infants, and fluid losses may be profound and life-threatening. In older children, loose stools may be mild or only intermittent, and in adults there may be little diarrhea, but the main symptoms are cramping abdominal pains and bloating. Abdominal distention may be prominent, especially in infants, who may also have recurrent vomiting. Weight loss in affected infants is common (Burman et al., 1978; Cornblath et al., 1963; Fanaroff & Martin, 1997; Komrower, 1980; Scriver et al., 1995a).

The risk of further sequelae is high, especially in infants. Dehydration may be complicated by metabolic acidosis. Large amounts of bicarbonate are secreted into the intestinal lumen to neutralize the contents and hydrogen ions produced by bacterial fermentation of the carbohydrate (Burman et al., 1978). Untreated lactose intolerance in infancy can lead to a more generalized malabsorption of other sugars, nitrogen compounds, and fats, with further impairment of nutrition (Burman et al., 1978; Cornblath & Schwartz, 1966; Wapnir, 1985; Winick, 1979).

In the diagnosis of carbohydrate disorders, there may be a positive family history of symptoms suggesting a primary carbohydrate malabsorption. The most important information is obtained from a detailed dietary history, linking the symptoms to carbohydrate ingestion. For infants, this requires full knowledge of the composition of infant formulas and weaning foods. The nurse has a pivotal role in obtaining a detailed dietary history from the parents and relating these findings to the clinical presentation (Schmidt, 1989).

The clinical response to dietary restriction is at times the last confirmatory evidence of a carbohydrate intolerance. Clinically, many infants with carbohydrate intolerance are too ill to justify formal challenges or to have detailed invasive investigations. An empirical diagnosis based on the history, clinical manifestations, and stool examination results in the prescription of lactose-free, disaccharide-free, or even carbohydrate-free diets (Winick, 1979). The diagnosis is confirmed later after stabilization and recovery. The nurse is often a key player in the investigation, diagnosis, evaluation, and management of these disorders.

The examination of stools of infants with suspected carbohydrate disorders includes the measurement of reducing substances, glucose, carbohydrate chromatography, pH, and organic acid content (Burman et al., 1978; Cornblath & Schwartz, 1966; Schmidt, 1989; Wapnir, 1985; Winick, 1979). The indices for carbohydrate intolerance in infants with diarrhea include concentrations of the reducing substances of more than 0.25 percent, 1+ glucose, and a stool pH of less than 6.0 (Wallach, 1983). All tests must be performed on the liquid portion of fresh stool specimens, preferably collected on nonabsorbent material. Formed stools are unlikely to contain significant amounts of sugars. It is necessary to perform the tests immediately, because fecal bacteria hydrolyze sugars very rapidly at room temperature and because pH decreases and lactic acid content increases quickly (Burman et al., 1978; Wapnir, 1985). All stools must be tested, because some specimens may be carbohydrate-free even in infants with severe intolerance (Burman et al., 1978).

Tests for reducing substances of stool are very useful but can yield false-positive and false-negative results. Antibiotic therapy and type of sugar in the diet must be considered in interpreting the results of the measurements of pH and sugar in stools. Fecal pH is influenced by the degree of colonic fermentation of unabsorbed carbohydrate. A pH less than 6 is frequently found in infants with fermentative diarrhea, but higher values do not exclude the diagnosis. The fecal pH is dependent on the bacterial fermentation of carbohydrates, and any factor modifying this relationship may alter stool pH without influencing the capacity to tolerate carbohydrates (Wapnir, 1985). False-positive results can be caused by nonabsorbable sugars such as lactulose or plant hexoses; oligosaccharides of bacterial origin and noncarbohydrate substances may be present without any sugar intolerance. Sugars such as lactose, sucrose, glucose, and galactose may be found in healthy neonates. For these reasons, carbohydrate chromatography may be necessary for testing the significance of the stool-reducing substances. When the detailed dietary description is compared with the results of this test, the type of carbohydrate malabsorption can be accurately determined (Burman et al., 1978).

The observed response to an oral sugar load is one of the standard tests of carbohydrate malabsorption. The shape of the blood sugar curve after ingestion is a measure of absorption, whereas the symptoms after ingestion (coupled with stool examination) indicate clinical intolerance (Burman et al., 1978; Scriver et al., 1995a; Wapnir, 1985). It is frequently the responsibility of the nurse to assess the infant throughout the carbohydrate oral challenge test, obtain frequent blood and stool specimens, and evaluate the infant's clinical response.

Breath tests have also been used in the diagnosis of carbohydrate malabsorption. If $^{14}CO_2$ is recovered in the breath after oral ingestion of ^{14}C-radiolabeled compound, at least a portion of the compound has been absorbed and metabolized (Burman et al., 1978). Although the research in this area is encouraging, there are theoretical disadvantages, including time of gastric emptying, glucose intermediary metabolism, the proportion of sugar that is absorbed, and fermentation of unabsorbed ^{14}C sugar, that may occur. Lastly, ^{14}C is unacceptable for use in children because of its radioactivity (Burman et al., 1978).

Hydrogen breath tests do not require the use of radiolabeled compounds. The amount of hydrogen excreted in the breath correlates well with the amount produced in the intestine by fermentation of carbohydrates. The proximal small intestine is the site of carbohydrate absorption, and is not normally colonized by H_2-producing bacteria. Breath concentration of hydrogen after an oral load of sugar is therefore a measure of the degree of malabsorption (Burman et al., 1978). It is independent of gastric emptying and intermediary glucose metabolism and does not involve the use of radioisotopes. Breath hydrogen measurement is the most accurate, sensitive, and specific indirect test for detecting lactose deficiency. In premature infants, results of laboratory tests of carbohydrate absorption, such as breath hydrogen, are frequently "abnormal" and have limited usefulness in the clinical management of these infants (Wapnir, 1985). Breath analysis is used for full-term neonates and older infants.

Disorders of Galactose Metabolism

- Three inherited abnormalities of galactose metabolism are known. They are transmitted by autosomal recessive inheritance.
- The metabolic disorders result from a deficiency of galactokinase, galactose-1-phosphate uridyltransferase, or uridine diphosphate galactose 4-epimerase, the enzymes of the pathway converting galactose to glucose.
- Galactokinase deficiency has mild clinical symptoms, resulting mainly in cataracts.
- Galactose-1-phosphate uridyltransferase deficiency is charac-

terized by failure to thrive, vomiting, liver disease, cataracts, and developmental delay. Long-term complications in transferase-deficient patients may occur despite a lactose-free diet. These consist of poor growth, speech abnormality, mental deficiency, neurologic syndromes, and ovarian failure in females. The pathophysiology of both the acute toxicity syndromes and the long-term complications is uncertain.

- Two forms of uridine diphosphate galactose 4-epimerase deficiency have been identified. One is benign and is detected by screening procedures that assay red blood cell galactose-1-phosphate. The other is clinically similar to transferase deficiency and responds to a restriction of dietary galactose. In this condition, some dietary galactose is necessary for the formation of uridine diphosphate galactose, which is essential in various metabolic processes.

Most galactose in the diet is in the form of the disaccharide lactose, which is synthesized in the mammary gland from glucose. Lactose is the primary carbohydrate source for nursing mammals and provides approximately 40 percent of the energy in human milk (Winick, 1979).

Lactose digestion is initiated by the hydrolysis of the disaccharide into absorbable monosaccharides glucose and galactose. Hydrolysis of lactose by the galactosidase lactase occurs in the brush border of the small intestine.

The main pathway of galactose metabolism is the conversion of galactose to glucose, which requires several enzymatic steps. In the normal pathway of galactose metabolism, galactose is phosphorylated with ATP to form galactose-1-phosphate. The galactose-1-phosphate reacts with uridine diphosphate (UDP-) glucose catalyzed by galactose-1-phosphate uridyltransferase to produce two products: glucose-1-phosphate and UDP-galactose. Classic galactosemia results from a block in this step. The UDP-galactose formed is converted to UDP-glucose by UDP-galactose 4-epimerase. The UDP-glucose formed can then serve as a substrate for the transferase reaction. These reactions function in a cyclic manner until all of the galactose-1-phosphate entering the pathway from galactose is converted to glucose-1-phosphate and subsequently to glucose (Scriver et al., 1995a).

When no galactose is introduced to the pathway from an external source, protective processes do exist to produce galactose and its metabolites, which are critical to the formation of complex lipids and glycoprotein. Glucose-1-phosphate reacts with UTP via UDP-glucose pyrophosphorylase activity to form UDP-glucose, which can then be epimerized to form UDP-galactose. Epimerase maintains an equilibrium between UDP-glucose and UDP-galactose in nearly all cells. The UDP-galactose formed can also be a source of cellular galactose-1-phosphate and galactose. Free galactose is also produced by turnover of glycolipids and glycoproteins (Scriver et al., 1995a).

If galactose is unable to be metabolized as a result of a deficiency or inefficiency of galactokinase, transferase, or epimerase, two alternative pathways are available. Galactose can be reduced to galactitol by aldolase reductase or oxidized to galactonate by an oxidase or dehydrogenase (Scriver et al., 1995a).

Hereditary Galactokinase Deficiency

This autosomal recessive disorder of galactose metabolism is caused by a deficiency in the enzyme galactokinase. The incidence of galactokinase deficiency varies from 1 in 40,000 to 1 in 155,000 across European populations (Ampola, 1982; Burman et al., 1978; Cohn & Roth, 1983; Hammersen & Bickel, 1982; Levy & Hammersen, 1978; Scriver et al., 1995a; Wapnir, 1985; Winick, 1979). The difference in occurrence is unexplained, although genetic heterogeneity may be one factor. Racially determined galactokinase polymorphism has been detected in North American blacks, in whom the red blood cells are less active than in whites (Levy & Hammersen, 1978).

The absence of clinical symptoms in the newborn period and the appearance of cataracts in older patients on unrestricted diets differentiate this disorder from transferase deficiency. Because galactokinase-deficient newborns are asymptomatic or develop cataracts as the first and only abnormality, the diagnosis in early infancy depends on the routine screening of blood and urine for galactose.

The diagnosis of galactokinase deficiency can be made by the finding of normal amounts of galactose-1-phosphate uridyltransferase and an absence of galactokinase in the red blood cells (Gitzelmann, 1967; Scriver et al., 1995a). High blood galactose levels are best detected after milk feedings. The presence of reducing substances in the urine may be identified as galactose. The urine of any newborn with cataracts should be examined for sugar with a method that does not use glucose oxidase, and there should be an assay of blood for the defect.

Galactokinase-deficient adults are not mentally deficient, although the visual deprivation caused by the cataract formation may affect psychomotor development. Galatokinase-deficient individuals have no aversion to milk and experience no discomfort from drinking it. They are asymptomatic, with the exception of cataracts that appear in infancy. If milk intake is high, they excrete substantial amounts of galactose and galactitol, and after an oral galactose load, the blood galactose level rises excessively (Ampola, 1982; Cockburn & Gitzelmann, 1980; Crawford et al., 1982; Galjaard, 1980; Levy & Hammersen, 1978; Lloyd & Scriver, 1985; Scriver et al., 1995a; Winick, 1979).

The nuclear cataracts develop as a result of an accumulation of galactitol in the lens. The trapped galactitol causes swelling and disruption of lens fibers. The formation of cataracts is caused by a complex sequence of events, including disturbances in the balance of water, electrolytes, amino acids, proteins, energy-rich phosphates, and reduced glutathione (Crawford et al., 1982; Scriver et al., 1995a). Treatment of galactokinase deficiency with a galactose exclusion diet must be continued throughout life. Minute amounts of galactose may be tolerated by these patients; however, in infants with galactose-1-phosphate uridyltransferase deficiency, no amount of galactose is tolerated (Levy & Hammersen, 1978; Winick, 1979).

Hereditary Galactose-1-Phosphate Uridyltransferase Deficiency

This autosomal recessive disorder results from a deficiency of galactose-1-phosphate uridyltransferase, which catalyzes the metabolism of galactose-1-phosphate to galactose to uridine diphosphate (Ampola, 1982; Burman et al., 1978; Galjaard, 1980; Levy & Hammersen, 1978; Wapnir, 1985; Winick, 1979). Incidence rates vary widely but are estimated at approximately 1 in 155,000 (Burman et al., 1978). The absence of transferase activity of erythrocytes is the basis for diagnosing galactosemia (Levy & Hammersen, 1978; Scriver et al., 1995a). The enzyme deficiency can also be demonstrated in many other tissues such as cultured skin fibroblasts and in cultured amniotic fluid. Heterozygotes have approximately one half of normal enzyme activity in their red blood cells (Burman et al., 1978; Levy & Hammersen, 1978; Scriver et al., 1995a).

Infants with galactosemia have normal birth weights but fail to gain weight after they start ingesting milk. Usually symptoms appear in the second half of the first week of life and include jaundice, vomiting, and diarrhea (Ampola, 1982; Burman et al., 1978; Levy & Hammersen, 1978; Wapnir, 1985; Winick, 1979). The jaundice and unconjugated hyperbilirubinemia are often associated with severe hemolysis, mimicking erythroblastosis fetalis. Many of the affected newborns receive exchange transfusions before diagnosis. Nuclear cataracts appear within days or weeks and become irreversible within weeks of their appearance (Ampola, 1982; Burman et al., 1978; Levy & Hammersen, 1978; Scriver et al., 1995a). If milk feedings continue, the disease usually progresses, resulting in abnormal liver function, hepatomegaly, cirrhosis, and death. Occasionally a patient presents, not with failure to thrive, but rather with motor retardation, hepatomegaly, and cataracts several months after birth. There also appears to be a high frequency of *E. coli* sepsis and neonatal death in infants with transferase deficiency galactosemia (Levy et al., 1977), probably because of inhibition of leukocyte bactericidal activity (Litchfield & Wells, 1978). Therefore, neonates with *E. coli* sepsis and older infants with cataracts should be suspected of having galactosemia and be tested for the enzyme deficiency (Scriver et al., 1995a).

The presumptive diagnosis of galactosemia may be made from the identification of galactose in urine and blood. The finding of reducing substance in the urine that does not react with glucose oxidase reagents, such as Clinistix, is consistent with the presence of galactose (Levy & Hammersen, 1978). However lactose, fructose, and pentose may also yield a positive result. Although this is a useful, noninvasive screening test, it is important to note that normal newborns may excrete up to 60 mg of galactose per deciliter in the first 5 days of life, and this level may be detected for up to 2 weeks in premature infants (Dahlqvist & Svenningsen, 1969).

Thirty-eight states have established screening for galactosemia in newborns (Scriver et al., 1995a). The disorder can be diagnosed with a simple filter paper blood specimen in a manner similar to that used to detect PKU (Benson, 1983; Bickel, 1980; Cockburn & Gitzelmann, 1980; Cohn & Roth, 1983; Hammersen & Bickel, 1982; Komrower, 1980; LeGrys, 1984; Levy & Hammersen, 1978; Wapnir, 1985). A complete protocol for the detection of all disorders of galactose metabolism has been described (Bowring & Brown, 1986). Because of widespread screening of newborns, many patients have been diagnosed early in the course of the disease and with proper diet management have avoided the acute toxic effects of galactosemia.

The outcome for infants with galactosemia is dependent on the early diagnosis and treatment of this disorder. In general, the clinical manifestations of the disorder are reversed a few weeks after initiation of appropriate treatment, but the long-term outcome and intellectual development are uncertain. Follow-up of galactosemic individuals has shown that many have developed very well, whereas others have had more severe problems involving growth, development, brain function, and, in females, ovarian dysfunction (Ampola, 1982; Burman et al., 1978; Komrower, 1980; Levy & Hammersen, 1978; Lloyd & Scriver, 1985; Scriver et al., 1995a; Winick, 1979).

The causes of variability in response to treatment require further study. Family differences related to genetic or sociologic factors may account for some of these findings. Another determinant for outcome is the age at which diagnosis was made; the outcome is more favorable if the infant is treated early. Furthermore, galactose-1-phosphate accumulates in the cord blood of infants born to galactosemic mothers, despite the mothers' being on restricted lactose intake throughout pregnancy (Ampola, 1982; Burman et al., 1978; Levy & Hammersen, 1978; Scriver et al., 1995a). Thus it can be inferred that the intrauterine environment is unfavorable to the homozygous fetus, resulting in irreversible prenatal damage to the brain and/or ovary.

Hereditary Uridine Diphosphate Galactose 4-Epimerase Deficiency

This disorder, inherited as a recessive trait, is caused by the absence of UDP-galactose 4-epimerase in the blood. The incidence has been estimated to be 1 in 23,000 in Japan, where screening programs were established (Misumi et al., 1981).

Two forms of UDP-galactose 4-epimerase deficiency exist. The benign condition, which is more common, results from the absence of UDP-galactose 4-epimerase in the blood. The only metabolic consequence of galactose ingestion is the elevation of galactose-1-phosphate in red blood cells, without any further red blood cell abnormality (Scriver et al., 1995a).

In contrast, a severe form exists in which UDP-galactose 4-epimerase activity is absent in liver and other tissues as well as in red blood cells. The clinical manifestation is similar to that of transferase deficiency, which presents with jaundice, vomiting, weight loss, hepatomegaly, aminoaciduria, and galactosuria (Henderson et al., 1983; Scriver et al., 1995a).

The treatment of this disorder requires a different approach than in transferase deficiency. Because epimerase forms UDP-galactose from UDP-glucose, a complete absence of galactose in the diet and lack of the formation of UDP-galactose via transferase would have serious results. Complex carbohydrates and galactolipids that require UDP-galactose for synthesis would not be formed. Hence, therapy includes providing small amounts of dietary galactose that does not produce toxicity but is adequate for galactoprotein and galactolipid synthesis (Scriver et al., 1995a).

Disorders of Fructose Metabolism

- Fructose is an important source of carbohydrate in the human diet. Fructose is metabolized predominantly in the liver, kidney, and small intestine and to a lesser extent in adipose tissue.
- Three inherited abnormalities of fructose metabolism are known, and all are inherited as autosomal recessive traits.
- Essential fructosuria is a benign, asymptomatic disorder caused by the absence of fructokinase, resulting in hyperfructosemia and fructosuria.
- Hereditary fructose intolerance is characterized by hypoglycemia and vomiting after the ingestion of fructose. In infants, prolonged fructose ingestion leads to poor feeding, vomiting, jaundice, hepatomegaly, hemorrhage, and potentially hepatic failure and death. The disorder results from a deficiency of fructose-1-phosphate aldolase in the liver, kidney cortex, and small intestine. Hypoglycemia after fructose ingestion is caused by fructose-1-phosphate inhibiting glycogenolysis and gluconeogenesis. Patients remain healthy on a diet free of fructose and sucrose.

Hereditary fructose 1,6-diphosphatase deficiency is characterized by episodes of hyperventilation, apnea, hypoglycemia, ketosis, and lactic acidosis. Gluconeogenesis is severely impaired as a result of the enzyme defect, leading to accumulation of amino acids, lactate, and ketones (gluconeogenic precursors) as liver glycogen stores are depleted. Beyond early childhood, patients develop normally and become more tolerant of fasting.

Fructose is a major food constituent in human nutrition, occurring in some fruits and vegetables and honey. It is also a component of the disaccharide sucrose, which is used extensively as sweetening additives for food, medications, and even infant formulas. Its consumption has steadily increased since the 1960s, during which it has gained popularity for clinical purposes.

Fructose is metabolized in two ways in the human body. After ingestion, it is in part assimilated into glucose in the intestine by phosphorylation by fructokinase to fructose-1-phosphate (Benson, 1983; Burman et al., 1978; Cornblath et al., 1963; Cornblath & Schwartz, 1966; Komrower, 1980; Lloyd & Scriver, 1985; Scriver et al., 1995a; Wapnir, 1985; Winick, 1979). The greater part reaches the liver, where it is extracted and rapidly phosphorylated to fructose-1-phosphate. Fructaldolase then splits fructose-1-phosphate into two triodes that may be used for energy by entering the tricarboxylic acid (TCA) cycle or may be condensed to fructose-1,6-diphosphate and used for glucose or glycogen formation (Benson, 1983; Burman et al., 1978; Komrower, 1980; Lloyd & Scriver, 1985; Scriver et al., 1995a; Wapnir, 1985). A small part of fructose passes through the liver and is transported to other tissues, such as adipose or muscle tissue, where it is metabolized to fructose-6-phosphate by the enzyme hexokinase (Burman et al., 1978; Scriver et al., 1995a). In the kidney, fructose is metabolized in the same way as in the intestine and the liver. Three inherited enzyme defects are known in the fructose pathway: (1) deficiency of fructokinase or essential fructosuria; (2) deficiency of fructaldolase B, or hereditary fructose intolerance; and (3) deficiency of fructose-1,6-diphosphatase.

Hereditary Fructose Intolerance

Hereditary fructose intolerance is inherited as an autosomal recessive trait and has an estimated incidence of 1:20,000 (Burman et al., 1978). Once thought to be very rare, it has become evident that hereditary fructose intolerance is more common. The disorder occurs as a result of a deficiency in fructose-1-phosphate aldolase activity in homozygotes. Fructose intake results in the accumulation of fructose-1-phosphate in the liver, kidney, and small intestine as a result of the inability of the defective aldolase B to split it. In heterozygotes, the fructose-1-phosphate aldolase activity is reported to be normal (Burman et al., 1978; Scriver et al., 1995a).

In infants with hereditary fructose intolerance, the appearance and severity of symptoms depend on the intake of fructose. In the absence of fructose (e.g., with breastfeeding), no metabolic derangement occurs. With the intake of sucrose in the form of fruits and vegetables at weaning, the first symptoms are observed. The younger the child, the more severe the reaction to dietary fructose, and this reaction may be life-threatening.

Older children and infants develop an aversion to sweets and protect themselves from most or all exposure to the noxious sugar. If they consume fructose repeatedly in small amounts, a milder but chronic form of hereditary fructose intolerance is observed. The clinical form of hereditary fructose intolerance is observed. The clinical manifestations of an acute ingestion include sweating, trembling, dizziness, nausea, vomiting, apathy, lethargy, coma, and convulsions. Chronic exposure results in clinical manifestations that include failure to thrive, vomiting, poor feeding, jaundice, hepatomegaly, cirrhosis, edema, ascites, and hemorrhages (Burman et al., 1978; Scriver et al., 1995a). Thus the two organs most involved are those in which there is a considerable pathway to metabolize fructose: the liver and the kidney.

Laboratory findings in infants with hereditary fructose intolerance include signs of liver dysfunction. Results of tests for serum transaminase levels, prothrombin time, serum protein levels, plasma methionine levels, and/or tyrosine levels are abnormal. Disturbed renal function may also be present and is manifested by melituria, proteinuria, hyperaminoaciduria, and acidosis. Derangements of intermediate metabolism are mirrored by lowered levels of serum phosphorus and potassium, fructosuria, organic aciduria, and metabolic acidosis. Morphologic study of liver tissue in infants with hereditary fructose intolerance has revealed fatty changes with vacuolization, fibrosis, and formation of bile ductules (Burman et al., 1978; Scriver et al., 1995a).

Diagnosis of hereditary fructose intolerance is suspected from a detailed nutritional history and clinical manifestations. The nonspecific nature of the clinical manifestations requires that other metabolic disorders (such as tyrosinosis, glycogenesis), hepatitis, liver cirrhosis, or liver tumor need to be considered. Pyloric stenosis may be suggested when vomiting is the primary symptom. Septicemia or intrauterine infection may clinically manifest in the same way as hereditary fructose intolerance, especially if clotting disturbances and hematologic changes are obvious.

The diagnosis is confirmed by a fructose tolerance test or the enzyme assay in liver tissue or intestinal mucosa. The fructose tolerance test entails a single intravenous dose of fructose and is more conclusive than the oral route (Burman et al., 1978; LeGrys, 1984; Scriver et al., 1995a). The oral fructose tolerance test is no longer used because it causes very severe GI symptoms. The parenteral fructose challenge results in a rapid decrease in fructose, associated with an increase in serum magnesium and uric acid levels and a decrease in serum phosphorus and glucose levels. The maximum effects are seen 40 minutes after the fructose injection (Burman et al., 1978; LeGrys, 1984; Scriver et al., 1995a). Once the diagnosis is established, treatment must be started immediately with a fructose-free diet. There is nearly immediate clearance of symptoms and signs, with the exception of hepatomegaly, which may persist for many months, although liver size decreases slowly (Burman et al., 1978; Winick, 1979). Fatty changes of hepatocytes have occasionally been seen many months after initiation of treatment. In young infants with severe liver damage, immediate withdrawal of fructose from the diet and infusions do not guarantee survival. Severe liver dysfunction may lead to hemorrhagic diastases and fatal liver failure (Burman et al., 1978; Scriver et al., 1995a).

Fructose-1,6-Diphosphate Deficiency

Fructose-1,6-diphosphate deficiency is an extremely rare disease that is inherited as an autosomal recessive trait (Ampola, 1982; Burman et al., 1978; Scriver et al., 1995a; Wapnir, 1985). The incidence of this disease is difficult to estimate because of the rarity of reported cases. The deficiency of fructose-1,6-diphosphatase, a key enzyme of gluconeogenesis, hinders the endogenous formation of glucose from lactate, alanine, and glycerol. Administration of these substances and of fructose causes, not a rise in blood glucose level, but immediate hypoglycemia and lactic acidosis (Burman et al., 1978; Scriver et al., 1995a). Because newborns depend on gluconeogenesis in the first few days, symptoms tend to occur during this period in infants with fructose-1,6-diphosphate deficiency.

Clinical manifestations are often triggered by infections and include symptoms of metabolic acidosis and acute hypoglycemia: hyperventilation, shock, apnea, trembling, lethargy, loss of consciousness, and convulsions (Ampola, 1982; Burman et al., 1978; Scriver et al., 1995a). Acute episodes are dramatic and life-threatening but may be promptly overcome by glucose infusions and bicarbonate. During the intervals between acute episodes, mild hyperventilation and lactic acidosis persist, but their severity depends on the frequency of food intake (Burman et al., 1978; Winick, 1979). During childhood, hepatomegaly, slight muscular hypotonia, and hyperreflexia are common. Intellectual development seems unimpaired.

Abnormal laboratory findings include hypoglycemia, severe acidosis (pH of 7.1 or less), excessive lactic acid in serum and urine, pyruvic acidemia, high values of free fatty acids in serum, increased alanine, and ketone bodies in serum and urine (Burman et al., 1978; LeGrys, 1984; Scriver et al., 1995a). In contrast to hereditary fructose intolerance, disturbances of liver function, renal tubular dysfunction, and hematologic changes are rarely observed in fructose-1,6-diphosphate deficiency (Burman et al., 1978; Scriver et al., 1995a). Prolonged fasting induces the typical biochemical derangements of hypoglycemia and lactic acidosis. In establishment of the diagnosis, fructose-1,6-diphosphate deficiency must be distinguished from other inherited disorders of gluconeogenesis or ketotic acidemia. Tolerance tests with fructose or alanine may prove helpful for clinical evaluation (Burman et al., 1978; LeGrys, 1984; Scriver et al., 1995a). Oral fructose loading should not be performed until hereditary fructose intolerance is excluded, because of the severe hypoglycemia and gastrointestinal side effects that may ensue in such patients. Definitive diagnosis is obtained by the in vitro demonstration of enzyme deficiency in a liver biopsy. The expression of enzyme activity varies from absent to partial defects, but fasting hypoglycemia is always present (Burman et al., 1978; Scriver et al., 1995a). Biopsy specimens may also be obtained from the intestine or kidneys.

Long-term treatment consists of frequent meals and the restriction of fructose and sorbitol. Dietary fat should be partly restricted. Avoidance of fasting, especially during febrile infections, is probably more important than fructose restriction for long-term management (Burman et al., 1978; Scriver et al., 1995a).

Nurses need to know that many milk formulas for infant nutrition, such as Isomil and Alimentum, contain fructose and sucrose, which are harmful to infants with hereditary fructose intolerance or fructose-1,6-diphosphate deficiency. Most endangered are newborns and young infants. Some glucose substitutes, such as fructose, sucrose, or sorbitol, used either for parenteral nutrition or for the treatment of cerebral edema, cause great danger to these infants (Burman et al., 1978; Scriver et al., 1995a).

Carbohydrate Malabsorption in the Intestinal Brush Border

- There are three inherited disorders of the intestinal membrane. They are rare autosomal recessive abnormalities.
- Clinical manifestation includes severe watery diarrhea and dehydration after birth, after weaning, or after starch dextrins have been added to the diet.
- These three intestinal brush border disorders are congenital lactase deficiency, sucrase-isomaltase deficiency, and congenital glucose-galactose malabsorption.

Chronic diarrhea and other digestive symptoms occur in a variety of inborn errors of metabolism. A number of diseases in pediatrics manifest with feeding difficulties, chronic vomiting, failure to thrive, recurrent infections, osteopenia, and generalized hypotonia in the presence of chronic diarrhea. Therefore, inborn errors of metabolism are easily misdiagnosed as milk intolerance; chronic ear, nose and throat infections; celiac disease; pyloric stenosis; immunodeficiency; or diverse intestinal problems (Scriver et al., 1995a). An infant with severe watery diarrhea and dehydration must be closely evaluated in the context of a possible inborn error of metabolism.

Congenital Glucose–Galactose Malabsorption

This autosomal recessive disorder results in severe gastrointestinal symptoms after the ingestion of milk in the neonatal period. Renal tubular reabsorption of glucose is also impaired, resulting in glycosuria. Unless glucose- and galactose-containing foods are withdrawn from the diet, the condition can be fatal. In vivo and in vitro studies have demonstrated defective or complete absence of sodium-coupled mucosal uptake of glucose in affected infants (Burman et al., 1978). Absorption of fructose, xylose, and the amino acids leucine and alanine is intact. An artificial milk with fructose as the only carbohydrate forms a satisfactory basis of early dietary treatment (Burman et al., 1978; Winick, 1979). The defect is thought to lie at the brush border level of the cell, but the precise molecular defect has not yet been defined. As in some other congenital disorders of carbohydrate intolerance, a limited dietary tolerance to offending carbohydrates develops with increasing age, but some form of lifelong dietary restriction is required (Scriver et al., 1995a; Winick, 1979).

Glycogen Storage Diseases

- All proteins involved in the synthesis or degradation of glycogen or its regulation have been discovered to cause some type of glycogen storage disease. In these disorders, the quantity or the quality of glycogen is abnormal. The different types of glycogen storage diseases have been categorized by numeric type in the chronologic order of the identification of the disorder.
- The most seriously affected tissues are liver and muscle—the tissues with the most abundant quantities of glycogen. The liver is responsible for maintaining plasma glucose via its regulation of carbohydrate metabolism. Thus glycogen storage diseases have hepatomegaly and hypoglycemia as the most common presenting features. Because the role of glycogen in muscle is to provide substrates that enable the ATP generation necessary for muscle contraction, the predominant features of glycogen storage diseases that primarily affect the muscle are muscle cramps, exercise intolerance, susceptibility to fatigue, and progressive weakness.
- Type Ia glycogen storage disease (von Gierke's disease) results from a deficiency of glucose-6-phosphatase activity in the liver, kidney, and intestinal mucosa. Excessive accumulation of glycogen occurs in these tissues. The clinical manifestations of this disorder include growth retardation, hepatomegaly, hypoglycemia, lactic acidemia, hyperuricemia, and hyperlipidemia. A variant caused by the transport of glucose-6-phosphate (type Ib) has the additional findings of neutropenia and impaired neutrophil function, resulting in recurrent bacterial infections and gastrointestinal ulceration. Defects in microsomal phosphate or pyrophosphate transport (type Ic) and in microsomal glucose transport (type Id) have been identified.
- In the past, type I glycogen storage disease was associated with a high mortality. The morbid manifestations in the survivors included gout, hepatic adenomas, osteoporosis, renal disease, and short stature. The use of continuous nocturnal feedings of glucose or orally administered uncooked cornstarch are effective for sustaining the metabolic indexes of adequate therapy. With early diagnosis and initiation of therapy, the prognosis for type I glycogen storage disease has markedly improved. Normal growth and pubertal development can now be achieved, and many patients who have survived to adulthood have no evidence of hepatic adenomas or symptoms of gout.
- Type II glycogen storage disease (Pompe's disease), is caused by a deficiency of lysosomal acid α-glucosidase. It is the prototype of a lysosomal storage disease that results from inherited inborn errors of metabolism.
- Type III glycogen storage disease results from a defect in the glycogen debranching enzyme activity. A deficiency in this enzyme impairs the release of glucose from glycogen but not from gluconeogenesis. The glycogen that accumulates resembles dextrin. Patients with type III glycogen storage disease have both liver and muscle involvement (type IIIa). A small percentage of patients have only liver involvement (type IIIb) without apparent muscle disease. During infancy, both forms of type III disease resemble type I disease, with hepatomegaly, hypoglycemia, hyperlipidemia, and growth retardation as clinical manifestations. However, in type III disease, the blood lactate and uric acid levels are normal, and increases in hepatic transaminases are prominent. The hepatic symptoms actually improve with age. Overt liver cirrhosis is rare. In patients with muscle involvement (type IIIa), muscle weakness increases with age and is manifested by progressive weakness and distal muscle wasting. There may be ventricular hypertrophy and electrocardiographic abnormalities. Treatment is symptomatic. Cornstarch supplements, frequent meals high in carbohydrates, or nocturnal continuous gastric feedings are effective in treating hypoglycemia. There is no effective treatment for the progressive myopathy or cardiomyopathy.

- Type IV glycogen storage disease results from a deficiency of branching enzyme activity that causes the accumulation of glycogen with unbranched, long, outer chains in the tissues. This form, when present, usually appears in the first year of life with hepatomegaly and failure to thrive. Hypoglycemia is rare. Progressive liver cirrhosis with portal hypertension, ascites, esophageal varices, and death occurs before the age of 5 years. Liver transplantation may be an effective treatment for the hepatic manifestations. However, because type IV disease affects other tissues, the long-term success of liver transplantation is not yet known.
- Type V glycogen storage disease (McArdle's disease), results from a deficiency of muscle phosphorylase activity. Symptoms usually appear in adulthood and manifest as exercise intolerance, muscle cramps, and myoglobinuria. Avoidance of exercise prevents the symptoms, and there is no need for specific therapy.
- Type VI glycogen storage disease is a heterogeneous group of disorders caused by a deficiency of the liver phosphorylase system. Clinical manifestations occur in early childhood with hepatomegaly and growth retardation. Mild hypoglycemia and hyperlipidemia are occasionally found. Lactic acid and uric acid levels are normal. Treatment is symptomatic and includes frequent feedings and a high-carbohydrate diet. These disorders are considered benign forms of glycogen storage diseases, and most patients do not require any therapy. The prognosis is good; adult patients have normal stature and minimal hepatomegaly. This disorder is inherited as an X-linked pattern, in contrast to the other glycogen storage diseases, which are transmitted in an autosomal recessive manner.
- Type VII glycogen storage disease is caused by a deficiency of muscle phosphofructokinase activity. The clinical manifestations include exercise intolerance, muscle cramps, and myoglobinuria, similar to type V glycogen storage disease. However, in type VII glycogen storage disease, there is usually a compensated hemolytic anemia, early-onset myogenic hyperuricemia, and a glucose-induced exertional fatigue.

Since the initial reports of a patient with a glycogen storage defect in 1928, a variety of glycogen storage diseases have been described. Nearly all proteins involved in the synthesis or degradation of glycogen and its regulation have been discovered to cause some inheritable form of glycogen storage disease (Scriver et al., 1995a) (Fig. 25–3).

Glycogen storage diseases have been classified in several ways. The original classification of glycogen storage diseases was described by G. T. Cori in 1958 as types I, II, III, and IV (Burman et al., 1978; Chen & Burchell, 1995). Glycogen storage diseases have also been classified by the recognition of the enzymatic defect or by the distinct clinical and biochemical features of the disorder. Currently, glycogen storage diseases are classified by numeric type in the chronologic order of the identification of the disorder (Chen & Burchell, 1995; Scriver et al., 1995a).

Liver and muscle have abundant amounts of glycogen and are therefore the most commonly and seriously affected tissues. The essential role of the liver in the regulation of carbohydrate metabolism and glucose homeostasis results in the usual presenting features of glycogen storage diseases—hypoglycemia and hepatomegaly. The types of glycogen storage diseases predominantly affecting the liver are type I (glucose-6-phosphatase), type III (debrancher), type IV (brancher), and type VI (liver phosphorylase and phosphorylase kinase). The hepatic glycogen storage diseases vary in the age at onset, progression, other organ involvement, and the clinical severity of the disorder (Chen & Burchell, 1995).

The role of glycogen in muscle is to provide substrates to enable ATP generation necessary for muscle contraction. Glycogen storage diseases that affect primarily the muscle can be divided into two groups: type II (acid α-glucosidase), a lysosomal enzyme deficiency, and type V (muscle phosphorylase deficiency), characterized by muscle fatigue and weakness (Chen & Burchell, 1995).

The glycogen storage diseases have one biochemical feature in common: abnormal storage of glycogen. This abnormality is more often an increase, but sometimes a decrease, and the glycogen may have normal or abnormal structure. Many other secondary biochemical changes may occur, such as hypoglycemia and changes in blood lipid components and lactate levels (Ampola, 1982; Burman et al., 1978; Scriver et al., 1995a).

The glycogen storage diseases show an overall frequency of approximately 1 in 20,000 to 1 in 25,000 live births, and almost all cases are autosomally inherited (Burman et al., 1978; Chen & Burchell, 1995). However, there are some exceptions to this pattern; autosomal recessive and sex-linked forms of type VI glycogen storage disease have been described (Burman et al., 1978; Chen & Burchell, 1995). Types I, II, III, and VI are the most common glycogen storage diseases and account for 90 percent of all cases.

Within the group of glycogen storage diseases, varying degrees of clinical severity exist. For example, types II and IV are almost invariably lethal within the first 3 to 12 months of life, whereas types III and V are often relatively mild (Burman et al., 1978; Chen & Burchell, 1995; Scriver et al., 1995a). Varying degrees of severity exist even within the same enzyme defect. This variation is particularly marked in type I (glucose-6-phosphatase deficiency [G6PD]), in which symptoms may vary from severe to relatively mild. The physical symptoms for the group of glycogen storage diseases are very similar to hepatomegaly, with a large protruding abdomen whose size is in sharp contrast to the thin extremities. Often there is psychomotor delay in the first years of life. There is distinct growth retardation, which is especially striking in children with G6PD. The most prominent features of the metabolic disturbance are hypoglycemia, acidosis with elevated blood lactate levels, fasting ketosis, hyperlipemia, and hyperuricemia (Ampola, 1982; Benson, 1983; Burman et al., 1978; Chen & Burchell, 1995; Galjaard, 1980; Komrower, 1980; Scriver et al., 1995a). Despite the similarity of physical symptoms, the metabolic abnormalities are highly dependent on the underlying type of enzyme defect.

Definitive diagnosis rests on the direct enzyme assay from suitable tissue. The tissues most suitable for enzymologic examination are usually liver or muscle but may include leukocytes or erythrocytes or fibroblasts (Chen & Burchell, 1995; LeGrys, 1984). Prenatal diagnosis is possible for some forms of the disorders (LeGrys, 1984; Scriver et al., 1995a). The most direct approach to establishing a definitive diagnosis is by enzyme assay of a liver biopsy or a leukocyte preparation (Ampola, 1982; Burman et al., 1978; Chen & Burchell, 1995; LeGrys, 1984; Scriver et al., 1995a). Early definitive diagnosis of these disorders is of practical importance for the management of affected infants, because management differs for each type of enzyme deficiency.

Hypoglycemia is the most common and most severe in infants with type I glycogen storage disease caused by debranching enzyme deficiency (Burman et al., 1978; Chen & Burchell, 1995; Scriver et al., 1995a) (see Fig. 25–3). There is almost complete dependence on exogenous glucose, because glucose production from glycogenolysis and gluconeogenesis is blocked. Frequent feedings with an ample supply of glucose are needed. The addition of starches into the diet has a twofold effect: It results in delayed gastric emptying time and serves as an extra source of fuel, thus saving glucose (Chen & Burchell, 1995; Winick, 1979). Affected infants can utilize all types of sugars, because they can easily convert galactose and fructose into glucose; however, they nonetheless require frequent high-carbohydrate feedings during the first year of life. These individuals have an enhanced rate of gluconeogenesis from protein and benefit from extra protein,

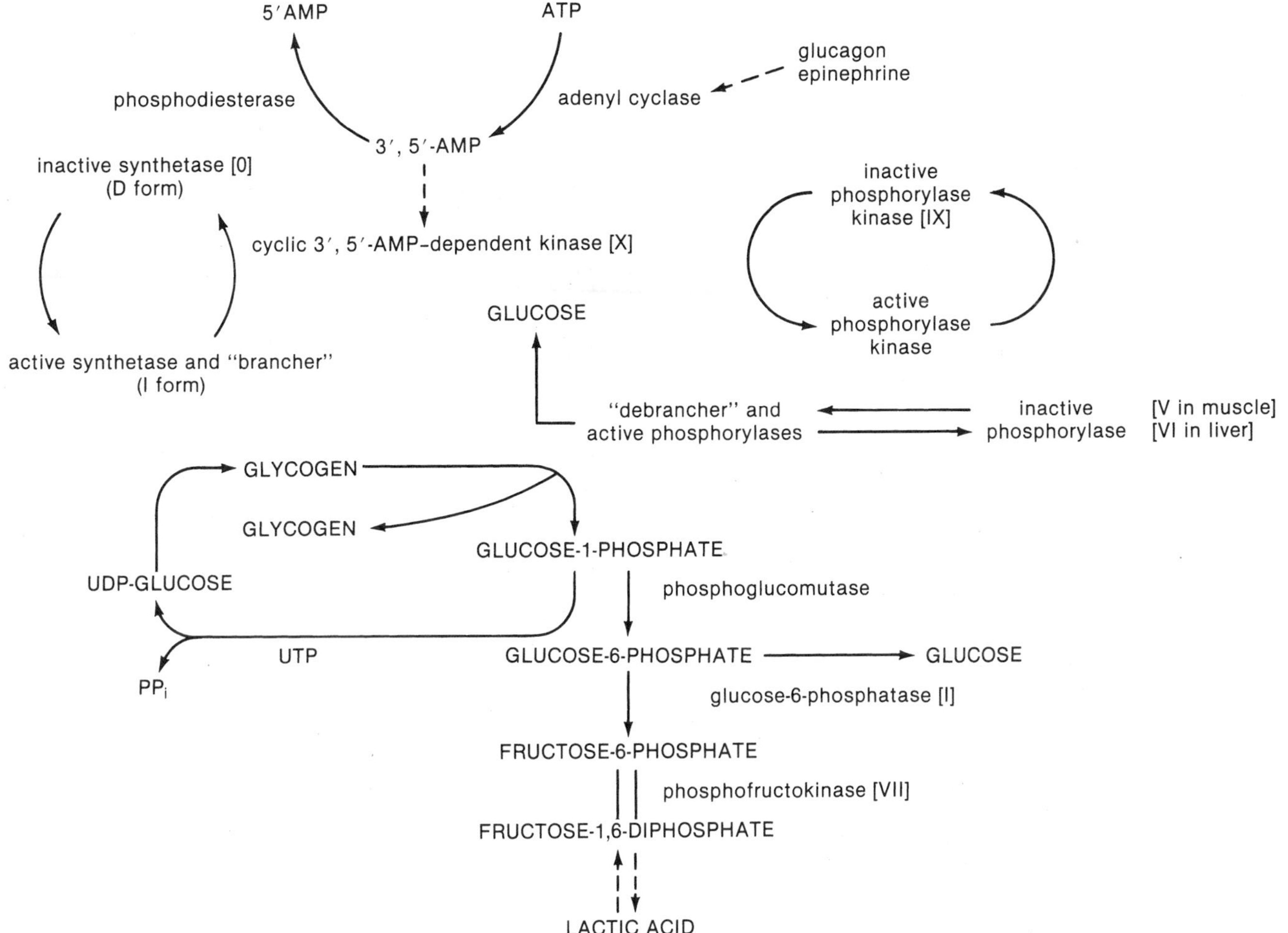

FIGURE 25–3. A summary of glycogen metabolism. Enzymes responsible for the various disorders of glycogen metabolism are noted with brackets. AMP, adenosine monophosphate; ATP, adenosine triphosphate; PP_i, inorganic pyrophosphate; UTP, uridine triphosphate.

particularly a high-protein feeding at bedtime (Chen & Burchell, 1995). Phosphorylase-deficient patients have only mild symptoms of hypoglycemia and do not require any special dietary provisions (Benson, 1983; Burman et al., 1978; Chen & Burchell, 1995; Scriver et al., 1995a; Winick, 1979).

Severe acidosis occurs only in glucose 6-phosphatase deficiency (type I), whereas fasting ketosis is most pronounced in debranching enzyme and virtually absent in G6PD (Burman et al., 1978; Chen & Burchell, 1995). In infants with G6PD (type I), the administration of oral sucrose and lactose results in enhanced lactate production, inasmuch as the galactose from lactose and the fructose from sucrose cannot be converted to glucose (Burman et al., 1978; Chen & Burchell, 1995; Scriver et al., 1995a). Therefore, lactose and particularly sucrose are restricted in the diet, which then consists largely of glucose and starch as sources of carbohydrate (Winick, 1979). Fasting ketosis is striking in individuals with debranching enzyme deficiency and within normal limits in infants with G6PD. The results of fasting ketosis in phosphorylase-deficient children have been variable. Dietary management to prevent excessive ketosis is the same as for hypoglycemia (Burman et al., 1978; Chen & Burchell, 1995; Winick, 1979).

It is not known whether the hyperlipidemia observed in these disorders involves an increased risk of atherosclerosis in adult life. However, it is desirable to attempt to reduce the hyperlipidemia. Dietary measures have had little effect on the hyperlipidemia in patients with G6PD (Burman et al., 1978; Chen & Burchell, 1995; Winick, 1979). In debranching enzyme- and phosphorylase-deficient children, there is a reduction achieved by a combination of a low carbohydrate content in the diet and the use of polyunsaturated fatty acids such as corn oil. Diets high in carbohydrate increase the lipid levels in the blood (Winick, 1979).

Hyperuricemia is a serious complication seen in patients with G6PD who survive the precarious first years of life. The long-standing elevated blood uric acid levels may result in gout and, more serious, renal damage as a result of hyperuricemia. The tendency toward hyperuricemia is suppressed at an early age. The use of allopurinol, a xanthine oxidase inhibitor, prevents the conversion of precursors into uric acid and results in a significant decrease in blood uric acid levels and the resolution of uric acid tophi (Burman et al., 1978; Chen & Burchell, 1995; Crawford et al., 1982; Scriver et al., 1995a; Wapnir, 1985; Winick, 1979).

The use of nocturnal nasogastric drip feedings has yielded some improvement in the growth patterns of infants with G6PD. The steady infusion of glucose is thought to diminish lactate production and result in decreased lactic acidosis. An additional benefit of the nocturnal nasogastric feedings is an improvement in the blood lipid profile of these patients (Burman et al., 1978; Chen & Burchell, 1995; Winick, 1979). Additional information about G6PD is given later in this chapter.

Liver transplantation has been performed in several patients with the hepatic manifestations of glycogen storage disease (type I). The hypoglycemia and the biochemical abnormalities were corrected after transplantation, and growth improved. However, liver transplantation should be performed only after all other management efforts have failed or if there is malignant transformation of an adenoma (Chen & Burchell, 1995).

Since the early 1990s, advances in the understanding of the molecular basis of the regulation of the enzymes have been used to improve the diagnosis and the prediction of the clinical outcome of the various genetic deficiencies. It is hoped that in the future, molecular studies will lead to the development of gene therapy for the more severe disorders.

AMINO ACID METABOLISM

Amino acids play a major role as constituents of intracellular and extracellular proteins. Some amino acids cannot be synthesized at rates that are sufficient to enable normal development, and these essential amino acids have to be derived from exogenous sources such as dietary protein and nonprotein nitrogen. Estimates of the daily requirements of these essential amino acids (isoleucine, leucine, lysine, methionine, phenylalanine, threonine, tryptophan, and valine) have been made. Although histidine is not an essential amino acid, its presence is essential for the normal growth of the infant (Nyhan, 1984).

Alanine, arginine, asparagine, aspartic acid, cysteine, glutamic acid, glutamine, glycine, histidine, proline, serine, and tyrosine can be synthesized from a reduced form of nitrogen and a carbon skeleton. Major sources of the carbon chain are f(α)-ketoglutarate, pyruvate, and oxaloacetate, and the reduced form of nitrogen becomes available from recycling of other compounds (Nyhan, 1984).

The detailed pathways of amino acid metabolism are beyond the scope of this discussion. However, for the purpose of this chapter, two facts are important: (1) The fetus is a rapidly growing organism supplied by its mother with all the necessary amino acids, which it uses to build up its body tissues; and (2) probably only minor amounts of amino acids are used by the fetus for purposes other than growth (Ampola, 1982; Nyhan, 1984; Scriver et al., 1995a; Stave, 1978).

The deposition of nitrogen during the perinatal period is greater than at any other time of life. The magnitude of protein synthesis can be demonstrated by the nitrogen content of the fetus, which is 0.4 g at 6 weeks' gestation, increases to 15 g by 20 weeks, and by full-term gestation is 500 g (Stave, 1978). In the early postnatal months, this trend of nitrogen deposition continues.

The synthesis of any protein is a complex multistep process that results in macromolecule formation from the 20 individual amino acids in a specific sequence that is under genetic control. There are two basic steps of all protein synthesis: (1) DNA that has the genetic code for the protein makes RNA; and (2) RNA makes the protein from cytosolic amino acids. All cellular constituents are continuously being degraded and replaced. In the perinatal period, the marked accumulation of protein occurs because synthesis is accomplished by the placental transport of amino acids and the rate of synthesis exceeds that of degradation. The process of birth temporarily interrupts the high rate of protein synthesis in the fetus, regardless of maturity. This disruption in protein synthesis is caused by a shift in the constant nutrient supply of the placenta to the inadequate and sporadic intake of the first days of life and results in a negative nitrogen balance (Stave, 1978).

GI digestion and absorption of released amino acids are well developed in neonates. This is evidenced even in small preterm infants by the total stool nitrogen content, which does not exceed 15 percent of intake. Nitrogen is retained with avidity, and the amount retained is proportional to the intake (Nyhan, 1984; Stave, 1978). In contrast to adults, in whom the effect is only transient, a high-protein intake results in high protein retention in neonates. Therefore, amino acid levels represent a net balance between a number of different processes, including (1) the amount available from the diet; (2) the amount used for tissue repair and growth; (3) the amount used for specific purposes; (4) the amount excreted in the urine; and (5) the amount remaining that must be metabolized. When an inborn error of protein metabolism is investigated, these factors merit consideration (Ampola, 1982; Blaskovics et al., 1974; Cohn & Roth, 1983; Nyhan, 1984; Scriver et al., 1995a; Wapnir, 1985).

Disorders of Amino Acid Metabolism

Disorders of amino acid metabolism may involve a specific enzyme disorder affecting amino acid metabolism, specific deficiencies in one of the intestinal absorption and renal tubular reabsorption systems, or the intralysosomal accumulation of an amino acid (Nyhan, 1984). Although there are only 20 amino acids, they undergo a multitude of reactions such as hydroxylation, oxidation, transamination, methylation, and coupling, and a metabolic disorder can result when one of these processes is disrupted. Examples of these types of amino acid disorders are discussed in the following section.

The Hyperphenylalaninemias

- The hyperphenylalaninemias are disorders of phenylalanine hydroxylation. The minimum requirements for a normal reaction are phenylalanine hydroxylase (PAH), oxygen, *L*-phenylalanine, and tetrahydrobiopterin (BH4) cofactor. For the pterin cofactor to function as a catalyst, dihydropterin reductase (DHPR) and reduced pyridine nucleotide are required. Other enzymes are also involved in recycling BH4, which is an obligatory component of hydrolase function.
- Hyperphenylalaninemia, defined as plasma phenylalanine levels above 2 mg/dl (120 μmol), is a heterogeneous disease caused by mutations at the genetic sites that encode components of the hydroxylation reaction. The known and putative forms involve (1) primary deficiency in PAH activity (PKU and nonphenylketonuria [non-PKU]); (2) impaired synthesis of BH4 as a result of enzyme deficiency; and, (3) impaired recycling of BH4 as a result of deficient activity of DPHR or other putative enzyme systems.
- The associated diseases are autosomal recessive. Two conditions are necessary to cause clinical manifestations: the genetic mutation and exposure to *L*-phenylalanine. In the BH4-deficient forms, mutation alone is the principal cause of the disease. Patients with PKU have plasma values greater than 1000 μmol; in patients with non-PKU hyperphenylalaninemia, values are less than those of PKU-affected infants. PKU is a disease carrying impaired cognitive and neurophysiologic consequences; non-PKU hyperphenylalaninemia signifies less clinical harm, and it may be a benign condition. The BH4-deficient forms of the hyperphenylalaninemias have no categoric degree of hyperphenylalanine; they impair two other hydroxylation reactions involving tyrosine and tryptophan and the synthesis of the corresponding neurotransmitter derivatives (L-dopa and 5-hydroxytryptophan). Pathogenesis of the brain disorder in the different hyperphenylalaninemias involves the effects of phenylalanine on essential cellular processes in the brain, notably myelination, protein synthesis, and the consequences of deficient neurotransmitter supply.
- The genes that encode the components of the hydroxylation reaction are at various stages of analysis in normal and mutant genomes. Loci on chromosomes 4, 12, and 14 have been identified as having a role in the hydroxylation reactions associated with hyperphenylalaninemia.
- Treatment requires restoration of blood phenylalanine levels

to values as near normal as possible for as long as possible throughout life. Available data indicate that any deviation from this policy may incur a cost in neurophysiologic function and brain myelination in classic PKU-affected individuals. Whether it also applies to non-PKU hyperphenylalaninemia is unclear but current opinion is shifting toward prudent (pretreatment) options contrary to the past policy of no treatment. The BH4-deficient forms of hyperphenylalaninemias necessitate adjunct therapy that includes supplements of L-dopa and 5-hydroxytryptophan; BH4 in disorders of the cofactor synthesis; and supplements of folinic acid in DHPR deficiency.

- The overall incidence of hyperphenylalaninemia is approximately 100 cases per 1,000,000 live births among white and Asian individuals. There is geographic and ethnic variation in the incidence of classic PKU (from 5 to 375 cases per 1,000,000 live births).
- Non-PKU is less prevalent than PKU and it shows less variation in the incidence (15 to 75 cases per 1,000,000 live births). The BH4-deficient forms are panethnic and pangeographic. Their overall incidence is approximately 1 to 2 cases per 1,000,000 live births.
- Neonatal screening is the best method of screening for hyperphenylalaninemia. Both classification of the phenotype or disease (diagnosis) and case finding of BH4 deficiency require measurement of phenylalanine, pterins (neopterin, biopterin, and BH4), and neurotransmitter derivatives in plasma and urine. Activity of the mutant enzyme can be assessed either directly by measurement in a population of cells, such as hepatocytes, or indirectly by DNA analysis, enzymatic assay, and measurement of metabolites in amniotic fluid in all forms of hyperphenylalaninemia.
- Maternal hyperphenylalaninemia causes fetal pathology that compromises growth and causes congenital malformations, including microcephaly and mental retardation in the offspring. It occurs as a result of excessive intrauterine phenylalanine exposure from the positive transplacental gradient. Women with hyperphenylalaninemia require preconceptional reproductive counseling and should receive treatment for and be in strict control of the phenylalanine levels before conception and throughout pregnancy. A normal outcome is possible with meticulous care.

Hyperphenylalaninemia is a generic term for a disease distinguished by a phenylalanine level persistently above its normal plasma values. The metabolic dysfunction can have clinical consequences, depending on its pathogenesis and degree. The associated diseases are named by the deficient enzyme; for example, PKU is hyperphenylalaninemia resulting from total or nearly total deficiency of PAH activity. Different mutations at the PAH site can cause a lesser degree of hyperphenylalaninemia (non-PKU hyperphenylalaninemia). The distinction between these two hyperphenylalaninemias is arbitrary and rests with the higher plasma phenylalanine values greater than 16.5 mg/dl (1000 μmol) and lower tolerance for dietary phenylalanine (less than 500 mg/dl in classic PKU).

The disorders associated with the synthesis or maintenance of BH4 are important in two additional hydroxylation reactions involving *L*-tryptophan and *L*-tyrosine, notably in the brain. The hydroxylated derivatives of these substrates, 5-hydroxytryptophan and L-dopa, are the precursors to serotonin and catecholamines and are neurotransmitters that influence brain development and function. Thus the diagnosis of these variants is relevant for prognosis and treatment of every infant with hyperphenylalaninemia.

PKU and Non-PKU Forms of Hyperphenylalaninemia

PKU is perhaps the best known specific enzyme deficiency that results in a metabolic encephalopathy (Scriver et al., 1995a). The incidence of PKU varies from 1 in 4500 live births in Northern Ireland to 1 in 61,000 live births in Japan (Ampola, 1982; Benson, 1983; Bickel et al., 1980; Blaskovics et al., 1974; Koch et al., 1993; Nyhan, 1984; Scriver et al., 1995a, 1995b). The average incidence of PKU in the United States ranges from 100 to 120 per 1,000,000 live births (Ampola, 1982; Koch et al., 1993; Nyhan, 1984; Scriver et al., 1995a, 1995b; Wapnir, 1985). The disease affects primarily people of Western and Central European descent; it is rare in blacks and in non-European populations (Ampola, 1982; Benson, 1983; Bickel et al., 1980; Nyhan, 1984; Scriver et al., 1995a, 1995b). PKU is an autosomal recessive trait with equal sex distribution and results in a deficiency of the enzyme PAH, which is found primarily in the liver (Scriver et al., 1995a, 1995b). This enzyme is one participant along with DHPR in the complex conversion of phenylalanine to tyrosine (Ampola, 1982; Benson, 1983; Bickel et al., 1980; Blaskovics et al., 1974; Nyhan, 1984; Scriver et al., 1995a, 1995b) (Fig. 25–4). Whereas PAH enzyme deficiency is a hepatic disease, the major clinical effect of the associated metabolic hyperphenylalaninemia is on brain function. The variant metabolic disease is thus the cause of the neurotoxicity of disorders of PAH activity. In disorders of BH4 synthesis and maintenance, there are indirect effects (through abnormal phenylalanine metabolism) and direct effects (by impairing tryptophan and tyrosine hydroxylations) on brain development and function.

PKU is characterized by serum phenylalanine levels greater than 25 mg/dl (1500 μmol), whereas the normal level is less than 2 mg/dl (120 μmol); by normal serum tyrosine levels; and by urinary excretion of phenylpyruvic and orthohydroxyphenylacetic acids when normal protein dietary conditions exist (Ampola, 1982; Benson, 1983; Bickel et al., 1980; Blaskovics et al., 1974; LeGrys, 1984; Nyhan, 1984; Scriver et al., 1995a, 1995b; Wapnir, 1985). PAH deficiency may be expressed in greater or lesser (to completely absent) amounts (Ampola, 1982; Nyhan, 1984; Scriver et al., 1995a, 1995b; Smith & Wolffe, 1976; Smith & the Medical Research Council Working Party on PKU, 1993; Svensson et al., 1994; Wapnir, 1985). In classic PKU, PAH is itself inactive, with less than 1 percent normal activity (Nyhan, 1984). In the absence of PAH, the enzymes that convert phenylalanine into phenylethylamine and phenylpyruvic acid are present and result in increasing concentrations of these compounds in the urine (Ampola, 1982; Benson, 1983; Bickel et al., 1980; Blaskovics et al., 1974; Koch et al., 1993; LeGrys, 1984; Nyhan, 1984; Paul et al., 1980; Scriver et al., 1995a, 1995b; Smith & Wolffe, 1976; Svensson et al., 1994; Winick, 1979).

There are no abnormal metabolites in PKU, only normal metabolites in abnormal amounts. With regard to neurotoxicity, phenylalanine is itself the villain. Induced high plasma values are associated with measurable acute impairment of higher integrative functions and with abnormal electroencephalograms (EEGs) (Ludolph et al., 1992). Both urine dopamine excretion and plasma L-dopa levels correlate inversely with plasma phenylalanine levels and positively with measures of brain dysfunction. Magnetic resonance imaging (MRI) and spectroscopy studies have demonstrated that higher plasma phenylalanine levels alter brain chemistry when plasma levels exceed 22.5 mg/dl (1300 μmol) (Azen et al., 1991; Battistini et al., 1991; Bick et al., 1991; Cleary et al., 1994; Hommes, 1991; Ramus et al., 1993).

Chronic levels of phenylalanine that exceed 20 mg/dl (1200 μmol) result in central nervous system damage, and some experts believe that individuals with phenylalanine levels chronically elevated at greater than 12 to 15 mg/dl (720 to 900 μmol) are also at risk for central nervous system damage (Ampola, 1982; Azen et al., 1991; Benson, 1983; Bick et al., 1991; Bickel, 1980; Blaskovics et al., 1974; Hommes, 1991; Koch et al., 1993; Nyhan, 1984; Scriver et al., 1995a, 1995b).

The threshold value for neurotoxicity in the acute effect may not correspond to the value associated with chronic neurotoxicity.

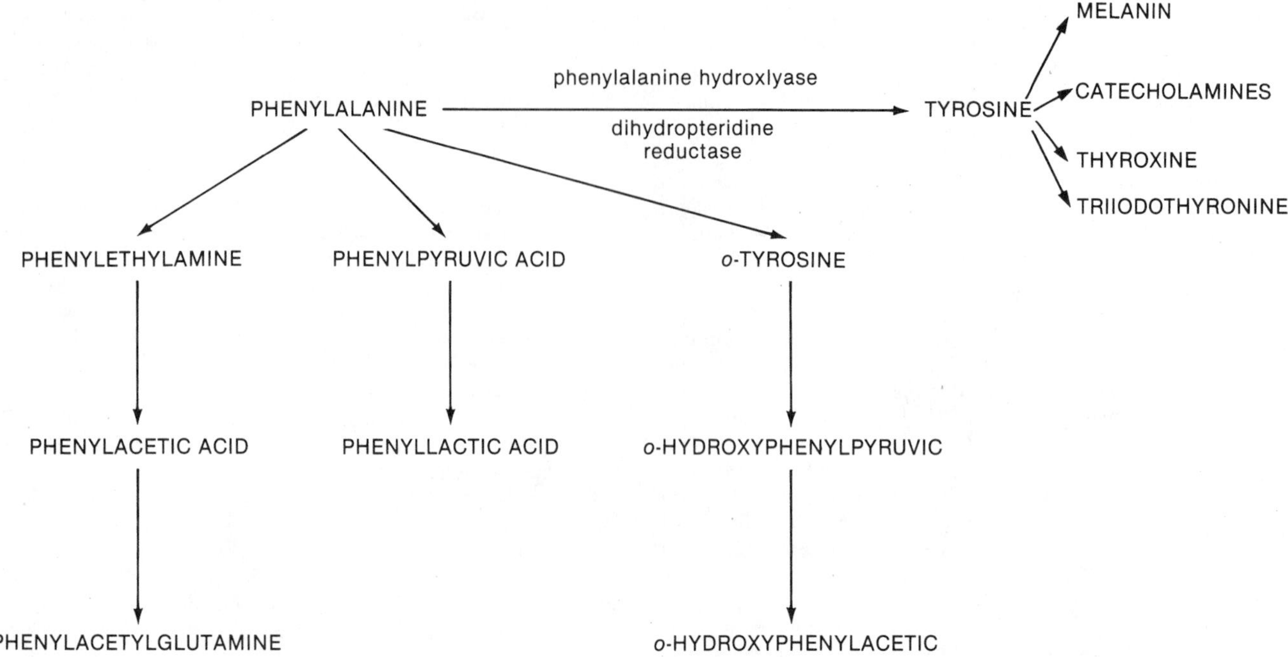

FIGURE 25–4. The conversion of phenylalanine to tyrosine. Phenylalanine hydroxylase, an enzyme found primarily in the liver, is one participant in the complex conversion of phenylalanine to tyrosine. A second enzyme, dihydropteridine reductase, also participates in the reaction but requires the reduced pteridine cofactor tetrahydrobiopterin.

Chronic neurotoxicity can manifest itself in at least two ways. First, it may occur in the brain white matter, where changes visible on MRI are more prevalent than the overt neurologic dysfunction. These findings are being discovered in patients, presumed to be well treated, who have only modest, chronic elevations of plasma phenylalanine less than 10 mg/dl (600 μmol) (Azen et al., 1991; Battistini et al., 1991; Cleary et al., 1994; Hommes, 1991; Koch et al., 1993). Second, in the IQ scores of the treated PKU patients, the values are distributed below the normal range despite good long-term control of plasma phenylalanine in the range of 1 to 5 mg/dl (60 to 300 μmol) (Azen et al., 1991; Costello et al., 1994; Koch et al., 1993; Smith & Beasley, 1988).

These findings are disturbing and significant. The data suggests that the neurotoxic threshold value for phenylalanine is different for the acute and chronic effects on the brain. The degree of any postnatal (or fetal) hyperphenylalaninemia could cause irreversible changes in brain structure (myelin) and function (cognition). If hyperphenylalaninemia recurs later in life, such as when treatment is terminated after satisfactory brain development has been achieved in the early-treated PKU patient or during bouts of intercurrent illnesses, reversible chemical changes will again appear. If the neurotoxic effect persists, irreversible changes in the white matter with deterioration in cognitive function could then follow (Koch et al., 1993; Scriver et al., 1995a, 1995b).

Overt clinical manifestations occur in untreated PKU-affected infants. Symptoms are virtually absent in the untreated non-PKU infants. The early diagnosis and treatment of the newborn with hyperphenylalaninemia has made the classic PKU disease manifestations a matter of historical rather than common occurrence. However, symptoms of classic PKU are still occasionally reported, and they achieve greater relevance as patients terminate treatment for one reason or another.

Clinical manifestations vary, depending on the expression of enzyme activity (Svensson et al., 1994). In the first weeks of life, digestive problems and vomiting may lead to the false diagnosis of pyloric stenosis. In untreated infants, there is normal mentation at birth, which over time progressively deteriorates. A delay in psychomotor development or a regression in development occurs after several months of age. After the first year, the intelligence quotient (IQ) of an untreated infant may be below 20; fewer than 4 percent have an IQ greater than 50 (Ampola, 1982; Azen et al., 1991; Benson, 1983; Bickel et al., 1980; Blaskovics et al., 1974; Nyhan, 1984; Pitt & Danks, 1991; Ramus et al., 1993; Scriver et al., 1995a, 1995b; Wapnir, 1985). There may be myoclonic or grand mal seizures in approximately 25 percent of the patients after the first few months, and 80 percent of patients have EEG abnormalities (Ludolph et al., 1992; Nyhan, 1984; Scriver et al., 1995a, 1995b; Wapnir, 1985). In a report that described the natural history of symptoms over 22 years in 51 patients with untreated PKU, 25 percent developed epilepsy, 50 percent were profoundly retarded (IQ, <35), approximately 50 percent were moderately retarded (IQ, 37 to 67), and 5 percent had an IQ higher than 68. The mean phenylalanine levels in this group ranged from 20 to 29 mg/dl (1180 to 1694 μmol) (Pitt & Danks, 1991).

Other clinical manifestations are cited in the literature. A direct cause-and-effect relationship may be difficult to determine secondary to the relatively few number of PKU individuals, although some degree of agoraphobia (Waisbren & Levy, 1991) seems to be a newly recognized and prevalent symptom. Individuals affected by PKU have hypopigmentation of hair, skin, and irises as a result of the decreased production of melanin. Eczema in early childhood is common (Blaskovics et al., 1974; Nyhan, 1984; Scriver et al., 1995a, 1995b). The urine has a musty odor resulting from the excretion of phenylacetic acid (Blaskovics et al., 1974; Nyhan, 1984; Paul et al., 1980; Scriver et al., 1995a, 1995b).

Behavior of these children may be hyperactive and aggressive, which may be indistinguishable from the behavior of children with autism or various childhood psychoses (Bickel, 1980; Bickel et al., 1954; Hommes, 1991; Koch et al., 1993; Pitt & Danks, 1991; Scriver et al., 1995a, 1995b; Smith & Beasley, 1988). These children exhibit constant agitation and show abnormal movements. There is unceasing movement of hands and fingers, and there may be violent anteroposterior contortions of the trunk. Neurologic examination reveals hypertonia, exaggerated tendon reflexes, and trembling with a clumsy, rigid walk (Ampola, 1982; Benson, 1983; Blaskovics et al., 1974; Galjaard, 1980; Komrower, 1980; Nyhan, 1984; Scriver et al., 1995a, 1995b; Wapnir, 1985).

On pathologic examination, the brain is low in weight and has a reduced myelin content (Hommes, 1991; Nyhan, 1984; Scriver et al., 1995a, 1995b). MRI changes in patients with PKU are compatible with disturbances in the water content of the white matter; the severity of the abnormality strongly correlates with the current phenylalanine level at the time of imaging (Battistini et al., 1991; Bick et al., 1991; Cleary et al., 1994; Hommes, 1991). The abnormal MRI changes are reversible if they are of recent onset and reflect greater turnover of myelin during states of hyperphenylalaninemia. In the context of cognitive development and brain function, hyperphenylalaninemia may alter the patterns of neuronal connections and result in a decreased number of permanent synaptic connections (Bick et al., 1991; Hommes, 1991). Neuropsychological studies demonstrate prolonged central motor conduction time, prolonged visual evoked potentials, and impaired peripheral sensory nerve conduction. MRI changes have not been strongly correlated to IQ scores (Azen et al., 1991; Bick et al., 1991; Cleary et al., 1994; Costello et al., 1994; Hommes, 1991; Koch et al., 1993; Ludolph et al., 1992). Many comparison studies of intellectual and neuropsychological measures have been performed with adults affected by PKU and with their unaffected control siblings. Early diagnosed and treated adults had normal intelligence, attention, and complex visual constructual ability (Azen et al., 1991; Costello et al., 1994; Koch et al., 1993; Ramus et al., 1993; Ris et al., 1994). Intellectual outcome is best predicted by the degree of early neurologic insult, whereas performance on novel problem-solving was best predicted by current phenylalanine level. These results provide further convincing evidence that treatment should be continued well into adulthood (Ris et al., 1994) and perhaps for life (Battistini et al., 1991; Koch et al., 1993; Scriver et al., 1995a, 1995b).

The goal of screening for hyperphenylalaninemia is early medical intervention. The goal of diagnosis is correct medical intervention. The screening for PKU occurs when the infant's blood is collected as dried spots on filter paper and is screened by use of bacterial inhibition, chromatographic, fluorometric assays, enzymatic assays, or tandem mass spectrometry (Ampola, 1982; Benson, 1983; Bickel et al., 1980; Blaskovics et al., 1974; Chace et al., 1993; Cockburn & Gitzelmann, 1980; Doherty et al., 1991; LeGrys, 1984; Nyhan, 1984; Qu et al., 1991; Scriver et al., 1995a, 1995b; Wapnir, 1985). Phenylalanine in dried blood spots on filter paper, properly stored, is stable for years. The microbiologic and chromatographic methods are semiquantitative, with limitations of accuracy at lower phenylalanine concentrations. The fluorometric assay is fully quantitative down to and into the normal range.

A crucial characteristic of a screening test is its sensitivity: the ability to minimize the frequency of false-negative test results. The timing of the sample collection and the threshold value are thus critical in the accuracy of the screening test. The PKU screening test is done after birth, and thus the capillary blood phenylalanine level in affected cases is lower the closer the day of testing is to the day of birth. Therefore, the sensitivity of the test could be impaired when it is done on the first or second day of life rather than on day three or four. The greatest risk of false-negative test results occurs if testing is performed before 24 hours of age (Holtzman et al., 1986; Irons, 1993; LeGrys, 1984; McCabe & McCabe, 1983; Natowicz & Alper, 1991; Nyhan, 1984; Scriver, 1982; Scriver et al., 1995a).

New birthing practices and early discharges from birthing units has created challenges for neonatal screening practices. Routine follow-up or repeat testing of early discharged infants with negative first results would be financially prohibitive and inefficient. To convert the test methodology from microbiologic or chromatographic (semiquantitative) to fluorometric (fully quantitative) has technical merits but would require a massive reorganization of most screening programs in the United States, inasmuch as only a few currently employ a fluorometric assay method. The threshold value to signify hyperphenylalaninemia has been lowered to improve sensitivity. If the critical value of 2 mg/dl is used for screening, few infants with true PKU will be missed (Doherty et al., 1991; Holtzman et al., 1986; Irons, 1993; McCabe & McCabe, 1983; Natowicz & Alper, 1991; Scriver et al., 1995a, 1995b). While accepting a tolerable increase in the rate of false-positive results, the lower threshold will prevent the occurrence of many false-negative results that occurred with the early discharge of normal newborns. Currently, only one case of PKU is missed for every 70 detected in America (Holtzman et al., 1986; Scriver et al., 1995a, 1995b). The cause for this can be errors of compliance and procedure (McCabe & McCabe, 1983) as well as biologic variation in the postnatal rise of phenylalanine (Scriver et al., 1995a, 1995b). False results, either positive or negative, may also arise from technical factors such as ampicillin contamination of the sample, total parenteral nutrition with some amino acid solutions, and even the lot variability of the filter paper (McCabe & McCabe, 1983). In affected newborns, the plasma level of phenylalanine increases after commencement of normal feedings. By the fourth or fifth day, infants with classic PKU have phenylalanine levels 10 to 20 times normal (Ampola, 1982; Bickel et al., 1980; Blaskovics et al., 1974; Doherty et al., 1991; Nyhan, 1984; Scriver et al., 1995a, 1995b). Most of these affected newborns are detected after 1 day of adequate protein intake, even if the screening method used detects at least 4 mg/dl of phenylalanine (Doherty et al., 1991; Irons, 1993; Natowicz & Alper, 1991; Nyhan, 1984; Scriver et al., 1995a, 1995b).

Enhanced urinary excretion of phenylpyruvic acid (indicative of PKU) produces a blue-green color when urine is mixed (1:1) with 5 percent ferric chloride solution. Phenistix (Ames Laboratories, Elkhart, IN) was an early method used in PKU screening (Paul et al., 1980). However, in many infants with PKU, the urine test does not become positive for at least several weeks after birth despite markedly elevated serum phenylalanine levels. This occurs because the enzyme that converts phenylalanine to phenylpyruvic acid is often delayed in its appearance. Therefore, PKU screening should not depend on the urine test for phenylpyruvic acid (Bickel et al., 1980; Blaskovics et al., 1974; LeGrys, 1984; Nyhan, 1984; Paul et al., 1980; Scriver et al., 1995a, 1995b).

A positive neonatal screening test identifies an infant with hyperphenylalaninemia. The diagnostic test identifies the cause of the hyperphenylalaninemia in that particular infant. Some infants with a positive first screening test have brief and transient hyperphenylalaninemia of no further clinical significance; the majority have persistent hyperphenylalaninemia. Among those infants, hyperphenylalaninemia is caused predominantly (>97 percent) by a deficiency of PAH. Approximately 1 to 3 percent of infants with hyperphenylalaninemia have impaired synthesis or recycling of BH4. These cases require specific treatment to offset the BH4 deficiency. Because plasma phenylalanine levels alone do not distinguish between the BH4-impaired and BH4-sufficient forms of hyperphenylalaninemia, every case of persistent hyperphenylalaninemia must be investigated further to determine metabolism of BH4 (Bickel et al., 1980; Blaskovics et al., 1974; LeGrys, 1984; Nyhan, 1984; Scriver et al., 1995a, 1995b; Wapnir, 1985) (Fig. 25–5).

Diagnostic tests in the newborn include the direct measurement of plasma phenylalanine and the plasma phenylalanine response to BH4. There are no reliable phenylalanine metabolites, and phenylalanine loading tests are not recommended in the newborn. Three days of protein feeding at normal volumes has been used in older subjects to classify the type of PKU. Tests for pterin metabolites are reliably done only in laboratories with

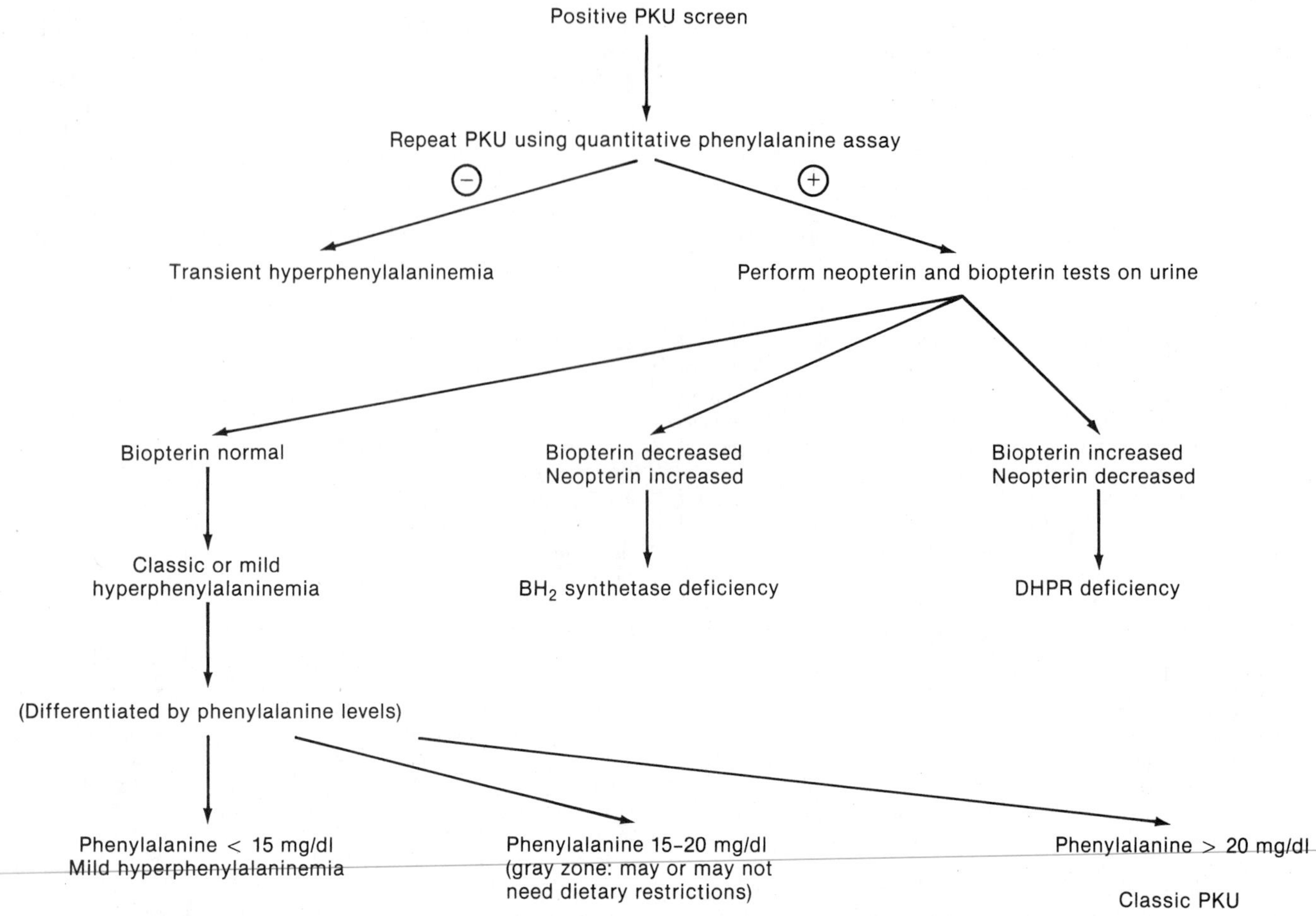

FIGURE 25–5. Verification of phenylketonuria (PKU) diagnosis. BH_2, dihydropteridine; DHPR, dihydropteridine reductase.

expertise in this assay. The pterin tests are measured from dried blood spots on filter paper. Total activity was formerly assayed by its cofactor effect on phenylalanine hydroxylation in vitro. "Activity" of these two assays is high in untreated cases with ambient hyperphenylalaninemia and intact BH4 synthesis; it is low in disorders of BH4 homeostasis. Normal values of phenylalanine are less than 150 μmol in neonates and less than 120 μmol in older subjects. In the phenylalanine response to BH4, the BH4 is given orally at a time when the phenylalanine level is elevated, and a fall in the phenylalanine level indicates BH4 deficiency.

Diagnostic tests can also be performed at the enzyme level. Direct measurement of PAH activity requires liver biopsy (Bickel, 1980; Blaskovics et al., 1974; LeGrys, 1984; Nyhan, 1984; Scriver et al., 1995a, 1995b). Dihydrobiopterin reductase (DHPR) activity is measured in many tissues, including liver, skin fibroblasts, amniocytes, erythrocytes, leukocytes, platelets, and dried blood on filter paper (Bickel, 1980; Blaskovics et al., 1974; LeGrys, 1984; Nyhan, 1984; Scriver et al., 1995a, 1995b). Complex DNA analysis with use of venous blood, dried blood spots, buccal cells, and cultures of skin fibroblasts can be performed to analyze the mutation. The indications for prenatal diagnosis are not trivial in hyperphenylalaninemia. Treatment under some conditions may be difficult to obtain or administer, and prognosis for a normal outcome is not certain in all cases. Analysis of amniocytes, chorionic villus samples, amniotic fluid, and fetal erythrocytes have been performed to diagnose and classify the type of PKU prenatally (Scriver et al., 1995a, 1995b).

Once the diagnosis has been established, the treatment consists of early and competent management of a low-phenylalanine diet, which has been feasible since the 1950s (Ampola, 1982; Bickel, 1980; Blaskovics et al., 1974; Clark, 1992; Nyhan, 1984; Scriver et al., 1995a, 1995b; Thomas, 1992; Winick, 1979). Optimally, treatment of PKU requires (1) early onset of treatment within the first month after birth; (2) continuous treatment throughout childhood, adolescence, and adulthood, and certainly preconceptionally in PKU-affected women; and (3) restriction of phenylalanine intake to amounts sufficient to hold plasma phenylalanine values as close to the normal range (4 to 8 mg/dl, or 250 to 500 μmol) as possible. Phenylalanine tolerance varies according to the infant and the severity of the enzyme deficiency (Svensson et al., 1994; Winick, 1979). Atypical forms of PKU result in a variable amount of PAH activity, resulting in a higher tolerance for phenylalanine in the diet, and are associated with less severe mental retardation. These atypical forms of the disease are also autosomal recessive and may necessitate dietary restriction of phenylalanine (Bickel, 1980; Blaskovics et al., 1974; Costello et al., 1994; Galjaard, 1980; Nyhan, 1984; Scriver et al., 1995a, 1995b; Wapnir, 1985).

Protein intake cannot be reduced sufficiently to prevent the hyperphenylalaninemia without causing deficiencies of other essential amino acids. PKU infants are consumers with special needs, and they need selective restriction of phenylalanine intake. The tolerance for dietary phenylalanine to maintain "nontoxic" phenylalanine levels in young PKU patients is 25 percent of normal or less (approximately 250 to 500 mg of phenylalanine per day) (Bickel et al., 1954; Clark, 1992; Scriver et al., 1995a, 1995b; Thomas, 1992). A semisynthetic diet low in phenylalanine and adequate in other nutrients is used to treat PKU patients. Several commercial products consisting of modified protein hydrolysates or mixtures of free amino acids provide the essential amino acids in suitable proportions. The nutritional composition of these products is vastly different from that of human milk.

Because phenylalanine is an essential amino acid, small amounts of natural protein sources must be added to the diet to ensure minimal phenylalanine levels (Clark, 1992; Thomas, 1992; Winick, 1979). Complete restriction of all phenylalanine from the diet results in phenylalanine deficiency, manifested by anemia, growth retardation, cutaneous lesions, and mental deficiency. Phenylalanine deficiency is as detrimental as elevated levels of that amino acid (Ampola, 1982; Bickel, 1980; Blaskovics et al., 1974; Clark, 1992; Crawford et al., 1982; Fanaroff & Martin, 1997; Nyhan, 1984; Scriver et al., 1995a, 1995b; Thomas, 1992; Winick, 1979).

The dietary mode of treatment has its pitfalls. Transient hyperphenylalaninemia, followed by hypophenylalaninemia, is a hazard during overtreatment of PKU. This occurs when phenylalanine is used for anabolic needs when the normal protein synthesis is impaired by a deficiency of other essential nutrients. Adjustments of phenylalanine and protein intake are a challenge during bouts of intercurrent illnesses or in the growing preterm infant with PKU. Breast milk has been given safely as a supplement to the low-phenylalanine formula used in infancy. Both the long-term hypophenylalaninemia during excessive treatment and the persistent hyperphenylalaninemia during treatment have adverse consequences. The poor gustatory properties of the commercial diets are likely to affect compliance adversely. Close follow-up is essential for these infants because phenylalanine levels can become elevated when tissue catabolism releases amino acids into the blood (Ampola, 1982; Clark, 1992; Dixon & Leonard, 1992; Falk et al., 1994; Scriver et al., 1995a, 1995b; Wapnir, 1985). Thus parents must be aware of the first signs of illness in their infant and decrease the phenylalanine in the diet even further to prevent its toxic accumulation. In addition, during periods of anabolism and growth, dietary phenylalanine will need to be increased to prevent hypophenylalaninemia.

Aspartame is a popular artificial sweetener that, upon hydrolysis in the intestines, releases free *L*-phenylalanine, *L*-aspartic acid, and methanol. Its use comprises approximately 12 percent of the total sweeteners consumed. Its wide availability makes it a relevant hazard in the dietary management of PKU patients. For example, a quart of aspartame-sweetened flavored drink contains 280 mg of phenylalanine, or half of the daily allowance for phenylalanine. Thus PKU homozygote patients and their families must be meticulously cautious about reading product labels and adjusting diet accordingly.

The aspartame hazard for pregnant PKU heterozygotes is still debated. Newer studies have compared large-bolus ingestions of aspartame in normal subjects and heterozygotes. There was no significant disturbance of blood phenylalanine, tyrosine, and large amino acid levels in response to the load. Aspartame intake above the 90th percentile (the equivalent of drinking 24 twelve-ounce servings of aspartame-sweetened beverage over 8 hours) increased the blood phenylalanine level by less than 1 mg/dl (40 μmol) in the heterozygotes 30 minutes after ingestion, a trivial change (Trefz et al., 1994).

Controlled trials of treatment by selective restriction of phenylalanine intake on infants have never been attempted. Information regarding the effectiveness of this therapy is empirically derived from case reports of alternative dietary regimens in which the infant developed classic PKU symptoms and in never-treated PKU patients who still have the neuropsychological manifestations of the disease. In contrast, patients treated meticulously after neonatal diagnosis are essentially free of the classical IQ deterioration. Retrospective evidence to support these findings is substantial (Ampola, 1982; Azen et al., 1991; Bickel et al., 1954; Clark, 1992; Crawford et al., 1982; Holtzman et al., 1975; Komrower, 1980; Lloyd & Scriver, 1985; Ludolph et al., 1992; Nyhan, 1984; Pitt & Danks, 1991; Ramus et al., 1993; Ris et al., 1994; Scriver et al., 1995a, 1995b; Smith & Beasley, 1988; Smith & Wolffe, 1976; Thomas, 1992; Williamson et al., 1977; Winick, 1979). One study compared the IQ scores of 28 PKU-affected late-treated and early-treated sibling pairs. The study demonstrated that the difference in IQ scores between the early-treated siblings (all IQs > 80) and their late-treated siblings (mean IQ = 45; range, 30 to 81) was significant. A comparison of the IQ scores between the early-treated sibling and their nonaffected siblings revealed that the mean IQ scores were 94 and 99, respectively (Smith & Wolffe, 1976).

The Northern American Collaborative Study has been evaluating the outcome of early-treated PKU cases. The study found that early treatment was compatible with attainment of a normal IQ score, results which have been confirmed by several other investigators (Azen et al., 1991; Clark & Cockburn, 1991; Costello et al., 1994; Koch et al., 1984; Ludolph et al., 1992; Pitt & Danks, 1991; Scriver et al., 1995a, 1995b; Smith & Beasley, 1988). IQ score correlates positively with the age at which dietary treatment was stopped and the mean parental IQ score and negatively with the age at which treatment had begun and on the plasma values during treatment. The best IQ scores and psychological test scores were obtained by the patients treated earliest and the longest and in whom the plasma phenylalanine levels were less than 15 mg/dl (900 μmol) throughout life. In addition to changes in IQ scores, treated PKU patients have measurable deficits in their performance of conceptual, visuospatial, and language-related tasks and in reading and arithmetic skills. Despite these deficits, early-treated PKU-affected persons function well in daily life. Thus the response to early treatment for PKU has established that (1) early treatment can ameliorate the clinical impact of the disease; (2) early-treated children have a mean IQ score approximately 0.5 standard deviation below the scores for the unaffected siblings and population norms; (3) a high proportion of early-treated subjects (not just those of poorly treated cases) exhibited some degree of intellectual impairment attributable to events in early childhood rather than to later relaxation or termination of treatment; and (4) most early-treated PKU-affected children function within the broad range of ability and attend regular schools.

There has been a long-term concern that premature termination of treatment might impair later neurologic function. Early comparative studies (performed in the 1950s) of the effects of continued versus terminated dietary treatment showed that there was a decrease in IQ scores after treatment was discontinued (Holtzman et al., 1975; Winick, 1979). Subsequent studies clearly confirmed these initial results, more in some patients than in others (Koch et al., 1993; Potocnik & Widhalm, 1994; Scriver et al., 1995a, 1995b; Smith et al., 1991; Thomas, 1992). The effects of treatment termination are apparent in more than IQ score. They can also appear as deviant EEG findings, decreased neurotransmitter levels, impaired vigilance, and impaired reaction times. Behavioral problems have been reported as occurring more frequently with termination rather than with relaxation of treatment (Ludolph et al., 1992; Potocnik & Widhalm, 1994; Scriver et al., 1995a, 1995b; Smith et al., 1991; Thomas, 1992).

Although IQ and cognitive function have been the foci of past research, much of the current research focuses on the abnormalities of brain white matter revealed by MRI. The changes reflect abnormal myelin synthesis or demyelination (Bick et al., 1991; Cleary et al., 1994). The significance of the MRI changes is unclear inasmuch as they have been demonstrated in continuously well-treated individuals and seem to be more severe in patients with a history of poor control of phenylalanine levels. There is also evidence that MRI changes and overt neurologic deterioration can both improve when dietary treatment is reinstated and when plasma phenylalanine levels return to normal (Battistini et al., 1991; Ris et al., 1994). Although MRI changes seem to be much more common than overt neurologic changes and more prevalent than measurable psychological deficits in treated and post-treated PKU patients, the association with long-term hyperphenylalaninemia seems undeniable. It may no longer be possible to cite non-PKU hyperphenylalaninemia to illustrate normal cognitive function in the presence of modest increases in phenylalanine. In reality, there may be no threshold value for blood phenylalanine at which the brain escapes some effect of persistent elevations in phenylalanine. The outcome of treatment correlates with the quality of treatment and its success in normalizing the blood phenylalanine level.

The Maternal PKU collaborative study investigated the effects of nutrient intake on pregnancy outcome (Koch et al., 1993; Matalon et al., 1991; Rossiter & Johnson, 1992). The study found that 80 percent of the fetuses could be adversely affected and demonstrated that women affected by PKU who reach childbearing age should adhere strictly to dietary restrictions regarding phenylalanine. The normal transplacental gradient favors the fetus from early pregnancy onward, with the fetal-to-maternal ratio of phenylalanine in the range of 1.5:1 to 2.9:1 (Acosta & Wright, 1992; Ampola, 1982; Benson, 1983; Bickel, 1980; Blaskovics et al., 1974; Clark & Cockburn, 1991; Fanaroff & Martin, 1997; Fisch et al., 1993; Hanley et al., 1987; Koch et al., 1993; Matalon et al., 1991; Nyhan, 1984; Scriver et al., 1995a, 1995b; Stern & Vert, 1987; Wapnir, 1985; Winick, 1979). Thus fetal phenylalanine level cannot be accurately predicted from the corresponding maternal level, except that it is at least as high or perhaps nearly three times as high as the maternal level. Therefore, the goal is to keep the maternal plasma phenylalanine level as near normal as possible, as early as possible in the pregnancy. If the low-phenylalanine diet has been stopped, it is essential in preconceptional teaching that the mother realize the need to restart diet restrictions before a pregnancy.

Elevated maternal phenylalanine levels greater than 15 mg/dl (900 μmol) have been associated with increased risk for offspring of cardiac defects, prenatal and postnatal growth retardation, microcephaly, and permanently impaired mentality in heterozygous infants (Ampola, 1982; Benson, 1983; Bickel, 1980; Blaskovics et al., 1974; Koch et al., 1993; Levy et al., 1992; Nyhan, 1984; Scriver et al., 1995a, 1995b; Wapnir, 1985). The degree of impaired mentality in infants is in proportion to the degree of elevated maternal phenylalanine. Thus a genetically normal infant is affected if the maternal diet is not closely followed. When these heterozygous infants are tested for PKU with normal neonatal screening, the excess serum phenylalanine has already been cleared from the infant's blood and the test result is normal (Bickel, 1980; LeGrys, 1984; Fanaroff & Martin, 1997; Nyhan, 1984; Scriver et al., 1995a, 1995b). In that case, the cause of the infant's impairment may be difficult to isolate if the maternal PKU status is unknown. Routine screening of infant cord blood for phenylalanine identifies some of these PKU-affected mothers who did not resume dietary restrictions; however, the damage to the infants has already occurred. Some authors advocate the routine screening of maternal urine for phenylpyruvic acid early in pregnancy to detect PKU-affected women; however, even early identification and subsequent control of elevated maternal serum phenylalanine levels may not be enough to avoid the mental impairment of the infant (Bickel, 1980; Blaskovics et al., 1974; LeGrys, 1984; Levy et al., 1992; Nyhan, 1984; Scriver et al., 1995a, 1995b).

Every PKU-affected woman of childbearing years should remain on a low-phenylalanine diet and have low serum phenylalanine levels before conception (Bickel, 1980; Blaskovics et al., 1974; LeGrys, 1984; Nyhan, 1984; Scriver et al., 1995a, 1995b; Wapnir, 1985). During pregnancy, the serum phenylalanine levels should be less than 8 mg/dl (500 μmol) to maximize neonatal outcome (Ampola, 1982; Bickel, 1980; Blaskovics et al., 1974; Clark & Cockburn, 1991; Evans & Shulman, 1991; Gregory, 1992; Hanley et al., 1987; Koch et al., 1993; Matalon et al., 1991; Nyhan, 1984; Rossiter & Johnson, 1992; Scriver et al., 1995a, 1995b; Wapnir, 1985). The use of maternal surrogates or "gestational carriers" has been advocated by at least one investigator for some women affected by PKU to minimize the fetal exposure to any elevation in phenylalanine in utero (Fisch et al., 1993).

In addition to dietary therapy, alternative modes of treatment are theoretically possible in PKU. Enzyme "replacement" is possible through the use of heterologous partial liver transplantation or implantation of normal hepatocytes. This could replace the deviant or missing PAH activity and would constitute "multigene" therapy. No activity on this front has been reported in the literature.

The most promising surrogate enzyme replacement is bacterial phenylalanine ammonia lyase. After ingestion, it converts phenylalanine to a nontoxic derivative, plus an equivalent amount of ammonia. It does not require a cofactor. In animal research, this enzyme replacement was much more effective in lowering the elevated phenylalanine levels than was a low-phenylalanine diet (Bourget & Chang, 1985). Further research in this area may be limited by the extremely high cost of this enzyme.

The limitations and inadequacies of conventional diet therapy and the absence of any significant steps in enzyme replacement therapy and new knowledge on the molecular basis of PKU mutations have made investigators consider specific gene therapy. Promise lies in implanting a normal PAH gene in place of, or in addition to, the mutant cells of a PKU patient. An expressible PKU gene is available, as is the method for delivering the incoming normal gene into the cell. Integration of the gene into the nuclear genome of the target cell is likely, and there is assurance that it will be expressed and transmitted to daughter cells. This research is currently being conducted on animal models, but no human research has been attempted (Scriver et al., 1995a, 1995b).

Hyperphenylalaninemia Caused by Defects of BH4 Recycling

The hydroxylation of phenylalanine, tyrosine, and tryptophan is catalyzed by three enzymes, each pterin-dependent. Accordingly, it was anticipated that some patients would have persistent elevations of phenylalanine with neurologic deficits related to decreased neurotransmitter derivatives of tyrosine and tryptophan. Careful investigation of the progressive neurologic disorders in these patients with hyperphenylalaninemia, despite seemingly well controlled on diet therapy, revealed that there were two etiologies. In some cases, the cause was attributed to impaired recycling of BH4 as a result of DHPR deficiency and in some cases, the cause was attributed to impaired BH4 cofactor synthesis. The incidence among all cases of hyperphenylalaninemia is 1 to 3 cases per 1,000,000 births with worldwide occurrence and no evidence for regional or ethnic clusters (Medical Research Council Steering Committee for MRC/DHSS PKU Register, 1981; Scriver et al., 1995a, 1995b).

Procedures for the early identification of BH4-deficient patients has become an integral part of all neonatal screening programs for three reasons: (1) cases of BH4 deficiency cannot be distinguished from other forms of neonatal hyperphenylalaninemia by the blood values alone; (2) conventional treatment of PKU is inadequate; and (3) until BH4-deficient forms of hyperphenylalaninemia have been excluded, there is uncertainty about the cause of the elevated phenylalanine, choice of treatment, and the prognosis (Blaskovics et al., 1974; Blau et al., 1992; Clark, 1992; Doherty et al., 1991; Durand-Zaleski et al., 1992; Scriver et al., 1995a, 1995b)

Since the first reports of BH4 deficient forms of hyperphenylalaninemia were published in 1975, the DHPR gene has been cloned, the mutations on chromosome 4 characterized, and heterogeneity at the levels of the genotype and phenotype have been established. The condition is autosomal recessive (Kaufman, 1992a, 1992b; Scriver et al., 1995a, 1995b; Smith & the Medical Research Council Working Party on PKU, 1993).

The treatment goals are to minimize the hyperphenylalaninemia, correct the neurotransmitter deficiency, and maintain folate homeostasis. The low phenylalanine diet is recommended to maintain plasma phenylalanine levels in the near normal range. This diet avoids the interruption of neurotransmitter synthesis by the excessive phenylalanine in vivo and prevents the other effects of phenylalanine on the brain (Kaufman, 1992a, 1992b; Thomas, 1992). Because DHPR is necessary to maintain amounts of cofactor for synthesis of amines from tyrosine and tryptophan, replacement of these neurotransmitters is likely to be effective in DHPR deficiency. L-dopa and 5-hydroxytryptophan are given around the clock in order to restore normal circadian metabolism. The effectiveness of treatment is inversely related to the age at which it begins. Treatment with BH4 is not practical because in the absence of DHPR to recycle the BH4, catalytic amounts of BH4 cannot be maintained by the body. It is thought that BH4 also plays a role in folate metabolism, which is also deficient in these patients. Thus supplementation with folinic acid is part of the normal treatment. The objective is to achieve cerebrospinal fluid (CSF) concentrations of tetrahydrofolate in the high normal range and to prevent demyelination and other signs of cortical dysgenesis (Kaufman, 1992a, 1992b; Scriver et al., 1995a, 1995b; Thomas, 1992; Wapnir, 1985; Winick, 1979).

Hyperphenylalaninemia Caused by Defects of BH4 Synthesis

Insufficient supply of endogenous BH4 cofactor impairs the hydrolase function. It was recognized early as the cause of hyperphenylalaninemia in "atypical PKU." The clinical signs and symptoms are parkinsonian in nature. There is characteristic truncal hypotonia and increased limb tone with pronated hand postures. Difficulty in swallowing, ocular spasms, somnolence, irritability, hyperthermia, seizures, and impaired neuropsychological development are all present clinically (Cerone et al., 1986).

Replacement of BH4 abolishes the hyperphenylalaninemia, and daily treatment with BH4 is required. As the enzyme dihydrobiopterin is present in adequate amounts, the replaced BH4 can be "recycled" more effectively and adequate BH4 levels can be achieved. BH4 replacement is expensive and is available from only one source, in Switzerland. Replacement of dopamine and serotonin is necessary to abolish the central nervous system symptoms because BH4 does not penetrate the blood–brain barrier. Replacement is achieved with L-dopa and 5-hydroxytryptophan to restore the neurotransmitter levels; fine adjustments of dosage and schedule are needed to restore circadian rhythms. For reasons yet unknown, the response to treatment is variable. Postnatal treatment may be too late if the fetal phenotype has already affected central nervous system development (Cerone et al., 1986; Kaufman, 1992a, 1992b; Scriver et al., 1995a, 1995b).

The Hypertyrosinemias

- In humans, tyrosine is obtained from two sources: dietary intake and hydroxylation of phenylalanine. Degradation of tyrosine occurs primarily in the liver and is both glucogenic and ketogenic. The rate of tyrosine degradation is, for the most part, determined by the activity of tyrosine aminotransferase (TAT).
- Most inborn errors of tyrosine catabolism produce hypertyrosinemia. Hypertyrosinemia may also occur in various acquired conditions, including severe hepatocellular disease.
- Hepatorenal hypertyrosinemia, or type I tyrosinemia, is an autosomal recessive disease caused by a deficiency of fumarylacetoacetate hydrolase (FAH). Symptoms are highly variable and include acute liver failure, cirrhosis, hepatocellular carcinoma, renal Fanconi's syndrome, glomerulosclerosis, and crises of peripheral neuropathy. In untreated patients, the tyrosine levels are elevated. The presence of increased levels of succinylacetone in plasma or urine is diagnostic for this condition. There may be a partial response to dietary restriction of tyrosine and phenylalanine in many patients. Hepatic transplantation cures the liver manifestations and prevents further neurologic crises. Treatment with 2-(2-nitro-4-trifluoromethylbenzoyl)-1,3-cyclohexanedione (NTBC), an inhibitor of 4-hydroxyphenylpyruvate dioxygenase (pHPPD), has been reported to cause a marked improvement in hepatic and renal function. The mutant gene responsible for the FAH deficiency has been mapped to chromosome 15. Mutational heterogeneity in FAH activity has been found among patients from the French Canadian province of Quebec and among the Scandinavian populations, both of which have a higher incidence of this disease than does the general world population.
- Type II tyrosinemia is a deficiency of the enzyme TAT, which results in oculocutaneous tyrosinemia. The ocular and cutaneous symptoms are characterized by palmoplantar keratosis and painful corneal erosions associated with photophobia. Half of the reported patients have mental retardation. The ocular and cutaneous symptoms respond to dietary restriction of tyrosine and phenylalanine.
- Type III tyrosinemia results in three different conditions associated with dysfunction of the enzyme pHPPD: primary pHPPD deficiency, hawkinsinuria, and transient tyrosinemia of the newborn.
- Primary pHPPD deficiency has been described rarely in the literature. The two case reports were neurologically abnormal. Biochemically, the patients demonstrated hypertyrosinemia and elevated urinary excretion of 4-hydroxyphenyl derivatives.
- Hawkinsinuria is an autosomal dominant condition putatively caused by dysfunction of pHPPD. It results in acidosis and failure to thrive in infancy. Hypertyrosinemia is minimal or absent. The urinary excretion of hawkinsin, an amino acid thought to be an intermediate of the pHPPD reaction, is diagnostic for this condition. Symptoms may respond to dietary protein restriction and to the administration of ascorbate.
- Transient tyrosinemia of the newborn results from a combination of pHPPD immaturity, elevated tyrosine and phenylalanine intake, and a relative ascorbate deficiency.
- Improvement is spontaneous but can be accelerated by the administration of ascorbate and by dietary protein restriction, especially of tyrosine and phenylalanine. Most children with transient tyrosinemia are asymptomatic and recover without adverse effects on development. However, the adverse consequences of this disorder has not been eliminated in all cases.

Tyrosine is derived either from hydrolysis of dietary or tissue protein or from hydroxylation of phenylalanine and thus is considered a semiessential amino acid. Tyrosine is the starting point of synthetic pathways leading to the synthesis of catecholamines, thyroid hormone, and the melanin pigment. However, the major fate of tyrosine is to be incorporated into proteins or degraded for its component molecules. The degradation occurs in the cytosol of the hepatocytes. In the presence of elevated tyrosine levels, degradation is controlled by the activity of TAT (Kvittingen, 1991; Scriver et al., 1995a, 1995b).

Typical plasma tyrosine levels in normal subjects range from 25 to 103 μmol in the newborn and 35 to 90 μmol in the adult. Urinary levels range from 6 to 55 μmol per mmol of creatinine in the newborn and 2 to 23 in the adult. A fetal-to-maternal gradient is present, fetal plasma tyrosine level being approximately two times higher than maternal levels. In the adult, tyrosine is efficiently (97 to 99 percent) reabsorbed by the renal tubules. The transamination product of tyrosine, 4-hydroxyphenylpyruvate (pHPP) is found in low concentration in the plasma and is actively cleared by the renal tubules. As pHPP accumulates, related products are excreted and form part of the basis for diagnostic testing for this disorder (Goldsmith, 1983b; Kvittingen, 1991; Scriver et al., 1995a, 1995b).

The enzymes mediating the metabolism of tyrosine are still being investigated. The normal activity of the first enzyme, TAT, is usually one half to one third that of the second enzyme, pHPP, which, in turn, is one half to one tenth that of the last enzymes of tyrosine catabolism, maleylacetoacetate (MAA) isomerase and FAH (Berger et al., 1983; Scriver et al., 1995a, 1995b).

Plasma tyrosine levels are usually quantified by ion-exchange amino acid chromatography. For purposes of neonatal screening, spectrophotometric or bacteriologic (Guthrie) assays can be used. PHPP and its derivatives can be analyzed by gas chromatography-mass spectrometry. Succinylacetone levels are often determined enzymatically or with gas chromatography–mass spectrometry technique (Coskun et al., 1991; Kvittingen, 1991; Scriver et al., 1995a, 1995b).

Hypertyrosinemia can result from several inherited and acquired conditions, including transient tyrosinemia of the newborn, inborn errors of tyrosine catabolism, severe hepatocellular disease, hyperthyroidism, and scurvy. Most of these causes can be diagnosed by clinical history, physical examination, and readily available laboratory tests. Transient tyrosinemia of the newborn, severe hepatocellular disease, and inborn errors of tyrosine catabolism are the most common causes of hypertyrosinemia.

The most difficult clinical problem with hypertyrosinemia is in the context of hepatic dysfunction. It must be determined whether the elevated tyrosine levels are caused by primary hepatorenal tyrosinemia or whether the tyrosine levels are elevated as a result of secondary hepatocellular dysfunction. The determination of plasma amino acids is not diagnostic in these patients because both tyrosine and methionine can be nonspecifically elevated in cirrhosis and in acute liver failure.

The presence of renal tubular dysfunction in patients with hepatocellular failure is consistent with hepatorenal tyrosinemia but is also seen in other inherited metabolic diseases such as galactosemia, hereditary fructose intolerance, certain lactic acidoses, and glycogen storage diseases. The presence of a family history suggestive of tyrosinemia is helpful in the diagnosis. The presence of high levels of succinylacetone in blood or urine establishes the diagnosis (Coskun et al., 1991; Kvittingen, 1991; Scriver et al., 1995a, 1995b).

A practical consideration is that plasma levels of tyrosine and of several other amino acids can be mildly elevated in nonfasting subjects. Repeated amino acid analyses by chromatography should be obtained before investigation for hypertyrosinemia, especially if the patient has none of the other symptoms associated with the metabolic disorders of tyrosine catabolism. Some disorders of tyrosine catabolism and its branch pathways are not associated with hypertyrosinemia, and 4-hydroxyphenylic derivatives of tyrosine can be found in increasing amounts in patients with primary liver disease. Urinary 4-hydroxyphenylacetate is commonly of gut bacterial origin and may be increased in malabsorption. Last, patients receiving certain parenteral nutritional solutions containing *N*-acetyltyrosine may excrete large amounts of this compound (Coskun et al., 1991; Kvittingen, 1991; Scriver et al., 1995a, 1995b).

Hepatorenal Tyrosinemia: Fumarylacetoacetate Hydrolase Deficiency (Tyrosinemia Type I)

Hepatorenal tyrosinemia is a clinically severe inborn error of metabolism that affects principally the liver, kidney, and peripheral nerves and results from a deficiency of FAH. The mechanism by which the hepatic and renal symptoms of tyrosinemia arise is unknown, and many questions in the areas of pathophysiology and treatment remain unanswered. Advances in the confirmation of the enzymatic deficiency, cloning of the human FAH gene, new medical and surgical therapies, and development of an animal model of the disease will no doubt have an explosive impact on this disease in the future.

In contrast to other inborn errors of amino acid metabolism in which the metabolites preceding the enzymatic blocked enzyme are excreted in high levels, in FAH deficiency, the preceding compounds upstream from the block, MAA and fumarylacetoacetate (FAA), have not been isolated as circulating or excreted metabolites. It therefore is speculated that these reactive metabolites may be compartmentalized in tyrosinemia, causing damage within single cells (Kvittingen, 1991; Scriver et al., 1995a, 1995b).

A secondary deficiency of hepatic pHPPD activity (usually from 0 to 30 percent of normal activity) is an important factor in hepatorenal tyrosinemia and, at first, was thought to be the etiology of the disease. The mechanism of pHPPD inactivation is unknown, but it may occur as a result of the abnormal sulfhydryl metabolism observed in hepatorenal tyrosinemia. Research has indicated that inactivation of pHPPD may serve a protective function in this disorder (Lindblad et al., 1977) by reducing the production of FAA and other tyrosine derivatives downstream. Lindstedt and colleagues found a correlation between the severity of the clinical manifestations of the disease and the degree of residual hepatic pHPPD activity. The administration of NTBC, which is a potent inhibitor of pHPPD, has been associated with improvement in the hepatic and renal function of these patients (Lindstedt et al., 1992).

A deficiency of methionine adenosyltransferase (MAT) explains the hypermethioninemia seen in many tyrosinemic children. This sulfhydryl-containing enzyme has multiple distinct forms and mediates the major pathway of methionine catabolism. FAA inhibits one form of this enzyme, but the clinical relevance of this observation has yet to be explored (Berger et al., 1983). The significance of hypermethioninemia in hepatorenal tyrosinemia, other than as an approximate index of hepatic function, is uncertain. Patients with an isolated deficiency of MAT have normal development and no liver dysfunction, despite elevated methionine levels (Berger et al., 1983), which suggests that the hypermethionine levels in hepatorenal tyrosinemia may be well tolerated.

The best established pathophysiologic mechanism in hepatorenal tyrosinemia is the role of succinylacetone in the acute episodes of porphyria-like peripheral neuropathy. Succinylacetone is the most potent known inhibitor of the porphyrin synthetic enzyme δ-aminolevulinic acid (δ-ALA) dehydratase (Sassa & Kappas, 1983). This compound is excreted in very high levels in children with hepatorenal tyrosinemia and has been demonstrated to be neurotoxic (Kvittingen, 1991; Moore & Meredith, 1976), and evidence supports the theory that it is responsible for the neurologic crises of hepatorenal tyrosinemia.

Succinylacetone has other effects at high concentrations, including inhibition of renal tubular transport and heme synthesis (Roth et al., 1991) and inhibition of cell growth and immune function (Tschudy et al., 1982). How these effects influence the clinical symptoms is unknown.

Hepatorenal tyrosinemia is an autosomal recessive trait. Obligatory heterozygotes (parents of the affected offspring) have approximately 50 percent of normal enzyme activity and yet are asymptomatic and have normal levels of tyrosine-related metabolites (Scriver et al., 1995a, 1995b).

There are two population clusters of hepatorenal hypertyrosinemia: in a small French Canadian province of Quebec and in Scandinavia. The population genetics suggest that the mutant gene was introduced into Canada by founder couples settling the region who may have originated from northern France and were related to one another. The overall incidence of hepatorenal tyrosinemia in Quebec is 1 in 16,786 live births. The incidence in Scandinavia is approximately 1 in 100,000 live births, and this incidence is higher than elsewhere in the world, in which it is estimated to be approximately 1 in 150,000 live births. Lack of French Canadian or Scandinavian ancestry does not exclude the diagnosis (Scriver et al., 1995a, 1995b).

Neonatal screening for hepatorenal tyrosinemia has been available since the 1970s. Initially, screening for tyrosine levels was done, but the disadvantage was that the elevated tyrosine levels overlapped those found in transient neonatal tyrosinemia. Currently, screening is accomplished through the use of the parameters that are abnormal in hepatorenal tyrosinemia, such as methionine, succinylacetone, or δ-ALA dehydratase levels (Holme & Lindstedt, 1992; Kvittingen, 1991; Kvittingen & Brodtkorb, 1986; Scriver et al., 1995a, 1995b).

In Quebec, blood succinylacetone has been screened along with tyrosine since the 1980s. A threshold of 248 μmol (4.5 mg/dl) is selected as the cutoff level for tyrosine, and approximately 2.4 percent of neonates born in Quebec currently have levels that exceed this amount. This low cutoff value and the high specificity of the succinylacetone marker are believed to have permitted complete detection of all affected newborns while eliminating false-negative results. In Quebec, the average age at follow-up for affected newborns is 20 days (Scriver et al., 1995a, 1995b).

In the United States, six states (Alaska, Georgia, Idaho, Maryland, Nevada, and Oregon) screen for neonatal tyrosinemia by using blood tyrosine levels with an initial threshold value of 331 μmol (6 mg/dl), 10 percent of newborns being recalled for further testing. Currently the threshold value has been increased to 663 μmol (12 mg/dl), with a recall rate of 0.1 percent. In Georgia, none of the patients with hepatorenal tyrosinemia have been identified by neonatal screening, although one case of oculocutaneous tyrosinemia and five cases of prolonged severe transient neonatal hypertyrosinemia have been detected since 1978. Several children were identified as having secondary hypertyrosinemia from unrecognized hepatocellular disease or feeding errors (Coskun et al., 1991; Kvittingen, 1991; Scriver et al., 1995a, 1995b). In the other states, the proportion of newborns with tyrosine levels above the threshold value of 331 μmol (6 mg/dl) is approximately 0.12 percent. A new screening method entailing use of δ-ALA dehydratase is being investigated and should detect FAH deficiency, succinylacetone accumulation, and inhibition of δ-ALA dehydratase deficiency. The decision to initiate neonatal screening for hepatorenal tyrosinemia involves many factors, including the impact of presymptomatic detection on the family, the incidence of the disease, and the marginal increase in cost of the procedure.

Hepatorenal tyrosinemia should be suspected in any newborn with evidence of hepatocellular disease, cirrhosis, or decreased synthetic function (especially perturbed coagulation) for which the cause is not evident. The presence of hypophosphatemic rickets and other renal tubular diseases or of typical neurologic crises also suggests the diagnosis (Coskun et al., 1991; Kvittingen, 1991).

In symptomatic patients, plasma tyrosine levels are usually elevated to a variable degree but may be affected by a low-protein diet and are found in many other disorders of amino acids metabolism. The demonstration of increased amounts of succinylacetone in blood or urine is pathognomonic for hepatorenal tyrosinemia. FAH enzymatic analysis should be assayed with the use of lymphocytes, erythrocytes, or hepatocytes. Enzyme analysis must be interpreted in the context of the patient's clinical and biochemical findings (Coskun et al., 1991; Kvittingen, 1991; Scriver et al., 1995a, 1995b).

Prenatal diagnosis is available through three methods: determination of succinylacetone in amniotic fluid, FAH assay, and molecular analysis in amniocytes. In general, the assay of succinylacetone in amniotic fluid has been an excellent means of prenatal diagnosis in 36 pregnancies at risk among French Canadians (Jakobs et al., 1990; Kvittingen, 1991; Kvittingen & Brodtkorb, 1986; Ploos van Amstel et al., 1994).

The hepatic manifestations of hepatorenal tyrosinemia include acute decompensations, chronic cirrhosis, and hepatocellular carcinoma. Approximately 69 percent of deaths were attributed to liver failure and coagulopathy, and 16 percent were attributable to hepatocellular carcinoma. It is important to remember that these conditions are not exclusive and may coexist (Kvittingen, 1991; Pitkanen et al., 1994; Scriver et al., 1995a, 1995b).

The liver profile of a patient with hepatorenal tyrosinemia is characterized by a marked decrease in synthetic function with markedly reduced clotting factors in comparison with other parameters of hepatic function. Prothrombin and partial thromboplastin times may be markedly prolonged. Vitamin K administration does not correct this abnormality. Serum transaminase levels are variable and may be normal or only slightly elevated. Of the most commonly measured hepatic function tests, serum bilirubin is the least sensitive indicator of dysfunction, and jaundice is rare in the early phases of this disease (Kvittingen, 1991; Scriver et al., 1995a, 1995b).

A hepatic crisis may be precipitated by infections or other catabolic conditions. Ascites and GI bleeding are common. Hepatomegaly is present in variable degrees. A "boiled cabbage" odor may be detectable. Elevations of plasma tyrosine, methionine, and other amino acids may be observed during hepatic crises. Renal tubular function may deteriorate during these episodes. Although some crises spontaneously resolve, some progress to complete liver failure and hepatic encephalopathy. Between crises, there is mild hepatomegaly, with normal or mildly elevated transaminases and normal bilirubin. In severe episodes, transaminases rapidly and markedly increase, hyperbilirubinemia may develop, and the alpha-fetoprotein level is elevated (100,000 to 400,000 ng/ml) (Pitkanen et al., 1994; Salt et al., 1992; Scriver et al., 1995a, 1995b).

Cirrhosis eventually develops in all patients, and the risk of hepatocellular carcinoma is extremely high in hepatorenal tyrosinemia. The incidence of hepatocellular carcinoma has been reported to range from approximately 17 to 37 percent (Pitkanen et al., 1994; Salt et al., 1992). Hepatocellular carcinoma has been reported to develop in infants as young as 21 months. Hepatic nodules develop with cirrhosis, and there is no reliable, noninvasive way to determine their malignant nature. Although their presence is worrisome, most nodules are, in fact, benign. However, a high degree of suspicion should be maintained when there is a significant rise in transaminase levels from baseline in the absence of a liver crisis.

The neurologic crises of hepatorenal tyrosinemia are acute episodes of peripheral neuropathy, followed by a recovery phase. The acute period is dominated by painful parathesias, autonomic signs (tachycardia, hypertension, and ileus) and sometimes progressive paralysis (Coskun et al., 1991; Moore & Meredith, 1976). A period of recovery follows. The painful crises are preceded by a minor infection and associated with irritability, decreased activity, and often vomiting. There is extreme hyperextension of the trunk and neck, which can be mistaken for opisthotonos or meningitis and for tonic convulsions, but the patient is conscious. Of importance is that the mental development of these children is normal and that during these crises, their mental function is not diminished. The excruciating pain, the abnormal, striking postures, and frequent self-mutilation makes these crises very dramatic and disturbing for all involved. The active phase usually lasts from 1 to 7 days. Weakness and paralysis may develop, and mechanical ventilation may be required for respiratory muscle weakness. Recovery is possible, even after prolonged ventilation for respiratory insufficiency. Patients with repetitive severe crises may have some degree of chronic muscle weakness. The neurologic crises are not associated with exacerbation of liver dysfunction. Plasma transaminase levels, prothrombin times, and plasma bilirubin level are unchanged from baseline values between crises (Scriver et al., 1995a, 1995b).

Several other complications may occur during this time. Tongue lacerations, severe bruxism, vomiting, and ileus complicate the nutritional management of these patients. Marked hyponatremia, hypophosphatemia, and hypokalemia occur especially in children with renal tubular dysfunction. Neurologic crises are a major cause of morbidity. There is an appreciable risk of death from respiratory insufficiency. All tyrosinemic patients who are ill need to be closely monitored for signs of neurologic deterioration. Respiratory insufficiency occurs rapidly, and thus children with impending neurologic crisis should be hospitalized for continuous monitoring of respiratory function during the acute phase (Coskun et al., 1991; Halvorsen et al., 1988; Scriver et al., 1995a, 1995b).

Some degree of renal involvement is always present in children with hepatorenal tyrosinemia, with signs ranging from mild tubular dysfunction to overt renal failure. Both tubular function and glomerular function may be affected. The severity of tubular dysfunction is variable and is exacerbated during episodes of decompensation. Clinically, hypophosphatemic rickets develops in hepatorenal tyrosinemia caused principally by tubular losses of phosphorus. There may also be renal tubular acidosis, aminoaciduria, and glycosuria. Nephromegaly and nephrocalcinosis may occur frequently (Coskun et al., 1991; Scriver et al., 1995a, 1995b).

Pancreatic islet cell hypertrophy associated with hypoglycemia has been reported. The relationship between pancreatic function and acute liver failure is uncertain. Hypertrophic cardiomyopathy, macrosomia, and ataxia have also been reported (Giardini et al., 1983; Lindblad et al., 1987; Moore & Meredith, 1976; Scriver et al., 1995a, 1995b).

Management of hepatorenal tyrosinemia is difficult because of the lack of reliable biologic parameters of good metabolic control. Although medical management can slow the progression of the disease, the patients are at risk for liver failure, hepatocellular carcinoma, and neurologic crises.

Diet therapy has long been used in the early management of this disorder. Dietary restriction of phenylalanine and tyrosine has been demonstrated to improve renal dysfunction (Aronson et al., 1968; Halvorsen & Gjessing, 1964; Jagenburg et al., 1972; Mini Symposium on Tyrosinemia, 1990; Wong et al., 1967). Any acute increase in tyrosine or phenylalanine intake results in increased tyrosine metabolites downstream and places the patient at risk for acute liver decompensation. When the diagnosis of hypertyrosinemia is made in the newborn, tyrosine levels are elevated but decline after 24 to 48 hours of feeding with tyrosine-free formula. After the tyrosine levels decline sufficiently, tyrosine and phenylalanine are added in the form of breast milk or formula. The rate of reintroduction depends on the clinical state of the child and the plasma levels of tyrosine. After the acute phase, the intake of phenylalanine and tyrosine is titrated according to the infant's growth and metabolic needs. Treatment is individualized according to the evaluation of the child's metabolic state and individual requirements for tyrosine and for phenylalanine. Maintaining plasma tyrosine levels within the normal range ensures adequate growth. An important goal of therapy is to avoid catabolic stress and to stimulate anabolism with adequate dietary intake of energy and nutrients. When catabolic stress occurs, the tyrosine and phenylalanine are reduced early in the course of the event and return to normal when anabolism resumes.

The renal tubular disease usually improves to some extent with dietary therapy. Vitamin D–resistant rickets is the primary dysfunction in tyrosinemia. Nephrocalcinosis may develop, and some children may require alkali for renal tubular acidosis. There is no specific therapy for the deterioration in glomerular function seen in some patients (Aronson et al., 1968; Halvorsen et al., 1988; Roth et al., 1991; Scriver et al., 1995a, 1995b).

The management of liver disease in hepatorenal tyrosinemia has followed the traditional regimens of reducing the offending protein during periods of crises and providing adequate sustenance for growth. Despite seemingly good control of diet, hepatic symptoms often progress to cirrhosis and failure or the development of hepatocellular carcinoma. The use of early liver transplantation has completely changed the therapeutic approach to this disease. Liver transplantation is performed on younger and smaller infants and preferably should be performed before the development of acute liver failure and hepatocellular carcinoma. Liver transplantation still carries a 10 to 15 percent mortality rate, and the child must face a lifetime of immunosuppressive therapy with cyclosporine. For the stable patient, elective transplantation should be timed in consideration of the current quality of life, liver status, risk of acute hepatic or neurologic decompensation, and the experience of the local pediatric liver transplantation team (Freese et al., 1991; Salt et al., 1992; Sokal et al., 1992).

In two studies, patients with hepatorenal hypertyrosinemia were administered NTBC, a potent inhibitor of pHPPD (Heubi, 1993; Lindstedt et al., 1992). Marked improvements were seen in levels of urinary succinylacetone and δ-ALA excretions, erythrocyte δ-ALA dehydratase values, serum alpha-fetoprotein levels, coagulation factors, and the indexes of renal tubular function. The early studies are promising, and NTBC is predicted to diminish or eliminate the neurologic crises of hepatorenal tyrosinemia and to slow the progression of the hepatic and renal disease (Heubi, 1993; Lindstedt et al., 1992; Scriver et al., 1995a, 1995b).

Oculocutaneous Tyrosinemia: Tyrosine Aminotransferase Deficiency (Tyrosinemia Type II)

Oculocutaneous tyrosinemia is caused by the autosomal recessive deficiency of tyrosine aminotransferase (TAT). Males and females are equally affected. Consanguinity of the parents has been present in at least 20 cases. The disease affects the skin, ocular cornea, and the central nervous system. It is also known as Richner-Hart syndrome and keratosis palmoplantaris with corneal dystrophy. The disorder occurs in populations of many different ethnic and geographic origins, including Italian, German, French, Swiss, Spanish, Norwegian, American, Canadian, Australian, Arabic, Lebanese, and Japanese persons and Turkish Ashkenazi Jews (Campbell et al., 1967; Scriver et al., 1995a).

The corneal disease is thought to result from the deposition of tyrosine into the corneal epithelial cells. The tyrosine crystallizes and disrupts these cells and their lysosomes and initiates an inflammatory response (Gipson et al., 1975). In contrast, neither tyrosine crystal formation nor disruption of lysosomes has been demonstrated in the skin lesions. It has been suggested that excessive amounts of intracellular tyrosine could enhance cross-links between aggregated tonofilaments and modulate the number and stability of microtubules. Both mechanical and regional factors play a role in the confinement of the lesions to the palmar and plantar surfaces (Chitayat et al., 1992; Goldsmith, 1983a; Paige et al., 1993).

The time of onset of ophthalmologic symptoms is highly variable, ranging from the first day of life to 38 years of age (Chitayat et al., 1992). Skin manifestations usually start after the first year of life but may occur as early as 6 months of age. Ocular and cutaneous lesions may manifest individually or together, and the symptoms can vary among members of an individual family. Ocular lesions manifest as lacrimation, photophobia, redness, and pain. Typically, the symptoms wax and wane. On examination, there are usually central dendritic corneal erosions. Conjunctivitis may be seen, and neovascularization may be prominent. Long-term consequences include corneal opacities, decreased visual acuity, cornea plana, astigmatism, strabismus, amblyopia, and glaucoma (Chitayat et al., 1992; Gipson et al., 1975; Goldsmith, 1983a; Paige et al., 1993).

Cutaneous lesions are painful, nonpruritic, hyperkeratotic plaques on the palmar and plantar surfaces. Blistering may precede plaque formation, which has a predilection for the fingertips and the hypothenar and thenar eminencies. Hyperkeratotic lesions elsewhere have been reported, and leukokeratosis of the tongue may occur. Hyperhidrosis may be associated with hyperkeratosis. Hyperpigmentation is not associated with this disease. Pain may prevent ambulation (Goldsmith, 1983a; Paige et al., 1993; Scriver et al., 1995a).

A variable degree of mental retardation occurs in less than half of the patients. It is not known whether cytosolic TAT deficiency can manifest only as a neurologic disease. There are reports of correlations between plasma tyrosine levels and degree of retardation, convulsions, and microcephaly (Chitayat et al., 1992; Paige et al., 1993).

In a patient with the typical manifestations, the diagnosis of oculocutaneous tyrosinemia is established by the finding of hypertyrosinemia. Plasma phenylalanine level is normal, and urinary excretion of tyrosine metabolites is abnormal. It is rarely necessary to perform a liver biopsy to confirm the TAT deficiency. Preclinical detection and treatment should be possible when neonatal screening for hypertyrosinemia is available (Campbell et al., 1967; Scriver et al., 1995a).

Treatment consists of dietary restriction of tyrosine and phenylalanine to a degree sufficient to achieve a resolution of eye and skin symptoms. There is no consensus about the optimal level of tyrosine. To optimize growth and to meet other nutritional requirements, a commercial low-phenylalanine, low-tyrosine formula is used. The eye and skin lesions resolve a few weeks after diet therapy has started but recur if the dietary restriction is stopped (Halvorsen et al., 1988; Paige et al., 1993; Scriver et al., 1995a). The fetal effects of maternal oculocutaneous tyrosinemia are not well known. Two children of an untreated mother had microphthalmia and psychomotor retardation. There are other reports of children with mental retardation and seizures (Francis et al., 1992). Careful dietary control of maternal plasma tyrosine levels should be considered during pregnancy in light of these reports of neurologically affected offspring (Francis et al., 1992).

Deficiency of 4-Hydroxyphenylpyruvate Dioxygenase (Type III Tyrosinemia)

At least three conditions are caused by a dysfunction of pHPPD: primary deficiency of pHPPD, hawkinsinuria of the newborn, and transient tyrosinemia of the newborn. In most cases, the dysfunction of pHPPD is apparently compatible with normal development and function. The biochemical abnormalities respond well to therapy.

Primary Deficiency of pHPPD. Primary deficiency of pHPPD is a rare disorder that has been documented in the literature only twice. The first patient was a girl, who had neither hepatorenal or oculocutaneous symptoms. She was apparently well until she experienced an episode of ataxia at 17 months, which disappeared over the next few days. Mild ataxia reoccurred with a tyrosine loading dose, resulting in hypertyrosinemia. However, subsequent development was normal despite administration of a normal diet and persistent hypertyrosinemia. The second patient, born of a brother–sister mating, had convulsions, cerebral atrophy, and decreased myelination. He died of accidental causes at 3½ months (Giardini et al., 1983; Origuchi et al., 1982; Scriver et al., 1995a).

Hepatic histologic findings were normal in the first patient and showed fatty degeneration in the second. The second case showed a dramatic decrease in tyrosine level after restriction of intake. Both patients had tyrosinemia and markedly increased amounts of pHPP derivatives. The origin of the neurologic symptoms is unclear in the second patient. pHPPD deficiency may be compatible with normal development in some cases, but the incidence and mode of neurologic complications are not well understood (Giardini et al., 1983; Origuchi et al., 1982; Scriver et al., 1995a).

Hawkinsinuria. First reported in the literature in 1975, this rare disorder is known to have become symptomatic in only four children. The amino acid responsible for this condition is (2-*L*-cystein-S-yl-1,4-dihydroxycyclohex-5en-1-yl)-acetic acid, or hawkinsin, named after the first family in which the disorder was described. It is thought to be an intermediate metabolite of tyrosine. The exact molecular basis of hawkinsinuria is unknown (Borden et al., 1992; Nyhan, 1984; Scriver et al., 1995a).

The small number of patients with hawkinsinuria may reflect its benign nature under conditions of normal protein intake, which may seldom lead to medical consultation. Symptoms of the reported cases have documented failure to thrive after weaning from breast milk or when fed with commercial formula. Metabolic acidosis is reported. Symptoms abated when low-protein feedings and ascorbic acid were reinstituted. After several weeks of therapy, the diets were discontinued gradually and the patients remained asymptomatic. Commercial formula with a composition similar to that of breast milk may also be effective in control of the symptoms (Borden et al., 1992). Manifestations of hawkinsinuria are not known outside of infancy. It would be of some interest to monitor the affected newborns for evidence of acidosis and hemolysis at times of metabolic stress.

Transient Tyrosinemia of the Newborn. Transient tyrosinemia is the most common disorder of amino acid metabolism in humans. It is thought to result from an imbalance of tyrosine catabolism and the activity of pHPPD, which matures late in the newborn. Risk factors for the development of this disorder include prematurity, a high protein intake, and an insufficient vitamin C intake (Nyhan, 1984; Rice et al., 1989; Wong et al., 1967).

In the fetus and newborn, pHPPD activity is low and pHPP and its derivatives are excreted at high levels. The rapidity of the response suggests that pHPPD is present in the inactivated state in the hepatocyte. Because of the generally benign nature of transient tyrosinemia and the localization of pHPPD in liver and kidney, enzymatic studies have not been performed in humans. A role for genetic factors in pHPPD maturation is plausible but unproven. Prematurity, insufficient vitamin C intake, and a high protein intake are the most important predisposing factors. In the past, most children with transient tyrosinemia of the newborn had received cow's milk, and protein intake was greater than 5 g/kg/day. Diets with less than 3 g/kg/day were protective (Light et al., 1966; Mathews & Partington, 1964; Rice et al., 1989; Wong et al., 1967).

The diagnosis for this disorder is made when there is isolated hypertyrosinemia in an asymptomatic neonate, which responds to ascorbic acid administration or resolves spontaneously on a normal diet. Typically, the hypertyrosinemia peaks before 14 days and resolves by 1 month. Urinary 4-hydroxyphenyl derivatives are excreted at increased levels. Biochemical abnormalities respond rapidly to ascorbic acid administration (Light et al., 1966; Mathews & Partington, 1964; Rice et al., 1989; Wong et al., 1967). Together with the absence of liver, renal, or cutaneous signs, the biochemical abnormalities that respond to ascorbic acid administration distinguish transient tyrosinemia from other disorders described in this chapter.

The incidence of hypertyrosinemia has changed with feeding practices of newborns over the decades. During the 1960s up to 10 percent of full-term and 30 to 50 percent of preterm infants were reported to develop hypertyrosinemia. Since then, the feeding practices have shifted from cow's milk to lower protein–based formulas or breast milk, and the mean protein intake has decreased (Rice et al., 1989; Scriver et al., 1995a).

Although transient tyrosinemia is probably benign, it is prudent to restrict protein intake to 2g/kg/day and to administer ascorbic acid to newborns identified with this disorder, in order to normalize plasma tyrosine as quickly as possible. If the infant is breast-fed, breast milk feedings should be supplemented with vitamin C. Serum tyrosine begins to decrease within hours of ascorbic acid administration. If the clinical examination is normal and there is no family history compatible with hepatorenal tyrosinemia, the infant can be monitored as an outpatient for the repeated measurement of tyrosine levels with ascorbic acid supplements (Scriver et al., 1995a).

Disorders of Histidine Metabolism

- There are two known disorders of histidine metabolism: histidinemia and urocanic aciduria. Histidinemia is an autosomal recessive trait and is caused by a defect in histidase, which catalyzes the conversion of histidine to urocanic acid. This enzyme is most readily identified in the stratum corneum of the skin. As a result of the metabolic block, there is an increased concentration of histidine in the blood, urine, and CSF and a decreased concentration of urocanic acid in the blood and the skin. There are increased histidine metabolites in the urine. Histidinemia seems to be benign in most persons, although some reports of neurologic dysfunction exist. Urocanic aciduria is an autosomal recessive disorder. The enzyme urocanase is defective and cannot catalyze the conversion of urocanic acid to imidazolonepropionic acid. In this apparently benign disorder, an increase in urinary urocanic acid is the only known metabolic aberration.
- Initially discovered in 1961, histidinemia has been found to be the most frequent and well-known disorders of histidine metabolism. In various world locations where neonatal screening is routinely performed, the incidence is found to be 1 in 11,500 live births among more than 20 million screened infants. The incidence is particularly high in Japan with reports as high as 1 in 8000 live births. The prominence of this disorder prompted a study of histidase, which is found primarily in liver and skin.
- The deficiency of urocanic acid in histidinemia may have implications for the putative functions of urocanic acid as a natural sunscreen against ultraviolet light and as a mediator of ultraviolet light–induced immunosuppression.
- Atypical histidinemia is a biochemically milder form of this disorder, perhaps accounting for a substantial minority of cases of histidinemia. Affected patients are reported to be clinically normal with higher skin histidase activities and lower histidine levels and metabolites than in the classic disorder.
- Maternal histidinemia is most likely benign.
- Histidinuria without histidinemia has been reported. All patients had substantially reduced renal tubular reabsorption of histidine, with normal reabsorption of other amino acids. Four of the five were mentally retarded and two had myoclonic seizures, but an association between histidinuria and central nervous system lesions has not been established. This disorder is probably transmitted as an autosomal recessive trait.
- Urocanic aciduria has been reported in at least eight children; four discovered by specific testing have been mentally retarded. The four discovered as a result of neonatal screening have been neurologically normal, which suggests that the mental retardation may not be related to the metabolic disorder.

The primary disorder of histidine metabolism is histidase deficiency resulting in increased serum levels of histidine. This inborn error of metabolism blocks the conversion of histidine to urocanic acid, resulting in accumulations of histidine and histidine metabolites as well as a deficiency of urocanic acid. Whether histidine is an essential amino acid or not has been debated, although it seems clear that histidine is essential for the human infant. Withdrawal of histidine from the diet of young infants results in a reduced rate of weight gain and a fall in nitrogen retention (Snyderman et al., 1963). In addition, a rash resembling infantile eczema develops (Snyderman, 1965). During the treatment of these patients with a low-histidine diet, the blood histidine level is lowered in direct response to the dietary changes. The effect of low dietary histidine on older children and adults remains uncertain. If histidine biosynthesis occurs, it may be sufficient only for basic physiologic needs and may be insufficient for needs of growth or physiologic stress (Stifel & Herman, 1972). Thus it appears that histidine would be an essential amino acid for infants, growing children, and perhaps adults.

Although endogenous histidine synthesis remains to be fully described, the metabolic pathway and catabolism of histidine is well known. The major pathway is through urocanic acid to glutamic acid through a sequence of reactions catalyzed by four enzymes (Fig. 25–6). The first step in this pathway is the nonoxidative deamination of *L*-histidine to trans-urocanic acid by histidase (histidine ammonia-lyase). This enzyme is found primarily in the liver and skin (Furuta et al., 1992; Meister, 1965; Peterkofsky, 1962). There are differences reported in the expression of histidase in these two tissues. In the liver, urocanic acid is an intermediate in the conversion of histidine to glutamic acid, whereas in the skin, it accumulates and may function as an ultraviolet protectant and immunoregulator (Scriver et al., 1995a). The second step in the sequential reaction requires the cytosolic enzyme urocanase, which catalyzes the nonoxidative conversion of trans-urocanic acid to imidazolonepropionic acid. Urocanase is deficient in patients with urocanic aciduria. Urocanase activity has been found only in the liver; there is no detectable activity in the skin, and this accounts for the accumulation of urocanic acid in the skin. The third step in the enzymatic sequence is the conversion of imidazolonepropionic acid to formiminoglutamic acid, an important step that links histidine catabolism to folate metabolism. The enzyme responsible for this conversion is imidazolonepropionic acid hydrolase. The fourth step in the enzymatic conversion is the formation of formiminotetrahydrofolic acid from formiminoglutamic acid catalyzed by the enzyme formiminotransferase. Tetrahydrofolic acid is required for this reaction, and glutamic acid is liberated (Levy, 1985; Levy et al., 1995; Scriver et al., 1995a).

Histidinemia is an autosomal recessive trait. The human histidase gene has been mapped to a location on chromosome 12. The characteristic finding in histidinemia is increased serum concentration of blood histidine, varying from 290 to 1420 μmol (normal range, 70 to 120 μmol) (Levy, 1985; Levy et al., 1974). The level varies, with the highest values at age 1 year and slightly lower values in older children and adults. The variation of levels also reflect dietary protein (histidine) intake and the degree of metabolic block (Kuroda et al., 1980). Urine histidine is also increased in affected persons, probably reflecting overflow from the blood (Levy, 1985). In contrast to inborn errors of metabolism with devastating neurologic consequences in which the CSF-to-plasma ratio is markedly elevated, as in nonketotic hyperglycinemia, histidine is found in the CSF in a normal CSF-to-plasma ratio. Yet, the CSF-to-plasma ratio is normal in some other neurologically devastating inborn errors of metabolism such as PKU (Snyderman et al., 1981).

The children identified during the first decade after the discovery of histidinemia had speech disorders and mental retardation. However, since selective screening of impaired individuals was

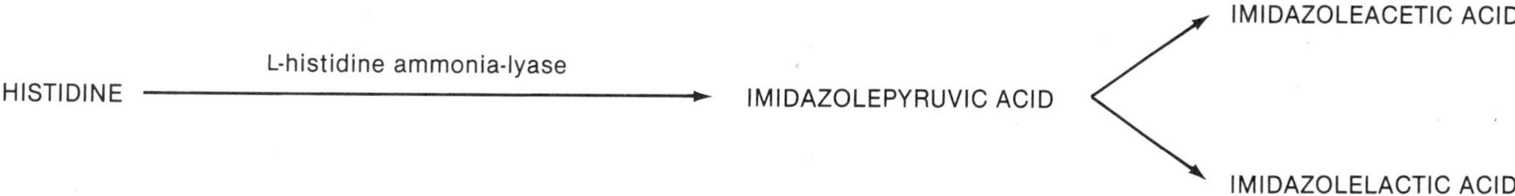

FIGURE 25–6. The metabolism of histidine. In histidinemia, the enzyme histidine ammonia-lyase is deficient. The normally minor degradative pathway by which imidazolepyruvic acid is converted to imidazolelactic and imidazoleacetic acids is enhanced in this disorder.

replaced with widespread population screening for this disorder, quite a few persons were found to have histidinemia and normal intelligence and normal speech, which suggests that histidinemia might actually be benign and that the clinical abnormalities reported initially were coincidental with rather than caused by the genetic disorder. Several prospective follow-up studies of neonates screened for histidinemia in Massachusetts, Japan, and Los Angeles support the view that histidinemia does not cause disease (Alfi et al., 1978; Levy et al., 1974).

The diagnosis of histidinemia is based on finding an elevation of histidine in the blood and increased excretion of histidine in the urine. The urinary metabolite imidazolepyruvic acid can usually be detected by the ferric chloride method. The green color is very similar to that observed with urine from a subject with PKU.

Because 99 percent of histidinemic patients apparently do not require treatment and only 1 percent might benefit, treatment is rarely a consideration. Histidase has been encapsulated for potential use as enzyme replacement therapy (Khanna & Chang, 1990).

Before routine neonatal screening, histidinemia was thought to be a very rare inborn disorder. Neonatal screening dramatically altered this view and demonstrated that histidinemia is one of the most frequent metabolic disorders (Levy, 1973a, 1973b). Neonatal screening identifies infants with elevated blood histidine (Alm et al., 1981; Amador & Carter, 1986; Tada et al., 1984). False-positive results in the bacterial assay for histidine can occur as a result of increased phenylalanine in phenylketonuric infants. Reported incidences of histidinemia vary from 1 in 8000 live births to 1 in 90,000 live births (Amador & Carter, 1986). The wide range of incidence may reflect differing sensitivities of screening methods rather than true population differences.

The recognition that maternal hyperphenylalaninemia causes fetal damage has led to the interest in other maternal inborn errors and fetal consequences. Because maternal histidinemia is such a frequent metabolic disorder, considerable interest has been generated. Various reports in the literature have examined the offspring of histidinemic mothers (Armstrong, 1975; Bruckman et al., 1970; Levy & Benjamin, 1985; Lyon et al., 1974; Matsuda et al., 1983; Tada et al., 1982). The offspring have generally been normal and have not had microcephaly, mental retardation, or congenital anomalies, as seen in the offspring of mothers with PKU. Thus there is no conclusive evidence that there is an adverse fetal effect from maternal histidinemia.

Histidinuria

There are rare reports in the literature of children with increased urinary histidine excretion with low or normal blood histidine levels. Four of the five reported children were mentally retarded (Kamoun et al., 1981; Nyhan & Hilton, 1992; Sabater et al., 1976). The children were tested because of their retardation; thus the increased urinary histidine may be an incidental finding and not causal. Although histidase levels were not measured, all the children had normal blood histidine levels, none excreted histidine metabolites, and it was therefore unlikely that histidase was deficient. Three children had a slow response to histidine loading, which suggests that the etiology may be a defect in intestinal transport or a renal defect (Nyhan & Hilton, 1992).

Urocanic Aciduria

The four children reported in the literature with urocanic aciduria have been mentally retarded, and three have had growth retardation. Biochemical studies are consistent with a defect in urocanase. The level of urocanic acid in the urine was up to 50 times the normal amount. Histidine loading aggravated the condition and increased the urinary excretion of urocanic acid. The presence of urocanase deficiency was proven in three patients and all patients had abnormalities after histidine loading (Kalafatic et al., 1980).

The mental retardation might not be related to the metabolic disorder. All of the patients were referred as a result of an investigation into their mental retardation. Four other patients have been identified with neonatal screening (Lemieux et al., 1988; Swenson et al., 1992) and they have maintained normal development without diet or other therapy. Thus it is likely that urocanic aciduria is benign and that the mental retardation described in reported cases is coincidental rather than causal. The incidence is more frequent than the reports indicate, inasmuch as the disorder may escape detection by the conventional investigative methods. Urocanic acid is ninhydrin-negative and therefore is not identified by amino acid analysis. It is also not soluble in ethyl acetate, the usual solvent employed in organic acid extraction of urine. Autosomal recessive transmission is the most likely mode of inheritance.

Nonketotic Hyperglycinemia

- Nonketotic hyperglycinemia is an inborn error of glycine degradation in which large amounts of glycine accumulate in all tissues, including the central nervous system. The diagnosis is established by calculating the CSF-to-plasma ratio of glycine. A value greater than 0.08 is diagnostic. The diagnosis is confirmed by measuring the activity of the glycine cleavage enzyme system in liver tissue.
- The neonatal form of the disease is the most common manifestation, occurring within the first few days of life. Lethargy, pronounced hypotonia, and myoclonic jerking progressing to apnea and often death occur. In the infants who do regain spontaneous respiration, intractable seizures and profound mental retardation develop.
- In the infantile form of the disease, the patients develop symptoms later in life. The typical manifestation is the development of seizures and various degrees of mental retardation after a period of apparently normal development. Affected patients may be asymptomatic up to the age of 6 months.
- A transient form of hyperglycinemia has been described in newborns with symptoms indistinguishable from those of the neonatal form. The elevated glycine levels are identical to those found in the neonatal form but return to normal by 8 weeks of age.
- Glycine is a neurotransmitter. It functions to inhibit the neurotransmission in the spinal cord, and it is excitatory in the cortex. Excessive stimulation of the cortical brain is thought to be responsible for the seizures and brain damage.
- The primary metabolic defect is in the glycine enzyme cleav-

age system found within the mitochondria. The glycine cleavage enzyme system consists of four components: a pyridoxal phosphate–dependent glycine decarboxylase (P protein); a lipoic acid–containing hydrogen carrier protein (H protein); a tetrahydrofolate-dependent protein (T protein); and lipoamide dehydrogenase (L protein). In the neonatal form of the disease, the P protein is defective. Metabolic variations in this disease may reflect defects in the T, H, or L proteins.

- The gene for the P protein has been mapped to chromosome 9. Nonketotic hyperglycinemia is inherited as an autosomal recessive trait. The incidence is increased in northern Finland, where a genetic mutation in one common ancestor has resulted in an incidence of 1 in 12,000 births, in comparison with an overall incidence of 1 in 55,000 in Finland. Prenatal diagnosis is possible with chorionic villus sampling.
- No effective treatment exists. Experimental studies are focused on decreasing the glycine concentration in tissues and blocking the effect of glycine in the cortex to reduce the seizure threshold.

Glycine is a simple amino acid. An average adult diet contains approximately 3 to 5 g of glycine per day, and the rate of glycine turnover is about 1 g/kg/day (Scriver & Rosenberg, 1973). It is also endogenously synthesized from serine and can be converted to glucose via pyruvate (Fig. 25–7). Normal glycine tissue levels have been established (Scriver et al., 1975; Scriver et al., 1995a). Glycine is an important constituent of protein, providing more than a fourth of the amino acid residues of abundant structural proteins such as collagen, elastin, and gelatin. Glycine also has an important synthetic role in metabolism, and it is incorporated into purines, creatine, and porphyrins (Scriver et al., 1995a).

Most synaptic neurotransmission in the brain is carried out by the amino acids glutamate, γ-aminobutyric acid (GABA), and glycine as neurotransmitters (Greenamyre, 1986). The most prominent excitatory neurotransmitter is glutamate, whereas GABA is the most prominent inhibitory neurotransmitter (Cooper et al., 1991). Glycine plays an inhibitory role in the spinal cord and mediating excitatory neurotransmission in the cerebral cortex and the forebrain (Agamanolis et al., 1993; Ascher & Johnson, 1989; Krnjevic, 1974; Probst et al., 1986).

Neonatal Nonketotic Hyperglycinemia

This is the most common form of the disease, and patients present in a strikingly similar manner. The patients typically are products of normal, uncomplicated pregnancies with appropriate growth in all parameters at birth. No external congenital anomalies are present. The symptom-free interval ranges from 6 hours to 8 days; 66 percent of the patients become symptomatic by 48 hours (Dalla Bernardina et al., 1979). There is a progressive development of hypotonia, lethargy, and refusal to feed. Wandering eye movements and increased deep tendon reflexes are present. As the encephalopathy progresses to coma, frequent segmental myoclonic jerks, apneic episodes, and hiccups develop. Most infants require assisted ventilation in the first weeks of life (Scriver et al., 1995a).

In view of the severe neurologic manifestation of this disorder, newborns with nonketotic hyperglycinemia have remarkably normal findings on routine laboratory studies. Hematologic parameters are normal without evidence of sepsis, anemia, or thrombocytopenia. The electrolytes are normal, without metabolic acidosis. The anion gap is normal. Respiratory acidosis may be present if ventilation is inadequate. Urine organic acids are normal. The only consistent metabolic abnormality is elevation of glycine concentration in urine, plasma, and CSF.

The diagnosis is established by determining the CSF-to-plasma ratio of glycine (Perry et al., 1975; Scriver et al., 1995a). Plasma concentrations of glycine in this disorder range from high normal to values eight times the normal mean and four times the upper normal limit. Urinary glycine levels are usually increased but may be difficult to interpret because of the physiologic hyperglycinuria seen in the newborn period. Thus screening urine for glycine is not useful in the diagnosis. The CSF concentration of glycine is elevated (15 to 30 times normal) to a much greater extent than the plasma levels. A CSF-to-plasma ratio higher than 0.08 is considered diagnostic of nonketotic hyperglycinemia. The normal CSF-to-plasma ratio of glycine is consistently less than 0.02. In patients with atypical nonketotic hyperglycinemia, ratios approximate 0.09, whereas in neonatal patients, ratios range from 0.2 to 0.3 (Scriver et al., 1995a). Definitive diagnosis can be established by measuring the glycine cleavage enzyme system activity of liver tissue. This procedure requires a liver biopsy and is not feasible in critically ill neonates.

Despite neonatal intensive care, approximately 30 percent of these patients die in the neonatal period. Those who survive usually regain spontaneous respiration by three weeks of age, and survival is reported to range from several months to 22 years. Most patients regain the ability to suck, but many must be gavage-fed. Untreated patients develop intractable seizures by age 12 months but rarely before 3 months. The seizure pattern evolves with the initial development of myoclonic jerks, progressing to infantile spasms, partial motor seizures, and/or tonic extension. Severe psychomotor retardation and little adaptive or social behavior is the usual outcome. Spastic quadriplegia replaces the initial hypotonia (Scriver et al., 1995a).

EEGs progress from an early initial burst-suppression pattern to a hypsarrhythmia pattern later. The EEG usually does not correlate to the clinical findings. After 1 year of age, the sleep–wake EEG patterns differ. During sleep, hypsarrhythmia pattern is routine, but the awake tracing reveals a slow background with lack of normal wake and sleep components and frequent independent multifocal spike discharges (Scriver et al., 1995a). All patients have prolonged latencies on the auditory evoked responses, which suggests a slowing of the conduction system along the brain stem auditory pathway (Markland et al., 1982).

There is some speculation that patients with nonketotic hyperglycinemia may experience prenatal brain injury. The corpus callosum is abnormally thinned or completely absent, and there is an abnormal gyral pattern in many subjects studied with computed tomography or at autopsy (Dobyns, 1989). Although not a specific finding for nonketotic hyperglycinemia, it represents a poor prognosis (Scriver et al., 1995a). There are reports that mothers of infants with nonketotic hyperglycemia observe abnormal fetal movements described as persistent hiccups (Von Wendt et al., 1981).

At autopsy, infants with this disorder have spongiform degeneration of the white matter, which is normally well-myelinated at birth (Dobyns, 1989; Scher et al., 1986). There is diffuse vacuolation of the myelin. If death occurs after the neonatal period, areas that normally myelinate have thin myelin. It may be likely

$$\text{GLYCINE} \xrightarrow{\text{serine methyltransferase}} CO_2 + NH_4 + \text{HYDROXYMETHYLTETRAHYDROFOLIC ACID}$$

FIGURE 25–7. The catabolism of glycine to serine. Glycine is the simplest of the amino acids and is involved in a variety of synthetic reactions, including protein synthesis. The interconversion of glycine to serine is the most important pathway in the catabolism of this amino acid and is thought to be responsible for glycine encephalopathy.

that the imbalance of amino acid transmitters in the brain is responsible for interfering with normal myelin synthesis.

There have been several case reports of infants who meet the diagnostic criteria for nonketotic hyperglycinemia but who did not present with the disorder during the neonatal period. Infantile nonketotic hyperglycinemia occurs after a variable interval of normal development and growth until about 6 months of age. In the infantile form, the usual manifestation is seizures, and the infants tend to be spared the severe hypotonia and profound apnea that is typical of the neonatal form of the disease. Their survival rate is higher and the degree of mental retardation, although significant, is not as pronounced.

Five case reports of transient nonketotic hyperglycinemia have been described (Eyskens et al., 1992). With the initial presentation, these infants are indistinguishable from those with the neonatal form, with elevated CSF-to-plasma ratios and a burst-suppression pattern of EEG. By 2 to 8 weeks of age, the plasma and CSF glycine levels return to normal. Four of the five patients had no apparent neurologic sequelae at ages 6 months to 4 years (Eyskens et al., 1992; Schiffman et al., 1989), but one was severely retarded with white matter degeneration noted on MRI. The etiology of this disorder is presumably related to immaturity of the glycine cleavage enzyme system in both the liver and the brain. Genetic evidence is lacking as to the transmission of this rare disorder.

Several strategies have been attempted to ameliorate the intractable seizures and relentless brain damage seen in the disorder of neonatal nonketotic hyperglycinemia. No approach has consistently been proved effective. Reduction of tissue glycine levels by initiating glycine-free or glycine-and-serine-free diets resulted in reduced tissue glycine levels but had no effect on seizure frequency or developmental progress (Langan & Pueschel, 1983; Scriver et al., 1995a; Tada, 1987). Benzoate to reduce the tissue glycine levels has been used extensively. Therapy with benzoate reduces CSF glycine levels, improves arousal, and decreases the seizure frequency but has not improved developmental progress (Langan & Pueschel, 1983; Scriver et al., 1975, 1995a).

Because hyperglycinemia results in seizures related to an excitotoxic mechanism, conventional anticonvulsant therapy with phenobarbital and phenytoin, which act by enhancing inhibition, has not been effective in treating these seizures. Valproate may be specifically contraindicated in this disorder because it interferes with the glycine cleavage enzyme system activity in the liver in patients without nonketotic hyperglycinemia.

Use of antagonists of the cerebral excitatory receptor of glycine has been studied with varying reports of success. Strychnine and ketamine, which block the glycine excitatory receptor, have been used but are limited by their duration of action, route of administration, or potential to worsen the seizures and exacerbate brain damage (Scriver et al., 1995a). The use of dextromethorphan may be promising. Dextromethorphan, used at high doses, is an antagonist to the glycine excitatory receptor. In one report (Schmitt et al., 1993) dextromethorphan was used at 10 times the tussive dose in a 9-week-old infant. The patient's seizures (myoclonic jerks and flexor spasms) stopped, and the EEG normalized. At 6 months of age the dextromethorphan was stopped for 24 hours, and somnolence, hypotonia, and myoclonic jerks progressing to flexor spasms developed. The EEG showed multifocal spikes superimposed over extremely slowed background activity. Reintroduction of dextromethorphan resulted in recovery over 24 hours (Schmitt et al., 1993). However, other patients have been treated with a combination of benzoate and dextromethorphan without dramatic results in developmental progress (Scriver et al., 1995a).

The different therapeutic trials involve very small numbers of patients. Before any further progress in treatment, the molecular basis for the disease variability among individual patients must be more firmly established. Then more stringent methods will be required in order to study the various therapies to allow accurate assessment of clinical effect.

Disorders of Transsulfuration of Amino Acids

The transsulfuration pathway converts the sulfur atom of methionine into the sulfur atom of cysteine. This pathway is the chief route of disposal of methionine and explains why cysteine is not an essential amino acid in humans. Two additional metabolic sequences are also involved: the transmethylation reaction, by which the methyl group of methionine is ultimately transferred to form any of a host of methylated compounds, and the reformation of methionine by methylation of homocystine (Nyhan, 1984). At least nine specific genetic disorders that affect this metabolic pathway have been recognized. Only three disorders are discussed here: MAT deficiency, cystathionine β-synthase (CBS) deficiency, and γ-cystathionase deficiency.

Increased methionine levels are found in a number of metabolic disorders such as hereditary fructose intolerance, tyrosinemia, and homocystinuria (Nyhan, 1984). Methionine is also increased in preterm infants, because of the delayed appearance of degradation enzymes, and in infants fed a high-methionine formula (Ampola, 1982; Wapnir, 1985; Winick, 1979). Neonatal hepatitis also results in an elevated methionine level. Hereditary fructose intolerance and tyrosinemia have already been discussed.

- A deficiency of MAT has been found in newborns screened for hypermethioninemia. All were clinically well at ages ranging up to 38 years. Residual hepatic MAT activity was present in varying amounts, and the MAT activity in tissues other than the liver were normal.
- CBS deficiency is the most frequently encountered cause of homocystinuria. Homocystine, methionine and homocystine metabolites accumulate in the body or are excreted in the urine. Dislocation of the optic lens, osteoporosis, thinning and lengthening of the long bones, mental retardation, and thromboembolism are the most common clinical features.
- CBS deficiency is an autosomal recessive trait with considerable genetic heterogeneity. CBS activity may range from 0% to a small percentage of residual activity. The presence of a small amount of residual activity may be a necessary condition required for clinical responsiveness to pyridoxine administration. Pyridoxine-responsive patients have more slowly developing or milder manifestations of the disease.
- The frequency of CBS deficiency detected by neonatal screening for hypermethioninemia is 1 in 344,000 live births.
- The management of CBS-deficient patients involves the amelioration of the characteristic biochemical abnormalities with the use of low-methionine, cystine-supplemented diets. If the patient is pyridoxine-responsive, treatment with pyridoxine should be ordered. Dietary restriction in the newborn period has been shown to prevent mental retardation and, possibly, to decrease the incidence of seizures. Pyridoxine treatment has been shown to decrease the incidence of initial thromboembolic events.
- γ-Cystathionase deficiency leads to persistent excretion of large amounts of cystathionine in the urine and accumulation of cystathionine in body tissues and fluids. No clinical abnormalities are characteristically associated with this disorder. The deficiency is inherited as an autosomal recessive trait and likely has considerable genetic heterogeneity.

The pertinent reactions of the transsulfuration pathway and related areas are found in Figure 25–8. At least nine specific genetic disorders have been recognized from defects in the reactions shown. The discussion is limited to MAT deficiency, CBS deficiency, and γ-cystathionase deficiency.

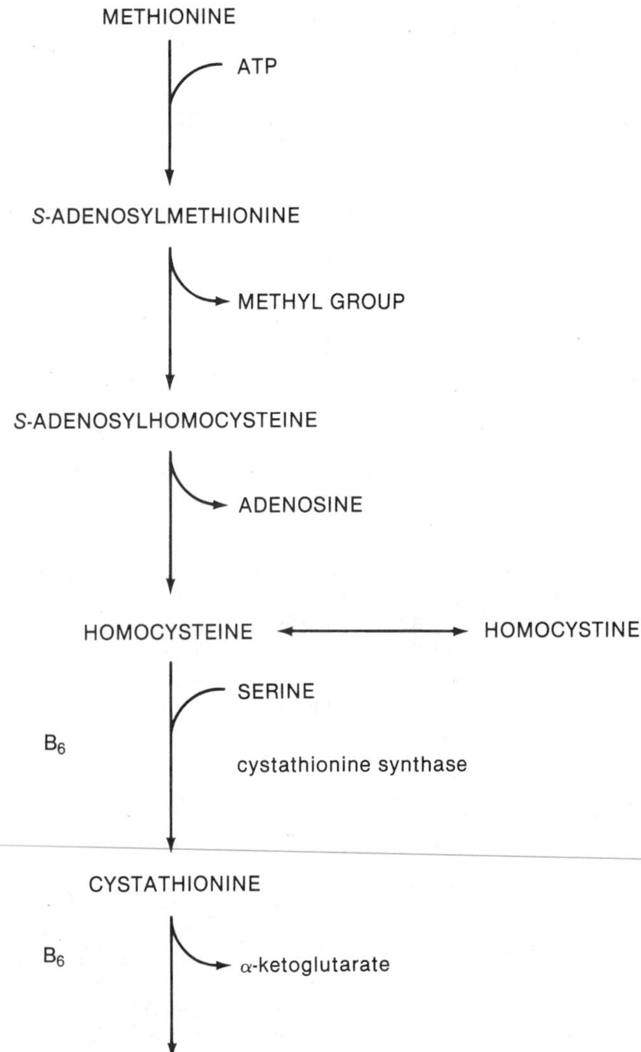

FIGURE 25–8. The development of homocystinuria. The primary defect is in the enzyme cystathionine β-synthase, which catalyzes the formation of cystathionine from serine and homocysteine. ATP, adenosine triphosphate.

Hepatic Methionine Adenosyltransferase Deficiency

Neonatal screening has detected a number of patients with hypermethioninemia associated with deficient MAT activity in the liver (Mudd et al., 1995). Plasma levels of methionine are 250 to 1270 μmol (upper limit of normal is approximately 30 μmol). When methionine intake is severely restricted, the level of hypermethioninemia drops only to about 400 μmol. When extracts of liver tissue were analyzed for MAT activity, only 8 to 18 percent of mean control values for MAT activity were found when the patient's methionine levels were high and up to 30 percent of control values were found at lower concentrations of plasma methionine (Mudd et al., 1995). MAT activity in other tissues was also assayed and found to be no different from control values. Thus hepatic enzyme activity of MAT is under separate genetic control from nonhepatic tissues.

Clinically, patients with proven or suspected defects of hepatic MAT activity have been virtually normal. The oldest patient recorded was 38 years old and well physically and mentally. His only complaint was the odor of his breath, caused by the presence of unusually large amounts of dimethylsulfide (Gahl et al., 1988). He was a long-distance runner with normal muscle mass (Gahl et al., 1987). The remaining patients were clinically well physically, developmentally, and mentally at ages 7 to 18 years (Gahl et al., 1988) on unrestricted diets. All patients were free of hepatic disease (Gahl et al., 1987, 1988).

Cystathionine β-Synthase Deficiency

This disease was first identified in 1962 and it is now recognized as CBS deficiency. Since that time, the clinical manifestations and the enzymatic defect have been identified. CBS deficiency is inherited as an autosomal recessive trait. Obligate heterozygous individuals have had 22 to 47 percent of mean control values for CBS activity in liver cells, skin fibroblasts, and lymphocytes (Mudd et al., 1995).

The metabolic consequence of deficient CBS activity is a tendency for homocystine to accumulate within the cell. The cell tends to export homocystine, and the plasma has abnormal concentrations of a variety of homocystine derivatives. CBS-deficient patients have an increase in protein-bound homocystine as well as non-protein–bound homocystine. The protein-bound homocystine may be the more sensitive indicator of an elevation of total plasma homocystine moieties (Mudd et al., 1995).

A second characteristic of CBS deficiency is the presence of abnormal concentrations of methionine in plasma. Under fasting conditions, the normal person's plasma contains less than 30 μmol of methionine. Untreated CBS-deficient patients have been reported to have fasting methionine levels as high as 2000 μmol (Mudd et al., 1995), presumably because of the high rate of methylation of elevated homocystine. Abnormal accumulations of methionine and homocystine occur in plasma and in other body fluids such as the aqueous humor and CSF (Tada et al., 1967). Renal tubular reabsorption of methionine is very efficient, and even with moderate elevations of plasma methionine, the urinary excretion may be within normal limits. Homocystine is absorbed less well, and in cases of severe untreated CBS deficiency, more than 1 mmol of homocystine may be excreted daily (Mudd et al., 1995).

In 1967 the first reports of the effect of high doses of pyridoxine in CBS-deficient individuals was described (Barber & Spaeth, 1969). These doses resulted in decreases of plasma methionine to normal and virtual elimination of homocystine from plasma and urine. During the response to pyridoxine, there are decreases in a number of additional compounds proximal to the block at CBS and increases in the number of compounds distal to the block (Mudd et al., 1995). Some CBS-deficient patients, however, are not responsive to pyridoxine. The pyridoxine-induced response is not due to correction of a pre-existing vitamin B_6 deficiency or to an alleviation of a defect in vitamin B_6 metabolism (Barber & Spaeth, 1969; Mudd et al., 1995). The biochemical response to pyridoxine may not occur in folate-depleted patients until after folate replenishment (Morrow & Barness, 1972; Wilcken & Turner, 1973), and such depletion may explain the apparent failure of some patients to respond to pyridoxine therapy.

The metabolic response to pyridoxine in CBS-deficient patients is not uniform. Some patients continue to have a slight elevation in plasma or urinary homocystine, whereas others do not (Mudd et al., 1995). Even patients who do respond well are not restored to biochemical normality, continuing to have abnormal rises of plasma and urinary homocystine after methionine loads, delayed restoration of plasma methionine to basal conditions, and maximal capacities for transsulfuration far below normal (Mudd et al., 1985, 1995). Pyridoxine responsiveness is constant among sibships (Mudd et al., 1995), indicating not only that the capacity to respond to pyridoxine is genetically determined but also that the degree of responsiveness is genetically determined and may be linked to the defective enzyme itself. There is evidence of a strong correlation between the presence of residual enzyme activity of CBS and clinical responsiveness to pyridoxine and between the absence of residual activity and nonresponsiveness (de Franchis et al., 1994; Mudd et al., 1995). Thus it seems that pyridoxine responsiveness is based on the presence of a small residual activity of CBS.

Homocystinuria due to CBS deficiency is accompanied by an abundance of clinical manifestations, in which four organ systems show major involvement: the eye and the vascular, skeletal, and central nervous systems. Other organ systems, including liver, skin, and hair, may also be involved. The risk that a manifestation of the disease will develop increases with age. If the individual is pyridoxine-responsive, the manifestations are usually milder.

The most consistent finding in CBS deficiency is ectopia lentis (dislocation of the ocular lens). Dislocation of the lens is usually in a downward direction and rarely occurs before age 2 (Mudd et al., 1995). After 2 years of age, the frequency of lens dislocation increases, so that by age 38, only 3 percent of untreated patients have intact lenses (Mudd et al., 1985). Along with the dislocation of the lens, a marked myopia develops when the lens begins to loosen and worsens as the subluxation progresses. In addition, acute pupillary block glaucoma, optic atrophy, retinal degeneration and detachment, cataracts, and corneal abnormalities are highly prevalent in this disorder (Mudd et al., 1995).

The most consistent skeletal manifestation, osteoporosis, occurs in the spine followed by the long bones. In at least 50 percent of untreated patients, osteoporosis is detectable by the end of the second decade of life (Brill et al., 1974). As a result of the spinal osteoporosis, vertebral collapse and scoliosis are common. Additional skeletal manifestations include increased length of the long bones; irregular, widened metaphyses; growth arrest lines; pes cavus; and high, arched palate (Brill et al., 1974; Mudd et al., 1995).

The primary vascular clinical manifestation, thromboembolism, is the major cause of morbidity and death in patients with CBS deficiency. Vascular occlusion can occur in any vessel at any age. In an international survey, 158 patients were reported to have had 253 thromboembolitic events (Mudd et al., 1985). Among these events, 51 percent occurred in peripheral veins (32 of which involved pulmonary embolism), 32 percent were cerebrovascular accidents, 11 percent affected peripheral arteries, 4 percent resulted in myocardial infarctions, and 2 percent were nonspecific. Complications of thromboembolism include optic atrophy, hemiparesis, cor pulmonale, renal hypertension, seizures, and focal neurologic damage (Mudd et al., 1995). The manifestation of vascular thromboembolism depends on age and pyridoxine responsiveness. Untreated pyridoxine-responsive patients are at little risk until about 12 years of age, with increasing risk thereafter, so that by age 20 years the cumulative risk for a thromboembolitic event is about 25 percent. Untreated pyridoxine-nonresponsive patient had a cumulative risk of 25 percent by 15 years of age (McCully, 1993; Rubba et al., 1990). The risk factors are based on the clinically apparent thromboembolic events. Efforts at ultrasonic detection of vascular disease have documented early vascular disease even in the absence of symptoms of ischemia (Rubba et al., 1990).

The most frequent clinical manifestation of the central nervous system in CBS deficiency is mental retardation, often manifesting as developmental delay during the first and second years of life. The IQ scores of untreated patients vary widely, ranging from 10 to 138, with the median approximately 64. The distribution of pyridoxine-responsive patients was shifted toward the higher IQ scores (median 78), in comparison with that for pyridoxine-nonresponsive patients (median 56). Twenty-one percent of infants with CBS deficiency untreated from early infancy have seizures, most frequently of grand mal type (Ludolph et al., 1991; Mudd et al., 1985, 1995). Abnormal EEGs have been reported. Signs of focal neurologic signs and hemiparesis suggest a cerebrovascular event (Ludolph et al., 1991; Mudd et al., 1985, 1995).

The presence of one or more of the typical signs and symptoms may lead to a suspicion of CBS deficiency, but definitive diagnosis is based on the presence of certain biochemical abnormalities. The most consistent biochemical abnormality is homocystinuria (Mudd et al., 1995). The presence of homocystine is suspected when the urinary cyanide–nitroprusside reaction is positive. Because this test also detects other disulfide compounds, homocystine must be specifically identified.

False-negative results can occur in tests for homocystinuria. Pyridoxine-responsive forms of CBS deficiency may have a marked response to even very small amounts of supplemental folate therapy (as little as one vitamin tablet daily) and thus may escape detection. Before testing, any supplemental vitamins should be discontinued for 2 to 4 weeks, and the amount of folate intake should be calculated on the basis of diet history (Morrow & Barness, 1972).

The presence of homocystinuria alone is not sufficient to establish the diagnosis of CBS deficiency. Homocystinuria is a nonspecific symptom; homocystine is excreted in other inborn errors of metabolism, and consequently serum amino acid analysis should be performed. In CBS deficiency, amino acid analysis should reveal hyperhomocystinemia and a markedly reduced concentration of cystine. Frequently, an increased level of methionine is also found. Direct enzyme analysis assayed from liver biopsy samples, cultured skin fibroblasts, or lymphocytes confirms the diagnosis (Burke et al., 1992; Mudd et al., 1995; Thuy & Nyhan, 1992; Uhlendorf & Mudd, 1968).

Medical management of CBS deficiency is aimed at (1) control or elimination of biochemical abnormalities with the goals of preventing clinical disease, halting the progression of existing clinical defects, and ameliorating the clinical manifestations that may be reversible and (2) supportive treatment of complications. Whenever possible, treatment should begin before the onset of complications, because many may cause irreversible damage. Thus, maximal benefit of therapy is obtained when the disorder is detected in the neonatal period either from neonatal screening or by family history (Burke et al., 1992).

The administration of pyridoxine has been effective in reducing or eliminating the biochemical abnormalities in many patients with pyridoxine-responsive CBS deficiency (Barber & Spaeth, 1969). The doses of pyridoxine have varied widely, and some patients have a dose–response correlation (Wilcken & Turner, 1973). The effectiveness of pyridoxine in preventing initial clinically detectable thromboembolytic events has been established (Mudd et al., 1985). For prevention of thromboembolism alone, pyridoxine treatment is strongly indicated for pyridoxine-responsive patients at any age. A similar analysis has also documented a decreased frequency of lens dislocation among the pyridoxine-responsive patients who were treated with pyridoxine (Mudd et al., 1985, 1995). In addition, there is evidence that behavior and IQ scores have improved in several late-treated pyridoxine-responsive patients (Grobe, 1980; Ludolph et al., 1991).

Folate deficiency is found in this disorder and may have to be replenished in order to effect a pyridoxine response. In other patients, folate therapy alone may be enough or may be used in combination with vitamin B_{12} and pyridoxine to achieve the lower concentrations of homocystine (Barber & Spaeth, 1969; Morrow & Barness, 1972; Mudd et al., 1995).

Vitamin therapy alone for CBS-deficient patients responsive to pyridoxine may not be as effective at reducing the biochemical abnormalities as when it is combined with a methionine-restricted diet. Even patients with maximal pyridoxine responsiveness have a reduced tolerance to methionine, and such patients may exhibit episodic increases in methionine or homocystine concentrations after protein intake (Acosta & Elsas, 1976). Therefore, the use of methionine-restricted diets or small, frequent feedings may be prudent.

The great majority of CBS-deficient patients detected by neonatal screening have been treated with diets low in methionine to reduce the accumulation of methionine and homocystine and supplemented with *L*-cystine to provide at least some of this amino acid. Current commercially available diets are based on a methionine-free synthetic mixture supplemented with *L*-cystine. The methionine requirement is met with the addition of small amounts of milk and later by the addition of low-protein foods in carefully controlled quantities. The amount of dietary protein is regulated by the maintenance of blood methionine levels within the normal range and by the absence of homocystine in the urine and blood (Acosta & Elsas, 1976). Methionine restriction, started from early infancy, has been shown to prevent or delay a number of serious complications of this disorder. Most patients detected by neonatal screening have been pyridoxine-nonresponsive, and thus the data is more convincing. In an international survey, the mean IQ score for early-treated, pyridoxine-nonresponsive patients was 94 ± 4, approximately 35 points above the mean IQ of late-treated pyridoxine-nonresponsive patients (Mudd et al., 1985). Early dietary treatment also tends to delay or prevent lens dislocation in some patients and may prevent seizures (Mudd et al., 1985). Early-treated patients are still too young to evaluate for the effect on thromboembolism and osteoporosis (Mudd et al., 1995). Treatment may be indicated for newborns who are responsive to pyridoxine along with a methionine-restricted diet.

The patients detected after the newborn period who are nonresponsive to pyridoxine therapy represent the greatest challenge to treatment. Compliance with a methionine-restricted diet is difficult to achieve in older children. When accepted and maintained, there is evidence of improvement in the biochemical abnormalities (Mudd et al., 1995), and results appear promising in terms of prevention of thromboembolic events (Acosta & Elsas, 1976; McCully, 1993). There is also anecdotal evidence of improved school performance (Grobe, 1980).

To date, most screening of newborns for CBS deficiency have relied on the detection of hypermethioninemia. The currently available data for prevalence rates for this disorder vary widely from 1 in 58,000 live births in Ireland to 1 in 889,000 live births in Japan. The current cumulative rate of detection is 1 in 344,000 live births worldwide, which may be an underestimate of its frequency. Hypermethioninemia may not be detected during the time when the newborn blood for screening is obtained because current feeding practices have provided lower protein intakes since the 1970s (Mudd et al., 1995).

An alternative to screening newborns for hypermethioninemia to identify CBS deficiency is to attempt to detect abnormal levels of homocystine in blood or urine. To date, no specific or reliable test has been firmly established for use as a tool for routine neonatal screening (Thuy & Nyhan, 1992). Prenatal diagnosis of CBS deficiency is feasible in the first and second trimesters of pregnancy through the use of extracts of cells cultured from amniotic fluid to detect the activity of CBS (Burke et al., 1992; Uhlendorf & Mudd, 1968).

γ-Cystathionase Deficiency

Deficient activity of γ-cystathionase has been reported in several patients who presented with cystathioninuria. In addition to an increased urinary excretion of cystathionine, this amino acid accumulated and was present in elevated concentrations in the body fluids and tissues. γ-cystathionine deficiency provided the first evidence in which a major biochemical abnormality caused by a defined enzyme defect was clearly shown to be alleviated by the administration of large doses of pyridoxine. The majority of these patients respond to pyridoxine with significant decreases in urinary cystathionine excretion.

The search for clinical manifestations of γ-cystathionine deficiency followed discovery of this disorder in a mentally retarded adult. The initial searches for cystathionuric patients concentrated on the mentally retarded population and the resulting ascertainment bias may have fostered the belief that this disorder was a cause of mental abnormalities (Ludolph et al., 1991; Mudd et al., 1995). In addition to mental abnormalities, a wide variety of other disorders have been found in these patients. Among these are convulsions, hypoplastic genitalia, acromegaly, thrombocytopenia, nephrocalcinosis, nephrogenic diabetes insipidus, and insulin-dependent diabetes mellitus. Strong evidence suggests, however, that it is doubtful that any clinical abnormalities result specifically from γ-cystathionase deficiency alone (Mudd et al., 1995).

Diagnosis can be demonstrated by the presence of cystathionine in the urine by amino acid chromatography. Plasma should also be analyzed for amino acids by using a suitable technique. In γ-cystathionase deficiency, amino acid chromatography demonstrates that an elevated level of cystathioninuria can occur transiently in the newborn, in association with liver disease, neuroblastoma, and hepatoblastoma and in vitamin B_6 deficiency (Mudd et al., 1995). When cystathioninuria has been established as persistent and apparently the primary disorder, a trial of oral pyridoxine supplementation should be performed to establish whether the condition is pyridoxine-responsive. Definitive diagnosis can be confirmed by liver biopsy to assay γ-cystathionase activity, but this may be controversial in a disorder considered by many clinicians to be probably benign. Enzymatic analysis of cultured lymphocytes is an alternative means of diagnosis (Mudd et al., 1995).

Because many clinicians consider γ-cystathionase deficiency a benign disorder, no specific management is indicated. For patients responsive to pyridoxine, oral pyridoxine can be administered with the goal of eliminating or significantly reducing the cystathioninemia and cystathioninuria.

Amino Acid Disorders That Involve Defects in Membrane Transport Systems

Cystinuria

- Cystinuria is a defect of the amino acid transport affecting the epithelial cells of the renal tubule and the GI tract. The defective transport of cystine, lysine, arginine, and ornithine is transmitted as an autosomal recessive trait. The heterozygous state may reflect true recessive or incompletely recessive inheritance. In the latter, the affected amino acids are excreted in urine in quantities greater than normal but less than in the homozygous state.
- The intestinal defect is demonstrated by oral loading tests and by intestinal perfusion studies. The dibasic amino acids can be absorbed by cystinuric subjects in a normal manner as dipeptides.
- The renal lesions of all four amino acids and the mixed disulfide of cystine-homocystine is demonstrated by clearance studies. The clearance of cystine in adults with cystinuria is frequently greater than the glomerular filtration rate (GFR), which suggests active secretion. Affected kidneys have demonstrated a defect in the transport system for the dibasic amino acids but not for cystine. Cystine and the dibasic amino acids appear to share the low-saturation, high-affinity renal cortical transport system that is probably defective in the cystinuric kidney. There is probably an interaction of cystine and the dibasic amino acids at the luminal membrane of the renal tubule cells; such an interaction may play an important role in the regulation of cystine transport into renal cortical cells.
- Cystinuria is expressed clinically as urinary tract calculus disease. Cystine stones are formed, and cystine crystals ap-

pear in the urine. Diagnosis may be pursued by testing urine with nitroprusside, electrophoresis, or column amino acid analysis. Stones generally form when cystine is excreted at rates greater than 300 mg of cystine per gram of creatinine in acid urine. Cystinuric patients are susceptible to all complications of stone disease. Treatment is aimed at reducing the concentration of cystine in urine by increasing urine volume, increasing cystine solubility by alkalinizing urine, and reducing cystine excretion by the use of drugs.

Cystinuria is a heritable disorder of amino acid transport affecting the epithelial cells of the renal tubules and gastrointestinal tract. The disease is expressed clinically by the formation of calculi in the urinary tract, with the potential for obstruction, infections, and ultimately renal insufficiency. The disease is characterized primarily by the precipitation of cystine, the least soluble of the naturally occurring amino acids, but lysine, arginine, ornithine, and cystine-homocystine are also found in excess in the urine (Scriver et al., 1995a).

Although cystinuria is thought to be a rare disease because of the estimated frequency of 1 to 20,000 live births in England and 1 to 100,000 live births in Sweden, there are populations in which homozygous cystinuria is relatively common. Among Israeli Jews of Libyan origin, the incidence has been estimated to be 1 in 2500 live births (Crawhall et al., 1969; Weinberger et al., 1974). Neonatal screening programs have estimated the frequency to be 1 in 2000 live births in England, 1 in 4000 live births in Australia, and 1 in 15,000 live births in the United States. According to Levy (1973a, 1973b), who summarized the results of neonatal screening, the overall frequency is 1 in 7000 live births, making cystinuria one of the most common inherited disorders. Although the disease affects both sexes equally, males are more severely affected and have a higher mortality rate. The higher mortality among males is most likely a function of male anatomy and urethral obstruction. Clinical manifestations may appear as early as the first year of life or as late as the ninth decade; the most common time for symptoms appears to be the second and third decades of life. Renal colic is the most common symptom and may be associated with obstruction, infection, and eventual loss of function. Occasionally, infection, hypertension, and renal failure are the reasons for seeking medical care, and the diagnosis of cystinuria is made subsequently (Scriver et al., 1995a).

The diagnosis of cystinuria should be considered in every patient with urinary tract calculi or with symptoms suggestive of calculi. Microscopic evaluation of urine sediment for typical cystine crystals is the simplest diagnostic procedure. Acidification of the urine with acetic acid may precipitate cystine crystals that were not visible in a fresh urine specimen. The cyanide–nitroprusside test has been widely applied as a chemical screening procedure. The lower limit of sensitivity of the reaction is 75 to 125 mg of cystine per gram of creatinine, permitting easy identification of homozygous stone formers, but the heterozygotes who may excrete less than that amount may be missed. Because crystalluria occurs with a variety of inborn errors of metabolism, patients with a positive cyanide–nitroprusside test result should be further studied for identification of urinary amino acids with thin-layer chromatography or electrophoresis. Urinary cystine can be measured quantitatively by high-performance liquid chromatography (Scriver et al., 1995a).

Cystinuria is a classic example of a disorder of renal tubular function. Normally, amino acids are filtered and are almost entirely reabsorbed in the proximal nephron. The reabsorptive mechanism has a maximal capacity that is exceeded in certain disorders. In most cases of aminoaciduria, an extrarenal defect leads to the accumulation of an amino acid in the plasma, which is then filtered in amounts exceeding the normal capacity of the nephron for reabsorption. These are not disorders of tubular function. When excessive loss occurs in the presence of normal or low amino acid plasma levels, the reabsorptive capacity of the renal tubule is diminished and tubular dysfunction exists. In cystinuria, excessive urinary losses of cystine and dibasic amino acids occur with normal or less than normal plasma levels of the affected amino acids.

When an amino acid is ingested, absorption occurs, and the unabsorbed amino acid is used by intestinal flora. The less the amino acid is absorbed, the lower the blood levels after eating, and the greater are the levels of the bacterial breakdown products in the stool and perhaps also in the plasma and urine. If bacterial flora are suppressed, the nonabsorbed amino acid should be demonstrable in the stool. The discovery of impaired intestinal amino acid transport from feeding experiments showed that some patients had total impairment of cystine, lysine, and arginine accumulation in the intestinal mucosa cells, others had small but detectable cystine transport but no dibasic amino acid transport, and still a third group had normal or slightly impaired cystine uptake and demonstrable but diminished lysine and arginine accumulation (Rosenberg et al., 1966). The intestinal transport studies confirm that cystine and dibasic amino acids share a common transport system. In the intestinal mucosa there is evidence of only a single shared system, which in many patients is completely defective in its function (Rosenberg et al., 1966; Scriver et al., 1995a). That system corresponds to the low-saturation, high-affinity shared component demonstrated in renal brush border membranes (McNamara et al., 1981). An important difference is that lysine transport by the cystinuric kidney is only partially impaired (Fox et al., 1964). Although the intestinal defect may be of little clinical importance, it has served as an extremely sensitive genetic marker and has paved the way for a new genetic classification of cystinuria (Scriver et al., 1995a).

If cystine were not so insoluble, cystinuria would be a metabolic oddity of no clinical significance except under conditions of critical limitation of protein intake. Treatment, therefore, is designed to reduce the excretion and improve the solubility of cystine. Therapeutic approaches are divided into three categories: (1) dietary restriction aimed at reducing cystine production and excretion; (2) attempts to increase the solubility of cystine; and (3) attempts to convert cystine to a more soluble compound. Surgical therapy may be required and involves (1) dissolving calculi by irrigation, lithotripsy, or lithotomy and (2) renal transplantation.

Dietary therapy has been instituted in cystinuria. Cystine production arises from the essential amino acid methionine, and numerous attempts have been made to design a diet low in methionine and yet adequate for nutritional purposes. The results of such diets are extremely variable (Zinneman & Jones, 1966). High sodium intake increases amino acid excretion in patients with cystinuria. Low-sodium diets have been shown to decrease cystine excretion in a number of patients and have been recommended as a therapeutic strategy in cystinuric patients (Peces et al., 1991).

At urinary pH values below 7.5, about 300 mg of cystine per liter of urine will be in solution. Increasing urine volume provides a progressive reduction in urinary cystine concentration and reduces the likelihood of precipitation. Many cystinuric patients excrete 1 g of cystine per day and thus would need to ingest more than 4 liters of fluid per day. Cystine solubility is also improved by an alkaline urine pH, but it does not substantially improve until the urine pH is greater than 7.5. Because the maximum possible urine pH is approximately 8, there is little leeway in the alkalinizing program. A regimen of citrate, bicarbonate, and carbonic anhydrase inhibitors has been used along with large fluid volumes early in the therapeutic regimen.

For patients who continue to form and pass stones despite diet therapy, increased fluid volumes, and urinary alkalinization, pharmacotherapy may be instituted to help to alter cystine solubility. The use of D-penicillamine, through a disulfide exchange reaction, converts cystine into cysteine–penicillamine, which is significantly more soluble than cystine. On adequate penicillamine therapy, cystine excretion is kept below 200 mg per gram of creatinine, a level at which stone formation is minimal. Although effective in preventing and dissolving cystine stones, penicillamine produces certain undesirable side effects, including allergic reactions, arthralgias, nephrotic syndrome, and pancytopenia. Proteinuria occurs after several months of therapy. The proteinuria usually clears after discontinuation of the drug but recurs when the drug is restarted. Penicillamine is also associated with dermatologic changes and increased copper excretion. Because of the significant side effects of penicillamine therapy, its use should be reserved for patients in whom more conservative therapy has failed or who have lost one kidney from cystine stone disease. Mercaptopropionylglycine (MPG) and captopril have also been used in the treatment of cystinuria. MPG has a mechanism of action similar to that of penicillamine and less frequent side effects. Initially used to treat the hypertension associated with this disorder, captopril was found to convert cystine to cysteine-captopril, which has a greater solubility. The fall in cystine excretion may take a period of several weeks of therapy. Drug therapy aimed at improving cystine solubility has raised many questions that are yet unanswered (Scriver et al., 1995a).

Glutamine administered orally has been reported to reduce the excretion of cystine in cystinuria. This effect is limited to patients in whom cystinuria is exacerbated by a high-sodium diet. Glutamine lowers cystine excretion to the level seen with a low-sodium intake. In patients with a low-sodium intake, glutamine has no further effect on cystine excretion. Thus glutamine appears to have no therapeutic benefit beyond what can be achieved by a low-sodium diet (Peces et al., 1991; Scriver et al., 1995a).

Surgical approaches may be required if conservative therapy and pharmacotherapy fail to prevent renal calculi formation. Cystine stones can be dissolved by irrigation of the urinary tract by supercutaneous nephrostomy urethral catheters. Irrigation with an alkaline solution of penicillamine or tromethamine has been successful in dissolving cystine stones in 1 week to several months. Although infection may be a complication, this procedure may prevent more invasive surgery.

Lithotripsy has been used in cystinuric patients to fracture the stones for easier dissolution with alkalizing solutions, but these stones are not as readily pulverized as are other stones. Although patients may retain stone fragments and require additional lithotripsy, this procedure has markedly decreased the need for muscle-splitting lithotomy. Stones causing obstruction or intractable pain still necessitate lithotomy as a form of treatment.

Occasionally cystinuria causes sufficient renal injury to lead to chronic renal failure. In these rare circumstances, renal transplantation is an effective cure. Because the defect in cystinuria resides in the transport epithelium of the affected individual, a kidney from a noncystinuric donor should remain disease free (Scriver et al., 1995a).

Hartnup Disease

- Hartnup disease is an autosomal recessive impairment of neutral amino acid transport limited to the kidneys and small intestine. It is postulated that the disease results from a genetic defect in the specific carrier for neutral amino acid transport across the brush border membrane of renal and intestinal epithelium. The diagnostic feature is the marked neutral aminoaciduria. Most affected persons also exhibit increased excretion of indolic compounds. These indolic compounds arise from the intestine from bacterial degradation of unabsorbed tryptophan. Reduced intestinal absorption of tryptophan and increased tryptophan loss in the urine leads to reduced availability of tryptophan for the synthesis of niacin.
- Pellagra-like clinical features have been described in patients with this disease. Some affected patients have also been mentally retarded to some degree. Treatment with nicotinamide has been associated with clearing of the rash and, on occasion, disappearance of ataxia. This has lead researchers to suggest that the clinical manifestations are caused by niacin deficiency.
- Most subjects identified by neonatal screening, as well as affected siblings of probands, have remained clinically well without treatment. Clinical expression of the disease depends on the genetic defect, the predisposition to low amino acid levels, and environmental influences such as poor diet or diarrhea.
- The renal and intestinal defects are not always expressed concordantly.
- Maternal Hartnup disease is probably benign to the fetus and to the pregnancy.

Hartnup disease is a familial disorder of renal and intestinal amino acid transport. Its constant feature is a specific hyperaminoaciduria that is caused by a diminished capacity for renal reabsorption of a group of neutral amino acids that share a common, defective transport system. In most affected persons, there is also a reduced intestinal absorption of at least some of the neutral amino acids, notably tryptophan. Hartnup disease is one of the most common of the hyperaminoacidurias. The combined neonatal screening experience worldwide identified 116 affected infants among approximately 3.5 million screened, or an incidence of 1 in 30,000. The prevalence of Hartnup disease seems to be slightly lower than that of cystinuria, both of which are about half as frequent as PKU. Most patients with Hartnup disease and cystinuria remain asymptomatic, but symptoms occur when certain factors are present (Scriver et al., 1995a).

The diagnosis of Hartnup disease is based on biochemical rather than clinical abnormalities. The characteristic pattern of neutral hyperaminoaciduria is the one constant feature. The pattern of urinary amino acid, rather than the total amino acid excretion, is the determining factor. A simple two-dimensional paper or thin-layer chromatographic system with location reagents for amino acids reveals this pattern, as does quantitative amino acid analysis. The amino acid pattern results from the defect in the renal transport mechanism. The feces contain increased free amino acids, which results from the defect in the intestinal transport of amino acids. The intestinal defect also accounts for the presence of indoles in the urine. Defective absorption of tryptophan allows bacterial enzymes to degrade tryptophan, releasing indole and related metabolites for absorption and further degradation within the body (Scriver et al., 1995a).

Infants identified by neonatal screening have almost always remained clinically normal, which suggests that Hartnup disease is usually benign. Nonetheless, some patients with Hartnup disease develop clinical abnormalities. The usual combination of a photosensitive rash and neuropsychiatric manifestations has been more often associated with Hartnup disease than would be expected from coincidence. The wide clinical spectrum of symptoms is explained by the interaction of the monogenic transport defect with polygenic and environmental factors. When these factors are aberrant, disease results. Thus the cause of Hartnup disease is multifactorial; otherwise the transport disorder alone is apparently benign (Scriver et al., 1995a).

The most frequent clinical abnormality is a pellagra-like rash. It has been noted as early as 10 days of age to as late as 13 years (Haim et al., 1978; Somasundaram & Papakumari, 1973; Strobel et al., 1978). The photosensitive rash has appeared as severe sunburn, and the patients begin to avoid the sun. After exposure to sunlight, blisters form much more readily than in normal persons. The rash forms only on sun-exposed surfaces. In some patients, the rash is pruritic (Strobel et al., 1978) or has had the appearance of eczema (Baron et al., 1956). After the acute erythematous phase, the skin frequently desquamates, exposing areas of depigmentation. Subsequently, the skin becomes dry and scaly with peripheral depigmentation (Scriver et al., 1995a).

Intermittent ataxia has been the next most common symptom reported among affected patients. The ataxia has usually appeared in the form of unsteadiness while standing and as an unsteady, wide-based gait. It is frequently accompanied by other abnormalities such as nystagmus, diplopia, and tremors, which suggests a cerebellar origin. The most striking feature of the ataxia is its intermittent character. In most cases, it is present for only a few days or less at one time and then spontaneously disappears. Precipitating factors in the ataxic episodes have usually not been identifiable. Although the first two patients identified were mentally retarded, there is no convincing data to suggest that persons with Hartnup disease generally have developmental delay or decreased cognitive abilities (Levy, 1995).

Other neurologic symptoms have been reported in patients with Hartnup disease, including increased muscle tone and deep tendon reflexes, pyramidal signs, and EEG abnormalities. All patients with abnormal EEG findings had other neurologic abnormalities such as anxiety and irritability, ataxia, and mental retardation. On the other hand, reports of normal EEGs in affected persons with profound neurologic disease have also been recorded (Hersov & Rodnight, 1960; Schmidtke et al., 1992). Most of the clinically affected Hartnup patients have had no psychiatric disturbances. However, there are reports in the literature documenting the marked emotional instability with depression, severe anxiety, nervousness, confusion, meaningless utterances, daytime bruxism, and markedly aggressive behavior of some affected persons (Hersov & Rodnight, 1960; Scriver et al., 1995a). These disturbances have always been episodic and frequently are accompanied by ataxia.

Neurologic imaging have been performed on several patients affected with Hartnup disease with variable findings. Cranial computed tomographic scans showed a calcified area in the frontal, subcortical region in an adult with neuropsychiatric illness (Mori et al., 1989) and minor brain atrophy in a child with progressive encephalopathy (Schmidtke et al., 1992), but they have also been normal in a child with neurologic disease (Darras et al., 1989).

The only rational treatment for this disorder is administration of nicotinic acid or nicotinamide to patients who have signs suggesting a deficiency of this vitamin. Oral ingestion of 50 to 300 mg/day of this vitamin has cleared the rash in many instances (Halvorsen & Halvorsen, 1963). Several investigators have reported cessation of ataxia and amelioration of psychotic-type behavior (Halvorsen & Halvorsen, 1963; Hersov & Rodnight, 1960; Scriver et al., 1995a). In addition to nicotinamide, a high-protein diet or protein supplements may be beneficial in some cases, particularly for patients with low plasma amino acids in whom symptomatic Hartnup episodes might be prevented (Jepson, 1978; Levy, 1995).

The efficacy of treatment is difficult to evaluate. Because the clinical abnormalities have generally been intermittent, their disappearance in most cases cannot be clearly designated as a therapeutic result. Furthermore, treatment with nicotinamide has not always achieved the desired result. However, it seems that patients with Hartnup disease should be given at least a trial of nicotinamide therapy (Levy, 1995).

Eleven offspring from four women with Hartnup disease have been reported (Mahon & Levy, 1986; Pomeroy et al., 1968; Shih et al., 1984). Of the cases reported in the literature, most of the offspring are clinically normal, and none has had Hartnup disease (Mahon & Levy, 1986). From these reports, it seems likely that Hartnup disease does not adversely affect pregnancy and is harmless to the fetus. In one pregnancy, the ratios between maternal and umbilical vein amino acids at delivery were normal, which suggests that the neutral amino acid defect is not expressed in the placenta when the mother has Hartnup disease (Mahon & Levy, 1986).

Urea Cycle Enzymes and the Congenital Hyperammonemias

- The urea cycle consists of a series of biochemical reactions and has two roles in metabolism. To prevent the accumulation of toxic nitrogenous compounds, the urea cycle incorporates nitrogen not used for net biosynthetic purposes into urea, which is the waste nitrogen product in humans. The urea cycle also contains several of the biochemical reactions required for the de novo synthesis of arginine.
- Five well-documented diseases have been described, each representing a defect in the biosynthesis of one of the normally expressed enzymes of the urea cycle. Four of these five diseases—deficiencies of carbamyl phosphate synthetase (CPS), ornithine transcarbamylase (OTC), argininosuccinic acid synthetase (AS), and argininosuccinase (AL)—are characterized by signs and symptoms induced by the accumulation of precursors of urea, principally ammonium and glutamine. The most dramatic clinical manifestation of these four diseases occurs in full-term infants with no obstetrical risk factors who appear normal for 24 to 48 hours and then exhibit progressive lethargy, hypothermia, and apnea all related to very high plasma ammonium levels. The encephalopathy is characterized by brain edema and swollen astrocytes. The intraglial accumulation of glutamine results in osmotic shifts of water into the cell and is thought to be responsible for the neuropathology. These four diseases may also manifest later in infancy, childhood, or adulthood with episodic mental status changes associated with lethargy and behavioral changes.
- A fifth disease, argininase deficiency, is characterized by a clinical picture consisting of progressive spastic quadriplegia and mental retardation; symptomatic hyperammonemia occurs neither as severely nor as commonly as in the other four diseases.
- OTC deficiency is inherited as an X-linked disorder; the other four diseases are inherited as autosomal recessive traits. Carrier status of OTC mutations in women can be determined by allopurinol-induced orotidinuria.
- For fetuses at risk, antenatal diagnosis is available by a number of methods, particular to each disease, including enzyme analysis of fibroblasts cultured from amniocytes, in utero liver biopsy, and DNA techniques.
- Treatment requires restriction of protein intake and activation of other pathways of waste nitrogen synthesis and excretion. For patients deficient in CPS, OTC, and AS, treatment with sodium phenylbutyrate activates the synthesis of phenylacetylglutamine, which serves as a waste nitrogen product. For patients deficient in AS and AL, supplementation of the diet with arginine promotes the synthesis of citrulline in the former and argininosuccinate in the latter, both of which serve as nitrogen waste products.

The urea cycle serves two purposes: (1) It contains the biochemical reactions required for the de novo biosynthesis and degradation of arginine; and (2) it incorporates nitrogen atoms not retained for the net biosynthetic purposes into urea, which serves as a waste nitrogen product. Urea cycle enzyme activity has been documented in the human fetus by 10 to 13 weeks of gestation. At 20 weeks of gestation, enzyme activity is similar to that found at birth, which may be 50 to 90 percent of adult levels (Baig et al., 1992).

The enzymes, substrates, and cofactors required for ureagenesis are described in Figure 25–9. CPS is a mitochondrial enzyme

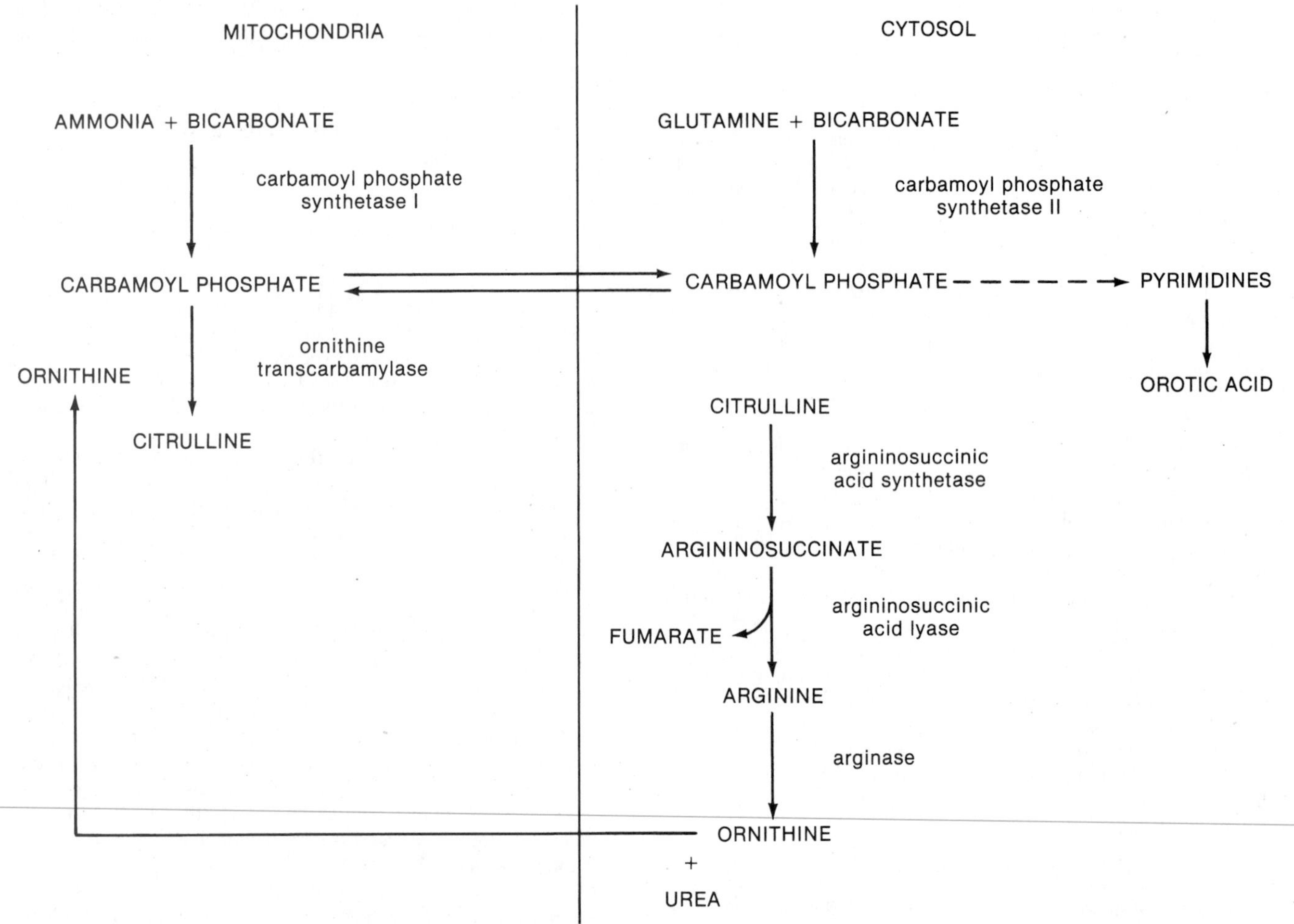

FIGURE 25–9. The urea cycle. Enzymes that are responsible for inborn errors of the urea cycle include carbamyl phosphate synthetase I (CPS I), ornithine transcarbamylase (OTC), argininosuccinic acid synthetase, argininosuccinic acid lyase, arginase, and carbamyl phosphate synthetase II (CPS II).

that catalyzes the biosynthesis of carbamyl phosphate from ammonium and bicarbonate. *N*-acetylglutamate (NAG) is a cofactor for this enzyme and may be an important regulator of ureagenesis. OTC is also a mitochondrial enzyme that catalyzes the biosynthesis of citrulline from ornithine and carbamyl phosphate. Citrulline is exported into the cytosol, where it condenses with aspartate via AS to form argininosuccinate, which is cleaved to arginine and fumarate by AL. Arginine is subsequently hydrolyzed by arginase to urea and ornithine, the latter again to be transcarbamylated to citrulline.

Although mutant enzymes are mainly characterized by a reduction of activity under all conditions, a number of other biochemical characteristics have been reported principally for OTC. OTC activity may be affected by pH, temperature, and the presence of specific substrates (Tedesco & Mellman, 1967).

The clinical manifestations in CPS, OTC, AS, and AL deficiencies are virtually identical but to greatly varying degrees within and among these diseases. The clinical manifestations may appear in the neonatal period and be fatal, or they may appear any time thereafter with varying degrees of severity. The similarity of clinical manifestation is related to the hyperammonemia, which is common to all these disorders. Their variability is principally a function of the different enzyme activities responsible for them. The variability in severity may also be related to other factors as well as to the metabolic consequences of the various enzyme deficiencies. For example, AL of a degree similar to OTC deficiency may not be as severe a disease because newly synthesized argininosuccinate may serve as a nitrogen waste product. Exceptions to this rule exist in female carriers of OTC deficiency who carry an OTC-mutant allele on one X chromosome. Variability of expression in such females depends on the proportion of hepatocytes in which the normal (or mutant) allele is on the active X chromosome. The other diseases—CPS, AS, and AL deficiencies—are inherited as autosomal recessive characteristics. These diseases can be distinguished from one another only by appropriate laboratory studies. A pedigree with evidence of X-linked transmission suggests a diagnosis of OTC deficiency. AL deficiency has two distinguishing features: severe hepatomegaly in the early-onset neonatal form and a hair abnormality in the late-onset form.

The Neonatal-Onset Group

The clinical course of the neonatal group of these diseases is monotonous in its regularity. The infant, almost always the product of a full-term normal pregnancy with no known prenatal or perinatal risk factors and with normal labor and delivery, appears to be normal for at least 24 hours. Sometime between 24 and 48 hours of life, the infant becomes lethargic and requires stimulation for feeding. Within hours, additional signs and symptoms may develop, including vomiting, increasing lethargy, hypothermia, and hyperventilation. The symptoms are often misinterpreted as signs of pulmonary disease or sepsis despite the lack of risk factors. The work-up for pulmonary disease and sepsis is unrevealing. Other routine laboratory studies are uninformative except for serum urea nitrogen, which may be as low as 1 mg/dl. Without intervention, the infant becomes comatose, requiring mechanical ventilation. A diagnosis of intracranial hemorrhage is often considered if a bulging fontanel and increasing head size are noted. However, a computed tomographic scan or ultrasound scan reveals only cerebral edema. If the plasma ammonium level is not measured, the infant's death is ascribed to sepsis, intracranial hemorrhage, or some other disease associated with prematurity despite the infant's being full-term. Unfortunately, the family history is often neglected. A history of consanguinity, neonatal sibling deaths, or neonatal male deaths on pedigree is frequently overlooked, only to be discovered after a diagnosis has been made (Scriver et al., 1995a).

The finding of an increased plasma ammonium level directs diagnostic efforts toward an inborn error of metabolism. The differential diagnosis of hyperammonemia in a neonate is limited to urea cycle enzyme deficiencies, transient hyperammonemia of the newborn, and herpes simplex. By combining the clinical characteristics with the plasma amino acid values and urinary orotate excretion, transient hyperammonemia of the newborn, the organic acidemias, and the individual urea cycle enzyme defects can be distinguished from one another (Brusilow & Horwich, 1995).

Plasma amino acid analysis provides sufficient information to make a confident diagnosis of a deficiency of AS or AL. The former is characterized by plasma citrulline levels between 1000 and 5000 μmol (normal levels, 10 to 20 μmol). The latter is characterized by the presence of high concentrations of argininosuccinate and its anhydrides, neither of which are normally found in the plasma. Plasma citrulline levels are always moderately elevated in AL deficiency (100 to 300 μmol) (Brusilow & Horwich, 1995; Tedesco & Mellman, 1967).

Because citrulline is a product of CPS and OTC, it is undetectable in plasma after 24 hours of life in hyperammonemic patients deficient in one of these enzymes. CPS and OTC can usually be distinguished by the level of urinary orotate; high levels occur in OTC deficiency as a consequence of diversion of accumulated mitochondrial CPS to the cytosolic pyrimidine synthetic pathway. Other pyrimidines, including uracil, uridine, and pseudouridine, have been found in the urine of patients with OTC deficiency (Brusilow & Horwich, 1995; Van Gennip et al., 1980; Webster et al., 1981). Other plasma amino acid abnormalities include increased plasma glutamine levels and decreased plasma levels of ornithine and arginine (Brusilow & Horwich, 1995).

The diagnosis of CPS deficiency is usually made by exclusion. However, because this diagnosis implies a lifetime commitment to an artificial diet and burdensome medication, it is appropriate to measure CPS activity in hepatocytes obtained from percutaneous liver biopsy. Attempts to make a diagnosis of symptomatic urea cycle defects by discontinuing therapy or protein loading is now strongly discouraged (Brusilow & Horwich, 1995). The risks of hyperammonemic coma far outweigh the risks from liver biopsy.

Although patients with propionic acidemia and methylmalonic acidemia have clinical manifestations similar to those in patients with urea cycle defects, there are usually three features that distinguish them: acidosis with ketosis, high plasma glycine levels, and abnormal urinary metabolites that can be detected by gas chromatography (Brusilow & Horwich, 1995). Although the number of identified inborn errors of metabolism associated with hyperammonemia is increasing, careful clinical assessment with appropriate laboratory studies of plasma and urine should provide the information required to make the diagnosis (Scriver et al., 1995a).

The Late-Onset Group

Among the four types of deficiencies (CPS, OTC, AS, and AL), there are few phenotypic differences. The variability of onset, severity, and degree of residual enzyme activity is similar among the four enzyme deficiencies. Some cases manifest during the first year of life; others, as late as adulthood (Brusilow & Horwich, 1995; MacLeod et al., 1972; Oizumi et al., 1984; Yudkoff et al., 1980). In infants, these episodes may be associated with weaning from breast milk or low-protein formula to cow's milk. In older children or adults, the episodes may be triggered by high-protein meals. Infection may precipitate symptoms in all patients, and in many, no cause can be identified as the trigger for the episode. The milder episodes often abate with cessation of protein intake and/or intravenous infusion of glucose. Older patients tend to self-select a low-protein diet (Scriver et al., 1995a).

Patients with urea cycle disorders rarely develop neurologic manifestations of apnea, seizures, or loss of consciousness abruptly unless they have sustained brain damage during previous episodes of hyperammonemia. Usually the hyperammonemia results in the appearance of symptoms such as seizures attributed to dysfunction of the cerebral cortex over several days (Brusilow & Horwich, 1995).

The major symptoms of these episodes of hyperammonemia include vomiting and abnormal mental status manifested by lethargy, irritability, combativeness, agitation, disorientation, ataxia, and somnolence often progressing to coma. Seizures, delayed physical growth, and developmental delay are common, although there are reports of normal development (Rowe et al., 1988). In addition to hyperammonemia, routine laboratory studies reveal a respiratory alkalosis. Diagnostic delay and error are common; the median age at diagnosis is 16 months. Symptoms have been wrongly attributed to gastroenteritis, colic, hyperactivity, encephalitis, Reye's syndrome, epilepsy, anicteric hepatitis, drug toxicity, and child abuse (Hilty et al., 1974; Rowe et al., 1988). For patients with hyperammonemia encephalopathy who do not have severe liver disease, the differential diagnosis includes CPS, OTC, AS, and AL deficiencies; the hyperammonemia, hyperornithinemia, and homocitrullinemia syndrome (HHH); lysinuric protein intolerance (LPI); the organic acidemias; and Reye's syndrome.

Plasma amino acid analysis diagnoses AS deficiency (citrulline levels > 1500 μmol), AL deficiency (high concentrations of argininosuccinate and its anhydrides and citrulline levels of 100 to 300 μmol), and the HHH syndrome (high concentrations of ornithine and homocitrulline). The organic acidemias are suggested if there is metabolic acidosis, and gas chromatography of the urine defines the specific organic acid disorder.

Late-onset CPS deficiency and OTC deficiency cannot be distinguished by amino acid analysis. OTC deficiency is characterized by large increases in urinary orotic acid. Thus, urinary orotic acid measurements are needed to distinguish between these two disorders. Measurement of hepatic CPS and OTC activity is definitive for the CPS deficiency, but it may be ambiguous for the OTC deficiency in women because the liver is a mosaic of hepatocytes, each which may express differing enzyme activities. If the OTC enzyme activity is consistently low among biopsy samples, the diagnosis can be assisted by these data. If the levels are higher, the data are ambiguous and are not helpful in establishing the diagnosis of OTC deficiency (Brusilow & Horwich, 1995).

The goal of therapy for urea cycle defects is to provide a diet sufficient in protein, arginine, and energy to promote growth and development while preventing the metabolic consequences of hyperammonemia and hyperglutaminemia. Successful therapy is measured by growth and nutritional assessment and maintenance of normal plasma ammonia and glutamine levels. Measurement of plasma glutamine levels are the best guide of whether therapy is effective because these levels appear to be a harbinger of hyperammonemia (Maestri et al., 1992a, 1992b) and they may reflect the fundamental pathology of hyperammonemic encephalopathy. Glutamine may represent a storage form of nitrogen that can offer substantial short-term buffering of ammonium. When this mechanism is saturated, as evidenced by high plasma glutamine levels, plasma ammonium levels rapidly increase to encephalopathic levels (Brusilow, 1991).

In designing therapy for hyperammonemia, three components of nitrogen metabolism should be considered: nitrogen intake, nitrogen retention in protein (which varies with the growth rate), and nitrogen excretion. Early recommendations for therapy included the dietary manipulation of nitrogen to reduce the requirement for waste nitrogen synthesis via the urea cycle. This was accomplished with the use of low-protein diets, essential amino acid diets, or a combination (Brusilow et al., 1979). These approaches failed for patients with severe enzyme deficiencies. The explanation for these dietary failures resides in the mechanism for nitrogen retention and balance. When nitrogen intake falls below the threshold for growth, nitrogen degradation occurs and a negative nitrogen balance develops. There must be a mechanism for excreting the nitrogen not retained for growth. In patients with some degree of ureagenetic capacity, there is some degree of nitrogen tolerance. For patients who have no residual ureagenetic capacity, some other pathway of waste nitrogen excretion is necessary to prevent nitrogen accumulation. In addition, dietary nitrogen tolerance in patients with defective ureagenesis is greater during the first months of life than in later years because the requirement for urea synthesis in the rapidly growing infant is only 19 percent of nitrogen, in comparison with over 80 percent in children and adults (Brusilow, 1991; Scriver et al., 1995a).

Because argininosuccinic acid contains the same two nitrogen atoms destined for urea synthesis, and because its renal clearance is the same as the GFR, argininosuccinate may serve as a nitrogen waste product in patients with argininosuccinate deficiency. To promote argininosuccinate biosynthesis, it is necessary to provide large amounts of exogenous arginine because the major pathway for arginine biosynthesis is defective via AL. Although ornithine may be synthesized via ornithine aminotransferase, the reaction greatly favors ornithine degradation, and ornithine cannot be sufficiently supplied to permit adequate argininosuccinic acid synthesis. With this new pathway of waste nitrogen synthesis, these patients can tolerate greater amounts of dietary protein per day. Neither high-dose arginine therapy nor the resulting high levels of argininosuccinate have been harmful in long-term studies (Maestri et al., 1992b; Scriver et al., 1995a).

Unlike the treatment of AS deficiency or AL deficiency, in which nitrogen-rich intermediates can be exploited as nitrogen waste products, therapy for CPS and OTC deficiencies must rely on activation of latent biochemical pathways whose products serve as substitutes for urea. In the past, the administration of benzoate or phenylacetic acid resulted in decreased urea excretion. The decreased excretion is accounted for by the increased hippurate nitrogen and phenylacetylglutamine nitrogen in the urine. The net result of benzoate and phenylacetate administration is a flux of nitrogen from the usual urea precursors—ammonium, alanine, and glutamate—to glycine or glutamine, after which they are conjugated to yield hippurate and phenylacetylglutamine (Maestri et al., 1992a, 1992b).

Despite the establishment of new pathways of waste nitrogen synthesis and excretion, some dietary manipulation of nitrogen intake is necessary to reduce the requirement for waste nitrogen synthesis for patients with the neonatal forms of CPS and OTC deficiencies. The current recommendation is one half of the dietary nitrogen from food protein and one half from essential amino acids. The essential amino acids are important in that they provide high-quality nitrogen intake and contain only 11 percent nitrogen, in comparison with the 16 percent nitrogen found in food protein. The diet is supplemented with citrulline, which serves as a source of arginine but has one less nitrogen atom that is contributed to the free amino acid pool than does arginine. In patients with late-onset disease, arginine is acceptable as a substitute for citrulline because of the increased nitrogen tolerance of these patients. As growth rate slows and protein accretion declines with age, the nitrogen tolerance of patients with CPS and OTC decreases. The quantity of dietary protein may then have to be adjusted to minimum levels compatible with growth (Brusilow et al., 1979; Brusilow & Horwich, 1995; Maestri et al., 1992a, 1992b).

The therapy of AS deficiency exploits citrulline as a waste nitrogen product similar to that used in AL deficiency. The diet is supplemented with arginine to stimulate citrulline synthesis and excretion. As a waste nitrogen product, citrulline has only one nitrogen atom, and its renal clearance is 20 percent of the GFR. When phenylbutyrate is added to supplementary dietary arginine, sufficient waste nitrogen capacity is achieved to permit a natural diet with limited protein intake (Maestri et al., 1992a, 1992b).

Although allogenic orthotopic liver transplantation has been performed for inborn errors of metabolism, the indications for transplantation have been for global liver failure. The use of liver transplantation as a form of enzyme replacement therapy is an option for patients with the neonatal forms of CPS and OTC deficiencies (Todo et al., 1992).

After thorough discussion of the neurodevelopmental outcome with the parents, treatment of neonates with hyperammonemic coma should be accomplished by hemodialysis. This procedure results in a decrease in plasma ammonium concentrations within a few hours, in comparison with peritoneal dialysis or arteriovenous filtration, which may require up to 24 hours. Hemodialysis is also 10 times more efficient at clearing ammonium and amino acids than is peritoneal dialysis or arteriovenous filtration. Because exchange transfusions remove toxins only from the vascular space, they should not be used to clear the ammonium and amino acids that are distributed throughout the total body water space. Dialysis has its greatest effect at removing the major nitrogen accumulation product glutamine. Prompt and repeated hemodialysis appears to be the most effective method of rapidly reducing the plasma ammonium levels seen in comatose neonates. As plasma ammonium levels reach three to four times the upper limit of normal, treatment with intravenous benzoate and phenylacetate, followed by oral sodium phenylbutyrate, is recommended. Arginine should be included in the daily fluid requirement of patients with CPS, OTC, and AS deficiencies (Brusilow & Horwich, 1995).

Most patients with late-onset urea cycle disorders who have had documented evidence of one or more episodes of hyperammonemic encephalopathy suffer some degree of brain damage or die (Brusilow & Finkelstien, 1993; Msall et al., 1984). Thus the goals of treatment of patients with late-onset disease are similar to those described earlier for the more severe forms of the disease: normal growth; maintenance of normal plasma levels of ammonium, glutamine, and arginine in OTC-deficient heterozygotes; and, the absence of orotic aciduria. In mild cases, it may be possible to maintain metabolic control by using dietary means alone, but the use of phenylbutyrate confers special advantages on patients with residual ureagenetic activity. The administration of phenylbutyrate provides an additional pathway for nitrogen excretion: It suppresses residual endogenous urea synthesis, which then is available as a reserve waste nitrogen pathway (Brusilow et al., 1979; Brusilow, 1991; Maestri et al., 1992b).

The outcome of therapy for hyperammonemias is complicated by the evolution of drug therapy, dietary protocols and supplements, and more aggressive and readily available treatment for hyperammonemic coma. Notwithstanding these reservations, the outcome reports suggest that high-dose monotherapy with phenylbutyrate combined with dietary therapy offers the best chance of survival (Scriver et al., 1995a). All patients rescued from neonatal hyperammonemic coma are brain-damaged, with significant reductions in IQ scores and a high incidence of cerebral palsy. Early and aggressive treatment results in better neurodevelopmental outcome (Brusilow & Finkelstien, 1993; Msall et al., 1984).

All five inborn errors of ureagenesis can be diagnosed antenatally. The techniques for doing so vary widely with the disorder and include measurement of an abnormal metabolite in amniotic fluid, analysis of DNA from chorionic villus or amniocytes, and enzyme or in utero liver biopsies (Brusilow & Horwich, 1995).

Screening newborn infants for urea cycle defects is indicated if the following three purposes can be fulfilled: (1) Neonates should be identified sufficiently early in the course of the disease so that prompt therapy will prevent permanent neurologic damage; (2) screening should be sensitive enough to detect milder forms of the disease; and, (3) screening should provide useful genetic information. For the neonatal forms of the disease, it is unlikely that screening is useful for therapeutic purposes. In view of the delay in the availability of the test results and the rapidity of onset of symptoms of the disease, it is likely that the permanent brain damage secondary to hyperammonemia cannot be confidently prevented. In addition, the sensitivities of the available screening methods may not be able to detect the diseases in asymptomatic neonates. Although neonatal screening may ultimately be shown to have a role in acute metabolic diseases, at present there is no substitute for a nurse, nurse practitioner, or physician who is keenly aware that all full-term neonates with nonspecific symptoms are candidates for symptomatic inborn errors of metabolism.

Disorders of Branched-Chain Amino and Keto Acids: Maple Syrup Urine Disease

- MSUD, or branched-chain ketoaciduria, is caused by a deficiency in the activity of the branched-chain α-keto acid dehydrogenase (BCKAD) complex. This metabolic block results in the accumulation of branched-chain amino acids (BCAAs) leucine, isoleucine and valine and the corresponding branched-chain α-keto acids (BCKAs). MSUD is divided into five phenotypic classes (classic, intermediate, intermittent, thiamine-responsive, and dihydrolipoyl dehydrogenase [E3]–deficient) on the basis of the clinical manifestation and biochemical responses to thiamine administration. Classic MSUD is characterized by a neonatal onset of encephalopathy and is the most severe and common form. Patients with variant forms of MSUD generally have the initial symptoms by 2 years of age. The levels of BCAA, especially leucine, are greatly increased in plasma and urine. Activity of BCKAD complex in skin fibroblasts or lymphoblast cultures is reduced and ranges from less than 2 percent of normal in the classic form to 30 percent of normal in the variant forms. The E3-deficient MSUD entails a combined deficiency of BCKAD, pyruvate dehydrogenase (PDH), and α-ketoglutarate dehydrogenase complexes.
- MSUD is an autosomal recessive disorder of panethnic distribution. The worldwide incidence is 1 per 185,000 live births, according to routine screening of 26.8 million newborns. In the inbred Old Order Mennonite population of Lancaster and Lebanon counties in Pennsylvania, MSUD occurs in approximately 1 in 176 newborns.
- The BCAAs constitute about 35 percent of the indispensable amino acids in muscle and 40 percent of the preformed amino acids required by humans. The catabolic pathways for BCAAs begin with the transport of these amino acids into cells, where they undergo reversible transamination by isoforms of the branched-chain aminotransferase to produce BCKAs. Leucine is catabolized to α-ketoisocaproate, isoleucine is catabolized into α-keto-beta-methylvalerate, and valine is catabolized into α-ketoisovalerate. Oxidative decarboxylation of the BCKA is catalyzed by the single BCKAD multienzyme complex generating the respective branched-chain acyl coenzyme A (CoA) that are further metabolized into separate pathways. The end products of leucine catabolism are acetyl CoA and acetoacetate. Valine yields succinyl CoA, and isoleucine produces acetyl CoA and succinyl CoA. BCAAs are the precursors for fatty acids and cholesterol synthesis through acetyl CoA. These amino acids are also substrates for energy production via succinyl CoA and acetoacetate.
- The oxidation of BCAA occurs primarily in the liver, kidney, heart, and adipose tissue. There is evidence that transamination is the rate-limiting step in the catabolism of BCAA in the liver, where aminotransferase activity is low. In extrahepatic tissues, oxidative decarboxylation of the α-keto acids is the rate-limiting step. A significant portion of BCKAs appears to originate from the skeletal muscle and circulates to the liver, where it is oxidized.
- The human BCKAD genes have been located on different chromosomes, including chromosomes 1, 6, 7, and 19. The genomic structure, including the regulatory and promoter regions of the genes of the BCKAD complex, has been characterized.
- The majority of untreated classic patients die within the early months of life from recurrent metabolic crisis and neurologic deterioration. Treatment involves both long-term dietary management and aggressive intervention during acute metabolic decompensation. Advances in both aspects of treatment have considerably decreased the morbidity, mortality rate, and length of individual hospitalization for patients since the mid-1980s. The age at diagnosis and the subsequent metabolic control are the most important determinants of long-term outcome. Patients in whom treatment is initiated after 10 days of age rarely achieve normal intellect.
- There have been successful pregnancies in classic MSUD patients. The major concerns are the stress of pregnancy on the metabolic homeostasis and the rapidly changing nutritional requirements during the course of pregnancy. These parameters require intensive monitoring.

Three essential amino acids—leucine, isoleucine, and valine—are classified as BCAAs. BCAAs constitute about 35 percent of the essential amino acids in muscle and 40 percent of the preformed amino acids required by humans. The fates of the carbon skeletons of BCAAs include incorporation into proteins and oxidative degradation in mitochondria. The catabolism of BCAAs have nutritional, biochemical, and clinical significance. After ingestion of protein, the BCAAs contribute to more than 60 percent of the increase in amino acid concentration in human blood (Wahren et al., 1976). BCAAs are metabolized in skeletal muscle as an alternative fuel source and are also actively metabolized in the kidney, heart, adipose tissue, and brain (Goodman, 1977; Odessey & Goldberg, 1972). In the liver, the BCKAs derived from BCAAs are rapidly catabolized to yield ketone bodies and succinyl CoA. Adipose tissue and muscle use acetyl CoA produced from leucine for the synthesis of long-chain fatty acids and cholesterol. Leucine also appears to have an important role in promoting protein synthesis, inhibiting its degradation, and stimulating insulin secretion (Yalow & Berson, 1960). Clinically, BCAA infusions counteract the catabolic state observed in sepsis and severe trauma. In patients with liver cirrhosis, hepatic encephalopathy, and chronic renal failure, plasma BCAA levels are decreased. Dietary supplementation with BCAAs or BCKAs restores nitrogen balance and ameliorates the pathophysiologic disturbances.

MSUD was first described in the mid-1950s as four cases of familial cerebral degenerative disease with onset within the first week of life, urine that had an odor resembling maple syrup, and death occurring within 3 months. MSUD results from greatly elevated levels of leucine, isoleucine, and valine (Westall et al., 1957). Later reports described variant forms of MSUD whose clinical manifestations were milder and whose symptoms were episodic and related to infection, increased dietary protein, and stress (Dancis et al., 1967). Attempts at dietary therapy were initiated but were largely unsuccessful (Dent & Westall, 1961). In 1964, Snyderman described a more rigorous and successful dietary therapy by restriction of BCAAs (Snyderman et al., 1964). In 1971, Scriver and associates reported a new thiamine-responsive form of MSUD in which the hyperaminoacidemia was completely corrected by thiamine in pharmacologic doses without recourse to dietary restrictions. This early phase of the history of MSUD defined the phenotypes, identified the metabolic block, and devised dietary treatment. Subsequently, the genetic control of this metabolic disease has been intensively investigated. On the basis of the clinical manifestation and biochemical responses to thiamine administration, MSUD can be divided into five clinical and biochemical phenotypes: classic, intermediate, intermittent, thiamine-responsive, and dihydrolipoyl dehydrogenase–deficient MSUD.

Classic MSUD. MSUD with a neonatal onset of encephalopathy is now considered the most severe and most common form of this disease. The levels of the BCAAs, especially leucine, are greatly increased in the blood, CSF, and urine, and the presence of alloisoleucine is diagnostic of MSUD. In classic MSUD, 50 percent or more of the BCKAs are derived from leucine. The activity of the BCKAD complex in skin fibroblasts or lymphocytes is usually less than 2 percent of normal. Affected newborns appear normal at birth, and symptoms usually develop between 4 and 7 days of age. Breastfeeding may delay onset to the second week of life. Lethargy and poor sucking with little interest in feeding are usually the first signs. This is followed by weight loss and progressive neurologic signs of altering hypotonia and hypertonia with dystonic extension of the arms resembling decerebrate posturing. Ketosis and the maple syrup or burnt-sugar odor become obvious at this time. Seizures and coma ensue, leading to death if left untreated. The majority of patients die within the first months of life from recurrent metabolic crisis or neurologic deterioration, often precipitated by infection or other stresses such as vaccination or surgery. Sudden death has been reported within the first week of life (Hallock et al., 1969) in two patients. Surviving patients suffer from severe neurologic damage, including mental retardation, spasticity or hypotonia, and occasionally cortical blindness. Although early treatment has greatly improved the outlook for these infants, there can be complications. Sudden onset of transient ataxia lasting 30 minutes to 1 hour has occurred even in patients with good metabolic control. During ketonemia, older patients have experienced visual hallucinations. Even with treatment, some patients have died from uncontrollable brain edema (Chuang & Shih, 1995; Riviello et al., 1991; Scriver et al., 1995a; Treacy et al., 1992).

Intermediate MSUD. Patients with the intermediate form of MSUD have persistent elevations of BCAAs and neurologic impairment but have no catastrophic illness in the neonatal period. Many do not have episodes of acute metabolic decompensation. The residual enzyme activity ranges from 3 to 30 percent of normal. About 20 patients have been reported to have intermediate MSUD. Diagnosis is most common between ages 5 months and 7 years, during evaluation for developmental delay and seizures. Several patients have had episodes of ketoacidosis, but acute encephalopathy was rare (Chuang & Shih, 1995).

Intermittent MSUD. Patients with the intermittent form of MSUD show normal early development, with normal growth and intelligence. However, they are at risk for acute metabolic decompensation during stressful situations. While they are asymptomatic, the laboratory data, including plasma BCAA levels, are normal. Activity of BCKAD complex in these patients ranges from 5 to 20 percent of normal. Many cases of intermittent MSUD have been reported. The initial symptoms generally appear between 5 months and 2 years of age in association with otitis media or other infection, but they may appear as late as the fifth decade of life (Chuang & Shih, 1995). Episodes of acute behavioral change and unsteady gait may progress to seizures and stupor or coma. The amino acid and organic acid profiles at these times are characteristic of MSUD. Death has occurred during these episodes of metabolic decompensation.

Thiamine-Responsive MSUD. A number of putative thiamine-responsive patients have been reported (Scriver et al., 1971). In general, these patients do not have acute neonatal illness, and their early clinical course has been similar to that of intermediate MSUD. Scriver described the first case, of a girl who had developmental delay at 11 months of age. Her plasma BCAA concentrations were found to be five times greater than normal, and alloisoleucine was detected. These levels fell abruptly to normal on a constant protein diet and after thiamine administration and rebounded during the two trials of thiamine withdrawal (Scriver et al., 1971). A combined treatment of protein restriction and thiamine supplementation was continued, and her BCAA levels were maintained over the years. Measurement of skin fibroblast BCKAD complex activity revealed 30 to 40 percent of normal activity. Other reports of patients with thiamine-responsive MSUD exist in the literature (Chuang & Shih, 1995). Thiamine-responsive patients are heterogeneous in their response to treatment, and a wide range of dosages have been administered with limited success. None have been treated with thiamine alone; all patients have been treated with a combination of low (BCAA) protein diet and thiamine for metabolic control (Scriver et al., 1995a).

Dihydrolipoyl Dehydrogenase (E3)–Deficient MSUD. E3 deficiency is a rare disorder, and only a handful of patients have been described (Matalon et al., 1984). The clinical phenotype is similar to that of intermediate MSUD but is accompanied by severe lactic acidosis. The urine organic acid profile exhibits abnormalities of both MSUD and lactic acidosis. Lactate, pyruvate, α-ketoglutarate, α-hydroxyisovalerate, and α-hydroxyglutarate are all increased. BCAAs are mildly to moderately elevated in the plasma, in comparison with those of classic MSUD patients. E3-deficient patients have a combined deficiency of the BCKAs, pyruvate, and α-ketoglutarate dehydrogenase complexes. The first few months of life are relatively uneventful. A brief metabolic acidosis has been observed in two patients. After the development of persistent lactic acidosis between the ages of 8 weeks and 6 months, the course is marked by progressive neurologic deterioration, including hypotonia, developmental delay, and movement disorder. Neuropathologic studies showed loss of myelin and the appearance of cavitation in discrete areas of the basal ganglia. The results of several treatment protocols that included pharmacologic doses of thiamine, biotin, and lipoic acid and dietary restriction of fat and BCAAs have been disappointing (Matalon et al., 1984; Scriver et al., 1995a).

MSUD is an autosomal recessive disorder. The worldwide frequency is approximately 1 in 185,000 live births based on frequency data from 26.8 million newborns. This frequency includes all forms of MSUD. In countries where consanguineous marriage is common (Saudi Arabia, Spain, Turkey, and India), the frequency is higher. MSUD is also highly prevalent in the inbred populations of the Old Order Mennonites of Lancaster and Lebanon counties in Pennsylvania, occurring in approximately 1 in 176 newborns (Marshall & DiGeorge, 1981).

Screening for MSUD is performed in 24 states in the United States and in at least 18 countries (Danner & Elsas, 1989). The Guthrie bacterial inhibition assay detects the increased leucine in blood spots. In states that screen for MSUD, a blood leucine level greater than 4 mg/dl or a level of 3 to 4 mg/dl (305 μmol) in the first 24 hours of life mandates immediate telephone contact with the infant's pediatrician. Infants with classic MSUD, the intermediate form, and E3 deficiency can usually be identified in the newborn period. Infants with the intermediate variety tend to have lower leucine levels than those with classic MSUD and may be missed. It is unlikely that infants with the intermittent form can be identified, because their blood BCAA levels are normal when asymptomatic. No cases of thiamine-responsive MSUD have been detected by neonatal screening.

When the newborn exhibits symptoms, the diagnosis can be made easily by amino acid analysis or organic acid profiling. The BCAAs are greatly increased in blood, CSF, and urine, and the presence of alloisoleucine is pathognomic for MSUD. This metabolite of leucine has delayed clearance, remains elevated in the plasma for several days after an episode of metabolic decompensation, and is detectable in classic MSUD at all times. Plasma alanine levels are low, and the ratios of blood to CSF BCAAs and BCKAs are reduced in encephalopathic infants (Dent & Westall, 1961). The urine 2,4-dinitrophenylhydrazine (DNPH) test is a simple test for α-keto acids and is useful in screening. Acidification of the urine enhances its maple syrup odor (Scriver et al., 1995a).

Gas chromatography–mass spectroscopy analysis of urine or plasma organic acids produces characteristic profiles when the infant is symptomatic. The metabolic profile of an infant with the intermittent form of MSUD is normal during remission. In older patients, transient elevations of BCAAs without the appearance of alloisoleucine may occur after several days of fasting and should not be mistaken for a form of MSUD. Mild to moderate elevations in the BCAAs in association with increases in lactate, pyruvate, α-ketoglutarate, and the BCKAs and their hydroxy derivatives are diagnostic for E3 deficiency (Danner & Elsas, 1989).

A close linear relationship exists between elevated BCAA and BCKA levels in plasma in MSUD patients, and adequate monitoring may be accomplished by determination of plasma BCAAs (Scriver et al., 1995a). Early detection is possible in patients at high risk for the disorder, such as siblings of affected patients, by using quantitative analysis of amino acids from plasma. Characteristic elevations in leucine and the appearance of alloisoleucine can be seen as early as 24 hours of life, regardless of the type of feeding.

Urine metabolic screening is less sensitive than plasma amino acid analysis for the early detection of MSUD. Changes in urinary amino acids may be minimal even when plasma amino acids are two to four times normal. A distinctive odor of maple syrup or burnt sugar is detectable on a wet diaper of young affected infants. The urine of normal infants may be mistaken for having unusual odors, depending on the use of spices and curry in the maternal diet of breastfeeding mothers (Danner & Elsas, 1989).

Enzymatic analysis for the direct determination of activity can be accomplished by obtaining cells for culture. Postmortem material is largely unsatisfactory in this disorder because of instability of the BCKAD complex. Currently, only skin fibroblasts and lymphoblasts are suitable for diagnostic studies because they are relatively homogeneous cell populations.

Prenatal diagnosis is accomplished by using cultured amniotic fluid cells, direct analysis of tissue from chorionic sampling, and cultured chorionic cells (Kleijer et al., 1985). The BCKAD complex activity in cultured amniocytes and chorionic villi is in the same range as skin fibroblasts. With the development of DNA diagnostic techniques, the detection of known mutations in fetuses at risk should be possible in the future. Attempts to achieve prenatal diagnosis of MSUD by determining the concentrations of BCAA and the α-keto acids and their corresponding α-hydroxy acids in amniotic fluid were unsuccessful (Dancis, 1972).

The neuropathology of MSUD involves the white matter. The spongy changes in the white matter and delayed myelination are not specific to MSUD and are seen in other metabolic disorders. Severe cerebral edema is found in patients who died during an acute metabolic crisis. In untreated cases, myelin deficiency and striking spongy degeneration of the white matter are prominent findings. A delay in myelination occurs mainly in the tracts normally myelinated after birth. The pyramidal tracts of the spinal cord, the myelin around the dentate nuclei, the corpus callosum, and the cerebral hemispheres are most affected. In treated patients, the neuropathology may be similar but of a lesser degree, or the examination may yield normal findings (Treacy et al., 1992).

The management of MSUD requires the restriction of the specific amino acids to that required for growth and development. This minimizes the accumulation of intermediates that damage organs, particularly the nervous system. In MSUD patients, an increase in plasma leucine is associated with the appearance of neurologic symptoms, whereas increased isoleucine is associated with an intensified odor of maple syrup in the urine. An increased valine level does not seem to have any clinical affects. Thus leucine and its keto acid are considered the neurotoxic metabolites in MSUD, and the plasma leucine concentration is an important parameter in monitoring treatment. There are two aspects to the treatment: long-term dietary management and therapy during acute metabolic crisis (Danner & Elsas, 1989). The principles of dietary management are to normalize the concentrations of blood BCAAs by limiting the intake of these three amino acids while simultaneously providing nutrition adequate to maintain growth and development. A trial of thiamine therapy is advised for every patient in order to determine thiamine responsiveness (Scriver et al., 1995a). Dietary therapy must be continued throughout the patient's life. Commercial diets are available and consist of BCAA-free formula with an amino acid intake of 2 to 3 g/kg/day. The requirement for leucine is met by the addition of a calculated amount of standard formula for infants or dietary protein for older children and adults. The isoleucine and valine concentration in natural food is low in relation to leucine, and supplementation of these free amino acids is necessary to maintain normal plasma levels. Plasma BCAA levels should be kept as close to normal as possible to minimize the neurotoxic effects. Plasma BCAA levels may have to be monitored weekly during the first 6 months of life, and the monitoring may be extended if there is good metabolic control and the infant is thriving (Chuang & Shih, 1995).

It is well known that infection has particularly deleterious effects on the metabolic status in MSUD. It often precipitates acute decompensation. During infection, and occasionally during the incubation period, tolerance of protein is lower, and endogenous BCAAs from protein catabolism are increased. The plasma BCAAs and BCKAs rise to toxic levels. Behavioral changes and loss of appetite are often the first signs of metabolic disturbance. Immediate reduction in dietary protein and substitution of BCAA-free synthetic formulas and protein-free foods are instituted to ensure adequate calorie intake. Nutritional changes are intended to promote anabolism and prevent the rise in BCAAs and BCKAs to toxic levels. Prompt treatment of the infection also prevents further deterioration (Scriver et al., 1995a).

Acute metabolic decompensation associated with infections leads to acute deterioration in cerebral function. This is a life-threatening condition and aggressive therapy is imperative. Clinical improvement is not possible until tissue catabolism is reversed.

There are three aspects to treatment of an acute metabolic crisis: rapid removal of the toxic metabolite, nutritional support, and minimizing the catabolic state and promoting anabolism.

Removal of toxic metabolites was initially performed by exchange transfusion with limited success. The effects were transient, and rebound occurred frequently. Peritoneal dialysis is currently the preferred method of initially removing toxic metabolites. The advantage of peritoneal dialysis is that it is relatively simple to perform and there is significant improvement in neurologic status in a few hours. A needle can be inserted into the peritoneum to initiate dialysis while a comatose patient is transported from an outlying hospital to a medical center. Studies have suggested that hemodialysis may be more effective than peritoneal dialysis in reducing the BCAA and BCKA levels (Danner & Elsas, 1989; Chuang & Shih, 1995). The disadvantage of hemodialysis is that it requires specialized equipment and a specially trained team. Continuous arteriovenous filtration has also been used in the treatment of acute metabolic crisis in MSUD. There are technical limitations to this technique, and not all medical centers have the expertise to perform this procedure. All of these procedures are invasive and can decrease the plasma leucine levels to approximately 1 mmol but are minimally effective below that level. They are useful in the initial treatment of severe metabolic decompensation. The choice of the procedure depends on the availability and expertise at each institution (Wendel, 1984).

Parenteral nutrition therapy for MSUD has been developed. The preparation consists of BCAA-free *L*–amino acid mixture in combination with glucose, lipid, electrolytes, and vitamins to provide balanced nutrition. The plasma concentrations of isoleucine and valine decrease faster than does that of leucine during treatment and must be supplemented after 1 to 2 days of therapy. An alternative nutritional approach to the treatment of MSUD is the stimulation of anabolism with insulin and growth hormone or the prevention of catabolism with high-calorie continuous nasogastric feeding (Parini et al., 1991; Wendel, 1984).

Liver transplantation has been successfully performed in a well-controlled patient with hepatic insufficiency and metabolic decompensation caused by fulminant hepatitis A infection. The plasma BCAA levels fell to normal levels dramatically, and this was able to be maintained on a normal diet. Alloisoleucine was still detectable, most likely from skeletal muscle production (Chuang & Shih, 1995).

MSUD is a suitable disease for attempting gene therapy, because increasing the enzyme activity by even a small percentage may alter the phenotype from the classic form to the intermittent form of the disease. A stable gene transfer into MSUD cells has been reported (Koyata et al., 1993). Stable chromosomal integration and persistent restoration of the BCKAD complex activity were achieved. This may represent the first step for developing gene therapy in animal models and subsequently in humans with MSUD.

Advances since the 1980s have significantly decreased the morbidity and mortality rates among patients with MSUD. The team approach to management and parental understanding and cooperation are essential for successful metabolic control. The outcome after treatment in more than 150 patients with classic MSUD and more than 25 patients with the variant forms of MSUD have now been reported (Kaplan et al., 1991; Naughton et al., 1982; Treacy et al., 1992). Most patients were diagnosed by neonatal screening or were diagnosed by laboratory testing on the basis of clinical suspicion. A small number were prospectively treated because of affected siblings. Approximately one third of the classic MSUD patients had IQ scores greater than 90, and one third had scores between 70 and 90. These patients score higher on verbal aspects of the examination than on the performance aspects. Short attention span and minor learning disabilities were observed even in patients treated soon after birth. Poor intellectual outcome is often associated with neurologic sequelae such as spasticity and quadriplegia (Naughton et al., 1982). Approximately one fifth of the classic MSUD patients died, the majority during acute metabolic decompensations precipitated by infections. The cerebral edema that develops during these crises and the recovery phases can be fatal, especially in preschool-aged patients (Treacy et al., 1992). Acute metabolic encephalopathy is less likely to occur after age 5 or 6 years. Older patients tolerate stress better, particularly if effective biochemical control is maintained (Danner & Elsas, 1989).

The most important determinants of long-term outcome for patients with MSUD are the age at diagnosis and the subsequent course of the disease. Treatment initiated before 10 days of age yields the best results, and only a few patients treated after 14 days of age achieved normal intelligence (Kaplan et al., 1991). Diagnosis during infancy is usually associated with a milder neonatal course. The impact and the degree of severity of the acute neonatal form of the disease and the subsequent metabolic complications are unfortunately difficult to quantify and predict.

Organic Acidemias: Disorders of Propionate and Methylmalonate Metabolism

- Propionyl CoA is formed by the catabolism of several essential amino acids, odd-chain fatty acids, and cholesterol. It is metabolized primarily by enzymatic conversion to methylmalonyl CoA, which is subsequently converted into succinyl CoA. This metabolic sequence is dependent on the activity of several enzymes: propionyl CoA carboxylase, methylmalonic CoA racemase, and methylmalonic CoA mutase. Propionyl CoA requires biotin as a cofactor, while methylmalonyl CoA mutase requires a cobalamin (vitamin B_{12}) coenzyme: adenosylcobalamin.
- Propionyl CoA carboxylase is composed of nonidentical subunits (alpha and beta) with biotin binding occurring only on the alpha subunit. The alpha subunit is regulated by a gene found on chromosome 13, whereas the beta subunit is regulated by a gene located on chromosome 3. Methylmalonyl CoA mutase has two identical subunits regulated by a gene on chromosome 6.
- Isolated deficiency of propionyl CoA carboxylase is a major cause of ketotic hyperglycinemia syndrome. It results from the accumulation of propionate in the blood and of 3-hydroxypropionate, methylcitrate, triglycine, and unusual ketone bodies in urine. Clinically, the disorder is characterized by severe metabolic ketoacidosis, which often appears in the neonatal period and for which reversal requires vigorous alkali therapy and protein restriction. Oral antibiotic therapy to reduce gut propionate production may also be useful.
- Inherited deficiency of methylmalonic CoA mutase activity is caused by gene mutations at many different loci. Neonatal or infantile metabolic ketoacidosis is the clinical hallmark of isolated methylmalonic CoA mutase deficiency. Cells may have zero mutase activity, or the mutase may be structurally altered when it was synthesized and has a decreased affinity and reduced stability for adenosylcobalamin. Affected infants exhibit methylmalonic acidemia and methylmalonic aciduria that does not respond to cobalamin supplementation but can be treated with dietary protein restriction. Oral antibiotic therapy may also be useful.
- Abnormalities of adenosylcobalamin synthesis leads to impaired methylmalonyl CoA mutase activity and the clinical manifestations identical to that seen in methylmalonic CoA mutase deficiency. In most but not all affected infants, large pharmacologic doses of cyanocobalamin produce a distinct

reduction in methylmalonate accumulation and offer an valuable adjunct to dietary protein restriction.

- All of the disorders of propionate and methylmalonate metabolism for which there are adequate data are inherited as autosomal recessive traits. There is considerable genetic heterogeneity of the phenotype even among siblings.
- Prenatal diagnosis of propionyl CoA carboxylase deficiency, methylmalonyl CoA mutase deficiency, and defective synthesis of adenosylcobalamin has been accomplished by assays of cells from chorionic villi biopsy, cultured amniotic fluid cells, and chemical determinations on amniotic fluid or maternal urine.

Methylmalonic acid and its immediate precursor, propionic acid, are detectable in only trace amounts in normal human blood, urine, and CFS. These compounds are derived from the catabolism of lipid and protein. Catabolism of the branched-chain amino acid isoleucine leads to the formation of propionyl CoA, as does the degradation of methionine, valine, and threonine. Catabolism of these amino acids accounts for the much of the propionate production. Other sources of propionate include beta-oxidation of odd-chain fatty acids. Degradation of the side chain of cholesterol also leads to the synthesis of propionyl CoA, but the relative contribution of propionate from this source is minimal. Intestinal flora may contribute more than 20 percent of the propionate production (Fenton & Rosenberg, 1995; Tanaka et al., 1975).

Methylmalonyl CoA is synthesized essentially only from propionyl CoA as an intermediate in the formation of succinate from propionate by the hepatocytes. Three enzymes are responsible for the conversion of propionyl CoA to succinyl CoA. The first involves the carboxylation of propionyl CoA to methylmalonyl CoA, which requires the catalyst propionyl CoA carboxylase. The D-isomer of methylmalonyl CoA is produced in this reaction and must be converted to the L form of the isomer by another enzyme, methylmalonyl CoA racemase. The third reaction is catalyzed by methylmalonyl CoA mutase which converts *L*-methylmalonyl CoA to succinyl CoA. Succinyl CoA enters the tricarboxylic acid cycle, in which it is ultimately converted to pyruvate by way of oxaloacetate (Fenton & Rosenberg, 1995) (Fig. 25–10).

Propionic Acidemias

Propionic acidemia refers to a heterogenous group of inborn metabolic disorders that result in the accumulation of propionic acid in the blood. It may result from a primary deficiency of propionic CoA carboxylase or from abnormalities of biotin metabolism that lead to the deficiency of the multiple biotin-dependent carboxylases (Fenton & Rosenberg, 1995).

Symptoms appear in the neonatal period with severe metabolic acidosis manifested by the refusal to feed, vomiting, lethargy, and hypotonia; dehydration, seizures, and hepatomegaly occur less commonly (Nyhan et al., 1972). Other patients have presented later, either with encephalopathy or episodic ketoacidosis or with developmental retardation unassociated with attacks of ketosis or acidosis. There are reports of still other children with almost a complete absence of propionyl CoA carboxylase activity who have had no clinical abnormalities and were identified only during family studies (Kuhara et al., 1988).

The clinical course of symptomatic patients is characterized by repeated relapses usually precipitated by excessive protein intake, constipation, or infection. Control of the condition is difficult to achieve, and neurologic sequelae have been commonly encountered. The most prominent neurologic sequelae include developmental delay, focal and generalized seizures, cerebral atrophy, and EEG abnormalities (Fenton & Rosenberg, 1995; Nyhan et al., 1972). Dystonia, severe chorea, and pyramidal signs are common in patients who survive longer. Leukopenia and thrombocytopenia, perhaps caused by the accumulation of toxic metabolites, are not uncommon (Fenton & Rosenberg, 1995).

A defect in the carboxylation of propionate explains many of the findings reported in this disorder. This enzymatic block would be expected to lead to an increased concentration of propionate in the blood and an inability of leukocytes to catabolize propionate to carbon dioxide. Because isoleucine, valine, threonine, and methionine are precursors of propionate, such a block should lead to an intolerance of protein and the specific amino acids. When propionyl CoA carboxylation is blocked, the synthesis of long odd-chain fatty acids is augmented because propionyl CoA is the primary substrate for these compounds. The mechanism for the hyperglycinemia and hyperammonemia observed in infants with this disorder probably reflects inhibition of the mitochondrial glycine cleavage enzyme and of carbamyl phosphate synthetase I (CPS I), respectively, by the accumulated organic acids or their CoA esters (Fenton & Rosenberg, 1995). There is another pathway or defect in the carboxylation of propionate, which occurs as a result of inhibition of cytosol action or carbamyl phosphate synthetase II (CPS II). The result again is an accumulation of organic acids of CoA esters.

A defect in propionate carboxylation must be considered in any infant in whom ketosis or acidosis develops in the neonatal period. Other inborn errors of metabolism must be ruled out, as must the more common causes of acidosis in the neonatal period. Determinations of propionic acid and its metabolites in blood and urine and studies of propionyl CoA carboxylase activity in leukocytes or fibroblast extracts are required for definitive diagnosis (Fenton & Rosenberg, 1995). The enzymatic test is the only definitive test, inasmuch as propionate accumulation can also occur in patients with defects in methylmalonate metabolism. The cord blood can be used to test high-risk infants.

A low-protein diet or a diet selectively reduced in the content of propionate precursors appears to be the best treatment for this disorder at this time. Dietary management minimizes the number of attacks of ketoacidosis but does not necessarily eliminate them or enable normal development. Because fasting has been shown to increase the number of propionate metabolites, frequent feedings are recommended (Thompson & Chalmers, 1990). Attacks of ketoacidosis should be promptly and aggressively treated by withdrawing all dietary protein and administering sodium bicarbonate parenterally. In order to prevent catabolism, glucose should be administered. Attacks that are accompanied by hyperammonemia should be treated with peritoneal or hemodialysis. Each critically ill infant requires total parenteral nutrition formulated specifically for the metabolic abnormality (Fenton & Rosenberg, 1995). Because propionyl CoA carboxylase requires biotin as a coenzyme and because some patients' cells have shown a biotin-dependent increase in enzyme activity (Wolf, 1980), it is possible that some patients may improve with biotin supplementation. Although no patient with propionyl CoA carboxylase activity has been demonstrated to have a response to biotin, a dramatic response can be seen in patients in whom the propionyl CoA carboxylase deficiency is part of a constellation now called "multiple carboxylase deficiency" (Scriver et al., 1995a).

Two other therapies are currently being investigated in the treatment of propionic acidemia. The administration of *L*-carnitine has been suggested to reverse the putative carnitine deficiency in these patients. *L*-carnitine reduces the ketogenic response to the fasting state (Wolff et al., 1986). No long-term treatment studies with *L*-carnitine have been completed. The recognition that gut bacteria may substantially contribute to propionate production has led to the suggestion that specific antimicrobiologic therapy may be of clinical benefit by reducing the total amount of propionate in the tissues. Metronidazole has been reported to reduce fecal propionate significantly and decrease the anaerobic bacterial count. Plasma propionate levels fell by 50 to 60 percent, and the urinary excretion of propionate metabolites

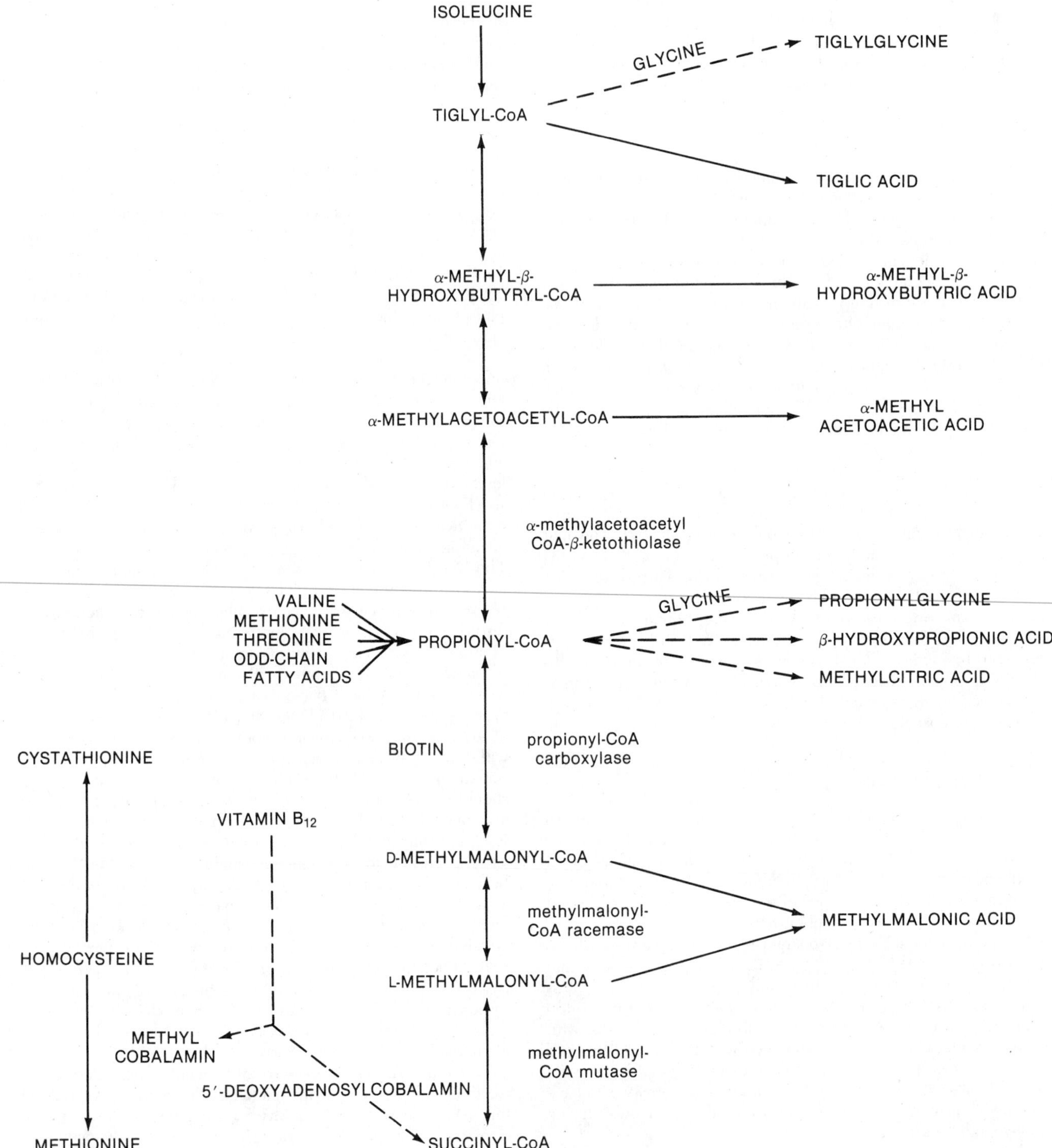

FIGURE 25–10. Isoleucine catabolism. Inborn errors in the catabolism of isoleucine result in various types of organic acidemias: Alpha-methylacetoacetyl CoA beta-ketothiolase deficiency, propionicacidemia, biotin-responsive multiple carboxylase deficiency, and methylmalonic acidemias.

was also reduced by an average of 34 percent (Thompson et al., 1990). Further study is required in order to establish whether such therapies improve the management of acute episodes of metabolic decompensation or provide any long-term benefit.

With the advances in the medical management of this disorder, the life expectancy has improved and has led to the survival of women with propionic acidemia into their childbearing years. One report has documented an uneventful pregnancy and delivery in a mildly affected woman treated with a low-protein diet and *L*-carnitine supplementation (Van Calcar et al., 1992). Other such pregnancies are more likely to occur in the future and should be managed according to each individual's metabolic needs.

Methylmalonic Acidemias

There are many different biochemical bases for inherited forms of methylmalonic acidemia: two distinct defects in the mutase enzyme, two distinct defects of adenosylcobalamin synthesis, and three distinct defects of both adenosylcobalamin and methylcobalamin synthesis (Fenton & Rosenberg, 1995). This discussion is limited to the disorders associated with a deficiency of methylmalonyl CoA mutase.

More than 100 cases of isolated mutase deficiency in children have been documented. The most common clinical manifestation includes lethargy, failure to thrive, recurrent vomiting, dehydration, respiratory distress, and muscular hypotonia (Fenton & Rosenberg, 1995; Matsui et al., 1983). Less commonly, the disorder manifests as developmental retardation, hepatomegaly, or coma. Patients with the least enzymatic activity present earlier, usually within the first week of life, than those with some residual activity, who present later in the neonatal period.

The laboratory findings of methylmalonic acidemia include normal serum cobalamin levels and metabolic acidosis, with blood pH values as low as 6.9 and serum bicarbonate levels as low as 5 mEq/L. Ketonemia or ketonuria is present in 80 percent of the cases, and hyperammonemia is only slightly less common. Leukopenia and thrombocytopenia are present in more than half of the patients (Matsui et al., 1983). There are also reports of cases of persons with mutase deficiency who had an accumulation of methylmalonic acid in the blood and urine but had no symptoms. At diagnosis, these patients ranged in age from 18 months to 13 years and had been subsequently monitored for 7 years, during which time at least some remained symptom-free (Fenton & Rosenberg, 1995).

The deficiency of methylmalonyl CoA mutase results in a primary block in the conversion of methylmalonyl CoA to succinyl CoA and explains the accumulation of methylmalonate in blood and urine; the augmentation of methylmalonate excretion; the precipitation of ketosis by protein, amino acids, or propionate; and the excretion of long-chain ketones formed in the catabolism of branched-chain amino acids. The acidosis may result from the inhibition of pyruvate carboxylase by methylmalonyl CoA. This would interrupt gluconeogenesis and lead to hypoglycemia and indirectly to the catabolism of lipid, with ketosis and acidosis. The mechanism for the hyperglycinemia and hyperammonemia observed in infants with this disorder probably reflects inhibition of the mitochondrial glycine cleavage enzyme and of CPS I, respectively, by the accumulated organic acids or their CoA esters (Fenton & Rosenberg, 1995).

The diagnosis of methylmalonic acidemia must be considered in any infant in whom acidosis and ketosis develop after birth. After other sources of neonatal acidosis and infantile ketosis have been eliminated, blood and urine assays for methylmalonate must be obtained. If excessive amounts of methylmalonate are found in the urine, cobalamin deficiency can be determined from a direct measurement of serum cobalamin. The specific enzymatic block can then be determined by cell cultures and extracts. Prenatal diagnosis is accomplished by measurement of methylmalonate in amniotic fluid and maternal urine in midpregnancy and by studies of mutase activity and cobalamin metabolism in cultured amniotic fluid cells (Ampola et al., 1975).

Two treatment protocols for children with methylmalonic acidemia exist and should be employed in tandem. A protein-restricted diet or a diet restricted in amino acid precursors of methylmalonate should be instituted as soon as life-threatening problems such as ketoacidosis, hypoglycemia, and hyperammonemia have been addressed. Supplementary cobalamin should be instituted as soon as the diagnosis of methylmalonic acidemia is seriously considered (Fenton & Rosenberg, 1995). Such measures have been shown to decrease the levels of methylmalonic and propionic acid. As is the case with propionic acidemia, the administration of *L*-carnitine has been shown to improve the clinical symptoms. Oral antibiotic therapy has been shown to improve appetite, decrease vomiting, increase growth, improve behavior, and decrease the number and severity of acidotic episodes (Scriver et al., 1995a).

The response to supplementary cobalamin and the long-term outcome in affected patients depend on the nature of the biochemical abnormality causing the methylmalonic acidemia. The long-term outcome for affected patients with complete absence of enzyme activity is poorest, with the highest rate of mortality and highest degree of neurologic impairment. The affected patients who were responsive to cobalamin administration had the best long-term outcome (Shevell et al., 1993).

Prenatal therapy has been documented in a woman carrying a fetus with cobalamin-responsive methylmalonic acidemia. Administration of cobalamin to the mother resulted in a decrease in maternal excretion of methylmalonate (van der Meer et al., 1990). The value of this therapy over one that is instituted postnatally has yet to be established.

Preliminary steps are being taken toward somatic gene therapy for mutase deficiency (Stankovics et al., 1992). In addition to the usual issues that surround gene therapy, two questions remain unanswered: (1) How much activity must be restored to normalize the biochemical hallmarks of the disease? (2) Does correction of the defect in the liver lead to reversal of the pathologic changes in other organ systems? Future research is directed at investigating these issues.

Lactic Acidemia: Disorders of Pyruvate Carboxylase and PDH

- Lactic acid that circulates in the body is the product of the anaerobic metabolism of glucose that takes place primarily in red blood cells, skin, kidney medulla, and white skeletal muscle. Some of it is oxidized by red muscle and kidney cortex, but the bulk is taken up by the liver and made into glucose. Lactate is always produced by the reduction of pyruvate through lactate dehydrogenase (LDH) and is always removed by a reversal of this process. The oxidation of pyruvate proceeds through PDH, the tricarboxylic acid (Krebs') cycle, and the respiratory chain. Anaerobic use proceeds primarily through pyruvate carboxylase. A defect in any of these pathways may lead to inadequate removal of pyruvate and lactate from the circulation, and lactic acidemia results.
- Deficiency of PDH complex is the most common of the disorders leading to lactic acidemia. It may be caused by a defect in the E1, E2, E3, X-lipoate, or PDH phosphatase component of the complex. The most common of these is the defect in the E1 component. The clinical manifestation of this disorder is a graded spectrum from most severe to least severe. In its most severe form, overwhelming lactic

acidosis is present at birth, and death occurs the neonatal period. In the second form of the disorder, the lactic acidemia is moderate, but there is quite profound psychomotor retardation with increasing age and, in many patients, concomitant damage to the basal ganglia and brain stem, leading to death in infancy. In the third form of the disorder, found only in males, there are carbohydrate-induced ataxic episodes coupled with mild developmental delay.

- The E1 defects are caused by mutations in the E1 alpha gene, which is X-linked. Males and females are equally affected, even though only one X chromosome in females carries the mutation. Thus, this disorder is classified as X-linked dominant.
- The E2 and protein X-lipoate defects are rare and result in severe psychomotor retardation.
- The E3 lipoamide dehydrogenase defect leads to deficient activity not only in the PDH complex but also in the α-ketoglutarate and branched-chain keto acid dehydrogenase complexes. PDH phosphatase deficiency has been documented in four cases. The most common pathologic feature of deficiency of PDH complex is the development of cystic lesions in the cerebral cortex, basal ganglia, and brain stem.
- Pyruvate carboxylase deficiency has two clinical forms. In the simple form of the disease, the patient presents in the first few months of life with a mild to moderate lactic acidemia and delayed development. Survivors have severe mental retardation. These patients are thought to have some residual enzyme activity. In the more complex form of the disease, the patient presents soon after birth with severe lactic acidemia accompanied by hyperammonemia, citrullinemia, and hyperlysinemia. These patients are thought to have no residual enzyme activity and rarely survive beyond 3 months of age. In a single case, the patient presented with only episodic attacks of lactic acidosis and with no psychomotor retardation.

Several inborn errors of metabolism manifest with acidosis in which the major contributor to the anion gap is lactate. Other inborn errors of metabolism entail elevated blood lactate levels on either a long- or short-term basis. For the most part, these elevated lactate levels are secondary, such as is seen in propionic acidemia, methymalonic acidemia, and the fatty acid oxidation defects. This is caused by the interference with CoA metabolism and its importance in the function of the PDH complex. These secondary lactic acidemias are distinguished by the presence of unusual organic acids in the urine. Excessive lactic acid is also present in many nongenetic conditions such as asphyxia and ischemia. To understand how lactic acid accumulates, it is necessary to review lactate metabolism.

In the fed state, the liver uses a percentage of ingested carbohydrate for a variety of purposes such as glycogen synthesis, energy provision, and lipogenesis, leaving the remainder to be used by peripheral tissues. Hepatic gluconeogenesis uses lactate as a substrate to produce glucose. The hepatic output of glucose is not oxidized to CO_2 and H_2O but rather is converted in glycolytic tissues back into lactate and released into the circulation. Small amounts of lactic acid are released from brain and white muscle, and much of this lactate is reconverted into glucose in the liver, with a small amount being oxidized by red muscle. This conversion of glucose to lactate in the periphery and reconversion of lactate to glucose in the liver is called the Cori cycle, and it is this cycle that is responsible for the turnover of lactate in the body fluids. An estimated 50 to 90 percent of the ingested carbohydrate that is oxidized to CO_2 and H_2O is used by the brain, the proportion being higher in infants and lower in adults (Robinson, 1995).

In the fasting state, major changes occur in the metabolism of glucose. Fatty acids are substituted as the major fuel for muscle and liver. A major new carbohydrate source from muscle breakdown is available in the form of amino acids (mostly alanine) as gluconeogenic precursors. Last, glycerol derived from triglyceride breakdown contributes to gluconeogenesis. The activity of the Cori cycle and oxidation of glucose remain unchanged in the early phases of fasting. However, as fasting continues, the reliance of the brain on carbohydrate fuels decreases as ketone body oxidation is substituted as a source of energy (Robinson, 1995). This process slows the process of muscle breakdown characteristic of the early phases of fasting and conserves lean body mass. Because infants have a relatively large ratio of brain to lean body mass, they are more prone to the development of hypoglycemia in the fasting state. In the fasting state, the brain is the major site of oxidation of glucose produced in the liver. As a result of the brain's dependence on glucose as fuel, the activity of the PDH complex, the tricarboxylic acid cycle, and the respiratory chain are essential to the normal working of the human central nervous system (Scriver et al., 1995a). Normal liver pyruvate carboxylase and phosphoenolpyruvate carboxykinase function are essential for the maintenance of glucose output in the fasting state.

If the oxygen supply is adequate, most cells derive their energy requirements from the oxidation of pyruvate, fatty acids, or ketone bodies via the tricarboxylic acid cycle. Some tissues, however, preferentially derive their energy supply from glycolytic activity, which produces pyruvic and lactic acids as end products. Some tissues, such as blood, have few (in white blood cells) to zero mitochondria (in red blood cells), and thus glycosis is obligatory. Other tissues have a high glycolytic activity that acts to suppress the oxidative metabolism. In tissues that are highly oxidative, such as the liver, red muscle, and the kidney cortex, the products of oxidative phosphorylation act to suppress the activity of the glycolytic pathway.

In the normal person, the blood lactate level is between 1 and 2 mmol and does not change appreciably with fasting, feeding, or simple infectious diseases. CSF lactate levels are similar with an upper limit of normal of 2.2 mmol. The normal range of blood and CFS pyruvate levels vary between 40 and 150 μmol, with a lactate:pyruvate ratio between 10:1 and 25:1 (Robinson, 1995).

Disorders of the Pyruvate Dehydrogenase Complex

There are now five components in which defects have been documented to lead to the deficiency of the PDH complex. A profile of enzymatic activity of each of the five enzyme components to the PDH complex can be developed for each patient suspected of having PDH deficiency. Patients have been described with defects in the E1 PDH, E2 transactylase, and the E3 lipoyl dehydrogenase enzymes, as well as in the X-component and in PDH phosphatase.

E1, or Pyruvate Decarboxylase, Deficiency. The severity of the disease is a function of the severity of the lactic acidemia. The most severely affected infants die before the age of 6 months, have low residual enzyme activity of the PDH complex, and chronic, severe lactic acidemia (Robinson & Sherwood, 1984). Another group of patients have mild to moderate lactic acidemia and do not experience major acid–base disturbances except for short periods, usually concurrent with infections. These patients were discovered only after they presented for the investigation for developmental delay. Neuropathologically, these infants had cystic lesions in the basal ganglia and brain stems, cerebral atrophy, agenesis of the corpus callosum, and cysts in the cerebral hemispheres. The third group of patients have a milder form of the disease in which there is either chronic or episodic ataxia (Falk et al., 1976; Kodama et al., 1983). Often the ataxia is carbohydrate induced, and these infants do well on ketogenic diets (Falk et al., 1976). All these patients are males and have lactic acid levels that are not greatly elevated (Robinson & Sherwood, 1984). Some have normal IQs, but others have varying degrees of mental retardation. The neuropathologic lesions seen in the more severely affected patients are completely absent in some of the more mildly affected patients and are slow to develop in others. The variability in clinical manifestations in patients with similar percentages of residual enzyme activity is currently unexplained. There is a lack of correlation of the in vitro enzyme data with the clinical spectrum of disease (Scriver et al., 1995a).

Facial dysmorphism is a characteristic of PDH complex deficiency (Robinson & Sherwood, 1984), and its features resemble those of fetal alcohol syndrome. Typically, a long, narrow head with frontal bossing, an upturned nose, long philtrum, and flared nostrils are present. The parallel with fetal alcohol syndrome occurs as a result of a common mechanism. In fetal alcohol syndrome, acetaldehyde from the maternal circulation inhibits the fetal PDH activity, causing the malformations. In PDH complex deficiency, the endogenous low activity of the complex in the fetus causes the same facial malformations (Robinson & Sherwood, 1984; Scriver et al., 1995a).

A partial deficit in PDH complex activity would have to be compensated for by excess glycolysis and excess lactic acid production in tissues with high energy demand. Chronic situations arising from this problem may lead to neuronal cell death because of either localized lactic acidosis or intracellular ATP depletion or both (Scriver et al., 1995a). Thus, necrotic lesions develop where there is heavy energy demand or decreased perfusion of tissue, resulting in the localized and generalized neuropathology seen in this disorder.

The use of a high-fat, low-carbohydrate diet that is ketogenic has resulted in the clinical improvement and increased stability of several patients (Falk et al., 1976). The provision of ketone bodies as an alternative oxidative substrate to pyruvate for brain mitochondria appears to compensate for the PDH complex deficiency.

Defects in the E2 and X Components of the Pyruvate Dehydrogenase Complex. Three patients have been described with these defects. One patient with 24 percent PDH complex residual activity presented at 2 weeks of age with hyperammonemia and lactic acidosis and eventually died at 3.5 years with profound psychomotor retardation. E2 transacetylase activity was measured at only 32 percent, whereas that of E1 and E3 were normal (Robinson et al., 1990). This patient had normal E1 and E3 proteins, absence of E2, and a reduced amount of protein X. Another case of severe psychomotor retardation and lactic acidosis was reported in a Turkish male infant. This patient had blood lactate levels that ranged from 6 to 9 mmol and had absence of protein X with decreased E1 and E2. Other case reports that document psychomotor retardation along with a decreased or mutant protein X suggest that protein X participates in the overall reaction of the PDH complex and that its absence results in a deficit of catalytic activity (Robinson et al., 1990).

Deficiency of E3 or Lipoamide Dehydrogenase: Combined α-Keto Acid Dehydrogenase Complex Deficiency. Of the six cases reported in the literature, none presented at birth, but lactic acidemia became apparent at a few months of age. E3 is a common component to both the PDH and α-keto acid dehydrogenase complexes. The fact that all complexes are deficient is consistent with the fact that elevations of pyruvate, lactate, α-ketoglutarate, and branched-chain amino acids are found in the blood from these patients. The branched-chain amino acids are not elevated to the extent seen in classic MSUD. Neuropathology of the brain reveals myelin loss and cavitation in discrete areas of the basal ganglia, thalamus, and brain stem. The cerebral cortex is free of pathology (Robinson, 1995).

Deficiency of Pyruvate Dehydrogenase Phosphate. This is a rare disorder putatively caused by a decrease in PDH phosphate, which removes phosphate from E1 serine residues (Scriver et al., 1995a). The enzyme can be only indirectly measured in patients' tissues. Patients typically present early in the neonatal period with unremitting lactic acidosis and the development of the characteristic neuropathologic cystic lesions described previously. The development of a direct measurement of this enzyme should increase the knowledge of this disorder in the upcoming years.

Disorders of the Pyruvate Carboxylase Complex

Pyruvate carboxylase is the first enzyme in the gluconeogenic pathway; it is activated in conditions in which fatty acids are mobilized and acetyl CoA is generated. It has binding sites for ATP, HCO_3^-, and acetyl CoA and is almost totally dependent on the presence of acetyl CoA for activity. Pyruvate carboxylase is the major regulatory enzyme in the pathway of gluconeogenesis, being regulated by the acetyl CoA:CoA and ATP:adenosine diphosphate (ADP) ratios in liver mitochondria. The liver and kidney have the highest concentrations of pyruvate carboxylase, but it is also found in lesser amounts in other tissues such as brain, muscle, adiposites, and fibroblasts, in which it plays a role in maintenance of intermediates for the citric acid cycle (Scriver et al., 1995a).

Patients with documented pyruvate carboxylase deficiency usually present in the neonatal period or in early infancy with lactic acidemia and psychomotor retardation. The earlier the manifestation of the disorder, the more severe the enzyme deficit and the shorter the survival (usually less than 3 months). More severely affected patients have a more complex biochemical disturbance with lactic acidemia, hyperammonemia, citrullinemia, and hyperlysinemia (Robinson, 1995).

The pathology associated with pyruvate carboxylase deficiency has been documented primarily in the liver and brain. Hepatomegaly is apparently caused by lipid droplet accumulation in the hepatocytes. Histologic study of the liver has also revealed hyperplasia of endoplasmic reticulum of the hepatocyte and abnormal hepatic mitochondria. The central nervous system pathology consists of very poor myelination and paucity of neurons in the cerebral cortex, gliosis, ventricular enlargement, thinning of the corpus callosum, and proliferation of astrocytes (Atkin et al., 1979; Saudubray et al., 1976; Scriver et al., 1995a). Additional findings include cavitated infarcts of the cerebral cortex and diffuse vacuolization of kidney tubules (Atkin et al., 1979). The pathologic appearance of the brain suggests that myelination is not taking place and neuronal death is occurring, resulting in developmental arrest of the brain. Thus, pyruvate carboxylase is essential for normal brain development.

The patient with lactic acidemia presents one of the more difficult diagnostic problems in genetics. It is important to assemble as much biochemical and pathologic information as possible on the patient and analyze the signs and symptoms to pinpoint the diagnosis. The initial measurements should include blood lactate, pyruvate, 3-hydroxybutyrate, acetoacetate, quantitative serum amino acids, urine organic acids, fasting blood glucose, lactate, and 3-hydroxybutyrate. Establishing a diagnosis by biochemical assay of enzymes in skin fibroblasts, lymphoblasts, and liver biopsies or by DNA analysis is a complex process. Because testing procedures are a difficult and lengthy process, treatment regimens may be instituted on the basis of clinical observations, if caution is exercised by monitoring for adverse affects.

Metabolic Errors That Affect Blood and Blood-Forming Tissue: Pyruvate Kinase and Glucose-6-Phosphatase Deficiencies

Human red blood cells are devoid of nuclei and cytoplasmic organelles. This structure simplifies their physiology but simultaneously restricts their metabolic capacities and their ability to adapt to changing environmental conditions. The unique properties of hemoglobin allow it to mediate gas transport and exchange without expending energy. However, the maintenance of membrane plasticity depends on an adequate source of high-energy phosphate, specifically ATP, which is also necessary for a number of other essential cell functions. These include maintenance of ionic fluxes in opposition to the electrochemical gradient, preservation or generation of membrane components and intracellular nucleotides, synthesis of glutathione, and initiation and maintenance of glycolysis itself. In addition, reducing energy is required for preserving the functional valance of hemoglobin iron and for protecting enzyme and structural proteins from irreversible oxidative denaturation (Tanaka & Paglia, 1995).

Energy requirements of the red blood cells are fulfilled almost entirely by the metabolism of glucose, with the consequent generation and storage of high-energy phosphates, principally ATP, or as reducing equivalents in the form of glutathione (GSH) and pyridine nucleotides (NADH and NADPH). Glucose is assimilated by facilitated transport and phosphorylated by hexokinase, providing a common substrate for either anaerobic glycolysis through the Embden-Meyerhof pathway or for oxidative glycolysis via the hexose monophosphate (HMP) shunt. Normally, the anaerobic pathway predominates by a factor of 10, but oxidant stimulation of HMP shunt activity can reverse the ratio (Paglia, 1994).

Anaerobic glycolysis in the red blood cell is regulated by the kinase-mediated enzymatic reactions, principally phosphofructokinase, hexokinase, and pyruvate kinase. These enzymes are sensitive to a multitude of feedback regulators, including substrates, products, cofactors, intermediates, and electrolyte and hydrogen ion concentration. Fixation of inorganic phosphate occurs at the glyceraldehyde-3-phosphate dehydrogenase step, allowing generation and subsequent transfer of high-energy phosphate to ADP. This results in a net gain of two molecules of ATP for every one of catabolized glucose. The 1,3-phosphodiester can revert to a low-energy state by a mutation to 2,3-diphosphoglycerate, which comprises one half to two thirds of all organic phosphates in the erythrocyte and has an important regulatory influence on hemoglobin affinity (Benesch & Benesch, 1969). Diversion through this pathway bypasses an ATP-generating step but simultaneously contributes to a large reservoir of potential substrate for pyruvate kinase, thus providing a sensitive regulator to optimize ATP:ADP ratios. The pyridine nucleotide (NAD^+/NADH) cycled by anaerobic glycolysis is an essential cofactor in methemoglobin reduction via cytochrome b_5 reductase.

During oxidative glycolysis, HMP shunt activity serves to maintain high concentrations of reduced GSH, a cysteine-containing compound with a very low oxidation potential, allowing it to protect other cellular proteins from oxidant damage by serving as a sacrificial reductant. $NADP^+$ is the obligate cofactor for each dehydrogenase reaction in the shunt, and the $NADP^+$:NADPH ratio provides the principal regulator of glucose catabolism via this pathway. HMP shunt activity can be stimulated 20- to 30-fold or more in response to oxidant challenge (Tanaka & Paglia, 1995).

Glucose is oxidized at the 1-carbon position, generating CO_2 and ribulose 5-phosphate, which can be modified and recombined into two intermediates of anaerobic glycolysis. One of the intermediates, fructose-6-phosphate, can undergo isomerization back to glucose-6-phosphate, providing additional substrate for recycling back through the HMP shunt if the $NADP^+$:NADPH ratio compels it to do so (Tanaka & Paglia, 1995).

On the basis of the known physiologic functions of these two major pathways, defective enzymes in either can be expected to interfere with erythrocyte metabolism with predictable results. Enzyme defects of anaerobic glycolysis result in increased concentrations of glycolytic intermediates proximal to the defective enzyme, impaired production of ATP, and chronic hemolysis with its characteristic clinical sequelae. In contrast, enzyme defects of the HMP shunt are more often characterized by susceptibility to oxidant stresses, including acute episodic hemolysis in otherwise hematologically normal individuals. G6PD deficiency is the model of the latter group of disorders and pyruvate kinase is for the former.

Pyruvate Kinase Deficiency

- Pyruvate kinase deficiency is the most common enzyme defect of anaerobic glycolysis that results in a hereditary hemolytic anemia. This disorder has been documented to occur worldwide and is characterized by lifelong chronic hemolysis of variable severity. Splenectomy often results in amelioration of the hemolytic process in more severely affected patients. The defective pyruvate kinase enzyme in affected erythrocytes results in increased concentrations of 2,3-diphosphoglycerate and decreased ATP, in relation to cells of comparable age.
- Pyruvate kinase deficiency is inherited as an autosomal recessive trait. Heterozygous carriers usually have 40 to 60 percent of the normal red blood cell pyruvate kinase activity, and they do not have any significant hematologic or clinical abnormalities. In the absence of consanguinity, clinically affected patients are usually compound heterozygotes with two mutant alleles. Thus they have two intracellular mixtures of defective pyruvate kinase enzymes, which complicates the interpretation of the biochemical data. Genes encoding the principal natural pyruvate kinase enzymes have been identified, as have several mutations resulting in hemolytic anemia.

Pyruvate kinase deficiency and G6PD deficiency are the two most common red blood cell enzyme defects associated with chronic hemolytic anemia and are equally prevalent in the population (Mentzer, 1993; Valentine et al., 1989). In contrast, all the other enzyme defects combined account for less than 20 percent of such cases and thus are not discussed in this chapter.

Pyruvate kinase deficiency occurs equally in males and females. It has been most commonly reported in the kindreds of northern Europe, but it is also found throughout the United States, Canada, Japan, Western Europe, Southeast Asia, Australia, and New Zealand. Pyruvate kinase deficiency has also been reported in Mexicans, Arabs, Filipinos, Africans, American Blacks, and in patients with partial American Indian ancestry. The Amish in western Pennsylvania have a particularly high prevalence of a severe form of the disease (Bowman et al., 1965).

Pyruvate kinase deficiency is transmitted as an autosomal recessive trait with clinical consequences occurring in only homozygotes or compound heterozygotes. In rare instances, however, heterozygotes are hematologically normal. In affected patients, the primary clinical manifestation is chronic hemolytic anemia varying in severity from asymptomatic and fully compensated to life-threatening cases with lifelong transfusion requirements (Valentine et al., 1989). The latter often present with neonatal anemia and jaundice, necessitating exchange transfusions.

Pyruvate kinase deficiency has no distinguishing or pathognomonic features. Individuals affected by pyruvate kinase deficiency usually manifest the hallmarks of a chronic hemolytic process: variable degrees of jaundice, slight to moderate splenomegaly, and increased numbers of gallstones. In most cases, the anemia and jaundice are apparent in infancy or early childhood, if not in the neonatal period. In rare instances, cases escape detection until adulthood (Tanaka & Paglia, 1995).

Early onset of symptoms is characteristic of more severe forms of the disorder, and late onset is typical of milder cases. Milder cases may be asymptomatic, and diagnosis may emerge during evaluation of pregnancy or acute illness. Thus there is a full spectrum of clinical severity. The most severe cases necessitate multiple transfusions or even splenectomy in early childhood in order to maintain acceptable hemoglobin levels. Beyond early childhood or after splenectomy, transfusion requirements often diminish, and hemoglobin concentrations tend to stabilize 1 to 3 g/dl higher. Lower hemoglobin levels are better tolerated because of decreased oxygen affinity induced by characteristically elevated concentrations of red blood cell 2,3-diphosphoglycerate activity (Fanning & Hinkle, 1985).

Chronic hemolysis is exacerbated by pregnancy or acute illnesses, especially viral infections (Fanning & Hinkle, 1985). Pregnancy may be well tolerated but may necessitate transfusions in some patients in whom previous transfusions were rare or unnecessary. Parvo-like viruses have been reported in association with aplastic crisis in pyruvate kinase deficiency (Duncan et al., 1983). Other clinical effects of pyruvate kinase deficiency include growth retardation and frontal bossing, although general neurodevelopment is not impaired. After splenectomy, growth and development may be enhanced in severely affected children. Rare complications include kernicterus (Bowman et al., 1965), hydrops fetalis (Hennekam et al., 1990), chronic leg ulcers, acute pancreatitis secondary to biliary tract disease, iron overload, splenic abscess, and spinal cord compression from extramedullary hematopoiesis (Rutgers et al., 1979).

Red blood cell morphologic abnormalities are not a prominent feature of pyruvate kinase deficiency. Milder cases may exhibit only macrocytosis and a few smaller, irregularly contracted or spiculated cells. All these findings are more prevalent when the disease is severe, particularly after splenectomy, when siderocytes, target cells, and Howell-Jolly bodies become more prominent (Tanaka & Paglia, 1995). These findings, however, are nonspecific. The anemia is variable in severity but is usually normochromic and macrocytic. Splenectomy often results in a paradoxic rise in the reticulocyte count, frequently as high as 40 to 70 percent, but this is not a pathognomonic finding. Hemoglobin concentrations range from 6 to 12 g/dl, and hematocrit ranges from 17 to 37 percent. Hemoglobin is of the adult type (AA), and hemoglobins F and A2 are within normal limits. Leukocyte and platelet counts are normal to slightly increased (Mentzer, 1993; Valentine et al., 1989).

Erythrocyte osmotic fragility test results are normal, and the antiglobulin (Coombs') test result is negative. Erythrocyte life span is moderately to severely shortened. The spleen sequesters and destroys many pyruvate kinase–deficient reticulocytes as a result of their decreased deformability (Nathan et al., 1968). Although the reticulocyte possesses the advantage of a highly efficient ATP generation through mitochondrial oxidative phosphorylation, that process is greatly suppressed in the acidotic and hypoxemic environment of the spleen. Splenectomy permits longer survival of these newly formed cells; thus the reticulocyte count may paradoxically rise after splenectomy even though the anemia is less severe (Keitt, 1966). The liver is also a major site of pyruvate kinase–deficient red blood cell destruction. Leukocytes and platelets do not share the enzyme defect, and so their cell counts are unaffected (Tanaka & Paglia, 1995).

Pyruvate kinase deficiency is not associated with any other organ dysfunction. Indirect hyperbilirubinemia occurs in proportion to the severity of hemolysis, and fecal urobilinogen excretion is accordingly increased. Although the liver shares the abnormality, its function is not impaired sufficiently to alter standard hepatic function tests. This is because of the ongoing ability of the hepatocytes to synthesize the enzyme, a process not available to the red blood cell. Compensatory erythrocyte hyperplasia may expand marrow spaces to produce radiographic changes characteristic of more severe anemia (Valentine et al., 1989).

Definitive diagnosis of pyruvate kinase deficiency requires demonstration of specific red blood cell enzyme abnormalities. Erythrocyte enzyme deficiency may range from 5 to 25 percent of normal in affected patients and 40 to 60 percent in heterozygous carriers, who remain hematologically normal. Care must be taken with laboratory assays to be certain that erythrocyte preparations are free of leukocytes, because white blood cells have 300 times more pyruvate kinase activity than do erythrocytes on a per cell basis. Reticulocytes and young erythrocytes have disproportionately more pyruvate kinase activity than older red blood cell populations, which must be considered in the interpretation of in vitro assays (Tanaka & Paglia, 1995).

Glucose-6-Phosphate Dehydrogenase Deficiency

- G6PD is an enzyme found in all cells that catalyzes the first step in the HMP pathway. It produces NADPH, which is required for reactions of various biosynthetic pathways as well as the preservation and regeneration of the reduced form of glutathione. Because catalase and glutathione are essential for detoxification of hydrogen peroxide, the defense of cells against this compound depends ultimately and heavily on G6PD. This is especially true of red blood cells, which are exquisitely sensitive to oxidative damage and in which other NADPH-producing enzymes are lacking.
- The gene that encodes the protein for G6PD has been mapped to the long arm of the X chromosome. Therefore, one of the two G6PD alleles is subject to inactivation in females.
- G6PD deficiency is the most commonly known red blood cell enzyme deficit. It is estimated to affect over 400 million people worldwide. The highest incidences are found in tropical Africa, in the Middle East, in tropical and subtropical Asia, in some areas of the Mediterranean, and in Papua New Guinea. The prevalence rates vary in these geographic regions from 5 to 25 percent.
- The most common clinical manifestations are neonatal jaundice and acute hemolytic anemia. In some cases the hyperbilirubinemia is severe enough to cause permanent neurologic sequelae or death. The active hemolytic anemia is triggered by a number of drugs, by infections, or by the ingestion of fava beans. In a proportion of cases, the hemolysis can be life-threatening. The mechanism of hemolysis is thought to occur as a result of the inability of red blood cells to withstand the oxidative damage produced, directly or indirectly, by the triggering agent. Red blood cell destruction is largely intravascular, and therefore hemoglobinuria is present. Between episodes of hemolytic anemia, most G6PD-deficient persons are asymptomatic. A very small proportion of G6PD-deficient persons have a chronic hemolytic disorder, which might be quite severe.

G6PD deficiency is genetically heterogeneous. Numerous different variants have been reported on the basis of diverse biochemical characteristics. This diversity suggests that these variants result from many allelic mutations in the G6PD gene seen in the different parts of the world where this abnormality is prevalent. Genetic heterogeneity also explains the diversity of clinical manifestations.

Clinical manifestations of G6PD deficiency have been known for centuries. Pythagoras, the Greek mathematician, warned his followers against the dangers of eating fava beans; at the turn of the twentieth century, Italian physicians described the clinical manifestations of favism (Beutler, 1993; Luzzatto & Mehta, 1995).

Because of the erratic response to the consumption of fava beans, the genetic inheritance pattern was difficult to establish, and the disorder was first attributed to allergies or a toxic reaction. The fact that certain drugs caused a hemolytic reaction in susceptible persons was not recognized until the 1950s. Observant practitioners during this time did notice that this condition tended to run in families. In 1956, the discovery of the low levels of G6PD in the red blood cells of these affected patients began the biochemical investigation into this disorder. Since the 1960s, the biochemical basis and clinical manifestations of G6PD deficiency have been established. More recently, the molecular structure of the normal gene and various mutations have been defined.

G6PD is the first step in the intermediary metabolism of glucose-6-phosphate to pentose phosphate in the HMP pathway. G6PD produces NADPH, the coenzyme that is the main hydrogen donor for numerous enzymatic reactions involved in biosynthetic pathways and in protecting cells against oxidative damage (Luzzatto & Mehta, 1995).

The majority of individuals with G6PD deficiency are asymptomatic and go through life unaware of the genetic abnormality. The only common clinical manifestation is acute hemolysis, which may be rapidly compensated and often remains undetected. Clinical manifestations of the disorder result from an interaction of the molecular properties of each G6PD molecular variant, exogenous factors, and genetic factors for the population. G6PD deficiency can cause clinical pathology, including drug-induced hemolysis, infection-induced hemolysis, favism, neonatal jaundice, and chronic nonspherocytic hemolytic anemia.

G6PD deficiency was discovered as a direct consequence of investigations into the development of hemolysis in patients who had received primaquine (Beutler et al., 1954; Carson et al., 1956), which in other persons causes no red blood cell destruction. Subsequently, G6PD deficiency has become the prototype of hemolytic episodes arising from a unique interaction between genetic and exogenous factors. Clinical hemolysis and jaundice typically begin within 1 to 2 days of the exposure to the drug (Tarlov et al., 1962). Hemolysis is largely intravascular and associated with hemoglobinuria. The anemia worsens until the seventh or eighth day. Heinz bodies are characteristically found in peripheral blood. An increase in the reticulocyte count begins, and the hemoglobin level begins to recover on the eighth to tenth day. A self-limited course is characteristic with some G6PD variants because the newly produced cells have a higher amount of G6PD activity and therefore are less susceptible than the older cells, which are selectively destroyed (Luzzatto & Mehta, 1995; Tarlov et al., 1962). A more protracted hemolysis occurs with a high drug dosage or in patients with severe G6PD deficiency.

Beutler (1978) analyzed the data for drug interactions and hemolysis in G6PD-deficient individuals. There is strong evidence for a relatively short list of drugs that trigger hemolysis, including antimalarials (primaquine, pamaquine, pentaquine), sulfonamides (sulfanilamide, sulfacetamide, sulfapyridine, sulfamethoxazole), sulfones (thiazosulfone, dapsone), nitrofurans (nitrofurantoin), antipyretics (acetanilid), and other drugs and chemicals (naphthalene, trinitrotoluene, toluidine blue). Drugs that have a possible association with hemolytic episodes include chloroquine, sulfamethoxypyridazine, sulfadimetine, sulfamerazine, aspirin, ciprofloxacin, norfloxacin, chloramphenicol, and vitamin K analogues. Drugs that have a doubtful association with hemolytic episodes include quinine, sulfadiazine, acetaminophen, probenecid, phenacetin, PAS, L-dopa, and dimercaprol (Beutler, 1978, 1984; Luzzatto & Mehta, 1995).

A number of inherited and acquired factors influence an individual's susceptibility to, and the severity of, drug-induced hemolysis. The inherited factors include the metabolic integrity of the erythrocyte, the precise nature of the enzyme defect, and genetic differences in pharmacodynamics. The acquired factors include the drug dose, absorption, metabolism, and excretion of the drug; the presence of additional oxidative stress such as infection; the effect of the drug on enzyme activity; the pre-existing hemoglobin level; and the age distribution of red blood cell population (Beutler, 1984; Burka et al., 1966).

Infection is the most common cause of hemolysis in G6PD-deficient persons who live outside the areas where favism is prevalent. The severity and clinical consequences of hemolysis are influenced by a number of factors, including concurrent administration of oxidant drugs, the pre-existing level of hemoglobin, hepatic function, and age. Various bacterial, viral, and rickettsial infections have been reported as precipitants, but most important are infectious hepatitis, pneumonia, and typhoid fever (Beutler, 1993; Burka et al., 1966). Gastrointestinal and respiratory viral infections are reported to cause more severe hemolysis in children (Shannon & Buchanan, 1982). Hemolysis is more common in children with G6PD deficiency who develop hepatitis than in normal children, but the degree and the duration of jaundice is out of proportion to the degree of hemolysis. This suggests that the jaundice is of hepatocellular origin (Beutler, 1993).

Favism is a condition described as an episode of acute hemolysis after ingestion of broad (fava) beans. It has occurred on an epidemic scale in areas now known to have an increased prevalence of G6PD deficiency (the Mediterranean, Middle East, Far East, and North Africa). This geographic region correlates to the area where fava beans are customary in the diet. Not all G6PD-deficient persons are sensitive to fava beans, and even those who are show remarkable variability from one exposure to the next. It is thought that there is an additional, as yet unidentified, factor responsible for the variable hemolytic response to fava bean ingestion. Clinically, favism presents with sudden onset of acute hemolysis within 24 to 48 hours after ingesting the beans. Pallor and hemoglobinuria are hallmarks of this disorder. Jaundice is always present, but because not all the hemolysis is intravascular, the bilirubin level is less than in hemolytic attacks triggered by drugs or infection. The hemolysis is severe, and the amount of hemoglobinuria is increased. Therefore, the amount of hemoglobin catabolism is reduced, leaving less hemoglobin to be recycled by the liver. The mainstay of prevention is avoidance of fava beans. Neonatal screening and health education is essential in communities with a high prevalence rate for G6PD. Supportive treatment of red blood cell transfusions is necessary in severe cases. The administration of desferrioxamine, which reduces the iron-dependent formation of damaging oxygen radicals, is being investigated (Khalifa et al., 1989).

G6PD is the most common red blood cell enzyme deficiency that results in neonatal jaundice. Jaundice appears by 1 to 4 days of age, at about the same time as or slightly earlier than physiologic jaundice and later than blood group isoimmunization. Reports of abnormal red blood cell morphology, mild anemia, and reticulocytosis suggest an element of hemolysis, but impaired hepatic function, similar to that seen in normal neonates, may well be the major cause in both premature and full-term G6PD-deficient infants (Luzzatto & Mehta, 1995).

The jaundice seen in G6PD-deficient infants shows a wide variation in its frequency and severity in different populations. Thus in endemic areas where G6PD is prevalent, it is the major cause of neonatal jaundice. Although kernicterus is a rare complication, the most common cause of it in Africa and Southeast Asia is G6PD deficiency (Ifekwunigwe & Luzzatto, 1966). The cause of this variability is not completely understood, and both genetic and environmental factors are likely to be important. The severity of neonatal jaundice does not correlate to the G6PD activity of the red blood cells. Management of neonatal jaundice generally includes avoiding oxidant drugs and promptly treating hypoxia, sepsis, and acidosis in newborns. Specific measures include the elimination of mothballs, prophylactic administration of phenobarbital, and exchange transfusion. Phototherapy was once thought to be contraindicated in infants with G6PD because it was thought to decrease riboflavin levels and decrease its antioxidant activity. Several studies have shown that phototherapy is indeed effective in reducing the level of unconjugated bilirubin and should remain as the mainstay of the treatment of neonatal jaundice whenever the bilirubin level is not so high as to warrant an exchange transfusion (Beutler, 1993; Burka et al., 1966; Luzzatto & Mehta, 1995).

Although a slight degree of chronic hemolysis accompanies G6PD deficiency, most affected persons experience significant hemolysis and anemia only under conditions of oxidant stress. The degree of chronic hemolysis is variable, depending on the type of G6PD variant. Such variants have been described in many parts of the world (almost always in males), regardless of the type of G6PD endemic to the area. The degree of enzyme deficiency may be severe, and detailed biochemical characterization of the residual enzyme is often made more difficult because of its instability. In rare cases associated with granulocyte dysfunction, hemolysis may be made worse by the increased susceptibility to infections (Luzzatto & Mehta, 1995). Sometimes the chronic hemolysis may arise from an association of mild G6PD deficiency with an unrelated, genetically transmitted erythrocyte abnormality such as pyruvate kinase deficiency or congenital spherocytosis (Rattazzi et al., 1971).

Clinically, affected persons have a history of neonatal jaundice, often requiring an exchange transfusion. A history of infection or drug-induced hemolysis is also common. Gallstones may be a prominent feature. Splenomegaly is usually but not always present. Although occasionally the hemoglobin level is normal and the hemolysis is well compensated, oxidant stress can lead to a dramatic fall in the hemoglobin level. The red blood cell half-life is shortened to 2 to 17 days, and all patients have a reticulocytosis from 4 to 34 percent (Rattazzi et al., 1971). Occasionally, the degree of reticulocytosis is out of proportion to the length of red blood cell half-life. Red blood cells usually do not show abnormal osmotic fragility. In contrast to the acute hemolysis, the hemolysis in chronic hemolytic anemia is only partially intravascular, and studies have shown increased red blood cell sequestration in the liver and spleen (Luzzatto & Mehta, 1995). Management of these patients has included the use of vitamin E (an antioxidant) and splenectomy. There are conflicting reports of the efficacy of both of these management therapies (Johnson et al., 1983; Tanaka & Beutler, 1969).

The diagnosis of G6PD is relatively easy. Careful attention must be paid to the method and the interpretation of the results. Prenatal diagnosis is reported (Beutler et al., 1992). The wide geographic distribution of the disorder and high prevalence among developing countries makes it important to adopt tests that are simple and inexpensive. The actual enzyme activity of G6PD, not the amount of G6PD protein, should be measured. The level of G6PD activity is greater in younger erythrocytes than in older ones. Thus reticulocytosis may lead to a false normal result. Because of red blood cell mosaicism arising from random X chromosome inactivation in females, heterozygotes have a mixture of normal and G6PD-deficient cells. The proportion of the two cell types can vary enormously, ranging from completely normal activity to complete deficiency. In this case, microscopic evaluation of the individual cells on a slide is necessary. All of the existing methods for determining G6PD activity depend essentially on the production of NADPH. The direct enzyme assay gives a quantitative measurement, and a number of other procedures provide convenient screening tests, aiming to classify individuals as only G6PD normal or G6PD-deficient (Luzzatto & Mehta, 1995).

LIPID METABOLISM

Lipids are a heterogeneous group of substances that can be extracted from tissues. There are three main classes of lipids—fatty acids, triglycerides, and phospholipids—that function as insulation and an energy source and to provide structure to cell membranes. Fat insulation consists mainly of triglycerides packed densely into adiposites. Triglycerides are hydrolyzed into fatty acids and glycerol, which serve as an energy source. Phospholipids provide an important component of all cellular membranes.

Fatty Acids. The sources of fatty acids in the blood are the supply of fat in the diet and the release of fatty acids from adipose tissue. In suckling infants, there is a high level of fatty acids in the blood, and there is greater fatty acid use at this time than at any time before birth or after weaning (Ampola, 1982; Stave, 1978; Wapnir, 1985). Fatty acids are synthesized in two metabolic pathways: malonyl-CoA and reversal of β-oxidation. The rate of fatty acid synthesis is greater in the fetus than in the adult. This rate of fatty acid synthesis decreases rapidly after birth, possibly in relation to the accumulation of some metabolite (glycerol, fatty acids, and acyl-CoA) and the rise in the rate of gluconeogenesis, which decreases the availability of citrate (Stave, 1978; Wapnir, 1985). Fatty acid oxidation occurs in the mitochondria. As opposed to the passive, gradient-dependent transport across cell membranes, fatty acids must be converted from acyl-CoA to acylcarnitine to be transported across the mitochondrial membrane. Once inside the mitochondrion, the acylcarnitine is reassembled into acyl-CoA and oxidized (Scriver et al., 1995a, 1995b; Stave, 1978).

Oxidation of fatty acids requires more oxygen than does oxidation of carbohydrates. After birth, fatty acid oxidation is greatly enhanced. In brown fat, fatty acid oxidation is completely dependent on the presence of carnitine and ATP. Carnitine is also important for acetate oxidation and for optimum ketone production by liver mitochondria. Lysine is the precursor of carnitine, and when protein ingestion is severely limited, there may also be a carnitine deficiency (Scriver et al., 1995a; Scriver et al., 1995b; Stave, 1978).

The liver lacks the enzyme needed for the transfer of CoA from succinyl-CoA to acetoacetate. Thus the final products of fatty acid oxidation in the liver are the ketone bodies: acetoacetic acid, β-hydroxybutyric acid, and acetone. The rate of ketone body production is dependent on the supply of fatty acids to the liver. Fatty acids from the blood enter the liver in large amounts after birth. In the liver, the fatty acids are broken down into ketone bodies, which are then transported to other tissues and organs, where they serve as a source of energy (Stave, 1978).

Triglycerides. The triglyceride blood level is dependent on fat absorption from the intestines, the release of triglycerides from the liver, and the removal of triglycerides from the blood. Triglycerides cannot serve as an immediate energy source because they must first be hydrolyzed into fatty acids and glycerol. In the blood, triglycerides are transported as lipoproteins and are removed from the blood by many tissues. After birth, chylomicrons appear in the blood 1 to 3 days after feedings have been initiated (Stave, 1978). The major storage site of triglycerides is adipose tissue.

Lipogenesis is the process in which fatty acids combine with CoA to form acyl-CoA. Three molecules of acyl-CoA and glycerol-3-phosphate combine to form a triglyceride molecule. Lipolysis is not a reversal of the synthetic process. The rate of fatty acid synthesis depends on a sufficient supply of glycerol-3-phosphate. If fatty acid levels accumulate, the excess acyl-CoA inhibits further fatty acid synthesis and glycolytic reactions. In lipolysis, triglycerides are hydrolyzed by tissue lipases into fatty acids and glycerol. Glycerol-3-phosphate arises by phosphorylation of glycerol by glycerol kinase. The glycerol released from adipose tissue during lipolysis can be used for energy only after being phosphorylated (Stave, 1978).

Phospholipids. Phospholipids are any lipid molecules that contain a radical derived from phosphoric acid. Phospholipids are an important part of cell walls and cell particle membranes, myelin sheaths, and lung secretions. The composition of fatty acids in phospholipids changes considerably with age and in various organs. Fatty acid composition of phospholipids is less dependent on dietary changes than is that of triglycerides.

The metabolism of fatty acids cannot be discussed without an understanding of the relationships between glucose and fatty acid metabolism. There exist several control points at which it is determined whether glucose or fatty acids will be predominantly synthesized or oxidized. For example, glucose synthesis is promoted by fatty acid oxidation. A high-fat diet enhances gluconeogenesis and fatty acid oxidation and results in a decrease in lipid synthesis. The elevated level of fatty acids supplied to the newborn after birth is responsible for the decreased rate of glycolysis in the liver and the brain, the increased rate of acetoacetate formation, the decreased rate of fatty acid synthesis in the liver, and the postnatal increase in the rate of gluconeogenesis (Ampola, 1982; Wapnir, 1985). After birth, the rate of fatty acid oxidation and ketone body formation increases dramatically as a result of sympathetic stimulation of lipolysis in adipose tissue and the resulting increased fatty acid delivery to the liver.

Disorders of Lipid Metabolism

Disorders of lipid metabolism may affect any component of fatty acid, triglyceride, or phospholipid synthesis or degradation. Disorders of lipid metabolism may also affect β-oxidation of fatty acids in the mitochondria. General clinical manifestations of a lipid metabolic disorder include vomiting, changes in level of consciousness, metabolic acidosis, odor of sweaty feet, severe hypoglycemia without ketosis, hyperammonemia, and hepatic and/or muscular lipid accumulation. These clinical manifestations may occur acutely after birth or intermittently. The fulminant neonatal course is rapidly fatal.

Lipoprotein Disorders: Abetalipoproteinemia, Familial Combined Hyperlipidemia, and Tangier Disease

Very low density lipoproteins (VLDLs) and chylomicrons, which transport triglycerides to the peripheral tissues in the blood, are major lipoprotein secretory products of the liver and intestine. Each class of these lipoproteins contains a protein of high molecular weight (a β-lipoprotein) that is essential for the secretion of the lipoprotein particle and that has a high affinity for lipids, remaining with the lipoprotein complex throughout its metabolic processing in plasma or lymph. Familial β-lipoprotein deficiencies represent one of several classes of lipoproteins that are absent or are present in abnormally low concentrations in the plasma. The three most common types of disorders are abetalipoproteinemia, familial combined hyperlipidemia, and Tangier disease.

- The single structural gene for β-lipoproteins is responsible for the synthesis of the two types of lipoproteins found in humans. The predominant β-lipoprotein of VLDLs and low-density lipoproteins (LDLs) is apo B-100. The predominant type of apo B in chylomicrons is apo B-48. Several disorders result from the abnormal secretion of apo B containing lipoproteins.
- Abetalipoproteinemia is an autosomal recessive disorder characterized by the virtual absence of VLDLs and LDLs from plasma. Fat malabsorption is severe, and triglycerides accumulate in erythrocytes and in the liver. Acanthocytosis of erythrocytes is common. Spinocerebellar ataxia, peripheral neuropathy, degenerative pigmentary retinopathy, and ceroid myopathy all appear to be secondary to defects of transport of tocopherol in blood. Intracellular accumulation of β-lipoprotein results from an impairment in the assembly or secretion of triglyceride-rich proteins. The absence of activity of microsomal triglyceride transfer protein, a factor critical to the lipidation of B proteins, was the first recognized defect in lipoprotein deficiencies. Treatment involves (1) the restriction of dietary fat to prevent steatorrhea and (2) supplementation with tocopherol to prevent progression of the neuromuscular and retinal degenerative disease.
- Clinical manifestations of hypobetalipoproteinemia are indistinguishable from those of abetalipoproteinemia in the homozygous state: acanthocytosis, neuromuscular disability, and malabsorption. Clinically, this disorder is distinguished from recessive abetalipoproteinemia by the appearance of hypolipidemia in heterozygotes. The defects that underlie this disorder involve the gene for apo B. A number of mutations that involve secretion of a truncated form of the apo B protein, abnormal rate of apo B protein synthesis, or removal from the blood have been identified.
- Chylomicron retention disease is characterized by fat malabsorption and the absence of chylomicrons in plasma after fat ingestion. Acanthocytosis and neurologic manifestations occur in some patients. Large numbers of nascent chylomicrons crowd the enterocyte, which results from a specific defect in the secretion of chylomicrons. High levels of apo B 100 have been found in the cytoplasm and the endoplasmic reticulum of the enterocyte.
- Familial combined hyperlipidemia is probably the most prevalent genetically determined disorder of lipoproteins. It significantly increases the risk of coronary arthrosclerosis. It is recognized as an autosomal dominant trait with high penetrance that leads to high levels of apo B 100 and elevated levels of VLDLs, LDLs, or both in plasma.

Abetalipoproteinemia

This autosomal disorder occurs as a result of the absence of apolipoprotein B and is characterized by very low plasma cholesterol and triglyceride levels. It has a higher incidence among Ashkenazic Jews, who constitute 25 percent of those affected (Ampola, 1982; Bickel, 1980; Scriver et al., 1995a). It affects males more frequently than females, and heterozygotes are in good health. The clinical manifestations develop shortly after birth, with fat malabsorption, acanthocytosis, pigmented retinitis, and ataxia (Kane & Havel, 1995).

Malabsorption of fat is a central pathologic feature of abetalipoproteinemia. Steatorrhea occurs after birth and is associated with malabsorption of the fat-soluble vitamins A, D, E, and K. Affected infants are poor feeders and have frequent vomiting and voluminous steatorrheic stools, which result in somatic underdevelopment and failure to thrive. Hepatic steatosis occurs with severe disturbances in plasma lipid levels, which are less than 50 percent of normal. Triglyceride levels are often undetectable, phospholipid levels are lowered by 75 percent, and the cholesterol level is often less than 0.025 g/L. Unlike vitamins A and K, in which modest supplementation achieves normal plasma levels, the transport of tocopherol is severely limited in this disorder. The abnormal lipoproteins of abetalipoproteinemia appear incapable of incorporating normal amounts of vitamin E even in the presence of relatively large supplements. Massive supplementation, however, somehow increases the flux into the body, eventually increasing the vitamin E levels in adipose tissue appreciably (Kane & Havel, 1995). The intestinal villi are normal but the mucosa has a yellow discoloration that results from a greatly increased lipid content. Electron microscopy has demonstrated an increase in lipid droplets in the cells, even if no fat has been ingested for days (Kane & Havel, 1995). Despite the inability of the liver to secrete VLDLs, abnormalities of liver function are uncommon.

Severe anemia develops secondary to abnormally shaped erythrocytes. Red blood cell survival is frequently shortened, and hyperbilirubinemia has been described. Reticulocytosis and erythroid hyperplasia occurs in many patients, which suggests that erythropoiesis is not notably impaired. Acanthocytosis is not found in the bone marrow, which suggests that the membrane changes leading to the malformation are acquired by contact with the plasma (Kane & Havel, 1995).

There is ocular involvement, which manifests as retinitis pigmentosa, decreased visual acuity, nystagmus, and ophthalmoplegia. The more severe cases of retinopathy occur in patients with the more severe neurologic impairment, which suggests a common mechanism. Major pathologic features are the loss of photoreceptors, loss of pigmented epithelium, and relative preservation of submacular pigmented epithelium (Kane & Havel, 1995). These retinal changes closely resemble the retinopathy of vitamin E deficiency. Deficiency of vitamin A may also contribute to the retinopathy, and some patients benefit from additional supplementation. The time of onset of symptoms is variable. Compromise of visual acuity may occur during the first decade, although many patients are asymptomatic until adulthood. Loss of night or color vision is frequently a presenting sign. Patients are often unaware of the slow progression of the ophthalmologic disease. Nystagmus and complete loss of vision can occur. Neuropathy affects the oculomotor nerve and results in ophthalmoplegia (Kane & Havel, 1995).

The most characteristic degenerative sites in the nervous system are the large sensory neurons of the spinal ganglia and their heavily myelinated axons. There is a progressive neuropathy and extensive demyelination of these areas. The first neurologic signs are diminution in the intensity of the deep tendon reflexes, which may occur in the first few years of life. Vibratory sense and proprioception tend to be lost progressively, and an ataxic gait develops. Neurologic problems are evident in 35 percent of the children by 10 years of age. By 20 years of age, mild to severe ataxia and intellectual deficits are present (Ampola, 1982; Bickel, 1980; Kane & Havel, 1995; Wapnir, 1985). Untreated patients are unable to stand by the third decade. Muscle contractions are common, leading to pes cavus, pes equinovarus, and kyphoscoliosis. Muscle weakness is a frequent feature of this disorder. The clinical determination that myopathy is present tends to be obscured by the frequent presence of degenerative peripheral neuropathy. Cardiomyopathy may lead to death early in the second decade of life (Kane & Havel, 1995). Slow neuromuscular development has been recorded in a number of cases. Attributing the developmental delay to this disorder is difficult because specific neuropathologic cerebral disease is lacking. In addition, slow neurologic development is common in infants who have steatorrhea and fail to thrive and may reflect nutritional deficiencies. Furthermore, because many patients with this disorder are products of consanguineous matings, other rare inborn errors may be responsible for the mental retardation.

The diagnosis of this disorder is suggested by the absence of apolipoprotein B, low serum cholesterol levels, low triglyceride levels, and plasma that is devoid of chylomicrons (LeGrys, 1984). In addition, there are low levels of vitamins A, E, and K, folic acid, and iron (Ampola, 1982; Bickel, 1980; Kane & Havel, 1995).

Treatment includes early dietary restriction of long-chain triglycerides to control the gastrointestinal symptoms. Fatty acids derived from medium-chain triglycerides do not require the formation of chylomicrons for absorption. They are transported mainly by albumin as free fatty acids via the hepatic portal system and serve as energy substrate for the liver but are not necessary nutrients. Hepatic function should be monitored in affected patients receiving medium-chain triglyceride supplements. Infant formula should contain medium-chain triglycerides (Winick, 1979). Prolonged observation of vitamin E supplementation has concluded that such supplementation does inhibit the progression of the neurologic disease and probably leads to the regression of symptoms even if it is started in adulthood (Kane & Havel, 1995). The retinopathy may be prevented if therapy is started early, or it may be stabilized if disease is already present when therapy is started. The myopathy is also reversed with vitamin E therapy (Kane & Havel, 1995). Treatment requires large doses (1000 to 10,000 mg/day) of oral vitamin E until the reliability and safety of parenteral preparations are established. Initiation of vitamin E therapy before the appearance of neurologic symptoms prevents them. If vitamin A and carotene levels are low, additional supplementation may be of benefit. Because vitamin D has its own transport mechanism and because the symptoms of vitamin D deficiency are not associated with this disorder, no specific supplementation is necessary. Supplementation with vitamin K should be given if bruising, bleeding, or hypoprothrombinemia is present (Kane & Havel, 1995).

Familial Combined Hyperlipidemia

Familial combined hyperlipidemia was identified as a disease in studies of the survivors of myocardial infarction and their relatives. Three patterns of lipoprotein distribution were recognized: elevated plasma levels of VLDLs, of LDLs, or of a combination of both. The pattern may change over time in an affected individual or within a family. Family pedigrees are compatible with an autosomal dominant pattern. Although seen in childhood, the manifestations are limited until about the third decade of life. Plasma triglyceride levels tend to remain between 200 to 400 mg/dl but may be much higher. LDL levels are usually greater than 100 mg/dl. Most affected family members have apo B levels greater than 85 mg/dl. Xanthoma formation is less common than in heterozygous familial hypercholesterolemia at similar LDL levels. The prevalence of familial combined hyperlipidemia is estimated at 1 to 2 percent of the population in North America and Europe. Treatment goals include the achievement of ideal body weight in addition to the restriction of cholesterol and saturated fats. Hypercholesterolemia appears to respond well to treatment with hydroxymethylglutaryl (HMG)–CoA reductase inhibitors. Triglycerides levels respond to a lesser extent. The addition of nicotinic acid often reduces the VLDL levels dramatically and appears to have a synergistic effect on LDL levels. The use of bile acid–binding resins alone frequently increases the triglyceride level. The combined regimen of bile acid–binding resins and nicotinic acid is often very effective.

Tangier Disease

- Tangier disease is characterized by a severe deficiency or absence of normal high-density lipoproteins (HDLs) in plasma and results in the accumulation of cholesterol esters in many tissues throughout the body, such as tonsils, the liver, the spleen, the thymus, lymph nodes, intestinal mucosa, peripheral nerves, and the cornea.
- Clinical manifestations include hyperplastic, orange tonsils; splenomegaly; and relapsing neuropathy. HDL deficiency and low plasma cholesterol concentration accompanied by normal or elevated triglyceride levels in combination with hyperplastic adenoidal tissue is pathognomonic. Despite the HDL deficiency, there is only a minimal risk of myocardial infarction.
- Plasma apo-I concentration is less than 3 percent that of controls, and the small amount of HDL in Tangier plasma differs from that in normal plasma. Levels of chylomicron remnants and VLDLs are very abnormal.

- Heterozygotes are asymptomatic and have half-normal concentrations of HDLs, apo-I, and apo-II.

The molecular basis for the disease is still unknown but is likely related to a defect in the pathway in intracellular lipid transfer processes. There is no specific treatment for Tangier disease.

This extremely rare autosomal recessive disorder is characterized by severe deficiency of plasma LDL and the accumulation of cholesterol esters in a variety of tissues (Ampola, 1982; Assman et al., 1995; Cohn & Roth, 1983; Scriver et al., 1995a; Wapnir, 1985). There is abnormal metabolism of apolipoprotein A, which results in hypercatabolism of high-density lipoprotein constituents. Clinical manifestations include tonsillar hypertrophy with yellow-orange bands. Other organs such as the spleen, thymus, intestinal mucosa, skin, liver, and lymphatic ganglia also hypertrophy (Assman et al., 1995). Other manifestations reported with Tangier disease include hemolysis and hemolytic anemia. The altered erythrocyte morphology is caused by the decrease in cholesterol and increase in phosphatidylcholine in the red blood cell membranes. Ocular abnormalities include corneal opacifications, ectropion, retinal pigment mottling and diplopia. Peripheral neuropathy occurs and is thought to result from abnormal lipid deposition in Schwann cells. Although it may be asymptomatic, relapses are common and occasionally devastating. Weakness, paresthesias, increased sweating, diplopia, ocular nerve palsies, diminished or absent deep tendon reflexes, muscle atrophy, and loss of pain and temperature sensation may occur. Most patients have some degree of neuromuscular dysfunction, although symptoms may be subtle and transient (Assman et al., 1995).

Despite HDL deficiency and despite very elevated cholesterol ester accumulation in tissues, there does not appear to be an increased risk for atherosclerosis in these patients. No evidence of coronary artery disease or vascular disease has been reported in patients less than 40 years of age. Documented evidence of cardiovascular and cerebrovascular disease has been reported in patients over 40 years of age, but these patients also had additional risk factors such as obesity, smoking, and hypertension (Assman et al., 1995).

Familial Hyperlipoproteinemia: Familial Lipoprotein Lipase Deficiency

These disorders are characterized by a marked elevation of cholesterol, triglycerides, or both, and of LDLs, which may increase the risk of accelerating atherosclerosis.

- Familial lipoprotein lipase deficiency is one of three disorders in which chylomicrons accumulate in the plasma. Chylomicronemia can also occur in persons with common familial forms of hypertriglyceridemia who also have an acquired cause of hypertriglyceridemia such as untreated diabetes mellitus, estrogen or antihypertensive drug therapy, or alcohol use.
- Familial lipoprotein lipase deficiency is a rare autosomal recessive disorder characterized by massive accumulation of chylomicrons in plasma and a corresponding increase in the plasma triglyceride concentration. The concentration of VLDL may be normal.
- The disease is usually detected in childhood on the basis of repeated episodes of abdominal pain, recurrent attacks of pancreatitis, eruptive cutaneous xanthomatosis, and hepatosplenomegaly. The severity of the symptoms is directly related to the degree of hyperchylomicronemia, which in turn is related to dietary fat intake.
- More than 30 structural defects in the lipoprotein lipase gene are associated with lipoprotein lipase defects. This lipolytic enzyme is present on the vascular endothelial cells of extrahepatic tissues and is essential for hydrolysis of chylomicron and VLDL triglycerides to provide free fatty acids to tissues for energy.
- Diagnosis is based on low or absence of enzyme activity and confirmed by demonstrating the defect in the structure of the lipoprotein lipase gene. The disorder is not associated with atherosclerotic vascular disease, but recurrent pancreatitis may threaten the patient's life.
- Restriction of dietary fat to less than 20 g/day is usually sufficient to reduce plasma triglyceride levels and to keep the patient free from symptoms. Available lipid-lowering drugs are not effective.
- Heterozygotes exhibit a 50 percent decrease in lipoprotein lipase but have normal or only slightly abnormal plasma lipid levels.

This autosomal recessive disorder occurs as a result of decreased extrahepatic activity of lipoprotein lipase, which catalyzes the removal of triglyceride-rich lipoprotein from the blood. It is associated with an elevation of levels of chylomicrons, cholesterol, and triglycerides in the serum (Brunzell, 1995; Cohn & Roth, 1983; Scriver et al., 1995a; Wapnir, 1985). Heterozygotes have elevated serum triglyceride levels (LeGrys, 1984; Scriver et al., 1995a). The clinical manifestations are usually detected late in the first decade, but some are detected as early as infancy or as late as the fourth decade of life (Brunzell, 1995).

In infancy, splenomegaly, anorexia, colicky pain, failure to thrive, and malaise are common. At all ages the most common symptom is episodic abdominal pain. Young patients learn to prevent abdominal pain by avoiding foods with high fat content. In older individuals, abdominal pain from pancreatitis is common and may be life-threatening. The pancreatitis is usually of acute onset and is often recurrent, occasionally leading to total pancreatic necrosis and death. Mild fat malabsorption can occur. The pain varies from mild to incapacitating. Serum and urine amylase levels may be normal or elevated in pancreatitis from hyperchylomicronemia. Hepatomegaly is commonly encountered; splenomegaly is less commonly documented. The hard, enlarged spleen can return to normal size within 1 week of lowering the triglyceride levels in patients with lipoprotein lipase deficiency who are placed on a very low fat diet.

Painless yellow xanthomas develop in skin creases and other pressure areas when the serum cholesterol is greater than 2000 mg/dl (Brunzell, 1995; LeGrys, 1984). The lesions result from extravascular phagocytosis of chylomicrons by macrophages in the skin and reflect the chronic hyperchylomicronemia. The xanthomas are localized over the buttocks, knees, and extensor surfaces of the arms. They may become generalized and are usually not tender except when they are continually traumatized. When the plasma triglyceride levels are lowered, the xanthomas clear over the course of several months. Recurrent or persistent xanthomas indicate that therapy to lower triglyceride levels is ineffective.

The diagnosis of this disorder can be made when there are a marked increase in chylomicrons; normal or decreased levels of high-density, low-density, and very low density lipoproteins; and increased serum cholesterol and triglyceride levels. In the chylomicron fraction of blood, triglyceride levels may rise to 2500 to 29,000 mg/dl, and serum cholesterol may not increase until triglyceride levels are over 3000 mg/dl (Brunzell, 1995; LeGrys, 1984). The diagnosis can be confirmed when the removal of dietary fat results in the dramatic fall of triglyceride and cholesterol levels (Brunzell, 1995; Winick, 1979). Despite a markedly elevated serum cholesterol level in this disorder, there is no increased risk for atherosclerosis (Ampola, 1982; Brunzell, 1995; Wapnir, 1985). In the past, many affected patients died of pancreatitis at an early age. However, with the improved recognition of the disease, the avoidance of unnecessary surgery, and the maintenance of a low-fat diet, these patients can lead a fairly normal life.

Familial Cholesterolemia

- Familial hypercholesterolemia is characterized by an elevated concentration of LDL, deposition of LDL-derived cholesterol in tendons and skin, and autosomal dominant inheritance.
- Heterozygotes number approximately 1 in 500 persons, making familial hypercholesterolemia among the most common inborn errors of metabolism. Heterozygotes have twofold elevations in plasma cholesterol (350 to 550 mg/dl) from birth. Tendon xanthomas and coronary atherosclerosis develop after ages 20 and 30, respectively.
- Homozygotes are more severely affected and number about one in one million persons. They have severe hypercholesterolemia (650 to 1000 mg/dl). Cutaneous xanthomas appear in the first 4 years of life. Coronary heart disease begins in childhood and frequently causes death from myocardial infarction before age 20.
- The primary defect is an inability of the LDL receptors to bind with circulating LDL. When LDL receptors are deficient, the rate of removal of LDL from plasma declines, and the level of LDL rises in inverse proportion to the receptor number. The excess plasma LDL is deposited in scavenger cells and other cell types, producing xanthomas and atheromas.
- The LDL receptor gene has been mapped to chromosome 19. Five classes of mutations at the LDL receptor locus have been identified. Each class has been subdivided into multiple alleles, and more than 150 different mutant alleles have been described.
- Heterozygotes have one normal and one mutant allele; their cells are able to take up LDL at approximately half the normal rate. Homozygotes show a total or near total absence of LDL binding.
- Treatment is directed at lowering plasma LDL. In heterozygotes, the most effective therapy is the administration of drugs that stimulate the single normal gene to produce additional messenger RNA for the LDL receptor, such as through the combined administration of a bile acid–binding resin and an inhibitor of HMG-CoA reductase. These drugs enhance LDL receptor activity in the liver, which in turn increases LDL catabolism and decreases LDL production. Homozygotes with two nonfunctional genes are resistant to drugs that work by stimulating LDL receptors. Effective treatment can lead to a reduced rate or slower progression of coronary artery disease.

This autosomal dominant disorder occurs as a result of a complete lack of LDL cell membrane receptors and is characterized clinically by a lifelong elevation in the concentration of LDL cholesterol in the blood, leading to premature coronary heart disease. This disorder was the first genetic disease recognized to cause myocardial infarctions (Cohn & Roth, 1983; Goldstein et al., 1995; Wapnir, 1985).

Normally, LDL cholesterol binds to cell surface membrane receptors and only cholesterol is taken into the cell. Cholesterol, once inside the cell, inhibits an enzyme that is essential for further cholesterol synthesis. Thus, in this disorder, cholesterol production is not inhibited, and serum LDL cholesterol levels rise. Clinical manifestations of xanthomas are present in all homozygotes by 4 years of age and may be present at birth. There is early, generalized atherosclerosis and cardiovascular death as early as 5 to 20 years of age. In heterozygotes, symptoms of coronary artery disease occur by 30 years of age and may be associated with joint pain, polyarthritis, and cardiac murmurs (Cohn & Roth, 1983; Goldstein et al., 1995; Wapnir, 1985). The diagnosis of this disorder is suggested by serum cholesterol levels greater than 650 ml/dl in homozygotes and 300 ml/dl in heterozygotes, with an elevation in levels of LDL (LeGrys, 1984). The definitive diagnosis occurs when LDL receptor function is measured in cultured skin fibroblasts (LeGrys, 1984). The treatment of this disorder with drugs and a diet low in saturated fat and cholesterol has met with very limited success to date (Winick, 1979). Drastic surgery to create a portal caval shunt or sustained plasmapheresis has not been successful in long-term studies (Goldstein et al., 1995; Scriver et al., 1995a; Wapnir, 1985). Cholestyramine and other bile acid sequestrants have had some success with nicotinic acid and fenofibrate (Winick, 1979).

Prenatal diagnosis can be accomplished by functional assays for quantitative assessment of LDL receptor activity in cultured amniotic fluid cells, measurement of cholesterol level on fetal cord blood obtained at 24 weeks of gestation or by chorionic villi samples taken at 8 weeks of gestation. Diagnosis is confirmed by skin fibroblast cultures of aborted fetuses. Neonatal diagnosis is made by measuring the cord blood LDL cholesterol level in infants born to a parent known to carry the familial hypercholesterolemia gene defect. Neonatal cord blood screening is not a reliable means of screening heterozygotes in the general population, because, as with adults, the majority of infants with elevated LDL cholesterol levels do not have familial hypercholesterolemia.

Treatment of heterozygotes exploits the feedback regulatory system that controls the transcription of the single normal LDL gene. When the demand for cholesterol is increased, normal and heterozygote cells produce an increased number of LDL receptors as a result of enhanced transcription. The acid-binding resins (cholestyramine and cholestipol) were the first class of drugs to exploit this mechanism. These agents have been used since the mid-1960s to lower LDL cholesterol by 15 to 20 percent in heterozygous hypercholesterolemic states. The liver compensates for the cholesterol deficiency by increasing the synthesis of cholesterol. Currently, bile acid sequestrants are used along with pharmacologic agents that decrease hepatic cholesterol synthesis. Lovastatin and chemically modified versions have become available for human therapy. In animal models, these drugs block cholesterol synthesis and elicit two compensatory mechanisms: (1) hepatocytes synthesize increased amounts of HMG-CoA reductase, and (2) they synthesize increased numbers of LDL receptors via transcriptional induction. The plasma levels fall as a result of the increased number of LDL receptors. Combined therapy of cholestyramine and lovastatin have decreased the plasma LDL levels by 50 percent (Goldstein et al., 1995).

Surgically created partial ileal bypass prevents bile salt reabsorption and produces essentially the same therapeutic effect in heterozygotes as does cholestyramine (Goldstein et al., 1995). The major drawbacks are frequent bowel movements, overt diarrhea, kidney stones, gallstones, and symptomatic bowel obstruction.

Dietary restriction of cholesterol to 150 mg/day is recommended for every person with hypercholesterolemia. Total fat intake should also be limited, and intake of saturated fats should be severely restricted. An important consideration in the treatment of familial hypercholesterolemia is the need to identify and treat affected family members. All first- and second-degree relatives should have plasma cholesterol determinations, followed by drug or diet therapy as indicated.

Therapy for familial hypercholesterolemia homozygotes differs from that of the heterozygotes in that they are resistant to the therapies just discussed. Because the homozygotes do not have LDL receptors, the number of these receptors cannot be enhanced by messenger RNA transcription induction, dietary changes, ileal bypass or bile acid sequestrants. If the LDL receptor is partially functional, the patient should be aggressively treated with a combination of bile acid–binding agent, an HMG-

CoA reductase inhibitor, and nicotinic acid in addition to strict dietary measures.

Surgical portacaval shunts have been used on a limited number of patients aged 2.5 to 35 years, resulting in a reduction in cholesterol from 25 to 50 percent. Regression of xanthomas occurs commonly as the cholesterol is lowered, and regression of aortic stenotic lesions and stabilization and regression of coronary artery disease have been documented (Goldstein et al., 1995). Portacaval shunt surgery is not associated with a significant enough reduction in LDL cholesterol to be used as the sole therapy for these patients.

The most successful approach for homozygotes is the direct removal of LDL cholesterol by the use of a continuous-flow blood cell separator that exchanges the patient's plasma with normal plasma or albumin. If the procedure is repeated every 1 to 2 weeks and combined with oral nicotinic acid, the mean plasma cholesterol can be reduced by about 50 percent on a long-term basis (Goldstein et al., 1995). This therapy produces regression of xanthomas and some amelioration of coronary artery disease and has been reported to extend the life span of affected persons by 5.5 years. More recently, plasma exchange has been replaced with LDL pheresis. In this method, the plasma is passed in a continuous manner extracorporeally over columns that remove VLDLs, LDLs, and intermediate-density lipoproteins but do not absorb HDLs or other plasma proteins. After the procedure, the fall in LDL cholesterol is about 70 percent, which increases to prepheresis levels in 1 week. Angiographic regression of coronary artery disease has been reported in about 50 percent of patients treated long term (Goldstein et al., 1995).

Liver transplantation has been performed on a limited number of homozygotes. The first was a 6-year-old girl who had a cholesterol level of 1000 mg/dl and had had repeated myocardial infarctions. After receiving the liver transplant, her cholesterol level fell to the 200 to 300 mg/dl range. Thirteen months after transplantation, she started lovastatin treatment, and her LDL cholesterol fell even further to 150 mg/dl. Thus liver transplantation not only lowered her cholesterol level but also restored responsiveness to lovastatin, the action of which requires an LDL receptor gene (Goldstein et al., 1995). Liver transplantation has been performed in five patients, four of whom recovered from transplant surgery. In all the survivors, the transplanted liver decreased the LDL cholesterol significantly. These results underscore the importance of hepatic LDL receptors and has emphasized the potential value of a direct gene therapy approach in which a normal LDL receptor gene is delivered to hepatocytes in vivo (Goldstein et al., 1995).

DISORDERS OF LYSOSOMAL ENZYMES

Gangliosidoses

Several types of gangliosidoses manifest in infancy with progressive encephalopathies and psychomotor deterioration, retinal lesions, and a particular neuronal alteration.

GM_1 Gangliosidoses

This autosomal recessive disorder results from a deficiency of hydrolase ganglioside GM_1 β-galactosidase (acid β-galactosidase), which normally uses ganglioside GM_1 and galactose-containing glycoproteins as substrates (Scriver et al., 1995a). As a result of this enzyme deficiency, ganglioside GM_1 that is normal in composition accumulates in the gray matter of the brain and in lesser amounts in the liver (Ampola, 1982; Cohn & Roth, 1983; Scriver et al., 1995a; Wapnir, 1985). Galactose-containing glycoprotein also accumulates in the liver (Ampola, 1982; Wapnir, 1985). The clinical manifestations are often evident at birth, with edema affecting the face and extremities and occasionally with ascites. There is a poor appetite, weak sucking, ineffective swallowing, and subnormal weight gain. After several months, facial dysmorphism is apparent, with enlarged skull, large forehead, coarse facial features, flattened nose, low-set ears, macroglossia, and hypertelorism. There is progressive psychomotor deterioration. The infant has a dull expression, is hypoactive and hypotonic, and never learns to sit independently. Tonic-clonic seizures may develop. Hepatomegaly is present (Ampola, 1982; Benson, 1983; Cohn & Roth, 1983; Scriver et al., 1995a; Wapnir, 1985). On ophthalmologic examination there is a cherry-red macular spot in 50 percent of these patients (Ampola, 1982; Scriver et al., 1995a; Wapnir, 1985). Affected patients who survive beyond the first year manifest decerebrate rigidity, blindness, deafness, spastic quadriplegia, and poor responsiveness to all external stimuli. Death usually occurs by age 3 years. Diagnosis of this disorder can be made by examination of bone marrow, liver, or spleen for the presence of foamy histiocytes (LeGrys, 1984; Scriver et al., 1995a). Prenatal diagnosis is possible. No treatment is available.

GM_2 Gangliosidoses

- The GM_2 gangliosidoses are a group of inherited disorders caused by excessive intralysosomal accumulation of ganglioside GM_2, particularly in neuronal cells. Enzymatic hydrolysis of ganglioside GM_2 requires a substrate-specific cofactor. There are two isoenzymes of β-hexosaminidase. Defects in any of the three genes that regulate the synthesis of these proteins result in the accumulation of gangliosides in the cell. Only Tay-Sachs disease is discussed.
- Clinical phenotypes in the GM_2 gangliosidoses vary widely, ranging from an infantile-onset form with rapidly progressive neurodegenerative disease that culminates in death before age 4 years (Tay-Sachs) to later-onset, subacute or chronic forms with more slowly progressive neurologic conditions compatible with survival into childhood or adolescence or with long-term survival. Chronic forms include several manifestations, including progressive dystonia, spinocellular degeneration, motor neuron disease, and psychosis.
- At least 54 genetic mutations have been described. Most mutations are associated with the severe, infantile-onset disease. The subacute and chronic forms of the disease are associated with variable low levels of residual enzyme activity, with the level of activity correlating to the severity of the disease.
- All GM_2 gangliosidoses exhibit an autosomal recessive inheritance pattern. The defective genes have been mapped to chromosome 15 (hexosaminidase A [HEX A]) and chromosome 5 (hexosaminidase B [HEX B] and GM_2 activator/cofactor). Heterozygotes for any of the defects are completely asymptomatic. The availability of rapid and inexpensive methods for identifying heterozygotes for HEX A defects has made large-scale screening programs for family and population carriers possible. When combined with DNA-based diagnostics, the type of mutation (acute, subacute, or chronic) can be identified.
- In the non-Jewish population, the incidences are approximately 6 in 1000 for HEX A and 36 in 10,000 of HEX B mutations. Of these mutations, about 35 percent are characterized by the acute, infantile type of disease and 5 percent characterized by the chronic form.
- Among the Ashkenazi Jews of North America and in Israel, a heterozygote frequency of 33 in 1000 was found for HEX A mutations, 95 percent of which were characterized as the infantile or acute form of the disease. Extensive genetic counseling and monitoring of at-risk pregnancies has reduced the incidence of Tay-Sachs disease in the Ashkenazi population by 90 percent.

- Specific therapy for GM_2 gangliosidoses is not available. All HEX A deficiency disorders can be diagnosed prenatally from amniotic fluid, cultured amniotic fluid cells, or chorionic villus biopsy specimens.

The autosomal recessive disorder more commonly known as Tay-Sachs disease results from a deficiency of HEX A. Two hexosaminidase enzymes—A and B—are present in all normal tissues except red blood cells. The deficiency of HEX A results in the accumulation of its substrate, ganglioside GM_2, in enormous amounts in the cerebrum. The amount of ganglioside GM_2 in the visceral organs is not significantly increased (Scriver et al., 1995a, 1995b). This disorder is most prevalent among Ashkenazic Jews, with an incidence of 1 in 3600 live births versus the non-Jewish population incidence of 1 in 360,000 live births (Ampola, 1982; Benson, 1983; Cohn & Roth, 1983; Gravel et al., 1995; Scriver et al., 1995a; Wapnir, 1985).

The clinical manifestations of this disorder appear shortly after birth with an exaggerated startle reaction to sharp sounds. Audiogenic myoclonia is very characteristic of this disorder. By 3 months of age, there is evidence of motor weakness that progresses. Although affected infants may learn to sit and crawl, they never learn to walk. After the first year, there is poor muscle tone, rapid mental and motor deterioration, ineffective swallowing, and generalized paresis. Ophthalmologic examination reveals an infiltrated cream-colored macula with a central cherry-red spot. By 16 months, macrocephaly develops from the cerebral gliosis, and the ventricles are enlarged. By 18 months, there is evidence of progressive sensory deficits leading to blindness and deafness. Subsequently, seizures, spasticity, and decerebrate rigidity develop. The infant's facial appearance is "doll-like," with pale pink translucent skin, long eyelashes, and fine hair. Deglutitional complications and infections lead to death by the age of 2 to 5 years (Ampola, 1982; Benson, 1983; Bickel, 1980; Cohn & Roth, 1983; Gravel et al., 1995; Wapnir, 1985).

The diagnosis of this disorder can be made by determining the levels of HEX A and HEX B in cord blood (LeGrys, 1984). To identify carriers of the mutation, the enzyme can be assayed from venous blood. However, this enzyme increases after the eighth week of pregnancy in general, and so screening should be accomplished before pregnancy. In addition, the carrier test is not reliable in women who are taking oral contraceptives or who have diabetes, hepatitis, an acute myocardial infarction, pancreatitis, or rheumatoid arthritis (LeGrys, 1984). Definitive diagnosis of carrier state or true disorder is made by enzyme assay from blood leukocytes (LeGrys, 1984; Scriver et al., 1995a) or by DNA diagnostics (Gravel et al., 1995). The only treatment for this disorder is prevention by carrier identification.

Sphingomyelin Lipidoses: Niemann-Pick Disease (Types A and B)

- Types A and B Niemann-Pick disease (NPD) are lysosomal storage disorders that result from the deficient activity of acid sphingomyelinase (ASM). Type A NPD is a fatal disorder of infancy characterized by failure to thrive, hepatomegaly, and a rapidly progressive neurodegenerative course that leads to death by the age of 2 to 3 years. In contrast, type B NPD is a variable disorder usually diagnosed in childhood by the presence of hepatomegaly. Most type B patients have little to no neurologic impairment and survive into adulthood. In severely affected type B patients, progressive pulmonary infiltration causes pulmonary insufficiency and lifestyle changes.
- The pathologic hallmark of types A and B NPD is the lipid-laden foam cell often referred to as the "Niemann-Pick cell." These cells result from the accumulation of sphingomyelin and other lipids in the monocyte–macrophage system, which is the primary pathologic site of the disease.
- Type A NPD patients have less than 5 percent of normal ASM activity in their cells and tissues. Type B NPD patients, who have milder disease, may have residual enzyme activity that ranges from 5 to 10 percent of normal.
- Both types A and B NPD are inherited as autosomal recessive traits. Type A NPD has a high incidence among Ashkenazic Jews in comparison with the general population. The frequency of disease among this population is approximately 1 in 120 live births with a carrier frequency of 1 in 60.
- The ASM gene has been mapped to chromosome 11. Twelve mutations that result in types A and B NPD have been identified in the ASM gene.
- The diagnosis of types A and B can be made by enzymatic determination of ASM activity in cell or tissue extracts. Heterozygote detection requires molecular studies. Prenatal diagnosis by enzymatic and/or molecular analysis has been accomplished through chorionic villi sampling and cultured amniocytes.
- There is no specific therapy for type A and B NPD. At the present time, research is directed at enzyme replacement and gene transfer in type B NPD.

NPD types A and B are two separate diseases of cellular sphingomyelin metabolism, which vary in onset, rate of progression, and neurologic symptoms. Sphingomyelin is a constituent of cellular membranes and also occurs in extracellular lipoproteins. In visceral organs, it constitutes 5 to 10 percent of the total phospholipid content; in erythrocytes, plasma, and white matter of the brain, this percentage is more than 20 percent. Because of the wide distribution of sphingomyelin in the body, a defect in the catabolism of this substance results in severe visceral and neuronal abnormalities. The increase in sphingomyelin content in visceral organs is more pronounced in patients with type A than in those with type B disease. Accumulation of sphingomyelin in the nervous system has not been demonstrated in patients with type B (Ampola, 1982; Schuchman & Desnick, 1995; Wapnir, 1985).

This autosomal recessive disorder occurs as a result of decreased activity (from 0 to 9 percent of normal) of ASM, an enzyme that catalyzes the breakdown of sphingomyelin (Ampola, 1982; Bickel, 1980; Cohn & Roth, 1983; Schuchman & Desnick, 1995; Wapnir, 1985). Sphingomyelin accumulates progressively in the central nervous system and visceral organs. Clinical manifestations of this disorder include jaundice, generalized edema, progressive developmental delay, failure to thrive, hepatosplenomegaly, and feeding difficulties, which lead to emaciation. Often the abdomen is protuberant and extremities are osteoporotic and thin. In 50 percent of affected infants, a cherry-red spot in the macular region is evident on ophthalmologic examination. Progressive neurologic deterioration with progressive loss of motor and intellectual function interferes with feeding, swallowing, and breathing. General muscular hypotonia, weak tendon reflexes, progressive deterioration, and recurrent respiratory infections are observed after the first months. Subsequently, seizures develop, and death occurs by 3 years of age (Ampola, 1982; Benson, 1983; Cohn & Roth, 1983; Schuchman & Desnick, 1995; Wapnir, 1985). In some instances, the onset of symptoms may occur after a period of relatively normal development. The diagnosis of this disorder is accomplished by a bone marrow aspiration to evaluate for large, foamy histiocytes and a specific enzyme assay for acid sphingomyelinase (LeGrys, 1984) and molecular studies of tissue to determine heterozygotes. Like Tay-Sachs disease, this disorder has a higher frequency among Ashkenazic Jews. No specific treatment is available (Schuchman & Desnick, 1995; Wapnir, 1985).

NPD type B does not involve the central nervous system but does entail abnormal accumulation of sphingomyelin in the viscera and 5 to 10 percent of normal activity of acid sphingomyelinase (Ampola, 1982; Cohn & Roth, 1983; Schuchman & Desnick, 1995; Wapnir, 1985). The visceral manifestations include hepatosplenomegaly, interstitial pulmonary infiltrates, and a predisposition to respiratory infections and repeated pneumothoraces. Children with NPD type B may develop normally during several years before the hepatosplenomegaly is detected. No neurologic abnormalities are found, the fundi are normal, and the intellectual development has been undisturbed. Marked hepatosplenomegaly persists, and there is a prolongation of the prothrombin time (Schuchman & Desnick, 1995).

Cellular Cholesterol Lipidoses: Niemann-Pick Disease (Type C)

- NPD type C is an autosomal recessive lipidosis that results from an error in cellular trafficking of exogenous cholesterol that is associated with the lysosomal accumulation of unesterified cholesterol. This disorder is biochemically distinct from NPD types A and B. Most patients with NPD type C have progressive neurologic disease and hepatic damage.
- The clinical manifestations in NPD type C are varied. Patients most commonly present in late childhood with variable degrees of hepatosplenomegaly, ophthalmoplegia, progressive ataxia, dystonia, and dementia. Death occurs in the second decade. This disorder may also manifest in the neonatal period with fatal liver disease or in the infantile period with hypotonia and developmental delay. The clinical manifestations may also appear as late as adulthood, in which psychosis and dementia predominate as symptoms.
- There is a panethnic distribution of NPD type C. Genetic isolates have been described in Nova Scotia (formerly called NPD type D) and southern Colorado. Despite the variable clinical manifestations, studies have not shown genetic heterogeneity.
- NPD type C is as least as frequent as types A and B combined. The true prevalence of the disease is underestimated because of the lack of a definitive diagnostic test before the discovery of the abnormalities of cellular cholesterol processing.
- Foam cells are present in many tissues and are not specific for NPD type C. Foam cells may be absent in patients lacking visceromegaly.
- The primary molecular defect in NPD type C is unknown. Unesterified cholesterol, sphingomyelin, phospholipids, and glycolipids are stored in excess in the liver and spleen. Glycolipids are elevated in the brain.
- The diagnosis of NPD type C requires both measurement of cellular cholesterol esterification and documentation of filipin–cholesterol staining in cultured fibroblasts during LDL uptake.
- Symptomatic treatment of seizures, dystonia, and cataplexy is effective in many patients with NPD type C. Various drug protocols have been used to lower hepatic cholesterol levels, but it is not known whether this therapy influences the neurologic progression of the disease.

NPD type C has a later onset than types A and B of neurologic manifestations, which occur at 3 to 4 years of age. The initial manifestations include spasticity, ataxia, loss of speech, grand mal seizures, and moderate visceromegaly. In the following years, intellectual functions are lost, and neurologic abnormalities become more pronounced. Urinary incontinence develops, as do seizures and the inability to walk; after a period of vegetative existence, the patients die. There is less severe accumulation of sphingomyelin than in other types of NPD, and acid sphingomyelinase activity in tissues is often paradoxically normal. Death occurs by 5 to 15 years of age (Ampola, 1982; Cohn & Roth, 1983; Pentchev et al., 1995; Scriver et al., 1995a; Wapnir, 1985).

PURINE METABOLIC DISORDERS

Hypoxanthine–Guanine Phosphoribosyltransferase Deficiency: Lesch-Nyhan Syndrome

- Lesch-Nyhan syndrome is caused by a complete deficiency of hypoxanthine–guanine phosphoribosyltransferase (HPRT), a purine salvage enzyme. The disease is characterized by hyperuricemia, choreoathetosis, spasticity, mental retardation, and compulsive self-mutilation. Patients with a partial deficiency of HPRT have hyperuricemia and gouty arthritis but are generally spared the neurologic consequences of Lesch-Nyhan syndrome.
- Patients with Lesch-Nyhan syndrome are clinically normal at birth. By 6 months of age, developmental delay is evident. Choreoathetoid movements begin within the first year. Self-mutilation is present in most patients and may begin as early as 6 months or as late as 16 years. Gouty arthritis in patients with partial HPRT deficiency develops during adulthood.
- The HPRT enzyme is expressed in all tissues at low levels except in the basal ganglia, in which the levels are higher, presumably because the rate of de novo purine synthesis is low.
- The human HPRT gene lies on the X chromosome. The genetic lesions that lead to HPRT deficiency are heterogeneous. DNA mutation techniques are used in the diagnosis of affected males and for the determination of carrier status of asymptomatic females. Tissues can be analyzed for the presence or absence of HPRT activity.
- Treatment with allopurinol, an inhibitor of xanthine oxidase, reduces serum uric acid levels and prevents most of the symptoms associated with hyperuricemia. There is no effective therapy for the neurologic complications of Lesch-Nyhan syndrome.

Lesch-Nyhan syndrome is an X-linked recessive disorder that occurs as a result of a deficiency of hypoxanthine–guanine phosphoribosyltransferase, an enzyme necessary for purine metabolism. Hypoxanthine deficiency prevents the conversion of hypoxanthine into nucleotide inosinic acid, and guanine phosphoribosyltransferase deficiency prevents the conversion of guanine into the nucleotide guanylic acid (Ampola, 1982; Cohn & Roth, 1983; Mikanagi et al., 1988; Rossiter & Caskey, 1995; Wapnir, 1985). These two enzymatic deficiencies result in an enhanced rate of conversion to uric acid. The hyperuricemia causes hyperuricuria, uric acid lithiasis, and uric acid tophi.

Clinical manifestations at birth may include clubfeet and congenital hip dislocation caused by spasticity in utero. Occasionally, the first clinical sign is the presence of sandy orange crystals in the infant's diapers. When this disorder is present, the uric acid level is usually greater than 9 mg/dl. Uric acid crystalluria leads to symptomatic nephrolithiasis and azotemia. Renal complications may lead to renal insufficiency and renal failure. Bony demineralization and partial osteopenia occur. Increased blood uric acid causes urate stones to develop in the urinary tract and urate tophi in subcutaneous tissues and joints (Ampola, 1982; Cohn & Roth, 1983; Mikanagi et al., 1988; Rossiter & Caskey, 1995; Wapnir, 1985).

The clinical course of neurologic impairment is fairly well defined in Lesch-Nyhan syndrome. After unremarkable prenatal and birth histories, delayed motor development becomes evident by 3 to 4 months (Ampola, 1982; Rossiter & Caskey, 1995; Wapnir, 1985). Frequent vomiting, hypotonia, and respiratory difficulty develop. Pyramidal signs appear and include hyperreflexia, extensor plantar reflexes, sustained ankle clonus, and scissoring. Extrapyramidal signs develop between 8 and 12 months of age, as evidenced by dystonia, chorea, and fine athetoid movements of the head and feet. The electromyogram is normal. During the second and third years of life, finger-chewing, lip-biting, tooth-grinding, and increased spasticity are easily recognized. Growth retardation occurs in all cases. IQ scores have been reported in the range of 40 to 80 on conventional testing. The EEG can be normal or show diffuse slowing. More than 50 percent of affected patients have seizures and bilateral cortical atrophy with developmental delay. There is compulsive self-mutilation such as biting associated with tissue loss between 2 and 16 years of age, which is aggravated during stress. Patients begin by biting their lips, buccal mucosa, or fingers, and the destructive urge is often so severe that arm restraints or dental extraction is necessary to prevent serious injury. The mutilation differs from that seen occasionally in other mentally retarded persons: In Lesch-Nyhan patients, there is a loss of tissue around the mouth or hands, as opposed to hypertrophy or callous formation. These patients display aggression toward other people, such as hitting and spitting, and opisthotonic posturing. Aggression towards others is usually followed by remorse. Death usually occurs in the second or third decade from pneumonia, aspiration, or chronic renal failure (Mikanagi et al., 1988; Rossiter & Caskey, 1995).

Diagnosis can be made by enzymatic assay from leukocytes or cultured skin fibroblasts (LeGrys, 1984; Mikanagi et al., 1988) or DNA-based mutation detection techniques (Rossiter & Caskey, 1995). Variable activity of these enzymes alters the severity of the disorder. Treatment with allopurinol, a xanthine oxidase inhibitor, can prevent the nephropathy by decreasing uric acid levels to within the normal range. Treatment with allopurinol results in the excretion of large amounts of xanthine and hypoxanthine, which are relatively insoluble. Thus the dose must be titrated carefully, and fluid intake must be greatly increased to minimize the likelihood of xanthine stone formation. Allopurinol does not reverse the central nervous system dysfunction. Although diazepam, phenobarbital, levodopa, and haloperidol have shown some benefit in some patients, no therapy has proved to be universally effective. To prevent self-mutilation and aggression, the use of restraints and behavior modification has had some success (Mikanagi et al., 1988; Rossiter & Caskey, 1995). At present, gene therapy is being investigated as a potential treatment for Lesch-Nyhan patients. The devastating nature of the disease, the lack of therapeutic options, and the development of efficient gene transfer techniques have made this disease a candidate for gene therapy. The HPRT gene has been transferred into HPRT-deficient cells in animal models. The use of this therapy in humans has yet to be accomplished (Rossiter & Caskey, 1995).

Hereditary Xanthinuria

- A deficiency of the enzyme xanthine dehydrogenase results in the inability to degrade purine bases hypoxanthine and xanthine to uric acid, the normal end product of purine metabolism in humans. Xanthine and hypoxanthine accumulate in place of uric acid in plasma and urine. Xanthine is excreted; hypoxanthine is recycled by a salvage pathway. Excess xanthine in the defect is derived from guanine nucleotide catabolism; guanine is converted to xanthine via the enzyme guanase.
- The clinical manifestations of classical xanthinuria relate to the extreme insolubility of the purine base xanthine and its high renal clearance. The disease may manifest in the neonatal period as renal damage caused by xanthine calculi. The renal damage may be severe, leading to renal failure and death.
- Whereas classical xanthinuria results from a deficiency of xanthine dehydrogenase, a second type of xanthinuria results from a deficiency of three enzymes—xanthine dehydrogenase, sulfite oxidase, and aldehyde oxidase—which have a common (and, in this case, deficient) molybdenum cofactor. This disorder manifests in the neonatal period with intractable seizures and is not discussed further.
- Xanthine dehydrogenase is concentrated predominantly in the liver and intestinal mucosa. This mutant enzyme has not yet been studied on the molecular level; however, complementary DNA for the human enzyme has been cloned. The gene locus for xanthine dehydrogenase has been linked to chromosome 2.
- The genetic defect in classical xanthinuria and the cofactor deficiency is inherited as an autosomal recessive trait. Heterozygotes for the classical defect have 50 percent of the normal enzyme activity with normal uric acid levels.
- No specific treatments have proved successful for these patients; however, a high fluid intake and avoidance of purine-rich foods may be of benefit.

This autosomal recessive disorder occurs as a result of a deficiency of xanthine dehydrogenase, an enzyme that catalyzes the oxidation of hypoxanthine to xanthine and of xanthine into uric acid (Mikanagi et al., 1988; Scriver et al., 1995a; Wapnir, 1985). It is characterized by excessive urinary excretion of xanthine, which is extremely insoluble. The clinical manifestations of this disorder are variable. Approximately 20 percent of the affected persons are asymptomatic, whereas others have xanthine urinary tract calculi, myopathy, and arthropathy; males represent two thirds of the cases. The symptoms, which may begin at birth, include persistent emesis, poor weight gain, irritability, hematuria, urinary tract infection, renal colic, crystalluria, urolithiasis, and acute renal failure. The severity of the disease may lead to nephrectomy or terminal uremia. There may be cramping after exercise, and myopathy and polyarthritis may be present (Ampola, 1982; Cohn & Roth, 1983; Mikanagi et al., 1988; Scriver et al., 1995a; Wapnir, 1985); these features are presumably caused by deposition of xanthine crystals in skeletal muscle. Whereas the renal symptoms tend to occur in childhood, the myopathy and arthropathy tend to occur later in life.

In the absence of urolithiasis, the diagnosis of this disorder is difficult in the newborn who exhibits acute renal failure. Renal ultrasonography can detect the presence of crystal urolithiasis and should be performed in all infants who exhibit hematuria and acute renal failure not attributable to perfusion injury. The diagnosis of this disorder is suggested by very low serum uric acid levels (usually below 1 mg/dl) (Scriver et al., 1995a; Wapnir, 1985). The ratio of xanthine to hypoxanthine is significantly elevated (LeGrys, 1984; Lloyd & Scriver, 1985; Scriver et al., 1995a). In the urine, uric acid excretion is decreased and xanthine is increased (LeGrys, 1984; Paul et al., 1980; Scriver et al., 1995a). Because the enzyme is not expressed in all tissues, confirmation of enzyme deficiency is accomplished through liver or intestinal mucosal biopsy. Prenatal diagnosis is available, although not required for classical xanthinuria, and chorionic villus or amniotic fluid sampling will detect cofactor deficiency.

Treatment of classic xanthinuria includes a high fluid intake and restriction of dietary purine to prevent stone formation (Mikanagi et al., 1988; Scriver et al., 1995a; Winick, 1979). Because of the poor solubility of xanthine at any pH, alkalization of the urine is relatively ineffective at preventing stone formation. Vigorous exercise should be avoided. Lithotripsy or lithotomy may be required if obstructive nephropathy develops.

Pyrimidine Metabolic Disorders

Hereditary Orotic Aciduria

- Pyrimidines, along with purines, are the building blocks of DNA and RNA. Like purines, pyrimidines have two routes of nucleotide formation: the de novo pathway, which begins with ribose phosphate, amino acids, CO_2, and ammonia, and the salvage pathway, which scavenges free bases and nucleosides back to nucleotides. The de novo and salvage pathways are balanced and connected through the enzymes that degrade the nucleotides.

- There are four defects of pyrimidine metabolism: hereditary orotic aciduria, pyrimidine 5′-nucleotase deficiency, dihydropyrimidine dehydrogenase deficiency, and dihydropyrimidinuria. Only hereditary orotic aciduria is discussed in this section.
- The end product of purine metabolism is uric acid, which is easily recognized and quantified. There is no equivalent end product in pyrimidine metabolism.
- Hereditary orotic aciduria results from a defect in the de novo pathway. It is an autosomal recessive disorder that results from a severe deficiency of the last two enzyme activities of the pathway. Although two enzymes are affected in this disorder, they are regulated by a single polypeptide encoded by a single gene localized to chromosome 3.
- Only 15 cases of hereditary orotic aciduria have been reported in the literature. All patients have had macrocytic hypochromic megaloblastic anemia and orotic acid crystalluria. Treatment with uridine has resulted in clinical improvement in most patients. Other clinical manifestations of the disorder include crystal lithiasis, cardiac malformations, and strabismus. Infections are a problem in some patients with various alterations of immune function. Mild intellectual impairment has not been a constant feature before treatment.

This extremely rare autosomal recessive disorder occurs as a result of the deficiency of the last two sequential enzymes in the pyrimidine pathway: orotate phosphoribosyltransferase and orotidine-5′-phosphate decarboxylase. Orotate phosphoribosyltransferase converts orotic acid into orotidine-5′-phosphate, and orotidine-5′-phosphate converts orotidine 5′-phosphate into uridine-5′-phosphate (Ampola, 1982; Ogata, 1986; Webster et al., 1995). Affected persons are totally dependent on exogenous sources of pyrimidines for survival. The clinical manifestations appear in infancy, with failure to thrive and retarded growth and development. There is bilateral strabismus, and hair is fine and dry. Splenomegaly may be present, as is megaloblastic anemia. Orotic acid crystals in the urine may result in urinary tract obstruction (Mikanagi et al., 1988; Webster et al., 1995; Wapnir, 1985).

The diagnosis of this disorder is made by screening the urine for orotic acids (LeGrys, 1984; Paul et al., 1980; Webster et al., 1995). In this disorder, orotic acid excretion is 1000 times higher than normal (Mikanagi et al., 1988; Wapnir, 1985; Webster et al., 1995). Hematologically, there are hypochromia, anisocytosis, poikilocytosis, erythroid hyperplasia, and atypical megaloblastic changes in the bone marrow (LeGrys, 1984; Webster et al., 1995). The definitive diagnosis is made by enzymatic assay of red blood cells, white blood cells, or cultured skin fibroblasts (LeGrys, 1984; Mikanagi et al., 1988; Webster et al., 1995).

Treatment with glucocorticoids leads to hematologic improvement in a few patients, although there are no changes in bone marrow (Mikanagi et al., 1988). Pyrimidine replacement with the nucleotide uridine is the treatment of choice and leads to hematologic remission and normal growth and development if initiated early (Mikanagi et al., 1988; Webster et al., 1995). Several women with hereditary orotic aciduria have had a number of pregnancies. The reports in the literature suggest that uridine is not teratogenic and that pregnancy is well tolerated. The dose of uridine must be adjusted to maintain an affected woman's normal nonpregnant hemoglobin level and amount of orotic acid excretion.

Treatment with uridine does reverse the megaloblastic anemia and reduce the amount of orotic acid excretion; however, it is not necessarily an indication that the effects of the metabolic defect have been eliminated in other tissues. Long-term prognosis of survival into early adult life is excellent in the majority of treated cases and even in some in whom treatment was delayed (Webster et al., 1995).

CONCLUSION

Many metabolic disorders have become identifiable in the prenatal and postnatal periods; thus the demand for early screening for these disorders has become greater. It is therefore extremely important that both the general public and the medical community intelligently evaluate each disorder in terms of the need for and desirability of screening. Such an evaluation must be based on both humanistic and economic considerations.

Neonatal screening programs must be revised on the basis of changing priorities of the importance of screening a disease in a given population. Such a program evaluation is necessary in order to eliminate screening for disorders with less severe consequences or disorders that occur very rarely, whereas disorders with more severe consequences and those with greater frequency should be included. Expanded and revised neonatal screening will provide the tools for improved preventive health measures as well as for genetic counseling in the areas of greatest need in each specific population. The use of gene therapy to replace or augment the substrate or enzyme that is missing offers hope in the future. At present, however, early neonatal detection is the best weapon against iatrogenic or long-term sequelae if any correction of the metabolic dysfunction can be made. From the discussion, it is obvious that the management of newborns with inborn errors of metabolism requires collaboration among the physician, nurse, family, geneticist, neurologist, ophthalmologist, endocrinologist, teacher, nutritionist, and social worker.

REFERENCES

Acosta, P. B., & Elsas, L. J. III. (1976). *Dietary management of inherited metabolic disease: Phenylketonuria, galactosemia, tyrosinemia, homocystinuria, maple syrup urine disease*. Atlanta: ACELMU.

Acosta, P. B., & Wright, J. L. (1992). Nurse's role in preventing birth defects in offspring of women with phenylketonuria [Review]. *Journal of Obstetric, Gynecologic, and Neonatal Nursing, 21*(4), 270–276.

Agamanolis, D. P., Potter, J. L., & Lungren, D. W. (1993). Neonatal glycine encephalopathy: Biochemical and neuropathologic findings. *Pediatric Neurology, 9*(2), 140–143.

Alfi, O. S., Shaw, K. N. F., Fishler, K., & Wenz, E. (1978). Histidinemia: Follow-up of 13 patients. *American Journal of Clinical Genetics, 30*, 20A.

Alm, J., Holmgren, G., Larsson, A., & Schimpfessel, L. (1981). Histidinemia in Sweden. Report on a neonatal screening programme. *Clinical Genetics, 20*(3), 229–233.

Amador, P. S., & Carter, T. P. (1986). Historical review of newborn screening in New York state: Twenty years' experience. In T. P. Carter & A. M. Willey (Eds.), *Genetic disease, screening and management* (pp. 343–358). New York: A. R. Liss.

Ampola, M. G. (1982). *Metabolic diseases in pediatric practice*. Boston: Little, Brown.

Ampola, M. G., Mahoney, M. J., Nakamura, E., & Tanaka, K. (1975). Prenatal therapy of a patient with vitamin B_{12} responsive methylmalonic acidemia. *New England Journal of Medicine, 293*(7), 313–317.

Armstrong, M. D. (1975). Maternal histidinemia [Letter]. *Archives of Disease in Childhood, 50*(10), 831–832.

Aronson, S., Emgelson, G., Jagenburg, R., & Palmgren, B. (1968). Long-term dietary treatment of tyrosinosis. *Journal of Pediatrics, 72*(5), 620–627.

Ascher, P., & Johnson, P. W. (1989). The NMDA receptor, its channel and its modulation by glycine. In J. C. Watkins & G. L. Collingridge (Eds.), *The NMDA receptor*. Oxford, UK: Oxford University Press.

Assman, G., von Eckardstein, A., & Brewer, H. B. (1995). Familial high density lipoprotein deficiency: Tangier disease. In C. R. Scriver, A. L. Beaudet, W. S. Sly, & D. Valle (Eds.), *The metabolic and molecular bases of inherited metabolic disease* (7th ed., 2053–2072). New York: McGraw-Hill.

Atkin, B. M., Buist, N. R., Utter, M. F., et al. (1979). Pyruvate carboxylase deficiency and lactic acidosis in a retarded child without Leigh's disease. *Pediatric Research, 13*(2), 109–116.

Azen, C. G., Koch, R., Friedman, E. G., et al. (1991). Intellectual development in 12 year old children treated for PKU. *American Journal of Disease of Children, 145*(1), 35–39.

Baig, M. M. A., Swamy, H. M., Hassan, S. I., et al. (1992). Studies on the urea cycle enzyme levels in the human fetal liver at different gestational ages. *Pediatric Research, 31*, 143.

Ballard, R. A., Vinocur, B., Reynolds, J. W., et al. (1978). Transient hyperammonemia in the preterm infant. *New England Journal of Medicine, 299*(17), 920–925.

Barber, G. W., & Spaeth, G. L. (1969). The successful treatment of homocystinuria with pyridoxine. *Journal of Pediatrics, 75*(3), 463–478.

Baron, D. N., Dent, C. E., Harris, H., et al. (1956). Hereditary pellagra-like skin rash with temporary cerebellar ataxia. Constant renal aminoaciduria and other bizarre biochemical features. *Lancet, 2*, 421.

Battistini, S., De Stefano, N., Parlanti, S., & Federico, A. (1991). Unexpected white matter changes in an early treated PKU case and improvement after dietary treatment. *Functional Neurology, 6*(2), 177–180.

Benesch, R., & Benesch, R. E. (1969). Intracellular organic phosphates as regulators of oxygen release by haemoglobin in medicine. *Nature, 221*(181), 618–622.

Benson, P. F. (1983). *Screening and management of potentially treatable genetic metabolic disorders*. Boston: MTP Press.

Berger, R., van Faassen, H., & Smith, G. P. (1983). Biochemical studies on the enzymatic deficiencies in hereditary tyrosinemia. *Clinica Chimica Acta, 134*(1–2), 129–141.

Beutler, E. (1978). Glucose-6-phosphate deficiency. In E. Beutler (Ed.), *Hemolytic anemia in disorders of red cell metabolism*. New York: Plenum.

Beutler, E. (1984). Sensitivity to drug-induced hemolytic anemia in glucose-6-phosphate dehydrogenase deficiency. In S. Omenn & H. V. Gelboin (Eds.), *Genetic variability in responses to chemical exposure* (Barnbury Report 16). Cold Spring Harbor, NY: Cold Spring Harbor Laboratory.

Beutler, E. (1993). Study of glucose-6-phosphate dehydrogenase: History and molecular biology. *American Journal of Hematology, 42*(1), 53–58.

Beutler, E., Dern, R. J., & Alving, A. S. (1954). The hemolytic effect of primaquine: IV. The relationship of cell age to hemolysis. *Journal of Laboratory and Clinical Medicine, 44*, 439.

Beutler, E., Kuhl, W., Fox, M., et al. (1992). Prenatal diagnosis of glucose-6-phosphate dehydrogenase deficiency. *Acta Haematologica, 87*(1–2), 103–104.

Bick, U., Fahrendorf, G., Ludoph, A. C., et al. (1991). Disturbed myelination in patients with treated hyperphenylalaninemia: Evaluation with MRI. *European Journal of Pediatrics, 150*(3), 185–189.

Bickel, H. (1980). Rationale of neonatal screening for inborn errors of metabolism. In H. Bickel, R. Guthrie, & G. Hammersen (Eds.), *Neonatal screening for inborn errors of metabolism* (pp. 1–6). New York: Springer-Verlag.

Bickel, H., Gerrard, J. W., & Hickmans, E. M. (1954). Influence of phenylalanine intake on the chemistry and behaviour of a phenylketonuric child. *Acta Paediatrica, 43*, 64–77.

Bickel, H., Guthrie, R., & Hammersen, G. (1980). *Neonatal screening for inborn errors of metabolism*. New York: Springer-Verlag.

Bier, D. M., Arnold, K. J., Sherman, W. R., et al. (1977). In vivo measurement of glucose and alanine metabolism with stable isotope tracers. *Diabetes, 26*(11), 1005–1015.

Blaskovics, M. E., Schaeffler, G. E., & Hack, S. (1974). Phenylalaninemia: Differential diagnosis. *Archives of Disease in Childhood, 49*(11), 835–843.

Blau, N., Kierat, L., Heizmann, C. W., et al. (1992). Screening for tetrahydrobiopterin deficiency in newborns using dried urine on filter paper. *Journal of Inherited Metabolic Disease, 15*(3), 402–404.

Borden, M., Holm, J., Leslie, J., et al. (1992). Hawkinsinuria in two families. *American Journal of Medical Genetics, 44*(1), 52–56.

Bourget, L., & Chang, T. M. (1985). Phenylalanine ammonia-lyase immobilized in semipermeable microcapsules for enzyme replacement in phenylketonuria. *FEBS Letters, 180*(1), 5–8.

Bowman, H. S., McKusick, V. A., Dronamraju, K. R. (1965). Pyruvate kinase deficient hemolytic anemia in an Amish isolate. *American Journal of Human Genetics, 17*, 1.

Bowring, F. G., & Brown, A. R. (1986). Development of a protocol for newborn screening for disorders of the galactose metabolic pathway. *Journal of Inherited Metabolic Disease, 9*(1), 99–104.

Brill, P. W., Mitty, H. A., & Gaull, G. E. (1974). Homocystinuria due to cystathionine synthase deficiency: Clinical and roentgenologic correlations. *American Journal of Roentgenology, Radium Therapy & Nuclear Medicine, 121*(1), 45–54.

Bruckman, C., Berry, H. K., & Dasenbrock, R. J. (1970). Histidinemia in two successive generations. *American Journal of Disease of Children, 119*(3), 221–227.

Brunzell, J. D. (1995). Familial lipoprotein lipase deficiency and other causes of the chylomicronemia syndrome. In C. R. Scriver, A. L. Beaudet, W. S. Sly, & D. Valle (Eds.), *The metabolic and molecular bases of inherited metabolic disease* (7th ed., 1913–1932). New York: McGraw-Hill.

Brusilow, S. W. (1991). Treatment of urea cycle disorders. In R. J. Desnick (Ed.), *Treatment of genetic disease*. New York: Churchill Livingstone.

Brusilow, S., Batshaw, M., & Walser, M. (1979). Use of ketoacids in inborn errors of urea synthesis. In M. Winick (Ed.), *Nutritional management of genetic disorders*. New York: John Wiley.

Brusilow, S. W., & Finkelstien, J. E. (1993). Restoration of nitrogen homeostasis in a man with partial ornithine transcarbamylase deficiency. *Metabolism, 42*(10), 1336–1339.

Brusilow, S. W., & Horwich, A. L. (1995). Urea cycle enzymes. In C. R. Scriver, A. L. Beaudet, W. S. Sly, & D. Valle (Eds.), *The metabolic and molecular bases of inherited metabolic disease* (7th ed., pp. 1187–1232). New York: McGraw-Hill.

Burka, E. R., Weaver, Z., & Marks, P. A. (1966). Clinical spectrum of hemolytic anemia associated with glucose-6-phosphate deficiency. *Annals of Internal Medicine, 64*, 817.

Burke, G., Robinson, K., Refsum, H., et al. (1992). Intrauterine growth retardation, perinatal death, and maternal homocysteine levels. *New England Journal of Medicine, 326*(1), 69.

Burman, D., Holton, J. B., & Pennock, C. A. (Eds.). (1978). *Inherited disorders of carbohydrate metabolism*. Baltimore: University Park Press.

Campbell, R. A., Bruist, N. R. M., & Jacinto, J. D. (1967). Supertyrosinemia, tyrosine aminotransferase deficiency: Congenital anomalies and mental retardation. *Proceedings of the Society for Pediatric Research, 80*.

Carson, P. E., Flanagan, C. L., Ickes, C. E., & Alving, A. (1956). Enzymatic deficiency in primaquine-sensitive erythrocytes. *Science, 124*, 484.

Cerone, R., Scalisi, S., Cotellessa, M., et al. (1986). Dihydropterin reductase deficiency. Clinical, biochemical and therapeutic effects. *Journal of Inherited Metabolic Disease, 9*(Suppl. 2), 244.

Chace, D. H., Milligton, D. S., Terada, N., et al. (1993). Rapid diagnosis of phenylketonuria by quantitative analysis for phenylalanine and tyrosine in neonatal blood spots by tandem mass spectroscopy. *Clinica Chemica, 39*(l), 66–71.

Chen, Y., & Burchell, A. (1995). Glycogen storage disease. In C. R. Scriver, A. L. Beaudet, W. S. Sly, & D. Valle (Eds.), *The metabolic and molecular bases of inherited metabolic disease* (7th ed., 935–966). New York: McGraw-Hill.

Chitayat, D., Balbul, A., Hani, V., et al. (1992). Hereditary tyrosinemia type II in a consanguineous Ashkenazi Jewish family: Intrafamilial variation in phenotype; absence of parental phenotype effects on the fetus. *Journal Inherited Metabolic Disease, 15*(2), 198–203.

Chuang, D. T., & Shih, V. E. (1995). Disorders of branched chain amino acid and keto acid metabolism. In C. R. Scriver, A. L. Beaudet, W. S. Sly, & D. Valle (Eds.), *The metabolic and molecular bases of inherited metabolic disease* (7th ed., pp. 1239–1278). New York: McGraw-Hill.

Clark, B. J., & Cockburn, F. (1991). Management of inborn errors of metabolism during pregnancy. *Acta Paediatrica Scandinavica, 373*(Suppl.), 43–52.

Clark, B. J. (1992). After a positive Guthrie—What's next? Dietary management for the child with phenylketonuria. *European Journal of Clinical Nutrition, 46*(Suppl. 1), S33–S39.

Cleary, M. A., Walter, J. H., Wraith, J. E., et al. (1994). Magnetic resonance imaging of the brain in phenylketonuria. *Lancet, 344*(8915), 87–90.

Cockburn, F., & Gitzelmann, R. (1980). *Inborn errors of metabolism in humans*. New York: A. R. Liss.

Cohn, R., & Roth, K. (1983). *Metabolic disease: A guide to early recognition*. Philadelphia: W. B. Saunders.

Cooper, J. R., Bloom, F. E., & Roth, R. H. (1991). *The biochemical basis of neuropharmacology.* New York: Oxford University Press.

Cornblath, M., & Schwartz, R. (1966). *Disorders of carbohydrate metabolism in infancy.* Philadelphia: W. B. Saunders.

Cornblath, M., Wybregt, S. H., & Bacens, G. S. (1963). Studies of carbohydrate metabolism in the newborn infant. *Pediatrics, 32,* 1007.

Coskun, T., Ozalp, I., Kocak, N., et al. (1991). Type I hereditary tyrosinemia: Presentation of 11 cases. *Journal of Inherited Metabolic Disease 14*(5), 765.

Costello, P. M., Beasley, M. G., Tillotson, S. L., & Smith, I. (1994). Intelligence in mild atypical phenylketonuria. *European Journal of Pediatrics, 153*(4), 260–263.

Crawford, M. d'A., Gibbs, D. A., & Watts, R. W. E. (Eds.). (1982). *Advances in the treatment of inborn errors of metabolism.* New York: John Wiley.

Crawhall, J. C., Purkiss, P., Watts, R. W. E., & Young, E. P. (1969). The excretion of amino acids by cystinuric patients and their relatives. *Annals of Human Genetics, 33*(2), 149–169.

Dahlqvist, A., & Svenningsen, N. W. (1969). Galactose in the urine of newborn infants. *Journal of Pediatrics, 75*(3), 454–462.

Dalla Bernardina, B., Aicardi, J., Goutieres, F., & Plouin, P. (1979). Glycine encephalopathy. *Neuropediatrie, 10*(3), 209–225.

Dancis, J. (1972). Maple syrup urine disease and congenital hyperuricemia. In A. Dorfman (Ed.), *Antenatal diagnosis.* Chicago: University of Chicago Press.

Dancis, J., Hutler, J., & Rolkones, T. (1967). Intermittent branched chain ketonuria: A variant of maple syrup urine disease. *New England Journal of Medicine, 276,* 84.

Danner, D. J., & Elsas, L. J. II. (1989). Disorders of branched chain amino acids metabolism. In C. R. Scriver, A. L. Beaudet, W. S. Sly, & D. Valle (Eds.), *The metabolic basis of inherited disease* (6th ed). New York: McGraw-Hill.

Darras, B. T., Ampola, M. G., Dietz, W. H., & Gilmore, H. E. (1989). Intermittent dystonia in Hartnup disease. *Pediatric Neurology, 5*(2), 118–120.

de Franchis, R., Kozich, V., McInnes, R. R., & Kraus, J. P. (1994). Identical genotypes in siblings with different homocystinuric phenotypes: Identification of three mutations in cystathionine beta-synthase using an improved bacterial expression system. *Human Molecular Genetics, 3*(7), 1103.

Dent, C. E., & Westall, R. G. (1961). Studies in maple syrup urine disease. *Archives of Disease in Childhood, 36,* 259.

Dhondt, J. L., Farriaux, J. P., Sailly, J. C., & LeBrun, T. (1991). Economic evaluation of cost-benefit ratio of neonatal screening for phenylketonuria and hypothyroidism. *Journal of Inherited Metabolic Disease, 14*(4), 633–639.

Dixon, M. A., & Leonard, J. V. (1992). Intercurrent illness in inborn errors of intermediary metabolism. *Archives of Disease in Childhood, 67*(11), 1387–1391.

Dobyns, W. B. (1989). Agenesis of the corpus callosum and gyral malformations are frequent manifestations of nonketotic hyperglycinemia. *Neurology, 39*(6), 817–820.

Doherty, L. B., Rohr, F. J., & Levy, H. L. (1991). Detection of phenylketonuria in the very early newborn blood specimen. *Pediatrics, 87*(2), 240–244.

Duncan, J. R., Potter, C. B., Cappellini, M. D., et al. (1983). Aplastic crisis due to parvovirus infection in pyruvate kinase deficiency. *Lancet, 2*(8340), 14–16.

Duran, M., Dorland, L., De Bree, P. K., & Berger, R. (1994). Selective screening for amino acid disorders. *European Journal of Pediatrics, 153*(7, Suppl. 1), S33–S37.

Durand-Zaleski, I., Saudubray, J. M., Kamoun, P. P., & Blum-Boisgard, C. (1992). Inborn errors of amino acid metabolism. The best strategy for their diagnosis. *International Journal of Technology Assessment Health Care, 8*(3), 471–478.

Evans, M. I., & Schulman, J. D. (1991). In utero treatment of fetal metabolic disorders. *Clinical Obstetrics and Gynecology, 34*(2), 268–276.

Eyskens, F. J. M., Van Dororn, J. W. D., & Marien, P. (1992). Neurologic sequelae in transient nonketotic hyperglycinemia of the neonate. *Journal of Pediatrics, 121*(4), 620.

Falk, R. E., Cederbaum, S. D., Blass, J. P., et al. (1976). Ketonic diet in the management of pyruvate dehydrogenase deficiency. *Pediatrics, 58*(5), 713–721.

Falk, M. C., Knight, J. F., Roy, L. P., et al. (1994). Continuous venovenous hemofiltration in the acute treatment of inborn errors of metabolism. *Pediatric Nephrology, 8*(3), 330–333.

Fanaroff, A., & Martin, R. (Eds.). (1997). *Neonatal-perinatal medicine. Diseases of the fetus and infant* (6th ed.). St. Louis: Mosby–Year Book.

Fanning, J., & Hinkle, R. S. (1985). Pyruvate kinase deficiency hemolytic anemia: Two successful pregnancy outcomes. *American Journal of Obstetrics and Gynecology, 153,* 313.

Fenton, W. A., & Rosenberg, L. E. (1995). Disorders of propionate and methylmalonate metabolism. In C. R. Scriver, A. L. Beaudet, W. S. Sly, & D. Valle (Eds.), *The metabolic and molecular bases of inherited metabolic disease* (7th ed., pp. 1423–1450). New York: McGraw-Hill.

Fisch, R. O., Tagatz, G., & Stassart, J. P. (1993). Gestational carrier—A reproductive haven for offspring of mothers with phenylketonuria (PKU): An alternative therapy for maternal PKU [Review]. *Journal of Inherited Metabolic Disease, 16*(6), 957–961.

Fost, N. (1992). Ethical implications of screening asymptomatic individuals. *FASEB Journal, 6*(10), 2813–2817.

Fox, M., Thier, S., Rosenberg, L. E., et al. (1964). Evidence against a single renal transport defect in cystinuria. *New England Journal of Medicine, 270,* 556.

Francis, D. E. M., Kirby, D. M., & Thompson, G. N. (1992). Maternal tyrosinemia type II: Management and successful outcome. *European Journal of Pediatrics, 151*(3), 196–199.

Freese, D. K., Tuchman, M., Schwarzenberg, S. J., et al. (1991). Early liver transplantation is indicated for tyrosinemia type I. *Journal of Pediatric Gastroenterology and Nutrition, 13*(1), 10–15.

Furuta, T., Takahashi, H., Shibasaki, H., & Kasuya, Y. (1992). Reversible stepwise mechanism involving a carbonion intermediate in the elimination of ammonia from L-histidine catalyzed by histidine ammonia-lyase. *Journal of Biological Chemistry, 267*(18), 12600–12605.

Gahl, W. A., Finkelstein, J. D., Mullen, K. D., et al. (1987). Hepatic methionine adenosyltransferase deficiency in a 31-year-old man. *American Journal of Human Genetics, 40*(1), 39–49.

Gahl, W. A., Bernardini, I., Finkelstien, J. D., et al. (1988). Transsulfuration in an adult with hepatic methionine adenosyltransferase deficiency. *Journal of Clinical Investigation, 81*(2), 390–397.

Galjaard, H. (1980). *Genetic metabolic diseases.* New York: Elsevier/North Holland Biomedical Press.

Giardini, O., Cantini, A., Kennaway, N. G., & D'Eufemia, P. (1983). Chronic tyrosinemia associated with 4-hydroxyphenylpruvate dioxygenase deficiency with acute intermittent ataxia and without visceral and bone marrow involvement. *Pediatric Research, 17*(1), 25–29.

Gipson, I. K., Burns, R. P., & Wolfe-Lande, J. D. (1975). Crystals in corneal epithelial lesions of tyrosine-fed rats. *Investigative Ophthalmology, 14*(12), 937–941.

Gitzelmann, R. (1967). Hereditary galactokinase deficiency, a newly recognized cause of juvenile cataracts. *Pediatric Research, 1,* 14.

Goldsmith, L. A. (1983a). Tyrosinemia type II: Lessons in molecular pathophysiology [Review]. *Pediatric Dermatology, 1*(1), 25–34.

Goldsmith, L. A. (1983b). Tyrosinemia and related disorders. In J. B. Stanbury, J. B. Wyngaarden, D. S. Fredrickson, et al. (Eds.), *The metabolic basis of inherited disease* (5th ed., p. 287). New York: McGraw-Hill.

Goldstein, J. L., Hobbs, H. H., & Brown, M. S. (1995). Familial hypercholesterolemia. In C. R. Scriver, A. L. Beaudet, W. S. Sly, & D. Valle (Eds.), *The metabolic basis of inherited disease* (7th ed., pp. 1981–2030). New York: McGraw-Hill.

Goodman, H. M. (1977). Site of action of insulin in promoting leucine utilization in adipose tissue. *American Journal of Physiology, 223*(2), E97–E103.

Gravel, R. A., Clarke, J., Kaback, M. M., et al. (1995). The GM_2 gangliosidoses. In C. R. Scriver, A. L. Beaudet, W. S. Sly, & D. Valle (Eds.), *The metabolic basis of inherited disease* (7th ed., pp. 2839–2882). New York: McGraw-Hill.

Greenamyre, J. T. (1986). The role of glutamate in neurotransmission and in neurologic disease. *Archives of Neurology, 43*(10), 1058–1063.

Gregory, J. W. (1992). Antenatal diagnosis of inborn errors of metabolism [Letter]. *Archives of Disease in Childhood, 67*(l), 152.

Grobe, H. (1980). Homocystinuria (cystathionine synthase deficiency): Results of treatment in late diagnosed patients. *European Journal of Pediatrics, 135*(2), 199–203.

Haim, S., Gilhar, A., & Cohen, A. (1978). Cutaneous manifestations associated with aminoaciduria. Report of two cases. *Dermatologica, 156*(4), 244–250.

Hallock, J., Morrow, G. III, Karp, L. A., & Barness, L. A. (1969).

Postmortem diagnosis of metabolic disorders. The finding of maple syrup urine disease in a case of sudden and unexpected death in infancy. *American Journal of Disease of Children, 118*(4), 649.

Halvorsen, K., & Halvorsen, S. (1963). Hartnup disease. *Pediatrics, 31,* 29.

Halvorsen, S., & Gjessing, L. R. (1964). Studies on tyrosinosis: 1. Effect of low tyrosine and low phenylalanine diet. *British Medical Journal, 2,* 1171.

Halvorsen, S., Kvittingen, E. A., & Flatmark, A. (1988). Outcome of therapy of hereditary tyrosinemia. *Acta Pediatrica Japonica, 30*(4), 425–428.

Hammersen, G., & Bickel, H. (1982, August 16–21). *Proceedings of the International Meeting on Neonatal Screening* (p. 128), Tokyo.

Hanley, W. B., Clarke, J. T., & Schoonkey, T. W. (1987). Maternal phenylketonuria (PKU)—A review [Review]. *Clinical Biochemistry, 20*(3), 149–156.

Henderson, M. J., Holton, J. B., & MacFaul, R. (1983). Further observations in a case of uridine diphosphate galactose-4-epimerase deficiency with a severe clinical presentation. *Journal of Inherited Metabolic Disease, 6*(1), 17–20.

Hennekam, R. C., Beemer, F. A., Cats, B. P., et al. (1990). Hydrops fetalis associated with red cell pyruvate kinase deficiency. *Genetic Counseling, 1*(6), 75–79.

Hersov, L. A., & Rodnight, R. (1960). Hartnup disease in psychiatric practice: Clinical and biochemical features of three cases. *Journal of Neurology Neurosurgery Psychiatry, 23,* 40.

Heubi, J. E. (1993). Promising new treatment for type I tyrosinemia. *Journal of Pediatric Gastroenterology and Nutrition, 17*(3), 340.

Hilty, M. D., Romshe, C. A., & Delamater, P. V. (1974). Reye's syndrome and hyperaminoaciduria. *Journal of Pediatrics, 84*(3), 362–365.

Holme, E., & Lindstedt, S. (1992). Neonatal screen for hereditary tyrosinemia type I. *Lancet, 340*(8823), 850.

Holtzman, C., Slazyk, W. E., Cordero, J. F., & Hannon, W. H. (1986). Descriptive etiology of missed cases of phenylketonuria (PKU) and congenital hypothyroidism. *Pediatrics, 78*(4), 553–558.

Holtzman, N. A. (1992). The diffusion of new genetic tests for predicting disease. *FASEB Journal, 6*(10), 2806–2812.

Holtzman, N. A., Welcher, D. W., & Mellits, E. D. (1975). Termination of restricted diet in children with PKU: A randomized controlled study. *New England Journal of Medicine, 293,* 1121.

Hommes, F. A. (1991). On the mechanism of permanent brain dysfunction in hyperphenylalaninemia. *Biochemical Medicine and Metabolic Biology, 46*(3), 277–287.

Ifekwunigwe, A. E., & Luzzatto, L. (1966). Kernicterus in G6PD deficiency. *Lancet, 1,* 667.

Irons, M. (1993). Screening for metabolic disorders. How are we doing? *Pediatric Clinics of North America, 40*(5), 1073–1085.

Jagenburg, B. R., Lindblad, B., Magnus de Mare, J. M., & Rodjer, S. (1972). Hereditary tyrosinemia: Metabolic studies in a patient with partial *P*-hydroxyphenylpyruvate hydroxylase activity. *Journal of Pediatrics, 80*(6), 994–1004.

Jakobs, C., Stellaard, K., Kvittingen, E. A., et al. (1990). First trimester prenatal diagnosis of tyrosinemia type I by amniotic fluid succinylacetone determination. *Prenatal Diagnosis, 10*(2), 133–134.

Jepson, J. B. (1978). Hartnup disease. In J. B. Stanbury, J. B. Wyngaarden, & D. S. Fredrickson (Eds.), *The metabolic basis of inherited disease* (4th ed). New York: McGraw-Hill.

Johnson, G. J., Vatassery, G. T., Finkel, B., & Allen, D. W. (1983). High-dose vitamin E does not decrease the rate of chronic hemolysis in G6PD deficiency. *New England Journal of Medicine, 308*(17), 1014–1017.

Kalafatic, Z., Lipovac, K., Jezerinac, Z., et al. (1980). A liver urocanase deficiency. *Metabolism: Clinical and Experimental, 29*(11), 1013–1019.

Kamoun, P. P., Parvy, P., Cathelineau, L., & Meyer, B. (1981). Renal histidinuria. *Journal of Inherited Metabolic Disease, 4*(4), 217–219.

Kane, J. P., & Havel, R. J. (1995). Disorders of the biogenesis and secretion of lipoproteins containing the B apoproteins. In C. R. Scriver, A. L. Beaudet, W. S. Sly, & D. Valle (Eds.), *The metabolic basis of inherited disease* (7th ed., pp. 1853–1886). New York: McGraw-Hill.

Kaplan, P., Mazur, A., Field, M., et al. (1991). Intellectual outcome in children with maple syrup urine disease. *Journal of Pediatrics, 119*(1, Part 1), 46–50.

Kaufman, S. (1992a). Novel aspects of metabolism and function of tetrahydrobiopterin. *Journal of Nutrition Science and Vitaminology* (Special Issue), 492–496.

Kaufman, S. (1992b). Biopterin responsive hyperphenylalaninemia. *Journal of Nutrition Science and Vitaminology* (Special Issue), 601–606.

Keitt, A. S. (1966). Pyruvate kinase deficiency and related disorders of red cell glycolysis [Review]. *American Journal of Medicine, 41*(5), 762–785.

Khalifa, A. S., El-Alfy, M. S., Mokhtar, G., et al. (1989). Effect of desferrioxamine B on hemolysis in glucose-6-phosphate dehydrogenase deficiency. *Acta Haematologica, 82*(3), 113–116.

Khanna, R., & Chang, T. M. (1990). Characterization of L-histidine ammonia-lyase immobilized by microencapsulation in artificial cells: Preparation, kinetics, stability, and in vitro depletion of histidine. *International Journal of Artificial Organs, 13*(3), 189–195.

Kleijer, W. J., Horsman, D., Mancini, G. M., et al. (1985). First-trimester diagnosis of maple syrup urine disease on intact chorionic villi [Letter]. *New England Journal of Medicine, 313*(25), 1608.

Koch, R., Azen, C., Friedman, E. G., & Williamson, M. L. (1984). Paired comparisons between early treated PKU children and their matched sibling controls on intelligence and school achievement test results at eight years of age. *Journal of Inherited Metabolic Disease, 7*(2), 86–90.

Koch, R., Levy, H. L., Matalon, R., et al. (1993). The North American Collaborative Study of Maternal Phenylketonuria. Status Report 1993. *American Journal of Diseases of Children, 147*(11), 1224–1230.

Kodama, S., Yagi, R., Ninomiya, M., et al. (1983). The effect of a high fat diet on pyruvate decarboxylase deficiency without central nervous system involvement. *Brain and Development, 5*(4), 381–389.

Komrower, G. M. (1980). Inborn errors of metabolism. *Pediatrics in Review, 2*(6), 175–181.

Koyata, H., Cox, R. P., & Chuang, D. T. (1993). Stable correction of maple syrup urine disease in cells from a Mennonite patient by retroviral-mediated gene transfer. *Biochemical Journal, 295*(Part 3), 635–639.

Krnjevic, K. (1974). Chemical nature of synaptic neurotransmission in vertebrates. *Physiological Reviews, 54,* 418.

Kuhara, T., Inoue, Y., & Matsumoto, I. (1988). Urinary acid profiles of asymptomatic propionyl CoA carboxylase deficiency [Letter]. *Journal of Pediatrics, 113*(4), 787.

Kuroda, Y., Ogawa, T., Ito, M., et al. (1980). Relationship between skin histidase activity and blood histamine response to histidine intake in patients with histidinemia. *Journal of Pediatrics, 97*(2), 269–272.

Kvittingen, E. A. (1991). Tyrosinemia type I—An update. *Journal of Inherited Metabolic Disease, 14*(4), 554.

Kvittingen, E. A., & Brodtkorb, E. (1986). The pre- and post-natal diagnosis of tyrosinemia type 1 and the detection of the carrier state by assay of fumarylacetoacetate. *Scandinavian Journal of Clinical and Laboratory Investigation* (Suppl. 184), 35–40.

Langan, T., & Pueschel, S. M. (1983). Nonketotic hyperglycinemia: Clinical, biochemical, and therapeutic considerations. *Current Problems in Pediatrics, 13*(3), 1–30.

LeGrys, V. (1984). *The laboratory diagnosis of selected inborn errors of metabolism.* New York: Praeger.

Lemieux, B., Auray-Blais, C., Giguere, R., et al. (1988). Newborn urine screening experience with over one million infants in Quebec network of genetic medicine. *Journal of Inherited Metabolic Disease, 11*(1), 45.

Levy, H. L. (1973a). Genetic screening [Review]. *Advances in Human Genetics, 4,* 1–104.

Levy, H. L. (1973b). Genetic screening. In H. Harris & K. Hirschorn (Eds.), *Advances in human genetics.* New York: Plenum.

Levy, H. L. (1989). Effect of mutation on maternal-fetal metabolic homeostasis: Maternal aminoacidopathies. In J. K. Lloyd & C. R. Scriver (Eds.), *Genetic and metabolic disease in pediatrics.* London: Butterworths.

Levy, H. L. (1995). Hartnup disorder. In C. R. Scriver, A. L. Beaudet, W. S. Sly, & D. Valle (Eds.), *The metabolic basis of inherited disease* (7th ed., pp. 3629–3642). New York: McGraw-Hill.

Levy, H. L., & Benjamin, R. (1985). Maternal histidinemia: Study of families identified by routine cord blood screening. *Pediatric Research, 19,* 250A.

Levy, H., & Hammersen, G. (1978). Newborn screening for galactosemia and other galactose metabolic defects. *Journal of Pediatrics, 92*(6), 871–877.

Levy, H. L., Lobbregt, D., Sansaricq, C., & Snyderman, S. E. (1992). Comparison of phenylketonuric and nonphenylketonuric sibs from untreated pregnancies in a mother with phenylketonuria. *American Journal of Medical Genetics, 44*(4), 439–442.

Levy, H. L., Sepe, S. J., Shih, V. E., et al. (1977). Sepsis due to *Escherichia coli* in neonates with galactosemia. *New England Journal of Medicine, 297*(15), 823–825.

Levy, H. L., Shih, V. E., & Madigan, P. M. (1974). Routine newborn screening for histidinemia. Clinical and biochemical results. *New England Journal of Medicine, 291*(230), 1214–1219.

Levy, H. L., Taylor, R. G., & McInnes, R. R. (1995). Disorders of histidine metabolism. In C. R. Scriver, A. L. Beaudet, W. S. Sly, & D. Valle (Eds.), *The metabolic basis of inherited disease* (7th ed., pp. 1107–1124). New York: McGraw-Hill.

Light, I. J., Berry, H. K., & Sutherland, J. M. (1966). Aminoaciduria of prematurity. *American Journal of Diseases of Children, 112*(3), 229–236.

Lindblad, B., Fallstrom, S. P., Hoyer, S., et al. (1987). Cardiomyopathy in fumarylacetoacetate hydrolase deficiency. *Journal of Inherited Metabolic Disease, 10,* 319.

Lindblad, B., Lindstedt, S., & Steen, G. (1977). On the enzyme defects in hereditary tyrosinemia. *Proceedings of the National Academy of Sciences of the United States of America, 74*(10), 4641–4645.

Lindstedt, S., Holme, E., Lock, E. A., et al. (1992). Treatment of hereditary tyrosinemia type I by inhibition of 4-hydroxyphenylpyruvate-dioxygenase. *Lancet, 340*(8823), 813–817.

Litchfield, W. J., & Wells, W. W. (1978). Effects of galactose on free radical reactions of polymorphonuclear leukocytes. *Archives of Biochemistry and Biophysics, 188*(1), 26–30.

Lloyd, J. K., & Scriver, C. R. (Eds.). (1985). *Genetic and metabolic disease in pediatrics*. London: Butterworths.

Ludolph, A. C., Ullrich, K., Bick, U., et al. (1991). Functional and morphological deficits in late-treated patients with homocystinuria: A clinical, electrophysiologic and MRI study. *Acta Neurologica Scandinavica, 83*(3), 161.

Ludolph, A. C., Ullrich, K., Nedjat, S., et al. (1992). Neurologic outcome in 22 treated adolescents with hyperphenylketonuria. A clinical and electrophysiological study. *Acta Neurologica Scandinavica, 85*(4), 243–248.

Luzzatto, L., & Mehta, A. (1995). Glucose-6-phosphate dehydrogenase deficiency. In C. R. Scriver, A. L. Beaudet, W. S. Sly, & D. Valle (Eds.), *The metabolic basis of inherited disease* (7th ed., pp. 3367–3398). New York: McGraw-Hill.

Lyon, I. C., Gardner, R. J., & Veale, A. M. (1974). Maternal histidinaemia. *Archives of Disease in Childhood, 49*(7), 581–583.

MacLeod, P., Mackenzie, S., & Scriver, C. R. (1972). Partial ornithine carbamyl transferase deficiency: An inborn error of the urea cycle presenting as orotic aciduria in a male infant. *Canadian Medical Association Journal, 107*(5), 405–408.

Maestri, N. E., Hauser, E. R., Bartholomew, D., & Brusilow, S. W. (1992a). Prospective treatment of urea cycle disorders. *Journal of Pediatrics, 119*(6), 923.

Maestri, N. E., McGowan, K. D., & Brusilow, S. W. (1992b). Plasma glutamine concentration: A guide for the management of urea cycle disorders. *Journal of Pediatrics, 121*(2), 259–261.

Mahon, B. E., & Levy, H. L. (1986). Maternal Hartnup disorder. *American Journal of Medical Genetics, 24*(3), 513–518.

Markland, O. N., Garg, B. P., & Brandt, I. K. (1982). Nonketotic hyperglycinemia: EEG and evoked potentials. *Abnormal Neurology, 32,* 151.

Marshall, L., & DiGeorge, A. (1981). Maple syrup urine disease in the Old Order Mennonites. *American Journal of Human Genetics, 33,* 139A.

Matalon, R., Stumpf, D. A., Michals, K., et al. (1984). Lipoamide dehydrogenase deficiency with primary lactic acidosis: Favorable response to treatment with oral lipoic acid. *Journal of Pediatrics, 104*(1), 65–69.

Matalon, R., Michals, K., Azen, C., et al. (1991). Maternal PKU Collaborative Study: The effect of nutrient intake on pregnancy outcome. *Journal of Inherited Metabolic Disease, 14*(3), 371–374.

Mathews, J., & Partington, M. W. (1964). The plasma tyrosine levels of premature babies. *Archives of Disease in Childhood, 39,* 371.

Matsuda, I., Nagata, N., & Endo, F. (1983). A family with histidinemic parents [Letter]. *Journal of Pediatrics, 103*(1), 169.

Matsui, S. M., Mahoney, M. J., & Rosenberg, L. E. (1983). The natural history of the methylmalonic acidemias. *New England Journal of Medicine, 308*(15), 857–861.

McCabe, E. R., & McCabe, L. (1983). Screening for PKU in sick or premature infants [Letter]. *Journal of Pediatrics, 103*(3), 502–503.

McCully, K. S. (1993). Chemical pathology of homocystine. *Annals of Clinical Laboratory Science, 23*(6), 477.

McNamara, P. D., Pepe, L. M., & Segal, S. (1981). Cystine uptake by rat renal brush-border vesicles. *Biochemical Journal, 194*(2), 443–449.

Medical Research Council Steering Committee for MRC/DHSS PKU Register. (1981). Routine neonatal screening for PKU in the United Kingdom from 1964–1978. *British Medical Journal Clinical Research Edition, 282*(6277), 1680–1684.

Meister, A. (1965). *Biochemistry of the amino acids* (2nd ed.). New York: Academic Press.

Mentzer, W. C., Jr. (1993). Pyruvate kinase deficiency and related disorders of red cell glycolysis. In D. G. Nathan & F. A. Oski (Eds.), *Hematology of infants and childhood* (4th ed). Philadelphia: W. B. Saunders.

Mikanagi, K., Nishioka, K., & Kelley, W. N. (Eds.). (1988). *Purine and pyrimidine metabolism in man IV. Part A: Clinical and molecular biology.* New York: Plenum.

Mini symposium on tyrosinemia. (1990). *American Journal of Human Genetics, 47*(2), 302–342.

Missiou-Tsagaraki, S. (1992). Screening for glucose-6-phosphate dehydrogenase deficiency as a preventative measure: Prevalence among 1,286,000 Greek newborn infants. *Journal of Pediatrics, 119*(2), 293–299.

Misumi, H., Wada, H., Kawakakami, M., et al. (1981). Detection of UDP-galactose-4-epimerase deficiency in a galactosemia screening program. *Clinical Chimica Acta, 116*(6), 101–105.

Moore, M. R., & Meredith, P. A. (1976). The association of delta-aminolevulinic acid with the neurological and behavioral effects of lead exposure. In E. H. Delbert (Ed.), *Conference on Trace Substances in Environmental Health* (p. 363). Columbia: University of Missouri Press.

Mori, E., Yamadori, A., Tsutsumi, A., & Kyotani, Y. (1989). Adult-onset Hartnup disease presenting with neuropsychiatric symptoms but without skin lesions [Japanese]. *Rinsho Shinkeigaka—Clinical Neurology, 29*(6), 687–692.

Morrow, G. III, & Barness, L. A. (1972). Combined vitamin responsiveness in homocystinuria. *Journal of Pediatrics, 81*(5), 946–954.

Msall, M., Batshaw, M. L., Suss, R., et al. (1984). Neurologic outcome in children with inborn errors of urea cycle enzymopathies. *New England Journal of Medicine, 310*(23), 1500–1505.

Mudd, S. H., Skovby, F., Levy, H. L., et al. (1985). The natural history of homocystinuria due to cystathionine beta-synthetase deficiency. *American Journal of Human Genetics, 37*(1), 1–31.

Mudd, S. H., Levy, H. L., & Skovby, F. (1995). Disorders of transsulfuration. In C. P. Scriver, A. L. Beaudet, W. S. Sly, & D. Valle (Eds.), *The metabolic basis of inherited disease* (7th ed., pp. 1279–1328). New York: McGraw-Hill.

Nathan, D. G., Oski, F. A., Miller, D. R., & Gardner, F. H. (1968). Life-span and organ sequestration of the red cells in pyruvate kinase deficiency. *New England Journal of Medicine, 278*(2), 73–81.

Natowicz, M. R., & Alper, J. S. (1991). Genetic screening: Triumphs, problems, and controversies. *Journal of Public Health Policy, 12*(4), 475–491.

Naughton, E. R., Jenkins, J., Francis, D. E., & Leonard, J. V. (1982). Outcome of maple syrup urine disease. *Archives of Disease in Childhood, 57*(12), 918–921.

Nyhan, W. L. (1984). Hawkinsinuria. In W. L. Nyhan (Ed.), *Abnormalities in amino acid metabolism in clinical medicine* (p. 187). Norwalk, CT: Appleton-Century-Crofts.

Nyhan, W. L., Ando, T., & Rasmussen, K. (1972). Ketotic hyperglycinemia. In J. Stern & C. J. Toothill, C. (Eds.), *Organic acidurias.* London: Churchill Livingstone.

Nyhan, W. L., & Hilton, S. (1992). Histidinuria: Defective transport of histidine. *American Journal of Medical Genetics, 44*(5), 558–561.

Odessey, R., & Goldberg, A. L. (1972). Oxidation of leucine by rat skeletal muscle. *American Journal of Physiology, 223*(6), 1376–1383.

Ogata, E. (1986). Carbohydrate metabolism in the fetus and neonate and altered neonatal glucoregulation. *Pediatric Clinics of North America, 33*(l), 35–45.

Oizumi, J., Ng, W. G., Koch, R., et al. (1984). Partial ornithine transcarbamylase deficiency associated with recurrent hyperammonemia, lethargy and depressed sensorium. *Clinical Genetics, 25*(6), 538–542.

Origuchi, Y., Endo, F., Kitano, A., et al. (1982). Sural nerve lesions in a case of hypertyrosinemia. *Brain Development, 4*(6), 463–468.

Paige, D. G., Clayton, P., Bowron, A., & Harper, J. I. (1993). Richner-Hanhart syndrome (oculocutaneous tyrosinaemia). *Journal of the Royal Society of Medicine, 85*(12), 759–760.

Paglia, D. E. (1994). Biochemistry of the red cell. In R. Hoffman, E. J. Benz, Jr., S. J. Shattil, et al. (Eds.), *Hematology: Basic principles and practice* (2nd ed). New York: Churchill Livingstone.

Parini, R., Sereni, L. P., & Bagozzi, D. C. (1991). Continuous feeding as the only treatment in neonatal maple syrup urine disease. *Society for the Study of Inborn Errors of Metabolism Annual Symposium.*

Paul, T. D., Naylor, E. W., & Guthrie, R. (1980). Urine screening for metabolic disease in newborn infants. *Journal of Pediatrics, 96*(4), 653–656.

Peces, R., Sanchez, L., Gorostidi, M., & Alvarez, J. (1991). Effects of variation of sodium intake on cystinuria. *Nephron, 57*(4), 421–423.

Pentchev, P. G., Vanier, M. T., Suzuki, K., & Patterson, M. C. (1995). Niemann-Pick disease type C: A cellular cholesterol lipoidoses. In C. R. Scriver, A. L. Beaudet, W. S. Sly, & D. Valle (Eds.), *The metabolic basis of inherited disease* (7th ed., pp. 2625–2640). New York: McGraw-Hill.

Perry, T. L., Urquhart, N., Maclean, J., et al. (1975). Nonketotic hyperglycinemia. *New England Journal of Medicine, 292*(24), 1269–1273.

Peterkofsky, A. (1962). The mechanism of action of histidase: Aminoenzyme formation and partial reactions. *Journal of Biological Chemistry, 237,* 787.

Pitkanen, S., Salo, M. K., Kusela, P., et al. (1994). Serum levels of oncofetal markers CA 125, CA 19-9 and alpha-fetoprotein in children with hereditary tyrosinemia type I. *Pediatric Research, 35*(2), 205.

Pitt, D. B., & Danks, D. M. (1991). The natural history of untreated phenylketonuria over 20 years. *Journal of Pediatrics and Child Health, 27*(3), 189–190.

Ploos van Amstel, J. K., Jansen, R. P., Verjaal, M., et al. (1994). Prenatal diagnosis of type I hereditary tyrosinemia. *Lancet, 344*(8918), 336.

Pomeroy, J., Efron, M. L., Dayman, J., & Hoefnagel, D. (1968). Hartnup disease in a New England family. *New England Journal of Medicine, 278*(22), 1214–1216.

Potocnik, U., & Widhalm, K. (1994). Long-term follow-up of children with classical phenylketonuria after diet discontinuation: A review [Review]. *Journal of the American College of Nutrition, 13*(3), 232–236.

Probst, A., Cortes, R., & Palacios, J. M. (1986). The distribution of glycine receptors in the human brain. A light microscopic autoradiographic study using [3H] strychnine. *Neuroscience, 17*(1), 11–35.

Qu, Y., Miller, J. B., Slocum, R. H., & Shapira, E. (1991). Rapid automated quantitation of isoleucine, leucine, tyrosine and phenylalanine from dried filter paper specimens. *Clinica Chimica Acta, 203*(2–3), 191–197.

Ramus, S. J., Forrest, S. M., Pitt, D. B., et al. (1993). Comparison of genotype and intellectual phenotype in untreated PKU patients. *Journal of Medical Genetics, 30*(5), 401–405.

Rattazzi, M. C., Corash, L. M., Van Zanen, G. E., et al. (1971). G6PD deficiency and chronic hemolysis: Four new mutants—Relationships between clinical syndrome and enzyme kinetics. *Blood, 38*(2), 205–218.

Rice, D. N., Houston, I. B., Lyon, I. C., et al. (1989). Transient neonatal tyrosinaemia. *Journal of Inherited Metabolic Disease, 12*(1), 13–22.

Ris, M. D., Williams, S. E., Hunt, M. M., et al. (1994). Early treated phenylketonuria: Adult neuropsychologic outcome. *Journal of Pediatrics, 124*(3), 388–392.

Riviello, J. J. Jr., Rezvani, I., DiGeorge, A. M., & Foley, C. M. (1991). Cerebral edema causing death in children with maple syrup urine disease. *Journal of Pediatrics, 1*(1, Part 1), 42–45.

Robinson, B. H. (1995). Lactic acidemia. In C. R. Scriver, A. L. Beaudet, W. S. Sly, & D. Valle (Eds.), *The metabolic basis of inherited disease* (7th ed., pp. 1479–1500). New York: McGraw-Hill.

Robinson, B. H., MacKay, N., Petrova-Benedict, R., et al. (1990). Defects in the E2 lipoyl transacetylase and the X-lipoyl containing component of the pyruvate dehydrogenase complex in patients with lactic acidemia. *Journal of Clinical Investigation, 85*(6), 1821–1824.

Robinson, B. H., & Sherwood, W. G. (1984). Lactic acidemia, the prevalence of pyruvate decarboxylase deficiency. *Journal of Inherited Metabolic Disease, 7*(Suppl. 1), 69–73.

Rosenberg, L. E., Downing, S., Durant, J. L., & Segal, S. (1966). Cystinuria: Biochemical evidence of three genetically distinct genetic diseases. *Journal of Clinical Investigation, 45*(3), 365–371.

Rossiter, J. P., & Johnson, T. R. (1992). Management of genetic disorders during pregnancy. *Obstetrics and Gynecology Clinics of North America, 19*(4), 801–813.

Rossiter, B. J., & Caskey, C. T. (1995). Hypoxanthine-guanine phosphoribosyltransferase deficiency: Lesch-Nyhan syndrome and gout. In C. R. Scriver, A. L. Beaudet, W. S. Sly, & D. Valle (Eds.), *The metabolic basis of inherited disease* (7th ed., pp. 1679–1706). New York: McGraw-Hill.

Roth, K. S., Carter, B. E., & Higgins, E. S. (1991). Succinylacetone effects on renal tubular phosphate metabolism: A model for experimental renal Fanconi syndrome. *Proceedings of the Society for Experimental Biology and Medicine, 196*(4), 428–431.

Rowe, P. C., Valle, D., & Brusilow, S. W. (1988). Inborn errors of metabolism in children referred with Reye's syndrome. *Journal of the American Medical Association, 260*(21), 3167–3170.

Rubba, P., Faccenda, F., Pauciullo, P., et al. (1990). Early signs of vascular disease in homocystinuria: A noninvasive study by ultrasound method in eight families with cystathionine-beta-synthase deficiency. *Metabolism: Clinical and Experimental, 39*(11), 1191–1195.

Rutgers, M. J., Van der Lugt, P. J., & Van Turnhout, J. M. (1979). Spinal cord compression by extramedullary hematopoietic tissue in pyruvate kinase deficiency-caused hemolytic anemia. *Neurology, 29,* 510.

Sabater, J., Ferre, C., Puliol, M., & Maya, A. (1976). A renal and intestinal histidine transport deficiency found in two mentally retarded children. *Clinical Genetics, 9*(2), 117–124.

Salt, A., Barnes, N. D., Rolles, K., et al. (1992). Liver transplantation in tyrosinemia type I: The dilemma of timing the operation. *Acta Paediatria, 81*(5), 449–452.

Sassa, S., & Kappas, A. (1983). Hereditary tyrosinemia and the heme biosynthetic pathway. Profound inhibition of delta-aminolevulinic acid dehydratase activity by succinylacetone. *Journal of Clinical Investigation, 71*(3), 625–634.

Saudubray, J. M., Marsac, C., Cathelineau, C. L., et al. (1976). Neonatal congenital lactic acidosis with pyruvate carboxylase deficiency in two siblings. *Acta Paediatrica Scandinavica, 65*(6), 717–724.

Scher, M. S., Bergman, I., Ahdab-Barmada, M., & Fria, T. (1986). Neurophysiology and anatomical correlations in neonatal nonketotic hyperglycinemia. *Neuropediatrics, 17*(3), 137–143.

Schiffman, R., Kaye, E. M., Willis, J. K. III, et al. (1989). Transient neonatal hyperglycinemia. *Annals of Neurology, 25*(2), 201–203.

Schmidt, K. (1989). A primer to the inborn error of metabolism for perinatal and neonatal nurses. *Journal of Perinatal-Neonatal Nursing, 2*(4), 60–71.

Schmidtke, K., Endres, W., Roscher, A., et al. (1992). Hartnup syndrome, progressive encephalopathy and allo-albuminemia. *European Journal of Pediatrics, 151*(12), 899–903.

Schmitt, B., Steinmann, B., Gitzelmann, R., et al. (1993). Nonketotic hyperglycinemia: Clinical and electrophysiological effects of dextromethorphan, an antagonist of the NMDA receptor. *Neurology, 43*(2), 421–424.

Schuchman, E. H., & Desnick, R. J. (1995). Niemann-Pick disease types A and B: Acid sphingomyelinase deficiencies. In C. R. Scriver, A. L. Beaudet, W. S. Sly, & D. Valle (Eds.), *The metabolic basis of inherited disease* (7th ed., pp. 2601–2624). New York: McGraw-Hill.

Scriver, C. R. (1982). Screening for medical interventions: The PKU experience in human genetics. *Progress in Clinical Biological Research, 103*(Part B), 437–445.

Scriver, C. R., Beaudet, A. L., Sly, W. S., & Valle, D. (Eds.). (1995a). *The metabolic basis of inherited disease* (7th ed.). New York: McGraw-Hill.

Scriver, C. R., Kaufman, S., Eisensmith, R. C., & Woo, S. L. C. (1995b). The hyperphenylalaninemias. In C. R. Scriver, A. L. Beaudet, W. S. Sly, & D. Valle (Eds.), *The metabolic basis of inherited disease* (7th ed., pp. 1015–1076). New York: McGraw-Hill.

Scriver, C. R., Mackenzie, S., Clow, C. L., & Delvin, E. (1971). Thiamine-responsive maple-syrup-urine disease. *Lancet, 1*(694), 310–312.

Scriver, C. R., & Rosenberg, L. E. (1973). *Gycine, in amino acid metabolism and its disorders.* Philadelphia: W. B. Saunders.

Scriver, C. R., White, A., Sprague, W., & Horwood, S. P. (1975). Plasma—CSF glycine ratios in normal and nonketotic hyperglycemic subjects [Letter]. *New England Journal of Medicine, 293*(15), 778.

Shannon, K., & Buchanan, G. R. (1982). Severe hemolytic anemia in black children with glucose-6-phosphate dehydrogenase deficiency. *Pediatrics, 70*(3), 364–369.

Shaw, D., MacLeod, P. M., & Applegarth, D. A. (1991). Recurrent abortion and amino acid abnormalities. *Journal of Inherited Metabolic Disease, 14*(5), 851.

Shevell, M. I., Matiaszuk, N., Ledley, F. D., & Rosenblatt, D. S. (1993). Varying neurological phenotypes among muto and mut- patients with methymalonylCoA mutase deficiency. *American Journal of Medical Genetics, 45*(15), 619–624.

Shih, V. E., Coulombe, J. T., Wadman, S. K., et al. (1984). Occurrences of methylmalonic aciduria and Hartnup disorder in the same family. *Clinical Genetics, 26*(3), 216–220.

Shuman, R. M., Leech, R. W., & Scott, C. R. (1978). The neuropathology of the nonketotic and ketotic hyperglycinemias: Three cases. *Neurology, 28*(2), 139–146.

Smith, I., & Beasley, M. (1988). Intelligence and behavior in children with early treated PKU. *European Journal of Clinical Nutrition, 43*(Suppl. 1), 1–5.

Smith, I., Beasley, M., & Ades, A. E. (1991). Effect of intelligence of relaxing the low phenylalanine diet in phenylketonuria. *Archives of Disease in Childhood, 66*(3), 311–316.

Smith, I., & the Medical Research Council Working Party on PKU. (1993). PKU due to PAH deficiency: An unfolding story. *British Medical Journal, 306*, 115.

Smith, I., & Wolffe, O. H. (1976). Natural history of PKU and the influence of early treatment. *Lancet, 12*, 540.

Snyderman, S. (1965). The histidine requirements in infants. In R. Kluthe & N. R. Katz (Eds.), *Histidine: Metabolism, clinical aspects, therapeutic use.* Stuttgart: Georg Thieme.

Snyderman, S. E., Boyer, A., Roitman, E., et al. (1963). The histidine requirement of the infant. *Pediatrics, 31*, 786.

Snyderman, S. E., Norton, P. M., Roitman, E., & Holt, L. E., Jr. (1964). Maple syrup urine disease with particular reference to dietotherapy. *Pediatrics, 34*, 454.

Snyderman, S. E., Sansaricq, C., Norton, P. M., & Castro, J. V. (1981). Plasma and cerebral spinal fluid amino acid concentrations in phenylketonuria during the newborn period. *Journal of Pediatrics, 99*(1), 63–67.

Sokal, E. M., Bustos, R., Van Hoof, F., & Otte, J. B. (1992). Liver transplantation for hereditary tyrosinemia—Early transplantation following the patient's stabilization. *Transplantation, 54*(4), 937.

Somasundaram, O., & Papakumari, M. (1973). Hartnup disease. A report on two siblings. *Indian Journal of Pediatrics, 10*(7), 455–472.

Stankovics, J., Andrews, E., Wu, G., & Ledley, F. D. (1992). Overexpression of human methylmalonyl CoA mutase in mouse liver after in vivo gene delivery using asialoglycoprotein complexes. *American Journal of Human Genetics, 51*, A177.

Stave, U. (Ed.). (1978). *Perinatal physiology.* New York: Plenum.

Stern, L., & Vert, P. (Eds.). (1987). *Neonatal medicine.* New York: Masson.

Stifel, F. B., & Herman, R. H. (1972). Is histidine an essential amino acid in man? [Review]. *American Journal of Clinical Nutrition, 25*(2), 182–185.

Strobel, M., Fall, M., Kuakuvi, N., et al. (1978). Maladie de Hartnup. *Bulletin de la Societe Medicale d Afrique Naire de Langue Francaise, 23*(2), 118–123.

Svensson, E., Iselius, L., & Hagenfeldt, L. (1994). Severity of mutation in the phenylalanine hydrolase gene influences phenylalanine metabolism in phenylketonuria and hyperphenylalaninemia heterozygotes. *Journal of Inherited Metabolic Disease, 17*(2), 215–222.

Swenson, E. F., Walraven, C., & Levy, H. L. (1992). *A 25 year experience with newborn screening.* Paper presented at the 9th National Neonatal Screening Symposium, Raleigh, NC, April 7–11, 1992.

Tada, K. (1987). Nonketotic hyperglycinemia: Clinical and metabolic aspects. *Enzyme, 38*(1–4), 27–35.

Tada, K., Tateda, H., Arashima, S., et al. (1982). Intellectual development in patients with untreated histidinemia. A collaborative study group of neonatal screening for inborn errors of metabolism in Japan. *Journal of Pediatrics, 101*(4), 562–563.

Tada, K., Tateda, H., Arashima, S., et al. (1984). Follow-up study of a nation-wide neonatal metabolic screening program in Japan. A collaborative study group of neonatal screening for inborn errors of metabolism in Japan. *European Journal of Pediatrics, 142*(3), 204–207.

Tada, K., Yoshida, T., Hirono, H., & Arakawa, T. (1967). Homocystinuria: Amino acid pattern of the liver. *Tohoku Journal of Experimental Medicine, 92*(4), 325–332.

Tanaka, K., Armitage, I. M., Ramsdell, H. S., et al. (1975). Valine metabolism in methylmalonicacidemia using nuclear magnetic resonance: Propionate as an obligate intermediate. *Proceedings of the National Academy of Sciences of the United States of America, 72*(9), 3692–3696.

Tanaka, K. R., & Beutler, E. (1969). Hereditary hemolytic anemia due to glucose-6-phosphate dehydrogenase Torrance: A new variant. *Journal of Laboratory Clinical Medicine, 73*(4), 657–667.

Tanaka, K. R., & Paglia, D. E. (1995). Pyruvate kinase and other red cell enzymopathies of the erythrocyte. In C. R. Scriver, A. L. Beaudet, W. S. Sly, & D. Valle (Eds.), *The metabolic basis of inherited disease* (7th ed., pp. 3485–3512). New York: McGraw-Hill.

Tarlov, A. R., Brewer, G. J., Carson, P. E., & Alving, A. S. (1962). Primaquine sensitivity—Glucose-6-phosphate dehydrogenase deficiency. *Archives of Internal Medicine, 109*, 209.

Tedesco, T. A., & Mellman, W. J. (1967). Argininosuccinate synthesis activity and citrulline metabolism in cells cultured from a citrullinemic subject. *Proceedings of the National Academy of Sciences of the United States of America, 57*, 829.

Thomas, E. (1992). Dietary management of inborn errors of amino acid metabolism with protein modified diets. *Journal of Child Neurology, 7*(Suppl.), S92–S111.

Thompson, G. N., Butt, W. W., Shann, F. A., et al. (1991). Continuous venovenous hemofiltration in the management of acute decompensation in inborn errors of metabolism. *Journal of Pediatrics, 118*(6), 879–884.

Thompson, G. N., & Chalmers, R. A. (1990). Increased urinary metabolite excretion during fasting in disorders of propionate metabolism. *Pediatric Research, 27*(4, Part 1), 413–416.

Thompson, G. N., Chalmers, R. A., Walter, J. H., et al. (1990). The use of metronidazole in management of methylmalonic and propionic acidemias. *European Journal of Pediatrics, 149*(11), 792–796.

Thuy, L. P., & Nyhan, W. L. (1992). A screening method for cystine and homocystine in urine. *Clinica Chimica Acta, 211*(3), 175–179.

Todo, S., Starzl, T. E., Tzakis, A., et al. (1992). Orthotopic liver transplantation for urea cycle enzyme deficiency. *Hepatology, 15*(3), 419–422.

Treacy, E., Clow, C. L., Reade, T. R., et al. (1992). Maple syrup urine disease: Interventions between branched chain amino-, oxo-, and hydroxyacids; implications for treatment; associations with central nervous system dysmyelination. *Journal Inherited Metabolic Disease, 15*(1), 121–135.

Trefz, F., de Sonneville, L., Matthis, P., et al. (1994). Neuropsychological and biochemical investigations in heterozygotes for phenylketonuria during ingestion of high dose aspartame. *Human Genetics, 93*(4), 369–374.

Tschudy, D. P., Hess, R. A., Frykholm, B. C., & Blaese, R. M. (1982). Immunosuppressive activity of succinylacetone. *Journal of Laboratory Clinical Medicine, 99*(4), 526–532.

Uhlendorf, B. W., & Mudd, S. H. (1968). Cystathionine synthase in tissue culture derived from human skin: Enzyme defect in homocystinuria. *Science, 160*(831), 1007–1009.

Valentine, W. N., Tanaka, K. R., & Paglia, D. E. (1989). Pyruvate kinase and other enzyme deficiency disorders of the erythrocyte. In C. R. Scriver, A. L. Beaudet, W. S. Sly, & D. Valle (Eds.), *The metabolic basis of inherited disease* (6th ed). New York: McGraw-Hill.

Van Calcar, S. C., Harding, C. O., Davidson, S. R., et al. (1992). Case reports of successful pregnancy in women with maple syrup urine disease and propionic acidemia. *American Journal of Medical Genetics, 44*(5), 641–646.

van der Meer, S. B., Spaapen, L. J., Fowler, B., et al. (1990). Prenatal treatment of a patient with vitamin B_{12}-responsive methylmalonic acidemia. *Journal of Pediatrics, 117*(6), 923–926.

Van Gennip, A. H., Van Bree-Blom, E. J., Grift, J., et al. (1980). Urinary purines and pyrimidines in patients with hyperammonemia of various origins. *Clinica Chimica Acta, 104*(2), 227–239.

Von Wendt, L., Simila, S., Saukkonen, A.-C., et al. (1981). Prenatal brain damage in nonketotic hyperglycinemia. *American Journal of Diseases of Children, 135*(11), 1072.

Wahren, J., Felig, P., & Hagenfeldt, L. (1976). Effect of protein ingestion on splanchnic and leg metabolism in normal men and in patients with diabetes mellitus. *Journal of Clinical Investigation, 57*(4), 987–999.

Waisbren, S. E., & Levy, H. L. (1991). Agoraphobia in PKU. *Journal of Inherited Metabolic Disease, 14*(5), 755–764.

Wallach, J. (1983). *Interpretation of pediatric tests.* Boston: Little, Brown.

Wapnir, R. A. (1985). *Congenital metabolic diseases: Diagnosis and treatment.* New York: Marcel Dekker.

Webster, D. R., Becroft, D. M. O., & Suttle, D. P. (1995). Hereditary orotic aciduria and other disorders of pyrimidine metabolism. In C. R. Scriver, A. L. Beaudet, W. S. Sly, & D. Valle (Eds.), *The metabolic basis of inherited disease* (7th ed., pp. 1799–1840). New York: McGraw-Hill.

Webster, D. R., Simmons, H. A., Barry, D. M., & Becroft, D. M. (1981). Pyrimidine and purine metabolites in ornithine carbamyl transferase deficiency. *Journal of Inherited Metabolic Disease, 4*(1), 27–31.

Weinberger A., Sperling, O., Rabinovitz, M., et al. (1974). High frequency of cystinuria among Jews of Libyan origin. *Human Heredity, 24*(5–6), 568–572.

Wendel, U. (1984). Acute and long-term treatment of children with maple syrup urine disease. In S. A. Adibi, W. Fekl, U. Langenbeck, & P. Schauder (Eds.), *Branched chain amino and ketoacids in health and disease*. Basel, Switzerland: Karger.

Westall, R. G., Dancis, J., & Miller, S. (1957). Maple syrup urine disease. *American Journal of Disease in Children, 94,* 571.

Wilcken, B., & Turner, B. (1973). Homocystinuria: Reduced folate levels during pyridoxine treatment. *Archives of Disease in Childhood, 48*(1), 58–62.

Williamson, M., Dobson, J. C., & Koch, R. (1977). Collaborative study of children treated for phenylketonuria: Study design. *Pediatrics, 60*(6), 815–821.

Winick, M. (Ed.). (1979). *Nutritional management of genetic disorders.* New York: John Wiley.

Wolf, B. (1980). Reassessment of biotin-responsiveness in "unresponsive" propionyl CoA carboxylase deficiency. *Journal of Pediatrics, 97*(6), 964–966.

Wolff, J. A., Carroll, J. E., Thuy, L. P., et al. (1986). Carnitine reduces ketogenesis in patients with disorders of propionate metabolism. *Lancet, 1*(8476), 289–291.

Wong, P. W., Lambert, A. M., & Komrower, G. M. (1967). Tyrosinemia and tyrosyluria in infancy. *Developmental Medicine Child Neurology,* 9(5), 551–562.

Wu, J. T. (1991). Screening for inborn errors of amino acid metabolism [Review]. *Annals of Clinical Laboratory Science, 21*(2), 123–142.

Yalow, R. S., & Berson, S. A. (1960). Immunoassay of endogenous plasma insulin in man. *Journal of Clinical Investigation, 39,* 1157.

Yudkoff, M., Yang, W., Snodgrass, P. J., & Segal, S. (1980) Ornithine transcarbamylase deficiency in a boy with normal development. *Journal of Pediatrics, 96*(3, Part 1), 441–443.

Zinneman, H. H., & Jones, J. E. (1966). Dietary methionine and its influence on cystine excretion in patients. *Metabolism: Clinical and Experimental, 15*(10), 915–921.

CHAPTER 26

Assessment and Management of Endocrine Dysfunction

VIVIAN GAMBLIAN KIM BIVENS KIMBERLY S. BURTON
CAROLINE HOELL KISTLER TRACEY A. KLEEMAN CYNTHIA PROWS

RESEARCH AGENDA

Which factors in the perinatal period are related to the development of growth hormone (GH) deficiency in the neonate?

Is there a relationship between perinatal trauma and GH deficiency?

Is the premature infant at greater risk for GH deficiency than is the full-term infant?

Is there a relationship between transient hypothyroidism in a premature infant and the development of thyroid problems in later life?

Is there a relationship between respiratory distress syndrome (RDS) and an infant of a diabetic mother?

What are the risk factors for the development of ambiguous genitalia?

What is the relationship between heredity and environment in endocrine abnormalities in the fetus?

VIGNETTE

Timothy was born at 35 weeks' gestation to a 27-year-old primigravida. The mother's history was significant for Graves' disease, treated years before by subtotal thyroidectomy. The mother was maintained on Synthroid (levothyroxine sodium), with dosages varying between 0.05 and 0.15 mg daily. During the last month of pregnancy, a dosage of 0.05 mg/day was held steady.

Labor progressed quickly: 4 hours and 25 minutes. Rupture of the membranes revealed meconium-stained fluid. The infant experienced tachycardia during labor, but no other distress signs were noted. Timothy did well with suctioning on the perineum, and the cords appeared clear on laryngoscopic visualization by the pediatrician. Blow-by O_2 was given to improve the pale color.

On arrival in the nursery, the infant was assessed. Initial vital signs were temperature, 38°C; pulse, 180 bpm; respirations, tachypneic with clear breath sounds; peripheral blood pressure, slightly elevated at 67/35. Timothy had good muscle tone and demonstrated irritability when examined. Blood glucose was normal. He was weaned to room air, which he tolerated easily. An abnormal physical finding was exophthalmos, a bulging of the eyes along with edematous eyelids. Possible neonatal thyrotoxicosis was diagnosed.

At 3 hours of age, Timothy's respiratory rate increased to 90, and his O_2 saturation values decreased to 86 percent from his previously better readings. Gases indicated hypoxemia, so 30 percent O_2 per head hood was reinstated. His pale color and lab values improved quickly. Timothy's prematurity may have been sufficient cause for his tachypnea and O_2 requirement; however, chest x-ray films indicated that all lung fields were clear, with cardiothymic silhouette enlargement.

Timothy's tachycardia continued in the 160s to 170s range. His temperature remained at about 38°C. To determine whether the problem was thyroid based, an ECG was ordered and TSH, T_3, T_4, and CBC with differential were drawn; however, blood, urine, and gastric aspirates were sent for culture, in case infection was a possibility.

All infection indicators returned negative. However, Timothy's T_3 returned low, and T_4 measured greater than three times the normal level. It was decided by the endocrinology consult that Timothy's problem was indeed neonatal thyrotoxicosis. A plan was made to treat him with propylthiouracil (PTU) in split doses three times per day until levels stabilized.

Supportive nursing care included respiratory support with Oxy-Hood and status monitoring. Temperature regulation measures and monitoring were important owing to Timothy's hypermetabolic state. Cardiac monitoring for arrhythmias was continued. Of particular importance was fluid and electrolyte homeostasis, so accurate I&O calculations every 4 hours and daily weights were instituted. IV fluids for both fluid and caloric support were continued until PTU treatment was effective. Nutrition and feeding needs were very challenging because of Timothy's increased respiratory rate, constant level of fatigue, irritability when disturbed, and tendency to vomit. Diarrhea, leading to decreased nutrient and medication absorption, was a problem for several days prior to and at the beginning of his PTU therapy. Skin care became necessary in addition to the intensification of fluid balance and nutrition interventions. Decreased stimulation techniques were used to increase rest, decrease irritability and vomiting, and improve feeding behaviors and volumes. We took Timothy into a dimly lit feeding room away from the noise and lights of the NICU. Eye care with lubricating drops was begun to prevent corneal damage, as Timothy's eyelids did not close completely over his bulging eyes.

With stabilization of Timothy's thyroid function, discharge preparation became a focus. Techniques for administering his medication, as well as signs and symptoms to indicate thyroid or medication instability, were taught to his parents. They understood that the appropriate dosage would have to be adjusted as Timothy grew, and that he would be dependent on thyroid-suppressive treatment for the duration of his life. Eye care was practiced gingerly by the parents. Both understood and competently demonstrated well baby care, as they had often been involved with care during their visits to Timothy's bedside. The mother had more difficulty working with her baby to get the necessary medication doses "down the hatch." She became frustrated easily and often verbalized guilt related to the passage of thyroid problems to her son. The nursing team worked intensively with her, providing support, encouragement, and guidance for feeding techniques. Timothy was discharged at 3 weeks of age, and a home visit was scheduled for the next day to follow his progress and assist the parents with any further questions or concerns.

Joyce M. Dohme

Alterations in the endocrine system are common during the neonatal period. Unfortunately, these dysfunctions are normally complex, affecting other or all body systems. This chapter highlights the most common endocrine problems: (1) GH deficiency or excess, (2) syndrome of inappropriate antidiuretic hormone (SIADH), (3) hypothyroidism, (4) hyperthyroidism, (5) infant of a diabetic mother, (6) ambiguous genitalia, and (7) cystic fibrosis. The discussion begins with a review of the endocrine system, its organs, and the hormones it produces that regulate endocrine function.

PHYSIOLOGY OF THE ENDOCRINE SYSTEM

In utero, the placenta acts as the major endocrine organ, producing precursors for hormones, allowing movement of hormones across the membrane from maternal circulation to fetal circulation, and promoting steroid synthesis. Human chorionic gonadotropin (hCG), human chorionic somatomammotropin, human placental lactogen, and progesterone are the main hormones produced by the placenta. Early in fetal development, the organs of the endocrine system begin to take shape.

The endocrine system comprises several organs: the hypothalamus; the pituitary, pineal, thyroid, parathyroid, and adrenal glands; the gonads; and the pancreatic islet cells. The pituitary gland is composed of two main parts: the adenohypophysis (anterior pituitary) and the neurohypophysis (posterior pituitary). The pituitary begins to function at 8 to 9 weeks' gestation. The thyroid gland and its accompanying cells begin to secrete triiodothyronine (T_3) and thyroxine (T_4) and trap iodine by 11 to 12 weeks' gestation. T_3 and T_4 regulate thyrotropin-releasing hormone (TRH) by blocking its synthesis and the fetal secretion of thyroid-stimulating hormone (TSH). TSH cannot cross the placenta, but TRH can. The presence of hCG also effectively reduces TSH action. During the second half of gestation, the parathyroid gland and the chief and oxyphil cells form. The adrenal glands arise owing to the migration of neural crest cells. These cells are also responsible for innervation of the bowel and formation of the midline fusion. The adrenal medulla develops primarily from the neural cells. The cells in this region differentiate to produce norepinephrine- and epinephrine-secreting cells. The adrenal cortex's growth peaks at 16 weeks' gestation, with a gradual regression over the remainder of gestation and the first 6 months of postnatal life. At 16 weeks' gestation, the adrenal gland is actually larger than the metanephric kidney. The adrenal glands are capable of steroid synthesis by 8 weeks' gestation, even though the peak growth period extends over another 8 weeks.

The pancreas is one of the major endocrine organs; the islets of Langerhans constitute its endocrine portion. The islets of Langerhans contain alpha, beta, C, and delta cells. The alpha cells, which are present at 10 weeks' gestation, produce glucagon. The precursors of the beta cells, present by 13 weeks' gestation, produce insulin. The beta cells are fully functional by 14 to 16 weeks' gestation. The ability of the fetus to produce insulin is important because maternal insulin does not cross the placental barrier. The C cells and delta cells of the pancreas are derived from neural crest cells. Their function is not well delineated.

In addition to the major endocrine organs, other cells aid endocrine regulation. Endocrine cells are present throughout the gastrointestinal and respiratory systems and the brain; they are called *amine precursor uptake and decarboxylation cells* or *gastroenteropancreatic cells*. These cells are responsible for the secretion of peptide hormones. Gastrin cells, which are found in the regions of the pylorus and duodenum, secrete the hormone gastrin. Enterochromaffin cells, located in the gastric area, secrete serotonin. The delta cells—in the islets of Langerhans, the gastric area, and the small intestines—are responsible for the secretion of somatostatin. These hormones, along with the hormones produced in the hypothalamus, serve as the principal controls for a variety of metabolic activities within the human body. Hormone actions vary widely in type of action and rapidity of effect, with some effects occurring in seconds and others over a period of hours, weeks, or years.

The endocrine, or hormonal, system uses chemical substances (hormones) that are produced and secreted by a cell or group of cells into body fluids. The result is physiologic control of other cells and cell function. *Local hormones*, thus named because of their specific local effects, include acetylcholine, secretin, cholecystokinin, and many others. In contrast, *general hormones* are secreted by specific endocrine glands and are transported via the systemic circulation to distant points at which the physiologic action occurs. Some general hormones affect many body tissues, as does GH, which is secreted by the adenohypophysis, and thyroid hormone, which is secreted by the thyroid gland. The majority of general hormones, however, exert their effect only on specific target tissues.

Chemistry of Hormones

Chemically, endocrine hormones may be described as proteins, derivatives of amino acids, peptides, or steroids (Table 26–1). Most protein hormones link directly with nuclear DNA. They have long, complex chains, unlike the short chains of the peptides. Generally, peptide and protein hormones act rapidly, within seconds to minutes. Thyroid hormone and epinephrine and norepinephrine from the adrenal medulla are amino acids derived from tyrosine. They enter the cell membrane by combining with a specific receptor; their purpose is protein synthesis.

TABLE 26–1 Chemistry of Hormones

Hormone Origin	Protein	Peptides	Amino Acid Derivatives	Steroids
Pancreas	X			
Anterior pituitary	X			
Thyroid			X	
Adrenal medulla			X	
Posterior pituitary		X		
Adrenal cortex				X
Ovary				X
Testis				X

Steroids are secreted by the gonads and the adrenal cortex, which are derived from the mesenchymal layer of the embryo. Typically, the action of steroid hormones occurs slowly, over a period of hours or days. The action of steroid hormones causes protein synthesis in target cells, which then act as enzymes or carrier proteins to activate other cells.

Hormonal Control by Negative Feedback

The phenomenon by which endocrine hormones maintain appropriate levels of secretion is known as negative feedback. The hypothalamus is responsible for releasing hormones that move to the anterior pituitary by way of a hypothalamic-hypophyseal (pituitary) portal system. This system is not fully functional until about 15 weeks' gestation.

The releasing hormones act as stimulants on the adenohypophysis (anterior pituitary) to produce a specific trophic hormone. This hormone, in turn, acts as an inductor to stimulate a specific endocrine gland to produce yet another hormone that acts on a specific target organ. This mechanism produces a cascade effect.

In general, the specific hormone is secreted until the physiologic effect is achieved. At that point, information is transmitted that causes the producing gland to stop secretion. A critical blood level of a specific hormone is the determining factor that tells the hypothalamus to stop secreting releasing factors. Conversely, undersecretion results in decreased physiologic effects of the hormone. This feedback mechanism signals the need to secrete more hormone to again produce the appropriate physiologic response.

Mechanisms of Hormonal Action

Hormones affect the function of target tissues in a number of ways. They may alter the cellular chemistry, adjust the cell membrane permeability, or act on the cell as a whole. Some hormones stimulate adenosine 3′,5′-cyclic monophosphate (cAMP) to be formed in the cell. cAMP then triggers hormonal effects within the cell, acting as a "second messenger" for hormone mediation. See Table 26–2 for a list of hormones affected by cAMP.

Another intracellular hormonal mediator (or second messenger) is cyclic guanosine monophosphate (cGMP), which is similar to cAMP in structure and action, except that it contains the base guanine rather than adenine. Prostaglandins may also act as a type of intracellular hormonal mediator.

Hormone interaction with target tissues is dependent on the cell's recognition, via receptor sites, of specific hormones. This recognition is thought to be related to hormone receptor binding. The receptors may be membrane bound, cytoplasmic, or intranuclear. A receptor, by definition, is a cellular molecule that is highly selective in its affinity for a particular hormone. The result of the receptor's binding with a given hormone is regulated by the hormone. Thus, the hormone acts as a catalyst, or initiator, in the process but not as a participant per se.

Membrane receptors for hormones are specific in that the hormone binds with high affinity. However, other agonists and antagonists may also bind with the receptors. Numerous chemical and pharmacologic agents act as agonists or antagonists at the membrane receptor level. Hormone membrane receptors act to trigger the "first" message. The hormone itself triggers the "second" message, which culminates in the desired specific cellular event.

As mentioned, two types of second messengers are cAMP and cGMP. The action of cAMP is cell-specific. Both cAMP and cGMP act on cell protein kinases. Some hormone actions appear to attain their desired effect by reducing cAMP. The ratio of cAMP to cGMP appears to produce a metabolic balance. Hormones may also alter cell membrane permeability for certain substances. For example, insulin acts to facilitate glucose entry into certain cells.

TABLE 26–2 Hormones Affected by Cyclic Adenosine Monophosphate

Adrenocorticotropic hormone	Glucagon
Thyroid-stimulating hormone	Vasopressin
Luteinizing hormone	Secretin
Follicle-stimulating hormone	Catecholamines
Parathyroid hormone	Hypothalamic releasing factors

Intracellular Receptors

Some hormones (e.g., thyroid hormone) have receptors in the cell nucleus or within the cytosol. Many factors determine the intracellular binding of hormones. Only cells with specific receptors respond to the hormone. Additionally, intracellular hormone–receptor interactions are concentration dependent, have a limited period of effectiveness, and are reversible. It is believed that the hormone–receptor interaction triggers a regulatory protein that induces a specific change in the cell's DNA, ultimately causing a change in the genetic transcription that is necessary for protein synthesis.

ALTERATIONS IN THE ENDOCRINE SYSTEM

Growth Hormone

Human growth hormone (hGH) is a protein consisting of 191 amino acid residues. It is encoded by a gene located on the long arm of chromosome 17 (Rimoin, 1990). GH (somatotropin) is secreted from somatotroph cells in the anterior portion of the pituitary gland (Wallis, 1988).

GH is secreted in pulses rather than in a continuous manner. Secretion is under the control of two hypothalamic peptides: growth hormone–releasing factor (GHRF) and somatostatin (Gelato et al., 1987). GHRF stimulates the release of GH from the anterior pituitary gland. GHRF is thought to play a significant role in the magnitude of GH secretion. Somatostatin, in contrast, inhibits GH release and is thought to be the primary cause for the timing and duration of GH pulsatile release (Argente & Chowen, 1994).

The actions of GH influence growth rate (Hindmarsh et al., 1991). Proliferation and differentiation of various cells are affected by GH. Uptake of GH by liver and skeletal muscle cells improves amino acid transport and protein synthesis. Liver cells increase glucose output and produce insulin-like growth factors called *somatomedins*. The insulin-like growth factors, which are in synergy with GH, appear to stimulate skeletal growth. An anti-insulin effect occurs in muscle (Ganong, 1985; Wallis, 1988). In fact, GH has been used in the treatment of hyperinsulinemia (Hocking et al., 1986). Metabolism of carbohydrates is improved and circulating free fatty acid lipids are increased in the presence of GH (Ganong, 1985; Wallis, 1988).

As early as 10 weeks after conception, GH can be detected in the fetal anterior pituitary gland. High levels of GH in the cord blood of neonates have a fetal origin because GH does not cross the placental barrier. Concentrations of GH in full-term and premature newborns have not been statistically different (Bona et al., 1994). Despite high levels, GH seems to have little effect on gestational size. Rather, somatomedins appear to play a bigger role in fetal tissue growth and differentiation (Bona et al., 1994).

Based on studies of rat pups, Schanberg and Field (1987) suggested that certain tactile-kinesthetic stimulation may encourage GH release and protein synthesis in very small preterm neonates. Weight gain and awake active periods appear to improve when preterm infants are given appropriate stimulation. In all infants, a rapid decline of GH occurs 1 to 2 weeks postnatally; however, throughout the first 8 weeks of life, these levels are persistently higher than those in adults (Lanes et al., 1989).

Growth Hormone Deficiency

Pathophysiology

GH deficiency is not thought to be the root cause of the majority of short stature cases in humans. When GH and related hormones are involved, the cause of deficiency is variable (Wallis, 1988).

Various defects produce low levels or the absence of GH. For example, a defect of the hypothalamus limits stimulation of the pituitary to release GH. Developmental or degenerative lesions of the pituitary also prohibit GH secretion. The somatotrophs may be unable to produce GH if the gene response for its production is defective. Under such circumstances, target organs may be unable to respond to hormonal stimulation. Lastly, the hormone itself may be abnormal and rendered useless (Rimoin, 1990; Wallis, 1988).

Clinical Manifestations

To remain within the scope of this text, only clinical manifestations of neonatal and early infancy GH deficiency are described. Although GH deficiency can, in some cases, lead to short stature in childhood and beyond, it is not necessarily responsible for intrauterine growth retardation or small for gestational age neonates. Comparison of levels measured directly on cord and venous blood in neonates of average for gestational age and small for gestational age indicate that GH can be higher in small for gestational age neonates during the first 3 days of life. This higher level may be due to a resistance at the level of the hGH receptor or a insulin-like growth factor-1 synthesis defect (Varvarigou et al., 1994).

Neonates. Neonates with isolated GH deficiency can have height and birth weight within normal range (Herber & Kay, 1987).

The neonate with isolated GH deficiency often presents with persistent hypoglycemia, the mechanism of which is not clearly defined but which may be related to the production of insulin-like growth factors (somatomedins). Micropenis in the male is also a characteristic sometimes associated with GH deficiency (Herber & Milner, 1984).

Infants. Infants younger than 6 months of age often present with failure to thrive, poor feeding, and subnormal height velocity. Hypoglycemia may also be present in this age group (Herber & Milner, 1984). A thorough history and physical examination includes assessing the infant for pallor, lethargy, and excessive perspiration, which are also signs of GH deficiency.

GH deficiency can be a part of many different disorders. Any condition that disrupts GH production, stimulation, secretion, or tissue response can result in deficiency. For example, a neonate with congenital absence of the anterior pituitary gland manifests signs and symptoms like those in isolated GH deficiency. In addition, many other glands and hormones are affected because the pituitary is the master endocrine gland. Clinical features include early lethargy, hyperbilirubinemia, a minute penis in males, hypoplastic gonads and thyroid, hypoglycemia, cyanosis, convulsions, and circulatory collapse. Autosomal recessive inheritance has been suggested in this disorder (Rimoin, 1990).

Septo-optic dysplasia is a sporadic condition in which dwarfism with documented GH deficiency occurs. This developmental anomaly can involve defects in the brain, optic tract, and pituitary. An association of optic disk hypoplasia with an absent septum pellucidum was first described. Neonates with severe disease may present with hypoglycemia, hypotonia, prolonged jaundice, microphallus, and seizures. The young infant may present with defective vision, hypotonia, behavioral delay, and seizures (Rimoin, 1990).

Risk Factors

The incidence of GH deficiency has been quoted to be as high as 1 in 4000 and as low as 1 in 30,000 live births. This discrepancy has been thought to be due to missed diagnoses resulting from professional oversight rather than lack of parental concern (Vimpani et al., 1981). GH deficiency appears to be more prevalent in boys than in girls, with an incidence of 2:1 to as much as 4:1. However, these ratios reflect GH deficiency diagnosed throughout childhood and adolescence. Researchers propose that the ratios reflect the probability that boys are more likely than girls to seek medical attention for short stature (Herber & Kay, 1987).

There have been conflicting reports about whether perinatal trauma is a significant risk factor for GH deficiency. A study by Herber and Kay (1987) did not reveal a significant relationship between traumatic deliveries and subsequent GH deficiency. Breech deliveries were not studied separately in this research; however, other researchers report that patients with GH deficiency were more likely to have presented in a noncephalic fetal position. It is postulated that perinatal trauma or difficulty compromises the blood supply to the pituitary gland, which can result in deficient GH secretion (Aetiology of growth hormone deficiency, 1988).

Differential Diagnosis

There are several ways to diagnose GH deficiency. Direct measurement of GH is the first; however, the pulsatile nature of the hormone makes random measurements of little value. Maximal secretory levels must be stimulated either physiologically or pharmacologically and then measured. Attempts to characterize GH secretion in premature infants by quantifying urinary GH excretion also is inadequate. Immature renal proximal tubular function in both preterm and full-term neonates does not allow urine GH levels to depict endogenous GH secretion adequately (Tsukahara et al., 1993). It has been observed that the level of insulin-like growth factors is constant throughout the day, and low levels are seen in the majority of children with GH deficiency. However, many other factors influence circulating insulin-like growth factors; consequently, they have limited screening and diagnostic value for deficient GH (Lee & Rosenfeld, 1987). Work has also been done with GHRF. It is used to evaluate the GH-releasing capacity of the anterior pituitary gland. L-Dopa, glucagon, or propranolol combined with GHRF can also be used to evaluate hypothalamic function (Shimano et al., 1985).

Collaborative Management

Nurses caring for neonates with isolated GH deficiency manifested by persistent hypoglycemia should monitor vital signs and laboratory values closely. The nurse is an ideal person to ensure coordinated care from multiple disciplines. Parents need to be kept well informed throughout hospitalization. They may require encouragement and education about how to ask questions, assert their needs, and be their child's advocate. Current support systems for parents should be evaluated, and any necessary alterations suggested. If there is a suspected genetic cause of the deficiency, the family needs referral to a genetic center for evaluation and counseling.

Parents need to be taught how to give biosynthetic parenteral GH and any other medication that must be administered. Such teaching includes not only how and when to give medication but also how to recognize adverse side effects and signs and symptoms of toxicity. They also need telephone numbers of the local poison control center and health care professionals. Hormone replacement is a long-term need. The importance of compliance with medication therapy may need to be stressed repeatedly.

Recent reports indicate that treatment with biosynthetic human GH causes transient decreases in the percentage of B lymphocytes and T lymphocytes (Rapaport et al., 1991). For this reason, parents must be instructed to notify the physician in charge of GH replacement therapy if their neonate is having significant problems with recurring infections.

TABLE 26–3 Permeability in Presence of Antidiuretic Hormone

	Permeability			Active Transport of Na
	H_2O	Urea	NaCl	
Loop of Henle				
Thin descending limb	4+	+	±	0
Thin ascending limb	0	3+	4+	0
Thick ascending limb	0	±	±	4+
Distal convoluted tubule	±	±	±	3+
Collecting tubule				
Cortical portion	3+*	0	±	2+
Outer medullary portion	3+*	0	±	1+
Intermedullary portion	3+	3+	±	1+

*Values indicated by asterisks are in the presence of vasopressin. These values are 1+ in absence of vasopressin.

Adapted from Kokko, J. P. (1979, February). Renal concentrating and diluting mechanisms. *Hospital Practice, 14*(2), 113. Used with permission.

Syndrome of Inappropriate Antidiuretic Hormone

The survival rate of infants at high risk has greatly increased; the need for optimal management has increased concurrently. Infants with RDS and pulmonary disease, periventricular or intraventricular hemorrhage, meningitis, or perinatal asphyxia are at greatest risk for the development of problems associated with antidiuretic hormone (ADH) and renal function, affecting fluid and electrolyte imbalances. Fluid and electrolyte balance is one of the most critical and challenging issues faced in the neonatal intensive care unit environment. The goal of homeostasis of all physiologic functions requires a strong understanding of the neonate's complex body systems in order that supportive therapy may be successful.

The endocrine system, along with the autonomic nervous system, functions to maintain metabolic stability by compensating during times of stress, such as in the case of asphyxia. The kidney carries out the role of maintaining fluid and electrolyte balance by means of hormonal feedback mechanisms in response to osmoreceptors.

Physiology of Antidiuretic Hormone

ADH, or vasopressin (arginine vasopressin), is a hormone produced by the hypothalamus and stored in the anterior pituitary gland. It is normally secreted in physiologic states when there is an increase in serum osmolality. The primary function of ADH is to control fluid and electrolyte balance. It contributes to the adaptation to changes in intravascular (extracellular) volume by regulating renal clearance of free water (Weise & Zaritsky, 1987). ADH allows the renal distal tubules to absorb water from the collecting ducts and consequently decrease urine output. Specialized osmoreceptors in the anterior hypothalamus control the release of ADH in response to plasma osmolality. ADH also exerts a modest vasopressor effect on baroreceptors in the left atrium and carotid sinus, causing vasoconstriction in response to hypotension. Under normal conditions, the response of the kidney to plasma hypo-osmolality is to concentrate the urine maximally (Table 26–3; Fig. 26–1) (Kinzie, 1987). Hence, disorders that affect the release and actions of ADH are indicative of ineffective maintenance and balance of fluid and electrolytes.

Clinical Manifestations

SIADH is a condition in which there is increased secretion of ADH, which leads to water retention when there is already a low serum osmolar state or relative fluid overload. In this situation, the continued reabsorption of free water leads to plasma hypo-osmolality, hyponatremia, and expanded intravascular volume. Increased plasma volume results in an increased glomerular filtration rate and increased fractional excretion of sodium, further decreasing the sodium concentration (Kinzie, 1987). Signs and symptoms associated with SIADH secretion are indicative of water retention or edema. The most classic signs are low serum osmolality and hyponatremia accompanied by high urine osmolality.

Risk Factors

In the newborn population, the most frequent cause of inappropriate ADH secretion is asphyxia, with signs including low

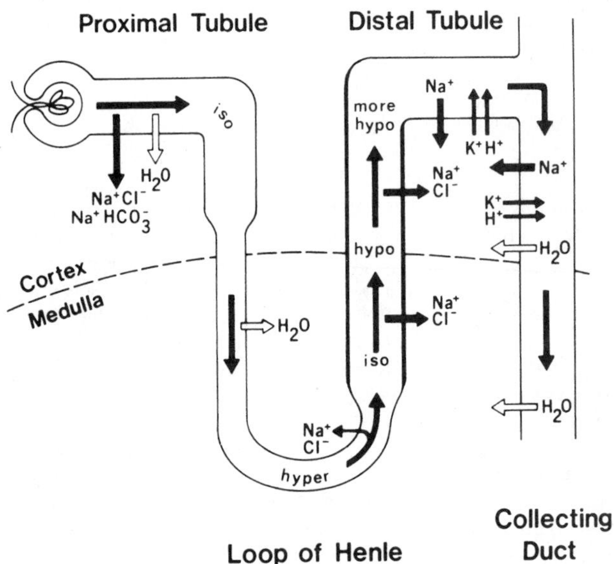

FIGURE 26–1. Tubular reabsorption and secretion. Summary of changes in the osmolality of tubular fluid in various parts of the nephron. The thickened wall of the ascending limb of the loop of Henle indicates relative impermeability of the tubular epithelium to water. In the presence of vasopressin, the fluid in the collecting ducts becomes hypertonic, whereas in the absence of this hormone, the fluid remains hypotonic throughout the collecting duct. Aldosterone promotes reabsorption of Na^+ and secretion of H^+ and K^+ in the distal convoluted tubule. (From Cannon, P. J. [1977]. The kidney in heart failure. *New England Journal of Medicine, 296*[1], 26–32. Reprinted with permission.)

serum osmolality; low serum potassium, chloride, and calcium levels; high urinary sodium levels in the face of severe hyponatremia; decreased free water clearance; and elevated urine specific gravity. SIADH has been reported in both term and preterm infants in association with meningitis, pneumonia, hypoplasia of the anterior pituitary and idiopathic vasopressin secretion, surgical repair of a patent ductus arteriosus, pneumothorax, pain, positive pressure ventilation, periventricular-intraventricular hemorrhage, and, as mentioned, perinatal asphyxia (Fig. 26–2) (Klaus & Fanaroff, 1993).

Differential Diagnosis

The diagnosis of SIADH assumes that there is normal cardiac output as well as normal renal, adrenal, and thyroid function. Therefore, these systems must first be evaluated for normal function before a diagnosis of SIADH can be made. It is based on laboratory findings and the clinical manifestations listed previously.

Collaborative Management

SIADH can mimic and be confused with clinical symptoms of other disorders and is often difficult to diagnose. Collaborative management of the clinical manifestations through early recognition and detection is essential in promoting recovery. The nurse must be familiar with the various conditions that place the neonate at risk for the development of SIADH. Interventions are therefore related to finely tuned assessment skills, with close attention to perinatal history, physical examination, and evaluation of laboratory and clinical data.

A vicious circle ensues if attempts are made to treat the hyponatremia and fluid imbalance with administration of sodium chloride infusions, because this intervention not only can exacerbate the hypervolemia but also can correct the hyponatremia only briefly because the sodium is quickly lost in the urine. The treatment of choice is fluid restriction, which decreases the availability of free water. Exceptions are if the serum sodium level is less than approximately 120 mEq/L or if neurologic signs such as seizures are present. More rapid elevation of serum tonicity may be achieved with furosemide (Lasix), 1 mg/kg intravenously every 6 hours, whereas urinary sodium is replaced milliequivalent for milliequivalent with hypertonic saline (3 percent solution). This therapy results in accelerated loss of free water with no net change in total body sodium. Fluid restriction alone should be relied on only after the serum sodium level exceeds 120 mEq/L (Cloherty & Stark, 1991).

Overall responsibility involves a high degree of sensitivity to infants at risk. The signs of SIADH include the following (values vary according to institution):

Hyponatremia	Serum sodium levels <135 mEq
Serum hypo-osmolality	Serum osmolality <275 mOsm
Urine hyperosmolality	Urine osmolality >1000 mOsm
High urine sodium	Urine sodium levels > 220 mEq/ 24 hours

Appropriate collaborative actions or interventions include (1) monitoring urine output, (2) maintaining intravenous fluids, (3) monitoring urine specific gravity and dipsticks with every void every 4 hours, (4) monitoring laboratory data and documenting the results of the renal panel serum and urine osmolarity and urine electrolytes, (5) notifying the physician or nurse practitioner of urine volumes exceeding the fluid intake and adjusting the intravenous fluids accordingly, and (6) monitoring for signs and symptoms of water intoxication. The signs and symptoms of water intoxication include irritability, lethargy, seizure activity, or a change in neurologic examination results or reflex activity. Bringing the delicate fluid and electrolyte balance of the infant with water intoxication back into control presents a challenge. It requires a diligent effort at collaborative care.

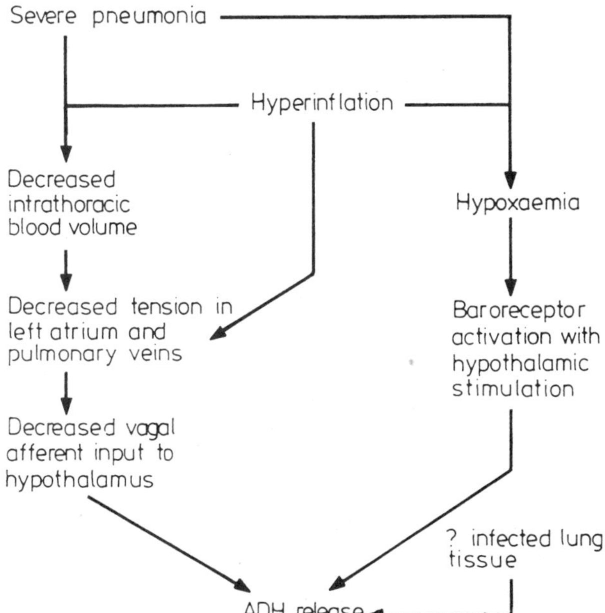

FIGURE 26–2. Possible mechanism of origin for syndrome of inappropriate antidiuretic hormone, ruling out pneumonia. (From Rivers, R. P. A., Forsling, M. L., & Oliver, R. P. [1981]. Inappropriate secretion of ADH in infants with respiratory infections. *Archives of Disease in Childhood,* 56[5], 361. Reprinted with permission.)

Thyroid Gland

Development

The first endocrine gland to appear during embryologic development is the thyroid gland. It begins to develop about 25 days after conception. The thyroid evolves from a thickening of epithelial cells at the base of the tongue. As the embryo grows and elongates, the thyroid gland grows a downward duct called a *diverticulum.* The diverticulum divides into the right and left lobes, which are connected by an isthmus that lies anterior to the developing second and third tracheal ring. By 7 weeks' gestation, the thyroid gland has reached its anatomic position in the neck (Moore & Persaud, 1993).

The thyroid gland is an H-shaped structure located below the larynx in the anterior middle portion of the neck. It is composed of many sac-like structures called *follicles.* These follicles are filled with a secretory substance called *colloid,* which consists largely of a glycoprotein–iodine complex, thyroglobulin.

Function

Thyroid function is apparent by 11 to 12 weeks' gestation. The thyroid has the ability at this time to accumulate and concentrate the iodine that is being produced. Synthesis of T_4 and iodine occur by 14 weeks' gestation. Secretion of the thyroid hormones is under hypothalamic pituitary control. The hypothalamus secretes TRH, which promotes release of TSH from the pituitary gland. TSH, in turn, stimulates the production of the actual thyroid hormones.

Physiologic Action of Thyroid Hormones

The principal functions of the thyroid gland are to synthesize, store, and release the thyroid hormones T_3 and T_4 into the circulating blood. T_3 and T_4 can be studied together because T_4 is the prohormone (stimulating hormone) for T_3. T_3, however, accounts for only 20 percent of the thyroid hormones in the blood.

The thyroid hormones stimulate the rate of cellular oxidation, which leads to a higher oxygen consumption and production of heat. The thyroid hormones affect protein, carbohydrate, and calcium metabolism. They also incorporate creatinine into the phosphocreatine cycle.

Transport of Hormones

Nearly all the thyroid hormones in the blood stream are transported by binding to three major proteins: thyroxine-binding globulin (TBG), thyroxine-binding prealbumin, and albumin. The binding of thyroid hormones by serum proteins is important for both physiologic and clinical reasons. Changes in binding protein concentrations or binding affinity can drastically change the total concentration of T_3 and T_4 measured in the serum. When TBG, thyroxine-binding prealbumin, and albumin are normally present in the blood, they serve to reduce the unbound (free) thyroid hormones. Since it is the free hormone fraction that is metabolically active, these binding proteins can exert a major influence on the thyroid gland. However, increases or decreases in serum T_3 or T_4 cannot be said to reflect an alteration in thyroid function until both the T_4-binding capacity and the level of free hormones have been estimated. These binding proteins appear to be involved in the transport of the thyroid hormones but not in facilitating transfer of these hormones into the cell (Walfish & Tseng, 1989).

Factors Altering Thyroid Hormone–Binding Capacity

In humans, TBG may be congenitally absent, reduced, or even elevated. Alterations in TBG levels can be sporadic or familial. Pedigree studies have shown that the TBG resides on the X chromosome. There is no male-to-male transmission; female offspring or affected males are carriers of this trait, and affected males show full expression of this defect.

Thyroid Hormone Levels in Newborns

The delivery process in the healthy, full-term infant creates a transient increase in TSH, which is believed to be mediated by TRH secretion in response to the cold extrauterine environment and ligation of the umbilical cord. This is accompanied by a sudden rise in T_3 and T_4 levels, followed by a decline over the next several days (Walfish & Tseng, 1989).

Neonatal serum TSH increases from mean cord serum values of 9 μU/ml to a mean peak of 85 μU/ml within 30 minutes after delivery. The placenta is impermeable to the passage of thyroid hormones from mother to fetus. Thus, the fetal hypothalamic pituitary–thyroid system appears to be independent of the maternal system. However, TRH is capable of crossing the placental barrier, thus producing some effects on the fetus. One of these effects is suppression of the fetal thyroid hormone production. With this knowledge, mass screening programs for recognition of neonatal hypothyroidism have been established and used on cord blood or neonatal heel blood.

Thyroid Screening. T_3 levels have been found to be increased in amniotic fluid early in pregnancy and to decrease gradually to cord serum concentrations, which are still higher than maternal values at term. The possible use of amniotic fluid T_3 or cord serum as a diagnostic tool has been proposed (Malvaux, 1981).

Premature infants frequently have low levels of T_4 when compared with the normal range for full-term infants. This condition is referred to as transient hypothyroidism. Serious illness is also associated with low T_4 values. In infants with gestations of less than 30 weeks, low levels of TBG may be present. After 30 weeks, TBG has reached the level present at term and therefore does not account for low levels of T_4 (Fanaroff & Martin, 1997). Cord blood levels of T_4 range from 6 to 15 μg/dl (Goetzman & Wennberg, 1991).

Thyroid Function Tests. Total T_4 ranges from 7.1 to 22.7 mg/dl during the first few months of life. Values vary in infants and children. Values accepted as within normal limits also vary by institution.

Congenital Hypothyroidism

Pathophysiology

Abnormal embryologic development of the thyroid gland is most frequently the cause of congenital hypothyroidism, which includes the absence of the thyroid gland or the lack of development of the thyroid (ectopic) (Malvaux, 1981).

Clinical Manifestations

The infant is usually more than 42 weeks' gestational age with a birth weight greater than 4000 g and may have a large posterior fontanelle owing to delayed ossification. There may also be respiratory difficulty from goiter compression. Hypothermia is another concern because thyroid hormones assist in thermoregulation. The infant may appear lethargic and hypotonic and have difficulty feeding as well as delayed passage of meconium. Abdominal distention may be present because of slowed gastric and intestinal motility. There may be an elongated nasal bridge, enlarged tongue, and hoarse cry. These symptoms are directly related to the function of the thyroid and its effect, along with GH, on (1) bone maturation, (2) calcium regulation, (3) temperature regulation, and (4) metabolic rate. A general slowdown of body functions occurs, including a shutdown or slowdown in terms of temperature.

Differential Diagnosis

To make a diagnosis of congenital hypothyroidism, blood is drawn for determination of serum T_3, T_4, and TSH levels. Most institutions use the filter paper spot technique, whereby a capillary blood sample from the heel is taken and placed on round filter paper, measuring T_4 levels. Approximately one third of all measurements are low and blood must be drawn again to confirm an abnormal TSH level. Another diagnostic aid is long bone radiographs. These are used to determine if the characteristic pattern of scattered bone growth centers are visible; if so, this is indicative of hypothyroidism. This picture is in contrast to one central location of growth normally found at the epiphyseal plate.

Collaborative Management

The goal of treatment is to establish a euthyroid state as soon as possible. Two types of thyroid hormones are available; one derived from the extracts of pork and beef is not used as frequently as is synthetic thyroid hormones. Thyroid extracts contain 0.21 percent iodide. Synthetic hormones are available as a sodium salt of L-thyroxine (levothyroxine sodium) and L-triiodothyronine (liothyronine sodium). The latter is more potent than the former, and its intestinal absorption is more complete. The metabolic effects appear and disappear rapidly. In the long run, it is preferable to use levothyroxine because the effects are longer lasting (blood TSH levels remain constant), and thus it need be given orally only twice a day. The cost of the synthetic hormone, which was once high, is now much reduced. The dose of thyroid hormone prescribed should be adequate to regulate metabolic functions. The T_4 level should increase rapidly to ensure a euthyroid level of this hormone. The dose of levothyroxine during the newborn period is 8 to 10 μg/kg/day for most full-term infants (Goetzman & Wennberg, 1991). The prognosis for mental development has been correlated with the onset of hormone replacement therapy (Malvaux, 1981). Delay in instituting hormone replacement therapy or noncompliance with its administration leads to mental retardation. Parents and caregivers need to be informed of the dire consequences associated with the infants not receiving their medication.

Over the first few days after the initiation of replacement therapy, observations must be made for cardiac problems. Cardiac failure or arrhythmias are possible. The infant becomes more active and body temperature normalizes as therapeutic levels are reached. Observation of growth is crucial because it can be the only indicator that treatment is truly successful.

Before medication is deemed effective, metabolic demand is decreased. Thus, the activity of the infant may be reduced because of fatigue and weakness. Constipation may result owing to decreased peristaltic action. The infant may become edematous secondary to infiltration of fluid into interstitial tissues. Cold intolerance may also develop, leading to discomfort.

Congenital Hyperthyroidism

Neonatal hyperthyroidism is serious and potentially life-threatening. The infant may be born with a very small goiter or even a small thyroid gland. Serum T_4 levels may be low, normal, or even high at birth, depending on the degree of in utero thyroid suppression. Most often, this neonatal thyrotoxicosis is due to maternal Graves' disease. The condition may be temporary in the neonatal period (Becks & Burrow, 1990).

Infant of a Hyperthyroid Mother

Maternal hyperthyroidism is present in 1 in 500 pregnancies (Becks & Burrow, 1990). This hyperthyroidism creates a great threat to the unborn fetus, with an increase in spontaneous abortions as well as premature births (Parks, 1981). After the first trimester, the maternal-fetal pituitary–thyroid axes are independent. T_3, T_4, and TSH do not cross the placenta, but antibodies in the form of immunoglobulin G do cross the placental barrier. These antibodies act on the thyroid gland of the fetus, causing thyroid function and GH to be increased. The hyperthyroid state occurs as the passage of these antibodies increases during the second and third trimesters of pregnancy. Maternal antithyroid medications and stable iodine can also affect the fetus and neonate (Becks & Burrow, 1990). These substances, although effective therapy for both mother and fetus because they cross the placenta, can also affect the fetus adversely. Therefore, the use of stable iodine in pregnant women is contraindicated because of the blockage of fetal thyroid hormone release, which, in turn, leads to hypothyroidism and goiter. Excess dosage of maternal antithyroid medications is also likely to cause fetal and neonatal hypothyroidism.

Differential Diagnosis

The diagnosis of fetal and neonatal hyperthyroidism is determined by the presence of maternal thyroid-stimulating antibodies and clinical manifestations (Becks & Burrow, 1990).

Clinical Manifestations

Heart rates of 160 bpm or greater, goiter, intrauterine growth retardation, mature bone growth greater than expected for gestational age, and craniosynostosis are the common signs and symptoms of hyperthyroidism (Becks & Burrow, 1990).

Treatment

The overall objective of therapy is to restore and maintain a euthyroid state. This can be achieved in a variety of ways. No single therapy is ideal. One technique is to use medications that interfere with thyroid hormone synthesis. Methimazole and carbimazole are used throughout the United States. These drugs decrease the active transport of iodine into the thyroid gland. Propranolol is given to the severely hyperthyroid infant to reduce heart rate and lessen tremors. This drug is generally used in the first week of replacement therapy.

If medical treatment is not chosen as a mode to restore the infant to a euthyroid state, or is not effective, surgical removal of part or all of the thyroid gland is possible. However, hypothyroidism may result even if only a small portion of the thyroid is removed.

Radioiodine treatment is another alternative treatment. Beta emissions cause local tissue damage. The radiation dose given is dependent on the individual mass and geometry of the thyroid gland. Reservations about the use of radioiodine therapy in children relate to concerns about the development of thyroid carcinoma or leukemia during adulthood. Damage to the thymus gland, a major immune organ in the neonate, is possible, which leaves the neonate vulnerable to infections.

Collaborative Management

The disease process of hyperthyroidism results in increased metabolic demands (Avery et al., 1994). These infants need a higher caloric intake, often greater than 180 kcal/kg/day (up from about 100 to 120 kcal/kg/day) to maintain positive growth. Providing adequate nutrition with sufficient caloric intake is essential to the well-being of these infants. Propranolol may be used to decrease the heart rate and to combat the occurrence of heart failure (Avery et al., 1994).

These neonates also experience fatigue and exhaustion owing to the hypermetabolic state and use of energy stores (Parks, 1981). Diarrhea may result because of increased peristalsis, thus leading to even more loss of nutrients as well as fluids. Heat intolerance and profound diaphoresis are side effects of the increased basal metabolic rate. Another feature of these infants is an eye malformation called exophthalmos. This condition is a concern because of the inability of the infant's eyelid to close completely. The cornea dries, and abrasions are possible from normal eye and lid movements. Lubricating drops or ointment should be used to protect the eye from damage.

It is essential that accurate intake and output be documented every 4 hours and that weights be obtained daily in these infants. Head circumference and growth curve determinations should be performed at least weekly. The parents need to understand that thyroid therapy for either hypothyroidism or hyperthyroidism is a lifelong commitment.

Diabetes

Infant of a Diabetic Mother

Maternal Considerations. During pregnancy, a woman experiences increasing levels of estrogen and progesterone. This hormonal increase stimulates pancreatic beta cell hyperplasia and increases the secretion of insulin. This pancreatic beta cell hyperplasia continues as the pregnancy progresses. Pregnant women with diabetes also experience these hormonal changes, making it more difficult to manage their glucose levels (Hoskins, 1990).

Gestational diabetes occurs during pregnancy and is usually self-limited to the pregnancy. It occurs in 2 to 3 percent of pregnancies (Sills & Rapaport, 1994). Proper screening during pregnancy is essential for all women in order to monitor accurately for glucose intolerance. One must be aware of certain risk factors that may predispose a woman to gestational diabetes. These risk factors include a previous pregnancy with gestational diabetes, obesity, or a previous infant macrosomatia seen by ultrasonography, maternal glycosuria, or uterine size larger than normal for gestational date.

The severity of maternal diabetes and the duration of the disease contribute to how the infant may be affected. The severity of maternal diabetes can be determined by using White's (1974) Classification of the Disease Process:

A Gestational diabetic; controlled by diet
B Onset after age 20; duration > 10 years
C Onset age 10 to 19; duration 10 to 19 years
D Onset before age 10; duration < 20 years; retinitis; hypertension; calcification in the lower extremities
F Nephropathy
R Malignant retinitis

No matter what the maternal class is, the fetus is at risk for many problems. These problems include spontaneous abortion, stillbirth, cephalopelvic disproportion (CPD), asphyxia, respiratory distress, hypoglycemia, macrosomatia, congenital anomalies, hypocalcemia, hypomagnesemia, hyperbilirubinemia, and polycythemia. The morbidity of these problems can be diminished with good prenatal care and proper glucose regulation during the antenatal and intrapartum periods. Maintaining glucose control before conception or early in the pregnancy is essential for the woman with insulin-dependent diabetes mellitus. This control offers the infant a better chance for a positive outcome. One of the major neonatal problems is a labile glucose level.

Fetal and Neonatal Risks

HYPOGLYCEMIA. Hypoglycemia is signified by a blood glucose level less than 40 mg/dl for the term infant and less than 20 mg/dl for the preterm infant. The fetus is exposed to large amounts of glucose, as maternal glucose readily crosses the placenta. Knip and associates (1983) noted that the glucose content of the amniotic fluid in diabetic women is higher than normal. The reason for this increase is that insulin is a larger molecule than glucose and it does not cross the placenta easily, so maternal glucose levels are mirrored with the neonatal system and amniotic fluid.

This maternal hyperglycemia leads to fetal hyperglycemia. Since maternal insulin does not cross the placenta, elevated glucose levels stimulate the fetal pancreas to secrete insulin. This stimulation also leads to hyperplasia of the beta cells and increased production of insulin, which continues after delivery. Insulin is the main growth hormone for the fetus, so this hyperinsulinemia leads to fat accumulation and macrosomatia (Hoskins, 1990).

Because of this hyperinsulinism and then the loss of maternal glucose at delivery, the infant can become hypoglycemic within a few hours after delivery and must be monitored closely. Common signs of hypoglycemia are jitteriness, cyanosis, irritability, seizures, and apnea. Serum glucose levels need to be monitored frequently. Giving the infant early feedings or intravenous fluids to maintain a proper glucose level may be necessary.

MACROSOMATIA. According to Schwartz and associates (1994), despite better control of glucose levels in the pregnant woman with diabetes, macrosomatia (birth weight >4 kg for a term infant) continues to occur at a high rate. It is felt that this is a result of fetal hyperinsulinemia.

The infant of a diabetic mother has a characteristic appearance. These infants are large for gestational age with increased adipose tissue, have a full face liberally covered with vernix, and are plethoric. The placenta and umbilical cord are also large.

Growth acceleration is especially apparent in infants of mothers with poorly controlled diabetes. These infants have a smaller head circumference:weight ratio and a larger weight:length ratio. Woods and colleagues (1980) found that the body proportions were appropriate in infants of mothers with well-controlled diabetes. They also observed that all infants of diabetic mothers presented with hairy pinna but that it is more distinct in infants of mothers with poorly controlled diabetes.

Infants of diabetic mothers can experience CPD, leading to difficult deliveries secondary to their size. Birth trauma includes brachial plexus trauma, fractured clavicle, facial palsy, shoulder dystocia, asphyxia, and subdural hemorrhage. One must also be prepared for birth asphyxia resulting from CPD. The mother's ability to deliver vaginally must be assessed and cesarean section performed for CPD to avert complications.

RESPIRATORY DISTRESS SYNDROME. Also known as hyaline membrane disease, RDS is a disease in which there is a decreased amount of surfactant. This lack of surfactant leads to alveolar collapse and an inability to ventilate adequately. Pulmonary surfactant is a lipoprotein produced by alveolar type II epithelial cells. After formation, it is secreted into the alveolar space, where it forms a film that covers the alveolar surface and creates the needed surface tension to maintain alveolar expansion.

Recent research has shown that the pregnant diabetic woman may have a disorder in the production of the lipoprotein. Lung development in the infant of a diabetic mother is related to the pregnant woman's glucose control during the pregnancy (Zapata et al., 1994). According to Neufeld (1987), hyperinsulinemia influences the fetal lung maturity in infants of diabetic mothers by inhibiting the fetal lung synthesis of surfactant.

Zapata and associates (1994) conducted a study looking at the association between the presence of hypoglycemic episodes and fetal lung maturity. They found a significant association between episodes of hypoglycemia during the pregnancy and improved fetal lung maturity. The hypoglycemia acts as a stressor and accelerates the maturation of the fetal lung.

Early literature documented that respiratory distress occurred frequently in infants of diabetic mothers. Perelman (1983) suggested that in the case of poorly controlled diabetes in the mother, respiratory distress is almost inevitable for the infant because of impaired maturation of the lungs.

More recent literature and studies have shown that with advances and proper management of diabetic mothers and their infants, RDS is not as much a problem as it once was. Mimouni and colleagues (1987) studied 127 pregnant diabetic women and their newborn infants using a comprehensive computer base. In this study, 127 infants of diabetic mothers were matched to 127 infants of nondiabetic mothers. Specific matching criteria for respiratory status, sex, gestational age, and race were used. Impressions based on the matching criteria revealed no overall significant difference. They concluded that with current practice and management, RDS is not a direct risk factor of diabetes.

One still must be aware of the chance for respiratory distress. Some women with poor diabetes control or poor prenatal care

are at risk for having infants with RDS secondary to surfactant deficiency and not gestational age.

HYPOCALCEMIA AND HYPOMAGNESEMIA. Hypocalcemia and hypomagnesemia are major metabolic problems exhibited by infants of diabetic mothers. The incidence is related to the severity of the maternal diabetes; both problems must be followed closely. The symptoms are similar to those seen with hypoglycemia (Perelman, 1983).

Hypocalcemia develops within the first 3 days of life and is seen primarily in the infant of the insulin-dependent diabetic mother. It is thought that hypocalcemia may be secondary to decreased hypoparathyroid functioning resulting from hypomagnesemia. The infant should be observed for hypocalcemia and hypomagnesemia and treated as needed (Cowett & Schwartz, 1982).

HYPERBILIRUBINEMIA AND POLYCYTHEMIA. Hyperbilirubinemia is a common occurrence in the infant of a diabetic mother. Most infants of diabetic mothers have the unconjugated form of bilirubin circulating in their systems. This finding suggests an impairment of the glucuronidation system (Neufeld, 1987). Hyperbilirubinemia may also be related to decreased albumin levels, leaving less albumin available for binding bilirubin.

Polycythemia is also frequently observed in infants of diabetic mothers. The infant with polycythemia may exhibit signs and symptoms such as jitteriness, tachypnea, cyanosis, priapism, and oliguria. Treatment is usually a partial exchange transfusion using normal saline, plasma protein fraction (Plasmanate), or 5 percent albumin (Cowett & Schwartz, 1982).

A complication of polycythemia that occurs frequently in infants of diabetic mothers is renal vein thrombosis. Signs include hematuria and a palpable renal mass. Renal vein thrombosis is usually treated medically, but on rare occasions a nephrectomy may be required (Neufeld, 1987).

CONGENITAL ANOMALIES. The most significant source of morbidity and mortality in the infant of a diabetic mother is major congenital anomalies. It is thought that hyperglucosemia occurring early in pregnancy is teratogenic (Rose et al., 1988). Preconceptual glucose control is essential because anomalies may occur before the woman knows she is pregnant. Many of these defects occur before the seventh week of gestation as a result of maternal hyperglycemia, which inhibits cellular mitosis, resulting in anomalies (Hitti et al., 1994; Hoskins, 1990; Novak & Robinson, 1994).

Rose and associates (1988) found a correlation between the occurrence of congenital anomalies and high glycosylated hemoglobin levels. The most common anomalies involve the cardiac, musculoskeletal, and central nervous systems. The occurrence of congenital heart disease in the infant of a diabetic mother can be as high as five times that of normal infants. Atrial or ventricular septal defects, transposition of the great vessels, and coarctation of the aorta are the most common heart lesions seen.

Hitti and associates (1994) found an increase in the frequency of skeletal malformations. These infants are at risk for delayed ossification and osseous defects. Caudal regression syndrome is a common malformation, as is agenesis or hypoplasia of the femur. Central nervous system anomalies include hydrocephalus, meningomyelocele, and anencephaly. These areas of development are usually completed by the seventh week after conception (Perelman, 1983).

Another congenital defect is the small left colon syndrome. This syndrome does not occur very often, and there is not much known about it. A possible cause is a spasm of the ileum as a result of high glucagon levels (Kenner et al., 1988). It usually resolves spontaneously early in the neonate's life without the need for surgical intervention (Cowett & Schwartz, 1982). Maintaining hydration and gastric decompression is necessary, as is monitoring for infection. Once feedings are initiated, the infant should be observed closely for bowel obstruction.

Collaborative Management. The nurse, in collaboration with the health care team, needs to observe the infant of a diabetic mother closely after delivery to provide quick intervention if problems arise. The infant of a diabetic mother must be monitored for signs and symptoms of hypoglycemia to prevent adverse effects on the central nervous system. These include jitteriness, extreme hunger (sucking vigorously on hands and fingers), diaphoresis, cyanosis, tachypnea, lethargy, seizures, and apnea. Serum glucose levels must be monitored frequently until they are stable at 80 to 120 mg/dl. After delivery, the glucose level must be monitored at least every hour until it has stabilized. Perelman (1983) identifies hypoglycemia as glucose levels less than 30 mg/dl for the term infant, 20 mg/dl for the preterm infant, and 40 mg/dl for any infant who is showing signs and symptoms of hypoglycemia. If the infant's condition is stable, early feedings should be given. Intravenous fluids of 10 percent dextrose in water at 6 to 8 mg/kg/minute should be started for the infant unable to take oral feedings. If the glucose levels remain low, administering an intravenous bolus of dextrose may be necessary with a concentration no greater than $D_{10}W$. Administration of more concentrated dextrose solutions may cause rebound hypoglycemia.

The infant should be monitored for any signs of birth trauma, such as brachial plexus damage or a fractured clavicle, especially in the macrosomic infant. If decreased movement is noted in an arm or if the infant cries when an extremity is moved, a radiograph should be obtained to look for a fracture. If a fracture is present, the affected extremity should be stabilized and an orthopedic consultation obtained. Bottle feeding may be difficult for the macrosomic infant. These infants have weaker reflex functioning and poor motor behavior during the first 2 days of life (Pressler, 1991).

When caring for an infant of a diabetic mother in whom there was poor glucose control during pregnancy, the nurse should be observant for the possibility of respiratory distress. Treatment should be the same as for other infants with RDS. No special considerations for treatment are needed.

The infant also needs to be monitored for hypocalcemia and hypomagnesemia. The signs, such as jitteriness or lethargy, usually appear within the first 3 days of life and are similar to those seen in hypoglycemia (see Chapter 22, Fluids, Electrolytes, Vitamins, and Trace Minerals: Basis of Ingestion, Digestion, Elimination, and Metabolism). If these signs persist after glucose levels are stabilized, blood levels of calcium and magnesium should be obtained and supplementation given as needed.

A spun hematocrit should be carried out to assess for polycythemia. A partial exchange transfusion may need to be performed for a central hematocrit greater than 65 percent. The infant may need to be given phototherapy for treatment of hyperbilirubinemia. The infant also needs to be monitored for any congenital anomalies. Appropriate actions should be taken depending on the type of anomaly.

Many of the problems that occur are transient and resolve within a few days. For infants who are affected more severely, it is imperative that the parents be given the support and education needed for these problems. Counseling on further pregnancies may also be required.

Many problems can occur with infants of diabetic mothers. Proper screening, good prenatal care, and aggressive management of maternal diabetes decreases morbidity and mortality in these infants.

Ambiguous Genitalia

When the sperm fertilizes the ovum at conception, the genetic sex of the embryo is determined. However, during the first 7 weeks of gestation, the primitive gonads contain both ovarian (cortical) and testicular (medullary) components (Avery et al., 1994), creating a "bipotential environment" in which either gender's characteristics may emerge. This initial stage of "sexual indifference" lasts until the seventh week of gestation, when the gonads, which are the future testes or ovaries, begin to acquire sexual characteristics (Moore & Persaud, 1993). The determining factor in sexual differentiation involves not only genetic information contained within the original X and Y sex chromosome combination but also a number of additional components, including hormonal and environmental influences. Failure to achieve sexual differentiation owing to defective gene expression or abnormal external influences, or both, may result in the congenital anomaly of ambiguous genitalia (Penny, 1990). This anomaly may occur as a single manifestation or as part of a larger syndrome.

Although most conditions resulting in ambiguous genitalia are not life-threatening (with the exception of the salt-wasting form of congenital adrenal hyperplasia), it is vitally important that early diagnosis be made and treatment instituted to minimize any negative sequelae and maximize outcome. Prolonged delay in intervention can lead to serious consequences for both patient and family. To gain a better understanding of ambiguous genitalia, it is helpful to know the normal development and sexual differentiation of the embryo.

Normal Embryologic Development and Sexual Differentiation

Normal sexual differentiation is contingent on the successful development of the genital system. Development and differentiation occur at three levels: the gonads, the internal genital ducts, and the external genitalia (Fig. 26–3). This orderly sequence of events takes place early in fetal development.

Near the fifth week of gestation, the gonads begin to develop with primordial germ cell migration to the urogenital ridge. The indifferent gonad consists of both male germ cells at the inner medullary position and female germ cells at the outer cortical position. The chromosomal sex determined at fertilization directs the development of the gonad into either a testis or an ovary (Hamblin et al., 1989). The medulla differentiates into a testis, whereas the cortex regresses in an embryo with XY chromosomal makeup; the cortex differentiates into an ovary, whereas the medulla regresses in an XX chromosomal embryo.

At 7 to 8 weeks of gestation, the fetus possesses two pairs of genital ducts: the mesonephric (or wolffian) ducts and the paramesonephric (or mullerian) ducts. Development of these ducts into male or female internal structures is dependent on the release or nonrelease of specific hormones, respectively. At this time, the male testes produce and release two hormones: a masculinizing androgen hormone (testosterone) and a mullerian-inhibiting substance (MIS). Testosterone stimulates the development of the mesonephric ducts to form the male genital tract, including the epididymis, vas deferens, seminal vesicles, and ejaculatory ducts. The MIS causes regression of the paramesonephric ducts, which would have developed into female reproductive structures. In the absence of these hormones, the female fetus develops the paramesonephric ducts into female internal genitalia, including fallopian tubes, uterus, cervix, and upper vagina. In addition, the mesonephric ducts regress in the female fetus (Hamblin et al., 1989; Mazur, 1983; Moore & Persaud, 1993). Thus, the male testis is active in producing hormones for sexual differentiation, whereas the female ovary has a passive role in sexual differentiation.

During the 7th through 16th weeks of gestation, the external genitalia differentiate. In the presence of testosterone in the male fetus, virilization of the genital tubercle occurs, producing a penis. The ureteral folds fuse and form the anterior urethra while the genital swellings fuse and form the scrotum. The urogenital sinus develops to form the prostate. In the absence of testosterone in the female fetus, the genital swellings form the labia minora and labia majora, respectively. The urogenital sinus develops to form the lower vagina (Hamblin et al., 1989).

It is important to emphasize that sexual differentiation of both internal and external genitalia occurs in a fixed sequence at specific critical periods of development. If there are abnormal circulating androgens during the differentiation period of the female external genitalia, varying degrees of virilization may occur, resulting in urogenital sinus fusion and clitoral enlargement (Shapiro et al., 1989). In addition, lack of substantial MIS hormone in the male fetus may not adequately suppress the paramesonephric ducts, and subsequent female internal structures may develop.

It is evident that a wide variety of sexual differentiation abnormalities may occur in the fetus. Some conditions result in evident ambiguous genitalia at birth, whereas others may not be detected until puberty. Basic knowledge of these categories aids the nurse in the assessment and management of these individuals.

Abnormal Sexual Differentiation

The more common disorders of sexual differentiation can be categorized into two generalized groups: congenital adrenal hy-

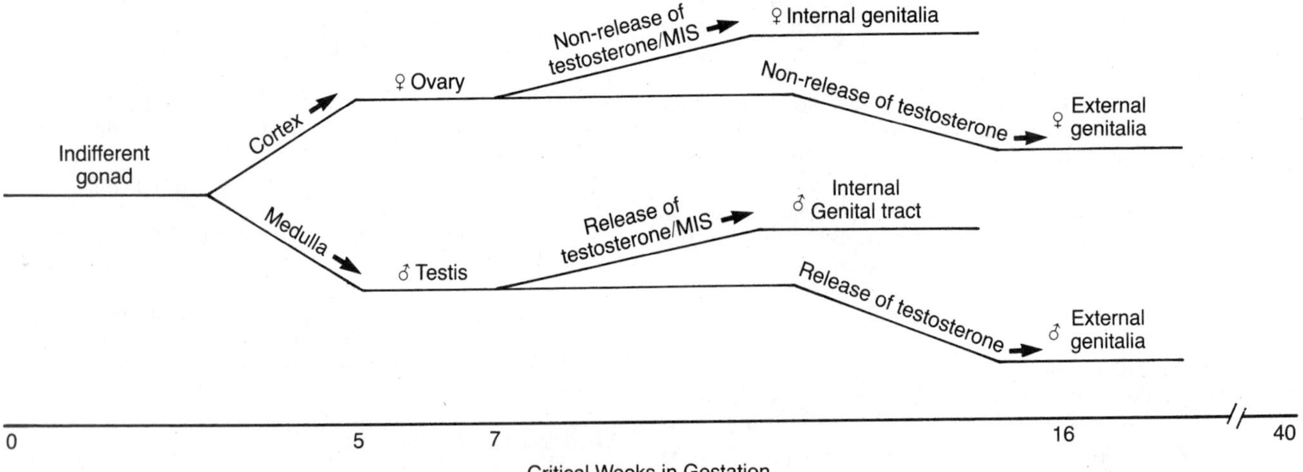

FIGURE 26–3. Sexual differentiation in the developing fetus.

perplasia (CAH) and disorders of gonadal differentiation (Table 26–4). The most common cause of ambiguous genitalia in the newborn is CAH, but not all patients with the disorder show sexual ambiguity. The same is true for disorders of gonadal differentiation.

Congenital Adrenal Hyperplasia

CAH is an autosomal recessive inborn error of metabolism that affects male and female fetuses equally. It is estimated that from 1 in 5000 to 1 in 15,000 births result in CAH. Affected female infants often present with some degree of virilization of the external genitalia, but the internal female structures remain normal. Conversely, few male infants show any genital anomalies and the condition may go unrecognized until later infancy or childhood (Griffin & Wilson, 1986; Shapiro et al., 1989).

PATHOPHYSIOLOGY

The adrenal cortex consists of three regions: the outer zona glomerulosa, the middle fasciculata, and the inner zona reticularis, which adjoins the adrenal medulla. The reticularis, however, does not complete differentiation until about 3 years of age. There are three classes of hormones produced by the adrenal gland: mineralocorticoids, glucocorticoids, and sex steroids. Specific enzymes are necessary for the biosynthesis of these hormones. Adrenocorticotropic hormone (ACTH) stimulates the adrenal gland to produce the steroids. When sufficient quantities are released into the blood stream, ACTH is turned off by a negative feedback mechanism (Mininberg et al., 1982; New et al., 1990).

Many forms of CAH exist. Abnormally high ACTH levels with low plasma cortisol levels are pathognomonic of all forms of CAH. Each type is the result of a separate enzyme deficiency necessary for production of a particular steroid. No matter which form of CAH is operating, a deficiency in cortisol results. This deficiency, in turn, prohibits the natural negative feedback loop necessary to turn off pituitary secretion of ACTH. Thus, ACTH continues to stimulate the adrenal gland to synthesize and secrete deficient steroids, and adrenal hyperplasia ensues (Kelnar, 1993; Miller & Levine, 1987; Mininberg et al., 1982).

The types and symptoms of CAH depend on which steroids are deficient and which are produced in excess (Miller & Levine, 1987). To remain within the scope of this text, only the types of CAH typically detected in the neonatal period or early infancy are discussed.

CAH may be separated into three categories: rare enzyme defects, nonclassic forms, and classic forms. The rare enzyme defects may be incompatible with life and are thus rarely seen clinically. The nonclassic forms are usually hidden at birth, with no major developmental abnormalities noted. If signs of the disorder appear at all, they are typically seen later in life. One of the classic forms of CAH, 21-hydroxylase deficiency, is the most common autosomal recessive disorder in humans (New et al., 1990). Although the nonclassic forms of CAH are more prevalent in the general population, the classic forms are expressed most commonly in the neonatal population.

TABLE 26–4 Sexual Differentiation

- I. Congenital adrenal hyperplasia
  - A. Rare enzyme defects
  - B. Nonclassic forms
    - 1. Nonclassic 21-hydroxylase deficiency
  - C. Classic 21-hydroxylase deficiency
- II. Disorders of gonadal differentiation
  - A. Phenotypic females with abnormal differentiation
    - 1. Turner's syndrome
    - 2. Swyer's syndrome
  - B. Phenotypic males with abnormal differentiation
    - 1. Klinefelter's syndrome
    - 2. XX males
  - C. Sexual ambiguity with gonadal dysgenesis
    - 1. Male pseudohermaphroditism
    - 2. True hermaphroditism
    - 3. Leydig cell hypoplasia
    - 4. Testicular regression syndrome

CLINICAL MANIFESTATIONS AND RISK FACTORS IN 21-HYDROXYLASE DEFICIENCY. CAH due to 21-hydroxylase deficiency accounts for 90 to 95 percent of all cases of CAH (Mininberg et al., 1982; New, 1988). The severe form occurs in 1 in 5000 to 1 in 14,000 births. A milder form is present in 0.3 percent of whites and in 1 to 3 percent of European Jews (Kalaitzoglou & New, 1993; White et al., 1986). The mutated gene responsible for 21-hydroxylase deficiency is located within the HLA complex of genes on the short arm of chromosome 6. Many of the gene deletions that result in 21-hydroxylase deficiency are associated with the haplotype HLA-B47;DR7 (Kalaitzoglou & New, 1993).

CAH due to 21-hydroxylase deficiency results in a build-up of 17-hydroxyprogesterone that is not converted to 11-deoxycortisol. Without sufficient circulating cortisol, the negative feedback loop to the hypothalamus and pituitary does not operate. Increasing amounts of ACTH continue to be secreted, resulting in high levels of circulating androgens. Excess circulating androgens lead to progressive virilism, which begins during prenatal development. Female neonates can present with mild clitoral enlargement with or without labioscrotal folds or, in severe cases, with a penile urethra (Kalaitzoglou & New, 1993). Premature female neonates are at risk for delayed diagnosis because prominent clitoris and electrolyte imbalance caused by renal immaturity are not uncommon (Cruz et al., 1995). The increased testosterone does not, however, interfere with normal development of internal genitalia, uterus, or fallopian tubes. Consequently, virilized females have the potential for a normal female reproductive life, complete with childbearing. Androgen excess also contributes to initial rapid skeletal growth with early closure of the epiphyses and consequent short adult stature.

Males with 21-hydroxylase deficiency often appear normal at birth. An enlarged penis with small testicles may be present. The disorder may go unrecognized until precocious puberty develops during later infancy or early childhood. This condition may be seen in the development of early pubic hair, advanced muscular development, and rapid growth. Infertility may result without treatment (New & Josso, 1988).

The classic form of 21-hydroxylase deficiency is the most common presenting CAH disorder. Twenty-five percent of affected newborns have a simple virilizing form. Seventy-five percent of patients with classic 21-hydroxylase deficiency are unable to synthesize adequate aldosterone, which is a necessary component for the transport of sodium ions across cell membranes (New et al., 1990). A defect in aldosterone biosynthesis results in the inability of the distal and collecting tubules of the kidney to reabsorb sodium. Salt wasting occurs and creates high urinary sodium levels. Serum sodium levels drop while serum potassium levels rise. In an effort to increase levels of aldosterone, large amounts of renin are released into the plasma. As a result, circulating angiotensin II is also increased. Despite high levels of the natural vasoconstrictor, blood pressure falls, presumably owing to down-regulation of angiotensin receptors in vascular smooth muscle. Patients with this form of CAH may die in the neonatal period as a result of hyponatremic shock (Ganong, 1985; New, 1988). Rapid diagnosis with accurate treatment is clearly an important goal for these newborns.

A reliable screening test developed in 1977 uses capillary blood obtained through a heel prick to test for classic 21-hydroxylase deficiency (Pang et al., 1977). Blood spots routinely collected for newborn screening can be used to detect the 17-hydroxyprogesterone concentration. Benefits to earlier diagnosis and treatment include prevention of severe adrenal crisis, postnatal growth acceleration, and premature pubarche. Although false-positive results in preterm, sick, or low birth weight infants have been reported, it is interesting to note that the male:female ratio of affected individuals detected by screening programs was 1:1. Published case surveys of CAH detected because of symptoms repeatedly report a higher prevalence in females than in males (Cicognani, 1992). Male infants with the salt-wasting form of CAH may die early in infancy without the cause being identified. Also, in male patients with the simple virilizing form of CAH, the disorder may be diagnosed later in life or not at all.

Treatment involves replacing deficient cortisol with hydrocortisone or a similar synthetic substitute, such as dexamethasone. In addition, mineralocorticoid replacement is necessary in the salt-wasting form (New & Josso, 1988). The goal of hormone replacement therapy is to prevent adrenal crisis, achieve normal growth and development, and suppress excessive androgen production (Einaudi et al., 1993). Supplemental medication must be taken for the duration of the patient's life (DiGrande, 1984). Surgical repair of ambiguous genitalia may also be indicated.

3-HYDROXYSTEROID DEHYDROGENASE DEFICIENCY OF CONGENITAL ADRENAL HYPERPLASIA. 3-Hydroxysteroid dehydrogenase deficiency is also due to recessive genes that have been mapped to the short arm of chromosome 1. Testosterone, aldosterone, and cortisol levels are all reduced. Males have incomplete prenatal genital development resulting from decreased androgen synthesis in the testes as well as in the adrenal gland. Females can experience mild masculinization because of the increased production of a weak androgen that is produced before the deficient enzyme in the hormone biosynthesis pathway of the adrenal gland. The majority of patients with 3-hydroxysteroid dehydrogenase deficiency have varying degrees of salt wasting owing to insufficient aldosterone levels (Kalaitzoglou & New, 1993; Miller & Levine, 1987; New et al., 1990).

11-HYDROXYLASE DEFICIENCY. The second most common form of CAH is 11-hydroxylase deficiency. The recessive genes involved in this disorder are located on the long arm of chromosome 8. Unlike the other two forms of CAH described, 11-hydroxylase deficiency is distinguished by hypertension, hypokalemia, and sodium retention in the majority of patients. 11-Deoxycortisol is not converted to cortisol and deoxycorticosterone is usually not converted to corticosterone. Again, because there is deficient cortisol, which acts as a negative feedback to turn off adrenal production of steroids, excess prenatal androgen secretion results in female virilization with normal internal female reproductive organs (Kalaitzoglou & New, 1993; New, 1988; New et al., 1990).

17-HYDROXYLASE AND 17,20-LYASE DEFICIENCY. A defect in the microsomal enzyme $P450_{c17}$, which catalyzes both 17-hydroxylase and 17,20-lyase, is present in both the adrenals and gonads. Consequently, a reduction in all androgens and estrogens results. Males present with pseudohermaphroditism and gynecomastia. Females express infantile genitalia. Neither male nor female adolescents experience pubertal changes. Hypertension and hypokalemia may develop because of elevated concentrations of deoxycorticosterone. The recessive gene for the $P450_{c17}$ enzyme has been mapped to chromosome 10 (Kalaitzoglou & New, 1993).

COLLABORATIVE MANAGEMENT

NEWBORNS. The degree of female virilization is not indicative of the degree of adrenal insufficiency (New et al., 1990). A newborn with ambiguous genitalia must be evaluated by an endocrinologist and geneticist. Serum hormone concentrations must be determined and blood for chromosomal analysis must be drawn. The neonate with confirmed CAH needs to be closely monitored during the first few weeks of life for signs of acute adrenal insufficiency. Replacement hormone therapy may be started when CAH is suspected. At the latest, it needs to be started once a diagnosis is made. Eventually, virilized females can undergo surgical correction (Miller & Levine, 1987; New, 1988).

Recently, there has been emphasis placed on prenatal diagnosis and treatment of CAH resulting from 21-hydroxylase deficiency. The goal is to avoid corrective genital surgery after birth by preventing virilization of females. Oral dexamethasone or hydrocortisone is administered to the pregnant mother as early as possible during the first trimester. A chorionic villus sampling, performed between 8 and 12 weeks' gestation, or amniocentesis, performed between 14 and 18 weeks' gestation, can be used for DNA analysis and gender determination (Kuller et al., 1996).

If the fetus is a male or an unaffected female, the mother can discontinue treatment. Therapy is continued to term if the fetus is an affected female. It is thought that the extra glucocorticoid in the maternal circulation crosses the placenta and thus provides negative feedback for fetal ACTH secretion. Hyperplasia of the adrenal gland along with oversecretion of androgens can then be circumvented (Loeuille et al., 1990; Pang et al., 1990). Reported maternal side effects have typically been mild and reversible: weight gain, hypertension, edema, and mood swings. However, with higher doses of 1 to 1.5 mg/day, maternal side effects have been more severe: excessive weight gain, glucose intolerance, facial hirsutism, marked cushingoid features, hypertension, and mood swings (Kelnar, 1993).

The effectiveness of prenatal treatment has been variable. Several explanations have been postulated. The dosage of glucocorticoids may have been inadequate or the onset of treatment may have been late. Exogenous cortisol appears to have a high affinity for serum corticosteroid-binding globulin. A portion of exogenous dexamethasone is thought to be catalyzed by the placenta. The amount of exogenous glucocorticoids reaching the fetus is also hypothesized to be influenced by maternal metabolism. Another factor limiting the success of exogenous glucocorticoid administration is that fetal adrenal function is believed to be regulated by other factors in addition to ACTH. Lastly, the fetal ACTH–glucocorticoid feedback mechanism may not be sufficiently developed during early gestation (Pang et al., 1990).

PARENTS. The parents of a newborn with CAH-induced ambiguous genitalia require immediate information about questionable sex assignment. Naming their child is postponed until the sex can be genetically determined. Explanations about the cause and treatment must be simple and concise and require repeated reinforcement as the child grows. Health care providers should refer to the neonate as "baby," "infant," or "child." It must be emphasized that virilized females possess normal internal reproductive organs and that external genitalia can be surgically corrected.

Parents need time to verbalize their feelings. Because CAH is recessively inherited, parents often feel guilt for having given their child "bad genes" and "causing" their infant's condition. The nurse needs to emphasize that the parents have no control over the genes their newborn received. Parents need to know that every person has some altered genes that can cause genetic anomalies. Every person has a background risk of 2 to 3 percent for having a child with a birth defect. Therefore, the parents are not somehow different or "defective" because they transmitted an altered gene to their offspring.

Parents may experience anger and disappointment over the loss of their prenatal ideas and dreams of a perfect child. Their child's "normal features" need to be emphasized. Any concerns about their child growing up as a masculine female, feminine male, or homosexual owing to the ambiguous genitalia should be discussed openly to allow parents an opportunity for catharsis.

Nurses need to encourage parent–infant activities that promote bonding. Parents may also require help accessing current support systems and obtaining new support persons or agencies as needed.

The parents must be taught medication administration and schedules. Compliance must be stressed and the need for lifelong hormone replacement therapy emphasized. Parents also need to be familiarized with signs and symptoms of dehydration. Frequent and regular evaluation of affected infants is necessary to monitor and adjust the dosage of cortisone when ACTH suppression may be inadequate. Certain stressors, such as illness, trauma, and surgery, may trigger an adrenal crisis requiring medication adjustment (DiGrande, 1984).

Disorders of Gonadal Differentiation

Disorders of gonadal differentiation involve abnormal combinations of the sex chromosomes X and Y. Basic descriptions of these disorders can be classified into three separate categories based on phenotypic expression or the observable characteristics of the individual.

The first general category involves phenotypic females with abnormal gonadal differentiation. Two specific types include Turner's syndrome and Swyer's syndrome. Individuals with Turner's syndrome have a 45,X genotype with characteristic congenital anomalies that include skeletal defects, webbing of the neck, lymphedema of the hands and feet at birth, and shortened stature in adulthood. The gonads are eventually reduced to fibrous streaks, which leads to primary amenorrhea, sexual infantilism, and infertility (New & Josso, 1988). Recognition of the syndrome before puberty may be accomplished by obtaining a karyotype of the chromosomal set. The incidence of Turner's syndrome is 1 in 2200 female births (Wiedemann et al., 1989). Treatment involves sex hormone (estrogen) replacement therapy at puberty and subsequent low-dose maintenance estrogen administration (New & Josso, 1988; Ross et al., 1983).

Swyer's syndrome, like Turner's syndrome, often presents at puberty with primary amenorrhea. Streak gonads are seen but without the congenital anomalies that accompany Turner's syndrome. The karyotype may reveal a 46,XX or 46,XY genotype. Treatment involves hormone replacement therapy and exploratory surgery to remove streak gonads.

The second general category consists of phenotypic males with abnormal gonadal differentiation. Two types include Klinefelter's syndrome and XX male phenotypes.

The karyotype of individuals with Klinefelter's syndrome shows one additional X chromosome. Mosaic combinations (usually 46,XY, 47,XXY) may also be possible. Adult XXY males present with small testes, sterile seminiferous tubules, and gynecomastia owing to lowered testosterone levels. Mental retardation may also be seen. Diagnosis is made through Barr screening to determine the sex chromosomal arrangement. Treatment includes testosterone replacement therapy in individuals with postpuberal hypogonadism (New & Josso, 1988).

XX male phenotypes have testicular development in the absence of a Y chromosome. Individuals usually present with infertility problems. The disorder may be genetically inherited by either dominant (Kasdan et al., 1973) or recessive (De la Chapelle et al., 1978) autosomal genes.

The third general category comprises sexually ambiguous individuals with gonadal dysgenesis. Identifiable types include (1) male pseudohermaphroditism, (2) true hermaphroditism, (3) Leydig cell hypoplasia, and (4) testicular regression syndrome.

Individuals with pseudohermaphroditism with mixed gonadal dysgenesis have impaired testicular function, which leads to early fetal testicular dysgenesis. Sexual ambiguity is seen with the presence of one or two testes, hypospadias, cryptorchidism, and an intact uterus. There is an increased risk of gonadal tumors. In addition, Turner's syndrome–like characteristics may be seen. The sex of rearing is preferably female if the syndrome is diagnosed in infancy and treated at an early age, usually younger than 2 years. If the child is older, sex reassignment may impair the individual psychologically. Thus, it is better to correct the hypospadias and cryptorchidism surgically, remove gonadal streaks, and monitor for tumor development. Testosterone hormone replacement should be provided at puberty, and the individual should retain his male gender (New & Josso, 1988).

True hermaphrodites possess both testicular and ovarian tissue, often combined in the same gonad, called an ovotestis. The newborn presents with ambiguous genitalia and abnormal internal anatomic structures. Although internal testicular tissue usually degenerates, the ovarian tissue remains functional, and thus fertility may be possible in the female sex. For this reason, female is the desired sex of rearing. Treatment involves surgical removal of internal organs contradictory to the desired sex.

Leydig cell hypoplasia and embryonic testicular regression syndrome are both rare occurrences. Sexual ambiguity is often seen, and these disorders may be genetically transmitted.

Additional Causes of Ambiguous Genitalia

In addition to the causes of ambiguous genitalia previously discussed, certain forms may be be caused by other, less common factors. They include maternal exposure to androgens, 5α-reductase deficiency, and end-organ androgen insensitivity (Hamblin et al., 1989). Maternal exposure to androgens may be either exogenous (through the use of certain prescribed oral contraceptives) or endogenous (by increased circulating androgens resulting from a maternal tumor).

Strategies in Assessment

Any neonate presenting with ambiguous genitalia, regardless of the severity, should be thoroughly evaluated. It is a critical problem that needs both medical and social intervention. Assessment of the newborn with ambiguous genitalia includes a complete family history and physical examination, followed by a thorough diagnostic evaluation.

Family History. A complete history begins with the construction of a family pedigree. A pedigree is a diagram identifying all family members, their relationship to the affected individual, and their personal health history with emphasis on specific hereditary conditions. Genetics plays an important part in individuals with ambiguous genitalia and should be investigated carefully. In addition, special attention should be directed to the mother and her prenatal and reproductive history. "Maternal ingestion of potentially androgenic substances (including certain forms of oral contraception) during pregnancy; a family history of maternal aunts with sterility, amenorrhea, or an inguinal hernia containing a gonad; or an unexplained infant death in the neonatal period" may assist in establishing a diagnosis (Hamblin et al., 1989).

Physical Examination. Specific physical findings that are seen with sexual ambiguity include (1) a structure that resembles an enlarged clitoris or a micropenis with hypospadias, (2) partial fusion of the labioscrotal folds, and (3) absence of gonads or one palpable gonad in the incomplete scrotum of a term infant (Mazur, 1983). Downward bowing of the penile-clitoral structure, called chordee, can also be present. Varying degrees of ambiguity may be seen, depending on the severity of the disorder.

Whenever a physical examination reveals ambiguous genitalia, further diagnostic evaluation is essential. Major medical centers often have a comprehensive team to conduct a diagnostic evaluation of these infants (Castiglia, 1989).

Diagnostic Evaluation. The goals of the diagnostic evaluation in the infant presenting with sexual ambiguity are to determine the cause of the abnormality and to develop an appropriate plan of care. It should be explained to the parents that although their infant was born with sexual organs that appear underdeveloped or unfinished, a thorough evaluation can help define the extent of the condition and determine the most effective strategy to complete the unfinished sex organs (Mazur, 1983).

A comprehensive diagnostic evaluation involves three areas of testing: (1) measurement of the circulating hormones, (2) analysis of the chromosomes, and (3) visualization of the internal organs.

First, measurement of the circulating hormones identifies the presence of abnormal levels. Evaluating specific hormone levels can be accomplished through measurement of urinary 17-ketosteroids and blood pregnanetriol levels. Elevation of these hormonal levels may indicate CAH. These levels may also be assessed prenatally via the amniotic fluid to identify an affected fetus (Frasier et al., 1974; Pang et al., 1977). However, it should be noted that affected males may not have abnormal amniotic fluid levels (Frasier et al., 1974; Pang et al., 1977).

Infants with ambiguous genitalia in which CAH has been ruled out may be evaluated further with serum testosterone measurement and an hCG stimulation test. Performed between 2 and 9 weeks of age, these tests can help determine the integrity of the hypothalamic-pituitary axis in male infants and can identify the presence of testicular tissue in infants with ambiguous genitalia (Ismail et al., 1989).

Second, analysis of the chromosomes determines the chromosomal or genetic sex of the infant. Complete chromosomal analysis can be performed through the establishment of a karyotype. In the past, attempts were made to identify the chromosomal sex of the infant immediately through analysis of buccal smears, which is currently considered ineffective because no information is provided about the structure or possible mosaicism of the chromosomes (Castiglia, 1989).

Advances in genetics (Erickson et al., 1990) have provided information about the sex-determining gene, zinc finger Y, which can be identified on part of the Y chromosome with the use of a probe. The probe can determine the integrity of the gene and can be useful in the diagnosis for an infant with ambiguous genitalia.

Third, visualization of the internal organs provides a comprehensive picture of the anatomic structures involved in an infant with abnormal sexual differentiation. Pelvic ultrasonography is an important diagnostic tool for determining the presence of a uterus or urogenital sinus, or both. Contrast studies (genitography) may further clarify the presence of a urogenital sinus. Magnetic resonance imaging can be useful in identifying the presence of undescended testes. Endoscopy of the urogenital sinus may determine the presence of a small or abnormal vagina. Laparotomy or laparoscopy and gonadal biopsy in the infant is controversial owing to the limited availability of smaller-sized instruments. These procedures should be performed only in infants who require removal of the gonads, such as true hermaphrodites and infants with mixed gonadal dysgenesis (Hamblin et al., 1989).

After the infant with ambiguous genitalia has been thoroughly assessed and a diagnosis has been made, a collaborative team approach to managing the infant must be established to optimize successful intervention.

Collaborative Management

Medical Management. The focus of medical management for an infant presenting with ambiguous genitalia involves assessment and diagnosis of the disorder, as well as physical stabilization of the neonate experiencing a salt-wasting adrenal crisis from CAH. Explanations and support for the family are critical. A comprehensive medical and surgical plan of care should be established by the primary physician and conveyed clearly to all persons involved with the infant's care.

A determination as to the desired sex of rearing should be made through the extensive diagnostic process. Gender assignment is based on the infant's anatomy (Hamblin et al., 1989), with less emphasis on the chromosomal sex or the prospect for future fertility except in females with CAH. It is usually more difficult to masculinize than to feminize an affected individual. Therefore, only those infants with a satisfactory phallic structure, typically greater than 2 cm in length from the symphysis pubis to the tip, should be considered candidates for male sex assignment. An adequate phallic structure responds to testosterone replacement therapy, whereas an inadequate phallic structure does not (Penny, 1990). The infant with a micropenis assigned the female gender requires surgical correction of the external genitalia, gonadectomy, estrogen supplementation therapy at puberty as well as maintenance therapy in adulthood, and possible additional surgery for the construction of a neovagina (Castiglia, 1989; Rock & Jones, 1989).

It is extremely important to establish the sex of the affected individual as early as possible, preferably no later than 2 years of age. Early sex determination, within 3 to 6 months after birth, may be helpful so that reconstructive surgery can be undertaken that is appropriate for the selected sex.

Nursing Management. Nursing care for the infant presenting with ambiguous genitalia can be challenging. To develop an effective plan of care, the nurse must establish three levels of concern on which to focus. These levels include immediate, midrange, and long-term needs and goals (see section on CAH for details of management).

The immediate needs and goals of the newborn with ambiguous genitalia involve the potential for a life-threatening adrenal crisis, as may be seen in the neonate with salt-wasting CAH. The primary goal is directed toward achieving an elevation of circulating cortisol and replacement of sodium and water deficits. Fluid and electrolyte status and circulating cortisol levels should be monitored carefully. (See Chapter 22, Fluids, Electrolytes, Vitamins, and Trace Minerals: Basis of Ingestion, Digestion, Elimination, and Metabolism.)

The midrange needs and goals of the sexually ambiguous infant relate to the assessment and diagnosis of the disorder that led to the ambiguous genitalia. The nurse may assist in obtaining the family history as well as performing a thorough physical examination of the neonate. In addition, the nurse may draw blood for measurement of hormonal levels and chromosome analysis. Although not directly involved in diagnostic evaluation, the nurse may assist with certain procedures such as pelvic ultrasonography or magnetic resonance imaging. The goal is to provide primary care for the neonate and support for the family while an investigation for a diagnosis is made.

The needs and goals of the infant at the long-term level pertain to the therapeutic intervention developed to manage the disorder and correct the ambiguous genitalia. As this may cover an extended period, the nurse involved in a long-term primary health care setting is in an excellent position to provide continuity of care. The primary goal is to supply information and support for the affected individual and the family.

At all three levels at which the nurse develops a plan of care, parental involvement is extremely important. Ideally, a primary nurse should be responsible for the care and education provided to the infant and family. The nurse needs to coordinate the specialists involved with the patient so that the family understands all the information that is given to them. The role of the nurse working with the family is to deliver knowledgeable, factual information adjusted to the parents' level of comprehension, clarify misconceptions they may have, and reinforce family teaching (Mazur, 1983).

Parents often wonder about the risk of recurrence, which, in fact, depends on the actual diagnosis of their affected child. In the more common classic 21-hydroxylase deficiency of CAH, there is a 25 percent risk of a subsequent affected sibling (Shapiro et al., 1989). The parents should undergo genetic counseling to determine the risk in subsequent childbearing.

Families may benefit from a referral to social services to assist them with available community resources. Support groups may be established so that families and affected individuals can gain confidence in knowing that they are not alone in dealing with the disorder.

Little nursing research has been conducted in the area of sexual ambiguity. Most nursing literature involves case study presentations with subsequent descriptions of management of care. Recent genetic research has centered on identification and interpretation of the sex-determining gene. Further research is needed in the area of genetics as well as on the identification of additional risk factors for ambiguous genitalia.

The nurse working with neonates usually does not encounter ambiguous genitalia on a daily basis. In addition, certain presentations of ambiguous genitalia can be subtle, as there may be varying degrees of expression. Knowledge and understanding of basic neonatal embryology, sexual differentiation, and sexual ambiguity can be beneficial to the nurse, who may be in a position to be the first to identify the infant presenting with ambiguous genitalia.

Cystic Fibrosis

Cystic fibrosis (CF), formerly known as mucoviscidosis or CF of the pancreas, is an inherited, chronic, progressive, metabolic disorder affecting the exocrine glands, or the mucus-secreting glands, of the body. Classic CF is characterized by chronic pulmonary infection, pancreatic insufficiency, and increased salt loss through the sweat glands.

Pathophysiology

The gene responsible for CF is the cystic fibrosis transmembrane conductance regulator (CFTR) gene and is a mutation on the long arm of human chromosome 7 (Riordan et al., 1989). In approximately 75 percent of patients, three base pairs that code for the amino acid phenylalanine are deleted, causing the gene to code for a defective protein in the cell. This three-base deletion is designated as the ΔF508 mutation because the deletion lies in the 508th position of the polypeptide chain (Riordan et al., 1989). Researchers believe that the defective protein is one of a class of proteins within the cell membrane that is involved in the movement of ions across the cell membrane. The primary defect appears to be an alteration in the transport of chloride ions, leading to excessive salt content within the sweat and the production of thick mucus secretions in the intestinal and respiratory tracts (Hilman, 1989).

Seventy-five percent of individuals with CF have at least one gene with the ΔF508 deletion. In some individuals, both genes are affected, whereas others (approximately 50 percent) have a second gene with a different mutation. To date, more than 400 mutations in the CFTR gene have been identified (Dean & Santis, 1994). The fact that there are many mutations that cause CF may partially explain the large patient-to-patient variability seen in the presentation, manifestations, and degree of severity of the disease. Currently, researchers are working on the correlation between specific mutations (genotype) and clinical characteristics (phenotype)(Dean & Santis, 1994). For example, ΔF508 homozygosity is strongly associated with pancreatic insufficiency (Cystic Fibrosis Genotype-Phenotype Consortium, 1993), whereas some other mutations are associated with normal pancreatic function.

Pulmonary disease probably begins with the development of mucus plugging or obstruction of small airways. Eventually, the patient experiences chronic inflammation and obstruction of larger airways. As the patient is colonized with bacteria, infection sets in. Repeated infection and inflammation leads to structural changes in the airway, consisting of damage to respiratory epithelium, supporting structures' airway wall, and pulmonary vasculature. Repeated exacerbations can result in bronchiectasis and pulmonary fibrosis. Pulmonary parenchymal changes cause an increase in pulmonary vascular resistance, leading to pulmonary hypertension, cor pulmonale, and cardiorespiratory failure (Hilman, 1989).

The course of CF is chronic and progressive, characterized by frequent respiratory infections with *Haemophilus influenzae, Staphylococcus aureus*, and *Pseudomonas aeruginosa. Burkholderia cepacia* (formerly *Pseudomonas cepacia*) is seen less commonly but may be associated with greater morbidity and mortality than *P. aeruginosa* colonization.

Hyperinflation or emphysema due to partial airway obstruction, and patchy areas of atelectasis due to complete airway obstruction, are early radiographic findings. Characteristically, patients exhibit generalized nodulocystic shadowing and increased bronchial markings. Destructive changes within the airways eventually lead to severe bronchiectasis with a "honeycomb" appearance of the lung on radiograph (Hilman, 1989).

Risk Factors

CF is the most common fatal genetic disorder affecting whites. It is inherited as a recessive condition with a carrier frequency of 1 in 20. The incidence of CF in the United States is approximately 1 in 2000 individuals of European ancestry. The incidence in the black population is 1 in 17,000 (Kulczycki & Schauf, 1974); it is estimated to be much less common in Asians and Native Americans (Wood et al., 1976).

Clinical Manifestations

Most patients present with a combination of recurrent respiratory infections, abnormal stools, and failure to thrive. Less common presentations are intestinal obstruction (such as meconium ileus), rectal prolapse, nasal polyps, prolonged neonatal jaundice, hyponatremic-hypochloremic dehydration, and hypoproteinemia.

Pulmonary disease is usually a major clinical problem for the patient with CF later in life, but it can also present in the neonatal period. Recent studies using bronchoscopy in infants with CF indicate that inflammation and air trapping may be present at birth, especially in infants colonized with *P. aeruginosa* (Rosenfeld et al., 1994). The most constant symptom of pulmonary involvement is a cough that is initially dry and later becomes productive and increased at night. Decreased exercise tolerance, tachypnea, retractions, flaring, and an increased anteroposterior diameter of the chest are common signs. Crackles and wheezes may be heard on auscultation. Digital clubbing may be apparent, depending on the severity of the pulmonary disease. As the disease progresses, pulmonary exacerbations caused by viral and bacterial infections are common and may develop into pneumonia. Once generalized bronchiectasis is evident, the clinical course steadily progresses with frequent exacerbations and eventually respiratory failure, cor pulmonale, and death (Wood et al., 1976).

Pancreatic insufficiency dominates the clinical picture in the majority of neonates and infants with CF. Between 80 and 90 percent of patients suffer from pancreatic insufficiency, which is apparent at birth (Orenstein, 1989). The pancreas produces enzymes for digestion that pass through the pancreatic duct to the small intestine. In CF, the pancreatic duct becomes obstructed with thick mucus, which does not allow the passage of enzymes. This obstruction leads to fibrosis and destruction of the pancreas. Consequently, food (predominantly proteins and fats) cannot be digested and absorbed normally, leading to signs and symptoms of malnutrition. Absorption of the fat-soluble vitamins, A, D, E, and K, is therefore impaired. Clinical manifestations include frequent, bulky, loose, greasy stools (steatorrhea) and poor growth.

Approximately 10 to 20 percent of newborns with CF present with meconium ileus, which is a functional bowel obstruction due to large quantities of thick meconium in the small and large intestine. This obstruction presents between 24 and 48 hours of age with abdominal distention, vomiting, and failure to pass meconium. Occasionally, meconium may escape into the peritoneum through a perforation and cause meconium peritonitis (Orenstein, 1989). The patient with CF may have many other complications that need to be assessed (Table 26–5).

Differential Diagnosis

The diagnosis of CF is based on a combination of typical clinical signs and symptoms as well as a positive sweat test. The accepted method to confirm the diagnosis of CF is the Gibson-Cooke sweat test. This method uses pilocarpine iontophoresis with quantitative analysis of chloride (Gibson & Cooke, 1959), and it is more than 90 percent sensitive (Hilman, 1989). A sweat chloride concentration of greater than 60 mEq/L is diagnostic in children; 70 mg of sweat is needed to obtain an accurate result. Sweat testing in the newborn period is difficult, as infants may not produce sufficient quantities of sweat. If a sufficient quantity is collected, the results are as valid as in older individuals (Orenstein, 1989).

The most common cause of a false-positive sweat test is laboratory error. False-positive results can also be found in malnutrition, adrenal insufficiency, ectodermal dysplasia, nephrogenic diabetes insipidus, hypothyroidism, and mucopolysaccharidosis. False-negative results can occur in the presence of edema and hypoproteinemia (Wood et al., 1976).

DNA analysis can be performed on buccal smears (cheek cell smears) of infants weighing less than 8 pounds or when sufficient sweat is unobtainable. This test is 90 percent sensitive for the North American white population (Richards et al., 1992).

Prenatal testing for CF includes DNA analysis of chorionic villus samples during the first trimester (8 to 10 weeks) or amniotic fluid samples collected after 14 weeks. If a positive family history of CF exists, the risk can usually be assessed in the fetus by testing through mutation analysis or restriction fragment length polymorphism markers to determine haplotype. The most appropriate type of testing is dependent on each individual's situation. Thus, the patient or family is referred to a geneticist for assessment.

In general, newborn screening programs are not used in the United States. Assays of meconium albumin were once used with 85 percent sensitivity, because infants with pancreatic insufficiency due to CF have elevated levels of protein in the stool. Another screening test is the immunoreactive trypsin assay, which is performed on a dried blood spot. A newborn with CF can have extremely high levels of plasma trypsinogen compared with normal infants. This elevation is presumed to occur because of pancreatic duct obstruction. The rationale for newborn screening is that early diagnosis may lead to earlier treatment, thereby reducing the morbidity and mortality associated with CF. However, screening is not accepted worldwide because an improvement in outcome is not clearly demonstrated in relationship to earlier diagnosis (Waters et al., 1990) and there is no screening method available that detects at least 90 percent of affected individuals.

TABLE 26–5 Complications of Cystic Fibrosis

Respiratory
Recurrent pneumonia
Recurrent bronchiolitis
Atelectasis/emphysema
Pansinusitis
Haemophilus influenzae, Staphylococcus aureus, Pseudomonas aeruginosa, and *Burkholderia cepacia* (formerly *Pseudomonas cepacia*) infection
Pneumothorax
Hemoptysis (usually self-limiting and associated with pulmonary exacerbation)

Gastrointestinal
Meconium ileus (10%–20%)
Malabsorption/steatorrhea due to pancreatic insufficiency (80%)
Failure to thrive with a weight and/or height less than fifth percentile
Rectal prolapse (5%)
Biliary cirrhosis (3%–5%)
Meconium ileus equivalent (seen in the older child and associated with a partial bowel obstruction from thick stool and secretions)
Intussusception
Fat-soluble vitamin deficiencies
Hypoproteinemia/edema

Miscellaneous
Nasal polyps (20%)
Heat prostration with hyponatremia/hypochloremia dehydration
Azoospermia
Digital clubbing/hypertrophic pulmonary osteoarthropathy
Diabetes mellitus (3%–5%)

Collaborative Management

There is still no cure for CF. Care revolves around preventing the progression of the disease and treating the symptoms. The comprehensive management of CF requires input from an interdisciplinary team within a CF center following the standards and guidelines recommended by the Cystic Fibrosis Foundation.

Team members usually include a pulmonologist, gastroenterologist, nurse, social worker, nutritionist, respiratory therapist, and physical therapist. Practitioners of other disciplines, such as psychology, genetics, and internal medicine, may be required.

The first goal of therapy is to minimize pulmonary infections and prevent the progression of disease. This goal is accomplished by using mucus clearance techniques such as chest physiotherapy and postural drainage. In older children, other methods, such as flutter devices and positive expiratory pressure valves, are used. Occasionally, aerosols or bronchodilators and mucolytic agents are used in combination with chest physiotherapy. In children older than 5 years, rhDNase (Pulmozyme) is used as an aerosol to reduce the viscosity of mucus secretions by breaking down the DNA (Shak et al., 1990). Oral or intravenous antibiotics are used during respiratory exacerbations to help decrease bacterial colonization and minimize inflammation. High-dose ibuprofen, used in children between 5 and 13 years of age, acts to reduce inflammation of the lung tissue to slow the progression of lung disease (Konstan et al., 1995). Supplemental oxygen becomes necessary when hypoxemia occurs.

Double lung transplantation may be an option in end-stage disease. It has been performed successfully in a relatively small number of CF patients. Survival is 62 percent at 1 year and 51 percent at 2 years (Registry, 1992).

A second goal of therapy is to assure adequate nutrition. The aim of nutritional therapy is to foster normal growth and development while contributing to the general health of the individual. Data suggest that lung function and exercise capacity may improve with optimal nutritional management.

Pancreatic enzyme replacement therapy is used to replace the enzymes that normally reach the intestine via the pancreatic duct. A diet high in calories (120 to 150 percent of the recommended daily allowance) and protein (200 percent of the recommended daily allowance) is needed, along with vitamin supplementation, with emphasis on the fat-soluble vitamins (A, D, E, and K) in a water-soluble form. The diet prescription varies among individuals. With appropriate enzyme replacement, neonates are successfully fed popular infant formulas or breast milk. However, infants are often prescribed an elemental or predigested formula such as Pregestimil or Portagen, especially if the infant is nutritionally deprived at the time of diagnosis. To meet an individual's nutritional goals, an increased calorie per ounce of formula may be given (e.g., 24 or 27 kcal/oz).

Individuals may also receive feedings via nasogastric, gastrostomy, or jejunostomy tubes if oral intake is poor. A thorough nutritional assessment is an important component of a patient's treatment.

A third goal of treatment is to facilitate family coping skills and adaptation to a condition that is lifelong. Families are confronted by enormous psychological stresses, financial obligations, and time burdens. The nurse can assist in the adjustment process, and referral to the social worker or psychologist may be indicated. Families can be referred to a genetic specialist for genetic counseling and future planning.

In the majority of cases, a diagnosis of CF is made in the first year of life. Therefore, the neonatal nurse must be alert to the signs and symptoms of respiratory and nutritional problems that are associated with CF. For nursing management of meconium ileus, see Chapter 24, Assessment and Management of Gastrointestinal Dysfunction.

If an infant is suspected of having CF, the nurse assists in making a referral to the CF clinic and collaborates with the nurse on the CF team to help coordinate efforts and avoid confusing the family with conflicting information. He or she can allay parents' fears about the sweat test by explaining how the test is performed and letting the parents know when the results will be available. After the diagnosis is confirmed and the team physician or nurse initiates the educational process, the nurse provides support and facilitates the adaptation process. He or she provides written and verbal information and assesses the family's understanding of the diagnosis. The nurse also provides clarification regarding the diagnosis, genetic issues, therapy, home management, medications, equipment, normal growth and development, and follow-up routine. As a patient advocate, the nurse refers a family to their local Cystic Fibrosis Foundation and parent support group and assists the family in locating community information, service, and support resources as well as funding sources. The nurse enables and empowers the family of a child newly diagnosed with CF by providing opportunities for the family to acquire the necessary knowledge and skills so that they can become competent and independent. A nurse sensitive to family needs helps a family understand what CF means to them and how to incorporate it into their lifestyle. The nurse portrays a hopeful and positive outlook so that parents feel encouraged and able to help their child lead a full and happy life.

Prognosis

Since CF was first recognized as a clinical syndrome in the mid-1940s, treatment has improved considerably, resulting in greater longevity and quality of life for individuals with CF. Survival statistics are improving steadily, and the median age of survival is now approaching 30 years of age (Cystic Fibrosis Genotype-Phenotype Consortium, 1993; Cystic Fibrosis Foundation, 1994). It is estimated that the life expectancy of children with CF diagnosed today is 40 to 50 years (Fitzsimmons, 1993). Therefore, it is important for a family to treat children with CF as normally as possible and to plan for education, career, marriage, and other long-term goals as with any other child.

CONCLUSION

The endocrine system is a highly complex structure, and its function touches on every other body system. It is not surprising that neonates with alterations in endocrine function require an accurate and thorough head-to-toe assessment.

REFERENCES

Aetiology of growth hormone deficiency [Letter]. (1988). *Archives of Disease in Childhood, 63*(2), 219–220.

Argente, J., & Chowen, J. A. (1994). Neuroendocrinology of growth hormone secretion. *Growth Genetics & Hormones, 10*(2), 1–5.

Avery, G. B., Fletcher, M. A., & MacDonald, M. G. (Eds.). (1994). *Neonatology: Pathophysiology and management of the newborn* (4th ed.). Philadelphia: J. B. Lippincott.

Becks, G. P., & Burrow, G. N. (1990). Thyrotoxicosis in pregnancy. In N. M. Nelson (Ed.), *Current therapy in neonatal-perinatal medicine 2* (pp. 108–111). Philadelphia: B. C. Decker.

Bona, G., Aquili, C., Ravanini, P., et al. (1994). Growth hormone, insulin-like growth factor-I and somatostatin in human fetus, newborn, mother plasma and amniotic fluid. *Panminerva Medica, 36*(1), 5–12.

Castiglia, P. T. (1989). Ambiguous genitalia. *Journal of Pediatric Health Care, 3*(6), 319–321.

Cicognani, A. (1992). The experience of neonatal screening for congenital adrenal hyperplasia. *Hormone Research, 37*(Suppl. 3), 34–38.

Cloherty, J. P., & Stark, A. R. (Eds.). (1991). *Manual of neonatal care* (3rd ed.). Boston: Little, Brown.

Cowett, R. M., & Schwartz, R. (1982). The infant of the diabetic mother. *Pediatric Clinics of North America, 29*(5), 1213–1231.

Cruz, T. V. D., MacMillan, D. R., Browning, R. M., & Stewart, D. L. (1995). Delayed diagnosis of congenital adrenal hyperplasia in a premature female infant. *Journal of Kentucky Medical Association, 93*(1), 19–21.

Cystic Fibrosis Foundation. (1989). Gene that causes cystic fibrosis identified. *Commitment*, pp. 1–8.

Cystic Fibrosis Foundation. (1994). Patient Registry 1993, Annual Data Report, Bethesda, MD.

Cystic Fibrosis Genotype-Phenotype Consortium. (1993). Correlation between genotype and phenotype in patients with cystic fibrosis. *New England Journal of Medicine, 329*(18), 1308–1313.

Dean, M., & Santis, G. (1994). Heterogeneity in the severity of cystic fibrosis and the role of CFTR gene mutations. *Human Genetics, 9*(4), 364–368.

De la Chapelle, A., Koo, G. C., & Wachtel, S. S. (1978). Recessive sex-determining genes in human XX male syndrome. *Cell, 15*(3), 837.

DiGrande, A. (1984). The child born with ambiguous genitalia: Family assessment and nursing intervention. *Issues in Comprehensive Pediatric Nursing, 7*(6), 307–318.

Einaudi, S., Lala, R., Corrias, A., et al. (1993). Auxological and biochemical parameters in assessing treatment of infants and toddlers with congenital adrenal hyperplasia due to 21-hydroxylase deficiency. *Journal of Pediatric Endocrinology, 6*(2), 173–178.

Erickson, R. P., Verga, V., & Dasouki, M. (1990). Use of a probe for the putative sex determining gene, zinc finger Y, in the study of patients with ambiguous genitalia and XY gonadal dysgenesis. *American Journal of Medical Genetics, 36*(2), 232–236.

Fanaroff, A. A., & Martin, R. J. (Eds.). (1997). *Neonatal-perinatal medicine* (6th ed.). St. Louis: Mosby–Year Book.

Fitzsimmons, S. C. (1993). The changing epidemiology of cystic fibrosis. *Journal of Pediatrics, 122*(1), 1–9.

Frasier, S. D., Weiss, B. A., & Horton, R. (1974). Amniotic fluid testosterone: Implications for the prenatal diagnosis of congenital adrenal hyperplasia. *Journal of Pediatrics, 8*(5), 738.

Ganong, W. F. (1985). *Review of medical physiology* (12th ed.). Los Altos, CA: Lange Medical Publications.

Gelato, M. C., Malozowski, S., Pescovitz, O. H., et al. (1987). Growth hormone–releasing hormone: Therapeutic perspectives. *Pediatrician, 14*(3), 162–167.

Gibson, L., & Cooke, R. (1959). A test for concentration of electrolytes in sweat in cystic fibrosis of the pancreas utilizing pilocarpine by iontophoresis. *Pediatrics, 23,* 545–549.

Goetzman, B. W., & Wennberg, R. P. (1991). *Neonatal intensive care handbook* (2nd ed.). St. Louis: Mosby–Year Book.

Griffin, J. E., & Wilson, J. D. (1986). Disorders of sexual differentiation. In P. C. Walsh, R. F. Gittes, A. D. Perlmutter, & T. A. Stamey (Eds.), *Campbell's urology* (5th ed.). Philadelphia: W. B. Saunders.

Hamblin, J. E., Assimos, D. G., & Kroovand, R. L. (1989). Pediatric urology. *Primary Care, 16*(4), 889–904.

Herber, S. M., & Kay, R. (1987). Aetiology of growth hormone deficiency. *Archives of Disease in Childhood, 62*(7), 735–736.

Herber, S. M., & Milner, D. G. (1984). Growth hormone deficiency presenting under age 2 years. *Archives of Disease in Childhood, 59*(6), 557–560.

Hilman, B. (1989). Cystic fibrosis—changing concepts. *Schumpert Medical Quarterly, 7,* 345–370.

Hindmarsh, P. C., Bridges, N. A., & Brook, C. G. D. (1991). Wider indications for treatment with biosynthetic human growth hormone in children. *Clinical Endocrinology, 34*(5), 417–427.

Hitti, I. F., Glasberg, S. S., Huggins-Jones, D., & Sabet, R. (1994). Bilateral femoral hypoplasia and maternal diabetes mellitus. *Pediatric Pathology, 14*(4), 567–574.

Hocking, M. D., Newell, S. J., & Rayner, P. H. W. (1986). Use of human growth hormone in treatment of nesidioblastosis in a neonate. *Archives of Disease in Childhood, 61*(7), 706–707.

Hoskins, S. K. (1990). Nursing care of the infant of a diabetic mother. *Neonatal Network, 9*(4), 39–46.

Ismail, A. A., Walker, P. L., Macfaul, R., & Gindal, B. (1989). Diagnostic value of serum testosterone measurement in infancy: Two case reports. *Annals of Clinical Biochemistry, 26*(Part 3), 259–261.

Kalaitzoglou, G., & New, M. I. (1993). Congenital adrenal hyperplasia: Molecular insights learned from patients. *Receptor, 3*(3), 211–222.

Kasdan, H., Nankin, H. R., Troen, P., et al. (1973). Paternal transmission of maleness in XX human beings. *New England Journal of Medicine, 288*(11), 539–545.

Kelnar, C. J. H. (1993). Congenital adrenal hyperplasia (CAH)—The place for prenatal treatment and neonatal screening. *Early Human Development, 35*(2), 81–90.

Kenner, C., Harjo, J., & Brueggemeyer, A. (Eds.). (1988). *Neonatal surgery: A nursing perspective.* New York: Grune & Stratton.

Kinzie, B. J. (1987). Management of the syndrome of inappropriate secretion of antidiuretic hormone. *Clinical Pharmacy, 6*(8), 625–633.

Klaus, M. H., & Fanaroff, A. A. (1993). *Care of the high-risk neonate* (4th ed.). Philadelphia: W. B. Saunders.

Knip, M., Lautala, P., Leppäluoto, J., et al. (1983). Relation of enteroinsular hormones at birth to macrosomia and neonatal hypoglycemia in infants of diabetic mothers. *Journal of Pediatrics, 103*(4), 603–611.

Konstan, M., Byard, P., Hoppel, C., & Davis, P. (1995). Effect of high-dose ibuprofen in patients with cystic fibrosis. *New England Journal of Medicine, 332*(13), 848–854.

Kulczycki, L., & Schauf, V. (1974). Cystic fibrosis in blacks in Washington, D.C.: Incidence and characteristics. *American Journal of Diseases of Children, 127*(1), 64.

Kuller, J. A., Chescheir, N. C., & Cefalo, R. C. (Eds.). (1996). *Prenatal diagnosis & reproductive genetics.* Philadelphia: J. B. Lippincott.

Lanes, R., Nieto, C., Bruguera, C., et al. (1989). Growth hormone release in response to growth hormone–releasing hormone in term and preterm neonates. *Biology of the Neonate, 56*(5), 252–256.

Lee, P. D. K., & Rosenfeld, R. G. (1987). Clinical utility of insulin-like growth factor assays. *Pediatrician, 14*(3), 154–161.

Loeuille, G. A., David, M., & Forest, M. G. (1990). Prenatal treatment of congenital adrenal hyperplasia: Report of a new case. *European Journal of Pediatrics, 149*(4), 237–240.

Malvaux, P. (1981). Hypothyroidism. In Brook C. (Ed.), *Clinical paediatric endocrinology* (pp. 329–336). London: Blackwell Scientific Publications.

Mazur, T. (1983). Ambiguous genitalia: Detection and counseling. *Pediatric Nursing, 9*(6), 417–422, 431.

Miller, W. L., & Levine, L. S. (1987). Molecular and clinical advances in congenital adrenal hyperplasia. *Journal of Pediatrics, 111*(1), 1–17.

Mimouni, F., Miodovnik, M., Whitsett, J. A., et al. (1987). Respiratory distress syndrome in infants of diabetic mothers in the 1980s: No direct adverse effect of maternal diabetes with modern management. *Obstetrics and Gynecology, 69*(2), 191–195.

Mininberg, D. T., Levine, L. S., & New, M. I. (1982). Current concepts in congenital adrenal hyperplasia. In T. V. N. Persaud (Ed.), *Advances in the study of birth defects: Genetic disorders, syndromology and prenatal diagnosis* (Vol. 5, pp. 181–196). New York: Alan R. Liss.

Moore, K. L., & Persaud, T. V. N. (1993). *Before we are born: Basic embryology and birth defects* (4th ed.). Philadelphia: W. B. Saunders.

Neufeld, N. D. (1987). Infants of diabetic mothers: Prenatal care and outcomes for the infant. *Mount Sinai Journal of Medicine, 54*(3), 266–271.

New, M. (1988). Congenital adrenal hyperplasia. *Biochemical Society Transactions, 16*(5), 691–694.

New, M. I., & Josso, N. (1988). Disorders of gonadal differentiation and CAH. *Endocrinology and Metabolism Clinics of North America, 17*(2), 339–366.

New, M. I., White, P. C., Speiser, P. W., et al. (1990). Congenital adrenal hyperplasia. In A. E. H. Emery & D. L. Rimoin (Eds.), *Principles and practice of medical genetics* (Vol. 2., pp. 1559–1586). Edinburgh: Churchill Livingstone.

Novak, R. W., & Robinson, H. B. (1994). Coincident DiGeorge anomaly and renal agenesis and its relation to maternal diabetes. *American Journal of Medicine Genetics, 50*(4), 311–312.

Orenstein, D. (1989). *Cystic fibrosis: A guide for patient and family.* New York: Raven Press.

Pang, S., Hotchkiss, J., Drash, A. L., et al. (1977). Microfilter paper method for 17 alpha-progesterone radioimmunoassay: Its application for rapid screening for congenital adrenal hyperplasia. *Journal of Clinical Endocrinology and Metabolism, 4*(5), 1003.

Pang, S., Pollack, M. S., Marshall, R. N., & Immken, L. (1990). Prenatal treatment of congenital adrenal hyperplasia due to 21-hydroxylase deficiency. *New England Journal of Medicine, 322*(2), 111–115.

Parks, J. S. (1981). Hyperthyroidism. In C. Brook (Ed.), *Clinical paediatric endocrinology* (pp. 340–361). London: Blackwell Scientific Publications.

Penny, R. (1990). Ambiguous genitalia [Editorial]. *American Journal of Diseases of Children, 144*(7), 753.

Perelman, R. H. (1983). The infant of the diabetic mother. *Primary Care, 10*(4), 751–760.

Pressler, J. L. (1991). Strategies useful in caring for macrosomic newborns. *Journal of Pediatric Nursing, 6*(3), 149–153.

Rapaport, R., Petersen, B., Skuza, K. A., et al. (1991). Immune functions during treatment of growth hormone–deficient children with biosynthetic human growth hormone. *Clinical Pediatrics, 30*(1), 22–27.

Registry (1992). The registry of the International Society for Heart and Lung Transplantation: Ninth official report—1992. *Journal of Heart and Lung Transplantation, 11*(4, Part 1), 599–606.

Richards, B., Skoletsky, J., Shuber, A., et al. (1992). Multiplex PCR amplification from the CFTR gene using DNA prepared from buccal brushes/swabs. *Human Molecular Genetics*, *2*(2), 159–163.

Rimoin, D. L. (1990). Genetic disorders of the pituitary gland. In A. E. Emery & D. L. Rimoin (Eds.), *Principles and practice of medical genetics* (Vol. 2, pp. 1461–1488). Edinburgh: Churchill Livingstone.

Riordan, J., Rommens, J., Kerem, B., et al. (1989). Identification of the cystic fibrosis gene: Cloning and characterization of complementary DNA. *Science, 245*(4922), 1066–1073.

Rock, J. A., & Jones, H. W., Jr. (1989). Construction of a neovagina for patients with a flat perineum. *American Journal of Obstetrics and Gynecology, 160*(4), 845–853.

Rose, B. I., Graff, S., Spencer, R., et al. (1988). Major congenital anomalies in infants and glycosylated hemoglobin levels in insulin-requiring diabetic mothers. *Journal of Perinatology, 8*(4), 309–311.

Rosenfeld, M., Ramsey, B., Redding, G., et al. (1994). Changes in pulmonary function associated with pseudomonal respiratory colonization in infants with cystic fibrosis. *Pediatric Pulmonology, 10*(Suppl.), 262. [Poster abstract 298 presented at 8th annual North American Cystic Fibrosis Conference. Orlando, FL, October 20–23.]

Ross, J. L., Cassorla, F. G., Skerda, M. C., et al. (1983). A preliminary study of the effect of estrogen dose on growth in Turner's syndrome. *New England Journal of Medicine, 309*(18), 1104.

Schanberg, S. M., & Field, T. M. (1987). Sensory deprivation stress and supplemental stimulation in the rat pup and preterm human neonate. *Child Development, 58*(6), 1431–1447.

Schwartz, R., Gruppuso, P. A., Petzold, K., et al. (1994). Hyperinsulinemia and macrosomia in the fetus of the diabetic mother. *Diabetes Care, 17*(7), 640–648.

Shak, S., Capon, D., Hellmiss, R., et al. (1990). Recombinant human DNase I reduces the viscosity of cystic fibrosis sputum. *Proceedings of the National Academy of Sciences USA, 87*, 9188–9192.

Shapiro, E., Santiago, J. V., & Crane, J. P. (1989). Prenatal fetal adrenal suppression following in utero diagnosis of CAH. *Journal of Urology, 142*(Part 2), 663–666.

Shimano, S., Suzuki, S., Nagashima, K., et al. (1985). Growth hormone response to growth hormone releasing factor in neonates. *Biology of the Neonate, 47*(6), 367–370.

Sills, I. N., & Rapaport, R. (1994). New-onset IDDM presenting with diabetic ketoacidosis in a pregnant adolescent. *Diabetes Care, 17*(8), 904–905.

Tsukahara, H., Fujii, Y., Kuriyama, M., et al. (1993). Urinary growth hormone excretion in preterm neonates. *Biology of the Neonate, 63*(1), 8–13.

Varvarigou, A., Vagenakis, A. G., Makri, M., & Beratis, N. G. (1994). Growth hormone, insulin-like growth factor-1 and prolactin in small for gestational age neonates. *Biology of the Neonate, 65*(2), 94–102.

Vimpani, G. V., Vimpani, A. F., Pocock, S. J., & Farquhar, J. W. (1981). Differences in physical characteristics, perinatal histories, and social backgrounds between children with growth hormone deficiency and constitutional short stature. *Archives of Disease in Childhood, 56*(2), 922–928.

Walfish, P. G., & Tseng, K. H. (1989). Thyroid physiology and pathology. In R. Collu, J. Duchame, & H. Guyda (Eds.), *Pediatric endocrinology* (pp. 367–375). New York: Raven Press.

Wallis, M. (1988). The molecular basis of growth hormone deficiency. *Molecular Aspects of Medicine, 10*(5), 429–509.

Waters, D., Dorney, S., Gaskin, K., et al. (1990). Pancreatic function in infants identified as having cystic fibrosis in a neonatal screening program. *New England Journal of Medicine, 322*(5), 303–308.

Weise, K., & Zaritsky, A. (1987). Endocrine manifestations of critical illness in the child. *Pediatric Clinics of North America, 34*(1), 119–130.

Wiedemann, H.-R., Kunze, J., Grosse, F.-R., & Dibbern, H. (1989). *Atlas of clinical syndromes: A visual aid to diagnosis* (2nd ed.). St. Louis: Mosby–Year Book.

White, P. (1974). Diabetes mellitus in pregnancy. *Clinics in Perinatology, 1*(2), 331–347.

White, P. C., New, M. I., & Dupont, B. (1986). Structure of human steroid 21-hydroxylase genes. *Proceedings of the National Academy of Sciences USA, 83*(14), 5111–5115.

Wood, R., Boat, T., & Doershuk, C. (1976). Cystic fibrosis. *American Review of Respiratory Disease, 113*(6), 833–878.

Woods, D. L., Malan, A. F., & Coetzee, E. J. (1980). Intra-uterine growth in infants of diabetic mothers. *South African Medical Journal, 58*(11), 441–443.

Zapata, A., Grande, C., & Hernandez-Garcia, J. M. (1994). Influence of metabolism control of pregnant diabetics on fetal lung maturity. *Scandinavian Journal of Clinical & Laboratory Investigation, 54*(16), 431–434.

CHAPTER 27

Assessment and Management of Immunologic Dysfunction

JUDY WRIGHT LOTT CAROLE KENNER

RESEARCH AGENDA

What factors influence the development of the neonatal immune system?

What maternal factors put the neonate at risk for immunologic dysfunction?

What are the effects of passive maternal immunity on the development of neonatal immunologic problems?

What is the effect of shorter hospital stays on the incidence of early and late neonatal sepsis?

What is the role of immunotherapy in improving mortality and morbidity of neonates?

Are there new methods to reduce transmission of infection?

VIGNETTE

Tommy was a 2.4-kg male born at 37 weeks' gestation to a 33-year-old, G2 PO>1 0-positive female, with prenatal care beginning at 8 weeks. Pregnancy was complicated by preterm labor at 7 months and vaginitis (treated with erythromycin and ampicillin) in the second trimester. At term, Mrs. G presented in active labor with membranes ruptured for 16 hours. At the time of admission, her temperature was 101.2°F. Upon placement of the fetal monitor, the infant was noted to have decelerations and decreased to absent variability; therefore, an emergency C-section was performed.

Tommy required minimal resuscitation, involving blow-by oxygen and bulb suction. Apgars were 8(1) and 9(5). He was then taken to the normal newborn nursery.

Tommy was doing well until 2 days later when mild respiratory distress developed. His axillary temperature was 38.6°C. He was taken to the special care nursery. After a complete sepsis work-up, he was started on ampicillin and gentamicin. His temperature continued to elevate. The respiratory distress worsened. His respiratory rate fluctuated between 70 and 100 with retractions. He required increased oxygen and had a cardiac murmur. Initial labs showed development of a base deficit in the capillary blood gas.

Physical exam findings included lethargy; pale pink coloring in head-hood oxygen; skin intact with multiple petechiae; HEENT grossly normal; chest significant for retractions; tachypnea; breath sounds bilaterally equal with rales; regular rate with systolic murmur present; good capillary refill; abdomen soft, not tense, but distended with hepatosplenomegaly and no masses; and irritability.

During the next 3 days, Tommy's respiratory status deteriorated to the point that intubation and assisted ventilation were required. Fluid restriction was unsuccessful because of DIC. Tommy needed so many units of packed red blood cells, platelets, and fresh-frozen plasma that his fluid status was difficult to manage. He became progressively less responsive. A head ultrasound showed significant cranial hemorrhaging. Tommy's parents reached a very difficult decision: to remove Tommy from the ventilator and allow him to die peacefully. He died in his mother's arms at 5 days of age.

Tracey A. Kleeman

The primary function of the immune system is to protect the body from harm caused by infection from invading microorganisms such as bacteria, viruses, fungi, protozoa, and parasites. During gestation, the healthy fetus grows and develops within the usually protective environment of the mother's uterus. During and after birth, however, the neonate is exposed to a wide variety of microorganisms. The neonate's extrauterine existence is contingent upon an equilibrium between its own host defense mechanisms and the hostile microorganisms in its environment.

Even though the host defense mechanisms begin to develop early during gestation, many of these mechanisms do not function at the time of birth—even in the term neonate—as efficiently as in older infants, children, or adults. This immaturity of the complex immune system becomes apparent in light of the relatively high prevalence of infectious disease that occurs during the perinatal period as well as the increased prevalence of neonatal infection caused by agents considered to be of low pathogenicity (Yoder & Polin, 1997). Although the cells of the fetal and neonatal immune system are not fully developed, they show a remarkable ability to respond to the environment. Yet, humans at these early stages of development are susceptible to injury either caused directly by immunologic mechanisms or imposed by infectious microbes that overwhelm the relatively immature and inexperienced immune system (Bellanti et al., 1994). These processes form the foundation for the prevention, diagnosis, and treatment of neonatal infectious diseases.

GENERAL DEVELOPMENT OF THE IMMUNE SYSTEM

The immune response is characterized as a sequence of adaptive cellular responses to threats from a dynamic and potentially hostile environment. Three levels of host adaptation to the environment, as described by Bellanti and colleagues (1994), are in progressive order as follows:

1. Phylogeny (species). From an evolutionary standpoint, the effect of a hostile microenvironment has provided the particular pressures leading to the survival of existing life forms within the species that are best adapted to that environment.
2. Ontogeny (individual). In the developing fetus, the microenvironment in which undifferentiated precursor cells exist provides another type of inductive environment, which allows the full expression of immunity within the developing infant. The best selected form resulting from this level is the immunologically mature individual.
3. Induction (cellular). The highest level is the molecular environment in which immunologically reactive cells exist, providing the inductive stimulus leading to the proliferative and differentiative events frequently associated with cellular immune responses. The best-adapted form for this environment may be the establishment of memory cells.

Even though the cells and functions that make up the immune system appear early in gestation, some of them are activated only after birth, as the neonate begins to interact with the external environment. In intrauterine infections, however, the environment of the fetus may be so changed that activation of some of these cells and functions may begin in utero.

EMBRYOLOGIC DEVELOPMENT OF THE IMMUNE SYSTEM

Host defense mechanisms may be separated into two major categories: nonspecific mechanisms and specific mechanisms:

1. The *nonspecific* mechanisms, which include physical barriers, chemical barriers, phagocytosis, the inflammatory response, and amplification systems, including complement, function effectively without necessitating prior exposure to a microorganism or its antigens.
2. The *specific* mechanisms, consisting of the cell-mediated (T cell) and humoral or antibody–mediated (B cell) immune responses, operate most effectively with prior exposure to the infective agent or its antigens.

Both the nonspecific and the specific mechanisms are closely interrelated and interdependent. The body defends against infection by preventing access to pathogenic microorganisms by mechanical barriers, including intact skin and mucus and other body fluids, such as tears, saliva, and urine, which protect the epithelial surfaces. Phagocytes, which arise from the bone marrow stem cells, engulf particles, including infectious agents, and internalize and destroy them. *Chemotaxis* is the process by which phagocytes are attracted to the site of infection.

Phagocytosis, or cell-eating, is the most primitive of the host defense mechanisms. Although the most important phagocytic cells are the polymorphonuclear leukocytes, other cells, including monocytes and the nonmobile phagocytic cells of the reticuloendothelial system, are also involved in phagocytosis (Yoder & Polin, 1992). Specific phase defects in some areas of phagocytic function have been recognized in normal neonates, suggesting that the newborn may be compromised because of its deficiencies in both cellular and humoral factors involved in the process of phagocytosis. Under certain conditions, both in vitro and in vivo, neonatal polymorphonuclear leukocytes demonstrate less phagocytic capability than those of adults (Bellanti et al., 1994).

Inflammatory Response

Inflammation is the body's response to injury; it consists of three reactions:

- Increased blood supply to the area
- Increased capillary permeability
- Migration of leukocytes (polymorphonuclear neutrophils) and macrophages out of the capillaries into surrounding tissues

A spectrum of cellular and systemic events are activated upon invasion by microbes as tissue injury occurs; the host attempts to restore and maintain homeostasis, and this constitutes the inflammatory response. The acute inflammatory response is characterized by blood vessel dilatation and the accumulation of white blood cells (WBCs) and fluid. Shortly thereafter, neutrophilic granulocytes appear, which phagocytize and kill pathogenic microbes. The ensuing febrile reaction, resulting from increased metabolic activity probably related to the release of endogenous pyrogens from the host's WBCs, is underdeveloped in the neonate; thus, fever is not a significant sign of infection during the neonatal period. Likewise, an increase in WBCs and sedimentation rate, which is often associated with bacterial infection in older infants, children, and adults, is infrequent in neonates (Bellanti et al., 1994). There are, however, some signs of inflammatory responses seen in newborns, including an increase in total numbers of band (immature neutrophil) forms as well as activation of the coagulation system with disseminated intravascular coagulation (DIC). The deficiency of complement components, as well as the deficiency of some coagulation factors (i.e., vitamin K–dependent factors), contributes to the diminished inflammatory response of neonates.

Humoral Immunity

Complement System

The complement system consists of approximately 20 serum proteins that interact with each other and with other components of the immune system. The complement system assists the immunologically specific effects of antibody by the opsonization and lysis of red blood cells and bacteria.

The functions of the complement system are (1) cell activation, (2) cytolysis of target cells, and (3) opsonization of cells to facilitate phagocytosis of bacteria.

When activated, the complement system creates a cascade effect with amplification that works to "complement" antibody activity in destroying bacteria and to rid the body of antigen–antibody complexes. In so doing, the complement system induces an inflammatory response. Synthesis of most complement components begins early in fetal development, as early as 5 weeks' gestation, and is not related to the presence of antigen. Reasonable quantities appear in the serum at 12 to 14 weeks' gestation, remain at these somewhat low levels until about 26 to 28 weeks' gestation, and then markedly increase, so that, at term, total complement titers are at least half of the corresponding levels in adults. The concentration of complement decreases slightly after birth and recovers by 3 weeks of age; this may indicate that antigen stimulation may be involved in the induction of complement synthesis (Bellanti et al., 1994). Little is known regarding the biologic activities of this system in the neonate despite its significant role in the natural resistance to infection.

Immunoglobulins

Immunoglobulins (antibodies) are a group of glycoproteins in the serum and tissue fluids of all mammals. Immunoglobulins are produced when the host's lymphoid system comes into contact with immunogenic foreign molecules (antigens); they bind specifically to the antigen that induced their formation. There are five classes of immunoglobulins:

1. Immunoglobulin G (IgG) is the major immunoglobulin in

normal human serum. It makes up approximately 70 to 75 percent of the total immunoglobulin pool. IgG is distributed evenly between the intravascular and extravascular pools. It is the major antibody of secondary immune responses and the exclusive antitoxin class. Maternal IgG is transported across the placenta only during the last trimester.
2. Immunoglobulin M (IgM) makes up approximately 10 percent of the immunoglobulin pool. It is confined primarily to the intravascular pool. IgM is the predominant early antibody; it is frequently directed against antigenically complex infectious organisms. IgM is produced by the fetus in response to intrauterine infection.
3. Immunoglobulin A (IgA) makes up approximately 15 to 20 percent of the immunoglobulin pool. It is the predominant immunoglobulin in seromucous secretions such as saliva, tracheobronchial secretions, colostrum, milk, and genitourinary secretions. Secretory IgA is abundant in seromucous secretions and is protected from proteolysis by combination with another protein (the secretory component).
4. Immunoglobulin D (IgD) makes up less than 1 percent of the total plasma immunoglobulins, but it is present in large quantities on the membrane of many circulating B lymphocytes. The precise biologic function of IgD is not known; it may be involved in antigen-triggered lymphocyte differentiation.
5. Immunoglobulin E (IgE) is a trace serum immunoglobulin found on the surface membrane of basophils and mast cells in all individuals. It may function in active immunity to helminths; more commonly, it is associated with immediate hypersensitivity diseases such as asthma and fever.

Cellular Immunity

Leukocytes

Leukocytes, or WBCs, are nucleated cells that protect the body against infection. There are three types of leukocytes: (1) granulocytes, which include neutrophils, eosinophils, and basophils; (2) monocytes; and (3) lymphocytes.

Granulocytes, or polymorphonuclear leukocytes, are produced in the bone marrow. They evolve from myeloblasts into myelocytes and, finally, into mature granulocytes. The types of granulocytes are differentiated by cell-staining techniques. Neutrophils can leave the blood circulation and enter the tissues, where they ingest foreign substances and bacteria through phagocytosis. These cells are called phagocytes. Eosinophils are also phagocytes because they ingest and destroy antigen–antibody complexes. The function of the basophils is not fully known. Basophils appear to act similarly to the mast cells found in connective tissue, releasing histamine (bronchoconstrictor) and heparin (anticoagulant). Monocytes arise from the bone marrow and develop into macrophages, which are phagocytic. Monocytes ingest foreign particles and fragmented cells. Lymphocytes originate in such lymphogenous sites as bone marrow, lymph nodes, spleen, liver, thymus, subepithelial lymphoid tissue, and connective tissue.

Lymphocytes develop from lymphoblasts or other lymphocytes. Lymphocytes are involved in cellular immunity and antibody formation. There are two different types of lymphocytes: T lymphocytes and B lymphocytes. T lymphocytes (T cells) are involved in cell-mediated immunity, and B lymphocytes (B cells) produce antibodies. Infections stimulate the increased production and maturation of lymphocytes. Generally, the number of WBCs produced depends on the body's need for them. Infection, tissue damage, or presence of viral agents stimulates the production and circulation of leukocytes.

Granulocytes and monocytes arise from a common stem cell, or colony-forming unit (G-CSF and M-CSF, respectively). The eosinophil has a separate stem cell (CFU-Eo). The three types of granulocytes develop through the following similar stages: myeloblast, promyelocyte, myelocyte, metamyelocyte, band, and polymorphonuclear neutrophil or mature segmented neutrophil. In the routine differential count, the different stages of the eosinophils and basophils are not identified, they are just counted as eosinophils and basophils. The neutrophil stages are always identified.

Neutrophil Kinetics

As the myeloblast develops into the mature, segmented neutrophil, the myeloblast, promyelocyte, and myelocyte undergo cell division. These cells constitute the mitotic pool and generally undergo a total of three to five cell divisions over 6 to 7 days. During the promyelocyte stage, the cell produces nonspecific granules. The number of granules per cell decreases with each cell division. At the myelocyte stage, the cell produces specific granules.

In the metamyelocyte stage, mitosis is not possible. The metamyelocyte matures for approximately 7 to 8 days in the storage pool. The number of bands and segmented neutrophils in the storage pool is approximately 15 times the number in the peripheral blood, and the mitotic pool is approximately one third the size of the storage pool.

The release of mature segmented neutrophils into the peripheral blood is not completely understood, but appears to be a selective release. It is thought that substances such as colony-stimulating factor and granulopoietin regulate granulocyte production and control the movement of granulocytes from the bone marrow to the blood.

When the mature segmented neutrophils leave the storage pool, approximately 50 percent of the neutrophils circulate freely in the circulating pool. The other 50 percent adhere to the walls of the vessels and constitute the marginal pool. The cells in the marginal pool are not included in the WBC count, so the differential represents only half the number present. The cells constantly change between the circulating and marginal pools.

The mature segmented neutrophils are released first, along with a small percentage of bands. When the demand for neutrophils increases, more mature segmented neutrophils are released. If the demand is still not met, increased numbers of bands are released from the storage pool into the peripheral blood, reflecting an increased percentage of bands. A ratio of bands to segmented neutrophils greater than 0:3 or of immature neutrophils to total neutrophils equal to or greater than 0:2 should create suspicion of infection.

The neutrophils in the peripheral blood are replaced 2½ times every 24 hours. Neutrophils do not return to the bone marrow. From the marginal pool, neutrophils randomly enter tissues and body cavities, where they carry out their major function of stopping or retarding the action of foreign material or infectious agents by (1) moving into the area of inflammation or infection (2) phagocytizing foreign material, and (3) killing and digesting foreign material. The neutrophils are generally the first phagocytic cell to reach infected areas, followed by monocytes.

Eosinophils

Eosinophils are primarily tissue cells. They leave the blood and move into the tissues, where they localize in areas exposed to the external environment (e.g., skin, lungs, and gastrointestinal tract). Once in tissues, eosinophils do not return to the blood.

Eosinophils are metabolically more active than neutrophils, although their function is not clearly known. Eosinophils are capable of phagocytizing foreign material and antigen–antibody complexes, but this is not thought to be their primary function.

Eosinophils are thought to be anti-inflammatory cells because they modulate reactions in which basophils and mast cells are active. Eosinophils also help defend against helminths (parasites) by attaching to the parasite and releasing toxic substances.

Basophils

Basophils develop from a cell similar to the myeloblast, although the specific stem cell has not been identified. The function of basophils is not fully understood. Basophils exhibit chemotaxis and some phagocytosis. Basophil granules contain peroxidase, histamine, and heparin. Basophils synthesize an eosinophil chemotactic factor, a slow-reacting substance of anaphylaxis, and platelet-activating factor.

Basophils appear to participate in immediate hypersensitivity reactions and are involved in some delayed hypersensitivity reactions. Basophil membranes bind IgE. When specific antigens react with the membrane-bound IgE, degranulation occurs, and the contents of the basophil granules are released into the surrounding area. This response releases the eosinophil chemotactic factor and causes accumulation of eosinophils in the area.

Mast Cells

Mast cells are similar to basophils. They are found in the thymus, spleen, and bone marrow. Mast cells are of mesenchymal origin. The mast cell is slightly larger than the basophil and contains serotonin and some proteolytic enzymes in addition to the contents of the basophil.

Monocytes

The monocyte originates from the same committed stem cell as the neutrophil. The precursor of the monocyte is the promonocyte (sometimes called the myelomonoblast). The monocyte is considered an immature cell. The promonocyte is less phagocytic and less motile than the monocyte. After formation, the promonocyte undergoes 2 to 2½ mitotic divisions in approximately 2 days. The monocyte differentiates in the tissues into macrophages.

Monocytes and macrophages are motile, capable of chemotaxis, able to move through blood vessel walls, and able to migrate to areas of inflammation. They respond to migration-inhibiting factor, produced by the T lymphocytes to immobilize macrophages, and to chemotactic inhibitors. The monocyte and macrophage are capable of phagocytosis and pinocytosis. Monocyte production (hence, circulation) is increased in inflammation. The functions of the monocyte in providing immunity are as follows:

- Acts as a defense mechanism against intracellular parasites, including certain bacteria, fungi, and protozoa
- Removes damaged and old cells, plasma protein, and plasma lipids
- Participates in iron metabolism
- Processes antigen information for lymphocytes
- Produces and secretes various substances, including lysosomal enzymes, acid phosphatase, proteinase, collagenase, plasminogen activator, thromboplastin, platelet-activating factors, complement factors, and interferons

Colony-Stimulating Factors

Stem cells that are found in the fetal and neonatal immune tissue, primarily in the bone marrow, differentiate during development into myeloid and lymphoid stem cells. These colony-forming units or cells then become committed to a specific pathway of further maturation and development. Further development is a result of stimulating factors that cause colonies of cells to divide rapidly. These factors, then, are referred to as colony-stimulating factors. The colony-stimulating factors regulate hematopoiesis. Granulocyte–monocyte colony-stimulating factors (GM-CSFs) and granulocyte colony-stimulating factors (G-CSFs) are the two main types currently identified. Under their influence, the neutrophil storage pool is induced to release neutrophils and then enhance chemotaxis and bacteria-killing actions of the neutrophils. Thus, they contribute to phagocytosis of the nonspecific immune system. GM-CSF and G-CSF are produced naturally by fetal and neonatal tissue, but each can be administered postnatally in recombinant forms.

The environment plays a key role in the continued production of effective phagocytes and granulocytes. The site of granulopoiesis requires either a stimulating factor by itself or contact with another cell that may act as a regulator or receptor of other cells. Many authors refer to the need for an adherent layer of cells, consisting of "fibroblast-like cells, macrophages, reticular adventitial cells, adipocytes, and endothelial cells," which, in turn, synthesize proteins in the form of "collagen, fibronectin, thrombonectin, hemonectin, and glycosaminoglycans" (Stockman & DeAlarcon, 1992). The major component of interest in neonatal immunocompetency is fibronectin. Fibronectin is a glycoprotein whose action is not completely understood. One known action is as an opsonin that coats bacteria and enhances phagocytosis. Located within the neutrophils and neutrophil storage pools, fibronectin is carried by the polymorphonuclear leukocytes to the site of invasion by a foreign substance (Polin, 1990). Fibronectin appears to have a role in the regulation of vascular permeability of the surrounding tissue. The implication is that microvascular integrity and permeability are also regulated by its presence. This action of fibronectin may have adverse effects, such as development of capillary leak syndrome, which is often associated with overwhelming sepsis as well as respiratory distress syndrome. It is theorized that fibronectin may also be responsible for the build-up of fibrinous tissue in the pulmonary tree, often associated with chronic lung changes in the neonate. Thus, alveolar macrophages most likely produce fibronectin (Polin, 1990).

The locus for fibronectin is chromosome 2. Fibronectin levels continue to increase over the first few weeks of postnatal life, increasing the neonate's ability to fight bacterial infections. Plasma concentration in term infants is approximately 220 mg/ml. Levels are reduced in the premature infant as they are in the presence of respiratory distress syndrome, sepsis, malnutrition, or asphyxia. Fibronectin contains binding sites for *Staphylococcus aureus*, *Streptococcus pyogenes*, and *Treponema pallidum*. It may also facilitate binding of *Escherichia coli*. After an infection, fibronectin levels reduce to normal in approximately 5 days (Polin, 1990). Fibronectin administration is used experimentally to enhance the immunocompetence of the infected neonate.

Lymphocytes

Lymphocytes are produced by the lymph nodes, spleen, thymus, and bone marrow. Mature lymphocytes appear in the peripheral blood in varying sizes. The lymphocytes are classified as small, medium, or large. They are vital to the immune system. Lymphocytes function in the production of circulating antibodies and in the expression of cellular immunity. Antibodies are a class of molecules produced by B lymphocytes, which act as flexible adaptors between the infectious agent and phagocytes. Any particular antibody molecule can bind to only one type of infectious agent. Antibodies attach to antigens.

The mature lymphocyte has little or no endoplasmic reticulum, has only a small Golgi apparatus, possesses only a few mitochondria, and has ribosomes that are free and in clusters. Peripherally circulating lymphocytes include B, T, and null lymphocytes. The distinction is based on function and immunologic (cell surface) criteria; they are not morphologically distinguishable on peripheral blood smear. There are two main classes of lymphocytes: B lymphocytes and T lymphocytes.

B Lymphocytes

The B lymphocytes, derived from the bone marrow, were first discovered in birds (bursa of Fabricius). The B lymphocyte migrates from the bone marrow to the peripheral lymphatic tissues, where it interacts with antigens and differentiates into a plasma cell that secretes immunoglobulins for defense against infection (humoral immunity).

B lymphocytes are programmed to produce a specific antibody in response to an encounter with an antigen, after which they can interlock and mark the antigen for destruction. B lymphocytes originate from hematopoietic stem cells, and their development occurs in a progression of stages that are based on morphology and functional criteria. B-lymphocyte differentiation begins in the fetal liver around the eighth week of gestation, when the appearance of pre–B lymphocytes starts. Soon thereafter, the cells migrate from the liver and are maintained in the bone marrow. At this point, the B lymphocytes are immature; they express surface IgM but are extremely susceptible to inactivation by antigen binding. At 13 weeks' gestation, most B lymphocytes can produce both IgM and IgD. B lymphocytes are first observed in the peripheral blood at 12 weeks' gestation and are essentially at the level of term neonates by 15 weeks' gestation. IgG that is passively transferred from the mother's circulation is seen as early as the fourth week of gestation, but no other immunoglobulin is able to cross the placenta (Xanthou, 1987). Term newborns probably have a full repertoire of B lymphocytes that are capable of synthesizing each type of immunoglobulin. Yet, neonates fail to respond effectively to all antigens, and their response to protein antigens is mainly IgM production and a slow response as compared with the IgG response in adults. Most of these B lymphocytes remain fixed in lymph nodes and spleen, whereas some seem to recirculate.

T Lymphocytes

T lymphocytes are crucial in regulating the elaborate immune system, and, in particular, cytotoxic T lymphocytes can directly attack body cells that are infected. Most of the lymphocytes appearing in the thymus originate from hematopoietic stem cells; they enter the thymus about the eighth week of gestation and are induced into lymphoid differentiation. During cellular maturation, many lymphocytes die, whereas others migrate to the thymic medulla. Mature T lymphocytes migrate from the thymus and circulate through the lymphatics and vasculature. These circulating T lymphocytes are long-lived, perhaps up to 10 years, explaining the phenomenon of no immediate immunologic deficit upon removal of the thymus. After birth of the neonate, the thymus plays an ever-changing role in proportion to body size. It is largest during fetal development and continues to grow during childhood; involution begins at the time of puberty.

Generally, T lymphocytes acquire immunocompetence early in fetal development, although T lymphocyte–mediated suppression of immune responsiveness is slightly higher in neonates as compared with adults. Neonatal T lymphocytes invoke increased spontaneous suppressor activity and suppressor effects for natural killer (NK) cell activity (Bellanti et al., 1994). In addition, T lymphocyte cytotoxicity in the newborn is less than that in adults. This lesser cytotoxicity may increase the severity of viral infections during the neonatal period and may prevent graft-versus-host disease in response to maternal cells transferred to the fetus. A low T-lymphocyte function may occur as a result of neonatal viral infection, hyperbilirubinemia, steroid therapy, or maternal medications (Bellanti et al., 1994).

T lymphocytes mature in the thymus and then travel to the peripheral tissues, where they interact with antigens to form specific effector cells, which act in delayed hypersensitivity reactions, suppression of tumors, graft rejection, and against some intracellular organisms (cellular immunity). The T lymphocytes may also assist in regulating both humoral and cellular immune responses.

T lymphocytes secrete interleukins that stimulate further production of T and B lymphocytes. Interleukin-2 (IL-2) is considered a T-cell growth factor. IL-2 is one type of cytokine. Cytokines include tumor necrosis factor (TNF), IL-2, and interleukin-6 (IL-6). These are produced by monocytes and macrophages (Witek-Janusek & Cusack, 1994). Infants who are truly septic have high plasma levels of TNF and IL-6. Cytokines are being researched for their potential role in treatment of sepsis. Interferon is a related factor that is released by T lymphocytes, which, in turn, stimulate B-lymphocyte growth and release of other cytokines (Witek-Janusek & Cusack, 1994). The importance of interferon is its role in viral inhibition.

A third population of lymphocytes, called null lymphocytes, lacks the characteristics of the mature T and B lymphocytes and are termed null lymphocytes. The NK lymphocytes are thought to be in this group of cells. NK cells are leukocytes capable of recognizing cell-surface changes on virally infected cells. NK cells bind to these infected cells and kill them.

Interferon, produced by virally infected cells and by lymphocytes, activates NK cells to induce a state of viral resistance in unaffected tissue cells. This state is the first line of resistance against many viruses. Acute phase proteins are serum proteins that increase rapidly in concentration (up to 100 times) following infection. C-reactive protein is an acute phase protein that binds to the C protein of pneumococci. C-reactive protein promotes the binding of complement, which facilitates its uptake by phagocytes; this process is known as opsonization.

Lymphocytes first appear in fetal tissue at approximately 40 days' gestation, and there is a rapid increase in the blood level until 25 weeks' gestation (175 days). By the time of their birth, both term and preterm neonates have lymphocyte counts ranging from 3700 to 10,000/mm^3, reflecting the absolute lymphocytosis during the neonatal period. The majority of lymphocytes are long-lived, with a life span of approximately 4 years. Some may live up to 10 years. Approximately 15 percent of the total number live for only 3 to 4 days.

MATERNAL-FETAL-NEONATAL RELATIONSHIPS

The development of the immune system in the fetus and newborn cannot be studied in isolation from its maternal influences. The ability of the mother's body to tolerate the fetus during pregnancy, rather than rejecting it as a foreign body, is not well understood. It is well documented that maternal blood with immunocompetent lymphocytes does circulate in contact with fetal cells, that both fetal and maternal cells are exchanged through the placenta, and that humoral and cellular immunity to fetal antigens develops in the mother (Xanthou, 1987). The predominant transfer of antibody occurs by way of passage of IgG from the maternal to the fetal circulation by an active transport process. Such immunity is transient; nevertheless, it may provide protection during a vulnerable time of life. Although this passive antibody may protect the newborn, this process may interfere with active antibody synthesis after immunization. Secretory IgA in breast milk may also interfere with successful immunization, particularly with live polio virus, by neutralization of virus by antibody in the gastrointestinal tract. Maternal antibodies may have other harmful effects on the newborn.

Inherited Newborn Immunodeficiencies

Phagocytic Disorders

Neutropenia (low neutrophil count) is the most common sign of phagocytic dysfunction and is easily detected by a simple complete blood count with differential. Neutropenia can be further worked up by bone marrow examination, blood smear examination, and other specific tests such as the dye test for chronic granulomatous disease. Defects in neutrophil chemotaxis, described in patients with recurrent abscesses, can be evaluated by special tests.

Disorders of Antibody Formation

Evaluation of antibody-mediated immunity begins with quantitative immunoglobulins; however, because most of the neonate's immunoglobulin is maternal, this test is not particularly helpful during the first 3 months of life. IgM elevation in the cord blood may indicate intrauterine infection, however, and elevations of both IgM and IgA suggest maternal-fetal bleeding (Yoder & Polin, 1992). Studies of circulating B lymphocytes should be performed in infants with immunoglobulin deficiency. Some infants who cannot make immunoglobulins do have circulating B lymphocytes, but these cannot differentiate into plasma cells and secrete immunoglobulins or antibodies, as is common in patients with acquired agammaglobulinemia (called common variable immunodeficiency) (Yoder & Polin, 1997).

T-Lymphocyte Immunodeficiency

Because T lymphocytes constitute the vast majority of the circulating peripheral lymphocyte population, lymphopenia is seen when the number of T lymphocytes is decreased. Delayed hypersensitivity skin reactions are not elicited in patients with cell-mediated immunodeficiency. But, because such positive reactions require both a competent T-lymphocyte immunity and exposure to the specific antigens used, few neonates can mount a response in the first 6 months of life. Therefore, other tests of lymphocyte responses are necessary to diagnose those infants with T-lymphocyte abnormalities, such as DiGeorge syndrome and severe combined immunodeficiency disease (SCID).

Severe Combined Immunodeficiency Disease

SCID refers to a group of disorders characterized by the absence of both T-lymphocyte and B-lymphocyte immunity. This congenital absence of cell-mediated and antibody-mediated immunity causes a profound susceptibility to a broad range of bacterial, viral, protozoal, and fungal infections. In infants with this complex, symptoms of life-threatening infection usually develop during the first 3 months of life, and the infants often die quickly without immunologic reconstitution. There is some speculation from work on the Human Genome Project that at least one form of SCID may be an inborn error of metabolism that can potentially be successfully treated in utero (Bellanti et al., 1994).

Complement Disorder

Both persistent and transient deficiencies of components of serum complement have been reported. The usual serum screening for complement levels of serum proteins detects defects in the classic pathway but does not ascertain deficiencies in the alternative pathways.

ASSESSMENT OF THE IMMUNE SYSTEM

Evaluation of the neonatal immune system is challenging, encompassing the dynamic, rapidly evolving, adaptive, and changing boundaries of the neonate in response to its modifications in relation to the internal and external environment.

Subjective Data

A carefully detailed history, with particular emphasis on the family background and the pregnancy, is imperative. Areas to be covered in the history include family history of immune diseases, previous stillbirths or newborn deaths in the family, infections during pregnancy, maternal medications, previous diseases in the mother, and prior isoimmunization of the mother.

Objective Data

A meticulous physical examination of the neonate, in conjunction with the history, should provide a solid basis for interpretation of further objective data, including laboratory data.

Diagnostic Work-up

Because of the differences in the developmental status of the neonate's host defense mechanisms and the lack of exposure to antigens, the laboratory and clinical evaluation of the function of these mechanisms is slightly different from that performed for older children and adults. All host defense systems, including phagocytic, complement, antibody, and cell-mediated immunity, should be thoroughly evaluated. Initial screening tests should be performed, moving on to more definitive testing to establish a specific diagnosis. The definitive tests may be available only at a tertiary care center specializing in immunologic disorders.

INFECTION IN THE NEONATE

Identifying and caring for the infected newborn can be one of the greatest challenges in nursing. Nurses are often the first to recognize that there is something wrong with an infant, leading to investigation of the symptoms. Usually, treatment is begun once a presumptive diagnosis of infection is made.

Clinical Manifestations

Some of the signs and symptoms that are identified in an infected newborn are listed in Table 27–1. Hypothermia, the inability of the neonate to maintain temperature in the neutral thermal zone (usually between 97.7°F and 99°F axillary), may be an indication of the onset of a serious infection. Newborns traditionally do not have the febrile mechanisms intact. Premature infants often present with a low body temperature as illness ensues. Hyperthermia can occur in term newborns, with temperatures of more than 100.1°F, but it is relatively rare in preterm infants.

An infected infant often presents with lethargy, poor feeding, and perhaps a poor Moro reflex. The infant may eat well in the morning, but by evening sucks on nipples poorly or has residuals if being gavage fed. A newborn with infection may have abdominal distention, delayed gastric emptying time, and perhaps diarrhea or loose green or brown stools. Over a longer period, it

TABLE 27–1 Signs and Symptoms of Neonatal Infection

Clinical	
General	*Gastrointestinal*
Poor feeding	Diarrhea
Irritability	Hematochezia
Lethargy	Abdominal distention
Temperature instability	Emesis
Skin	Aspirates
Petechiae	*CNS*
Pustulosis	Hypotonia
Sclerema	Seizures
Edema	Poor spontaneous movement
Jaundice	*Circulatory*
Respiratory	Bradycardia/tachycardia
Grunting	Hypotension
Nasal flaring	Cyanosis
Intercostal retractions	Decreased perfusion
Tachypnea/apnea	
Laboratory Values	
White blood cell count	
Neutrophils	<5000 cells/mm^3, neutropenia >25,000 cells/mm^3, neutrophilia
Absolute neutrophil count (neutrophil and bands)	<1800 cells/mm^3 (during first week)
Immature: total neutrophil ratio	≥0:2
Platelet count	<100,000, thrombocytopenia
Cerebrospinal fluid	
Protein	150–200 mg/L (term) 300 mg/L (preterm)
Glucose	50–60% or more of blood glucose level

Adapted with permission from Lott, J. W., & Kilb, J. R. (1992). The selection of antibacterial agents for treatment of neonatal sepsis. *Neonatal Pharmacology Quarterly, 1*(1), 19–29.

may be identified that a particular infant has poor weight gain. Hypoglycemia or hyperglycemia, as well as glycosuria, is often present in an infected infant who is unable to compensate for the overload of an invasion of infectious organisms. Small preterm infants who are infected often present early with problems handling glucose loads.

Vascular perfusion is typically decreased when an infant is infected. Often, a sick neonate appears gray, mottled, or ashen in color. A sick infant may have poor perfusion and hypotension. Infants can present as cyanotic and can develop petechiae and, potentially, thrombocytopenia. Infections can cause DIC, thereby affecting the prothrombin time, partial thromboplastin time, and split fibrin product laboratory values of the newborn. Neonates may exhibit a hemolytic anemia, thereby significantly decreasing oxygen-carrying capacity, especially in the tiny preterm infant.

Apnea in a term infant in the first few hours of life can be a serious sign of inability to regulate the brain's respiratory center. Respiratory distress can be an early sign of pneumonia and must be considered carefully. A preterm infant who demonstrates apnea in the first 24 hours of life is likely to be infected with foreign organisms. Shock can be a sudden clinical sign of fulminant sepsis and necessitates immediate and aggressive intervention to restore adequate circulation. (Cairo et al., 1987; Levy & O'Rourke, 1995).

Unexplained bradycardia may be a signal of possible sepsis. Sclerema and sudden purpura, rash, or petechiae are also early signs of sepsis.

A complete blood count can provide initial clues for diagnosis of infection. An infected infant may demonstrate leukopenia, especially neutropenia with a cell count of polymorphonuclear leukocytes less than 5000/mm^3, or the infant may have a large number of immature leukocytes (>25,000 cells/mm^3), in particular, bands, with the band to leukocyte ratio greater than 0:2.

Indications of bacterial infection include the following:

- Increased total neutrophils—neutrophilia
- Decreased total neutrophils—neutropenia
- Increased immature forms (bands, metamyelocytes, sometimes promyelocytes, and myeloblasts)
- Increased band to segmented neutrophil ratio equal to or greater than 0:3 or immature neutrophils to total neutrophils greater than or equal to 0:2
- Presence of Döhle bodies (aggregates of reticuloendothelial system)
- Presence of vacuoles in nucleus
- Toxic granules in cell

Other symptoms of sepsis in the newborn include jaundice, hepatosplenomegaly, and irritability. The diagnosis of sepsis in a newborn is very difficult to make and is most often based on clinical findings.

Risk Factors

Prematurity is a primary risk factor for infection. Premature infants are far more likely to be jeopardized by the invasion of foreign agents. Because of being born prematurely, these infants have deficient passive transmission of maternal antibodies, developed by exposure to antigens and subsequent creation of an antibody defense system. Also, the cellular immune system is not well developed in the preterm infant exhibiting decreased phagocytic cellular defenses.

Prolonged rupture of the fetal membranes (PROM) is a well-known risk factor for the development of infection. The fetus is at increased risk because the break in the amniotic sac provides a pathway for the migration of organisms up the vaginal vault. The current trend of permitting PROM to persist in the presence of a preterm fetus creates the potential environment for bacterial proliferation and subsequent neonatal infection. PROM lasting longer than 24 hours is considered in the evaluation of infants for potential for infection.

A mother with a fever or illness before delivery can pass the infection on to her infant. If maternal temperature is 101°F at delivery, a sepsis workup is indicated. Maternal cervical or amniotic fluid cultures may be helpful to determine the causative agent. If the maternal illness suggests viral infection, neonatal viral cultures should be drawn. Early identification of causative agents in the mother may help in the management of the infant, by allowing faster identification of the microorganism and initiation of appropriate antimicrobial therapy.

The presence of foul-smelling amniotic fluid is an indication for neonatal antimicrobial therapy in symptomatic infants. Routine blood cultures and a complete blood count with differential is indicated for identification of neonatal infection. Under these circumstances, the placenta should be sent for pathologic evaluation.

Other risk factors known to be associated with neonatal infection are antenatal or intrapartal asphyxia, iatrogenic complications of treatment modalities, and postnatal invasive procedures. A predisposition of tiny low birth weight babies placed on indomethacin therapy for treatment of patent ductus arteriosus to develop sepsis has been observed (Herson et al., 1988). (See Chapter 44, Iatrogenic Complications of the Neonatal Intensive Care Unit.) Stress in any form inhibits the newborn's ability to fight infection by increasing the metabolic rate, thus requiring more oxygen and energy to support or sustain the body's vital functions. If the newborn is severely compromised and the oxygen levels continue to be low, regional tissue damage can result. Ischemic or necrotic areas in the lungs, heart, brain, or gastrointestinal system provide a receptive environment for colonization and overgrowth of normal bacterial flora. This overgrowth of bacteria is one of the most common sources of neonatal sepsis. Damaged tissue can be repaired only if the infectious process is reversed and adequate tissue perfusion is restored (Herson et al., 1988).

There are several known maternal factors associated with neonatal sepsis and infection: low socioeconomic status, malnutrition, no prenatal care, substance abuse, PROM (before 37 weeks' gestation or at the start of labor), presence of a urinary tract infection at delivery, peripartum infection, clinical amnionitis, and general bacterial colonization.

Neonatal risk factors include antenatal stress, intrapartal stress (perinatal asphyxia), congenital anomalies, male sex, multiple gestations, concurrent neonatal disease processes, prematurity, immaturity of the immune system, invasive admission procedures, and antimicrobial therapies.

Differential Diagnosis

The microorganisms responsible for neonatal infection have changed over the past 60 years, and there are marked regional variations (Table 27–2). Microorganisms commonly responsible for early-onset infection include streptococci, *Listeria monocytogenes,* and gram-negative enteric rods. Late-onset infections are most often caused by staphylococci, *Pseudomonas,* or *Bacteroides fragilis* (anaerobes) (Table 27–3). After the neonate is 7 days of age, nosocomial microorganisms should be considered. These microorganisms include *Staphylococcus epidermidis,* particularly when invasive medical devices, such as endotracheal tubes and arterial lines, have been used; *S. aureus* (common skin contaminant); and the spectrum of gram-negative bacilli, including *Klebsiella, Pseudomonas, Serratia,* and *E. coli.* Hospitalized preterm infants are often affected by repeated episodes of sepsis. Many of these episodes are termed presumed or suspected sepsis because no microorganism is recovered and cultured, despite clinical evidence of infection, which responds to therapy.

A high index of suspicion of infection resulting in early identification of the microorganism and institution of therapy provide the best outcome. The evaluation for infection generally includes a complete blood count with differential, platelet count, and blood, urine, and cerebrospinal fluid (CSF) cultures. Gram stain of the CSF can give an indication of the type of microorganism responsible for the infection. Cell count and protein and glucose levels of the CSF may also indicate the presence of infection. A chest radiograph is performed to detect pneumonia. Other tests that may be useful include latex agglutination or counterimmunoelectrophoresis of urine or CSF, erythrocyte sedimentation rate, and acute phase proteins. Other nonspecific findings, such as hypoglycemia, hypocalcemia, thrombocytopenia, hyponatremia, and metabolic acidosis, may also be present. Definitive diagnosis is based on recovery of a microorganism in blood, CSF, urine, or other body fluids (see Table 27–1).

TABLE 27–2 Historical Review of Neonatal Sepsis

Decade	Predominant Microorganism
1930s	Group A streptococcus
1940s	Group A streptococcus *Escherichia coli*
1950s	*Staphylococcus aureus* *Staphylococcus epidermidis* Group B streptococcus
1960s	*E. coli* Group B streptococcus
1970s	Group B streptococcus
1980s	Group B streptococcus *S. epidermidis*
1990s	?

Used with permission from Lott, J. W., & Kilb, J. R. (1992). The selection of antibacterial agents for treatment of neonatal sepsis. *Neonatal Pharmacology Quarterly, 1*(1), 19–29.

TABLE 27–3 Microorganisms Causing Neonatal Sepsis

Gram Positive	Gram Negative
Cocci	
Streptococcus	*Neisseria meningitidis*
Group A	*Neisseria gonorrhoeae*
Group B	*Branhamella catarrhalis*
Group D	
Pneumococci	
Staphylococcus aureus (coagulase positive)	
Staphylococcus epidermidis (coagulase negative)	
Rods	
Listeria monocytogenes	Enterobacteriaceae*
Corynebacterium diphtheriae	*Escherichia coli*
Bacillus cereus	*Klebsiella*
Anaerobes	*Shigella*
Clostridium difficile	*Proteus*
Clostridium perfringens	*Salmonella*
Clostridium botulinum	*Serratia*
Clostridium tetani	*Citrobacter*
	Haemophilus influenzae
	Pseudomonas
	Anaerobes
	Bacteroides fragilis

*Also called coliforms.

Used with permission from Lott, J. W., & Kilb, J. R. (1992). The selection of antibacterial agents for treatment of neonatal sepsis. *Neonatal Pharmacology Quarterly, 1*(1), 19–29.

Prognosis

The introduction of broad-spectrum antimicrobials dramatically improved the prognosis for infection; however, infection still accounts for significant morbidity and mortality in the neonatal period. The incidence of neonatal infection is approximately one in 1000 live births in full-term neonates and approximately 160 in 1000 in very low birth weight infants. More than 30 percent of all neonatal deaths are attributed to infection. Fifty percent of all neonatal deaths that occur on the first day of life are caused by infection. Even with aggressive therapy, the mortality rate for early-onset group B streptococcal infection approaches 100 percent. Major complications of infection include respiratory distress, shock, acidosis, DIC, and meningitis.

Collaborative Management

Collaborative management for an infected infant focuses on ventilatory support, oxygen therapy, correction of acidosis, immune therapy, volume expanders, extracorporeal membrane oxygenation if persistent pulmonary hypertension is present, and antimicrobial agents. The exact management plan is based on individual signs, symptoms, and laboratory findings.

Antimicrobials

The selection of antimicrobials is based on the microorganism present and the infant's response to therapy. Infectious microorganisms are divided into two broad classes: gram positive and gram negative. The shape of the microorganism categorizes it as either a coccus or a rod. Generally, the gram-positive organisms respond to broad-spectrum antibiotics, such as penicillin analogues and first-generation cephalosporins (beta-lactamases), and the beta-lactamase penicillins. The gram-negative microorganisms are most often susceptible to aminoglycosides, cephalosporins, and chloramphenicol. Tests must be run to determine the specific sensitivity of a microorganism to the antimicrobial selected.

Most gram-positive cocci respond to penicillin, unless the microorganism produces beta-lactamase (or penicillinase). The beta-lactamase destroys the penicillin. *S. aureus* is a beta-lactamase–producing microorganism and is therefore not usually responsive to penicillin. A group of semisynthetic penicillins with added side chains are used for treatment of *S. aureus* sepsis. Of this group, nafcillin and oxacillin are most often used. Other similar drugs are methicillin, dicloxacillin, and cloxacillin. First-generation cephalosporins, such as cefazolin, cephalexin, and cephalothin, are also resistant to beta-lactamase.

S. epidermidis and *S. aureus* strains may be resistant to penicillin, semisynthetic penicillins, and cephalosporins. Methicillin-resistant *S. aureus* is unresponsive to semisynthetic penicillins. In this case, vancomycin is the drug of choice. It may also be used for *S. epidermidis* and sepsis related to foreign bodies or invasive procedures.

Third-generation cephalosporins are used to treat gram-negative cocci that are penicillin and methicillin resistant. *L. monocytogenes,* a gram-positive rod, is most successfully treated with ampicillin. Aminoglycosides or third-generation cephalosporins are the drugs of choice for gram-negative enteric rods. Some gram-negative rods are classified according to their lactose fermentation ability. The lactose fermenters are *E. coli* and *Klebsiella.* They are sensitive to aminoglycosides and third-generation cephalosporins. *Shigella* and *Salmonella* are nonlactose fermenters, which respond well to ampicillin and third-generation cephalosporins.

Haemophilus influenzae is usually sensitive to ampicillin and third-generation cephalosporins, although some strains are ampicillin resistant. *Pseudomonas* requires the following combination therapy: aminoglycoside and antipseudomonas penicillin such as azlocillin, carbenicillin, imipenem, mezlocillin, piperacillin, and ticarcillin.

Anaerobes are a subset of gram-negative and gram-positive rods. Two anaerobes associated with sepsis are *Bacteroides* and *Clostridium. Bacteroides* is susceptible to metronidazole, clindamycin, chloramphenicol, and some of the newer beta-lactamases, such as imipenem and ampicillin with sulbactam. *Clostridium* is usually susceptible to penicillin.

A combination of ampicillin and gentamicin is useful for antibacterial action against streptococci, *L. monocytogenes,* and gram-negative enteric rods. This combination of antimicrobials has a synergistic effect, increasing the efficacy of either drug therapy used by itself. Additional therapy or selection of other agents is necessary if staphylococcal infection is suspected, if *Pseudomonas* or *Bacteroides* (most often iatrogenically acquired) is present, if there is an outbreak of resistant organisms, or if prolonged ampicillin and gentamicin therapy has been used. Antibacterial agents must be reevaluated after completion of cultures and sensitivity testing (Lott & Kilb, 1992). See Table 27–4 for common antimicrobial agents and their dosages.

TABLE 27–4 Selected Antimicrobial Agents and Their Dosages

Antimicrobial Agent	Dosage
Penicillin G	Sepsis 25,000–50,000 IU/kg/dose q 12 hours <7 days q 8 hours <7 days q 6 hours >7 days Group B streptococcus Higher dose + aminoglycoside
Ampicillin	Sepsis 100–200 mg/kg/dose q 8–12 hours <7 days q 6–8 hours >7 days Meningitis 200–400 mg/kg/dose q 8–12 hours <7 days q 6–8 hours >7 days
Methicillin	25–50 mg/kg/dose IV q 8–12 hours <7 days q 6–8 hours >7 days
Gentamicin	<7 days postnatal age ≤29 weeks: 2.5 mg/kg/dose q 24 hours 30–34 weeks: 3 mg/kg/dose q 24 hours ≥35 weeks: 2.5 mg/kg/dose q 12 hours >7 days postnatal age ≤29 weeks: 3.0 mg/kg/dose q 24 hours 30–34 weeks: 2.5 mg/kg/dose q 12 hours ≥35 weeks: 2.5 mg/kg/dose q 8 hours
Vancomycin	≤29 weeks: 18 mg/kg/dose q 24 hours 30–36 weeks: 15 mg/kg/dose q 12 hours 37–44 weeks: 10 mg/kg/dose q 8 hours ≥45 weeks: 10 mg/kg/dose q 6 hours

q, every.
Adapted with permission from Lott, J. W., & Kilb, J. R. (1992). The selection of antibacterial agents for treatment of neonatal sepsis. *Neonatal Pharmacology Quarterly, 1*(1), 19–29.

TYPES OF NEONATAL INFECTION

This section briefly describes the types of microorganisms causing neonatal infection and their clinical manifestations, diagnosis, and collaborative management. The discussion includes both congenitally acquired and nosocomially acquired infections caused by bacterial, viral, fungal, and protozoal organisms.

Congenital Infections

The microorganisms most often responsible for congenitally acquired infections have been grouped together as the TORCH infections. These include *t*oxoplasmosis, *o*thers, *r*ubella, *c*ytomegalovirus (CMV), and *h*erpes. The "others" category includes various microorganisms that have been responsible for congenital infections. However, the list of microorganisms implicated in congenital infections has grown, so the acronym is no longer inclusive. Nevertheless, it is still used to mean all infections acquired by the fetus in utero.

Toxoplasmosis

The importance of the parasite *Toxoplasma gondii* was discovered by perinatal health care workers in the 1980s. *Toxoplasma* is a pathogen that is ever present in nature. Perinatal transmission takes place when the mother contracts the protozoa and the subsequent protozoemia transmits the organism transplacentally to the fetus. The microorganisms then invade and multiply within the placenta and eventually enter the fetal circulation.

The life cycle of *Toxoplasma* is complicated. The predominant host of this organism is the ordinary house cat; however, other animals can serve as hosts. There are significant differences in the prevalence rates of this microorganism throughout the world (Remington et al., 1995). The tissue cyst form of the microorganism persists in the flesh of animals, such as cattle and sheep. The oocyte form of the parasite persists in soil contaminated by cat feces. Thus, congenital toxoplasmosis is known to be transmitted from undercooked meat or food or from fomites in cat feces (Carter & Frank, 1986). In the United States, approximately 20 to 70 percent of the population has been exposed to this protozoa. The exact incidence varies according to geographic area. As with any infectious microorganism, the greatest concern is that a nonimmune pregnant woman would become exposed to this agent during fetal organogenesis (weeks 4 to 8 of gestation), which might result in congenital anomalies.

Clinical Manifestations

Acute toxoplasmosis in a pregnant woman often goes undetected and undiagnosed. Clinical questioning after the identification of an infected infant often leads to reflection and memories of a period of enlarged lymph nodes and fatigue but no fever. Women sometimes report a mononucleosis-like syndrome that may have a febrile course, with malaise, headache, fatigue, sore throat, and sore muscles. These symptoms may persist up to 6 months (Daffos et al., 1988).

In an infant, toxoplasmosis can manifest with hydrocephalus, chorioretinitis, and intracranial calcification. There is a wide variety of clinical signs in the scope of the disease. A normal picture at birth, or even severe erythroblastosis, hydrops fetalis, and other clinical signs, can occur (Remington et al., 1995).

Neurologic signs similar to encephalitis (e.g., convulsions, bulging fontanelles, nystagmus, and abnormal increase in circumference of the head) may be the only significant presentation of this clinical problem. If the infant receives treatment, signs and symptoms may disappear, allowing normal cerebral growth and development.

Mild cases of the disease can easily go unrecognized in the newborn. Signs and symptoms of delayed onset of disease in premature infants include severe central nervous system or eye lesions appearing at 3 months of age.

In term infants, delayed disease may occur in the first 2 months of life and is usually more mild. Clinical signs may be generalized sepsis, enlarged liver and spleen, late-onset jaundice, enlarged lymph nodes, or late-onset central nervous system problems, including hydrocephalus and eye lesions. Infants with congenital toxoplasmosis may have new lesions appearing until age 5 years (Koppe et al., 1986).

Collaborative Management

The best and most effective treatment is prevention and early recognition. The cost effectiveness of pregnancy serology screening depends on the costs of the tests and the estimated cost of treating the infection if identified early. At present in the United States, screening is done erratically and there are no particular screening standards.

Counseling education for the prevention of toxoplasmosis should focus on avoidance of raw meat and use of gloves during feline litterbox handling and during gardening in what may be contaminated soil.

Treatment for congenital toxoplasmosis is pyrimethamine plus sulfonamides. The suggested dose is 1 mg/kg/day orally, with a maximum dose of 25 mg/day. Duration of treatment is varied, depending on the presentation of the congenital disease. Sulfonamides (sulfadiazine or trisulfapyrimidine) are given in doses of 85 mg/kg/day (two divided oral doses). Spiramycin can be given, 100 mg/kg/day orally in two doses every other month, as an alternative treatment. These drugs are potentially toxic and need close monitoring (Remington et al., 1995).

Toxoplasmosis is one of the most common causes of deafness. The Collaborative Perinatal Project found a doubling in the frequency of deafness in infants of mothers with the antibody for toxoplasmosis. There was a 60 percent increase in microcephaly and a 30 percent increase in low intelligence quotients (less than 70) in relation to high antibody levels in mothers (Remington et al., 1995).

Nursing Management

Nursing management is supportive and dependent on the severity of the infection. Neurologic impairment at birth can be significant, requiring ventilation and seizure control. Documented positive infants should be cared for by nonpregnant personnel.

Rubella

In 1941, N. McAlister Gregg described 78 patients with congenital cataracts. Most of these patients were small for gestational age, had feeding difficulties, and had congenital heart problems. A history of German measles during pregnancy was found in 68 of the cases (87 percent). Much of the current knowledge about the effects of congenital rubella was established by Gregg's report on these patients (Gregg, 1941). It has been further established that the rubella virus can be responsible for other destructive events. The infection has an impact on number of miscarriages, abortions, and stillborns and on fetal development (South & Sever, 1985).

With the advent of vaccination, rubella was almost eradicated. The number of infected infants was at its lowest in the United States in 1988 (Centers for Disease Control [CDC], 1989). This trend is no longer true. Failure to immunize many young children has resulted in an increase in rubella incidence. Therefore, despite a national immunization program, at least 10 percent of women of childbearing age are vulnerable to the virus, particularly the wild virus, because either they have not been immunized or they have not acquired immunity from the infection themselves. Rubella outbreaks have been reported all over the United States. In 1964, 12,500,000 adult cases of infection and 20,000 cases of congenital infection were reported to the CDC. In 1987a, 306 adult cases of infection and six cases of congenital infection were reported. In 1988, 221 adult cases and one congenital case were reported (CDC, 1989). Thus, there has been a change in the epidemiology of the infection over the past 25 years.

Clinical Manifestations

The typical presentation of the rubella virus is mild, with malaise, low-grade fever, headache, and conjunctivitis. In 1 to 5 days, a macular rash appears on the face and usually disappears after 3 to 4 days. Natural viremia is necessary for placental and fetal rubella infection. Most cases occur following primary disease. Frequently, skin rashes that resemble rubella may occur as a result of adenovirus, enterovirus, or other respiratory virus infections. Laboratory titers are recommended to confirm the diagnosis of rubella infection.

A fetus infected with rubella often has cardiac defects and deafness. The central nervous system seems particularly vulnerable to the rubella virus, especially if the virus is acquired before the first 16 weeks of gestation. Congenital rubella syndrome is described by the CDC as hearing loss, mental retardation, cardiac malformations, and eye defects.

The rubella virus can slow cell replication. This causes intrauterine growth retardation and a failure of cell differentiation during fetal organ formation. Tissue damage also seems to occur from the inflammatory response to the infection or is even possibly an autoimmune reaction. Myocarditis, pneumonitis, hepatosplenomegaly, and vascular stenosis can also be present because of these processes. As is seen with other severe congenital infections, signs and symptoms may continue to develop until the patient is 10 to 20 years of age. Late clinical signs of this disease include insulin-dependent diabetes, thyroid abnormalities, hypoadrenalism, hearing loss, and eye damage (Sever et al., 1985).

Differential Diagnosis

The possibility of subclinical infection with rubella highlights the need for laboratory confirmation. Clinical confirmation of rubella isolation is obtainable in approximately 4 to 6 weeks. The detection of rubella antibody confirms the presence of the infection. Rubella-specific IgG persists for life and can be detected by enzyme immunoassay. With confirmed serologic results, the risk of fetal damage after 16 weeks' gestation appears to be small (Munro et al., 1987).

Demonstration of rubella-specific IgM in fetal blood obtained by cordocentesis has been used to establish diagnosis in utero. Chorionic villus sampling has also demonstrated recovery of the virus during the first trimester (Enders & Jonatha, 1987; Kuller et al., 1996).

Collaborative Management

All infants should be vaccinated against rubella at 15 months of age. Also, women who do not have detectable IgG rubella antibody and are of childbearing age (and not pregnant) should be immunized (CDC, 1984a). After immunization, they should avoid pregnancy for at least 3 months to decrease the risk for development of rubella syndrome in the fetus. Health care workers who may be inadvertently exposed to rubella should be immunized if they do not have immune titers. If a woman receives rubella vaccine and has recently received blood products or RhoGAM (RhIG), the vaccine may not trigger an immune response because blood products and RhoGAM have pooled sera that may contain antibodies against rubella. Thus, the woman's body does not produce antibodies. These women should have titers drawn 6 weeks after vaccination or at most 3 months after vaccination.

In more than 500 women who were accidentally immunized against rubella while pregnant, there were no cases of congenital rubella syndrome. Rubella vaccination is not recommended during pregnancy, yet the risks to the fetus have been determined to be negligible and an inadvertent rubella vaccination by itself is not considered an indication for termination of pregnancy.

Currently, treatment in the nursery of the rubella-infected infant is rare. Therapy for identified problems, such as respiratory, cardiac, or neurologic deficits, is supportive and there is no specific recommended therapy. Caretakers should have known immune titers and not be pregnant. Rubella-specific IgM can usually accurately identify these infants. Persistent shedding of the virus may last until 1 year of life; thus, pregnant women should avoid contact with these patients. Follow-up care for surgical corrections of heart defects and cataracts as well as special schooling may be needed for these infants.

Cytomegalovirus

Infection with CMV, a member of the herpes family, is common. CMV is a DNA virus covered with a glycoprotein coat that closely resembles the herpes and varicella-zoster viruses. By adulthood, most people have been exposed to CMV and antibodies have developed to it. CMV infection is more prevalent in lower socioeconomic groups and is especially common in developing countries. In the United States, women of childbearing age from lower socioeconomic groups have an incidence of infection of approximately 6 percent, whereas those from higher socioeconomic groups have an incidence of approximately 2 percent. CMV may lie dormant, with periods of exacerbation followed by remission. During remission, the patient is asymptomatic, but the virus is shed (Stagno, 1995). The virus is usually transmitted person to person through body fluids and secretions. Blood, urine, breast milk, cervical mucus, semen, and saliva harbor CMV. The virus can cause an infectious mononucleosis-like syndrome, with general malaise, liver complications, fever, and general fatigue. Perinatal transmission can occur within 2 to 3 days of infection by transplacental crossing of the organism. The fetus can also contract the virus intrapartally while descending through the birth canal from infected maternal cervical secretions. CMV can also be transmitted through infected breast milk (Nelson & Grossman, 1986).

Clinical Manifestations

More damage occurs to the fetus when the exposure to and acquisition of CMV occur from a primary lesion. Congenital CMV occurs in approximately 0.2 to 2.2 percent of all newborn infants. Primary lesions cause intrauterine growth retardation, microcephaly, periventricular calcifications, deafness, blindness, congenital cataracts, profound mental retardation, hepatosplenomegaly, and jaundice. A characteristic pattern of petechiae, called "blueberry muffin" syndrome, is associated with congenital CMV. Approximately 26 percent of severely infected infants die. Severe complications at birth are seen in approximately 5 percent of congenital infections. Sequelae develop in 5 to 15 percent of asymptomatic infected infants and in 90 percent of symptomatic infected infants (Stagno, 1995). Recurrent CMV infections are not as severe because of partial antibody protection from previous exposure. The American Academy of Pediatrics (1994) reports the incidence of neonatal complications to be 5 to 10 percent for hearing loss, 2 percent for chorioretinitis, and less than 1 percent for mental retardation.

Diagnosis

Suspicious clinical findings or obstetric history warrant further investigation for CMV infection. Urine culture for CMV is the most rapid and sensitive indicator of infection. IgG and IgM antibody titers should also be measured. Elevated IgM levels alone denote exposure to CMV but are not diagnostic because there is no method to determine the timing of the exposure. Elevated neonatal IgG titers indicate perinatally acquired CMV infection. A negative maternal IgG titer and a positive neonatal IgG titer indicate postnatal transmission. Experimentally, elevated rheumatoid factors may provide evidence to support the diagnosis of CMV in subclinical cases (Stagno, 1995).

Prevention

Transmission of CMV via infected blood products has been significantly decreased through the use of CMV-negative donors or irradiation of blood products. Premature and low birth weight infants are especially vulnerable to the infusion of this virus in blood products (Gilbert et al., 1989). The best method of prevention is the institution of universal precautions, including good handwashing techniques.

Collaborative Management

Newborns with CMV infection exhibit a wide range of symptoms. General supportive therapy is based on the presence of these clinical manifestations. Specific therapy for CMV is still in the experimental stage but includes immunoglobulin therapy, vaccines, and chemotherapy. Intravenous immunoglobulin therapy provides passive immunity to at-risk infants but not to those already infected. Two live attenuated vaccines for CMV have been developed and tested on renal transplant patients. Theoretically, these vaccines would be useful preconceptually or perinatally to prevent vertical transmission; however, only limited research has been done with this population. Chemotherapy offers the most promise for treatment of neonatal CMV infection; however, clinically, it has not been shown to be effective in improving outcome. Chemotherapeutic agents under investigation include idoxuridine, 5-fluoro-2′-deoxyuridine, cytosine arabinoside, adenine arabinoside, acyclovir, leukocyte interferon, interferon stimulators, and ganciclovir. Toxicity and immunosuppression associated with these agents raise concern about widespread neonatal use (Stagno, 1995).

Syphilis

The microorganism *T. pallidum* has persisted as a threat to perinatal patients over the past 400 years. Despite available therapy for the past 40 years, many women do not receive adequate treatment for primary or secondary infections. In addition, the virus is known to lie dormant, much like the herpes family of viruses. Currently, the incidence of syphilis is increasing, owing to an increase in substance abuse, sexual practices involving multiple partners, and human immunodeficiency virus (HIV)-positive immunocompromised individuals, who act as reservoirs for *T. pallidum.* Consequently, there has been a resurgence of congenital infections. Recent worldwide concern regarding the role of genital ulcers in conjunction with HIV infection has created great concern for eradication of sexually transmitted diseases.

The diagnosis of antepartum syphilis is most often made by screening at the first prenatal visit. Screening usually involves the use of the Venereal Disease Research Laboratory (VDRL) test or rapid plasma reagin (RPR) test, each of which measures anticardiolipin antibody. These tests are reactive in almost 80 percent of patients with secondary or early latent (less than 1 year duration) primary syphilis. A definitive diagnosis can be made with an elevated VDRL or RPR accompanied by a positive *T. pallidum* fluoroantibody test or a reactive serologic test for *T. pallidum* in the CSF. Condylomata lata, bony changes, or snuffles in the presence of a positive serologic test are diagnostic (Ingall et al., 1995).

Untreated syphilis adversely affects pregnancy outcome. Vertical transmission of treponemas can occur at any time during pregnancy. The microorganisms can cause preterm labor, PROM, stillbirth, congenital infection, or neonatal death. In one study done in Miami, the overall rate of cases of congenital syphilis was 18.4 in 10,000 births, which was a threefold increase from 1986 to 1988. Liveborn infants had lower birth weights 21 percent of the time, and 34 percent of infected women delivered stillborns. The perinatal mortality rate in this study was high—464 in 1000 births (Ricci et al., 1989). Current untreated secondary infection causes the greatest risk of damage to the fetus, particularly if infection occurs during the period of organogenesis. Late untreated syphilis in the mother usually results in delivery of an unsymptomatic infant who needs treatment in the newborn nursery.

Reports state that, between 1983 and 1985, 437 infants in the United States were delivered with congenital syphilis. The mean age of acquiring prenatal care was 22 weeks' gestation, and at least half of the cases were preventable, because they were results of failure of initial or third-trimester screening (Ingall et al., 1995).

Clinical Manifestations

When newborns acquire syphilis from hematogenous spread across the placenta, the effects are on the major organ systems of the fetus, especially the central nervous system. Common presentations of the infected infant are hepatosplenomegaly, jaundice, low birth weight, intrauterine growth retardation, anemia, and osteochondritis. There is often a bilateral superficial peeling of the skin (desquamation) on the neonatal palms and soles. Nonimmune hydrops is a common presentation in congenital syphilis (Chawla et al, 1988). The symptoms of perinatal syphilis are similar to those of any other viral infection that spreads hematogenously from the mother to the placenta and on to the developing fetus (Ingall et al., 1995).

Differential Diagnosis

A lumbar puncture for CSF analysis and radiographs of the long bones facilitate the definitive diagnosis of syphilis in the neonate. Congenital neurosyphilis is always a consideration, and the CSF should be examined for the presence of spirochetes. Radiologic changes such as osteochondritis (a blurring of the epiphyseal borders) demonstrate recent fetal infection (within 5 weeks), and periostitis represents prolonged involvement, probably within 16 weeks or second-trimester infection.

Stillborn infants should be examined by whole-body radiographic study and autopsy if possible. Spirochetes can be visualized by special staining techniques (Ingall et al., 1995)

Interpretation of serologic tests for syphilis on serum obtained from cord blood is complicated because of the transplacental transfer of maternal IgG antibody. VDRL titers at least two dilutions higher than maternal VDRL titers indicate probable fetal infection.

Prognosis

Infants with syphilis should receive the same amount of follow-up as normal infants. Serologic measurements can be made at follow-up visits at 1, 2, 3, 6, and 12 months of age. The infection can be effectively treated, but the physiologic and developmental prognosis depends on the degree of organ damage sustained during fetal development.

Collaborative Management

The recommended treatment for a newborn presumed to be infected with congenital syphilis is aqueous penicillin G. In many perinatal centers, the presence of a positive VDRL in a neonate dictates treatment as if positive for syphilis. If neonatal clinical manifestations are highly suspicious for syphilis and there is a positive VDRL but the titer is not significantly higher than the maternal titer, syphilis treatment should be instituted. A newborn with an antibody titer four times or more higher than the maternal level should be treated as if a definitive diagnosis has been obtained. To prevent neurosyphilis, the infant should be given aqueous penicillin G, 100,000 to 150,000 units/kg intravenously in two or three divided doses for at least 10 to 14 days, or 50,000 units/kg/day of procaine penicillin in a daily dose for 10 to 14 days.

For asymptomatic infants whose mothers were treated adequately during pregnancy, treatment is not necessary unless follow-up cannot be ensured. Some clinicians recommend a single dose of benzathine penicillin, 50,000 units/kg intramuscularly in a single dose if the infant is not likely to be followed up. If maternal treatment did not include penicillin and if neonatal follow-up is likely to be unreliable, the neonate is given a full 10-day course.

Isolation of an infant with suspicious symptoms may be necessary until appropriate treatment is given. There is a definite role for nursing education and support in the treatment of an infant exposed to syphilis. The 10- to 14-day course of penicillin treatment may lead to the establishment of a trusting relationship between the nurse and family, thus providing opportunity to give more information regarding sexual risk factors. Families often need encouragement and support to get treatment for other sexual partners and to obtain other necessary medical evaluations (such as HIV screening or drug counseling).

Herpes Simplex Virus

Herpes simplex virus (HSV) is a member of a family of large DNA viruses. They contain linear, double strands of DNA. The herpes family also includes CMV, varicella-zoster, and Epstein-Barr virus. HSV possesses the quality of "latency," whereby the virus can persist in a latent state for a period of time and then be reactivated by certain stimuli. A strand of the viral DNA persists in an infected individual for a lifetime; thus, the virus maintains a "foothold" in its host. Clinical experiences demonstrate that, after primary HSV infection, at the site of the infection (perhaps an oral or genital site), the microorganism invades the sensory nerve endings and remains there. The more severe the primary infection, as determined by the size and extent of the skin lesion, the more likely are frequent recurrences.

Potential stimuli for HSV reactivation include periods of stress, emotional trauma, and prolonged exposure to the sun. Maintenance of the latency state and recurrence of the virus are topics of intense current research. There are many unanswered questions about what triggers latency and about the cofactors for reactivation of the virus.

Maternal HSV is usually the source of neonatal infection. The risk of neonatal infection is estimated to be 5 percent if it is recurrent herpes and higher if it is a primary infection (Arvin, 1988).

Recurrent infections are the most common problem in pregnancy. Transmission of the infection to the fetus can be caused by passage through infected genital secretions in the intrapartum period or by ascending infection from the vaginal vault via ruptured (or not) membranes. Many women can be asymptomatic and still be shedding HSV. Although primary infection is less common, it causes the most severe neonatal disease, most likely including central nervous system problems, disseminated disease into other organ systems, and probable death. The incidence of intrapartum transmission with a primary infection is approximately 40 to 50 percent. Many neonatal complications such as prematurity, intrauterine retardation, and respiratory distress syndrome can potentiate the neonate's illness, limiting the ability to fight off HSV (Prober et al., 1988). There is a broad range of severity of neonatal infection, from severe to benign and asymptomatic, but the incidence of neonatal herpes is approximately 1500 to 2000 cases per year (Overall, 1994). Susceptibility of the newborn to HSV is increased because there is a lack of passively acquired maternal antibody in some infants. The failure of newborns to control HSV may also be related to decreased production of or response to interferon or perhaps to decreased production of cellular cytotoxic immune mechanisms (Brown et al., 1987).

Clinical Manifestations

Acquisition of HSV in utero can result in spontaneous abortion, preterm birth, or a normal baby. Manifestations of the disease are broad; the clinical presentation of the congenital acquisition of the infection includes skin vesicles or scarring, hypopigmentation, chorioretinitis, microcephaly, and hydranencephaly. There are three categories of neonatal patients. The first category includes patients with localized infections of the skin, eyes, or mouth. The second category includes patients with encephalitis. In this group, neurologic sequelae occur in approximately 50 percent. Approximately one third of these patients do not have skin vesicles, and they are identified by history alone. CSF is positive for the virus in 25 to 40 percent of these cases. Presence of cells and increased protein are very common in the CSF of patients with encephalitis, and they die if not treated. The third category of neonatal patients includes those with disseminated disease characterized by irritability, seizures, respiratory distress, jaundice, DIC, shock, and other symptoms of viral and bacterial sepsis. All major neonatal organs may be involved. Liver and the adrenals are the most common reservoirs for the virus. The central nervous system is involved in 70 to 90 percent of affected neonates. In more than 20 percent of the newborns with disseminated disease, skin vesicles do not develop, making identification of positive infants more difficult (Whitley & Arvin, 1995).

Differential Diagnosis

Laboratory tests are the most common way to differentiate HSV infection from other bacterial and viral infections. The most rapid method includes a cytologic examination. Routine cultures should be obtained from any vesicle on the skin, oropharyngeal or eye secretions, or stool. Viral typing is done for epidemiologic purposes only. HSV types I and II are the most commonly known. Type I has been most closely associated with any herpes found outside the genital area; type II is commonly referred to as genital herpes. However, either type can occur almost anywhere in the body. Treatment does not differ for these different viral types.

Risk Factors

Intrapartal transmission is more likely to occur in the presence of ruptured membranes. Other risk factors include intrauterine fetal monitoring and fetal scalp sampling. It is not recommended that women infected with HSV be monitored by these methods. Transmission from mother to infant from an infected breast lesion has been reported. Transmission has also been documented from oral lesions.

Prevention

Presence of maternal active HSV genital lesions is a contraindication to vaginal delivery. If the membranes have been ruptured 4 hours or longer, cesarean section may or may not prevent transmission to the neonate. Haddad and colleagues (1993) reported a study of use of oral acyclovir during the third trimester of pregnancy in women with a history of genital type II herpes. The hypothesis was that acyclovir would cause asymptomatic viral shedding and decrease fetal or neonatal transmission. The findings did not support the hypothesis. Postnatal nosocomial transmission is greatly reduced with good handwashing techniques and universal precautions.

Collaborative Management

The most recent methods of treatment include the antiviral drugs acyclovir and vidarabine. The results of these methods of therapy and treatment are reported in the National Institute of Allergy and Infectious Diseases (NIAID) Joint Collaborative Antiviral Study. These drugs have potentially influenced neonatal morbidity and mortality from disseminated disease and encephalitis.

Vidarabine is usually given intravenously in dosages of 15 to 30 mg/kg/day over a 12-hour period for 10 to 14 days. It has been reported that newborns receiving the higher dosages of 30 mg/kg/day seem to progress to less serious forms of the disease. In some circumstances, longer periods of treatment may be necessary, because infants can have either a clinical recurrence or a clinical progression of the disease.

Acyclovir, a relatively new antiviral agent undergoing clinical study has recently become the recommended mode of therapy. Acyclovir appears to be very helpful in decreasing the frequency of the reactivation of the virus, particularly in the treatment of herpes simplex encephalitis. Acyclovir is a selective inhibitor of viral replication and thus has few side effects. The recommended dosage is 30 mg/kg/day intravenously divided over 8 hours. Duration of therapy is 10 to 14 days.

Early identification and intervention are essential, because early institution of antiviral therapy has been shown to improve outcome and decrease sequelae (Whitley et al., 1988). Newborns with eye involvement should be given topical antiviral agents such as trifluridine, 1 drop every 2 hours, as well as intravenous therapy. Vidarabine and acyclovir are potent drugs with a potential for toxicity. Neonatal therapeutic ranges for these drugs have not been established. Monitoring of the infant's physiologic status is necessary to detect potential side effects. Infected infants must be isolated, because viral shedding provides a reservoir for infecting other infants in the nursery.

HSV continues to be a life-threatening neonatal infection in the United States. There is growing concern about transmission of the virus to unborn children with the concomitant increase in genital herpes as a sexually transmitted disease. It is important for all health care providers in the perinatal arena to maintain a high index of suspicion in infants whose symptoms may be compatible with HSV infection. Early identification allows prompt treatment or necessary continued observation or both. Continued research may produce a more rapid method of virus identification and perhaps a safe and effective vaccine. Prevention of neonatal HSV depends on improved knowledge regarding the factors of virus transmission between mother and infant. Appropriate use of cesarean section in women with active genital herpes is an important management step (Johnson, 1986).

Primary nursing responsibilities in the management of a family with HSV infection are education and support. Mothers should be educated as to the mode, methods, and possible origins of the HSV, and concerns should be addressed regarding potential transmission to newborns. Nurses are often the first to document a mother's comment that she "had a small bump or blister and fever" right before her infant was born. Careful history taking and thorough questioning can often identify potentially infected patients early. With the diagnosis of genital herpes and subsequent monitoring procedures, families often feel stigmatized as well as anxious. Parents and responsible family members need education and support. Mothers with a history of genital HSV should be investigated for findings of active infection during the prepartum period. The definition of an active lesion includes one of the following at birth:

1. Positive viral culture of a lesion
2. Positive fluorescent antibody test
3. Presence of skin vesicles or lesions
4. Cytologic screen with identified HSV markers

All family members with active lesions anywhere on the body should be taught careful handwashing techniques to use before handling the baby. Any person with an oral HSV infection who handles the infant must wash well, wear a mask, and not kiss the infant anywhere until the lesions are completely crusted over and healed.

A common nursing concern is whether a mother with active genital herpes should be isolated. Transmission occurs with direct contact with the infected lesion. There must be thorough handwashing before handling the infant and after touching the genital area. The risks for transmission are unknown, but they are low. Hospital personnel usually gown and glove until viral status is known. Positive cultures at birth may just reflect colonization and cultures should be repeated at 24 to 48 hours. If these are positive, the infant is considered to be positive for infection. Breastfeeding is contraindicated if the mother has a lesion on her breast. Infants are not isolated unless they themselves are infected. Many nurseries have guidelines regarding a 24- to 48-hour observation period to check cultures on an infant who was delivered vaginally through an infected genital area. An uninfected child does not require prolonged hospitalization, and, upon discharge, the family needs information and education. Families should be informed that immediate medical consultation should be obtained with the development of major findings, including malaise, irritability, fever, temperature instability, respiratory distress, apnea, large abdomen or liver, sudden changes in skin color, new skin vesicles, lesions on the mucous membranes, or conjunctivitis. Sudden onset of systemic disease in a small recovering preterm infant can include DIC and shock. Skin lesions are often absent in these severe cases, which may delay diagnosis.

Varicella

Varicella is the member of the herpesvirus family that commonly causes chickenpox as well as varicella-zoster. Most women of childbearing age in the United States have been exposed to or have contracted this virus, yet women from other parts of the world may not be seropositive. Incidence of this virus in pregnant women is very low, probably approximately 0.5 in 10,000 pregnancies (Gershon, 1995)

Symptoms of varicella are usually present 10 to 20 days after exposure and include fever, malaise, and an itchy rash. The maculopapular rash eventually forms vesicles and crusts over. Potential complications include pneumonia, encephalitis, arthritis, and bacterial cellulitis. If the virus is contracted early in pregnancy, the damage is likely to be cutaneous, musculoskeletal, neurologic, and ocular. Infants can have intrauterine growth retardation, microcephaly, cerebellar and cortical atrophy, cataracts, and chorioretinitis (Freij & Sever, 1988). Viral infection in the last 3 weeks of pregnancy affects one in four newborns. The severity of neonatal disease is determined by the timing of the exposure. Infections are generally severe if contracted within 4 days before and 2 days after delivery. Severe viral respiratory distress with significantly depleted maternal passive antibody transmission puts the infant at an even greater risk for other complications. When maternal varicella infection occurs 5 to 21 days before delivery, the newborn has a much milder course of the disease and appears more capable of fighting the infection. This milder course is probably due to passive immunity transmitted to the infant via maternally derived antibodies.

The diagnosis of varicella is made by isolation of HSV. Strict isolation of identified infants or of those whose symptoms are highly suspicious for infection is necessary. Vidarabine or acyclovir can be used for treatment of severe disease in newborns. Varicella-zoster immune globulin (VZIG) can be given to newborns to decrease the severity of infection in those exposed (CDC, 1984b).

Prevention

Typically, if a mother has contracted varicella infection late in pregnancy, other persons, such as health care workers, family members, or other newborns, may have been exposed. Exposed susceptible persons should be protected with VZIG. A live attenuated varicella vaccine approved by the Food and Drug Administration is produced by Merck & Co., Inc. (Clark, 1995). There is skepticism among pediatricians as to the efficacy of using the vaccine rather than allowing a usually benign childhood illness to occur. For women of childbearing age who have not contracted varicella, however, the vaccine may be advocated rather than allowing the women to risk contraction of the disease during pregnancy.

Gonorrhea

Neisseria gonorrhoeae is a species of small gram-negative diploid bacteria. They are diploid because they grow in pairs. Infection with this organism is seen most frequently in young adults, aged 15 to 24 years. There are approximately 1 million new cases of gonorrhea each year. In females, infection is asymptomatic, which compromises detection of the disease. The organism is easily transmitted by infected tissue and secretions from the cervix, pharynx, urethra, or rectum. The incubation period is approximately 2 to 7 days. Pelvic inflammatory disease is often caused by the organism.

Clinical Manifestations

Gonorrhea infections are often mild but often cause blockage of the fallopian tubes. Perhaps 50 percent of women are asymptomatic with an infected cervix. In a pregnant woman, gonorrheal colonization of the cervix can cause inflammation and weakening of the fetal membranes and early rupture. Chorioamnionitis with *N. gonorrhoeae* as the causative organism can occur in the antepartum period and during labor and delivery; it is also related to increased risk of postpartum endometritis.

Disseminated gonococcal infection may present during pregnancy, causing arthritis, tendinitis, general aching, fever, and malaise. A previous history of gonorrhea presents a strong possibility that it may recur during pregnancy. Sexual partners should be screened and given treatment, because reinfection after treatment is common.

Gonococcal conjunctivitis in the newborn has historically been a risk from transmission via the birth canal. Prophylaxis has been mandated by law in the United States, and silver nitrate 1 percent solution or erythromycin is administered in both eyes of the neonate at birth. Fetal scalp electrodes have been identified as a potential method of organism transmission to the fetus. *N. gonorrhoeae* has been isolated from scalp abscesses, gastric and pharyngeal aspirates, conjunctival aspirates, and other blood and body fluids. Maternal and neonatal risks from exposure to the gonorrheal microorganism are significant and make it particularly important to screen for gonorrhea during pregnancy. Infected women have a higher incidence of premature labor, PROM, and infectious complications (Fletcher & Gordon, 1990).

Prevention

Use of silver nitrate solution or erythromycin for prevention of gonococcal ophthalmia neonatorum is one of the early achievements in preventive medicine. Routine prophylaxis is mandated by law in the United States and has made a significant difference in the treatment of ocular disease. Chlamydia conjunctivitis has become far more common than gonococcal conjunctivitis in the neonate because of the continual screening for gonorrhea and the routine use of silver nitrate. Erythromycin ointment in both eyes is a more common prophylactic practice, because it covers both gonococcal and chlamydial organisms (Hammerschlag et al., 1989).

Collaborative Management: Mother

The appropriate treatment for a pregnant woman includes ceftriaxone, 250 mg intramuscularly once, plus erythromycin, 500 mg orally four times a day for 7 days (CDC, 1987b). If gastrointestinal side effects are too severe, amoxicillin can be used (Majeroini, 1994). Follow-up, per the CDC, requires cervical and rectal cultures for *N. gonorrhoeae* be obtained 4 to 7 days after treatment. Ideally, pregnant women should also receive treatment for chlamydia infection. In the nonpregnant woman, treatment with doxycycline, ofloxacin, and azithromycin is effective but their use in pregnancy is not advised. Azithromycin has not been tested in pregnant women, but, if proven safe, only one dose would be required for effective treatment (Majeroini, 1994).

Collaborative Management: Neonate

Infants who are delivered by an infected, untreated mother are usually given a complete sepsis work-up, including a lumbar puncture, and placed on ampicillin and gentamicin therapy. If cultures confirm the presence of the microorganism and resistance is an issue, then infants should be treated with ceftriaxone, 25 to 50 mg/kg/day intravenously or intramuscularly in single doses, or cefotaxime, 25 mg/kg intravenously or intramuscularly every 12 hours (CDC, 1989).

Education and support regarding the origin of the infectious agent are important in the treatment of gonorrhea. Sexual partners of infected persons should be encouraged to seek testing and appropriate antibiotic treatment for chlamydia as well as gonorrhea (Gutman & Holmes, 1995).

Hepatitis B Virus

The hepatitis B virus (HBV) is fairly large, approximately 42 mm in diameter. It is a double-stranded DNA-containing virus. Exposure to infected blood and body fluids, percutaneous introduction of blood, and administration of infected blood products are the principal routes of transmission. Contamination or infection of wounds can easily transmit the disease. The virus is fairly strong and is able to live on inanimate objects or fomites. Deactivation requires at least 1 minute in boiling water and extended autoclaving time.

In the adult, HBV infection produces systemic illness with general malaise, jaundice, anorexia, and nausea. Early stages of the disease may include fever, rash, and sore joints. Health care workers have historically been particularly vulnerable to this virus because of their repeated exposures to contaminated blood and body fluids and needle sticks. A carrier state of HBV can precipitate chronic liver disease (Lott & Kenner, 1994a; 1994b). In certain areas of the world, such as Africa, Southeast Asia, and the Pacific Rim, the virus is considered endemic. In these areas, carrier rates are estimated to be 35 percent. Approximately 40 percent of these carriers have been identified as having been perinatally infected (Gabbe et al., 1986).

Hepatitis B surface antigen (HB_sAg) is an important test in assessing a woman's risk of transmitting HBV to her unborn child. The presence of HB_sAg and hepatitis B e antigen (HB_eAg) is the best indication of infectiousness. It is currently recommended that all pregnant women be screened at their first prenatal visit for HB_sAg and HB_eAg to prevent prenatal transmission (ACIP, 1990).

Infection early in pregnancy with HBV causes a 50 percent risk of neonatal HBV infection. Ninety percent of infants born to women who are positive for both HB_sAg and HB_eAg are at risk for development of HBV infection by their first birthday if they are not given treatment. Infants born to women who are positive for HB_sAg but negative for HB_eAg have lower rates of perinatal infection (20 percent) (Lee et al., 1986). Infants who do not receive treatment are likely to become carriers, which may eventually lead to primary hepatocellular carcinoma (Lott & Kenner, 1994a, 1994b).

Treatment for these infants should be HBV vaccine along with hepatitis B immunoglobulin. For neonates whose mothers are

HB_sAg positive or exposed, HBV vaccine, 0.5 ml (10 μg/ml), should be given intramuscularly in the anterolateral thigh at or within 24 hours of birth. Immunoglobulin (0.5 ml) should be given concurrently at a separate site. Vaccination should be repeated at 1 and 6 months: 0.5 ml; booster injections are suggested at 12 months and may need repeating at 5-year intervals (American Academy of Pediatrics, 1992). The vaccine can be used in infants who have been exposed to HIV. There is usually an immune response in these infants despite an altered CD4 count. The response does appear to be somewhat diminished (Rutstein et al., 1994).

Vertical transmission of HBV may occur during vaginal delivery. The sharing of bodily secretions during sexual intercourse can result in disease transmission also. HBV has a long incubation period—50 to 190 days, average 90 days. Current recommendations are for all pregnant women to be screened initially and again before delivery. Screening is essential to identify potential risk for perinatal transmission and for protection of those who are exposed to antigen-positive blood. Family clustering of HBV has been identified through spread via household contact.

Clinical Manifestations

Prematurity, low birth weight, and hyperbilirubinemia are clinical signs of HBV infection. Hepatosplenomegaly is also a common presenting symptom in an infant infected with a virus. An infant infected with HBV can be asymptomatic or present with a picture of fulminant sepsis.

Risk Factors

Pregnant women in high-risk categories (i.e., they are known to have sexual contact with HBV-infected persons) should be screened so that appropriate follow-up can be provided. Persons in certain ethnic groups, such as Asians (Taiwanese especially) and Australian aborigines; intravenous drug users; and health professionals are at risk for the development of HBV. Individuals living in poor sanitary conditions are also at risk (Lott & Kenner, 1994a, 1994b).

Collaborative Management and Prevention

Vaccination is recommended for individuals who are at risk for exposure to HBV, including health care workers, family members of chronic carriers, persons with large numbers of heterosexual partners, and intravenous drug users. Hb_sAg protein is administered to the deltoid muscle once, and then again 1 month and 6 months later.

If the mother's antigen status is unknown at delivery, titers should be drawn and the woman should be vaccinated if the result is Hb_sAg positive. If the test results are unavailable or cannot be obtained, the neonate should be treated as if the mother were positive. It is estimated that the cost of preventing one case of neonatal HBV infection is $3000 (Schalm et al., 1989). At an annual national birth rate of 3.5 million, a national policy of routine antepartum screening of all pregnant women would result in an annual net savings of more than $105 million. Thus, in high-risk groups, as many as 140 cases of acute neonatal hepatitis and 1400 cases of chronic liver disease would be prevented yearly, per 100,000 pregnant women, at a net yearly savings of $765 million (Arevalo & Washington, 1988).

Proper and prompt identification of women in high-risk groups and knowledge of HBV status are important in the delivery room to determine whether the infant is at risk for infection. In accordance with universal infection control measures, appropriate barriers are used to protect health care workers from blood and body secretions. Delivery room and nursery personnel should always wear gloves when handling any new infant. The infant of a mother with confirmed HBV infection should be bathed with soap and water immediately, with special attention to removing all blood and secretions present on the skin and hair. The infant may be breastfed (unless the mother's nipples are cracked) and cared for routinely.

Human Papillomavirus

Genital warts, or condylomata acuminata, are caused by human papillomavirus (HPV). HPV is a double-stranded DNA virus. Two specific strains of HPV have been identified as causing venereal warts and thus are of concern as sexually transmitted viruses. The incidence of this disease has increased rapidly since the 1980s, along with that of other sexually transmitted diseases. The time lag between exposure and infection can be up to 6 months (Bennett, 1987). Symptoms of HPV infection include warty growths on the vagina, cervix, vulva, perineum, buttocks, or inner thigh. The presence of these warts can be extremely uncomfortable during vaginal delivery. Intrapartal transmission is possible if genital warts are visible. Current maternal treatment to prevent transmission includes carbon dioxide laser therapy and 85 percent trichloroacetic acid. Condyloma in 31 of 32 women (97 percent) was controlled with this combination therapy. The incidence of maternal-to-newborn transmission is approximately 2 percent with this treatment (Schwartz et al., 1988). Newborns can contract a respiratory or laryngeal papillomatosis from infection with this virus.

Prenatal treatment is associated with low complication and recurrence rate. The treatment alleviates the need for a cesarean delivery. Examination, treatment, and follow-up of sexual partners are important aspects of treatment, because 50 percent of partners are infected (Bourcier & Seidler, 1987).

Clinical Manifestations

Laryngeal papillomatosis causes newborns to have a "weak cry" or hoarseness. The expected incidence of laryngeal papilloma in an infant born to a woman with untreated HPV is approximately 78 percent (Arvin & Maldonado, 1995). The newborn may have stridor or other respiratory symptoms.

Collaborative Management

Education and counseling of mothers and their partners are the primary concerns in the treatment of condyloma. Patients are instructed about methods of transmission and methods to decrease transmission. Emotional support is important, because venereal disease is extremely painful and demoralizing. Condyloma lesions have a high recurrence rate (70 percent). Early identification of newborns at risk for laryngeal papillomas is important to prevent respiratory complications. Newborns experiencing respiratory distress and stridor should be evaluated for laryngeal papillomas. Supportive ventilatory therapy may be needed.

There may be long-term complications from perinatal transmission of HPV, for example, one area of research is the study of increased risk of cervical cancer in females who were exposed in utero (Pakarian et al., 1994). The relationship between HPV and cancer of the cervix and vulva has been studied (Bennett, 1987).

Chlamydia

Chlamydia is a genus of bacteria that grows between cells. Chlamydial infection is one of the most common sexually transmitted diseases. Probably 50 percent of infected women of childbearing age are asymptomatic. Studies have shown that the infected population comprises sexually active women between 18 and 35 years of age having a high school education or less and three or more sexual partners in the previous 3 months (Phillips et al., 1989). The infection can present as cervicitis, salpingitis, urethritis, or pelvic inflammatory disease.

Chlamydia trachomatis infection has been identified as causing a significant increase in the incidence of PROM, the number of low birth weight babies, and the rate of infant mortality (Ryan et al., 1990). Thus, screening pregnant women for chlamydia is important. Treatment with erythromycin or clindamycin may prevent transmission to the newborn.

Clinical Manifestations

Chlamydia conjunctivitis can present in the newborn with a very watery discharge that may progress to purulent exudate. Application of erythromycin ointment at birth for ocular prophylaxis successfully treats both chlamydial and gonococcal conjunctivitis. Pneumonia can occur in newborns who have contracted chlamydia from their mother's genital tract. The incubation period is anywhere from 5 days to 3 to 4 months. Typical presentation is tachypnea, barrel chest, and an increased oxygen requirement. The infant may have interstitial infiltrations, hepatosplenomegaly, and increased eosinophils. In a prospective study of chlamydia, there was a 16 percent incidence of pneumonia in infants identified as being at risk for chlamydial infection (Schachter & Grossman, 1995).

Diagnosis of chlamydial infections is based on physical and laboratory examination; in cases of conjunctivitis, Giemsa-stained conjunctival scrapings provide a method of direct fluorescent antibody testing. The definitive diagnosis for chlamydial pneumonia is made by culture of the respiratory tract or identification of high levels of IgM antibodies to chlamydia.

Collaborative Management and Prevention

Treatment of chlamydia infection in the newborn is usually with ampicillin and gentamicin if the infant's work-up is for generic sepsis. Once the chlamydia organism is identified, more specific treatment is with erythromycin for 10 to 14 days.

If chlamydia is confirmed in a pregnant woman and treated, her sexual partners also require treatment. Rapid screening and diagnosis can be made using monoclonal antibodies, and some laboratories offer a chlamydia test called Chlamydiazyme, which gives results very quickly, allowing appropriate treatment to be initiated early. Positive results indicate the need for treatment, but negative results indicate that repeated screening is needed.

Education and counseling regarding the method of transmission of chlamydia are important. This organism may be present for many years in the female genital tract and produce no symptoms. The organism does not respond to partial treatment; an infected woman and all her sexual partners must receive full treatment as soon as possible. Men should wear condoms during sexual relations to prevent transmission. Without treatment, the severe complications for the woman include pelvic inflammatory disease, ectopic pregnancy, and endometritis. The common newborn complication is pneumonia. Supportive ventilation in the newborn is usually necessary.

Bacterial Infections

Group B Streptococcus

Group B beta-hemolytic streptococci were unknown to the perinatal scene until the early 1970s when they replaced *E. coli* as the single most common agent associated with bacterial meningitis during the first 2 months of life. The incidence of infection with group B streptococci has increased over the past 10 years, and they frequently cause postpartum infections in otherwise normal mothers (Gaffney & Salinger, 1987). Use of a rapid screening test to identify colonized mothers and intrapartum treatment with ampicillin have been shown to reduce vertical transmission (Morales et al., 1986).

The number of newborn deaths associated with either early onset (prior to the first week of life) or late onset continues to be high, particularly in high-risk urban centers. Potential for permanent neurologic sequelae for infant survivors of meningeal infections is approximately 15 percent (Baker & Edwards, 1995). The mortality rate of infected newborns is also estimated to be 15 percent (Opal et al., 1988).

Pathophysiology

Streptococcus is a gram-positive diplococcus with an ultrastructure similar to that of other gram-positive cocci. It was classified as hemolytic because of its double zone of hemolysis surrounding colonies on blood agar plates. Culture of body fluids, such as blood, urine, CSF, and other secretions, is the most common method of identifying group B streptococci. Counterelectrophoresis and latex agglutination are rapid assays that enable a presumptive diagnosis before cultures are returned. Rapid identification of the group B streptococcus organism is important in treating colonized pregnant women and in the early diagnosis and treatment of infection in the sick, unstable septic infant. To accurately predict maternal colonization with group B streptococci, both vaginal and rectal areas should be cultured on more than one occasion (Minkoff & Mead, 1986).

Clinical Manifestations

Group B streptococcus has been identified as a relatively common cause of midgestational fetal loss in women who experience vaginal hemorrhage, PROM, fetal membrane infection, and spontaneous abortion. The rate of stillbirth is reported to be as high as 61 percent in association with these bacteria. Early-onset neonatal infections with group B streptococcus can be asymptomatic or can manifest with severe symptoms of respiratory distress and shock, which can rapidly progress to death (Klein & Marcy, 1995).

Early-onset group B streptococcus infection usually appears within the first 24 hours of life and is most common in premature infants. Infants who weigh 1000 g or less usually present with congenital pneumonia. The most common presentations are pneumonia and meningitis. Signs of respiratory distress, apnea, grunting, tachypnea, and cyanosis are common. Hypotension is found in 25 percent of newborns with group B streptococcus infection; these infants are at risk for cardiopulmonary collapse. Nonspecific signs of sepsis include lethargy, poor feeding, temperature instability, abdominal distention, pallor, tachycardia, and jaundice. Experienced health care professionals may observe that the neonate "just doesn't look right," which is sometimes a critical point for early detection and implementation of therapy.

Overwhelming group B streptococcal septicemia is often compounded by meningitis. Lumbar puncture and examination of the CSF is the only way to exclude meningeal involvement and therefore is an important part of the workup. Seizures may occur in infants with group B streptococcal meningitis. Low birth weight infants have been identified as particularly vulnerable, but a study in Texas revealed a high incidence of infection in term newborns (Baker & Edwards, 1995). These infants had no risk factors for sepsis; therefore, there was a delay in identification and treatment. The mortality rate in these term newborns was 14 percent (Baker & Edwards, 1995).

Late-Onset Infection

Late-onset infection with group B streptococcus usually occurs in term newborns 7 days to 12 weeks of age. The fatality rate is less than that with early-onset infection, but meningitis is a common complication. In one study of 292 neonates with meningitis, 26 percent died in the hospital (Wald et al., 1986). Of the survivors, 25 to 50 percent had permanent neurologic damage, varying in severity from mild handicaps to severe impairment. Complications include global or profound mental retardation, spastic quadriplegia, cortical blindness, deafness, uncontrolled seizures, hydrocephalus, and diabetes insipidus. Thus, early treatment is an important part of the prevention of long-term serious sequelae. An infant with a positive blood culture can often be asymptomatic initially. The diagnosis of group B streptococcal infection is complicated because signs and symptoms of neonatal infection are not specific and symptoms may represent other conditions of the neonate. For example, apnea may be a symptom of central nervous system immaturity in the preterm neonate, but it is also associated with infection. The health care professional must maintain a high index of suspicion for infection in all conditions involving the neonate. Therefore, infection must be considered in the differential diagnosis of many problems found. Screening tests, such as complete blood count with differential, are often used to identify the need for further evaluation for sepsis. Abnormal results indicate the necessity for definitive testing and implementation of antimicrobial therapy.

Collaborative Management

Regional and institutional differences in infectious agents must be considered in the selection of antimicrobial therapy. Before culture results are returned, a broad-spectrum penicillin and an aminoglycoside are started to provide coverage for the most prevalent microorganisms causing infection. Generally, ampicillin and gentamicin are selected until culture results and sensitivities are available. Group B streptococcus is generally very sensitive to penicillin G, and, in many institutions, it is substituted for ampicillin once the diagnosis is made. See Table 27–4 for dosages.

Therapy is maintained for 7 to 10 days for sepsis and 14 to 21 days for meningitis. The lumbar puncture may be repeated midway or at the end of therapy to ensure that there are no microorganisms remaining in the CSF.

Fluid management, volume expansion, and appropriate antimicrobial therapy are the key components of nursing care. Infants with group B streptococcal infection are often very labile and do not tolerate frequent interventions. Minimal handling is sometimes required for their care.

Baker and Edwards (1995) recommended the active immunization of all women of childbearing age, either before pregnancy or late in pregnancy (at approximately 7 months' gestation). Passive transmission of antibodies to the newborn occur via the placenta; however, women often deliver infants prematurely, before the successful transmission of appropriate protective antibodies. Therefore, this concept is still being investigated. The cost of developing a suitable vaccine would probably be less than the cost of the care required by the critically ill newborn and the chronically ill, debilitated, severely handicapped newborn.

Staphylococcus

From the 1950s to the 1970s, coagulase-positive *S. aureus* was the main organism identified as a pathogen in hospitals. In the 1980s, coagulase-negative organisms, in particular *S. epidermidis,* were discovered to be equally important. These organisms have caused many serious and even fatal infections in newborns.

Ill neonates and premature infants who are already immunocompromised are particularly vulnerable to infections. Any open skin lesions, surgical incisions, or puncture wounds secondary to diagnostic tests or procedures are conducive to bacterial growth, especially *S. aureus* or *S. epidermidis* (Howells & Jones, 1988). Nosocomial infections may also be transmitted to the neonate via contaminated articles or on the hands of health professionals. Overgrowth of *S. epidermidis* may occur in nurseries where an attempt has been made to reduce colonization of *S. aureus.* Resistant organisms pose a threat to preterm infants who require extensive invasive treatments. They are particularly susceptible to colonization with coagulase-negative staphylococci or even methicillin-resistant *S. aureus* (Reboli et al., 1989).

Staphylococci release endotoxins that have systemic effects. One of these effects is alteration of the skin's protective layer. Scalded skin syndrome is one of the most dramatic results of these endotoxins. Integumentary dysfunction secondary to staphylococcal infection is discussed in Chapter 32, Assessment and Management of Integumentary Dysfunction.

Collaborative Management

Management and supportive therapy for staphylococcal infection are initially the same as for infection with group B streptococci. Antimicrobial therapy begins with ampicillin and gentamicin. Once definitive cultures and sensitivities are available and if the organism is ampicillin resistant, the drug of choice is one of the synthetic penicillins: oxacillin, methicillin, cloxacillin, dicloxacillin, or nafcillin. If the organism is methicillin resistant, the best available drug is vancomycin (Lott, 1994).

Escherichia coli

E. coli is a gram-negative, non–spore-forming motile rod. It is a normal inhabitant of the gastrointestinal tract and the most common cause of gram-negative sepsis in the newborn. Colonization of the gastrointestinal tract with *E. coli* occurs postnatally through environmental exposure and enteral feedings.

Listeria monocytogenes

L. monocytogenes has been recognized as a cause of perinatal complications since the early 1900s. It is found in birds and mammals, including domestic and farm animals. It is found in unpasteurized milk, soil, and fecal material. *Listeria* infection appears to be underdiagnosed and an underreported cause of congenital sepsis. A study done at the University of Southern California looked at 20 mother-infant pairs from whom *Listeria* was isolated in the prior 10 years. Antepartum factors such as high maternal leukocyte count, fetal tachycardia, decreased fetal heart rate variability, and absence of intrapartum fetal heart rate accelerations were identified in the history of the newborns diagnosed with congenital *Listeria* infection (Boucher & Yonekura, 1986).

The incidence of *Listeria* infection in the United States is unknown, and the route of transmission is unclear. Investigators of recent outbreaks, however, have shown that the infection can be foodborne. In a study that examined United States hospital discharge data from 1980 to 1982, it was determined that the incidence of listeriosis in newborns was 568 per 1 million of the population per year (Ciesielski et al., 1988). The number of fetal deaths caused by *Listeria* is unknown.

Clinical Manifestations

A mother infected with *Listeria* commonly has flu-like symptoms, including malaise, fever, chills, diarrhea, and back pain. It is also possible to contract the infection and remain asymptomatic or have only minor symptoms. This organism has been identified as a cause of spontaneous abortion (Lennon et al., 1984).

If contracted between 17 and 28 weeks' gestation, *Listeria* can cause fetal death or premature birth of an acutely ill newborn who may die hours later. However, early maternal treatment with intravenous ampicillin and gentamicin has been associated with normal newborn outcome (Bortolussi & Schlechi, 1995). Infection late in pregnancy may cause the infant to be born with a congenital infection, usually pneumonia. Mortality rates are high but are usually related to the amount of prematurity. Late-onset listeriosis, which can occur up to 4 weeks after delivery, can easily result in meningitis. A term newborn with listeriosis has less chance of dying but often suffers complications of hydrocephalus and mental retardation (Visintine et al., 1977). However, in either preterm or term neonates in whom meningitis develops, there is a 70 percent mortality rate if treatment is delayed (Bortolussi & Schlechi, 1995).

Newborns infected with *Listeria* may be born prematurely and be meconium stained, exhibit apnea and flaccidity, have a papular erythematous skin rash and hepatosplenomegaly, and be poor feeders (Visintine et al., 1977). Preterm birth associated with meconium staining should always be considered suspicious for listeriosis.

Collaborative Management

Intrapartum administration of antibiotics may decrease fetal morbidity and mortality rates. Ampicillin in combination with an aminoglycoside is the most common treatment. Investigators have shown that newborn survival rates are significantly different if the mother as well as the infant receives treatment (71 percent versus 29 percent) (Bortolussi & Schlechi, 1995).

Careful handwashing is a very important aspect of caring for the infant infected with *Listeria.* Institutional policy may require that the infant be isolated for the first 24 hours of life, until the antibiotics are on board. The mother's urine, stool, and lochia should be cultured, and, if positive, she should be given ampicillin.

Listeriosis often presents suddenly in the last trimester of pregnancy, precipitating an unexpected preterm delivery. Extensive emotional support may be necessary for the mother and family.

Neonatal Meningitis

Pathophysiology

Meningitis can be a sequela of newborn sepsis. The incidence of neonatal sepsis is reported to be 1 to 8.1 in 1000 live births (Klein & Marcy, 1995). The incidence of meningitis associated with newborn sepsis is thought to be approximately 25 percent of those presenting with sepsis. Meningitis is a more common complication of late-onset sepsis. The morbidity rate is higher for preterm infants than for term infants. Morbidity of survivors of infection with gram-negative bacilli or group B streptococci approaches 20 to 50 percent. These complications include mental and motor problems, seizure disorders, hydrocephalus, hearing loss, blindness, and abnormal speech patterns (Wald et al., 1986).

In most cases, meningitis results from bacteremia. Thus, an inoculation of organisms may pass the blood–brain barrier and infect the CSF. Cytologic tests on the CSF can identify the presence of an inflammatory response. A Gram stain of the CSF fluid should be prepared and other appropriate cultures obtained. High CSF protein and low glucose levels are also indicators of meningitis. See Table 27–1 for additional information.

Clinical Manifestations

Initially, the infant with meningitis presents with signs and symptoms of generalized sepsis. In addition, the meningeal irritation results in increased irritability, crying, increased intracranial pressure leading to bulging fontanelles, lethargy, tremors or twitching, seizure activity, vomiting, alterations in consciousness, and diminished muscle tone. Focal signs include hemiparesis, horizontal deviation of the eyes, and some cranial nerve involvement (Klein & Marcy, 1995).

Risk Factors

The National Institutes of Health sponsored a Collaborative Perinatal Project Study, which found that low birth weight infants are three times more likely to acquire meningitis than term infants (Niswander & Gordon, 1972; Overall, 1970).

In one study, meningitis was 17 times more frequent in the low birth weight groups. It seems that the smaller the baby, the more frequent the signs and symptoms of sepsis and meningitis. Very low birth weight infants, weighing less than 750 g, have been identified as having high rates of sepsis and other complications (La Gamma et al., 1983).

It appears that male infants are more vulnerable to sepsis and meningitis. There has been a suggestion regarding a sex-linked factor, that is, that a particular gene located on the X chromosome is involved with the function of the thymus or with synthesis of immunoglobulin to defend the newborn host (Schlegel & Bellante, 1969). Female infants have lower rates of respiratory distress syndrome and lower rates of most congenital infections (Portillo & Sullivan, 1979).

Geography and socioeconomic factors are influential in patterns of neonatal disease. These differences probably reflect populations served, including unique cultural activities and sexual practices, as well as local customs. It probably also reflects different treatment patterns in local nurseries and variations of antimicrobial selections.

Prognosis

Brain abscess is associated with a poor prognosis; approximately 50 percent of affected patients die. Destruction of brain tissues, hemorrhages, and infarcts causing necrosis to vital brain cells may cause extensive brain damage, leading to death or poor neurologic outcomes. With the introduction of ultrasonography and computerized tomography, brain abscesses are being identified earlier (Renier et al., 1988).

Collaborative Management

The selection of antimicrobial therapy for meningitis is based on the causative microorganism. Supportive therapy is necessary for the newborn with meningitis. Acute observation and monitoring of vital signs and activity level are crucial. Infants who become critically ill with meningitis may deteriorate quickly and need rapid, acute interventions. Infants often require long-term antibiotic therapy, and, often, venous access is a problem. Placement of a percutaneous line for parenteral nutrition may be necessary. Families need educational and emotional support during the long-term hospitalizations, particularly if complications develop.

Viral Agents

Respiratory Syncytial Virus

Respiratory syncytial virus (RSV) is an infection usually found in older infants. It is thought that maternal antibodies protect infants for the first few weeks of life, but as passive immunity diminishes, these infants become more vulnerable. Premature infants, already immunocompromised, are more susceptible to the virus during their long-term hospitalizations.

Clinical Manifestations

An infant who is infected with RSV before 4 weeks of age may be asymptomatic or may have an upper respiratory infection with fever, bronchiolitis, apnea, or pneumonia. There may be a definite need for assisted ventilation, and deaths have occurred in rapidly fulminating disease, for which there is little available treatment. Small preterm infants who are already in significant pulmonary and cardiac jeopardy with respiratory distress syndrome or bronchopulmonary dysplasia are especially susceptible to development of severe infections. Nosocomial transmission of the virus between caretakers is possible; such transmission appears to result in less severe infection. The first clinical signs of transmission include a clear nasal discharge at approximately 10 to 52 days of life, followed by cough and wheezing. Radiologic changes compatible with pneumonia may also be found.

Treatment and Prevention

Good handwashing is extremely important in the prevention of transmission of RSV between critically ill patients. It has been shown that RSV-infected secretions can remain viable for up to 6 hours on countertops, 45 minutes on cloth gowns and paper tissues, and 20 minutes on skin (Hall et al., 1980). Thus, all infected infants should be cared for in cohort. Caretakers should be consistently assigned to decrease transmission rates. Gown and glove precautions can significantly reduce nosocomial transmission of RSV (LeClair et al., 1987).

Any infant with a runny nose, nasal congestion, or unexplained apnea should be considered for isolation and be investigated for RSV infection. Attention should be specific for those infants older than 4 weeks of corrected age. Specific cultures and screens should be performed because specific treatment is available if RSV is found.

Collaborative Management

Treatment for identified RSV pneumonia is ribavirin. Ribavirin administration should be closely monitored by those who have been trained appropriately (American Academy of Pediatrics, 1987; Outwater et al., 1988). Ribavirin can be administered safely to infants receiving mechanical ventilation and to infants in an oxygen hood. Specific safety precautions should be taken to protect the caretaker, because ribavirin has been identified as being potentially teratogenic (Prows, 1989). Protective measures include wearing a gown, gloves, and mask when in direct contact with the particles or mist containing ribavirin. Ideally, no pregnant woman would take care of an infant with RSV who is receiving ribavirin. Close monitoring of the pulmonary status, including the use of oxygen and mechanical ventilation, may be necessary. Isolation of the infected infant from other infants who could potentially be infected is important; the usual method for isolation is to minimize risk of the spread of the airborne virus and ribavirin particles.

Adenovirus and Rotavirus

Adenoviruses can be enteric and are very small; rotaviruses are approximately 70 nm in size. Both these categories of organisms can cause significant viral gastroenteritis and are considered medically important because of their ability to cause neonatal diarrhea. Breastfeeding, with the transmission of secretory IgA, is thought to be one of the best protections against illness caused by adenovirus or rotavirus (Welsh & May, 1979). Animal data support the theory that breastmilk provides immunologic protection from sepsis when the gastrointestinal system is involved, as long as there is no existent endotoxemia. This protection may be related to the presence of secretory IgA or the presence of naturally occurring lactobacilli and *E. coli* in greater numbers in the gut when breastmilk rather than commercial formula is given (Witek-Janusek & Ratmeyer, 1991).

Rotavirus is a double-stranded RNA virus that has a wheel-like appearance under electron microscope. Rotavirus, like other acute diarrhea diseases in general, is uncommon in neonates. Infants are usually at greater risk at 3 or 4 months of age. Yet, with prolonged length of stay in a neonatal intensive care unit (NICU), nosocomial transmission is possible.

In newborn nurseries, attack rates are unpredictable. Within the same city, attack rates among infants may show dramatic variations in different hospitals and different years.

Once introduced, the virus is able to spread steadily until changes in admission policies or nursing practices stop the cycle. Exactly how the virus is introduced and transmitted is uncertain. Some of the ways a newborn could acquire infection include the following: (1) ingestion of viral particles at or shortly before the time of delivery, (2) transfer of virus from infants or toddlers excreting the virus, via hands of nursery personnel or parents, (3) transmission by direct contact with adults or older children excreting the virus, (4) infection by airborne or droplet particles, (5) infection by fomites, and (6) ingestion of contaminated foods or formula.

Transfer of particles from infant to infant on the hands of nursery and medical staff is probably the most common means of viral spread (Duffy et al., 1986).

Clinical Manifestations

An infected newborn can be asymptomatic or may have severe gastrointestinal problems. Early signs of illness include lethargy, irritability, and poor feeding, usually followed by the passage of watery yellow or green stools that are free of blood but contain mucus. Vomiting and slight fever may accompany the diarrhea for a time. Rotavirus has been identified as a potential cause of necrotizing enterocolitis (Rotbart et al., 1988). Specific methods of virus detection include radioimmunoassay, immunofluorescence, latex agglutination, and enzyme-linked immunosorbent assay. Some nurseries use the commercially available product Rotozyme II, which is quick and effective.

Collaborative Management

The primary goal of treatment is to provide supportive electrolytes and fluid management. Minimizing the fluid and electrolyte losses resulting from diarrhea is the key component of care. Persistent or recurrent diarrhea with the use of milk-based formulas or breast milk demands further investigation of carbohydrate intolerance or cow's milk intolerance. Some critically ill infants who may have reduced gastrointestinal absorptive surface (short bowel syndrome) or severe mucosal damage may require an elemental diet or parenteral nutrition.

Handwashing after each contact with the affected infant remains the single most important method of preventing the spread of the infection. Rotaviruses and adenoviruses are often excreted in an infant's stool 2 or 3 days before the illness is recognized. The isolation of an infant with diarrhea is often too late to prevent cross-contamination. Infants in whom gastroenteritis develops should be moved out of the nursery area if there are adequate facilities. The use of an incubator is helpful, because it may be a reminder that appropriate gowning and gloving are necessary before the infant can be handled. Encouraging the rooming of infants with their mothers can be helpful in containing nursery epidemics.

Several live orally administered rotavirus vaccines are being tested for their effectiveness in young infants (Losonsky et al., 1988). Also, milk containing concentrates of immunoglobulin prepared from rotavirus-hyperimmunized cows has been fed to infants hospitalized for acute rotavirus gastroenteritis. This practice appears to reduce excretion of the virus significantly and has prevented rotavirus diarrhea outbreaks in nurseries (Hilpert et al., 1987).

Fungal Agents

Candida albicans

Candida species is a fungus that is frequently found in humans, and *C. albicans* is the most prevalent form in neonates. *Candida* organisms are oval yeast-like cells that can bud to reproduce. *C. albicans* produces endotoxins, hemolysis, pyrogens, and proteolytic enzymes that are damaging to tissues (Kotloff et al., 1989). Early recognition and treatment of fungal sepsis are imperative to prevent severe central nervous system complications and death.

Prolonged broad-spectrum antibiotic treatment for small premature infants may predispose infants to *Candida* overgrowth in the gastrointestinal tract. This overgrowth may predispose the infant to disseminated fungemia. Administration of hyperalimentation, frequent use of indwelling venous lines, and invasive procedures may also predispose the infant to *C. albicans* infection. One study has identified previous antibiotic therapy and assisted ventilation as the major factors that correlated to *Candida* sepsis (Kotloff et al., 1989).

Clinical Manifestations

The newborn infected with *C. albicans* presents a picture similar to that of any septic infant. These newborns present with serious clinical signs of sepsis, often worsening with no presence of positive cultures. The infant is typically 20 to 30 days of age, has difficulties with oral feeds, depends on hyperalimentation, and has been given multiple courses of antibiotics. The infant may have respiratory distress, abdominal distention, guaiac-positive stools, carbohydrate intolerance, candiduria, temperature instability, and hypotension (Miller, 1995).

Differential Diagnosis

A positive *Candida* culture should never be considered a contaminated specimen. Intermittently positive cultures may reflect transient candidemia, and, usually, removal of any indwelling catheters and lines and changing of antibiotic therapy may be indicated. In symptomatic low birth weight infants with positive systemic cultures, treatment should begin pending culture results.

Collaborative Management

The most effective drug for treatment of *C. albicans* infection is amphotericin B. This toxic, potent antifungal agent must be used cautiously. The initial dose is 0.1 to 0.3 mg/kg given intravenously over a period of 2 to 6 hours. The maintenance dosage is 0.5 to 1.0 mg/kg/day over 2 to 6 hours. Lower doses are started until higher doses can be tolerated. Increments of 0.1 mg/kg/day are used to increase the daily dose slowly. Many infants tolerate a total dose of 20 mg/kg if titrated over approximately 1 month. Often, if organ involvement is minimal, infants can be successfully given lower doses. If meningitis is suspected, 5-fluorouracil (5-FU) may be used. This antifungal agent acts to inhibit DNA synthesis so that *Candida* replication cannot occur.

Kidney toxicity is a major side effect of amphotericin B therapy because it causes renal vasoconstriction and decreases both renal blood flow and glomerular filtration rate. This damage can result in hyponatremia, hypokalemia, increased blood urea nitrogen, and increased creatinine, as well as acidosis. If the medication makes the patient oliguric, most physicians recommend stopping the drug until the next day. Thrombocytopenia, granulocytopenia, fever, nausea, and vomiting are the common side effects associated with amphotericin B. One major side effect of 5-FU is bone marrow depression, resulting in a decreased platelet count.

Because of the insidious onset of candidiasis, the septic infant who is not responding to traditional antibiotic treatment may have *Candida*. Catheter tips at intravenous sites and percutaneous lines should be changed and cultured. Urine can easily be cultured for the presence of *Candida*. Thrush and monilial rashes are indicative of candidiasis. These can easily be treated with oral and local antifungal agents.

Monitoring of infants receiving amphotericin B is challenging, because infants may have reactions to this medication. Blood pressure should be monitored every half hour, and urine output should be followed up closely. Vital signs and laboratory work, including liver enzyme tests, should be followed up daily to detect early signs of neonatal toxicity.

Human Immunodeficiency Virus

HIV is discussed in Chapter 42, Neonatal Acquired Immunodeficiency Syndrome: Human Immunodeficiency Virus Infection and Acquired Immunodeficiency Syndrome in the Infant.

Nosocomial Infections

Both colonization and infection are nosocomial events, meaning "of or related to a hospital." The common meaning of the term nosocomial is "hospital acquired." Nursery-acquired infections are reported to the Centers for Disease Control, which has a National Nosocomial Infections Surveillance System (Garner et al., 1988).

The incidence of nosocomial infections in NICUs is 5 to 25 percent (Donowitz, 1989). Infants who are critically ill and remain in a pathogen-filled environment are often in jeopardy because of their prolonged length of stay in the hospital. The mortality rate associated with these infections is between 5 and 20 percent, depending on the geographic area and specific birth weight groups (Kotloff et al., 1989).

Coagulase-negative staphylococcus has been identified as a major cause of nosocomial infections. Low birth weight, multiple gestation, and prolonged hospitalization are significant factors for nosocomial infection. Yeast infections often occur if previous antibiotic therapy has been given. This infection is also associated with colonization of vascular catheters, assisted ventilation, and necrotizing enterocolitis (Kotloff et al., 1989).

Nursery epidemics can be caused by gram-negative and gram-positive or viral organisms because they have (1) the ability to colonize or infect human skin or the gastrointestinal tract, (2) the ability to be carried from person to person by hand contact, and (3) characteristics that allow existence on hands of personnel or in fluids or on inanimate objects, including intravenous fluids, respiratory support equipment, solutions used for medications, disinfectants, and banked breast milk.

Resistance to antibiotics is a serious problem in many NICUs, particularly with gram-negative enteric pathogens. Aminoglycoside resistance is a problem in many urban nurseries, as is colonization and infection with methicillin-resistant *S. aureus*. Respiratory infections with RSV, influenza virus, parainfluenza virus, rhinovirus, and echovirus occur in many nurseries. These are more difficult to identify and thus more difficult to report. CMV infection has been reported as a transfusion-related problem in low birth weight infants, thus prompting the current policy of using CMV-screened blood donors (Lamberson et al., 1988). Hepatitis A infection has also been reported as a transfusion-related problem that may develop in infants and staff in NICUs (Azimi et al., 1986). Hepatitis C has been linked to use of immunoglobulins such as Gammagard by Baxter (Burton, 1995). Almost any organism given the right environment and support can become a nosocomially transmitted infection.

Infection Control Policies

Policies and procedures in nurseries should be set up by the hospital infection control committee based on the recommendations of the American Academy of Pediatrics and the CDC. The significance of these policies to newborns should be detailed in a hospital policy book. The following topics should be covered: (1) ocular prophylaxis, (2) skin and cord care, (3) nursery staff, (4) nursery design and environment, (5) handwashing, (6) staff apparel, (7) isolation, (8) visitors, (9) employee health, and (10) epidemic control (Donowitz, 1989).

CONCLUSION

This chapter presents an overview of the function and development of the components of the neonatal immune system. Many factors place the neonate at high risk for infection. The nurse is in a unique role to implement methods for prevention of infection in nurseries, to detect early signs and symptoms of infection, and to participate in infection control. A better understanding of the neonatal immune system, methods of perinatal acquisition of organisms, common microorganisms, signs and symptoms of infections, and appropriate therapy provides the nurse with a sound basis for management of care as well as the development of hospital infection control policies for the NICU.

REFERENCES

Advisory Committee on Immunization Practices. (1990). Protection against viral hepatitis. *Morbidity and Mortality Weekly Report, 39*(RR-2).

American Academy of Pediatrics. (1994). *Report of the Committee on Infectious Diseases: The red book.* Elk Grove Village, IL: American Academy of Pediatrics.

American Academy of Pediatrics. Committee on Infectious Diseases. (1987). Ribavirin therapy of respiratory syncytial virus. *Pediatrics, 79*(3), 475–478.

American Academy of Pediatrics. (1992). Universal hepatitis B immunization. Policy statement. *AAP News, 8*(2), 13–15, 22.

Arevalo, J. A., & Washington, A. E. (1988). Cost-effectiveness of prenatal screening and immunization for hepatitis B virus. *Journal of the American Medical Association, 259*(3), 365–369.

Arvin, A. (1988). Antiviral treatment of herpes simplex infection in neonates and pregnant women. *Journal of the American Academy of Dermatology, 18*(1P-2), 200–203.

Arvin, A. M., & Maldonado, Y. A. (1995). Other viral infections of the fetus and newborn. In J. S. Remington & J. O. Klein (Eds.), *Infectious diseases of the fetus and newborn infant* (4th ed., pp. 745–756). Philadelphia: W. B. Saunders.

Azimi, P. H., Roberto, R. R., Guralnik, J., et al. (1986). Transfusion acquired hepatitis A in a premature infant with secondary nosocomial spread in an intensive care nursery. *American Journal of Diseases of Children, 140*(1), 23–27.

Baker, C. J., & Edwards, M. S. (1995). Group B streptococcal infection. In J. S. Remington & J. O. Klein (Eds.), *Infectious diseases of the fetus and newborn infant* (4th ed., pp. 980–1054). Philadelphia: W. B. Saunders.

Bellanti, J. A., Pung, Y-H., & Zeligs, B. J. (1994). Immunology. In G. B. Avery, M. A. Fletcher, & M. G. MacDonald (Eds.), *Neonatology: Pathophysiology and management of the newborn* (4th ed., pp. 1000–1029). Philadelphia: J. B. Lippincott.

Bennett, E. C. (1987). Sexually transmitted diseases. *NAACOG Newsletter, 14*(8).

Bortolussi, R., & Schlechi, W. F. (1995). Listeriosis. In J. S. Remington & J. O. Klein (Eds.), *Infectious diseases of the fetus and newborn infant* (4th ed., pp. 1055–1073) Philadelphia: W. B. Saunders.

Boucher, M., & Yonekura, M. L. (1986). Perinatal listeriosis (early onset), correlation of antenatal manifestations and neonatal outcome. *Obstetrics and Gynecology, 68*(5), 593–597.

Bourcier, K. M., & Seidler, A. J. (1987). Chlamydia and condylomata acuminata: An update for the nurse practitioner. *Journal of Obstetric, Gynecologic, and Neonatal Nursing, 16*(1), 17–22.

Brown, Z. A., Vontver, L. A., Benedetti, J., et al. (1987). Effects on infants of a first episode of genital herpes during pregnancy. *New England Journal of Medicine, 317*(20), 1246–1251.

Burton, T. M. (1995). A drug from Baxter is said to have posed a risk of hepatitis. *The Wall Street Journal, LXXVI*(194), July, 20, A1, A7.

Cairo, M. S., Worcester, C., Rucker, R., et al. (1987). Role of circulating complement and polymorphonuclear leukocyte transfusion in treatment and outcome in critically ill neonates with sepsis. *Journal of Pediatrics, 110*(6), 935–941.

Carter, A. O., & Frank, J. W. (1986). Congenital toxoplasmosis, epidemiology, features and control. *Canadian Medical Association, 135*(6), 618–623.

Centers for Disease Control. (1984a). Rubella prevention. *Morbidity and Mortality Weekly Report, 33*(84), 301.

Centers for Disease Control. (1984b). Varicella zoster immune globulin for the prevention of chicken pox. *Morbidity and Mortality Weekly Report, 33*(84), 301.

Centers for Disease Control. (1987a). Congenital rubella—United States (1984, 1986). *Morbidity and Mortality Weekly Report, 36*(12), 664–671.

Centers for Disease Control. (1987b). Progress toward achieving the national 1988 objectives for sexually transmitted disease. *Morbidity and Mortality Weekly Report, 36*(12).

Centers for Disease Control. (1989). Sexually transmitted disease treatment guidelines. *Morbidity and Mortality Weekly Report, 38*(58).

Chawla, V., Pandit, P. B., & Nkrumah, F. K. (1988). Congenital syphilis in the newborn. *Archives of Disease in Childhood, 63*(11), 1393–1394.

Ciesielski, C. A., Hightower, A. W., Parsons, S. K., & Broome, C. V. (1988). Listeriosis in the United States, 1980–1982. *Archives of Internal Medicine, 148*(6), 1416–1419.

Clark, G. (1995). Varicella vaccine approved. *AAP News, 11*(4), 1, 10.

Daffos, F., Forestier, F., Capella-Pavlovsky, M., et al. (1988). Prenatal management of 746 pregnancies at risk for congenital toxoplasmosis. *New England Journal of Medicine, 318*, 271–275.

Donowitz, L. G. (1989). Nosocomial infection in neonatal intensive care units. *American Journal of Infection Control, 17*(5), 250–257.

Duffy, L. C., Riepenoff-Talty, M., Byers, T. E., et al. (1986). Modulation of rotavirus enteritis during breast feeding. *American Journal of Diseases of Children, 140*(11), 1164.

Enders, G., & Jonatha, W. (1987). Prenatal diagnosis of intrauterine rubella. *Infection, 15*(3), 162–164.

Fletcher, J. E., Jr., & Gordon, R. C. (1990). Perinatal transmission of bacterially sexually transmitted disease. Syphilis and gonorrhea. *Journal of Family Practice, 30*(4, Part I), 448–456.

Freij, B. J., & Sever, J. L. (1988). Herpesvirus infections in pregnancy: Risks to embryo, fetus and neonate. *Clinics in Perinatology, 15*(2), 203–231.

Gabbe, S. E., Neibyl, J. R., & Simpson, J. L. (Eds.). (1986). *Obstetrics: Normal problem pregnancies.* New York: Churchill Livingstone.

Gaffney, S. E., & Salinger, L. (1987). Group B streptococcus. The pregnant woman and her neonate. *Journal of Obstetric, Gynecologic, and Neonatal Nursing, 16*(2), 91–96.

Garner, J. S., Jarvis, W. R., Emori, T. G., et al. (1988). CDC definitions for nosocomial infections. *American Journal of Infection Control, 16*, 128–140.

Gershon, A. A. (1995). Chickenpox, measles, and mumps. In J. S. Remington & J. O. Klein (Eds.), *Infectious diseases of the fetus and newborn infant* (4th ed., pp. 565–618). Philadelphia: W. B. Saunders.

Gilbert, G. L., Hayes, K., Hudson, I. L., & James, J. (1989). Prevention of transfusion-acquired cytomegalovirus infection in infants by blood filtration to remove leucocytes. *Lancet, 1*(8649), 1228–1231.

Gregg, N. M. (1941). Congenital cataract following German measles in the mother. *Transactions of the Ophthalmological Society of Australia, 3*, 35.

Gutman, L. T., & Holmes, K. K. (1995). Gonococcal infection. In J. S.

Remington & J. O. Klein (Eds.), *Infectious diseases of the fetus and newborn infant* (4th ed., pp. 1087–1104). Philadelphia: W. B. Saunders.

Haddad, J., Langer, B., Astruc, D., et al. (1993). Oral acyclovir and recurrent genital herpes during late pregnancy. *Obstetrics & Gynecology, 82*(1), 102–104.

Hall, C. B., Douglas, R. G., Jr., & German, J. M. (1980). Possible transmission by families for respiratory syncytial virus. *Journal of Infectious Diseases, 141*(1), 98–102.

Hammerschlag, M. R., Cummings, L., Roblin, P. M., et al. (1989). Efficacy of neonatal ocular prophylaxis for the prevention of chlamydial and gonococcal conjunctivitis. *New England Journal of Medicine, 320*(12), 769–772.

Herson, V. C., Krause, P. J., Eisenfeld, L. I., et al. (1988). Indomethacin-associated sepsis in very low birth weight infants. *American Journal of Diseases of Children, 142*(5), 555–558.

Hilpert, H., Brüssow, H., Mietens, L., et al. (1987). Use of bovine milk concentrate containing antibody to rotavirus to treat rotavirus gastroenteritis in infants. *Journal of Infectious Diseases, 156*(1), 158–166.

Howells, C. H., & Jones, H. E. (1988). Neonatalogy—then and now. Neonatal sepsis (1960). Two outbreaks of neonatal skin sepsis caused by *Staphylococcus aureus*, phage type 71. *Archives of Disease in Childhood, 63*(12), 1506.

Ingall, E., Sanchez, P. J., & Musher, D. (1995). Syphilis. In J. S. Remington & J. O. Klein (Eds.), *Infectious diseases of the fetus and newborn infant* (4th ed., pp. 529–564). Philadelphia: W. B. Saunders.

Johnson, R. E. (1986). Genital herpes and pregnancy. *American Family Physician, 33*(3), 167–171.

Koppe, J. G., Loewer-Sieger, D. H., & de Roever-Bonnet, H. (1986). Results of 20 year following of congenital toxoplasmosis. *Lancet, 1*(8475), 2594–2596.

Klein, R. O., & Marcy, S. M. (1995). Bacterial sepsis and meningitis. In J. S. Remington & J. O. Klein (Eds.), *Infectious diseases of the fetus and newborn infant* (4th ed., pp. 835–890). Philadelphia: W. B. Saunders.

Kotloff, K. L., Blackmon, L. R., Tenney, J. H., et al. (1989). Nosocomial sepsis in the neonatal intensive care unit. *Southern Medical Journal, 82*(6), 699–704.

Kuller, J. A., Chescheir, N. C. & Cefalo, R. C. (Eds.). (1996). *Prenatal diagnosis & reproductive genetics.* Philadelphia: J. B. Lippincott.

La Gamma, E. F., Drusin, L. M., Mackles, A. W., et al. (1983). Neonatal infections: An important determinant of late NICU mortality in infants less than 100 grams at birth. *American Journal of Diseases of Children, 137*(9), 838–841.

Lamberson, H. V., Jr., McMillian, J. A., Weiner, L. B., et al. (1988). Prevention of transfusion-associated cytomegalovirus infection in neonates by screening blood donors for IgM to CMV. *Journal of Infectious Diseases, 157*(4), 820–823.

LeClair, J. M., Freeman, J., Sullivan, B. F., et al. (1987). Prevention of nosocomial respiratory syncytial virus infections through compliance with glove and gown precautions. *New England Journal of Medicine,* 317(6), 329–334.

Lee, S. D., Lo, K. J., Wu, J. C., et al. (1986). Prevention of maternal-infant hepatitis B virus transmission by immunization: The role of serum hepatitis B virus DNA. *Hepatology, 6*(3), 369–373.

Lennon, D., Lewis, B., Mantall, C., et al. (1984). Epidemic perinatal listeriosis. *Pediatric Infectious Disease Journal, 3*(1), 30–34.

Levy, F. H., & O'Rourke, P. P. (1995). Topics in pediatric critical care. In S. L. Barnhart & M. P. Czervinske (Eds.), *Perinatal and pediatric respiratory care* (pp. 548–570). Philadelphia: W. B. Saunders.

Losonsky, G. A., Rennels, M. B., Lim, Y., et al. (1988). Systemic and mucosal immune response to rhesus rotavirus vaccine MMU 18006. *Pediatric Infectious Disease Journal, 7*(6), 388–393.

Lott, J. W. (1994). *Neonatal infection: Assessment, diagnosis, and management.* Petaluma, CA: NICU INK.

Lott, J. W., & Kenner, C. (1994a). Keeping up with neonatal infections: Designer bugs. *MCN, American Journal of Maternal Child Nursing, 19*(4, Part I), 207–213.

Lott, J. W., & Kenner, C. (1994b). Keeping up with neonatal infection: Designer bugs. *MCN, American Journal of Maternal Child Nursing, 19*(5, Part II), 264–271.

Lott, J. W., & Kilb, J. R. (1992). The selection of antibacterial agents for treatment of neonatal sepsis or Which drug kills which bug? *Neonatal Pharmacology Quarterly, 1*(1), 19–29.

Majeroini, B. A. (1994). Chlamydial cervicitis: Complications and new treatment options. *American Family Physician, 49*(8), 1825–1829, 1832.

Miller, M. J. (1995). Fungal infections. In J. S. Remington & J. O. Klein (Eds.), *Infectious diseases of the fetus and newborn infant* (4th ed., pp. 703–744). Philadelphia: W. B. Saunders.

Minkoff, H., & Mead, P. (1986). An obstetric approach to prevention of early onset group B beta-hemolytic streptococcal sepsis. *American Journal of Obstetrics and Gynecology, 154*(5), 973–977.

Morales, W. J., Lim, D. V., & Walsh, A. F. (1986). Prevention of neonatal group B streptococcal sepsis by the uses of a rapid screening test and selective intrapartum chemotherapy. *American Journal of Obstetrics and Gynecology, 155*(5), 979–983.

Munro, N. D., Sheppard, S., Smithells, R. W., et al. (1987). Temporal relations between maternal rubella and congenital defects. *Lancet, 2*(8552), 201–204.

Nelson, B. I., & Grossman, J., II. (1986). Perinatal infections. In S. E. Gabbe, J. R. Neible, & J. L. Simpson (Eds.), *Obstetrics: Normal and problem pregnancies.* New York: Churchill Livingstone.

Niswander, K. R., & Gordon, M. (1972). The women and their pregnancies: The Collaborative Perinatal Study of the National Institute of Neurological Diseases and Stroke. *U.S. Department of Health, Education and Welfare Publication No. NIH 73–379.*

Opal, S. M., Cross, A., Palmer, M., & Almazen, R. (1988). Group B streptococcal sepsis in adults and infants. Contrasts and comparisons. *Archives of Internal Medicine, 148*(3), 641–645.

Outwater, K. M., Messner, H. C., & Peterson, M. B. (1988). Ribavirin administration to infants receiving mechanical ventilation. *American Journal of Diseases of Children, 142*(5), 512–515.

Overall, J. C., Jr. (1970). Neonatal bacterial meningitis. *Journal of Pediatrics, 76*(4), 499–511.

Overall, J. C., Jr. (1994). Herpes simplex virus infection of the fetus and newborn. *Pediatric Annals, 23*(3), 131–136.

Pakarian, F., Kaye, J., Cason, J., et al. (1994). Cancer associated human papillomaviruses: Perinatal transmission and persistence. *British Journal of Obstetrics and Gynaecology, 101*(6) 514–517.

Phillips, R. S., Hanff, P. A., Holmes, M. D., et al. (1989). *Chlamydia trachomatis* cervical infection in women seeking routine gynecological care: Criteria for selective testing. *American Journal of Medicine, 86*(5), 515–520.

Polin, R. A. (1990). Role of fibronectin in disease of newborn infants and children. *Reviews of Infectious Diseases, 12*(Suppl. 4), S428–S438.

Portillo, D. T., & Sullivan, J. L. (1979). Immunological basis for superior survival of females. *American Journal of Diseases of Children, 133*(12), 1251–1253.

Prober, C. G., Hensleigh, P. A., Boucher, F. D., et al. (1988). Use of routine viral cultures at delivery to identify neonates exposed to herpes simplex virus. *New England Journal of Medicine, 318*(14), 887–891.

Prows, C. A. (1989). Ribavirin risks in reproduction—how great are they? *MCN, American Journal of Maternal Child Nursing, 14*(6), 400–404.

Reboli, A. C., John, J. R., Jr., & Levkoff, A. H. (1989). Epidemic methicillin-gentamicin resistant *Staphylococcus aureus* in a neonatal intensive care unit. *American Journal of Diseases of Children, 143*(1), 34–39.

Remington, J. S., McLeod, R., & Desmonts, G. (1995). Toxoplasmosis. In J. S. Remington & J. O. Klein (Eds.), *Infectious diseases of the fetus and newborn infant* (4th ed., pp. 140–267). Philadelphia: W. B. Saunders.

Renier, D., Flandin, C., Hirsch, E. E., & Hirsch, J. F. (1988). Brain abscesses in neonates. A study of 30 cases. *Journal of Neurosurgery,* 69(6), 877–882.

Ricci, J. M., Fojaco, R. M., & O'Sullivan, M. J. (1989). Congenital syphilis. The University of Miami Jackson Memorial Medical Center experience (1986–1988). *Obstetrics and Gynecology, 74,* 687–693.

Rotbart, H. A., Nelson, W. L., Glode, M. P., et al. (1988). Neonatal rotavirus-associated necrotizing enterocolitis: Case control study and prospective surveillance during an outbreak. *Journal of Pediatrics, 112*(1), 87–93.

Rutstein, R. M., Rudy, B., Codispoti, C., & Watson, B. (1994). Response to hepatitis B immunization by infants exposed to HIV. *AIDS, 8*(9), 1281–1284.

Ryan, G. M., Jr., Adbella, T. N., McNeeley, S. G., et al. (1990). *Chlamydia trachomatis* infection in pregnancy and effect of treatment on outcome. *American Journal of Obstetrics and Gynecology, 162*(1), 34–39.

Schachter, J., & Grossman, M. (1995). Chlamydia. In J. S. Remington & J. O. Klein (Eds.), *Infectious diseases of the fetus and newborn infant* (4th ed., pp. 657–667). Philadelphia: W. B. Saunders.

Schalm, S. W., Mazel, J. A., deGast, G. C., et al. (1989). Prevention of hepatitis B infection in newborns through mass screening and delayed vaccination of all infants of mothers with hepatitis B surface antigen. *Pediatrics, 83*(6), 1041–1048.

Schlegel, R. J., & Bellante, J. A. (1969). Increased susceptibility of males to infection. *Lancet,* 2(625), 826–827.

Schwartz, D. B., Greenberg, M. D., Daould, Y., & Reid, R. (1988). Genital condylomas in pregnancy: Use of trichloroacetic acid and laser therapy. *American Journal of Obstetrics and Gynecology, 158*(6, Part 1), 1407–1416.

Sever, J. L., Smith, M. A., & Shaver, K. A. (1985). Delayed manifestations of congenital rubella. *Reviews of Infectious Diseases,* 7(Suppl. 1), S164–S169.

South, M. A., & Sever, J. L. (1985). Teratogen update: The congenital rubella syndrome. *Teratology, 31*(2), 297–307.

Stagno, S. (1995). Cytomegalovirus. In J. S. Remington & J. O. Klein (Eds.), *Infectious diseases of the fetus and newborn infant* (4th ed., pp. 312–353). Philadelphia: W. B. Saunders.

Stockman, J. A., & DeAlarcon, P. A. (1992). Hematopoiesis and granulopoiesis. In R. A. Polin & W. W. Fox (Eds.), *Fetal and neonatal physiology* (Vol. 2, pp. 1327–1380). Philadelphia: W. B. Saunders.

Visintine, A. M., Oleske, J. M., & Nahmias, A. J. (1977). Infection in infants and children. *American Journal of Diseases of Children, 131*(4), 393–397.

Wald, E. R., Bergman, I., Taylor, H. G., et al. (1986). Long-term outcome of group B streptococcal meningitis. *Pediatrics, 77*(2), 217–221.

Welsh, J. K., & May, J. T. (1979). Anti-infective properties of breast milk. *Journal of Pediatrics, 94*(1), 1–9.

Whitley, R. J., & Arvin, A. M.(1995). Herpes simplex virus infections. In J. S. Remington & J. O. Klein (Eds.), *Infectious diseases of the fetus and newborn infant* (4th ed., pp. 354–376). Philadelphia: W. B. Saunders.

Whitley, R. J., Corey, L., Arvin, A., et al. (1988). Changing presentation of herpes simplex virus infection in neonates. *Journal of Infectious Diseases, 158*(1), 109–116.

Witek-Janusek, L., & Cusack, C. (1994). Neonatal sepsis: Confronting the challenge. *Critical Care Nursing Clinics of North America,* 6(2), 405–419.

Witek-Janusek, L., & Ratmeyer, J. K. (1991). Sepsis in the young rat: Maternal milk protects during cecal ligation and puncture sepsis but not during endotoxemia. *Circulatory Shock, 33*(4), 200–206.

Yoder, M. C., & Polin, R. A. (1997). Developmental Immunology. In A. A. Fanaroff & R. J. Martin (Eds.), *Neonatal-perinatal medicine: Diseases of the fetus and infant* (6th ed., pp. 685–716). St. Louis: Mosby–Year Book.

CHAPTER 28

Assessment and Management of Hematologic Dysfunction

NANCY SHAW

RESEARCH AGENDA

What are the fetal and neonatal risk factors that influence the development of neonatal hematologic problems?

What is the risk of acquiring HIV from neonatal blood transfusions?

Does the timing of cord clamping after birth have an effect on the neonatal hematocrit?

Is direct fetal peritoneal transfusion as effective as fetal transfusions through the umbilical vessels in treating erythroblastosis fetalis in utero?

VIGNETTE

"Nothing's happening!" I thought desperately. "*What* is wrong with this baby?"

I had been called to the delivery of Mrs. Q at 39 weeks' gestation. Although the pregnancy had been uncomplicated for this primigravida, late and deep variable decelerations were noted on L & D admission. An amniotomy was done, which revealed thick particulate meconium in the fluid. Scalp electrode heart rate tracings confirmed that all decelerations had slow return to a baseline rate of approximately 100 and were characterized by minimal variability. No cord was palpable. Because positional changes, oxygen, and a fluid bolus had not remedied the pattern, a decision was made to deliver by C-section.

The pediatrician, Dr. N, and I were ready. At birth, the baby was pale white, apneic, and poorly perfused. The vocal cords were checked by laryngoscopy and found to be clear of meconium. Positive-pressure ventilation with 100 percent O_2 was then provided at a rate of 60 breaths per minute. I scored the initial Apgar at 2. Cardiac compressions were necessary because heart rate was 50 bpm. After 1 minute, this little boy was still slow to respond. Dr. N quickly intubated and gave intratracheal epinephrine. An umbilical vein line was placed, and 30 ml of plasma protein fraction was slowly infused. A second bolus of 10 ml was given 5 minutes later. Five milliequivalents of bicarbonate was administered twice. The slow pulse increased significantly (from 50 bpm to 90 bpm). Compressions were stopped. Still, improvement was sparing: respirations and neurologic responses lagged. "*What* is wrong with this baby?" I wondered. I noted the Apgars of 4 (5) and 5 (10).

I thought back to other resuscitations in which the infant had been slow to respond to the standard resuscitation protocol. Two cases that quickly came to mind had resulted from acute fetal blood loss, one after the insertion of a solid intrauterine pressure catheter and one after a bloody amniocentesis tap in a mother with immune thrombocytopenic purpura. But in both these cases, there had been obvious fetal bleeding before delivery. No overt or hidden bleeding had been discovered in this case.

Just then, the initial laboratory results were returning from the first blood draw from the umbilical vein catheter: pH, 7.1; Chemstrip, 30; hematocrit, 26 percent. "There it is!" I thought. "But why?" Dr. N jumped at the same time I did. "We need some O-negative un-crossmatched packed cells or blood, whatever's faster," he ordered.

Baby boy Q was holding steady. Before the cells arrived, we gave a 10 percent dextrose in water bolus, followed by a similar maintenance solution in the peripheral IV line. I obtained a peripheral blood pressure (52/18), which was within satisfactory limits, and oxygen saturation value was at 86 percent.

The packed cells arrived, and a total of 30 ml was infused in 15 minutes. Shortly after the infusion began, the oxygen saturation value began to rise. After the cells were completely infused, the infant's neurologic signs began to improve. Leg flexion was noted, some response to pain became apparent, and Baby Q attempted some breaths on his own. As we began to withdraw the 100 percent positive-pressure ventilation, I rated a 30-minute Apgar of 7. We transferred him to the NICU and gave report. As I left him, the nursing staff was beginning to wean the blow-by O_2 percentage.

I found Dr. N. "What happened to this baby? He responded as if there had been acute blood loss, but there was no fetal bleeding evident in this case."

He shrugged. "I'm just guessing here," he said. "Mother is Rh-negative, father is Rh-positive. I'm placing bets that the baby is Rh-positive. There must have been a fetal-to-maternal bleed during the pregnancy that sensitized the mother. She probably developed antibodies that crossed the placenta and destroyed fetal red blood cells. That is why his hematocrit was low. Because most oxygen is transported bound to hemoglobin, his severe anemia caused him to be very slow to respond to resuscitation."

"But mother received Rh immune globulin at 28 weeks' gestation, and this is her first pregnancy," I said, searching the prenatal information.

"I saw that," he stated. "I really can't explain it. Perhaps the fetal-to-maternal transfusion was large enough to tie up the entire dose, plus sensitize her to the Rh-positive factor. The obstetrician will order a Kleihauer test on the mother to check for the presence of Rh antibodies. That will give us our answer."

Baby Q improved during several weeks. He required additional transfusions of red blood cells and continuing therapy for persistent hypoglycemia. Feedings were begun late and increased slowly to avoid stressing the gastrointestinal system, which probably suffered some tissue damage because of the low hematocrit.

Mrs. Q's Kleihauer test result was positive, verifying Dr. N's guess. On an exam, an area was found on the placenta where a tear had occurred, which theoretically could have allowed a fetal-to-maternal transfusion of the necessary volume to have produced maternal sensitization despite the prenatal Rh immune globulin dose.

Baby Q was discharged from the NICU about 3 weeks after his birth, breathing and feeding well. His persistent problems of anemia and hypoglycemia were resolved. Dr. N will observe him to determine whether any long-term medical or developmental sequelae will result from his traumatic birth experience.

Joyce M. Dohme

Invasion of the endometrium by the primitive placenta permits simple diffusion of nutrients, which provides the initial nutritional support needed by the newly fertilized ovum. Because the developing embryo requires a large and consistent source of sustenance, it quickly outgrows the nutrients available in the surface lining of the endometrium and the rate at which simple diffusion can supply these needs. Consequently, development of an efficient form of nutrient transport, such as that provided by circulating blood, is of utmost importance for continued growth of the embryo and explains the early embryologic appearance of the hematologic and cardiovascular systems. Activation of these two systems supplies nutrition to the embryo and fetal membranes at the interface between fetal and maternal circulations through passive and active diffusion, active transport, and pinocytosis (Page et al., 1981). Although blood begins to circulate by the third to fifth week of gestation, the cardiovascular and hematologic systems undergo refinement in the following months.

This chapter outlines the embryologic development of the hematopoietic system. It also describes the more common neonatal hematologic problems and associated high-risk factors along with collaborative management strategies.

EMBRYOLOGIC DEVELOPMENT OF THE HEMATOPOIETIC SYSTEM

The hematopoietic system is characterized by the presence of pluripotent stem cells that differentiate into the multiple forms of circulating blood cells: red blood cells (RBCs), white blood cells (WBCs), and platelets. Hematopoiesis is a continuous process that involves cell maturation and destruction, followed by new cell production. Gestational age and postnatal age influence this maturational process and govern the individual cell constituents, activity, and site of production. Characteristics of the neonatal erythrocyte leave the preterm and term infant susceptible to problems associated with hemolysis, including immature hepatic response to erythrocyte destruction, and the effects of shortened erythrocyte life span as seen in physiologic neonatal anemia and anemia of the premature infant. Besides these maturational influences, pre-existing maternal diseases and intrauterine abnormalities can affect RBC function and production, resulting in increased oxygen and nutritional requirements of the growing fetus.

The production of platelets and clotting factors is also a function of gestational age. Although some factors are deficient at birth, several factors and platelets are present in concentrations similar to adult values. However, many of these components are functionally different from those of the adult, possibly owing to impaired activity or limited ability to respond to increased needs. Coagulation dysfunction in the newborn may also be the result of genetic abnormalities (e.g., X-linked hemophilia), pre-existing maternal illness (e.g., immune thrombocytopenic purpura), or infection (e.g., disseminated intravascular coagulation).

Production and function of WBCs are also affected by gestational age. This subject is covered in more detail in Chapter 27, Assessment and Management of Immunologic Dysfunction.

Primitive Vascular Formation

Angiogenesis, the development of blood vessels, begins in the fertilized ovum during the third week of gestation. Vessels begin to form in the yolk sac in response to the relative paucity of nutrition available to the rapidly growing embryo. Angiogenesis is initially observed between the two cell layers of the yolk sac, the extraembryonic mesoderm and extraembryonic endoderm. These two layers are produced by the same cells that give rise to the placenta and fetal membranes. Vascular formation involves mesenchymal cells, located in the extraembryonic mesoderm, that possess the ability to differentiate into various types of tissue.

Some of these mesenchymal cells differentiate into primitive vascular cells called angioblasts, which aggregate and give rise to blood islands. The blood islands quickly develop an inner cavity around which the angioblasts arrange themselves, forming the primitive endothelial lining of the newly formed vessels. These vessels then fuse and extend to create the vascular system for the yolk sac that will eventually become incorporated into the primitive gut. The angioblasts of the endothelial lining begin production of primitive plasma and blood cells (hemocytoblasts) shortly after vascular formation (de Alarcon, 1988).

Blood vessel formation in the connecting stalk and chorion begins at the same time that angiogenesis starts in the yolk sac. Blood cell formation, or hematopoiesis, can be identified in the connecting stalk and chorion by the third week and proceeds in the same manner as in the yolk sac (Moore & Persaud, 1993). The vessels in the connecting stalk become the umbilical vessels that indirectly link the embryo to maternal circulation through the placenta; vessels in the chorion give rise to the vasculature of fetal membranes and villi of the placenta. The formation of blood islands in the yolk sac regresses at the end of the second month of gestation, at which time hematopoiesis primarily becomes the function of the liver (Tuchmann-Duplessis et al., 1975).

Blood vessel formation in the embryo lags behind that of the yolk sac by approximately 2 days, but plasma and blood cell production in the embryo does not begin until the fifth week of gestation (Moore & Persaud, 1993). Vascular development starts in the middle layer of the trilaminar (three-layered) embryo. This middle layer, the intraembryonic mesoderm, is composed of mesenchymal cells that form the vasculature of the fetal circulatory system. This vascular complex eventually fuses with the vasculature developing in the yolk sac and connecting stalk at approximately the fourth week of gestation (Fig. 28–1). When fusion occurs and blood circulation is established, primitive erythropoiesis becomes noticeable in the hepatic vascular spaces (de Alarcon, 1988).

Development of Hematopoietic Function

Blood cell production in the embryo and fetus progresses through three phases: the mesoblastic (megaloblastic), hepatic, and myeloid periods (Fig. 28–2). Each phase is marked by alterations in cell composition and changes in the major site of produc-

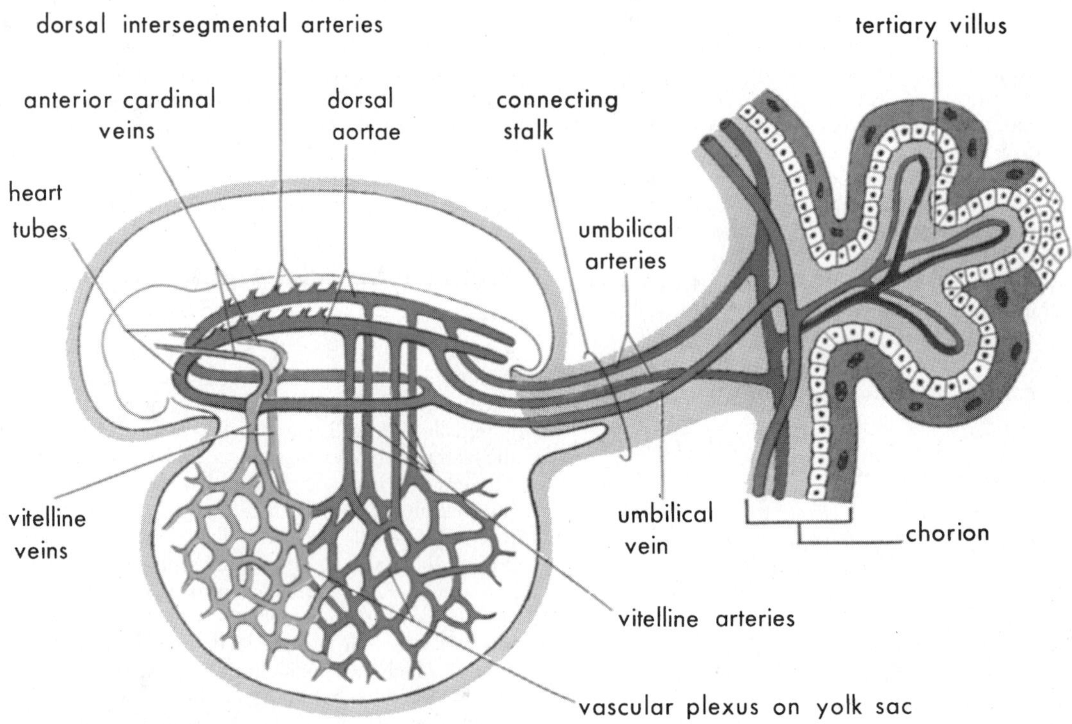

FIGURE 28–1. The developing vasculature of the yolk sac, connecting stalk, chorion, and embryo eventually fuse and connect the circulations of the embryo and fetal membranes. This union provides for delivery of nutrients and removal of waste products in the embryo and its supporting structures. (From Moore, K., & Persaud, T. [1993]. *The developing human* [5th ed., p. 65]. Philadelphia: W. B. Saunders.)

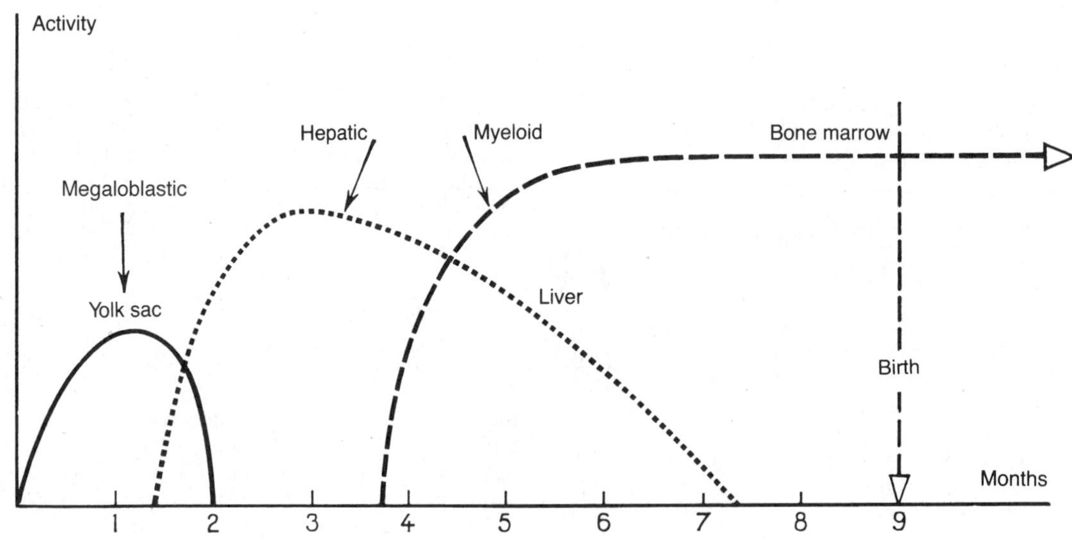

FIGURE 28–2. Hematopoiesis progresses through three phases during embryonic and fetal life, with each new production period overlapping the previous phase. The initial phase is the megaloblastic (mesoblastic) period, which begins in the yolk sac of the developing embryo. It is quickly replaced by the hepatic period, which marks the liver as the major site of hematopoiesis until the bone marrow takes over production during the myeloid period. (From Rothstein, G. [1993]. Origin and development of blood and blood forming tissues. In G. Lee, T. Bithell, J. Foerster, et al. [Eds.], *Wintrobe's clinical hematology: Vol. I* [9th ed., p. 55]. Philadelphia: Lea & Febiger.)

tion. The mesoblastic period is characterized by blood cell production in the yolk sac; during the hepatic period, the liver is the major site of hematopoiesis; and in the myeloid period, the bone marrow is the major manufacturer.

Mesoblastic Period

Formation of vasculature and blood cells from mesenchymal tissue occurs during the first stage of hematopoiesis, known as the mesoblastic period. Primitive hematopoietic tissue consists of cells called hemocytoblasts, which are derived from the endothelial cells (angioblasts) of blood vessels developing in the embryo and fetal membranes. Although most of these cells differentiate into primitive erythrocytes, they can give rise to WBCs and megakaryocytes as well (Sieff & Nathan, 1993).

Hepatic Period

At approximately the fifth to sixth week of gestation, the megaloblastic period ends and the hepatic period begins. This period marks the beginning of the embryonic liver as the major source of blood cells, with concurrent cell formation occurring in the spleen and lymph nodes. Hepatic hematopoiesis involves the production of blood cells from multipotent stem cells that have either migrated from the yolk sac through the blood into the liver or arisen independently from another line of stem cells (Djaldetti, 1979; Petti et al., 1985). These multipotent stem cells exhibit several significant characteristics: (1) a variable capacity for self-renewal, (2) the potential to differentiate into different cell lines, and (3) the ability to repopulate. As they produce and divide in the liver parenchyma, these cells undergo a process of maturation that reduces their ability to self-replicate and forces commitment to a specific cell line. Hematopoietic stem cells are considered the common progenitors of erythrocytes, lymphocytes, granulocytes, monocytes, and megakaryocytes. Hematopoietic stem cells continue to reproduce throughout a person's life, but the available number of stem cells decreases with age. These stem cells are the basis for cord banks that are coming into vogue in the United States. Umbilical cords can be saved and stored for future use in the case of childhood cancers or other immune problems (McMillan, 1996). Ethical and practical dilemmas are associated with these cord banks. There is even a national network for cord banking. This trend is not likely to change in the near future. Its importance in immunotherapy or the treatment of hematologic disorders remains to be seen.

The hepatic phase marks the onset of production of specific cell lines. During this stage, a portion of the stem cells begin to form erythrocytes (normoblasts) that develop into more mature forms with increasing gestational age (Brown, 1988a). Another line of stem cells differentiates into leukocytes, which can be identified in the embryo at 5 to 7 weeks of gestation. Leukocytes, however, have several sites of production besides the liver parenchyma, including various connective tissues such as the meninges, mesentery, and stromal cells of the lymph plexus (Oski & Naiman, 1982c). Between the 7th and 10th weeks of gestation, lymphopoiesis is also observed in the gut, thymus, and associated lymphoid tissue. Megakaryocytes, the precursors of platelets, are present in the yolk sac and liver at 5 to 6 weeks' gestation, and platelets can be identified in the blood at approximately 11 weeks.

Myeloid Period

The liver remains the chief organ of hematopoiesis until it is gradually replaced by the bone marrow. This period, known as the myeloid period of hematopoiesis, begins at the fourth month of gestation and becomes quantitatively important by the sixth month. During the last 3 months of gestation, the bone marrow is the chief source of blood cell production; extramedullary sources of hematopoiesis generally cease by the first postnatal month (Oski, 1993). The bone marrow is primarily composed of blood vessels occupying cartilage lacunae that become invested with hematopoietic stem cells. Theoretically, these cells either have migrated from the liver to the bone marrow through the blood or have arisen from an independent source of stem cells. The volume of marrow occupied by hematopoietic tissue continues to increase until term.

The production of all blood cells escalates during the myeloid period. Mature RBCs produced by the marrow appear about 1 week after marrow development and are present in significant quantities at 17 weeks' gestation. In the final 2 months of gestation, the RBC production per kilogram of body weight in the fetus is three to four times greater than in the adult. Concurrent with myeloid RBC production, leukocyte production begins in the bone marrow of the clavicle. Stem cells in the clavicular marrow differentiate to form two separate populations of lymphocytes, T (thymus) cells and B (bone marrow) cells. Other forms of leukocytes (granulocytes and monocytes) develop after the lymphocyte. Although relatively few granulocytes are present during the first half of gestation, their concentration rapidly increases during the last trimester; monocytes are apparent during the fifth fetal month. The increase in bone marrow production of megakaryocytes parallels increasing gestational age. However, after 27 weeks' gestation, platelet counts are similar regardless of gestational age.

Erythrocyte Maturation

RBCs undergo specific changes in their composition and concentration during the three stages of hematopoiesis (Fig. 28–3). The production of the mature RBC is a complex process involving initial differentiation of hematopoietic stem cells into RBC precursors and further transition through multiple stages of maturation.

Megaloblastic Period

Hemocytoblasts, arising from the endothelial cells of the primitive blood vessels during the mesoblastic period, give rise to primitive nucleated RBCs called megaloblasts or megalocytes. The megalocytic form of erythrocyte contains an embryonic form of hemoglobin, the first of three sequential embryonic forms. Megalocytes do not progress into more mature forms but remain primitive blood cells.

Hepatic and Myeloid Periods

When the liver becomes the predominant source of erythrocyte production, a definitive line of RBCs is formed that progresses through several phases of refinement before reaching maturation. This progression is identical in the bone marrow when it assumes erythrocyte production. Control over erythropoiesis during early fetal life is uncertain, but erythropoietin appears to exert great control over RBC production late in gestation. Erythropoietin stimulates stem cells to become committed progenitors of the erythrocyte (Fig. 28–4). Stem cells in the liver and bone marrow differentiate into early and late erythroid burst-forming units (BFU-E) and erythroid colony-forming units (CFU-E). The CFU-E differentiate into normoblasts, which must divide several more times and accrue hemoglobin before becoming mature erythrocytes. When the hemoglobin concentration of the normoblasts reaches 34 percent, the nuclei are extruded and the cells become reticulocytes. About 1 to 2 days later, reticulocytes become mature RBCs.

At 10 weeks' gestation, hemoglobin synthesis changes from the

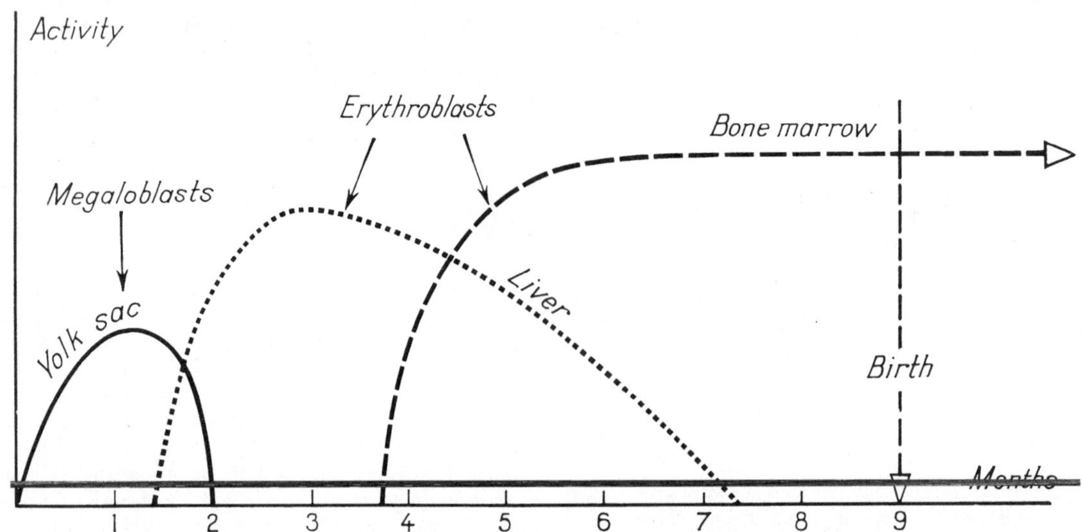

FIGURE 28–3. Erythropoiesis, the development of RBCs, begins with the production of hemocytoblasts from the endothelial cells of the primitive blood vessels. Hemocytoblasts are then converted into megaloblasts, and finally megalocytes, during the megaloblastic period. When the liver becomes invested with hematopoietic stem cells, some of these stem cells are stimulated by erythropoietin to become erythroblasts and subsequently erythrocytes. At approximately 4 months' gestation, the production of RBCs gradually becomes the responsibility of the bone marrow, signaling the beginning of the myeloid period of RBC production. (From Rothstein, G. [1993]. Origin and development of blood and blood forming tissues. In G. Lee, T. Bithell, J. Foerster, et al. [Eds.], *Wintrobe's clinical hematology: Vol. I* [9th ed., p. 55]. Philadelphia: Lea & Febiger.)

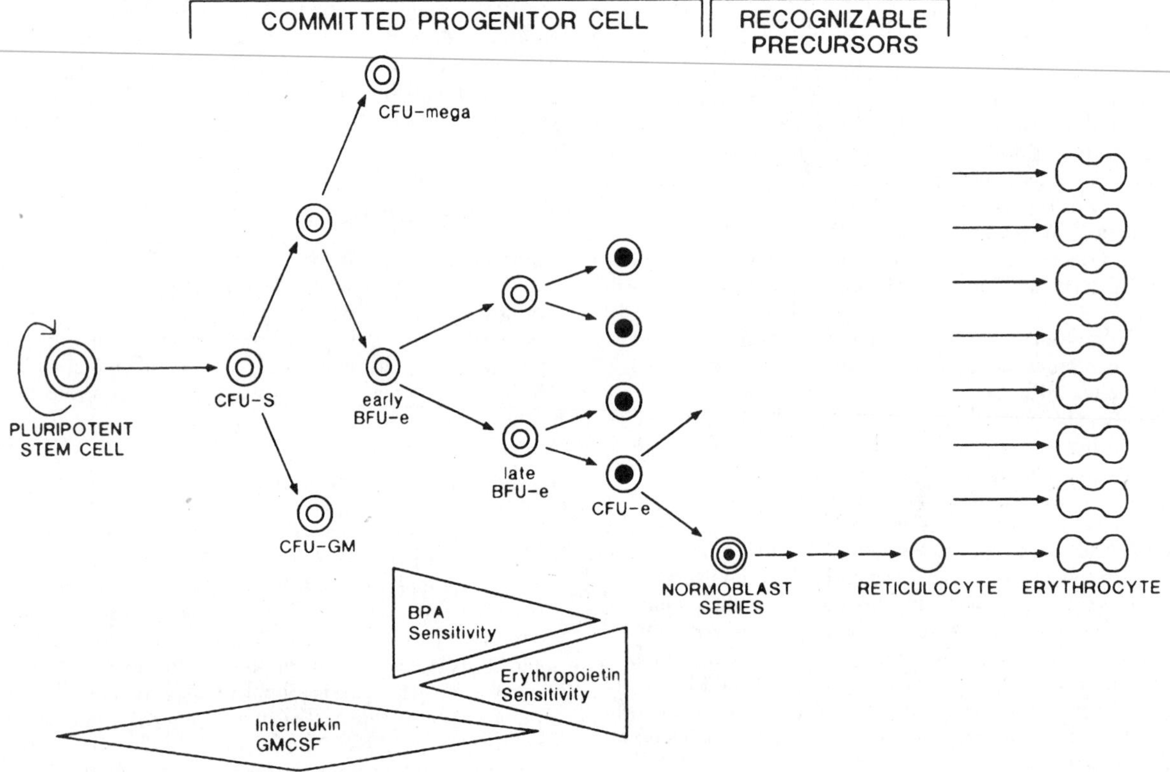

FIGURE 28–4. Hematopoietic stem cells stimulated to become erythrocytes initially develop into early and late erythroid burst-forming units (BFU-E) and erythroid colony-forming units (CFU-E). These progenitor cells progress to form the erythrocyte precursor, the normoblast. Multiple divisions and alterations of the normoblast lead to the development of the reticulocyte. When the reticulocyte extrudes its nucleus, it normally moves out of the liver or bone marrow, the predominant sites of its production, and into the blood. BPA, burst-promoting activity; CFU-GM, colony-forming unit–granulocyte–macrophage; CFU-S, colony-forming unit–spleen; GMCSF, granulocyte–macrophage colony-stimulating factor. (From Brown, M. [1988]. Fetal and neonatal erythropoiesis. In J. Stockman & C. Pochedly [Eds.], *Development and neonatal hematology* [pp. 39–56]. New York: Raven Press.)

embryonic to the fetal form (hemoglobin F). The mechanisms by which stem cells and progenitor cells perform this changeover remain uncertain.

Although low levels of a third form of hemoglobin, adult hemoglobin (hemoglobin A), are detectable at this time, hemoglobin F remains the predominant form during fetal development. At 30 weeks' gestation, 90 to 100 percent of hemoglobin is the fetal form; the remainder is hemoglobin A. Between 30 and 32 weeks, the percentage of hemoglobin F starts to decrease (Bard & Prosmanne, 1982). Fifty to 75 percent of RBCs contain fetal hemoglobin at 40 weeks' gestation, 5 to 8 percent at 6 months of age, and 1 percent at 1 year of age (Bard, 1975).

Each type of hemoglobin has properties that make it valuable at the time of its synthesis. Each has a different affinity for oxygen that varies its uptake and release to the tissue (Fig. 28–5). Fetal hemoglobin has a high affinity for oxygen, binding it more readily at the intervillous spaces in the placenta when fetal Po_2 averages between 25 and 30 mm Hg. Adult hemoglobin has a decreased affinity for oxygen. This decreased affinity allows easier release of oxygen to the tissues when metabolic needs are high and the lungs are functional.

Erythropoietin

Factors affecting RBC production are still unclear, but erythropoietin appears to exert great control over erythropoiesis during late gestation. This circulating glycoprotein hormone, whose gene is located on the seventh chromosome, is an obligate growth factor in the development of both BFU-E and CFU-E, progenitors of the RBC. Whereas the adult kidney produces 90 to 95 percent of erythropoietin, the fetal liver is considered the predominant site of production throughout most of gestation.

The major stimulus for erythropoietin release is decreased tissue oxygenation. In the absence of erythropoietin, hypoxia has no effect on the production of RBCs. However, if erythropoietin production is intact, hypoxia stimulates a rapid increase in erythropoietin levels, which remain elevated until hypoxia no longer exists. Although the liver is less responsive to hypoxia than the kidney is, production of erythropoietin in the fetus and newborn increases within minutes to hours after a precipitating event such as hypoxia. It acts by directly stimulating the CFU-E to differentiate into RBC precursors, accelerating their passage through the various maturational stages. Although erythropoietin levels increase rapidly, no change in the number of erythrocytes is noted for approximately 5 days after a hypoxic stress. However, when erythropoietin stimulates production of RBCs in excess of normal, the RBCs are released into the circulation before they have reached maturity (i.e., as reticulocytes). This maturation is reflected in an elevated reticulocyte count.

Other factors affecting erythropoietin production besides hypoxia are testosterone, estrogen, thyroid hormone, prostaglandins, and lipoproteins. Erythropoietin levels are also increased in cases of maternal hypoxemia, smallness for gestational age, and poor placental function. Cord blood levels are normally elevated, in comparison with adult values, but drop dramatically to almost undetectable levels in the newborn. Thus, the healthy newborn produces few RBCs in the first few weeks of life because the hypoxic stimuli of low fetal Po_2 levels are no longer present. Erythropoietin levels do not increase in the term infant until 8 to 10 weeks of age, when tissue hypoxia due to anemia is sensed by the kidneys.

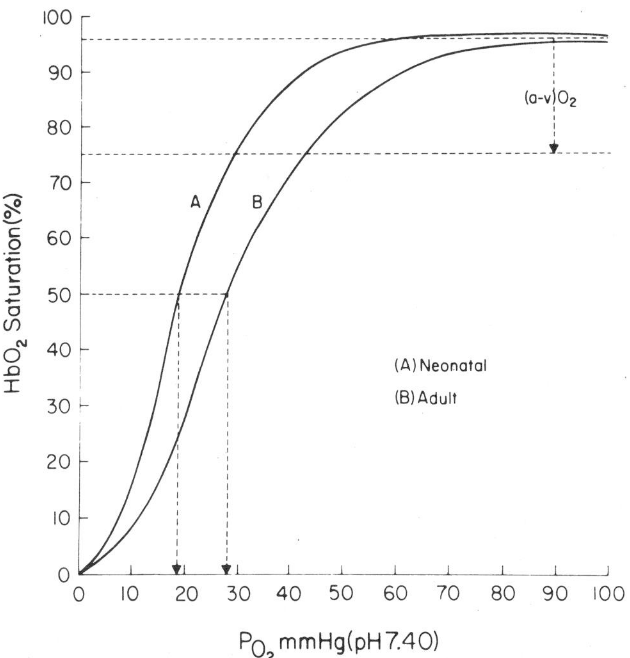

FIGURE 28–5. The affinity for oxygen (i.e., the ability of the hemoglobin molecule to bind and hold the oxygen molecule) is markedly different between fetal and adult hemoglobin. Fetal hemoglobin has a greater affinity for oxygen. It is able to bind to oxygen more readily at the intervillous spaces of the placenta, a property that is useful in the low Po_2 environment of the fetus. Adult hemoglobin has a decreased affinity for oxygen, which allows easier release of oxygen to the tissue when metabolic needs are greater than those of the fetus. (From Sacks, L., & Delivoria-Papadopoulos, M. [1984]. Hemoglobin-oxygen interactions. *Seminars in Perinatology, 8,* 168–183.)

NORMAL HEMATOLOGIC VALUES IN THE NEWBORN

Factors Affecting Laboratory Values

Normal blood values found shortly after birth reflect a time of maximal change. Table 28–1 summarizes these changes on the basis of the increase in gestational and postnatal age. Blood values at birth depend on (1) the timing of cord clamping, (2) the infant's gestational age, (3) the blood sampling site, and (4) the technique used to obtain adequate blood flow. Blood volume in the newborn can be significantly influenced by the timing of cord clamping and the positional differences between the infant and the level of the placenta at the time of clamping. Complete emptying of placental vessels before clamping can increase blood volume by 61 percent (Usher et al., 1963; Yao et al., 1969); one quarter of the placental transfusion occurs within the first 15 seconds, and half of the transfusion is complete by 1 minute.

Average blood volume is approximately 85 ml/kg of body weight in the term infant, whereas it can average 90 to 105 ml/kg in the preterm infant. The younger the gestational age of the infant, the greater the blood volume per kilogram (Usher et al., 1975). Hemoglobin concentration and hematocrit are also functions of gestational age, especially in infants born before 32 weeks' gestation. The average mean hemoglobin concentration at 26 to 30 weeks is 13.4 g/dl, with an average mean hematocrit of 41.5 percent (Johnson, 1993). In the term infant, mean hemoglobin values range between 16.5 and 18.5 g/dl, with mean hematocrit values between 51 and 56 percent. Mean hemoglobin values in postmature infants are higher than in the term infant, possibly caused by progressive placental dysfunction and oxygen deficit, which stimulates erythropoietin release.

It is important to consider sampling site and quality of blood flow in interpreting laboratory values. Capillary blood has 20 percent higher hemoglobin levels than venous blood. This differ-

TABLE 28–1 Normal Fetal (26 to 30 Weeks' Gestation) and Neonatal (28 Weeks' Gestation to Term) Blood Values—Age-Specific Indices

Age	Hgb (g/dL) (Mean − 2 SD)	Hct (%) (Mean − 2 SD)	MCV (fL) (Mean − 2 SD)	MCHC (g/dL) (Mean − 2 SD)	Retic (%)	WBC/mm³ × 1000 (Mean + 2 SD)	Platelets (10³/mm) (Mean + 2 SD)
26–30 wk Gestation*	13.4 (11)	41.5 (34.9)	118.2 (106.7)	37.9 (30.6)	—	44 (2.7)	254 (180–327)
28 wk	14.5	45	120	31.0	5–10	—	275
32 wk	15.0	47	118	32.0	3–10	—	290
Term† (cord)	16.5 (13.5)	51 (42)	108 (98)	33.0 (30.0)	3–7	18.1 (9–30)‡	290
1–3 days	18.5 (14.5)	56 (45)	108 95	33.0 (29.0)	1.8–4.6	18.9 (9.4–34)	192
2 wk	16.6 (13.4)	53 (41)	105 (88)	31.4 (28.1)	0.1–1.7	11.4 (5–20)	252

*Values are from fetal samplings.
†Younger than 1 month, capillary hemoglobin exceeds venous: 1 hour, 3.6-g difference; 5 days, 2.2-g difference; 3 weeks, 1.1-g difference.
‡Mean (95% confidence limits).
Hgb, hemoglobin; Hct, hematocrit; MCV, mean corpuscular volume; MCHC, mean corpuscular hemoglobin concentration; retic, recticulocyte percentage of erythrocytes; WBC, white blood cells.
Modified from Johnson, K. (1993). *Harriet Lane handbook* (13th ed., p. 231). St. Louis: Mosby–Year Book.

ence between capillary and venous samples can be minimized by warming the extremities before a blood draw to enhance peripheral perfusion. Although this allows better spontaneous blood flow, discarding the first few drops obtained on a capillary draw also improves the accuracy of the sample. When the venous route is used for sampling, poor blood flow through small-bore needles enhances the possibility of hemolysis, which can lead to sampling errors. Greater accuracy can be obtained by using the largest bore needle possible for a blood draw and removing the needle from the syringe before placing the sample in the specimen container.

Fetal and Neonatal Blood Components

The life span of the RBC in the fetus and newborn is much shorter than the 120 days of the adult erythrocyte. The term newborn's erythrocyte can last 60 to 70 days, the preterm infant's 35 to 50 days (Oski, 1993; Stockman, 1988). One theoretical reason for this difference in life spans between adult and infant RBCs is the decreased deformability of the neonatal erythrocyte. Because of its larger size and cylindric shape, the neonatal erythrocyte is more prone to destruction in the narrow sinusoids of the spleen.

The mean RBC count in the term newborn is in the range of 5.1 to 5.3 million/ml, with an elevated reticulocyte count of 3 to 7 percent during the first 24 to 48 hours of life (Johnson, 1993; Zaizov & Matoth, 1976). Mean RBC counts in the premature infant range from 4.6 to 5.3 million/ml, with a greater number of circulating immature RBCs reflected in a higher reticulocyte count (3 to 10 percent). The reticulocyte count falls abruptly to about 1 percent by the first week of life, and erythropoietin drops to low, often undetectable, levels in both groups of infants.

WBC counts depend on gestational and postnatal age; a wide range of leukocyte counts, predominantly neutrophils (bands, segmented neutrophils, and metamyelocytes), are present in newborn infants. The normal mean WBC count at birth is 4400/mm³ in the preterm infant and 30,000/mm³ in the term infant. During the first 12 hours of life, the WBC count rises, reaches a plateau, and then slowly declines. Neutrophil counts in the term infant average about 11,000/mm³ at this time, remaining constant from day 3 to the end of the first month of life (Fig. 28–6). The neutrophil count averages about 8000/mm³ in infants less than 37 weeks of gestation and about 6000/mm³ in infants less than 32 weeks. By day 4 of life, no difference is noted between the various gestational age groups. In well newborns, the average number of bands, a form of immature neutrophil, is 10 percent of the total WBC count. Neutrophil counts can be lowered by conditions such as maternal hypertension, intraventricular hemorrhage, hemolytic disease, and infection. As the newborn increases in age, WBC composition changes. The number of lymphocytes increases, whereas the monocyte count remains low.

Sampling site must be taken into consideration in evaluating the WBC count at birth. When peripheral venous and arterial samples are compared with capillary samples, venous samples have an 82 percent correlation with the values obtained by capillary sampling, and arterial samples have a 77 percent correlation with capillary sample results (Christensen & Rothstein, 1979).

Because immature RBCs still maintain their nuclei and are relatively high in number for the first 4 days of life, they can be incorrectly counted in the total WBC count. Therefore, the WBC count needs to be corrected to adjust for any nucleated RBCs (NRBCs). This correction is usually done automatically by the hematology laboratory when the blood slide is read. If the count is not automatically adjusted, this can easily be done by multiplying the total WBC count by the percentage of NRBCs observed and subtracting this sum from the total WBC count:

$$\text{adjusted WBC count} = \text{total WBC count} - (\text{total WBC count} \times \text{NRBCs})$$

Platelet counts in the newborn do not vary much in relation to gestational age (Sell & Corrigan, 1973). From 27 to 40 weeks' gestation, counts are similar, with the range of normal being 215,000 to 378,000/mm³. Platelet counts less than 150,000/mm³ are considered thrombocytopenic (Hathaway & Bonnar, 1978).

Assessment of Hematologic Function

Because infants respond to a variety of problems in a similar manner, many clinical findings such as hypoglycemia, hypocalcemia, hypothermia, apnea, bradycardia, cyanosis, lethargy, and poor feeding warrant at least a complete blood count (CBC) as an initial evaluation tool in determining the possibility of a hematologic reason for these symptoms. In the presence of active bleeding, platelet counts, clotting studies, and levels of fibrinogen and fibrinolytic split products or fibrin degradation products can shed light on the type of blood dyscrasia present and the most therapeutic approach to the problem. All these studies provide a way to monitor and evaluate the applied therapies. Laboratory

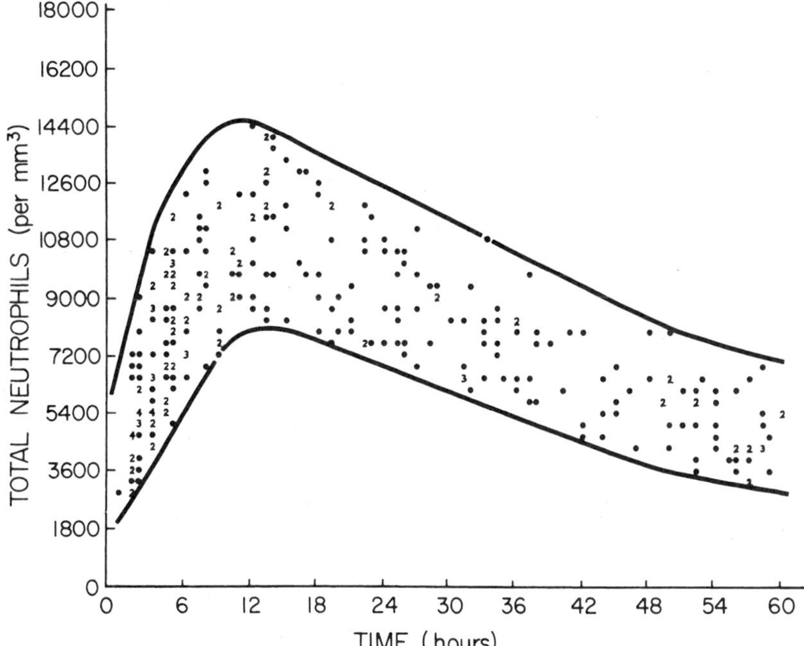

FIGURE 28–6. The normal range of the neutrophil count changes dramatically during the first 3 days of life. The range then stabilizes and remains constant for a short time. The neutrophil count initially rises during the first 12 hours of life, reaches a plateau, and then begins a slow decline. (From Manroe, B., Weinberg, A., Rosenfeld, C., & Browne, R. [1979]. The neonatal blood count in health and disease. I. Reference values for neutrophilic cells. *Journal of Pediatrics, 95,* 89.)

data are most helpful, however, when they are employed in association with astute observation and physical assessment skills.

Several physical findings can determine well-being and homeostasis of the hematologic system (Table 28–2). Presence of cutaneous abnormalities such as hematomas, abrasions, petechiae, and bleeding should alert one to the possibility of a hematologic abnormality. Hepatosplenomegaly can also herald the presence of abnormal breakdown of RBCs. Hepatosplenomegaly concurrent with hyperbilirubinemia and hemolysis can signal the presence of alloimmune problems (e.g., Rh and ABO incompatibilities) or acquired, congenital, and postnatal infections (e.g., cytomegalovirus infection, toxoplasmosis, herpes simplex, and hepatitis).

HEMATOLOGIC DYSFUNCTION IN THE NEONATE

Blood Group Incompatibilities

Blood group incompatibilities were first discovered in the Rh system in the 1940s, and the test for detection of antibody-coated RBCs was devised by Coombs in 1946. Before the introduction of Rh immune globulin (RhIG) or RhoGAM in 1964, Rh incompatibility accounted for one third of all blood group incompatibilities. Since the use of RhIG, the frequency of Rh incompatibility has dropped significantly and ABO has become the main blood group incompatibility, with sensitization occurring in 3 percent of all infants. Both involve maternal antibody response to fetal antigen, leading to RBC destruction by hemolysis. Rh antibody response is elicited on exposure to antigen and does not exist spontaneously, whereas anti-A and anti-B antibodies occur naturally. These entities also differ in the severity with which they affect the fetus and newborn as well as in the method of treatment.

Other minor blood groupings (e.g., Kell, C, E, Duffy, and Kidd) can also cause incompatibilities resulting in hyperbilirubinemia, but Rh and ABO incompatibilities are the most common, being responsible for 98 percent of all cases of blood group incompatibilities. There are 400 known RBC antigens that can induce antibody production. Some of these antibodies are induced after transfusion therapy with incompatible blood, whereas others occur in response to the transfer of incompatible fetal blood cells into maternal circulation during pregnancy.

TABLE 28–2 Physical Findings Helpful in Evaluating the Integrity of the Hematologic System

Obvious blood loss—hemorrhage	Ecchymosis
Pallor	Jaundice
Plethora	Hepatosplenomegaly
Petechiae	Hematomas

ABO Incompatibility

Antigens or agglutinogens, present on the RBC surface of each blood type, react with antibodies or agglutinins found in the plasma of opposing blood types. Of the 30 common antigens involved in antigen–antibody reactions, the ABO antigens are one of two groups most likely to be a problem, the other being the Rh group (Guyton, 1996a). The four major blood types are A, B, O, and AB. Antigens A and B occur on the surface of RBCs in the majority of the population, making A and B the most common blood types. Antibodies to the antigens of different blood types occur naturally in the plasma (Table 28–3). For example, type A blood has A antigens on the cell surface but has circulating anti-

TABLE 28–3 Blood Groups and Their Constituent Antigens (Agglutinogens) and Antibodies (Agglutinins)

Genotypes	Blood Groups	Agglutinogens	Agglutinins
OO	O	—	Anti-A and anti-B
OA or AA	A	A	Anti-B
OB or BB	B	B	Anti-A
AB	AB	A and B	—

From Guyton, A. (1991). Blood groups; transfusion; tissue and organ transplantation. *Textbook of medical physiology* (8th ed., p. 386). Philadelphia: W. B. Saunders.

B antibodies in the plasma. Type B blood has just the opposite, B antigens on the cell surface and anti-A antibodies in the plasma. AB blood has A and B antigens on the cell surface and neither antibody in the plasma, whereas O type has neither antigen on the cell surface and both anti-A and anti-B antibodies in the plasma. Unlike antigens, which are usually polypeptides and complex proteins, antibodies are immunoglobulins (mostly IgG and IgM).

With antigen and antibody in harmony, no RBC destruction occurs; but when a conflicting antibody is introduced into the circulation, RBC destruction may occur. RBCs have multiple binding sites to which opposing antibodies can attach. An antibody is capable of simultaneously attaching to several RBCs, thus creating a clump of cells. This clumping of cells, known as agglutination, can cause occlusion of small vessels and impair local circulation and tissue oxygenation. Fetal RBCs coated with antibodies attract phagocytes and macrophages that eventually destroy these agglutinated RBCs, usually through hemolysis by the reticuloendothelial cells in the spleen. Hemolysis can occur without preliminary agglutination, but it is a more delayed process because the body must first activate its complement system. High antibody titers (hemolysins) are required to stimulate this system, which causes the release of proteolytic enzymes that rupture the cell membrane.

In a transfusion reaction, when opposing blood types are mixed, the donor's RBCs are agglutinated, whereas the recipient's blood cells tend to be protected. The plasma portion of donor blood that contains antibodies becomes diluted by the recipient's blood volume, thus decreasing the available titer of donor antibodies in the recipient's circulation. However, recipient antibody titers are adequate to destroy the donor RBCs by agglutination and hemolysis or by hemolysis alone. This situation is what occurs in the case of ABO incompatibility. In this entity, the maternal blood type is usually O, containing anti-A and anti-B antibodies in the serum, whereas the fetus or newborn is type A or B. Although incompatibility can occur between A and B types, it is not seen as frequently as AO or BO because of the globulin composition of the antibodies. In the O-type mother, the antibodies are usually IgG and can cross the placenta, whereas the antibodies of the type A or B mother are frequently IgM, which are too large to cross the placenta.

When transplacental hemorrhage (TPH) occurs between ABO-incompatible mother and fetus, fetal blood entering the maternal circulation undergoes agglutination and hemolysis by maternal antibodies. This rapid response prevents the development of antibodies to other antigens present on fetal RBCs, because a time lapse is required for activation of the immune system. Consequently, fetal RBCs that are Rh-positive in addition to being type A or B are destroyed by naturally occurring anti-A or anti-B antibodies before any other maternal antibodies to Rh factor (anti-D) can be produced. This naturally occurring phenomenon provides the basis for the use of RhIG, in which extrinsic anti-D destroys fetal cells before the maternal antibody system can be activated.

In spite of this destruction of fetal RBCs, maternal anti-A or anti-B antibodies of the IgG form can freely cross the placenta and adhere to RBCs in the fetal circulation. For this reason, ABO incompatibility can occur in the first pregnancy (40 to 50 percent of total occurrences involve primigravidas) because TPH and inoculation of the mother by foreign fetal blood are not necessary for the development of these naturally occurring antibodies (Oski & Naiman, 1982b). The A and B antigens on the fetal and neonatal RBCs are not well developed, so only a small amount of antibodies actually attaches to the antigen. Other body tissues also have antigen sites to which some of the circulating antibodies can adhere, thereby decreasing the potential for RBC destruction. The resulting small amounts of IgG in the plasma do not stimulate activation of the complement system, so hemolysis is minimal. This lack of stimulation of the complement system may explain why only 3 to 20 percent of infants become symptomatic of the 15 to 22 percent who are ABO incompatible with their mothers (Bowman, 1988; Mollison, 1984; Ozolek et al., 1994).

Erythrocyte antibodies are not usually present in the circulating blood until 2 to 8 months of postnatal age. Antibody production then increases, reaching a maximal titer at 8 to 10 years of age (Guyton, 1996a). The newborn becomes inoculated with A and B antigens after birth through the ingestion of food and resulting bacterial colonization. This initiates production of anti-A or anti-B antibodies that will circulate in the plasma, depending on the antigens present on the RBCs.

Clinical Manifestations

The chief symptom of ABO incompatibility is jaundice within the first 24 hours of life (Maisels, 1990); 90 percent of all affected infants are female. Hemolysis and anemia are minimal, although signs of a mildly compensated hemolytic state are reflected in certain CBC values. On peripheral blood smear, there may be evidence of spherocytes, which are RBCs lacking the normal central pallor and biconcave, disk-like shape of the normal RBC. Because they are smaller in size, spherocytes appear thicker than the normal RBC. These physical characteristics result in abnormal fragility under osmotic stress. Spherocytes are not distensible or compressible owing to lack of the normal amount of loose cell membrane. Thus, they are more susceptible to destruction in the splenic sinusoids.

Additional laboratory findings include a positive direct Coombs' test result in 3 to 32 percent of the cases (Glader & Naiman, 1991; Ozolek et al., 1994) and positive results of both direct and indirect Coombs' tests in 80 percent of the cases when microtechniques are used (Seibel & Gross, 1987). The direct Coombs' test is a measurement of the presence of antibody on the RBC surface; the indirect Coombs' test is a measurement of antibody in the serum. ABO incompatibility can also be identified by the performance of an eluate test, which involves washing the RBCs of the newborn and testing the wash for the presence of anti-A or anti-B antibodies.

On physical examination, hepatosplenomegaly can be observed, a reflection of extramedullary erythropoiesis generated by the fetus in response to significant hemolysis. In an effort to compensate for increased cell destruction, the liver and spleen continue to manufacture RBCs for a longer time than is usually seen in the fetus and newborn. Engorgement of the splenic sinusoids by hemolyzed RBCs also contributes to splenomegaly.

Treatment

Because the antibodies involved in ABO incompatibility occur naturally, the elimination of this type of incompatibility is virtually impossible. However, its effects on the fetus and newborn are much less dramatic and life threatening than those of Rh incompatibility. Consequently, amniocentesis and monitoring of amniotic fluid bilirubin levels, intrauterine transfusions, and early delivery are not usually necessary. However, the problems associated with postnatal bilirubin clearance can exist, with phototherapy and possibly exchange transfusion becoming part of the repertoire of care. These two modalities of care are discussed in further detail later in this chapter.

Rh Incompatibility

Incompatibilities involving the Rh system are the second most common alloimmune problem, but the severity of complications far surpasses that of ABO incompatibility. There are three Rh gene loci with the capability of producing five recognized antigens in the Rh complex: C, D, E, c, and e. The d antigen is considered an absence of antigen D because it cannot be isolated at present. Each individual has a paired set of these factors, having inherited a single set of either C or c, D or d, and E or e from each parent. There exists a predilection toward three particular combinations, two Rh-positive (CDe, cDE) and one Rh-negative (cde). Of these six factors, the two involved in Rh determination are D and d. The D antigen is most prevalent; its presence on the RBC indicates an Rh-positive cell, whereas its absence indicates an Rh-negative cell. Because of single-set inheritance from each parent, the potential for three different combinations of paired antigens exists: one pair being both d (Rh-negative, homozygous), another pair being both D (Rh-positive, homozygous), and the third pair being a combination of d and D (Rh-positive, heterozygous).

The Rh antigen can be detected as early as 38 days of gestation on the fetal RBC and is completely developed during fetal life. This antigen is necessary for normal function of the RBC membrane and, unlike A and B antigens, is confined exclusively to the RBC. Antibodies never occur naturally in the Rh system; exposure to the antigen is necessary to produce antibodies. Such exposure is thought to occur through maternal inoculation with fetal RBCs by TPH or undetectable hemorrhage during labor, abortion, ectopic pregnancy, or amniocentesis.

Spontaneous TPH occurs during 50 to 75 percent of all pregnancies (Bowman, 1988), with the greatest and most severe occurrence at the time of delivery. At this time, fetal RBCs are passed into maternal circulation, where antibodies develop in response to any RBC antigen the mother does not possess. The risk for immunization depends on the ABO status of both mother and fetus and the size of the hemorrhage. On the basis of blood type, the risk for maternal Rh immunization in an ABO-compatible Rh-negative mother and Rh-positive fetus is 16 percent, whereas an ABO-incompatible pregnancy with an Rh-negative mother and Rh-positive fetus runs a 1.5 to 2 percent risk with each pregnancy (Woodrow, 1970). If the hemorrhage is less than 0.1 ml RBCs, the risk for immunization is 3 percent. If the hemorrhage is greater than 5 ml, the risk increases to 50 to 65 percent (Bowman, 1988).

The maternal Rh antibody is slow to develop and, at first, may consist exclusively of IgM, which cannot cross the placenta because of its molecular size. This is followed by the production of IgG, which can cross the placenta into fetal circulation. The maximal concentration of the IgG form of antibody occurs within 2 to 4 months after termination of the first sensitizing pregnancy (Guyton, 1996a). If initial immunization occurs shortly before or at the time of delivery, the first Rh-positive infant born to such a mother may trigger the initial antibody response but will not be affected. However, subsequent exposure to RBCs of Rh-positive fetuses produces a rapid antibody response that consists mostly of IgG. This response does affect these fetuses, by antibody attachment to antigen sites on the fetal RBCs. The antibody coating of the RBCs forms the basis for a positive result of the direct Coombs' test. The affected RBCs undergo agglutination, phagocytosis, and eventually extravascular hemolysis in the spleen. The by-products of hemolysis, especially bilirubin, pass through the placenta into the maternal circulation to be metabolized and conjugated by the maternal liver. The rate of destruction of fetal RBCs depends on the amount of anti-D antibodies present on the cells, the effectiveness of anti-D antibodies in promoting phagocytosis, and the capability of the reticuloendothelial system of the spleen to remove antibody-coated cells (Zipursky & Bowman, 1993).

Erythroblastosis Fetalis

Hemolysis in the fetus due to Rh incompatibility results in the disease known as erythroblastosis fetalis (EBF); the major consequences are anemia and hyperbilirubinemia. The name is derived from the presence of immature circulating RBCs (erythroblasts), which are forced into the circulation of affected fetuses to compensate for rapid destruction of fetal blood cells. The severity of the disease depends on the degree of hemolysis and the ability of the fetus's erythropoietic system to counteract the ensuing anemia. In an attempt to compensate for rapid destruction, the fetus continues to use extramedullary organs, such as the liver and spleen, that would normally have ceased RBC production after the seventh month of gestation (Tuchmann-Duplessis et al., 1975).

Clinical Manifestations

The clinical manifestations of EBF are similar to ABO incompatibility but are often more intense (Table 28–4). Jaundice results from an exaggerated rise in bilirubin, with the premature infant exhibiting an even earlier rise and a more prolonged period of elevation. Hepatosplenomegaly can be found on physical examination along with varying degrees of hydrops. Hydrops fetalis is the presence of severe total body edema often accompanied by ascites and pleural effusions. Although the pathogenesis is unclear, it is theorized to be due to a combination of congestive heart failure and intrauterine hypoxia from severe anemia, portal and umbilical venous hypertension caused by hepatic hematopoiesis, and low plasma colloid osmotic pressure induced by hypoalbuminemia. Low serum albumin levels are a consequence of altered hepatic synthesis, which may be due to local cellular necrosis and compromised intrahepatic circulation (Phibbs et al., 1974). All of these factors can lead to portal and venous hypertension and edema (Bowman, 1988). The more severe the anemia and hypoalbuminemia, the greater the extravasation of fluid into the tissue.

Altered hepatic synthesis can impair production of vitamin K and vitamin K–dependent clotting factors, which can lead to

TABLE 28–4 Comparison of Features Seen in Rh and ABO Incompatibility

	Rh Incompatibility	ABO Incompatibility
Blood Group Setup		
Mother	Negative	O
Infant	Positive	A or B
Type of Antibody	Incomplete (7S)	Immune (7S)
Clinical Aspects		
Occurrence in firstborn	5%	40%–50%
Predictable severity in subsequent pregnancies	Usually	No
Stillbirth or hydrops	Frequent	Rare
Severe anemia	Frequent	Rare
Degree of jaundice	+ + +	+
Hepatosplenomegaly	+ + +	+
Laboratory Findings		
Direct Coombs' test (infant)	+	+ or 0
Maternal antibodies	Always present	Not clear-cut
Spherocytes	0	+
Treatment		
Need for antenatal measures	Yes	No
Exchange transfusion		
Frequency	Approximately $\frac{2}{3}$	Approximately $\frac{1}{10}$
Donor blood type	Rh-negative Group-specific, when possible	Rh, same as infant Group O only
Occurrence of late anemia	Common	Rare

From Maisels, M. (1975). Neonatal jaundice. In G. Avery (Ed.), *Neonatology* (p. 393). Philadelphia: J. B. Lippincott.

hemorrhage in these infants. The presence of petechiae and prolonged bleeding from cord and blood sampling sites may be initial signs of clotting abnormalities.

Hypoglycemia, secondary to hyperplasia of the pancreatic islet cells, is also associated with EBF. Products of RBC hemolysis are theorized to inactivate circulating insulin, thus promoting increased insulin release and subsequent pancreatic beta cell hyperplasia. Another theory suggests that potassium or amino acids released from hemolyzed cells may directly stimulate insulin production or indirectly produce this effect by increasing glucagon secretion (Oski & Naiman, 1982b). Low blood glucose levels and elevated plasma insulin levels are present in approximately one third of surviving erythroblastotic infants.

Antenatal Therapy

ANTENATAL SCREENING

Adequate antenatal care is important in safeguarding the fetus potentially affected by EBF. Proper screening of any pregnant woman at her first prenatal visit is essential and should include blood type and Rh factor. If the mother is Rh-negative, the father's blood type should also be ascertained. If the father is Rh-positive, it becomes essential to determine the presence of Rh immunization by Coombs' testing, specifically the indirect Coombs' test. In addition to blood typing, a concise obstetrical history regarding any previous spontaneous or therapeutic abortions, or delivery of an affected infant, is important to ensure appropriate management of the present pregnancy. Women who are sensitized require more surveillance throughout their pregnancy in comparison to their unsensitized counterparts, and women who have previously given birth to affected infants require the greatest degree of care.

RhIG THERAPY

Unsensitized Rh-negative mothers can benefit from antenatal and postpartum administration of RhIG. Before the inception of RhIG in 1964 when the first clinical trials were conducted, the frequency of Rh immunization was 7 to 8 percent in ABO-compatible pregnancies and 1 percent in ABO-incompatible pregnancies, with close to 50 percent of all perinatal deaths attributable to EBF (Allen et al., 1950). With the use of RhIG after delivery, the frequency of Rh immunization was dramatically decreased to 1 to 1.8 percent. Because sensitization was known to occur without evidence of TPH at the time of delivery, the question of antenatal sensitization in response to frequent, small, and undetectable hemorrhage before or during labor was raised. For this reason, antenatal RhIG was initiated to eliminate such cases of alloimmunization. Antenatal administration has further decreased the frequency to as low as 0.1 percent (Chavez et al., 1991; Sacher & Queenan, 1987). However, there will always be pregnancies in which RhIG fails to suppress the formation of antibodies or when its administration is not feasible. Immunization is not effective if sensitization occurs before initial antenatal screening or if RhIG dosage is inadequate to neutralize a massive TPH. For these reasons, it is estimated that the occurrence cannot be reduced beyond 4 in 10,000 pregnancies, despite the use of RhIG (Bowman, 1988).

RhIG adheres to any Rh-positive fetal RBCs that have invaded the maternal circulation. Agglutination, hemolysis, and removal of these foreign RBCs occur before the maternal immune system can recognize the invasion and develop antibodies that would transplacentally cross into the fetus. In the initial preclinical trials in 1963 (Clarke et al., 1963), rapid clearing of invading fetal RBCs was noted after the injection of anti-D antibodies, indicating that this form of immunosuppression involves the entire blood cell and not merely the Rh antigen present on the cell. It is theorized that RhIG may also suppress the antigen-induced response of B cells to produce antibodies by increasing the production of suppressor T cells. The anti-D from RhIG does enter the fetal circulation, but it does not seem to cause significant hemolysis.

Because it is common practice to administer RhIG and rubella vaccine together, one caution stated in the manufacturer's insert for rubella vaccine should be noted. When a mother receives RhIG or blood products along with the rubella vaccine, the vaccine may be inactivated by antibodies against rubella present in the donor sera (Edgar & Hambling, 1977; Govoni & Hayes, 1988; McEvoy, 1990). Donor sera antibodies provide passive immunity and can block the response of the mother's own immune system to the vaccine. As with any type of passive immunity, the mother's protection tends to be transient, and she may remain vulnerable to rubella. Rubella titers should be repeated 6 to 8 weeks after the simultaneous administration of RhIG and rubella vaccine to verify protection.

Several obstetrical conditions can increase the risk for sensitization by increasing the chances for TPH. Some of these problems necessitating RhIG prophylaxis include the following:

1. Therapeutic or spontaneous abortion beyond 7 to 8 weeks' gestation; there is an increased frequency of TPH in therapeutic abortion, with potentially 3 of 30 women being sensitized.
2. Amniocentesis, which has a 10 percent chance of causing TPH.
3. Ectopic pregnancies or hydatidiform moles.
4. Abdominal trauma.

Failure to receive RhIG after such occurrences may place these women at risk for sensitization and may explain already elevated titers of anti-D in their blood. The American College of Obstetricians and Gynecologists recommends a dose of 50 μg for high-risk situations that arise before 13 weeks' gestation and 300 μg after 13 weeks' gestation.

In the at-risk, Rh-negative mother with low antibody titers on the initial prenatal screen, repeated titers are recommended at 28 weeks' gestation (Scott & Branch, 1994). If titers remain low at this time, an injection of RhIG (300 μg) is recommended. A single dose given at 28 weeks' gestation is 94 percent effective in preventing maternal sensitization (Sacher & Queenan, 1987). Titers need not be repeated until delivery, at which time a second dose of 300 μg is given if titers are low. Some caregivers test earlier (18 to 20 weeks' gestation) and repeat titers monthly (Bowman, 1994).

RhIG has a half-life of 25 to 27 days and is effective for approximately 2 weeks after antigen exposure. The timing of its administration after delivery is important and the recommendation is within 72 hours of delivery. The postdelivery dosage allows a maximal estimated fetal transfusion of 30 ml, which leaves 1 percent of postpartum mothers without full coverage (Ness et al., 1987). If massive TPH is suspected, the dose of RhIG may need to be increased to provide adequate amounts of anti-D antibodies. Testing maternal blood for the presence of RBCs with fetal hemoglobin after the administration of RhIG can help determine whether any additional amount is needed.

Because TPH has the greatest chance of occurring at the time of delivery, maximal antibody titers may not be reached for several months after termination of a pregnancy. All unsensitized Rh-negative mothers, especially those experiencing cesarean section, breech delivery, twin pregnancy, toxemia, placental abruption or previa, or transverse lie, should be monitored carefully after delivery for elevated antibody titers.

AMNIOCENTESIS

Elevation of maternal anti-D antibody titers during a pregnancy indicates alloimmunization and excludes further use of RhIG. In a first sensitized gestation, impact on the fetus tends to be mild. These pregnancies can be managed with monthly titers and serial ultrasound examinations to evaluate the fetus for signs of ascites and soft tissue edema. If titers remain low and ultrasound findings

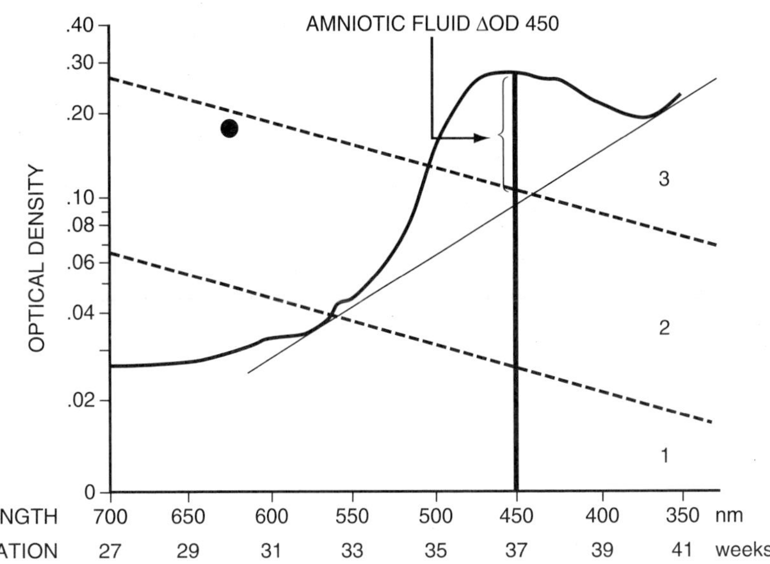

FIGURE 28–7. The spectral absorption curve of amniotic fluid obtained by amniocentesis is plotted against a graph that depicts the normal optical density (OD) of amniotic fluid. Values that fall in zone 1 are considered normal. The presence of indirect bilirubin in the amniotic fluid increases the optical density at the 450 nm point of the wavelength. The amount of bilirubin present can be indirectly measured by calculating the optical density rise in comparison with normal values. This change from the norm is called the optical density (now termed *absorbance*). Severity of hemolysis is then classified as moderate (zone 2) or severe (zone 3). (From Bowman, J. [1986]. Haemolytic disease of the newborn. In N. Robertson [Ed.], *A textbook of neonatology* [pp. 469–483]. Edinburgh: Churchill Livingstone.)

are normal, pregnancy can continue to near term without further testing. Subsequent pregnancies with Rh-incompatible fetuses, however, lead to more adverse fetal effects, whereas maternal antibody titers become less predictive of fetal well-being. Amniocentesis becomes a consideration when antenatal maternal blood titers indicate significant sensitization has occurred.

Amniocentesis is done to extract amniotic fluid samples for evaluation of bilirubin levels. Amniotic fluid develops a xanthochromic appearance as bilirubin is released during RBC destruction and is an indirect reflection of the degree of fetal anemia. Bilirubin is theorized to find its way into amniotic fluid by passing from the fetal plasma through the membrane covering the umbilical cord. Amniotic fluid bilirubin levels are determined by measuring the optical density (OD) (now termed absorbance) of amniotic fluid at 450 nm (Liley, 1961), because actual levels are minuscule and difficult to measure. The OD of amniotic fluid as determined by spectrophotometry normally forms a straight line between 350 and 700 nm. When bilirubin is present, a large bulge appears at 450 nm (Fig. 28–7). The difference between the height of the bulge and the normal line (OD) indicates the amount of bilirubin in the amniotic fluid. Results are expressed as levels, which are then divided into three zones of severity. Zone 1 (0.04 mg/dl) is considered normal; zone 2 (greater than 0.1 mg/dl) indicates Rh hemolytic disease; and zone 3 (levels in excess of 0.8 mg/dl) is indicative of imminent fetal demise within 7 to 10 days. If zone 3 is reached in an advanced pregnancy (i.e., 31 to 33 weeks) and a reasonable lung maturation is present, preterm delivery may be indicated after an attempt to enhance lung maturation with maternal steroid therapy. If high zone 2 to zone 3 is reached between 23 and 31 weeks' gestation, intrauterine transfusion may be necessary to maintain the fetus until further maturation occurs.

The reliability of spectrophotometry and the Liley curve has come into question. The original bilirubin OD graphs were based on gestational ages greater than 27 weeks. Because amniotic fluid bilirubin levels rise with increasing gestational age, peak at 23 to 24 weeks' gestation, and then decline, the original Liley curves cannot simply be extrapolated downward. Investigators have modified the original Liley curve (Fig. 28–8) in an effort to use amniotic fluid OD in pregnancies as early as 16 weeks' gestation (Bowman, 1992). Poor correlation between amniotic fluid bilirubin levels obtained during the second trimester and actual fetal hematocrits has been reported (Nicolaides et al., 1986). However, with the use of chloroform extraction and assessment of value trends in the midzone, the Liley curve has been found reliable by other investigators in identifying the severely affected fetus (Spinnato et al., 1991).

Amniocentesis is also beneficial in determining fetal blood type and can be performed at an earlier gestational age than direct fetal sampling. Clinical use of polymerase chain reaction on amniocytes obtained during amniocentesis has been investigated and appears successful in accurately determining fetal blood type (Fisk et al., 1994).

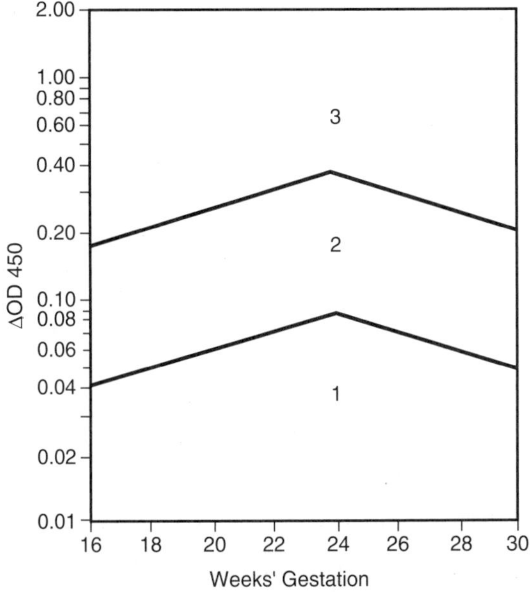

FIGURE 28–8. Modification of the original Liley optical density graph allows more accurate interpretation of amniotic fluid bilirubin levels in the premature infant less than 26 weeks' gestation. This modification compensates for the natural increase in amniotic fluid bilirubin levels during the second trimester and a natural decrease in amniotic fluid at approximately 24 weeks' gestation. (From Bowman, J. [1992]. Rhesus haemolyticus disease. In N. Wald [Ed.], *Antenatal and neonatal screening* [2nd ed.]. Oxford: Oxford University Press.)

Timing of the initial amniocentesis depends on the previous obstetrical history and maternal titers. An indirect Coombs' titer of 1:16 or more is considered a critical level and warrants performance of this procedure as early as 16 to 18 weeks' gestation. The fetus less than 16 weeks' gestation is rarely affected, possibly because antibodies do not cross the placenta before this time. In high-risk pregnancies with severely affected fetuses, amniocentesis is usually performed every 1 to 3 weeks. Amniotic fluid OD is 95 percent accurate in predicting the severity of hemolysis if serial measurements are done and the last measurement is performed after 26 to 27 weeks' gestation (Bowman, 1994).

The risks involved in amniocentesis are fetal demise, premature rupture of membranes, and increase in the frequency of TPH by 8.4 percent (Mennuti et al., 1980). Mothers undergoing amniocentesis in midtrimester or later should receive 300 μg of RhIG after each procedure.

CORDOCENTESIS

Introduced in the 1980s, this technique involves cannulation of an umbilical vessel to obtain blood samples for determining the severity of fetal hemolytic disease and to perform fetal transfusions. Cordocentesis is useful during times when fetal sampling and transfusion are needed, but the procedure is usually not feasible before 18 weeks' gestation. It more accurately determines the degree of fetal anemia and has better predictive abilities than amniocentesis. However, the risks are higher than in amniocentesis. Although fetal loss for both procedures is low, there is an increased risk for TPH accompanied by increased antibody titers in mothers undergoing this procedure. Titers can increase by as much as 40 percent when the transplacental approach is used (Kuller et al., 1996; Weiner et al., 1991). In addition to fetal loss and TPH, other adverse effects of cordocentesis are amnionitis and premature rupture of membranes.

INTRAUTERINE TRANSFUSIONS

Intrauterine transfusions are usually deemed necessary to salvage an immature fetus so compromised by EBF that death may occur secondary to circulatory collapse before 34 weeks' gestation. The fetus is capable of compensating for anemia with adequate acid–base balance until the hematocrit drops to a value below 50 percent of normal. With improved techniques and the advent of ultrasonography, survival rates have improved dramatically. The overall survival rate was 34 percent in 1969, increasing to 60 to 70 percent by the late 1970s. In the 1980s, survival rates increased to 89 percent in cases without hydrops and 54 percent when hydrops was present. In the 1990s, the overall survival rate is 88 to 96 percent (Tannirandorn & Rodeck, 1991; Weiner et al., 1991), with survival of hydropic infants ranging from 66 to 85 percent (Ney et al., 1991; Tannirandorn & Rodeck, 1991). Potential risks of intrauterine transfusion include maternal and fetal complications inherent in the performance of an amniocentesis as well as graft-versus-host phenomenon in the fetus from transfusion of lymphocytes, which can be modified through the use of irradiated blood.

Intrauterine transfusion involves the instillation of packed RBCs with a hematocrit of approximately 90 percent into the fetal peritoneal cavity (intraperitoneal transfusion [IPT]) or into the umbilical vein or artery (intravascular transfusion [IVT]). Type-specific RBCs are used if the fetal blood type is known and no ABO incompatibility exists; if fetal blood type is unknown, O-negative RBCs are used.

In IPT, 80 percent of the cells injected into the fetal peritoneal cavity are absorbed into the venous circulation through the right lymphatic duct and into the subdiaphragmatic lymph vessels. Approximately 10 to 13 percent of the blood cells are absorbed every 24 hours, with complete absorption taking 8 to 10 days. Absorption is ineffective in the presence of ascites and may be too lengthy to prevent fetal demise if a fetus is severely hydropic, moribund, or not breathing. If IPT must be done in a hydropic fetus, 20 to 30 ml of ascitic fluid in excess of the planned infusion may need to be removed from the peritoneal cavity before infusion. Because the fetal hematocrit is not usually raised to the desired level with one transfusion, another is given in 9 to 14 days and then every 3 to 4 weeks until delivery. The volume of blood infused depends on gestational age, and the dosage can be calculated in the following manner:

$$(\text{gestational age in weeks} - 20) \times 10 = \text{ml of blood}$$

Instillation of RBCs into the fetal peritoneal cavity consists of the following steps done while constantly monitoring fetal heart tones:

1. Ultrasound localization of placenta and fetal peritoneal cavity;
2. Insertion of needle, usually 16-gauge, into the fetal peritoneal cavity, through which an epidural catheter is threaded;
3. Insertion of contrast medium through the catheter and radiographic verification of placement in the peritoneal cavity;
4. Infusion of RBCs into the peritoneal cavity at a rate of 10 ml every 3 to 5 minutes.

Direct IVT employing the umbilical vein and artery is performed by use of ultrasonography (Fig. 28–9). Amniocentesis is done after the preceding steps for IPT; in addition, fetal umbilical vessels are then located by ultrasonography. After the catheter tip is determined to be intravascular by contrast study, fetal blood samples for laboratory analysis are drawn and donor blood is then infused directly into the fetal circulation. The umbilical vein is preferred over the umbilical artery because there is less occurrence of fetal bradycardia during the transfusion. Blood is infused at a rate of 10 ml every 1 to 2 minutes, with the total volume usually reaching 50 ml/kg. Fewer complications are reported when the increase in umbilical venous pressure during and after the transfusion is held to a maximum of 10 mm Hg (Hallak et al., 1992). This procedure may need to be repeated every 2 to 3 days to achieve the desired hematocrit of 40 to 45 percent. After this hematocrit level is achieved, subsequent transfusions are timed to keep the hematocrit above 25 to 30 percent. This may require an IVT every 2 to 4 weeks.

In a comparison of these two methods by Harman and associates (1990), IVT seemed to have less associated mortality and morbidity than IPT. In a group of fetuses undergoing IVT versus IPT, survival was 91 versus 66 percent; 5-minute Apgar scores were higher (greater than 7 in 14 versus 38 percent); and vaginal deliveries were more frequently accomplished (83 versus 50 percent) in the IVT group. In a comparison of sensorineural outcome, fetuses undergoing IVT also fared better than their counterparts undergoing IPT (Doyle et al., 1993). For these reasons, IVT is the preferred choice of transfusion site in the severely affected infant. If IPT and IVT are impossible to perform, intracardiac infusion may be the only feasible route available to save a moribund fetus.

PRENATAL PHARMACOLOGIC AGENTS TO CONTROL HEMOLYSIS

Attempts to suppress antibody action on fetal RBCs or to improve bilirubin conjugation and elimination through antenatal use of medications in the Rh-sensitized mother have not proved beneficial. Some of these pharmacologic agents are phenobarbital, promethazine, corticosteroids, and D-positive erythrocyte membrane (EMOT). None of these is routinely in use at present.

Collaborative Postnatal Management of the Erythroblastotic Infant

On delivery of an infant with EBF, assessment of the cardiorespiratory status is of utmost importance. As the result of ascites,

Needle placement in IUIVT

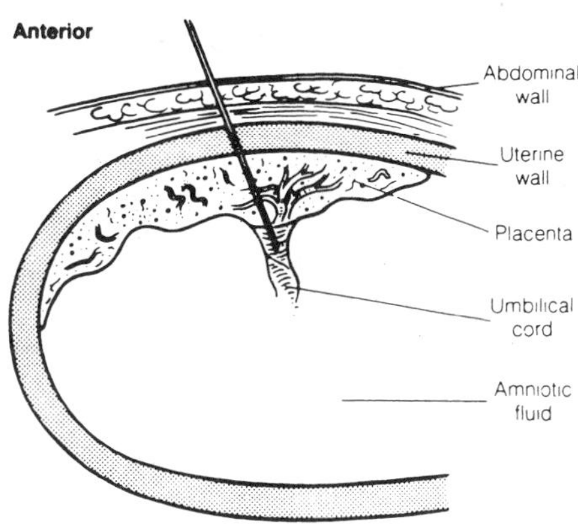

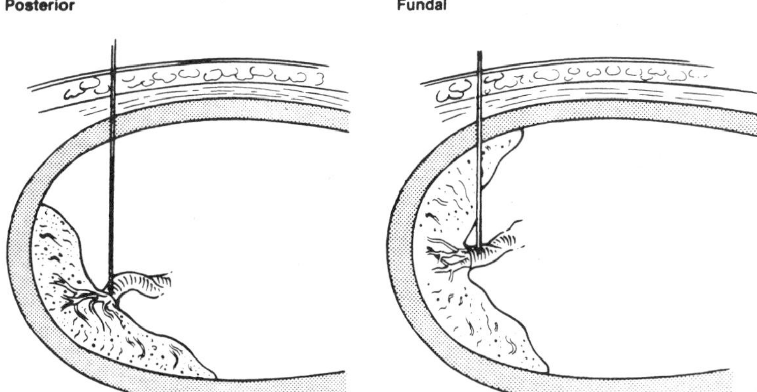

FIGURE 28–9. Direct intravascular transfusion (IVT) involves cannulation of the umbilical cord and placement of the needle in either the vein or the artery. Ultrasonography is used to locate the placenta and to verify appropriate needle placement. Packed RBCs are then transfused directly into the fetal intravascular compartment. (From Scott, J., & Branch, D. [1994]. Immunologic disorders in pregnancy. In J. Scott, P. DiSaia, C. Hammond, & W. Spellacy [Eds.], *Danforth's obstetrics and gynecology* [7th ed., pp. 393–408]. Philadelphia: J. B. Lippincott.)

pleural effusions, and circulatory collapse, these infants often require stabilization of the airway by intubation and mechanical ventilation. When peritoneal or pleural fluid prevents adequate chest excursion, it may be necessary to perform a paracentesis to remove fluid from the abdominal cavity and a thoracentesis, or chest tube insertion, to drain excess pleural fluid.

Delivery of an infant shortly after intrauterine transfusion may not allow adequate time for absorption of blood from the peritoneal cavity. The unabsorbed portion could lead to decreased lung expansion, resulting in respiratory failure or restricted mechanical ventilation. Such infants may require paracentesis for the removal of blood from the peritoneal cavity.

After the initiation of respiratory support, the infant should be assessed for adequacy of circulating blood volume. If the infant is severely hydropic, the inevitable anemia needs to be corrected with transfusions of packed RBCs, because an exchange transfusion may not be tolerated until the intravascular RBC volume is replenished. Transfusion is accomplished with use of O-negative or type-specific Rh-negative blood crossmatched against maternal blood. Initial use of a single-volume or partial exchange may offer a degree of cardiovascular stability before a double-volume exchange is attempted. Congestive heart failure, not present at the time of intravascular volume depletion, may become apparent as the infant is transfused. Oftentimes, the severely affected infant may benefit from digitalization and diuretic therapy.

Damage to the liver during gestation can adversely affect the coagulation factors in such infants, making them prone to bleeding disorders. This damage can intensify any hyperbilirubinemia present, because the hepatic substances required for conjugation may also be impaired. Laboratory evaluation of the infant affected by EBF should consist of liver function studies, hematocrits, and evaluation of coagulation status.

Nursing care of the infant affected by EBF involves scrupulous attention to the infant's cardiorespiratory status and vital signs. Positioning the infant in a manner that decreases abdominal pressure on the diaphragm allows better chest expansion. Maintenance of normal P_{O_2} and avoidance of overventilation may prevent barotrauma to lungs already compromised by pleural effusions. The lungs may be hypoplastic if their growth has been sufficiently compromised by hydrops in utero, making ventilation difficult and predisposing the infant to extraventilatory air.

All of these infants require careful monitoring of vital signs and blood volume status. Vital signs are usually assessed every hour until the infant's condition has stabilized. Hematocrits and bilirubin levels should be checked frequently during the first few hours and days of life to maintain adequate circulating blood volumes and to prevent toxic levels of bilirubin by timely initiation of therapy. If the cord bilirubin levels are significantly elevated, exchange transfusion may be necessary shortly after birth. If bilirubin levels do not require immediate exchange, blood levels should be checked every 4 to 8 hours, depending on the initial cord blood levels and subsequent rate of rise. In Rh incompatibility, exchange is imminent if the rate of rise exceeds 1 mg/h for the first 6 hours of life. The interval of blood sampling for bilirubin may be increased to 6 to 12 hours after the first 48 hours of life.

The major therapies used to control excessive unconjugated bilirubin levels are similar for all problems resulting in elevated bilirubin levels. Phototherapy and exchange transfusion remain the most frequently used therapies and are discussed later.

Analysis of Laboratory Data

The following laboratory data can be helpful in the diagnosis and treatment of EBF:

1. Mother's and infant's blood and Rh types.
2. Coombs' reactivity: The infant's RBCs are coated with anti-D antibodies, resulting in a positive direct Coombs' test result; on occasion, the heavy coating of neonatal RBCs with antibody can lead to a false Rh typing (Rh-negative); if the direct Coombs' test result is positive, the infant should be considered Rh-positive.
3. Infant's hematocrit, reticulocyte count, and RBC morphologic characteristics: The presence of immature cells or spherocytes assists in distinguishing Rh from ABO incompatibility.
4. Plasma bilirubin levels: The initial cord blood bilirubin level and the rate of rise determine the appropriate timing of any exchange transfusion needed to control bilirubin levels.

Cord bilirubin levels are closely associated with the severity of disease and mortality rate. There are three forms of circulating bilirubin: (1) direct or conjugated, (2) indirect, and (3) free. Measurement of direct bilirubin identifies the amount of conjugated bilirubin that will react directly with van den Bergh's reagent. The unconjugated portion of bilirubin is bound to albumin and is lipid soluble. It does not react with van den Bergh's reagent until it is combined with alcohol, thus the term indirect bilirubin. Free bilirubin is not attached to albumin and can easily cross the blood–brain barrier, causing the damage seen in kernicterus. All three measurements become important in the evaluation of the hyperbilirubinemic infant.

Bilirubin Metabolism and Hyperbilirubinemia

Bilirubin production begins as early as 12 weeks' gestation. It is the primary degradation product of hemoglobin, although 20 to 30 percent is derived from nonerythroid sources such as tissue heme. Bilirubin is produced after completion of the natural life span of the RBC, but ineffective erythropoiesis or premature destruction of blood cells can increase its production. In RBC destruction, the aging or hemolyzed RBC membrane ruptures, releasing hemoglobin that is phagocytosed by macrophages. The hemoglobin molecule then splits into a heme portion and a globin portion. Bilirubin is derived from the degradation of the heme ring in the heme portion that binds to heme oxygenase. The ferric heme breaks down to the ferrous form and then is cleaved to form carbon monoxide and biliverdin. Biliverdin is further reduced to form bilirubin, and carbon monoxide joins with heme to form carboxyhemoglobin.

Although bilirubin is found in stool and amniotic fluid, the major route of elimination in the fetus is through the placenta. For this reason, bilirubin must be retained in the form that allows its passage into maternal circulation. Consequently, the enzyme systems found in the fetus enhance the retention of bilirubin in the unconjugated form. It is the persistence of some of these fetal mechanisms during the newborn period that can contribute to jaundice. The plasma concentrations of bilirubin are usually low in the fetus, except in cases of severe hemolytic disease. All bilirubin in the cord blood of the fetus is of the unconjugated variety that is effectively metabolized, conjugated, and excreted by the maternal liver and gallbladder. The mean cord blood bilirubin concentration in the infant unaffected by hemolytic disease is 1.8 mg/dl, regardless of the gestational age or weight of the infant.

As the production of bilirubin exceeds the newborn liver's capacity to conjugate and eliminate it, plasma levels begin to rise rapidly. Jaundice becomes noticeable when the serum concentration reaches three times the normal amount present in the serum. The conjunctivae become visibly jaundiced at serum levels of more than 2.5 mg/dl. In the full-term infant, jaundice usually becomes apparent within 2 to 4 days after birth and lasts until the sixth day, reaching a peak concentration of 6 to 7 mg/dl. Although infants born at 37 weeks' gestation or more are considered term, they are more likely to reach or exceed serum bilirubin levels of 13 mg/dl or higher than are those infants born at 40 weeks' gestation (Gale et al., 1990; Linn et al., 1985; Maisels et al., 1988). The preterm infant has cord blood levels similar to those of the term infant, but peak levels are higher, jaundice lasts longer, and levels peak later, at 5 to 7 days. Sixty-three percent of preterm infants reach levels of 10 to 19 mg/dl, and 22 percent reach levels greater than 15 mg/dl.

Although the neonatal liver's conjugating mechanisms are reduced during the first few days of life, it possesses the ability to metabolize and excrete two thirds to three quarters of the bilirubin circulating throughout the body. Initially, bilirubin is transported in the plasma, bound to albumin at two sites: (1) a primary binding site that has a strong bond and (2) a secondary site that has a weak bond. When available albumin binding sites are saturated, bilirubin then circulates freely in the plasma. It is this portion of unconjugated bilirubin that can migrate into brain cells, causing damage known as kernicterus. The occurrence of kernicterus is related to the amount of diffusible, loosely bound bilirubin and availability of albumin binding sites.

When bilirubin reaches the liver, it is transferred from plasma albumin, across the cell membrane of the liver, and into the liver cell (Fig. 28–10). Two proteins, Y and Z, also called ligands, affect bilirubin transfer from plasma to liver. Here it is either stored in the cell cytoplasm or removed from the ligands and conjugated in the hepatic endoplasmic reticulum. Conjugation is essential for the excretion of bilirubin into bile. Eighty percent of bilirubin is conjugated with glucuronic acid, becoming bilirubin glucuronide. Glucuronosyltransferase is the important hepatic enzyme required for the production of bilirubin glucuronide. Ninety-five percent of bilirubin glucuronide is excreted into bile and subsequently into the intestine (Oski & Naiman, 1982b).

The effective excretion of bilirubin from the intestine depends on the length of time needed for the passage of stool and on the presence of substances that break down conjugated bilirubin. The newborn may have decreased bowel motility and delayed meconium passage that allow longer exposure of stool to the enzyme responsible for breakdown of conjugated bilirubin, bilirubin glucuronidase. This enzyme, coupled with the newborn's lack of intestinal flora required for bilirubin reduction to urobilinogen, converts the conjugated form to the unconjugated form that is then resorbed by the intestine.

Kernicterus

When albumin binding sites are filled, increased amounts of free bilirubin are available for passage into the central nervous system (CNS). Free bilirubin easily crosses the blood–brain barrier and is transferred into the brain cells, causing obvious yellow staining of the brain tissue (kernicterus) that is similar to its effect on the skin. The areas of the brain usually affected by the staining are the hypothalamus, dentate nucleus, and cerebellum. Kernicterus is associated with varying degrees of neurologic damage, but a direct correlation between serum bilirubin levels and the severity of involvement cannot be drawn.

Many factors can influence the bilirubin binding capacity and increase the risk for kernicterus at lower bilirubin levels. Some of these factors are as follows:

1. The total amount of available serum albumin: Premature infants normally experience a relative hypoproteinemia and have fewer albumin binding sites available for free bilirubin.

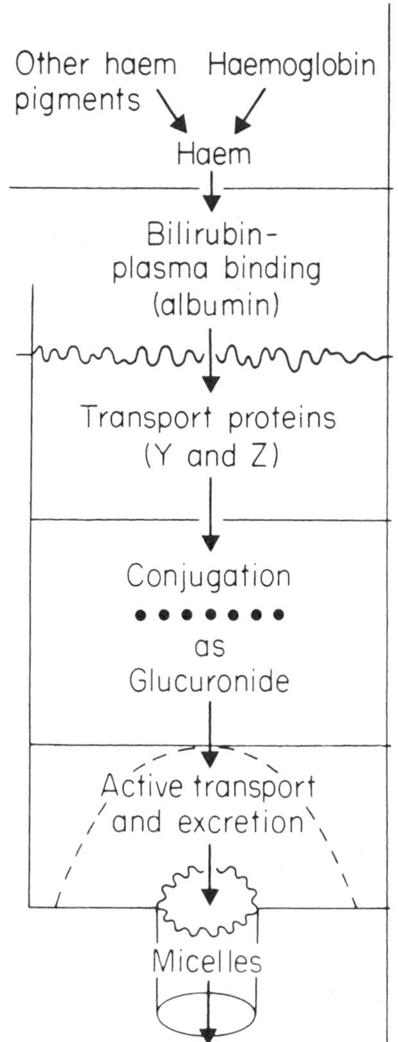

FIGURE 28–10. Unconjugated bilirubin, bound to plasma albumin, is absorbed into the hepatic cell through the membrane, which separates it from the albumin molecule. Bilirubin immediately combines with one of two proteins found inside the hepatic cell, Y protein and Z protein. It eventually becomes separated from these two proteins and conjugated to other substances, mostly glucuronic acid, to form excretable bilirubin. (From Sherlock, S. [1985]. Jaundice. In S. Sherlock [Ed.], *Diseases of the liver and biliary system* [7th ed., p. 201]. Oxford: Blackwell Scientific Publications.)

2. The presence of other substances competing for available binding sites: Certain drugs, such as sulfisoxazole, salicylates, and sodium benzoate, compete with bilirubin for binding sites or replace bilirubin loosely attached to binding sites.
3. Acidosis and hypoxia: Increased production of hydrogen ions and implementation of anaerobic metabolism can impede bilirubin binding. Albumin's ability to bind bilirubin drops to half its potential at a serum pH of 7.1, with free fatty acids produced during anaerobic metabolism competing for albumin binding sites (Bowman, 1988). When acidosis and hypoxia, which can open the blood–brain barrier, are concurrently present in a sick infant, such an infant can be exposed to kernicterus at much lower serum bilirubin levels. Evidence also suggests that tests evaluating bilirubin binding capacity, rather than serum bilirubin concentrations, have a better correlation with the appearance of subsequent CNS abnormalities (Brodersen, 1980; Wennberg & Hance, 1986).

Clinical Manifestations

Kernicterus usually becomes evident during the first 5 days of life. The signs of its presence include lethargy or irritability, hypotonia, paralysis of upward gaze, high-pitched cry, poor eating, opisthotonic posturing, and spasticity. It is also associated with deafness, cerebral palsy, and tooth enamel abnormalities. The overall risk for kernicterus is 50 percent if serum bilirubin levels are 30 mg/dl or greater and 10 percent if levels are between 20 and 25 mg/dl. Prevention of elevated levels of free bilirubin is the major way that kernicterus can be eliminated. This prevention may require phototherapy for the slowly rising levels but will almost certainly demand exchange transfusion if the rise is rapid and marked.

Common Nonimmune Causes of Hyperbilirubinemia

Elevated bilirubin levels within the first 24 hours of life or levels that exceed 12 mg/dl are not considered physiologic and deserve investigation. Many conditions other than blood group incompatibilities can cause jaundice in the newborn. The majority of commonly seen problems result in elevated unconjugated rather than conjugated bilirubin levels. These pathologic conditions can be classified as (1) problems causing increased RBC breakdown, such as sepsis, drug reactions, and extravascular blood; (2) problems that interfere with bilirubin conjugation, such as breast milk jaundice, drug interactions, hypothyroidism, hypoxia, and asphyxia; or (3) problems causing abnormal bilirubin excretion, such as bowel obstruction. However, the single factor most implicated in hyperbilirubinemia is prematurity, with the severity of jaundice directly correlated to decreasing gestational age. The premature infant is theorized to be subject to a combination of increased RBC breakdown secondary to decreased RBC life span and impaired bilirubin conjugation due to liver immaturity.

Increased Red Blood Cell Breakdown

Several problems that arise in the perinatal period are associated with excessive and premature destruction of the RBC by hemolysis. Neonatal bacterial and viral infections and intrauterine viral infections, especially those of the TORCH complex (toxoplasmosis, other agents, rubella, cytomegalovirus, and herpes simplex), have been implicated in the hemolytic destruction of the RBC. Certain medications, such as the synthetic analogues of vitamin K or large doses of natural vitamin K, also induce RBC destruction. Other conditions prevalent in the premature and term newborn can result in the extravasation of large quantities of blood (e.g., cephalhematoma and pulmonary or intracerebral hemorrhages). These extravascular collections of blood cells must undergo hemolysis to be resorbed by the body. Significant hemolysis, regardless of the cause, increases the bilirubin load on a metabolically immature neonatal liver. This increased load often results in hyperbilirubinemia in the newborn.

Interference With Bilirubin Conjugation

Breast Milk Jaundice

Breast milk jaundice affects approximately 2 to 4 percent of all breastfed babies; symptoms become apparent at 3 to 5 days of life. Bilirubin levels can reach 12 to 20 mg/dl between 8 and 15 days and may remain elevated for as long as 2 months (Maisels, 1990). The jaundice is believed to be caused by substances present in breast milk that either interfere with bilirubin conjugation or increase enterohepatic circulation, resulting in resorption of bilirubin from the intestine.

Two substances found in breast milk, pregnanediol and fatty acids, inhibit glucuronosyltransferase, the enzyme necessary for bilirubin conjugation in the liver. Another substance present in breast milk, β-glucuronidase, enhances the breakdown of conjugated bilirubin, deposited in the intestine as bile, before it can be eliminated in the stool. Conjugated bilirubin is then broken down to the unconjugated form and resorbed by the small and large bowel. Unconjugated bilirubin diffuses easily into the blood supply of the bowel, where it is redistributed into the circulation.

When breastfeeding is discontinued, the bilirubin level falls within 24 to 48 hours, decreasing to half its previous peak level by 48 hours. With resumption of breastfeeding, the bilirubin level will again start to rise, but at a much slower pace (Maisels, 1990). Interruption of breastfeeding is not recommended; instead, continued and frequent breastfeeding is encouraged. However, the health care provider has the option to supplement nursing with formula or to interrupt breastfeeding and substitute formula, depending on the degree of bilirubin level elevation. Supplementation of nursing with water or glucose water does not appear to have any effect on bilirubin levels in healthy term infants (Nicoll et al., 1982).

Drugs Interfering With Bilirubin Conjugation

Certain medications ingested by the mother and transplacentally passed to the fetus, such as salicylates and sulfa preparations, can interfere with the ability of albumin to bind bilirubin. Administration of these drugs to the newborn can produce the same effect. Other medications, such as sodium benzoate, a commonly used preservative, compete with bilirubin for albumin binding sites.

Hypothyroidism

Twenty percent of all infants with hypothyroidism have elevated bilirubin levels lasting 3 to 4 weeks, with normalization of levels requiring up to 4 months. The suspected mechanism for jaundice is theorized to be a delay in glucuronosyltransferase synthesis or impairment of hepatic proteins that bind bilirubin and remove it from the plasma. The plasma membrane of liver cells may also be altered, resulting in decreased bilirubin influx into the hepatic cells.

Acidosis and Hypoxia

As previously stated in the discussion regarding kernicterus, a drop in serum pH alters albumin's ability to bind bilirubin. The accompanying increase in free fatty acid production promotes competition between fatty acids and bilirubin for binding sites. In animal models, respiratory acidosis but not metabolic acidosis increases movement of bilirubin across the blood–brain barrier (Bratlid et al., 1984; Burgess et al., 1985).

Abnormal Bilirubin Excretion

Any disease state resulting in abnormal bilirubin excretion can raise serum bilirubin levels significantly. This is seen in hepatic dysfunction secondary to such entities as hypoxia or asphyxia, bowel obstruction, ileus, and congestive heart failure. These conditions have a tendency, however, to elevate both the conjugated and the unconjugated bilirubin levels. Decreased bowel motility associated with these conditions provides an increased time for β-glucuronidase, naturally present in the gut, to act on conjugated bilirubin in the stool. This enzymatic reaction converts conjugated bilirubin into the unconjugated form, which is resorbed into the

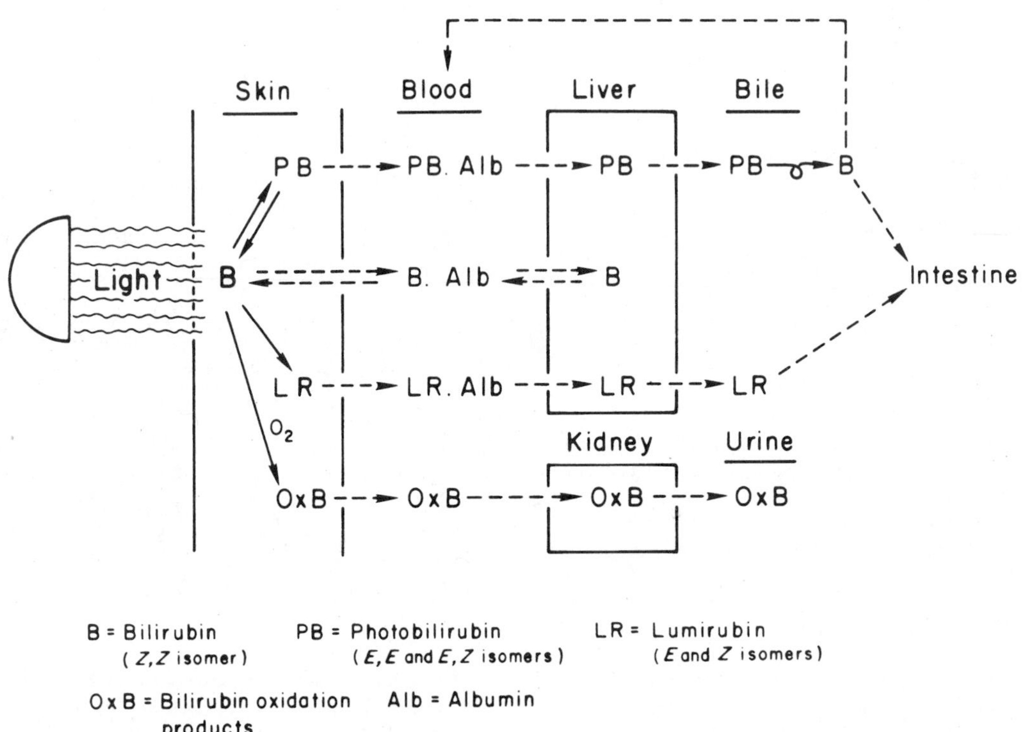

FIGURE 28–11. The mechanisms of phototherapy include both photo-oxidation and photoisomerization. In photo-oxidation, bilirubin is oxidized into colorless products that are excreted in the urine. The more significant contribution to bilirubin breakdown, photoisomerization, involves the conversion of naturally occurring bilirubin into water-soluble isomers. One isomer, photobilirubin, is eliminated through the stool, whereas lumirubin (lumibilirubin) is eliminated through urine and bile. (From McDonaugh, A., & Lightner, D. [1985]. Like a shriveled blood orange—bilirubin, jaundice and phototherapy. *Pediatrics,* 75[3], 443–455.)

intravascular compartment through the enterohepatic circulation. Direct hepatocellular damage associated with cholestasis and bacterial and viral infections can further impair the liver's ability to metabolize bilirubin.

Treatment of Hyperbilirubinemia

Phototherapy

The actual mechanisms by which phototherapy reduces unconjugated bilirubin and the exact mode of bilirubin excretion are not clearly understood (McDonagh & Lightner, 1985). Photo-oxidation and photoisomerization are the two mechanisms theorized to change bilirubin into water-soluble and excretable forms (Fig. 28–11). Photo-oxidation involves the oxidation of bilirubin pigment deposited in the skin and its conversion into colorless products that can be excreted into the urine. Of the total body bilirubin concentration, 15 percent can undergo photodegradation through oxidation. Photoisomerization involves the conversion of bilirubin polymers present in the skin into excretable isomers. When the natural form of bilirubin is exposed to blue light at certain wavelengths, it undergoes photoisomerization. This changes it from a tetrapyrrole, a lipid-soluble substance, into two water-soluble isomers. One isomer is excreted into bile without undergoing conjugation. Once this unstable isomer is incorporated into bile, it must be promptly eliminated from the gastrointestinal tract as a component of stool or it may revert back to its natural form. A small portion of this isomer is usually reabsorbed from the gut and recirculated into the plasma. The second isomer, lumibilirubin, is a stable water-soluble form of bilirubin that is eliminated through urine and bile (Knox et al., 1985).

Phototherapy is also thought to enhance the hepatic excretion of unconjugated bilirubin and to increase bowel transit time. With the initiation of early phototherapy, a 20 to 35 percent reduction in serum bilirubin concentrations is noted by day 2 of life, with a reduction of 41 to 55 percent by day 4. This reduction is more significant than the naturally occurring drop in the untreated infant.

Although no significant adverse effects are known to be attributed to the use of phototherapy, it is not without associated side effects. Some of these problems include dermal rash, lethargy, abdominal distention, possible eye damage, dehydration due to increased insensible water loss through the skin and digestive tract, thrombocytopenia, hypocalcemia, and secretory diarrhea possibly due to a temporary intestinal lactose deficiency. Another effect of phototherapy seen in infants having a significant direct bilirubin component is the "bronze baby" syndrome (Kopelman et al., 1972). This syndrome is theorized to be due to skin deposition of a photoproduct of bilirubin decomposition, possibly copper porphyrins, that causes bronzing of the skin and urine. Although no harmful effects can be attributed to the bronzing, it can last for several weeks to several months and is somewhat alarming to parents.

Phototherapy is not adequate therapy for a rapidly rising bilirubin level, but it is effective in the treatment of moderate hyperbilirubinemia that has not reached or exceeded levels known to be associated with kernicterus. Intensive phototherapy can produce a decline of only 1 to 2 mg/dl of total serum bilirubin within 4 to 6 hours (Bergman et al., 1994). It is also beneficial in reducing the need for exchange transfusions after 12 hours of age (Ebbesen, 1979). This time lapse is a reflection of the length of exposure necessary for phototherapy to exhibit its effectiveness. The American Academy of Pediatrics (Bergman et al., 1994) adopted a new set of guidelines for the initiation of phototherapy and exchange transfusion in the term, healthy newborn (Table 28–5). Suggested bilirubin levels for initiation of therapy based on birth weight, including very low birth weight, are found on a chart devised by King and Jung (1990) (Fig. 28–12). Recommended levels for the use of phototherapy or exchange transfusion must be adjusted downward in the presence of prematurity, acidosis, hypoxia, respiratory distress, asphyxia, and neurologic decompensation (Fig. 28–13).

Although administration of intravenous immune globulin (IVIG) to the mother has produced contradictory results (Chitkara et al., 1990; de la Camara et al., 1988), its administration to infants with Rh hemolytic disease may be beneficial (Rubo et al., 1992). When IVIG was given to a group of infants with Rh incompatibility, it was associated with a reduction in the rate of exchange transfusion to 12.5 percent in comparison to 69 percent in the control group. It is hypothesized that IVIG may interfere with receptors in the reticuloendothelium that are required to induce hemolysis. The optimal dosage still needs to be determined, but 500 mg/kg was administered in the study by Rubo and associates.

On the other hand, administration of albumin to an infant undergoing phototherapy may reduce the amount of bilirubin available in the skin for photoisomerization. In an attempt to saturate the increased available albumin binding sites, free bilirubin is drawn into the vascular compartment from the skin, where phototherapy exerts its effect. For this reason, use of albumin in the infant undergoing phototherapy should be carefully weighed.

Collaborative Management

Infants requiring phototherapy benefit most from blue light in the wavelength range at which photoisomerization occurs most efficiently, that is, 420 to 460 nm. In addition to appropriate wavelength, effective illumination must also be maintained. Spectroradiometric readings of 4 to 6 $\mu W/cm^2/nm$ are considered in

TABLE 28–5 Total Serum Bilirubin Levels and Recommended Therapy in Healthy Term Newborns

	Total Serum Bilirubin Level, mg/dL (μmol/L)			
Age, Hours	***Consider Phototherapy***	***Phototherapy***	***Exchange Transfusion if Intensive Phototherapy Fails***	***Exchange Transfusion and Intensive Phototherapy***
≤24	—	—	—	—
25–48	≥12 (170)	≥15 (260)	≥20 (340)	≥25 (430)
49–72	≥15 (260)	≥18 (310)	≥25 (430)	≥30 (510)
>72	≥17 (290)	≥20 (340)	≥25 (430)	≥30 (510)

From Bergman D., Cooley, J., Coombs, J., et al. (1994). American Academy of Pediatrics. Practice parameter: Management of hyperbilirubinemia in the healthy term newborn. *Pediatrics, 94*(4, Part 1), 558–561.

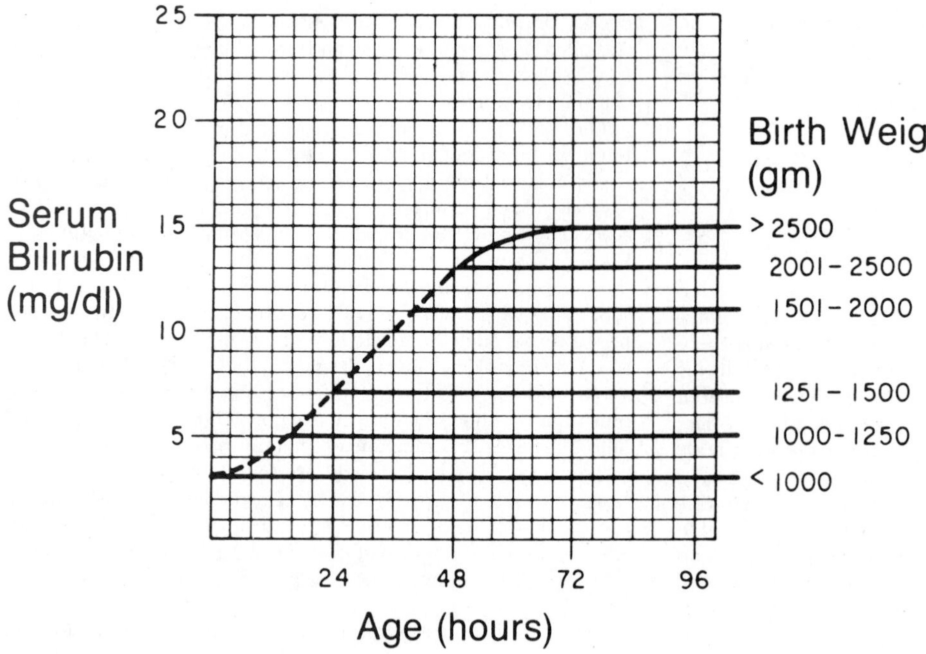

FIGURE 28–12. Suggested bilirubin levels for initiation of phototherapy in infants of various birth weights and postnatal ages. (From King, J., & Jung, A. [1990]. Phototherapy. In N. Nelson [Ed.], *Current therapy in neonatal-perinatal medicine* [p. 461]. Philadelphia: B. C. Decker.)

the effective therapeutic range. For optimal therapy, phototherapy units should be checked by nursing or bioengineering staff for adequate light levels with a radiometer before phototherapy is initiated and every 8 to 12 hours while lights are in use.

Because the effects of prolonged exposure to phototherapy lights can potentially cause retinal damage, infants undergoing phototherapy require eye protection. Phototherapy units and eye protection should be periodically removed throughout the day, however, to provide the infant with visual stimulation and interaction with parents and caregivers. The nursing staff should also be aware that they may experience headaches from prolonged exposure to phototherapy lights.

Infants undergoing phototherapy require temperature stabilization appropriate for their size and overall condition. A larger infant who is basically well can be nursed in an open crib; but the sick, premature, or low birth weight infant requires temperature control through the use of open warmers or closed incubators. Adequate fluid intake and compensatory fluid adjustments for increased insensible water loss may be required to prevent dehydration in these infants. While the infant is receiving photother-

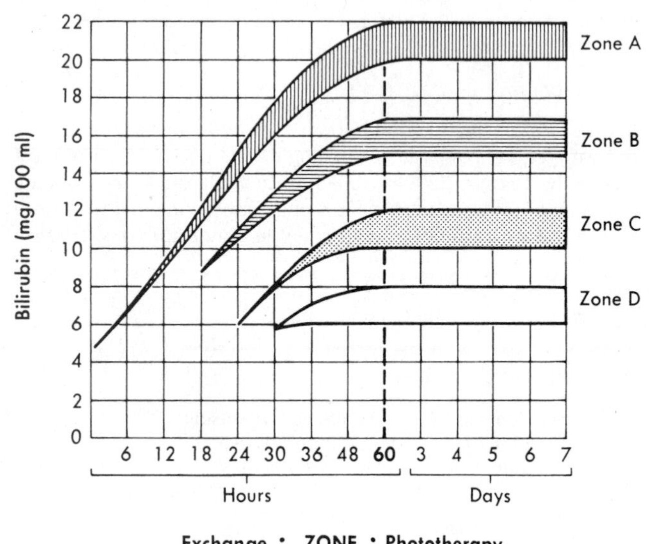

FIGURE 28–13. The rate of increase of bilirubin levels, gestational age, and the newborn's general condition determine the form of treatment for hyperbilirubinemia and the rapidity of its initiation. This chart is a useful guideline for the initiation of phototherapy or exchange transfusion in hyperbilirubinemic infants. (From Pernoll, M., Benda, G., & Babson, S. [1986]. Neonatal hyperbilirubinemia and prevention of kernicterus. *Diagnosis and management of the fetus and neonate at risk* [5th ed., p. 278]. St. Louis: C. V. Mosby.)

apy, bilirubin levels must be monitored frequently to assess the need for exchange transfusion and effectiveness of therapy. Because phototherapy lights can alter blood bilirubin results, the lights should be turned off during blood draws for serum bilirubin determinations.

Many hyperbilirubinemic infants who are healthy and not in need of thermoregulation or exchange transfusion can easily be cared for at home. Their parents must have access to home phototherapy equipment and a medical supply company to service the equipment as well as the support of their medical caregiver. If the infant can remain normothermic in an open crib without clothing, home phototherapy should be considered a cost-effective alternative to hospitalization. The same precautions regarding protective eye covering and adequate fluid intake must be observed in these infants. Required frequent blood samples for bilirubin levels can be drawn on a daily basis at the physician's office or neighborhood hospital laboratory or by a home health care worker.

Pharmacologic Agents

Phenobarbital is thought to accelerate bilirubin excretion by increasing its uptake and conjugation by the liver and increasing its excretion by enhancing bile flow. However, no increased benefit is noted that cannot be achieved with phototherapy alone. No medications have been approved in the United States as therapy for the inhibition of bilirubin synthesis, but clinical trials have preliminarily shown that metalloporphyrin may be effective in controlling hyperbilirubinemia in the term and preterm infant. Metalloporphyrins are inhibitors of heme oxygenase, the enzyme involved in the degradation of heme to biliverdin, an intermediate in the synthesis of bilirubin. Tin-mesoporphyrin and tin-protoporphyrin are the two heme oxygenase inhibitors used in clinical trials as a prophylaxis and as treatment (Kappas et al., 1988; Valaes et al., 1994). Although these studies have shown beneficial effects, they are still in the initial stages.

Exchange Transfusion

If bilirubin levels start to approach those associated with kernicterus in spite of phototherapy, exchange transfusion may be necessary to protect the CNS status of the jaundiced infant. The object of this procedure is to remove bilirubin and the antibody-coated RBCs from the newborn's circulation. In addition, an exchange transfusion removes some of the circulating maternal antibodies and Rh-positive fetal RBCs and normalizes the hematocrit. After a single-volume exchange, 75 percent of the newborn's RBC mass is removed; a double-volume exchange removes 85 to 90 percent of the cells (Valaes, 1963). However, bilirubin removal is much less effective; only 25 percent of the infant's total body bilirubin is removed during a double-volume exchange. This probably occurs because the major portion of bilirubin is in the extravascular compartment, an area not affected by the exchange of blood volume. Rebound in bilirubin levels occurs within 1 hour of the exchange, with post-transfusion levels rising as high as 55 percent of pre-exchange values (Valaes, 1963).

Although EBF remains the main condition requiring the use of exchange transfusion, this procedure can also be used in cases of sepsis to reduce levels of circulating endotoxins while supplying needed neutrophils and in anemia-induced congestive heart failure to re-establish a normal hematocrit without further volume overloading of the infant. The mortality rate for exchange transfusions is 1 percent. This rate includes death during the procedure or within 6 hours after its completion but excludes hydropic, kernicteric, or moribund infants (Gartner & Lee, 1992).

The following criteria are used to determine the need for and timing of exchange transfusions, particularly in infants with EBF (Bergman et al., 1994; Bowman, 1988):

1. Cord blood bilirubin level greater than 4.5 mg/dl in term infants and 3.5 mg/dl in preterm infants.
2. Hemoglobin level less than 8 g/dl and bilirubin level greater than 6 mg/dl within 1 hour of delivery in a term infant.
3. Hemoglobin level less than 11.5 g/dl and bilirubin level greater than 3.5 mg/dl within 1 hour of delivery in a preterm infant.
4. Increase in bilirubin levels by 0.5 mg/dl/h despite phototherapy.
5. Bilirubin level greater than 20 to 25 mg/dl in an uncompromised term infant (see Table 28–5), 18 mg/dl in the high-risk term newborn, and 10 to 18 mg/dl in the preterm infant, depending on gestational age and condition (Table 28–6).
6. Bilirubin level greater than 10 to 17 mg/dl in the stressed or very immature preterm infant, 10 to 12 mg/dl if hypoxia and acidosis are present.

Identical criteria are used to determine the need for repeated exchange transfusion.

Preparation of an Infant for an Exchange Transfusion

The infant undergoing an exchange transfusion should be prepared in a manner that produces the most benefit from the procedure without exposure to unnecessary risks. A double-volume exchange is usually done as soon as the need arises and the infant's condition permits. There are several ways in which an exchange can be done. The most common methods use umbilical artery catheters and umbilical vein catheters, although central venous and peripheral arterial lines can also be used. One procedure uses the intermittent push–pull method in which an aliquot of the infant's blood is withdrawn and replaced with an aliquot of donor blood. This can be done with use of one or two indwelling lines. Another method is the constant infusion of donor blood through the umbilical or peripheral vein and the constant withdrawal of the infant's blood through an umbilical artery. This method provides for more consistent arterial blood pressure. When peripheral arterial lines are used, blood can be withdrawn from them but should be returned by a central or peripheral venous line to prevent arterial spasm and clotting of the line.

The placement of the umbilical vein catheter is important to the provision of adequate splanchnic blood flow to the bowel. Infusion of large quantities of blood containing desaturated hemoglobin could result in ischemic injury to the bowel wall mucosa, with subsequent necrosis and sloughing of the mucosa. Such injury can predispose the infant to bowel wall ischemia, necrotizing enterocolitis, and perforation. Proper placement of

TABLE 28–6 Maximal Total Serum Bilirubin Concentration Allowed Before Exchange Transfusion

	Total Serum Bilirubin Concentration (mg/dL)	
Birth Weight Category (g)	***Uncomplicated Course***	***Complicated Course***
<1000	10	10
1000 to 1249	13	10
1250 to 1499	15	13
1500 to 1999	17	15
2000 to 2500	18	17
2500 and up	25	20

From Gartner, L., & Lee, K. (1992). Jaundice and liver disease. In A. Fanaroff & R. Martin (Eds.), *Behrman's neonatal-perinatal medicine: Vol. II* (5th ed., p. 1093). St. Louis: Mosby–Year Book.

the umbilical vein catheter above the diaphragm would decrease the potential risk for ischemic injury, but passing the catheter beyond the liver still generates the risk for liver damage and cardiac arrhythmias.

Before and during an exchange, albumin can be administered to infants considered to have low reserves of albumin binding sites (Bowman, 1988). Its administration is thought to provide more available binding sites for circulating free bilirubin and bilirubin deposited in the extravascular compartment. Theoretically, albumin should implement movement of bilirubin into the intravascular space, where it can be removed during an exchange transfusion. The recommended dosage is 1 g/kg of 25% albumin administered 1 to 2 hours before the exchange. Because intravascular albumin rapidly equilibrates with the extravascular compartment, its administration could potentially increase the amount of bilirubin pulled out of the plasma and into the tissue. For this reason, albumin administration before or during an exchange remains controversial. In the presence of severe anemia, hydrops, or congestive heart failure, use of albumin is contraindicated.

Selection of Blood Products

Selection and preparation of blood products are aimed at (1) decreasing antigen–antibody reaction, thus preventing hemolysis and additional bilirubin production; (2) removing toxic substances or endotoxins; (3) substituting a higher, more efficient circulating RBC volume for a low RBC mass; and (4) preventing biochemical imbalances caused by blood products during the exchange transfusion.

When exchange is imperative shortly after birth, O-negative blood crossmatched against the mother is usually used. The cells may need to be partially packed if anemia is significant and congestive heart failure is present. If exchange is not urgent, the blood used in Rh incompatibility can be type specific and Rh-negative. If the exchange is done for ABO incompatibility, O-type Rh-specific or low-titer (low anti-A and anti-B) O-type cells suspended in AB plasma can be used. Infants who are immunocompromised or have received intrauterine transfusions and are at risk for graft-versus-host reaction or who are born in areas where the incidence of cytomegalovirus infection is high should be exchanged with irradiated blood. This eliminates the possibility of giving WBCs, particularly lymphocytes, in the transfused blood.

Blood used for exchange transfusion should be as fresh as possible, preferably less than 48 hours old, to prevent problems associated with elevated potassium levels. When blood is older than 72 hours, the membrane of the RBC becomes more permeable, allowing intracellular potassium to leak out of the cell. In time, this phenomenon, coupled with normal RBC hemolysis, increases the amount of potassium in banked blood. Problems with arrhythmias and sudden cardiac death have been attributed to elevated potassium levels in transfused blood (Baumgart & Kim, 1988). If blood less than 48 hours old is not available, reconstituting RBC concentrates less than 7 days old with fresh frozen plasma is an alternative. This preparation not only ensures adequate oxygen-carrying capacity of the RBC but also provides a greater measure of safety in regard to potassium levels compared with whole blood older than 48 hours. It is also recommended that RBC concentrates older than 4 days be washed to further remove excess potassium.

Because of the unpredictable nature of potassium levels in banked blood, it is advisable to measure the level in the donor blood before its use. In one study measuring banked blood preserved with citrate–phosphate–dextrose (CPD), 21 percent of 28 units less than 4 days old had potassium levels of 11 mEq/L or higher (Scanlon & Krakaur, 1980). However, receiving blood with an elevated potassium content may not necessarily increase the serum potassium levels of these infants from their pretransfusion levels (Barnard et al., 1980).

Physiologic Effects of Exchange Transfusion

Exchange transfusion has a marked effect on the cardiovascular status and the intravascular compartment, which is reflected in pressure changes, volume fluctuations, and biochemical balance.

INTRAVASCULAR PRESSURE AND VOLUME CHANGES

Significant fluctuation in blood pressure and heart rate can occur during an exchange transfusion; rapid blood withdrawal causes greater pressure drops (Aranda & Sweet, 1977). With slow blood exchange—3 minutes for one exchange cycle (withdrawal and replacement of an aliquot)—the blood pressure drops but returns to baseline during the infusion cycle. However, in a rapid exchange cycle lasting 45 to 60 seconds, the pressure drops, then rises, but does not return to baseline. At aliquots of 5 ml/kg every 3 minutes, an average exchange should take approximately 100 to 110 minutes.

Because cardiac return and output drop during hypotension, the risk for decreased ileocolonic blood flow due to sustained arterial hypotension exists during an exchange transfusion. When an umbilical vein catheter is used for blood infusion, a rise in portal venous pressure during the injection phase can also result in diminished colonic blood flow at the end of injection (Touloukian et al., 1973). Regardless of the cause of gut hypoperfusion, ischemic damage of the intestinal mucosa can occur, resulting in necrotizing enterocolitis and perforation (Aranda & Sweet, 1977). Difficult or traumatic insertion or prolonged placement of the umbilical vein catheter can also lead to thrombosis of the portal vein and infection.

Because changes in mean arterial and intracranial pressures seem to parallel each other, exchange transfusion can also affect cerebral blood flow (Bada et al., 1979). When arterial pressure decreases in response to blood withdrawal and increases in response to infusion, intracranial pressure changes accordingly, a reflection of the immature autoregulatory mechanisms of neonatal cerebral blood flow. Marked fluctuations in intracranial pressure, especially in the preterm infant, can predispose these infants to the risk for intraventricular and intracerebral hemorrhage.

ELECTROCARDIOGRAM CHANGES

During exchange transfusion, cardiac conduction abnormalities can occur. The precise reasons for these electrocardiogram changes are unclear because several causative factors are concurrently present. Placement of the umbilical vein catheter, changes in blood volume due to removal and infusion of blood, and fluctuations in blood pressure can contribute to the occurrence of arrhythmias or electrocardiographic changes. The most common problems encountered include P wave elevation, tachycardia, bradycardia, ST segment changes, and abnormal QRS complex.

METABOLIC DISTURBANCES

The common anticoagulants used to preserve banked blood are ACD (acid–citrate–dextrose), CPD, CPD–adenine, and heparin. Heparin is not widely used because it has a limited shelf life and predisposes its receiver to a state of hypocoagulability. However, it does not cause rebound hypoglycemia, acidosis, and hypocalcemia seen with use of the other three preparations. The citrate found in blood preserved with ACD and CPD binds calcium, and if it is not metabolized quickly, as is the case in the preterm or seriously ill infant, it can lead to acidosis and hypocalcemia. Blood preserved with CPD and CPD–adenine is actually used more frequently because it contains half the acid load of ACD-preserved blood. Blood preserved with CPD–adenine has the longest shelf life.

Controversy regarding the use of calcium supplementation and correction of acidosis during an exchange still exists (Baumgart & Kim, 1988). Although the total serum calcium level may be lowered, the ionized calcium level does not change during an exchange transfusion (Baumgart & Kim, 1988). However, if the initial ionized calcium level is low or drops during the exchange, or if electrocardiographic symptoms of hypocalcemia occur, administration of 100 to 200 mg of calcium gluconate is recommended. Blood calcium levels are only transiently raised by the administration of calcium supplements (Fig. 28–14).

Excess heating of blood during an exchange produces hemolysis, resulting in elevated serum potassium levels. If the hemolysis is severe, it may produce effects similar to a transfusion reaction and could lead to death. High serum potassium levels can also cause arrhythmias and cardiac arrest. Potassium levels should be monitored closely before, during, and after exchange. In the infant who is already hyperkalemic, it may be beneficial to screen the donor blood for its potassium level before the transfusion is started.

Because the dextrose concentration used in blood preservation is equivalent to 300 mg of glucose per liter of blood, rebound hypoglycemia can occur shortly after completion of an exchange transfusion. The compensatory insulin release requires adequate supplemental glucose if hypoglycemia is to be avoided. Blood glucose levels should be monitored during and after the exchange.

ALTERATION OF PHARMACOKINETICS

Exchange transfusion alters blood levels of certain medications. The two determining factors are the timing of doses in relation to the start of the exchange and the rate of metabolism of the medication. The following medications were evaluated for the percentage of decrease after single-volume and double-volume exchanges (Lackner, 1982):

Drug	Single (percentage loss)	Double (percentage loss)
Ampicillin	7.7	14.2
Gentamicin	5.2	10.1
Digoxin	1.2	2.4
Phenobarbital	6.4	12.3
Vancomycin	5.7	11.0

Medications with altered blood levels as a consequence of exchange transfusion should be scheduled for administration after completion of the exchange. Drug levels may prove helpful in determining the need for supplemental medication doses.

HEMATOLOGIC CHANGES

In the term newborn, the neutrophil count drops during the early phase of exchange transfusion but rises rapidly within hours after completion of the procedure (Phibbs, 1970). This phenomenon also occurs in the preterm infant, but the subsequent rise is more gradual (Prindull & Prindull, 1970). The neutrophil increase does not seem to be bone marrow–mediated in either group, because there is no increase in the immature forms of neutrophils (Mantalenaki-Asfi et al., 1975). The increase is suspected to occur through the release of neutrophils from storage pools or from demargination of cells from the vascular walls.

Collaborative Management of the Infant Undergoing an Exchange Transfusion

In addition to the general nursing care required by a sick infant, specific stabilization procedures are necessary for a successful exchange transfusion. A sample protocol for required care during an exchange is presented in Table 28–7; the salient points are summarized here.

1. The infant should be in the most stable cardiorespiratory status possible. This includes maintenance of an adequate airway, stable blood gas values reflecting adequate ventilation, and continuous monitoring of vital signs.
2. The infant should be placed in an open warmer with continuous monitoring of temperature to ensure adequate thermoregulation during the procedure. To prevent dislodgment of catheters and intravenous lines or contamination of the sterile field, the infant's extremities should be restrained. Drapes should be placed in a manner that permits observation of the infant without compromising warmth or sterility.
3. Pre-exchange laboratory data should include blood type and crossmatch; direct and indirect Coombs' tests; electrolyte determinations; bilirubin, calcium, and glucose levels; and hematocrit. All blood work except type, crossmatch, and

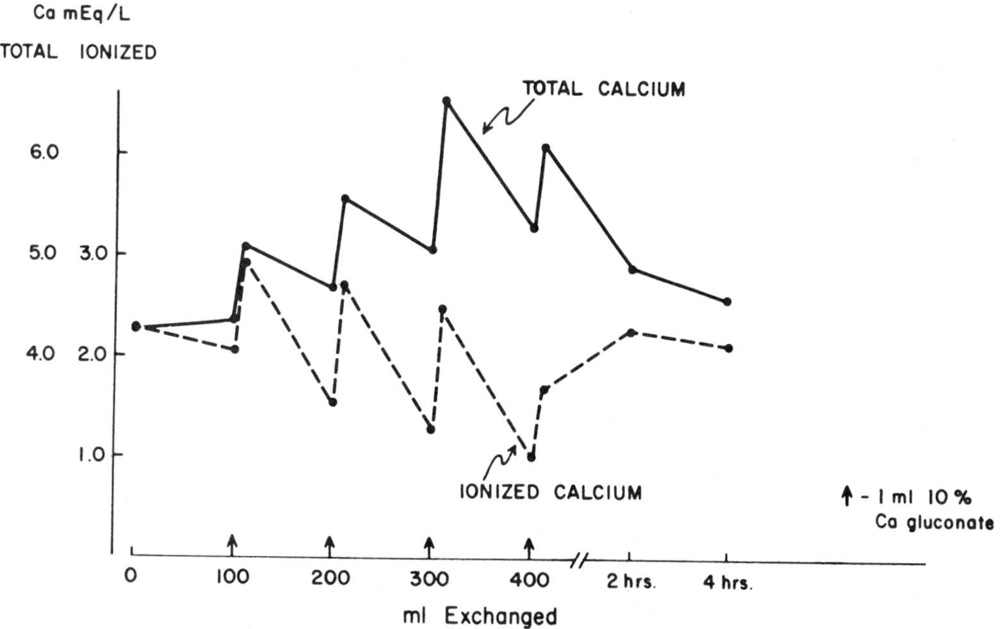

FIGURE 28–14. The administration of calcium gluconate during exchange transfusion temporarily increases the ionized calcium level, but this response is not sustained. (From Maisels, M., Li, T., Piechockin, J., & Werthman, M. W. [1974]. The effect of exchange transfusion on serum ionized calcium. *Pediatrics, 53,* 683.)

TABLE 28–7 Nursing Procedure for Care of an Infant During an Exchange Transfusion

Patient Care Services Primary Children's Medical Center

Procedure	
Section: Unit 7–Specialized Care	
Title: Procedure for Exchange Transfusion	
Origination date: April 1978 Review dates: 3/80, 12/82, 3/83, 5/86, 4/89, 11/91, 4/95 OSHA Classification: I	Author: Protocol Committee Reviewer: Protocol Committee

Purpose

To outline the nursing responsibilities during an exchange transfusion

Supportive Data

Indications for an exchange transfusion:

- To regulate antibody–antigen levels
- To remove toxins significantly concentrated in the blood and not otherwise removable
- To correct life-threatening electrolyte and fluid imbalance
- To regulage the level and type of hemoglobin
- To treat coagulation defects not remedied by single-component replacement

The infant should be NPO at least 3 hours before the procedure with hydration by a separate intravenous line. If the patient has not been NPO for 3 hours, an oral-gastric tube must be placed and any stomach contents aspirated back. A type and crossmatch for 1 unit of whole blood should be ready. The physician or neonatal nurse practitioner inserts a line for the exchange transfusion. The normal range for warmer blood with our blood-warming unit is 36.5°C to 37.5°C. If this range is exceeded, the alarm will sound, and the machine should be exchanged with another from Central Supply. If the tubing has been filled with blood, it cannot be transferred to a new machine. It will leak in the process. New tubing is needed for a new blood-warming unit.

The first aliquot of blood withdrawn is usually sent for bilirubin and miscellaneous laboratory determinations. The volume exchanged is usually 160 mL/kg in full-term infants and 180 mL/kg in premature infants in passes of 5 to 10 mL (double-volume exchange). The final aliquot of blood out can be used for bilirubin, hematocrit, and other laboratory tests as ordered.

Equipment List

- Open warmer and skin temperature probe
- 1 unit whole blood typed and crossmatched to the patient
- Blood warmer and tubing (from Central Supply)
- Exchange transfusion tray
- Equipment for umbilical artery or umbilical vein catheter insertion
- Cardiac monitor

Content

- Follow universal precautions.
- Place nasogastric tube if needed.
- Immobilize extremities during the procedure.
- Turn the blood warmer on. Push the on/off toggle switch past "on" to check the alarm. Hold the switch in this position a few seconds. A beep will sound and an "A" will flash on the screen. If these alarm functions do not work, obtain another blood warmer.
- Unlatch doors—open carefully.
- Remove blood-warming set from package and insert into warmer. (Directions for tubing insertion are detailed on the back of the tubing package and in the hospital *General Nursing Procedure Book*.) The tubing must be in the warmer and the latch closed before blood is run through the tubing.
- Attach male end of blood-warming tubing to extension tube of stopcock assembly from transfusion tray.
- Attach separate extension tube to stopcock assembly and hang down into waste blood container (included in transfusion tray).
- Monitor vital signs every 15 minutes for the first hour, then every 30 minutes for the next 3 hours. These are recorded on the transfusion record. The infant's general condition is monitored continuously during the procedure by the nurse.
- Notify the physician or neonatal nurse practitioner performing the exchange transfusion when each 100 mL of blood has been exchanged.

Documentation

Document the following on the transfusion record sheet.

- Vital signs
- Aliquots of blood in and out
- Laboratory specimens

Document the following in nursing notes and flow sheet:

- Preparations before the exchange
- How the patient tolerated the procedure
- Presence or absence of complications

Exceptions/Complications

The possibilities of complications during exchange transfusions are numerous; therefore, the following is a list of possible complications and possible reasons for them.

- Heart failure—due to transfusion overload if blood volume is miscalculated.
- Cardiac arrest—due to hyperkalemia or hypocalcemia. Citrate added to donor blood as an anticoagulant combines with ionized calcium to produce hypocalcemia. After 100 mL of blood has been exchanged, calcium gluconate (96 mg/mL) may be given to counteract the effects of calcium binding by the preservative.
- Irregular cardiac rhythm—due to contact of catheter tip with myocardium or caused by rapid injection of blood directly into the heart when the catheter is in too deeply, infusion with unwarmed blood, or electrolyte imbalance.
- Air embolus—due to large amounts of air sucked into the catheter if the infant gasps deeply when an umbilical vein catheter is used and the catheter is placed within the thorax or air bubbles are injected during the procedure.
- Perforation of umbilical vein or artery—during attempts to force passage of the catheter.
- Bacterial infection—due to poor technique or contaminated donor blood.
- Acidemia—due to the fact that the pH of donor blood is often 6.8 or less.
- Hyperglycemia followed by hypoglycemia—donor blood contains dextrose, which may lead to hyperglycemia, followed by hypoglycemia when dextrose is used up by the infant's system. Implications are to check dextrose frequently and observe for signs and symptoms of hyperglycemia or hypoglycemia. A peripheral intravenous line may be needed throughout the procedure to prevent a drop in blood glucose levels during the exchange. Monitor glucose level every hour for 4 hours after the exchange as ordered. Feedings may be resumed 4 hours after transfusion if the infant is stable.
- Transfusion reaction—especially when untyped and unmatched blood is given. Rare in newborns. Watch for temperature elevation, rash, and dark urine.

References

Fletcher, M. A., & MacDonald, M. G. (1993). *Atlas of procedures in neonatology*. Philadelphia: J. B. Lippincott.

Goetzman, B. W., & Wennberg, R. P. (1991). *Neonatal intensive care handbook* (2nd ed.). St. Louis: Mosby–Year Book.

Sherman-Streeter, N. (1986). *High risk neonatal care*. Rockville: Aspen.

Modified from Primary Children's Medical Center. (1995). *Nursing procedure manual*. Salt Lake City, UT.

Coombs' tests should be repeated midway through and at the completion of the exchange.

4. Necessary catheters and lines should be placed and kept patent with appropriate intravenous fluids until the procedure begins. Most central venous, umbilical artery catheter, and umbilical vein catheter lines can be kept open with 5 or 10 percent dextrose solutions. Normal saline or 0.45 percent saline solutions can be infused through peripheral arterial lines. The addition of calcium and electrolytes should be dictated by the infant's metabolic status.
5. Blood administration sets should be assembled and placed on a blood warmer set at the manufacturer's recommended temperature. If a blood warmer is not used, donor blood should be allowed to reach room temperature before use. Parental consent for blood transfusion and exchange transfusion should be obtained beforehand.
6. Vital signs should be taken before the procedure begins and at 15-minute intervals thereafter. Cardiorespiratory and blood pressure monitoring should be continuous throughout the procedure. If the infant is on a ventilator or receiving oxygen, transcutaneous carbon dioxide and saturation monitors should be used, with blood gas sampling before, during, and after the procedure. The infant should be carefully observed for any signs of congestive failure, respiratory or circulatory deterioration, or adverse blood reactions.
7. Accurate tally of blood withdrawal and infusion and medication administration during the procedure should be kept. Blood is usually exchanged in aliquots of 10 to 20 ml for a term infant and 5 to 10 ml for a severely anemic, hydropic, or preterm infant.
8. Readjustment of medication schedules, based on completion time of the exchange, may be required. Drug levels may be needed to evaluate this.
9. The infant will require the resumption of phototherapy and observation of postprocedural vital signs every 15 minutes for approximately 2 hours or until stable.

Anemia

Pathophysiology

During the neonatal period, several abnormalities can evoke both acute and chronic anemia in the newborn. These forms of anemia often precede, and are independent of, the natural propensity toward physiologic anemia that exists as a common entity among all infants, both term and preterm. The most common conditions that can trigger the presence of these pathologic anemias are acute or chronic episodes of hemorrhage, acute or chronic RBC destruction and hemolysis, and blood sampling for laboratory analysis.

The presence of anemia, defined in RBC volume rather than by hematocrit, is associated with increased mortality rates in both term and preterm infants. RBC volume is determined by multiplying the blood volume per kilogram times the hematocrit. The average blood volume of the term newborn is estimated at 82 to 85 ml/kg; blood volume in the preterm infant approaches 100 ml/kg as gestational age decreases (Brown, 1988b). The following is a sample calculation of RBC volume in an 800-g infant with 100 ml/kg blood volume and hematocrit of 25 percent:

$$100 \times 0.25 = 25 \text{ ml/kg RBC volume}$$

On the basis of a study by Faxelius and colleagues (1977), it is estimated that 25 percent of all infants admitted to the neonatal intensive care unit (NICU) have RBC volumes less than 25 ml/kg. In the overall population of infants admitted to the NICU with such low blood volumes, the mortality rate is 58 percent, compared with 20 percent in infants with RBC volumes greater than 25 ml/kg. In infants less than 1500 g with blood volumes less than 25 ml/kg, the mortality rate rises to 89 percent.

Clinical Manifestations

Acute Anemia

The physical presentation of acute anemia is more intense than that seen in the chronic form, because the causes of acute anemia (Table 28–8) are more emergent, life threatening, and disruptive to the homeostasis of the infant. The resulting cardiovascular collapse, followed closely by respiratory failure, can overwhelm the neonate who possesses only marginal reserves. Immediate intervention and replacement of lost intravascular volume are often required to achieve stabilization. An infant experiencing an acute anemic episode, with hemorrhage being the most common cause, exhibits symptoms reflecting compromise of the cardiorespiratory system: shock, poor peripheral perfusion, poor respiratory effort or respiratory distress, tachycardia, pallor, lethargy, and hypotension. Before signs of acute anemia become apparent, the hemoglobin level needs to precipitously fall to a level of less than 12 g/dl (Oski, 1993).

TABLE 28–8 Causes of Acute Anemia in the Newborn

Obstetrical Accidents, Malformations of the Placenta and Cord
Rupture of a normal umbilical cord
Precipitous delivery
Entanglement
Hematoma of the cord or placenta
Rupture of an abnormal umbilical cord
Varices
Aneurysm
Rupture of anomalous vessels
Aberrant vessel
Velamentous insertion
Communicating vessels in multilobed placenta
Incision of placenta during cesarean section
Placenta previa
Abruptio placentae
Occult Hemorrhage Before Birth
Fetoplacental
Tight nuchal cord
Cesarean section
Placental hematoma
Fetomaternal
Traumatic amniocentesis
After external cephalic version, manual removal of placenta, use of oxytocin
Spontaneous
Chorioangioma of the placenta
Choriocarcinoma
Twin-to-twin
Chronic
Acute
Internal Hemorrhage
Intracranial
Giant cephalhematoma, subgaleal, caput succedaneum
Adrenal
Retroperitoneal
Ruptured liver, ruptured spleen
Pulmonary
Iatrogenic Blood Loss

From Oski, F., & Naiman, J. (1982). Anemia in the neonatal period. In F. Oski & J. Naiman (Eds.), *Hematologic problems in the newborn* (p. 57). Philadelphia: W. B. Saunders.

Acute blood loss results in a recognizable sequence of symptoms based on the amount of volume loss (Oski & Naiman, 1982a):

- 7.5 to 15 percent volume loss: Little change is noted in heart rate and blood pressure, but the stroke volume and subsequent cardiac output are decreased. Peripheral vasoconstriction occurs, resulting in decreased blood flow to skeletal muscles, gut, and carcass.
- 20 to 25 percent volume loss: Hypotension and shock become apparent. Cardiac output is decreased, and peripheral vasoconstriction is present. Low tissue oxygen levels and acidosis become apparent.

Chronic Anemia

Prolonged or chronic anemia may not require rapid intravascular volume expansion, but it is by no means completely benign (Table 28–9), as in the case of EBF or chronic twin-to-twin transfusion. In both of these conditions, infants may require removal of intravascular volume and replacement with volume of a higher hematocrit before stabilization is achieved. Because these infants have had considerable time to adjust to chronic blood loss or hemolysis, the changes in vital signs may reflect poor oxygen-carrying capacity rather than hypovolemia. On physical examination, pallor is usually accompanied by hepatosplenomegaly, a reflection of the body's attempt to compensate for blood loss through extramedullary hematopoiesis. The blood smear may also reflect the long-standing nature of the problem; RBCs appear hypochromic and small, and the number of immature RBCs is increased.

TABLE 28–9 Causes of Chronic Anemia in the Newborn

Immune
- Rh incompatibility
- ABO incompatibility
- Minor blood group incompatibility
- Maternal autoimmune hemolytic anemia
- Drug-induced hemolytic anemia

Infection
- Bacterial sepsis
- Congenital infections
  - Syphilis
  - Malaria
  - Cytomegalovirus
  - Rubella
  - Toxoplasmosis
  - Disseminated herpes

Disseminated intravascular coagulation

Macroangiopathic and microangiopathic hemolytic anemias
- Cavernous hemangioma
- Large-vessel thrombi
- Renal artery stenosis
- Severe coarctation of aorta

Galactosemia

Prolonged or recurrent acidosis of a metabolic or respiratory nature

Hereditary disorders of the red cell membrane
- Hereditary spherocytosis
- Hereditary elliptocytosis
- Hereditary stomatocytosis
- Other rare membrane disorders

Pyknocytosis

Red cell enzyme deficiencies
- Most common are glucose-6-phosphate dehydrogenase deficiency, pyruvate kinase deficiency, 5′-nucleotidase deficiency, and glucose-6-phosphate isomerase deficiency

Alpha-thalassemia syndrome

Alpha chain structural abnormalities

Gamma-thalassemia syndromes

Gamma chain structural abnormalities

From Oski, F., & Naiman, J. (1982). Anemia in the neonatal period. In F. Oski & J. Naiman (Eds.), *Hematologic problems in the newborn* (p. 74). Philadelphia: W. B. Saunders.

Common Causes of Pathologic Anemia in the Newborn

Hemorrhage

Fetal-Maternal Transfusion Caused by Transplacental Hemorrhage

This phenomenon occurs in approximately 50 to 75 percent of all pregnancies and can be an acute or chronic process (Bowman, 1988; Jones, 1969). An estimated 5.6 percent of pregnancies involve a fetal-maternal transfusion in the range of 11 to 30 ml of blood; another 1 percent involve an exchange of more than 30 ml (Ness et al., 1987). Fetal-maternal transfusions can be documented by the presence of fetal cells in maternal circulation with use of the erythrocyte rosette test and the Kleihauer-Betke acid elution test for fetal hemoglobin in maternal blood. The erythrocyte rosette test specifically detects fetal RBCs. The Kleihauer-Betke test consists of an acid wash of a maternal blood smear followed by staining. Fetal hemoglobin resists elution from intact RBCs in an acid solution. Intact cells containing fetal hemoglobin can be distinguished microscopically from adult erythrocytes. Presence of stained erythrocytes suggests contamination of maternal blood by fetal blood. This test is useful in identifying fetal RBCs in the mother's blood, provided that no underlying condition increases the amount of fetal hemoglobin in the mother's blood.

Twin-to-Twin Transfusion

This phenomenon, which can be both acute and chronic, occurs in 15 to 33 percent of all monochorionic (monozygotic) twins, in which the placentas tend to be fused. The anastomosis is usually between an artery of one placenta and the vein of the other, although vascular connections may be artery-to-artery or vein-to-vein (Oski & Naiman, 1982a, 1982d). In the chronic form of twin-to-twin transfusion, the size difference between twins can be helpful in determining the donor and the recipient. When the weight difference exceeds 20 percent, the smaller twin is always the donor (Tan et al., 1979). When the weight difference is less than 20 percent, either twin may be the donor. In such cases, hematocrit values provide help in determining donor and recipient. The donor twin is anemic, and the blood count reflects increased hematopoiesis as evidenced by an elevated reticulocyte count and increased numbers of immature RBCs. The recipient develops polycythemia but can exhibit signs of congestive heart failure and pulmonary or systemic hypertension. On analysis of laboratory data, there is usually a 5 g/dl difference between donor and recipient hemoglobin values. Stillbirths are common in twin-to-twin transfusion, with both twins being at risk.

Obstetrical Accidents

Many obstetrical problems, especially those occurring before labor and delivery, can result in chronic as well as acute blood loss. Long-standing problems, such as placenta previa or partial abruption, usually result in anemia. However, acute hemorrhage rather than anemia is the case in problems occurring at the time of delivery. Examples are severe abruption, severing of the placenta during cesarean section, or umbilical cord rupture due to sudden tension on a short or tangled cord. A tight nuchal cord can also decrease blood volume in a newborn by approximately

20 percent (Cashore & Usher, 1973). Holding a newly delivered infant above the placenta can also reduce the hematocrit and blood volume because of the gravitational drainage of blood from the newborn into the placenta.

Internal Hemorrhages

A drop in hematocrit during the first 24 to 72 hours that is not associated with hyperbilirubinemia is usually attributed to internal hemorrhage. Bleeding can occur in various parts of the body secondary to birth trauma or pre-existing anomalies. The areas of potential hemorrhage in the head include the subdural, subarachnoid, intraventricular, intracranial, and subperiosteal spaces. Infants can lose an estimated 10 to 15 percent of their blood during an intraventricular or intracranial hemorrhage. In cases of traumatic delivery or vacuum extraction, extensive scalp bleeding can result in significant blood loss that can be estimated by measuring the increase in the head circumference. Each centimeter of increase represents an estimated 38 ml of blood lost from the intravascular compartment. Hemorrhage can also occur into the liver, kidneys, spleen, or retroperitoneal space in association with traumatic and breech deliveries. Hepatic rupture occurs in approximately 1.2 to 5.6 percent of stillbirths and neonatal deaths; half of the hemorrhages are subcapsular. Infants with this disorder tend to be stable for 24 to 48 hours, then suddenly deteriorate. This deterioration seems to coincide with rupture of the capsule and hemoperitoneum. Hepatic rupture carries a poor prognosis, but rapid surgery preceded by multiple transfusions can save the infant. Splenic rupture is associated with severe EBF and should be suspected at the time of exchange transfusion if the central venous pressure is low rather than elevated. Signs of splenic rupture include scrotal swelling and peritoneal effusion without free air. Adrenal hemorrhage is seen more frequently in the infant of a diabetic mother and prediabetic mother and is characterized by the presence of a flank mass with bluish discoloration of the overlying skin.

Red Blood Cell Destruction and Hemolysis

Maternal-Fetal Blood Group Incompatibilities

Isoimmunization, as in ABO and Rh incompatibility, is responsible for the majority of cases of neonatal hemolysis. Decreased RBC life span resulting from hemolysis is usually associated with a rise in bilirubin level, 1 g of hemoglobin yielding 35 mg of bilirubin (Lemberge & Legge, 1949).

Acquired Defects of the Red Blood Cells

This hemolytic problem is seen in bacterial sepsis and viral infections, especially of the TORCH variety. Drug-induced RBC destruction, due to either maternal ingestion or direct administration of the drug to the newborn, is another common cause of hemolysis.

Congenital Defects of the Red Blood Cells

Defects resulting in destruction of the RBC can involve the cell membrane, enzymatic system, or hemoglobin component, as in glucose-6-phosphate dehydrogenase deficiency, thalassemia, and hereditary spherocytosis. Although these conditions can cause hemolysis in the newborn period, they are rare diseases.

Blood Sampling

Blood loss secondary to sampling is one of the two most frequent causes of chronic anemia in infants, the other being physiologic anemia of the newborn and premature infant. Among two groups of preterm infants admitted to NICUs, the average blood loss from sampling during the first 4 to 6 weeks of life was 46 to 50 ml/kg; severity of illness correlated with the amount of blood removed for sampling (Blanchette & Zipursky, 1984; Obladen et al., 1988). Prudent blood sampling may eliminate unnecessary blood volume depletion and decrease the need for replacement transfusion therapy. Accurate recording of blood lost to sampling can prove beneficial in the assessment of the circulatory status and volume needs of the sick infant.

Differential Diagnosis

History

Acute and chronic anemia can often be distinguished from each other and from other problems by analyzing the family history for the presence of anemia or jaundice. The maternal history should be carefully examined for evidence of drug ingestion during pregnancy that may affect RBC life span or production, bleeding during the pregnancy or labor, or other incidents surrounding the delivery that may contribute to blood loss in the newborn.

Laboratory Data

The type of anemia can often be identified on the basis of laboratory studies that evaluate RBC content and form.

1. Hematocrit and hemoglobin levels can define the type as well as the degree of anemia. Unlike in chronic anemia, blood loss during acute hemorrhage is rapid, with little evidence of compensatory hematopoiesis. RBCs are normal in size and have a normal hemoglobin mass, with no significant increase in the number of immature RBCs. Hemoglobin values may not initially reflect hemorrhage because the intravascular volume contracts and masks volume loss. It may take several hours for intravascular equilibration to occur before the hemoglobin accurately reflects the extent of the hemorrhage. The site of hemoglobin or hematocrit sampling is important in obtaining accurate information, because capillary sticks on an infant in shock reflect venous stasis. A more accurate sample at this time would be from an arterial or venous source.
2. Reticulocyte counts are useful in differentiating chronic and acute forms of anemia. Increased numbers of immature RBCs reflect the degree of hematopoietic activity in response to anemia. Increased hematopoiesis requires a time lapse between the occurrence of anemia and stimulation of the hematopoietic centers.
3. Peripheral blood smears are helpful in evaluating iron content and the size and shape of the RBC, which vary in different forms of anemia.
4. Blood typing, Rh determination, and Coombs' testing can help identify blood group incompatibilities as causes of anemia.

Treatment

Management of Acute Anemia

Stabilization of an infant with acute anemia includes the following:

1. Basic resuscitation of the infant experiencing precipitous blood loss often includes stabilization of the airway by means of intubation and ventilation.
2. Rapid line placement for fluid replacement, volume expansion, and blood sampling may necessitate use of the umbilical vein or artery. Central venous pressure can be helpful in

assessing the degree of volume loss and the quantity of needed replacement.

3. If acute volume expansion is required, low-titer type O-negative blood, plasma, albumin, or saline can initially be used in increments of 10 to 20 ml/kg until a type and crossmatch is available. If the infant responds to bolus infusion, this may indicate that hemorrhage is of an obstetrical nature and may justify repetition of another fluid bolus. Failure to respond may indicate ongoing internal hemorrhage.
4. Laboratory tests and physical examination should be initiated after stabilization of the infant to determine the cause of anemia and to rectify the problem.
5. Examination of the placenta, and maternal blood sample testing for the presence of fetal hemoglobin, may prove useful in determining the cause of the blood loss.

Collaborative Management of the Infant With Acute Anemia

As with all newborns, the principles of care that include the provision of warmth, monitoring of vital signs, and ongoing assessment and accurate determination of intake and output are essential to the well-being of the infant who has suffered acute blood loss. After initial stabilization, nursing care must include modifications that either eliminate recurrence of precipitous events or prevent further blood loss. Adequate knowledge of the principles and procedures surrounding volume expansion and use of blood products is required for providing safe care to such infants. A review of the use of blood products can be found at the conclusion of this chapter.

Collaborative Management of the Infant With Chronic Anemia

The major focus of therapy for the infant with chronic anemia is control or elimination of its cause. Several forms of anemia in term and preterm infants are linked to dietary deficiencies that can be eradicated by replacement therapy. Chronic forms of anemia requiring symptomatic therapy can also be treated with transfusion therapy and erythropoietin.

Dietary Supplementation

Three major dietary factors affecting RBC production are iron, folate, and vitamin E. Because all three increase in amount with increasing gestational age, premature birth predisposes the immature infant to anemia due to insufficiency.

In the newborn infant without benefit of iron supplementation, the hematopoiesis necessary to maintain a normal hemoglobin level depletes iron reserves by the time birth weight is doubled. Various factors can further contribute to subsequent iron deficiency anemia, such as low birth weight; low initial hemoglobin levels; and blood loss through trauma, hemorrhage, or sampling. In the term infant, exhaustion of iron reserves normally occurs by 20 to 24 weeks' postnatal age, but this happens much earlier in the preterm infant. Because iron stores needed for hemoglobin production are present in insufficient quantities at birth in the premature infant, these infants require supplementation during the first 2 to 4 months to prevent iron deficiency anemia.

Iron depletion, in any gestational age group, first becomes evident in decreased serum ferritin levels, a measure of accumulated iron stores, and in the disappearance of stainable iron from the bone marrow. Subsequent decrease in mean corpuscular volume of the RBC (i.e., the size of the RBC) is then followed by a drop in hemoglobin level. Although prophylactic iron supplementation will not prevent the initial fall in hemoglobin, administration of 1 to 2 mg/kg/day of supplemental iron should supply term and preterm infants with adequate reserves; 3 to 6 mg/kg/day is recommended in the iron-deficient infant or the infant receiving erythropoietin.

The relationship between serum ferritin levels and the administration of multiple transfusions to a population of newborn infants was evaluated to determine iron supplementation needs in this group. In a study by Arad and associates (1988), serum ferritin levels were measured in four groups of infants: (1) preterm infants transfused in excess of 100 ml of packed cells, (2) preterm infants transfused with less than 100 ml, (3) nontransfused preterm infants, and (4) nontransfused term infants. At 4 to 5 months of age, the preterm infants receiving more than 100 ml of RBCs had the highest ferritin levels of all four groups. This would suggest that low birth weight infants receiving large volumes of RBCs may amass iron stores sufficient for new RBC production during the first 4 to 5 months without the need for additional iron supplementation.

Folate is the generic description for folic acid and its related compounds. Folate is a component of the B-complex vitamins involved in the maturation of RBCs, particularly the synthesis of DNA, which controls nuclear maturation and division. Because bone marrow is among the body's most rapidly growing and proliferative tissue, its ability to produce RBCs is reduced during folic acid deficiency, producing a megaloblastic anemia. Folate is present in high quantities at birth in both term and preterm infants, but levels drop rapidly, especially in the low birth weight infant. It is estimated that approximately 68 percent of infants less than 1700 g have subnormal levels of folate at 1 to 3 months of age (Blanchette et al., 1994). However, only a few infants actually develop anemia. Human milk and soy-based products contain an adequate amount of natural folate, but commonly used commercial products must be artificially enriched. Premature infant formulas are adequately enriched to satisfy a premature infant's folate needs, provided that intake is sufficient. Because folate is absorbed in the duodenum and jejunum, any disease condition or medication that has an impact on the absorptive surface of these areas can impair folate absorption. A dosage of 50 μg/day is recommended to prevent folate deficiency in the premature infant (Goetzman & Wennberg, 1991).

Vitamin E, an antioxidant, is valuable in protecting the RBC membrane from destruction due to lipid peroxidation (Brown, 1988b). Deficiency of this nutrient shortens the life span of the cell by exposing the unprotected, unsaturated membrane lipids to peroxidation and hemolysis. Infants are born in a state of relative vitamin E deficiency that is more intense in the smaller and more premature infants. Vitamin E is required in increasing amounts as the intake of polyunsaturated fatty acids increases. Deficiency becomes apparent in infants of birth weights less than 1500 g at approximately 4 to 6 weeks of age, resulting in decreased hemoglobin levels ranging from 7 to 10 g/dl. Administration of iron supplementation in the presence of this deficiency intensifies the hemolytic response. Signs and symptoms, as with many neonatal diseases, mimic those of other disease entities that occur in the neonatal period. One of the more obvious symptoms is edema of the feet, lower extremities, and scrotal area. The RBC form may vary, but abnormalities usually include fragmented or irregularly shaped cells, presence of spherocytes, and thrombocytopenia. Treatment consists of 25 IU of vitamin E per day for 6 to 8 weeks for preterm infants (Goetzman & Wennberg, 1991).

Transfusion Therapy

Of preterm infants admitted to a NICU, approximately 90 percent receive one transfusion in the first 6 weeks of life; 50 percent receive cumulative transfusions in excess of their total circulating RBC mass (Blanchette & Zipursky, 1984; Levy et al., 1993). In determining which infants may need subsequent transfusions after the first 2 weeks of life, gestational age less than 30 weeks is the best predictor, regardless of severity of illness, number of transfusions during the first week, complications, or hematocrit at birth (Brown et al., 1990). Only 14 percent of infants more than 30 weeks' gestation require transfusions after 2 weeks of age.

Although the critically ill infant is generally maintained with a hematocrit of greater than 40 percent (Dear, 1984), the benefits of transfusion therapy in the convalescent infant remain controversial. When the effects of transfusion therapy in the convalescent infant are studied, the elimination of symptoms attributed to anemia is not a consistent finding. In premature infants with hematocrits less than 30 percent, apnea, bradycardia, dyspnea, feeding difficulties, poor weight gain despite good calorie intake, lethargy, tachypnea, tachycardia, and increased cardiac output and oxygen consumption appear to be relieved by transfusion therapy in some studies (DeMaio et al., 1986; Joshi et al., 1987). However, in a study by Keyes and colleagues (1989), there seemed to be no overall relationship between hematocrit values ranging from 19 to 64 percent and respiratory rate, heart rate, or the occurrence of apnea and bradycardia. In addition, there was no significant or predictable effect on any of these parameters after transfusion therapy. In a study by Blank and associates (1984), no change in the frequency of apnea or in weight gain was noted in infants with hemoglobin levels maintained at 10 g/dl or greater. Yet another study suggested that volume expansion may be the major factor in the elimination of abnormal respiratory patterns, not an increase in oxygen supply from increased hemoglobin levels (Bifano et al., 1992).

In light of all the controversy surrounding transfusions, evidence of impaired tissue oxygenation remains the ultimate criterion for the use of blood products. Lactic acid levels may prove helpful in determining which infants may benefit from transfusion therapy (Izraeli et al., 1993; Ross et al., 1989). When the oxygen-carrying capacity of hemoglobin is insufficient for tissue needs, anaerobic metabolism occurs, leading to excess lactic acid production. Monitoring lactic acid levels and transfusing only those infants with elevated levels may aid in establishing more sound criteria for transfusion therapy.

Several methods of blood preparation and use have been evaluated to minimize donor exposure and decrease the potential for transmitted disease. Studies suggest that packed RBCs with a shelf life of greater than 5 days, and up to 42 days, are safe for use in neonatal transfusions (Cook et al., 1993; Lee et al., 1995; Liu et al., 1994; Patten et al., 1991). This finding, combined with use of a sterile connection device allowing multiple aseptic entries into a unit of blood, would permit use of a designated unit for each infant at risk for multiple transfusions, thereby significantly reducing donor exposure (Lee et al., 1995; Liu et al., 1994).

Blood administered to the newborn is often irradiated, which causes cell membrane disruption and potassium leakage from the cell in time. The decision by the U.S. Food and Drug Administration to change its recommendations for the maximal storage time of irradiated blood from 42 to 28 days affects the length of use of a designated unit (Quinnan, 1993). Although older blood appears safe to administer, it is not recommended for rapid transfusions, administration of large aliquots, exchange transfusions, or treatment of coagulopathies.

An effective way to minimize donor exposure is through the establishment of transfusion criteria. These guidelines help determine which infants would benefit from transfusion on the basis of symptoms, hematocrit levels, and degree of illness.

Recombinant Human Erythropoietin Therapy

Cloning of the human erythropoietin (HuEPO) gene in 1985 resulted in the production of large quantities of HuEPO for use as an exogenous stimulant of erythroid progenitor cells in patients with anemia. The principal action of HuEPO is on the hematopoietic stem cells housed in the bone marrow that have been designated the colony-forming units–erythrocyte (CFU-E), the precursors of the RBC (Fig. 28–15). Studies from the United States and England have demonstrated the use of recombinant erythropoietin to be an effective replacement for transfusion therapy in raising the hemoglobin level in hyporegenerative anemia and end-stage renal disease (Eschbach et al., 1987; Winearls et al., 1986). Further studies of preterm infants have demonstrated that HuEPO maintains the hematocrit level during the phase of normal anemia of the premature infant, with good proliferation of erythroid progenitor cells in response to HuEPO (Rhondeau et al., 1988; Ross et al., 1989; Shannon et al., 1987).

HuEPO has not attained recognition as a standard of care for anemia of prematurity because clinical trials are still in progress to determine ideal dosages, appropriate timing of therapy, and effectiveness in infants of low and very low birth weight. Preliminary data suggest that preterm infants less than 34 weeks' gestation respond to HuEPO with increased blood levels of erythropoietin, reticulocytes, and RBC volume 2 to 3 weeks after the initiation of therapy (Halperin et al., 1989). The effective dose of HuEPO required to enhance erythropoiesis in the premature infant ranges from 300 to 1400 U/kg/week (Maier et al., 1994; Messer et al., 1993; Meyer et al., 1994; Ohls et al., 1995; Shannon et al., 1995).

HuEPO has been evaluated for its effectiveness as an alternative to transfusion therapy for treatment of anemia in premature infants resulting from (1) blood sampling, with administration beginning within the first 2 days of life (Maier et al., 1994; Ohls et al., 1995); (2) physiologic anemia of prematurity, with therapy starting at 1 to 4 weeks of age (Emmerson et al., 1993; Messer et al., 1993; Meyer et al., 1994; Shannon et al., 1995); and (3)

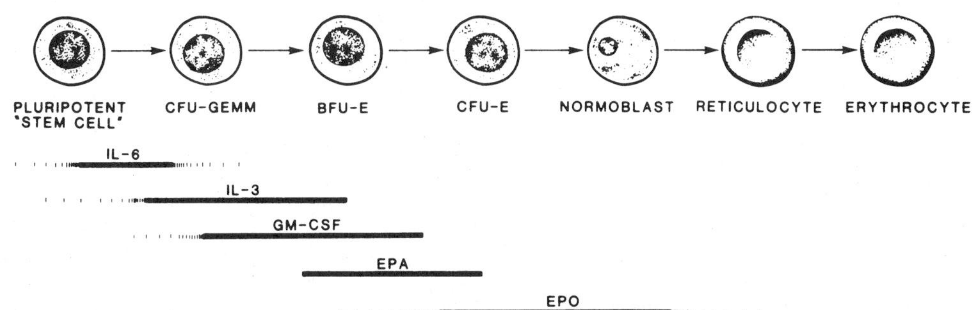

FIGURE 28–15. The principal action of human recombinant erythropoietin is on the derivatives of the hematopoietic stem cells in the bone marrow that have been designated colony-forming units–erythrocyte (CFU-E), the precursors of the red blood cell (RBC). CFU-GEMM, colony-forming units–granulocytes, erythroid cells, macrophages, and megakaryocytes; BFU-E, burst-forming units–erythrocyte; IL-6, interleukin-6; IL-3, interleukin-3; GM-CSF, granulocyte–macrophage colony-stimulating factor; EPA, erythroid potentiating activity; EPO, erythropoietin. (From Christensen, R. [1989]. Recombinant erythropoietic growth factors as an alternative to erythrocyte transfusion for patients with "anemia of prematurity." *Pediatrics, 83,* 793–796.)

anemia of bronchopulmonary dysplasia, with treatment starting at 3 months of age (Ohls et al., 1993).

Serum ferritin levels decrease rapidly after the initiation of HuEPO therapy in infants with normal pretreatment ferritin levels, in spite of prophylactic iron supplementation of 2 mg/kg/day. This predisposition to the development of iron deficiency anemia underlines the need for increased iron supplementation in infants treated with HuEPO. Transient thrombocytosis shortly after the initiation of therapy and transient neutropenia lasting as long as 2 months after the discontinuation of therapy have also been documented. It has been postulated that this phenomenon is due to a stimulant effect of HuEPO on megakaryocyte progenitors and a negative effect on granulocyte–monocyte progenitor cells.

If HuEPO proves effective in raising hematocrits without causing significant untoward effects, it is projected that it may eliminate the need for one third of all transfusions in premature infants (Brown et al., 1990).

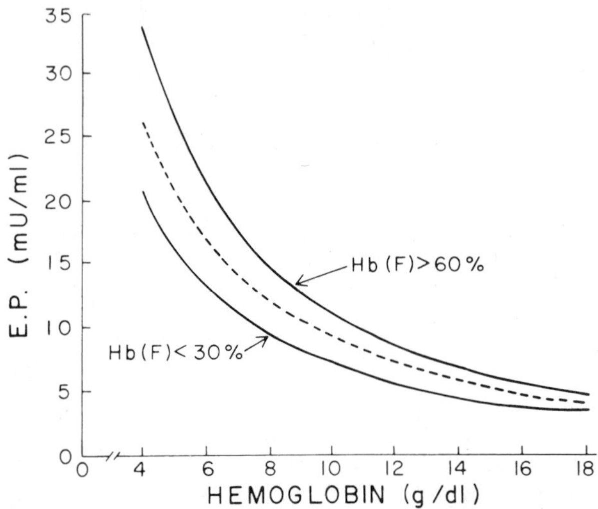

FIGURE 28–17. Because of the differences in oxygen affinity between adult and fetal hemoglobin, variations in the percentage of available fetal hemoglobin (F) affect erythropoietin levels. Improved oxygen uptake but decreased unloading at the tissue level is associated with hemoglobin F. Therefore, the stimulus for erythropoietin production is decreased when lower concentrations of hemoglobin F are present (<30 percent). When higher concentrations (60 percent) of hemoglobin F are present, the stimulus response is an increase in erythropoietin production. At identical total hemoglobin levels, the stimulus for erythropoietin production is increased whenever the percentage of fetal hemoglobin exceeds the adult norm. (From Stockman, J., Garcia, F., & Oski, F. [1977]. The anemia of infancy and the anemia of prematurity. Factors governing the erythropoietin response. *New England Journal of Medicine, 296,* 647.)

Physiologic Anemia of the Newborn and Anemia of the Premature Infant

Shortly after birth, the physiologic regulator of RBC production, erythropoietin, falls to barely perceptible levels because the relative intrauterine hypoxia that stimulates its release is no longer present. Erythropoietin levels remain low until another hypoxic stimulus occurs, one created by the normal drop in hemoglobin level in physiologic anemia of the newborn. This drop in hemoglobin level is due to decreased marrow production of RBCs secondary to diminished circulating erythropoietin levels, shorter life span of the neonatal RBC with destruction of fetal hemoglobin, and hemodilution caused by growth.

The drop in hemoglobin, prompting the postnatal rise in erythropoietin, is directly correlated with the infant's gestational age and birth weight (Fig. 28–16). The smaller and more immature infant reaches a lower nadir at an earlier postnatal age. The hemoglobin level in the term newborn reaches a nadir of 11.4 g/dl ± 0.9 in the first 2 to 3 months of life (Stockman, 1988). It plateaus at this level for approximately 2 more months and then gradually increases. Although there is no significant difference in cord blood hemoglobin levels between term infants and preterm infants born after 32 weeks' gestation, the drop in hemoglobin level occurs earlier in the preterm infant, is more precipitous, and reaches a lower nadir. Starting at 2 weeks of age, the preterm infant has a drop in hemoglobin level of 1 g/dl/wk for the first several weeks; the nadir at 6 to 8 weeks of age is 2 to 3 g/dl lower than that of the term infant. An infant weighing 1000 to 1500 g at birth will have a low mean hemoglobin of 8 g/dl at 4 to 6 weeks of age.

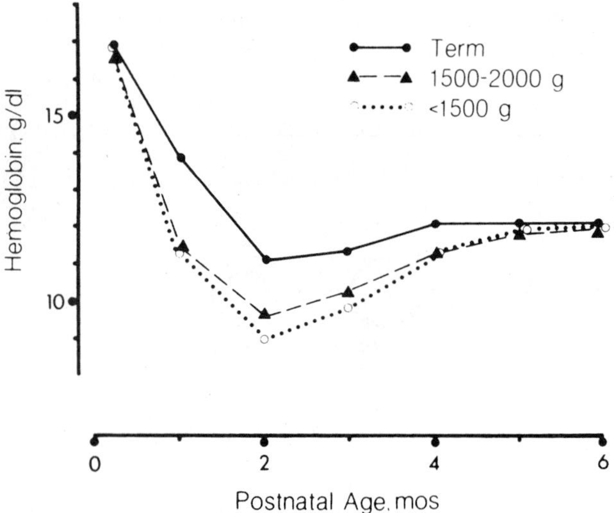

FIGURE 28–16. Gestational age and birth weight are directly correlated with the timing of the postnatal drop in hemoglobin as well as with the nadir of the drop. Shown here are the differences seen between term infants and two groups of preterm infants weighing 1500 to 2000 g and less than 1500 g. (From Brown, M. [1988]. Physiologic anemia of infancy: Normal red cell values and physiology of neonatal erythropoiesis. In J. Stockman & C. Pochedly [Eds.], *Developmental and neonatal hematology* [p. 262]. New York: Raven Press.)

Infants who have undergone exchange transfusion or multiple transfusions also have a greater fall in hemoglobin level in the first 3 months of life. This phenomenon may theoretically be due to improved oxygen delivery to tissue associated with the replacement of fetal with adult hemoglobin (Stockman, 1988). Adult hemoglobin has less affinity for oxygen because of the structural difference of the globin portion of the hemoglobin molecule. This, coupled with the increased amount of 2,3-bisphosphoglycerate present in the blood, allows adult hemoglobin to release oxygen to the tissue more easily. Improved tissue oxygenation effectively lowers serum erythropoietin levels (Fig. 28–17), resulting in decreased RBC production. Consequently, an infant undergoing exchange transfusion or frequent transfusions has improved tissue oxygenation and a decreased erythropoietin level.

In addition to the change in hemoglobin form, the predominant site of erythropoietin production during fetal life moves from the liver to the kidney. The hepatic production of erythropoietin in response to hypoxia is not as rapid as the kidney's response, an adjustment that actually spares the fetus from polycythemia in utero. However, persistence of this hepatic pathway after premature birth may explain why the premature infant has a lower nadir for a longer time in comparison with the term infant. Although erythropoietin levels are decreased in the early newborn period, the erythroid progenitor cells in the bone marrow are exceedingly sensitive to erythropoietin and respond rapidly as blood levels increase. The normal erythropoietin level in infants beyond the newborn period is 10 to 20 mU/ml.

Physiologic anemia does not usually require any form of treatment. With good nutrition, the hemoglobin level in the term infant should start to rise by 3 months of age. With adequate nutrition and iron supplementation, the hemoglobin level in the preterm infant should start to increase by 5 months of age, eventually attaining hemoglobin values comparable to those of the term infant. It is the preterm infant with symptomatic anemia of prematurity who poses the question of transfusion versus HuEPO therapy, a question that has not been conclusively answered.

Polycythemia

Pathophysiology

Polycythemia, defined as a peripheral venous hematocrit of greater than 65 percent, occurs in 4 to 5 percent of the total population of newborns, in 2 to 4 percent of term infants appropriate for gestational age, and in 10 to 15 percent of infants small for gestational age and large for gestational age. It has not been observed, however, in infants less than 34 weeks' gestation. Although the fetus lives in a low Po_2 environment that should induce a polycythemic response, it protects itself by limiting hematocrit levels to less than 60 percent. This may be a function of slower fetal hepatic response to hypoxia compared with rapid renal response after birth. The average hematocrit on the first day of life is approximately 50 percent in the term infant and the preterm infant greater than 32 weeks' gestation and 45 percent in the preterm infant less than 32 weeks' gestation. During the first 4 to 12 hours of life, hemoglobin and hematocrit values tend to rise and then equilibrate, especially in infants receiving large placental transfusions (Ramamurthy & Berlanga, 1987; Shohat et al., 1984).

Hematocrit values vary considerably depending on the sampling site, particularly during the early newborn period when peripheral circulation may be somewhat sluggish. Infants younger than 1 day of age either lack or have diminished cutaneous vasoregulatory mechanisms that decrease peripheral perfusion (Norman et al., 1992). Polycythemia further impairs peripheral circulation by increasing blood viscosity and decreasing flow rate. As blood viscosity increases, vascular resistance increases in the peripheral circulation and the microcirculation of the capillaries throughout the body. In comparison to venous samples, capillary samples are 5 to 15 percent higher, and umbilical vessel or arterial samples are 6 to 8 percent lower.

Three major factors determine blood viscosity: hematocrit, plasma viscosity (osmolality), and deformability of the RBC. With hematocrit levels less than 60 to 65 percent, blood viscosity increases in a linear fashion, but viscosity exponentially increases at higher hematocrit levels. Variations in the components of plasma affect blood viscosity, independent of the hematocrit. Abnormal composition of plasma protein, electrolytes, and other metabolites can either decrease or increase plasma viscosity. Such an increase in the presence of a high hematocrit further raises blood viscosity and decreases blood flow rate. The ability of cells to modify their shape to successfully traverse the peripheral vascular bed and microcirculation also contributes to blood flow rate. The degree of deformability of the cell determines its ability to pass through small vascular spaces. The more deformable the cell, the quicker its passage. Less deformable cells can increase blood viscosity by occluding small vessels and enhancing sludging in the microcirculation, leading to thrombosis and tissue ischemia.

In a study by Black and Lubchenco (1979) of term infants affected by hyperviscosity, 32 percent of these infants had significant neurologic sequelae, with spastic diplegia and hypotonia the most common manifestations. Thirty percent had fine motor abnormalities, which included tremors. In a matched group of infants without hyperviscosity, only 6 percent showed any neurologic abnormalities. Asymptomatic infants with hyperviscosity also demonstrated a greater frequency of subsequent neurologic sequelae in comparison with the normal population. The authors noted that outcome of infants with polycythemia secondary to long-standing intrauterine hypoxia was different from that of infants with polycythemia secondary to a large placental transfusion, regardless of treatment.

There are two major types of polycythemia: (1) the active form, due to the production of an excessive number of RBCs in response to hypoxic and other poorly defined stimuli; and (2) the passive form, caused by RBC transfusion to an infant secondary to maternal-fetal transfusion, twin-to-twin transfusion, or delayed cord clamping.

Active Polycythemia

Tissue hypoxia, regardless of cause, elicits an increase in erythropoietin that stimulates RBC production. In the fetus, erythropoietin is produced initially by the liver and then by the kidney, mimicking the adult production site. The kidney's potential to release erythropoietin is effective by 34 weeks' gestation (Halvorsen & Finne, 1968). At this time, a renal erythropoietic factor reacts with a substance in the plasma to produce the RBC stimulating factor, erythropoietin. Tissue hypoxia adjacent to the renal tubules, where erythropoietin is theorized to be produced, is the potent stimulator of this factor's release.

Many factors can lead to tissue hypoxia associated with the active form of polycythemia. Some of them are

1. Maternal factors resulting in decreased placental blood flow
   - Pregnancy-induced hypertension
   - Increased maternal age
   - Maternal renal or heart disease
   - Severe maternal diabetes—hematocrit values of 64 percent or more are found in 42 percent of infants of a diabetic mother and 30 percent of gestational infants of a diabetic mother
   - Oligohydramnios
   - Maternal smoking—the mechanism is theorized to be production of carbon monoxide that crosses the placenta and induces a state of tissue hypoxia in the fetus
2. Placental factors
   - Placental infarction
   - Placenta previa
   - Viral infections, especially TORCH
   - Postmaturity
   - Placental dysfunction resulting in small for gestational age infant
3. Fetal syndromes
   - Trisomies 13, 18, and 21
   - Beckwith-Wiedemann

Passive Polycythemia

Passive polycythemia is a result of increased fetal blood volume due to maternal-fetal transfusion; twin-to-twin transfusion, with one twin being polycythemic and the other anemic; or delayed cord clamping. A diagnosis of maternal-fetal transfusion can be considered when (1) the infant's blood is found to contain larger amounts than expected of adult hemoglobin, IgA, or IgM; (2)

RBCs in the infant's blood have maternal blood group antigens, if the mother's and infant's blood groups are different; or (3) XX cells are found in an XY infant. In twin-to-twin transfusion, morbidity and mortality are comparable in both groups of affected infants, with one twin being anemic and the other polycythemic. By far, however, the most common cause of fetal transfusion is delayed cord clamping with positioning of the newborn below the level of the placenta. Delayed cord clamping can increase the circulating volume by as much as 60 percent and can raise the hematocrit value by 10 percent (Usher et al., 1963).

Clinical Manifestations

Symptoms of polycythemic hyperviscosity are usually evident within the first few days after birth and reflect compromise of various organ systems. The most commonly seen findings are

1. Neurologic
   - Lethargy
   - Hypotonia
   - Tremulousness
   - Exaggerated startle
   - Poor suck
   - Vomiting
   - Seizures
   - Apnea
2. Cardiovascular
   - Plethora
   - Cardiomegaly
   - Electrocardiogram changes: right and left atrial hypertrophy, right ventricular hypertrophy
3. Respiratory
   - Respiratory distress
   - Central cyanosis
   - Pleural effusions
   - Pulmonary congestion and edema
4. Hematologic
   - Thrombocytopenia
   - Elevated reticulocytes
   - Hepatosplenomegaly
5. Metabolic
   - Hypocalcemia
   - Hyperbilirubinemia
   - Hypoglycemia

Hypoglycemia found in conjunction with polycythemia can be a reflection of (1) increased glucose consumption by an overabundant number of RBCs; (2) increased cerebral extraction of glucose secondary to hypoxia; (3) a state of hyperinsulinemia caused by increased erythropoietin levels; or (4) decreased hepatic glucose production due to sluggish hepatic circulation. Hyperbilirubinemia associated with polycythemia is a reflection of increased by-products of RBC destruction.

The severe complications of polycythemia center around the increased resistance to blood flow related to hyperviscosity, with circulation to all organ systems being impaired because of sluggish flow. Pulmonary blood flow can be dramatically compromised, resulting in pulmonary hypertension, retained lung fluid, and respiratory distress syndrome. Taxation of the heart by an increased vascular load can lead to congestive heart failure and left-to-right shunting across the foramen ovale or ductus arteriosus. Sludging of blood in the microcirculation of the kidney can lead to renal vein thrombosis and renal failure. Impairment of blood flow to the bowel can lead to necrotizing enterocolitis.

Treatment

Although the majority of infants with polycythemia are asymptomatic or minimally symptomatic, the level of the hematocrit and the presence of symptoms, even if minimal, should form the basis of treatment. Because hematocrit levels of 65 percent can lead to neurologic abnormalities and levels of 75 percent or more are always associated with neurologic changes, a venous hematocrit of 65 percent or greater should be considered for treatment by partial exchange transfusion.

Partial exchange causes dramatic improvement in the symptomatic infant, relieving congestive failure and improving CNS function. It also corrects hypoglycemia, relieves respiratory distress and cyanosis, and improves renal function. In a prophylactic clinical trial, partial exchange was noted to improve the clinical and radiographic course of polycythemic infants within 24 hours. Although the treated infants were initially clinically abnormal in comparison to the control group, they were less symptomatic than the untreated group at 3 days of age. At the end of 2 weeks, the untreated group was still abnormal, whereas the treated and control groups were not significantly different. At 8 months of age, the untreated group remained neurologically abnormal (Goldberg et al., 1976; Hakanson, 1981). However, other studies failed to support these findings, revealing no difference between treated, untreated, and control groups at 8 months of age (Van der Elst et al., 1980).

Partial exchange transfusion should be done as the venous hematocrit (Hct) approaches 65 percent and as symptoms appear. Five percent albumin or crystalloid is suggested as replacement for the removed aliquot of blood. With the advent of stricter precautions for prevention of viral transmission by blood products, use of fresh frozen plasma would not seem advisable. The formula for calculating the partial replacement of blood volume is

$$\text{Replacement volume} = \frac{\text{observed Hct} - \text{desired Hct}}{\text{observed Hct}} \times \text{blood volume}$$

Collaborative Management

The care of any newborn infant should include a screening hematocrit for polycythemia by 12 hours of age. This enables detection of any infant with polycythemia and allows adequate observation before symptoms become apparent. Because the initial sample is usually obtained by heel stick or finger stick, detection of a high value should be followed by venipuncture confirmation. The infant should be kept adequately hydrated and closely monitored for hypoglycemia and hypocalcemia. A hematocrit value of greater than 65 percent should prompt careful observation of the infant for any symptoms associated with hyperviscosity. If symptoms appear, the infant should undergo partial exchange transfusion. During the partial exchange, the same care given during a single-volume or double-volume exchange transfusion should be provided.

Coagulopathies in the Newborn Period

Coagulation disorders are present in approximately 1 percent of all admissions to newborn nurseries, with the frequency being much higher in the sick term or preterm infant. In one study, 40 percent of all infant deaths in the NICU were associated with hemorrhage or thrombosis at autopsy (Hathaway & Bonnar, 1978). Bleeding disorders affecting the newborn can be classified as (1) intensification of existing transient deficiencies of the coagulation mechanism, (2) disturbances of coagulation associated with certain disease states, (3) inherited deficiencies, or (4) abnormalities of platelets or vascular structures.

Development of Hemostasis and Coagulation

Embryologic Development of Coagulation Factors and Platelets

The components involved in blood coagulation and fibrinolysis (dissolution of a formed clot) are produced in the liver, vascular wall, and tissue during early fetal life. Many of the clotting factors (procoagulants) and anticoagulants (inhibitors) can be identified during the 8th to 12th weeks of gestation. However, procoagulants, anticoagulants, and the substances responsible for dissolution of a clot, fibrinolytics, do not increase in number and function or reach adult levels simultaneously (Tables 28–10, 28–11, and 28–12). Some components increase with increasing gestational age, whereas others achieve normal adult levels several weeks to months before the fetus reaches term. Still other components do not achieve normal adult levels until several weeks to months after birth. Although the function of coagulation factors and anticoagulants in the fetus is not identical to that in an older child or adult, initial vascular response to injury, by release of tissue thromboplastin, is functional in the fetus as early as 8 weeks.

Another major coagulation component, the megakaryocyte, which develops from pluripotent hematopoietic stem cells, can be identified in the embryonic yolk sac at 5 to 6 weeks' gestation. The site of megakaryocyte production changes with either migration of stem cells from the yolk sac or formation of a new colony of stem cells in the fetal liver, spleen, and, subsequently, bone marrow. These platelet precursors are identifiable in the fetal liver by 6 weeks' gestation. Two distinct phases of hepatic thrombopoiesis produce two different types of megakaryocytes. Those produced during the early phase are less differentiated and smaller than the adult form, whereas megakaryocytes produced during the late phase more closely resemble the adult form in size and nuclear characteristics (Emura et al., 1983). True adult-sized megakaryocytes do not develop until the end of the first year of life (Izumi et al., 1983).

Megakaryocytes develop thin cytoplasmic projections that can penetrate and cross the endothelium of the organ in which they are being produced, eventually coming into contact with a blood

TABLE 28–10 Normal Blood Levels of Coagulation Factors in Fetuses 19 to 27 Weeks' Gestation and Newborns 28 Weeks' Gestation to Term

Tests	19–27 Weeks (Mean ± SD)	28–31 Weeks, Mean (Boundary)	30–36 Weeks, Day 1 Mean (Boundary)	30–36 Weeks, Day 5 Mean (Boundary)	Full Term, Day 1 Mean (Boundary)	Full Term, Day 5 Mean (Boundary)
PT (s)	—	15.4 (14.6–16.9)	13.0 (10.6–16.2)	12.5 (10.0–15.3)	13.0 (10.1–15.9)	12.4 (10.0–15.3)
APTT (s)	—	108 (80–168)	53.6 (27.5–79.4)	50.5 (26.9–74.1)	42.9 (31.3–54.5)	42.6 (25.4–59.8)
TCT (s)	—	—	24.8 (19.2–30.4)	24.1 (18.8–29.4)	23.5 (19.0–28.3)	23.1 (18.0–29.2)
Fibrinogen (g/L)	1.00 ± 0.4	2.56 (1.60–5.50)	2.43 (1.50–3.73)	2.80 (1.60–4.18)	2.83 (1.67–3.99)	3.12 (1.62–4.62)
Factor II (U/ml)	0.12 ± 0.02	0.31 (0.19–0.54)	0.45 (0.20–0.77)	0.57 (0.29–0.85)	0.48 (0.26–0.70)	0.63 (0.33–0.93)
Factor V (U/ml)	0.41 ± 0.10	0.65 (0.43–0.80)	0.88 (0.41–1.44)	1.00 (0.46–1.54)	0.72 (0.34–1.08)	0.95 (0.45–1.45)
Factor VII (U/ml)	0.28 ± 0.04	0.37 (0.24–0.76)	0.67 (0.21–1.13)	0.84 (0.30–1.38)	0.66 (0.28–1.04)	0.89 (0.35–1.43)
Factor VIII (U/ml)	0.39 ± 0.14	0.79 (0.37–1.26)	1.11 (0.50–2.13)	1.15 (0.53–2.05)	1.00 (0.50–1.78)	0.88 (0.50–1.54)
vWF (U/ml)	0.64 ± 0.13	1.41 (0.83–2.23)	1.36 (0.78–2.10)	1.33 (0.72–2.19)	1.53 (0.50–2.87)	1.40 (0.50–2.54)
Factor IX (U/ml)	0.10 ± 0.01	0.18 (0.17–0.20)	0.35 (0.19–0.65)	0.42 (0.14–0.74)	0.53 (0.15–0.91)	0.53 (0.15–0.91)
Factor X (U/ml)	0.21 ± 0.03	0.36 (0.25–0.64)	0.41 (0.11–0.71)	0.51 (0.19–0.83)	0.40 (0.12–0.68)	0.49 (0.19–0.79)
Factor XI (U/ml)	—	0.23 (0.11–0.33)	0.30 (0.08–0.52)	0.41 (0.13–0.69)	0.38 (0.10–0.66)	0.55 (0.23–0.87)
Factor XII (U/ml)	0.22 ± 0.03	0.25 (0.05–0.35)	0.38 (0.10–0.66)	0.39 (0.09–0.69)	0.53 (0.13–0.93)	0.47 (0.11–0.83)
PK (U/ml)	—	0.26 (0.15–0.32)	0.33 (0.09–0.57)	0.45 (0.26–0.75)	0.37 (0.18–0.69)	0.48 (0.20–0.76)
HMWK (U/ml)	—	0.32 (0.19–0.52)	0.49 (0.09–0.89)	0.62 (0.24–1.00)	0.54 (0.06–1.02)	0.74 (0.16–1.32)
Factor XIIIa (U/ml)	—	—	0.70 (0.32–1.08)	1.01 (0.57–1.45)	0.79 (0.27–1.31)	0.94 (0.44–1.44)
Factor XIIIb (U/ml)	—	—	0.81 (0.35–1.27)	1.10 (0.68–1.58)	0.76 (0.30–1.22)	1.06 (0.32–1.80)
Plasminogen (U/ml)	—	—	1.70 (1.12–2.48)	1.91 (1.21–2.61)	1.95 ± 0.35 (44)	2.17 ± 0.38 (60)

PT, prothrombin time; APTT, activated partial thromboplastin time; TCT, thrombin clotting time; vWF, von Willebrand's factor; PK, prekallikrein; HMWK, high-molecular-weight kininogen.

Modified from Andrew, M., Paes, B., & Johnston, M. (1990). Development of the hemostatic system in the neonate and young infant. *American Journal of Pediatric Hematology/Oncology, 12*(1), 97–98; Andrew, M., Paes, B., Milner, R., et al. (1987). Development of the human coagulation system in the full-term infant. *Blood, 70*, 166; and Andrew, M., Paes, B., Milner, R., et al. (1988). Development of the human coagulation system in the healthy premature infant. *Blood, 72*, 1653.

TABLE 28–11 Normal Blood Levels of Coagulation Inhibitors in Newborns 30 Weeks' Gestation to Term

	30 to 36 Weeks' Gestation		Full Term	
Coagulation Inhibitors	***Day 1 Mean (Boundary)***	***Day 5 Mean (Boundary)***	***Day 1 Mean (Boundary)***	***Day 5 Mean (Boundary)***
ATIII (U/ml)	0.38 (0.14–0.62)	0.56 (0.30–0.82)	0.63 (0.39–0.87)	0.67 (0.41–0.93)
α_2-M (U/ml)	1.10 (0.56–1.82)	1.25 (0.71–1.77)	1.39 (0.95–1.83)	1.48 (0.98–1.98)
C1E-NH (U/ml)	0.65 (0.31–0.99)	0.83 (0.45–1.21)	0.72 (0.36–1.08)	0.90 (0.60–1.20)
α_1-AT (U/ml)	0.90 (0.36–1.44)	0.94 (0.42–1.46)	0.93 (0.49–1.37)	0.89 (0.49–1.29)
HCII (U/ml)	0.32 (0.10–0.60)	0.34 (0.10–0.69)	0.43 (0.10–0.93)	0.48 (0.10–0.96)
Protein C (U/ml)	0.28 (0.12–0.44)	0.31 (0.11–0.51)	0.35 (0.17–0.53)	0.42 (0.20–0.64)
Protein S (U/ml)	0.26 (0.14–0.38)	0.37 (0.13–0.61)	0.36 (0.12–0.60)	0.50 (0.22–0.78)

ATIII, antithrombin III; α_2-M, alpha$_2$-macroglobulin; C1E-INH, C1 esterase inhibitor; α_1-AT, alpha$_1$-antitrypsin; HCII, heparin cofactor II.
Modified from Andrew, M., Paes, B., Johnston, M. (1990). Development of the hemostatic system in the neonate and young infant. *American Journal of Pediatric Hematology/Oncology, 12*(1), 98–99; Andrew, M., Paes, B., Milner, R., et al. (1987). Development of the human coagulation system in the full-term infant. *Blood, 70*, 167; and Andrew, M., Paes, B., Milner, R., et al. (1988). Development of the human coagulation system in the healthy premature infant. *Blood, 72*, 1653.

vessel. These cytoplasmic projections then develop constrictions that pinch off the distal ends, resulting in fragments called platelets. Although erythropoietin and thrombopoietin are involved in the initial stem cell differentiation, the actual inducer of megakaryocyte fragmentation and platelet production is unknown. At 32 weeks' gestation, platelet levels are comparable to those of an adult, but platelet function is not.

Hemostasis

Hemostasis consists of a delicate and dynamic balance between factors that prevent exsanguination and those that keep the blood in a fluid form. The interrelationship among four distinct components helps ensure orderly hemostasis and fibrinolysis when vascular integrity is destroyed or interrupted. These four parts consist of the following.

Vascular Components. The components of the vascular wall affect the structure and function of damaged blood vessels. Vascular spasm is the first mechanism by which hemostasis is achieved in a damaged vessel.

Platelets and Their Activating Substances. Formation of a platelet plug is the second mechanism of hemostasis after vascular injury has occurred.

Coagulation or Plasma Factors. These factors consist of procoagulants and anticoagulants (inhibitors). Coagulation completes the hemostatic mechanism by strengthening the platelet plug.

Fibrinolytic Pathway. This pathway contributes to disintegration of the clot and re-establishment of normal circulatory flow. It consists of fibrinolytics (substances that lyse a fibrin clot) and inhibitors.

Initial Steps in Hemostasis

Vascular Spasm

Initial hemostasis in a ruptured blood vessel consists of vascular spasm, resulting from a combination of chemical mechanics, ner-

TABLE 28–12 Normal Blood Levels of Fibrinolytic Components in Premature and Term Newborns

	Premature Infants		Full-Term Infants	
Fibrinolytic Component	***Day 1 Mean (Boundary)***	***Day 5 Mean (Boundary)***	***Day 1 Mean (Boundary)***	***Day 5 Mean (Boundary)***
Plasminogen (U/ml)	1.70 (1.12–2.48)	1.91 (1.21–2.61)	1.95 (1.25–2.65)	2.17 (1.41–2.93)
TPA (ng/ml)	8.48 (3.00–16.70)	3.97 (2.00–6.93)	9.6 (5.0–18.9)	5.6 (4.0–10.0)
α_2-AP (U/ml)	0.78 (0.40–1.16)	0.81 (0.49–1.13)	0.85 (0.55–1.15)	1.00 (0.70–1.30)
PAI (U/ml)	5.4 (0.0–12.2)	2.5 (0.0–7.1)	6.4 (2.0–15.1)	2.3 (0.0–8.1)

TPA, tissue plasminogen activator; α_2-AP, alpha$_2$-antiplasmin; PAI, plasminogen activator inhibitor.
Modified from Andrew, M., Paes, B., Johnston, M. (1990). Development of the hemostatic system in the neonate and young infant. *American Journal of Pediatric Hematology/Oncology, 12*(1), 102–103.

vous reflexes, and localized muscle spasm (Guyton, 1991b). Although nervous reflexes are a response to pain, most of the vascular spasm is due to muscle contraction in the vessel wall secondary to direct injury. This vascular response to injury is present in an 8-week fetus, and at term it is the equivalent of adult norms in regard to capillary fragility and bleeding time (Feusner, 1980). This component is gestational age dependent and is evident in the increased capillary fragility exhibited by the preterm infant (Bleyer et al., 1971).

Formation of a Platelet Plug

Platelets coming into contact with an injured vascular wall adhere to the wall and form a platelet plug. This hemostatic plug constitutes the primary means of closure of small vascular holes at the capillary and small vessel level. The ability of platelets to adhere on contact to a denuded vascular wall requires a glycoprotein, von Willebrand's factor, that is synthesized by vascular endothelial cells and megakaryocytes. Von Willebrand's factor is complexed with Factor VIII (antihemophilic factor), and they circulate jointly.

In addition to adhesion, platelets have the ability to aggregate (stick to other platelets), forming large clumps. Aggregation is made possible by the platelet's ability to modify its shape and to secrete many biochemical substances (platelet release reaction) that enhance cohesion. When platelets and associated glycoproteins are activated by excess release of these biochemical substances during times of stress, fibrinogen receptors appear on the surface of the platelet. These receptors enhance the platelet's ability to bind fibrinogen, which in turn cross-links platelets in the process of platelet aggregation. This provides a tight mesh of clot around an injured vessel that controls bleeding (Fig. 28–18). After 32 weeks' gestation, average platelet counts are comparable to those of term infants and adults, but the ability of platelets to aggregate is diminished (Mull & Hathaway, 1970).

Coagulation

When bleeding cannot be controlled merely with a platelet plug, circulating plasma coagulation factors are triggered to form a network of fibrin that turns the existing plug into a hemostatic seal. Fibrin threads, necessary to clot formation, can develop within 15 to 20 seconds in the presence of normal coagulation factors. Within 3 to 6 minutes after vascular rupture, the entire opening is occluded by a clot; and within 30 to 60 minutes, the clot begins to retract, pulling the injured vascular portions together and further sealing the vascular end. This coagulation reaction involves several plasma proteins and three distinct phases. The first phase involves the formation of prothrombin activator, the second involves the activation of prothrombin to thrombin, and the third involves the conversion of soluble fibrinogen to fibrin (Guyton, 1996b).

PHASE I: FORMATION OF PROTHROMBIN ACTIVATOR

There are two separate pathways by which prothrombin activator can be generated, the intrinsic and extrinsic pathways. The intrinsic pathway is triggered by trauma or damage occurring inside the vessel or to the blood itself, and the extrinsic pathway is triggered by the production of tissue thromboplastin that is generated by vessel wall damage. This bimodal pathway can be interrupted or negated by a deficiency in platelets or any of the plasma coagulation factors or by the presence of inhibitors (anticoagulants) in the plasma. Selective activation of one of these pathways depends on the site of injury and the extent of its severity.

Of the two pathways, activation of the intrinsic pathway is

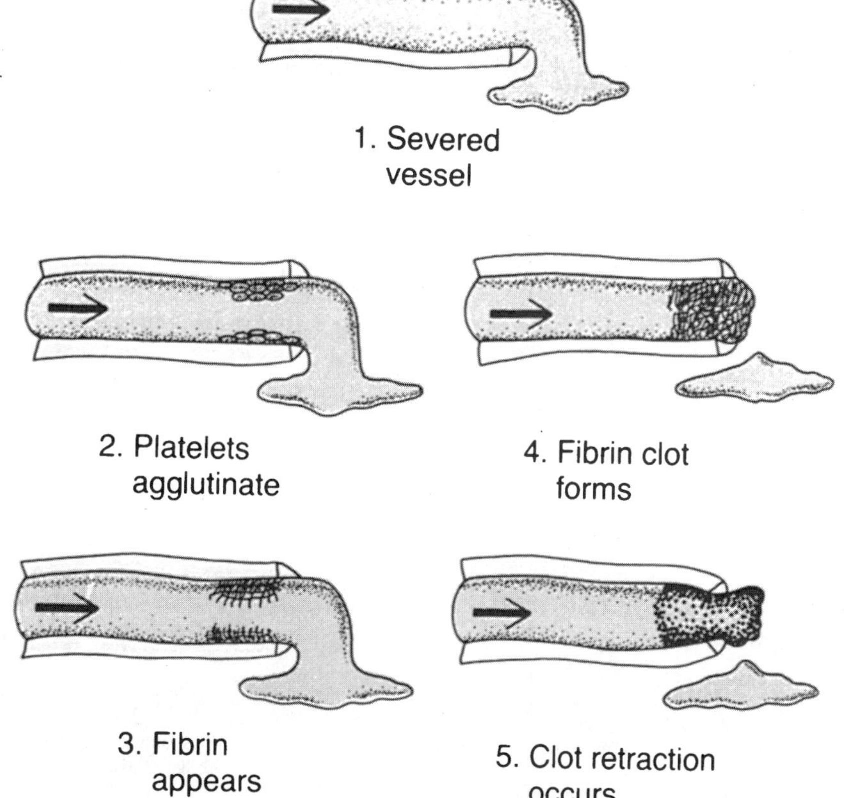

FIGURE 28–18. When vessel wall injury occurs, the initial clotting process begins with the formation of a platelet plug. Platelet activation stimulates fibrinogen receptors found on the surface of the platelets, which enhance their aggregation with other platelets and fibrinogen. The fibrin clot that forms will retract and occlude the damaged vascular wall. (From Guyton, A. [1991]. Hemostasis and blood coagulation. *Textbook of medical physiology* [8th ed., pp. 390–399]. Philadelphia: W. B. Saunders.)

slower because it lacks the major stimulus of the extrinsic pathway, which is tissue thromboplastin generated by vessel wall damage. The intrinsic pathway relies on blood trauma or injury within the vessel to alter platelets and plasma proteins and convert dormant factors (zymogens), naturally found in circulating blood, into active proteolytic enzymes (Fig. 28–19). Each activated enzyme subsequently reacts with the succeeding factor, changing it into its activated form. The steps of intrinsic activation of coagulation are as follows:

1. An activator (blood trauma, injury within the vessel, or contact with collagen) activates Factor XII, converting it to XIIa, while simultaneously damaging platelets, which causes a release of platelet phospholipids.
2. Factor XIIa, in conjunction with prekallikrein and high molar weight kininogen, activates Factor XI, converting it to XIa.
3. Factor XIa activates Factor IX, converting it to IXa.
4. Factor IXa, platelet phospholipid, and Factor VIII combine to activate Factor X, converting it to Xa.
5. Factor Xa combines with Factor V and platelet phospholipids to form prothrombin activator (prothrombinase), which releases thrombin from prothrombin. Calcium is required for this and the preceding two steps.

The extrinsic pathway can generate thrombin in a matter of seconds when injury occurs outside of the vascular space (Fig. 28–20). Tissue thromboplastin, composed of glycoproteins and phospholipids, is produced when tissue is injured. When plasma comes into contact with this substance, the initial intrinsic phases are bypassed and the following responses occur:

1. Tissue thromboplastin (Factor III) activates Factor VII to VIIa. These two factors then form a complex with glycoprotein that activates Factor X, converting it to Factor Xa.
2. Factor Xa forms complexes with phospholipids and Factor V, in the presence of calcium, to form prothrombin activator.

From this point on, the intrinsic and extrinsic pathways are identical, with both proceeding to phase II.

PHASE II: FORMATION OF THROMBIN

Prothrombin activator from either of the two pathways continues the clotting cascade by further influencing the breakdown of the unstable plasma protein, prothrombin. Prothrombin (Factor II) is synthesized by the liver, under the influence of vitamin K, along with the other factors that form the prothrombin complex (Factors VII, IX, and X). When acted on by prothrombin activator, prothrombin forms the potent coagulant thrombin. The newly formed thrombin stimulates completion of the third and final phase of coagulation.

PHASE III: FORMATION OF THE FIBRIN CLOT

Procoagulants. Thrombin promotes the conversion of fibrinogen (Factor I), a protein produced by the liver, into fibrin by splitting off two peptides from the soluble fibrinogen molecule. This exposes two sites to which other split fibrin molecules can

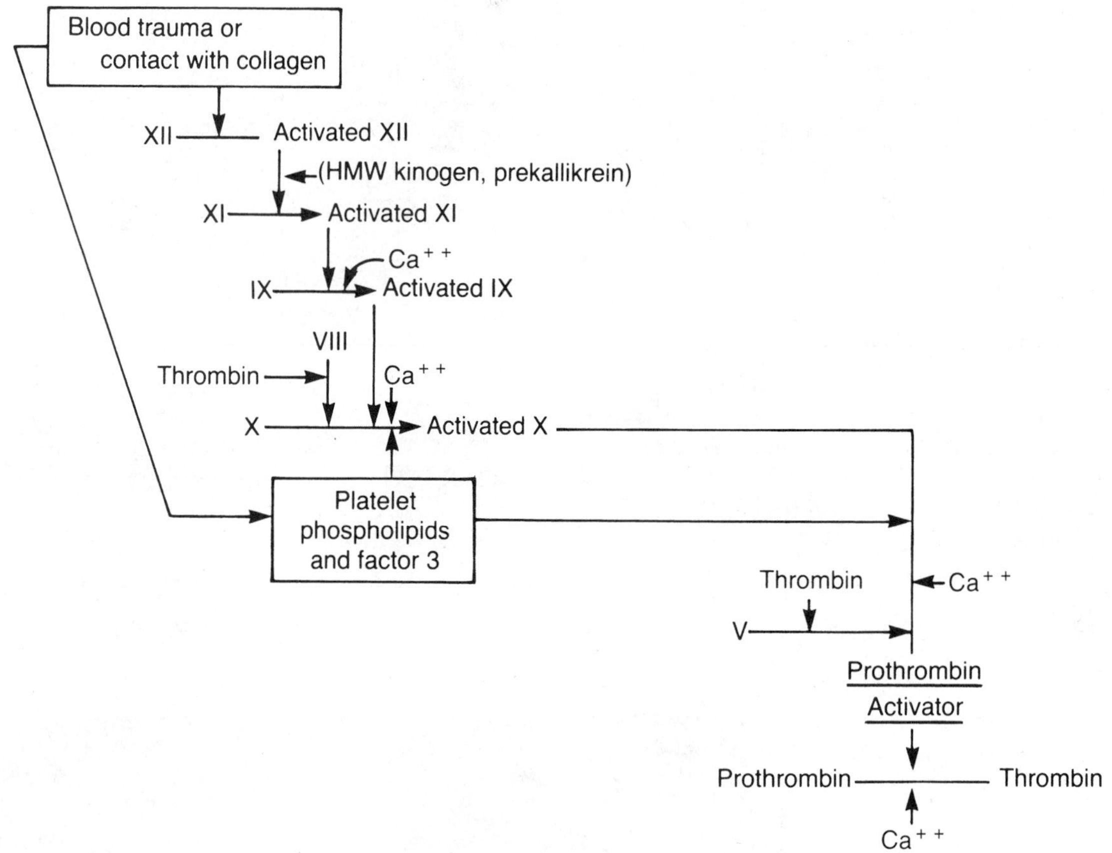

FIGURE 28–19. The intrinsic pathway for initiating the clotting cascade is activated by trauma to the blood, injury within the vessel, or contact with collagen. HMW, high molecular weight. (From Guyton, A. [1991]. Hemostasis and blood coagulation. *Textbook of medical physiology* [8th ed., pp. 390–399]. Philadelphia: W. B. Saunders.)

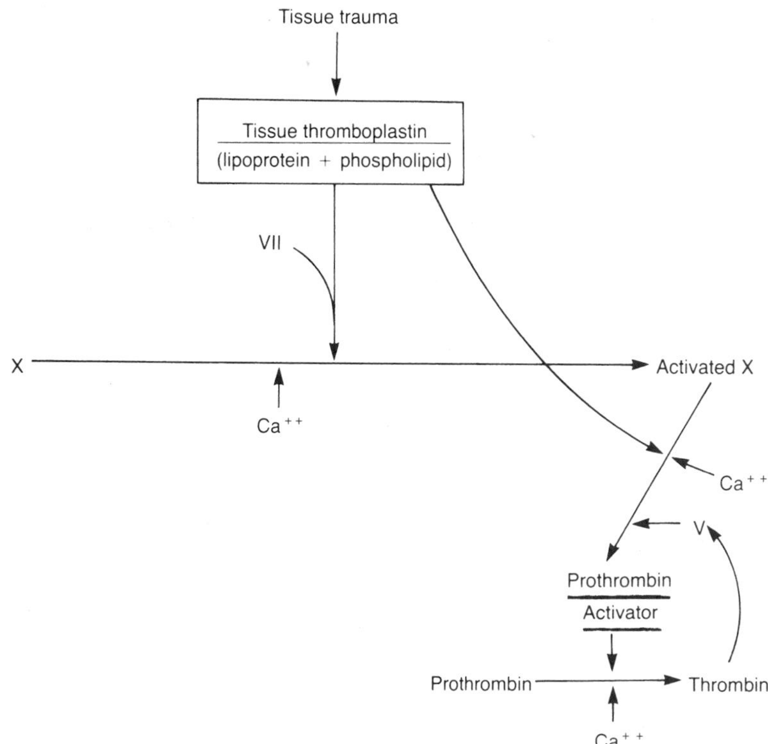

FIGURE 28–20. The extrinsic pathway for initiating the clotting cascade can generate thrombin rapidly owing to thromboplastin release from injured tissue. (From Guyton, A. [1991]. Hemostasis and blood coagulation. *Textbook of medical physiology* [8th ed., pp. 390–399]. Philadelphia: W. B. Saunders.)

link, forming an insoluble fibrin chain. Fibrin stabilizing factor (Factor XIII) further strengthens the tight bond of this developing fibrin mesh. Fibrin stabilizing factor is naturally found in the plasma and is also secreted by entrapped platelets. The forming fibrin clot begins to contract and retract with the help of platelets that have actin–myosin action, the same action by which a muscle works. Extension of the clot into the surrounding circulating blood promotes further thrombosis. Thrombin from the clot has the ability to cleave prothrombin into more thrombin and enhances the production of prothrombin activator, thus acting as a potent biofeedback system for perpetuation of the clotting cascade.

Anticoagulants. Throughout the entire coagulation pathway, the action of the activated enzymes is modulated at each stage by multiple and specific inhibitors (anticoagulants). Consequently, coagulation is a process of balance between coagulation factors and naturally occurring inhibitors. Some of these anticoagulants are endothelial surface factors that prevent coagulation until the vessel's endothelial wall is damaged. One such factor is the smoothness of the wall, which prevents any adherence and subsequent activation; another is the monomolecular layer of protein covering the wall, which repels plasma clotting factors and platelets.

Two inhibitors, $alpha_1$-antitrypsin and C1 esterase inhibitor, interfere with the coagulation factors involved in the initial activation of the intrinsic pathway. Thrombin acts as its own inhibitor by stimulating activation of protein C that in the presence of another vitamin K–dependent inhibitor, protein S, inactivates Factors V and VIII. Other inhibitors of thrombin formation include (1) fibrin threads formed during clot formation that absorb thrombin, thus removing it from circulation along with its potential for further coagulation; (2) $alpha_2$-macroglobulin that inhibits proteases, including thrombin; (3) antithrombin III that combines with thrombin, blocking the conversion of fibrinogen into fibrin; and (4) heparin cofactor II that removes several activated procoagulants. Both antithrombin III and heparin are produced in the precapillary connective tissue of the lungs and liver.

Fibrinolysis

Once a clot develops, it can be invaded by fibroblasts that lay down connective tissue throughout the clot or it can be dissolved. The process of dissolution occurs by activation of naturally occurring factors that lyse the clot. Fibrinolysis is activated simultaneously with stimulation of the coagulation system, with powerful but inactivated anticoagulants built right into the clot. One of these anticoagulants, plasminogen, is manufactured by the liver, kidneys, and eosinophils. Plasminogen, under the influence of thrombin, activated Factor XII, and tissue plasminogen activator, is converted into plasmin, a proteolytic enzyme that breaks down fibrin into fibrin split products. Plasmin not only digests the fibrin chains but also deactivates fibrinogen, Factor V, Factor VII, Factor XII, and prothrombin. However, plasmin can be inactivated by its inhibitor, $alpha_2$-antiplasmin, and tissue plasminogen activator can be inactivated by its inhibitor, plasminogen activator inhibitor.

Overall Development of Hemostasis

In summary, both term and preterm newborns have the ability to create a balance between transitory deficiencies in the amount and function of a variety of clotting factors, platelets, and anticoagulant factors. The homeostasis between clotting factors and anticoagulants places the newborn in a mildly hypercoagulable state at birth. Thus, the newborn has no greater tendency to bleed, but several differences in regard to coagulation components and reserves do exist in comparison with the older child and the adult. These differences include (1) gestational age–dependent variations in the concentrations of coagulation factors, anticoagulants, and fibrinolytics; (2) faster turnover rate of components; (3) slower rate of synthesis of components; and (4) limited ability to supply necessary components during times of increased need.

Common Coagulation Disorders in the Newborn

Hemorrhagic Disease of the Newborn

The majority of clotting factors, including those of the prothrombin complex, are produced by the liver. Adequate function of this complex requires the specific action of vitamin K, which is continuously synthesized by bacteria in the bowel. Vitamin K is not directly involved in the synthesis of these factors but is required for the conversion of precursor proteins produced by the liver into active factors having coagulant capabilities (Jackson & Suttu, 1977). Vitamin K is especially necessary for conversion of prothrombin binding sites into forms that can bind calcium, which is required for completion of many steps in the clotting cascade.

Vitamin K–dependent factors reach approximately 30 to 60 percent of adult levels in the cord blood of term infants but quickly drop to half that amount if the infant is not given vitamin K. Because these factors are gestational age dependent, the more premature the infant, the lower the levels at birth. The exaggerated drop after birth may be due to poor placental transfer of maternal vitamin K, immature liver function, and delayed synthesis of vitamin K by the bowel. These factors slowly rise but do not reach normal adult levels until approximately 9 months of age. Administration of approximately 25 μg (0.025 mg) of vitamin K can prevent this decline and normalize the prothrombin time (Aballi & DeLamerens, 1962).

Hemorrhage occurring during the early neonatal period that can be attributed to a deficiency of vitamin K–dependent factors is classified as hemorrhagic disease of the newborn, of which there are three identified forms. The first and least common consists of bleeding within the first 24 hours of life, usually associated with maternal anticonvulsant therapy. It is theorized that anticonvulsants may induce fetal hepatic enzymes involved in the degradation of already low levels of fetal vitamin K. Early neonatal bleeding cannot be prevented by postnatal administration of vitamin K. Daily antenatal administration of large doses of oral vitamin K (10 mg) to mothers receiving anticonvulsant therapy for at least 10 days before delivery was found to be beneficial to the newborn (Anai et al., 1993). Vitamin K crosses the placenta, elevating newborn levels of vitamin K for 10 days after birth, with the increase in levels correlating with timing of the last prenatal dose.

Early or classic hemorrhagic disease usually occurs during the first 2 to 5 days of life and manifests itself as generalized and, occasionally, dramatic bleeding. The most common sites are the gastrointestinal tract, umbilicus, circumcision site, skin, and internal organs. The late form of hemorrhagic disease, occurring after the first week of life, is more devastating than the early form because of the increased occurrence of intracranial hemorrhage, approaching a 63 percent risk (Bhanchet et al., 1977). Mortality can be as high as 14 percent with subsequent permanent neurologic sequelae in 24 percent (Loughnan & McDougall, 1993). Both early and late hemorrhagic disease of the newborn are intensified in breastfed infants.

Definitive diagnosis includes a history of lack of vitamin K prophylaxis at birth and a prolonged prothrombin time (Fig. 28–21), which measures the prothrombin complex clotting factors consisting of Factors II, VII, IX, and X. A recently developed test, PIVKA-II (protein induced by vitamin K absence or antagonist–II), is useful in identifying proteins induced by vitamin K deficiency that appear in the plasma of vitamin K–deficient infants. These proteins consist of the inert and functionally defective precursors of prothrombin that are produced when vitamin K levels are deficient.

Several factors can predispose an infant to hemorrhagic disease of the newborn. Almost all of these factors involve some form of hepatic dysfunction. The most obvious predisposing factor is failure of an infant to receive prophylactic vitamin K postnatally. Other risk factors include maternal ingestion of anticonvulsants and coumarin anticoagulants (which interfere with the action of the prothrombin complex factors), birth asphyxia, prolonged labor, and breastfeeding. Human milk contains a lower vitamin K content than cow's milk. Infants receiving a commercial formula for 24 hours have prothrombin times similar to those of infants receiving vitamin K after birth (Keenan et al., 1971). Infants having hepatic dysfunction or bowel malabsorption, although not found strictly in the early neonatal period, can develop vitamin K deficiency in spite of having received prophylaxis at birth. Such disorders as chronic diarrhea, biliary atresia, hepatitis, cystic fibrosis, and prolonged parenteral nutrition do not allow adequate vitamin K production and can result in low prothrombin complex factors. These infants benefit from weekly vitamin K supplementation of 1 mg intramuscularly (Goetzman & Wennberg, 1991). This is the dose recommended by the American Academy of Pediatrics (1993) for postnatal newborn prophylaxis. The suggested preparation for administration to the newborn is the natural aqueous solution of vitamin K, rather than the synthetic preparation, which can cause hemolysis. Because of hepatic immaturity and inability to effectively synthesize clotting factors, the preterm infant's response to vitamin K is not as predictable as that of the term infant.

Controversy over the use of intramuscular versus oral prophylaxis still continues, with conflicting data. Intramuscular administration of vitamin K has been associated with an increased risk for childhood cancers in one retrospective study (Golding et al., 1990, 1992), but this has been refuted in three other studies from Sweden (Ekelund et al., 1993), the United States (Klebanoff et al., 1993), and Denmark (Olsen et al., 1994). Use of one or two oral doses of vitamin K as an effective treatment is also disputed, with several studies finding decreasing vitamin K levels (Hathaway et al., 1991; McNinch et al., 1985) and increasing PIVKA-II levels (Motohara et al., 1987) in newborns older than 1 week. Research is still ongoing to determine adequate timing and number of oral doses of vitamin K as well as to develop an adequate oral preparation. Alternative therapies are also being investigated with use of antenatal maternal dosing to prevent antenatal intraventricular hemorrhage and postnatal maternal dosing as prophylaxis in the breastfed infant.

Active bleeding due to hemorrhagic disease of the newborn may require blood replacement or the use of fresh frozen plasma for immediate clotting factor replacement.

Hemophilia

Classic hemophilia (hemophilia A) is the most commonly inherited coagulation abnormality, accounting for 90 percent of all genetically linked coagulopathies and 85 percent of all hemophilias. It is passed from mother to son as an X-linked trait and is caused by Factor VIII deficiency. Factor VIII has two components: a large glycoprotein called von Willebrand's factor, which is required for proper platelet adhesion; and a small procoagulant protein, the antihemophilic factor, which is defective in hemophilia A. Hemophilia A involves the production of structurally and functionally ineffective clotting factors, as opposed to a deficiency in quantity.

The concentration of circulating antihemophilic factor in the serum determines the severity of the disease. Levels of 1 to 2

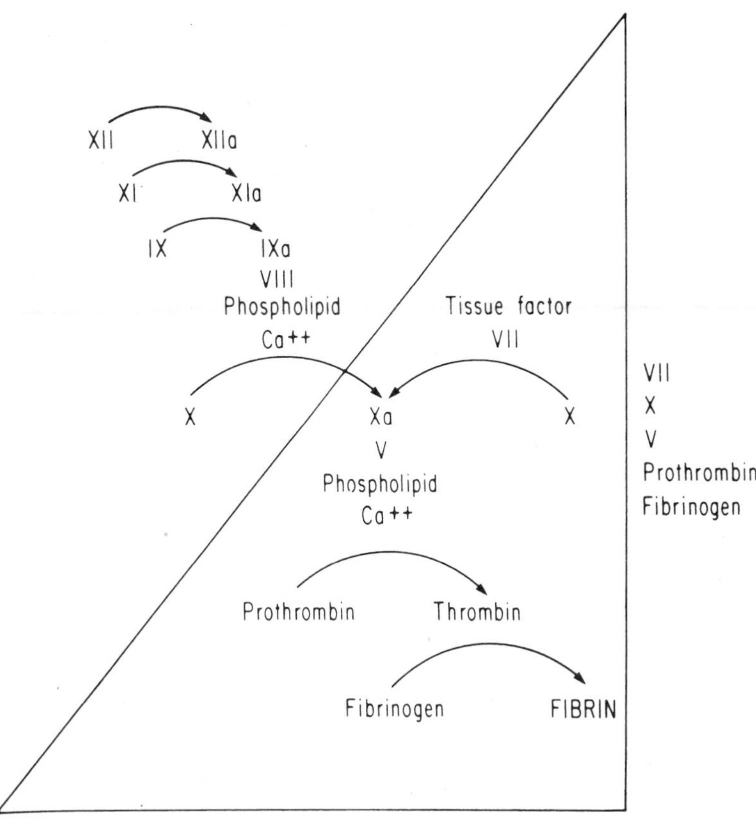

FIGURE 28–21. The prothrombin time measures the prothrombin complex consisting of Factors II (prothrombin), VII, IX, and X. These factors depend on vitamin K for their synthesis. The prothrombin time is also a measurement of the extrinsic pathway of coagulation. (From Lusher, J. [1987]. Diseases of coagulation: The fluid phase. In D. Nathan & F. Oski [Eds.], *Hematology of infancy and childhood* [3rd ed., p. 1298]. Philadelphia: W. B. Saunders.)

percent are associated with severe disease, 2 to 5 percent with moderate disease, and greater than 5 percent with mild disease, a level at which active bleeding rarely occurs. In a retrospective study of hemophiliacs, approximately 44 percent of a group of severe hemophiliacs were symptomatic during the first week of life, whereas only 14 percent of a mildly affected group displayed any bleeding during the first 7 days of life (Schulman, 1962).

Infants affected with hemophilia have a prolonged partial thromboplastin time, but the prothrombin time, thrombin time, and platelet count are relatively normal. The major symptom of hemophilia consists of bleeding, with the most common areas being the circumcision site, scalp, umbilicus, and brain (Baehner & Strauss, 1966). Not all severe hemophiliacs bleed after circumcision in the early newborn period. The reason for this is not known, but it has been suggested that tissue thromboplastin release, caused by the circumcision clamp on the foreskin, may initiate the extrinsic pathway and clotting cascade, thus preventing excessive bleeding.

Diagnosis

Prenatal diagnosis is feasible, but results are not always accurate. Diagnosis involves the measurement of the ratio of factor antigen to coagulant antigen on blood samples of fetuses greater than 20 weeks' gestation.

Treatment

Treatment consists of raising the defective or deficient factor to a level that will prevent bleeding. In hemophilia A, the concentration of antihemophilic factor is raised to a level of 20 percent. It is suggested that use of factor concentrates be avoided, but if they must be used, a pasteurized form should be used to decrease the risk for transmittable viral diseases such as hepatitis and human immunodeficiency virus (HIV) infection. Acquired immunodeficiency syndrome (AIDS) is now the second most frequent cause of death in the hemophiliac. The suggested mode of therapy is the use of cryoprecipitate in the dose of 10 U/kg. Each unit per kilogram raises the antihemophilic factor level by 1.5 to 2 percent; a bag of cryoprecipitate contains 80 U. Two alternative methods of treatment that raise both components of Factor VIII twofold to threefold are 1-desamino-8-D-arginine-vasopressin (DDAVP) as an injection and desmopressin acetate as a nasal spray. The effectiveness and applicability to the newborn of these two therapies are still unknown, but at present, they are not recommended for treatment if the antihemophilic factor level is less than 5 percent or in infants younger than 11 months of age.

Thrombocytopenia

The normal range of platelets is 150,000 to 450,000/mm^3; the average count in the newborn is approximately 250,000/mm^3 (Aballi et al., 1968). Platelet counts less than 150,000/mm^3 are considered abnormal and should be subject to investigation for a possible pathologic process. Although 14 percent of all preterm infants and 4 percent of all term infants are thrombocytopenic, with platelet counts less than 150,000/mm^3, not all of these infants are ill.

Thrombocytopenia is the most common bleeding disorder in the newborn; 20 percent of all NICU admissions have platelet counts of less than 50,000/mm^3, and 80 percent of sick infants have counts of less than 100,000/mm^3. However, the pathogenesis of the thrombocytopenia can be determined in only 60 percent of these infants. Abnormalities of the platelet count are due to either increased destruction or decreased production, with the underlying cause being mediated by maternal, placental, neonatal, or iatrogenic factors. In the majority of thrombocytopenic newborns, platelet counts are low as a result of increased destruction rather than bone marrow depression. Overall mortality for infants with thrombocytopenia is 34 percent; 22 percent of these infants exhibit a bleeding diathesis (Mehta et al., 1980). Infants with a platelet count of less than 20,000/mm^3 are at particularly high risk for bleeding.

Maternal Factors

Thrombocytopenia is the most common form of hemostatic problem present during pregnancy; 5 to 7 percent of healthy mothers have platelet counts less than 150,000/mm^3 (Burrows & Kelton, 1988). Some of the maternal factors associated with thrombocytopenia are

1. Maternal drug ingestion, such as chloramphenicol, hydralazine, tolbutamide, and thiazides;
2. Maternal eclampsia and hypertension;
3. Placental infarction;
4. Immune-mediated maternal platelet antibodies.

IMMUNE-MEDIATED MATERNAL PLATELET ANTIBODIES

Idiopathic Thrombocytopenia. Eighty percent of immune-mediated thrombocytopenia, in which maternal antibodies cause destruction of platelets, is caused by the autoimmune form or maternal idiopathic thrombocytopenic purpura (ITP). ITP is a pre-existing condition in which maternal lymphocytes produce IgG antiplatelet antibodies that attack maternal platelets. These antibodies are specifically directed at platelet antigen and bind to platelets. These platelets are then phagocytosed by cells carrying a specific receptor, the Fc receptor. The greatest number of cells with this receptor are found in the reticuloendothelial system of the spleen.

Because IgG can cross the placenta, fetal platelets can also be destroyed by the transplacental passage of platelet antibodies, resulting in thrombocytopenia in the fetus and newborn. The mortality rate is 1 to 10 percent in these affected infants, with postnatal persistence of this condition for as long as 4 months (Burrows, 1995; Plunket, 1987).

Neonatal Alloimmune Thrombocytopenia. The remaining 20 percent of immune-mediated thrombocytopenias are caused by an alloimmune (isoimmune) reaction in which maternal antibodies are produced against foreign fetal platelets while maternal platelet levels remain normal. This reaction occurs when fetal platelets possessing an antigen not found on maternal platelets pass into maternal circulation and is similar to the mechanism behind Rh incompatibility. Unlike Rh incompatibility, alloimmune thrombocytopenia affects 33 to 50 percent of first pregnancies (Reznikoff-Etievant, 1988). The mother develops IgG antibodies that eventually cross into fetal circulation, resulting in platelet destruction. The $P1^{A1}$ alloantibodies are responsible for 50 to 80 percent of neonates with alloimmune thrombocytopenia (von dem Borne et al., 1980). This phenomenon occurs in approximately 1:2000 to 1:3000 live births (Taaning & Skibsted, 1990). The mortality rate of 10 to 15 percent in isoimmune thrombocytopenia is higher than that in ITP, because bleeding tends to be more severe. The frequency of intracranial hemorrhage in utero is reported to be as high as 10 to 15 percent (Mueller-Eckhardt et al., 1989), with the majority occurring between 30 and 35 weeks' gestation. The treatment consists of transfusion of maternal platelets, exchange transfusion, and the use of IVIG in the dosage of 400 mg/kg during 5 days (Suarez & Anderson, 1986). Platelets usually normalize in the newborn by age 4 weeks.

ANTENATAL TREATMENT

Antenatal treatment is not universally agreed on, but several sources suggest the use of corticosteroids 1 to 2 weeks before delivery and the administration of multiple aliquots of IVIG within 7 to 9 days of delivery. Steroids and IVIG are theorized to work in similar fashion by (1) decreasing the production of antiplatelet antibodies, (2) interfering with antibody attachment to the surface of the platelets, and (3) decreasing platelet destruction by interfering with phagocytic receptors in the reticuloendothelial system.

Serious bleeding during labor and delivery occurs only in infants with platelet counts less than 50,000/mm^3 (Scott et al., 1980). Scalp sampling in fetuses of mothers with ITP and delivery by cesarean section of those infants with levels of less than 50,000/mm^3 are recommended.

POSTNATAL TREATMENT OF THE NEONATE

Postnatal treatment consists of platelet transfusion, exchange transfusion with blood less than 2 days old, steroid therapy (prednisone, 1 to 5 mg/kg/day) (Goetzman & Wennberg, 1991), and IVIG. The major difference in therapy between ITP and alloimmune thrombocytopenia is the use of washed, irradiated, maternal platelets in infants with alloimmune thrombocytopenia.

Neonatal Factors

Neonatal factors associated with thrombocytopenia include the following (Mehta et al., 1980):

1. Asphyxia.
2. Apgar scores of less than 7 in 70 percent of infants.
3. Disseminated intravascular coagulation—16 percent.
4. Exchange transfusion—12 percent.
5. Infection—52 to 77 percent (Mondanlou & Ortiz, 1981; Zipursky & Jaber, 1978).
6. Smallness for gestational age.
7. Necrotizing enterocolitis—90 percent (Hutter et al., 1976).
8. Hyperbilirubinemia and phototherapy.
9. Meconium aspiration.
10. Cold injury.
11. Polycythemia.
12. Pulmonary hypertension.
13. Cardiopulmonary bypass for heart surgery—reduces platelets by 70 percent (Kern et al., 1992).

Treatment of thrombocytopenia due to neonatal factors consists initially of amelioration of the underlying problem, followed by symptomatic treatment with platelet transfusion. Transfusion therapy should be considered if platelet counts are in the range of 50,000 to 100,000/mm^3 and active bleeding is present. Platelet transfusion should be considered at levels of less than 50,000/mm^3 even if active bleeding is not present. In estimating the rise in platelets after transfusion, the following formula is a helpful calculation:

$\frac{1}{10}$ of the volume (in ml) of a unit of platelets per kg of weight raises the platelet count by 50,000/mm^3

Disseminated Intravascular Coagulation

Disseminated intravascular coagulation is marked by a generalized deficiency in coagulation factors and platelets that leaves the infant predisposed to hemorrhage. Because this condition is triggered by a pre-existing illness and does not occur independently, treatment consists of identification and resolution of the underlying problem. The most common factors associated with bleeding that occurs secondary to disseminated intravascular coagulation are obstetrical complications, respiratory distress syndrome, hypoxia, hypotension, and sepsis. Occasionally, thrombosis of large vessels can trap platelets and consume an amount of clotting factors sufficient to cause disseminated intravascular coagulation. Mortality rates reach 60 to 80 percent in infants with disseminated intravascular coagulation who experience severe bleeding (Oski & Naiman, 1982a, 1982c, 1982d).

The hematologic picture of disseminated intravascular coagulation (Table 28–13) reflects a depletion of platelets, prothrombin, fibrinogen, Factor V, Factor VIII, and Factor XIII. The prothrombin time and partial thromboplastin time are prolonged and are not corrected with the addition of fresh frozen plasma to the blood sample. The fibrinolytic system is also stimulated and is evident by the presence of degradation products of fibrinolysis (i.e., fibrin degradation products or fibrinolytic split products).

Successful treatment of disseminated intravascular coagulation depends on the ability to alleviate the underlying cause. Palliative treatment consists of replacement of deficient clotting factors and platelets and exchange transfusion. Heparin is infrequently used and only with the occurrence of large-vessel thrombosis. It is administered as an initial bolus of 50 U/kg followed by 15 to 25 U/kg/h (Young & Magnum, 1997).

Differential Diagnosis of Newborn Coagulopathies

Analysis of multiple factors can often help in identifying a specific coagulopathy affecting an infant. Careful evaluation of these factors can pinpoint the correct diagnosis and influence the choice of therapy or intervention to be used. Some factors that aid in the differential diagnosis are

1. Familial history of a bleeding disorder such as hemophilia.
2. Maternal history of a bleeding disorder, as in autoimmune thrombocytopenia.
3. Obstetrical history suggesting a possible abnormality, as in maternal alloimmunization or hypofibrinogenemia.
4. Adverse neonatal history, such as the presence of hypoxia or asphyxia;
5. Failure to administer prophylactic vitamin K at birth.
6. Physical manifestations of a bleeding disorder, such as obvious bleeding, the presence or absence of petechiae or ecchymosis, and the overall condition of the infant.
7. Laboratory data that identify specific abnormalities, such as specific coagulation factor deficiencies; thrombocytopenia; and prolonged prothrombin time, partial thromboplastin time, and clotting times.

Collaborative Management of a Coagulopathy

Care of an infant with a bleeding diathesis should be aimed at the prevention of further injury or bleeding. Prevention of injury to fragile tissue and limitation of blood draws from sites other than central catheters are of great importance in the infant who lacks adequate clotting factors to control bleeding. Appropriate administration of platelets, clotting factors, or blood products requires the correct equipment, the correct method of administration, and conscientious monitoring of vital signs to ensure effective therapy without causing further harm to the infant. Wise decisions regarding replacement blood products are now important in light of the severe and potentially lethal sequelae of acquired infection. Monitoring laboratory tests to determine ongoing needs and the efficacy of therapy continues to be an important need throughout the infant's entire course of therapy.

In administering blood or blood products, the infant must be continuously evaluated for signs of fluid overload and untoward reaction. Although blood reactions are rare in the newborn, they tend to occur within the first 15 minutes of blood or blood product administration and are manifested as rashes, tachycardia, hypertension, hematuria, cyanosis, and hyperthermia. Throughout the acute course of illness, the nurse must also keep a continual tally of blood loss from blood draws, making medical personnel aware of blood depletion as it approaches 10 percent of the infant's blood volume. An infant should be able to tolerate this degree of blood loss but may become symptomatic when losses exceed this amount. Symptoms include metabolic acidosis, hypotension, poor perfusion, tachycardia, cyanosis, and shock.

TABLE 28–13 Hematologic Picture of Disseminated Intravascular Coagulation

Features	Disseminated Intravascular Coagulation
Uniformity of clotting defect	Variable
Capillary fragility	Usually abnormal
Bleeding time	Often prolonged
Clotting time	Variable
One-stage prothrombin	Moderately prolonged
Partial thromboplastin time	Prolonged
Fibrin degradation products	Present
Factor V	Decreased
Fibrinogen	Often decreased
Platelets	Often decreased
Red cell fragmentation	Usually present
Response to vitamin K	Diminished or absent
Associated disease	Severe, may include sepsis, hypoxia, acidosis, or obstetrical accident
Previous history	Associated diseases; vitamin K given

From Oski, F. (1976). Hematological problems. In G. Avery (Ed.), *Neonatology* (p. 408). Philadelphia: J. B. Lippincott.

Blood and Blood Component Therapy

Commonly Used Blood Products

Whole Blood. This product is not used for routine volume expansion because of the hematocrit dilution that occurs. It is used in surgical procedures requiring large volumes of blood for replacement, for exchange transfusions, and for priming heart–lung oxygenators for extracorporeal membrane oxygenation.

Packed Red Blood Cells. Blood is "hard-spun" to concentrate cells and allow the supernatant to be removed. As the result of this form of preparation, less volume can be administered. Packed RBCs can be reconstituted with normal saline, 5 percent albumin, or fresh frozen plasma. Packed RBCs can be used in exchange transfusions or in the treatment of anemia in the acutely ill or symptomatic convalescent infant.

Washed Red Blood Cells. For additional protection, RBCs can be washed to remove as much of the plasma, nonviable RBCs, WBCs, and metabolic wastes as possible. To further eliminate the possibility of a graft-versus-host reaction, cells can be irradiated with 5000 rad of radiation. This prevents T-lymphocyte proliferation and, when done in conjunction with washing, can remove up to 95 percent of T lymphocytes.

Frozen Deglycerolized Red Cells. Frozen storage of deglycerolized RBCs allows preservation of rare units of blood, but the cost of preparation increases considerably. In addition, this product tends to have a higher potassium content and hemoglobin concentration. Centrifuging it, removing the supernatant, and diluting it to the desired hematocrit tend to control these problems.

Fresh Frozen Plasma. A whole unit of fresh frozen plasma can be thawed, but once entered, it is good for only 6 hours. If, however, it is packaged in aliquots such as a quad pack before freezing and then thawed, the quad pack unit is good for 24

hours once it is thawed. Fresh frozen plasma provides a rich source of coagulation factors, containing 1 IU/ml of all clotting factors; 10 to 15 ml/kg raises the overall level of clotting factor activity by 20 to 30 percent. Fresh frozen plasma can often normalize a prolonged prothrombin time and partial thromboplastin time in the newborn having a generalized deficiency in quantity and activity of available clotting factors.

Platelets. The number of platelets available for circulation after transfusion depends on the storage time. In transfusions using platelet bags less than 7 days old, the rise in platelet levels is comparable to the rise seen with the use of fresh platelets. Use of packs older than 7 days achieves only 70 percent of the rise seen with the use of fresh platelets. Platelets can also be concentrated by centrifuge if smaller volumes are required. One caveat to remember: platelets require a special administration set for proper infusion.

Granulocytes. Granulocytes, used for infusion in septic infants with severe neutropenia, are prepared from fresh donor blood through the process of plasmapheresis. WBCs are removed from the unit of blood, but a large number of RBCs remain. For this reason, the donor unit needs to be typed and crossmatched to the infant for type and Rh compatibility. WBCs are usually irradiated to eliminate donor T cells to prevent graft-versus-host responses.

Cryoprecipitate. This form of plasma preparation is rich in Factor VIII, Factor XIII, and fibrinogen and is useful in the treatment of hemophilia. Because it is a single-donor collection, the risk for infection is lower than in pooled substances.

Factor Concentrates. Factor concentrates are used as specific therapy for identified factor deficiencies. They are obtained from pooled plasma and expose the recipient to multiple donors, thereby increasing the potential for infection, especially with hepatitis B, cytomegalovirus, and AIDS. Eighty percent of hepatitis B can be identified by the third-generation screening tests, and blood screening for cytomegalovirus is also available. Because the risk for transmission of HIV is increased by pooled concentrates, it is now recommended that concentrates be treated with heat, solvent, steam, detergent, or ultraviolet light to kill any potential virus. At present, it is unclear whether such treatment alters or inactivates the clotting activity of factor concentrates.

CONCLUSION

The development of the blood cells formed from the pluripotent stem cells begins early in fetal development and becomes more sophisticated as the human organism matures. This maturation continues after birth and throughout adult life. The newborn and premature infant possess substantial hematologic capabilities but are hampered by their inability to compensate as well as the older child and adult on exposure to significant stress. Their ability to adequately maintain themselves during a steady state, however, must be acknowledged.

Many abnormalities in the hematologic system can result from congenital, acquired, perinatal, and postnatal factors. Some of these disturbances occur because of maturational deficiencies, congenital defects, or acquired disease states. The newborn has a limited repertoire with which to respond to and compensate for any such abnormalities.

Treatment of these abnormalities depends on the abnormality itself, but symptomatic treatment often plays a major role in therapy. Because of the potentially lethal outcome of some of the acquired illnesses contracted from contaminated blood sources, the use of blood and blood products must be carefully analyzed for its appropriateness.

REFERENCES

Aballi, A., & DeLamerens, S. (1962). Coagulation changes in neonatal period and early infancy. *Pediatric Clinics of North America, 9,* 785–817.

Aballi, A. J., Puapondh, Y. A., & Desposito, F. (1968). Platelet counts in thriving premature infants. *Pediatrics, 42*(4), 685–689.

Allen, F., Diamond, L., & Vaughan, V., III. (1950). Erythroblastosis fetalis; prevention of kernicterus. *American Journal of Diseases of Children, 80,* 779.

American Academy of Pediatrics. (1993). *Guidelines to perinatal care* (3rd ed.). Elk Grove Village, IL: Author.

Anai, T., Hirota, Y., Yoshimatsu, J., et al. (1993). Can prenatal vitamin K_1 (phylloquinone) supplementation replace prophylaxis at birth? *Obstetrics and Gynecology, 81*(2), 251–253.

Arad, I., Konijn, A. M., Linder, N. A., et al. (1988). Serum ferritin levels in preterm infants after multiple blood transfusions. *American Journal of Perinatology, 5*(1), 40–43.

Aranda, J. V., & Sweet, A. V. (1977). Alterations in blood pressure during exchange transfusion. *Archives of Disease in Childhood, 52*(7), 545–548.

Bada, H. S., Chua, C., Salmon, J. H., & Hajjar, W. (1979). Changes in intracranial pressure during exchange transfusion. *Journal of Pediatrics, 94*(1), 129–132.

Baehner, R. L., & Strauss, H. S. (1966). Hemophilia in the first year of life. *New England Journal of Medicine, 275*(10), 524–528.

Bard, H. (1975). The postnatal decline of hemoglobin F synthesis in normal full term infants. *Journal of Clinical Investigations, 55*(2), 395–398.

Bard, H., & Prosmanne, J. (1982). Postnatal fetal and adult hemoglobin synthesis in preterm infants whose birth weight was less than 1,000 grams. *Journal of Clinical Investigations, 70*(1), 50–52.

Barnard, D. R., Chapman, R. G., Simmons, M. A., & Hathaway, W. E. (1980). Blood for use in exchange transfusion in the newborn. *Transfusion, 20*(4), 401–408.

Baumgart, S., & Kim, H. (1988). Blood component therapy in the neonate. In J. Stockman & C. Pochedly (Eds.), *Developmental and neonatal hematology* (pp. 199–222). New York: Raven Press.

Bergman, D., Cooley, J., Coombs, J., et al. (1994). American Academy of Pediatrics. Practice parameter: Management of hyperbilirubinemia in the healthy term newborn. *Pediatrics, 94*(4, Part 1), 558–561.

Bhanchet, P., Tuchinda, S., Hathirat, P., et al. (1977). A bleeding syndrome in infants due to acquired prothrombin complex deficiency. *Clinical Pediatrics, 16*(11), 992–998.

Bifano, E. M., Smith, F., & Borer, J. (1992). Relationship between determinants of oxygen delivery and respiratory abnormalities in preterm infants with anemia. *Journal of Pediatrics, 120*(2, Part 1), 292–296.

Black, V. D., & Lubchenco, L. O. (1979). Neurologic and developmental sequelae of neonatal hyperviscosity. *Clinical Research, 27,* 123A.

Blanchette, V., Doyle, J., Schmidt, B., & Zipursky, A. (1994). Anemias. In G. Avery, M. Fletcher, & M. MacDonald (Eds.), *Neonatology* (4th ed., pp. 952–999). Philadelphia: J. B. Lippincott.

Blank, J. P., Sheagren, T. G., Vajaria, J., et al. (1984). The role of RBC transfusion in the premature infant. *American Journal of Diseases of Children, 138*(9), 831–833.

Bleyer, W. A., Hakami, N., & Shepard, T. H. (1971). The development of hemostasis in the human fetus and newborn infant. *Journal of Pediatrics, 79*(5), 838–853.

Bowman, J. (1988). Alloimmune hemolytic disease of the neonate. In J. Stockman & C. Pochedly (Eds.), *Developmental and neonatal hematology* (pp. 223–248). New York: Raven Press.

Bowman, J. (1992). Rhesus haemolyticus disease. In N. Wald (Ed.), *Antenatal and neonatal screening* (2nd ed.). Oxford: Oxford University Press.

Bowman, J. (1994). Maternal blood group immunization. In R. Creasy & R. Resnik (Eds.), *Maternal-fetal medicine: Principles and practice* (3rd ed., pp. 714–757). Philadelphia: W. B. Saunders.

Bratlid, D., Cashore, W. J., & Oh, W. (1984). Effect of acidosis on bilirubin deposition in rat brain. *Pediatrics, 73*(4), 431–434.

Brodersen, R. (1980). Bilirubin transport in the newborn infant, reviewed with relation to kernicterus [Review]. *Journal of Pediatrics, 96*(3, Part 1), 349–356.

Brown, M. (1988a). Fetal and neonatal erythropoiesis. In J. Stockman & C. Pochedly (Eds.), *Developmental and neonatal hematology* (pp. 39–56). New York: Raven Press.

Brown, M. (1988b). Physiologic anemia of infancy: Normal red cell values and physiology of neonatal erythropoiesis. In J. Stockman & C. Pochedly (Eds.), *Developmental and neonatal hematology* (p. 262). New York: Raven Press.

Brown, M. S., Berman, E. R., & Luckey, D. (1990). Prediction of the need for transfusion during anemia of prematurity. *Journal of Pediatrics, 116*(5), 773–778.

Burgess, G. H., Oh, W., Bratlid, D., et al. (1985). The effects of brain blood flow on brain bilirubin deposition in newborn piglets. *Pediatric Research, 19*(7), 691–696.

Burrows, R. (1995). Perinatal thrombocytopenia. In E. Bifano & R. Ehrenkrantz (Eds.), *Clinics in Perinatology: Perinatal hematology* (Vol. 22, pp. 779–799). Philadelphia: W. B. Saunders.

Burrows, R. F., & Kelton, J. G. (1988). Incidentally detected thrombocytopenia in healthy mothers and their infants. *New England Journal of Medicine, 319*(3), 142–145.

Cashore, W. J., & Usher, R. H. (1973). Hypovolemia resulting from a tight nuchal cord at birth. *Pediatric Research, 7,* 399.

Chavez, G. F., Mulinare, J., & Edmonds, L. (1991). Epidemiology of Rh hemolytic disease of the newborn in the United States. *Journal of the American Medical Association, 265*(24), 3270–3274.

Chitkara, U., Bussel, J., Alvarez, M., et al. (1990). High-dose intravenous gamma globulin: Does it have a role in the treatment of severe erythroblastosis fetalis? *Obstetrics and Gynecology, 76*(4), 703–708.

Christensen, R. D., & Rothstein, G. (1979). Pitfalls in the interpretation of leukocyte counts of newborn infants. *American Journal of Clinical Pathology, 72*(4), 608–611.

Clarke, C., Donohue, W., McConnell, R., et al. (1963). Further experimental studies in the prevention of Rh hemolytic disease. *British Medical Journal, 1,* 979–989.

Cook, S., Gunter, J., & Wissel, M. (1993). Effective use of a strategy using assigned red cell units to limit donor exposure for neonatal patients. *Transfusion, 33*(5), 379–383.

de Alarcon, P. (1988). Thrombopoiesis in the fetus and newborn. In J. Stockman & C. Pochedly (Eds.), *Developmental and neonatal hematology* (pp. 103–130). New York: Raven Press.

Dear, P. (1984). Blood transfusion in the preterm infant [Editorial]. *Archives of Disease in Childhood, 59*(4), 296–298.

de la Camara, C., Arrieta, R., Gonzalez, A., et al. (1988). High-dose intravenous immunoglobulin as the sole prenatal treatment for severe Rh immunization. *New England Journal of Medicine, 318*(8), 519–520.

DeMaio, J. G., Harris, M. C., & Spitzer, A. R. (1986). The response of apnea of prematurity to transfusion therapy. *Pediatric Research, 20,* 389A.

Djaldetti, M. (1979). Hemopoietic events in human embryonic spleens at early gestational stages. *Biology of the Neonate, 36*(3–4), 133–144.

Doyle, L. W., Kelly, E. A., Rickards, A. L., et al. (1993). Sensorineural outcome at 2 years for survivors of erythroblastosis treated with fetal intravascular transfusions. *Obstetrics and Gynecology, 81*(6), 931–935.

Ebbesen, F. (1979). Superiority of intensive phototherapy—blue double light—in rhesus hemolytic disease. *European Journal of Pediatrics, 130*(4), 279–284.

Edgar, W. M., & Hambling, M. H. (1977). Rubella vaccination and anti-D immunoglobulin administration in the puerperium. *British Journal of Obstetrics and Gynaecology, 84*(10), 754–757.

Ekelund, H., Finnstrom, O., Gunnarskog, J., et al. (1993). Administration of vitamin K_1 to newborn infants and childhood cancer. *British Medical Journal, 307,* 89–91.

Emmerson, A. J., Coles, H. J., Stern, C. M., & Pearson, T. C. (1993). Double blind trial of recombinant human erythropoietin in preterm infants. *Archives of Disease in Childhood, 68*(3, Spec. No.), 291–296.

Emura, I., Sekiya, M., & Ohnishi, Y. (1983). Two types of immature megakaryocyte series in the human fetal liver. *Archivum Histologicum Japonicum, 46*(1), 103–114.

Eschbach, J. W., Egrie, J. C., Downing, M. R., et al. (1987). Correction of the anemia of end-stage renal disease with recombinant human erythropoietin. Results of a combined phase I and II clinical trial. *New England Journal of Medicine, 316*(2), 73–78.

Faxelius, G., Raye, J., Gutberlet, R., et al. (1977). Red cell volume measurements and acute blood loss in high-risk newborn infants. *Journal of Pediatrics, 90*(2), 273–281.

Feusner, J. H. (1980). Normal and abnormal bleeding times in neonates and young children utilizing a full standardized template technique. *American Journal of Clinical Pathology, 74*(1), 73–76.

Fisk, N. M., Bennett, P., Warwick, R. M., et al. (1994). Clinical utility of fetal RhD typing in alloimmunized pregnancies by means of polymerase chain reaction on amniocytes or chorionic villi. *Journal of American Obstetrics and Gynecology, 171*(1), 50–54.

Gale, R., Seidman, D. S., Dollberg, S., & Stevenson, D. (1990). Epidemiology of neonatal jaundice in the Jerusalem population. *Journal of Pediatric Gastroenterology and Nutrition, 10*(1), 82–86.

Gartner, L. M., & Lee, K. (1992). Jaundice and liver disease: Part I. Unconjugated hyperbilirubinemia. In A. Fanaroff & R. Martin (Eds.), *Behrman's neonatal-perinatal medicine* (5th ed., pp. 1075–1103). St. Louis: C. V. Mosby.

Glader, B. E., & Naiman, J. L. (1991). Erythrocyte disorders in infancy. In H. W. Taeusch, R. A. Ballard, & M. E. Avery (Eds.), *Schaffer and Avery's diseases of the newborn* (6th ed., pp. 798–827). Philadelphia: W. B. Saunders.

Goetzman, B. W., & Wennberg, R. P. (1991). *Neonatal intensive care handbook* (2nd ed.). St. Louis: Mosby–Year Book.

Goldberg, K. E., Lubchenco, L. O., & Guggenheim, M. (1976). Sequelae of neonatal hyperviscosity. *Pediatric Research, 10,* 448.

Golding, J., Greenwood, R., Birmingham, K., & Mott, M. (1992). Childhood cancer, intramuscular vitamin K, and pethidine given during labor. *British Medical Journal, 305*(6849), 341–346.

Golding, J., Paterson, M., & Kinlen, L. (1990). Factors associated with childhood cancer in a national cohort study. *British Journal of Cancer, 62*(2), 304–308.

Govoni, L. E., & Hayes, J. E. (1988). *Drugs and nursing implications* (5th ed.). Norwalk, CT: Appleton & Lange.

Guyton, A. (1996a). Blood groups; transfusions; tissue and organ transplantation. In A. Guyton, *Textbook of medical physiology* (9th ed., pp. 457–462). Philadelphia: W. B. Saunders.

Guyton, A. (1996b). Hemostasis and blood coagulation. In A. Guyton, *Textbook of medical physiology* (9th ed., pp. 463–472). Philadelphia: W. B. Saunders.

Hakanson, O. (1981). Neonatal hyperviscosity syndrome: Long term benefit of partial plasma exchange transfusion. *Pediatric Research, 15,* 449.

Hallak, M., Moise, K. J., Jr., Hesketh, D. E., et al. (1992). Intravascular transfusion of fetuses with rhesus incompatibility: Prediction of fetal outcome by changes in umbilical venous pressure. *Obstetrics and Gynecology, 80*(2), 286–290.

Halperin, D. S., Wacher, P., Lacourt, G., et al. (1989). Response of premature anemic infants to subcutaneous recombinant erythropoietin (Abstract). *Molecular Biotheraphy, 1,* 64.

Halvorsen, S., & Finne, P. (1968). Erythropoietin production in the human fetus and newborn. *Annals of the New York Academy of Sciences, 149*(1), 576–577.

Harman, C. R., Bowman, J. M., Manning, F. A., & Menticoglou, S. M. (1990). Intrauterine transfusion—intraperitoneal versus intravascular approach: A case-control comparison. *American Journal of Obstetrics and Gynecology, 162*(4), 1053–1059.

Hathaway, W., & Bonnar, J. (1978). Coagulation and hemostasis: General considerations. In W. Hathaway & J. Bonnar (Eds.), *Perinatal coagulation* (pp. 1–26). New York: Grune & Stratton.

Hathaway, W. E., Isarangukura, P. B., Mahasandana, C., et al. (1991). Comparison of oral and parenteral vitamin K prophylaxis for prevention of late hemorrhagic disease of the newborn. *Journal of Pediatrics, 119*(3), 461–464.

Hutter, J. J., Jr., Hathaway, W. E., & Wayne, E. R. (1976). Hematologic abnormalities in severe neonatal necrotizing enterocolitis. *Journal of Pediatrics, 88*(6), 1026–1031.

Izraeli, S., Ben-Sira, L., Harell, D., et al. (1993). Lactic acid as a predictor for erythrocyte transfusion in healthy preterm infants with anemia of prematurity. *Journal of Pediatrics, 122*(4), 629–631.

Izumi, T., Kawahami, M., Enzan, H., & Ohkita, T. (1983). The size of megakaryocytes in human fetal, infantile, and adult hematopoiesis. *Hiroshima Journal of Medical Science, 32*(3), 257–260.

Jackson, C. M., & Suttu, J. W. (1977). Recent developments in understanding the mechanism of vitamin K and vitamin K–antagonist drug action and the consequences of vitamin K action in blood coagulation. *Progress in Hematology, 10,* 333–359.

Johnson, K. (1993). *Harriet Lane handbook* (13th ed., p. 231). St. Louis: C. V. Mosby.

Jones, W. R. (1969). The application of the Kleihauer technique to fetal blood. *Australian and New Zealand Journal of Obstetrics and Gynaecology, 9*(1), 33–36.

Joshi, A., Gerhardt, T., Shandloff, P., & Bancalari, E. (1987). Blood transfusion effects on the respiratory pattern of preterm infants. *Pediatrics, 80*(1), 79–84.

Kappas, A., Drummond, G. S., Manola, T., et al. (1988). Sn-protoporphyrin use in the management of hyperbilirubinemia in term newborns with direct Coombs-positive ABO incompatibility. *Pediatrics, 81*(4), 485–497.

Keenan, W. J., Jewett, T., & Glueck, H. I. (1971). Role of feeding and vitamin K in hypoprothrombinemia of the newborn. *American Journal of Diseases of Children, 121*(4), 271–277.

Kern, F. H., Morana, N. J., Sears, J. J., & Hickey, P. R. (1992). Coagulation defects in neonates during cardiopulmonary bypass. *Annals of Thoracic Surgery, 54*(3), 541–546.

Keyes, W. G., Donohue, P. K., Spivak, J. L., et al. (1989). Assessing the need for transfusion of premature infants and the role of hematocrit, clinical signs and erythropoietin level. *Pediatrics, 84*(3), 412–417.

King, J., & Jung, A. (1990). Phototherapy. In N. Nelson (Ed.), *Current therapy in neonatal-perinatal medicine* (p. 461). Philadelphia: B. C. Decker.

Klebanoff, M. A., Read, J. S., Mills, J. L., & Shiono, P. H. (1993). The risk of childhood cancer after neonatal exposure to vitamin K. *New England Journal of Medicine, 329*(13), 905–908.

Knox, I., Ennever, J. F., & Speck, W. T. (1985). Urinary excretion of an isomer of bilirubin during phototherapy. *Pediatric Research, 19*(2), 198–201.

Kopelman, A. E., Brown, R. S., & Odell, G. B. (1972). The "bronze" baby syndrome: A complication of phototherapy. *Journal of Pediatrics, 81*(3), 466–472.

Kuller, J. A., Chescheir, N. C., & Cefalo, R. C. (Eds.). (1996). *Prenatal diagnosis and reproductive genetics.* Philadelphia: J. B. Lippincott.

Lackner, T. (1982). Drug replacement following exchange transfusion. *Journal of Pediatrics, 100*(5), 811–814.

Lee, D. A., Slagle, T. A., Jackson, T. M., & Evans, C. S. (1995). Reducing blood donor exposures in low birth weight infants by the use of older, unwashed packed red blood cells. *Journal of Pediatrics, 126*(2), 280–286.

Lemberge, R., & Legge, J. (1949). *Hematin compounds and bile pigments.* New York: Intersciences Publishers.

Levy, G. J., Strauss, R. G., Hume, H., et al. (1993). National survey of neonatal transfusion practices: I. Red blood cell therapy. *Pediatrics, 91*(3), 523–529.

Liley, A. (1961). Liquor amnii analysis in management of pregnancy complicated by rhesus immunization. *American Journal of Obstetrics and Gynecology, 82,* 1359–1371.

Linn, S., Schoenbaum, S. C., Monson, R. R., et al. (1985). Epidemiology of neonatal hyperbilirubinemia. *Pediatrics, 75*(4), 770–774.

Liu, E. A., Mannino, F. L., & Lane, T. A. (1994). Prospective, randomized trial of the safety and efficacy of a limited donor exposure transfusion program for premature neonates. *Journal of Pediatrics, 125*(1), 92–96.

Loughnan, P., & McDougall, P. (1993). Epidemiology of late onset haemorrhagic disease: A pooled data analysis. *Journal of Paediatrics and Child Health, 29*(3), 177–181.

Maier, R. F., Obladen, M., Scigalla, P., et al. (1994). The effect of epoetin beta (recombinant human erythropoietin) on the need for transfusion in very-low-birth-weight infants. *New England Journal of Medicine, 330*(17), 1173–1178.

Maisels, M. (1990). Hyperbilirubinemia. In N. M. Nelson (Ed.), *Current therapy in neonatal-perinatal medicine* (2nd ed., pp. 258–262). Philadelphia: B. C. Decker.

Maisels, M. J., Gifford, K., Antle, C., & Lieb, G. R. (1988). Jaundice in the healthy newborn infant: A new approach to an old problem. *Pediatrics, 81*(4), 505–511.

Mantalenaki-Asfi, K., Morphis, L., Nicolopoulos, D., & Matsaniotis, N. (1975). Influence of exchange transfusion on the development of serum immunoglobulins. *Journal of Pediatrics, 87*(3), 396–399.

McDonagh, A. F., & Lightner, D. A. (1985). "Like a shriveled blood orange"—bilirubin, jaundice, and phototherapy. *Pediatrics, 75*(3), 443–455.

McEvoy, G. K. (Ed.). (1990). *American Hospital Formulary Service (AHFS) drug information.* Bethesda, MD: American Society of Hospital Pharmacists.

McMillan, M. P. (1996). Banking on cord blood. *Journal of Obstetric, Gynecologic, and Neonatal Nursing, 25*(2), 115.

McNinch, A. W., Upton, C., Samuels, M., et al. (1985). Plasma concentrations after oral or intramuscular vitamin K_1 in neonates. *Archives of Diseases in Childhood, 60*(9), 814–818.

Mehta, P., Vasa, R., Neumann, L., & Karpatkin, M. (1980). Thrombocytopenia in the high-risk infant. *Journal of Pediatrics, 97*(5), 791–794.

Mennuti, M. T., Brummond, W., Crombleholme, W. R., et al. (1980). Fetal-maternal bleeding associated with amniocentesis. *Obstetrics and Gynecology, 55*(1), 48–54.

Messer, J., Haddad, J., Donato, L., et al. (1993). Early treatment of premature infants with recombinant human erythropoietin. *Pediatrics, 92*(4), 519–523.

Meyer, M. P., Meyer, J. H., Commerford, A., et al. (1994). Recombinant human erythropoietin in the treatment of the anemia of prematurity: Results of a double-blind, placebo-controlled study. *Pediatrics, 93*(6, Part 1), 918–923.

Mollison, P. (1984). *Blood transfusion in clinical medicine* (7th ed., p. 675). Oxford: Blackwell Scientific Publications.

Mondanlou, H. D., & Ortiz, O. B. (1981). Thrombocytopenia in neonatal infection. *Clinical Pediatrics, 20*(6), 402–407.

Moore, K., & Persaud, T. (1993). Formation of the human embryo. In K. Moore & T. Persaud, *The developing human* (5th ed., pp. 53–69). Philadelphia: W. B. Saunders.

Motohara, K., Endo, F., & Matsuda, I. (1987). Screening for late neonatal vitamin K deficiency by acarboxylprothrombin in dried blood spots. *Archives of Diseases in Childhood, 62*(4), 370–375.

Mueller-Eckhardt, C., Kiefel, V., Grubert, A., et al. (1989). Three hundred and forty-eight cases of suspected neonatal alloimmune thrombocytopenia. *Lancet, 1*(8634), 363–366.

Mull, M., & Hathaway, W. (1970). Altered platelet function in newborns. *Pediatric Research, 4,* 229.

Ness, P. M., Baldwin, M. L., & Niebyl, J. R. (1987). Clinical high-risk designation does not predict excess fetal-maternal hemorrhage. *American Journal of Obstetrics and Gynecology, 156*(1), 154–158.

Ney, J. A., Socol, M. C., Dooley, S. L., et al. (1991). Perinatal outcome following intravascular transfusion in severely isoimmunized fetuses. *International Journal of Gynecology and Obstetrics, 35*(1), 41–46.

Nicolaides, K. H., Rodeck, C. H., Mibashan, R. S., & Kemp, J. R. (1986). Have Liley charts outlived their usefulness? *American Journal of Obstetrics and Gynecology, 155*(1), 90–94.

Nicoll, A., Ginsburg, R., & Tripp, J. H. (1982). Supplementary feeding and jaundice in newborns. *Acta Paediatrica Scandinavica, 71*(5), 759–761.

Norman, M., Fagrell, B., & Herin, P. (1992). Effects of neonatal polycythemia and hemodilution on capillary perfusion. *Journal of Pediatrics, 121*(1), 103–108.

Obladen, M., Sachsenweger, M., & Stahnke, M. (1988). Blood sampling in very low birth weight infants receiving different levels of intensive care. *European Journal of Pediatrics, 147*(4), 399–404.

Ohls, R. K., Hunter, D. D., & Christensen, R. D. (1993). A randomized, double-blind, placebo-controlled trial of recombinant erythropoietin in treatment of the anemia of bronchopulmonary dysplasia. *Journal of Pediatrics, 123*(6), 996–1000.

Ohls, R. K., Osborne, K. A., & Christensen, R. D. (1995). Efficacy and cost analysis of treating very low birth weight infants with erythropoietin during their first two weeks of life: A randomized, placebo-controlled trial. *Journal of Pediatrics, 126*(3), 421–426.

Olsen, J. H., Hertz, H., Blinkenberg, K., & Verder, H. (1994). Vitamin K regimens and incidence of childhood cancer in Denmark. *British Medical Journal, 308*(6933), 895–896.

Oski, F. (1993). The erythrocyte and its disorders. In D. Nathan & F. Oski (Eds.), *Hematology of infancy and childhood* (3rd ed., pp. 18–43). Philadelphia: W. B. Saunders.

Oski, F., & Naiman, J. (1982a). Anemia in the neonatal period. In F. Oski & J. Naiman (Eds.), *Hematologic problems in the newborn: Vol. IV. Major problems in clinical pediatrics* (3rd ed., pp. 56–86). Philadelphia: W. B. Saunders.

Oski, F., & Naiman J. (1982b). Erythroblastosis fetalis. In F. Oski & J. Naiman (Eds.), *Hematologic problems in the newborn: Vol. IV. Major problems in clinical pediatrics* (3rd ed., pp. 283–346). Philadelphia: W. B. Saunders.

Oski, F., & Naiman, J. (1982c). Normal blood values in the newborn period. In F. Oski & J. Naiman, *Hematologic problems in the newborn: Vol. IV. Major problems in clinical pediatrics* (3rd ed., pp. 1–31). Philadelphia: W. B. Saunders.

Oski, F., & Naiman., J. (1982d). Polycythemia and hyperviscosity in the neonatal period. In F. Oski & J. Naiman, *Hematologic problems in the*

newborn: Vol. IV. Major problems in clinical pediatrics (3rd ed., pp. 87–96). Philadelphia: W. B. Saunders.
Ozolek, J. A., Watchko, J. F., & Mimouni, F. (1994). Prevalence and lack of clinical significance of blood group incompatibility in mothers with blood type A or B. *Journal of Pediatrics, 125*(1), 87–91.
Page, E., Villee, C., & Villee, D. (1981). *Human reproduction: Essentials of reproductive and perinatal medicine* (3rd ed.). Philadelphia: W. B. Saunders.
Patten, E., Robbins, M., Vincent, J., et al. (1991). Use of red blood cells older than five days for neonatal transfusion. *Journal of Perinatology, 11*(1), 37–40.
Petti, S., Testa, U., Migliaccio, A. R., et al. (1985). Embryonic hemopoiesis in human liver: Morphologic aspects at sequential stages of ontogenic development. *Progress in Clinical Biological Research, 193,* 57–71.
Phibbs, R. (1970). Response of newborn infants to leukocyte depletion during exchange transfusion. *Biology of the Neonate, 15,* 112–122.
Phibbs, R. H., Johnson, P., & Tooley, W. H. (1974). Cardiorespiratory status of erythroblastotic infants: II. Blood volume, hematocrit, and serum albumin concentration in relation to hydrops fetalis. *Pediatrics, 53*(1), 13–23.
Plunket, D. (1987). Bleeding syndromes of the newborn. In D. Kasprisin & N. Luban (Eds.), *Pediatric transfusion medicine* (Vol. I, pp. 53–68). Boca Raton, FL: CRC Press.
Prindull, G., & Prindull, B. (1970). Leukocyte reserves of newborn infants. I. Observations during exchange transfusions. *Blut, 21*(2), 79–86.
Quinnan, G. (1993). *Recommendations regarding license amendments and procedures for gamma irradiation of blood products.* Washington, DC: U.S. Department of Health and Human Services, Center for Biologics Evaluation and Research, Food and Drug Administration.
Ramamurthy, R. S., & Berlanga, M. (1987). Postnatal alteration in hematocrit and viscosity in normal and polycythemic infants. *Journal of Pediatrics, 110*(6), 929–934.
Reznikoff-Etievant, M. F. (1988). Management of alloimmune neonatal and antenatal thrombocytopenia [Review]. *Vox Sanguinis, 55*(4), 193–201.
Rhondeau, S. M., Christensen, R. D., Ross, M. P., et al. (1988). Responsiveness to recombinant human erythropoietin of marrow erythroid progenitors from infants with the "anemia of prematurity." *Journal of Pediatrics, 112*(6), 935–940.
Ross, M. P., Christensen, R. D., Rothstein, G., et al. (1989). A randomized trial to develop criteria for administering erythrocyte transfusions to anemic preterm infants 1 to 3 months of age. *Journal of Perinatology, 9*(3), 246–253.
Rubo, J., Albrecht, K., Lasch, P., et al. (1992). High-dose intravenous immune globulin therapy for hyperbilirubinemia caused by Rh hemolytic disease. *Journal of Pediatrics, 121*(1), 93–97.
Sacher, R., & Queenan, J. (1987). Hemolytic disease of the newborn: Antenatal and prophylactic management. In D. Kasprisin & N. Luban (Eds), *Pediatric transfusion medicine* (Vol. 1, pp. 23–42). Boca Raton, FL: CRC Press.
Scanlon, J. W., & Krakaur, R. (1980). Hyperkalemia following exchange transfusion. *Journal of Pediatrics, 96*(1), 108–110.
Schulman, I. (1962). Pediatric aspects of the mild hemophilias. *Medical Clinics of North America, 46,* 93–105.
Scott, J., & Branch, D. (1994). Immunologic disorders in pregnancy. In J. Scott, P. DiSaia, C. Hammond, & W. Spellacy (Eds.), *Danforth's obstetrics and gynecology* (7th ed., pp. 393–408). Philadelphia: J. B. Lippincott.
Scott, J. R., Cruikshank, D. P., Kochenour, N. K., et al. (1980). Fetal platelet counts in the obstetric management of immunologic thrombocytopenia purpura. *American Journal of Obstetrics and Gynecology, 136*(4), 495–499.
Seibel, M., & Gross, S. (1987). Exchange transfusion in the neonate. In D. Kasprisin & N. Luban (Eds.), *Pediatric transfusion medicine* (Vol. 1, pp. 43–52). Boca Raton, FL: CRC Press.
Sell, E. J., & Corrigan, J. J., Jr. (1973). Platelet counts, fibrinogen concentrations and factor V and factor VIII levels in healthy infants according to gestational age. *Journal of Pediatrics, 82*(6), 1028–1032.
Shannon, K. M., Keith, J. F., III, Mentzer, W. C., et al. (1995). Recombinant human erythropoietin stimulates erythropoiesis and reduces erythrocyte transfusions in very low birth weight preterm infants. *Pediatrics, 95*(1), 1–8.
Shannon, K. M., Naylor, G. S., Torkildson, J. C., et al. (1987). Circulating erythroid progenitors in the anemia of prematurity. *New England Journal of Medicine, 317*(12), 728–733.
Shohat, M., Merlob, P., & Reisner, S. H. (1984). Neonatal polycythemia. 1. Early diagnosis and incidence relating to time of sampling. *Pediatrics, 73*(1), 7–10.
Sieff, C., & Nathan, D. (1993). The anatomy and physiology of hematopoiesis. In D. Nathan & F. Oski (Eds.), *Hematology of infancy and childhood* (3rd ed., pp. 156–215). Philadelphia: W. B. Saunders.
Spinnato, J. A., Ralston, K. K., Greenwell, E. R., et al. (1991). Amniotic fluid bilirubin and fetal hemolytic disease. *American Journal of Obstetrics and Gynecology, 165*(4, Part 1), 1030–1035.
Stockman, J. (1988). Physiology of the neonate as it relates to transfusion therapy. In D. Kasprisin & N. Luban (Eds.), *Pediatric transfusion medicine* (pp. 1–22). Boca Raton, FL: CRC Press.
Suarez, C. R., & Anderson, C. (1986). High-dose intravenous gamma globulin in neonatal immune thrombocytopenia. *Pediatric Research, 20,* 393A.
Taaning, E., & Skibsted, L. (1990). The frequency of platelet alloantibodies in pregnant women and the occurrence and management of neonatal alloimmune thrombocytopenia purpura. *Obstetrics and Gynecology Survey, 45*(8), 521–525.
Tan, K. L., Tan, R., Tan, S. H., & Tan, A. M. (1979). The twin transfusion syndrome. Clinical observations on 35 affected pairs. *Clinical Pediatrics, 18*(2), 111–114.
Tannirandorn, Y., & Rodeck, C. H. (1991). Management of immune haemolytic disease in the fetus [Review]. *Blood Review, 5*(1), 1–14.
Toloukian, R. J., Kadar, A., & Spencer, R. P. (1973). The gastrointestinal complications of umbilical venous exchange transfusion—a clinical and experimental study. *Pediatrics, 51*(1), 36–43.
Tuchmann-Duplessis, H., David, G., & Haegel, P. (1975). Circulatory system. In H. Tuchmann, G. David, & P. Haegel (Eds.), *Illustrated human embryology: Vol. 2. Organogenesis* (pp. 104–137). New York: Springer-Verlag.
Usher, R. H., Saigal, S., O'Neil, A., et al. (1975). Estimation of red blood cell volume in premature infants with and without respiratory distress syndrome. *Biology of the Neonate, 26*(3–4), 241–248.
Usher, R., Shepard, M., & Lind, J. (1963). The blood volume of the newborn infant and placental transfusion. *Acta Paediatrica Scandinavica, 52,* 497–512.
Valaes, T. (1963). Bilirubin distribution and dynamics of bilirubin removal by exchange transfusion. *Acta Paediatrica Scandinavica, 52*(Suppl.), 604–605.
Valaes, T., Petmezaki, S., Henschke, C., et al. (1994). Control of jaundice in preterm newborns by an inhibitor of bilirubin production: Studies with tin-mesoporphyrin. *Pediatrics, 93*(1), 1–11.
Van der Elst, C., Molteno, C., Malan, A., & Heese, N. (1980). The management of polycythemia in the newborn infant. *Early Human Development, 4,* 393–403.
von dem Borne, A., von Reisz, E., Verheugt, H., et al. (1980). Bak[a], a new platelet-specific antigen involved in neonatal alloimmune thrombocytopenia. *Vox Sanguinis, 39,* 113–120.
Weiner, C. P., Wenstrom, K. D., Sipes, S. S., & Williamson, R. A. (1991). Risk factors for cordocentesis and fetal intravascular transfusion. *American Journal of Obstetrics and Gynecology, 165*(4, Part 1), 1020–1025.
Wennberg, R., & Hance, A. (1986). Experimental bilirubin encephalopathy: Importance of total bilirubin, protein binding, and blood-brain barrier. *Pediatric Research, 20,* 789–792.
Winearls, C. G., Oliver, D. O., Pippard, M. J., et al. (1986). Effect of human erythropoietin derived from recombinant human DNA on the anemia of patients maintained by chronic haemodialysis. *Lancet, 2*(8517), 1175–1177.
Woodrow, J. (1970). Rh immunization and its prevention. In K. Jensen & S. Killman (Eds.), *Series Haemologica* (Vol. 3, pp. 29–46). Baltimore: Williams & Wilkins.
Yao, A. C., Lind, J., Tiisala, R., & Michelsson, K. (1969). Placental transfusion in the premature infant with observation on clinical course and outcome. *Acta Paediatrica Scandinavica, 58*(6), 561–566.
Young, T., & Mangum, B. (1997). *Neofax* (5th ed.). Columbus, OH: Ross Laboratories.
Zaizov, R., & Matoth, Y. (1976). Red cell values on the first postnatal day during the last 16 weeks of gestational age. *American Journal of Hematology, 1*(2), 276–278.
Zipursky, A., & Bowman, J. (1993). Isoimmune hemolytic diseases. In D. Nathan & F. Oski (Eds.), *Hematology of infancy and childhood* (3rd ed., pp. 44–73). Philadelphia: W. B. Saunders.
Zipursky, A., & Jaber, H. M. (1978). The haematology of bacterial infection in newborn infants. *Clinics in Haematology, 7*(1), 173–193.

CHAPTER 29

Assessment and Management of Neurologic Dysfunction

SUSAN TUCKER BLACKBURN

RESEARCH AGENDA

What are the effects of nursing activities on cerebral hemodynamics and pressure relationships?

What interventions reduce the risk or severity of intraventricular hemorrhage in preterm infants?

What effect do new technologies, such as extracorporeal membrane oxygenation and high-frequency jet ventilation, have on long-term neurologic outcome?

What collaborative management interventions support positive neurologic development?

VIGNETTE

Mrs. O barely made it to the hospital in time. Her membranes had ruptured at home, revealing meconium-stained fluid, and labor progressed rapidly. Little Jack O was born by spontaneous vaginal delivery in the ER of a local hospital. Mom and baby were transferred to the labor and delivery unit after initial stabilization. Jack had some initial jitteriness and hypoglycemia, so he was kept in the transitional care nursery for observation. Early q 3-hour feedings were initiated.

My shift started at 3 P.M. By this time, Jack's preprandial glucoses were above 40 mg/dl, and all hypoglycemic symptoms had resolved except for a little irritability. After my initial assessment and review of Jack's plan of care, I rolled his crib out to see mom. I introduced myself to Mrs. O and then assessed her level of understanding. As she cuddled Jack closely, she said, "Judy told me that his initial blood sugar was a little low and that you would continue to follow these for awhile before his feedings. She told me that his levels were now normal and that it's common to see this in newborns."

"Yes, it can be fairly common," I restated. "However, we will still follow his glucose levels closely over the next 12 hours. You will want to feed him every 3 hours for now. We will draw the glucose levels before the feedings since this is the time that we would be able to detect his lowest level. Your pediatrician will be here to examine him in a few hours."

Jack fed eagerly and was later returned to the nursery for another glucose level (40 mg/dl). He was rooting around as if to say "I'm hungry," so I took him out for mom to feed. Twenty minutes later, Mrs. O called to ask me to come to her room—Jack was acting "funny." On my arrival, Jack was alert, pink, and resting quietly in mother's arms. Mrs. O stated that he had "raised his right arm above his head in a jerking motion and his right eye twitched and rolled back in his head." After reassuring her, I took Jack back to the nursery.

Under the bright lights, I noted Jack's color to be dusky around the lips. I provided free-flow O_2, placed an oximeter on his toe, and transferred him into our special care nursery. The oximeter dropped into the lower 80s when O_2 was slowly withdrawn. I then placed Jack in a 30 percent O_2 head hood and on a cardiac monitor while a nursing colleague paged the pediatrician, Dr. S. While waiting for his call, I completed my assessment and drew a glucose level (40 mg/dl). I then started an IV of $D_{10}W$ at 80 ml/kg/day according to protocol. Vital signs at this time were as follows: axillary temperature, 97.6°F; apical pulse, 120; respiratory rate, 40.

In the meantime, Dr. S was on his way. He arrived within 20 minutes. He reviewed the history and completed his exam of Jack while I described what had happened. While collaborating on our plan of care, Jack began exhibiting subtle signs of seizure activity: repetitive blinking of his eyes, tongue thrusting, and apnea. This activity progressed to clonic jerking of the right arm. Thirty milligrams of phenobarbital was immediately given IV push. The seizure lasted approximately 1 minute. During the seizure, respirations were slow and shallow, and Jack's color was slightly dusky. He slowly "pinked up" and became more active and alert. A septic work-up was completed, and the following serum labs were obtained: glucose, calcium, electrolytes, magnesium, hematocrit, and blood gases. My main goal at this time was to support and protect Jack during and after the seizures.

Jack continued to have seizures over the next hour, and another 30 mg of phenobarbital was given IV push. In the meantime, most of the lab work had come back negative. Something was definitely wrong, I thought to myself. Dr. S and I once again reviewed the perinatal history. "Why isn't the phenobarb working?" I questioned Dr. S. I knew that numerous disorders can cause seizures and that it was often difficult to pinpoint the cause. "I'll need to see the rest of the lab results," said Dr. S, a concerned look on his face. Jack's parents then came into the nursery and to his bedside. "I can't believe this is happening," Mrs. O said as tears rolled down her cheeks. I placed a comforting hand on hers.

Administration of anticonvulsants failed to control Jack's seizures. They continued to occur intermittently over the next few hours until he received 100 mg of pyridoxine IV. The seizures stopped immediately, a finding that was diagnostic of pyridoxine dependency. Jack was subsequently discharged and remained free of seizures on 50 mg of pyridoxine a day.

I saw Jack again 2 years later at our special care nursery

reunion. He looked wonderful. He was very shy as I knelt down to say "hi." Mrs. O stated that he continued to take the pyridoxine and had had no more seizures. So far, developmental testing had shown normal results. She told me that she was expecting another baby. About 6 months into this pregnancy, her fetus was diagnosed as having seizures in utero. From Jack's experience, pyridoxine-dependent seizures were suspected. Mrs. O said she began taking prescribed doses of pyridoxine and would continue throughout the pregnancy. "Just like Jack, this baby will need vitamin B_6 supplement throughout his whole life. I'm glad they could figure it out so quickly," she smiled. Our conversation ended abruptly as she chased after Jack, who was helping himself at the cookie table.

Marianne McGraw

The central nervous system (CNS) is one of the most complex systems in the human body. Normal function of the CNS is critical for the functioning of every organ in the body and the integration of organ systems for coordinated physiologic and neurobehavioral processes. Neurologic dysfunction during the neonatal period can arise from insults before, during, or after birth. These insults can affect the infant's ability to survive the perinatal and neonatal periods and can have implications for later developmental and cognitive outcome. Thus, alterations in neurologic function in the neonate have significant immediate and long-term consequences for the infant and family. Early recognition of infants at risk for neurologic dysfunction and prompt implementation of appropriate interventions are crucial for the survival of these infants and for the reduction of long-term morbidity.

This chapter examines the structural and functional development of the CNS in the embryo, fetus, and neonate and the basis for common congenital and developmental anomalies. Neurologic assessment of the neonate and related diagnostic techniques are also presented, as are selected pathophysiologic problems affecting the central and peripheral nervous systems. Neurologic problems that are examined herein include neonatal seizures, intracranial hemorrhage, hypoxic-ischemic encephalopathy (HIE), structural alterations, and birth injuries. Nursing and collaborative management of infants is described for each of these problems. Figure 29–1 illustrates the general structure of the CNS.

EMBRYOLOGIC DEVELOPMENT OF THE CENTRAL NERVOUS SYSTEM

The development of the CNS can be divided into six stages: (1) neurulation, (2) prosencephalic development, (3) neuronal proliferation, (4) neuronal migration, (5) organization, and (6) myelinization. These stages are overlapping, and development progresses at different rates in various sections of the CNS. Embryologic development of the CNS begins shortly after fertilization, and maturation continues after birth until adulthood. Thus, the CNS is one of the earliest systems to begin development and one of the last systems to mature completely. The stages and timing of CNS development are summarized in Table 29–1.

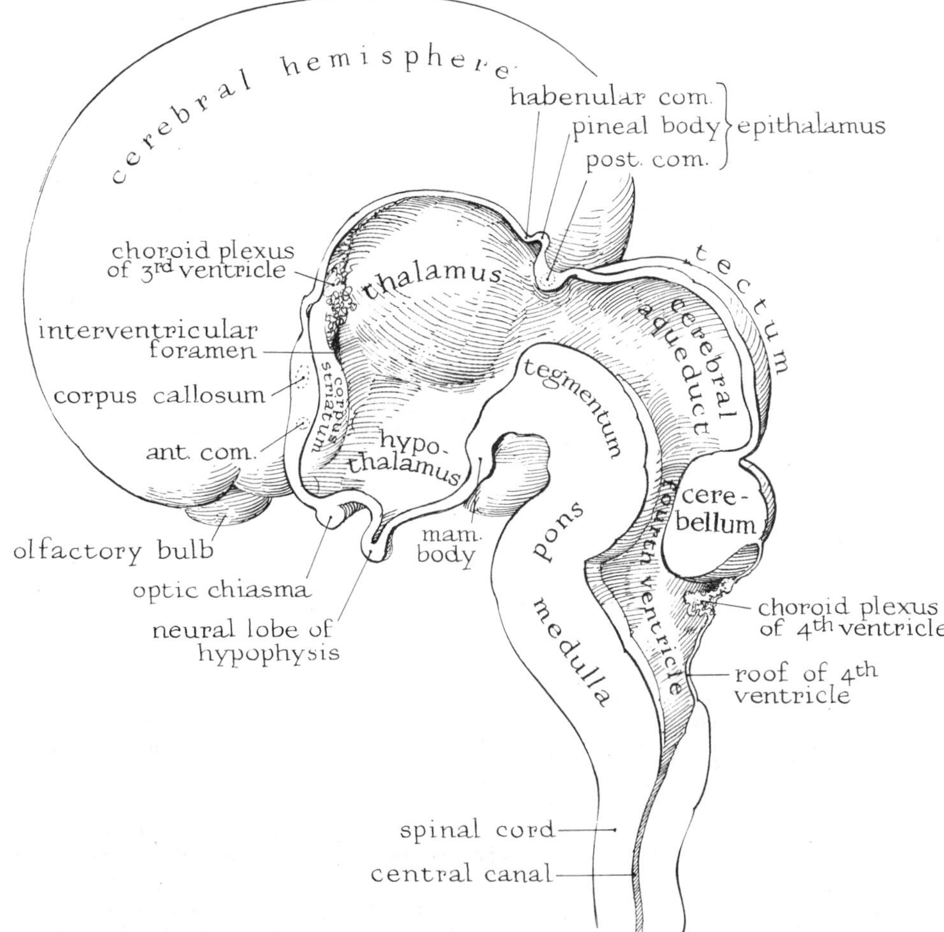

FIGURE 29–1. Gross topography of the central nervous system. (From Gilbert, S. G. [1989]. *Pictorial human embryology* [p. 114]. Seattle: University of Washington Press. Reprinted with permission.)

TABLE 29–1 Stages in the Development of the Central Nervous System and Related Developmental Defects

Stage	Peak Time Occurrence	Developmental Defects
Neurulation	3–4 weeks' gestation	Neural tube defects: anencephaly: encephalocele, spina bifida cystica (meningocele, meningomyelocele, myeloschisis), dermal sinus
Prosencephalic development	2–3 months' gestation	Holoprosencephaly, holotelencephaly
Neuronal proliferation	3–4 months' gestation	Microcephaly vera, macrocephaly, neurofibromatosis, other neurocutaneous disorders
Neuronal migration	3–5 months' gestation	Hypoplasia or agenesis of the corpus callosum, schizencephaly, lissencephaly, pachygyria, polymicrogyria
Organization	5 months' gestation to 1 year after birth	Alterations in brain development secondary to the effects of Down syndrome and trisomy 13-15, behavioral alterations, mental retardation
Myelinization	8 months' gestation to 1 year after birth	Brain hypoplasia, neurologic deficits

Modified from England, M. A. (1988). Normal development of the central nervous system. In M. I. Levene, M. J. Bennett, & J. Punt (Eds.), *Fetal and neonatal neurology and neurosurgery* (pp. 3–27). Edinburgh: Churchill Livingstone; Hill, A., & Volpe, J. J. (1989). *Fetal neurology*. New York: Raven Press; Volpe, J. J. (1987). *Neurology of the newborn* (2nd ed.). Philadelphia: W. B. Saunders.

Neurulation

Primary neurulation or dorsal induction occurs during the first 3 to 4 weeks of gestation. Formation of the primitive brain and spinal cord occurs during this period. The notochord acts as an inducer for formation of the CNS. The CNS arises as a thickening of the ectoderm on the dorsal portion of the embryo at about 18 days' gestation. This neuroectodermal thickening, known as the neural plate, lies cranially to the primitive streak and extends to the oropharyngeal membrane (Fig. 29–2*A*). The brain and spinal cord develop from the neural plate. The neural plate invaginates, forming the midline neural groove along the dorsal surface of the embryo. The parallel folds of tissue on either side of this groove are called the neural folds. The neural folds eventually form the forebrain, midbrain, and hindbrain, as well as the spinal cord.

By the end of the third postconceptual week, the neural folds move together and fuse to form the neural tube (Fig. 29–2*B*). The cranial portion of the lumen of the neural tube forms the ventricles; the caudal portion forms the central canal of the spinal cord. The tissues of the neural tube interact with surrounding mesoderm tissue (somites) to stimulate development of the bony structures of the CNS (i.e., the skull and vertebrae).

As the neural folds fuse, some of the neuroectodermal cells on the upper margins are not incorporated into the neural tube. These cells form the neural crest, which lies between the neural tube and the surface ectodermal layer. The neural crest tissue forms the peripheral nervous system, including cranial, spinal, and autonomic system ganglia and nerves, Schwann cells, melanocyte (pigment) cells, meninges, and skeletal and muscular components of the head (Moore & Persaud, 1993). The neural crest cells migrate away from the neural tube in a ventral and lateral direction (Fig. 29–3). These cells migrate and grow anteriorly to form the spinal and cranial nerves and posteriorly to form the ganglia of the cranial nerves and autonomic nervous system.

The neural folds do not fuse simultaneously. Closure of the neural tube begins near the future neck at the cerebrospinal junction in the area of the lower medulla, at about 22 days' gestation. Fusion proceeds in cephalic and caudal directions from this site. Fusion of the cranial portion forms the forebrain. For several days, the neural tube is fused toward the central area but is open at both ends. The end areas are known as the rostral (anterior) and the caudal (posterior) neuropores. These openings communicate with amniotic fluid. The rostral neuropore consists of dorsal and terminal lips. Closure occurs bidirectionally along these lips; failure of closure (anencephaly) is seen most often along the dorsal lip (O'Rahilly & Muller, 1994). The cranial end of the neural tube closes at 24 days' gestation. The caudal neuropore, which is in the future lumbosacral area, closes, in a rostrocaudal direction, at 26 days' gestation (O'Rahilly & Muller, 1994). Once both neuropores are closed, the neural tube is a closed, fluid-filled system that has no further connection to the amniotic cavity unless a defect is present. Failure of these neuropores to close gives rise to neural tube defects (NTDs). Because differentiation of the surrounding mesodermal tissue (somites) into vertebrae, cranium, and dura depends on interaction with the neural tube, NTDs involve not only the neural elements but also the bony structures and meninges (O'Rahilly & Muller, 1994).

Secondary neurulation involves two phases: canalization and regressive differentiation. These processes form the spinal cord caudally to the upper lumbar area. Development of the lower lumbar, sacral, and coccygeal areas begins at 28 to 32 days' gestation. These areas arise from a group of undifferentiated cells (caudal cell mass) at the caudal end of the neural tube. Vacuoles develop that gradually coalesce, enlarge, and contact the caudal end of the neural tube. This period of canalization continues until 7 weeks' gestation. Canalization is followed by a period of regressive differentiation, which lasts until after birth and is characterized by regression of much of the caudal cell mass (Volpe, 1995).

Disorders of Neurulation

Congenital anomalies that arise during the period of neurulation result from failure of neural tube closure. NTDs are usually accompanied by alterations in vertebral, meningeal, vascular, and dermal structures. These anomalies include anencephaly, myelomeningocele, encephalocele, and spina bifida occulta. NTDs arise from genetic factors, environmental factors, or both. The incidence is significantly higher in mothers with a poor diet and a low socioeconomic class (Wald, 1994). Most embryos with NTDs are lost early in pregnancy. The estimated incidence of NTDs at 26 days' gestation is 2.6 percent, versus 0.006 percent at term (Shiota, 1991).

The cellular basis for these defects is uncertain. One theory suggests that damage to the ectoderm results in a bleb of fluid in the neural cleft. This leads to embryonic scarring, which prevents the neural tube from fusing at that site (Brann & Schwartz, 1987). Recent evidence supports the importance of folic acid in neural tube closure (Scott et al., 1994; Wald, 1994). Folic acid supplementation at conception reduces the rate of NTDs by up to 70 percent (Wald, 1994). Folate is a cofactor for enzymes needed in DNA and RNA synthesis that is important in a cell's ability to methylate proteins, lipids, and myelin, and in the actions of other B vitamins. Folic acid may reduce the incidence of NTDs by

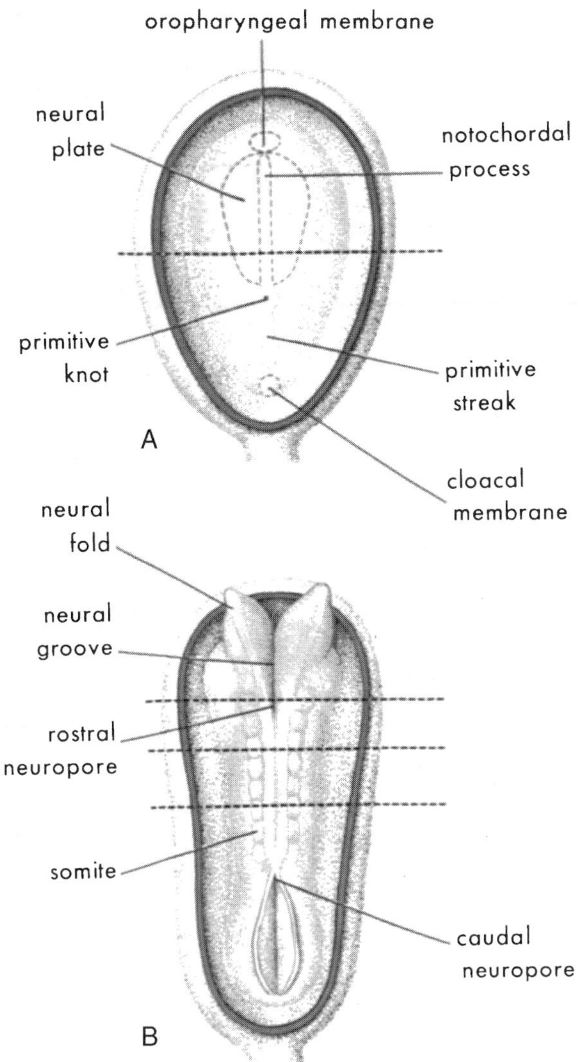

FIGURE 29–2. Embryologic development of the central nervous system. *A,* Formation of the neural plate. *B,* Closure of the neural tube. (From Moore, K. L., & Persaud, T. V. N. [1993]. *Before we are born: Essentials of embryology and birth defects embryology* [4th ed., p. 276]. Philadelphia: W. B. Saunders Co.)

correcting a deficiency or by overcoming a genetically induced metabolic block (Copp & Bernfield, 1994; Scott, et al., 1994). Current recommendations are that a woman increase her intake of folic acid from the time she begins considering conception up to 12 weeks of gestation. Dosage recommendations are that women with previous children with an NTD take a 4- to 5-mg/day supplement and that women with no previous history of an affected infant take a 0.4-mg/day supplement (Wald, 1994).

Anencephaly

Anencephaly is caused by failure of the anterior neural tube to fuse in the cranial area. The incidence of anencephaly has been declining with the advent of perinatal diagnosis and folic acid therapy; the overall frequency is 1 per 1000 live births (Paidas & Cohen, 1994). Because fusion of the neural tube in this area forms the forebrain, anencephalic infants have minimal development of brain tissue. The most common forms of this anomaly involve the forebrain and the upper brain stem. The brain tissue that does develop is poorly differentiated and becomes necrotic with exposure to amniotic fluid. This situation results in a mass of vascular tissue that has neuronal and glial elements and a choroid plexus that has a partial absence of the skull bones (Volpe & Hill, 1987). The mother may have hydramnios secondary to leakage of large amounts of cerebrospinal fluid (CSF) directly into the amniotic sac. Because anencephaly is caused by failure of the neural tube to close cranially, the alterations in development occur at 23 to 26 days' gestation (around the period of rostral neuropore closure).

Genetic and environmental factors appear to be involved in the development of this defect. Many anencephalic infants have other anomalies, the most consistent being adrenal hypoplasia secondary to pituitary dysfunction. Three fourths of these infants

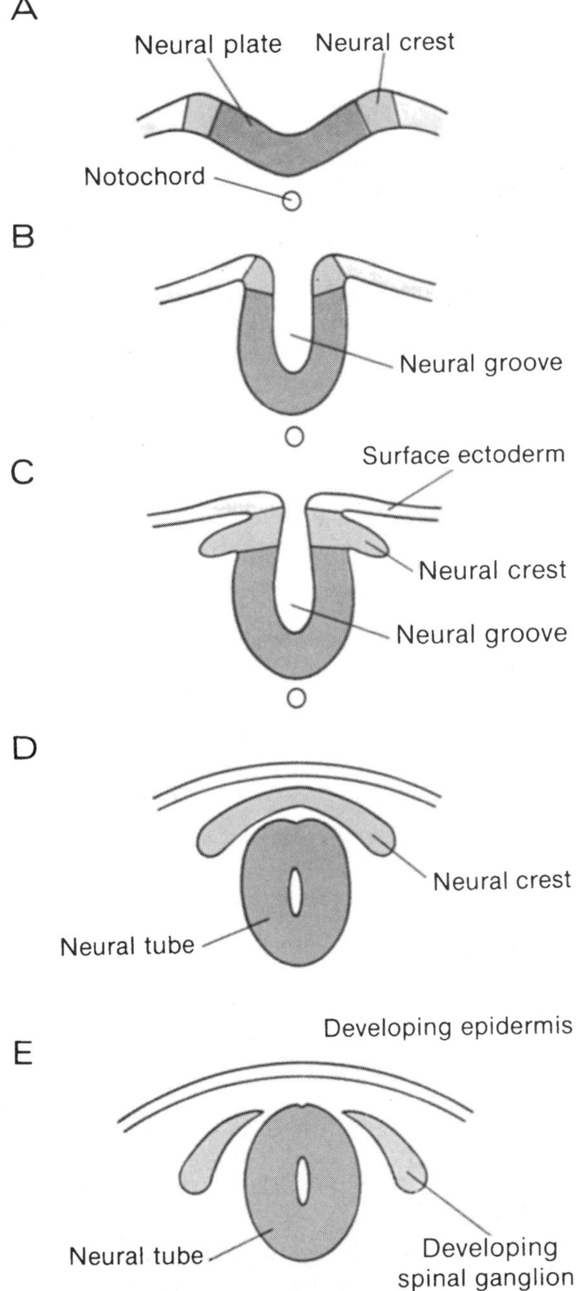

FIGURE 29–3. Formation of the neural crest. (From Moore, K. L., & Persaud, T. V. N. [1993]. *Before we are born: Essentials of embryology and birth defects* [4th ed., p. 53]. Philadelphia: W. B. Saunders Co.)

are stillborn; the remainder die during the neonatal period, with fewer than 20 percent still alive at 1 week (Volpe, 1995). Nursing management of infants with anencephaly is supportive, with provision of warmth and comfort until the infant dies. Families require emotional support and assistance in coping with their grief over the birth of an infant with a defect and the death of their infant (see Chapter 8, Bereavement: A State of Having Suffered a Loss). Anencephalic infants have been considered to be candidates for organ donation and have been kept alive for this purpose. This practice has raised many ethical issues (see Chapter 3, Ethical Aspects of Perinatal Care), including those related to keeping one infant alive for the good of another and criteria for determining brain death (Erlen, 1990; Diaz, 1993).

Encephalocele

Encephalocele has an incidence of 1 in 2000 births (Bellig, 1989). Encephaloceles, including craniomeningomyelocele, encephalomyelocele, and other forms of cranium bifida, arise from failure of closure of a portion of the neural tube in the anterior region. Although this defect can occur in any region, approximately three fourths occur in the occipital region. The sac protrudes from the back of the head or the base of the neck. The next most common area is the frontal region, and the orbit, nose, and/or nasopharynx is involved (Volpe, 1995; Volpe & Hill, 1987). Hydrocephalus occurs with 60 to 70 percent of occipital encephaloceles, owing to alterations in the posterior fossa. Hydrocephalus may be present at birth or may develop after repair of the encephalocele (Punt, 1988). Encephaloceles may occur in association with meningomyelocele.

The protruding sac varies considerably in size. The size of the external sac does not correlate with the presence of neural elements. For example, a large occipital sac may contain minimal neural tissue, whereas a small sac may contain parts of the cerebellum or accessory lobes; some occipital lesions have no neural elements in the sac (Miller, 1997; Milhorat & Miller, 1994). If the sac is leaking CSF at birth, immediate repair is necessary. If the defect is covered by skin, surgery may be delayed until a complete work-up, including skull radiography, computed tomography (CT) or cranial ultrasonography, and electroencephalography (EEG), can be performed. Surgical closure helps prevent infection and helps facilitate feeding and other care (Miller, 1997). If the infant is also hydrocephalic, a shunt is usually inserted 7 to 10 days after the encephalocele is repaired (Milhorat & Miller, 1994). In general, prognosis for these infants is poor if the sac contains significant brain tissue. Mortality and later outcome are significantly better for infants with anterior defects than for those with posterior defects (Brown & Sheridan-Pereira, 1992).

Collaborative Management

Collaborative management includes prevention of infection and trauma and positioning to avoid pressure on the defect. Promotion of normothermia is essential, especially in infants with CSF leakage, because these infants are at risk for thermoregulatory problems that result from evaporative losses. Postoperative management includes assessment of ventilation and perfusion, comfort measures, monitoring of neurologic and motor function, promotion of normothermia, prevention of infection, positioning to prevent pressure on the operative site, and monitoring of the site for CSF leakage.

Families of infants with an encephalocele need initial and ongoing support and counseling. Initial parental care involves assisting parents with the shock of the defect and its appearance and their grief over having an infant with an anomaly, and helping parents deal with the outcome implications of this defect. Nursing care also involves enhancing parent–infant interaction and involving the parents in the infant's care when they are ready (see Chapter 7, Sibling Adaptation to the Neonate, and Chapter 10, Fetal Development: Environmental Influences and Critical Periods). Teaching before discharge includes skin care, positioning, exercises, handling and feeding techniques, and activities to promote growth and development.

Spina Bifida

Spina bifida is a general term used to describe defects in closure of the neural tube that are associated with malformations of the spinal cord and vertebrae. Spina bifida arises from defects in closure of the caudal neuropore (open defects) or during secondary neurulation (closed defects). Defects range from minor malformations that have minimal clinical significance to major disorders that result in paraplegia or quadriplegia and loss of bladder and bowel control. The degree of sensory and motor neurologic deficit depends on the level and severity of the defect. The two major forms of spina bifida are spina bifida occulta and spina bifida cystica. Treatment of infants with spina bifida is discussed later in this chapter.

Spina bifida occulta occurs in 10 to 30 percent of the population. This disorder is a vertebral defect at L5, or S1, or both, that arises from failure of the vertebral arch to grow and fuse between 5 weeks' gestation and the early fetal period (Moore & Persaud, 1993). Spina bifida occulta is a defect in the formation of the caudal portion of the spinal cord (secondary neurulation). Most individuals with this defect have no problems, and the defect may be unrecognized. A few have underlying abnormalities of the spinal cord, or the nerve roots, or both; diastematomyelia (division of the spinal cord or nerve roots in an anteroposterior direction by a bony spicule or cartilaginous band); or dermoids or dermal sinuses (Brann & Schwartz, 1987). These abnormalities are usually manifested externally by a hemangioma, dimple, tuft of hair, or lipoma in the lower lumbar or sacral area.

Spina bifida cystica is a generic term for NTDs that are characterized by a cystic sac containing meninges, or spinal cord elements, or both, along with vertebral defects. The sac is covered by epithelium or a thin membrane. This defect occurs in approximately 1 in 1000 live births, and the incidence has decreased in recent years, similarly to anencephaly. The three main forms of spina bifida cystica are meningocele, myelomeningocele, and myeloschisis (Fig. 29–4). Spina bifida cystica can occur anywhere along the spinal column but is seen most often in the lumbar or lumbosacral area. A meningocele involves a sac that contains meninges and CSF, but the spinal cord and nerve roots are in their normal position. These infants usually have minimal residual neurologic deficit if the defect is covered with skin and if appropriate management is instituted early. A meningocele arises at 6 to 8 weeks' gestation (O'Rahilly & Muller, 1994).

Myelomeningocele is the most common form of spina bifida cystica. The sac contains spinal cord, or nerve roots, or both, in addition to meninges and CSF. During development, the nerve tissues become incorporated into the wall of the sac, impairing differentiation of nerve fibers (Moore & Persaud, 1993). Infants with myelomeningocele have neurologic deficit below the level of the sac. Approximately 80 percent of these malformations occur in the lumbar area, which is the final area of neural tube fusion. This defect occurs at 26 to 30 days' gestation (around the time of closure of the caudal neuropore) (Paidas & Cohen, 1994).

Myeloschisis is a severe defect in which no cystic covering exists, so the spinal cord is open and exposed. Myeloschisis is thought to arise from a local overgrowth of the neural plate, which prevents neural tube closure. This defect probably occurs between 18 and 23 days' gestation. The spinal cord in affected patients is a flattened mass of neural tissue. These infants have significant neurologic deficits and are at great risk for infection.

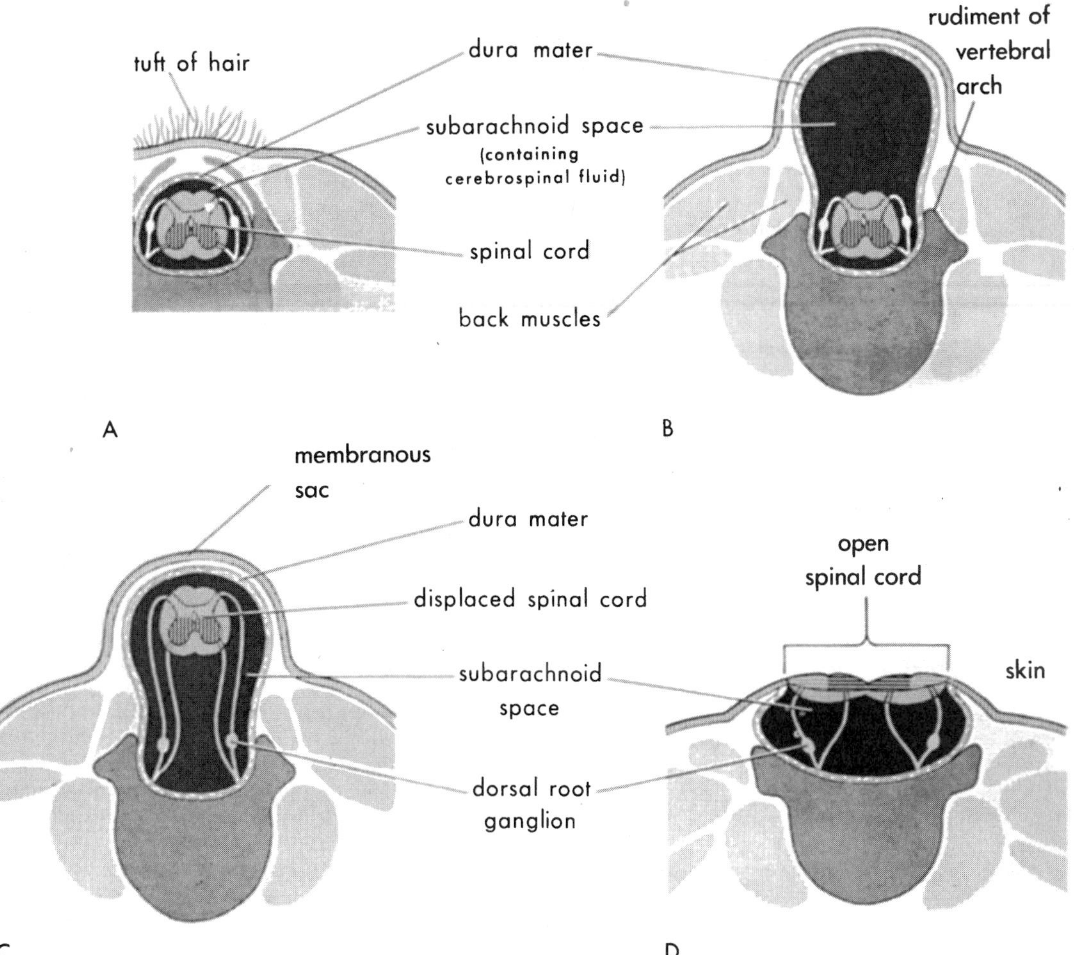

FIGURE 29–4. Different types of spina bifida. *A,* Spina bifida occulta. *B,* Spina bifida cystica: meningocele. *C,* Spina bifida cystica: myelomeningocele. *D,* Spina bifida cystica: myeloschisis. (From Moore, K. L., & Persaud, T. V. N. [1993]. *Before we are born: Essentials of embryology and birth defects* [4th ed., p. 284]. Philadelphia: W. B. Saunders Co.)

This defect can involve the entire length of the spinal cord and can occur in association with anencephaly (Moore & Persaud, 1993). Most infants with this defect are stillborn.

Another spinal cord defect is a spinal dermal sinus. A dermal sinus is a tract of squamous epithelium that connects to the dura mater. This defect is found in midline and corresponds to the location of the caudal or rostral neuropores. The more common defect occurs in the lumbosacral area and may be associated with a sacral dimple. Dermal sinus is occasionally recognized at birth, but it is more often diagnosed later, after repeated episodes of meningitis (Milhorat & Miller, 1994).

Prosencephalic Development

Prosencephalic development or ventral induction involves early development of the brain and ventricular system during the second to third month of gestation (peaking at 5 to 6 weeks). The brain develops from the cranial end of the neural tube beginning at the end of the fourth week. The peak period for prosencephalic development is 5 to 6 weeks' gestation. During this period, the three primary brain bulges (or vesicles) and cavities are formed, after fusion of the neural folds in the cranial area. Development of the face is associated with prosencephalic development of the CNS. As a result, alterations in brain development often result in facial malformations (Moore & Persaud, 1993).

The primary brain bulges are the forebrain (prosencephalon), the midbrain (mesencephalon), and the hindbrain (rhombencephalon). During the fifth week, the forebrain divides into two secondary vesicles, the telencephalon and diencephalon, and the hindbrain divides into the metencephalon and myelencephalon. The derivatives of each of these structures are illustrated in Figure 29–5. The fourth and third ventricles are formed from cavities within the rhombencephalon and diencephalon. These two ventricles are linked by the aqueduct of Sylvius. The lateral ventricles arise from cavities in the cerebral hemispheres and are connected to the third ventricle by the foramen of Monro (see Fig. 29–1). Early growth of the neural tube is most rapid in the forebrain region. In order for these structures to have space to grow, the neural tube bends at several points, forming the mesencephalic (midbrain area), cervical (junction of the hindbrain and spinal cord), and pontine flexures (Fig. 29–6).

Disorders of Prosencephalic Development

Malformations occurring during this period are generally thought to arise around the fifth to sixth weeks of gestation. Infants with these anomalies have a poor prognosis, and many are lost in early pregnancy or stillborn. Malformations of the forebrain include holoprosencephaly and holotelencephaly. Holoprosencephaly is an abnormality in cleavage of the hemispheres that arises from genetic or possibly environmental alterations. Failure of horizontal, transverse, and sagittal cleavages of the

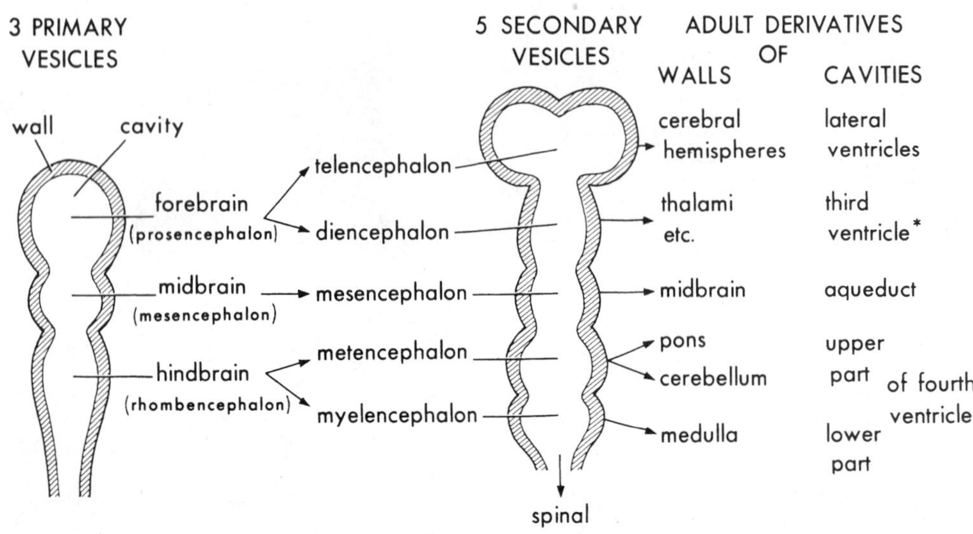

FIGURE 29–5. Derivatives of the primary brain vesicles in the fetus and adult. (From Moore, K. L., & Persaud, T. V. N. [1993]. *Before we are born: Essentials of embryology and birth defects* [4th ed., p. 287]. Philadelphia: W. B. Saunders Co.)

prosencephalon disrupts formation of the telencephalon and the diencephalon and its derivatives (see Fig. 29–5). The resultant brain has a single monoventricular cerebral mass that is enclosed by a membrane; aplasia of the optic tract with absence of the olfactory tracts and bulbs; corpus callosum; and supralimbic cortex. There may also be partial fusion of the basal ganglia, microcephaly, hydrocephaly, and facial anomalies (Lyon & Beaugerie, 1988; Volpe, 1995). The incidence ranges from 1 in 5200 (infants with abnormal chromosomes) to 1 in 53,400 (infants with normal chromosomes) live births (Paidas & Cohen, 1994). With holotelencephaly, the parts of the brain that develop from the telencephalon (see Fig. 29–5) form a single spheroid structure; the diencephalon and its derivatives are less affected.

Congenital hydrocephalus can also arise during this period. At about 6 weeks' gestation, three critical events occur related to the formation and circulation of CSF. These events are (1) development of secretory epithelium in the choroid plexus; (2) perforation of the roof of the fourth ventricle; and (3) formation of the subarachnoid space. Alterations in the second and third events give rise to a communicating form of hydrocephalus. This form is less common than obstructive (noncommunicating) hydrocephalus, which arises later in gestation (Lyon & Beaugerie, 1988; Volpe, 1995).

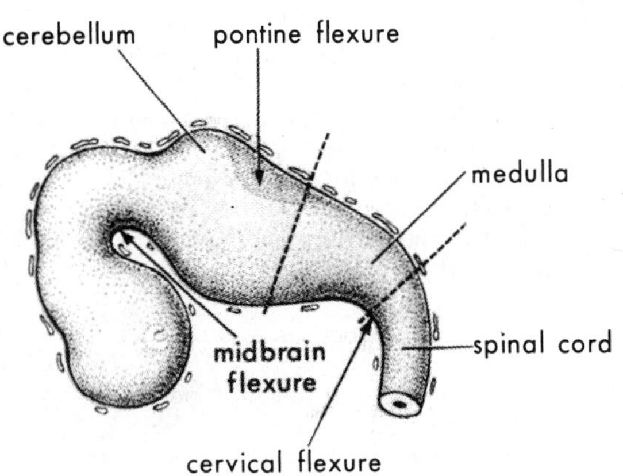

FIGURE 29–6. Development of the brain at the end of the fifth week, showing the primary divisions of the brain and the brain flexures. (From Moore, K. L., & Persaud, T. V. N. [1993]. *Before we are born: Essentials of embryology and birth defects* [4th ed., p. 287]. Philadelphia: W. B. Saunders Co.)

Neuronal Proliferation

Development of neurons and glial cells involves proliferation in the germinal matrix, migration (to final destination) in the next stage of CNS development, and differentiation (during the period of organization) of glial cells into specific cell types, alignment of neurons, and development of interneuron and glial-neuron relationships. The peak period of neuronal proliferation lasts from 2 to 4 months' gestation. During this stage, further development occurs in the subventricular and ventricular zones, where neurons and glial cells are derived from stem cells in the germinal matrix. The development of these cells can be studied by measuring changes in the amount of DNA, which correlates with cell numbers. Initial proliferation involves primarily neurons and radial glial cells (needed for neuron migration). Proliferation of other glial cells and their derivatives (astrocytes and oligodendrocytes) occurs intensively during the stage of organization at 5 to 8 months' gestation. During the most intense period of proliferation, before 32 to 34 weeks' gestation, the periventricular area receives a large proportion of the cerebral blood flow. This area is vulnerable to intraventricular hemorrhage in preterm infants.

Disorders of Neuronal Proliferation

Disorders of proliferation arise from inadequate or excessive proliferation of neuronal, glial, or glial cell derivatives. Because mature neurons are not able to divide, the eventual number of neurons is determined early in gestation. Insults may alter the stem cells (reducing the number of neurons or glial cells) or may alter cell growth (resulting in smaller cells) (Morgane et al., 1993). These disorders include micrencephaly vera, macrocephaly, and neurofibromatosis. Micrencephaly vera is associated with a small brain size (caused by decreased size of the proliferating units) that occurs at 2 to 4 months' gestation. It may occur as a result of insufficient proliferation, arrested cell growth, or excessive normal cell death. These infants often do not have marked neurologic deficits or seizures during the neonatal period, but later they are severely retarded. Micrencephaly vera may result from genetic causes (autosomal recessive or dominant, X-linked recessive, or translocation) or environmental factors (irradiation, metabolic alterations, or infections). Micrencephaly vera is found with maternal rubella, fetal alcohol syndrome, maternal cocaine use, and maternal phenylketonuria with elevated phenylalanine levels during pregnancy (Lyon & Beaugerie, 1988; Volpe, 1995).

Macrocephaly results in a large brain size from excessive proliferation of neuronal elements, or nonneuronal elements, or both. Macrocephaly is associated with genetic disorders (including Beckwith's syndrome), achondroplasia, and neurocutaneous disorders, such as neurofibromatosis. Neurofibromatosis involves excessive proliferation of nonneuronal elements in the CNS and mesodermal structures of the body, with cutaneous stigmata (Volpe, 1995). Onset is after neuronal proliferation at the time of glial cell proliferation during organization. About 40 percent of infants with neurofibromatosis have more than 5 café au lait cells of greater than 5 mm diameter at birth (Korf, 1992).

Neuronal Migration

The stage of neuronal migration, which has a peak time of 3 to 5 months' gestation, is characterized by the movement of millions of cells from their point of origin in the subependymal germinal matrix of the periventricular region (see Fig. 29–1) to their eventual loci within the cerebral cortex and the cerebellum. The process of neuronal migration is critical for the formation of the cortex, gyri, and deep nuclear structures. Development of the gyri and sulci follow a predictable pattern that is linked to gestational age (see Fig. 29–6) (Girard et al., 1995). At 21 to 25 weeks' gestation, the central ventricles are large and the brain agyric; gyral development begins by the end of this period.

The mechanisms that guide neuronal migration are not completely understood. Radial glial cells act as guides for migrating cells. These glial cells later transform into astrocytes (Volpe, 1995). The cerebral cortex has essentially achieved its full complement of neurons by 20 weeks' gestation. Later, migration predominantly involves glial cells.

Disorders of Neuronal Migration

Migration of neurons and glial cells can be altered by inborn errors or exogenous insults before or after birth. Alterations in migration can result in hypoplasia or agenesis of the corpus callosum, agenesis of a part of the cerebral wall (schizencephaly), or gyral anomalies (pachygyria, lissencephaly, polymicrogyria). The preterm infant may be especially vulnerable to gyral alterations. Rapid development of the gyri begins at 26 to 28 weeks' gestation and continues through the third trimester into the postbirth period. Development of gyri results in a marked increase in cerebral surface area (Volpe, 1995).

Organization

The peak time for organization is from about the fifth month of gestation to 1 year after birth. However, organizational processes continue for many years after birth, especially in the cerebellum. Some processes, such as synaptogenesis, continue until death. Organizational processes include (1) establishment of subplate neurons (which serve as transient "way stations" by providing a place of synaptic contact for axons that ascend from the thalamus and other areas whose connecting cortical neurons are not yet in place; (2) attainment of the proper alignment, orientation, and layering of cortical neurons; (3) arborization or differentiation and branching of axons and dendrites (Fig. 29–7); (4) differentiation of the glial cells; (5) development of synaptic connections ("wiring" of the brain); (6) balancing of excitatory and inhibitory synapses; and (7) cell death and selective elimination of neuronal processes (Volpe, 1995). This latter process is important in adjusting the size of individual neurons to their anticipated need and is an important component of brain plasticity in infants. Thus, in the developing brain, neuronal processes targeted for elimination can be saved if they are needed because of damage to other processes; thus, functional ability is preserved.

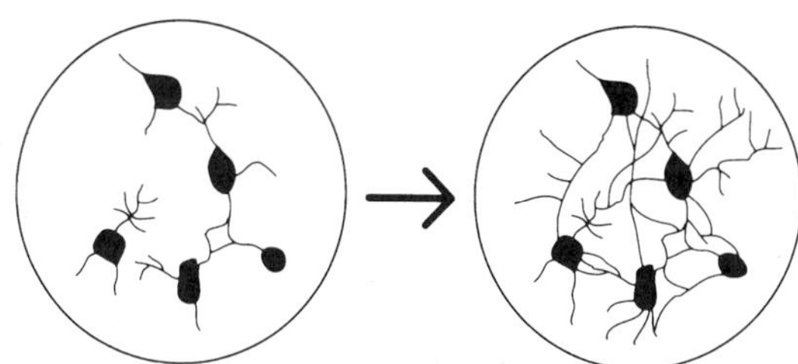

FIGURE 29–7. Schematic drawing illustrating dendritic arborization of early neurons. (From Bellig, L. L. [1989]. A window on the neonate's brain. *Neonatal Network*, 7[4], 13. Reprinted with permission.)

Disorders of Organization

Organization of the brain is susceptible to insults from inborn errors, abnormal chromosomes, and perinatal insults. These processes are particularly vulnerable in the preterm infant being cared for in an intensive care unit during this period. Alterations in arborization and wiring of the brain can lead to hypersensitivity, poorly modulated behavior, and all-or-nothing responses (see Chapter 49, Assessment and Management of Neonatal Neurobehavioral Development). Alterations in organization are seen in infants with Down syndrome, who have abnormal development of the axons and dendrites and altered synaptic formation, fragile X syndrome (the most common cause of inherited mental retardation in males), Angelman's syndrome (microdeletion of long arm of maternal chromosome 15), phenylketonuria, congenital rubella, and trisomy 13–15.

Myelinization

Myelinization begins during the second trimester of pregnancy, at about 20 weeks' gestation, and continues to adulthood. The peak time for myelinization is from 8 months' gestation to 1 year of age. The rate of myelinization varies in different parts of the nervous system. This process begins before birth in the peripheral areas—first in the peripheral motor and then in the peripheral sensory nerves. Myelinization also begins before birth in the CNS, moving upward from the brain stem. In the CNS, myelinization occurs first in the sensory and then in the motor areas. Myelinization of ascending pathways in the spinal cord, brain stem, and thalamus is completed by about 30 weeks' gestation, and myelinization from the thalamus to the cortex is completed by 37 weeks (Sarnat, 1984). This has implications for neonatal pain management (see Chapter 40, Indentification, Management, and Prevention of Pain in the Neonate). From birth to adulthood, myelinization proceeds within the cerebral hemispheres in conjunction with development of higher associative and sensory functions. Myelinization is important in most nerve tracts within the CNS because it insulates individual fibers to enhance specificity of connections; it increases the number of alternative pathways; and it markedly increases the speed of transmission (Sarnat, 1984).

This stage involves development of myelin sheaths around nerve fibers within the nervous system. The sheaths are formed by oligodendrocytes or Schwann cells (peripheral nerves). The lipoprotein plasma membranes of these cells wrap themselves around the nerve fibers for several layers. Myelinization of fiber tracts tends to occur before maturation of functional ability (Moore & Persaud, 1993).

Disorders of Myelinization

Myelinization is susceptible to damage from exogenous influences, particularly malnutrition, which can lead to a range of neurologic deficits in which hypoplasia of the cerebral white matter occurs. Primary hypoplasia of the white matter with vacuolization of the myelin occurs in postnatal malnutrition, congenital hypothyroidism, and amino and organic acidopathies, such as maple syrup urine disease, homocystinuria, and phenylketonuria (see Chapter 25, Assessment and Management of Metabolic Dysfunction). This defect in myelinization can lead to severe neurologic deficits in these infants (Volpe, 1995). Delayed myelinization has been noted in infants with severe, chronic fetal hypoxia or intrauterine growth restriction and in infants of diabetic mothers (Dambaka & Laure-Kamionowska, 1990).

ASSESSMENT OF NEUROLOGIC FUNCTION

Assessment of neurologic function is a collaborative process by nurses and other health care professionals. Assessment is an initial step in evaluating an infant's responses to transition to extrauterine life and the impact of perinatal events and pathophysiologic problems on the central and peripheral nervous systems. Assessment of neurologic function and identification of dysfunction encompass several components, each of which is described in this section. These components include history, physical examination, neurologic examination, laboratory tests, and other diagnostic techniques. Specific clinical signs associated with neurologic dysfunction are also discussed in this section.

History

Risk factors in the maternal, obstetrical, and neonatal history can be useful in identifying infants at risk for neurologic dysfunction and specific pathophysiologic factors. Specific risk factors for each problem discussed here are identified later in individual sections. General maternal or family historical factors that must be examined include family history of NTDs, chromosomal or genetic abnormalities or other malformations, maternal substance abuse, chronic maternal health problems, nutritional status, exposure to teratogens, outcome of previous pregnancies, and age.

Obstetrical risk factors include prematurity; postmaturity; placental problems, such as abruptio placentae and placenta previa; analgesia; anesthesia; and maternal problems, such as infection, hypertension, and substance abuse. Large for gestational age infants, prolonged or precipitate labor, forceps delivery, and abnormal presentation increase the risk of birth trauma and hemorrhage. Alterations in intrauterine growth and polyhydramnios may be present with an infant who has a CNS malformation. Fetal distress, perinatal asphyxia, and low Apgar scores are associated with intracranial hemorrhage and HIE.

Neurologic dysfunction can also arise from postnatal problems. Therefore, the infant's postbirth history is evaluated for status at birth and resuscitation required, asphyxia or hypoxic episodes, shock, hypoperfusion, hemorrhage, infection, and metabolic or electrolyte aberrations. The infant's record is also reviewed for the presence of clinical signs, such as seizures or alterations in activity, tone, and state, that are associated with neurologic dysfunction.

Physical Examination

A comprehensive physical examination is an important area of nursing assessment for any infant at risk for, or with evidence of, neurologic dysfunction. The physical examination is described in Chapter 17, Neonatal Assessment. Infants are examined for evidence of infection and birth trauma, such as ecchymosis, edema, lacerations, and fractures. Other parameters that are assessed include temperature, blood pressure, color, and respiratory pattern. Characteristics of the infant's cry, such as robustness, presence in response to aversive stimuli, and pitch, may also be useful. In addition, funduscopic examination may be performed in order to assess for chorioretinitis (associated with intrauterine viral infection), papilledema (seen with cerebral edema, although less reliably in neonates), and congenital anomalies (Amiel-Tison et al., 1986).

Specific parameters that are particularly important for the nurse to assess in infants with neurologic problems are (1) the head size, shape, and rate of growth; (2) sutures and fontanelles; (3) the presence of major and minor anomalies; and (4) the vertebral column. The first two are discussed below. Because CNS anomalies are often associated with other anomalies and syndromes, the infant is examined for the presence of major anomalies of body systems and for isolated or clustered minor malformations, such as low-set or abnormally shaped ears, micrognathia, and hypertelorism of the eyes. The vertebral column is inspected and palpated for evidence of NTDs. Signs that may indicate an underlying defect include hair tufts, dimples, and fistulae.

Head Size, Shape, and Rate of Growth

Monitoring and plotting of head circumference are basic components of health care for all infants, regardless of their gestation or health status. The largest circumference is measured, usually the occipitofrontal circumference, about 1 cm above the eyes. The measurement is plotted on the appropriate growth grid for the infant's sex and gestation (Fig. 29–8). The most accurate measurements are made with a metal or plastic tape that is marked in centimeters. Paper tapes tend to stretch and are less accurate but can be used for initial screening and for infants for whom there are no concerns regarding head size. The occipitofrontal circumference generally ranges from 32.6 to 37.2 cm in term infants (NAACOG, 1991). The head usually grows a maximum of 0.5 cm/week in term infants and 0.5 to 1 cm/week in preterm infants during the first weeks after birth (Amiel-Tison & Larroche, 1988).

Serial measurements must be made to identify alterations in rate of growth as well as size. Alterations in rate of growth are important because an infant may have a significant increase or decrease in head growth but still remain within the 10th to 90th percentiles on standard head-growth grids. Occipitofrontal circumference should be measured several times over the first days after birth to obtain an accurate baseline after molding and edema from birth have resolved. Head circumference is measured weekly on preterm or ill infants. More frequent measurements may be made if the infant is at risk for developing progressive ventricular dilation. Interrater and intrarater reliability can be a major problem in obtaining accurate head circumference measurement (Ifft et al., 1989). Development of a standardized protocol and regular assessment of reliability may alleviate this problem.

Head shape can also reflect perinatal events and specific anomalies. The head may be deformed by the forces of labor and delivery. These changes are transient and disappear within a few days. Infants with craniosynostosis (premature closure of one or more sutures) and hydrocephalus have abnormal head configurations.

Sutures and Fontanelles

The entire head is inspected and palpated, and each suture and fontanelle is assessed. The anterior fontanelle is assessed while the infant is in a quiet state and in a semiupright or sitting position. The fontanelle should be open, soft, and flat. Pulsation may be felt normally in a newborn but can be associated with increased blood pressure. A sunken or depressed fontanelle is seen with dehydration; a bulging fontanelle with increased intra-

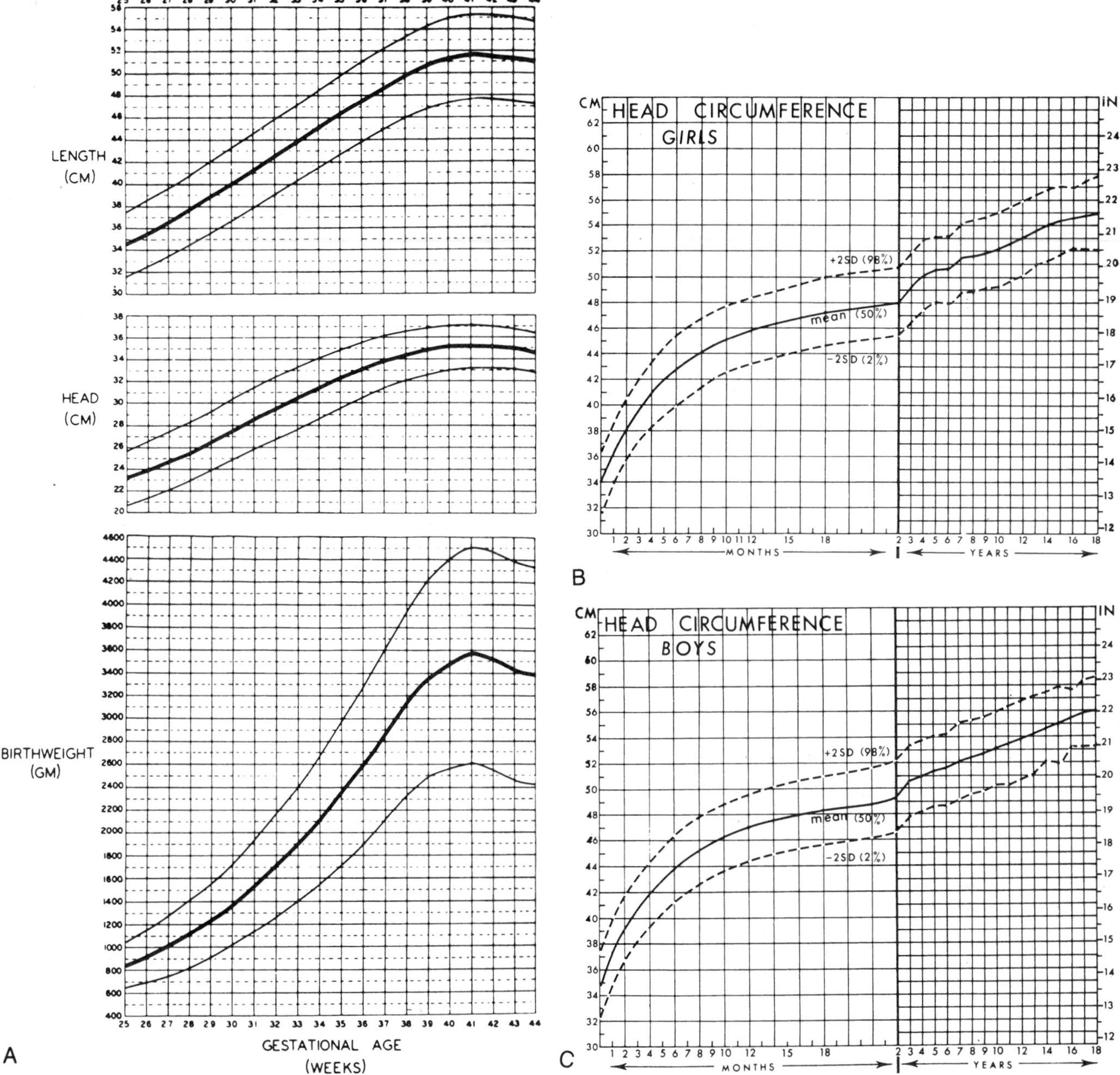

FIGURE 29–8. Charts for plotting head circumference. *A*, Intrauterine growth curves. *B* and *C*, Head circumference records for girls and boys, respectively. (*A*, From Klaus, M. H., & Fanaroff, A. A. [1986]. *Care of the high-risk neonate* [3rd ed., p. 424]. Philadelphia: W. B. Saunders Co.; as compiled from Usher, R., & McLean, F. [1969]. Intrauterine growth of liveborn Caucasian infants at sea level: Standard obtained in 7 dimensions of infants born between 25 and 44 weeks of gestation. *Journal of Pediatrics, 74,* 901. *B* and *C*, From Nellhaus, G. [1968]. Head circumference from birth to eighteen years. Practical composite international and interracial graphs. *Pediatrics, 41,* 106. Copyright American Academy of Pediatrics 1968. Reprinted with permission.)

cranial pressure (ICP). The anterior fontanelle is usually diamond shaped and may be small at birth if molding and overriding of the sutures are present; the size increases within a few days to the usual 3- to 4-cm long by 1- to 3-cm wide shape seen in term infants. The anterior fontanelle closes at 8 to 16 months of age. The anterior fontanelle may bulge slightly with increased tension when the infant cries and may be slightly depressed when the infant is placed in an upright position. The posterior fontanelle closes any time from 8 months' gestation to 2 months after birth. If it is open at birth, this fontanelle is 1 to 3 cm wide and has a triangular shape. Rarely, a "third fontanelle" may be palpated along the sagittal suture between the anterior and posterior fontanelles. This third fontanelle is not a true fontanelle but a defect in the parietal bone. It can be palpated in normal infants, but it is also seen in infants with Down syndrome or hypothyroidism.

A 4- to 5-mm separation of all of the sutures (Fig. 29–9), except the squamosal (temporoparietal) suture, is normal in the newborn. The squamosal suture should not be separated more than 2 to 3 mm. Overriding of the bones and molding from delivery may modify this finding in the first few days after birth. Abnormal findings include persistence of suture separation over time, increased separation of the sutures, and separation of the

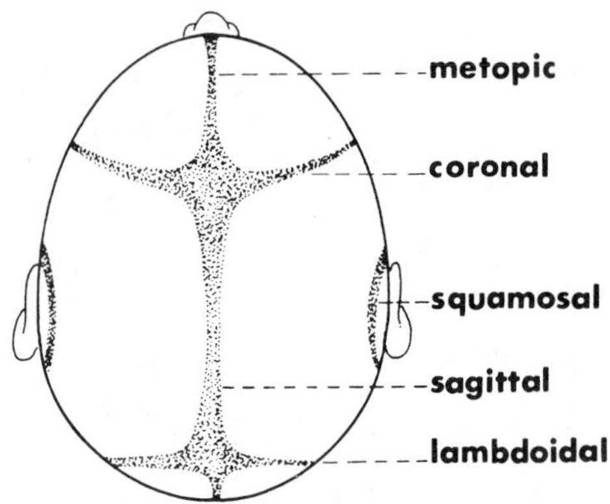

FIGURE 29–9. Cranial sutures. (From Amiel-Tison, C., Korobkin, R., & Klaus, M. H. [1986]. Neurologic problems. In M. H. Klaus & A. A. Fanaroff [Eds.], *Care of the high-risk neonate* [3rd ed., p. 360]. Philadelphia: W. B. Saunders Co.)

squamous suture by greater than 2 to 3 mm. With increased ICP, separation of the sutures occurs in a specific order: sagittal, coronal, metopic and lambdoidal, and squamosal. Thus, separation of the squamosal suture is the most clinically significant (Amiel-Tison & Larroche, 1988). The cranial bones are inspected and palpated so that fractures, extradural hemorrhage, edema, and areas of uneven ossification of the cranial bones or craniotabes can be identified.

Neurologic Examination

The neurologic examination is useful in evaluating the presence and extent of neurologic dysfunction in the neonate, in monitoring recovery, and as a prognostic indicator. Factors such as gestational age, health status, infant's state (see Chapter 49, Assessment and Management of Neonatal Neurobehavioral Development), medications, and timing of feedings must be considered in the interpretation of neurologic findings. Parameters that are examined in the assessment of neurologic status include level of consciousness, activity, tone, posture, reflexes, and evaluation of selected cranial nerves (Miller, 1997). The optimal state of the infant during a neurologic examination is quiet and alert. Specific assessment tools have been developed for the assessment of neuromotor function (Harris & Brady, 1986).

Clinical signs and symptoms of neurologic dysfunction in the neonate have been divided into three stages that are associated with prognosis for both survival and long-term developmental outcome (Amiel-Tison, 1978). Infants with minor manifestations (stage 1) may be hyperalert or have abnormal tone, but they are not stuporous or comatose, do not have seizures, and have normal primary reflexes. These infants tend to have a good prognosis. Moderate signs (stage 2), which are associated with variable outcomes, are CNS depression with or without one or more isolated seizures. Infants with severe manifestations (stage 3), including repeated seizures, altered consciousness, and abnormal tone, have a poor prognosis (Amiel-Tison & Larroche, 1988).

Level of Consciousness

Neurologic insults frequently alter the infant's level of consciousness. The level of consciousness may range from normal states of consciousness for gestation (see Chapter 48, Neonatal Sleep–Wake States) to hyperexcitability, irritability, lethargy, hyperalertness, and stupor or coma. The three clinical levels of consciousness that are most correlated to outcome are hyperalertness, lethargy, and stupor or coma (Finer et al., 1981; Sarnat & Sarnat, 1976). In the hyperalert state, the infant has an increased threshold to sensory stimulation, with wide-open eyes but with a decreased blink response and ability to fixate and follow (Amiel-Tison & Larroche, 1988). Lethargic infants respond to tactile and noxious stimuli, but their responses are delayed. The stuporous or obtunded infant's response is limited to noxious stimuli, whereas the comatose infant has no response to tactile or noxious stimuli (Miller, 1997). Hyperexcitability and irritability can be assessed by examining the infant's response to caregiving actions and medical procedures, state during intercaregiving intervals, and ability to use self-consoling maneuvers or to be soothed by others.

Activity, Posture, and Tone

Infant activity, tone, and general position are assessed, along with spontaneous positioning of the extremities and hands. The infant is first assessed while lying in a resting position. A frog-leg position while supine is seen in immature infants and in infants who have experienced severe asphyxia or who have major health problems or neuromuscular disorders (Miller, 1997). The quality and symmetry of activity with spontaneous and elicited movement are assessed. Alterations in symmetry of the trunk, face, and extremities at rest or with spontaneous movement suggest congenital anomalies, birth injury, or neurologic insult. Tight fisting is an abnormal sign. A cortical thumb (inside thumb on closure of the hand) may be normal, but it is abnormal if it is persistent. Opisthotonos and decerebrate or decorticate posturing (Table 29–2) may also occur.

Abnormal movements include seizure activity (described later), jitteriness, and tremors, although the last two findings are often normal. The characteristic movements seen with tremors in the neonate vary, depending on the underlying disorder. For example, tremors associated with metabolic problems are usually low-amplitude, high-frequency movements, whereas tremors associated with CNS problems are usually high-amplitude, low-frequency movements. Jitteriness is a common finding in infants, owing to lack of myelinization of pyramidal tracts. A major function of this tract is to inhibit spinal reflexes. In the neonate, these unmyelinated tracts respond in a mass way to central arousal with peripheral hyperexcitability. Tremors can be set off by spontaneous or elicited movement. Tremors can also be associated with metabolic abnormalities, asphyxia, or drug withdrawal. Tremors and jitteriness must be differentiated from seizures (Table 29–3).

Resting, passive, and active tone are assessed. Resting tone is evaluated by observation of the infant at rest in a supine position. Evaluation of passive tone involves examination of extensibility and involves maneuvers used in the neuromuscular component of gestational age assessment. The parameters usually examined include posture, dorsiflexion of the foot, scarf sign, passive movements of the arms, popliteal angle, and heel-to-ear maneuver (Fig. 29–10). Techniques to elicit these responses are described in Chapter 17 (Neonatal Assessment).

Assessment of active tone involves altering the posture of the infant in order to obtain directed motoric responses (Amiel-Tison & Larroche, 1988). Common maneuvers are righting reactions of the legs and trunk and examination of neck flexors and extensors (Fig. 29–11). Righting reactions are elicited by holding the infant upright with the feet on a firm surface. The ability of the infant to straighten his or her legs and trunk is assessed. Neck flexors and extensors are assessed using the pull-to-sit maneuver. For examination of neck flexors, the infant is pulled to a sitting position, and the tone and position of the head and neck are observed. Neck extensors are examined by use of a reverse pull-to-sit maneuver, that is, the infant is placed in a sitting position and moved backward toward the bed or examining table surface.

Strength may also be assessed. This parameter is difficult to evaluate in the newborn, and thus only a gross assessment can be obtained. Strength is affected by state, immaturity, and neuromuscular and neurologic problems. Strength of the upper extremities

TABLE 29–2 Clinical and Laboratory Features Useful in Differentiation of Tonic Seizures, Decorticate Posturing, Decerebrate Posturing, and Opisthotonos

Clinical Event	Duration	Provoked by External Stimuli	Leg Posture	Arm Posture	Trunk Posture	Change in Respiration	Ocular Position	Epileptic EEG Changes
Tonic seizure	Brief, intermittent	–	Extension	Flexed or extended	Usually arched (extended)	Apnea occasionally	Blinking, upward	Yes
Decorticate posturing	Brief, intermittent	+	Extension	Flexed, adducted, internal rotation; fisted	Extended	Typically none	Typically no change	No
Decerebrate posturing	Brief, intermittent	+	Extension	Extended, adducted, hyperpronated; fisted	Extended	Tachypnea, irregular breathing, apnea	Downward eye deviation; mydriasis	No
Opisthotonos	Prolonged, sustained posture	+/–	Extension	Variable; often extended	Marked prolonged arching	Typically none	Typically no change	No

From Clancy, R. R. (1983). Neonatal seizures. In R. A. Polin & F. Berg (Eds.), *Workbook in practical neonatology* (p. 132). Philadelphia: W. B. Saunders Co. Reprinted with permission.

POSTURE AND PASSIVE TONE FROM 28 TO 40 WEEKS GESTATIONAL AGE

Gestational age	28wk	30wk	32wk	34wk	36wk	38wk	40wk
Posture	Completely hypotonic	Beginning of flexion of the thigh at the hip	Stronger flexion	Frog-like attitude	Flexion of the 4 limbs	Hypertonic	Very hypertonic
Heel to ear maneuver							
Popliteal angle	150°	130°	110°	100°	100°	90°	80°
Dorsi-flexion angle of the foot			40-50°		20-30°		Premature reached 40w 40° Full term
Scarf-sign	Scarf sign complete with no resistance		Scarf sign more limited		Elbow slightly passes the midline		The elbow does not reach the midline
Return to flexion of forearm	Absent (Upper limbs very hypotonic lying in extension)			Absent (Flexion of forearms begins to appear when awake)	Present but weak, inhibited	Present, brisk, inhibited	Present, very strong not inhibited

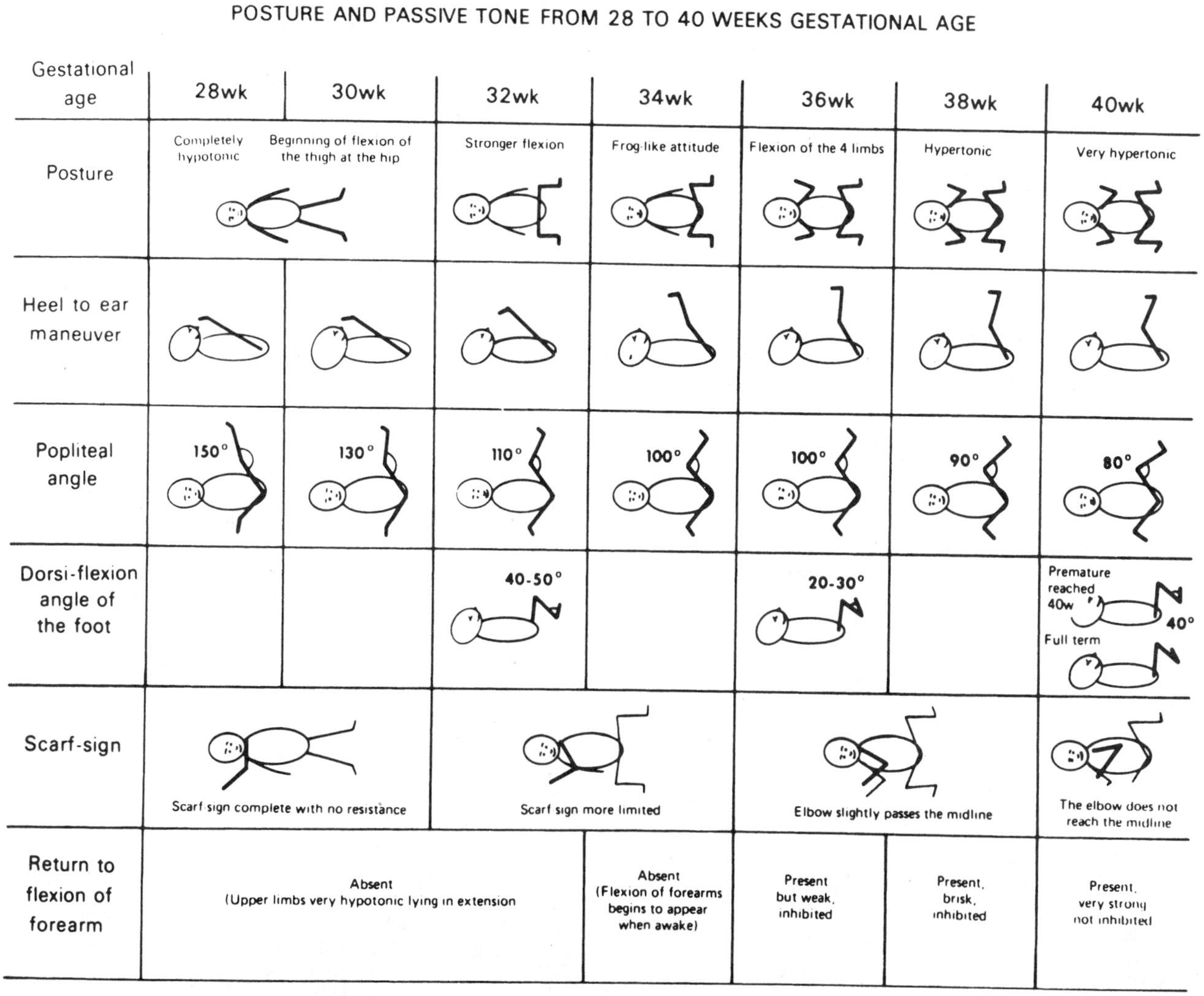

FIGURE 29–10. Posture and passive tone from 28 to 40 weeks of gestation. (From Rudolph, A. M., & Hoffman, J. [Eds.]. [1991]. *Rudolph's pediatrics* [19th ed., p. 178]. Norwalk, CT: Appleton & Lange. Reprinted with permission.)

ACTIVE TONE FROM 32 TO 40 WEEKS GESTATIONAL AGE

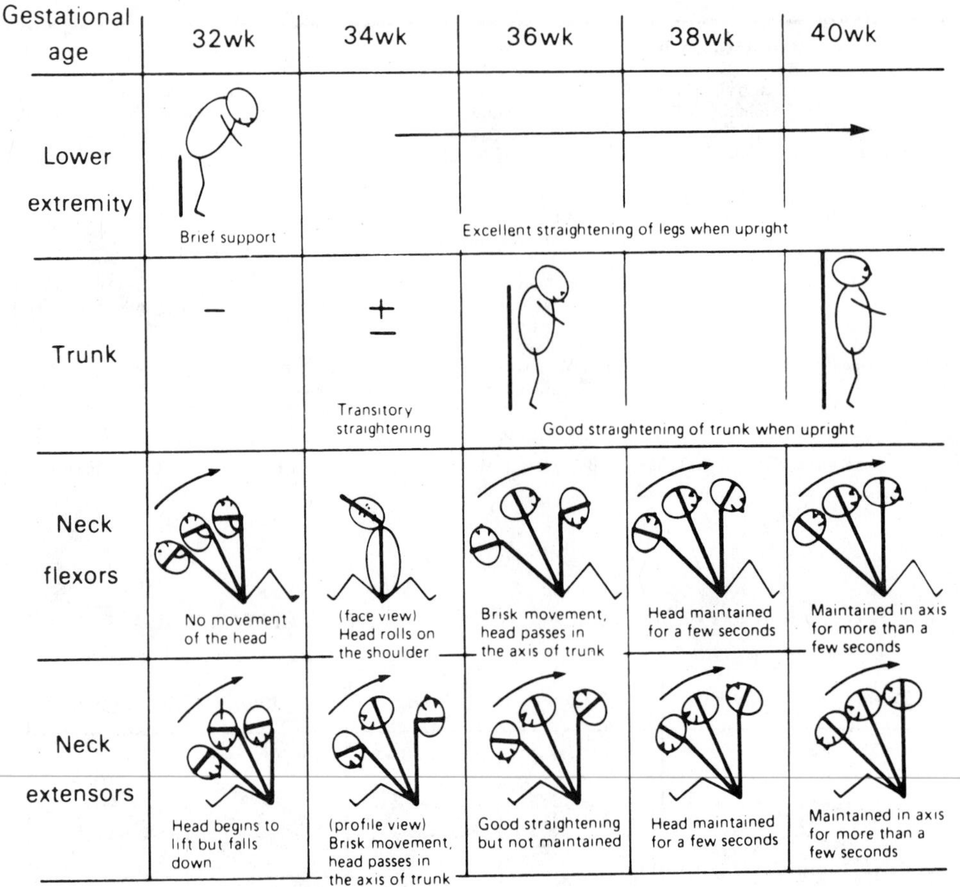

FIGURE 29–11. Active tone from 32 to 40 weeks of gestation. (From Rudolph, A. M., & Hoffman, J. [Eds.]. [1991]. *Rudolph's pediatrics* [19th ed., p. 179]. Norwalk, CT: Appleton & Lange. Reprinted with permission.)

and neck is assessed by eliciting the grasp reflex and pulling the infant to a sitting position. The righting reaction can be used to assess strength in the legs. Infants with peripheral nerve injuries, neuromuscular disorders, alterations at the neuromuscular junction, and spinal cord injuries tend to be hypotonic and have muscle weakness. Infants with CNS disturbances secondary to asphyxia, intracranial hemorrhage, Down syndrome, or metabolic disturbances tend to be hypotonic without muscle weakness (Amiel-Tison & Larroche, 1988; Miller, 1997). Hypertonia is seen less frequently than hypotonia in neonates with neurologic problems. Marked extensor hypotonia may be seen in association with severe hypoxic-ischemic injury, bacterial meningitis, or massive intraventricular hemorrhage (Volpe, 1995).

TABLE 29–3 Jitteriness Versus Seizures

Characteristic	Jitteriness	Seizures
Stimulus sensitive	Yes	No
Gaze or eye deviations	No	Yes
Predominant type of movement	Tremors	Clonic
Ceases with passive flexion	Yes	No

From Torrence, C. (1985, August). Neonatal seizures: Part I. *Neonatal Network, 4*, 12. Reprinted with permission.

Reflex Activity

Primary and tendon reflexes are assessed. In infants with neurologic dysfunction, these reflexes may be diminished, absent, or accentuated. The primary reflexes include sucking, grasping, crossed extension, automatic walking (stepping), and the Moro reflex. The primary reflexes are stereotypic responses for the first few months after birth. They should be present, symmetrical, and reproducible in the neonatal period and gradually disappear during infancy (Miller, 1997). These reflexes are affected by gestational age, but all are present to some degree by 28 to 32 weeks' gestation (Fig. 29–12). The tendon reflexes assessed in the neonate are the biceps, knee, and ankle jerk. All should be present and brisk. Ankle clonus is generally not a significant finding in the neonate.

Examination of Selected Cranial Nerves

Full cranial nerve assessment is generally not performed on the neonate. However, function of these nerves can be evaluated by use of several relatively simple maneuvers: fixation and following, pupillary responses, doll's eye response, hearing, vestibular response, and suck and swallow. These assessments and the usual findings are summarized in Table 29–4.

Clinical Signs Associated with Neurologic Dysfunction

Clinical manifestations of neurologic dysfunction can be specific or nonspecific or subtle. However, five types of clinical signs

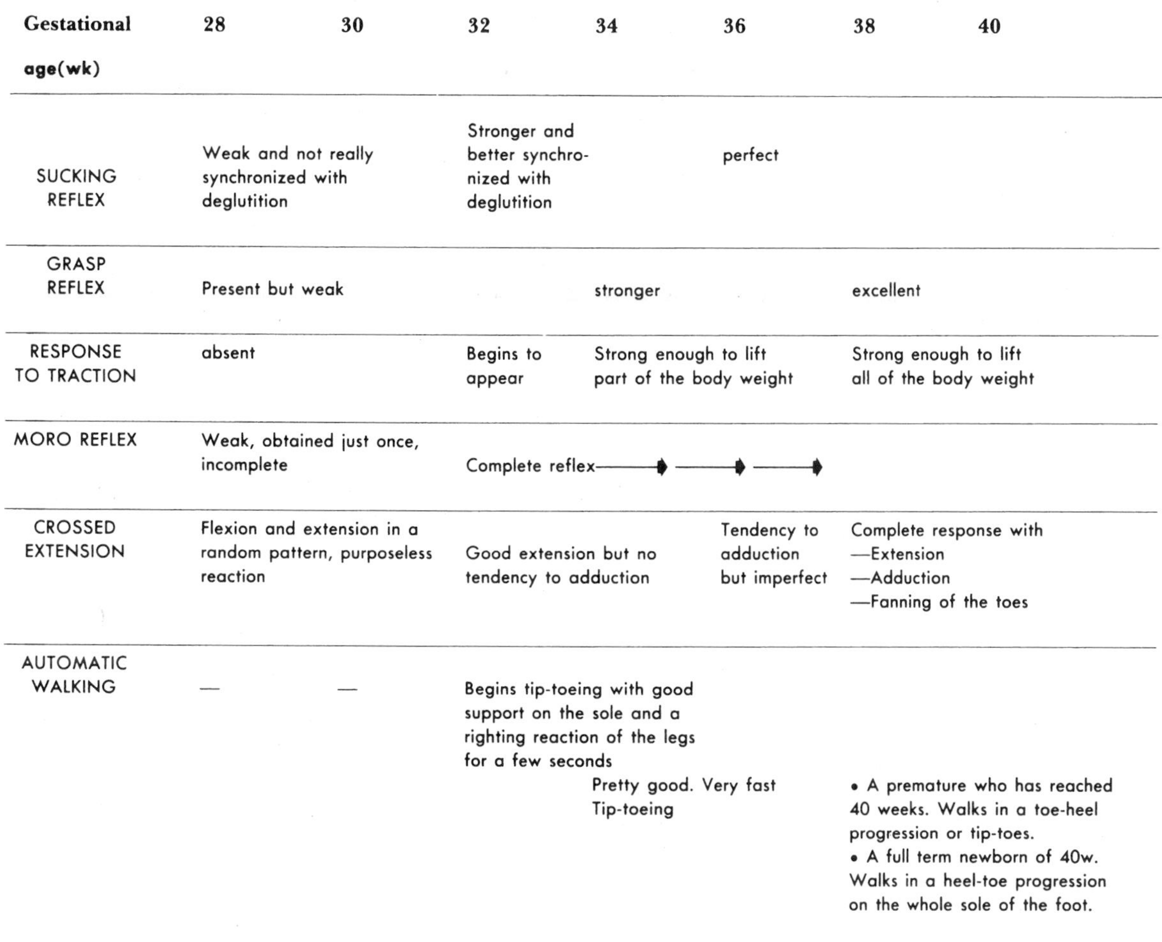

Gestational age(wk)	28	30	32	34	36	38	40
SUCKING REFLEX	Weak and not really synchronized with deglutition		Stronger and better synchronized with deglutition		perfect		
GRASP REFLEX	Present but weak			stronger		excellent	
RESPONSE TO TRACTION	absent		Begins to appear	Strong enough to lift part of the body weight		Strong enough to lift all of the body weight	
MORO REFLEX	Weak, obtained just once, incomplete		Complete reflex——→ ——→ ——→				
CROSSED EXTENSION	Flexion and extension in a random pattern, purposeless reaction		Good extension but no tendency to adduction		Tendency to adduction but imperfect	Complete response with —Extension —Adduction —Fanning of the toes	
AUTOMATIC WALKING	—	—	Begins tip-toeing with good support on the sole and a righting reaction of the legs for a few seconds	Pretty good. Very fast Tip-toeing		• A premature who has reached 40 weeks. Walks in a toe-heel progression or tip-toes. • A full term newborn of 40w. Walks in a heel-toe progression on the whole sole of the foot.	

FIGURE 29–12. Development of selected reflexes from 28 to 40 weeks of gestation. (From Rudolph, A. M., & Hoffman, J. [Eds.]. [1991]. *Rudolph's pediatrics* [19th ed., p. 178]. Norwalk, CT: Appleton & Lange. Reprinted with permission.)

are commonly seen in infants with neurologic problems: (1) CNS depression, (2) hyperirritability, (3) increased ICP, (4) seizure activity, and (5) movement alterations. Seizures are discussed later. Signs and symptoms of CNS depression, hyperirritability, increased ICP, and movement alterations are listed in Table 29–5.

Diagnostic Techniques

Diagnostic techniques that may be used with infants suspected of neurologic problems include neurophysiologic studies, radiographic assessment, structural brain imaging, measurement of cerebral blood flow, and measurement of ICP. These techniques are described in detail in Chapter 36 (Diagnostic Imaging) (radiologic assessment, ultrasonography, cerebral blood flow determination, radionucleotide assessment, magnetic resonance imaging [MRI]) and Chapter 37 (Diagnostic Tests and Laboratory Values) (CT, cerebral angiography, brain stem–evoked responses, EEG, lumbar puncture).

Laboratory tests are performed to assist in the diagnosis of specific neurologic disorders and to identify underlying causes. CSF is examined for signs of hemorrhage (increased red blood cells, increased protein, decreased glucose, and xanthochromia) and to rule out infection (Table 29–6). Xanthochromia is often a late sign and may reflect increased protein rather than blood (Clancy, 1983). If ICP is increased, this may be reflected by the pressure of the CSF on needle insertion. Other laboratory evaluations include hematocrit value, serum glucose level, electrolyte levels, blood gases, and acid-base status. A sepsis work-up or TORCH (toxoplasmosis, rubella, cytomegalovirus, and herpes simplex) screen (see Chapter 27, Assessment and Management of Immunologic Dysfunction) is performed if intrauterine infection or neonatal sepsis and meningitis are suspected. A genetic work-up and other metabolic studies are performed if inborn errors of metabolism or other inherited disorders are thought to be present.

Transillumination of the head has been used less frequently with the advent of ultrasonography and CT. A flashlight with a light-tight seal or a Chun-gun with a focused light is used in a dark room. The whole head is examined by placement of the light against different sections of the cranium. Abnormal diffusion of light with a ring of illumination around the light source, translucence of the entire skull, or a ring of light around the source in a localized area occurs when there is (1) an abnormal collection of fluid in the ventricles, subdural space, or scalp (intracranial hemorrhage, hydrocephalus, cephalhematoma, scalp edema) or (2) cerebral atrophy or cysts (hydranencephaly, ventricular enlargement with cortical mantles <1 cm thick, porencephaly). Small anomalies may result in negative findings on transillumination (Miller, 1997; Amiel-Tison & Larroche, 1988). If a flashlight is used, the ring of light should be less than 1 cm (<1.5 cm in the frontal area of the preterm infant). Gestational age norms are available for use with findings from Chun-gun transillumination (Vyhmeister et al., 1977).

Collaborative Management

Collaborative and nursing management specific to each type of neurologic dysfunction presented in this chapter are described in

TABLE 29–4 Nursing Assessment of Selected Cranial Nerves in the Newborn

Nerve	Assessment	Implications
Optic (II)	Blink in response to light (consistent by 28 weeks' gestation)	Visual system intact to the level of the superior colliculi (does not indicate visual cortex function)
	Fixation on object placed approximately 19 cm in front of infant's face (consistent by 32 weeks' gestation)	Presence of vision
	Follow with eyes and turning head (consistent by 37 weeks' gestation)	
	Examination of external eye	Evaluation of abnormalities, e.g., cataracts, irregularities of size or shape, microphthalmos, or scleral hemangiomas
	Funduscopic examination (set ophthalmoscope at −2 to −4 diopters)	Normal newborn optic disk is pale or grayish-white; observe for abnormalities, e.g., retinal hemorrhage or lesion
Oculomotor (III), trochlear (IV), and abducens (VI)	Pupillary reactivity (equal and responsive to light, which appears by 28 weeks' gestation and is consistent by 32 weeks)	Intact cranial nerve III; unequal or nonresponsive pupils in infants over 32 weeks' gestation associated with increased intracranial pressure or hemorrhage
	Doll's eye maneuver (vestibular response), which is present by 25 weeks' gestation (hold infant in an upright position at arm's length and rotate in both directions)	Stimulation of semicircular canals with impulses sent to the brain stem via nerves III, VI, and VII. Normal response is isotonic deviation of the eyes away from the direction of movement; lack of response is associated with brain stem dysfunction or excessive administration of sedatives such as phenobarbital; disconjugate eye movements and some nystagmoid movement are occasionally seen normally during the first 3 weeks
Trigeminal (V)	Elicit the corneal reflex (may not be reliable in newborn) or observe for a grimace on pinprick	Facial sensation (not usually done routinely, but may be useful with an infant with facial paralysis)
	Elicit sucking and ability of infant to bite down on examiner's finger	Masticatory power
Facial (VII)	Observe appearance and symmetry of face at rest and during spontaneous and elicited movement	Abnormalities associated with birth injury and cerebral insults
Acoustic (VIII)	Evaluate auditory function by noting response (blink or startle) to sudden loud noise (seen by 28 weeks' gestation) or (in more mature infants) by cessation of movement and turning to sound while in a quiet, alert state	This is a gross assessment of auditory function; thus, failure of the infant to respond while in a quiet, alert state in a quiet environment on repeated examinations indicates the need for examination of auditory function
Trigeminal (V), facial (VII), glossopharyngeal (IX), vagus (X), and hypoglossal (XII)	Evaluate sucking (V, VII, XII), swallowing (IX and X), and gag reflex (IX and X)	Impairment interferes with feeding and may indicate immaturity (see Chapter 24, Assessment and Management of Gastrointestinal Dysfunction) or be associated with cerebral insult

Data from Brann, A. W., & Schwartz, J. F. (1987). Central nervous system disturbances. In A. A. Fanaroff & R. J. Martin (Eds.), *Neonatal–perinatal medicine* (pp. 495–553). St. Louis: C. V. Mosby Co.; Volpe, J. J. (1987). *Neurology of the newborn* (2nd ed.). Philadelphia: W. B. Saunders Co.

TABLE 29–5 Clinical Manifestations of Central Nervous System Dysfunction

Alteration	Clinical Manifestations	Alteration	Clinical Manifestations
Central nervous system depression	Altered level of consciousness Weak, absent cry Weak, absent primary reflexes Poor feeding Decreased activity Decreased passive tone Decreased active tone Altered respirations	Increased intracranial pressure	Irritability Lethargy Increased head circumference Palpable sutures, especially squamous Bulging, tense fontanelle Increased extensor tone of neck Downward deviation of eyes Vomiting (late) Dilated head veins (late)
Hyperirritability	Sharp, excessive crying Hyperactivity Exaggerated passive tone Hypertonia Difficult to console Low sensory threshold	Seizures	See Table 29–8
		Movement alterations	Jitteriness, tremors (Table 29–3) Decerebrate posturing (Table 29–2) Decorticate posturing (Table 29–2) Opisthotonos (Table 29–2)

Data in part from Amiel-Tison, C., & Larroche, J. C. (1988). Brain development and neurological survey during the neonatal period. In L. Stern & P. Vert (Eds.), *Neonatal medicine* (pp. 245–267). New York: Masson Publishing USA.

TABLE 29–6 Evaluation of Cerebrospinal Fluid

CSF Finding	Appearance	
Normal	Clear and colorless	
Xanthochromia	Yellowish discoloration that may be due to ICH (discoloration by RBC pigments seen as early as 12 hours after hemorrhage), hyperbilirubinemia, with CSF protein content >150 mg/dl, or a normal variation	
Turbidity or cloudiness	Presence of cell counts >400/mm^3	
Pink or bloody	RBC count >6000 mm^3	
CSF Finding	**RBC Count**	
Normal	30 mm^3 (range up to 100 mm^3) with a nontraumatic tap	
Abnormal	>100 mm^3, associated with increased protein (protein increased 1 mg/dl per every 1000 RBC)	
Normal CSF Findings in Noninfected High-Risk Infants	**Term**	**Preterm**
WBC count (cells/mm^3)		
Range	0–32	0–29
Mean	8.2	9.0
Protein (mg/dl)		
Range	20–170	65–150
Mean	90	115
Glucose (mg/dl)		
Range	34–119	24–63
Mean	52	50
Ratio of CSF to blood glucose		
Range	44–248	55–105
Mean	81	74

CSF, cerebrospinal fluid; ICH, intracranial hemorrhage; RBC, red blood cell; WBC, white blood cell.

Modified from Sarff, L. D., Platt, L. H., & McCracken, G. H. (1976). Cerebrospinal fluid evaluation in neonates: Comparison of high risk infants with and without meningitis. *Journal of Pediatrics, 88,* 473; Clancy, R. R. (1983). Neonatal seizures. In R. A. Polin & F. Berg (Eds.), *Workbook in practical neonatology* (pp. 125–152). Philadelphia: W. B. Saunders Co.

later sections. In the nursing care of infants with neurologic dysfunction, however, common nursing diagnoses and related management that must be considered with all infants and their families can be identified. These include

1. Alteration in level of consciousness.
   a. Monitor infant state, activity, responsiveness, eye movements, head circumference, vital signs, seizure activity, and signs of increased ICP.
   b. Position to promote skin integrity, prevent contractures, and reduce ICP (head in midline and slightly elevated).
   c. Monitor fluid and electrolyte status.
   d. Maintain adequate ventilation and perfusion.
   e. Implement comfort measures (see Chapter 40, Identification, Management, and Prevention of Pain in the Neonate).
   f. Maintain an appropriate thermal environment.
   g. Reduce environmental stressors.
   h. Promote neurobehavioral stability.
2. Potential for injury related to trauma or infection.
   a. Maintain use of aseptic techniques.
   b. Use sterile technique when appropriate.
   c. Position to prevent contamination of defects or operative sites.
   d. Monitor for signs of localized infection or neonatal sepsis.
   e. Handle gently.
   f. Position to reduce potential of trauma or contamination.
3. Impairment of skin integrity.
   a. Position in alignment and change position.
   b. Use foam, sheepskin, lambskin, or waterbeds.
   c. Massage skin gently to stimulate circulation.
   d. Use appropriate skin care measures (see Chapter 32, Assessment and Management of Integumentary Dysfunction).
4. Alteration in comfort. Management is discussed in Chapter 40, Identification, Management, and Prevention of Pain in the Neonate.
5. Impaired mobility.
   a. Position in alignment and change position.
   b. Promote skin integrity.
   c. Use gentle range-of-motion exercises.
6. Alteration in thermoregulation. Management is discussed in Chapter 16, Neonatal Thermoregulation.
7. Alteration in nutrition. Management is discussed in Chapter 23 (Nutrition: Physiologic Basis of Metabolism and Management of Enteral and Parenteral Nutrition).
8. Promote neurobehavioral organization and development. Management is discussed in Chapter 49 (Assessment and Management of Neonatal Neurobehavioral Development).
9. Altered family processes. Management is discussed in Chapter 50 (Assessment and Management of the Transition to Home).
10. Grieving (family). Management is discussed in Chapter 8 (Bereavement: A State of Having Suffered a Loss).

TYPES OF NEUROLOGIC DYSFUNCTION

Seizures

Seizures are the most common neurologic sign seen during the neonatal period. Seizures are not a disease but a sign of underlying disease processes that have resulted in an acute disturbance within the brain (Volpe, 1995). If left untreated, these disorders can lead to permanent damage of the CNS or other tissues. Disease processes associated with seizures in the neonate include primary CNS disorders, asphyxia, systemic diseases, and metabolic insults. The reported incidence of neonatal seizures ranges from 0.15 percent in term infants to 22.7 percent in preterm infants (Bernes & Kaplan, 1994). Seizure activity may be an acute, recurrent, or chronic phenomenon. Neonatal seizures are usually acute and disappear within the first few weeks after birth. Recurrent or continuous seizures increase the risk of neurologic damage from the seizure activity itself (Bernes & Kaplan, 1994).

Pathophysiology

Seizures result from excessive, synchronous electrical discharge or depolarization within the brain that results in stereotypic, repetitive behaviors. Depolarization and repolarization of the nerves are produced by the movement of sodium (Na) and potassium (K) across the cell membrane. The inward migration of Na^+ results in depolarization; repolarization is produced by the outward migration of K^+. These processes require an energy-dependent pump and energy in the form of adenosine triphosphate (ATP).

The specific mechanism that causes neonatal seizures is unknown. Neonatal seizure might be the result of one or more of these mechanisms: (1) disturbances in energy production and the Na^+-K^+ pump, (2) altered neuronal membrane sodium permeability, and (3) imbalances in excitatory versus inhibitory neurotransmitter.

Disturbance in energy production with alterations in movement of Na^+ and K^+ across the neuronal membrane can lead to an imbalance between depolarization and repolarization. Thus, Na^+ movement (depolarization) is unbalanced by K^+ movement (repolarization). Alterations in energy production occur secondary to hypoxemia, ischemia, and hypoglycemia. Alterations in permeability of the neuronal membrane to sodium can occur with hypocalcemia. Calcium normally binds with proteins in the cell membrane to inhibit Na^+ movement. Decreased availability of calcium would increase inward movement of Na^+ and lead to depolarization. Hypomagnesemia also increases Na^+ membrane permeability. Alkalosis or hyponatremia can also lead to seizures via this mechanism.

Imbalances in neurotransmitter, resulting in a relative excess of excitatory (glutamate or acetylcholine) over inhibitory (gamma-aminobutyric acid) neurotransmitter, increases the rate of depolarization. This can occur as a result of either an excess of excitatory substance (associated with hypoxemia, ischemia, and hypoglycemia) or a deficiency of inhibitory substance. Pyridoxine deficiency leads to such events by depressing activity of the enzyme responsible for synthesis of gamma-aminobutyric acid. Excitatory inhibitors derived from ammonia are also increased in preterm infants who have excessive protein intakes or infants who have liver dysfunction after severe asphyxia (Bernes & Kaplan, 1994; Volpe, 1995).

Biochemical Effects of Seizures

Seizures result in increased energy expenditure by the organism. This leads to the following sequence of biochemical events: (1) breakdown of ATP to adenosine diphosphate with release of energy; (2) increased glycolysis, stimulated by adenosine diphosphate, with conversion of glycogen to glucose; (3) increased production of pyruvate, which is used by the mitochondria in ATP production; (4) increased oxygen and glucose consumption; (5) increased production of lactate from pyruvate, stimulated by increased adenosine diphosphate; and (6) lactate/H^+-stimulated local vasodilation increasing local blood flow and substrate availability (Volpe, 1995). The increased blood pressure associated with seizures also increases cerebral blood flow and substrate availability. These events are illustrated in Figure 29–13. Seizures result in a marked decrease in brain glucose concentrations because much of the available glucose is utilized by the cells to replenish ATP supplies.

Repetitive seizures in the neonate eventually alter brain lipid and protein metabolism as well as energy metabolism. This results in reduction in total brain DNA, RNA, protein, and cholesterol levels. These deficiencies lead to impairment of cellular proliferation, differentiation, and myelinization in animal models (Volpe, 1995). The effects in the human neonate are unclear but of concern. Brain damage due to seizure activity could be the result of alterations in protein metabolism or the energy supply, or it could be the result of damage from asphyxia or edema.

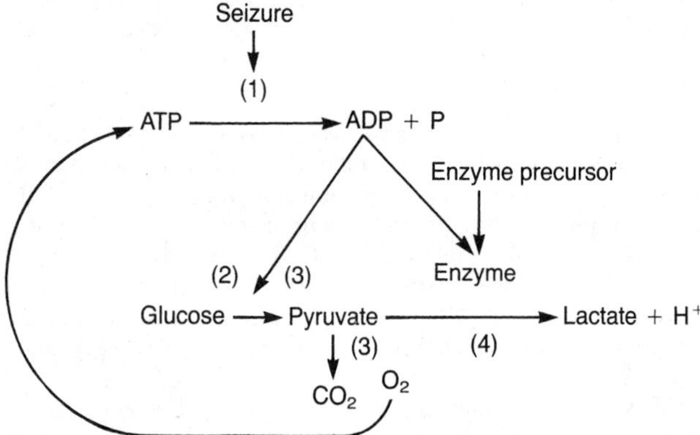

FIGURE 29–13. Biochemical effects of seizures. *1,* ↑ breakdown of adenosine triphosphate (ATP); *2,* ↑ glycolysis; *3,* ↑ oxygen and glucose consumption; *4,* ↑ production of lactate. ADP, adenosine diphosphate. (Modified from Volpe, J. J. [1987]. *Neurology of the newborn* [2nd ed., p. 131]. Philadelphia: W. B. Saunders Co.)

Seizures in Neonates Versus Older Children and Adults

Seizures are more common and of a different type in the neonate than in older individuals, owing to the developmental state of the neonate's brain. The peak time for organizational processes within the brain is from the fifth month of gestation to 1 year after birth. Thus, term, and especially preterm, infants have relatively immature brain organization at birth. This lack of organization results in an inability to propagate and sustain generalized seizures. For example, the neonate's brain lacks the arborization and synaptic connections (wiring) necessary for a firing neuron to recruit adjacent neurons to fire synchronously. Inadequate organization also leads to a slower response time to stimuli (Volpe, 1995). Therefore, the infant's neurons have difficulty firing rapidly and repetitively.

The neonate has more inhibitory than excitatory synapses. This is actually a protective mechanism because it reduces the chance that a generalized seizure will be propagated within the cerebral cortex. As a result, cortical seizures are rare in neonates (Brann & Schwartz, 1987; Volpe, 1995). Seizure activity in these infants is more likely to be generated in areas of the brain that are more mature. These areas include the temporal lobe and subcortical structures, especially in the limbic area. The limbic area, which is located in the gyrus area above the corpus callosum, is one of the oldest parts of the brain in terms of embryologic development. This area is involved with behaviors such as sucking, drooling, chewing, swallowing, oculomotor deviations, and apneic episodes. These behaviors are typical of those seen with subtle seizures in the neonate (Miller, 1997; Volpe, 1995).

Risk Factors

Seizures are a clinical manifestation associated with various underlying pathologic processes (Table 29–7). The two events that most often place the neonate at risk for seizures are perinatal asphyxia and metabolic disturbances, such as hypoglycemia and hypocalcemia. Other problems that increase the risk for seizures in the neonate include intracranial hemorrhage, infection (meningitis, congenital viral infections, viral encephalopathy), congenital anomalies of the CNS, and other metabolic disturbances, such as alkalosis, hypomagnesemia, hypernatremia, and hyponatremia. Less common causes of seizures are drug withdrawal from opiates or barbiturates, genetic disorders of amino and organic acid metabolism, kernicterus, hyperviscosity, and local anesthetic intoxication.

Differential Diagnosis

Seizures can be difficult to recognize in neonates because the clinical manifestations are often subtle; can be associated with other disorders or involve individual behaviors, such as grimacing, startles, sucking, and twitching; or can occur with minimal or no outward signs. In addition, the individual behaviors just mentioned are normally seen during active sleep (see Chapter 48, Neonatal Sleep–Wake States) and thus can also be benign.

Seizure and jitteriness may be confused in the neonate, although the predominant type of movement is different. With jitteriness, the predominant movements are tremors characterized by alternating rhythmic movements of equal rate and magnitude. Seizures that may be confused with jitteriness involve primarily clonic movements that have characteristic fast and slow components (Volpe, 1995). Differences between these phenomena are delineated in Table 29–3. Jitteriness sometimes occurs along with seizures in such disorders as hypoglycemia, and hypocalcemia and

TABLE 29–7 Major Causes of Neonatal Seizures

Cause and Frequency (% of Total)	Usual Age at Onset (Days)	Predominant Seizure Type	Relative Frequency PT	FT
Perinatal asphyxia (30% to 65%)	>1 (often 6–18 hours after birth); 90% in first 72 hours	Subtle (all), generalized tonic, multifocal clonic	+ + + +	+ + +
Intracranial hemorrhage				
IVH	1–4	Subtle progressing to tonic	+ + +	–
SAH	2–3	Any type	+ +	+
SDH	1–2	May be focal	+/–	+
Hypocalcemia (15%)				
Early	1–3	Usually focal or multifocal	+ + +	+/–
Late	4–7	Usually focal or multifocal	+ +	+
Hypoglycemia (10%)	1–2	Usually focal or multifocal	+ +	+/–
Infections (10% to 15%)				
Bacterial meningitis	4–7	Any type, may be tonic	+ +	+
Viral encephalopathy	2–15	Any type	+	+
Congenital viral	3–7	Tonic, myoclonic	+/–	+/–
CNS malformations <10%	2–10 (often not until several months of age)	Tonic, myoclonic	+	+/–
Drug withdrawal (rare)	3–34	Tonic or myoclonic	+/–	+/–
Local anesthetic intoxication* (uncommon)	<1 (1–6 hours after birth)	Tonic	+/–	+/–

*Caused by accidental injection of local anesthetics into the scalp during placement of paracervical, pudendal, or epidural blocks or during injection of local anesthetics at delivery.

+ + + +, most common; +, least common; –, not seen; PT, partial tremor; FT, focal tremor; IVH, intraventricular hemorrhage; SAH, subarachnoid hemorrhage; SDH, subdural hemorrhage; CNS, central nervous system.

Modified from Brown, J. K., & Minns, R. A. (1988). Seizure disorders. In M. I. Levene, M. J. Bennett, & J. Punt (Eds.), *Fetal and neonatal neurology and neurosurgery* (pp. 487–514). Edinburgh: Churchill Livingstone; Clancy, R. R. (1989). Neonatal seizures. In D. K. Stevenson & P. Sunshine (Eds.), *Fetal and neonatal brain injury* (pp. 123–140). Toronto: B. C. Decker; Torrence, C. (1985). Neonatal seizures: Part I. A developmental and clinical understanding. *Neonatal Network, 4*(1), 9–16; Torrence, C. (1985). Neonatal seizures: Part II. Recognition, treatment, and prognosis. *Neonatal Network, 4*(2), 21–2; Volpe, J. J. (1995). *Neurology of the newborn* (3rd. ed.). Philadelphia: W. B. Saunders Co.

after perinatal asphyxia. Tonic seizures are sometimes confused with decorticate posturing and opisthotonos (Clancy, 1983). Characteristics of each of these signs are summarized in Table 29–2.

Clinical Manifestations

Recognition of seizures in the neonatal period requires careful, ongoing assessment by the nurse of all infants at risk. Clinical manifestations of seizures in the neonate differ from those seen in older children and adults, owing to immaturity of the CNS. As a result, seizure manifestations tend to be subtler. Clinical manifestations may include abnormal movements or alterations in tone of the trunk or extremities; abnormal facial, oral, tongue, or ocular movements; and respiratory problems (Clancy, 1983; Gale, 1981). Specific examples of each of these are listed in Table 29–8. Status epilepticus in the neonate is defined as seizures that recur frequently within a short time interval before the infant recovers consciousness, or a prolonged single seizure (Amiel-Tison et al., 1986).

Types of Seizures

The types of seizures seen in the neonate are, in order of decreasing frequency, subtle, tonic, clonic (multifocal and focal), and myoclonic (Bernes & Kaplan, 1994; Volpe, 1995).

SUBTLE SEIZURES

Subtle seizures are the most common type of seizure seen in neonates, particularly among preterm infants. This type of seizure is often missed because the clinical manifestations are often difficult to recognize and distinguish from other events. The most common behaviors seen with subtle seizures are (1) tonic, horizontal deviations of the eyes with or without nystagmoid jerking; (2) repetitive blinking or fluttering of the eyelids; (3) drooling, sucking, and/or tongue thrusting; and (4) swimming or rowing movements of the arms with occasional bicycling movements of the legs (Bernes & Kaplan, 1994; Volpe, 1995). Apnea may occur but is usually the result of the underlying cause of the seizure rather than of the seizure per se and rarely occurs as an isolated seizure event (Bernes & Kaplan, 1994; Goldbarg & Yeh, 1991).

TONIC

The most common form of tonic seizures are generalized tonic seizures, which usually involve tonic extension of all of the extremities but are sometimes limited to one extremity or are manifested by tonic flexion of all limbs. Generalized tonic seizures can be confused with decorticate or decerebrate posturing (see Table 29–2). Other signs may include eye deviations, apnea, and occasional clonic movements. This type of seizure is the one seen most frequently in preterm infants, especially those with intraventricular hemorrhage and hypoxic-ischemic insults. Generalized tonic seizures are often accompanied by apnea or decerebrate-type postures or both. Occasionally focal tonic seizures may occur which are characterized by sustained asymmetrical posturing of the limbs, trunk, and/or neck. Focal tonic seizure activity may be difficult to differentiate from voluntary movement (Bernes & Kaplan, 1994; Goldbarg & Yeh, 1991).

CLONIC

Clonic seizures may be multifocal or focal. Because multifocal clonic (migratory) seizures involve the cortex, they are more characteristic of term infants but may occasionally be seen in older preterm infants. This type of seizure involves rhythmic, jerky clonic movements of one or more limbs that migrate to other parts of the body in a random fashion. Multifocal clonic seizures can be confused with jitteriness (see Table 29–3). These seizures are associated with diffuse hyperexcitability of the cortex,

TABLE 29–8 Clinical Manifestations of Seizures in the Neonate

Type of Manifestation	Specific Alterations
Abnormal movement or alterations of tone in the trunk and extremities	Clonic (generalized or multifocal, migratory)
	Altering hemiclonic
	Tonic (single extremity), extension of arms and legs ("decerebrate-like"), extension of legs and flexion of arms ("decorticate-like"), or generalized
	Myoclonic (isolated or general)
	Bicycling movements of legs
	Swimming/rowing arm movements
	Loss of tone with general flaccidity
Facial, oral, and tongue movements	Sucking
	Grimacing
	Twitching
	Chewing, swallowing, yawning
Ocular movements	Tonic horizontal eye deviation
	Staring, blinking
	Nystagmoid jerks
Respiratory manifestations	Apnea (usually preceded or accompanied by one or more subtle manifestations)
	Hyperpneic or stertorous breathing

Modified from Brann, A. W., & Schwartz, J. F. (1987). Central nervous system disturbances. In A. A. Fanaroff & R. J. Martin (Eds.), *Neonatal–perinatal medicine* (pp. 495–553). St. Louis: C. V. Mosby Co.; Clancy, R. R. (1983). Neonatal seizures. In R. A. Polin & F. Berg (Eds.), *Workbook in practical neonatology* (pp. 125–152). Philadelphia: W. B. Saunders Co.; Gale, E. (1981). Neonatal seizures. In R. Perez (Ed.), *Protocols for perinatal nursing practice* (pp. 385–390). St. Louis: C. V. Mosby Co.

such as occurs with metabolic derangements (Bernes & Kaplan, 1994). Focal clonic seizures are also seen more frequently in term than in preterm infants. This relatively uncommon form of seizure is characterized by localized clonic jerking that is usually confined to one limb or the face. Focal clonic seizures may be associated with focal traumatic CNS injuries, such as cerebral contusions and infarcts, or may be a response to a severe metabolic disturbance or asphyxia. These seizures are often seen in combination with other seizure types (Bernes & Kaplan, 1994; Goldbarg & Yeh, 1991).

MYOCLONIC

Myoclonic seizures are uncommon in infants and are rarely seen in preterm infants. These seizures are characterized by single or multiple sudden jerks with flexion of the upper (most common) or lower extremities and occasionally the trunk and neck. Myoclonic seizures are most often seen with inborn errors of metabolism or other metabolic problems.

Prognosis

Mortality in infants with seizures has decreased in recent years (from approximately 40 percent before 1969 to less than 10 to 20 percent currently). The risk for later developmental problems is 25 to 35 percent (Volpe, 1995). Preterm infants tend to recover more rapidly from a seizure than do term infants; however, mortality and later morbidity are higher in the preterm infant.

The prognosis for infants with seizures during the neonatal period is influenced by (1) the time of onset, (2) the cause of the seizure, (3) the interictal EEG results, and (4) the seizure frequency and duration (Bernes & Kaplan, 1994). Seizure onset at less than 48 hours after birth has a poorer prognosis, whereas seizure onset after 4 days generally has a good prognosis. Clonic seizures have a better prognosis than do the other types (Bernes & Kaplan, 1994). The EEG is a better prognostic sign in term than in preterm infants. Prognosis should not be based on a single EEG. Fewer than 10 percent of infants with a normal interictal EEG have neurologic sequelae.

Seizures are actually relatively difficult to produce and maintain in most newborn animals, including human infants, owing to CNS immaturity. Thus, the increased frequency of seizures during the neonatal period is thought to be due to the many severe pathologic events to which the neonate is exposed that have the potential to cause seizures. Seizures associated with severe birth asphyxia, grade III or IV intraventricular hemorrhage, herpes infection, some bacterial meningitis, and CNS malformations have the poorest prognosis. The best prognosis is seen in infants with seizures secondary to late hypocalcemia, hyponatremia, and uncomplicated subarachnoid hemorrhage. Other causes have a mixed prognosis (Bernes & Kaplan, 1994; Volpe, 1995).

The seizure itself, unless prolonged or repeated, probably causes little damage. As a result, CNS damage associated with neonatal seizures is usually secondary to underlying pathologic processes that are severe enough to cause a seizure. Repeated or prolonged seizures can lead to brain injury by altering cerebral blood flow and delivery of oxygen and nutrients, by depleting brain glucose and energy stores, and by interfering with ventilation (Volpe, 1995). The interaction of these events is summarized in Figure 29–14.

Collaborative Management

Management of neonatal seizures has two goals: (1) to determine and treat the underlying cause of the seizures and (2) to protect the infant from injury during and after the seizure. Determining the cause involves assessment of the perinatal and neonatal history, physical examination, laboratory evaluation, and other diagnostic studies. Previous events that may indicate the underlying cause include delivery history, bleeding, birth trauma, perinatal asphyxia, exposure to infectious agents and other teratogens, maternal substance abuse, and postbirth illnesses.

Physical examination includes evaluation of general health and neurologic status. Routine laboratory studies include electrolyte levels; glucose, calcium, magnesium, and blood urea nitrogen levels; hematocrit value, blood gases, and pH. A blood culture and lumbar puncture are also often performed. The lumbar puncture helps to rule out both infection and CNS bleeding. Other laboratory and diagnostic studies may include CT, ultrasonography, MRI, skull radiography, TORCH screening, amino acid screening (for inborn errors of metabolism), or EEG. An EEG may or may not be useful in determining the cause of the seizures, especially in preterm infants, but it can be used to localize the origin or to validate subtle seizure manifestations (Bernes & Kaplan, 1994). The results of an interictal EEG can provide information on prognosis, more so in a term than in a preterm infant. The timing of seizure onset and type of seizure can also help in determining the cause (see Table 29–7). An EEG for prognosis is often recommended 24 hours after seizure onset and again 5 days later (Amiel-Tison et al., 1986; Amiel-Tison & Larroche, 1988; Volpe, 1995).

Treatment of the underlying cause of the seizure is a priority for preventing further seizures and neurologic damage. Management of intracranial hemorrhage and CNS anomalies is discussed later in this chapter. Management of other disorders is discussed in detail in other chapters: perinatal asphyxia (Chapter 15, Resuscitation and Stabilization of the Neonate); metabolic and electrolyte problems (Chapter 22, Fluids, Electrolytes, Vitamins, and Trace Minerals; Chapter 25, Assessment and Management of Metabolic Dysfunction; Chapter 26, Assessment and Management of Endocrine Dysfunction); infections (Chapter 27, Assessment and Management of Immunologic Dysfunction); drug with-

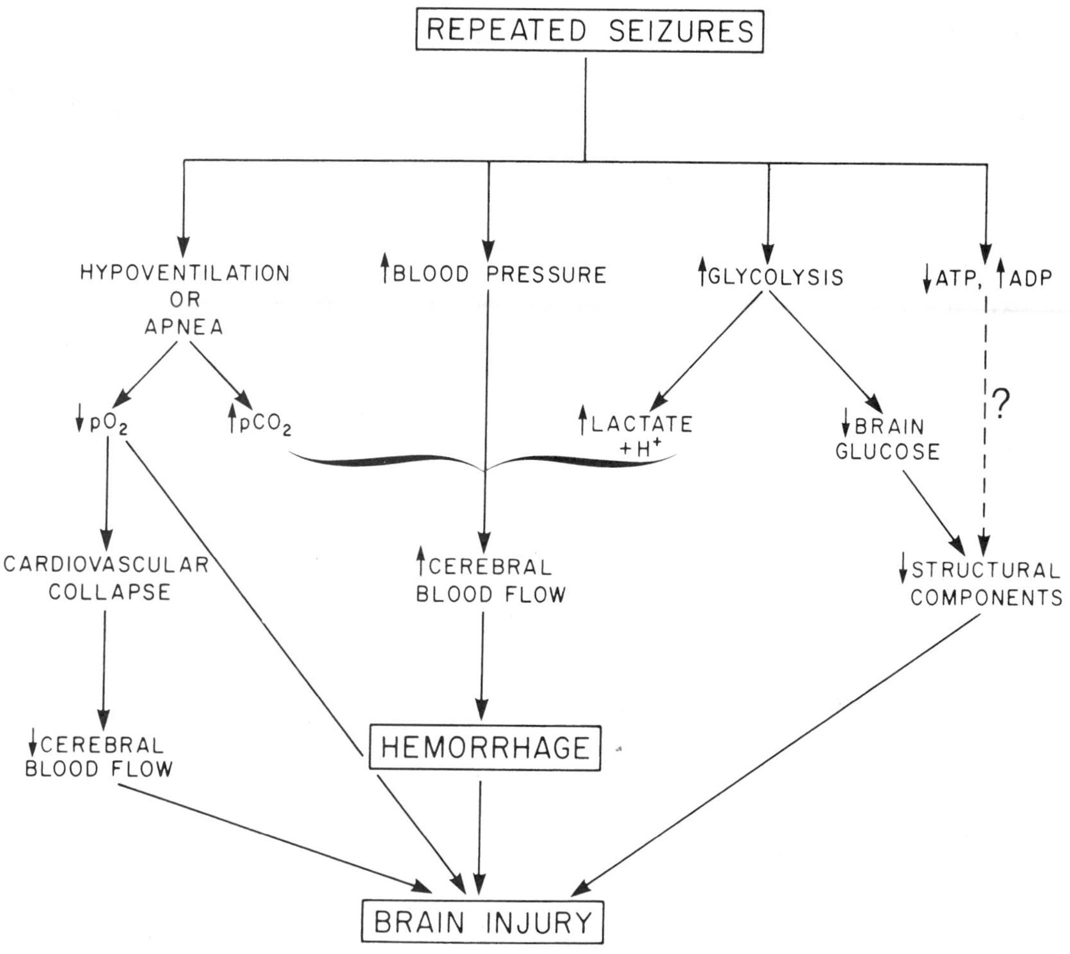

FIGURE 29–14. Mechanisms for brain injury with repeated seizures. ADP, adenosine diphosphate; ATP, adenosine triphosphate; Po_2, oxygen partial pressure; Pco_2, carbon dioxide partial pressure. (Modified from Volpe, J. J. [1987]. *Neurology of the newborn* [2nd ed., p. 146]. Philadelphia: W. B. Saunders Co.)

drawal (Chapter 45, The Drug-Exposed Neonate); and local anesthetic infiltration (Chapter 14, The Effects of Labor on the Fetus and Neonate).

Ongoing monitoring of blood gases, acid-base, serum glucose, and fluid and electrolyte status is important for any infant with seizures. Infants who are having seizures, regardless of their cause, need intravenous glucose because seizure activity depletes brain glucose and energy supplies (Wasterlain & Duffy, 1975). Alterations in oxygenation and acid-base status can occur as a complication of the apnea associated with a seizure or the physiologic consequences of seizure activity. Fluid and electrolyte management should be appropriate to the underlying cause of the seizures. For example, fluids are restricted initially in infants with cerebral edema and perinatal asphyxia (see Chapter 22, Fluids, Electrolytes, Vitamins, and Trace Minerals).

The issues of when to treat with anticonvulsant drugs and for how long are controversial. Some clinicians favor early aggressive therapy, whereas others do not because neonatal seizures often abate spontaneously. Recurrent or prolonged seizures require treatment with anticonvulsants to reduce the risk of brain injury. The most common anticonvulsant used in the neonate is phenobarbital. Other anticonvulsants used include phenytoin (Dilantin), diazepam, and lorazepam. General pharmacologic properties, dosages, and side effects of these drugs are discussed in Chapter 41 (Neonatal Pharmacology). Table 29–9 summarizes loading and maintenance doses for the treatment of neonatal seizures. Blood levels of these drugs must be monitored carefully to ensure therapeutic levels and prevent toxicity. Cardiovascular status and respiratory function must also be monitored. Administration of anticonvulsants may or may not be discontinued before discharge. Volpe (1995) indicates that anticonvulsant therapy can be discontinued if the infant has a normal neurologic examination and EEG and no brain lesions are seen on cranial imaging. If infants are receiving anticonvulsant therapy on discharge, they should be re-evaluated about 1 month later.

Nursing Management

The nurse is the individual most likely to observe seizure activity in the nursery. Therefore, nursing management focuses on recognizing and documenting seizure activity and protecting and supporting the infant during and after the seizure. Observing and documenting seizure activity involves noting and recording the following: the time the seizure begins and ends; the body parts involved (e.g., extremities, eyes, head); a description of motor movement; eye deviations; pupillary reactions; the respiratory status; the patient's color; the state and level of consciousness; and the postictal status (Gale, 1981).

Nursing interventions during a seizure vary with the severity, duration, and type of seizure. During the seizure, the nurse must ensure that the infant's airway is maintained, monitor vital signs, and assess for adequacy of respiration and heart rate to maintain ventilation and perfusion. To protect the infant from injury during the seizure, the nurse should not force anything into the infant's mouth or try to restrain the infant's extremities. The nurse should

TABLE 29–9 Treatment of Seizures with Anticonvulsant Drugs

Drug	Dose	Comments
Phenobarbital (drug of choice for neonatal seizures)	Loading: 10–20 mg/kg IV to maximum of 40 mg/kg Maintenance: 5–7 mg/kg in 2 divided doses beginning 12 hours after last loading dose	Therapeutic level: 20–25 μg/ml (obtain levels any time 1 hour after dose); respiratory depressant; incompatible with other drugs in solution
Phenytoin (added if seizures are not controlled by phenobarbital alone)	Loading: 10–20 mg/kg IV (no more rapidly than 10–20 mg/minute) Maintenance: 5–7 mg/kg in 1–2 doses/day beginning 12 hours after last loading dose	Therapeutic level: 15–20 μg/ml (obtain levels 1–10 hours after last loading or maintenance dose); incompatible with all other drugs, glucose, and pH <11.5; give slowly directly into vein; too-rapid administration causes dysrhythmias, bradycardia, hypotension, cardiovascular collapse, and/or respiratory distress
Diazepam	0.3 mg/kg IV (0.1–0.3 mg/kg/dose)	Sodium benzoate competes with bilirubin for albumin binding sites; potentiates jaundice, so kernicterus is possible at lower serum bilirubin levels
Pyridoxine	50–100 mg IV bolus	Pyridoxine (vitamin B_6) deficiency as cause of neonatal seizures is rare; seizures cease within 5 minutes after vitamin B_6 injection, if patient has deficiency
Lorazepam	0.05 mg/kg/dose IV over 2–5 minutes	Use justified in severely ill newborns with seizures that are nonresponsive to other drugs
Primidone	Loading: 15–20 mg PO Maintenance: 12–20 mg/kg/day	Use justified for refractory seizures; close monitoring of phenobarbital levels is necessary because levels increase after primidone loading and decrease precipitously with phenobarbital discontinuance
Valproic acid	Initial dose: 15–30 mg/kg/day PO, PR Maintenance: 15–60 mg/kg/day PO q 12 hours	Anticonvulsant for refractory neonatal seizures; complications include neutropenia, hepatic damage, and hyperammonemia

IV, intravenous; PO, by mouth; PR, through the rectum; q, every.
Modified from Merenstein, G. B., & Gardner, S. L. (1993). *Handbook of neonatal intensive care* (3rd. ed., p. 448). St. Louis: Mosby–Year Book.

try to turn the infant's head to the side, if possible. After the seizure, the infant's condition should be monitored, and supportive care should be provided so that ventilation, oxygenation, adequate fluids, glucose, and warmth are maintained. The nurse also assesses the infant for signs related to the events that can cause seizure activity in the neonate in order to help determine the cause of the seizure and prevent further seizures.

Nursing management also involves administering and monitoring anticonvulsants and interventions aimed at treating the underlying cause of the seizures. Because anticonvulsants can be respiratory, myocardial, and CNS depressants or can compete with bilirubin for albumin binding, cardiorespiratory status, color, and neurologic status are monitored in addition to drug effectiveness. Parent teaching includes helping the family to understand the cause and significance of the seizure or seizures and any diagnostic tests that are planned. Discharge teaching of parents includes recognition of seizure manifestations, care of the infant during and after a seizure, and administration of anticonvulsants (dosage and side effects) if administration of these drugs is to be continued after discharge.

Periventricular/Intraventricular Hemorrhage

Periventricular/intraventricular hemorrhage (P/IVH) is the most common type of intracranial hemorrhage seen in the neonatal period. P/IVH has been described as the most common and serious neurologic disorder of preterm infants. This type of hemorrhage is seen almost exclusively in preterm infants, particularly those born at less than 32 weeks' gestation, or weighing less than 1500 g, or both. The incidence in this group of infants has decreased and currently ranges from 15 to 20 percent (Volpe, 1995). The risk of P/IVH increases with decreasing gestational age. P/IVH occurs but is rare after 35 to 36 weeks' gestation, owing to involution of the subependymal germinal matrix and alterations in cerebral blood flow patterns after this time (de Vries et al., 1988b). On those rare occasions when P/IVH occurs in term infants, bleeding usually arises from the choroid plexus rather than from the germinal matrix. These infants are irritable and stuporous, and have focal or multifocal clonic seizures (Bernes & Kaplan, 1994).

Pathophysiology

The neuropathophysiology of P/IVH involves a complex interaction of intravascular, vascular, and extravascular factors. In infants less than 28 to 32 weeks' gestation, the hemorrhage generally arises from the subependymal germinal matrix at the head of the caudate nucleus near the foramen of Monro. In more mature infants, especially after a hypoxic-ischemic insult, the hemorrhage usually arises from the choroid plexus (Volpe & Hill, 1987).

The germinal matrix includes the tissue underlying the ependymal wall of the lateral ventricles. In 20 to 40 percent of preterm infants, the hemorrhage is confined to the subependymal area (Volpe & Hill, 1987). In the rest, the original hemorrhage ruptures into the lateral ventricles and then into the third and fourth ventricles. The blood eventually collects in the subarachnoid space of the posterior fossa, often extending into the basal cistern (see Fig. 29–1) (de Vries et al., 1988b). Rupture of the hemorrhage from the germinal matrix into the ventricles may serve a protective function by decompressing the hemorrhagic area and reducing further tissue destruction. Progressive ventricular dilation may occur as the result of obstruction of CSF flow by an obliterative arachnoiditis or as the result of blood clots at the level of the aqueduct of Sylvius or the foramen of Monro. With severe hemorrhages, the blood may dissect into the periventricular white matter.

Neuropathologic consequences of P/IVH include (1) destruction of the germinal matrix and its glial precursor cells, (2) infarction and necrosis of periventricular white matter, and (3) posthemorrhagic hydrocephalus. As the IVH moves from the germinal matrix area into the surrounding white matter, periventricular hemorrhagic infarction associated with intraparenchymal echodensities develops. The appearance of this parenchymal lesion is associated with increased mortality and neurodevelopmental sequelae (Perlman et al., 1993). Infants with P/IVH may also have periventricular leukomalacia (PVL). However, PVL is thought to arise as a consequence of hypoxic-ischemic injury and is not caused by the P/IVH per se (Volpe, 1995).

Pathogenic Factors

INTRAVASCULAR

Intravascular hemodynamic factors play a prominent role in the pathogenesis of P/IVH. These factors include distribution of blood to the periventricular region, pressure-passive cerebral blood flow, and venous hemodynamics. The early stages of CNS development that are characteristic of the preterm infant who is born at less than 32 to 33 weeks' gestation increase the risk of hemorrhage in the periventricular area.

Periventricular Blood Flow. The subependymal germinal matrix is a transient structure. It begins to thin at 23 to 24 weeks' gestation and has almost completely involuted by 36 weeks' gestation (Girard et al., 1995). This is the site where neuroectodermal cells that serve as precursors for neurons (before about 24 weeks' gestation) and glial cells develop. These cells subsequently migrate to their eventual locus in the cerebral cortex. Processes involved in the proliferation, differentiation, and migration of these cells result in an area that is highly vascularized and metabolically active. Before 32 weeks' gestation, a significant portion of the total cerebral blood flow goes to the periventricular germinal matrix, primarily to support neuroblast and glioblast mitotic activity and migration. Any factor that increases cerebral blood flow can result in overperfusion of the periventricular region. After 32 to 34 weeks' gestation, cell proliferation and migration decrease. The germinal matrix becomes less prominent and receives a smaller proportion of the cerebral blood supply. At this point, the greater proportion of blood flow is to the rapidly differentiating cerebral cortex.

Cerebral Autoregulation. The blood vessels of the brain are normally protected from marked alterations in flow by autoregulatory processes. If cerebral autoregulation is intact, the arterioles constrict or dilate to maintain a constant cerebral blood flow, despite fluctuations in systemic blood pressure. Asphyxia or hypoxemia in the neonate alters cerebral autoregulation. This alteration can lead to a pressure-passive system in which cerebral blood flow varies directly with arterial pressure. Subsequent alterations in systemic blood pressure, or cerebral blood flow, or both, are transmitted directly to the brain and, in particular, to the area receiving the greatest proportion of cerebral blood flow, that is, the fragile, thin-walled vessels of the germinal matrix. Thus, rapid fluctuations in systemic blood pressure or cerebral blood flow, that is, moving from increased to decreased flow and vice versa, also increase the risk of vessel rupture (de Vries et al., 1988b; Mullaart et al., 1994; Volpe, 1995). Altered hemodynamics with fluctuations in blood flow can occur with positive-pressure ventilation, rapid volume expansion, hypercapnia, and possibly decreased hematocrit and blood glucose values. Increased systemic blood pressure and, potentially, cerebral blood flow can also occur with caregiving events, handling, suctioning, and chest physical therapy (Funato et al., 1992; Goldberg et al., 1980; Shah et al., 1992; Volpe, 1995).

Venous Hemodynamics. Increased venous pressure, from events such as myocardial failure or positive-pressure ventilation, can also be transmitted directly to the capillaries of the germinal matrix. These events can impede cerebral venous return, leading to stasis and venous congestion, which then leads to increased venous pressure and vessel rupture. The point of vulnerability in the venous drainage system of the brain is at the level of the foramen of Monro and the caudate nucleus (usual site of P/IVH). At this location, a U-shaped turn exists in the venous drainage system where the confluence of the thalamostriate, terminal, and choroidal veins forms the internal cerebral vein, which empties into the great vein of Galen. This results in a sharp change in the direction of blood flow and predisposes to turbulent venous flow with stasis and thrombi formation and an area vulnerable to increased intravascular pressure (Volpe, 1995). In addition, the pliable skull of the preterm infant can easily be deformed, obstructing the major venous sinuses and increasing venous pressure (Cowan & Thorensen, 1985; Emery & Peabody, 1983; Kosmetatos & Williams, 1978).

VASCULAR

The capillary bed of the germinal matrix is immature, a quality that increases its vulnerability to rupture. The germinal matrix capillaries are large, irregular, thin-walled vessels described as "persistent immature vascular rete" (Pape & Wigglesworth, 1979). The capillary walls thicken with increasing gestational age. Fragility of these vessels is due in part to the lack of thickness and strength of the basement membrane and the lack of collagen and smooth muscle. With migration of the neuronal and glial cells and their derivatives, the germinal matrix undergoes involution. The immature capillary bed is remodeled into the definitive, mature capillary bed (Goldstein & Donn, 1984; Pape & Wigglesworth, 1979; Volpe, 1995).

The epithelial cells of these capillaries are dependent on oxidative metabolism and thus are easily injured by hypoxic events. This characteristic increases the likelihood of leakage or rupture if transmural pressure increases. Because these vessels require an adequate supply of oxygen for the maintenance of their functional integrity, decreased cerebral blood flow can lead to hypoxic-ischemic injury. These vessels are also susceptible to ischemia because they tend to lie in the vascular border zone or "watershed" area (see section on HIE). Thus, both increased and decreased cerebral blood flow can be involved in the pathogenesis of P/IVH.

EXTRAVASCULAR

The capillary bed of the highly vascularized germinal matrix is embedded in gelatinous material that is deficient in supportive mesenchymal elements, thus providing poor support for the fragile blood vessels. In addition, excessive fibrinolytic activity occurs in the periventricular area. As a result, a small initial bleed may not clot off and be localized, but rather may continue to enlarge and rupture into the ventricles, or the cerebral parenchyma, or both (Volpe, 1995).

Risk Factors

The overall major risk factors for P/IVH in the neonate are prematurity and hypoxic events interrelated with the anatomic and physiologic processes that make the periventricular site particularly vulnerable. From a clinical perspective, any perinatal or neonatal event that results in hypoxia or alters cerebral blood flow or intravascular pressure increases the risk of P/IVH. Perinatal events that can lead to fetal and neonatal hypoxia include maternal bleeding, fetal distress, perinatal asphyxia, prolonged labor, preterm labor, and abnormal presentations. Neonatal hypoxic events, such as respiratory distress, apnea, and hypotension, further increase the risk of intraventricular hemorrhage. The most consistent risk factors for P/IVH in the preterm infant are respiratory distress syndrome with severe hypoxia and mechanical ventilation (de Vries et al., 1988b).

Events associated with impeded venous return, or increased venous pressure, or both, include assisted ventilation, high positive inspiratory pressure, prolonged inspiratory duration, continuous positive airway pressure, and air leak. Venous pressure can also be increased by compression of the infant's skull during vaginal delivery, application of forceps, and use of constricting head bands (Carey, 1983; Cowan & Thorensen, 1985; Emery & Peabody, 1983; Kosmetatos & Williams, 1978). Rapid administration of hypertonic solutions, such as sodium bicarbonate and glucose; rapid volume expansion; hypernatremia; hypercarbia caregiving interventions; and environmental stress can increase cerebral blood flow (Funato et al., 1992; Goldberg et al., 1980; Kling, 1989; Lou et al., 1978; Papile et al., 1978; Shah et al., 1992). Hypercarbia causes cerebral vasodilation, thus increasing blood flow. Hypertonic solutions given rapidly or in a large bolus alter osmotic gradients between the brain and the blood. Repeated or prolonged seizures increase blood pressure and can lead to hypoxia. Alterations in the coagulation system increase the risk of an initial hemorrhage as well as extension of that hemorrhage or subsequent hemorrhages.

Differential Diagnosis

Periventricular/intraventricular hemorrhage usually occurs in preterm infants who have sustained some form of hypoxic insult. Many of these infants are ill with other problems. The clinical manifestations of this disorder are often nonspecific and are not well correlated with later positive evidence from CT of a bleed. Therefore, a high index of suspicion must be used along with careful monitoring of infants at risk.

Diagnosis is made by cranial ultrasonography or CT (see Chapter 36, Diagnostic Imaging). Ultrasonography is the preferred method because it can be performed at the patient's bedside and does not expose the infant to ionizing radiation. This procedure can be used to determine the presence and severity of a P/IVH and progression of the hemorrhage, and to monitor later complications such as PVL and progressive ventricular dilation.

Clinical Manifestations

More than 90 percent of infants with P/IVH bleed within the first 72 hours after birth; 50 percent of the bleeding occurs in the first 24 hours after birth (Volpe, 1995). Approximately 10 to 20 percent of infants observed serially with cranial ultrasonography after a bleed demonstrate progressive increases in the size of the hemorrhage over a 24- to 48-hour period (de Vries et al., 1988b). Late hemorrhages are seen after a few days or weeks in about 15 percent of infants. Late hemorrhages are seen primarily in preterm infants with severe, prolonged respiratory problems. A new hemorrhage or an extension of a previous one may develop in these infants. A P/IVH may also develop before birth in some infants (Wigglesworth, 1989).

The signs and symptoms of P/IVH are often nonspecific and subtle. The clinical signs that correlate most closely with CT evidence of hemorrhage are (1) a decreasing hematocrit value or a failure of the hematocrit value to increase after a transfusion; (2) a full anterior fontanelle; (3) changes in activity level; and (4) a decreased tone (Volpe, 1995). Other clinical signs that are associated with the presence of P/IVH are impaired visual tracking, increased tone of the lower limbs, neck flexor hypotonia, and brisk tendon reflexes (de Vries et al., 1988b).

Periventricular/intraventricular hemorrhage is classified into different types, according to the location and the severity of the hemorrhage. Several different systems have been proposed. One of the most common ones is illustrated in Table 29–10.

Laboratory evidence suggestive of P/IVH, in addition to a decreasing hematocrit value, are CSF findings indicative of hemorrhage: increased red blood cell levels, increased protein levels, decreased glucose levels, and xanthochromia (often a later finding and resulting from increased protein). Extremely low CSF glucose levels, or hypoglycorrhachia, can be found several days to a week (usually 5 to 15 days) after the hemorrhage in some infants. The CSF glucose level remains depressed for up to 2 to 3 months. The basis for this finding is unclear, but it may be caused by inhibition or alteration in glucose transport between the CNS and the CSF (Volpe, 1995).

Wide variations exist in the patterns of clinical manifestations seen in individual infants. Three clinical syndromes have been described: silent, catastrophic, and saltatory (Volpe, 1995). At one end of the continuum are most infants. These infants have only silent, subependymal bleeds with no clinical signs. The hemorrhage is discovered during routine ultrasonographic screening.

Catastrophic deterioration usually involves major hemorrhages that evolve rapidly over several minutes or hours. Clinical findings include stupor progressing to coma, respiratory distress progressing to apnea, generalized tonic seizures, decerebrate posturing, fixation of pupils to light, and flaccid quadriparesis. This clinical presentation is associated with a decreasing hematocrit value, bulging fontanelle, hypotension, bradycardia, alterations in temperature, hypoglycemia, and syndrome of inappropriate antidiuretic hormone (see Chapter 26, Assessment and Management of Endocrine Dysfunction, for a discussion of syndrome of inappropriate antidiuretic hormone). Infants with catastrophic hemorrhages have a high mortality and, if they survive, a poor prognosis for later development.

The saltatory pattern is associated with small hemorrhages that develop over hours to days. Signs and symptoms are usually subtle or silent and present irregularly. Clinical manifestations, if present, include alterations in level of consciousness or stupor, hypotonia, abnormal eye movements or positions, and altered mobility. An unexplained decrease in hematocrit value by 10 percent or more or failure of the hematocrit value to increase after a transfusion, even in the absence of other symptoms, suggests the possibility of a bleed. These infants generally survive. Later developmental outcome is variable, depending on the severity of the hemorrhage.

Prognosis

Mortality and morbidity are influenced by the severity and extent of the hemorrhage and the presence of associated problems, such as respiratory distress syndrome, perinatal asphyxia, and sepsis. Infants with a history of P/IVH are also at risk for development of posthemorrhagic ventricular dilation that can be

TABLE 29–10 Grading System for Periventricular Intraventricular Hemorrhage

Grade I	Subependymal (germinal matrix hemorrhage (SEH) only
Grade II	SEH with extension into normal-sized ventricles
Grade III	SEH with extension into dilated ventricles
Grade IV	Intraventricular hemorrhage with extension into brain parenchyma

From Papile, L., Burstein, J., Burstein, R., & Koffler, H. (1978). Incidence and evolution of subependymal and intraventricular hemorrhage: A study of infants with birth weights less than 1500 g. *Journal of Pediatrics*, 92, 529. Reprinted with permission.

either normopressive or associated with increased ICP. Infants with small or mild hemorrhages survive and generally have a good outcome, with a low incidence of major neurologic sequelae and posthemorrhagic ventricular dilation. Infants with moderate hemorrhages have a 5 to 20 percent mortality, and ventricular dilation develops in 15 to 25 percent of survivors and a risk of neurologic sequelae, such as cerebral palsy (CP), developmental retardation, sensory and attentional problems, learning disorders, and hydrocephalus, is present in 15 to 30 percent. Mortality in infants with severe hemorrhage averages 50 percent, with development of progressive ventricular dilation in 55 to 80 percent and neurologic sequelae in 35 to 90 percent (de Vries et al., 1988b; Volpe, 1995; Volpe & Hill, 1987). Although infants with severe hemorrhages tend to have significant motoric and cognitive deficits, some seem to escape significant long-term sequelae.

Collaborative Management

Many units have instituted routine ultrasonographic screening of infants at risk for P/IVH. Screening can identify infants with silent bleeds or bleeds associated with nonspecific, subtle symptoms. By identifying these vulnerable infants, interventions can be instituted to prevent new bleeds or extensions of existing ones. Management of P/IVH involves prevention of hemorrhage in infants at risk, acute care of infants with current bleeds, pharmacologic therapies, and management of posthemorrhagic ventricular dilation (Volpe, 1995).

Prevention begins in the perinatal period, with the prevention of preterm birth, perinatal asphyxia, and birth trauma. Ongoing assessment of fetal and neonatal oxygenation and perfusion is important, so that subtle alterations can be recognized and clinicians can intervene early to avoid cerebral hyperperfusion and stabilize cerebral blood flow and pressures. Prompt resuscitation at birth minimizes hypoxemia and hypercarbia, which can alter cerebral autoregulation. Hypertonic solutions and volume expanders are administered slowly, with careful monitoring of vital signs and color. This may be particularly important during delivery resuscitation and early stabilization efforts. Activities that can increase ICP or cause wide swings in arterial or venous pressure are avoided or minimized when possible, especially during the first 72 hours of life. Because seizures can alter cerebral blood flow and ICP, they must be recognized promptly and treated. Acute care of infants with bleeds focuses on monitoring and maintenance of oxygenation and perfusion to prevent further damage or extension of the bleed. Institution of guidelines to avoid factors associated with development of P/IVH were reported to reduce the incidence of this disorder by nearly one half by Szymonowicz and colleagues (1986).

Pharmacologic therapies, including phenobarbital, indomethacin, and vitamin E, have been tried prophylactically to reduce the incidence of hemorrhage or to prevent more severe bleeds, or neurologic damage, or both (Cooke, 1989; Kaempf et al., 1990; Ment et al., 1994a; Ment et al., 1994b). Research findings have been inconsistent. Additional research is needed regarding all of these agents.

Management of Progressive Ventricular Dilation

Progressive posthemorrhagic ventricular dilation is a common complication of P/IVH. Therefore, all infants with a history of P/IVH are observed with serial cranial ultrasonography. In most infants, ventricular dilation occurs slowly, without increased ICP (normopressive hydrocephalus). Ventricular growth spontaneously arrests in approximately half of these infants within about 30 days. The remaining infants continue to demonstrate ventricular dilation and increased ICP (Volpe, 1995).

Initial treatment of infants with normopressive hydrocephalus involves observation because in many, ventricular growth arrests spontaneously without treatment. Clinicians may use serial lumbar punctures to remove CSF and decrease ventricle size. Approximately 15 to 20 ml of CSF may be removed, with daily taps over a 1- to 3-week period. When the volume of CSF decreases to less than 5 ml for several days, the frequency of the taps is gradually decreased and then discontinued (Amiel-Tison et al., 1986; Volpe, 1995). Drugs to decrease CSF production have also been used, with variable results. These agents include carbonic anhydrase inhibitors, such as acetazolamide (Diamox) and furosemide, or osmotic agents, such as isosorbitol and glycerol. These agents require careful monitoring of serum potassium level, acid-base status, renal function, and hydration (Amiel-Tison & Larroche, 1988).

Progressive ventricular dilation with increasing ICP is managed with a ventriculoperitoneal shunt or, if the infant is too ill and/or small for surgery, with temporary ventricular drainage. Ventricular drainage can be accomplished by an external ventricular drain or a tunneled catheter attached to a subcutaneous reservoir (Volpe, 1995).

Nursing Management

Nursing management involves recognition of factors that increase the risk of P/IVH, interventions to reduce the risk of bleeding, and supportive care of infants with acute bleeds or posthemorrhagic ventricular dilation. Prevention or risk reduction begins in the perinatal period and is especially critical during the intrapartum period and the first 3 to 4 days after birth, the period of greatest vulnerability. Prevention and risk-reduction activities include interventions to avoid or reduce hypoxic or asphyxial events, to avoid rapid alterations in cerebral blood flow, to prevent fluctuations in systemic blood pressure, to prevent hyperosmolarity, and to prevent or minimize fluctuations in ICP. Specific nursing interventions to accomplish these goals are listed in Table 29–11.

These interventions are based on analysis of pathophysiologic events that are thought to be involved in the pathogenesis of P/IVH. Few investigations have been attempted to examine the effectiveness of specific interventions. Als and associates (1994) found that infants treated with individualized developmental care, as outlined in Chapter 49 (Assessment and Management of Neonatal Neurobehavioral Development), had a significantly decreased incidence of P/IVH and fewer severe hemorrhages than did infants treated with conventional care. Other studies suggested that the use of developmental interventions, such as containment or swaddling during aversive procedures such as endotracheal suctioning, may promote greater physiologic stability during these procedures and a more rapid return to baseline (Taquino & Blackburn, 1994).

Acute treatment of infants with P/IVH includes provision of physiologic support with maintenance of oxygenation, perfusion, normothermia, and normoglycemia. Physical manipulations and handling are minimized, as are environmental stressors, to reduce the risk of hypoxia and fluctuations in arterial blood pressure and in cerebral blood flow. The infant's position is also important. The infant can be placed prone or side lying. The head is positioned in midline or to the side, but without the neck's being flexed. The head of the bed can be slightly elevated. The Trendelenburg position is avoided. Vital signs, blood pressure, tone, activity, and level of consciousness are monitored frequently. Care of infants with progressive ventricular dilation is discussed in the section on hydrocephalus.

Parent care involves recognition and discussion of parental concerns about their infant's immediate and long-term prognosis and teaching regarding P/IVH, its implications, and management. The parents need to be shown how to interact with, and care for, the infant at risk for P/IVH in a developmentally appropriate manner, with the goal of promoting opportunities for interaction while minimizing stressful events. The nurse can model this type of care for parents and provide anticipatory guidance as to how

TABLE 29–11 Nursing Interventions to Reduce the Risks of Periventricular/Intraventricular Hemorrhage*

Nursing Care	Rationale
1. Position with head in midline and head of bed slightly elevated.	ICP is lowest with head in midline and head of bed elevated 30°. Turning the head sharply to the side causes an obstruction of the ipsilateral jugular vein and can increase ICP.
2. Avoid tight, encircling phototherapy masks.	Pressure on the occiput can increase ICP by impeding venous drainage.
3. Avoid rapid fluid infusions for volume expansion. • Know normal BP for infant's weight and age. • Suggest dopamine therapy to maintain BP if infant is not hypovolemic.	Rapid increases in intravascular volume can cause rupture of capillaries in germinal matrix. Risk may be increased if a history of hypoxia and hypotension exists. Even modest, abrupt increases in PB may cause P/IVH.
4. When $NaHCO_3$ therapy is necessary to correct a documented metabolic acidosis, slowly give dilute solution.	Role of $NaHCO_3$ unclear, but rapid infusions may cause elevations in CO_2, which could dilate cerebral vessels and contribute to a pressure-passive cerebral circulation.
5. Monitor BP diligently. Note fluctuating pattern in arterial pressure tracing in high-risk ventilated infants and inform physician.	Blood flow velocity in the anterior cerebral artery is reflected by the pattern of simultaneously recorded arterial BP. A fluctuating pattern is associated with the development of P/IVH and can be stabilized by pancuronium bromide.
6. Monitor closely for signs of pneumothorax, such as (a) increased mean BP, especially increases in diastolic BP (early); (b) increased heart rate; (c) changes in breath sounds, which may or may not be appreciated; (d) decreased Pa_{O_2}; (e) increased Pa_{CO_2}; (f) shift in cardiac point of maximum impulse; and (g) hypotension and bradycardia (late).	Pneumothorax frequently precedes P/IVH. The sum of hemodynamic changes caused by pneumothorax is flow under increased pressure in the germinal matrix capillaries. Changes in vital signs can be early indicators of pneumothorax.
7. Maintain temperature within neutral thermal range.	Hypothermia has been associated with P/IVH.
8. Suction only as needed.	Even brief (20-second) suctioning episodes can increase cerebral blood flow velocity, increase BP, increase ICP, and decrease oxygenation.
9. Avoid interventions that cause crying. • Consider long-term methods of achieving venous access to avoid frequent venipunctures. • Critically evaluate all manipulations and handling. • Use analgesics for stressful procedures.	Crying can impede venous return, increase cerebral blood volume, and compromise cerebral oxygenation in sick infants.
10. Maintain blood gas values within a normal range. • Use continuous noninvasive monitoring of oxygenation. • Adjust F_{IO_2}, as needed, to maintain Tc_{PO_2} or pulse oximeter values within desired range. • Avoid interventions that cause hypoxia.	Hypoxia and hypercapnia are associated with the development of P/IVH. These events increase cerebral blood flow and may impair the neonate's already limited ability to autoregulate the cerebral blood flow. Hypoxia can injure the germinal matrix capillary endothelium.

*Premature neonates are most vulnerable to P/IVH during the first 4 days of life, with approximately 50% of hemorrhages occurring in the first 24 hours. Attempts to minimize the risk of P/IVH should begin immediately after birth, even before the infant has reached the special care nursery.

ICP, intracranial pressure; BP, blood pressure; P/IVH, periventricular/intraventricular hemorrhage.

From Kling, P. (1989). Nursing interventions to decrease the risk of periventricular-intraventricular hemorrhage. *Journal of Obstetric, Gynecologic, and Neonatal Nursing, 18*, 457. Reprinted with permission.

the infant's needs and care will change as the infant matures (see Chapter 50, Assessment and Management of the Transition to Home). Parents can also be involved in developing and implementing a developmental plan of care for their infant in order to reduce environmental stressors.

Other Types of Intracranial Hemorrhage

In addition to P/IVH, several other clinically important types of intracranial hemorrhage exist in the neonate, including primary subarachnoid, subdural, and intracerebellar hemorrhage. These types arise from either trauma or hypoxia during the perinatal period.

Primary Subarachnoid Hemorrhage

Primary subarachnoid hemorrhage (SAH) is the most prevalent form of intracranial hemorrhage in neonates and the least clinically significant for most infants. SAH occurs in both preterm and term infants, but it is more common in preterm infants. SAH may occur alone (primary SAH) or as a secondary event with other forms of intracranial hemorrhage. For example, with P/IVH, blood moves into the subarachnoid space via the fourth ventricle.

Pathophysiology and Risk Factors

Primary SAH consists of bleeding into the subarachnoid space that is not secondary to subdural or intraventricular bleeding. In neonates, the source of the bleeding is venous blood; in older children and adults, SAH usually involves arterial blood. With primary SAH, blood leaks from the leptomeningeal plexus, bridging veins, or ruptured vessels in the subarachnoid space (de Vries et al., 1988a). This type of hemorrhage is associated with trauma or asphyxia. Trauma causing increased intravascular pressure and capillary rupture is the underlying causal event in most term infants with SAH. In preterm infants, SAH is usually the result of asphyxial events. Factors that place an infant at risk for SAH include birth trauma, prolonged labor, difficult delivery, fetal distress, and perinatal asphyxia.

Differential Diagnosis

Subarachnoid hemorrhage must be distinguished from other forms of intracranial hemorrhage and other neurologic problems. This differentiation can often be accomplished by evaluation of the infant's history and presentation, and, if the infant is having seizure activity, by the elimination of other causes of seizures. Blood in the CSF on lumbar puncture indicates the possibility of SAH, but true hemorrhage must be distinguished from a bloody tap. Ultrasonography and CT can also assist in confirming the diagnosis. CT may be more useful than ultrasonography (de Vries et al., 1988a).

Clinical Manifestations

Three clinical presentations have been described for infants with SAH (Volpe, 1995; Volpe & Hill, 1987). The most common occurs with preterm infants with a minor SAH. These infants are asymptomatic. The hemorrhage is discovered accidentally, that is, during a lumbar puncture as part of a sepsis work-up. In the second group, term or preterm infants may present at 2 to 3 days of age with isolated seizure activity (see Table 29–7) or preterm infants may occasionally present with apnea. Between seizures, the infant appears and acts healthy ("well baby with seizures"). Infants in both these groups survive and usually do well developmentally. The third type of presentation involves infants with a massive SAH that has a rapid and fatal course. This presentation is rare and is often associated with both a severe asphyxial event and birth trauma.

Prognosis

Generally, infants with SAH survive, and asymptomatic infants do well. Up to half of symptomatic infants with severe, sustained traumatic or hypoxic injury with further damage to the CNS have neurologic sequelae (Palmer & Donn, 1991). Hydrocephalus occasionally develops in infants with a history of SAH, owing to obstruction of CSF flow by adhesions. These infants should undergo repeat ultrasonography to monitor ventricular dilation.

Collaborative and Nursing Management

Collaborative and nursing management of these infants begins with efforts to avoid or reduce the risk of trauma and hypoxia during the perinatal period in order to reduce the risk for development of this type of hemorrhage. Infants with SAH are observed for seizures and other neurologic signs during the early neonatal period. Nursing care is primarily supportive and includes maintenance of oxygenation and perfusion and provision of warmth, fluids, and nutrients. Nursing management also involves helping the parents to understand the basis for, and the cause and prognosis of, SAH as well as the care of their infant. Occasionally, infants with massive, acute SAH may require a craniotomy.

Subdural Hemorrhage

Subdural hemorrhage (SDH) is more common in term than in preterm infants. The incidence of SDH has decreased markedly as a result of improvements in obstetrical care. This decrease has been particularly notable in term infants; therefore, some individuals report that the incidence of SDH in preterm infants is now similar to or higher than that in full-term infants (Tudehope & Vacca, 1988). Early recognition of SDH is critical for infants with severe bleeds who need surgical intervention.

Pathophysiology

Subdural hemorrhage in newborns is almost always caused by trauma during the perinatal period. Bleeding occurs between the dura and the arachnoid and can be unilateral or bilateral. The bleeding occurs over the cerebral hemispheres or posterior fossa with or without tentorium or falx cerebri lacerations (see Fig. 29–1). The cerebral hemispheres are the most common site for SDH. Bleeding usually occurs over the temporal convexity, with rupture of superficial cerebral veins or of "bridging" veins between the superomedial aspect of the cerebrum and the superior sagittal sinus. Because the superficial veins over the cerebrum are poorly developed in the preterm infant, this type of hemorrhage is seen less frequently in these infants. Bleeding over the posterior fossa involves bleeding below the tentorium and compression of the brain stem (see Fig. 29–1). Dural tears at the junction of the falx and tentorium near the attachment of the great vein of Galen are also associated with compression of the brain stem and midbrain (de Vries et al., 1988a).

Risk Factors

Risk factors include precipitous, prolonged, or difficult delivery, use of midforceps or high forceps, prematurity, cerebropelvic disproportion, and large for gestational age infants. SDH is seen more often in infants born to primiparas, possibly owing to the more rigid birth canal. Infants with abnormal presentations, such as breech, foot, brow, or face, are also at higher risk for SDH.

Differential Diagnosis

Subdural hemorrhage must be distinguished from other types of intracranial hemorrhage and neurologic problems. This differentiation can often be accomplished by evaluation of the infant's history and presentation and, if the infant is having seizure activity, by ruling out other causes of seizures. SDH over the cerebral hemispheres is often associated with SAH. SDH also occurs with extracranial hemorrhages, such as cephalhematoma and subgaleal, subconjunctival, and retinal hemorrhages; skull fractures; and brachial plexus or facial palsies (Tudehope & Vacca, 1988). Ultrasonography and CT can also assist in confirming the diagnosis. CT may be more useful than ultrasonography in infants with a small SDH (de Vries et al., 1988a). Lumbar punctures are not used to diagnose SDH, because of the risk of herniation (Volpe, 1995).

Clinical Manifestations

Clinical signs of SDH relate to the site of the bleeding and the severity of the hemorrhage. Three patterns are seen in infants with bleeding over the cerebral hemispheres (Volpe, 1995; Volpe & Hill, 1987). The first pattern is seen in most infants with SDH; they have a minor hemorrhage and are asymptomatic or have signs such as irritability and hyperalertness. In the second group, seizures develop during the first 2 to 3 days of life. These seizures are usually focal. Other neurologic signs may be absent or present and include hemiparesis, pupils that are unequal and respond sluggishly to light, full or tense fontanelle, bradycardia, and irregular respirations. The third pattern is seen in a few infants who have no or nonspecific signs in the neonatal period, but who have them at 4 weeks to 6 months of age. These infants generally present with increasing head size, owing to continued hematoma formation; poor feeding; failure to thrive; altered level of consciousness; and, occasionally, seizures from the chronic subdural effusion.

Infants with bleeding over the posterior fossa with tentorial lacerations usually present with abnormal neurologic signs from birth. Signs include stupor or coma, eye deviation, asymmetrical pupil size, altered pupillary response to light, tachypnea, bradycardia, and opisthotonos. As the clot enlarges, these infants rapidly deteriorate, with signs of shock appearing over minutes to hours. The infant becomes comatose, with fixed, dilated pupils and altered respirations and heart rate that culminate in respiratory arrest. Infants with small posterior fossa tears may have no clinical manifestations for the first 3 to 4 days of life. During this time, the clot is gradually enlarging until signs of increased ICP appear. As the brain stem becomes compressed, the infant's condition deteriorates, and oculomotor abnormalities, altered respiration, bradycardia, and seizures occur (Volpe, 1995).

Prognosis

The prognosis varies with the location and the severity of the hemorrhage. Infants with bleeding over the cerebral hemispheres who are asymptomatic do well, as do most infants who have transient seizures in the neonatal period if no associated cerebral injury is present. Most infants with bleeding over the posterior fossa and tentorium or falx cerebri die. In those that survive, severe hydrocephalus and neurologic sequelae usually develop.

Collaborative and Nursing Management

Subdural hemorrhage can often be prevented or its severity reduced by reducing trauma during the perinatal period. Treatment of infants who have bleeding over the cerebral hemispheres is supportive. Infants with a history of perinatal trauma or other risk factors are observed for seizures and other neurologic signs. Care is primarily supportive and includes maintenance of oxygenation and perfusion and provision of warmth, fluids, and nutrients. Nursing management also involves helping the parents to understand the basis for, and the cause and prognosis of, this type of hemorrhage as well as the care of their infant.

Symptomatic infants with bleeding over the temporal convexity and increased ICP may be treated with subdural taps to relieve the pressure. Subdural taps are not without risk and are not used unless the infant's condition progressively deteriorates. The SDH is first located by ultrasonography or CT to determine if the hematoma is accessible. Massive posterior fossa hemorrhage requires craniotomy and surgical aspiration of the clot (Amiel-Tison et al., 1986; de Vries et al., 1988a). Infants at risk for SDH should be monitored carefully over the first 4 to 6 months after birth for late signs of bleeding and hematoma formation. Monitoring of these infants includes observation of head size, growth, feeding, activity, level of consciousness, and presence or absence of seizures.

Intracerebellar Hemorrhage

Intracerebellar hemorrhage is rare and is thought to be the result of hypoxia. These hemorrhages occur in both term and preterm infants but are more common in preterm infants. Intracerebellar hemorrhage is seen during autopsy in infants with a history of perinatal asphyxia, or severe respiratory distress syndrome, or both, and P/IVH. Intracerebellar hemorrhage also occurs secondary to trauma, especially in very low birth weight infants. Mechanical deformation of the occiput during forceps or breech delivery and compression of the compliant skull during fixation of the head for caregiving procedures or with use of constrictive head bands are thought to be predisposing factors (Pape et al., 1976).

Two presentations have been described. Many infants are critically ill from birth, with rapidly progressive apnea, decreasing hematocrit value, and death within 24 to 36 hours. Other infants are less ill initially, and symptoms develop up to 2 to 3 weeks of age. Clinical manifestations include apnea, bradycardia, hoarse or high-pitched cry, eye deviations, opisthotonos, seizures, vomiting, hypotonia, and decreased or absent Moro reflex. In these infants, hydrocephalus often develops as early as the end of the first week after birth. Prognosis is poor in survivors, especially those who were born prematurely.

Hypoxic-Ischemic Encephalopathy

Hypoxic-ischemic encephalopathy occurs as a result of injury to the brain from a combination of systemic hypoxemia and decreased cerebral perfusion that leads to ischemia (de Vries et al., 1988c). The hypoxemia and ischemia may occur simultaneously or sequentially. Hypoxic-ischemic damage to the brain occurs in both preterm and term infants. The site of injury varies with maturational changes in the vascular anatomy and metabolic activity of the brain (Amiel-Tison et al., 1986). In the preterm infant younger than 32 to 34 weeks' gestational age, hypoxic-ischemic damage is usually associated with P/IVH. The incidence of severe forms of HIE have decreased markedly as a result of advances in perinatal care. The incidence of perinatal asphyxia in term infants ranges from 2.9 to 9 in 1000 births, with moderate-to-severe postasphyxial encephalopathy seen in approximately 1 in 1000 births (Levene, 1988b).

Pathophysiology

After 33 to 34 weeks' gestation, blood flow and brain metabolic activity become less prominent in the germinal matrix and periventricular area and shift to the cortical area. Thus, hypoxia and ischemia in older preterm and term infants are more likely to damage areas of the peripheral and dorsal cerebral cortex. Five types of lesions have been identified in infants with HIE: (1) selective neuronal necrosis, (2) status marmoratus of the neurons of the basal ganglia and thalamus with loss of neurons in these areas, (3) parasagittal cerebral injury, (4) PVL (primarily in preterm infants), and (5) focal or multifocal ischemic brain necrosis (Volpe, 1995).

The primary lesion for the hypoxic injury is necrosis of neurons in the cortices of the cerebrum and cerebellum, with damage to the gray matter at the depths of the sulci. Neurons of the brain stem may also be injured. Areas of necrosis may extend into the white matter and into the gray matter of the basal ganglia (Brann & Schwartz, 1987; Levene, 1988a, 1988b). The primary ischemic injury occurs in the posterior portion of the parasagittal region secondary to watershed or border-zone infarcts. The border zone is at the junctions of the anterior, middle, and posterior cerebral arteries and the superior and inferior cerebellar arteries. This area is farthest from the original source of the brain blood supply of the major cerebral vessels. Thus, with localized ischemia, such as occurs when the infant has systemic hypotension or hypoperfusion as a consequence of perinatal asphyxia, this is the area that receives the least amount of blood.

With asphyxia and systemic hypotension, cerebral perfusion is maintained at first by cerebral vasodilation and redistribution of blood flow to the brain from other organs. If the asphyxia continues, brain water balance and cerebral blood flow are altered, and ischemia and edema develop (Brann & Schwartz, 1987). Neurophysiologic activity is disrupted, owing to impairment of synaptic transmission from reduced synthesis and release of excitatory neurotransmitter, alteration in Na^+ and K^+-ATPase activity, and inability of the neurons to maintain electrical stability (Kjellmer, 1988).

After a hypoxic-ischemic insult, the entire cortex may initially be edematous, and further ischemic damage may occur as a result of compression of the cortex against the skull. Both cytotoxic and vasogenic edema may occur. Cytotoxic damage occurs when cells cannot eliminate metabolic water produced by glycolysis because of failure of cellular membrane pumps. Vasogenic damage occurs after localized damage to the vascular epithelium, with disruption of capillary tight junctions (Brann & Schwartz, 1987; Bernes & Kaplan, 1994; Levene, 1988a, 1988b; Novotny, 1989). This damage allows leakage of protein into the interstitial spaces, pulling intravascular fluid into this area. As a result, cerebral blood flow is further reduced, and ICP increases. A proposed model for the development of HIE is illustrated in Figure 29–15.

Permanent cerebral injury can occur with asphyxia. "Anoxia not only stops the machine, it wrecks the machinery" (Haldane, cited by Kjellmer, 1988). The potential mechanisms for cellular injury are acidosis, accumulation of cytotoxic amino acids, and generation of oxygen free radicals. Acidosis reduces brain oxygen uptake and impairs neurophysiologic activity and restoration of phosphates needed for the production of energy. Cytotoxic amino

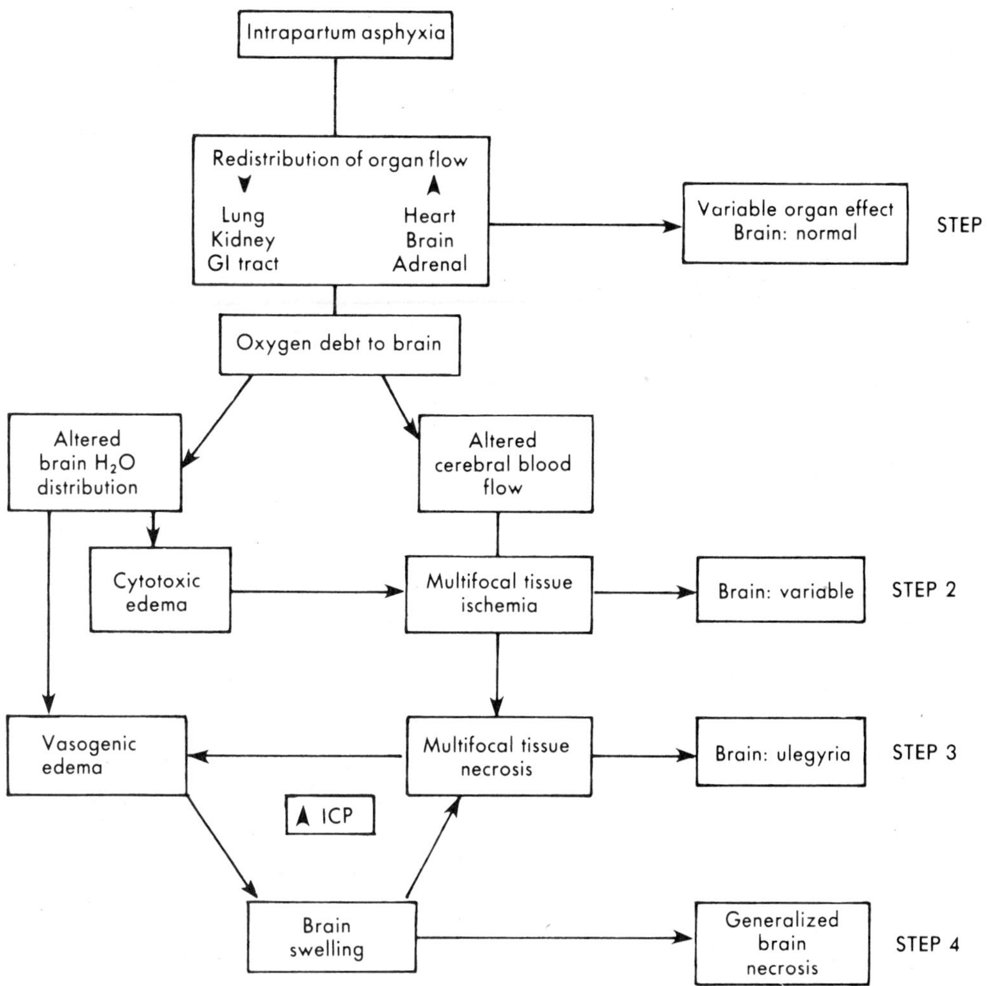

FIGURE 29–15. Proposed pathogenesis for the development of hypoxic-ischemic brain damage. GI, gastrointestinal; ICP, intracranial pressure. (Modified from Brann, A. W., & Schwartz, J. F. [1987]. Central nervous system disturbances. In A. A. Fanaroff & R. J. Martin [Eds.], *Neonatal-perinatal medicine* [p. 511]. St. Louis: C. V. Mosby Co.)

acids and oxygen free radicals interfere with cellular metabolism, inactivate cell enzymes, alter energy production, and interfere with the cell lipid membrane (Kjellmer, 1988).

Risk Factors

Hypoxic-ischemic encephalopathy may occur secondary to prenatal, intrapartal, or postnatal insults. Prenatal-intrapartal risk factors include fetal distress, perinatal asphyxia, abruptio placentae, placenta previa, maternal hypertension, prematurity, postmaturity, intrauterine growth retardation, prolapsed or nuchal cord, dystocia, and precipitate or prolonged labor. Injury during the postbirth period generally occurs in infants with a history of severe respiratory distress, persistent pulmonary hypertension, recurrent apnea, hypotension, or septic shock (Goldstein et al., 1989; Volpe & Hill, 1987).

Differential Diagnosis

Hypoxic-ischemic encephalopathy must be differentiated from other neurologic dysfunctions that result from trauma, infection, or CNS anomalies. A definitive work-up to define the type, extent, and location of the injury may include CT, cranial ultrasonography, brain stem auditory evoked potentials, MRI, EEG, and measurements of cerebral blood flow, ICP, and creatine kinase level (Amiel-Tison et al., 1986; Miller, 1997).

Clinical Manifestations

Hypoxic-ischemic encephalopathy in term or older preterm infants is usually found in infants with perinatal asphyxia. These infants often have low Apgar scores, decreased tone, and delay in onset of spontaneous respirations (Miller, 1997). Nonneurologic signs and symptoms related to the underlying perinatal asphyxia (see Chapter 15, Resuscitation and Stabilization of the Neonate) or another initial hypoxic-ischemic insult are discussed elsewhere. Most term infants with HIE demonstrate a characteristic pattern of neurologic findings over the first 72 hours of life. Neurologic findings in infants with HIE include seizures, altered level of consciousness, altered tone, altered activity, irregular respirations, apnea, poor or absent Moro's reflex, abnormal cry, poor suck, and altered pupillary responses and eye movements.

Sarnat and Sarnat (1976) developed a clinical grading system for infants with HIE (Table 29–12) that can be useful in evaluating infants and following the progression of their symptoms. According to Miller (1997), the three most significant neurologic findings in terms of severity of the injury and prediction of outcome are seizures, altered level of consciousness, and abnormal tone. Seizures occur in 30 to 60 percent of these infants, and the usual onset is 12 to 14 hours of age. The most common types of seizures are multifocal clonic seizures in term

TABLE 29–12 Clinical Grading System for Postasphyxial Encephalopathy in the Full-Term Newborn Infant

Neurologic Features	Stage 1	Stage 2	Stage 3
Level of consciousness	Hyperalert	Lethargic or obtunded	Stuporous
Neuromuscular control			
Muscle tone	Normal	Mild hypotonia	Flaccid
Posture	Mild distal flexion	Strong distal flexion	Intermittent decerebration
Stretch reflexes	Overactive	Overactive	Decreased or absent
Segmental myoclonus	Present	Present	Absent
Complex reflexes			
Suck	Weak	Weak or absent	Absent
Moro	Strong; low threshold	Weak; incomplete; high threshold	Absent
Oculovestibular	Normal	Overactive	Weak or absent
Tonic neck	Slight	Strong	Absent
Autonomic function	Generalized sympathetic	Generalized parasympathetic	Both systems depressed
Pupils	Mydriasis	Miosis	Variable; often unequal; poor light reflex
Heart rate	Tachycardia	Bradycardia	Variable
Bronchial and salivary secretions	Sparse	Profuse	Variable
Gastrointestinal motility	Normal or decreased	Increased; diarrhea	Variable
Seizures	None	Common: focal or multifocal	Uncommon (excluding decerebration)
Electroencephalogram findings	Normal (awake)	Early: low-voltage continuous delay and theta Later: periodic pattern (awake) Seizures: focal 1 to 1½ Hz spike and wave	Early: periodic pattern with isopotential phases Later: totally isopotential
Duration	Less than 24 hr	2–14 days	Hours to weeks

From Sarnat, H. B., & Sarnat, M. S. (1976). Neonatal encephalopathy following fetal distress. *Archives of Neurology, 33,* 696. Copyright 1976, American Medical Association. Reprinted with permission.

infants (see Table 29–7). Subtle seizures may occur as early as 2 to 6 hours after birth. Three clinical states (hyperalert, lethargy, and stupor or coma) have been described in these infants and have been correlated to outcome (Finer et al., 1981; Sarnat & Sarnat, 1976). Development of stupor or coma at any time or lethargy for more than 7 days was associated with the poorest prognosis.

Prognosis

The prognosis varies with the extent and the severity of the insult and the resulting brain injury. Prognosis ranges from death before or shortly after birth to severe neurologic impairment to minimal or no sequelae. Specific sequelae may not be apparent for several months or more. Some infants make a significant recovery, although the rate and degree of recovery are variable. The fetal and neonatal brain appears to be better able to withstand a hypoxic insult than does the adult brain. This protection is thought to be due to (1) the infant's ability to preserve cerebral circulation for longer periods, thus ensuring delivery of needed substrate; (2) decreased energy requirements, resulting from smaller neurons, less arborization, and fewer synapses; and (3) decreased oxygen dependency, resulting from lower metabolic demands (Kjellmer, 1988).

Sequelae of HIE in term infants are related to the site of injury (e.g., the cortex) and include mental retardation, microcephaly, cortical blindness, hearing deficits, and epilepsy. CP is more common in preterm infants than in term infants but does occur in term infants with HIE. In term infants, there is likely to be involvement of the upper extremities and speech as well as the lower extremities; most preterm infants primarily have involvement of the lower extremities. The risk of CP in term infants with early abnormal neurologic signs and seizures is 20 to 25 percent (Miller, 1997). The presence of tonic seizures during the first 24 hours after birth is significantly related to later neurologic problems (Bernes & Kaplan, 1994).

Collaborative Management

Infants with HIE have multiorgan and system problems arising from the original hypoxic-ischemic insult. As a result, management of these infants is complex and requires a coordinated team effort. Acute management of infants with HIE focuses on delivery room resuscitation; stabilization and management of the primary problem, usually perinatal asphyxia (see Chapter 14, The Effects of Labor on the Fetus and Neonate; and Chapter 15, Resuscitation and Stabilization of the Neonate); and related alterations in the cardiovascular, pulmonary, gastrointestinal, and renal systems. Management of these problems is discussed elsewhere. Seizures are treated promptly to prevent further alterations in ICP and cerebral blood flow.

Management of these infants in relation to neurologic problems focuses on elimination of the original hypoxia, alleviation of tissue hypoxia, and promotion of adequate cerebral perfusion and brain oxygenation (Miller, 1997). Interventions are directed toward establishing ventilation and adequate perfusion and preventing or minimizing hypotension, hypoxia, acidosis, and severe apneic and bradycardic episodes. Hyperoxia is also avoided because this state can result in cerebral vasoconstriction and decreased perfusion. Fluid management is critical not only for treating the cerebral edema but also because of alterations in renal function and problems such as acute tubular necrosis that frequently accompany moderate-to-severe forms of HIE (see Chapter 31, Assessment and Management of Genitourinary Dysfunction). Hypothermia to decrease metabolic rate is not recommended and can be dangerous to the newborn (Levene, 1988a, 1988b).

The infant's neurologic status is continually monitored and

documented, as are oxygenation, temperature, and blood pressure. Other parameters that are monitored include serum and urinary electrolyte levels and osmolality; blood urea nitrogen, serum creatinine, and glucose levels; and fluid and electrolyte balance. These infants are at risk for hypocalcemia (see Chapter 22, Fluids, Electrolytes, Vitamins, and Trace Minerals) secondary to release of excessive phosphorus from the breakdown of ATP that occurred to produce energy. This need for energy is in response to the stress induced by perinatal asphyxia. The excess phosphorus is also related to use of bicarbonate to correct acidosis induced by asphyxia.

Use of glucose infusions in the management of HIE is controversial, and conflicting evidence exists as to whether this is an effective or a dangerous therapy (Levene, 1988a, 1988b). Glucose administration may be therapeutic because glucose is the major substrate for brain metabolism. In addition, after perinatal asphyxia, an infant is at risk for hypoglycemia as a result of the depletion of stores from high energy demands. Concerns have been raised, however, that under anaerobic conditions, as occur with infants with perinatal asphyxia, glucose is converted to lactate, which may cause a localized metabolic acidosis and aggravate existing problems (Miller, 1997; Levene, 1988a, 1988b; Volpe & Hill, 1987). Blood glucose level should be closely monitored in infants with HIE, and any deviations should be treated promptly. Volpe and Hill (1987) recommended that blood glucose levels be maintained between 75 and 100 mg/dl.

Acute intracranial hypertension may be managed with osmotically active agents, such as mannitol or furosemide, barbiturates, and corticosteroids, as well as fluid restriction. Use of agents to reduce cerebral edema is controversial, and few data are available. Miller (1997) suggested that the usefulness of these agents varies with the type of edema. During the initial cytotoxic edema, management is directed toward decreasing localized increases in pressure with fluid restriction and decreasing energy requirements. Osmotically active agents, such as mannitol (0.25 to 1.0 g/kg of a 10 to 20 percent solution given intravenously every 6 hours) and furosemide (1.0 mg/kg given intravenously), may be used in the first 24 hours to reduce cerebral edema. Barbiturates and steroids are usually not particularly effective during this period.

During the period of vasogenic edema, management is directed toward reducing the increased ICP by fluid restriction, osmotic and diuretic agents, and possible use of steroids and barbiturates (Miller, 1997). If used, dexamethasone therapy is often started soon after birth, but it is not effective for 12 to 24 hours. This corticosteroid is given intramuscularly or intravenously, with a priming dose of 0.50 mg/kg, followed by 0.25 to 0.50 mg/kg/day for 5 to 7 days (Amiel-Tison & Larroche, 1988).

Barbiturates have also been proposed as a therapeutic measure to decrease cerebral metabolic rate, cerebral blood flow, and cerebral edema and to promote consumption of oxygen free radicals and modification of cell physiology. Barbiturates seem most effective when they are used before the hypoxic-ischemic event. The usefulness of these agents is debatable (Miller, 1997).

Nursing Management

Nursing management involves recognition of factors that increase the risk of further hypoxia, interventions to restore oxygenation, and supportive care of infants and their families. Nursing care activities include interventions to avoid or reduce hypoxic or asphyxial events, avoid rapid alterations in cerebral blood flow, prevent fluctuations in systemic blood pressure, prevent hyperosmolarity, and prevent or minimize fluctuations in ICP. The interventions listed in Table 29–11 to alter ICP and promote oxygenation in infants at risk for P/IVH can also be used with infants with HIE.

Nursing management involves promotion of oxygenation, perfusion, normothermia, and normoglycemia. Fluid status and intake and output are monitored to prevent fluid overload. The infant is monitored for hypoglycemia, hypocalcemia, and electrolyte disturbances. Fluctuations in systemic blood pressure with increased ICP and altered cerebral hemodynamics can occur as a result of caregiving or environmental stress. Therefore, developmental care of these infants (see Chapter 49, Assessment and Management of Neonatal Neurobehavioral Development) to reduce stress is essential. As the infant recovers, opportunities for sensory experiences are an important part of care. These experiences can be introduced slowly, as the infant can tolerate them without becoming stressed and overloaded. Chapter 49 describes guidelines for the provision of sensory input for high-risk infants.

Physiologic and neurologic status is monitored and documented at regular intervals. The infant is observed for changes in level of consciousness, tone, and activity and for evidence of seizures. Seizures are recognized and treated promptly to prevent further injury. Positioning and skin care (see Chapter 32, Assessment and Management of Integumentary Dysfunction, as well as Chapter 49) are important, especially for hypoactive, obtunded, or comatose infants.

Parents need initial and ongoing support in dealing with their infant's critical illness; the lack of infant responsiveness if the infant is hypoactive, stuporous, or comatose; the possibility of death; and the implications for later neurologic deficits. Parent teaching focuses on promoting an understanding of the infant's health status and care and providing anticipatory guidance regarding changes in the infant's state as well as outcome. The parents need to be shown how to interact with, and care for, their infant in a developmentally appropriate manner, with the goal of promoting opportunities for interaction while minimizing stressful events. The nurse can model this type of care for the parents and provide anticipatory guidance as to how the infant's needs and care will change as the infant matures (see Chapter 49). Parents can also be involved in developing and implementing a developmental plan of care for their infant.

Periventricular Leukomalacia

Periventricular leukomalacia is a form of hypoxic-ischemic injury and is the ischemic brain lesion most commonly seen in preterm infants. Leukomalacia means "softening of the white matter" (de Vries et al., 1988c). PVL is often associated with P/IVH, but it is a separate lesion that may also occur in the absence of P/IVH. PVL is a symmetric, nonhemorrhagic lesion caused by ischemia from alterations in arterial circulation. As the IVH moves from the germinal matrix area into the surrounding white matter, periventricular hemorrhagic infarction associated with intraparenchymal echodensities develops. Periventricular hemorrhagic infarction differs from PVL in that it is an asymmetrical, hemorrhagic lesion that primarily arises from alterations in the venous circulation (Volpe, 1995).

Pathophysiology

Periventricular leukomalacia begins with ischemic necrosis of the white matter dorsal and lateral to the external angles of the lateral ventricles, especially in the border zones areas (Miller, 1997). The border zone is the area farthest from the original source of the cerebral blood supply and thus is most susceptible to ischemic damage from decreased cerebral blood flow. PVL often extends into the cortical white matter. In up to 25 percent of infants, the PVL eventually becomes hemorrhagic, although this figure may be inflated by misdiagnosis of periventricular hemorrhagic infarction (Volpe, 1995). Pathologic changes begin with patchy areas of focal ischemic coagulation that may occur as early as 5 to 8 hours after the initial hypoxic-ischemic insult (de Vries et al., 1988c). This is followed within a few days by proliferation of macrophages and astrocytes along with endothelial and glial infiltration. Later changes include thinning of the white matter and liquefaction within the central portion of the necrotic area and cavitation, cystic changes, and decreased myelinization (de Vries et al., 1988c). Cerebral atrophy leads to expansion of the lateral ventricles and hydrocephalus.

Risk Factors

Periventricular leukomalacia occurs in both term and preterm infants. However, approximately 75 percent of infants with PVL are preterm. Risk factors include any event during the prenatal, intrapartal, or postbirth periods that results in cerebral ischemia. This includes perinatal asphyxia, P/IVH, hypoxia, hypercarbia, hypotension, cardiac arrest, and infection (with decreased blood flow from the action of endotoxins). The major risk factors are P/IVH in preterm infants and perinatal asphyxia and infection in term infants.

Differential Diagnosis and Clinical Manifestations

Periventricular leukomalacia is a compilation of prenatal or postnatal insults or both. It may develop in utero, during the first week after birth, or, most often, up to at least 40 weeks after birth (de Vries et al., 1988c; Wigglesworth, 1989). Often, no specific clinical findings are specific to PVL during the first weeks of life unless the damage is severe. Cranial ultrasonography can identify infants at risk for or with early signs of PVL (see section on prognosis). Infants at risk for PVL should undergo serial cranial ultrasonographic examinations and again at discharge, with follow-up occurring later (Miller, 1997). With severe damage, neuromotor abnormalities and signs of ventricular enlargement develop. As the infant matures, neurologic and motor deficits become apparent.

Prognosis

Infants with PVL may die in the neonatal period, usually from the original hypoxic or hemorrhagic insult rather than from PVL per se. Infants with PVL are at higher risk for later developmental problems and CP. Later outcome is related to the progression of the PVL abnormalities (Fazzi et al., 1992; Hagberg et al., 1993; Weisglas-Kuperus et al., 1992).

A wide range of outcomes have been reported for infants with periventricular echodensities seen on ultrasonogram. Infants without cystic lesions have a better prognosis, but up to half have been reported to have transient dystonia or other neurologic abnormalities (de Vries et al., 1988c).

The most prominent sequela in survivors, especially those who progress to cystic lesions, is spastic diplegia with or without hydrocephalus. Descending fibers from the motor cortex cross the affected area around the ventricles. Because the leg motor fibers are closest to the ventricles, spastic diplegia of the leg is the most common sequela (Fig. 29–16). If extension of the damage exists, arm involvement with spastic quadriplegia may occur. Damage to the optic radiations in this area leads to visual deficits (Bennett et al., 1990; Miller, 1997).

Collaborative Management

Initial management focuses on treatment of the primary insult and its attendant complications and prevention of further hypoxic-ischemic damage. This management involves preventing or minimizing hypotension, hypoxia, acidosis, and severe apneic and bradycardic episodes. Ultrasonography or CT is used serially to diagnose PVL and follow its progression in at-risk infants. Specific evidence of PVL on ultrasonography or CT may not be seen before cavitation, cerebral atrophy, and ventricular enlargement (Bennett et al., 1990).

Early changes may be transient in some infants and may resolve over a few weeks. In other infants, areas of increased density appear within 2 to 4 weeks, followed by development of cystic lesions. MRI can also be used to predict cystic changes (Bozynski et al., 1985; de Vries et al., 1988c). Later management involves care related to residual problems, such as spastic diplegia and hydrocephalus.

Nursing Management

Nursing interventions focus on acute management of the primary problem and supportive care for the infant and parents. Nurses have a major role in identifying signs of hypoxia and asphyxia and instituting interventions to prevent further ischemic damage. These interventions are similar to those described earlier and in Table 29–11. Environmental stressors may either increase the risk for development of P/IVH and subsequent PVL or cause associated developmental problems. Therefore, developmental and environmental interventions (see Chapter 49, Assessment and Management of Neonatal Neurobehavioral Development) are important aspects of nursing care.

Parents need initial and ongoing support in dealing with their

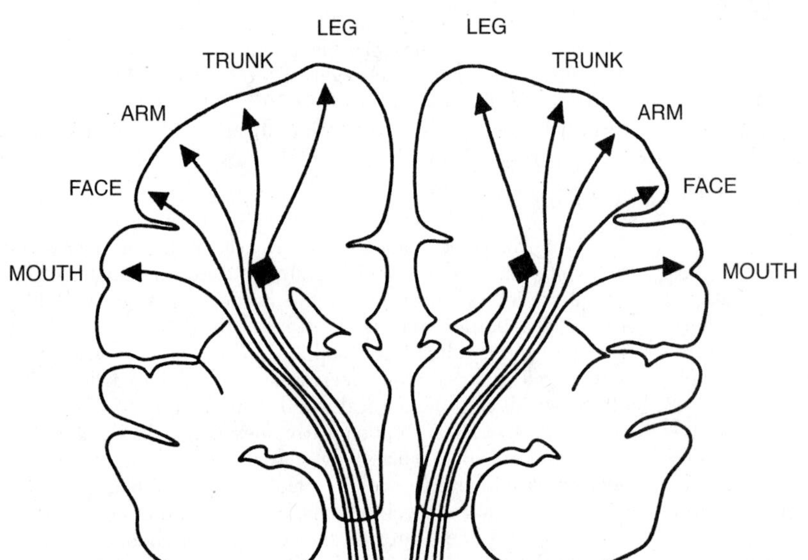

FIGURE 29-16. Schematic diagram of the corticospinal tracts from their origin in the motor cortex with descent past the periventricular region and into the internal capsule. The locus of PVL (marked with square boxes) and P/IVH in the preterm infant would be expected to affect, particularly, descending fibers for lower extremities more than laterally placed fibers for upper extremities. These fibers are more likely to be affected in HIE in the term infant. HIE, hypoxic-ischemic encephalopathy; P/IVH, periventricular/intraventricular hemorrhage; PVL, periventricular leukomalacia. (Modified from Volpe, J. J. [1995]. *Neurology of the newborn* [3rd ed.]. Philadelphia: W. B. Saunders Co.)

infant's illness and the risk of later neurologic problems. Parent teaching focuses on promoting an understanding of the infant's health status and care, as well as providing anticipatory guidance and follow-up care. The parents can be shown how to interact with, and care for, their infant in a developmentally appropriate manner to foster parent–infant interaction and to promote infant organization and development. The nurse can model this type of care for the parents and can provide anticipatory guidance as the infant's needs and care change (see Chapter 49, Assessment and Management of Neonatal Neurobehavioral Development).

Birth Injuries

Traumatic injury to the central or peripheral nervous system can occur during the perinatal or postnatal periods. Most of these injuries happen during the intrapartum period and may co-occur with perinatal asphyxia. The incidence of birth injury in the United States is 2 to 7 in 1000 live births; the incidence of neural injury is 0.22 in 1000 live births (Tudehope & Vacca, 1988). Perinatal events that are most frequently associated with birth injury include midforceps delivery, shoulder dystocia, low forceps delivery, birth weight of more than 3500 g, and second state of labor of greater than 60 minutes (Levine et al., 1984). The incidence of injury has decreased markedly in recent years as a result of improvement of obstetrical care and increased use of cesarean sections for abnormal presentations. However, birth injuries can also arise from trauma during a cesarean section or resuscitation.

Injuries that occur before the intrapartum period are usually caused by compression or pressure injuries from an unusual fetal position. The risk of injury to the central or peripheral nervous system is increased when malpresentation (especially breech), malposition, prolonged or precipitate labor, prematurity, multiple gestation, shoulder dystocia, macrosomia, and instrumental delivery occur. The most prevalent types of injury to the nervous system are extracranial hemorrhage, intracranial hemorrhage (described previously), skull fractures, spinal cord injury, and peripheral nerve injury (see Chapter 30, Assessment and Management of Musculoskeletal Dysfunction, for a discussion of birth trauma).

Extracranial Hemorrhage

Caput succedaneum and cephalhematoma are the most common types of birth injury, as well as the most benign. Caput succedaneum is characterized by soft, pitting, superficial edema that is several millimeters thick and overlies the presenting part in a vertex delivery. This edematous area lies above the periosteum and thus crosses suture lines. The edema consists of serum, or blood, or both. Infants with caput succedaneum may also have ecchymosis, petechiae, or purpura over the presenting part. Caput succedaneum occurs in infants after a spontaneous vertex delivery or after the use of a vacuum extractor. This type of extracranial hemorrhage requires no care other than parent teaching regarding its cause and significance. It resolves within a few days after birth with no sequelae.

Cephalhematoma occurs in 0.2 to 2.5 percent of newborns (Andre & Vert, 1987; Miller, 1997). It involves subperiosteal bleeding, usually over the parietal bone, but may occur over other cranial bones. Cephalhematoma is usually unilateral but can be bilateral. This type of hemorrhage is seen most frequently in males; after the use of forceps; after a prolonged, difficult delivery; and in infants born to primiparas. The characteristic finding is a firm, fluctuant mass that does not cross the suture lines. The mass often enlarges slightly by 2 to 3 days of age. Approximately 10 to 25 percent of cases have a linear skull fracture underlying the mass. Rarely, an infant may have a subdural or a subarachnoid hemorrhage.

A cephalhematoma can be distinguished from a caput succedaneum by the following characteristics: (1) it is limited to the periosteal area and thus does not cross suture lines; (2) ecchymosis is absent; (3) it increases in size over the first several days; and (4) it takes a longer time to resolve than a caput succedaneum (Miller, 1997). Caput succedaneum and cephalhematoma over the occipital bone must be differentiated from encephalocele. In contrast to extracranial hemorrhage, an encephalocele is characterized by pulsations, increased pressure (tenseness) with crying, and appearance of a bony defect on radiograph.

Infants with a cephalhematoma generally have no symptoms. Management includes parent teaching and monitoring for development of hyperbilirubinemia (see Chapter 28, Assessment and Management of Hematologic Dysfunction). Occasionally, an infant with a large cephalhematoma becomes anemic. These infants should also be monitored for symptoms of intracranial hemorrhage or skull fracture. Generally, cephalhematomas resolve between 2 weeks and 6 months of age, and most resolve by 6 weeks. Calcium deposits occasionally develop, and the swelling remains for 1 to 1½ years.

Skull Fracture

Two forms of skull fractures are seen in newborns: linear and depressed.

Pathophysiology and Risk Factors

Skull fractures occur in utero, during labor, with forceps delivery, or during a prolonged, difficult labor with compression and battering of the fetal skull against the maternal ischial spines, sacral promontory, or symphysis pubis (Miller, 1997; Tudehope & Vacca, 1988). The fetal skull is often able to tolerate mechanical stressors relatively well. This is because the fetal skull is flexible, malleable, poorly ossified, and less mineralized than the adult skull. Depressed fractures occur after forceps delivery but are occasionally seen after a vaginal or a cesarean birth. Compression of the skull causes a buckling of the inner table without a break in the continuity of the skull.

Differential Diagnosis and Clinical Manifestations

Linear fractures usually occur over the frontal or parietal bones. Linear fractures are often associated with extracranial hemorrhage and underlie 10 to 25 percent of cephalhematomas (Axton, 1966). This type of fracture is usually asymptomatic. Skull radiographs are required for the diagnosis. Intracranial hemorrhage rarely complicates linear fractures. Some infants may have underlying cerebral injury or may have a "growing fracture," which is a rare complication in which a dural tear allows the leptomeninges to extrude into the fracture site. A leptomeningeal cyst may develop in these infants. Enlargement of the cyst results in growth of the fracture and failure to fuse (Minarick & Beachy, 1989).

Rarely, a linear fracture occurs in the occipital bone at the base of the skull. This type of fracture is seen primarily after breech deliveries in which traction on a hyperextended spine occurs (Miller, 1997). An occipital fracture is associated with intracranial hemorrhage and meningeal tears. Infants present with shock, neurologic abnormalities, and leakage of CSF through their nose, or ears, or both.

A depressed skull fracture presents as a visible and palpable depression or dent in the skull, usually over the parietal area. These fractures are often described as resembling a ping-pong ball because the depression does not involve any loss of bone continuity. Unless underlying cerebral contusion or hemorrhage is present, no other signs or symptoms are seen.

Prognosis

Linear fractures heal spontaneously with no sequelae unless underlying cerebral damage or a growing fracture is present (Andre & Vert, 1987). Basal fractures are associated with high mortality and poor developmental outcome. Infants with depressed fractures that are small, or treated early, or both, have a good prognosis. Infants with large fractures, especially if treatment is delayed, have an increased risk of brain injury (Miller, 1997). Infants with concomitant brain damage underlying the fracture have a poorer outcome. Thus, unless a depressed fracture has lacerated the dura (a rare occurrence), neurologic deficits in these infants are usually caused by cerebral injury from the original trauma, or a hypoxic event, or both, rather than from the fracture per se (Minarick & Beachy, 1989; Tudehope & Vacca, 1988). Infants with skull fractures should undergo regular evaluation of growth and developmental status during infancy and early childhood.

Collaborative and Nursing Management

Diagnosis is confirmed with skull radiography or CT. Cranial ultrasonography or CT is performed to identify cerebral contusions or hemorrhage. Nursing assessment includes monitoring of these infants for signs of neurologic dysfunction, intracranial hemorrhage, meningitis, and seizures. These findings are rare. Parents are usually concerned over their infant's appearance (with a depressed fracture) and the possibility of brain damage. They need support and teaching. Controversies exist regarding whether these problems should be treated and which type of treatment should be used (Minarick & Beachy, 1989).

Infants with uncomplicated linear fractures require no special management. Follow-up skull radiographs are usually recommended so that a growing fracture and development of a leptomeningeal cyst can be ruled out. Infants with basal fractures are treated for shock and hemorrhage (see Chapter 28, Assessment and Management of Hematologic Dysfunction). If the infant has leakage of CSF, antibiotics are usually given prophylactically in order to prevent meningitis.

In some infants with a depressed fracture, the fracture elevates spontaneously within the first week. Most clinicians recommend manually elevating an uncomplicated depressed fracture that does not elevate spontaneously within a few days (Miller, 1997; Minarick & Beachy, 1989; Tudehope & Vacca, 1988). After this time, manual elevation is more difficult or impossible. Manual elevation can be accomplished by three methods. The clinician's thumbs can be placed on opposite margins of the depression, and gentle pressure is then applied toward the middle. Elevation can also be accomplished with a breast pump or vacuum extractor. A hand breast pump, with petroleum jelly around the rim to ensure a good seal, is placed over the depression, and gentle pressure is applied. Use of a vacuum extractor involves placing it over the depression and applying pressure at a setting of 0.2 to 0.5 kg/cm^2 for about 4 minutes (Miller, 1997).

If manual elevation fails or if the fracture is more severe, and bone fragments are in the cerebrum, neurologic deficits exist, or ICP is increased, surgical intervention is usually necessary. If surgery occurs early, the procedure can be performed by passing a blunt instrument through the anterior fontanelle. The instrument is passed extradural to the site of the fracture and applied to the base of the fracture to "pop" the area back into alignment. If surgery is delayed until after 10 days, craniotomy may be needed (Tudehope & Vacca, 1988).

Spinal Cord Injury

Spinal cord injuries usually occur in the midcervical to lower cervical and upper thoracic areas. Injury can occur at any point along the cord. Lower cervical to midthoracic injuries are usually seen associated with breech deliveries; midcervical to high cervical injuries, with vertex deliveries.

Pathophysiology

Spinal cord injuries result from excessive traction, rotation, and torsion of the vertebral column and neck. Injury usually does not result from compression, but rather from stretching of the spinal cord, which is less flexible than the bony vertebral column. The vertebral column and joints can stretch up to 5 cm, but the spinal cord can stretch only 6 to 8 mm without body disruption (Tudehope & Vacca, 1988). Damage to the spinal cord ranges from complete transection to laceration, edema, hemorrhage, and hematoma formation. Hemorrhage into the lining of the arteries may result in thrombosis, infarction, and ischemic cord damage.

Risk Factors

Spinal cord injuries occur most often in breech deliveries in which hyperextension of the head or version and extraction occur. This type of injury can also occur in infants with shoulder dystocia, with cord traction via the brachial plexus, or in a vertex secondary to torsional forces and rotation of the head (Tudehope & Vacca, 1988). Therefore, risk factors are breech delivery (major factor), dystocia, macrosomia, and cephalopelvic disproportion.

Differential Diagnosis

Infants who have severe injuries may initially appear similar to those who have experienced severe birth asphyxia. Other problems that can have similar presentation include spina bifida occulta, neuromuscular disorders, and tumors of the spinal cord.

Clinical Manifestations

Miller (1997) identified several clinical presentations seen in infants with spinal cord injury. Infants with partial spinal cord injury have subtle neurologic signs and variable degrees of spasticity. Infants with high cervical or brain stem injuries are either stillborn or die shortly after birth from respiratory depression, shock, and hypothermia. Infants with midcervical or upper cervical injury may be stillborn, born with marked respiratory depression, or present with respiratory depression with the neurologic injury going unrecognized until flaccidity, immobility of the legs, or urine retention, or all three, are noted. If born alive, these infants usually die within the first week, after development of progressive central respiratory depression that is often complicated by pneumonia. Other clinical findings in this group of infants include relaxation of the abdominal wall, absent sensation in the lower half of the body, absent deep tendon and spontaneous reflexes, brachial plexus injury (20 percent), and constipation. This group also includes infants with injuries at the C8 to T1 level. These infants usually survive. Infants with this type of injury may have a transient paraplegic paralysis at birth. Infants with mild injury may recover most or all of their function. Infants with moderate-to-severe damage are paraplegic or quadriplegic and have permanent neurologic damage.

Initially, the clinical manifestations are those of spinal cord shock with hypotonia, weakness, flaccid extremities, sensory deficits, relaxed abdominal muscles, diaphragmatic breathing, Horner's syndrome (ipsilateral ptosis, anhidrosis, and miosis), and a distended bladder. Infants with low cervical lesions have shallow, paradoxic respirations. These infants do not sweat. The skin over the affected area is dry and warm. Pin prick and deep tendon reflexes are absent. Areflexia may be noted over the upper and lower extremities in some infants. The degree of neurologic insult often cannot be accurately evaluated until after the infant has recovered from the initial period of spinal shock and any edema or hemorrhage has been reabsorbed (Minarick & Beachy, 1989). After several weeks or months, a paraplegic autonomic hyperreflexia develops that is characterized by periodic mass reflex response. This results in tonic spasms of extremities, spontaneous micturition, and profuse sweating over the paralyzed area.

Prognosis

The prognosis depends on the level and severity of the injury, but it is generally poor. Many infants with spinal cord injury will be stillborn or die shortly after birth, particularly those with midcervical to high cervical or brain stem injuries. Those that survive will have varying degrees of residual paralysis, respiratory problems, and bowel and bladder dysfunction, depending on the level of the injury. Most surviving infants have a spastic quadriplegia. Infants with involvement of the intercostal muscles and diaphragm will often be ventilator dependent.

Collaborative Management

At birth, the infant may be in shock and require delivery room resuscitation. Initial management focuses on stabilization; treatment of associated problems, such as perinatal asphyxia and hemorrhage; and management of respiratory depression. Infants with midcervical to upper cervical or brain stem lesions require assisted ventilation at birth or by 1 to 2 days after birth (Tudehope & Vacca, 1988). Parents are in shock initially and need time to grieve. They need ongoing support and teaching regarding the care of the infant. Ongoing management of these infants and their families requires a multidisciplinary team that includes nursing, medicine, neurology, neurosurgery, physical therapy, orthopedics, urology, social work, and psychology. Ultrasonography, CT, or MRI may be performed to determine the level and the extent of injury. Laminectomy is rarely useful and may affect later stability of the spine (Andre & Vert, 1987).

Nursing Management

Nursing management focuses on care of the infant and provision of support to the shocked, grieving parents. Care of the infant in the delivery room and neonatal intensive care unit involves initial stabilization, management related to accompanying perinatal asphyxia or hemorrhage, and promotion of ventilation. Ongoing management of these infants presents a major challenge to the nurse to support the infant and to prevent further complications.

Skin integrity over the paralyzed area must be maintained in order to prevent pressure areas and skin breakdown. Thermoregulation may be a problem because evaporative loss through the skin is reduced over the affected body parts in the initial period of the recovery process. The infant is positioned and repositioned regularly to promote normal alignment of body parts and prevent development of contractures and decubiti. Infants can be placed on soft foam, sheepskin, lambskin, or similar material, or on a waterbed, and their position should be changed every 2 to 3 hours. The affected areas should be kept clean and dry and massaged with gentle, passive range-of-motion exercises. These infants need meticulous bowel and bladder care to prevent urinary tract infection and skin excoriation. Glycerin suppositories at regular intervals can help normalize bowel function. Infants are also monitored for signs of respiratory infection and pneumonia. Parental teaching before discharge focuses on normal baby care issues and concerns as well as the special needs of a paralyzed infant.

Peripheral Nerve Injuries

Peripheral nerve injuries result from stretching, compression, twisting, hyperextension, or separation of nerve tissue (Andre & Vert, 1987). Injury can occur before, during, or after birth. Damage can range from neuropraxia (swelling of the nerve) to axonotmesis (complete peripheral degeneration with later total recovery) to neurotmesis (complete division of all structures) (Tudehope & Vacca, 1988). The more common sites affected are the brachial plexus and the facial, phrenic, radial, median, and sciatic nerves. This type of injury is seen predominantly in term or large for gestational age infants.

Injury to the radial nerve usually results from compression of the nerve resulting from fracture of the humerus during a breech delivery or from intrauterine compression of the arm. The infant has wrist drop with a normal grasp reflex. Recovery usually occurs over the first few weeks to months. Median and sciatic nerve injuries are generally postnatal iatrogenic events. Median nerve injury can be a complication of brachial or radial arterial punctures. These infants have decreased pincer grasp and thumb strength and a flexed fourth finger. Recovery is variable. Sciatic nerve injuries are often permanent. They arise from trauma from a misplaced intramuscular injection or from ischemia from an injection of hypertonic solutions into the gluteal muscle. Infants with this type of injury have decreased abduction and distal joint movement. Hip adduction, rotation, and flexion are unaffected (Minarick & Beachy, 1989; Tudehope & Vacca, 1988).

Facial Nerve Palsy

Facial nerve palsy is one of the most common types of peripheral nerve injuries. The incidence ranges from 1.3 to 7.5 in 1000 live births (Levine et al., 1984).

Pathophysiology and Risk Factors

Injury to the peripheral nerve is caused by trauma from oblique application of forceps, prolonged pressure on the nerve during labor from the maternal sacral promontory, or pressure from an abnormal fetal posture. Although some investigators have not found any differences in incidence between forceps and spontaneous vaginal deliveries, others have noted a correlation between the type of forceps and the incidence of injury (Hagadorn-Freathy et al., 1991). The facial nerve of the newborn is superficial after it emerges from the stylomastoid foramen. As a result, the nerve is vulnerable to compression injury at this site or as it transverses the ramus of the mandible. Injury can also be isolated to a peripheral nerve branch. The nerve branches most often involved are the temporofacial and cervicofacial. Three fourths of the injuries involve the left facies. Occasionally, central injury may occur associated with contralateral injury to the CNS that results from fracture of the temporal bone or intracranial hemorrhage (Andre & Vert, 1987; Miller, 1997). Because the prognosis is favorable, the injury appears to be caused by hemorrhage or edema into the nerve sheath rather than by disruption of the nerve fibers (Volpe, 1995).

Differential Diagnosis

Facial nerve paralysis must be distinguished from asymmetrical crying facies and nuclear agenesis. Asymmetrical crying facies results from absence of the depressor muscle of the angle of the mouth. These infants close their eyes normally when crying, but the mouth does not move down and out. They suck without dribbling. This disorder is generally benign. Nuclear agenesis (Möbius' syndrome) is a more severe disorder that is characterized by congenital paralysis of the facial muscles.

Clinical Manifestations

Clinical manifestations vary, depending on whether the injury is to the central nerve, the peripheral nerve, or the peripheral nerve branch. The complete peripheral nerve injury results in a unilateral inability of the infant to close the eye or open the mouth. The lower lip on the affected side does not depress during crying, nor does the forehead wrinkle. The affected side appears full and smooth, with obliteration of the nasolabial fold.

These infants dribble milk while feeding. Central injury usually results in a spastic paralysis of the lower portion of the face contralateral to the side of CNS injury, without involvement of the eyes or forehead. Peripheral nerve branch injury results in varying degrees of paralysis of the forehead, eye, or lower face, depending on the branch involved. The paralysis is apparent at birth or within 1 to 2 days after birth.

Prognosis

Almost all infants recover completely. Improvement is usually apparent by 1 to 3 weeks, and complete recovery occurs after several months in most infants. Infants with severe nerve regeneration have a longer recovery period and may occasionally require later cosmetic surgery. Nerve regeneration occurs at a rate of 2.5 cm/month.

Collaborative and Nursing Management

Nursing management involves parent counseling and teaching and prevention of complications. The eye on the affected side is patched, and 1 percent methylcellulose eye drops are instilled every 3 to 4 hours to prevent corneal damage. Dribbling with sucking can be a transient problem. If no improvement is noted by 7 to 10 days or further loss of function occurs, a neurosurgical consultation is usually recommended (Tudehope & Vacca, 1988). In infants with partial degeneration, physical therapy, massage, or electrical stimulation, or all three, may be used. The usefulness of these therapies is controversial and not well documented. Electromyography, nerve excitability, or nerve conduction latency examinations may be performed to evaluate the extent of the damage.

Brachial Plexus Palsy

Brachial plexus palsy involves injury of the C5 to C8 and T1 nerve roots and is seen almost exclusively in term infants. The incidence ranges from 0.5 to 1.9 in 1000 live births (Minarick & Beachy, 1989).

Pathophysiology and Risk Factors

Injury to the brachial plexus results from excessive lateral flexion, rotation, or traction on the neck (Tudehope & Vacca, 1988). The degree of injury is variable, ranging from edema and hemorrhage of the nerve sheath to avulsion of the nerve root from the spinal cord. With mild-to-moderate injury, the axons are shattered, but the nerve sheaths remain intact. This degree of intactness of the nerve sheaths promotes regeneration of the nerve by 2 to 3 months, with full recovery. Severe injuries result in radicular rupture or intraspinal tearing of the nerve and division of the nerve into radicles. If radicular rupture occurs, the root loses contact with the spinal cord. These injuries do not recover spontaneously (Andre & Vert, 1987).

Brachial plexus injuries are usually unilateral and on the left side. Fracture of the clavicle may occur in conjunction with this type of injury. Brachial plexus injury can be seen in uncomplicated deliveries but is often associated with large for gestational age infants, shoulder dystocia, breech and other abnormal presentations, and prolonged labor or difficult delivery.

Differential Diagnosis

Cerebral and spinal cord injuries can present with similar initial findings. Other disorders that should be considered include injury to the clavicle or humerus and to the soft tissues of the shoulder and upper arm.

Clinical Manifestations

Clinical manifestations vary with the location and severity of the injury. Signs of injury are usually apparent from birth but may be delayed for several days to a few weeks in some infants. The three major types of injury and their relative frequencies are (1) Erb-Duchenne palsy (85 to 90 percent), (2) Klumpke's palsy (1 to 3 percent), and (3) Erb-Duchenne-Klumpke palsy (7 to 9 percent).

Erb-Duchenne palsy results from injury to the C5 and C6 nerve roots. The shoulder and upper arm are involved, and denervation of the deltoid, supraspinous, biceps, and brachioradialis muscles occurs. The arm lies passively at the infant's side, abducted and internally rotated, and the forearm is pronated. The wrist and fingers are flexed. This posture is referred to as the "waiter's tip" position. The Moro reflex is absent, and the biceps and radial reflexes are diminished or absent on the affected side; the grasp reflex is normal. Occasionally, C4 roots are also affected, and an associated phrenic nerve (diaphragmatic) paralysis exists.

Klumpke's palsy involves the C8 to T1 roots, affecting the lower arm and hand, and denervation of the intrinsic muscles of the hand and flexors of the wrist and fingers exists. Cervical sympathetic fibers may also be affected; sweating and sensation are absent in the affected hand and arm. The infant holds the affected arm at the side of the thorax in a clawhand posture. The Moro and grasp reflexes are absent, and the triceps reflex is diminished or absent on the affected side; biceps and radial reflexes are present. If the T1 root is affected, the infant manifests Horner's syndrome (ipsilateral ptosis, anhidrosis, and miosis).

Erb-Duchenne-Klumpke palsy involves the entire arm and hand, owing to injury of the nerve roots of the brachial plexus from C5 to T1. This form of paralysis involves all the nerve fibers, and complete paralysis of the upper and lower arm and hand, flaccidity, and accompanying sensory, trophic, and circulatory changes occur (Tudehope & Vacca, 1988). Deep tendon and Moro's reflexes are all absent. If C4 roots are also affected, an associated phrenic nerve (diaphragmatic) paralysis occurs. Involvement of the T1 root leads to Horner's syndrome in about one third of these infants.

Prognosis

The prognosis depends on the level and severity of the injury. Approximately 80 to 90 percent of infants recover by 3 to 6 months with supportive care (Bennett & Harrold, 1976; Hardy, 1981). Some recovery is usually seen by 2 to 3 weeks of age. Lack of significant recovery by 3 months is associated with a high incidence of residual deficit (Boome & Kaye, 1988). Erb-Duchenne paralysis, the most common type of injury, has the best prognosis for full recovery. Infants with Erb-Duchenne-Klumpke paralysis are most likely to have residual paralysis. Residual functional deficits include alteration in abduction and external rotation of the shoulder; restricted movement of the elbow, forearm, and hand; and hand weakness (Boome & Kaye, 1988; Hardy, 1981). These functional impairments can lead to abnormal muscle development and arm growth.

Collaborative Management

Initial management focuses on protection of the arm until localized edema and pain are diminished. The affected arm is immobilized with shoulder and elbow splints to prevent contractures and further stretching of the plexus. After edema subsides, at about 7 to 10 days, physical therapy is gradually instituted, as the infant can tolerate it. Initially, the regimen may involve gentle, passive range-of-motion exercises. These infants have continued physical therapy consisting of massage and exercise over the first months until total or partial recovery occurs. Infants with brachial plexus injury should be evaluated for associated problems, including fractures and respiratory difficulty secondary to phrenic nerve paralysis.

If improvement is not noted within the first few months,

electromyography and nerve conduction studies are performed to determine the extent of the damage, to follow recovery, and to determine if surgical intervention is needed (Miller, 1997). Radicular ruptures can be repaired with microsurgical reconstruction, tendon transfers, and nerve grafts (Boome & Kaye, 1988). Surgery is considered if no improvement is seen by 3 months of age. Avulsion is not repairable.

Nursing Management

Infants with brachial plexus injuries often experience considerable pain during movement of the affected arm in the first few weeks after birth. Nursing management is directed at reducing passive and active movement of the arm and comfort measures. Interventions to reduce pain in neonates are described in Chapter 40 (Identification, Management, and Prevention of Pain in the Neonate). Splints are removed intermittently to reduce the risk of abduction contractures. The paralyzed arm is supported in a position of relaxation. Parent teaching regarding positioning, prevention of contractures, and exercise is essential.

Phrenic Nerve Palsy

Pathophysiology and Risk Factors

Phrenic nerve palsy is caused by injury of the cervical nerve roots at C3 to C5. The injury results from tearing of the nerve sheath, which is accompanied by edema and hemorrhage. Phrenic nerve palsy is frequently associated with Erb-Duchenne-Klumpke paralysis. Risk factors, especially breech delivery, are similar to those for brachial plexus injury. Damage of the phrenic nerve results in paralysis of the diaphragm. The injury is usually unilateral and on the right side.

Differential Diagnosis

Because the diaphragm is paralyzed, infants with phrenic nerve injury present with respiratory difficulty. This phenomenon must be differentiated from CNS, cardiac, and pulmonary problems. The differential diagnosis also includes neuromuscular disorders, such as myogenic dystonia. Diagnosis is confirmed by an elevated hemidiaphragm on radiography and paradoxic diaphragmatic movements on fluoroscopy (Tudehope & Vacca, 1988). Real-time ultrasonography, which can be performed at the infant's bedside, is also useful.

Clinical Manifestations

Infants with mild-to-moderate phrenic nerve injury may present with early respiratory difficulty, suggestive of hypoventilation, that stabilizes or improves. The infant may have recurrent episodes of cyanosis and dyspnea. The breathing pattern is altered. In these infants, breathing involves primarily thoracic movement with minimal or no abdominal excursions. Infants with complete avulsion or bilateral injuries have severe respiratory distress from birth, with tachypnea, apnea, and a weak cry (Miller, 1997).

Prognosis

A mortality rate of 10 to 20 percent has been reported, with complete recovery in 50 percent of survivors by 2 to 3 months of age (Tudehope & Vacca, 1988). Other infants recover clinically but have residual abnormalities of diaphragmatic movement on radiography.

Collaborative Management

Management focuses on promotion of ventilation and oxygenation. Infants may be placed on NPO (nothing by mouth) status initially, and feeding may be instituted as the infant's respiratory status improves. Infants with severe distress require positive-pressure ventilation or constant positive airway pressure for support until recovery occurs. The effectiveness of electrical pacing of the diaphragm is unclear and controversial. Some infants require prolonged assisted ventilation and may develop hypostatic pneumonia. Surgical plication of the diaphragm is performed if no improvement is noted or if the infant is still ventilator dependent at 4 to 6 weeks of age.

Nursing Management

The infant is positioned on the affected side. If the infant cannot be fed, adequate fluid and calories must be provided. Feeding is instituted gradually. Initially, the infant may need to be gavage fed. When oral feeding is started, the infant is fed slowly and is given ample opportunity for rest and monitoring of respiratory status. Because recovery takes several months, parents must be taught feeding, positioning, and comfort techniques. Nursing management of infants with respiratory problems is similar to that for any infant with respiratory distress (see Chapter 18, Assessment and Management of Respiratory Dysfunction). Developmental needs of infants requiring prolonged hospitalization must be met: sensory input and play activities appropriate to their maturity and health status must be provided.

Neurologic Structural Dysfunction

Neurologic structural dysfunctions arise as primary disorders resulting from alterations in developmental processes in the embryo or fetus or, in the case of some forms of hydrocephalus, from postnatal problems, such as intracranial hemorrhage or infection. This section focuses on the management of the two most common forms of neurologic structural abnormalities: NTDs and hydrocephalus.

Neural Tube Defects

Defects of the CNS occur in 2 to 3 in 1000 births, but the incidence in the United States is decreasing (Yen et al., 1992). Eighty percent of these defects result from failure of closure of the neural tube at either the cranial or the caudal ends (Moore & Persaud, 1993). NTDs include anencephaly, encephalocele, and spina bifida. Management of anencephaly, encephalocele, and spina bifida occulta are described in the section on embryologic development of the CNS. This section focuses on assessment and management of spina bifida cystica, especially myelomeningocele.

Pathophysiology

Neural tube defects arise from alterations in the closure of the neural tube and in the formation of the vertebrae. These processes and their alterations were described earlier. The three main forms of spina bifida cystica are meningocele, myelomeningocele, and myeloschisis (see Fig. 29–4). Spina bifida cystica can occur anywhere along the spinal column but is seen most often in the lumbar or lumbosacral area. A meningocele involves a sac that contains meninges and CSF, and the spinal cord and nerve roots are in their normal position. With myelomeningocele, which is the most common form of spina bifida cystica, the sac contains spinal cord, or nerve roots, or both, in addition to meninges and CSF. Myeloschisis is a severe defect in which no cystic covering exists, leaving the spinal cord open and exposed. The entire length of the spinal cord may be involved, and the infant may also be anencephalic (Moore & Persaud, 1993).

With myelomeningocele or myeloschisis, the spinal cord, or nerve roots, or both, are displaced dorsally; defects of the muscle and bony structures exist lateral to the defect. The lesions are covered with skin, or meninges, or both. If the sac is covered with meninges, risk of rupture exists during delivery, along with leakage of CSF and risk of infection and dehydration. Many infants also have an associated Arnold-Chiari malformation, with secondary aqueductal stenosis in 40 to 75 percent, that results in a noncommunicating form of hydrocephalus.

The Arnold-Chiari malformation is also a defect in neural tube closure. This malformation involves a group of anomalies, including displacement of the medulla, fourth ventricle, and lower cerebellum into the cervical canal; bony defects of the occiput, foramen magnum, and cervical vertebrae; and obstruction of the foramen magnum, leading to hydrocephalus. Infants with NTDs may also have cardiac, intestinal, orthopedic, and other neurologic anomalies (Milhorat & Miller, 1994). Common associated orthopedic anomalies are congenital dislocated hips and talipes equinovarus.

Risk Factors

Neural tube defects arise from genetic and environmental influences. They have a familial incidence and an increased genetic susceptibility. With one affected family member, the overall risk for defects in subsequent offspring in the United States is 2 to 3 percent, which doubles with two or more affected family members; the risk is increased if the previously affected offspring had a lesion at T11 or higher (Volpe, 1995). NTDs are seen more often in white than in black individuals and slightly more often in females than in males. The incidence is also higher with younger and older women, maternal diabetes, a history of miscarriages, and maternal exposure to drugs, such as valproic acid and aminopterin. Geographic and seasonal patterns are seen, and seasonal outbreaks have been reported in association with viral epidemics 8 to 9 months earlier (Paidas & Cohen, 1994).

Neural tube defects can be diagnosed prenatally via analysis of alpha-fetoprotein (AFP) and acetylcholinesterase levels in amniotic fluid and via fetal ultrasonography (see Chapter 9, Human Genetics). AFP is a major fetal glycoprotein, similar to albumin, that is produced in the fetal liver from 6 weeks of gestation. Concentrations of AFP peak at 13 to 15 weeks' gestation. AFP is found in fetal serum, CSF, and amniotic fluid. Normally, AFP concentration in CSF are 100 times higher than amniotic fluid concentrations, so when CSF leaks into the amniotic fluid, as occurs with an open NTD, amniotic fluid AFP levels are increased.

Amniotic fluid AFP can be measured by amniocentesis as early as 11 to 12 weeks with recent techniques for early amniotic fluid sampling (Kuller et al., 1996). Amniotic fluid analysis involves testing for AFP, acetylcholinesterase (increased in the presence of exposed neural tissue), and ratio of acetylcholinesterase to pseudocholinesterase (differentiates between NTDs and occult ventral wall defects) (Silver et al., 1989). Chorionic villus sampling is not useful for detecting increased AFP, because this protein is produced only in fetal tissues and not in the trophoblastic tissue. Because AFP level normally declines by 10 to 15 percent/week at midtrimester and because of laboratory differences, AFP levels are expressed in multiples of the normal median (MoM) for that lab and gestation. Most women with NTDs have AFP values of greater than 3.0 MoM (Cuckle, 1994). False-positive results are generally the result of blood contamination of the sample, fetal death, or other severe malformation. Increased AFP levels may also be found with open lesions (abdominal wall or skin defects), reduced amniotic fluid production (from renal agenesis or urethral obstruction), altered fetal swallowing (intestinal atresia), or altered protein breakdown (nephrosis) (Cuckle, 1994).

Amniocentesis is generally performed only if a specific indication exists, such as a family history of NTDs or advanced maternal age. Because AFP levels are easy to determine, they are usually obtained after all genetic amniocenteses, regardless of the original indication. Increased fetal AFP level can also be detected in maternal serum. Routine screening of all pregnant women for AFP has been instituted in many areas. If maternal serum AFP level is increased, an amniocentesis and/or fetal ultrasonography is performed to confirm the diagnosis. If the diagnosis can be confirmed by ultrasonography, amniocentesis may not be performed, unless chromosome analysis or other studies are also warranted. Maternal AFP determination is only a screening test because considerable overlap exists between levels in affected and those in unaffected pregnancies (Cuckle, 1994).

Leakage of CSF from the defect can lead to maternal hydramnios. Overdistention of the uterus by excessive accumulation of amniotic fluid can stimulate preterm labor. Thus, infants with NTDs may be preterm.

Differential Diagnosis and Clinical Manifestations

The defect may vary greatly in size but is apparent on examination of the infant. The protruding sac is usually in the lumbosacral area and is covered with skin or meninges. Fluid may be leaking from a partially or completely ruptured sac. Infants with this defect have altered tone and activity of the lower extremities and may assume a frog-like posture. If bowel and bladder involvement exists, dribbling of urine and feces may be noted. The neurologic deficit varies with the level of the defect. Sensory level generally tends to approximate the motor level but may be several segments lower, owing to differences in the pattern of innervation between sensory and motor fibers. Sensory level can be useful in predicting prognosis (Brann & Schwartz, 1987).

Infants with NTDs may have evidence of hydrocephalus at birth. Ultrasonography, CT, or MRI can be used to determine the size of the ventricular system, to rule out aqueductal stenosis and/or Arnold-Chiari malformation, and to monitor ventricular status and development of hydrocephalus. Renal dysfunction may develop, owing to recurring urinary tract infections. Hydronephrosis may be present at birth. An intravenous pyelogram may be obtained to evaluate renal status and presence of hydronephrosis (Miller, 1997).

Prognosis

Prognosis varies with the level and severity of the defect. Most infants with lesions lower than S1 will walk unaided; those with lesions higher than L2 will generally have some wheelchair dependency; bowel and bladder function are controlled at the level of S2-S4 (Volpe, 1995). However, these limitations are changing as a result of improved perinatal management and new technologies and aids, so more children are ambulatory now than previously. In addition, diagnosis before birth and delivery by elective cesarean section have been associated with prevention of sac rupture and improved motor function for the level of the lesion. Luthy and associates (1991) reported that delivery of these infants by cesarean section before the onset of labor (versus delivery by cesarean section after a period of labor) significantly reduced the incidence and the extent of paralysis and motor dysfunction and increased the likelihood of ambulation. Infants with the best prognosis are those with meningocele covered with skin. Infants with a myelomeningocele involving a small lumbosacral lesion, without accompanying hydrocephalus or other anomalies, have some degree of neurologic deficit. These infants may be paraplegic but have a good prognosis for eventual independent function. Infants with myeloschisis have a poor prognosis. Many of these infants die of sepsis in the neonatal period. Those that survive have severe neurologic impairments.

Prognosis has also improved with the current early and aggressive treatment of infants without major cerebral lesions, hemorrhage, infection, high spinal cord lesions, or advanced hydrocephalus. Thus, infants receiving early, aggressive treatment have a reported mortality of 14 percent by 3 to 7 years, and 74 percent of patients are ambulatory and 73 percent have an intelligence quotient of greater than 80 (Volpe, 1995).

Collaborative Management

Management of infants with NTDs, especially severe defects, is controversial and raises many ethical issues (see Chapter 3, Ethical Aspects of Perinatal Care). Decisions must be made in the immediate neonatal period regarding whether the defect should be closed surgically and how aggressively the infant will be managed. If all infants with NTDs are managed aggressively at birth, a proportion of them will survive but will have severe neurologic, motoric, renal, bowel, and bladder problems, causing significant psychological and economic stress to the family (Miller, 1997). Some feel that immediate surgical closure is not justified in infants with open, draining defects, severe hydrocephalus, or multiple anomalies and recommend that conservative, supportive care be used (Milhorat & Miller, 1994). Considerations in these decisions include the size and location of the defect, the prognosis, the presence of other anomalies, the availability of facilities for long-term care, the suffering of the infant, and the family dynamics and wishes (Brann & Schwartz, 1987). If the decision is made not to close the defect surgically, care is supportive. Some of these infants die in a few days to weeks, often as a result of infection, whereas others may survive for months or years, requiring long-term care.

For many infants with NTDs, immediate closure and aggressive care is the appropriate management. Unless the defect is severe or associated with multiple life-threatening anomalies, more than 90 percent of infants with myelomeningocele survive the neonatal period. If untreated, 15 to 30 percent survive and are left with increased deficit. Thus, immediate closure is the treatment of choice for most infants.

Immediate closure reduces the risk of infection and improves the prognosis by reducing further deterioration of the spinal cord and nerve tracts. Early closure also facilitates caregiving. Surgical closure is performed within the first 24 to 48 hours, and often in the first few hours after birth. A large defect may require several surgical procedures for complete closure to be achieved. If the defect is completely covered by epithelium, surgery may be delayed for a short period to further evaluate function. All infants with NTDs are evaluated and monitored for hydrocephalus. Urologic and renal function is also assessed on an ongoing basis. All infants with involvement of the spinal cord, or nerve roots, or both, require multidisciplinary follow-up and continuing care to deal with ongoing neurologic, urologic, orthopedic, and psychological problems.

Nursing Management

Immediate nursing management of an infant with NTDs includes stabilization and prevention of trauma or infection of the sac and its contents. The infant is monitored for signs of infection, including signs of sepsis or meningitis (see Chapter 27, Assessment and Management of Immunologic Dysfunction) and localized infection with redness or discharge from the sac. Warmth and hydration are provided, and fluid and electrolyte status is monitored. These infants are at increased risk for hypothermia and dehydration, owing to the open lesion that lacks the normal protective skin covering.

The infant is positioned prone or on the side to reduce tension on the sac. A roll between the legs at hip level assists in maintaining abduction of the legs; a foot roll is used to maintain the feet in a neutral position. Change of position from prone to side lying or side to side, as well as range-of-motion exercises, helps to prevent skin breakdown and contractures. Low Trendelenburg's position may be used to reduce CSF pressure on the sac. If the infant must be temporarily placed in a supine position for a procedure, a donut roll can be used to prevent pressure on the sac. Postoperative positioning also involves use of the prone or side-lying position, maintenance of body alignment, prevention of hip abduction, and prevention of pressure on the operative site with holding.

The sac must be kept sterile and free of fecal or urine contamination. Warm sterile saline dressings are often used on the sac itself. An alternative approach is to cover the sac with Telfa pads or another nonadherent dressing soaked in warm saline. Telfa pads are less likely than warm saline soaks or dressings to adhere to the lesion. The Telfa pad can be covered by dry pads and a sterile plastic drape (Silver et al., 1989). Meticulous skin care, consisting of keeping the skin clean and dry and removing urine and stool, helps prevent skin breakdown and infection. The timing and characteristics of urination and stool excretion are observed in order to assist in determining the degree of deficit.

Tone, spontaneous movement, range-of-motion, and reflex activity are assessed. Head circumference is monitored serially, and signs of increasing ICP noted. The infants have an intravenous drip and are placed on NPO status initially because surgery is usually performed within the first hours after birth. After surgery, the infants are also placed in a prone position initially until the surgical site heals. Skin care to prevent excoriation and contamination of the excision site continues to be critical during this period, as does prevention of contractures.

Families of infants with NTDs need initial and ongoing support and counseling. Initial parental care involves assisting parents with the shock of the defect and its appearance and with their grief over having an infant with an anomaly. Nursing care also involves enhancing parent–infant interaction and involving the parents in the infant's care when they are ready (see Chapter 7, Sibling Adaptation to the Neonate; and Chapter 10, Fetal Development: Environmental Influences and Critical Periods). Teaching before discharge includes skin care, positioning, exercises, handling and feeding techniques, and provision of activities to promote development. Many areas have spina bifida associations and parent-to-parent support programs to which parents can be referred for peer support.

Care of untreated infants is supportive, consisting of provision of warmth, hydration, and comfort. Decisions not to treat these types of infants, however, are controversial. A case of an infant with NTD was the basis for Baby Doe regulations. In any case, the birth of an infant with NTD is a difficult situation for the family as well as nurses and other staff (see Chapter 3, Ethical Aspects of Perinatal Care; and Chapter 4, Legal Aspects of Perinatal Care) that requires mutual understanding, support, and discussion of feelings.

Hydrocephalus

Hydrocephalus is the most common cause of head enlargement in the neonate. The incidence of this disorder is 3 to 4 in 1000 live births (Punt, 1988). It is caused by an abnormal accumulation of CSF in the ventricles and subarachnoid space. Hydrocephalus arises from alterations in circulation or production of CSF, owing to a congenital defect or postbirth problems, such as infection or hemorrhage.

Pathophysiology

Cerebrospinal fluid is produced in the choroid plexus at a rate of approximately 0.37 ml/minute (Miller, 1997). CSF then circulates from the lateral ventricles through the foramen of Monro to the third ventricle and via the aqueduct of Sylvius to the fourth ventricle. From here, CSF flows through the foramina of Luschka and Magendie, along the base of the brain, and around the hemispheres (see Fig. 29–1). CSF is absorbed by bulk flow through valves along the sagittal sinus. Although hydrocephalus can arise from overproduction of CSF by the choroid plexus, this cause is rare. Hydrocephalus almost always arises from an obstruction within the ventricular system (noncommunicating hydrocephalus) or external to the ventricles (communicating hydrocephalus).

Congenital hydrocephalus is usually associated with congenital malformations within the ventricular system proximal to the subarachnoid space. This is a noncommunicating form of hydrocephalus, that is, no free communication exists between the ventricles and the subarachnoid space. The most common malformations are stenosis of the aqueduct of Sylvius, Dandy-Walker syndrome, and Arnold-Chiari malformation. Aqueductal stenosis is the most common malformation associated with congenital hydrocephalus. The aqueduct is divided into many small channels that have varying amounts of occlusion (Miller, 1997). This abnormality is thought to arise at 15 to 17 weeks' gestation, as a result of an alteration in the normal constriction of the aqueduct that occurs during this period (Lyon & Beaugerie, 1988). Dandy-Walker syndrome is often associated with other CNS malformations. Infants with this defect have a cystic enlargement of the fourth ventricle, atresia of the foramina of Luschka and Magendie, and abnormal cerebellar development. The Arnold-Chiari malformation varies in severity and is often associated with NTDs.

Communicating hydrocephalus involves arachnoiditis with arachnoidal adhesions that arise after intracranial hemorrhage or postinfection inflammation in the fetal or neonatal periods. In this type of hydrocephalus, some degree of communication exists between the ventricles and the subarachnoid space. The most common cause of posthemorrhagic hydrocephalus in the newborn is P/IVH. This P/IVH results in an obliterative arachnoiditis in the posterior fossa, which impedes CSF flow from the fourth ventricle or through the subarachnoid space or cisterns. Hydrocephalus also occurs after meningitis, owing to impediment of CSF flow by fibrotic areas and adhesions at the exit of the fourth ventricle or in the subarachnoid space (Paidas & Cohen, 1994).

Hydrocephalus leads to progressive enlargement of the ventricles and compression of the cortex. Compression of the cortex may occur before clinical signs, such as changes in head size and separation of the sutures, are apparent. In the newborn, progressive ventricular dilation results in diffuse atrophy of the white matter and destruction of glial cells and axons, spongy edema of the periventricular area, and fibrosis of the choroid plexus. Neurons tend to be selectively spared (Milhorat & Miller, 1994).

Risk Factors

Risk factors vary with the type of hydrocephalus. Congenital hydrocephalus arises from genetic influences, or environmental influences, or both, during the period of embryonic or fetal development. Risk factors for hydrocephalus that develops after birth include intraventricular hemorrhage and other forms of intracranial hemorrhage, meningitis, and any factor that predisposes the infant to either intracranial bleeding or sepsis.

Differential Diagnosis

Hydrocephalus must be differentiated from other problems that are associated with increased or increasing head size. These include (Miller, 1997)

1. Subdural hemorrhage (described earlier).
2. Hydranencephaly, which is a congenital absence of the brain but with normal dura, scalp, and skull. This anomaly is probably caused by prenatal bilateral occlusion of the carotid arteries with reabsorption of the brain, or it may be caused by infection.
3. Porencephaly, a cystic cavitation of the brain that usually communicates with the ventricles or subarachnoid space. This anomaly probably arises from prenatal vascular occlusion with reabsorption of tissue and can occur along with hydrocephalus.
4. Arachnoid cysts that trap CSF in the pia-arachnoid and mimic hydrocephalus or, if they are found in the posterior fossa, compress the fossa and produce hydrocephalus.
5. Macrocephaly or enlargement of the brain, causing rapid head growth. This can be an isolated familial disorder or can be associated with disorders such as Tay-Sachs disease.
6. Normal head growth in a very low birth weight infant.
7. Malnutrition catch-up growth.
8. Small for gestational age infants who have a large head-to-body size.
9. Other disorders associated with an enlarged head in proportion to body size, such as achondroplasia and dwarfism.

Hydrocephalus can be differentiated from these disorders by transillumination, cranial ultrasonography (most common), MRI, and CT.

Clinical Manifestations

Often, few signs and symptoms of hydrocephalus are present in the neonate. Enlargement of the head may be noted at birth in infants with congenital hydrocephalus, or it may develop gradually. Posthemorrhagic and infection hydrocephalus develop after birth at varying times after the initial insult. Head size can increase without increases in ICP (normopressive hydrocephalus), owing to the neonate's soft, malleable skull and open sutures and fontanelles (Miller, 1997). A tense fontanelle may be noted when the infant is placed in an upright position. Progressive ventricular dilation may initially cause compression and damage to the cortex without causing any change in head size. The developing hydrocephalus may be apparent only on ultrasonographic examination. Transillumination findings are generally negative unless the cortical mantle is less than about 1 cm thick (Milhorat & Miller, 1994).

Head appearance may be altered, especially in congenital hydrocephalus with prominent frontal bones, a wide anterior cranium, or, in infants with Dandy-Walker syndrome, a large head with a prominent occiput (Amiel-Tison & Larroche, 1988). With aqueductal stenosis, the cranial vault is expanded and the posterior fossa is small, whereas in communicating hydrocephalus, the entire head is enlarged and all the sutures are separated (Milhorat & Miller, 1994). Signs of increased ICP, such as bulging anterior fontanelle, setting-sun sign, dilated scalp veins, and widely separated sutures, tend to be later findings. In normal infants, sutures should be separated only by a few millimeters in the first few days after birth because of overriding of the bones. Separation of the squamosal suture above the ear between the temporal and parietal bones is a good indicator of markedly increased ICP. Marked enlargement of the ventricles is associated with a "cracked pot" sound (Macewen's sign) on percussion of the head (Milhorat & Miller, 1994).

Prognosis

The prognosis depends on the cause of the hydrocephalus and the severity and the presence of associated problems. Prognosis tends to be better for infants with neonatal onset than for those with fetal onset. Infants with congenital hydrocephalus associated with NTDs or Dandy-Walker syndrome tend to have a high frequency of later neurologic problems, as do infants who have hydrocephalus after grade III or IV P/IVH or meningitis. On the other hand, infants with aqueductal stenosis as an isolated defect have a good prognosis.

Milhorat and Miller (1994) identified three groups of infants in terms of their prognosis. The first group is made up of infants who have progressive hydrocephalus with irreversible damage to the brain and other organs (often secondary to other anomalies). These infants have a poor prognosis for both survival and neurologic function. Shunting has little effect on prognosis. The infants in the second group have progressive hydrocephalus but do not have major anomalies or damage to other organ systems. With prompt treatment and shunting, these infants may have a good prognosis, depending on the severity of the hydrocephalus and the success of the therapy. The thickness of the cerebral mantle is somewhat predictive of outcome. Mantles at least 2 cm thick are associated with a good prognosis; mantles less than 1 cm thick are associated with a poor prognosis. Prognosis is variable for infants in whom mantle thickness is 1 to 2 cm (Paine, 1967).

The third group of infants are those whose hydrocephalus arrests. This phenomenon is rare with congenital hydrocephalus but is common in posthemorrhagic ventricular dilation. These infants need to continue to be observed for slow progression of normopressive hydrocephalus. Infants with arrested hydrocephalus have stable head sizes and normal psychomotor development for their age or stabilization or improvement of existing neurologic deficits (Milhorat & Miller, 1994).

Collaborative Management

Serial head circumference measurements are plotted on all infants at risk for progressive ventricular enlargement and hydrocephalus (see Fig. 29–8). The most accurate measurements are made by use of a metal tape marked in centimeters (rather than inches) (Amiel-Tison & Larroche, 1988). The rate of head growth is more critical than the absolute circumference.

Management can involve either surgical or medical therapy. Surgical management involves placement of a shunt to drain excess CSF. Other, less common, surgical procedures include removal of arachnoidal cysts or tumors or fenestration procedures for infants with Dandy-Walker syndrome.

A ventriculoperitoneal shunt is generally the shunt of choice in infants and children because this type is easier to insert, revise, and lengthen and has a lower risk of infection than does a ventriculoatrial shunt. One end of a radiopaque catheter is placed into the lateral ventricle, usually on the right side, and the other end is placed into the peritoneal cavity. The catheter contains a one-way valve that is palpable on the side of the head near the ear (Fig. 29–17).

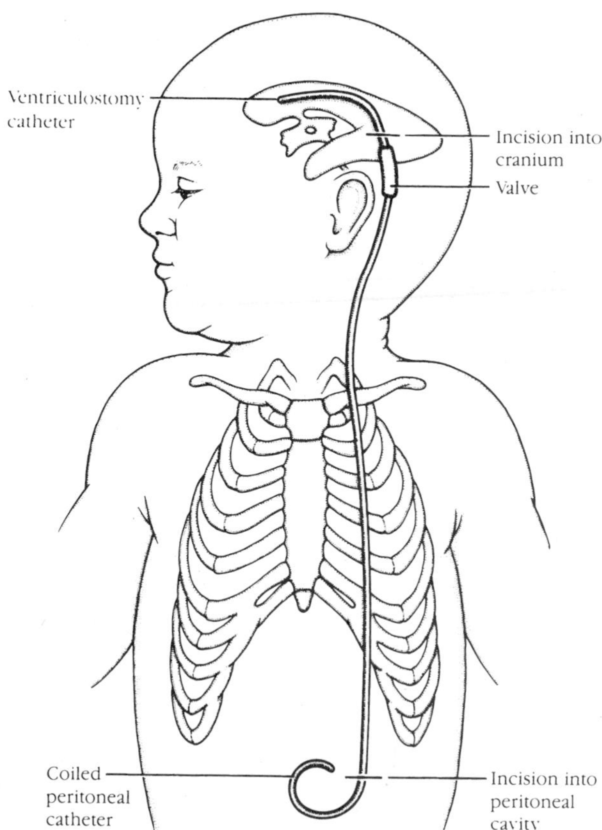

FIGURE 29–17. Ventriculoperitoneal shunt placement. (From Servonsky, J., & Opas, S. R. [1987]. *Nursing management of children* [p. 1297]. Boston: Jones & Bartlett Publishers. Reprinted with permission.)

The shunt needs multiple revisions during childhood for growth and for malfunctioning. In a term infant, revision of the shunt for growth can be anticipated at 3 to 4 years of age and at 10 to 13 years of age, when a permanent adult-length system is implanted. Preterm infants usually require an additional revision for growth at about 1 year of age (Milhorat & Miller, 1994). Major complications of ventriculoperitoneal shunts are infection and obstruction. Too-rapid drainage of CSF immediately after shunt insertion can lead to herniation of the brain or subdural hematoma.

The role of medical management is controversial. Infants with uncomplicated hydrocephalus may not need shunting if the hydrocephalus arrests. These infants are managed by close follow-up and monitoring of ventricular size and cortical mantle thickness with serial cranial ultrasonography. Medical therapy is used primarily with posthemorrhagic hydrocephalus, which is associated with spontaneous arrest in about 50 percent of infants. Serial lumbar punctures or pharmacologic agents (see section on P/IVH) to reduce CSF may be used while these infants are monitored for cessation of progressive ventricular dilation (Volpe, 1995). These therapies may also be used in infants who are too ill to tolerate surgery and shunt placement (Milhorat & Miller, 1994; Punt, 1988).

Nursing Management

Head circumference is monitored serially on all infants with, or at risk for, hydrocephalus. These infants are also monitored for signs of progressive ventricular enlargement and increased ICP. Skin care; use of soft foam, sheepskin, lambskin, or other materials that minimize pressure and excoriation; and regular change of position help prevent skin breakdown from pressure. The head of the hydrocephalic infant requires additional support, consisting of repositioning and holding. The infant may feed poorly and require small, frequent feedings. Irritability can be reduced by reduction of environmental stressors and institution of comforting measures (see Chapter 49, Assessment and Management of Neonatal Neurobehavioral Development).

After surgery, these infants are positioned on the side opposite the shunt, with the head of the bed flat or slightly elevated to prevent rapid loss of CSF and decompression. The valve should not be pumped unless this action is specifically ordered. The position can be rotated to supine every few hours in order to prevent skin breakdown. The skin should be kept clean and dry. The infant can also be placed on sheepskin or lambskin to prevent skin breakdown.

Shunted infants are observed for signs of localized or systemic infection, ileus, and shunt obstruction. Obstruction of the shunt leads to accumulation of CSF, enlargement of the head, and signs of increased ICP. Infection of the shunt may present as localized redness or drainage around the incision, temperature instability, altered activity, or poor feeding. Fluid status and intake and output are monitored, as are signs of dehydration from too rapid a loss of CSF. Signs of too-rapid decompression include a sunken fontanelle, agitation or restlessness, increased urine output, and electrolyte abnormalities. Management of infants with a ventriculoperitoneal shunt is summarized in Table 29–13.

Parent teaching before discharge includes care of the infant and shunt, including positioning and skin care. Parents must be comfortable in handling and caring for their infant before discharge. They should know signs of shunt malfunction, increased ICP, infection, and dehydration. Ongoing follow-up care of the

TABLE 29–13 Nursing Management of an Infant with a Ventriculoperitoneal Shunt

Purpose: To drain excess cerebrospinal fluid (CSF) from the ventricles into the peritoneum in order to relieve intracranial pressure, prevent further damage to the brain, and promote optimal outcome.

I. Positioning
   A. Place an unaffected side (may position on shunt side with "donut" over operative site once incision has healed). Keep head of bed flat to 15° to 30° to prevent too rapid fluid loss.
   B. Support head carefully when moving infant.
   C. Turn q 2 hr from unaffected side of head to back.

II. Shunt site
   A. Use strict aseptic technique when changing dressing.
   B. Pump shunt if and only as directed by neurosurgeon.
   C. Observe for fluid leakage around pump.

III. Observe and document all intake and output. Watch for symptoms of excessive drainage of CSF:
   A. Sunken fontanelle
   B. Increased urine output
   C. Increased sodium loss

IV. Observe, document, and report any seizure activity or paresis.

V. Observe for signs of ileus:
   A. Abdominal distention (serially measure abdominal girth)
   B. Absence of bowel sounds
   C. Loss of gastric content by emesis or through orogastric tube

VI. Perform range-of-motion exercises to all extremities.

VII. Observe and assess for symptoms of increased intracranial pressure (shunt failure):
   A. Increasing head circumference (measure head daily)
   B. Full and/or tense fontanelle
   C. Sutures palpable, more separated
   D. High-pitched, shrill cry
   E. Irritability/sleeplessness
   F. Vomiting
   G. Poor feeding
   H. Nystagmus
   I. Sunset sign of eyes
   J. Shiny scalp with distended vessels
   K. Hypotonia/hypertonia

VIII. Observe and assess for signs of infection:
   A. Redness or drainage at shunt site
   B. Hypothermia/hyperthermia
   C. Lethargy/irritability
   D. Poor feeding/weight gain
   E. Pallor

IX. Parent teaching
   A. Teach parents and give written copy of signs and symptoms of increased intracranial pressure, infection, and dehydration.
   B. Emphasize importance of notifying physician for any signs and symptoms.
   C. Demonstrate and receive return demonstration of proper head positioning (at rest, lifting, and carrying).
   D. Demonstrate and receive return demonstration of drug administration. Teach parents side effects of medications.
   E. Emphasize importance of follow-up medical care for assessment and medication adjustment.

From Merenstein, G. B., & Gardner, S. L. (1989). *Handbook of neonatal intensive care* (2nd ed., pp. 501–539). St. Louis: C. V. Mosby Co. Reprinted with permission.

infant and parental support are important. Parents may be referred to parent groups for peer support.

Cerebral Palsy

Cerebral palsy has been described as a "non-progressive, chronic disability, characterized by aberrant control of movement and posture, and appearing in early life" (Fawer & Calame, 1988). The incidence of CP is about 5 in 1000, with approximately 50 percent having mild, 40 percent having moderate, and 10 percent having severe disability.

Pathophysiology and Risk Factors

Cerebral palsy is a common sequela of perinatal disorders. Approximately 60 percent of CP arises from perinatal insults, 30 percent from prenatal events, and 10 percent from later insults. Risk factors include prematurity, perinatal asphyxia, periventricular hemorrhage, other hypoxic-ischemic events, prolonged or precipitate labor, and birth trauma. Spastic diplegia–type CP is the most common major neurologic handicap in infants born prematurely.

The primary problem in individuals with CP is lack of motor control that is caused by a central (brain) injury. This injury alters the integrative ability of the CNS in relation to motor function. The type of abnormality in movement and tone is related to the area of the brain that has been damaged. Damage to the cortex produces spasticity. Basal ganglia damage results in athetoid movements, whereas cerebellar insults are associated with ataxia.

The site of the lesion (see Figure 29–16), and thus the type of disability, varies with gestational age. In the preterm infant, the injury usually involves the white matter and the motor fibers of the lower extremities. Thus, preterm infants generally have a spastic diplegia, primarily of the legs, with normal or near-normal cognitive development because the gray matter of the cortex is not injured. The injury in term infants, usually from a hypoxic-ischemic insult, such as perinatal asphyxia, usually results from a parasagittal cortical lesion. This leads to involvement of the upper extremities, face, and tongue with impairment of speech. These infants often have a more severe involvement, with quadriplegia or hemiplegia, and are more likely to be mentally retarded.

Clinical Manifestations and Prognosis

Cerebral palsy is not diagnosed in the neonatal period. Manifestations become apparent over the first 3 to 18 months of age. Generally, the more severe the involvement, the earlier a specific diagnosis can be made. Thus, infants with quadriplegia are likely to be diagnosed within the first 3 to 6 months, whereas children with mild spastic diplegia affecting the legs may not be diagnosed until 12 to 18 months. Infants at risk or with subtle signs are treated with a high index of suspicion and are observed carefully. Transient dystonia is seen in many infants with birth weights of less than 1500 g during the first year. In a little over half of these infants, this dystonia resolves by about 12 months of age with no sequelae. In the remainder of infants with this problem, the dystonia either disappears but returns later or it persists with later diagnosis of CP. Transient dystonia has also been associated with later learning problems and hyperactivity (Amiel-Tison et al., 1983; Taeusch & Yogman, 1987).

Cerebral palsy causes impairment of coordination of muscle action; inability to maintain normal posture and balance; retention of primary reflexes; failure of automatic reactions, such as righting, equilibrium, and protective extension (parachute), to develop; and alterations in tone. Tone may be increased, decreased, or fluctuating. Impairment caused by CP ranges from mild to severe.

Atonic or flaccid tone results from failure of the muscles to respond to volitional stimuli, and automatic responses are absent. These children often become athetoid. Athetoid movements involve widely fluctuating muscle tone, from too high to too low. Contraction and fixture for precise, selective movements are lacking. Spasticity involves pathologic stretch responses in the affected body parts, increased activity of the deep tendon reflexes, hypertonia, scissor gait, hip flexion with adduction and internal rotation, and tendency toward toe walking. With excitement or increased effort, these children become more hypertonic.

Children with ataxia have good autonomic responses but low tone and improper grading of distance, giving them a clumsy appearance. They appear floppy and poorly balanced and coordinated. They may also have poor control of involuntary movements, leading to tremors. Individuals with CP may also have associated reactions, with widespread changes in tone in affected parts of the body that are not directly concerned with the movement the child is attempting. For example, as the child squeezes a ball with one hand, the other hand flexes.

Five general categories of CP are usually identified, depending on the type of motor abnormality and its distribution: (1) hemiplegia, (2) spastic quadriplegia or tetraplegia, (3) diplegia, (4) ataxia, and (5) dyskinetic CP (Ellison, 1984; Fawer & Calame, 1988; Ingram, 1984).

Hemiplegia is a unilateral spastic paresis. The arm is more likely to be involved than the leg. Spastic quadriplegia or tetraplegia (bilateral hemiplegia) involves the entire body. The upper body is more affected than the lower extremities. Head control is poor. Eye coordination and speech are also affected. Depending on the site of the injury, athetoid and ataxic movements may be present in addition to the spasticity.

Diplegia also involves the entire body, but the upper limbs are often markedly less involved than the lower extremities. Movement is predominantly spastic, but athetosis of the distal limbs may be noted. Head control and speech are not usually affected. Ataxia is characterized by hypotonia, poor coordination of voluntary movements, and impaired balance. Dyskinetic CP is characterized by involuntary movements and changes in tone that affect the trunk, the limbs, and the face (Fawer & Calame, 1988).

Infants with CP may have associated defects of speech, vision (uncoordinated eye movements, squinting, and lack of accommodation), and hearing (high-frequency deafness and agnosia). Many children with CP have normal cognitive function; however, the incidence of mental retardation is higher in this population. Other associated disorders include spatial agnosia, epilepsy, and psychological problems. The prognosis for independent function depends on the severity of the disability, the timing of the diagnosis, and the availability of appropriate therapy to prevent complications.

Collaborative and Nursing Management

Early recognition through careful monitoring of infants at risk for CP is critical for prompt diagnosis as evidence of this disability presents. Physical therapy is a primary discipline in providing ongoing assessment of motor behavior, movement patterns, postures, tone, reflex patterns, and motor development appropriate to the child's age. Treatment is directed at developing alternative pathways to achieve desired motor function, preventing development of contractures and other deformities, and preventing the child from using, and thus learning, abnormal movement patterns. Many systems of treatment exist: Temple-Fay, Doman-Delacato, Rood, Bobath neurodevelopmental, and proprioceptive neuromuscular facilitation. Treatment of high-risk infants is usually based on neurodevelopmental principles or their adaptations (Bly, 1981; Bobath, 1980). The goal of this type of therapy is "to provide the developing infant who exhibits symptomatology of central nervous system (CNS) impairment with the experience of normal patterns of posture and movement" (Piper et al., 1986, p. 304).

Therapy is usually started early, when abnormal patterns are seen, even if a specific diagnosis cannot yet be made. Early treatment is thought to reduce the degree of later deficit that results from development of abnormal patterns or deformities. Parents need to understand the problem and its prognosis and the importance of their active involvement in the child's therapy.

CONCLUSION

Infants with neurologic dysfunction present a significant challenge to the neonatal nurse. The nurse must respond to infants with life-threatening events, such as perinatal asphyxia and intracranial hemorrhage; transient problems, such as an isolated seizure; or chronic problems, such as NTDs. The nurse must also deal with her or his own responses and those of the families of infants who may die during the neonatal or early infancy periods or whose short-term and long-term outcome may be altered by the extent of neurologic insult. To optimally care for these infants and their families, the nurse must understand the basis for, and the implications of, specific types of neurologic dysfunction; must recognize clinical manifestations of these types of dysfunction; and must respond appropriately in concert with other health care professionals.

Nursing care of infants at risk for, or with, neurologic dysfunction involves assessment and monitoring of neurologic status and responses of the infant to the extrauterine environment and of subtle signs that may indicate a change in the infant's status. Nursing management of the infant involves activities to address alteration in level of consciousness, potential for injury related to trauma or infection, impairment of skin integrity, alterations in comfort, impaired mobility, alterations in thermoregulation, alterations in nutrition and fluid and electrolyte status, and promotion of neurobehavioral organization and development. The nurse must also assess family coping, interactive processes, knowledge, and grieving in order to assist the family in coping with the birth of an ill infant and, for many families, with the uncertainty or certainty of long-term neurologic deficits in their infant.

Additional research is needed to validate nursing interventions used with infants at risk for, or with, neurologic dysfunction. Many of the interventions currently used have no documented scientific basis as to their efficacy and effectiveness. Specific recommendations for research with this group of infants and their families include testing and evaluation of (1) specific nursing interventions to reduce the risk of P/IVH in very low birth weight infants; (2) developmental care strategies with both preterm and term infants with neurologic dysfunction; (3) interventions to enhance neurodevelopmental progress and outcome in infants with HIE, P/IVH, and PVL; (4) effects of different types of positioning on infants with specific types of neurologic dysfunction; (5) interventions to promote skin integrity in infants with impaired mobility and altered levels of consciousness; (6) interventions to support neuromuscular integrity in infants with impaired mobility and altered levels of consciousness; and (7) interventions to support family coping and functioning when an infant is born with or develops a neurologic problem.

REFERENCES

Als, H., Lawhon, G., Duffy, F. H., et al. (1994). Individualized developmental care for the very low birthweight preterm infant. Medical and neurofunctional effects. *Journal of the American Medical Association, 272*, 853–858.

Amiel-Tison, C. (1978). A method for neurological evaluation within the first year of life. *Ciba Foundation Symposium, 59*, 107–126.

Amiel-Tison, C., Dube, R., Garel, M., & Jequier, J. C. (1983). Late outcome after transient neuromotor abnormalities within the first year of life. In L. Stern, H. Bard, & B. Friis-Hansen (Eds.), *Intensive care IV* (pp. 247–258). New York: Masson Publishing USA.

Amiel-Tison, C., Korobkin, R., & Klaus, M. H. (1986). Neurologic problems. In M. H. Klaus & A. A. Fanaroff (Eds.), *Care of the high-risk neonate* (3rd ed., pp. 356–378). Philadelphia: W. B. Saunders Co.

Amiel-Tison, C., & Larroche, J. C. (1988). Brain development and neurological survey during the neonatal period. In L. Stern & P. Vert (Eds.), *Neonatal medicine* (pp. 245–267). New York: Masson Publishing USA.

Andre, M., & Vert, P. (1987). Birth injury. In L. Stern & P. Vert (Eds.), *Neonatal medicine* (pp. 176–190). New York: Masson Publishing USA.

Axton, J. H. (1966). Depressions of the skull in the newborn. *Nursing Mirror and Midwives Journal, 123*(5), 123–124.

Bellig, L. L. (1989). A window on the neonate's brain. *Neonatal Network, 7*(4), 13–20.

Bennett, F. C., Silver, G., Leung, E. J., & Mack, L. A. (1990). Periventricular echodensities detected by cranial ultrasonography: Usefulness in predicting neurodevelopmental outcome in low-birth-weight, preterm infants. *Pediatrics, 85*(3, Part 2), 400–404.

Bennett, G. C., & Harrold, A. J. (1976). Prognosis and early management of birth injuries to the brachial plexus. *British Medical Journal, 1*(6024), 1520–1521.

Bernes, S. M., & Kaplan, A. M. (1994). Evolution of neonatal seizures [Review]. *Pediatric Clinics of North America, 45*(5), 1069–1104.

Bly, L. (1981). The components of normal and abnormal movements during the first year of life. In D. E. Slaton (Ed.), *Development of movement in infancy.* Chapel Hill, NC: University of North Carolina.

Bobath, K. (1980). *A neurophysiological basis for the treatment of cerebral palsy.* London: Spastics International Medical Publications.

Boome, R. S., & Kaye, J. C. (1988). Obstetric traction injuries of the brachial plexus: Natural history, indications for surgical repair and results. *Journal of Bone and Joint Surgery. British Volume, 70*(4), 571–576.

Bozynski, M. E., Nelson, M. N., Matalon, T. A., et al. (1985). Cavitary periventricular leukomalacia: Incidence and short term outcome in infants weighing ≤1200 grams at birth. *Developmental Medicine and Child Neurology, 27*(5), 572–577.

Brown, M.S., & Sheridan-Pereira, M. (1992). Outlook for a child with a cephalocele. *Pediatrics, 90*(6), 914–919.

Carey, B. E. (1983). Intraventricular hemorrhage in the preterm infant [Review]. *Journal of Obstetric, Gynecologic, and Neonatal Nursing, 12*(3 Suppl.), 60S–68S.

Clancy, R. R. (1983). Neonatal seizures. In R. A. Polin & F. Berg (Eds.), *Workbook in practical neonatology* (pp. 125–152). Philadelphia: W. B. Saunders Co.

Cooke, R. (1989). The prevention and management of germinal layer hemorrhage and intraventricular hemorrhage. In J. S. Wigglesworth & K. Pape (Eds.), *Perinatal brain lesions* (pp. 191–217). Boston: Blackwell Scientific Publications.

Copp, A. J., & Bernfield, M. (1994). Etiology and pathogenesis of human neural tube defects: Insights from mouse models [Review]. *Current Opinions in Pediatrics, 6*(6), 624–631.

Cowan, F., & Thorensen, M. (1985). Changes in superior sagittal sinus blood velocities due to postural alterations and pressure on the head of the newborn infant. *Pediatrics, 75*(6), 1038–1047.

Cuckle, H. S. (1994). Screening for neural tube defects. *Ciba Foundation Symposium, 181,* 253–269.

Dambaka, M., & Laure-Kamionowska, M. (1990). Myelination as a parameter of normal and retarded brain maturation. *Brain Development, 12*(2), 214–220.

de Vries, L. S., Larroche, J. C., & Levene, M. I. (1988a). Intracranial haemorrhage and intraventricular haemorrhage. In M. I. Levene, M. J. Bennett, & J. Punt (Eds.), *Fetal and neonatal neurology and neurosurgery* (pp. 303–311). Edinburgh: Churchill Livingstone.

de Vries, L. S., Larroche, J. C., & Levene, M. I. (1988b). Germinal matrix haemorrhage and intraventricular haemorrhage. In M. I. Levene, M. J. Bennett, & J. Punt (Eds.), *Fetal and neonatal neurology and neurosurgery* (pp. 312–325). Edinburgh: Churchill Livingstone.

de Vries, L. S., Larroche, J. C., & Levene, M. I. (1988c). Cerebral ischemic lesions. In M. I. Levene, M. J. Bennett, & J. Punt (Eds.), *Fetal and neonatal neurology and neurosurgery* (pp. 326–338). Edinburgh: Churchill Livingstone.

Diaz, J. H. (1993). The anencephalic organ donor: A challenge to existing moral and statutory laws. *Critical Care Medicine, 21*(11), 1781–1786.

Ellison, P. H. (1984). Neurologic development of the high risk infant. *Clinics in Perinatology, 11*(1), 41–58.

Emery, J. R., & Peabody, J. L. (1983). Head position affects intracranial pressure in newborn infants. *Journal of Pediatrics, 103*(6), 950–953.

Erlen, J. A. (1990). Anencephalic infants as sources of organs: Issues and implications for nurses. *Journal of Obstetric, Gynecologic, and Neonatal Nursing, 19*(3), 249–254.

Fawer, C. L., & Calame, A. (1988). Assessment of neurodevelopmental outcome. In M. I. Levene, M. J. Bennett, & J. Punt (Eds.), *Fetal and neonatal neurology and neurosurgery* (pp. 71–88). Edinburgh: Churchill Livingstone.

Fazzi, E., Lanzi, G., Gerardo, A., et al. (1992). Neurodevelopmental outcome in very-low-birth-weight infants with or without periventricular haemorrhage and/or leukomalacia. *Acta Paediatrica, 81*(10), 808–811.

Finer, N. N., Robertson, C. M., Richards, R. T., et al. (1981). Hypoxic-ischemic encephalopathy in term infants: Perinatal factors and outcome. *Journal of Pediatrics, 98*(1), 112–117.

Funato, M., Tamai, H., Noma, K., Kurita, T., Kajimoto, Y., & Shimada, S. (1992). Clinical events associated with timing of intraventricular hemorrhage in preterm infants. *Journal of Pediatrics, 121*(4), 614–619.

Gale, E. (1981). Neonatal seizures. In R. Perez (Ed.), *Protocols for perinatal nursing practice* (pp. 385–390). St. Louis: C. V. Mosby Co.

Girard, N., Raybaud, C., & Poncet, M. (1995). In vivo MR study of brain maturation in normal fetuses. *American Journal of Neuroradiology, 16*(2), 407–413.

Goldbarg, H., & Yeh, T. F. (1991). Seizures. In T. F. Yeh (Ed.), *Neonatal therapeutics* (pp. 313–325). St. Louis: Mosby-Year Book.

Goldberg, R. N., Chung, D., Goldman, S. L., & Bancalari, E. (1980). The association of rapid volume expansion and intraventricular hemorrhage in the preterm infants. *Journal of Pediatrics, 96*(6), 1060–1063.

Goldstein, G. W., & Donn, S. M. (1984). Periventricular and intraventricular hemorrhages. In H. B. Sarnat (Ed.), *Topics in neonatal neurology* (pp. 83–108). New York: Grune & Stratton.

Goldstein, G. W., Johnston, M. V., Donn, S. M., & Custer, J. R. (1989). Birth asphyxia: Issues in neurologic management. In J. S. Wigglesworth & K. Pape (Eds.), *Perinatal brain lesions* (pp. 99–113). Boston: Blackwell Scientific Publications.

Hagadorn-Freathy, A. S., Yeomans, E. R., & Hankins, G. D. (1991). Validation of the 1988 ACOG forceps classification system. *Obstetrics and Gynecology, 77*(3), 356–360.

Hagberg, B., Hagberg, G., & Olow, L. (1993). The changing panorama of cerebral palsy in Sweden: VI. Prevalence and origin during the birth year period 1983–1986. *Acta Paediatrica, 82*(4), 387–393.

Hardy, A. E. (1981). Birth injuries of the brachial plexus: Incidence and prognosis. *Journal of Bone and Joint Surgery British Volume, 63*(1), 98–101.

Harris, S. R., & Brady, D. K. (1986). Infant neuromotor assessment instruments: A review. *Physical and Occupational Therapy in Pediatrics, 6*(3/4), 121–153.

Ifft, D. L., Engstrom, J. L., Meier, P. P., et al. (1989). Reliability of head circumference measurements for preterm infants. *Neonatal Network, 8*(3), 41–46.

Ingram, T. T. S. (1984). A historical review of the definition and classifications of cerebral palsies. *Clinics in Developmental Medicine, 87,* 1.

Kaempf, J. W., Porreco, R., Molina, R., et al. (1990). Antenatal phenobarbital for the prevention of periventricular and intraventricular hemorrhage: A double-blind, randomized, placebo-controlled, multihospital trial. *Journal of Pediatrics, 117*(6), 933–938.

Kjellmer, P. L. (1988). Prenatal and intrapartum asphyxia. In M. I. Levene, M. J. Bennett, & J. Punt (Eds.), *Fetal and neonatal neurology and neurosurgery* (pp. 357–369). Edinburgh: Churchill Livingstone.

Kling, P. (1989). Nursing interventions to decrease the risk of periventricular-intraventricular hemorrhage [Review]. *Journal of Obstetric, Gynecologic, and Neonatal Nursing, 18*(6), 457–464.

Korf, B. R. (1992). Diagnostic outcome in children with multiple cafe-au-lait spots. *Pediatrics, 90*(6), 924–927.

Kosmetatos, N., & Williams, M. (1978). Effect of positioning and head banding on intracranial pressure in the premature neonate. *Pediatric Research, 12,* 553.

Kuller, J. A., Chescheir, N. C. & Cefalo, R. C. (Eds.). (1996). *Prenatal diagnosis & reproductive genetics.* Philadelphia: J. B. Lippincott. Co.

Levene, M. I. (1988a). Management and outcome of birth asphyxia. In M. I. Levene, M. J. Bennett, & J. Punt (Eds.), *Fetal and neonatal neurology and neurosurgery* (pp. 383–391). Edinburgh: Churchill Livingstone.

Levene, M. I. (1988b). The asphyxiated newborn infants. In M. I. Levene, M. J. Bennett, & J. Punt (Eds.), *Fetal and neonatal neurology and neurosurgery* (pp. 371–382). Edinburgh: Churchill Livingstone.

Levine, M. G., Holroyde, J., Woods, J. R., Jr., et al. (1984). Birth trauma: Incidence and predisposing factors. *Obstetrics and Gynecology, 63*(6), 792–795.

Lou, H. C., Lassen, N. A., & Friis-Hanson, B. (1978). Decreased cerebral blood flow after administration of sodium bicarbonate in the distressed newborn infant. *Acta Neurologica Scandinavica, 57*(3), 239–247.

Luthy, D. A., Wardinsky, T., Shurtleff, D. B., et al. (1991). Cesarean section before the onset of labor and subsequent motor function in infants with meningomyelocele diagnosed antenatally. *New England Journal of Medicine, 324*(10), 662–666.

Lyon, G., & Beaugerie, A. (1988). Congenital developmental malformations. In M. I. Levene, M. J. Bennett, & J. Punt (Eds.), *Fetal and neonatal neurology and neurosurgery* (pp. 231–247). Edinburgh: Churchill Livingstone.

Ment, L. R., Oh, W., Ehrenkranz, R. A., et al. (1994a). Low dose indomethacin and prevention of intraventricular hemorrhage: A multicenter randomized trial. *Pediatrics, 93*(4), 543–550.

Ment, L. R., Oh, W., Ehrenkranz, R. A., Philip, A. G., et al. (1994b). Low dose indomethacin therapy and extension of intraventricular hemorrhage: A multicenter randomized trial. *Journal of Pediatrics, 124*(6), 951–955.

Merenstein, G., & Gardner, S. (1993). *Handbook of neonatal intensive care* (3rd ed.). St. Louis: C. V. Mosby Co.

Milhorat, T. H., & Miller, J. I. (1994). Neurosurgery. In G. B. Avery, M. A. Fletcher, & M. G. MacDonald (Eds.), *Neonatology: Pathophysiology and management of the newborn* (4th ed., pp. 1139–1163). Philadelphia: J. B. Lippincott Co.

Miller, G. (1997). Hypotonia and neuromuscular disease. In A. A. Fanaroff & R. J. Martin (Eds.), *Neonatal-perinatal medicine* (6th ed., pp. 911–923). St. Louis: Mosby–Year Book.

Minarick, C. J., & Beachy, P. (1989). Neurologic disorders. In G. B. Merenstein & S. L. Gardner (Eds.), *Handbook of neonatal intensive care* (2nd ed., pp. 501–530). St. Louis: C. V. Mosby Co.

Moore, K. L., & Persaud, T. V. N. (1993) *Before we are born: Essentials of embryology and birth defects* (4th ed.). Philadelphia: W. B. Saunders Co.

Morgane, P. J., Austin-LaFrance, R., Bronzino, J., et al. (1993). Prenatal malnutrition and development of the brain [Review]. *Neuroscience and Biobehavioral Reviews, 17*(1), 91–128.

Mullaart, R. A., Hopman, J. C., Rotteveel, J. J., et al. (1994). Cerebral blood flow fluctuations in neonatal respiratory distress and periventricular haemorrhage. *Early Human Development, 37*(3), 179–185.

NAACOG. (1991). *Physical assessment of the neonate. OGN practice resource.* Washington, DC: Author.

Novotny, E. J. (1989). Hypoxic-ischemic encephalopathy. In D. K. Stevenson & P. Sunshine (Eds.), *Fetal and neonatal brain injury* (pp. 141–145). Toronto: B. C. Decker.

O'Rahilly, R., & Muller, F. (1994). Neurulation in the normal human embryo [Review]. *Ciba Foundation Symposium, 181*, 70–82.

Paidas, M. J., & Cohen, A. (1994). Disorders of the central nervous system [Review]. *Seminars in Perinatology, 18*(4), 266–282.

Paine, R. S. (1967). Hydrocephalus [Review]. *Pediatric Clinics of North America, 14*(4), 779–796.

Palmer, T. W., & Donn, S. M. (1991). Symptomatic subarachnoid hemorrhage in the term newborn. *Journal of Perinatology, 11*(2), 112–116.

Pape, K. E., Armstrong, D. L., & Fitzhardinge, P. M. (1976). Central nervous system pathology associated with mask ventilation in the very low birthweight infant: A new etiology for intracerebellar hemorrhage. *Pediatrics, 58*(4), 473–483.

Pape, K. E., & Wigglesworth, J. S. (1979). *Haemorrhage, ischemia and the perinatal brain.* Philadelphia: J. B. Lippincott Co.

Papile, L., Burstein, J., Burstein, R., et al. (1978). Relationship of intravenous sodium bicarbonate infusions and cerebral intraventricular hemorrhage. *Journal of Pediatrics, 93*(5), 834–836.

Perlman, J. M., Rollins, N., Burns, D., & Risser, R. (1993). Relationship between periventricular intraparenchymal echodensities and germinal matrix-intraventricular hemorrhage in the very low birth weight neonate. *Pediatrics, 91*(2), 474–480.

Piper, M. C., Mazer, B. L., Hardy, S., & Doucette, C. (1986). Monitoring the effects of early physical therapy on the high risk infant: Preliminary results. *Pediatrics, 6*, 303.

Punt, J. (1988). Hydrocephalus. In M. I. Levene, M. J. Bennett, & J. Punt (Eds.), *Fetal and neonatal neurology and neurosurgery* (pp. 586–591). Edinburgh: Churchill Livingstone.

Sarff, L. D., Platt, L. H., & McCracken, G. H., Jr. (1976). Cerebrospinal fluid evaluation in neonates: Comparison of high-risk infants with and without meningitis. *Journal of Pediatrics, 88*(3), 473–477.

Sarnat, H. B. (1984). Anatomic and physiologic correlates of neurologic development in prematurity. In H. B. Sarnat (Ed.), *Topics in neonatal neurology* (pp. 1–25). New York: Grune & Stratton.

Sarnat, H. B., & Sarnat, M. S. (1976). Neonatal encephalopathy following fetal distress: A clinical and electroencephalographic study. *Archives of Neurology, 33*(10), 696–705.

Scott, J. M., Weir, D. G., Molloy, A., et al. (1994). Folic acid metabolism and mechanisms of neural tube defects [Review]. *Ciba Foundation Symposium, 181*, 180–187.

Shah, A. R., Kurth, C. D., Gwiazdowski, S. G., et al. (1992). Fluctuations in cerebral oxygenation and blood volume during endotracheal suctioning in premature infants. *Journal of Pediatrics, 120*(5), 769–774.

Shiota, K. (1991). Development and intrauterine fate of normal and abnormal human conceptuses. *Congenital Anomalies, 31*, 67.

Silver, R. K., Marzocchi, M., Farrell, E. E., & McLone, D. G. (1989). The perinatal management of central nervous system anomalies [Review]. *Clinics in Perinatology, 16*(4), 939–953.

Szymonowicz, W., Yu, V., Walker, A., & Wilson, F. (1986). Reduction in periventricular hemorrhage in preterm infants. *Archives of Diseases in Childhood, 61*(7), 661–665.

Taeusch, H. W., & Yogman, M. W. (1987). *Follow-up and management of the high risk infants.* Boston: Little, Brown & Co.

Taquino, L., & Blackburn, S. (1994). The effects of containment during suctioning and heel stick on physiological and behavioral responses of preterm infants. *Neonatal Network, 13*(7), 55.

Torrence, C. (1985a). Neonatal seizures: Part I. A developmental and clinical understanding. *Neonatal Network, 4*(1), 9–16.

Torrence, C. (1985b). Neonatal seizures: Part II. Recognition, treatment, and prognosis. *Neonatal Network, 4*(2), 21–28.

Tudehope, D. I., & Vacca, A. (1988). Traumatic injuries to the nervous system. In M. I. Levene, M. J. Bennett, & J. Punt (Eds.), *Fetal and neonatal neurology and neurosurgery* (pp. 393–404). Edinburgh: Churchill Livingstone.

Volpe, J. J. (1995). *Neurology of the newborn* (3rd ed.). Philadelphia: W. B. Saunders Co.

Volpe, J. J., & Hill, A. (1987). Neurologic disorders. In G. B. Avery (Ed.), *Neonatology: Pathophysiology and management of the newborn* (3rd ed., pp. 1073–1132). Philadelphia: J. B. Lippincott Co.

Vyhmeister, N., Schneider, S., & Cha C. (1977). Cranial transillumination norms of the premature infant. *Journal of Pediatrics, 91*(6), 980–982.

Wald, N. J. (1994). Folic acid and neural tube defects: The current evidence and implications for prevention [Review]. *Ciba Foundation Symposium, 181*, 192–208.

Wasterlain, C. G., & Duffy, T. E. (1975). Neonatal status epilepticus: Decrease in brain glucose without decrease in blood glucose. *Neurology, 25*, 365.

Weisglas-Kuperus, N., Baerts, W., Fetter, W., & Sauer, P. J. (1992). Neonatal cerebral ultrasound, neonatal neurology, and perinatal conditions as predictors of neurodevelopmental outcome in very low birthweight infants. *Early Human Development, 31*(2), 131–148.

Wigglesworth, J. S. (1989). Current problems in brain pathology in the perinatal period. In J. S. Wigglesworth & K. Pape (Eds.), *Perinatal brain lesions* (pp. 1–23). Boston: Blackwell Scientific Publications.

Yen, I. H., Khoury, M. J., Erickson, J. D., et al. (1992). The changing epidemiology of neural tube defects. United States, 1968–1989. *American Journal of Diseases of Children, 146*(7), 857–861.

CHAPTER 30

Assessment and Management of Musculoskeletal Dysfunction

JOYCE BUTLER

RESEARCH AGENDA

What are the parental perceptions of an infant with a musculoskeletal disorder?

How are growth and development affected by the diagnosis of a relatively mild musculoskeletal dysfunction such as clubfoot?

What effect does the stimulation of fetal movement via fetal physical therapy or stimulants such as caffeine have on the development of congenital contractures?

What are the common characteristics of subluxated hips that will spontaneously reduce without treatment?

What effect does a positive family history have on the incidence of clubfoot?

What is the impact of the diagnosis of birth trauma on maternal-infant interactions?

VIGNETTE

Working as a nurse in a newborn nursery while expecting my second child was a very long and anxious 9 months. As a nurse, I see so many of the tragic things that can happen to shatter the dream of the perfect baby every mother expects. I kept telling myself to focus on the happy outcomes, but the unfortunate ones always stood out in my mind.

After a basically uneventful pregnancy, my second child was delivered by C-section because of breech presentation. I can still recall the tears of joy and relief when I first saw the daughter I've always wanted. She looked so perfect! Nine months of worry disappeared—until the next morning when she was examined by her pediatrician. He discovered that she had a "hip click." X-rays were done to confirm the diagnosis. I knew exactly what this meant. My thoughts flashed back to a family, who, a few weeks before, was preparing to go home with their infant with the same condition. Their child was being treated with a Pavlik harness. I could recall thinking how hideous and cumbersome the appliance appeared and feeling sorry for the parents who had to deal with this problem. I had felt ineffective as a nurse because of the lack of support I could provide for this family. Now here was my daughter going through the same ordeal.

Talking with the orthopedic physician later that afternoon did not ease my anxiety. We were given all the statistics on the condition; females are affected five times more often than males, with breech presentation being an environmental factor. Our daughter had one hip that was "dislocatable"; the other was subluxated. The treatment was the same for both, the Pavlik harness. The harness was immediately applied and was to be left in place for a then undetermined length of time. The duration of treatment depended on when her joints would begin to "stabilize." The harness, which looks like parachute body gear with leg straps, holds the infant's legs in abduction to keep the head of the femur in correct alignment with the acetabulum. Frequent x-rays and checkups would be done to ensure that the treatment was effective. We were also told that there was a chance that the harness would not correct the problem and that surgery may be needed. Oh, and let's not forget that there was always the chance that my daughter would have difficulty walking. Add all this information together, combined with postoperative cesarean pain, changing hormones, and grief over the loss of the "perfect child," and you end up with overwhelming emotions of anxiety and grief. I recall worrying about any discomfort my daughter might be having, although I was assured that she had none. The harness just looked so uncomfortable! I worried that she might require more treatment than the harness could provide. I felt guilty that I somehow caused this condition. But most of all, I felt that her problem, compared with everything else that could have happened, was minor. Why couldn't I deal with this rationally? My daughter could have been born with a chronic or even fatal condition for which I would have gladly traded only a "hip click." But I guess new mothers have coped with enough and aren't always able to think rationally.

Despite how awful things appeared, my family and I did adjust. Bath time took twice as long as normal because the harness had to be worn at all times. I found disposable diapers more efficient than cloth, not only in changing, but in keeping the harness clean. There were no restrictions in positioning her, although she would be unable to roll over while in the harness. I wondered how this would affect her development. Probably the most difficult aspect of this ordeal was dealing with other people's reactions. Curious people would stop and stare, and an occasional one would ask, "What's wrong with your little girl?" This would always come at a time when I thought I was coping well, and a comment like that would reorient me to the fact that we were dealing with a problem with an uncertain outcome.

The day finally came 3½ months later when the treatment

was complete. The harness was removed! I can still remember the feeling I had when I held my little girl essentially for the first time without the harness. She was so soft and cuddly, and I could get so close to her with nothing between us. It was wonderful! She looked even more beautiful in her frilly pink dresses. She rolled over the first night without the brace. She walked without difficulty at 8½ months and hasn't stopped moving since! Most of my worries were left behind, although I still occasionally worry about all the x-rays to which she was exposed.

There have been several newborns in the nursery since then who have had the same problem as my daughter. I can easily put myself in the place of a mother of a child with any problem, whatever it may be, and better understand what they're going through. I hope I have helped those people to better understand and cope with their disappointments and to find comfort and strength from my experience.

Sandy Heim

Abnormalities of the neonatal musculoskeletal system may range from a subtle brachydactyly to a fatalistic form of osteogenesis imperfecta congenita. Causes range from uterine malpositioning of the fetus to autosomal dominant disorders. Regardless of the clinical significance, an overt structural defect can become the focus of parental attention.

Assessment of the musculoskeletal system, which can be fraught with normal variants, as well as knowledge of pathogenesis, sequelae, treatment, and prognoses for deformities of this system is imperative to the clinician. Delay in diagnosis and treatment may be implicated as a cause of a less than favorable outcome of the musculoskeletal deformity. Appropriate education of the family by the health care professional is often paramount to a beneficial outcome because many musculoskeletal disorders require compliance with long-term therapy.

The following are common terms that are used when discussing the musculoskeletal system:

1. *Valgus* refers to a deformity in which a body part is bent outward and away from the midline of the body; it is a part that is in abduction.
2. *Varus* implies a body part positioned inward, toward the midline of the body; it is a part that is in adduction.
3. *Talipes* refers to any one of various foot deformities.
4. *Reduction* is restoration to a normal position.
5. *Clinodactyly* is the medial or lateral deflection of one or more fingers.

Deformities of the musculoskeletal system create not only functional problems but, in some cases, visible defects as well. The type of dysfunction may greatly affect how the parent views the neonate and the infant's potential for positive growth and development.

This chapter outlines the common musculoskeletal dysfunctions seen during the neonatal period. In addition, it describes the collaborative management as well as the long-term implications of the functional and aesthetic problems encountered with musculoskeletal dysfunction.

EMBRYOLOGY

The embryonic period is characterized by maximal organogenesis and lasts from the end of the first week until the eighth week of gestation. The embryo originates from three cell layers, referred to as the ectoderm, endoderm, and mesoderm. The embryonic mesoderm gives rise to the articular, muscular, and skeletal systems.

The articular system, or joints, can be classified into three types: fibrous, cartilaginous, and synovial. Fibrous joints are those in which two bones are separated only by dense fibrous connective tissue, as seen in cranial sutures. Cartilaginous joints (such as the symphysis pubis) have hyaline cartilage or fibrocartilage between the two bony surfaces. The elbow and knee are examples of synovial joints. In these joints, the adjoining bone ends are covered with a thin cartilaginous layer and joined by a ligament lined with a synovial membrane. This synovial membrane secretes a lubricant referred to as synovial fluid, a source of nutrition for the articular cartilage. The articular system begins to develop during the sixth week of gestation, with functional joints being present by the end of the eighth week.

Groups of myotubes, the primordia of skeletal or striated muscle, are apparent by the end of the eighth week of gestation. As the myotubes enlarge, the appearance of myofilaments is evident in the interior regions. Growth of myofilaments leads to mature muscle fibers. Postnatal development of muscle fibers continues both in number and in size. Muscle development is dependent on proper innervation, evident at 8 to 10 weeks of gestation. Without this innervation, the muscles atrophy. Intrauterine fetal movements can be detected by the mother at 16 weeks of gestation.

The upper and lower limb buds first appear by the end of the fourth week of gestation. Sequential development progresses from limb buds, to hand and foot plates with digital rays, to hand and foot with separate digits at 8 weeks' gestation. The upper limbs develop more quickly than the lower limbs, and there is a lapse of several days between the development of the upper limbs and that of the lower limbs.

The skeleton develops by intramembranous bone formation and enchondral ossification. The vertebral column is initially of a cartilaginous form, with ossification beginning during the embryonic period and reaching completion in early adulthood. Ossification is evident in all long bones by 12 weeks' gestation.

Rapid cell division during organogenesis renders an organ vulnerable to any disturbance that might result in aberrant development. The most sensitive period for the development of major morphologic deformation of the limbs is from the beginning of the fourth until just shortly after the sixth week of gestation. Functional and minor morphologic abnormalities may occur any time during gestation. The skeletal system, because of its rapid growth through puberty, has a prolonged period of sensitivity.

ASSESSMENT

Astute systematic observation is the key tool for the clinician in assessing the neonatal musculoskeletal system. Visual inspection should begin in one body region, that is, cephalic or caudal, and progress along the body in an organized fashion. For the initial examination, the infant should be in a quiet resting state to assess posture, positioning, and identification of any overt anomalies. Active movement by the infant allows the clinician to view muscle tone and active ranges of motion. Manipulation is used to assess passive range of motion, including joint mobility. Radiologic studies as well as simple body measurements aid the clinician in the collection of evidence of covert musculoskeletal deformities.

In developing a differential diagnosis, the clinician must be aware that a combination of deformities presenting in a neonate may be a small part of a larger syndrome. Conversely, congenital anomalies presenting in combination in one infant may be a coincidental finding (Table 30–1).

TYPES OF MUSCULOSKELETAL DYSFUNCTION

Osteogenesis Imperfecta

Osteogenesis imperfecta (OI) is a connective tissue disorder with genetic origins. The primary pathophysiologic defect involves

TABLE 30–1 Common Musculoskeletal Conditions

Skeletal Dysplasias
Osteogenesis imperfecta
Achondroplasia
Arthrogryposis
Congenital hip dislocation
Limb Defects
Clubfoot
Syndactyly
Polydactyly
Amniotic band syndrome
Miscellaneous
Birth trauma
Torticollis

the collagen structure. Collagen (the major extracellular protein) formation fails to progress beyond the reticulin fiber stage. Further significant disruption in the collagen formation in OI includes a defect in cross-linking that results in decreased collagen stability (Francis et al., 1974). Even though osteoblastic activity appears normal, there is typically no collagen production (Follis, 1952). Any tissue containing collagen, such as sclerae, bones, ligaments, and teeth, may be affected.

Through various clinical, genetic, and biochemical studies, it has been determined that OI is of a heterogeneous nature; it may result from autosomal recessive or autosomal dominant disorders as well as from spontaneous mutations (Spitz, 1996). Clinical presentations of OI range from mild affectations to individuals with fatalistic prognoses.

Numerous attempts have been made to develop a taxonomy for OI. Because of limited knowledge as to the exact pathomechanics of the disease, however, a precise classification system remains elusive. The most widely used classification system was developed by Sillence and Danks in the late 1970s (Sillence & Danks, 1978). This system is a numerical classification based on clinical and genetic factors. There are four major groups: two are autosomal recessive and two are autosomal dominant. Two of the groups (OI types I and IV) are subdivided according to the absence or presence of dentin abnormalities (dentinogenesis imperfecta). Dentinogenesis imperfecta occurs when the dentin layer is affected concomitant with constriction of the pulp space (Lukinmaa et al., 1987). The clinical appearance of dentinogenesis imperfecta involves teeth that are grayish blue to brown in color. The teeth are typically worn down because there is decreased resistance to pressure. The deciduous teeth are more often affected than the permanent teeth. It is important to explain to the parents that the aesthetic appearance of the child may improve with the emergence of permanent teeth.

Osteogenesis Imperfecta Type I

OI type I is an autosomal dominant disorder. As with many other dominant disorders, there is variable penetrance. This means that the clinical appearance of affected individuals in the same family may range from mild to severe. Severe forms of OI present with early-onset fractures, and the frequency of fractures is increased. Other clinical features include severe hearing impairment, with an incidence of 40:1, and a majority of the affected individuals (75:1) report a preponderance for bruising. The sclera is often bluish as well.

OI type I is subdivided into types IA and IB. Type IA occurs without dentinogenesis imperfecta, whereas evidence of dentin abnormalities is seen in type IB.

The incidence of OI type I is 1 in 30,000 (Sillence et al., 1979a). The clinical presentation of this disorder is evident in the neonatal period in 10 percent of affected individuals. Fractures are the primary sign in neonates. Affected neonates typically have normal height and weight for their gestational age. Because of the progressive nature of kyphoscoliosis (a component of OI disorders), however, short stature develops in most affected persons.

Osteogenesis Imperfecta Type II

OI type II is an autosomal recessive disorder. It is an extremely severe OI disorder resulting in death either in the prenatal or neonatal period. Prenatal diagnosis is possible with this condition. Death occurs through damage to vital organs—brain, liver, and lungs—not protected by the fragile bony structures. The incidence has been reported as 1 in 62,487 (Sillence et al., 1979b).

Neonates affected with this disorder are typically small for gestational age and appear dwarf-like. The extremities are deformed and short as a result of multiple fractures and crumbling of the long bones. Chest radiographs exhibit beaded ribs with numerous fractures, both old and new. Blue sclera are characteristic features in both OI type I and OI type II. Blue sclera can be a normal finding in neonates, however, and cannot serve as a diagnostic criterion for this age group (Gertner & Root, 1990).

Trauma of birth exacts a further toll on the appearance of these infants, contributing to the maceration of the head and limbs. This form of OI is also referred to as the perinatal lethal form.

Osteogenesis Imperfecta Type III

OI type III is a rare, severe disorder with autosomal recessive inheritance patterns. Fractures may be present at birth, and the clinical course may simulate OI type II. Variations between types II and III are identified on physical examination. Neonates affected with OI type III have normal height and weight for gestational age at birth. Although there may be multiple rib fractures on chest radiograph, there is an absence of the beaded rib appearance. The long bones in OI type II are crumbled, whereas, in OI type III, the bones have multiple fractures and calcifications. The extremities do not usually appear deformed as in OI type II; however, individuals affected with OI type III have the shortest stature for all OI disorders. Mortality rates for children with OI type III are high because they have severe kyphoscoliosis (Sillence, 1981).

Osteogenesis Imperfecta Type IV

OI type IV is similar to type I in that it is an autosomal dominant disorder with variable penetrance. OI type IV is subdivided into types IVA and IVB, depending on the absence or presence of dentinogenesis imperfecta. OI type IV resembles types I and III in clinical presentation and course. Incidence rates for OI types III and IV have not yet been established.

Diagnosis

Accurate diagnosis of OI disorders is of primary concern for the affected individual and family. Recurrence rates and inheritance patterns vary among the recessive and dominant forms. There are also instances of OI resulting from spontaneous mutations.

Any of the forms of OI can be present at birth, although severity varies among the different types. In the milder cases, fractures in the neonatal period may result from birth trauma. Fractures are most abundant in the arms, legs, clavicles, and ribs. As the infant ages, the lower extremities are affected more frequently as a result of increased weight-bearing trauma.

Calcification is rapid in neonates, with callus formation usually occurring within 10 days. There does not appear to be a deficiency in callus formation in OI disorders; however, the callus is weaker than in normal individuals and predisposes the bone to further fractures in that area.

Multiple rib fractures in a neonate may prompt respiratory compromise, because the pain from the fracture thwarts the infant's breathing attempts. OI may be suspected when it is difficult to wean an infant from ventilatory support and other pathologic causes have been ruled out. In such cases, chest radiographs should be closely inspected for rib fractures and callus formation.

Case reports have identified newborns sustaining fractures of the femurs during routine examination of the hip for dysplasia. Paterson and colleagues (1992) reported eight cases of OI that were not recognized until either one or both femurs sustained fractures during hip examination. Of these eight cases, seven infants exhibited significant distress, immediately followed by prolonged crying, decreased movement of the extremity, or both.

Treatment

There is no treatment for the underlying pathologic cause of OI disorders. Therefore, management of OI centers around support and promotion of independence in terms of mobility, function, and social integration. Binder and associates (1993) discussed current rehabilitation strategies for children with OI. The children, aged 35 months to 10 years 10 months, were grouped according to physical and functional capacities. All children exhibited some degree of handicap, ranging from severe bowing of the extremities, joint contractures, and fractures to abnormal gait patterns. Rehabilitation techniques included active range of motion, strengthening exercises, stretching, and coordination exercises. Water activities appeared well tolerated, even in patients with severe affectations. The investigators demonstrated improved function in all children maintained with persistent, individualized therapy (Binder et al., 1993). Outcome appears enhanced when physical and occupational therapies are instituted promptly after birth, condition allowing.

Collaborative Management

In the neonatal period, infants with OI are managed according to clinical presentation and protocol for that particular gestational age. Health care professionals and the patient's family must handle the infant carefully. Padded splints for the extremities may help reduce the incidence of accidental fractures, and signs should be posted on the infant's bed to warn all individuals of the consequences of improper handling. As the infant grows, padded orthotic devices support the trunk and extremities to reduce the incidence of skeletal deformities, such as kyphoscoliosis.

Vascular checks of the casted or splinted extremity are required. A pink color of the capillary bed indicates adequate arterial flow, white (or pallor) symbolizes decreased or poor arterial flow, and cyanosis of the extremity indicates venous stasis. Although pulse checks may be helpful, the caregiver should realize that, by the time a pulse is absent, irreparable harm has probably occurred. For this reason, parents should be taught how to assess color and capillary refill rather than pulse palpation.

An infant with OI necessitates skin care in terms of positioning. Bedding should be such that discourages decubitus formation, because the infant may have minimal spontaneous movement secondary to pain from the fractures. It is wise for the caregiver to ask a colleague for assistance when repositioning these infants. Splints (e.g., rolled blankets or sandbags) placed beside the infant's chest stabilize the thoracic wall and potentiate effective ventilation. These splints are most effective in cases of multiple rib fractures.

Pain relief through medication and supportive measures should be considered for the infant. The infant may react to pain caused by multiple fractures through facial grimacing and crying upon movement. Alterations in vital signs (e.g., tachycardia, tachypnea, hypertension), irritability, and restlessness have also been attributed to pain in the neonate. (See Chapter 40, Identification, Management, and Prevention of Pain in the Neonate.)

Family education and support are integral components in the management of the neonate's care. Parents and other family members may be reluctant to hold and cuddle the infant for fear of causing additional fractures. The clinician should educate the family on proper handling of the infant. It should be stressed to the family that fractures are inevitable in the infant with OI.

Achondroplasia

Although the word achondroplasia was once used to describe any form of dwarfism, it is now recognized as one distinct type of dwarfism having characteristic features. Achondroplasia, the most common type of dwarfism, has an autosomal dominant pattern of inheritance. Most cases occur by spontaneous mutation. Achondroplasia occurs in 3 in 1 million live births (Gardner, 1977).

Other forms of dwarfism include hypochondroplasia, thanatophoric dwarfism, achondrogenesis, and short-rib polydactyly syndrome. Therefore, a differential diagnosis must be made as to which type of dwarfism is present and which treatment should be started.

Differential Diagnosis

The differential diagnosis of an infant with dwarfism includes achondroplasia, OI type II, thanatophoric dwarfism, and achondrogenesis. In achondroplasia, the patient has markedly shortened limbs and often bowing of the lower limbs, but radiographic studies do not show evidence of multiple fractures and long-bone crumbling as is seen in OI type II. Thanatophoric dwarfism and achondrogenesis, both typically fatal in the neonatal period, are characterized by an extremely narrow chest and marked defective ossification, respectively.

Clinical Manifestations

Achondroplasia is apparent at birth, unlike hypochondroplasia, which becomes clinically significant at 5 to 6 years of age. Characteristic features of achondroplasia include dwarfism with a disproportionately large head size resulting from an increased anteroposterior skull diameter; flattened nasal bridge with a prominent frontal region; short, broad hands; and a flattened anterior chest wall with costal flaring. Later, an exaggerated lumbar lordosis and increased muscular development become obvious. Intelligence is usually normal; however, a positive self-esteem may be difficult to establish.

Collaborative Management

Respiratory or ventilatory management of the severely affected achondroplastic dwarf is the primary concern. It can be challenging to support positive pulmonary functioning when there is reduced lung volume capacity within the narrow thorax. Mildly affected infants may compensate for decreased lung volume with a mild to moderate increase in the work of breathing. As the infant grows, this compensation becomes more difficult.

Compensatory mechanisms, such as increased work of breathing in the mildly affected achondroplastic dwarf, require that meticulous attention be paid to nutritional support of the increased energy needs. An infant exhibiting tachypnea or retractions must have increased caloric intake for positive growth to occur. If growth proceeds too rapidly, however, the infant's body mass may exceed the pulmonary capacity and decompensation may occur. Nutritionists may provide insights into the daily management of providing calories but not adding to the work of the infant.

Parental and family needs may be satisfied through education and collaboration with social services. Support groups specifically for parents of dwarfed infants are organized in many cities. From these groups, parents can gain a better perspective of the long-term development of their infant.

Long-Term Consequences of Achondroplasia

Complications of achondroplasia are primarily neurologic, involving the spinal nerves. Anatomic configuration of the intraspinal canal results in pressure on the cord and spinal nerves. This pressure produces chronic backache and, in the most severe scenario, paraplegia. Referrals to physical and occupational therapists along with long-term orthopedic follow-up can reduce some of the complications. If these changes in the spinal column do occur, the child is at greater risk for development of increased respiratory difficulties, mobility problems, self-concept and self-esteem concerns, physical pain, and central or peripheral nervous system neuropathies.

Because children with achondroplasia have a different appearance than their peers, any exaggeration of the condition can add to a faulty self-concept. As the child grows, it is important for both health professionals and parents to assess continually the personal image that is being formed in the child's mind. Positive support of parents during the neonatal period through comments about what the infant is doing and how the infant looks may provide a role model of positive behavior that the parents can emulate with the child.

Arthrogryposis

Historically, the term arthrogryposis (curved, hooked joint) has been used not only to provide a description of a clinical appearance but also as a diagnosis for various conditions. The one common denominator for conditions termed arthrogryposis is the presence of multiple congenital joint contractures. There are more than 150 known conditions in which multiple congenital contractures are the dominant feature, many of which are syndromes unrelated to a chromosomal or genetic problem (Clark & Eteson, 1991; Moessinger, 1983). The most common forms are autosomal dominant distal arthrogryposis, amyoplasia, multiple pterygium syndrome, and cerebro-oculo-facio-skeletal syndrome (Clark & Eteson, 1991). A less common form that is currently being examined by geneticists is Pena-Shokeir syndrome. Consequently, the name arthrogryposis multiplex congenita is often used to incorporate these many uses of the word.

An infant born with multiple congenital contractures may have either a specific syndrome or a chromosomal anomaly. It is important to achieve a precise diagnosis of the infant with multiple congenital contractures because recurrence risks vary among the different entities, and genetic counseling is dependent on knowledge of recurrences.

Arthrogryposis involves congenital, nonprogressive limitation of movement in two or more joints in different body areas (Hall, 1981). The deformity is primarily a result of fibrous and fatty changes in muscles secondary to decreased fetal movement. Although muscles undergo normal embryologic development, they are replaced by fibrous and fatty tissue after a reduction of normal fetal movement. The physiologic muscle changes subsequently produce contracted joints. Animal studies have produced congenital joint contractures by decreasing fetal movement through various processes (Drachman & Coulombre, 1962; Fuller, 1975; Moessinger, 1983). Ultimately, any process resulting in limited intrauterine movement by the fetus can lead to multiple congenital contractures (Hall, 1983). The severity of such contractures increases with a longer duration of limited movement. The earlier in fetal development that the limitation is imposed, the greater the severity of contractures. The causes of decreased fetal movement can be classified into three categories, which are listed in Table 30–2.

Incidence and Inheritance Patterns

The incidence of multiple congenital contractures is 1 in 3000 live births (Hall, 1989). Hall (1981) examined 350 infants and divided them into three categories based on the body areas affected by the contractures. This classification system, which is still in use, can provide a prognostic indicator for the clinician.

The first category primarily involves the limbs. Most affected infants are in this category, and otherwise they are normal. The second category primarily involves contractures in the limbs, but also involves other organ systems, predominantly the visceral organs. The third category involves multiple congenital contractures concurrent with central nervous system (CNS) dysfunction.

The first category can be subdivided into amyoplasia and distal arthrogryposis. Amyoplasia, a sporadic condition, is considered to be classic arthrogryposis. The sporadic nature of this condition refers to the lack of an identifiable inheritance pattern when a family history is examined. Thus, families with an affected member are not at increased risk for recurrence. Distal arthrogryposis is inherited by an autosomal dominant pattern (Clark & Eteson, 1991). Parents with an infant with distal arthrogryposis can have a risk calculation done by a genetics counselor to give them an idea of their potential for having another child with this same condition.

Two other types of arthrogryposis have an autosomal recessive inheritance pattern. The first is multiple pterygium syndrome, which consists of webbed, contracted fingers with later development of camptodactyly; micrognathia; low-set rotated ears; palpebral fissures that appear to have a downward slant; ptosis; rocker-bottom feet, much like those of an infant with trisomy 13 or 18;

TABLE 30–2 Etiology of Decreased Fetal Movement

Category	Examples
Myopathic	
Abnormal muscle function secondary to failure of muscle formation or degeneration	Congenital muscular dystrophy Absence of muscles
Neuropathic	
Abnormal nerve function or innervation; involving either CNS or peripheral nervous system	Drugs or toxins CNS malformations: decreased number of anterior horn cells
Abnormal connective tissue	Abnormal formation of bone, cartilage, tendons, or connective tissue
Mechanical Limitation	
Produces compression within the uterus	Twins Amniotic bands Oligohydramnios Uterine myomas

CNS, central nervous system.

possibly neck webbing; and possibly cleft palate (Clark & Eteson, 1991). The second syndrome is cerebro-oculo-facio-skeletal syndrome. It is associated with failure to thrive postnatally, microcephaly, intracranial calcifications, shortened palpebral fissures, and congenital cataracts (Clark & Eteson, 1991). These children usually die by school age.

Another form of arthrogryposis, which is very rare, is Pena-Shokeir syndrome. An infant with this syndrome has a short umbilical cord, pulmonary hypoplasia, intrauterine growth retardation, ankyloses, and camptodactyly (Clark & Eteson, 1991). The maternal history includes oligohydramnios and fetal akinesia, or decreased fetal movement. This condition may have an autosomal recessive inheritance pattern, but this has not been confirmed. This condition is the second most common condition involving multiple congenital contractures of the limbs. Distal arthrogryposis is an autosomal dominant disorder with variable penetrance (Hall et al., 1982).

Clinical Manifestations

On physical examination, amyoplasia has a typical appearance, with symmetric joint involvement, usually of all four limbs, and decreased muscle mass. Frequency of joint involvement increases from proximal to distal joints. Therefore, there is almost universal severe equinovarus deformity, and the wrists are typically flexed. The elbows and knees can be in a flexed or extended position; however, in most cases, both upper and lower extremities are in extension. There may be notable dimpling at the elbows and knees. Shoulders are internally rotated, and hips are frequently dislocated. Normal skin creases overlying the joints are absent, and the skin is tense and glossy.

The facies of an infant with amyoplasia are characterized by a round face and mild micrognathia. A midline hemangioma involving the eyes, nasal bridge, and forehead may be present and usually fades with time.

Newborn infants affected with amyoplasia are usually active but with decreased limb movement. They feed well, although positioning of the infant during feeding and routine baby care presents a challenge. Distal arthrogryposis primarily involves the hands and feet. On physical examination, the hands of the newborn with distal arthrogryposis have a typical appearance and thus are easily recognized. Hands are clenched, with the thumb flexed into the palm. Fingers cross over the thumb and palm, usually overlapping each other. This hand position resembles that of an infant with trisomy 18.

Collaborative Management

Excluding infants with concurrent CNS dysfunction, infants with multiple congenital contractures have excellent prognoses. The goal of collaborative management is to achieve and maintain an acceptable range of motion in the affected joints. With appropriate management, independent living is attainable for many individuals.

Physical therapy should be initiated early in the neonatal period. Collaboration with physical and occupational therapists should begin in the neonatal intensive care unit. In the past, infants with multiple congenital contractures were casted; however, this therapy was found to produce additional muscle atrophy secondary to the immobilization. Currently, physical therapy is used in conjunction with splinting when necessary.

Physical therapy is a lifetime process, and parents are taught the techniques to use with their child. Parental or family involvement is a key factor in the success of the physical therapy for these infants. Creativity on the part of the health care professional as well as the parents complements efforts to manipulate the rather rigid infant during feedings, sleeping, holding, and daily care activities. Parents may need referrals to agencies that can provide respite care or assistance from volunteers to carry out these physical therapies on a daily basis. The nurse may collaborate with social workers and financial counselors on behalf of the families for help with services and financing.

Research Findings

Based on the theory that multiple congenital contractures are a direct result of decreased fetal movement, researchers are examining ways to stimulate fetal movement for fetuses considered to be at high risk for the development of multiple congenital contractures. High-risk attributes include positive family history of arthrogryposis, maternal complaints of decreased fetal movement, oligohydramnios, and known or family history of muscle, nerve, CNS, or connective tissue abnormalities that might lead to decreased ability to move fetal body parts during development.

If in utero contractures occur because of fetal akinesia, then any stimulation of movement during development has the potential for preventing contracted joints. Stimulation could be in the form of intrauterine physical therapy and drugs such as caffeine to stimulate fetal activity.

Prognosis

The long-term prognosis for multiple congenital contractures depends on the extent of involvement. Hall (1981) reported a mortality rate of only 1 percent for infants affected primarily with limb involvement. Infants with limb and other organ involvement had a 7 percent mortality rate, whereas those with limb and CNS involvement experienced a 50 percent mortality rate.

Bianchi and Van Marter (1994) observed certain characteristics that placed the fetus in a high-risk category. These maternal/neonatal characteristics included a history of decreased fetal movements, hydramnios, contractures, micrognathia, and, on radiologic examination, thin ribs. Within a 10-year period, the researchers documented a 93 percent mortality rate (14 of 15) in infants with the diagnosis of arthrogryposis in the newborn period and requiring mechanical ventilation from birth.

Autopsies of the 14 infants revealed an equal distribution of CNS anomalies, neuropathies, and myopathies. The surviving infant initially given the diagnosis of arthrogryposis was ultimately determined to have myasthenia gravis (Bianchi & Van Marter, 1994).

Developmental Dysplasia of the Hip (DDH)

Developmental dysplasia (formerly called congenital dislocation) of the hip (DDH) refers to any manifestation of hip instability, ranging from subluxation to complete dislocation. DDH remains a common problem despite almost universal neonatal screening. Reports indicate success rates as high as 100 percent for the diagnosis of DDH in the neonatal period, yet these same reports also suggest that neonatal screening programs are ineffective (Robertson, 1984). Although controversy surrounds the usefulness of neonatal screening programs for the diagnosis of DDH, these programs have led to earlier diagnosis and treatment for many infants. Because some infants possess normal hip movement, some examinations may initially be normal, yet later exhibit abnormal hip development. Dysplastic hip screenings should be performed at routine health visits at 2 weeks and at 2, 4, 6, 9, and 12 months of age.

Incidence Rates and Risk Factors

There are various reports indicating the incidence of DDH. The incidence of DDH in the United States is approximately 10 in 1000 live births. In New York, Artz and associates (1975) reported the incidence of DDH to be 4.9 in 1000 in blacks and 15.5 in 1000 in whites. The incidence of DDH in Chinese children is almost nonexistent: 0.1 in 1000 (Hoaglund et al., 1981). However, Walker (1935) reported an incidence of 188.5 in 1000 for individuals in the Island Lake Regions in Manitoba.

Differences in incidence rates of DDH can be attributed to genetic, ethnic, and environmental influences. Other influential factors include the age of the infant at the time of examination, the expertise of the examiner, and the definition used by the examiner for the diagnosis of DDH.

There is an increased incidence of DDH in first-born children (Carter & Wilkinson, 1964). This increase may be due to the unstretched uterine and abdominal muscles, oligohydramnios, and the high association of fetal breech positioning in primigravidas. There is a definite preponderance toward DDH in female children. The ratio of occurrence of DDH in girls to boys is 6:1 (Bennett & MacEwen, 1989). Females account for 80 percent of all cases of DDH. Factors that may contribute to this finding include the fact that twice as many females as males present in the breech position, and, in females, there appears to be a heightened laxity in response to maternal relaxin hormones.

The breech position remains a major contributory factor to the development of DDH. Authors have reported that anywhere from 16 to 25 percent of affected infants are born in the breech presentation (Tachdjian, 1990a). Specific incidences of DDH in relationship to positioning are 0.7 percent for cephalic, 2 percent for footling, and 20 percent for single breech. The incidence of DDH for infants in the breech presentation is not altered by delivery methods. Breech-positioned infants delivered by cesarean section have the same predisposition to hip dislocation as those delivered vaginally (Artz et al., 1975).

The left hip is involved three times more frequently than the right hip. Approximately 60 percent of DDH is on the left side, 20 percent on the right side, and 20 percent bilateral (Tachdjian, 1990a). This finding is attributed to the tendency of the fetus to lie with its left thigh against the maternal sacrum. This position forces the left hip into a posture of flexion and adduction. Thus, the femoral head is covered more by the joint capsule than by the acetabulum.

For infants born with other musculoskeletal and congenital renal abnormalities, such as torticollis and Potter's association, the incidence of DDH is increased. Congenital renal abnormalities can result in fetal oliguria, subsequently producing oligohydramnios. (See Chapter 31, Assessment and Management of Genitourinary Dysfunction.) Oligohydramnios can cause postural deformities because of the mechanical pressure on the fetus (Tachdjian, 1990a). Torticollis, arthrogryposis, and metatarsus adductus are thought to result from intrauterine compression, as does DDH.

After 40 weeks' gestation, the femoral head in the normal infant is firmly seated in the acetabulum and remains positioned there by the surface tension of the synovial fluid. The hips of a normal infant are difficult to dislocate. Conversely, the infant with a dysplastic hip has a loosely fitting femoral head and acetabulum. Because of this pathophysiologic phenomenon, the femoral head can assume several abnormal positions in an infant with DDH. One such position is termed subluxation. Subluxation occurs when the femoral head can be moved to the edge of the acetabulum but not completely out of it. Another position is termed a dislocatable hip. A dislocatable hip exists when the femoral head can be displaced from the acetabulum by manipulation, but returns to the acetabulum afterward. The femoral head can also be found in a completely dislocated position at birth. Dislocated hips may or may not be reduced by manipulation.

DDH is a dynamic disorder that may improve or deteriorate with or without treatment. Thus, the joint may spontaneously dislocate and reduce (return to normal position) with normal neonatal movement. At the initial phase of the disorder, seen during the neonatal period, there is no other significant pathologic concern. With time, this simple mechanism progresses in complexity secondary to adaptive changes. DDH can eventually progress to either permanent reduction, complete dislocation, or dysplasia (abnormal development). More than 60 percent of infants with hip instability stabilize within the first week of life and 88 percent stabilize within the second month postnatally. Only 12 percent of infants with initial hip instability are considered to have DDH with potential for progression.

When complete dislocation occurs, pathologic changes occur to the femoral head, acetabulum, and ilium. This complete dislocation is due to the adaptive changes that occur in the adjacent tissue and bone. The long-term complication of dislocation, when adequate treatment has not occurred, is degenerative changes of both the femoral head and the acetabulum. Once adaptive changes occur, there is an increased risk for progressive degeneration despite treatment.

The subluxated hip, when not diagnosed in the neonatal period, is generally diagnosed at adolescence, when the strain of puberty and rapid growth spurts occur. With subluxation, the femoral head is laterally displaced and pushed upward into the joint; it is not completely out of the acetabulum. As the child grows and there is increased weight bearing, the femoral head slides around and moves to the joint's edge. Degenerative changes result from this continual sliding. Sclerosis of the underlying bone, loss of cartilage, and formation of degenerative cysts are the most common degenerative changes (Fanaroff & Martin, 1997).

Diagnosis and Clinical Manifestations

In the neonatal period, the Ortolani and Barlow maneuvers are useful in making the diagnosis of DDH. The Ortolani test is used to determine dislocation in the hip of a newborn, and the Barlow test is used to determine whether the hip is dislocatable (Barlow, 1962; Ortolani, 1976). In practice, both procedures are done in sequence. For examination, the infant is placed on a firm surface in the supine position. The infant should be relaxed and quiet. Only one hip should be examined at a time.

To perform the Ortolani test, the neonatal nurse specialist stabilizes the infant's pelvis with one hand and, with the other hand, grasps the infant's thigh on the side to be tested. The nurse's middle finger is located over the greater trochanter (lateral aspect of the upper thigh), and the thumb is across the knee. The nurse flexes the infant's hip to 90 degrees while bending the infant's knee. The infant's leg is then gently abducted with an anterior lift. In a positive Ortolani test, a "clunk" is heard with abduction. This clunk occurs as the dislocated femoral head slides over the posterior rim of the acetabulum and into the hip socket. Next, the hip is adducted, and, for the infant with DDH, a second clunk can be heard as the femoral head is displaced out of the acetabulum.

False-positive diagnoses of DDH have occurred when the examiner misinterprets a normal "click" (high-pitched sound) for a clunk. A click is not a sign of DDH. Clicks may be heard as a result of snapping of ligaments or tendons and are normal.

Barlow's test determines instability of the hip and identifies those hips that can be dislocated upon manipulation. Both hips and knees are flexed, with the hip to be tested in slight adduction. The examiner's middle finger remains positioned as for the Ortolani test, over the greater trochanter. However, the thumb is located over the medial aspect of the infant's lower thigh. Gentle pressure is exerted by the thumb posteriorly and laterally (down and out). For the infant with DDH, the femoral head can be felt to move out of the acetabulum with the typical clunk. The hip can then be reduced by the Ortolani maneuver or simply by releasing thumb pressure and abducting and flexing the hips.

When the femoral head is subluxated, the examiner may observe a sliding motion in the hip joint during physical examination. This sliding motion can be characteristic of an unstable hip joint. Most cases of unstable hips spontaneously resolve without treatment. Because there is no way to determine which hips will reduce and stabilize without treatment, it is best to treat all unstable hips.

The use of sonography is valuable for DDH detection but radiographic examination is not, because of the cartilaginous composition of the neonatal pelvis.

Collaborative Management

The goal of collaborative management is to achieve and maintain reduction of the unstable hip. The sooner treatment is implemented, the greater the chance for successful outcome. Various splinting devices are used to treat DDH in infants. Examples of splints include the Pavlik harness, von Rosen splint, Denis Browne hip adduction splint, and Frejka pillow splint. The most commonly used splint for neonates is the Pavlik harness.

The Pavlik harness allows for spontaneous hip and lower extremity movement while maintaining reduction of the hip joint. It can be worn comfortably during all aspects of normal newborn care, including diaper changes. The Pavlik harness can be adjusted for growth. It is indicated for use in newborns and infants up to 6 months of age. Use of the Pavlik harness is contraindicated for infants able to stand and for those infants in whom the hip joint is not reducible by manipulation, specifically the Ortolani procedure, because the infant may attempt to bear weight with the harness on, potentially pushing the hip out of alignment. This movement counteracts reduction of the hip joint. The greatest danger is that the child will become entangled in the parachute-like straps while attempting to push up to a standing position. It is possible for children to hang themselves in the straps.

A major factor influencing the success of the Pavlik harness is parental compliance with the treatment. One study (Corbett, 1988) that surveyed the parents of 22 infants undergoing treatment with a Pavlik harness reported that all parents removed the harness at some time. Most of the parents were able to reapply the harness without difficulty, whereas others were unable to reapply the harness correctly. Thus, parents were attempting to use the harness at least periodically but were not completely compliant with care instructions. Against medical advice, parents discontinued the harness for the following reasons: to ease bathing (75 percent), to facilitate transportation (25 percent), and to relieve their own frustration (10 percent). All parents reported difficulty with infant bathing, clothing, and transportation with the harness in place. There was universal lack of understanding on the part of the parents concerning their infant's disorder and treatment (Corbett, 1988). Results of the study emphasize the need for extensive parental education.

Parent and Family Education and Support

In addition to providing information regarding the pathology and treatment goals of DDH, the nurse should provide the parents with an opportunity to remove and reapply the harness while under supervision. Parental support groups can help parents adjust to the infant's temporary awkward condition. Parents should also be educated in the procedure used to reduce the dislocated hip because complete reduction must be achieved before the harness is applied.

Long-Term Consequences and Complications

As with most therapeutic treatments, the potential for iatrogenic complications exists. Complications observed following DDH treatment include avascular necrosis, redislocation, and acetabular dysplasia. Complications can result from either inadequate or overly aggressive treatment.

If the hip does not reduce after 2 to 3 weeks of splinting, alternative treatment modalities must be considered. Such alternatives include closed reduction with traction or open reduction with casting. A hip spica cast is most often used with these infants. Care then includes observance for poor pedal pulses, decreased peripheral circulation, pain, skin excoriation or abrasions, and possible development of respiratory infections resulting from decreased mobility. Parents should learn cast care, because the child is discharged with the cast in place.

Clubfoot

The classic clubfoot, talipes equinovarus, refers to a dysmorphic-appearing foot with hindfoot equinus, forefoot adduction, and midfoot supination. The term clubfoot may also be used to describe milder talipes conditions, including talipes calcaneus and talipes varus.

Foot deformities are among the most commonly occurring birth defects. Clubfoot has an incidence of 1 in 1000 live births. Males are affected nearly twice as often as females, and, in infants, with unilateral presentation, the majority appear on the right (Palmer et al., 1974; Wynne-Davies, 1964).

Mechanism of Development

The precise mechanism of development of clubfoot has not been irrefutably established. Some researchers allude to the theory of intrauterine malposition, whereas others, noting a higher incidence of clubfoot in families with a positive history of the disorder, ascribe it to a genetic cause (Fine et al., 1968; Macleod & Patriguin, 1974; Tachdjian, 1985). Gaining popularity is the theory that clubfoot is a multifactorial disorder involving a genetic predisposition coupled with environmental forces such as oligohydramnios, primiparity, macrosomia, and multiple fetuses (Palmer et al., 1974; Wynne-Davies, 1964).

Clinical Manifestations

Clubfoot deformities are apparent at birth. The skin overlying the lateral aspect of the foot may be taut, whereas the medial aspect may have increased skin folds. The affected foot may be smaller in size than a normal foot. In older children, the calf muscle may be noticeably decreased in size. Milder talipes conditions may be returned to the neutral position by manipulation.

Collaborative Management

Early diagnosis and treatment of clubfoot are essential. In the early newborn period, joints, muscles, and ligaments may be more compliant to corrective manipulation without surgical intervention. This may involve serial casting as frequently as 2- to 4-day intervals. As many as 50 percent of clubfoot deformities may require surgery. Difficulty with skin closure has been reported as a complication following correction of severe clubfoot. This is especially true if there has been prior surgery on the affected foot. Silver and associates (1993) reported successful skin closure in four children by using a tissue expander at the site 3 to 4 months before surgery. Special shoe splints or braces may be used toward the end of any successful treatment.

Parental education includes implementation of routine newborn care for an infant wearing either splints or bilateral casts. Problems and solutions associated with clothing, sleeping, feeding, and bathing should be addressed. Compliance by parents in using splints may vary. Because consistent treatment is necessary for a favorable outcome, health care professionals must explore parental feelings and actions while providing anticipatory guidance.

Syndactyly

Fusion, or webbing, between two digits is referred to as syndactyly. This condition is the most common anomaly of the hand, with an incidence of 1 in 2250 live births (Tachdjian, 1990b). Males are affected slightly more than females. Half of the time, both hands are involved in a symmetric presentation. Syndactyly of the fingers may be accompanied by syndactyly of the toes.

Mechanism of Development

Although most occurrences of syndactyly appear to be through spontaneous mutation, there have been reports of a familial predisposition, indicating an autosomal dominant pattern (Tachdjian, 1990b). Syndactyly may also be associated with a specific syndrome such as Apert's syndrome.

There are four classifications of syndactyly. Complete syndactyly occurs when the fusion is from the base to the tip of the digit. Fusion not extending to the tip of the digit is termed incomplete. Simple syndactyly refers to digits connected by skin and soft tissue. Fused digits involving an osseous connection is considered complex. Abnormal nerve and vessel configurations may accompany complex syndactyly.

Treatment

The type and timing of treatment of syndactyly depend on its classification. Surgery is directed toward promoting normal function and appearance. Fingers of unequal length should be separated within 6 to 12 months of age to prevent curvature of the longer finger deviated toward the shorter finger. If more than two adjacent digits are involved, surgery should be performed in stages to prevent vascular compromise of the middle digits.

Prognosis

Prognosis is favorable for normal function and appearance, except in cases of complex syndactyly involving not only bone but also vascular and nervous tissue. These cases may be associated with some loss of function postoperatively.

Collaborative Management

Parents of infants with syndactyly are instructed in physical therapy, specifically in massage of the interconnecting skin. This allows the webbed area to be stretched, thus allowing for easier repair.

Polydactyly

Polydactyly is any duplication of digits beyond the normal five. It is the second most common hand anomaly. Polydactyly is believed to be caused by duplication of a single embryonic bud. Blacks are affected 10 times more often than whites. Blacks more frequently have postaxial polydactyly (duplication of the little finger), whereas preaxial polydactyly (duplication of the thumb) occurs primarily in whites. In blacks, postaxial polydactyly is typically an isolated incidence, whereas, in whites, it is associated with syndromes and chromosomal anomalies. Central axial polydactyly is the duplication of the ring, long, or index finger. Central axial polydactyly is often associated with complex syndactyly.

Polydactyly may be further classified into three types. Type I is merely a rudimentary soft tissue mass connected by a pedicle. Treatment of this type involves simple excision, which is often done in the newborn nursery before discharge. Type II is a partial duplication with involvement of the phalanges. Type III, a rare occurrence, involves complete duplication of the metacarpal and phalanges.

Collaborative Management

Treatment of polydactyly types II and III centers around functional capacity first and appearance second. The infant is observed for which duplication is dominant and most functional, and efforts are made to remove the least functional counterpart. If both duplicated digits appear to be equally functional, surgery should then be used to promote aesthetic appearance. Reparative surgery should be completed by 3 years of age.

Amniotic Band Syndrome

Amniotic band syndrome, with an incidence ranging from 1 in 5000 to 1 in 15,000 live births, is characterized by uncommon, asymmetric fetal deformities (Ossipoff & Hall, 1977). Deformities that have been attributed to the amniotic band syndrome include congenital limb amputation, syndactyly, constriction bands, clubfoot, craniofacial defects such as cleft lip and palate, and visceral defects such as gastroschisis and omphalocele (Baraitser & Winter, 1996).

Mechanism of Development

Etiologic factors in the amniotic band syndrome are unclear. Part of the difficulty is that some of the same deformities that occur with this syndrome can also occur for other reasons. Thus, the exact cause of the deformities is not always identified. This area is in need of further research.

Diagnosis

Many clinicians believe that amniotic bands must be present for the diagnosis of amniotic band syndrome to be made. However, others believe that the presence of fetal deformities in a nonanatomic pattern, without obvious bands, is sufficient to establish the diagnosis of the syndrome. Congenital deformations, such as the visceral and craniofacial types, in the absence of amniotic bands may go undiagnosed as amniotic band syndrome because they could represent a faulty midline developmental pattern during the first trimester of pregnancy instead of the production of amniotic bands that constricted or restricted growth. Therefore, the true incidence of this syndrome may be much higher than it generally appears—not only because of the difficulty establishing a diagnosis but also because of the high mortality rate that exists during gestation. Amniotic band syndrome has been implicated in fetal deaths secondary to cord compression by the constricting bands (Kalousek & Bamfort, 1988).

In a series of 88 affected children, Light and Ogden (1993) found that digital amputations involving the hand were most common in the index, middle, and ring fingers. Syndactyly was also frequently associated with distal amputation. As was found in earlier clinical series, a 31 percent incidence of clubfoot deformity was seen in this population.

Pathophysiology

Two theories, endogenous and exogenous, exist to explain the cause of amniotic band syndrome (Lockwood et al., 1989). The endogenous theory postulates that the deformities are caused by an innate derangement of the primary embryonic cell layers from which the tissues and organs develop. The presence of amniotic bands, according to the endogenous theory, is a late development with no clinical significance.

The exogenous, and seemingly more popular, theory contends that early amniotic rupture allows the fetus to move into close approximation to the chorion by entering the chorionic cavity. The ruptured amnion then forms fibrous strings or bands. These bands can adhere to the skin, causing alterations of normal morphogenesis (e.g., cleft lip or palate, omphalocele), or disrupt the vascular integrity, resulting in gastroschisis. Amniotic bands have been found encircling normally developed structures, resulting in congenital amputations, constriction rings with lymphedema distal to the ring, and facial clefts in nonanatomic distribution. Postural deformities such as clubfoot are believed to be caused by the fetus' close approximation to the chorion. (See Chapter 10, Fetal Development: Environmental Influences and Critical Periods.)

Collaborative Management

Notwithstanding the inherent problems associated with omphaloceles, gastroschisis, encephaloceles, clubfoot, syndactyly, and facial clefts, the clinician must be attuned to the unique complications of constricting bands. Constricting bands are usually associated with edema distal to the band. The resulting edema and vascular compromise contribute to complications such as skin breakdown, necrosis, thromboemboli formation resulting from venostasis, and infection. Care should include frequent vascular checks to assess perfusion. Trauma and tissue breakdown are discouraged through positioning and skin care. Observation for localized areas of necrosis is stressed.

As with other aesthetically disappointing musculoskeletal disorders, the family requires emotional and psychological support as adjustment to and acceptance of the infant are allowed to occur. Parents may be fearful that an extremity will be lost because of necrotic tissue formation or infection. These fears may be justified, and the parents should be prepared for such a possibility. Complete surgical repair may not be possible during the infant's initial hospitalization, necessitating frequent hospitalizations during the early developing years. The delay in repair may necessitate that parents be taught to observe for vascular perfusion of an extremity, to recognize signs of infection, and to change dressings over open or healing areas. Preparation for discharge requires a multidisciplinary approach. The family may need surgical supplies, follow-up visitations by a home-visiting nurse, orthopedic or surgical consultations, pediatrician visits for general well-child care, and support of social or financial services to meet the long-term responsibilities of caring for their infant.

In addition, the nurse, working with the perinatal social worker, must attempt to provide opportunities for parent–infant bonding if the parents are to feel somewhat prepared for discharge. While the infant is still in the hospital, the parents must be encouraged to touch and talk to the infant and to participate in the infant's care. They must also be encouraged to verbalize their own feelings about their infant's condition. Every attempt should be made to attend to their fears, concerns, or misconceptions about the cause of their infant's problem. Only then will positive transition to home be possible.

Birth Trauma

Birth trauma encompasses both mechanical and asphyxial events occurring during delivery. This trauma may be due to pressure and distortion. Trauma can occur despite exemplary obstetrical care. Birth trauma occurs in approximately 2 to 7 in 1000 live births (Levine et al., 1984). A positive association exists between birth trauma and macrosomia, prematurity, breech presentation, dystocia, and cephalopelvic disproportion (Levine et al., 1984).

Clinical Manifestations

Birth trauma includes abrasions, ecchymoses, erythema, cephalhematomas, caput succedaneum, fractures (especially of the clavicle), brachial plexus damage, and nerve palsies. Clavicular fractures are the most common fractures diagnosed as birth trauma. Clavicles are at an increased risk for fractures during shoulder dystocias in a vertex presentation or with arms extended during a breech delivery (Fanaroff & Martin, 1997).

Physical examination findings related to birth trauma may appear only as bruising, abrasions, and petechiae that overlie the affected part. Further diagnostic methods should be used when the infant exhibits pain on movement, limited motion, and abnormal passive positioning of an extremity or head movement.

Skull fractures may present as cephalhematomas. Skull fractures are most often linear and typically involve the parietal bones (Menkes, 1991). Symptomatic evidence of a nondepressed skull fracture may resemble signs of increased intracranial pressure secondary to epidural hemorrhage. Usually, no treatment is indicated for asymptomatic skull fractures. Depressed skull fractures, however, may require elevation of the depressed area.

Vertebral fractures are incurred in difficult breech deliveries in which there may be longitudinal traction in combination with a twisting motion. These features frequently involve the seventh cervical and first thoracic vertebrae. Treatment depends on the extent of resultant nerve damage but frequently requires traction.

The most common nerve injury attributed to birth trauma is brachial plexus damage and resulting nerve palsy. This injury involves damage to the network of nerve fibers in the neck and shoulders referred to as the brachial plexus. Involvement may occur in the upper portion (Erb-Duchenne palsy), lower portion (Klumpke's paralysis), or both portions (complete brachial plexus palsy).

Erb-Duchenne paralysis is the most common form. The affected arm is limp and in a position of elbow extension and internal rotation. The Moro reflex is diminished, and the grasp reflex intact. Klumpke's paralysis involves paralysis of the hand and wrist. Complete brachial plexus paralysis results in paralysis of the entire arm.

Diagnosis

Diagnosis of birth trauma is based on physical assessment findings. These are usually fairly visible at birth or in the immediate postnatal period. Physical findings should be confirmed, when necessary, by radiologic evaluation to establish whether a fracture is present.

Collaborative Management

Treatment of birth trauma depends on the type and severity of the trauma. Often, supportive measures may be the only intervention required. For instance, brachial plexus injuries require immobilization in a neutral position using braces or splints. Passive range-of-motion exercises should be instituted at 7 to 10 days.

Clavicular fractures also respond to supportive management. Typically, the arm is held flexed and the elbow is held against the chest. This position limits movement, thereby decreasing pain and possible trauma to the site. Callus formation stabilizes the fracture by 10 days of age. A hard, palpable knot can often be felt with this callus formation.

Parent Education and Support

Diagnosing a disorder resulting from birth trauma can evoke anxiety in a parent. Birth trauma may connote thoughts of violence. The manner in which such information is taken from and conveyed to the family is important. Nonjudgmental, supportive care by health professionals along with consistent primary care by one individual may diminish some anxiety and allow the parents to establish trust. The mother may especially feel that she is to blame for the neonatal problem. Calm reassurance about the nature of the trauma is important. It also helps to allay fears that something was done incorrectly during the delivery process if parents understand that many of these injuries cannot be avoided or anticipated. Parental education is prerequisite if the parents are to understand the need for continued, long-term treatment, which many of these infants require. Many birth trauma injuries require long-term follow-up care by orthopedists, neurologists, or physical and occupational specialists. (For a complete discussion of birth trauma or injury, see Chapter 29, Assessment and Management of Neurologic Dysfunction.)

Congenital Muscular Torticollis

Congenital muscular torticollis, with an incidence of 0.4 percent of all live births, is another musculoskeletal deformity with unknown pathogenesis (Coventry & Harris, 1959). It is known to be primarily a disorder of the sternocleidomastoid muscle.

Pathophysiology

Several theories exist as to the cause of congenital torticollis, including genetics, abnormal uterine positioning, neurogenic disorders, and ischemic injury to the sternocleidomastoid muscle. Whatever the cause, this pathologic disorder consists of a fibrous contraction of the sternocleidomastoid muscle. Typically, the ipsilateral trapezius muscle is atrophic.

Diagnosis

Congenital torticollis can present within the neonatal period. Presentation may include a 1- to 3-cm hard, palpable mass in the neck on the affected side accompanied by an abnormal positioning of the head. Infants with congenital torticollis tilt the head to the affected side, and the chin is pointed upward in the opposite direction. Facial asymmetry may be a later appearing sign. The face and skull on the affected side appear smaller.

In children with untreated congenital torticollis, or in cases with torticollis unresponsive to therapy, the shoulder on the affected side is raised to compensate for the abnormal head positioning. This form of compensation may lead to cervical and lumbar scoliosis as well as chronic back pain.

Collaborative Management

Traditionally, physical therapy for congenital torticollis is instituted immediately. Because congenital torticollis may resolve naturally within the first year of life, surgery is typically delayed until after 1 year of age. Persistent congenital torticollis past 1 year of age should be surgically treated to prevent the compensatory complications described.

Physical therapists and orthopedic surgeons should be consulted to assist in the management and subsequent follow-up of these infants. Family members should be taught home physical therapy, which should be performed at least twice daily. Parents should be counseled regarding the possibility of a neck brace to be worn by the infant postoperatively. It is usually the nurse's responsibility to coordinate consultations and to prepare the family with discharge instructions. In addition, the nurse must determine whether the family lives in an area accessible to follow-up care. If not, a referral to social services or financial counseling may be needed so the family can participate in follow-up.

REFERENCES

Artz, T. D., Lim, W. N., Wilson, P. D., et al. (1975). Neonatal diagnosis, treatment, and related factors of congenital dislocation of the hip. *Clinical Orthopedics and Related Research, 110,* 112–136.

Baraitser, M., & Winter, R. M. (1996). *Color atlas of congenital malformation syndromes* (p. 83). St. Louis: Mosby-Wolfe.

Barlow, T. G. (1962). Early diagnosis and treatment of congenital dislocation of the hip. *Journal of Bone and Joint Surgery, 44B,* 292–301.

Bennett, J. T., & MacEwen, G. D. (1989). Congenital dislocation of the hip: Recent advances and current problems [Review]. *Clinical Orthopedics and Related Research, 247,* 15–21.

Bianchi, D. W., & Van Marter, L. J. (1994). An approach to ventilator-dependent neonates with arthrogryposis. *Pediatrics, 94*(5), 682–686.

Binder, H., Conway, A., & Gerber, L. H. (1993). Rehabilitation approaches to children with osteogenesis imperfecta: A ten-year experience. *Archives of Physical Medicine and Rehabilitation, 74,* 386–390.

Carter, C. O., & Wilkinson, J. A. (1964). Genetic and environmental factors in the etiology of congenital dislocation of the hip. *Clinical Orthopedics and Related Research, 33*(4), 119–128.

Clark, D. R., & Eteson, D. J. (1991). Congenital anomalies. In H. W. Taeusch, R. A. Ballard, & M. E. Avery (Eds.), *Schaffer and Avery's diseases of the newborn* (6th ed., pp. 159–191). Philadelphia: W. B. Saunders.

Corbett, D. (1988). Information needs of parents of a child in a Pavlik harness. *Orthopaedic Nursing, 7*(2), 20–23.

Coventry, M. B., & Harris, I. E. (1959). Congenital muscular torticollis in infancy. *Journal of Bone and Joint Surgery, 41,* 815.

Drachman, D. B., & Coulombre, A. (1962). Experimental clubfoot and arthrogryposis multiplex congenita. *Lancet, 2,* 523–526.

Fanaroff, A. A., & Martin, R. (Eds.) (1997). *Neonatal-perinatal medicine: Diseases of the fetus and infant* (6th ed.). St. Louis: Mosby–Year Book.

Fine, R. N., Gwinn, J. L., & Young, E. F. (1968). Smith-Lemli-Opitz syndrome: Radiologic and postmortem findings. *American Journal of Diseases of Children, 115*(4), 482–488.

Follis, R. H. (1952). Osteogenesis imperfecta congenita: A connective tissue diathesis. *Journal of Pediatrics, 41,* 713–721.

Francis, M. J., Smith, R., & Bauze, R. J. (1974). Instability of polymeric skin collagen in osteogenesis imperfecta. *British Medical Journal, 1*(905), 421–424.

Fuller, D. J. (1975). Immobilisation of foetal joints: A cause of progressive prenatal deformity. *Journal of Bone and Joint Surgery, 57B,* 115.

Gardner, R. J. M. (1977). A new estimate of the achondroplasia mutation rate. *Clinical Genetics, 11*(1), 31–38.

Gertner, J. M., & Root, L. (1990). Osteogenesis imperfecta. *Orthopedic Clinics of North America, 21,* 151–162.

Hall, J. G. (1981). An approach to congenital contractures (arthrogryposis) [Review]. *Pediatric Annals, 10*(7), 15–26.

Hall, J. G. (1983). Arthrogryposes (congenital contractures). In A. E. Emery & D. L. Rimoin (Eds.), *Principles and practice of medical genetics* (pp. 58–69). New York: Churchill Livingstone.

Hall, J. G. (1989). Arthrogryposis [Review]. *American Family Physician, 39*(1), 113–119.

Hall, J. G., Reed, S. D., & Greene, G. (1982). The distal arthrogryposes: Delineation of new entities—review and nosologic discussion [Review]. *American Journal of Medical Genetics, 11*(2), 185–239.

Hoaglund, F. T., Kalamchi, A., Poon, R., et al. (1981). Congenital hip dislocation and dysplasia in Southern Chinese. *International Orthopaedics, 4*(4), 243–246.

Kalousek, D. K., & Bamfort, H. S. (1988). Amnion rupture sequence in previable fetuses. *American Journal of Medical Genetics, 31*(1), 63–73.

Levine, M. G., Holroyde, J., Woods, J. R., Jr., et al. (1984). Birth trauma: Incidence and predisposing factors. *Obstetrics and Gynecology, 63*(6), 792–795.

Light, T. R., & Ogden, J. A. (1993). Congenital constriction band syndrome: Pathophysiology and treatment. *Yale Journal of Biology and Medicine, 66*(3), 143–155.

Lockwood, C., Ghidini, A., Romero, R., & Hobbins, J. C. (1989). Amniotic band syndrome: Reevaluation of its pathogenesis [Review]. *American Journal of Obstetrics and Gynecology, 160*(5, Part 1), 1030–1033.

Lukinmaa, P. L., Ranta, H., Ranta, K., & Kaitila, I. (1987). Dental findings in osteogenesis imperfecta: I. Occurrence and expression of type I dentinogenesis imperfecta. *Journal of Craniofacial Genetics and Developmental Biology, 7*(2), 115–125.

MacLeod, P., & Patriguin, H. (1974). The whistling face syndrome: Cranio-carpo-tarsal dysplasia. Report of a case and survey of the literature. *Clinical Pediatrics, 13*(2), 184–189.

Menkes, J. H. (1991). Perinatal central nervous system asphyxia and trauma. In H. W. Taeusch, R. A. Ballard, & M. E. Avery (Eds.), *Schaffer and Avery's diseases of the newborn* (6th ed., pp. 406–425). Philadelphia: W. B. Saunders.

Moessinger, A. C. (1983). Fetal akinesia deformation sequence: An animal model. *Pediatrics, 72*(6), 857–863.

Ortolani, M. (1976). Congenital hip dysplasia in the light of early and very early diagnosis. *Clinical Orthopedics and Related Research, 119,* 6–10.

Ossipoff, V., & Hall, B. D. (1977). Etiologic factors in the amniotic band syndrome: A study of 24 patients. *Birth Defects, 13,* 117–132.

Palmer, R. M., Conneally, P. M., & Yu, P. L. (1974). Studies of the inheritance of idiopathic talipes equinovarus. *Orthopedic Clinics of North America, 5,* 99–108.

Paterson, C. R., Beal, R. J., & Dent, J. A. (1992). Osteogenesis imperfecta: Fractures of the femur when testing for congenital dislocation of the hip. *British Medical Journal, 305*(6851), 464–466.

Robertson, N. R. C. (1984). Screening for congenital hip dislocation. *Lancet, 1,* 909–910.

Sillence, D. (1981). Osteogenesis imperfecta: An expanding panorama of variants. *Clinical Orthopedics and Related Research, 159,* 11–25.

Sillence, D., & Danks, D. (1978). The differentiation of genetically distinct varieties of osteogenesis imperfecta in the newborn period. *Clinical Research, 26,* 178A.

Sillence, D. O., Rimoin, D. L., & Danks, D. M. (1979a). Clinical variability in osteogenesis imperfecta: Variable expressivity or genetic heterogeneity. *Birth Defects, 15*(5B), 113–129.

Sillence, D. O., Senn, A., & Danks, D. M. (1979b). Genetic heterogeneity in osteogenesis imperfecta. *Journal of Medical Genetics, 16*(2), 101–116.

Silver, L., Grant, A. D., Atar, D., & Lehman, W. B. (1993). Use of tissue expansion in clubfoot surgery. *Foot and Ankle, 14*(3), 117–122.

Spitz, J. L. (1996). *Genodermatosis: A full-color clinical guide to genetic skin disorders.* Baltimore: Williams & Wilkins.

Tachdjian, M. (1985). Congenital deformities: Congenital talipes equinovarus. In M. Tachdjian (Ed.), *The child's foot* (pp. 139–170). Philadelphia: W. B. Saunders.

Tachdjian, M. (1990a). Congenital dysplasia of the hip: Embryology. In M. Tachdjian (Ed.), *Pediatric orthopedics* (Vol. 1, 2nd ed., pp. 297–312). Philadelphia: W. B. Saunders.

Tachdjian, M. (1990b). Syndactyly. In M. Tachdjian (Ed.), *Pediatric orthopedics* (Vol. 1, 2nd ed., pp. 222–236). Philadelphia: W. B. Saunders.

Walker, J. M. (1935). *A preliminary investigation of congenital hip disease in the Island Lake Reserve population.* Manitoba, Winnipeg, Canada: University of Manitoba.

Wynne-Davies, R. (1964). Family studies and cause of congenital clubfoot. *Journal of Bone and Joint Surgery, 46B,* 445–465.

CHAPTER 31

Assessment and Management of Genitourinary Dysfunction

CAROLE KENNER

RESEARCH AGENDA

Most nursing research in this area has centered on two areas: (1) the accuracy of obtaining urine specimens, and (2) the parental acceptance of the infant based on gender identity.

Does a difference in accuracy exist between urine specific gravities and laboratory dipstick samples for pH, blood, protein, glucose, bilirubin, and ketones obtained from bagged specimens versus disposable diapers? Two teams of nurse researchers have found no difference in the accuracy of the specimens obtained by either method (Reams & Deane, 1988; Suri, 1988). This research needs repeating because the superabsorbency of disposable diapers may alter the studies' findings.

How do parents react to the news of the prenatal detection of a genitourinary problem?

How does a genitourinary problem affect bonding in the neonatal period?

Under what conditions does pulmonary hypoplasia accompany oligohydramnios?

What is the determinant of the critical period for in utero correction of a fetal urinary problem?

What is the relationship between circumcision and frequency of urinary tract infections? Wiswell and associates (1987) found an increase in the incidence of urinary tract infections as the number of circumcisions decreased. This study needs to be replicated to determine the validity of their results.

What is the potential relationship between multicystic disease and the later appearance of Wilms' tumor?

What is the potential relationship between infertility and neonatal torsion?

Does inhaled furosemide therapy produce less electrolyte imbalance than conventional intravenous furosemide therapy?

VIGNETTE

The day's first new arrival in the nursery weighed in at 7 lb, 11 oz. Maternal history was notable for oligohydramnios found on biophysical profile testing. The baby was alert and active.

I began my assessment. David's pulse, respiration, and blood pressure were all within the normal range. However, his temperature in delivery had been 99.0°F, and now it was 100.0°F. His Apgar scores were 8 (1 minute) and 9 (5 minutes). Physical examination was essentially normal until I palpated his back. There I noted an enlargement or mass on his right flank. I asked a colleague to check my finding; she concurred.

When David's pediatrician arrived a short time later, she palpated the mass and felt that more tests were indicated. "Has he voided?" she asked. "Not yet," I replied. The doctor ordered vital signs q 4 hours, intake and output calculations, specific gravity with dipstick for protein, and blood determinations. I knew to check for changes in David's hydration status: signs of edema and skin turgor. The pediatrician ordered chest and abdominal x-rays and a renal ultrasound. A CBC with differential count was scheduled.

At that time, we went to speak with the parents. The pediatrician explained what we had found. "I suspect hydronephrosis." She described the mass she palpated in the baby's right flank and the tests that were ordered. "We need to find out why." She went on to inform them that their son would be moved to the special care nursery and that his hospital stay would probably be extended for several days longer than usual. The doctor was quiet as she waited for them to formulate their questions.

"When can I see my son?" his mother said anxiously.

"As soon as David is settled in the special care nursery, I'll come with a wheelchair to take you there. It will probably be about an hour or so before I am ready." I gave her a picture of David and the nursery telephone number.

The test results revealed a stricture of the right ureter. Urine was backing up into the right kidney. The left ureter and kidney were normal. The pediatrician and the consulting urologist decided to engage in expectant management with nutritional support.

For the next week, David was closely monitored. His parents were constantly at his bedside, despite encouragement for them to get some needed rest. They went home at night and returned by 10 o'clock in the morning with toys for their son. David's parents became very active in his care. They were taught normal infant behavior and development and baby care, such as diapering, bathing, and feeding. They loved performing these duties; they were parenting their child. David and his parents became part of the unit, part of the "team." Rapport between them and staff was open and good.

As David was monitored, his vital signs remained normal. His fever disappeared. His hydration level was normal; there were no signs of edema. He was alert and active. Gradually, his IV was attached to a heparin lock for antibiotics. Feedings were started slowly. David had a good appetite and enjoyed his bottles. His parents loved to hold him close and talk to him while they fed him. They talked about his toys, his kitty, and his room at home, and how much they wanted to take him there. They praised him with every ounce taken and every bubble returned. As feedings were increased and tolerated with good weight gain, his IV was discontinued.

On day 11, David was discharged from the hospital with instructions for nutritional supportive therapy. Close monitoring by the parents and the pediatrician for urinary tract infections or other problems stemming from the stricture would be important. Discharge instructions were given to the parents, who could barely listen because of their level of excitement. They could think of few questions to ask at that time. A home visit was planned for 2 days later to follow up on concerns that would arise in the interim.

Vicky Merritt

Alterations in the genitourinary (GU) system present a challenge to neonatal nurses. Management of infants experiencing a renal or genital complication requires a thorough understanding of normal anatomy and physiology of these two systems. Families must be included in the management of their infants because it is very frightening to be told that renal function is impaired or that a malformation in the reproductive tract exists. Parents have a difficult time dealing with their own sexual identity when infants with genital malformations are born. Parental support is necessary. Most problems of the genitalia are not life threatening; this is not always the case with renal problems.

Renal functioning in the premature infant may be very different from that in the sick full-term neonate. A thorough knowledge of renal physiology and embryologic development is essential for the assessment, planning, and implementation of nursing care.

Homeostasis of the newborn depends on a functioning renal system. Acid–base and fluid and electrolyte balance is partially regulated by the kidneys. The immature renal system responds slowly and erratically to physiologic changes and demands placed on it. The sick infant is often given drugs to stabilize other body systems, leaving the kidneys to filter and excrete massive doses of chemicals. As the infant becomes more compromised and circulation to the kidney declines, medications may easily reach toxic levels. The result is nephrotoxicity and further potential renal impairment. Many of the essential neonatal drugs, even when they are administered within therapeutic ranges, are nephrotoxic. Safe drug levels have not been established by long-term research.

Drug toxicity is not the only concern in renal functioning. Nutritional solutions, including formulas and hyperalimentation, may place a solute load on the kidneys that exceeds the renal threshold. This condition may result in a loss of nutrients and an imbalance of fluids and electrolytes.

Iatrogenic renal damage resulting from thrombus formation is a consequence of therapeutic interventions, such as arterial and umbilical line placement or continued use of these catheters, for either percutaneous or vascular catheterizations. Renal necrosis, renal vein thrombosis, and renal tubular acidosis are all examples of manifestations of procedural complications and other disease entities. Renal vein thrombosis is usually caused by umbilical or arterial line placement, birth trauma, hypoxia, dehydration, or hypotension or is a complication of maternal diabetes. It is characterized by thrombi formation within the renal vein, leading to obstruction and eventual necrosis. Renal tubular acidosis is preceded by metabolic acidosis and reflects the neonate's inability to respond to acid stress. The build-up of acid may occur when sodium bicarbonate is not adequately reabsorbed or hydrogen ions accumulate in the distal tubule.

Birth trauma can lead to physical kidney damage or damage to associated body systems, such as intracranial bleeding that alters levels of antidiuretic hormone, thereby resulting in impaired renal functioning. Hypoxia, metabolic and respiratory acidosis, and cold stress contribute to decreased renal blood flow. Hyperosmolar fluid loads stress the delicate functioning of the kidney. Alterations in tubular secretion and reabsorption may occur, leaving the infant struggling to achieve homeostasis. Neonatal anesthesia and shock are associated risk factors, the outcome of which is a hypotensive state at the level of the kidneys; this state results in altered renal perfusion. Use of drugs such as vasopressors to alter blood pressure also affects kidney perfusion. Altered kidney perfusion may be precipitated by congenital genetic syndromes, inborn errors of metabolism, or urinary obstruction. This type of renal tubular acidosis can be congenital or acquired. The other common form of renal tubular acidosis is related to metabolic acidosis in prematurity (Ingelfinger, 1985).

This chapter outlines the embryonic development and anatomy and physiology of the GU system and describes various GU neonatal conditions, including risk factors, differential diagnoses, medical treatment, and nursing management. The purpose is to provide the neonatal nurse with a comprehensive physiologic knowledge base from which a sound comprehensive plan of care can be formulated.

EMBRYOLOGIC DEVELOPMENT OF THE KIDNEY

During embryologic development, the kidney undergoes a series of three changes in formation: pronephros, mesonephros, and metanephros. The first stage of kidney development is the formation of the pronephros. The pronephros, which develops during the first month of gestation, is a rudimentary, nonfunctional form of the later permanent kidney. It gradually degenerates, contributing only a duct system for the next developmental stage.

The mesonephros is the second excretory organ to develop, appearing during the fourth to sixth week of gestation. It may or may not be transitorily functional. Simultaneously, the genitalia develop, thus creating a urogenital ridge between the developing kidney and the genitals. This stage contributes ducts and tubules that later degenerate, leaving only mesonephric and paramesonephric remnants in the female and the male (see section on development of the genital system later in this chapter).

The third and final stage of kidney development is the metanephros. It is this kidney that becomes the permanent, functional kidney. Kidney function with production of fetal urine is established by the eighth week of gestation. Fetal urine makes up a large percentage of the amniotic fluid. Thus, renal agenesis or obstructive renal pathology results in oligohydramnios. Because the fetus swallows and gastrointestinally absorbs amniotic fluid, obstruction or malformations of the GI system or central nervous system may result in polyhydramnios. Examples of such central nervous system or GI conditions are anencephaly, which renders the fetus incapable of effective swallowing or alteration in intestinal absorption, and tracheoesophageal fistula, which disrupts the passage and absorption of fluid through the GI system.

Rising from the mesoderm, the metanephros forms collecting ducts from the ureteric bud. The shaft of the bud forms the ureter. If this bud fails to grow, vital renal tissue will be missing, and development of the mesonephric duct may be retarded. For the male, such a deficiency results in no epididymis, vas deferens, seminal vesicles, or ejaculatory duct, because these structures are derived from the mesonephric duct itself or as a by-product of the duct's formation (Kaplan, 1994). An outgrowth of the ureteric bud is the renal pelvis, which subdivides first into the major and minor calices and finally into the collecting ducts or tubules, which number 1 to 3 million (Sadler, 1995). Fetal testosterone is believed to stimulate this growth. Thus, the collecting system for the kidney is evolved.

Kidney growth continues, and the renal artery continues to grow and branch. Small, fine arterial branches form at the ends of the collecting tubules. These arterial branches are called glomeruli and are the filter system of the kidney. The encapsulated end of the glomerulus is Bowman's capsule. The glomeruli, along with Bowman's capsule, are composed of layers of tissues, capillary endothelial cells, basement membrane, and epithelial cells (Vander, 1985). The glomerulus, Bowman's capsule, and tubules constitute a nephron, which is a part of the excretory system and the site of urine formation (Brion et al., 1994; Moore & Persaud, 1993). The process of nephron formation is called nephrogenesis. It begins at the end of the second month of gestation and continues until approximately the 34th week of gestation (Page et al., 1981). Nephrons multiply in the region of the medulla. Thus, the more premature the infant, the lower the glomerular filtration rate. A rate of less than 5 ml/minute/1.73 m^2 is common in a neonate of less than 27 weeks' gestation (Brion et al., 1994). Rates increase to more than 20 ml/minute/1.73 m^2 by the middle of the third trimester (Brion et al., 1994). In the neonatal period, glomerular capillary circumference is greater than that of the tubules, thus producing a decreased filtration at the level of the glomeruli. This filtration rate increases after birth, even in the premature infant. Although continued growth of the tubules is seen after birth, the tubules do not increase in number (Page et al., 1981). As a result of the increase in capillary circumference of tubules, by the age of 2 years, the glomerular filtration rate more closely resembles that of the adult.

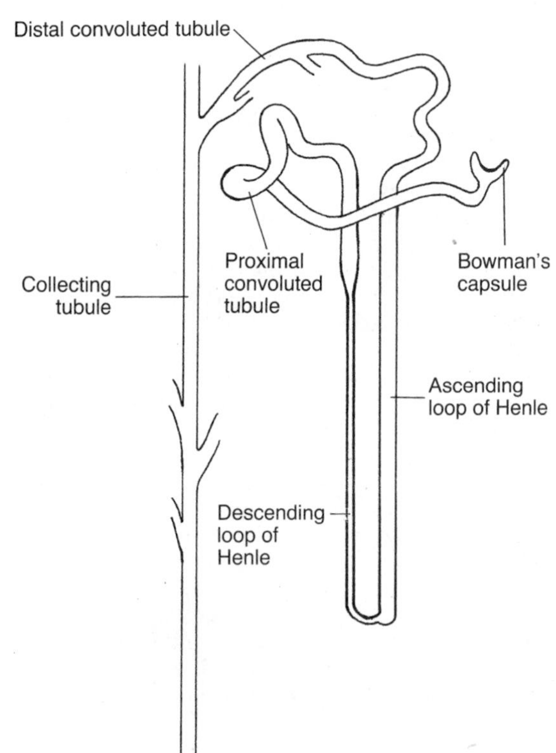

FIGURE 31–2. The loop of Henle.

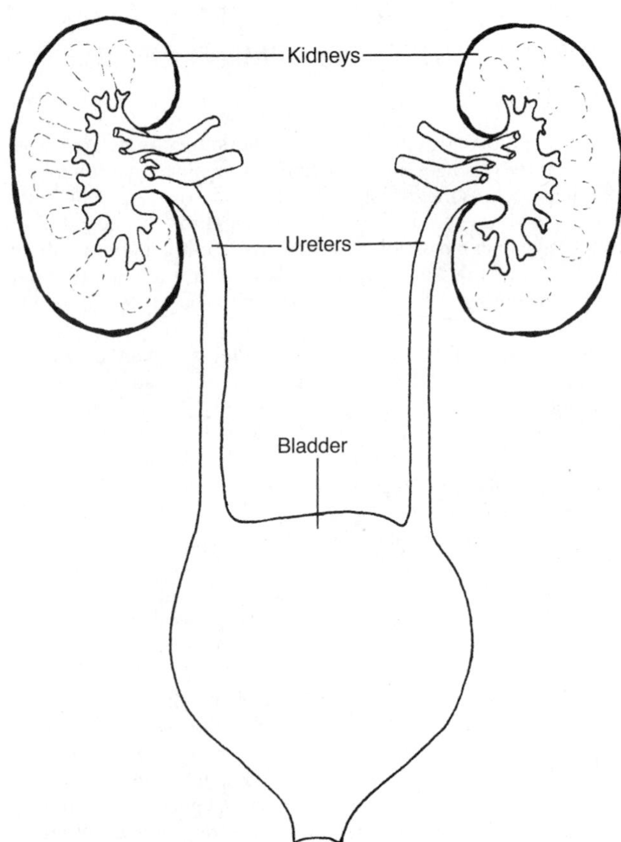

FIGURE 31–1. The genitourinary system.

The excretory portion of the renal system extends beyond the nephron. The distal end of the nephron's tubules is convoluted and communicates with a collecting tubule. Together, the two sets of tubules become convoluted, creating the proximal and the distal convoluted tubules and the loop of Henle (Figs. 31–1 and 31–2). In the neonate, the thin ascending portion, which controls reabsorption, is not fully formed, owing to the fact that nephron formation starts in the medullary area. By birth, it has extended from the medullary to the juxtamedullary area. The descending portion of the tubular system, which controls urine secretion, thus is more fully developed than the ascending segment at birth. Thus, the ability to concentrate urine is decreased in the newborn because urine secretion occurs readily but reabsorption is limited. Sometimes, this situation is referred to as a glomerular-tubular mismatch. This mismatch is a compensatory mechanism to conserve sodium chloride and rid the body of waste products (Baumgart, 1995). The implications for the preterm infant are an increased risk of extracellular fluid loss that results from the preterm infant's limited ability to rid the body of excess water from the hypertonic concentration of solutes in this extracellular fluid (Baumgart, 1995).

Initially, the kidney is located within the pelvic region. As the kidney grows, it makes a gradual ascent into its flank position or lumbothoracic area. This movement comes from the incurvation of the spinal column in the lumbosacral region. Blood supply to the ascending kidney changes from lower arteries that gradually regress to arteries that arise from the aorta. Now, the permanent kidney is complete and functional. Because the placenta functions as an excretory organ for the fetus, functional kidneys are not necessary during intrauterine life. Consequently, neonatal problems, such as aplastic, hypoplastic, and nonfunctioning kidneys, can occur.

To complete the formation of the urinary system, a bladder and urethra are produced. The cloacal portion of the hindgut is divided into the urogenital membrane and the anal membrane. The urorectal septum creates a compartmentalized cloaca consisting of the anorectal canal, or rectum, and the urogenital sinus (Sadler, 1995). From this urogenital sinus, the urethra and bladder arise. The primitive structures regress, fibrose, or become a part of the newly formed structures. Thus, the ureters dilate and open bilaterally into the urinary bladder as the ducts of the mesonephron are reabsorbed by the developing bladder. At the base of the umbilicus and the top of the bladder, the allantois narrows into a fibrous band called the urachus (Sadler, 1995). Sometimes, this urachus remains patent, causing a leakage of urine from the umbilical stump. This condition is referred to as a patent urachus or a urachal fistula. Variations of this abnormality include urachal cyst and urachal sinus (Sadler, 1995).

Differentiation of the urethra in the male and female fetus can be detected by 12 to 14 weeks' gestation. In the female, the upper portion of the urethra divides into two glands, the urethral and the paraurethral glands (Sadler, 1995). The male urethra grows with the prostatic urethral segment, giving rise to the prostatic gland.

PHYSIOLOGY OF KIDNEY FUNCTION

The kidney performs several critical functions for the neonate—(1) secretion, (2) reabsorption, and (3) excretion— which, in turn, regulate fluid and electrolyte balance, arterial blood pressure, and toxin levels in the body. These functions are all intimately tied to the formation of urine. This urine formation begins with renal blood flow. From the renal artery and into the afferent arteriole, plasma that is protein free is acted on by the glomeruli. Glomerular capillaries are permeable to small molecules or crystalloids, such as sodium, that are generally positively charged; however, large molecules called colloids cannot be filtered within the glomerular apparatus (Fig. 31–3). The most common colloids are plasma proteins. The size of these protein molecules creates a pressure gradient that results in colloidal osmotic or oncotic pressure. If these colloids are reduced in number, as is seen in alterations in the hepatic system, such as hepatitis and biliary atresia, a reduction of the oncotic pressure results. This pressure, coupled with the opposing hydraulic pressure within the glomeruli, determines the net filtration pressure of the capillaries (Vander, 1985). This net filtration pressure varies with the portion of the capillary being examined. Alterations in renal blood flow, in turn, alter the net filtration pressure. The reason for this effect is that the hydraulic pressure within the capillaries of the

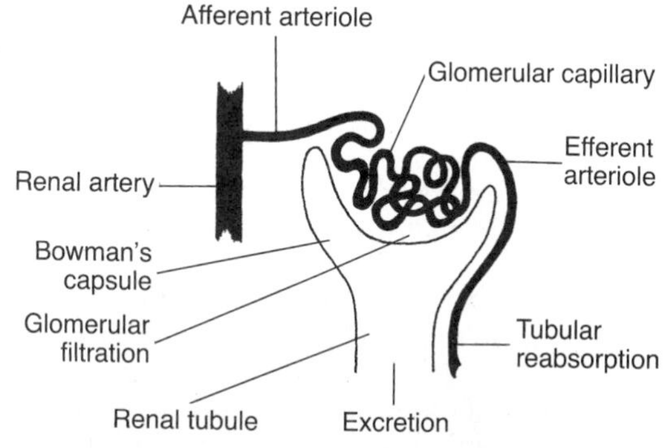

FIGURE 31–3. Glomerular apparatus.

glomeruli is dependent on renal arterial pressure. If renal arterial pressure decreases, the glomerular-capillary hydraulic pressure concurrently decreases. Constriction of the vessels leading into the glomerular capillary and increased resistance to blood flow into the capillary result in a lower hydraulic pressure at the level of the glomerular capillary, thus reducing the glomerular filtration rate (Vander, 1985). To control preterm labor, use of a beta-adrenergic antagonist, such as ritodrine hydrochloride, or a prostaglandin inhibitor, such as indomethacin, which readily crosses the placenta, can cause depression in the fetal glomerular perfusion and the glomerular filtration rate (Smith & Robillard, 1989). An obstruction in the urinary system also reduces the glomerular filtration rate. Hydraulic pressure within the capillary is dependent on blood flow.

Albumin is an exception to the filtration rule because it possesses a large molecular structure and passes through the filtration system, finding its way in small quantities into the urine. Positively charged particles find passage easier because the glomerular capillaries are composed of polyanions (Vander, 1985). Here, through the glomerular capillaries, plasma either is filtered into Bowman's capsule or leaves via the efferent arteriole and enters into the renal vein. This renal vein in turn leads to the tubule, where tubular secretion and, finally, either tubular excretion or absorption in the renal vein occur (see Fig. 31–3). Plasma that contains a high concentration of proteins that were impermeable to the filtration process possesses a higher oncotic pressure, or is more concentrated. Alteration in the permeability of the glomerular capillaries may result from inherent damage to the capillary, thus altering the pore size or changing the electrical charge within the membrane.

Tubular reabsorption, secretion, and excretion are closely tied together (see Fig. 31–2). These processes are concerned with the maintenance of the internal homeostasis. This maintenance depends on a flexible and dynamic reabsorption pattern that is responsive to other body systems.

Tubular reabsorption is the process that occurs via transport and diffusion of substances across a semipermeable membrane in the direction of the lumen into the epithelial lining of the tubule to the efferent arteriole (Vander, 1985). Many of the body's nutrients, electrolytes, and water are reabsorbed, thus achieving a balance for continued growth and normal physiologic function. Simple diffusion or passive transport involves movement of substances down a gradient, from an area of higher to an area of lower concentration, or according to polarization of the molecules, anions migrating toward cations. Active transport requires utilization of energy derived directly from adenosine triphosphate because the net movement of substances is against a gradient (Wodniak & Szwed, 1986). Molecular structures may link together to piggyback, or carry one another, across the membrane. Sodium first undergoes simple diffusion across the tubular membrane and then is transported via this mechanism of active transport by the sodium pump into the interstitial fluid (Wodniak & Szwed, 1986). Sodium filtration depends on the glomerular filtration rate. Thus, a higher glomerular filtration rate results in an increase in sodium reabsorption into the vascular space (Wodniak & Szwed, 1986). If the extracellular fluid volume increases, sodium reabsorption is decreased. Thus, the regulation of fluids and electrolytes is highly complex because sodium, in turn, influences other substances to move against their gradients.

Water follows the sodium ion across the membrane and into the capillary bed. This type of transport of a second substance is often referred to as secondary active transport (Vander, 1985). Simple facilitated diffusion is similar to active transport in that a carrier substance is used but the net movement is not against a gradient (Vander, 1985). Glucose is an example of a secondary substance that is carried with sodium across the membrane by secondary active transport. Glucose is reabsorbed by the proximal tubules, thus appearing in the urine only when the renal threshold or the maximal tubular transport capacity has been exceeded or the permeability of the filtering capillaries has been altered (Vander, 1985). Amino acids, water-soluble vitamins, and albumin and lactate are also transported in this fashion. Therefore, for example, inborn errors of metabolism may alter tubular reabsorption of amino acids. In contrast, creatinine, which passes through the tubule untouched, and to a lesser extent, urea (approximately 50 percent is reabsorbed, and some is secreted in the proximal tubule as well) are excreted and present in urine. Inulin, which resembles creatinine, is often used as a tag substance for testing the intactness of the kidney's filtering system and glomerular filtration rate. The creatinine clearance test is performed over the course of 1 minute to determine the amount of creatinine cleared (Vander, 1985; Wodniak & Szwed, 1986).

Tubular secretion is the process by which substances are moved from the epithelial lining of the tubule's capillaries into the interstitial fluid and finally into the lumen (Vander, 1985). Thus, the substances are secreted into the tubular lumen. Potassium and hydrogen undergo tubular secretion, as does para-aminohippurate (PAH). PAH is a unique substance that is secreted by the proximal tubules. PAH undergoes the filtration process within the glomerulus; however, it is generally not reabsorbed. Thus, PAH continues to move through the renal tubules so that it is effectively cleared via plasma movement within the kidney. The clearance of PAH is virtually 100 percent. By measurement of the renal clearance of PAH, the effective renal plasma flow is in fact determined. This is significant because measurement of the effective renal plasma flow is a direct way of determining the effectiveness of renal functioning (Vander, 1985).

Tubular excretion, the process by which substances enter into the filtrate that will eventually exit the body via urine, is linked with the secretion just described. Ions, such as potassium, that are secreted in the distal tubule (a portion is also reabsorbed in the proximal tubule) find their way into the urine when the body has no need for higher concentration levels. The excretion of potassium is influenced by the movement of hydrogen ions; thus, metabolic acidosis and alkalosis affect potassium levels. Hormones and drugs, especially diuretics, affect potassium movement. In the presence of aldosterone, potassium is secreted; thiazides, in contrast, result in potassium excretion. Other filtrates that show up in the urine are urea, creatinine, and other ions that are not needed by the body.

The regulation of fluids and electrolytes is an important function of the processes of tubular secretion, reabsorption, and excretion. Excretion of toxins, drugs, and other by-products of metabolism is also important and has been previously mentioned. However, the regulation of arterial blood pressure and the implications of the renin–angiotensin system need to be explained further. Renin is a substance that is found in high levels in the plasma. Newborns have a significantly higher renin level than that of their adult counterparts. This high level may be related to the neonate's altered glomerular filtration rate, vascular resistance, and renal blood flow. When renal blood flow is diminished as the result of a decrease in arterial pressure, the sympathetic nervous system, at the level of the kidney, responds to maintain homeostasis. Baroreceptors in the kidney sense the decrease in pressure and trigger renin secretion. Vander (1985) suggested that a decrease in the concentration of sodium and chloride ions (as would be the case when blood flow to the kidney glomeruli is decreased) may trigger the secretion. This secretion is a fairly complex process that depends on constriction of the afferent arterioles, decreases in glomerular-capillary hydrostatic pressure, and sodium secretion and reabsorption (Vander, 1985). Vander (1985) also suggested that alternative feedback mechanisms, in the form of antidiuretic hormone or vasopressin, which is a vasoconstrictor; potassium; and calcium all influence the renin activity by depressing its secretion.

Renal prostaglandins are postulated to also be involved in this process (Vander, 1985). They serve as strong vasodilators that may act on the renal blood vessels, thus increasing arterial blood flow and increasing the glomerular filtration rate. This action is in opposition to the hormone angiotensin II, which acts as a vasoconstrictor and stops or reduces renin secretion. The ultimate goal of the renin–angiotensin cycle is to maintain systemic blood flow adequately enough to supply the body's vital organs.

PHYSIOLOGIC DEVELOPMENT OF THE GENITALIA

Development and maturation of the fetal genital system represent the first step in gender identification. Although sexuality is determined at the time of fertilization, external characteristics are not present until the end of the second month of gestation. The formation of the gonads changes the fetus from a bisexual being. Ridges form in pairs along the mesonephros. These thickened areas or ridges are known as gonadal or genital ridges. Soon, fibrinous projections appear and extend into the mesenchymal tissue. These projections are called primary or primitive sex cords. At this developmental stage, the gonads are indifferent or undifferentiated according to sex. Each gonad contains mesonephric and paramesonephric ducts. The mesonephric duct evolves from the urogenital ridge. The upper portion communicates with the peritoneal cavity. At midline, the mesonephric and paramesonephric ducts join to form the uterovaginal canal. Invagination of the urogenital sinus ends in a protrusion called the mullerian (paramesonephric) tubercle (Sadler, 1995). During the sixth week of fetal development, primordial germ cells appear near the allantois along the wall of the yolk sac and begin their migratory journey from the hindgut to the genital ridges. These germ cells influence the development of the male and female gonads.

If an XX chromosome pair is present, the outer portion of the gonad, or the cortex, becomes an ovary, and the medullary portion degenerates (Moore & Persaud, 1993). Development of the ovary is slow, occurring in the 10th to 12th weeks of gestation. A primitive ovary forms initially and is called rete ovarii, a structure that eventually regresses, giving way to the permanent ovary. In the female, mitosis of the primordial follicles (groups of cells that form from the cortical cords and the germ cells) begins and is completed during fetal life. Development of oogonia, or female eggs, occurs only in utero. No new oogonia are produced postnatally.

If an XY chromosome pair is present, the opposite phenomenon occurs. The medullary portion becomes a testis cord, later forming the rete testis, which is grounded in epithelial tissue. As this cord grows, it separates from the epithelium, leaving a fibrinous, thick band of connective tissue known as the tunica albuginea (Sadler, 1995). The primary sex cords become seminiferous cords and, at puberty, patent tubules composed of sustentacular cells of Sertoli and spermatogonia. These seminiferous cords subdivide into branches called the ductuli efferentes testis. During the second trimester, mesenchymal cells called interstitial cells of Leydig appear. By the sixth month of gestation, the testis is matured enough to influence development of the external genitalia. In the male, a primitive connection between the mesonephros and the rete testis remains. It is called the mesonephric duct, or the ductus deferens (Sadler, 1995).

DIFFERENTIATION OF THE GENITALIA AND THE DUCT SYSTEM

Differentiation of the genitalia continues as the duct system and the external genitals flourish under hormonal influence. In the female, genital development is influenced by estrogen production coupled with the absence of androgens, in stimulating the formation of the clitoris from the phallus, the labia minora from the opened urogenital ridges, and the labia majora from the labioscrotal folds. A uterine tube or canal is evolved as the ovary descends slightly to just above the true pelvis. The posterior portion of the paramesonephric duct is stimulated by estrogen to develop into the uterine canal. The caudal portion of the paramesonephric ducts in a fused state creates two major structures, the uterus and the cervix. The caudal portion further fuses with endodermal cells and develops into a mullerian (paramesonephric) tubercle, thus forming the uterine tube. This tubercle stimulates the formation and canalization of the vagina by 18 to 20 weeks' gestation (Page et al., 1981). Enfolding of the peritoneal tissue occurs, creating the uterus's broad ligament, which subdivides the pelvic cavity into the uterorectal and the uterovesical pouches (Sadler, 1995). The hymen acts as a partition between the vaginal opening and the urogenital sinus.

In the male, the midkidney, or mesonephros, gradually diminishes, leaving a few rudimentary tubules under the influences of androgens and mullerian inhibiting substance that form the efferent testicular ducts. These ducts are in communication with the epididymal ducts. The ductus deferens forms from the tortuous epididymal ducts. This duct system is composed of smooth muscle that leads to an outgrowth or appendage, called the seminal vesicle, and finally into the most distal portion, called the ejaculatory duct. The male's external genitalia develop, as the phallic projection, which in the female creates the clitoris, continues to grow and form the penile organ. On the penis's ventral surface, the male urethral opening develops. Its formation is complete by 16 weeks' gestation. The patency and positioning of the urethral opening depend on the posterior-to-anterior progressive joining of the urogenital folds. The normal urethral position is midline, on the ventral surface of the glans penis. With the development of the male urethra comes Cowper's or bulbourethral glands, which form just below the prostatic portion of the urethra. This portion of the urethra swells and engulfs a portion of the mesenchymal tissue, forming the prostatic gland. Also, the scrotum forms, starting as outpouches of tissue (scrotal swelling), first found in the inguinal area and later located on either side of the urogenital folds anterior to the anal and peritoneal tissue.

The final stage of the development in the male is the descent of the testes. This process involves two simultaneous actions. First is the development of the gubernaculum testis. This occurs as the midkidney degenerates, leaving a rudimentary band of mesentery called the urogenital mesentery. This tissue band gradually fibroses, forming the caudal genital ligament. A portion of the ligament communicates with the developing scrotal swellings. This area is known as the inguinal region (Sadler, 1995). The product of these transformations is the gubernaculum testis. Simultaneously, in the female, the vaginal process is taking place. This process involves the differentiation of the inguinal region into the inguinal canal and the partitioning of the peritoneal cavity and the tunica vaginalis. Once this communication is no longer open, the testes begin to descend through the inguinal canals, moving from within the peritoneal cavity, reaching their final position in the scrotal sac at around 32 to 34 weeks of gestation (Moore & Persaud, 1993). The complete obliteration of the communication between the scrotal portion of the peritoneal cavity and the vaginal process occurs several months after birth.

ASSESSMENT OF THE UROGENITAL SYSTEM

History

It is imperative for neonates suspected of having urogenital problems to have a thorough familial history on record. Many of these problems have an inheritance pattern, which suggests genetic predisposition. The history should focus on any family members with anomalies of the GU system, cystic kidney disease, renal failure, or renal transplants or who have undergone dialysis. Do any family members have the fragile X syndrome or Turner's syndrome? Are there any abnormalities of the external genitalia, like hypospadias, ambiguous genitalia, or undescended testicles? Do any members have low-set ears or were they born with a single umbilical artery, both of which may be indicative of renal disorders?

Prenatal histories are important, too, because antepartal factors can predispose neonates to renal problems in particular. Presence of polyhydramnios or oligohydramnios or an increased fetal abdominal area on ultrasonography may be indicative of renal impairment or anomalies.

Neonatal history should include the following questions:

1. Has the infant undergone any hypoxic episodes that may result in delayed voiding? (The first voiding may occur in the delivery room or by 24 hours of life.)
2. Is the infant feeding? If so, is the fluid intake sufficient (120 to 160 ml/kg/day in the term infant)? (Requirements for the premature infant may be greater; however, this amount may not be achieved during the first 48 hours of life.)
3. Is the infant under treatment for jaundice? (Phototherapy increases fluid losses.)
4. Is the infant under a radiant warmer that increases insensible water loss?
5. Is the infant experiencing any frank hemorrhaging or increased GI losses, such as are caused by nasogastric suctioning, vomiting, and diarrhea?
6. What is the specific gravity of urine? (Normal range is 1.003 to 1.015.)
7. How old is the infant?
8. What is the gestational age?
9. Has micturition taken place? If so, at what age?

Physical Assessment

Physical examination should include inspection, palpation, and percussion. Auscultation is not generally useful for the renal system.

Inspection

Observation of the abdominal region is an important place to start. Is distention present? If so, is it unilateral or generalized? Is there urine from the umbilicus? Does the bladder appear distended? The abdominal musculature is relatively weak at birth, in comparison with the eventual state of the musculature several months after birth. Abdominal asymmetry is an abnormal finding. One congenital condition, called prune-belly syndrome, is characterized by an absence of muscle tone.

Next, the genital area is inspected. Peritoneal tissue leading to the anal opening should be intact and smooth in appearance. Any abnormal openings, depressions, or swellings should be noted. The anus is normally located midline and should be tested for patency by gentle insertion of a gloved, well-lubricated small finger. The anal wink, which is indicative of muscle tone, may be tested by gentle stroking of the anal tissue and observation for anal sphincter constriction. Inspection is also made for meconium or stool.

Male

If the infant is a full-term male, is the scrotal sac full, with rugae present? The premature male exhibits a generally flaccid, smooth scrotal sac. The coloration of the scrotal sac is important. It is generally darkly pigmented, without any bluish discoloration. A blue color may denote disruption of circulation to the area, and when coupled with dimpling, a torsion of the testicles must be suspected. The scrotum that is enlarged or very edematous may accompany a hydrocele (a trapping of fluid in the tunica vaginalis), or it may result from pressure on this tissue during the birth process, which is especially true in a breech birth. If a hydrocele is suspected, transillumination of the scrotum with a good light source, such as a transilluminator and a flashlight, helps determine the presence of fluid. On transillumination, fluid allows light to pass through it and shows as a highly lightened area.

The penis should be observed for length. Is it abnormally large or small in proportion to the gestational age and the rest of the body parts? If the penile structure is enlarged, a renal problem may be present. The penis is generally straight. Any downward incurvation, bowing, or chordee is most often associated with hypospadias. Priapism, or a constantly erect penis, is also an abnormal finding. The position of the urinary meatus is usually on the ventral portion, midline, of the glans penis. Alterations of this position result in dorsal or ventral placement anywhere along the shaft of the penis. This condition is known as epispadias if the urinary meatus is on the dorsum of the penis, or hypospadias if the opening is displaced along the ventral penile surface. If the male is uncircumcised, the foreskin is gently retracted for accurate observation. The foreskin must be returned to its unretracted state after inspection; otherwise, swelling with associated decreased circulation to the glans penis occurs. Observation of the urinary stream is important because this stream should be straight.

Female

In the full-term female, are the labia majora present and extending beyond the labia minora? Are the labia minora well formed? Is the clitoris present? (The clitoral tissue may be enlarged in both the full-term and the premature neonate.) If this infant is a premature female, the labia majora may well be smaller than the labia minora. The urinary meatus should be patent and anterior to the vaginal orifice. The vagina should be inspected for patency, and any vaginal secretions should be noted. A white milky vaginal secretion in the first few days of life, followed by pseudomenses or slight vaginal bleeding, is a normal finding.

Both Sexes

The urine is most often straw colored. Hematuria is a significant finding in either sex; it may denote infection, urinary obstruction, renal necrosis, renal thrombosis, trauma, traumatic suprapubic tap, or administration of hyperosmotic or nephrotoxic drugs. A urine dipstick test may be performed to determine the presence of blood in the urine. This test also indicates the presence of urinary protein. Blood is a protein; therefore, if blood is present, a positive protein test result should also be expected. This test requires that only one to two drops of urine be placed on the dipstick by a dropper, or the stick may be dipped into a specimen of urine. The results are obtained within 30 seconds to 1 minute after the stick is wet with urine. The exact timing for the most accurate reading is found on the bottles of the dipstick materials, based on the manufacturer's suggested clinical timing cycle.

The genital and peritoneal regions must be observed to make certain that a clear differentiation of the sexes is possible. If it is not, a genetics consult must be made.

Palpation

This portion of the physical examination is upsetting to the neonate, so it is best left until last. Percussion or auscultation may or may not be helpful. On palpation, the infant is best placed in a supine position. The examiner draws the infant's legs up with knees bent in the fetal position; this usually puts the infant at ease. In this position, the abdomen is gently palpated with a gradual downward movement, anteriorly to posteriorly. The kidneys may be felt on deep palpation. If palpation is not possible in this position, or if the infant starts crying, thus tensing the abdominal musculature, the palpation should be stopped and the infant repositioned. Another technique that is sometimes successful is placing the infant again in the supine position, with one hand placed along the flank area posteriorly while the other hand is poised anteriorly to gently begin palpation. This technique allows the examiner a chance to trap the kidney's pole between the two hands (ballottement).

The kidneys, which are located in the flank area, are bilaterally equal in size. The right kidney may be slightly lower than the left kidney, owing to the position of other abdominal organs. Ureters are not palpable unless they are grossly enlarged (Scanlon et al., 1979). No masses should be felt; however, if one is encountered, its position, mobility on palpation, and contour (either flat, lumpy, or depressed) must be accurately described. If Wilms' tumor is suspected, palpation should not be performed, because this maneuver may break the tumor into small fragments, leading to tumor seeding. Inguinal hernias may be found in either sex, although they are less common in females. Bladder distention or ureterocele sometimes exhibits a mobile mass.

Male

Palpation of the testes is another important part of the physical examination. The scrotal sac may be palpated by gentle pressing of the tissue between two fingers, one located on the anterior surface and the other on the posterior surface. Gentle movement of the fingers upward over the scrotum until the testes are detected bilaterally indicates if one or both testes are descended and where they are in relationship to the internal ring in the inguinal canal. The cremasteric reflex may be elicited at the same time by gentle stroking of the upper thigh or scrotal sac. A positive reflex is elicited when the testes recoil toward the inguinal canal (Scanlon et al., 1979).

Percussion

If bladder distention is palpated or observed, percussion should be performed. This technique is useful in determining whether fluid is filling the bladder, a situation denoted by a somewhat tympanic sound; if a solid mass is present, dullness is noted. Percussion may also be used over the entire abdominal region. Dullness is a normal finding at the right costal margin; this finding indicates the liver. Tympany is the high-pitched sound noted over the gastric bubble just at the left costal margin. Over the intestines, a semitympanic or more resonating sound is produced, depending on whether the neonate has been fed yet or not. If he or she has been fed, some intestinal gas may cause a tympanic sound; otherwise, if the infant is several days old and the GI tract has begun to colonize with bacteria, feces may be present, causing a duller sound on percussion. Even with the newly born neonate, meconium may be present in the intestines in sufficient quantities to produce a duller sound. This finding alone is not necessarily indicative of a problem. The intestines should be palpated and the abdomen inspected as well. Examination of the abdomen and intestinal area is discussed in depth in Chapter 24 (Assessment and Management of Gastrointestinal Dysfunction).

Related Findings

Neonates should be inspected for general characteristics that are highly suggestive of renal problems. Low-set ears and abnormal facies often accompany syndromes in which renal disorders are a component (Smith, 1988). Although the exact mechanism is not known, a minor anomaly such as a single umbilical artery is a common finding when renal problems are present (Smith, 1988).

Meningomyelocele and other neural tube defects may result in decreased or absent innervation to the bladder. The result may be a neurogenic bladder characterized by bladder distention. Ultimately, if untreated, the urinary stasis leads to urinary and cystic infection.

Potter's syndrome (now sometimes referred to as Potter's association because the features occur together more often than is likely just by chance) may be suspected in infants with a history of prenatal oligohydramnios. It can be detected on physical examination by abnormal facies, short neck, beak-like nose, ocular hypertelorism (wide-set eyes), micrognathia, and disproportionately large ears. It is also accompanied by multiple atresias, including anal, esophageal, and duodenal atresias. Internally, the vas deferens and seminal vesicles may be absent in the male, or the upper vagina and uterus may be absent in the female, and a concave sternum (due to hypoplastic lungs) may be present in either sex (Sanders, 1996). These findings are directly related to dehydration and compression of the fetus during development. The birth weight is usually low, and a breech delivery is common. Such an infant also has a maternal history of oligohydramnios because renal agenesis is the major disorder. Other syndromes that have associated renal and genital problems are listed in Table 31–1.

RISK FACTORS

Table 31–2 lists maternal, neonatal, and other risks associated with urogenital disorders. Specific risk factors for each of the urogenital dysfunctions are addressed in the appropriate sections.

DIAGNOSTIC WORK-UP

The diagnostic work-up for potential renal problems includes several diagnostic screening tests.

Urinalysis

One of the first steps in a urogenital work-up is urinalysis. Although leukocytes may be present as a result of vaginal drainage, infection should not be assumed unless bacteria are also present. Laundau and associates (1994) found that urinalysis is an effective initial screening for a differential diagnosis between acute pyelonephritis and lower urinary tract infection in neonates who display a fever. Variables normally assessed in urinalysis include pH, color, specific gravity, cells, odor, blood, and protein.

Urine Collection

Urine collection is a relatively simple procedure in the neonate. Several adhesive-backed collection bags are available. Skin lacerations are possible, however, from the use of such collection bags (see Chapter 32, Assessment and Management of Integumentary Dysfunction). Care is taken not to include the rectum or scrotum within the opening of the bag. Alternative collection systems can be used if sterile specimens are not required and accurate measurement of output is not needed. Cotton balls can be placed inside diapers to catch a small specimen for dipstick analysis or for measurement of specific gravity. Reams and Deane (1988) studied the use of bagged versus diaper specimens for urine specific gravity. They found that in regular-absorbency disposable diapers, the cotton lining could be removed and urine directly extracted, resulting in laboratory values as accurate as those of bagged urine specimens. The penis should not be left in urine, because infection and skin irritation as well as contamination of the specimen may occur. However, further nursing research is needed because many institutions are currently switching to super-absorbency disposable diapers. The super-absorbent material can potentially alter the results of the urine test. In male infants, test tubes or syringe barrels may be secured to the penis to collect small specimens. In female infants, a disposable diaper can be placed with the plastic side toward the infant to obtain a small pool of urine. For long-term collections, the use of a collection bag with connecting tubing can drain into a collection bottle. An active infant may require restraints to prevent the

TABLE 31–1 Syndromes Associated with the Development of Urogenital Disorders

Syndromes	Renal Component	Genital Component
Potter's association	Renal agenesis	Absence of vas deferens, seminal vesical, upper vagina, uterus
Meckel's syndrome	Polycystic kidneys	Ambiguous genitalia Hypoplastic phallus Cryptorchidism
Trisomy 21	Cystic kidneys and other renal anomalies	Hypoplastic penis and scrotum Cryptorchidism
Trisomy 18	Dysplastic renal system	Hypoplastic clitoris and labia minora Cryptorchidism
Turner's syndrome	Horseshoe kidney Duplications of the collecting system	Infantile genitalia
Prune-belly syndrome	Urinary tract dysplasia Bladder and ureter dilation Patent urachus	Cryptorchidism
Inborn errors of metabolism Galactosemia Tyrosinemia Glycogen storage (Gierke's) disease	Renal tubular dysfunction	
Adrenogenital syndrome		Masculinization of the female Incomplete masculinization of the male Clitoral hypertrophy Hypospadias Hypoplastic penis Cryptorchidism

TABLE 31–2 Risk Factors Associated With Genitourinary Dysfunction

Risk Factor	Urogenital Defect
Maternal	
Fetal alcohol syndrome	Hydronephrosis Hypospadias Small, rotated kidneys
Maternal cocaine use	Genitourinary anomalies
Rubella	Renal artery stenosis
Maternal diabetes	Renal tubular necrosis
Maternal hypertension	Renal tubular necrosis
Oligohydramnios	Renal agenesis
Positive familial history: Polycystic kidneys Renal transplants Medullary cystic disease Nephritis Tubular acidosis	Other similar renal anomalies
Neonatal	
Asphyxia	Renal tubular necrosis
Resuscitation	Renal tubular necrosis
Vascular catheterization	Renal vessel thrombosis
Birth and other trauma	Renal tubular necrosis Physical renal damage Renal hemorrhage Peritoneal lacerations
Polycythemia; dehydration	Renal vessel thrombosis Renal necrosis
Nephrotoxic drugs Gentamicin Hyperosmotic fluids Metabolic buffers Disseminated intravascular coagulation	
Other Defects	
Spina bifida	Urinary stasis
Meningomyelocele	Urinary stasis, infection
Compression of aorta	Acute renal failure
Abdominal wall defects	Multiple urogenital deformities

dislodgment of the bag, which would require the collection period to begin again.

Blood Urea Nitrogen and Creatinine

Another indicator of renal functioning is the determination of serum blood urea nitrogen (BUN) and creatinine level. Although not absolute indicators of long-term renal problems, these values can be used to identify and treat acute problems. During the first few days of life, BUN levels may not be greater than 20 mg/dl. Until this point, placental function has maintained normal serum fetal levels, which remain stable in the early newborn period. In many cases, dehydration can cause dramatic increases in serum levels to levels higher than adult norms. Ingestion of high protein loads may affect levels in infants with normal renal function. Creatinine levels in the newborn are near adult levels at birth, then decrease by 1 month of age. These levels, unless they are significantly increased, may not be a clear indicator of renal disease. Table 31–3 provides a summary of the differences in renal function between term and preterm infants.

Renal Clearance Tests

Renal clearance tests are of little value in the newborn. Although inulin clearance tests may be performed, other measurements may be more diagnostic in the newborn period.

Serum Chemistries

The measurement of serum chemistries plays a large role in assessing renal functioning. In the premature or compromised infant, serum electrolyte levels may indicate a wider range of problems than occurs in the healthy newborn. Dehydration, fluid overload, metabolic disorders, fluid-losing and electrolyte-losing disorders, and respiratory compromise all lead to alterations in serum electrolyte levels. High serum sodium levels may reflect severe dehydration, excessive fluid loss, or administration of high solute loads. Low sodium levels can occur with overhydration, the use of large amounts of free water, or inappropriate antidiuretic hormone secretion (Schreiner & Bradburn, 1988). Potassium losses are apparent with diuretic use and with episodes of diarrhea.

Urine Chemistries

By looking at serum electrolyte levels in comparison to urine, urine chemistries are helpful in determining fluid and electrolyte balance. If urine sodium levels are outside normal values, serum levels may still be normal. In this instance, the infant may be struggling to retain or secrete sodium in order to maintain homeostatic balance.

Adrenocorticosteroid Levels

In the infant with adrenogenital syndrome, adrenocorticosteroid levels can be helpful in determining the specific disorder and treatment. The most common form is 21-hydroxylase deficiency. In addition to physical evidence of deficiency on external genitalia examination, urine or plasma levels of 17-ketosteroids, pregnanediol, and 17α-hydroxyprogesterone are deficient (Goodman & Gorlin, 1983). The development of the adrenals is addressed in Chapter 26 (Assessment and Management of Endocrine Dysfunction).

Urine Culture

Urine culture in the newborn is used as an assessment for neonatal sepsis. Although urine infections are rare in the newborn, they can occur when urinary tract deformities are present or when organisms have been introduced to the sterile renal system via catheterization or suprapubic bladder taps. In many cases, clean-catch specimens are obtained by use of either sterile or clean infant specimen collectors. When organisms appear on a culture report, a repeat culture is usually performed. The presence of leukocytes may not be an indication of infection, especially in the female, owing to vaginal secretions.

Latex Agglutination Test

The latex agglutination test is used to detect antigens produced by bacteria such as group B streptococci (Goetzman & Wennberg, 1991). It should be used in conjunction with other tests, such as urine cultures, to aid in the accurate identification of a specific organism.

Suprapubic Tap

The performance of the suprapubic tap requires minimal equipment and time. The lower abdomen is prepared with an antimicrobial solution and allowed to dry. Palpation of the bladder is attempted, although it may not be felt in the neonate. If the infant has voided within the previous hour, the attempt should be delayed until the infant has a full bladder. If severe dehydration,

TABLE 31–3 Differences in Renal Function Between Term and Preterm Infants

	Preterm	Term
Creatinine clearance 1 week after birth (ml/min/1.73m²)	11 ± 5 (GA 25–28 wk) 15 ± 6 (GA 29–34 wk)	46 ± 15
Plasma creatinine 1 wk after birth (mg/dL)	1.4 ± 0.8 (GA 25–28 wk)	0.5 ± 0.1
Maximum urine osmolality (mOsm/kg H_2O)	400–700	600–900
Proteinuria (mg/m²/d)	88–377	68–309
Plasma bicarbonate (mEq/L)	19.5 ± 2.9	21.0 ± 1.8
Mean fractional excretion of sodium (%)	4 (GA <30 wk)	<2

GA, gestational age.
From Springate, J. E., Fildes, R. D., & Feld, L. G. (1987). Assessment of renal function in newborn infants. *Pediatrics in Review*, 9(2), 56. Reprinted with permission from *Pediatrics in Review*.

distention, or abdominal congenital anomalies are present, a suprapubic tap may not be warranted. A 3-ml syringe with an 18-gauge straight needle may be used. The needle is placed midline, 1 to 1½ cm above the symphysis pubis, and inserted perpendicularly or at a slight angle, pointing toward the head (Bradburn & Schreiner, 1988). Entry into the bladder is determined when resistance decreases as the needle is inserted. A slight traction on the plunger may be all that is necessary to aspirate urine into the syringe. If no urine is obtained on the first attempt, a second attempt should be delayed until sufficient urine build-up has occurred. Pressure should be applied over the puncture site until all evidence of bleeding has ceased.

This procedure may have complications. Uterine and bowel perforations, trauma to other portions of the renal system, and infection are known complications. The procedure is not recommended for any neonate with clotting disorders or known disseminated intravascular coagulation.

Specific Gravity

Specific gravity measurement in the newborn can be misleading in its interpretation. Normal levels often range from 1.003 to 1.015. A low specific gravity may appear normal yet may not be an accurate reflection of renal functioning, because the infant has a decreased ability to concentrate urine. High specific gravities often reflect dehydration versus high solute excretion. Excretion of glucose and protein in the urine may artificially increase the specific gravity in the newborn.

Radiologic Examination

Radiologic examination includes a range of tests available for determining anatomic and physiologic function. The injection of contrast material can be used to visualize kidney mass and ureter and bladder outline and to help determine the amount of functioning kidney. In the premature infant, contrast material should be used selectively because the solution is hyperosmolar and may lead to further renal compromise. In instances when an intravenous pyelogram is ineffective in determining structural outlines, retrograde instillation of dye may be used.

Radionuclide Evaluation

Radionuclide evaluation may be necessary if pyelographic studies do not indicate accurate renal mass. The amount of uptake and the timing of excretion both may indicate renal deficiencies. Excretion of the dye via the urinary tract should be handled according to institutional policy regarding radioactive waste.

Another radionuclide test is diuretic renography, which is used most often if hydronephrosis is suspected. A radioisotope injection is given, followed 15 minutes later by a diuretic injection. The diuretic facilitates the movement of the radioisotope through the renal system. The isotope's movement is tracked by a gamma computer. If a urinary obstruction is present, the isotope's progress is slowed or impeded, showing retention of the radioactive substance. If a dilation exists along the renal system, urine is retained at the uteropelvic junction until overflow occurs with diuretic action. The stretching of the muscle fibers at this point causes strong contractions to begin. Soon, the urine is released, thus rapidly moving the isotope along (about 20 minutes) and showing a sharp, immediate decline in isotope concentration. In a normal kidney, the isotope takes about 25 minutes to clear the system, and the isotope concentration gradually declines. Institutional variations in the selection of the diuretic and isotope exist. This procedure many be direct or indirect radionuclide cystography (Eggli & Tulchinsky, 1993). The direct type requires catheterization and instillation of radionuclear materials into the bladder. The indirect method consists of renal imaging that is performed serially. The radionuclear materials are injected intravenously, and the movement of the material is observed by serial imaging. Scintigraphic evaluation is a good method of evaluating urinary tract infection and vesicourethral reflux (Eggli & Tulchinsky, 1993).

Renal Ultrasonography

The safest and one of the most useful tests to determine renal anomalies is ultrasonography. Analysis can often determine differences in normal versus cystic tissue. Solid tumors and masses may be readily apparent. In most institutions, ultrasound examinations are performed before invasive studies are performed. In many cases, accurate and specific diagnosis may be determined from ultrasonography alone. It also has been found useful in cases of scrotal swelling that were assumed to be caused by torsion of the testicles but that were, however, actually caused by adrenal hemorrhage (Liu et al., 1994).

Another instance in which renal ultrasound should be used as a screening tool is the case of single umbilical artery (Bourke et al., 1994). Some of these infants (about a fivefold increase in renal anomalies over the general population) have renal anomalies that often result in vesicoureteric reflux. These anomalies were megaureter and abnormal positioning of one or both kidneys, dilation of ureters, and other morphologic abnormalities (Bourke et al., 1994). It is also helpful in determining uretic reflux because this dysfunction shows as a ballooning of the renal pelvis (Hiraoka et al., 1994).

Computed Tomography

Computed tomography can be helpful in locating major structures. Its use is limited in providing specific diagnoses, and the cost may be prohibitive in relation to other available testing methods.

Genetic Consultation

Genetic consultation is an important part of the care for the infant with genital abnormalities. Chromosome banding and karyotyping should be performed if the infant has a positive family history of GU anomalies or if a visible neonatal GU malformation is present. Chromosomal analysis may take several weeks before final reports are completed. Fetal chromosomal studies can be performed if a defect is suspected.

COLLABORATIVE AND NURSING MANAGEMENT

General Principles

Electrolyte Balance

Prevention of hyperkalemia is most important in the management of renal failure (see Chapter 22, Fluids, Electrolytes, Vitamins, and Trace Minerals). Potassium should never be added to an intravenous solution until an appropriate urine output has been established. When urine output decreases, serum electrolyte levels should be frequently monitored to prevent the overload of fluids and potassium. Excess potassium, whether through excess administration or extracellular shift, can often be controlled through the use of an exchange resin (sodium polystyrene sulfonate [Kayexalate]). Urine and serum chemistries should be monitored at least twice daily. Special attention should be paid to the serum potassium levels because hyperkalemia is a consequence of renal failure. If sodium polystyrene sulfonate is given via rectal suppository in order to reduce the potassium level, the nurse should observe the infant for cardiac arrhythmias. One milliequivalent of potassium is exchanged for each 2 to 3 mEq of sodium. The usual dosage is 1 g/kg, repeated every 4 to 6 hours (Kim & Mandell, 1988). If the serum potassium level is 7 mEq/L or more, Kim and Mandell suggested that 0.5 to 1.0 ml/kg of 10-percent calcium gluconate be given intravenously slowly over 1 to 3 minutes. Continuous electrocardiographic monitoring is required. This should be followed by 2 to 3 mEq/kg of sodium bicarbonate given intravenously, then 2 g/kg of 25-percent dextrose, and finally 0.5 to 1.0 U/kg of insulin intravenously (Kim & Mandell, 1988, p. 73). Placement of the infant on a cardiorespiratory monitor is essential. Electrocardiograms are necessary to detect any abnormal rhythms or patterns that result from alterations in potassium levels. Dialysis can be used to return the body to normal potassium levels, but the use of long-term dialysis in the neonate is limited. Hypokalemia may result if diuretics such as furosemide (Lasix) are used. Again, close observation is critical.

Furosemide is used to treat congestive heart failure as well as fluid balance problems caused by GU problems. One experimental therapy aimed at decreasing the incidence of electrolyte imbalance is nebulized furosemide. A single dose of 1 mg/kg of inhaled furosemide appears to be more effective than the intravenous route and has fewer side effects. Although this therapy is experimental, if side effects such as hypokalemia can be diminished, it certainly merits further investigation.

Fluid Volume and Nutritional Management

Aggressive fluid management may lead to fluid overload and hypertension, which often occur because of attempts to maintain adequate blood pressure levels or because sepsis and shock precipitate oliguria, which may have been treated aggressively with fluids. The use of antihypertensives and diuretics may be necessary to control blood pressure. Hydralazine, 0.2 to 0.5 mg/kg given intravenously or intramuscularly every 4 to 8 hours, or nitroprusside given intravenously, 0.5 μg/kg/minute, or diazoxide given intravenously, 1 to 3 mg/kg/dose, may be used (Kim & Mandell, 1988). The last two drugs should be used with extreme caution in the neonate because they are potent medications. Sodium levels should be checked because excess fluid dilutes extracellular sodium. No treatment is needed if the neonate is showing no signs of hyponatremia. Hypertonic saline solution should be used with caution because it can raise the intracranial pressure. The sodium is increased by use of the following formula (Kim & Mandell, 1988, p. 73):

$$\text{dose of Na (mEq)} = \text{weight (kg)} \times 5 \times 0.65$$

Nursing management involves the assessment and reporting of signs and symptoms. Fluid volume excess can be a problem. Daily or twice-daily weights should be obtained and recorded for a baseline determination of excessive fluid retention or loss. Accurate intake and output must be measured. This output may include the weighing of diapers. Urine specific gravity is checked every 4 hours. Fluid restriction may be important if hypovolemia is not a causative factor. This fluid restriction is based on insensible water loss in addition to the urinary output of the previous 24 hours (Ingelfinger, 1985). Alterations in fluids and electrolyte levels are another neonatal problem. Sodium, protein, and phosphorus restrictions may also be imposed, although if the infant is asymptomatic, such electrolyte restrictions are not necessary. A formula that is low in phosphorus may be given in the form of Similac PM 60/40 or SMA. However, the formula should be checked for the amount of potassium present because additional potassium may not be tolerated by the neonate who is already hyperkalemic (Ingelfinger, 1985).

Aluminum hydroxide, 60 mg/kg, can be used to bind phosphate in the intestines and lower the phosphorus levels to the normal range of 5 to 6 mg/dl (Kim & Mandell, 1988). Use of aluminum hydroxide to bind phosphorus in the intestines may be helpful. Calcium supplements can be used after phosphorus level is decreased. The calcium often stabilizes on its own. However, calcium supplementation may also be needed because the calcium level is affected by the phosphorus level. These levels are inversely proportional: as one increases, the other decreases. Calcium gluconate (10 percent) or carbonate may be given intravenously or orally at a dose of 50 to 100 g/kg/day (Kim & Mandell, 1988). Such supplementation should be instituted when the calcium level decreases to less than 6 mg/dl (Kim & Mandell, 1988). Calcium carbonate may help correct acidosis. One caveat, however, is that rapid administration of calcium can precipitate a cardiac arrest; thus, administration of this agent requires close observation by the nurse.

Dihydrotachysterol or vitamin D supplementation is also a useful adjunct for the correction of calcium levels because under its influence, calcium is shifted from the bones, freed, and absorbed by the body.

In addition to these concerns, positive growth and nutrition may be compromised. If a fluid restriction has been imposed, the caloric consumption must be increased without increasing fluid volume. Medium-chain triglyceride oil can be used to increase the fat content, or glucose polymers (Polycose) or Contolyte can be added in order to increase the carbohydrates. Hyperalimentation is a mode of nutrition needed by infants who are no longer capable of receiving enteral feedings (see Chapter 23, Nutrition: Physiologic Basis of Metabolism and Management of Enteral and Parenteral Nutrition). The overall goal of nutritional therapy is the preservation of a positive nitrogen balance and the avoidance of increases in nitrogenous waste products that can lead to further increases in urea nitrogen levels and uremia (Kim & Mandell, 1988).

Close monitoring of serum electrolyte and phosphorus and calcium levels is necessary, regardless of whether oral or intravenous electrolyte supplementation is being used. In addition, fluid shifts may occur secondary to fluid overload or a change in electrolyte balance, resulting in edema. Assessment for the presence of edema includes observation for periorbital edema, observation of dependent surfaces, and examination of the hands, feet, and scrotum. Pitting should be determined by gentle depression of a fingertip into the suspected edematous site. Caution should be taken around the ocular area because direct pressure on the eyeball may precipitate bradycardia. If ascites is present, the infant is gravely ill because this is a late sign of renal failure.

Skin Management

Skin integrity is a concern, especially when pitting edema is present. The infant's position should be changed every 2 hours because swelling may accumulate in the dependent regions. Skin around any operative site should be inspected with every dressing change for any signs of irritation or infection. The skin must be kept dry and clean to prevent skin breakdown and infection (see Chapter 32, Assessment and Management of Integumentary Dysfunction).

Respiratory Management

Respiratory compromise is common in the infant experiencing alterations in urinary elimination. During fetal life, insufficient amniotic fluid is linked to decreased development of the respiratory tree (see discussion on Potter's association). The chest may be small in comparison with the distended abdomen (Fig. 31–4).

The ability to use accessory muscles that help achieve effective respiration is lacking. This situation can lead to a decrease in ventilatory effort. In some cases, lung hypoplasia may result.

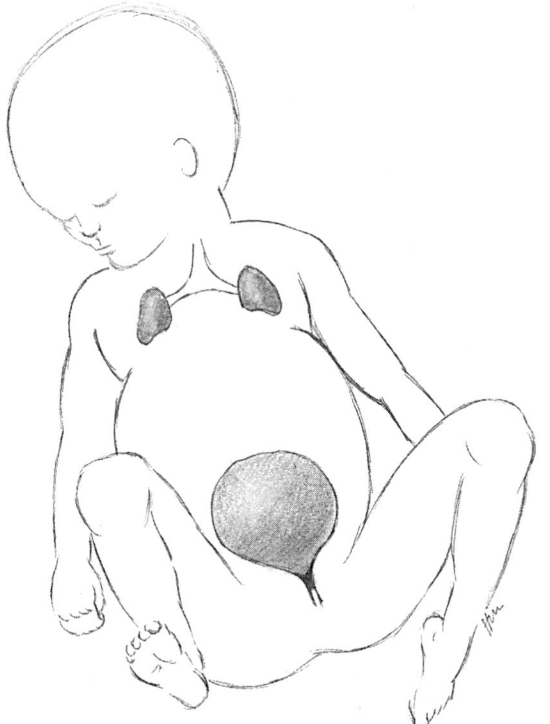

FIGURE 31–4. Urinary bladder obstruction with hypoplastic lungs.

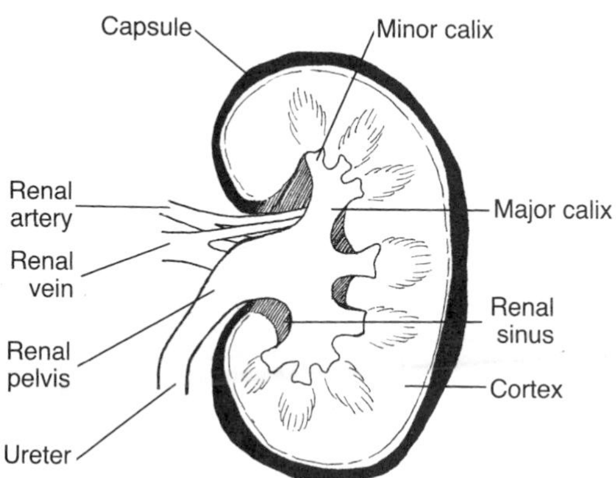

FIGURE 31–5. Kidney structure.

Before extensive therapy is initiated for the treatment of renal anomalies, careful evaluation of respiratory status should be performed (see Chapter 18, Assessment and Management of Respiratory Dysfunction, for a complete discussion of respiratory assessment). Measures to improve renal function should not be undertaken if respiratory capacity is insufficient to support life.

General Preoperative Management

Before surgery, the goal is to maintain the stability of the fluid and electrolyte balance and the hemodynamic status of the infant. Assessment for any signs of urinary tract infection, such as poor feeding, temperature instability, cyanosis, and any other detectable subtle change from the infant's baseline norm, should be performed because the infant should be infection free, if possible, before surgery.

General Postoperative Management

After surgery, nursing management is again focused on careful assessment and monitoring of the fluid and electrolyte status as well as the hemodynamic system, including blood pressure, pulse, and respiration of the infant. Accurate measurement of fluid intake and output is again critical. If poor renal function develops in one of the infant's kidneys, surgical placement of a nephrostomy tube is needed (Sugar & Firlit, 1988). This tube's insertion site is covered with a sterile dressing.

Because the renal system is a highly vascular system, the chance for bleeding or infection is great. After the insertion of a nephrostomy tube or tubes, pink-tinged urine or even urine with visible bloody streaks is common. These tubes should not be irrigated because they are located within the renal pelvis (Fig. 31–5). The tubes should be connected to a closed drainage system in order to maintain sterility. A clean dressing surrounding the tube should be used to maintain the position and protect the underlying skin. On removal of such tubes, urine leakage for as long as 48 hours is not unusual.

Maintenance of an aseptic suture line is important. Any dressings, especially over a nephrostomy site, should be closely observed for bleeding or drainage. An infant with a nephrostomy tube or who has undergone other renal surgery is at risk for infection. Broad-spectrum antibiotics, such as ampicillin and gentamicin, are useful. Use of trimethoprim-sulfamethoxazole (Bactrim) is appropriate in the infant older than 2 months of age and without severe renal impairment. This drug is specific to the bacteria that most often cause urinary tract infections.

A urinary stent may also be placed in the ureter to splint the site of the anastomosis that has been performed. Although no drainage is expected through this stent, a closed drainage system is necessary to protect the neonate from infection. The infant may have a Foley catheter as well. Eventually, the neonate may require a ureterostomy followed by a nephrectomy, if kidney function cannot be restored.

When urinary stents or suprapubic or nephrostomy tubes are used, it may be necessary to maintain the infant's position by placement in traction. Bryant's traction, a type of skin traction, may be used (Spindel et al., 1988).

Support to Parents

Parents may be extremely upset if their infant has had a nephrectomy. Removal of a kidney is frightening to them, especially with all the current media coverage on renal transplantation. The parents should be encouraged to express these concerns, and they must be given accurate information as to the prognosis for their infant. Use of the interdisciplinary team is essential. Collaboration among the neonatologist, pediatric urologist, nurse, clergy, social worker, and financial counselor helps the parents adjust to this frightening neonatal problem. If the infant is dying, early involvement by the clergy or other social support network—other parents, family, or friends—can ease the parents' pain of realizing that their child will not go home. The nurse should anticipate this need and act before a crisis occurs.

Nursing Considerations for the Protection of Health Professionals

The child who is born with cytomegalic inclusion disease sheds the virus in the urine for an unknown period of time, often years. The implications for nurses are twofold. When contracted by pregnant women, cytomegalovirus may result in damage to the central nervous system of the developing fetus. In the first trimester, exposure to cytomegalovirus sometimes results in miscarriage. Nurses who are of childbearing age must be cautious and use meticulous hand washing when caring for these infants. Gloves should be worn when diapers of any infant believed to be at risk for cytomegalovirus are changed. Good hand washing is essential after diaper changes and any type of urine testing.

Compromised newborns must also be protected against exposure to the virus because their immune system is not adequate to fight such an infection and it could result in death. Thus, cross-contamination is a vital consideration. Excretion–secretion precautions should be used in caring for neonates who are known to be cytomegalovirus-positive to ensure protection against accidental passage of the virus. Diapers should be disposed of at a bedside receptacle rather than at a receptacle across the nursery.

In addition, an infant with acquired immunodeficiency syndrome may be asymptomatic in the nursery; however, universal precautions should be used any time an infant is suspected to be at high risk for acquired immunodeficiency syndrome (see Chapter 42, Neonatal Acquired Immunodeficiency Syndrome).

The general principles of nursing management have been outlined. The remainder of the chapter addresses the most common GU neonatal problems.

URINARY TRACT INFECTION

Pathophysiology

Full-term neonates are at risk for developing any type of infection, owing to their immature immune status. The immune system has generally never been challenged by pathogens. In utero, the placenta acts as an effective barrier to many pathogens, bacterial and protozoan (Faden & Rosales, 1984). If the neonate is premature, stressed in utero or in extrauterine life, or has other congenital anomalies, the immune system is usually further depressed. Both the specific and the nonspecific immunity, as well as the complement system, are diminished, predisposing the newborn to difficulty in locating the source or the site of an infection and also in mounting an effective response to invasion.

The number of neutrophils and their phagocytic action are decreased. Fewer T-lymphocyte helper cells than suppressor cells exist, again contributing to compromise of the immune system. Monocytes are more effective than neonatal T lymphocytes. Although they confer some protection against bacteria, such as *Escherichia coli* and *Staphylococcus aureus*, they are not as effective against many viruses (Faden & Rosales, 1984). Maternal passive immunity plays a role in the depression of the neonate's immune system because maternal antibodies may respond to certain pathogens, thereby not allowing the neonatal system to be challenged. This factor lessens the infant's ability to respond, even on second invasion of the same pathogen. It is usually this second exposure that peaks the immune system, conferring enough immunity to fight infections. This secondary, or memory, response is the basis of booster injections for immunizations.

Gamma G immunoglobulin (IgG) is the immunoglobulin that is transferred most readily across the placenta. IgG effectively protects the infant against group A streptococcus and *Treponema pallidum* (Faden & Rosales, 1984). IgA is passed to the infant, even the premature infant, in small quantities in breast milk. Fibronectin is a glycoprotein that was recently found to be deficient in highly septic infants and premature infants. Therefore, it is believed to be bactericidal and increases the neonate's ability to fight such infections.

Urinary tract infections in neonates are not particularly common. Such neonatal infections are the result of iatrogenic factors or urinary malformation or obstructions. Bacteria may be introduced during procedures such as suprapubic bladder taps. These iatrogenic factors can be avoided if strict adherence to aseptic techniques is followed. Urinary obstructions along the renal or urinary pathways may cause urinary flow to be slowed or stopped. As a result, urinary stasis predisposes the neonate to bacterial colonization and ultimately bladder or urinary tract infections. Spinal or neural tube deformities like spina bifida or meningomyelocele are often accompanied by a neurogenic bladder, that is, one that lacks innervation; thus, urine flow is diminished. Urine builds up within the bladder, predisposing the infant to increased bacterial growth. The result is urinary and bladder infection (Faden & Rosales, 1984).

Common infectious agents responsible for urinary tract infections are gram-negative bacteria. These are most often introduced during urinary catheterization procedures. *E. coli* and group B streptococcus also may cause urinary tract infections. Seventy percent of all urinary tract infections are attributable to *E. coli*. This pathogen, along with group B streptococcus, is normally found in the female genital tract, especially in the vagina. Thus, infants are exposed to these agents during the birth process. These organisms may be found on the neonatal skin surface; thus, if a good cleansing preparation of the pubic area is performed before a suprapubic tap, for instance, the pathogens may be removed. *Klebsiella*, *Pseudomonas*, and *Proteus* species have also been implicated in urinary infections (Ingelfinger, 1985).

Fungal infections are becoming more common in neonates with long-term health problems who have required invasive procedures, and they may cause pyonephrosis. Nonsurgical treatment uses percutaneous nephrostomy tubes. This treatment is also useful for bacterial pyonephrosis. Bell and associates (1993) found that percutaneous nephrostomy tubes provided an effective method of diagnosing the exact fungal agent and of administering amphotericin B in conjunction with intravenous systemic amphotericin B and 5-fluorocytosine to combat *Candida albicans* and *Torulopsis glabrata* infections.

Clinical Manifestations

The clinical manifestations of a urinary tract infection are often subtle. The affected infant is often asymptomatic. Characteristics, if demonstrated, are temperature instability, poor feeding, cyanosis, abdominal distention, poor weight gain, hepatomegaly, jaundice, thrombocytopenia purpura, and fever; the infant may or may not have proteinuria (McCracken & Freij, 1987). These characteristics are a result of the immune system's response to infection. The nurse should report these signs to the medical team for further diagnostic work-up.

Because neonates have immature nonspecific and specific immune systems, localization of infection is not usually possible. General signs and symptoms of infection are commonly present. Nurses must perform an ongoing assessment of all newborns suspected of having any type of infection, including urinary tract infections.

Differential Diagnosis

In any neonate suspected of having a urinary tract infection, a blood culture should be obtained because overwhelming septicemia may be present (Ingelfinger, 1985). Other physical and internal anomalies must be considered whenever a urinary tract infection is suspected. Positive diagnosis of a urinary tract infection is made when a urine culture grows the causative agent.

Prognosis

The prognosis is generally good for an isolated urinary tract infection. However, the potential for serious complications is always present. Severe damage to the renal system could occur. Septicemia may be life threatening. The prognosis is directly dependent on the cause of such an infection. The exact cause of the infection must be determined as early as possible if complications are to be prevented.

Collaborative Management

Once a urinary infection is identified from the nursing or physician assessment and once the causative agent is known, appropriate antibiotic therapy must be started. Intravenous antibiotics are the treatment of choice. Because they are broad-spectrum antibiotics, ampicillin and gentamicin are the drugs of choice, unless the causative organism is not sensitive to these medications. Ampicillin is given at a dose of 100 mg/kg/day, and gentamicin is given at a dose of 3.5 to 7.5 mg/kg/day. These standardized neonatal dosages are dependent on functional kidneys and adequate urine output (1 ml/kg/hour). The physician or practitioner should be notified immediately if urinary output is diminished. Another drug that is particularly useful for urinary tract infections is trimethoprim-sulfamethoxazole. It is especially effective in treating infections that stem from group A beta-hemolytic streptococci, *E. coli, Proteus mirabilis,* and *Klebsiella, Staphylococcus,* and *Enterobacter* species. This sulfonamide is not recommended for use in infants younger than 2 months of age or in those with severe renal dysfunction (Deglin & Vallerand, 1988).

Intravenous pyelography and voiding cystourethrography should be performed after any trace of infection is gone. These tests are performed to ensure that no damage to the urinary tract exists. If the infection is a result of a suspected urinary or renal obstruction, further diagnostic studies must be performed. Again, preferably after the infection is cleared, radiologic testing and renal ultrasonography should be performed to determine if an obstruction or a deformity is present (Ingelfinger, 1985). Otherwise, the infant will experience recurrent urinary tract infections.

Collaborative and Nursing Management

A holistic assessment of the infant should be conducted. A review of the maternal and newborn history is essential. Any positive familial history of pyelonephritis or nephritis should be considered. Maternal infections, especially of the genital tract, should be noted. Neonatal procedures, such as suprapubic bladder taps, should be noted, along with the dates the procedures were performed. These dates give an estimation of the incubation time for possible pathogens.

A neonate with hepatomegaly, jaundice, or thrombocytopenia purpura may actually be exhibiting associated symptoms of urinary tract infections. Such an infant should be monitored closely for any baseline deviations and considered to potentially have a urinary tract infection.

Familial pyelonephritis is a risk factor for the development of neonatal renal dysfunction. However, pyelonephritis is not a common finding in the newborn period.

Careful assessment of the infant must include observation of fluctuations in temperature or the presence of fever. Temperature should be checked at least every 4 hours. If wide fluctuations are present or if a persistent temperature of greater than 37.5°C exists rectally, temperature checks should be made every 1 to 2 hours. If fever is present, tachycardia of greater than 160 beats per minute or tachypnea of greater than 60 breaths per minute may also occur. For the premature infant whose temperature is consistently less than 36.5 to 37°C, the baseline norm should be used for each individual infant. If the temperature is consistently greater than previous temperatures, a fever should be suspected.

If the infant has an indwelling urinary catheter, observation of the urine for cloudiness or hematuria should be noted. A urine culture should be sent any time a urinary tract infection is suspected. It should be noted in the patient's chart that hematuria may be present as the result of a traumatic catheterization or postsurgical trauma, especially that incurred during placement of nephrostomy tubes. Thus, hematuria alone is not a good indicator of urinary tract infection. A urine dipstick assessment may or may not be helpful, because proteinuria can be indicative of the presence of urinary bacteria. However, if hematuria is present, this finding is essentially useless because blood is a protein.

Observation of the infant's weight and ability to take feedings is important. Especially worrisome is a neonate who begins to progressively lose weight or does not feed as well as in the past. GI disturbances, such as vomiting and diarrhea, may also be suggestive of a urinary infection (Ingelfinger, 1985). It is imperative to have a good baseline of the typical feeding pattern and weight and thorough documentation of feeding and weight changes, because an infant's well-being must be measured against this baseline.

CIRCUMCISION

Historically, the practice of male circumcision has been based on the premise that this surgical procedure helped promote positive hygiene and prevent urinary tract infections. It was also believed that the circumcised male was less likely than an uncircumcised male to transmit sexual diseases to a partner. The American Academy of Pediatrics (1993) indicated that based on its current research findings, no absolute medical indication exists for this procedure. The removal of the prepuce, or foreskin, covering the glans penis may be performed in the delivery room or in the newborn nursery. The actual decision to circumcise is usually based on parental cultural values and beliefs.

Circumcision does make the cleansing of the penis and removal of smegma (the whitish secretions generally found lying underneath the foreskin) easier. Wiswell and colleagues (1987) found an increase in the incidence of urinary tract infections as the number of circumcisions declined. These findings were confirmed by Wiswell and Hachey (1993), in a study of 209,399 infants born in United States Army hospitals internationally from 1985 to 1990. They found that 550 females and 496 males were hospitalized for urinary tract infections during their first year of life. Uncircumcised male infants had 10 times more infections than circumcised male infants. These researchers also conducted a meta-analysis of studies regarding urinary tract infections and found that the rate of urinary tract infections was five to 89 times greater in uncircumcised infants than in circumcised infants (Wiswell & Hachey, 1993).

Circumcision does require surgical intervention and causes discomfort. Neonatal local anesthesia should be used to reduce the discomfort (Stang et al., 1988). Parents should be taught to observe the penis for any drainage or bleeding. They should receive an explanation about the Plastibell clamp, if it is left in place, including how long it will be on the penis and the fact that it will fall off. They need to be shown how to cleanse the penis without introducing bacteria.

ACUTE RENAL FAILURE

Pathophysiology

Acute renal failure is a diminishment or complete stoppage of kidney function. It can have many causes because any condition that potentially interferes with kidney function can lead to acute renal failure. It is most often associated with an accelerated production of vasoconstrictor prostaglandins, which result in vasoconstriction of the renal vessels. Thus, the blood flow through the kidneys is diminished, as is the glomerular filtration rate (Sadler, 1995). Acute renal failure has been estimated to affect as many as 25 percent of all neonates admitted to an intensive care unit (Brion et al., 1994).

Acute renal failure occurs in three forms: prerenal, intrarenal, and postrenal. Prerenal failure results from congenital conditions, such as cystic disease, aplasia, and nephrosis; acquired conditions, like clotting or necrosis; ischemia due to hypotension or hypoxia; nephrotoxic exposure that results from drug therapy (e.g., aminoglycosides, methicillin, and indomethacin); high-technology therapies, such as extracorporeal membrane oxygenation or use of contrast dye in radiologic testing; and miscellaneous conditions, such as acidosis, polycythemia, and urinary tract infection (John & Yeh, 1985; White et al., 1990).

In the prerenal type of renal failure, urine output in the neonate is directly influenced by perfusion of the kidneys. Hypoxia plays a large role in the development of the acute prerenal type of renal failure. Hypoxic episodes can occur antenatally, at the time of delivery, or during any point in the neonatal period. When blood pressure decreases, urine output decreases. In the neonate, hypotension can occur secondary to sepsis, cold stress, or hypovolemia. Thus, prerenal failure causes hypovolemia and hypoperfusion. Reversing the effects of hypovolemia and hypotension may prevent the occurrence of renal damage.

Intrarenal causes, such as acute tubular necrosis, use of maternal or neonatal nephrotoxic drugs, renal agenesis, pyelonephritis, nephritis, hypoplasia or dysplasia, and birth trauma, may result in renal failure (Fanaroff & Martin, 1997).

Postrenal failure is usually caused by congenital anomalies that obstruct the flow of urine. These anomalies include ureteropelvic junction and urethrovesical obstruction, prune-belly syndrome, and neurogenic bladder. A back-up of urine into the kidney pelvis inhibits the ability of the kidneys to function. If this condition persists, fluid permanently fills the tissue spaces. Damage can occur as early as the 16th to 18th weeks of gestation (Inturrisi et al., 1985). Hydronephrosis may be nonreversible, leading to renal failure in one or both kidneys. This condition can sometimes be diagnosed in the fetal period. Oliguria of the fetus leads to oligohydramnios, which may be detected on maternal physical examination. Familial tendency for some renal disorders may suggest that antenatal testing for fetal renal disease be performed in identified groups. Obstructive uropathies have been successfully treated in utero, thus preventing hydronephrosis (Golbus et al., 1985).

Persistent acute renal failure after the initial insult is related to tubular obstruction from cell debris. This decrease in blood flow leads to tubular damage and loss of sodium, resulting in release of renin and thereby decreasing the glomerular filtration rate. This situation becomes a vicious circle. The lack of renin release leads to a loss of sodium and water, which accounts for high-output failure (John & Yeh, 1985).

Acidosis may readily follow acute renal failure. Poor perfusion in neonates can lead to the build-up of organic acids. Respiratory compensation is slow and often inadequate, especially in an already compromised infant. The levels of other minerals and electrolytes must be carefully monitored. The prevention of toxic build-up products must be considered because severe renal failure may be difficult to treat. Table 31–4 provides a list of diagnostic indices for neonatal acute renal failure.

Risk Factors

Treatments such as mechanical ventilation and umbilical and femoral vessel catheterization may predispose the infant to renal failure because of renal vein and artery thrombosis. Birth injury, hypovolemia, and hypoxemia may compromise renal blood flow. Congenital causes of intrinsic renal failure include aplastic kidney, polycystic renal disease, necrosis, and maternal ingestion of nephrotoxic agents. Other infants at risk for renal disease include premature infants and infants with respiratory distress syndrome or trisomy defects and other genetic disorders. Prenatal exposure to indomethacin has been linked with renal insufficiency and acute renal failure in the first few days of postnatal life of the premature infant (Vanhaesebrouck et al., 1988).

Maternal use of certain drugs has also been implicated in the development of neonatal renal failure. Excessive use of acetaminophen can lead to nephrotoxic effects in the fetus. Lithium use is also considered to be potentially nephrotoxic in utero (Jain & Yeh, 1985).

Differential Diagnosis

Acute renal failure is a manifestation of many other problems, as stated in the pathophysiology section. The diagnosis is aimed at finding the causative agent and not just at determining the presence of acute renal failure. The specific diagnostic tests are determined by what the practitioner suspects is the contributing process. This hypothesis requires a thorough nursing assessment in conjunction with an aggressive medical work-up.

Clinical Manifestations

Decreased urine output, edema, and lethargy are clinical signs that may point to acute renal failure. Oliguria is the most significant sign of acute renal failure (John & Yeh, 1985). Edema is usually caused by fluid overload rather than by the condition itself. Hematuria and proteinuria are common signs of failure. Some neonates also present with abdominal distention or a flank mass. Because hypoperfusion of the kidneys may be common in the neonate, efforts should be made to determine the cause of the oliguria. In true renal failure, hematuria and hemoglobinuria may occur. Urinary-to-plasma osmolality ratio of 1.1 or less may indicate renal failure (John & Yeh, 1985). Renal compromise can be detected even in utero through fetal urine samples. The

TABLE 31–4 Diagnostic Indices in Neonatal Acute Renal Failure

	Prerenal Oliguria Without Renal Failure	Prerenal and Intrinsic Renal Failure
Serum findings		
Na	Normal or elevated	Low normal or elevated
K	Normal or elevated	Normal or elevated
BUN	Normal or elevated	Elevated
Creatinine	Normal or elevated	Elevated
Ca	Normal	Low
P	Normal	Normal or elevated
Urine findings		
RBC, protein, casts, and tubular cell casts	Usually absent	Present
Specific gravity	Increased	Low
Urine volume	Low	Low in 60%–80% (1 ml/kg/hr), normal or high in 40% (>2.4 ml/kg/hr)
Urine osmolarity (mOsm/kg water)	Increased >300–400	Decreased <300
Urine Na (mEq/L)	<30 mEq/L (preterm infant) <20 mEq/L	>30 mEq/L
Creatinine clearance	Normal or decreased	Decreased
U/P creatinine	>20:1	<10:1
U/P urea	>20:1	<10:1
U/P osmolarity	>1.5:1	<1.5:1
FE_{Na}%	<1% (term infant) <3% (preterm infant)	>2% (term infant) >3% (preterm infant)
RFI	<3%	>3%

FE_{Na} + excreted fraction of filtered sodium + $\frac{Una}{Ucr} \times \frac{Pcr}{PNa} \times 100$, where UNa = urinary sodium, Ucr = urinary creatinine, Pcr = plasma creatinine, and PNa = plasma sodium. PR = renal failure index = $\frac{UNa}{Ucr} \times Pcr$

U/P, urine:plasma ratio; RFI, renal failure index; BUN, blood urea nitrogen

Modified from John, E.G., & Yeh, T. F. (1985). Renal failure. In T. F. Yeh (Ed.), *Drug therapy in the neonate and small infant* (p. 279). Chicago: Year Book Medical Publishers. Reprinted with permission.

maximum fetal urine electrolyte levels considered within normal limits are sodium, 100 mEq/L; chloride, 90 mEq/L; and osmolality, 210 mOsm/kg (Grupe, 1987). Levels greater than these values are indicative of renal failure and poor prognosis. BUN levels and serum creatinine levels increase.

Urine output should be at least 1 ml/kg/hour. Urine output, at least initially, may be within normal limits (Brion, Satlin, & Edelmann, 1994). The use of diuretics may alter the results of urine tests, causing decreased specific gravity (dilute urine) and changes in urine electrolytes (increased loss of potassium with loop or thiazide diuretics and increased loss of chloride ions). Diuretic use should be documented when renal function studies are performed. Shock and volume depletion should always be evaluated when oliguria results. In the presence of open or draining congenital anomalies, hidden fluid losses may occur. Surgery to repair defects can lead to third spacing of fluids, leaving the infant further fluid compromised (see Table 31–3 for a brief review of the differences in renal function between term and preterm infants).

Complications of renal failure include hyperkalemia, volume overload, hyponatremia, hypertension, acidosis, hypocalcemia, hyperphosphatemia, nutritional problems, sepsis, anemia, and azotemia (increased level of nitrogenous waste products in the blood).

The blood pressure may at first be decreased, then rebound to an above-normal level. Hypertension, or a blood pressure of greater than 90/65 mm Hg in term infants, is often the result of fluid overload or increased secretion of renin and aldosterone.

Less common signs of renal failure are usually due to hypoxemia. Seizures, for example, may follow, as may intraventricular hemorrhage or cerebral edema. Hypoglycemia, uremia, or infection also can be manifestations of renal failure.

Prognosis

The prognosis of acute renal failure is solely dependent on the ability to treat the underlying problem. Early detection, sometimes even in utero, and treatment of acute renal failure guide the treatment course, possibly preventing life-threatening complications.

Collaborative Management

The treatment is aimed at preventing the long-term complications of acute renal failure. Symptomatic treatment is carried out until a definitive cause is determined and treated. Intravenous isotonic solution, 10 to 20 ml/kg given over 1 hour, is administered if no signs of heart failure are present. Mannitol and furosemide are given in order to prevent acute renal failure if the infant is believed to be at risk for its development. Dopamine may also be tried in low doses (John & Yeh, 1985).

Fluid replacement is limited to insensible loss and replacement of renal output. If the infant is acidotic, sodium bicarbonate is used instead of sodium chloride in the solution. Sodium bicarbonate should be used with caution because it is hypertonic and has been found to cause increases in intracranial pressure and resultant intraventricular hemorrhage. Hyponatremic acute renal failure is treated by fluid restriction. Peritoneal dialysis or hemodialysis should be used only in infants with severe congestive heart failure, fluid overload, or uremia. Peritoneal dialysis seems to be the method of choice in neonatal care. Either method can be used within the neonatal intensive care unit; however, expert professionals must be in charge of this procedure because close monitoring of the infant's status is needed. The cycle of dialysis infusion, dwell time, and release, as well as the accurate measurement of fluid intake and output and serum electrolyte levels, is critical. Exact parameters of dialysis are beyond the scope of this book.

Drugs with high sodium levels, such as carbenicillin, penicillin G, ampicillin, and cephalothin, or drugs diluted in sodium chloride should be used with caution in patients with renal failure because they may add to the problem of maintaining fluid and electrolyte balance.

Nursing care is aimed at maintaining fluid and electrolyte balance. It is also necessary to accurately calculate fluid intake and output to guard against fluid overload and resultant hypertension and edema. Nurses must remember, too, that potassium affects cardiac conduction. Therefore, because these neonates may experience hyperkalemia, all intake of potassium must be eliminated. This measure includes the use of only fresh blood for transfusions because the older the blood, the more likely the cells are to have broken down, releasing potassium. Calcium gluconate (10 percent) or calcium carbonate helps decrease the effect of potassium on the heart; dialysis may also be a necessary adjunct to standard therapy. Acidosis is inevitable and is complicated by the need to restrict sodium. Treatment for acidosis, however, is undertaken only when the infant is symptomatic.

Increased phosphorus and decreased calcium levels are treated by protein restriction. Calcium supplementation and phosphorus-binding substances may be needed. (See section on fluid volume and nutritional management in this chapter for specific information.)

Anemia is a potential consequence of renal failure. The infant's hematocrit value and hemoglobin level must be measured at least daily. Changes in the vital signs or color should be assessed so that subtle changes indicating anemia may be detected.

Hypertension that is secondary to fluid overload may be treated by sodium and fluid restriction. Antihypertensive agents may also be tried. Dialysis may be indicated if the condition is severe. These infants are prone to infections. Signs of infection should be watched for and reported to the physician or neonatal practitioner so that treatment is begun immediately.

Because the kidney is the clearinghouse for many drugs, the metabolism of drugs is altered when renal failure occurs. Aminoglycosides, penicillins, cephalosporins, theophylline, indomethacin, tolazoline, and magnesium should all be used with caution.

Nutritional needs for the infant are 1 to 1.5 g/kg/day of protein with 30 to 50 cal/kg/day. Vitamin D, vitamin B complex, and folic acid supplements may be needed. Vitamin A should be avoided. Breast milk, Similac PM 60/40, and SMA are recommended by some institutions because of their decreased sodium, potassium, and phosphorus loads.

Nursing Management

If the infant's condition continues to deteriorate and high BUN levels coupled with increasing ammonia levels are present, dialysis may be necessary. This procedure may be performed in the neonatal intensive care unit and requires one-on-one nursing care. The dialyzing cycle is dependent on the medical treatment being used and the severity of the condition. Nursing responsibility includes monitoring the equipment, monitoring the cycles if performed manually, performing clotting studies, and administering heparin and other drugs via the dialysis setup. Either hemodialysis or peritoneal dialysis may be performed. Catheter care includes maintenance of aseptic technique, prevention of hemorrhage and clotting, and observation of the insertion site for signs of infection or dislodgment. The nurse should observe for signs and symptoms of chemical imbalances during the entire dialysis procedure. Fluid shifts affecting blood pressure and electrolyte balance can occur rapidly, causing cardiac arrhythmias, muscle spasms, seizures, and shock.

POTTER'S ASSOCIATION (POTTER'S SYNDROME)

Pathophysiology

Potter's syndrome is an association of defects that begins with bilateral renal agenesis. For this reason, the term *syndrome* is generally being replaced by the word *association*. It occurs when the uretic bud fails to divide and develop, culminating in bilateral renal agenesis. Renal agenesis is the complete absence of the kidney. Because fetal urine is a major component of amniotic fluid, oligohydramnios is present. In the severest form, no amniotic fluid may be present. The developing fetal structures are compressed as a result of this lack of fluid, leading to the characteristic Potter facies (Sanders, 1996).

Clinical Manifestations

A typical appearance of the facies includes ears that are low set and malformed, micrognathia, "senile" appearance, wrinkled skin, parrot-beak nose, and eyes that are wide set with obvious epicanthal folds. Other associated defects include abnormal genital development, leg deformities, GI defects, and arthrogryposis, a condition associated with contractures of the extremities (see Chapter 30, Assessment and Management of Musculoskeletal Dysfunction, for a discussion of arthrogryposis).

The mother may go into premature labor. The infant with this syndrome may be stillborn. The infant is usually born in the breech position and is small for gestational age. In the absence of severe respiratory compromise, oliguria or anuria may be the only presenting symptoms.

Risk Factors

The incidence of Potter's association is approximately 1 in 10,000 births, with the condition being found predominantly in males (Goodman & Gorlin, 1983). Although no strong genetic predisposition exists, a multifactorial inheritance pattern has been suggested (Goodman & Gorlin, 1983). Evidence does exist that siblings of infants with Potter's association have a higher-than-average incidence of neural tube defects.

Differential Diagnosis

Potter's association is usually readily identifiable on direct observation because of its characteristic facies. Most often, no other diagnosis is even considered. Potter's association is also a part of the XYY syndrome.

Prognosis

The infant may die within the first several days of life, owing to lack of kidney tissue to support life. Because of the association of renal agenesis with lung hypoplasia, death often occurs as the result of respiratory insufficiency. The exact reason the lungs do not fully develop in the presence of renal agenesis has eluded researchers (Manning, 1987). Researchers have hypothesized that pulmonary development is dependent on adequate levels of amniotic fluid. This principle has been demonstrated in fetuses with esophageal atresia or another defect that interfered with fetal swallowing. Although the circulation of the amniotic fluid was disrupted, the amount of fluid was normal; therefore, lung development followed the usual course (Colodny, 1987). If the fluid was diminished or scanty, as with Potter's association, the pulmonary development was disrupted.

It is hypothesized that a mechanical element may be involved that stops or slows alveolar development. It may be that the fetal kidney secretes a substance that assists lung development. Researchers have demonstrated that when damage to the metanephros of the kidney occurs, the substance arginase is not produced (Colodny, 1987). Arginase is necessary for the conversion of ornithine to proline; the latter substance is required for mesenchymal development and thus the development of the bronchial and alveolar tree (Colodny, 1987). Owing to pulmonary hypoplasia that is irreversible, current treatment of neonates with Potter's association does not include renal transplantation or long-term dialysis.

Collaborative and Nursing Management

Focus on the parents is the most important aspect of nursing care. The parents need support and a chance to express their feelings. Denial and feelings of guilt are usual and are often a necessary defense mechanism in the first few days. The nurse must offer the parents the chance to see and hold their child, but some parents may fear attachment. This attitude must be accepted by the nurse. It is often helpful even after the infant's death to allow siblings to see and touch the infant. This strategy can be upsetting to the nurse but necessary for incorporation of the infant into a small child's reality. It may ease the parents' fear of talking about the death in front of their other children. Grandparents need support as well because they often feel guilt because they could not shield their children from this "hurt" (see Chapter 8, Bereavement: A State of Having Suffered a Loss, especially the section on grief and loss, for more specific information).

APLASTIC KIDNEY

Pathophysiology

When the uretic bud fails to form in utero, aplasia or absence of the kidney occurs. One kidney develops, but the other kidney does not. This is also called unilateral renal agenesis.

Risk Factors

The rate of occurrence may be as high as 1 in 500 births (Kaplan, 1994). It is most often associated with other structural defects, such as spinal deviations, especially scoliosis, imperforate anus, and, in the female, uterine and vaginal agenesis (Kaplan, 1994). No specific inheritance pattern is noted.

Clinical Manifestations

The infant may be asymptomatic if no renal disease is present in the unaffected kidney. Renal function of a single kidney is sufficient to support life. However, if the remaining kidney is dysfunctional, the infant may exhibit signs of renal problems. The exact symptoms exhibited are directly associated with the type of renal problem the infant is experiencing.

Differential Diagnosis

The differential diagnosis centers around the confirmation of the presence of a single kidney. This determination is best made by renal ultrasonography. If other kidney disease is suspected in the remaining kidney, testing would be dictated by the suspected dysfunction.

Prognosis

The prognosis for survival with a single kidney is excellent if the remaining kidney is disease free.

Collaborative and Nursing Management

The major focus of care is preparation of the infant and family for preliminary testing. If kidney function is not compromised, no nursing care beyond normal newborn care may be necessary. The sections on the specific disorders contain more information on nursing management to be implemented if kidney disease is found. This condition often goes undetected in the newborn period because no symptoms may be exhibited.

CYSTIC KIDNEY DISEASE

Pathophysiology

Cystic disease of the kidney involves replacement of normal kidney mass with cysts. The amount of cystic formation within each or both kidneys determines the severity of the disease. If the kidney is severely affected, ureteral agenesis may also occur. Cystic disease includes a variety of disorders, such as polycystic disease and multicystic disease.

Infantile polycystic disease is a genetic autosomal recessive disease. The cystic lesions occur in the collecting tubules. Cystic lesions may also occur in the liver, bile duct, and pancreas. Infantile polycystic disease generally involves both kidneys and has a poor prognosis. Adult-type polycystic disease is an autosomal dominant disease that is rarely seen in infants. When it occurs, it leads to serious renal compromise and death.

Multicystic kidney disease is a noninherited disorder. It usually follows an obstructive uropathy in utero and is most often unilateral. Back-up of urine causes the fluid-filled kidney mass to develop into cystic lesions.

Risk Factors

No specific risk factors exist for the development of this complex of dysfunctions. Polycystic kidney disease has an autosomal recessive inheritance pattern in the infant, whereas in the adult, it has an autosomal dominant inheritance pattern (Kaplan, 1994). Either of these types of family inheritance patterns should be considered a risk for the development of cystic kidney disease.

Clinical Manifestations

In the newborn, the abdomen may be enlarged and have an apparent palpable mass. The mass may not be perceived as a kidney, because the cystic lesions distort its normal shape. In single-kidney cystic disease, normal urine output is maintained. The affected kidney has a high potential for infection, owing to urinary stasis. Albuminuria occurs in polycystic kidney disease.

Differential Diagnosis

Cystic kidney disease must be differentiated from hydronephrosis, Wilms' tumor, and anatomic deformities. Palpation alone cannot lead to an accurate diagnosis. Ultrasonography and pyelography are necessary to differentiate between normal renal mass and cystic lesions. These tests should be delayed until the infant is 48 hours old to allow the neonate to become hydrated and to restore the fluid balance after birth. This delay helps in the detection of possible hydronephrosis or cystic kidney disease.

Voiding cystography should be performed in infants whom clinicians highly suspect have cystic disease. With cystic kidney disease, if one kidney is functional, the serum and urine chemistries may be normal. A renal scan helps differentiate between ureteropelvic junction obstruction and multicystic kidney disease. In multicystic kidney disease, the radioactive isotope is concentrated in a mass, whereas in ureteropelvic junction obstruction, the isotope continues on into the renal pelvis (King, 1988; Radhakrishnan, 1990).

Prognosis

The prognosis is poor for infantile polycystic disease. The prognosis for multicystic disease is directly dependent on the severity of kidney damage. In addition, infants with multicystic disease are at greater risk for later development of Wilms' tumor, a malignancy with a relatively poor prognosis. More research is needed in tracking this possible relationship.

Tissue hypertrophy in the contralateral, normal kidney begins at birth. This increase in renal tissue increases the functional ability of the kidney. Thus, the body compensates for the loss of one kidney.

Collaborative Management

Treatment entails complete or partial nephrectomy of the affected kidney. The treatment for single-kidney cystic disease is complete nephrectomy because the diseased kidney may continue to harbor infection. This infection may spread to the unaffected kidney. A partial nephrectomy may be performed if sufficient unaffected renal mass is found. If the cystic disease is the result of a ureteropelvic junction obstruction, pyeloplasty has been successful. In either case, the surgical intervention is followed by careful medical and nursing management.

Nursing Management

The health professional must thoroughly assess the infant for the presence of a mass, which is usually in the flank area. If Wilms' tumor is suspected, no palpation should be performed, because the tumor can break up and may be spread in this fashion. If urine output is normal, careful consideration of the fluid intake and output may not be necessary; if renal function is compromised, strict attention must be paid to fluid balance. Electrolyte status must be checked at least daily. Urine should be checked for the presence of albumin. Because hydronephrosis may be present, hematuria is also a consideration. Before surgery, a complete blood count with differential and a urine culture should be obtained because the infant is at risk for a urinary tract infection.

Hypertension has been documented in this condition. It is believed that the blood pressure change is related to decreased arterial renal perfusion and to concomitant elevations in renin levels (King, 1988). A nephrectomy reverses this trend.

If the infant undergoes a complete nephrectomy, strict adherence to aseptic technique must be followed. Because the infant is prone to infection, vital signs should be monitored at least every 2 to 4 hours after the immediate postoperative period. Any dressings should be inspected for the presence of bloody drainage or secretions. Initially, a small amount of bleeding at the site is common, but it should be short lived. No urine drainage should be noted on the dressing, because the entire kidney has been removed. Abdominal decompression is often necessary to prevent distention that could cause pressure and pull the suture line apart. If a nasogastric tube is in place, it should be irrigated with 2 ml of saline or air every 2 to 4 hours in order to maintain patency.

Feedings may be resumed once bowel sounds can be auscultated and the nasogastric tube has been removed. Feedings are usually tolerated 2 to 3 days after surgery.

PRUNE-BELLY SYNDROME (EAGLE-BARRETT SYNDROME)

Pathophysiology

An infant born with prune-belly syndrome has a congenital lack of appropriate abdominal musculature, undescended testicles, and urinary tract malformations (Sanders, 1996). The abdominal muscles may be so weakened that the abdominal region actually appears wrinkled, much like a prune's surface. It typically affects males; in females, the true syndrome does not exist (Short et al., 1985). Pseudohermaphroditism may be associated with prune-belly syndrome, or it may even be the diagnosis of record in the female (Chasnoff et al., 1988). The incidence rate is approximately 1 in every 50,000 births (Goodman & Gorlin, 1983). The associated urinary problems include an enlarged bladder and dilated, curved ureters. Dilation of the ureter is referred to as megaureter (primary reflux megaureter). This condition can be diagnosed before birth via ultrasonography (Cozzi et al., 1994). It is not always associated only with prune-belly syndrome but can be due to infection or other accompanying renal anomalies. Kidney development may have been diminished, thus resulting in hypoplastic kidneys. A patent urachus may also be associated with this anomaly (Tank & McCoy, 1983). Other associated problems include hip and feet deformities, respiratory insufficiency, imperforate anus, and cardiac anomalies. Owing to an imbalance of muscle pull, spinal deformities may occur.

No clear cause is known for prune-belly syndrome, but the defect may occur between the 23rd day and the 10th week of fetal development. During this time period, the bladder is taking shape and being separated from the allantois, and the abdominal wall is forming. The question arises as to whether the obstruction of the urethra causes back-up of urine, resulting in bladder distention and ultimately muscle deformity, or whether musculature defects lead to the obstructive uropathies (Fanaroff & Martin, 1997).

Risk Factors

No clear-cut genetic predisposition for this syndrome exists. The presence of oligohydramnios is suggestive of a renal problem. Ultrasound examination may reveal bladder distention and dilated ureters, again leading only to a highly suspicious status of the renal system. No other clear risk factors are known to precipitate this syndrome. Maternal use of cocaine, however, has been documented as a known teratogen that results in prune-belly syndrome, among other GU anomalies (Chasnoff et al., 1988; Rosenstein et al., 1990).

Clinical Manifestations

The musculature defect may be small or may cover the entire surface of the abdomen. Although all layers of musculature are present, the degree of development of these muscle layers varies. A thin layer of subcutaneous tissue, coupled with distention, gives the abdomen a wrinkled appearance. Cryptorchidism (undescended testes), prostatic urethral dilation, bladder distention, patent urachus, abdominal distention or protuberance, malrotation of the intestines, cardiac defects, congenital hip dysplasia and associated "click," and clubfoot (talipes equinovarus) are some of the other associated clinical findings. Not all of these other disorders are present in all infants, but they should be considered as potential problems.

Differential Diagnosis

Prune-belly syndrome may be obvious on observation. However, other conditions can result in abdominal distention and apparent weakened abdominal musculature. Any infant with severe uropathy and urethral obstruction may also demonstrate these signs. Differentiation should be made by palpation of bladder distention, as opposed to the finding of distended bowel loops. The latter would indicate an intestinal rather than a renal problem. Underlying renal disease must be distinguished from abdominal muscle defects with accompanying renal dysfunction. What must be determined is the exact nature of the renal problem, the degree to which renal function is compromised, and the other deformities that might also be present. The exact diagnosis can be made only when a demonstrable lack of abdominal musculature is present.

Appropriate diagnostic tests for a definitive determination of renal disease include abdominal radiography and renal ultrasonography, intravenous pyelography, voiding cystography, BUN level, and creatinine analysis (Brueggemeyer, 1988).

Prognosis

The prognosis is directly related to the degree of severity of the underlying renal dysfunction. As many as 50 percent of infants with prune-belly syndrome may die within the first 2 years of life if severe renal dysfunction or chronic renal failure is present (Goodman & Gorlin, 1983).

Collaborative Management

This triadic anomaly leads to severe urinary tract complications. The condition of the kidney can range from normal kidney mass to complete atresia. In many cases, dilation of the ureter, bladder, and urethra occurs, which may be caused by a lack of muscle fiber in the lining of the structures. The lack of muscle in the ureters leads to their elongation and distention. If obstruction occurs as a result of the tortuous nature of the ureters, surgical intervention may be necessary. Reimplantation or diversion may be necessary to prevent urine stasis and renal failure.

Obstruction of the urethra may be caused by angulation that results from a lack of musculature in the urethra or by an obstructive action that results from a distention of the enlarged prostatic urethra (Tank & McCoy, 1983). Surgical correction may not achieve bladder functioning, because bladder atonia persists.

This syndrome is accompanied by undescended testes. Orchiopexy may be performed. However, orchiopexy has not been found to improve fertility in the adult who has survived with prune-belly syndrome. Testosterone levels have been found to be adequate in two thirds of men studied (Griggs, 1982).

Catheterization should be performed by a skilled practitioner to prevent trauma to the distorted urethra and bladder. Bladder decompression is necessary for the prevention of stasis. Any severe abdominal distention and insufficient urinary output in the first day of life observed by the nurse should be evaluated by other members of the health care team to rule out the possibility of this syndrome. A large amount of urine may have accumulated in the fetal period, resulting in a greatly distended bladder. Renal dysplasia is common in more than 50 percent of the infants born with prune-belly syndrome (Griggs, 1982). Renal dysplasia is an abnormal development of the kidney or its associated structures. It is most commonly seen as aplastic kidneys and multicystic disease (Fanaroff & Martin, 1997).

If urine drainage is compromised, nephrostomy or ureterostomy diversion should be undertaken. Peristalsis may be absent or deficient. A vesicostomy may allow temporary drainage until extensive surgical intervention is tolerated by the infant. Long-term use of antimicrobial therapy may be necessary to prevent sepsis. In the presence of a patent urachus (fetal communication between the bladder and umbilicus), closure may not be necessary in the neonatal period if adequate drainage and prevention of infection can be maintained. If the bladder is distended, reduction cystoplasty is performed in order to relieve the tension on the bladder and to promote emptying (Hanna, 1989).

Long-term therapy includes exercise, use of abdominal binders, and reconstructive surgery. Although not curative, these methods provide some palliative benefit to the appearance and function of the distended and sagging abdomen.

The effects of renal damage that occur in the early stages of life require careful attention to fluid and electrolyte balance, removal of wastes, and adequate nutrition for growth and development. Growing children should be monitored for adequate growth and calcification of bones because both are dependent on good renal functioning. Frequent hospitalizations may be necessary during childhood. Parents need to be prepared for this and need to be assisted with financial as well as psychosocial support.

Nursing Management

The focus of nursing management is the maintenance of renal functioning. Fluid intake and output should be strictly measured and recorded. If an appliance is used, skin surfaces must be kept clean and dry. The use of adhesives may be necessary to prevent leakage around the stoma that results from skin folds and wrinkling. Turning and repositioning every 2 hours also helps decrease skin breakdown. Bladder decompression may be accomplished by intermittent catheterization or the Credé method. Use of the Credé method may be sufficient to empty the bladder. This method involves the practitioner's placing both hands under the infant's flank area and bringing the thumbs together at the umbilicus. Pressure is gently applied, and the thumbs are rolled downward from the umbilicus to the symphysis pubis.

If bladder distention and urinary retention continue to occur until the infant is discharged, parents must be taught a method of emptying the bladder. This may involve the Credé method or intermittent catheterization. Parents must be taught the signs and symptoms of a urinary tract infection; these are increased irritability accompanying urination, temperature instability, increase or decrease in urine output, and cloudy or foul-smelling urine. They must understand the importance of early detection and intervention to prevent long-term renal compromise. If a vesicostomy or other urinary diversion has been performed, specific instructions are necessary to prevent bladder contamination. The vesicostomy has been found to be an effective treatment to prevent urinary stasis and infection before reconstruction of this and other cloacal anomalies (Alexander & Kay, 1994). Stoma care is another aspect of parent education and discharge planning.

Lack of abdominal musculature also can lead to constipation, even in the newborn period. Long-term suppository use and bowel training may be necessary. Feedings should not promote distention and respiratory compromise. Parents should be well informed of dietary approaches to help promote appropriate GI functioning. Consideration for parental feelings must also center around the physical appearance of their baby. Because the American culture places great value on appearance, it may be difficult for parents to accept the loss of their "perfect" dream baby. Support is needed. A good strategy for increasing the parent–infant interaction is inclusion in caretaking procedures as the parents are ready.

EXSTROPHY OF THE BLADDER

Pathophysiology

In exstrophy of the bladder, the anterior abdominal wall fails to close at the point of the bladder (Sanders, 1996). During the first 4 weeks of gestation, the abdominal wall begins to fuse. When the mesenchymal cells fail to migrate over the abdomen, exstrophy results. A thin membrane forms over the abdominal contents, which may later rupture, leaving the bladder exposed.

Risk Factors

The incidence of this defect is 1 in 24,000 to 40,000 live births, with males being affected more than females (King, 1980; O'Donnell, 1984). Exact risk factors are not known, because exstrophy of the bladder is just one of many exstrophies of the cloacal membrane.

Clinical Manifestations

This condition is obvious on visual inspection. The bladder region appears open or uncovered. Because of the failure of the abdominal and anterior bladder wall to close, the posterior wall of the bladder is exposed. The implantation of the ureters may be visible as urine continues to pass from the orifices. A concomitant defect exists in the genitalia. In the male, the penis may be short, flat, and angulated. Epispadias may occur to the extent that proper sex identification may be difficult. In the female, the labia do not meet in the midline, and a divided clitoris exists. The defect may also include a prolapse of the rectum. This prolapse may occur through the abdominal wall defect, requiring an intestinal diversion. The failure of the pubic bones to meet anteriorly may lead to hip and leg deformities. Neurospinal defects, omphalocele, and other chromosomal abnormalities may occur with this defect.

Differential Diagnosis

The diagnosis of exstrophy of the bladder may be determined on visual inspection. However, the concomitantly occurring deformities, as mentioned previously, must be assessed.

Prognosis

The exact prognosis is directly related to the presence of other deformities. In and of itself, exstrophy of the bladder has a good prognosis for survival. However, the infant may have chronic problems. If this condition has been associated with intestinal problems that led to an ileostomy, the ileostomy may or may not be permanent, depending on the degree of severe intestinal malformation. As for the renal system, the infant may have a lifelong problem with incontinence. An ileal conduit may be permanent. Neurologic or orthopedic deformities require consultation from health care professionals in these specialties and again may result in chronic problems.

Collaborative Management

If the infant with exstrophy of the bladder must be transported to a tertiary center for treatment, the exstrophy is covered with plastic wrap or a similar material to protect the open area. Before surgical correction, the defect is covered with a petroleum dressing and sufficient gauze to absorb urine flow. This dressing should be changed when it becomes saturated; otherwise, skin irritation occurs. Skin is observed for extreme dryness because dryness promotes skin breakdown. Addition of humidification in the incubator helps prevent the drying. Diapers should be kept folded well below the defect if wound infections are to be avoided.

Urinary tract infection is uncommon if abdominal dressings are changed regularly. Some infants may not have the defect closed during initial hospitalization and require that dressings continue to be used at home. Parents must be taught the principles of skin management and the importance of the regularity of the changes as a method of preventing infection.

Primary closure of the defect is usually performed in the neonatal period. Some institutions perform a staged approach to closure and correction of genital defects. Closure in some cases may be delayed for a year or longer without serious complications. Before surgery is performed, broad-spectrum antibiotic therapy (ampicillin and gentamicin) is started to give protection against infections. This therapy is continued for at least 7 days after surgery because 42 percent of wound dehiscence is due to infections (Mesrobian, 1988). Strict observation of aseptic technique is essential. If infection is suspected, aggressive treatment should be started.

Surgical correction of the defect does not guarantee continence. In some cases, urinary diversion or use of ileal conduits may be necessary. In the infant with concomitant neurospinal defects, continence might never be achieved (O'Donnell, 1984). The nurse may need to coordinate follow-up by surgical, medical, and neurosurgical teams. Long-term follow-up may include the use of social services and financial counseling.

Nursing Management

Care of the infant with an exposed bladder includes protection as well as output measurement. Petroleum jelly–impregnated gauze should be used to protect the moist surface from trauma or drying. Preweighed gauze dressings can be used to collect and measure urine output. If accurate output measurement is not necessary, diapers may be used to collect urine drainage. If rectal prolapse has occurred through the abdominal defect, separate dressings should be maintained, if possible.

Parents should be told what to expect after surgery. Although closure of the abdominal defect may be accomplished in one stage, repair of the epispadias is performed when the child is older. If closure is delayed for a period of time, parents must be taught how to dress and care for the defect.

HYDRONEPHROSIS

Pathophysiology

Hydronephrosis is the accumulation of urine within the renal pelvis and calices to the point of overdistention. Hydronephrosis often follows obstruction of urine flow at the junction of the ureteropelvis, the ureterovesical valve, or the urethrovesical valve. The build-up of fluid that then accumulates in the kidney leads to distention of the renal pelvis and damage of the kidney mass. If only one ureter is affected, then damage occurs to that kidney only, leaving the other capable of supporting life. In some cases, hydronephrosis can be treated by removing the obstruction before permanent damage has occurred.

Prevention of hydronephrosis is possible in some circumstances. Fetal surgery is possible; this practice can relieve the obstruction in utero by placing a catheter into the bladder to drain the urine, thus preventing the infant from being born with permanently damaged kidneys (Figs. 31–6 and 31–7). After birth, definitive surgery is performed to correct the obstructive defect or to provide a diversion of urine flow. Early detection is necessary because damage to the kidneys may occur as early as the fourth month of gestation (see Chapter 38, Fetal Therapy).

Risk Factors

The presence of a urinary tract infection may result in an inflammatory response so severe that urinary obstruction and

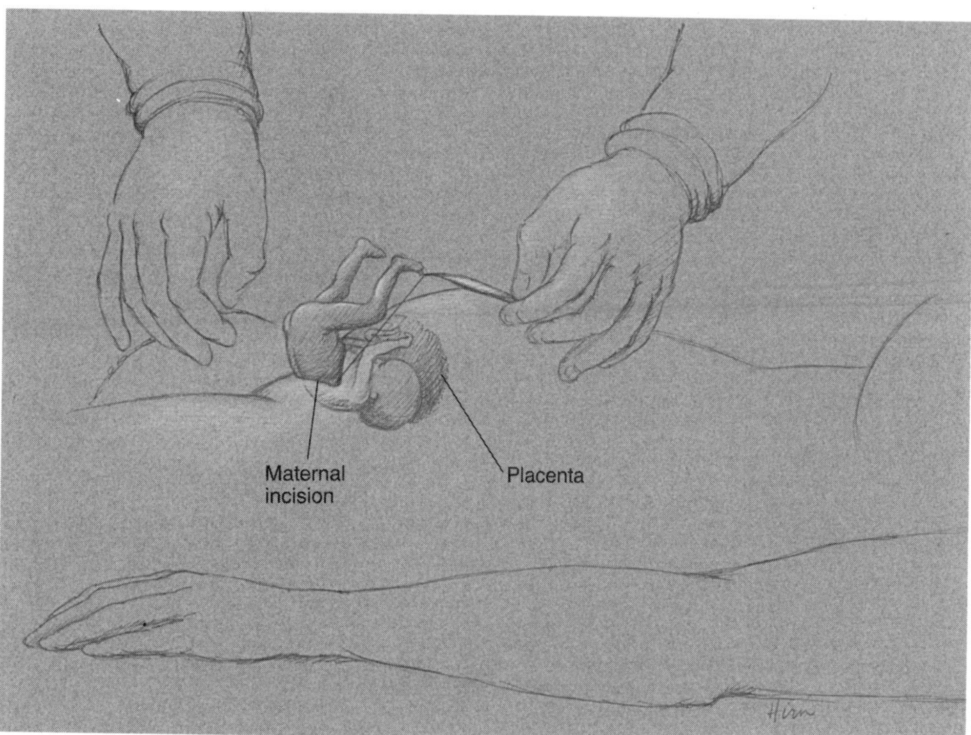

FIGURE 31–6. Fetal surgery to prevent hydronephrosis.

ultimately hydronephrosis occur. Renal or GU tumors or masses may precipitate this condition. Maternal oligohydramnios is suggestive of renal obstruction and may accompany hydronephrosis. Any factor or condition that potentially obstructs renal or urinary flow may contribute to the development of hydronephrosis.

Clinical Manifestations

In the newborn, hydronephrosis may be detected as a large, solid, palpable smooth mass at the region of the kidney. Urine output may be decreased or normal, depending on the amount of functioning kidney mass. If only one kidney is involved, urine output may be normal because a single kidney is sufficient for adequate removal of water and waste. Urinary tract infection often accompanies hydronephrosis, making fever and discomfort observable signs. Gross hematuria may be present and must be differentiated from the hematuria associated with Wilms' tumor and renal vein thrombosis.

Differential Diagnosis

Clinical diagnostic studies include pyelography, ultrasonography, and computed tomography. Intravenous pyelograms may not be definitive in that interpretation of the results could indicate nonexistence of the kidney because the fluid-filled mass does not readily pick up the dye. The kidney outline can be determined with retrograde pyelography. Before drastic reparative procedures are attempted, respiratory status must be assessed. During fetal life, oligohydramnios and distention of the abdomen can precipitate a cessation of growth of the respiratory tree. Renal surgery may be unnecessary for an infant whose respiratory status is insufficient to support life.

Because many different forms of abdominal masses may occur, it is essential that the origin of the mass be determined. This condition must be differentiated from cystic kidney disease, urogenital tumors, and renal vein thrombosis (Kaplan, 1994).

Prognosis

The prognosis for this condition depends on the underlying causative factor and the degree of severity of the permanent renal damage. If severe renal damage is present, the prognosis is grave. The more kidney damage present, the less likely the infant will survive. However, if only one ureter or kidney is affected, the other kidney should be able to support life.

Collaborative Management

Hydronephrosis is managed according to its cause. In the case of repairable obstructive uropathies, surgical treatment of the cause removes the source of the process, which may reverse itself in time. This correction is usually performed via pyeloplasty and nephrostomy tube insertion for drainage. If surgery is not required, nutritional support may be the only treatment necessary. The nurse should work with the nutritional support team to plan the course of care.

If irreversible damage has occurred to the entire kidney, nephrectomy may be necessary. The hydronephrotic kidney is a source for frequent urinary tract infections. Nephrectomy may be performed in the neonatal period to prevent the occurrence of infection, or it may be delayed until infection becomes a serious problem.

Nursing Management

Careful assessment is necessary for the infant who is thought to have hydronephrosis. First of all, the infant's respiratory status must be determined. The presence of cyanosis, grunting, nasal flaring, and retractions is important because the lungs may not have fully developed. The chest should be observed for any alterations in the anteroposterior diameter or asymmetry. Vital signs, including blood pressure, must be monitored at least every 4 hours and more frequently if they are unstable. The blood pressure is especially important because hypertension is common

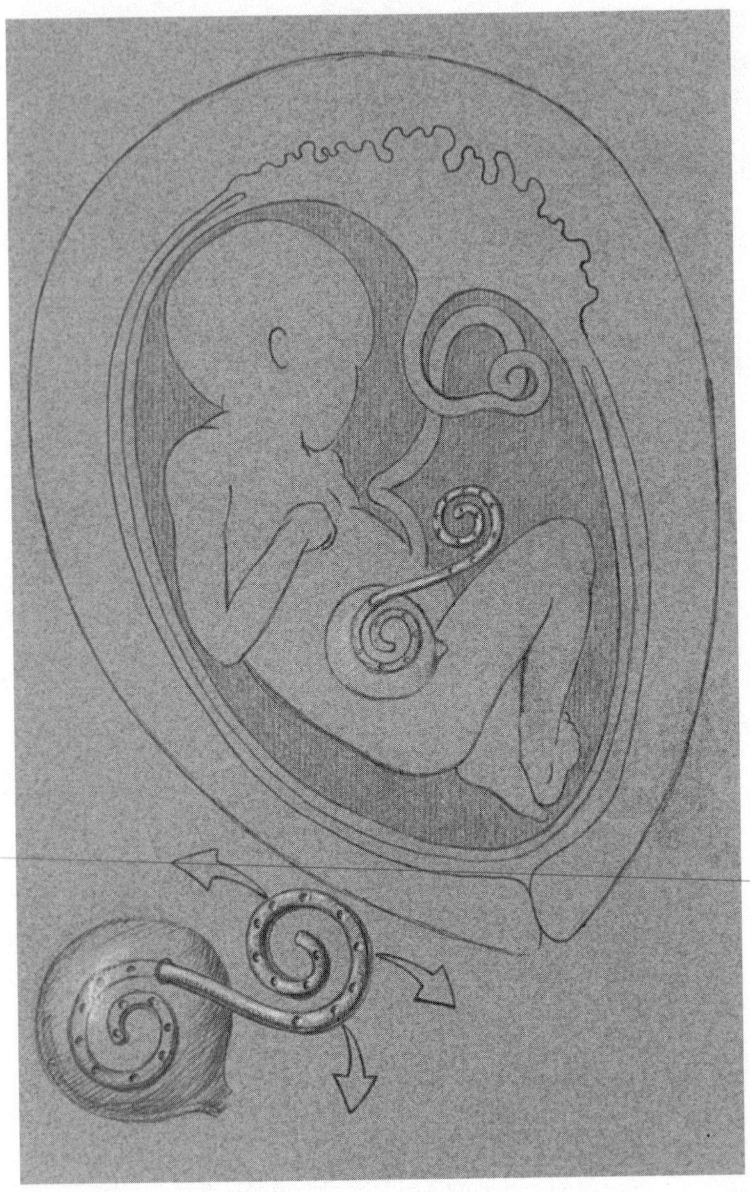

FIGURE 31–7. Placement of urinary catheter in utero.

in the infant with hydronephrosis. If hypertension is severe, antihypertensives may be given. Some institutions use intravenous hydralazine, intravenous diazoxide, or methyldopa. Use of any of these drugs requires extremely close monitoring of the cardiorespiratory system. Fluid and electrolyte status also must be carefully watched. Fluid intake and output should be recorded at least every 2 to 4 hours. Specific gravity may be checked every 4 to 8 hours. A urine dipstick assessment may be useful for determining the presence of protein or blood in the urine. Assessment of hydration status is important. The fontanelles should be observed to determine if they are sunken, dehydrated, or bulging. Skin turgor should demonstrate instant recoil.

The presence of any dependent or pitting edema should be checked for and recorded. The nurse often detects the early cues that an infant has hydronephrosis. If hydronephrosis is even suspected, the medical team must be notified so that early intervention and prevention of long-term complications can occur. Palpation of the abdomen is also helpful to determine if a mass is present.

After surgery, a nephrostomy or a urinary stent may be placed. These are connected to a closed drainage system.

URETERAL OBSTRUCTION

Pathophysiology

Ureteral obstruction occurs when the developing ureter fails to form a tube or the junction of the kidney pelvis or bladder is constricted. Most commonly, the obstruction occurs at the ureteral junction of the kidney pelvis; the second most common site is the junction of the bladder. Unilateral or bilateral obstructions may occur. The result is a back-up of urine into the affected kidney, resulting in a fluid-filled kidney. In some instances, complete obstruction does not occur, and minimal functioning persists until the child is older and symptomatology increases. Recurrent infection of the urinary tract should be investigated in the young child. The presence of static fluid in the kidney leads to permanent damage of renal tissue. The fluid may be contained in a sac or a cyst-like lesion on the ureter.

Risk Factors

The risk factors for the development of ureteral obstruction are actually the underlying causes of such an impingement. Cystic kidney disease, polycystic kidney disease, ureteropelvic junction obstruction, and urethral atresia are among the most common causes of this entity. Any one of these problems is considered to precipitate urethral obstruction.

Clinical Manifestations

An infant may be asymptomatic unless complete obstruction is present. Delayed voiding or failure to void may be signs. Hematuria may or may not be present. Because the presence of a blocked ureter may lead to hydronephrosis, an enlarged, palpable kidney may be the first indication of a problem.

Differential Diagnosis

It is essential that a determination be made regarding (1) whether urethral obstruction is occurring by itself as urethral atresia, (2) whether hydronephrosis or cystic or polycystic kidney disease is present, and (3) whether there is a ureteropelvic junction obstruction. A radiologic examination after renal scanning or ultrasonography helps definitely differentiate among these entities.

Prognosis

The prognosis is directly dependent on the severity of kidney damage. The less the damage, the greater the chances for survival if no other lethal conditions are present.

Collaborative Management

Correction or repair of the blocked ureter may lead to reversal of hydronephrosis. If permanent damage has occurred, nephrectomy may be performed. Once surgical correction is completed, long-term medical care is essential for the early detection of chronic renal problems. The nurse must educate parents about the need for this follow-up.

Nursing Management

The nurse must observe for signs of decreasing urine output. The infant may be edematous, making good skin care a high priority. Infection may be present and should be treated before any surgical intervention. For more specific management, see the section on hydronephrosis in this chapter.

HYDROCELE

Pathophysiology

Hydrocele, the collection of fluid in the scrotal sac, is a common finding in the neonate. During embryologic development, the coelom, or the peritoneal cavity, and the processus vaginalis freely communicate within the confines of the scrotum. At birth, this area is still open; however, during the first few months of postnatal life, this communicating space gradually closes. If small cysts develop along this closure, fluid may be secreted from them. This secretory process leads to the accumulation of fluid between the layers of the tunica vaginalis within the scrotal sac (Sadler, 1995). Thus, a hydrocele results.

Risk Factors

The premature infant and the infant who experiences increased abdominal pressure secondary to manual resuscitation and high ventilatory pressures are at risk for hydrocele. It occurs as fluid accumulation in the scrotal sac through failure of the processus vaginalis to close.

Clinical Manifestations

Fluid accumulation in the scrotum readily transilluminates with the use of a good light source. Palpation reveals no masses. Some infants may have a mass in the groin that fades when abdominal pressure is decreased, such as after an infant stops crying. This mass is most often associated with a hernia, but a hydrocele may exist also. If the defect is large enough, fluid may continue to shift from the abdomen into the scrotal sac and back into the abdomen. As abdominal pressure increases, the shift of fluid becomes unidirectional into the scrotal sac. When the defect is large, abdominal contents may also pass into the scrotal sac. This condition is called a congenital herniation or an inguinal hernia.

In rare instances, female infants may have fluid accumulation in the labia, causing edema. They may also experience herniation into the patent passageway, which is called the processus vaginalis.

Differential Diagnosis

Because the hydrocele may be asymptomatic, if it does not occur in conjunction with an inguinal hernia and is not large enough to create observable scrotal swelling, it may be difficult to detect. The "silk glove" test is useful in an older infant but is generally not useful in the neonatal period. In this test, the examiner places pressure on the peritoneal surfaces by rubbing gently on the scrotal tissue that follows the inguinal canal. If a hydrocele is present, the two distinct open layers of tissue should be felt sliding over each other. If the hydrocele is palpable, it feels smooth and is painless. In the neonate, direct observation and transillumination with a strong light source should reveal a lightened area of scrotum where the fluid has accumulated. Observation of the infant during a crying episode, in which the intra-abdominal pressure is the greatest, may also demonstrate a hydrocele or scrotal swelling. If scrotal swelling is detected, the nurse should report this finding immediately to the medical team.

The most important element of the differential diagnosis is distinguishing a hydrocele from an incarcerated inguinal hernia. This distinction can best be made by rectal examination and simultaneous palpation of the inguinal canal. If the examiner encounters loops of intestine near the vas deferens or the ductus deferens within the scrotal sac, an inguinal hernia is present.

Prognosis

The prognosis for infants with hydrocele is excellent.

Collaborative Management

The treatment for hydrocele involves removal of the fluid by the physician. The fluid may be aspirated, or actual tissue removal may be necessary to close the freely communicating space. Treatment is often not attempted until the infant is 1 year of age. Until the hydrocele is corrected, the nurse must observe the infant closely for signs of herniation. If any herniation is suspected or the bowel is believed to be incarcerated, surgical intervention is needed immediately.

Nursing Management

Hydrocele repair is usually not performed in the newborn stage, because resolution often occurs spontaneously. Parents must be taught the signs of herniation and incarceration before discharge. These signs are the presence of a lump found in the groin (this lump is especially noticeable when the infant is crying) and increased irritability on the part of the infant. They must understand the need to seek immediate medical attention if either of these symptoms appears. Careful attention must be paid to skin care of the edematous scrotum.

After surgery, the infant may experience abdominal distention that could place pressure on the suture line, pulling it apart. Therefore, the use of a nasogastric tube attached to low intermittent suction may be necessary. If a nasogastric tube is used, patency must be maintained by irrigation with 2 ml of air or saline every 2 to 4 hours. The infant should be placed in the side lying or supine position with the head turned to the side to prevent rubbing or pressure on the suture line. The bed should be flat. Maintenance of a dry sterile or waterproof occlusive dressing over the operative site is essential to prevent infection and skin breakdown. The perineum should be carefully cleaned after every void and stool.

TORSION OF THE TESTICLE

Pathophysiology

Torsion of the testicle occurs when the testis or sperm cord twists, restricting circulation to the testicle. If circulation is allowed to remain compromised, permanent damage to the testicle results. In the newborn, permanent damage may have resulted in utero, with consequent necrosis of the testicle. In the female, torsion of the fallopian tube may result in compromised circulation to the ovary.

Torsion in the neonate results when the descent of the testicle into the scrotal sac is complicated by twisting of the tunica vaginalis testis. This problem can be unilateral or bilateral.

Risk Factors

No specific risk factors are known. Torsion of the testicle is a common finding in the newborn period.

Clinical Manifestations

Common to many scrotal problems are enlargement and edema. In torsion, the scrotum is firm to the touch and is very tender. The mass itself does not transilluminate. The scrotum and the surrounding abdomen may show significant discoloration, being either plethoric or cyanotic.

Differential Diagnosis

Because of its similarities with other nonserious scrotal problems, torsion must always be considered in the diagnosis. The diagnosis is usually made on the basis of the presence of the discoloration of the scrotum and the nontransilluminating consistency of the scrotal sac.

Prognosis

The prognosis for survival is very good; however, maintenance of testicular function may not be possible.

Collaborative Management

The treatment is aimed at surgical relief of the twisting of the testicle. Correction can be performed either transscrotally or inguinally. Usually, if the torsion is severe, a simple orchidopexy may be performed (Kaplan, 1994). In certain instances, the twisted testis has been left in place to atrophy and necrose, in an attempt to preserve the function of the Leydig cells, to avoid testosterone therapy. This method of treatment is performed only sporadically in the neonate (Kaplan & Silber, 1988). However, infertility is a potential long-term complication of neonatal torsion. This is an area for future research.

Nursing Management

The focus of nursing care is on keeping the infant comfortable and as quiet as possible. The abdominal girth should be measured every 4 hours for any signs of distention. The scrotum must be inspected for edema, discoloration, and skin temperature. If the infant is experiencing vomiting because of abdominal distention, the use of a nasogastric tube attached to intermittent low suction may be necessary. The tube should be irrigated every 2 to 4 hours with 2 ml of saline or air in order to maintain patency. Positioning of the infant should be only on the back with head turned to the side or in a side-lying position because otherwise too much pressure may be placed on the abdominal and scrotal areas.

After surgery, the nursing care is centered around stability of the vital signs and prevention of infection. The respiratory status must be carefully assessed because abdominal distention may compromise the respiratory function. Nasopharyngeal suctioning may be necessary. The suture line is generally small but still requires aseptic technique. The site should be assessed for the presence of edema, drainage, or discoloration. A urinary drainage bag may be necessary to protect the skin and to prevent infection if excessive drainage is present.

INGUINAL HERNIA

Pathophysiology

Inguinal hernia is one of the most common surgical problems in the infant. It occurs more frequently in the premature infant.

Inguinal hernia occurs when the small intestine and gonads pass through the open processus vaginalis. In the female, the herniation may occur into soft tissue of the labia. Small hernias without complications may be allowed to close on their own. Often, hernia repair is deferred until the infant is older and can tolerate anesthesia. The matured premature infant must be closely observed for respiratory and cardiac compromise in the postoperative period because he or she is prone to apnea and bradycardia. When the intestines are caught within the processus, incarceration can occur. Vomiting and abdominal distention may indicate obstruction of the herniated intestine. Strangulation of the bowel and gonads occurs when the circulation becomes compromised. Necrosis may follow a few hours later.

Risk Factors

Right-sided hernias occur more often than left-sided ones, and bilateral hernias make up only a small percentage of occurrences. Males are commonly affected more than females, and a high incidence exists in the premature population. A rare genetic syndrome exists called deficiency of mullerian inhibition substance that results in a phenotypic male; however, a uterus and fallopian tube can be found in the scrotal sac (Snyder, 1988).

Clinical Manifestations

The inguinal hernia can be felt as a mass in the groin. In many cases, crying or increased abdominal pressure can exaggerate the hernia. In reducible hernias, the intestine can be gently manipulated back into the abdomen. Transillumination may not be helpful in diagnosis, because bowel air may be difficult to differentiate from a hydrocele.

Differential Diagnosis

In the differential diagnosis, an inguinal hernia occurring in isolation should be distinguished from one accompanying a hydrocele. Some experts do not believe that such a distinction is possible (Filston & Izant, 1985). A distinction should be made between a hydrocele and undescended testicles by scrotal examination for the presence of testes. A hydrocele may or may not be palpated, but a hernia appears as a lump or swelling within the groin. Another concern is whether or not the hernia is incarcerated. It is then necessary to perform a rectal examination and palpate the scrotum simultaneously. This examination reveals whether an intestinal loop is present in the scrotal sac versus a fluid-filled hydrocele.

A reducible hernia may be easily popped back into place, whereas an incarcerated hernia is thick and nonreducible. Radiologic studies may demonstrate the presence of intestinal gas within the scrotal sac (Filston & Izant, 1985).

Prognosis

The prognosis for survival is excellent in inguinal hernias.

Collaborative Management

Surgery is indicated in all inguinal hernias that do not resolve spontaneously. Surgical intervention is also required if strangulation or incarceration occurs. It involves repair of the hernia and separation of the hernia from the inguinal canal. The nurse must instruct the parents in recognizing symptoms of intestinal obstruction or protrusion of bowel loops through the hernia that do not reduce easily or become discolored. These symptoms indicate the need for immediate surgery.

Nursing Management

The focus of preoperative nursing care is on keeping the infant quiet and comfortable. If vomiting has occurred, the infant should be assessed for dehydration, and the fluid and electrolyte status should be monitored closely. After surgery, the aim is adherence to aseptic technique with regard to suture line maintenance. The infant should be placed in a side-lying or supine position with the head turned to the side to prevent disruption of the suture line. If abdominal distention is present, a nasogastric tube for decompression may be necessary. Operative dressings should be observed for any drainage and bleeding. They should be kept dry, and the underlying skin should be inspected for irritation or breakdown.

NEPHROBLASTOMA

Pathophysiology

The occurrence of malignant tumor in the neonate is rare. Wilms' tumor does occur in the young infant (Thompson & Cohen, 1996). Associated with Wilms' tumor are aniridia, GU tract defects, and hemihypertrophy. The presence of these signs in the neonate should alert the health care professional to the potential development of Wilms' tumor beyond the neonatal period.

Risk Factors

When hemihypertrophy is present, the infant may be at risk for nephroblastoma (Brion et al., 1994).

Clinical Manifestations

The usual finding is a smooth, solid abdominal or flank mass that is actually a renal mass. It may be accompanied by hypertension, owing to the possibility of renal artery stenosis. Fever is another common symptom of Wilms' tumor.

Differential Diagnosis

The diagnosis may be made on the basis of an intravenous pyelogram showing distorted renal calices, and on an abdominal radiograph, the mass will appear coarse (Filston & Izant, 1985). A chest radiograph should be taken to determine the presence of any lung metastatic lesions. This condition must be differentiated from other abdominal masses.

Prognosis

Although the prognosis is generally good, this may be because mesoblastic nephroma, a benign tumor, was mislabeled as Wilms' tumor. In the newborn period, metastasis may occur, making treatment difficult.

Nursing Management

The mass must not be palpated, because palpation may seed the tumor to other areas of the body. The major focus of nursing management, at least initially, is support of the parents. They may fear attachment to the infant. Otherwise, the neonatal nurse may not see an infant with Wilms' tumor, because it is often not diagnosed in the newborn period.

AMBIGUOUS GENITALIA

The most common cause of ambiguous genitalia is an adrenal problem. This neonatal problem is discussed in Chapter 26 (Assessment and Management of Endocrine Dysfunction).

CONCLUSION

The GU system is extremely important to the well-being of the neonate. This system not only distinguishes the sex or gender of the infant but also helps regulate the electrolyte, fluid, and acid–base balance of the physiologic system. Management includes assessment and treatment of problems with fluid volume excess; alterations in fluids and electrolytes, cardiac output, and breathing patterns; and changes in family processes. The neonatal nurse must achieve confidence in accurately assessing and managing this vital system.

REFERENCES

Alexander, F., & Kay, R. (1994). Cloacal anomalies: Role of vesicostomy. *Journal of Pediatric Surgery, 29*(1), 74–76.

American Academy of Pediatrics. (1993). *Guidelines for perinatal care* (3rd ed.). Washington, DC: American Academy of Pediatrics and American College of Obstetricians and Gynecologists.

Baumgart, S. (1995, March). *The very low birthweight infant and transition to the extrauterine environment: Fluids and electrolytes.* Paper presented at the National Association of Neonatal Nurses Baltimore Clinical Update, Baltimore, MD.

Bell, D. A., Rose, S. C., Starr, N. K., et al. (1993). Percutaneous nephrostomy for nonoperative management of fungal urinary tract infections. *Journal of Vascular and Interventional Radiology, 4*(2), 311–315.

Bourke, W. G., Clarke, T. A., Mathews, T. G., et al. (1994). Isolated single umbilical artery: The case for routine screening. *Archives of Disease in Childhood, 68*(5, Spec. No.), 600–601.

Bradburn, N. C., & Schreiner, R. L. (1988). Infectious diseases. In R. L. Schreiner & N. C. Bradburn (Eds.), *Care of the newborn* (2nd ed., pp. 119–131). New York: Raven Press.

Brion, L. P., Satlin, L. M., & Edelmann, C. M., Jr. (1994). Renal diseases. In G. B. Avery (Ed.), *Neonatology: Pathophysiology and management of the newborn* (4th ed., pp. 792–886). Philadelphia: W. B. Saunders.

Brueggemeyer, A. (1988). Alterations in the genitourinary system. In C. Kenner, J. Harjo, & A. Brueggemeyer (Eds.), *Neonatal surgery: A nursing perspective* (pp. 191–217). Orlando, FL: Grune & Stratton.

Chasnoff, I. J., Chisum, G. M., & Kaplan, W. E. (1988). Maternal cocaine use and genitourinary tract malformations. *Teratology, 37*(3), 201–204.

Colodny, A. H. (1987). Antenatal diagnosis and management of urinary abnormalities. *Pediatric Clinics of North America, 34*(5), 1365–1381.

Cozzi, F., Madonna, L., Maggi, E., et al. (1994). Management of primary megaureter in infancy. *Journal of Pediatric Surgery, 28*(8), 1031–1033.

Deglin, J. H., & Vallerand, A. H. (1988). *Davis's drug guide for nurses.* Philadelphia: F. A. Davis.

Eggli, D. F., & Tulchinsky, M. (1993). Scintigraphic evaluation of pediatric urinary tract infection. *Seminars in Nuclear Medicine, 23*(3), 199–218.

Faden, H., & Rosales, S. (1984). Infections in the compromised neonate. In P. L. Ocra (Ed.), *Neonatal infections: Nutritional and immunologic interactions* (pp. 185–202). Orlando, FL: Grune & Stratton.

Fanaroff, A. A., & Martin, R. J. (1997). *Neonatal-perinatal medicine: Diseases of the fetus and infant.* (6th ed.). St. Louis: Mosby–Year Book.

Filston, H. C., & Izant, R. (1985). *The surgical neonate: Evaluation and care* (2nd ed.). New York: Appleton-Century-Crofts.

Goetzman, B. W., & Wennberg, R. P. (1991). *Neonatal intensive care handbook.* St. Louis: C. V. Mosby.

Golbus, M. S., Filly, R. A., Callen, P. W., et al. (1985). Fetal urinary tract obstruction: Management and selection for treatment. *Seminars in Perinatology, 9*(2), 91–97.

Goodman, R., & Gorlin, R. (1983). *The malformed infant and child.* New York: Oxford University Press.

Griggs, C. (1982). What is the prune-belly syndrome? *American Journal of Maternal Child Nursing, 7*(4), 253–257.

Grupe, W. E. (1987). The dilemma of intrauterine diagnosis of congenital renal disease. *Pediatric Clinics of North America, 34*(3), 629–638.

Hanna, M. K. (1989). Megaureter. In L. R. King (Ed.), *Urologic surgery in neonates and young infants* (pp. 160–203). Philadelphia: W. B. Saunders.

Hiraoka, M., Kasuga, K., Hori, C., & Sudo, M. (1994). Ultrasonic indicators of ureteric reflux in the newborn. *The Lancet, 343*(8896), 519–520.

Ingelfinger, J. R. (1985). Renal conditions in the newborn period. In J. P. Cloherty & A. R. Stark (Eds.), *Manual of neonatal care* (2nd ed., pp. 377–394). Boston: Little, Brown.

Inturrisi, M., Perry, S. E., & May, K. A. (1985). Fetal surgery for congenital hydronephrosis. *Journal of Obstetric, Gynecologic, and Neonatal Nursing, 14*(4), 271–276.

Jain, R., & Yeh, T. F. (1985). Placental transfer of drugs. In T. F. Yeh (Ed.), *Drug therapy in the neonate and small infant* (pp. 21–29). Chicago: Year Book Medical Publishers.

John, G., & Yeh, T. F. (1985). Renal failure. In T. F. Yeh (Ed.), *Drug therapy in the neonate and small infant* (pp. 277–298). Chicago: Year Book Medical Publishers.

Kaplan, G. W. (1994). Structural abnormalities of the of the genitourinary system. In G. B. Avery, M. A. Fletcher, & M. G. MacDonald (Eds.), *Neonatology: Pathophysiology and management of the newborn* (4th. ed., pp. 887–913). Philadelphia: J. B. Lippincott.

Kaplan, G. W., & Silber, I. (1988). Neonatal torsion: To pex or not? In L. R. King (Ed.), *Urologic surgery in neonates and young infants* (pp. 386–395). Philadelphia: W. B. Saunders.

Kim, M. S., & Mandell, J. (1988). Renal function in the fetus and neonate. In L. R. King (Ed.), *Urologic surgery in neonates and young infants* (pp. 59–76). Philadelphia: W. B. Saunders.

King, L. (1980). Exstrophy of the bladder and epispadias. In J. Raffensperger (Ed.), *Pediatric surgery* (pp. 753–768). New York: Appleton-Century-Crofts.

King, L. R. (1988). The management of multicystic kidney and ureteropelvic junction obstruction. In L. R. King (Ed.), *Urologic surgery in neonates and young infants* (pp. 140–154). Philadelphia: W. B. Saunders.

Laundau, D., Turner, M. E., Brennan, J., & Majd, M. (1994). The value of urinalysis in differentiating acute pyelonephritis from lower urinary tract infection in febrile infants. *Pediatric Infectious Disease Journal, 13*(9), 777–781.

Liu, K. W., Ku, K. W., Cheung, K. L., & Chan, Y. L. (1994). Acute scrotal swelling: A sign of neonatal adrenal haemorrhage. *Journal of Paediatric Child Health, 30*, 368–369.

Manning, F. A. (1987). Fetal surgery for obstructive uropathy: Rational consideration. *American Journal of Kidney Diseases, 10*(4), 259–267.

McCracken, G., & Freij, B. T. (1987). Bacterial and viral infections of the newborn. In G. B. Avery (Ed.), *Neonatology: Pathophysiology and management of the newborn* (3rd ed., pp. 917–943). Philadelphia: J. B. Lippincott.

Mesrobian, J. G. J. (1988). Exstrophy of the bladder. In L. R. King (Ed.), *Urologic surgery in neonates and young infants* (pp. 265–290). Philadelphia: W. B. Saunders.

Moore, K. L., & Persaud, T. V. N. (1993). *The developing human: Clinically oriented embryology* (5th ed.). Philadelphia: W. B. Saunders.

O'Donnell, B. (1984). The lessons of 40 bladder exstrophies in 20 years. *Journal of Pediatric Surgery, 19*(5), 547–549.

Page, E., Villee, C., & Villee, D. (1981). *Human reproduction: Essentials of reproduction and perinatal medicine* (3rd ed.). Philadelphia: W. B. Saunders.

Radhakrishnan, J. R. (1990). Obstructive uropathy in the newborn. *Clinics in Perinatology, 17*(1), 215–239.

Reams, P. K., & Deane, D. M. (1988). Bagged versus diaper urine specimens and laboratory values. *Neonatal Network, 6*(6), 17–20.

Rosenstein, B. J., Wheeler, J. S., & Heid, P. L. (1990). Congenital renal abnormalities in infants with in utero cocaine exposure. *Journal of Urology, 144*(1), 110–112.

Sadler, T. W. (1995). *Langman's medical embryology* (7th ed.). Baltimore: Williams & Wilkins.

Sanders, R. C. (1996). *Structural fetal abnormalities: The total picture.* St. Louis: C. V. Mosby.

Scanlon, J. W., Nelson, T., Grylack, L. J., & Smith, Y. F. (1979). *A system of newborn physical examination.* Baltimore: University Park Press.

Schreiner, R. L., & Bradburn, N. C. (Eds.). (1988). *Care of the newborn* (2nd ed.). New York: Raven Press.

Short, K. L., Groff, D. B., & Cook, L. (1985). The concomitant presence of gastroschisis and prune belly syndrome in a twin. *Journal of Pediatric Surgery, 20*(2), 186–187.

Smith, D. L. (1988). *Recognizable patterns of malformations in development.* Philadelphia: W. B. Saunders.

Smith, F. G., & Robillard, J. E. (1989). Pathophysiology of fetal renal disease. *Seminars in Perinatology, 13*(4), 305–319.

Snyder, H. M. (1988). Management of ambiguous genitalia in the neonate. In L. R. King (Ed.), *Urologic surgery in neonates and young infants* (pp. 346–385). Philadelphia: W. B. Saunders.

Spindel, M. R., Winslow, B. H., & Jordan, G. H. (1988). The use of paraexstrophy flaps for urethral construction in neonatal girls with classical exstrophy. *Journal of Urology, 140*, 574–576.

Stang, H., Gunnar, M. R., Snellman, L., et al. (1988). Local anesthesia for neonatal circumcision. *Journal of the American Medical Association, 259*(10), 1507–1511.

Sugar, E. C., & Firlit, C. F. (1988). Management of cloacal exstrophy. *Urology, 32*(4), 320–322.

Suri, S. (1988). Simplifying urine collection from infants and children without losing accuracy. *American Journal of Maternal Child Nursing, 13*(6), 438–441.

Tank, E., & McCoy, G. (1983). Limited surgical intervention in the prune belly syndrome. *Journal of Pediatric Surgery, 18*(6), 688–691.

Thompson, D. G., & Cohen, D. G. (1996). Nursing management of the infant with a congenital malignancy. *Journal of Obstetric, Gynecologic, and Neonatal Nursing, 25*(1), 32–38.

Vander, A. J. (1985). *Renal physiology* (3rd ed.). New York: McGraw-Hill.

Vanhaesebrouck, P., Thiery, M., Leroy, J. G., et al. (1988). Oligohydramnios, renal insufficiency, and ileal perforation in preterm infants after intrauterine exposure to indomethacin. *Journal of Pediatrics, 113*(4), 738–743.

White, C., Richardson, C., & Raibstein, L. (1990). High-frequency ventilation and extracorporeal membrane oxygenation. *AACN Clinical Issues in Critical Care, 1*(2), 427–444.

Wiswell, T. E., Enzenauer, R. W., Holton, M. E., et al. (1987). Declining male to female sex ratio of urinary tract infections in early infancy. *Pediatrics, 79*(3), 338–342.

Wiswell, T. E., & Hachey, W. E. (1993). Urinary tract infections and the uncircumcised state: An update. *Clinical Pediatrics*, *32*(3), 130–134.

Wodniak, C., & Szwed, J. (1986). Fluid and electrolytes. In L. Abels (Ed.), *Critical care nursing: A physiologic approach*. St. Louis: C. V. Mosby.

CHAPTER 32

Assessment and Management of Integumentary Dysfunction

JOANNE McMANUS KULLER CAROLYN HOUSKA LUND

RESEARCH AGENDA

Does the presence of melanocytes in dark-skinned infants have an effect on the accuracy of transcutaneous bilirubin measurements?

Which soap or bathing practices result in the least irritation to neonatal skin?

Which adhesives result in the least disruption or trauma to neonatal skin or the stratum corneum?

What is the relationship between the use of either alcohol or povidone-iodine and skin trauma, alterations in surface (skin) pH, dryness, and efficacy as a decontaminating solution for the skin?

Which dressings are more effective in promoting moist healing of wounds?

What are the effects of different soaps on the pH and microbial colonization of the skin?

Does the use of humidity affect the maturation of epidermal barrier function?

What are the effects of various antimicrobial skin preparation agents on the barrier function of the skin?

VIGNETTE

You can get a very skewed perspective of childbearing by working in a NICU. Just to assure myself that normal people have normal babies, I contracted to teach prenatal classes. I very much enjoyed my experience: interacting with nice couples who enjoyed good outcomes. It was always fun to see them with their new babies and to listen to their birth experiences.

Bad things do happen to nice people, though. Julie is just one such person. I struck up a friendship with Julie and her husband, Mike, while they were attending one of my classes. It was Julie's first pregnancy, after several years of infertility testing and treatment. Julie and Mike were really looking forward to the birth of their child. They often stayed after class or talked to me during break.

Julie went into labor shortly before her due date. Labor progressed according to expectations, except that Julie revised her natural childbirth plans in favor of an epidural. After 5½ hours of labor, Julie gave birth to a robust (Apgars, 8[1] and 9[5]) 8-pound 3-ounce boy. Julie and Mike were delighted with their newborn, and Julie was able to begin nursing him in the delivery room.

On the baby's transfer to the admitting nursery, the delivery nurse noted that Travis looked normal except for some abrasions on several fingers and at the base of his umbilical cord. As the nursery nurse conducted Travis' admitting physical assessment, she noted bruising and an ulcerated area on the occiput. The fetal monitor scalp site appeared abraded. There were also several blisters on the upper gums.

The pediatrician was notified and suspected one of two possible causes: scalded skin syndrome due to a staphylococcal infection or epidermolysis bullosa, a familially inherited blistering skin disease. She ordered protective isolation with sterile linens and cloth diapers. Sterile gloves were to be worn during the newborn's care. No heel sticks were to be performed; minimal tape was to be used. She ordered gentle Betadine cleansing of the denuded areas, to be followed by Polysporin ointment. A CBC with differential and blood glucose was to be performed; blood and surface cultures must be sent for bacteria or herpesvirus discovery. Ampicillin and gentamicin were ordered, and a heparin well was inserted. A urine bag was put on Travis for a urine Wellcogen test. Blood was to be drawn for immunoglobulin electrophoresis.

Travis was put in an incubator and transferred to the NICU. As I cared for him over the next 2 weeks, blisters would form and break open, leaving denuded flesh, which would seep serosanguineous fluid. Blisters formed over all the pressure points: on the back and sides of his head, lips, gums, and tongue, and over his shoulder blades, elbows, chest, groin, thighs, and buttocks. Many blisters appeared on his fingers; he even lost several fingernails. The lesions appeared in different stages of breakdown and healing. They appeared open and raw for 4 days, during which time they would seep. They would then crust over and, if left undisturbed, would appear to heal slowly, from the edges inward. His plan of care included use of sheepskin and repositioning every hour.

Julie and Mike came frequently to the NICU to visit Travis. They were encouraged to hold him, and Travis continued to nurse well. When I asked how she was coping with all of this, Julie said, "I'm hoping a little cream can fix this."

All cultures were returned with negative findings. A dermatologist was called in to consult. He examined Travis and suspected a diagnosis of epidermolysis bullosa. A skin biopsy was scheduled for light and electron microscopic analysis to distinguish between the several types of this disease. This waiting period was a difficult time for Julie and Mike. They became involved in Travis's care, learning how to wash and apply ointment to their son's sores.

The day came for the test results to be back, and the dermatologist called for a family conference. The news was not good. The analysis indicated epidermolysis bullosa letalis. They were told that this is a relatively rare genetic disease. The blistering process would continue and increase in response to innocuous trauma and friction. There was no treatment and no cure. Travis would eventually die from fluid loss and infection.

"How long?" Julie managed to choke out.

"Could be several weeks, could be longer, depending on how he blisters and what kind of care he receives." He looked at them with understanding in his eyes. "No matter how well you care for him, you cannot prevent this from happening. You can strive to make him comfortable and give him a normal experience in his lifetime."

I stayed with them after the doctor had answered all their questions and left. The news was devastating. Julie and Mike cried. Their pain was so intense that I found myself crying, too. Not only was Travis to die, but the doctor had informed them that all future children they produced were also at risk.

It took several days for them to collect themselves, but Julie and Mike decided to take Travis home. I helped them prepare their home environment and plan for necessary medications and equipment. I taught them both how to clean and care for his lesions. We talked through any and all ideas about cutting down on friction and trauma to which Travis might be exposed. Because Julie felt that she needed someone to help her after Mike returned to work, I contacted a home care agency for a nurse to visit and help with Travis's care.

I kept in touch with the family. Travis did well until he started to crawl. Julie could not keep him from this highly desired activity. He would also pull toys and other objects to his face and cause trauma by chewing on them or bumping against them. Travis died at 8 months from sepsis, after a 2-week hospitalization for extensive skin excoriation and corneal sloughing. He expired in his parents' arms. Julie was both mentally and physically drained and sought counseling to deal with her feelings.

The story does have a nice ending. Several years later, Julie and Mike are the proud parents of a healthy set of twins, one of each sex. Julie obtained prenatal testing early in the pregnancy and was relieved to find out that Margot and Mark are not affected by the gene that causes epidermolysis bullosa.

Joyce M. Dohme

In neonatology, skin phenomena, along with other examination findings, are used to assess maturity, duration of pregnancy, and neonatal vitality. The skin is a major organ of the premature infant, making up 13 percent of the body weight, compared with 3 percent in adults (Klaus & Fanaroff, 1987). This large organ provides a barrier against infection, protects internal organs, contributes to temperature regulation and insensible water loss, stores fats, excretes electrolytes and water, and provides tactile sensory input. The sensations of touch, pressure, temperature, pain, and itch are received by millions of microscopic dermal nerve endings. As a means of communication, the skin is instrumental in early establishment of the mother–infant relationship (Montagu, 1971). Ashley Montagu believes that the quality of touch and stimulation that an infant receives is responsible for the infant's later responses to other people and to the environment. In this sense, it fulfills a task of vital importance, particularly in the area of maternal–child nursing (Dietel, 1978).

Nursing care practices that affect the fragile, underdeveloped skin of the premature infant present major concerns as well as dilemmas for care providers. Life support and monitoring equipment must be securely attached and frequently removed or replaced; this practice causes trauma to the skin. Numerous invasive procedures, such as vascular access, blood sampling, and chest tube insertion, are necessary but invade the skin's barrier. Because the skin of the premature infant makes up such a large percentage of body weight, trauma to skin can result in the diversion of an excessive proportion of caloric intake to the repair of this large organ. Other concerns about the effects of trauma to premature skin include the energy demands of electrolyte imbalances and increased evaporative heat loss through damaged skin and the risk of toxicity when substances are applied to the skin surface.

The single most significant concern, however, is infection. Because of trauma to the skin, large areas of the skin are portals to bacteria and fungus in an already immunocompromised host. Even common skin flora, such as coagulase-negative staphylococci and *Candida* species, can have serious pathogenic capabilities in these hosts and often enter the system through mucocutaneous inoculation (Baley & Silverman, 1988; Baley et al., 1986; D'Angio et al., 1989; Patrick, 1990; Patrick et al., 1989). Thus, significant morbidity and mortality can be attributed to practices that cause either trauma to skin or alterations in normal skin function.

Iatrogenically caused skin problems, including burns and caustic lesions from isopropyl alcohol (Schick & Milstein, 1981) and erythema and skin craters from transcutaneous oxygen monitoring, have been reported in the medical literature (Boyle & Oh, 1980; Golden, 1981). Increased skin permeability of preterm infants (Hey & Katz, 1969; Montagna et al., 1972; Nachman & Esterly, 1971) and percutaneous toxicity from drugs and chemicals (Pyati et al., 1977; West et al., 1981; Wester & Maibach, 1982) have also been well documented.

This chapter covers the development and structure of skin, the normal physiologic variations in newborn skin, and dermatologic diseases. This information is then incorporated into the nursing management of the neonatal skin.

SKIN STRUCTURE AND FUNCTION

All skin consists of three anatomically distinct layers: the epidermis, the dermis, and the subcutaneous tissue. The principal functional compartment of the epidermis is the stratum corneum epidermidis, the horny outer layer of the epidermis. It is primarily composed of closely packed dead cells that are being continually brushed off by clothing and washing. These exfoliated cells form part of the vernix caseosa, the cheese-like substance that covers and protects fetal skin. The bottom, living basal layer constantly replaces these cells. It takes approximately 26 days for cells from this layer to migrate up to the stratum corneum. Approximately 20 percent of an adult's protein requirement is needed for this purpose. Keratin-forming cells, which cornify the outer layer of the epidermis, and melanocytes are contained in the lower levels of the epidermis. Melanocytes begin producing melanin, or pigment, before birth and distribute it to the epidermal cells. Active pigmentary activity can be observed before birth in the epidermis of infants of dark-skinned races, but little evidence of such activity exists in white fetuses (Moore & Persaud, 1993).

The dermis lies directly under the epidermis and is 2 to 4 mm thick at birth. It is a closely woven layer of collagen, which is a fibrous protein, and elastin fibers. Many nerves and a rich supply of blood vessels are contained there. They nourish the skin cells and act as carriers of the sensations of heat, touch, pressure, and pain from the skin to the brain. Hair originates from deep in the dermis. Down-growths, called epidermal ridges, that extend into the developing dermis result from a proliferation of cells in the basal layer. These ridges are permanently established by the 17th week and produce ridges and grooves on the surface of the palms, including the fingers, and on the soles of the feet, including the toes. Determined genetically, this type of pattern constitutes the basis for the use of fingerprints in criminal investigations and medical genetics. Dermatoglyphics is the study of the pattern of these epidermal ridges. The presence of abnormal chromosome complements affects the development of the ridge patterns. For example, infants with Down syndrome exhibit distinctive hand and feet patterns that are of diagnostic value (Moore & Persaud, 1993).

The major component of the subcutaneous layer is fatty connective tissue. The subcutaneous fat functions as a heat insulator, a shock absorber, and a calorie reserve area. Fat accumulation occurs predominantly in the last trimester.

Sebaceous glands are found in both the dermis and the subcutaneous layer. Well-developed and potentially functional at birth, these glands have only minimal function until puberty. Sweat glands are also found in the dermis and the subcutaneous layer and are affected directly by external environmental temperature. In premature infants, sweat gland maturation occurs between 21 and 33 days of age. In term infants, this maturation occurs at about 5 days of age. Poor sweat production in the premature infant is caused by sweat gland immaturity. However, adult function in any infant is not achieved until the second or third year of life (Dietel, 1978).

Normal term infant skin is soft, wrinkled, velvety, and covered with vernix caseosa. Transformation of the fetal circulation is evident soon after the cord is cut, as the skin develops the intense red coloration that is characteristic of the newborn. This color may remain for hours. A bluish blotchiness may appear if the infant is exposed to a cool environment.

The insulating layer of vernix is usually lost during the first few days of life, owing to traditional newborn skin care. This results in a loss of insulation for the upper stratum corneum, which then peels off, resulting in skin with a grayish-white or yellowish hue. Visible desquamation of newborn skin comes to an end after about 7 days. Vernix, which has bactericidal property and protects the infant's skin, should be allowed to wear off at its own rate.

In comparison with that of the term infant, the premature infant's skin at birth is more transparent and gelatinous and tends to be free of wrinkles. Lanugo, which has been lost in the full-term infant, may be present in varying degrees and is one criterion used to estimate gestational age. Additionally, subcutaneous edema may be present—clinical evidence of a cutaneous excess of water and sodium (Solomon & Esterly, 1973). This edema decreases within the first few days of life, and the skin then lies loosely over the infant's entire body (Harmon & Steele, 1975).

The immaturity of the infant's skin is linked to the premature newborn's difficulty maintaining body temperature. A poorly developed fat supply and a large body surface area in relation to body weight add to this difficulty.

The skin of the full-term infant has a well-developed epidermis; the stratum corneum is structured to perform efficiently to controlling transepidermal water loss (TEWL) and prevent absorption of toxic substances, similar to the function of the adult epidermis (Holbrook, 1982). The premature infant, in contrast, has been shown to have a less well-developed stratum corneum, with infants less than 30 weeks' gestation having the least developed stratum corneum. This immaturity results in the premature infant's decreased capacity to resist particles, viruses, parasites, and bacteria in the external environment, leaving the infant readily susceptible to infection and irritation of the skin.

Transferring from the intrauterine aquatic environment to the external atmospheric environment stimulates and accelerates maturation of skin function. Holbrook (1982) reported that by 10 days' postnatal age or with increasing gestational age, the integrity of the premature infant's skin improves, approaching that of the term infant or adult. However, using light and transmission electron microscopy to examine skin samples received from infants who were 23 to 40 weeks' estimated gestational age (EGA), Nonato and Guy (1995) concluded that the epidermis develops between 23 to 24 weeks' EGA in utero; the epidermis and dermis are not mature by 1 month postnatal age in neonates less than 34 weeks' EGA; and the stratum corneum is still not fully developed after 8 weeks' postnatal age in neonates less than 34 weeks' EGA. Therefore, both gestational and postnatal age are important considerations in the management of neonatal skin.

Embryologic Development of Skin

The skin consists of two morphologically different layers, which are derived from two different germ layers. The epithelial structures (epidermis, pilosebaceous-apocrine unit, eccrine unit, and nails) are ectodermal derivatives. The ectoderm also gives rise to the hair, the teeth, and the sense organs of smell, taste, hearing, vision, and touch—everything involved with events occurring outside the organism. Mesenchymal structures (collagen, reticular, and elastic fibers; blood vessels; muscles; and fat) originate from mesoderm. These developments are outlined in Table 32–1.

The epidermis, which develops from the surface ectoderm, consists of one layer of undifferentiated cells in a 3-week-old embryo. By 4 weeks' gestational age, it has an inner germinative layer of cuboidal cells with dark, compact nuclei and an outer layer of slightly flatter cells covered by microvilli (Ackerman,

TABLE 32–1 Embryonic and Fetal Development of Skin

Embryonic period: undoubtedly the most important period of human development because the beginnings of all major external and internal structures develop.

Fetal period (9th week to birth): primarily concerned with growth and differentiation of tissue and organs that started to develop during the embryonic period.

Weeks of Gestation	
3	Epidermis, which develops from surface ectoderm, consists of one layer of cells.
5	Cutaneous nerves are detectable in embryonic dermis.
6–7	Periderm, a thin protective layer of flattened cells, is formed.
11	Collagen and elastic fibers are developing in the dermis. Epidermal ridges (fingerprints) are forming. Nails begin to develop at the tips of the digits.
13–16	Scalp hair patterning is determined.
17–20	Melanocytes migrate to the epidermal-dermal junction and begin to produce melanin. Skin is covered with vernix caseosa and lanugo. Keratin is accumulating in the epidermis.
21–25	Skin is wrinkled, translucent, and pink to red because blood in the capillaries has become visible.
26–29	Subcutaneous fat begins to be deposited and starts to smooth out the many wrinkles in the skin. Eccrine sweat glands are anatomically developed and found over the entire body; their function, however, is somewhat immature in the perinatal period.
30–34	Skin is pink and smooth. Fingernails reach fingertips. Lanugo begins to shed.
35–38	Fetuses are usually plump. Skin is usually white or bluish-pink. Toenails reach toe tips.

Data from Ackerman A. (1985). Structure and function of the skin. In S. Moschella & H. Hurley (Eds.), *Dermatology* (Vol. II, 2nd ed.). Philadelphia: W. B. Saunders Co.

1985). About the middle of the second month of gestation, some of the cells begin to be crowded to the surface, forming a thin, protective layer of flattened cells known as the periderm. The cells of this layer continually undergo keratinization and desquamation and are replaced by cells arising from the basal layer. The periderm is often called the epitrichial ("upon the hair") layer of the epidermis because the hairs that later grow up from the deeper layers are said not to penetrate this thin surface layer but to push it up on their growing tips, causing it to be cast off if it has not already disappeared (Ackerman, 1985). These exfoliated cells form part of the vernix caseosa.

During the later part of the second month, the epithelium tends to become thicker. This occurs (at first) by a staggering of the nuclei and the beginning of cell rearrangement, which leads rapidly to the formation of an intermediate layer between the flattened cells of the epitrichial layer and the basal layer adjacent to the underlying dermis. The cells of this intermediate layer tend to become enlarged and show a high degree of vacuolation. The basal layer of the epidermis is later called the stratum germinativum (Moore & Persaud, 1993).

At the end of the second month of gestation, the cutaneous nerves, which are detectable in embryonic dermis about the fifth week of gestation, appear to be functional, although the skin is primitive by comparison with that of an adult.

> When the embryo is less than an inch long crown to rump, and less than 8 weeks old, light stroking of the upper lip or wings of the nose will cause bending of the neck and trunk away from the source of stimulation. At this stage in its development the embryo has neither eyes nor ears.
>
> Montagu, 1971

At about 10 weeks' gestation, fingernail development begins at the tips of the digits. A thickened area of epithelium on the dorsum of each digit is the first sign of nail formation. Our nails are adaptations of the epidermis, homologous to the claws and hoofs of lower mammals, and are formed by a modified process of keratinization. Development of the fingernails is begun and completed (30 to 34 weeks) before that of the toenails (35 to 38 weeks).

By about 11 weeks' gestation, collagen and elastic connective tissue fibers begin to develop in the dermis. The epidermal-dermal junction, which has been smooth up to this time, now becomes wavy as epidermal thickenings grow down into the dermis of the palm and the soles of the feet. Dermal papillae develop in these dermal projections. Capillary loops develop in some dermal papillae, and Meissner's corpuscles, which are the sensory nerve endings of touch, form in others (Moore & Persaud, 1993). These epidermal ridges produce ridges and grooves in a genetically determined pattern and are the basis for fingerprinting and footprinting. The development of these ridges can be distinctly affected by the presence of abnormal chromosome complements (e.g., as occurs in Down syndrome). These ridges are permanently established by about 17 weeks' gestation.

During the third to fourth month of gestation, the stratum germinativum differentiates from the rest of the epithelium. These cells are termed the germinative layer because they undergo the repeated cell divisions that are responsible for the growth of the epidermis.

During the fourth month of gestation, the epithelium starts to become many cells thick, and keratin begins to accumulate in the cells above the stratum germinativum layer. Daughter cells from the basal layer are crowded upward and undergo progressive changes in each layer, finalizing in cornification. The thin stratum granulosum epidermidis, which contains keratohyalin granules, is the layer directly above the stratum germinativum. The next higher layer is the thin and clear stratum lucidum epidermidis, whose content is a fluid, eleidin, that replaces the granules. Above that is the keratinized multilayered stratum corneum epidermidis (Moore & Persaud, 1993). As the keratin accumulates in these cells, they become more and more sluggish and finally die, so that the surface layer of the epidermis is made up of tough, scale-like, dead cells that form a relatively impermeable membrane.

In areas such as the soles of the feet and the palms of the hands, where the skin is subjected to more than ordinary wear, the keratinization of the outer layer is much heavier than in the general body surface. Of interest, however, is that the greater thickness of palmar and plantar epidermis becomes evident in the embryo long before it is possible for these areas to have been subjected to any more wear than other parts of the skin. When the aforementioned layers are all completely differentiated, the structure of fetal epidermis resembles that of adult epidermis.

During the early fetal period, neural crest cells migrate into the dermis and differentiate into melanoblasts. At about 17 to 20 weeks of gestation, these melanoblasts differentiate into melanocytes, migrate to the epidermal-dermal border, and begin to produce melanin. Fetal melanocytes in white races contain little or no pigment, whereas in dark-skinned races, they produce melanin granules. The skin of black newborns is only a little darker than that of white newborns. The skin at the bases of the fingernails and toenails is often noticeably darker, however. The skin of black infants continues to darken after birth, as increased melanin production occurs in response to light. When melanocytes remain behind in the dermis, they appear bluish through the overlying cutaneous tissue and are called mongolian spots. Some believe that it is not the number of melanocytes present that is important, but rather their activity level. The hormone secreted by the pituitary gland that controls the clumping or dispersion of the melanin granules is melanocyte-stimulating hormone. Melanin is primarily responsible for skin coloration, but other factors that have an influence are carotene, circulation of blood in the skin capillaries, degree of oxygen saturation of hemoglobin, presence of bile pigment, and thickness of the epidermis (Harmon & Steele, 1975).

Around 20 weeks of gestation, the eyebrows, upper lip, and chin hair are first recognizable. On the general body surface, the hair makes its appearance about a month later. These fine hairs are called lanugo. As stated earlier, the emergence of this hair breaks off the periderm, and the periderm becomes one component of the vernix caseosa. The other components of vernix are sebum from the sebaceous glands, fetal hair, and desquamated cells from the amnion (Moore & Persaud, 1993). Vernix protects the epidermis against a macerating influence that would be exerted by the amniotic fluid and acts as a lubricant to prevent chafing injuries from the amnion as the growing fetus becomes progressively confined in its fluid-filled sac.

Between 21 and 24 weeks' gestation, the fetus's skin is wrinkled, translucent, and pinkish-red because blood in the capillaries has become visible. Head and lanugo hair are well developed in a 26- to 29-week fetus. At this same time, eccrine sweat glands are anatomically developed and are found over the entire body. Their function, however, is somewhat immature in the perinatal period (Dietel, 1978).

Brown adipose tissue cells begin to differentiate in the seventh month of gestation, and the accumulation of subcutaneous fat begins to smooth out the many skin wrinkles. Between the 30th and 34th week of gestation, the skin is pink and smooth, and the lanugo is beginning to shed. The fingernails reach the fingertips, but the distal part of the nail is still thin and soft (Moore & Persaud, 1993). During the last trimester of pregnancy, subcutaneous fat accumulates, and the fetus acquires a plump appearance. The composition of amniotic fluid tested at this time reflects skin function. The number of anucleated cells and keratinized lipid-containing skin flakes increases. The cytologic count of fat-laden cells is 10 percent at 36 to 38 weeks, and the finding of more than 20 percent of fat-laden cells is an indication of a mature fetus (West et al., 1981).

Developmental Variations

Several factors are responsible for the functional differences between premature and term infants' skin. These differences subside with increasing gestational and postnatal age (Table 32–2).

Skin Permeability

In comparison with that of a term infant, the skin of a premature infant is remarkably permeable. It appears that permeability correlates inversely with gestational age. Because of this increased skin permeability, which allows the infant to absorb greater quantities of topical medications than the adult, the preterm infant is at great risk for toxicity from topically applied drugs (West et al., 1981). The increased permeability of the premature infant's skin also favors cutaneous insensible water loss and heat dissipation and contributes to the difficulty the premature newborn experiences in maintaining body temperature (Rutter & Hull, 1979).

Iatrogenic injury secondary to the increased permeability of preterm infants' skin has occurred in the clinical setting. Hexachlorophene, 3 percent emulsion, was routinely used in hospital nurseries to prevent the growth of coagulase-positive staphylococci until studies associated such practice with central nervous system damage (Curley et al., 1971). Central nervous system problems associated with hexachlorophene toxicity include hypertoxicity, central nervous system irritability, seizures, twitching of extremities, and coma. In fatal cases of hexachlorophene toxicity, spongy degenerative vacuolating lesions of the brain and spinal cord have been found. The same washing procedure yielded much higher hexachlorophene blood levels in premature infants than in term infants. Kopelman (1973) concluded that dermal absorption of hexachlorophene was much greater in premature infants.

Liberal use of povidone-iodine as a preparatory agent before invasive procedures has been associated with high iodine levels, iodine goiter, and hypothyroidism in the newborn (Chabrolle & Rossier, 1978; Jackson & Sutherland, 1981; Pyati et al., 1977). These reports recommend that iodine-containing preparations be used with caution in full-term infants and be avoided in premature infants. It is important to be sure that the use of povidone-iodine does not lead to false diagnosis of a congenital hypothyroidism, because many neonatal hypothyroidism screening programs depend on an increased thyroid-stimulating value. If it is used to

TABLE 32–2 Structural Differences Between Infant and Adult Skin

	Premature	Full-term	Adult
Epidermis	Thinner cells compressed Fewer desmosomes Fewer layers of stratum corneum Melanin production low	Stratum corneum appears as adherent cell layers Melanin production low	Good resistance to penetration
Dermoepidermal junction	Fewer hemidesmosomes; less cohesion between layers		
Dermis	Fewer elastin fibers Thinner than in the adult	Fewer elastin fibers Thinner than in the adult	Full complement of elastin fibers
Eccrine glands	May be more typical of fetus than adult Ducts patent; secretory cells undifferentiated	Equivalent in structure to adult Denser distribution	Distribution less dense than in infant
Hair	Lanugo hair may be present Hair growth synchronous	Vellus hair characteristic Hair growth synchronous	Both vellus and terminal hairs Hair growth dyssynchronous
Sebaceous glands	Large and active	Large and active, but diminishing rapidly in both size and activity for several weeks after birth	Large and active
Nerve and vascular system	Not fully organized Most nerves are small in diameter, unmyelinated, sensory, and autonomic Unmyelinated nerves are typically fetal in structure Meissner's touch receptors not fully formed	Vascular system not fully organized until 3 months Cutaneous nerve network not fully developed, may continue to develop until puberty Most nerves are small in diameter, unmyelinated, sensory, and autonomic Meissner's touch receptors not fully formed	Adult pattern
Permeability	Highly permeable Higher penetrability of fat-soluble substances Greater absorption because of higher skin surface: body weight ratio	Good resistance to penetration Higher penetrability of fat-soluble substances Greater absorption because of higher skin surface: body weight ratio	Good resistance to penetration
Eccrine sweating	Reduced sweating capability, especially for first 13–24 days	Reduced sweating capability, especially for first 2–5 days	Full sweating capability
Photosensitivity	Melanin production low; will sunburn readily	Melanin production low; will sunburn readily	Sensitivity to sun depends on skin type
Related conditions	Reduced ability to ward off infection because of deficient immune system Low reactivity to allergens	Reduced ability to ward off infection Low reactivity to allergens	Readily sensitized to allergens

From Shalita, A. (1981). *Principles of infant skin care* (pp. 6–18). Skillman, NJ: Johnson & Johnson Baby Products. Reprinted with permission.

prepare skin surfaces, povidone-iodine should be completely washed off because it can reach high blood concentration levels in neonates (Pyati et al., 1977).

Several commonly used drugs and chemicals have been reported to cause percutaneous toxicity in infants; these include phenol, boric acid, salicylic acid, resorcinol, estrogens, corticosteroids, epinephrine, hexachlorophene, chlorhexidine, and lindane (West et al., 1981). In 18 cases of methemoglobinemia, a laundry rinse containing trichlorocarbanilide was reported as the likely source of the toxicity (Fisch et al., 1963). Its use is now contraindicated in hospital laundering by the American Academy of Pediatrics (American Academy of Pediatrics, 1977). Based on this information, all solutions topically applied to the infant's skin, especially to the premature infant's skin, during the first 2 to 3 weeks of life should be carefully evaluated as to their necessity and should be applied appropriately and sparingly if they are deemed beneficial to the infant's care.

Nachman and Esterly (1971) and Harpin and Rutter (1983) demonstrated the extraordinary permeability of premature infants' skin by applying phenylephrine (Neo-Synephrine 10 percent) ophthalmic solution to the skin of infants of various gestational ages. The result is a reduction in the cutaneous blood flow and a constriction of the vascular beds. They examined the rate of TEWL and the extent of blanching that occurred. A significant response occurred in both parameters in newborns of 28- to 34-week gestational age; this response diminished to almost no response in term infants (Figs. 32–1 and 32–2). Thickness of the stratum corneum, which is a function of maturity, was cited as the cause of the variations in the rates of permeability. The feasibility of using a percutaneous route to administer theophylline was tested by Evans and associates (1985) in an attempt to use the increased skin permeability of preterm infants to their advantage. Theophylline was readily absorbed in infants of less than 30 weeks' gestation, and therapeutic levels were achieved or maintained. As the epidermis matured with increasing postnatal age, a marked decline in absorption was observed.

Harpin and Rutter (1983) continued their study of skin permeability by measuring skin water loss and the blanching response to topical phenylephrine on normal and damaged skin. They found that the outermost layer of the dermis was stripped off when adhesive tape, monitoring probes, or electrodes were removed. This stripping resulted in increased drug absorption and water loss from these damaged areas (Figs. 32–3 and 32–4).

Hutchinson and colleagues (1963) speculated that the skin might be a route of oxygen entry and advocated the use of hyperbaric oxygen as one method of resuscitating asphyxiated infants. The skin of the very premature infant (<31 weeks' gestation) is readily permeable to oxygen and carbon dioxide, with rates of gas exchange between five and six times higher than those found in term infants (Evans & Rutter, 1986b). They estimated that if the infant were surrounded by an ambient oxygen concentration of 40 percent, approximately 13 percent of total resting oxygen consumption could pass through the skin. Close correlation was found between percutaneous gas exchange and TEWL, suggesting that in preterm infants, both these factors are controlled by epidermal barrier function. Again, younger premature infants (<29 to 30 weeks' gestation) had the highest degree of permeability and TEWL. In summary, clinical implica-

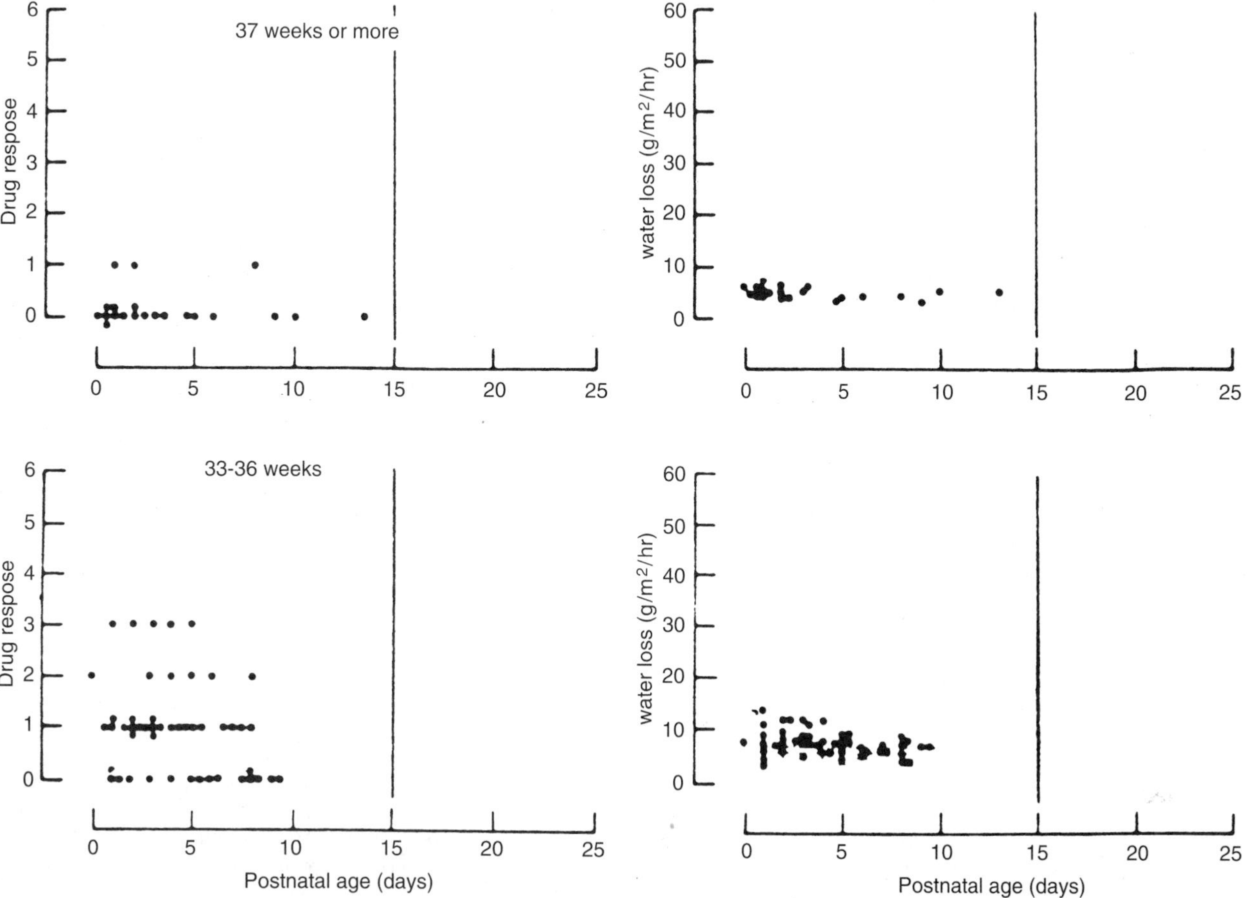

FIGURE 32–1. Drug response (blanching response to phenylephrine) and water loss from abdominal skin in infants of different gestational ages (>37 weeks and 33 to 36 weeks). (From Harpin, V.A., & Rutter, N. [1983]. Barrier properties of the newborn infant's skin. *Journal of Pediatrics, 102*(3), 419. Reprinted with permission.)

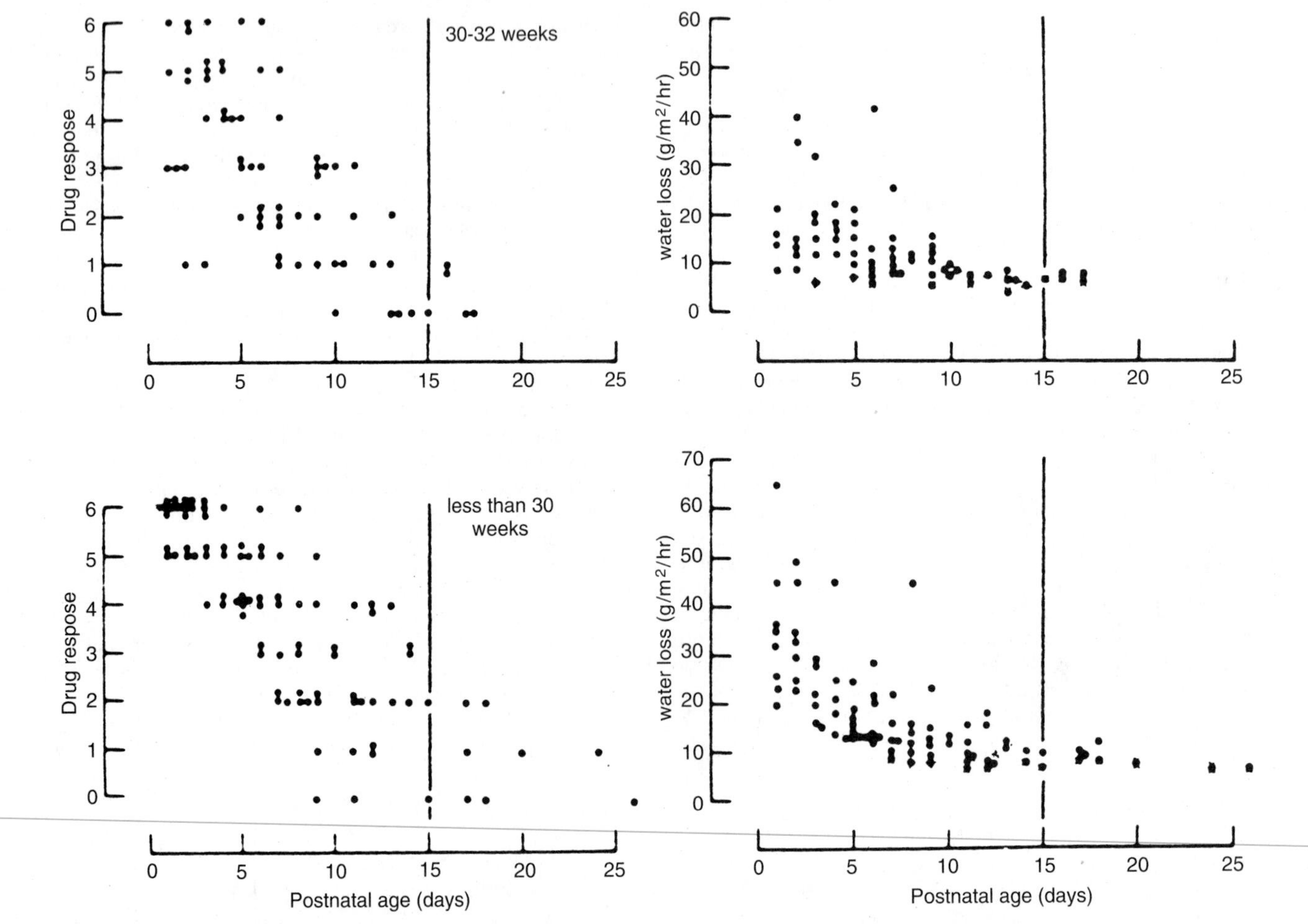

FIGURE 32–2. Drug response (blanching response to phenylephrine) and water loss from abdominal skin in infants of different gestational ages (30 to 32 weeks and <30 weeks). (From Harpin, V.A., & Rutter, N. [1983]. Barrier properties of the newborn infant's skin. *Journal of Pediatrics, 102*(3), 419. Reprinted with permission.)

tions for these differences are demonstrated by increased evaporative heat loss (Wheldon & Hull, 1983), increased fluid requirements (Lorenz et al., 1982), and risk for percutaneous toxicity from substances applied to the skin (Chabrolle & Rossier, 1978; Curley et al., 1971; Harpin & Rutter, 1982; Kopelman, 1973).

Dermal Instability

Collagen in the dermis increases with gestational age as the tendency toward water fixation and edema decreases (Dietel, 1978). The other component of the dermis, the elastin fibers, is formed mostly after birth and may not become fully mature until 3 years of age. This results in low resiliency in term infants and further reduced resiliency in premature infants (Shalita, 1981). To help prevent necrosis resulting from edema in the dermis, waterbeds, range-of-motion exercises, and routine turning should be used.

Diminished Cohesion

Another variation in the premature infant's skin structure and function is the diminished cohesion between the dermis and the epidermis. The junction of the epidermis and the dermis, which is normally connected by numerous fibrils, has fewer and more widely spaced fibrils in the premature infant than in term infants or adults (Fig. 32–5) (Holbrook, 1982). These fibrils become stronger with increasing gestational and postnatal age. Because the premature infant in the neonatal intensive care unit (NICU) is usually covered with some type of adhesive in order to secure intravenous lines, cardiorespiratory electrodes, endotracheal tubes, and umbilical artery catheters, the premature infant is at higher risk for blistering and a tendency toward stripping of the epidermis when adhesives are removed (Adamkin, 1977; Gordon & Montgomery, 1996). The cohesion between many of the currently used adhesives and the stratum corneum may be stronger than the bond between the dermis and the epidermis (Harpin & Rutter, 1983).

Thickness of the Stratum Corneum

The barrier function of the skin resides in the outermost layer of the epidermis, the stratum corneum. This barrier is composed of keratinocytes coated by intercellular lipids (Elias, 1983). The stratum corneum begins to develop in the fetus after 21 weeks' EGA (Holbrook, 1982). The stratum corneum in infants of 28 weeks' gestation consists of only a few cell layers and is markedly thinner than that of term infants. These findings correlate with the immaturity of barrier function of the stratum corneum; this immaturity is characterized by increased permeability (Harpin & Rutter, 1983; Nachman & Esterly, 1971) and increased TEWL (Cunico et al., 1977; Sedin et al., 1985).

By 32 to 34 weeks' EGA, the stratum corneum has developed sufficiently to offer slight protection (Evans and Rutter, 1986a,

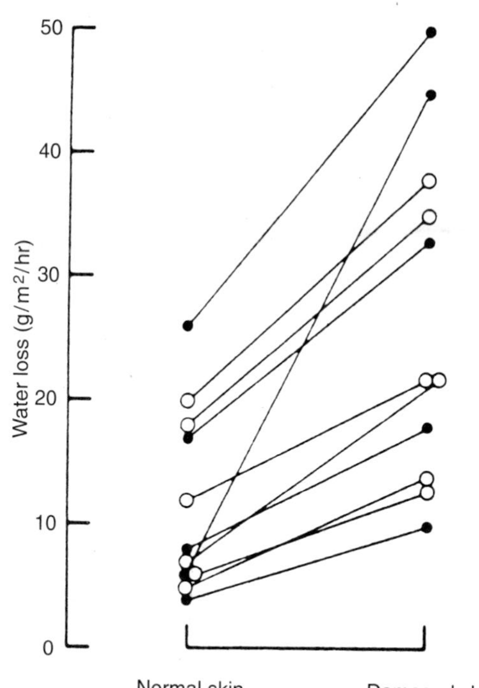

FIGURE 32–3. Water loss from normal and damaged skin. Skin damage caused by adhesive materials. ○, adhesive tape; ●, adhesive ring. (From Harpin, V.A., & Rutter, N. [1983]. Barrier properties of the newborn infant's skin. *Journal of Pediatrics, 102*(3), 419. Reprinted with permission.)

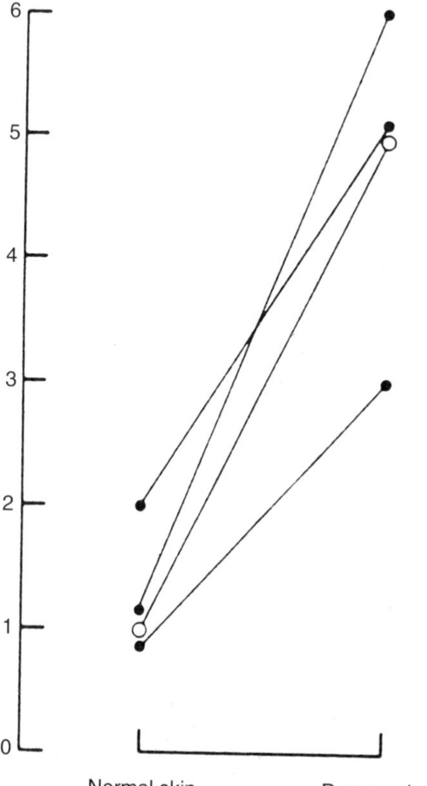

FIGURE 32–4. Drug response (blanching response to phenylephrine) from normal and damaged skin. Skin damage caused by adhesive materials. ○, adhesive tape; ●, adhesive ring. (From Harpin, V.A., & Rutter, N. [1983]. Barrier properties of the newborn infant's skin. *Journal of Pediatrics, 102*(3), 419. Reprinted with permission.)

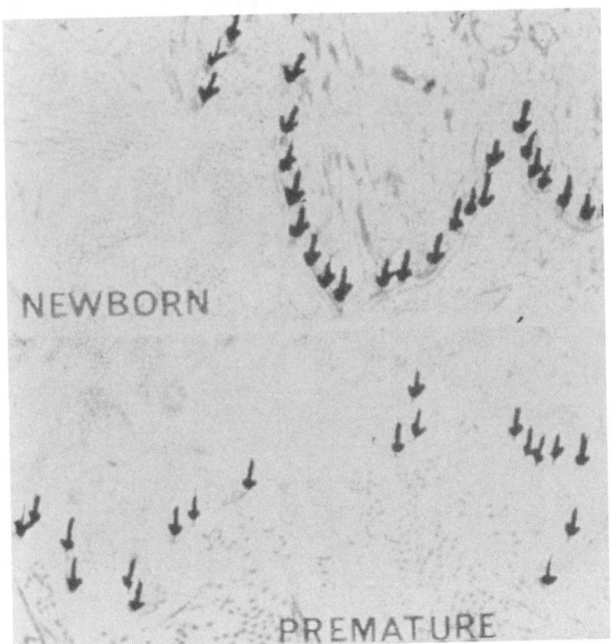

FIGURE 32–5. Connecting filaments between the dermis and epidermis. (From Holbrook, K.A. [1982]. A histological comparison of infant and adult skin. In H.I. Maibach & E.K. Boisits [Eds.], *Neonatal skin: Structure and function* [pp. 3–31]. New York: Marcel Dekker. Reprinted with permission.)

Harpin & Rutter, 1983). The full-term infant has a fully functional stratum corneum.

After birth, rapid postnatal maturation occurs, with thickening of the epidermis and development of the stratum corneum. The development of skin impermeability depends on the density and the thickness of the stratum corneum, which are functions of skin maturation.

Skin pH

Another developmental variation of infant skin resides in the functional capacity of the skin to form a surface pH of less than 5.0, which is the acid mantle. A skin surface pH of less than 5 is ordinarily seen in both children and adults, as documented extensively by Behrendt and Green (1971).

In the large number of term newborns studied, the skin was found to have a mean pH of 6.34 immediately after birth, based on combined data from the shoulder, axilla, and abdomen. Within 4 days, the pH decreased to a mean of 4.95, and between 7 and 30 days, it further decreased to 4.7 (Fig. 32–6). In a later study of 127 low birth weight infants, these authors documented that the mean pH decreased from 6.7 (day 1) to 5.04 (day 9). However, a different technique for measuring pH was used than in the previous study, so the absolute values for pH may not be comparable. They concluded that acidification of the skin is independent of gestational age.

An acidic skin surface is credited with having bactericidal qualities against some pathogens and serves in the defense against microorganisms (Behrendt & Green, 1971). Microbial colonization also begins immediately after birth. These bacteria exist and grow in a state of equilibrium that protects against pathogenic organisms (American Academy of Pediatrics, 1974). An increased skin pH, from acidic to neutral, can cause an increase in the total numbers of bacteria and a shift in the species present (Shalita, 1981). TEWL has also been shown to increase when the pH increases (Wilhelm & Maibach, 1990). Information regarding the effect of bathing or other skin care practices on skin surface pH in premature infants is not available, but the regeneration of the skin pH after washing with alkaline soap solutions takes longer than an hour in most normal newborns (Peck & Botwinick, 1964).

Melanin Production

Melanin's main function is to screen the skin from the sun's harmful rays by absorbing their radiant energy (Ackerman, 1985). Although melanin production and therefore pigmentation are lower during the neonatal period than later in life, certain areas, such as the linea alba, the areola, and the scrotum, are often deeply pigmented as a result of high circulating levels of maternal and placental hormones.

Melanin production in premature infants is even less than in term infants, placing them at greater risk for sunburn and the resulting damage to the barrier effectiveness of the skin that is caused by dehydration and desquamation of the epidermis (Shalita, 1981).

ASSESSMENT AND PHYSIOLOGIC VARIATIONS

Acrocyanosis, or peripheral cyanosis involving the hands, feet, and circumoral area, is a common finding in the newborn. It occurs because of sluggish blood flow in the feet and hands that results from limited development of the peripheral capillary circulation. Acrocyanosis usually resolves within the first few days of life but may reappear with cold stress.

Pallor is most commonly a sign of anemia, hypoxia, or poor peripheral perfusion that results from hypotension or infection. Meconium staining is caused by the passage of meconium in utero and usually requires at least 6 hours of meconium contact to stain the skin.

Jaundice, which occurs in 50 to 70 percent of newborns (Ziai et al., 1984), is a yellowing of the skin that develops because of the presence of indirect bilirubin in the blood. Bilirubin is normally processed by the liver and is eliminated in the urine and feces. In newborns, the body cannot eliminate bilirubin as fast as it is produced.

For visible staining of the skin and sclera, a bilirubin level of at least 5 mg/100 ml is required. The head-to-toe progression of jaundice over the body gives a crude estimate of the level of bilirubin.

Linea nigra is a line of increased pigmentation from the umbilicus to the genitals. This area of benign pigmentation may become less noticeable as the infant's skin darkens.

Mongolian spots are the pigmented lesions of the skin that are most frequently seen at birth. They are bluish-gray, irregular, bruise-like spots that are seen primarily over the sacrum and the buttocks but may extend over the back and shoulders (Fig. 32–7). They are caused by the presence of pigmented cells deep in the dermis. Most commonly seen in newborns with darkly pigmented skin, they are found in 90 percent of black, Asian, and Native American infants. They occur in 1 to 5 percent of white infants (Margileth, 1994). Although they look like bruises, they are harmless.

Lanugo is the fine downy hair that is most commonly seen over the back, shoulders, and facial areas of a premature newborn. It is shed at the seventh to eighth month of gestation and is one criterion used to estimate gestational age.

Milia are tiny epidermal cysts that develop in connection with the hair follicle and sebaceous gland. They are seen as small, white, pinhead-sized bumps that are scattered over the chin, cheeks, nose, and forehead of 25 to 40 percent of full-term babies (Avery et al., 1994). They spontaneously resolve within the first

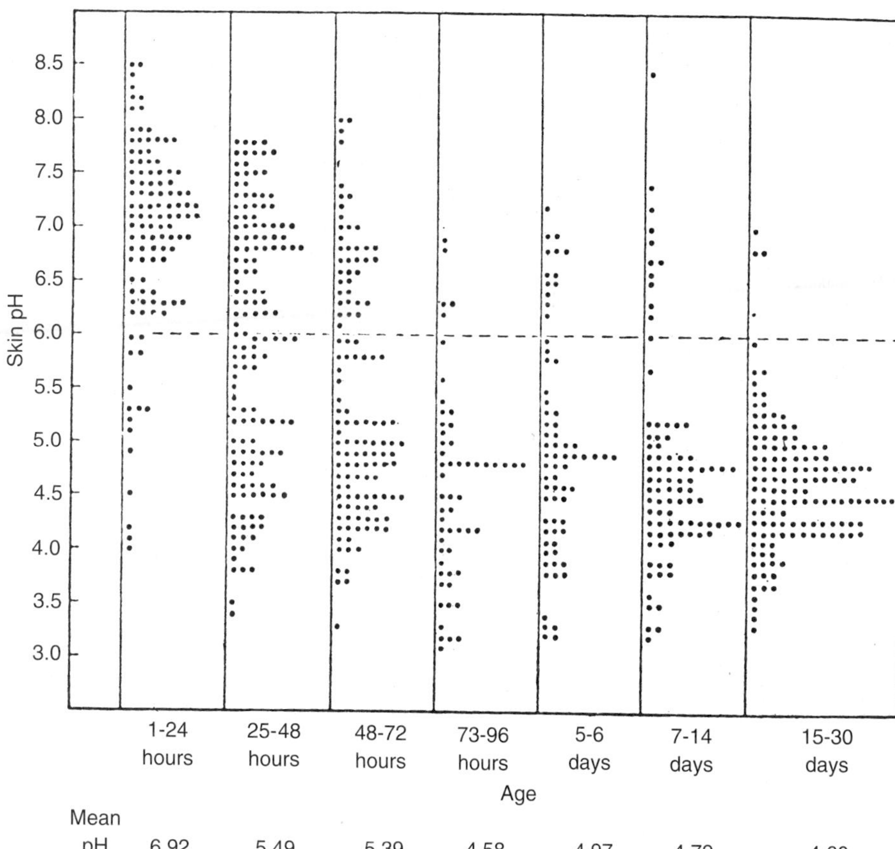

FIGURE 32–6. Patterns of skin pH from birth. (From Behrendt, H., & Green, M. [1971]. *Patterns of skin pH from birth through adolescence*. Springfield, IL: Charles C Thomas, Publishers. Reprinted with permission.)

month of life. Mothers should be instructed not to squeeze or prick these pimple-like spots. Milia can develop on the foreskin of infant boys; these are called epidermal inclusion cysts, or when they occur on the palate, they are called Epstein's pearls.

Miliaria is caused by the retention of sweat as a result of edema of the stratum corneum; this edema blocks eccrine pores, resulting in four types of miliaria: rubra (prickly heat), crystallina, pustulosa, and profunda (Arndt, 1978). Miliaria pustulosa and miliaria profunda are rarely seen in temperate climates. Miliaria rubra is commonly observed in infants exposed to excessive environmental temperatures with humidity. It appears as pink or white pimples with a little redness around them. They resolve when the infant is moved to cooler temperatures. Miliaria crystallina presents as clear, 1- to 2-mm superficial water blisters without inflammation (Margileth, 1994). The distribution and grouping of vesicles that contain no eosinophils help to differentiate them from erythema toxicum.

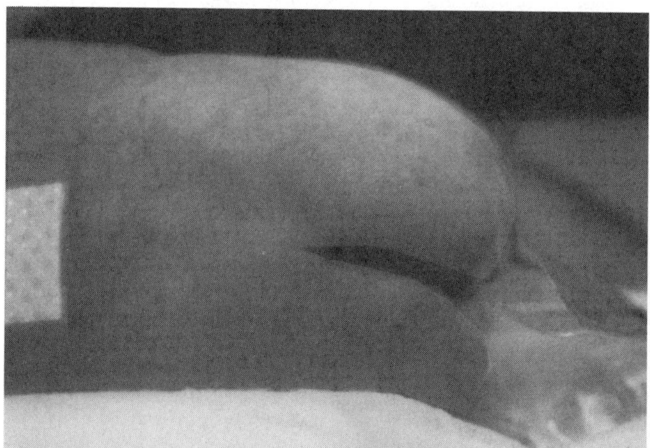

FIGURE 32–7. This mongolian spot, which is dark with an irregular border, is commonly located over the sacral area. (From Clark, D., & Thompson, J. [1986]. Dermatology of the newborn. Parts 1 and 2. In *Pathology of the neonate slide series* [Vol. III, No. 3]. Philadelphia: Wyeth-Ayerst Laboratories. Reprinted with permission.)

Harlequin color change is a dramatic but benign phenomenon in which the color on the dependent half of an infant in a side-lying position turns deep red while the upper half is pale. The color reverses when the infant is turned. Attributed to a temporary imbalance in the autonomic regulatory mechanism of the cutaneous vessels, this phenomenon is more common in low birth weight infants, whether well or sick (Solomon & Esterly, 1973).

Vernix caseosa is a grayish-white cheesy substance that is protective to the fetal skin while the fetus is in utero and helps the infant slide through the birth canal. The vernix covering diminishes as the fetus reaches term and is one determinant of gestational age.

Cutis marmorata, or mottling, is a normal physiologic vascular response to cool air. This generalized mottling reflects the infant's vasomotor instability (Esterly & Spraker, 1985). The marbling disappears with rewarming and is uncommon after several months of age. Mottling is often prominent in infants with Cornelia de Lange's syndrome and Down syndrome (Jones, 1988).

Erythema toxicum, the most common rash of newborns, usually occurs within 5 days of birth and affects 30 to 70 percent of term infants. It appears as small, firm, white, or pale yellow pustules with an erythematous margin (Fig. 32–8). It is most commonly found on the trunk, arms, and diaper area. It is less likely to occur on the face and is never found on the palms of the hands or the soles of the feet (Moschella & Hurley, 1985). Although the

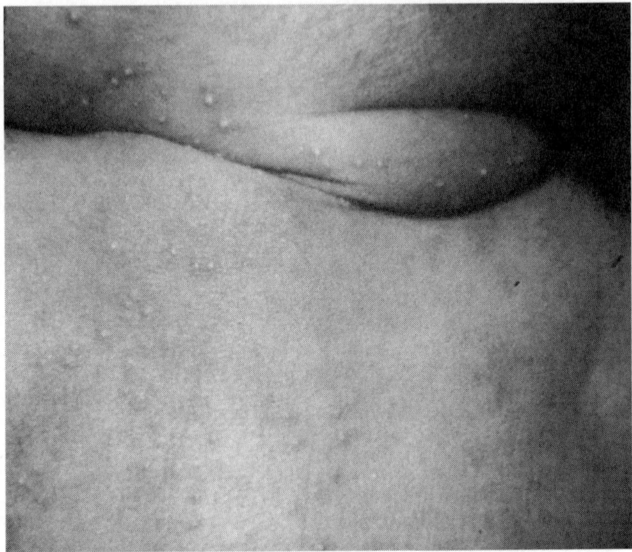

FIGURE 32–8. Erythema toxicum may not be present at birth; it most commonly occurs within the first 5 days of life and affects nearly 50 percent of full-term infants. The small pustules have an erythematous margin. (From Clark, D., & Thompson, J. [1986]. Dermatology of the newborn. Parts 1 and 2. In *Pathology of the neonate slide series* [Vol. III, No. 3]. Philadelphia: Wyeth-Ayerst Laboratories. Reprinted with permission.)

cause is unknown, it is believed to result from a sensitivity to the environment.

A smear and Wright's stain of the pustules reveal numerous infiltrates of eosinophils that are devoid of bacteria. The differential diagnosis includes transient neonatal pustular melanosis, candidiasis, staphylococcal pyoderma, and miliaria.

The cause of erythema toxicum is unknown, although a sensitivity to the environment is suspected. No treatment is necessary.

Acne neonatorum, or infantile acne, is caused by stimulation and dysfunction of the immature oil-producing (sebaceous) glands of the baby's face. The glands are stimulated by maternal hormones. Acne develops during the first or second postnatal month and is seen more frequently in boys.

Most infants require no treatment for the acne; daily cleansing with a mild soap and water is sufficient. Petrolatum, baby oils, and lotions should be avoided because the underlying problem is caused by the production of oily skin (Margileth, 1994).

Transient neonatal pustular melanosis is a lesion that is similar to miliaria but is present at birth, usually causing the infant to be unnecessarily isolated. It occurs most frequently on the face, the palms of the hands, and the soles of the feet. It is most commonly seen in black infants. If the lesions are ruptured, smeared on a slide, and stained, the contents are found to be amorphous debris. The lesion is neither infectious nor contagious. It is self-limiting and requires no treatment.

Sucking blisters that contain sterile, serous fluid may be seen on the thumb, index finger, or lip. Presumably, they are the result of vigorous sucking in utero and resolve without treatment.

Pigmentary Lesions

The causes of skin coloration can be seen in Table 32–3 (Nasemann et al., 1983).

Café au lait spots are irregularly shaped, oval lesions. Their color resembles coffee to which milk has been added. They should be noted on the newborn's initial physical examination, and if they are larger than 4 to 6 cm or if more than six are

TABLE 32–3 Materials That Contribute to Skin Color

	Exogenous	
Endogenous	***External***	***Internal***
Melanin Blood Bile products	Tattoos Other foreign objects (e.g., dirt from accidents) Silver nitrate, gentian violet (dermatologists and patients)	Acrotene—yellow Atabrine—yellow Clofazimine—reddish Silver, other metals—gray Phenothiazines—gray

From Nasemann, T., Sauerbrey, W., & Burgdorf, W. (1983). *Fundamentals of dermatology* (p. 19). New York: Springer-Verlag. Reprinted with permission.

present, a diagnosis of neurofibromatosis should be considered (Korones, 1986).

Hyperpigmentation that presents in a diffuse pattern is unusual in the newborn. When present, it may be caused by congenital Addison's disease, hepatic or biliary atresia, metabolic disease (Hartnup's disease, porphyria), nutritional disorders (pellagra, sprue), hereditary disorders (lentiginosis, melanism), or unknown causes (the bronze discoloration seen in Niemann-Pick disease). Hyperpigmentation of the labial folds with clitoral hypertrophy may result from the transplacental passage of androgens (Margileth, 1994).

Hypopigmentation presenting as a diffuse or localized loss of pigment in the neonate may be the result of metabolic (phenylketonuria), endocrine (Addison's), genetic (vitiligo, piebaldism, tuberous sclerosis, albinism), traumatic, or postinflammatory causes (Avery et al., 1994).

Piebaldism, or partial albinism, an autosomal dominant disorder that is present at birth, is easily detected in the dark-skinned infant. Off-white macules are seen on the scalp, widow's peak, and forehead, with extension to the base of the nose, trunk, and extremities. Differential diagnoses are Klein-Waardenburg syndrome, vitiligo, nevus anemicus, Addison's disease, and white macules of tuberous sclerosis. When illuminated with a Wood light, the amelanotic areas of piebaldism exhibit a brilliant whiteness (Margileth, 1994).

Albinism is a lack of pigmentation that may occur in any race. The incidence is approximately 1 in 5000 to 1 in 15,000 and is caused by an autosomal recessive gene (Margileth, 1994).

White leaf macules are the earliest cutaneous manifestations of tuberous sclerosis, an autosomal dominant neurocutaneous syndrome. They are variable in size and shape but most often resemble a mountain ash leaflet. They may be difficult to see in a newborn infant and may be more readily observed by examination with a Wood lamp, which heightens the contrast between the macule and normal skin. Normal infants occasionally have a single lesion, but the presence of one or more of these macules in an infant with neurologic problems strongly suggests the diagnosis of tuberous sclerosis. Skin biopsy is nondiagnostic. A careful family history, physical examination, and when appropriate, additional diagnostic studies are indicated in infants with these lesions (Ziai et al., 1984).

Lesions Related to the Birth Process

Caput succedaneum is a diffuse, generalized edema of the scalp that is caused by local pressure and trauma during labor. The borders are not well defined, and the swelling crosses suture lines (Kuller, 1990).

Cephalhematoma is a subperiosteal hemorrhage caused by the trauma of labor and delivery. The margins of the suture lines are clearly demarcated, and the swelling never crosses suture lines (Kuller, 1990).

Sclerema neonatorum may have the same cause and adipose tissue abnormality in the subcutaneous tissues as those noted in fat necrosis (Solomon & Esterly, 1973). However, sclerema more commonly affects the premature or debilitated infant. It is a diffuse hardening of the subcutaneous tissue that results in cold, nonpitting skin. Low environmental temperature alone can produce this injury. The extremities may be involved at first, but generalized involvement occurs within 3 to 4 days (Avery et al., 1994). Infants with this disorder are usually critically ill, but if they survive, the sclerematous changes rarely last beyond 2 weeks. Treatment is based on therapy for the underlying systemic disease, restoration of body temperature, and adequate nutrition.

Forceps marks are identified by their rounded contours and position. The bruised area should be checked for underlying tissue and nerve damage (Ziai et al., 1984).

Scalp lacerations can occur in many ways. A laceration can be caused by the placement of an internal monitoring lead or by the artificial rupture of membranes. A circular red or ecchymotic area may be caused by the use of a vacuum extractor. Any abraded area may serve as a portal of entry for infection (Korones, 1986); therefore, a scalp laceration should be carefully and continuously assessed for the presence of infection.

Subcutaneous fat necrosis is attributed to birth trauma, shock, asphyxia, and cold exposure. It is a sharply defined subcutaneous nodule that is produced by pressure against the bony pelvis or by the presence of forceps applied during the birth process (Korones, 1986). It is most commonly seen over the parietal bones and may have a deep reddish or purplish discoloration. The disease occurs in well infants and gradually reabsorbs over weeks to months if it is left alone. Residual atrophy or scarring is unusual (Ziai et al., 1984).

Internal fetal monitoring sites are at risk for infection, owing to the introduction of the maternal vaginal flora directly into the subcutaneous tissue of the fetus. Scalp abscesses caused by implantation of a fetal electrode are generally benign, self-limited occurrences. Rare instances have been reported of major complications, however, including significant areas of cellulitis, osteomyelitis, and sepsis (Freedman & Baltimore, 1990).

DERMATOLOGIC DISEASES

Diseases of the skin in newborns often present patterns that are different from the presentation of the same disease in adults. Therefore, a careful physical examination of the skin is necessary for an accurate dermatologic diagnosis to be made. All lesions should be described and their location and pattern noted.

Lesions can be classified as either primary or secondary. A primary lesion is the initial or principal lesion that is identified when the disease begins. A secondary lesion is one that ordinarily develops from a primary lesion. The classification of primary and secondary lesions according to site is listed in Table 32–4 (Nasemann et al., 1983).

A reduction in the newborn's cellular and humoral immune response easily explains their increased susceptibility to infectious diseases.

Terminology

Ecchymoses appear as black and blue bruises of varying sizes anywhere over the body. Primarily seen over the presenting part in a difficult vertex delivery or a vaginal breech delivery, ecchymosis is most frequently due to trauma associated with labor and delivery. It occurs more commonly in the fragile premature infant. This bruising, however, can be indicative of serious infection or bleeding disorders.

TABLE 32–4 Classification of Primary and Secondary Lesions According to Site

Primary Lesions*	Secondary Lesions†
Above the skin	
Papule	
Nodule	
Plaque	
Vesicle	
Bulla	
Pustule	Scale
Hive (wheal)	Crust
	Scar (hypertrophic)
In the skin (not palpable)	
Macule	Scar
Below the skin	Scar (atrophic)
	Erosion
	Excoriation
	Rhagades
	Ulcer
	Atrophy

*Note that all primary lesions rise above the surface, whereas many secondary lesions reflect skin loss.

†Occasionally secondary lesions present primarily; for example, some atrophies are primary.

From Nasemann, T., Sauerbrey, W., & Burgdorf, W. (1983). *Fundamentals of dermatology* (p. 16). New York: Springer-Verlag. Reprinted with permission.

Petechiae are pinpoint hemorrhagic areas, less than 1 mm, scattered over the upper trunk and face as a result of pressure during the descent and rotation of birth. Their incidence is increased when the umbilical cord has been around the neck or when the cervix clamps down after delivery of the head. They usually fade within 24 to 48 hours. If they continue to develop or are unusually numerous, a complete work-up for infection or bleeding disorders should be performed (Ziai et al., 1984).

Intracutaneous hemorrhage may be caused by thrombocytopenia, inherited disorders of coagulation, transient deficiency of vitamin K, disseminated intravascular coagulation, and trauma. Disseminated intravascular coagulation should be suspected in an acutely ill infant who has an intracutaneous hemorrhage. Thrombocytopenia and disorders of coagulation generally occur in infants who seem well otherwise. Thrombocytopenia should be suspected when the infant presents with general cutaneous petechiae. It frequently accompanies neonatal infections and is most commonly associated with the TORCH diseases (toxoplasmosis, rubella, cytomegalovirus, and herpes simplex) (Moschella & Hurley, 1985).

Ecchymoses and petechiae are purple discolorations caused by hemorrhage into the superficial skin layers. They do not disappear with blanching, because the blood is contained in the tissues.

Macules are nonpalpable, nonraised lesions less than 1 cm in diameter that are identified only by color change (Nasemann et al., 1983). They are seen in measles, rubella, scarlet fever, roseola, typhoid fever, and drug reactions.

Papules are superficial elevated solid lesions less than 1 cm in diameter. They are firm and not fluid filled (Nasemann et al., 1983). They may follow the macular stage in many eruptive diseases.

Vesicles are skin elevations that contain serous fluid (blisters). They are commonly seen with herpes simplex, insect bites, and poison ivy.

Pustules are localized accumulations of pus in or just beneath the epidermis. They are often centered around appendageal structures (e.g., hair follicles) and are usually caused by bacterial infections or skin abscesses. When a pustule breaks, the degree of crusting is more marked than occurs with the rupture of a vesicle (Nasemann et al., 1983).

Nodules are deep solid lesions larger than 1 cm in diameter. Nodules are similar to papules but are larger. Because of their size, they are more likely to have a dermal component than are papules.

Developmental Vascular Abnormalities

Angiomas or vascular nevi are common cutaneous congenital malformations seen during early infancy. Two major groups seen in children are the involuting and the noninvoluting vascular lesions, which may be flat (telangiectatic) or raised (hemangiomatous). The common involuting types include salmon patch, spider nevi (telangiectases), and strawberry and cavernous hemangiomas. Noninvoluting lesions, which are seen less commonly in newborns, are the port-wine stain and, rarely, the pyogenic granuloma (Margileth, 1994).

Pigmented Nevus

Pigmented nevi are benign tumors of the skin that contain nevus cells. Nevus cells can produce melanin and are closely related to melanocytes. In contrast to melanocytes, they tend to lie in groups or nests. Congenital pigmented nevi are different from pigmented nevi that arise later in that they are usually larger and more extensive. As the infant grows, the area becomes thicker and darker (Margileth, 1994).

Flat, junctional nevi are seen in about 1 percent of newborns. They are brown or black, and their size varies from one to several centimeters. When they are present at birth, they may be associated with neurofibromatosis, tuberous sclerosis, or bathing trunk nevi. Therapy is rarely needed, but lesions larger than 3 cm should be removed.

Giant Hairy Nevus

A giant hairy nevus is characterized by a pigmented, hairy, and softly infiltrated area. The color varies from pale brown to black. When the nevi are large, they tend to have a dermatomic distribution, and their location and size give them their name (e.g., bathing trunk nevus, vest nevus, shoulder stole nevus) (Fig. 32–9). On histologic examination of a biopsy specimen, the nevus cells are seen penetrating deeply into the dermis and subcutaneous tissue (Ziai et al., 1984).

When a giant nevus is situated on the head or neck, it may be associated with mental retardation, epilepsy, or hydrocephalus. Spina bifida or meningocele may occur when this nevus is present over the spine (Margileth, 1994). Other abnormalities that are sometimes associated with a giant pigmented nevus are clubfoot, hypertrophy or hypotrophy of the affected limb, and von Recklinghausen's disease (neurofibromatosis).

Besides being a cosmetic problem, the giant nevus is associated with a higher incidence of malignancy. Malignant melanomas develop in as many as 15 percent of these patients.

Collaborative Management

Management involves surgical excision of the entire lesion at or near puberty to prevent the development of skin cancer in the lesion (Rosen et al., 1983; Walton, 1971). Plastic surgical reconstruction may be needed if the excision is extensive.

Hemangiomas

Hemangioma of infancy is an angiomatous disorder characterized by the proliferation of capillary endothelium, with multilamination of the basement membrane and accumulation of mast cells, fibroblasts, and macrophages (Ezekowitz et al., 1992). Hemangioma is the most common tumor of infancy, occurring in up to 22 percent of preterm babies weighing less than 1000 and in 10 to 12 percent of white infants. Hemangiomas appear on 1 to 3 percent of infants at birth and develop on another 10 percent, usually within the first 3 to 4 weeks of life. When examined microscopically, hemangiomas are one of two kinds, capillary or cavernous (Korones, 1986). They most often appear in the skin as a single tumor, but multiple cutaneous lesions also occur, often with involvement of other organ systems.

The natural history of the hemangioma is characterized by their appearance during the first few weeks of life, rapid postnatal growth for 8 to 18 months (proliferative phase), followed by very slow but inevitable regression for the next 5 to 8 years (involutive phase). Hemangiomas completely resolve in more than 50 per-

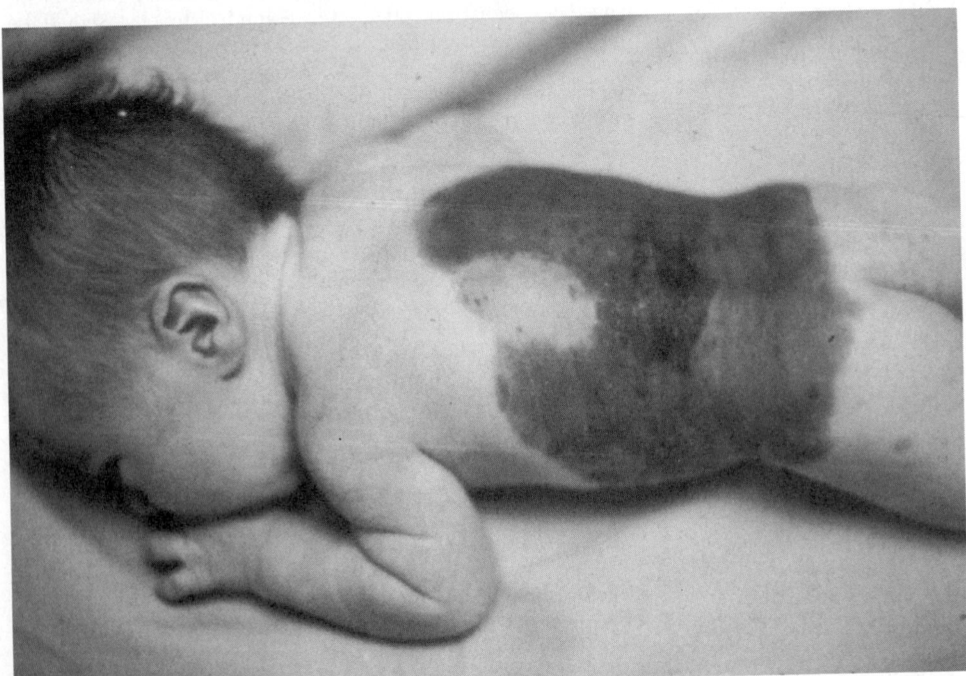

FIGURE 32–9. The giant pigmented hairy nevus of this infant involves the thorax, abdomen, and back and is commonly called a "bathing trunk" nevus. It is raised with fleshy elements and has a somewhat leathery texture. (From Clark, D., & Thompson, J. [1986]. Dermatology of the newborn. Parts 1 and 2. In *Pathology of the neonate slide series* [Vol. III, No. 4]. Philadelphia: Wyeth-Ayerst Laboratories. Reprinted with permission.)

cent of children by the age of 5 years of age and in more than 70 percent by 7 years of age, and continued improvement occurs in the remaining children until 10 to 12 years of age. The rate of regression does not seem to be related to the sex or age of the infant or to the site, size, or appearance of the hemangioma or the duration of the proliferative phase (Ezekowitz et al., 1992).

Strawberry hemangiomas consist of a dilated mass of capillaries in the dermal and subdermal layers that protrude above the skin surface. They are bright red, soft, compressible tumors that can appear anywhere on the body (Figs. 32–10 and 32–11). These marks require no treatment, and no permanent scars occur if the marks are left alone. However, when these lesions interfere with vital functions, such as vision, feeding, and respiration, intervention is required (Ziai et al., 1984).

Cavernous hemangiomas are more deeply situated in the skin than strawberry hemangiomas. They are bluish-red and feel spongy when touched.

Most hemangiomas are small, harmless birthmarks that involute to leave either normal or slightly blemished skin. However, even a small hemangioma can obstruct the airway or impair vision. A large hemangioma in the liver or an extensive cutaneous hemangioma can divert a considerable volume of blood through its extensive labyrinth of capillaries and produce high-output heart failure. The increased capillary endothelial surface that characterizes a giant hemangioma can also trap platelets and may cause thrombocytopenic coagulopathy (Kasabach-Merritt syndrome) (Ezekowitz et al., 1992).

A few hemangiomas grow to an alarming size or proliferate simultaneously in several organs, causing life-endangering conditions, such as soft tissue destruction, deformation or obstruction of vital structures, serious bleeding, congestive heart failure, and sepsis (Rosen et al., 1983; Morad et al., 1993). Large lesions can expand the skin, and even after they regress, they can result in excess slack skin, pigment changes, and a fibrofatty residuum (Enjolras et al., 1990).

In general, visceral hemangiomas denote a poor prognosis (Enjolras et al., 1990). Death is usually caused by heart failure. Laryngeal hemangiomas are the most common visceral vascular manifestation. Liver and gastrointestinal hemangiomas are extremely rare. Flow through extensive hemangiomas increases the total blood volume, causes hemodeviation, and disturbs the hemodynamic equilibrium. The hyperdynamic cardiovascular state of the hemangiomas decreases or shunts blood away from other tissues, resulting in hypoperfusion of other tissues. This hypoperfusion may cause brain hypoxia and acidosis, predisposing to the seizures seen in some cases. Close surveillance of the cardiovascular system is necessary to determine the proper time to begin digitalization (Enjolras et al., 1990).

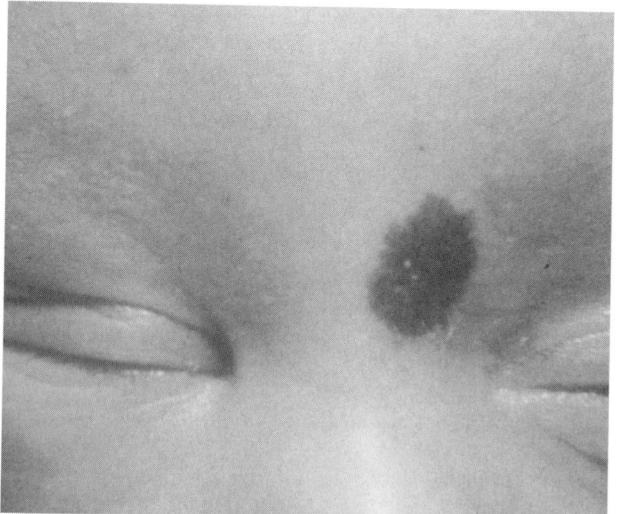

FIGURE 32–10. This photograph shows the early hemangioma of a premature infant. The infant was 28 weeks' gestation and had no hemangioma at birth. Approximately 5 weeks after birth, the first area of discoloration appeared. (From Clark, D., & Thompson, J. [1986]. Dermatology of the newborn. Parts 1 and 2. In *Pathology of the neonate slide series* [Vol. III, No. 3]. Philadelphia: Wyeth-Ayerst Laboratories. Reprinted with permission.)

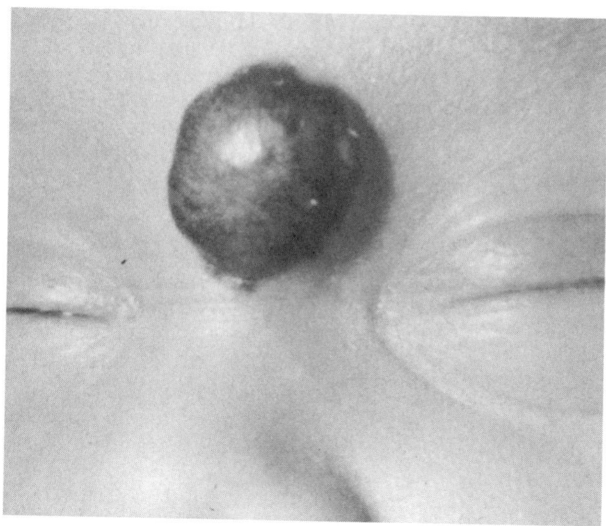

FIGURE 32–11. The same infant as in Figure 32–10. One month later, the hemangioma has grown considerably. The irregular surface with sharp demarcation is typical of strawberry hemangioma. This eventually enlarged to approximately twice the size as it appears in this photograph and then began to resolve. (From Clark, D., & Thompson, J. [1986]. Dermatology of the newborn. Parts 1 and 2. In *Pathology of the neonate slide series* [Vol. III, No. 3]. Philadelphia: Wyeth-Ayerst Laboratories. Reprinted with permission.)

Collaborative Management

Management of both strawberry and cavernous hemangiomas consists of a detailed history; close scrutiny of the lesion or lesions, including three-dimensional measurements; and evaluation of the growth pattern of the hemangioma. As involution progresses, the color gradually changes from grayish-pink to white or pink, and the tension of the lesion decreases. Ulcerated hemangiomas should be treated with topical antibiotics to prevent infection (Rosen et al., 1983).

While the cutaneous lesions are being monitored, the infant's clinical course and physical development must be closely observed for poor growth, altered cry, stridor, dyspnea, cyanosis, feeding difficulties, or swallowing impairment. If any abnormal sign or symptoms appear, such as tachycardia, heart murmur, hepatomegaly, and bruit heard over the liver, the infant should be examined for evidence of heart failure. Ultrasonography, echocardiography, and computed tomography may be needed (Enjolras et al., 1990).

In general, management consists of planned neglect, which is essential in avoiding disfiguring scars. Complications of therapy may be significant, but residual scarring after complete involution is uncommon. Hemangiomas located in exposed areas often cause great parental anxiety, which increases as the hemangioma grows. This anxiety often puts pressure on the physician to do something. However, the hemangioma should be left to regress spontaneously, and preconceived notions about birthmarks should be discussed with the family.

Enjolras and associates (1990) reviewed 25 infants with

"alarming hemangiomas"—a term used to categorize lesions that impair vital functions or cause life-threatening complications. A vascular mark was present at birth in 68 percent of these infants. Visceral hemangiomas are associated with cervicocephalic hemangiomas or with small hemangiomas scattered over the body. About a third of these life-threatening hemangiomas respond to treatment with corticosteroids, but for the others, no safe and effective treatment exists. The mortality rate can be as high as 54 percent for life-threatening visceral or hepatic hemangiomas and may be up to 30 to 40 percent with platelet-consumptive coagulopathy, despite the administration of steroids (Ezekowitz et al., 1992).

High-dose corticosteroid therapy is the primary means of controlling hemangiomas pharmacologically. These agents inhibit the activators of fibrinolysis in vessel walls, decrease plasminogen activator content of endothelium, and increase sensitivity to vasoactive amines, causing constriction of arterioles (Morad et al., 1993). When steroids fail, less conventional modalities, such as embolization, operative excision, and radiotherapy, are used.

Ezekowitz and colleagues (1992) evaluated the effects of daily subcutaneous injections of interferon alfa-2a (≦3 million units per square meter of body surface area) in 20 neonates and infants with life-threatening or vision-threatening hemangiomas that failed to respond to corticosteroid therapy. Their mechanisms of action includes inhibition of motility and proliferation of endothelial cells and interference with new capillary vessel formation, thereby preventing platelet trapping (Morad et al., 1993). These daily injections seemed to reduce the local and systemic complications and appeared to shorten the length of time to involution in 18 of the 20 neonates. Sustained therapy for 9 to 14 months appeared to be desirable because earlier withdrawal was followed by regrowth of the lesion that was halted and reversed by reintroduction of the drug. Interferon alfa therapy was not accompanied by toxic effects other than fever, and this occurred in all patients for the first week and responded to treatment with acetaminophen.

Morad and associates (1993) reported their limited use of tranexamic acid in the treatment of giant hemangiomas in three newborns. Tranexamic acid is a fibrinolytic inhibitor that exerts its effect through inhibition of plasminogen activator and plasmin and through inhibition of tumor vessel proliferation. One of the infants had a measurable response in the size of the hemangioma and the extent of the coagulopathy. The other two had progression of their lesions. It appears that tranexamic acid is an additional agent for treatment of giant hemangiomas, but its efficacy is limited. Further study of this treatment is needed to determine which patients may respond best.

Port-Wine Stain

Port-wine stain is a capillary angioma consisting of dilated and congested capillaries lying directly beneath the epidermis. It appears in approximately 3 of 1000 newborns. This birthmark appears pink at birth but gradually darkens to purple. Most commonly found on the face and neck, it is a permanent developmental defect. Although a port-wine stain is primarily a cosmetic problem, it is occasionally an indicator of a multisystem disorder, such as the Sturge-Weber syndrome or the Klippel-Trenaunay-Weber syndrome. The presence of convulsions, mental retardation, hemiplegia, or intracortical calcification suggests the presence of Sturge-Weber syndrome (Solomon & Esterly, 1973). An ophthalmologic examination is extremely important in these infants. A water-repellent cosmetic cream (e.g., Covermark, Retouch) effectively covers the mark. Because of the inability to properly match the skin color of the normal skin and the possibility of scar formation, tattooing cannot be recommended. Plastic surgical repair may be necessary in an older child because of the development of a thickened nodular surface. Laser beam therapy appears to be effective, and the best results are achieved when the child is near puberty (Apfelberg et al., 1978; Cosman, 1980).

Blistering Diseases

Epidermolysis Bullosa

Epidermolysis bullosa is a group of rare congenital blistering disorders, all of which are inherited (Ziai et al., 1984). They are considered mechanobullous diseases, meaning that trauma to, or friction on, the skin induces blister formation. The different varieties of epidermolysis bullosa are distinguished by the level of the skin at which the blister forms (Rosen et al., 1983). Pathologically, the disease is characterized by blister formation resembling that of second-degree burns after slight or innocuous trauma (Artnak et al., 1981). The underlying defect appears to be a lack of cellular glue in squamous epithelium, which is responsible for the maintenance of cellular integrity. Diagnostic studies should include a skin biopsy for light and electron microscopy.

This disease has been classified into two major subgroups: nonscarring and scarring epidermolysis bullosa (Watson, 1978). Four of the subtypes may occur at birth or in early infancy (Table 32–5) (Margileth, 1994). Nonscarring epidermolysis bullosa presents in two forms: epidermolysis bullosa letalis (Herlitz's disease), which is extremely rare, and epidermolysis bullosa simplex (EBS), which is common by comparison.

Epidermolysis bullosa simplex is the mildest form of epidermolysis bullosa. The lesions occur at the basal layer of epidermis and do not lead to scarring and hyperkeratosis. Usually present at birth, the vesicles and bullae appear over the joints and the bony protuberances and at sites subjected to repeated trauma (Hymes, 1983). The differential diagnosis may be aided by the absence of milia, which are commonly seen in the dystrophic types of epidermolysis bullosa.

In epidermolysis bullosa letalis, a rare autosomal recessive type of epidermolysis bullosa, severe generalized blistering is present at birth. Subsequent extensive denudation may be fatal in a few days to a few months, owing to fluid loss or sepsis. Histopathologically, a separation occurs between the plasma membrane of the basal cells and the basal lamina (Hymes, 1983).

Mild symptoms of dominant epidermolysis bullosa dystrophica may appear in early infancy but are not as severe as in the recessive forms, owing to the presence of a normal gene, which seems to reduce the severity of its manifestation. Moderately severe blisters are seen on the distal extremities and bony protuberances (Fig. 32–12). Some scar formation occurs, and the nails may be mildly dystrophic. Atrophy may occur with healing. Nikolsky's sign (the external skin layer is easily rubbed off by slight friction or injury) is present. Milia, due to a functional disorder of the sweat glands, are found on the rims of the ears, the dorsa of the hands, and the extensor surfaces of the arms and legs. The oral, anal, and esophageal mucosae are frequently involved. Some of the associated complications are dwarfism,

TABLE 32–5 Epidermolysis Bullosa

Nonscarring Types	
Epidermolysis bullosa simplex	Autosomal dominant
Epidermolysis bullosa letalis (junctional bullous)	Autosomal recessive
Scarring: Dermolytic Bullous Dermatosis	
Dominant dystrophic	Autosomal dominant
Recessive (polydysplastic) dystrophic	Autosomal recessive

From Margileth, A. (1987). Dermatologic conditions. In G. Avery (Ed.), *Neonatology: Pathophysiology and management of the newborn* (3rd ed., pp. 1230–1273). Philadelphia: J. B. Lippincott Co. Reprinted with permission.

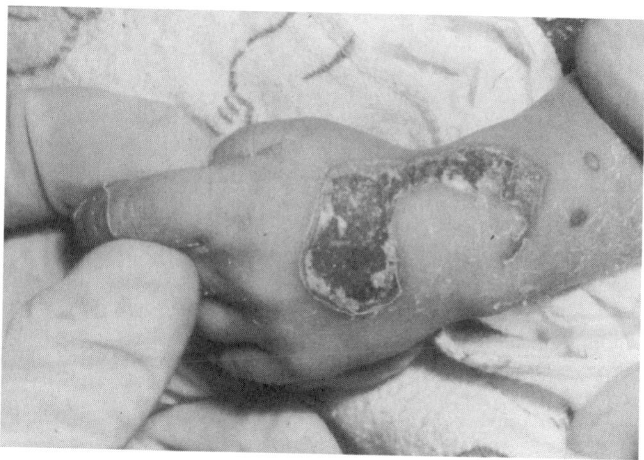

FIGURE 32–12. This photograph of epidermolysis bullosa shows the scaling broken bullae with underlying erythroderma. (From Clark, D., & Thompson, J. [1986]. Dermatology of the newborn. Parts 1 and 2. In *Pathology of the neonate slide series* [Vol. III, No. 4]. Philadelphia: Wyeth-Ayerst Laboratories. Reprinted with permission.)

pseudosyndactylism, contractures, claw-like hands, partial scalp alopecia, and absence of body hair (Hymes, 1983).

Recessive epidermolysis bullosa dystrophica is the most severe form of the disease. Generalized cutaneous and mucosal blistering begins at birth. Subsequent esophageal strictures result in anemia and growth retardation. The digits of the hands and feet become fused from scarring and develop claw-like deformities. The skin is atrophic and easily blistered, with frequent flexion contractures from scarring. The lesions appear to lie at the level of the basement membrane, and the epidermis is thickened and flat with hyperkeratosis (Artnak et al., 1981).

Complications include infections and hemolytic, nutritional, orthopedic, gastrointestinal, and psychiatric sequelae (Artnak et al., 1981). These vary, depending on the severity of the disease.

Collaborative Management

Nursing care centers around three main issues: (1) skin breakdown, (2) contractures, and (3) dysphagia.

Skin breakdown occurs after the rupture of bullae, reflecting the decrease in skin collagen. Preventive measures are directed toward alleviating skin excoriation. Clean, soft dressings may be helpful over bony pressure points. For secondary infection prevention, bacitracin ointment should be used after surgical soap cleansing is performed, two or three times daily. The use of emollients helps to avoid dry skin (Avery et al., 1994). Sterile gloves should be used for the application of all topical agents. Insensible water loss may be diminished through the use of cool, humidified air. Accurate intake and output are essential for fluid administration calculations.

From birth to 6 months of age, the environment is easy to control through the use of sheepskin, loose-fitting clothes, and mittens for the infant's hands and feet. Cloth diapers softened with fabric softener are preferred over rougher, disposable diapers. Any person handling the infant should avoid wearing jewelry.

Protection of the infant becomes more difficult once the infant is mobile. The infant should always wear long pants, and foam rubber pads sewn into the knees help avoid trauma during crawling.

Contractures may form quickly as scarring begins to occur. The pathologic increase in elastic skin fiber adds to this process (Hymes, 1983). Gentle range-of-motion exercises lessen contracture formation.

Dysphagia can occur from facial and pharyngeal scarring, which is secondary to erosions on the buccal mucosa, tongue, palate, esophagus, and pharynx (Hymes, 1983). Feedings should be performed slowly and carefully to avoid aspiration and to maintain adequate nutrition. The metabolic needs of these infants are high, owing to the continuous sloughing of epithelium, which results in large protein, fluid, and electrolyte losses (Artnak et al., 1981). Adding additional puncture holes to a nipple may help prevent oral mucosal trauma. If oral ulcerations do occur, several weeks of hyperalimentation and high-dose steroid therapy are instituted. Gavage feedings are discouraged, owing to the possibility of trauma.

It is essential that the family receive genetic counseling regarding the inheritance pattern associated with epidermolysis bullosa; a negative family history does not exclude its occurrence.

Infections of the Skin

Microbial colonization of the skin of the newborn begins immediately after birth. In general, the skin flora exist and grow in a state of equilibrium that protects against pathogenic organisms (American Academy of Pediatrics, 1974). The most common organisms found on the surface of the skin are coagulase-negative staphylococci. However, other microorganisms can also be found on the skin surface, including *Staphylococcus aureus*, diphtheroids, streptococci, and coliform bacteria; these are also considered to be part of the skin flora unless a specific skin infection is manifested by cutaneous lesions or other alterations in skin integrity. Skin infections and skin manifestations of systemic infection can be of bacterial, viral, or fungal origin. In this section, the various skin infections from each type of microorganism are discussed, along with implications for nursing care.

Bacterial

Staphylococcus aureus

Infections resulting from *S. aureus* are seen in newborns and can result in two types of skin lesions. Bullous impetigo of the newborn involves blisters that originate in the stratum corneum and are filled with clear or straw-colored fluid. These lesions appear after the first few days after delivery. There may be few or many blisters, dispersed widely over all areas of the body, that rupture easily, leaving denuded areas of skin. *S. aureus* is most commonly cultured, but other bacteria, such as group A streptococci and beta-hemolytic streptococci, are sometimes seen.

Collaborative Management

Medical and nursing management is focused on treatment of the affected infant and on prevention of the spread of infection to other infants because this condition is highly contagious. The treatment consists of either cleansing the lesions with antimicrobial solutions three or four times a day (Margileth, 1994) or applying saline or sterile water compresses, followed by antimicrobial ointment (Esterly & Solomon, 1995). Antibiotics may be administered if systemic infection is suspected. Fluid and electrolyte monitoring is necessary if the denuded areas cover a large surface or if the infant is of low birth weight. Isolation of the affected infant is necessary to prevent the spread of the infection throughout the nursery.

Scalded Skin Syndrome

S. aureus can also result in a severe bullous eruption called scalded skin syndrome. Initially, the infant's skin is bright red, resembling a scald, followed by the formation of large flaccid blisters that quickly progress to large sheets of skin being shed (Fig. 32–13). The entire epidermis is frequently shed during the course of this disease. The mechanism for this severe injury involves the production of an endotoxin, called exfoliatin, that causes the skin manifestations. Usually, the skin lesions do not culture positive for the responsible organism, so culturing the nasopharynx, blood, conjunctiva, and normal skin is recommended to recover the organism for appropriate sensitivity assessment (Esterly & Solomon, 1995).

Collaborative Management

Medical and nursing management also involves administration of the appropriate antibiotic regimen and supportive measures in terms of fluid and electrolytic replacement, prevention of secondary infection through the damaged epidermis, and comfort. Applying local antibiotic solutions or ointments is generally not necessary; keeping open skin areas clean and dry promotes healing and prevents secondary infection. The infant may be more comfortable in an incubator rather than in a radiant warmer; this is because the incubator is a convective heat source that does not have a direct cutaneous effect, whereas the radiant heat source heats directly through the skin. In addition, the radiant heat source may further increase the degree of insensible water loss through the damaged epidermis. Usually, a flaking process is observed on the skin during the healing process.

Listeria monocytogenes

Another bacterial skin disorder is listeriosis, caused by *L. monocytogenes*. This organism, which can cause severe systemic disease, can also result in a disseminated miliary granulomatosis in neonates (Esterly & Solomon, 1995). In some cases, miliary abscesses can occur; occasionally, more generalized erythema or petechiae may be present. Systemic listeriosis is a very severe infection, causing blood hemolysis and a high mortality rate. Prompt recognition and treatment with intravenous penicillin or ampicillin are indicated for the best prognosis. No direct skin therapy has been described as being necessary in this disease.

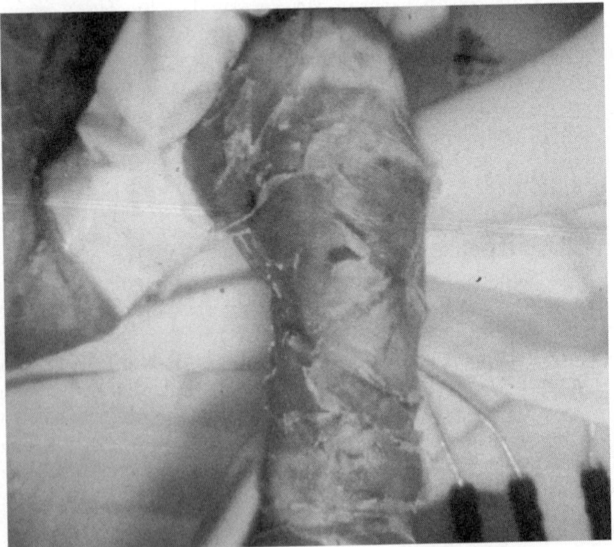

FIGURE 32–13. The peeling, scaling skin of this premature infant had an acute onset at approximately 2 weeks of age. This is the scalded skin syndrome resulting from *Staphylococcus aureus*. (From Clark, D., & Thompson, J. [1986]. Dermatology of the newborn. Parts 1 and 2. In *Pathology of the neonate slide series* [Vol. III, No. 4]. Philadelphia: Wyeth-Ayerst Laboratories. Reprinted with permission.)

Syphilis

Congenital syphilis is another bacterial infection that has skin manifestations. If the infant with congenital syphilis is not treated after birth, a maculopapular or bullous skin eruption develops between 2 and 6 weeks of age (Margileth, 1994). Sometimes, the bullous lesions may be observed at birth on the palms or the soles, signifying the presence of more severe disease. Fluid contained in the blisters contains spirochetes.

The lesions most commonly seen in congenital syphilis are copper-colored and maculopapular and are located on the soles and palms. In addition, open lesions may be present around the mouth, anus, or genitals, and a highly contagious nasal discharge is occasionally seen. If the syphilis remains untreated, the lesions regress in 1 to 3 months, leaving areas on the skin with either hyperpigmentation or hypopigmentation.

Collaborative Management

Medical and nursing management for the infant with congenital syphilis involves prompt, consistent administration of penicillin, usually a 10-day course. Titers are obtained over the next year at 3-month intervals, and a negative serologic finding is expected at 1 year. Care of the skin lesions is primarily directed toward preventing the spread of infection during the active phase of the illness, especially when bullous lesions or open areas are apparent. No direct topical therapies have been advocated in the literature.

Viral

Some of the viral infections that may result in cutaneous manifestations include several of the herpes conditions, cytomegalovirus, and rubella. Toxoplasmosis, which has cutaneous manifestations and is caused by a parasite, is also discussed in this section.

Herpes Simplex

Herpesvirus is a common concern in neonatal nurseries because certain types of herpes infection can be transmitted from infant to infant and are potentially serious pathogens. Herpes simplex is one of the most serious viral infections that affects newborns. Vesicles that occur on the skin with this disease vary; a few faint scars may be present, or actual vesicle formations may be present with either one large swelling or discrete groups of vesicles (Fig. 32–14). Vesicles may recede, then recur over months.

Collaborative Management

Medical and nursing management is centered primarily on early recognition and treatment with antiviral medication. The prognosis of systemic herpes simplex is extremely poor if encephalitis develops, with either death or severe mental retardation being the sequela. An important consideration in the care of infants with known or suspected herpes simplex infection is isolation from other patients in order to prevent transmission.

Varicella-zoster

Another viral infection with manifestation in the skin is varicella-zoster. Varicella-zoster infection is rare, but when it occurs in the first 10 days of life, it is generally thought to have been acquired in utero. The vesicular eruptions are the same as those in chickenpox acquired at any age. A mortality of 20 percent is associated with varicella infection in newborns, and certainly this infection poses a significant risk for the immunocompromised infants in premature and intensive care nurseries. No systemic medication or topical treatment is required for these lesions.

Occasionally scarring can occur. Strict isolation is absolutely necessary to protect other infants from exposure because this virus is airborne. Passive immunization of infants exposed to the affected infant may also be necessary.

Toxoplasmosis

Toxoplasmosis, which is caused by an intracellular parasite (*Toxoplasma gondii*), can be transmitted transplacentally and can result in systemic infection. Some infants may have a generalized maculopapular rash as well as hepatosplenomegaly, jaundice, fever, and anemia. The rash may progress to desquamation and hypopigmentation in very severe cases. Direct topical therapy is not reported to be necessary or efficacious; systemic therapy may be considered.

Cytomegalovirus and Rubella

Both cytomegalovirus and rubella have symptoms that are manifested in the skin. Petechial lesions can occur with both infections. These are the result of thrombocytopenia and usually disappear in 2 to 6 weeks. In severe rubella infection, and very rarely in cytomegalovirus, bluish-red papules that are 2 to 8 mm in diameter can occur on the head, trunk, and extremities (Fig. 32–15). This so-called blueberry muffin syndrome is the result of erythropoiesis in the dermis and usually subsides in 2 to 3 weeks. Neither of these lesions requires topical therapy. (For a complete discussion of infections, see Chapter 27, Assessment and Management of Immunologic Dysfunction.)

Fungal

Candida albicans infection is the primary fungal infection with cutaneous manifestations, although other strains, such as *Malassezia furfur*, can also potentially colonize the skin of term and preterm newborns, particularly those who are hospitalized in an intensive care nursery. Manifestations of infection with *Candida* species can range from diaper dermatitis or other localized skin or mucous membrane eruptions to systemic candidemia resulting in significant morbidity and mortality. *Candida* is not normally found in the skin flora of the newborn. The gastrointestinal system is the primary reservoir, but the skin may also be colonized during passage through a colonized vaginal canal. The incidence of *Candida* colonization is also increased with the frequent use of broad-spectrum antibiotics that alter normal skin flora in infants after delivery.

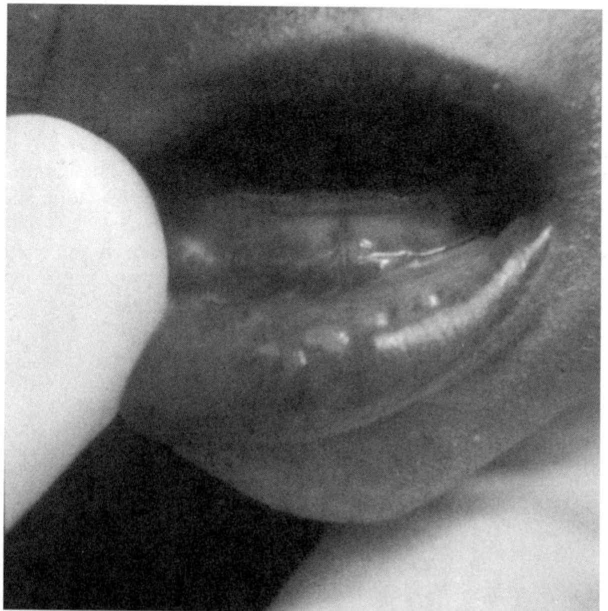

FIGURE 32–14. Herpes type II was cultured from these mucosal vesicles from an infant with localized infection. (From Clark, D. [1986]. Perinatal infections. In *Pathology of the neonate slide series* [Vol. I, No. 2]. Philadelphia: Wyeth-Ayerst Laboratories. Reprinted with permission.)

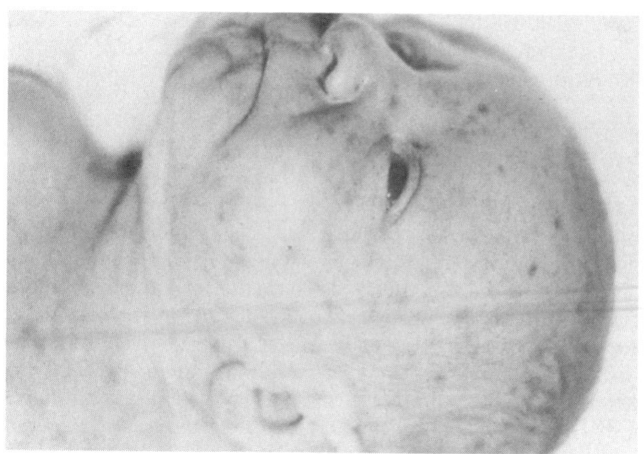

FIGURE 32–15. This is an example of the "blueberry muffin" syndrome, seen in an infant with congenital cytomegalovirus infection. The infant has multiple petechiae and purpura resulting from thrombocytopenia in this systemic infection. (From Clark, D., & Thompson, J. [1986]. Dermatology of the newborn. Parts 1 and 2. In *Pathology of the neonate slide series* [Vol. III, No. 4]. Philadelphia: Wyeth-Ayerst Laboratories. Reprinted with permission.)

In a recent study of 18 infants treated for systemic candidiasis, Baley and Silverman (1988) identified cutaneous involvement in most of the infants. Two different dermatologic conditions were identified. Eight infants had a diffuse burn-like dermatitis affecting large areas on the lower back, buttocks, chest, and abdomen; in a few infants, the axilla and groin were affected. Scaling followed the erythematous macular patches, and in one infant, severe desquamation developed that was similar to that seen in staphylococcal scalded skin syndrome. These infants did not have the satellite papules and pustules normally seen with *Candida* diaper dermatitis. The onset of the generalized rash occurred within the first 3 days of life in six infants and later in the others.

A monilial diaper rash was the other dermatologic condition seen by these investigators. This rash consisted of a red, scaling dermatitis in the groin, and the rash spread to other body parts. Only one infant in this study had systemic candidiasis without cutaneous manifestations.

Collaborative Management

Medical and nursing management of infants with systemic or local *Candida* infection involves topical therapy with antifungal creams and systemic antifungal medications if evidence of systemic infection exists. Yeast is sometimes difficult to culture; techniques include obtaining urine to look for hyphae or budding yeast, blood cultures, and skin scrapings prepared with potassium hydroxide and examined for pseudohyphae. Nursing observation in low birth weight infants for evidence of the diffuse burn-like dermatitis or a spreading monilial diaper rash is essential and may expedite the initiation of therapy for systemic candidiasis.

Scaling Disorders

A scaly appearance in the skin of a newborn can have a range of causes, from relatively benign to long term and potentially life-threatening. In this section, scaly skin due to postmaturity, essential fatty acid deficiency, congenital ichthyosis, and eczema is discussed, and areas of nursing management are determined.

Postmaturity

Many term infants born between 40 and 42 weeks' gestation experience a period of shedding or desquamation that is considered to be a normal physiologic process. Postmature infants born after 42 weeks' gestation may also have this appearance, but other characteristics are different. The postmature infant may have a lean appearance, with little subcutaneous fat; the weight is low in relationship to length. The skin resembles parchment paper and may literally peel off in sheets (Fig. 32–16). There may be staining of the fingernails with meconium, long fingernails, and long hair.

Skin care is not the major problem, nor is it the focus of medical or nursing management. Eventually, the skin underneath the peeling layers predominates; even during the period of desquamation, the skin functions well as a barrier because these infants have all the layers of stratum corneum of a term infant or adult. Aside from bathing with a mild soap initially, no lubrication is necessary during the period of desquamation. More careful attention is paid to the more compelling problems associated with postmaturity, such as hypoglycemia and meconium aspiration.

Essential Fatty Acid Deficiency

In some newborns who are unable to receive an adequate diet because of other illnesses or surgical condition, scaly dry skin may signify the development of essential fatty acid deficiency syndrome. Infants may be more prone to the development of this syndrome, especially if they are premature or postmature, owing to the decreased fat stores available.

The skin appearance in essential fatty acid deficiency includes a superficial scaling and, in some cases, desquamation. Later presentation may involve oozing and irritation in the neck, groin, or perianal region.

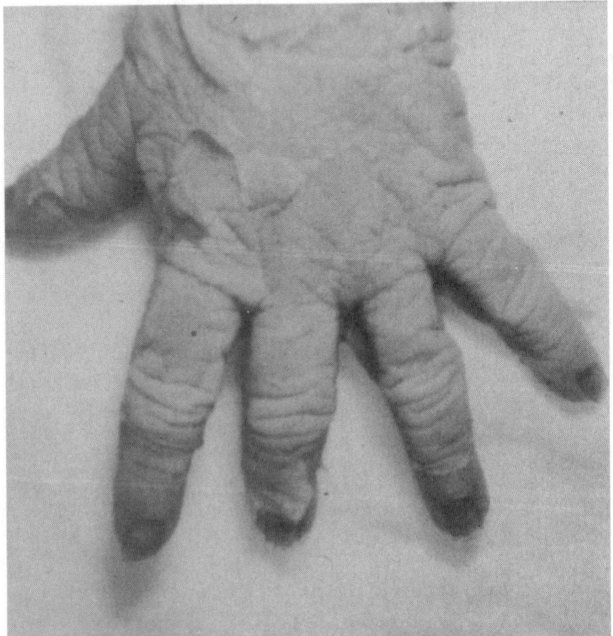

FIGURE 32–16. This is an example of a hand of a postmature infant. Notice the peeling of the skin, a common finding after 40 weeks' gestation.

This syndrome is sometimes confused with other conditions that cause scaling or other skin disruptions, including ichthyosis, acrodermatitis enteropathica, and candidal infection. Laboratory findings that confirm this diagnosis are decreased serum essential fatty acid levels, possibly in conjunction with thrombocytopenia and impaired platelet aggregation, because essential fatty acids are necessary to ensure platelet function (Friedman, 1980).

Collaborative Management

Medical and nursing management consists of replacement of essential fatty acids through the administration of intravenous lipid solutions or diet. Human breast milk and most infant formulas contain more than adequate amounts of essential fatty acids. However, if the gastrointestinal system is not functioning well in the digestion and absorption of nutrients, intravenous therapy is required.

Once skin symptoms are present, administration of intravenous lipid solution can reverse the process in 1 to 2 weeks. Dietary replacement takes longer and is effective only in the presence of healthy gastrointestinal function. Another useful adjunct to therapy is the topical administration of sunflower seed oil (which is rich in linoleic acid), which is then absorbed transdermally and raises serum levels of essential fatty acids over time.

Prevention of essential fatty acid deficiency is possible and should be the goal. Early administration of intravenous lipid solutions in the first weeks of life in a dose as low as 0.5 g/kg/day can prevent the development of essential fatty acid deficiency.

Ichthyosis

The most serious cause of scaly skin in the newborn is ichthyosis dermatosis. Four major types of ichthyosis exist: (1) X-linked ichthyosis, (2) lamellar ichthyosis, and (3) bullous congenital ichthyosiform erythroderma, which are present at birth, and (4) ichthyosis vulgaris, which usually appears after the third month of life. Terms commonly used to describe infants with ichthyosis may include harlequin fetus and collodion baby, but these terms do not define which form of ichthyosis is present.

In the X-linked type of ichthyosis, males are affected. Some female heterozygotes may exhibit mild scaling of the arms and lower extremities. Affected male newborns have large yellow or brown plaques that cover the whole body except the palms, soles, and midface and over joints. At birth, some affected males may appear scaly, whereas others are often called collodion babies.

Lamellar ichthyosis, formerly called nonbullous congenital ichthyosiform erythroderma, is an autosomal recessive disorder. Initially, affected newborns may have a bright red appearance, which rapidly progresses to desquamation; rarely is a collodion baby appearance present at birth. Later, scales develop that are yellow to brown and that may eventually become thick, horny plates. Although the prognosis is usually good, infants who are severely affected, the so-called harlequin fetuses, may die of sepsis or require extensive plastic surgery (Fig. 32–17).

In bullous congenital ichthyosiform erythroderma, autosomal dominance is the mode of heredity, so several family members may be affected. Large bullae are initially seen, as well as erythema and dry scaly skin; the blistering that recurs throughout childhood differentiates this form from the lamellar type. Extensive denuded areas of the skin can present a problem in the newborn as the blisters burst because secondary infections with *Streptococcus* or *Staphylococcus* can occur and are life-threatening.

Collaborative Management

Medical and nursing management of all forms of ichthyosis involves the continual use of topical therapies and prescription bathing techniques and the prevention of infection. Bathing may be necessary as often as twice daily with a water-dispersible bath

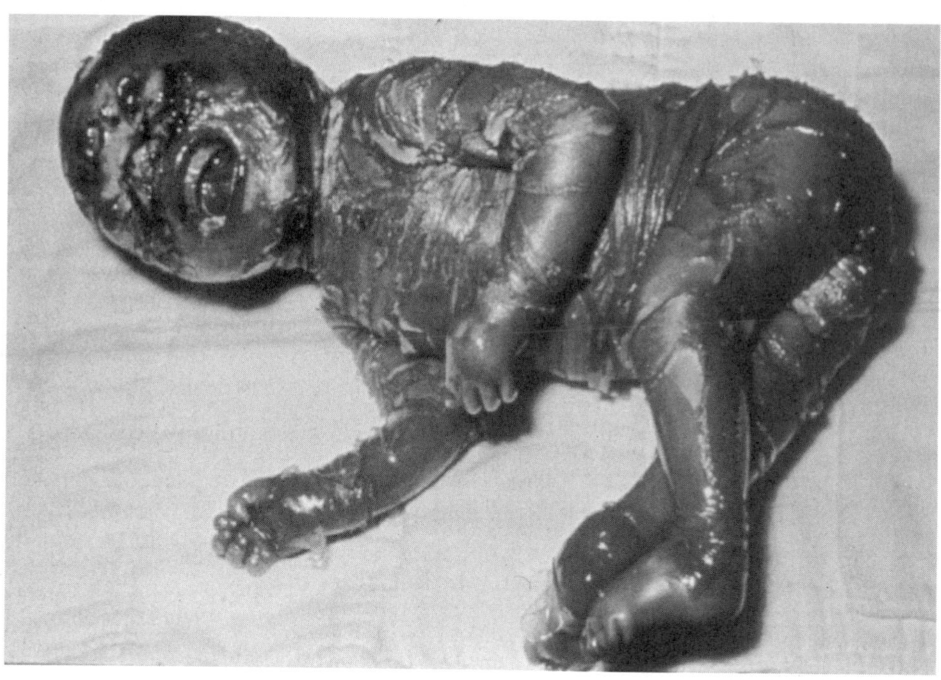

FIGURE 32–17. This harlequin infant is an example of the most severely affected ichthyotic infant. The skin is hard and thick, with deep crevices. Inelasticity of the skin results in fleshy deformities of joints and limbs. (From Clark, D., & Thompson, J. [1986]. Dermatology of the newborn. Parts 1 and 2. In *Pathology of the neonate slide series* [Vol. III, No. 4]. Philadelphia: Wyeth-Ayerst Laboratories. Reprinted with permission.)

oil, and soaps that are excessively drying or irritating should be avoided. In the bullous form, judicious use of antimicrobial bathing may be prescribed to reduce colonization, but this measure should be carefully performed to avoid toxicity from absorption of these substances through the skin. Ointments or creams that preserve moisturization, such as Aquaphor, are applied several times daily. At times, steroid ointments are used on a short-term basis, but only to treat irritant dermatitis, should it occur. In cases of bullous ichthyosis, systemic oral steroids are sometimes necessary to reduce the inflammatory process.

Infants with severe skin involvement from ichthyosis may require protective isolation if they are cared for in an intensive care nursery because of the higher risk of contact with nosocomial infections. Incubators may be useful for thermoregulation of these infants; incubators also provide a barrier to infection. Use of sterile linen and sterile gloves and other measures are needed if larger areas of denuded skin are present.

Comfort is another key nursing concern in the care of the infant who is significantly affected with ichthyosis. Fussy, irritable agitation may be seen, which is related to pruritus or inflammation. Some form of analgesia may help, although the topical therapies prescribed have the most direct effect. Some authors describe the use of diphenhydramine (Benadryl) if severe pruritus exists, but this would be very hard to determine in a neonate, who lacks verbal or fine motor skills to communicate this symptom. A trial of this medication with careful observation might be helpful in the case of a very frantic or irritable infant when other measures (e.g., topical treatment, pacifiers, feeding) are unsuccessful.

Working with the parents of an infant with ichthyosis has many facets. The appearance of the infant, especially if he or she is severely affected, could be shocking and traumatic to the parents and could require careful interventions. As with parents of infants with other congenital abnormalities, a period of shock, denial, and grief occurs over the loss of a perfect baby. In addition, the genetic nature of this disorder and the implications for future children must be comprehended. Parents of these infants need genetic counseling, support, and education as they come to terms with this disease.

Eczema

Eczema, which is a skin disorder that causes several degrees of skin irritation and has multiple causes, is rarely seen in the newborn period. It is more commonly seen after 2 months of age and involves an eruption that proceeds to the development of microvesicles and oozing, which later turns into scaling of the epidermis as this layer tries to regenerate rapidly. Lichenification, or thickening of the skin, which occurs in adult skin with eczema, is not seen in infants.

Primary irritants, such as saliva, feces, and some soaps or skin preparations, rather than allergies, are the usual causes of eczema in infants. It is important to have a good history of all products that have been applied to the skin to sort out the causes. If external agents have been ruled out, other diagnoses are considered, such as seborrheic dermatitis and Leiner's disease, which involves a total exfoliation of the entire body.

Collaborative Management

Medical and nursing treatment of eczema involves prevention by avoiding the primary irritant source, if it has been identified, or protection, as in the use of zinc oxide paste to the perianal area to prevent contact with feces. For more generalized eruptions, short-term therapy with topical 1-percent hydrocortisone cream may be used. Bathing should be carried out in tepid water with water-dispersible oil; use of irritating or drying soaps should be avoided. If large areas of skin are involved, thermoregulation may be a concern, especially in dry climates. Humidification may be desirable in some climates, especially during the summer months. Air conditioning may also be necessary during the summer months.

Discomfort is also a significant concern because infants with eczema may experience considerable pruritus. Topical therapy is generally the first consideration, followed by the judicious use of diphenhydramine in severe cases.

SKIN CARE PRACTICES

The most basic aspects of skin care for newborns include daily bath, lubrication with emollients, skin preparation with antimicrobial solutions, and use of adhesives for life support devices, monitoring of vital signs, and oxygenation, if the newborns are hospitalized. During all these practices, the skin of the newborn has the potential for trauma or alterations in normal barrier function and pH. The literature is reviewed to determine what is currently known about these daily practices and their impact on the skin of newborns.

Bathing

The purpose of bathing newborns has primarily been the reduction of antimicrobial colonization and removal of waste materials, as well as for general aesthetic reasons. Antimicrobial bathing has been the most extensively studied. Although effective in reducing colonization with S. *aureus* strains (Sarkany & Arnold, 1970), bathing with hexachlorophene has been abandoned or curtailed by most nurseries, owing to the toxicity associated with its absorption (American Academy of Pediatrics, 1977). Kopelman (1973) found the degree of absorption to be much greater in premature infants as well, so this practice is not considered safe by most clinicians. For antimicrobial bathing, chlorhexidine has replaced hexachlorophene in many settings. Studies reporting on results of the use of this agent found it to be effective for as long as 4 hours after bathing (Davies et al., 1977). Absorption of chlorhexidine has been shown to occur in both term and premature infants (Cowen et al., 1979), but toxicity from chlorhexidine has not yet been identified. In clinical practice many NICUs are reluctant to risk even potential toxicity from antimicrobial bathing in very small premature infants, so bathing only once or not at all with an antimicrobial soap is commonly seen.

Other soaps commonly used in routine bathing practices for premature infants are the same as soaps used for term infants and include so-called baby soaps, regular soaps (like Ivory), neutral pH soaps (like Neutrogena or Dove), and superfatted soaps (like Basis or Oilatum); occasionally, deodorant soaps (like Dial) are recommended for their antimicrobial properties (Morelli & Weston, 1987). Most experts agree that all soaps are at least mild irritants (Frosch & Kligman, 1979; Tupker et al., 1990a, 1990b), and that frequent soaping increases irritation. The exact properties of soaps that cause the irritation are not clear, however. The irritation studies have all been performed on adults; however, because soaps have minimal contact time with skin, most children can tolerate any soap without adverse effects (Morelli & Weston, 1987). This tolerance may not pertain to premature infants with immature skin development; the degree of irritation as well as the drying effects on the stratum corneum and the alterations in skin pH are not known but may have consequences for the ability of the premature infant's skin to function as a barrier and to maintain a normal acid surface. Therefore, both the type of soap and the frequency of bathing are considerations. Infrequent bathing with mild, neutral pH soaps may be beneficial.

Lubrication

Lubricants are commonly applied to the skin of premature infants in an effort to prevent or treat a dry or chapped appearance. The level of hydration in the stratum corneum is related to the ability of this layer to take up water and to its capacity to retain water (Thune et al., 1988). It has been shown that the water content of the stratum corneum is low in conditions such as psoriasis and eczema and also in aged skin (Potts et al., 1984; Tagami & Yoshikuni, 1985; Tagami et al., 1982). The water content of the stratum corneum of the premature infant is not known, nor is the effect of various lubrication methods on skin hydration.

The only study that has looked at the application of topical agents on the skin of premature infants was concerned with their effect on barrier function, specifically the ability of the stratum corneum to prevent the high levels of TEWL common in premature infants. Brice and associates (1981) initially tested five creams, three oils, and three greases on adult skin and measured TEWL with an evaporimeter; the only substance with a lasting "water-proofing" effect over a 4-hour period was soft paraffin, a mixture of petroleum hydrocarbons. They noted a less effective response with soft paraffin on newborn skin inside a warm incubator, so they elected to mix hard and soft paraffin to study the effect on TEWL in two premature infants, 26 and 32 weeks' gestation and less than 7 days of age. They report that skin water loss was immediately stopped at the sites of application, and that the effect was sustained for longer than 6 hours. They later applied paraffin to the overall skin surface in another three premature infants, 26 to 30 weeks' gestation, and calculated that skin water loss decreased by 50 percent.

In a later study comparing two methods of reducing skin water loss in premature infants, they found that both the paraffin method and the use of a plastic "bubble paper" blanket were equally efficacious and that each method had positive and negative effects. They reported that skin rashes developed in seven of the 22 infants treated with paraffin; the rashes ranged from mild to severe (Rutter & Hull, 1981).

It is unfortunate that Rutter and Hull did not test any of the other creams or oils on the premature infants' skin, because the effects seen on adult skin may not be generalizable to the immature stratum corneum of the premature infant. Also, because the investigators were interested primarily in an overall effect on total body skin water loss, the direct effects of skin lubrication on stratum corneum hydration, pH, and barrier function have not been reported on in premature infants, and potential positive or negative influences of products routinely used for lubrication in premature infants in the NICU are yet to be determined. If they are necessary for the prevention of excessive drying, chapping, or fissuring in the skin, lubricants should be selected that are relatively free of perfumes or dyes because these may be absorbed and may be contact irritants. Lubricants that may be helpful include Heb cream, which is used as a base in dermatologic preparations, and Eucerin cream. Others may also be used. Another concern about the use of lubricants is the potential to increase bacterial or fungal colonization if the lubricants are used frequently. However, there is currently no literature regarding this concern.

Antimicrobial Skin Solutions

The use of solutions to decontaminate skin before an invasive procedure, such as venipuncture, heel stick blood sampling, and umbilical catheter insertion, is considered to be necessary in premature and term infants in the NICU. However, the literature contains anecdotal reports documenting negative effects from these practices. Skin sloughing and blistering in a 27-week-gestation infant was described after the use of isopropyl alcohol pledgets instead of conduction paste under electrocardiographic leads (Schick & Milstein, 1981). Another infant, 25 weeks' gestation, sustained second- and third-degree burns to the buttocks from isopropyl alcohol poured over the umbilicus before umbilical catheter insertion. Another case of severe hemorrhagic skin necrosis and toxic blood alcohol levels was reported in a 27-week-gestation infant during the same type of procedure (Harpin & Rutter, 1982). These authors speculated that these changes resulted from direct damage to the epidermis. Despite these reports, alcohol pledgets are still found in any NICU and are used on premature infants. Even in the absence of catastrophic trauma, one might speculate that some degree of compromise to skin function occurs after the application of this solution.

Another common antimicrobial skin preparation used before invasive procedures is povidone-iodine solution. Instances of high iodine levels, iodine goiter, and hypothyroidism have been associated with liberal use of povidone-iodine as a preparatory agent before invasive procedures (Chabrolle & Rossier, 1978; Jackson &

Sutherland, 1981; Pyati et al., 1977). Some clinicians believe that this is sufficient reason to abandon the use of this solution in premature infants. However, the risk of introducing microorganisms through the skin during such procedures exists in these immunocompromised patients, and many continue to use povidone-iodine solution, advocating that it be removed completely with water as soon as possible after the procedure is completed.

The efficacy of decontamination with either solution is an important issue. A publication of the National Committee for Clinical Laboratory Standards recommends the use of alcohol rather than povidone-iodine, unless a blood culture is obtained that suggests better efficacy of povidone-iodine (NCCLS, 1986). A comparative study of preoperative skin decontamination showed a superior efficacy of alcohol, but the method of application was markedly different from that used for blood sampling (Rathburn et al., 1986). A recent study of 35 children (aged 2 to 14 years) and 35 adults showed that povidone-iodine provided more effective decontamination than alcohol (Choudhuri et al., 1990).

The effects of both alcohol and povidone-iodine on the skin of premature infants have not been described, in terms of trauma, alterations in surface pH, dryness, or efficacy. It would be useful to know the effects on skin properties as well as efficacy so that standards could be generated for which solution should be used and how it should be used with the least harmful effects.

Adhesive Application and Removal

Harpin and Rutter (1983) found that premature infants' skin beneath adhesive tape and the adhesive rings used to secure transcutaneous oxygen electrodes was stripped of the epidermal layer when the adhesive was removed. This resulted in increased TEWL and was proof that adhesive removal could have a significant effect on skin barrier function. Alterations in skin barrier function from removal of adhesives have been documented in adult skin after repeated strippings with tape; these findings have been used as a model for skin irritation in studies of other agents (Lo et al., 1990).

Many different adhesives and products used to enhance adhesion are currently in use in the NICU, where life support and monitoring devices must be securely attached to premature infants. Solvents such as Wisk and Dermasol have been used in many pediatric settings to prevent discomfort from adhesive removal but should not be used in premature infants because of the dangers of toxicity from their absorption.

The use of skin barriers, products that are placed between the skin and adhesive to either promote adhesion or protect the skin, has also been examined. A plastic polymer, spray-on dressing was examined by Evans and Rutter (1986b) and was found to reduce trauma, as measured by a lower TEWL, when used under the adhesive rings for transcutaneous oxygen monitors. Higher rates of water loss persisted for 12 to 16 hours after the standard adhesive rings were removed, and the authors noted no alterations in oxygen readings from the devices affixed in this manner. However, they did note a residue that built up over time and that was difficult to remove, and the potential absorption of this substance was not examined. Tincture of benzoin is also frequently used in adults, primarily to increase the adherence of adhesives and strengthen the epidermis. However, the bond between tape and epidermis created by benzoin may, in fact, be stronger than the bond between epidermis and dermis, especially on premature infants, and can result in increased epidermal stripping. Therefore, this barrier should be used judiciously, if at all, and probably not on premature infants during the early rapid phase of skin development that occurs after birth.

Cartlidge and Rutter (1987) later compared the effects on barrier function (measured by TEWL) of two different adhesive electrodes in 20 premature infants, 24 to 32 weeks' gestation and younger than 10 days of age. A conventional adhesive electrode and one with karaya gum adhesive were affixed to opposite sides of the chest and removed after 24 hours. The conventional adhesive removal resulted in an 80-percent change in TEWL from an adjacent untouched site; the karaya electrode removal caused less than a 5-percent change in TEWL from the untouched control site. Despite these impressive results, some evidence of skin irritation with the use of the karaya electrode available in the United States has been found. This irritation was probably not from traumatic removal but more likely was a sensitivity rash on the very immature infants on whom it was tried.

Other adhesives that may have promise for reducing skin trauma on removal from premature infants include pectin-based barriers, such as those used for stoma appliances, that have replaced similar karaya products, and hydrophilic gelled adhesives. In a systematic evaluation of the use of a pectin-based barrier, Hollihesive was used under tape (Fig. 32–18) to secure a variety of appliances in 45 newborns with a mean weight of 1571.6 g, a mean gestational age of 31.3 weeks, and a mean postnatal age of 7 days (Lund et al., 1986). In 199 applications and removals of Hollihesive, nine excoriations were visibly inspected and recorded. However, no control site was observed, and the use of visual observation is not adequate to discern important changes in barrier function. Similarly, the newer gelled adhesive products used in electrocardiographic leads, over temperature skin probes, and for phototherapy masks have seemed less traumatic by visual inspection but have not yet been studied by instrumentation to detect other important changes in skin function.

Although definitive research has not defined precise practices in regard to adhesive application and removal, the following practices used in many NICUs have proved to be beneficial in clinical practice. First, minimal use of tape is essential; tape can be backed with cotton, another piece of tape, or pectin-based barriers so that trauma on removal is reduced. When tape is removed, a slow, careful method with water-soaked cotton balls can be used successfully; alcohol pledgets are also sometimes used, but they can be drying and irritating to skin, so they should be avoided, especially in premature infants. Soft gauze wraps to secure pulse oximeter probes, hydrophilic gelled electrodes, and temperature probe covers also reduce trauma to the epidermis. The Newborn Skin Care Protocol at the end of the chapter outlines neonatal skin management.

CONTROL OF EVAPORATIVE WATER AND HEAT LOSS

Because of the poorly keratinized stratum corneum, which provides minimal resistance to the diffusion of water, the preterm infant is subjected to high insensible water loss that also results in low body temperatures during the first few days after birth. Characteristic skin factors that predispose infants to water loss include larger surface area in relation to body weight, thinner epidermis, increased water content, increased permeability, and increased blood supply that is closer to the skin surface (Loper, 1992).

Transepidermal water loss is directly correlated to gestational age and degree of maturation of the epidermal stratum corneum. Mature keratin, which is a major component of the tough, nonliving outer layer of the epidermis, is relatively water impermeable. Because keratin formation is directly related to gestational age, the extremely premature infant is at increased risk for increased evaporative losses. Water easily diffuses across the permeable skin barrier and evaporates. Keratinization and subsequent maturation of the epidermis occurs over the first 2 to 4 weeks of postnatal life and contributes to a reduction in evaporative loss (Thomas,

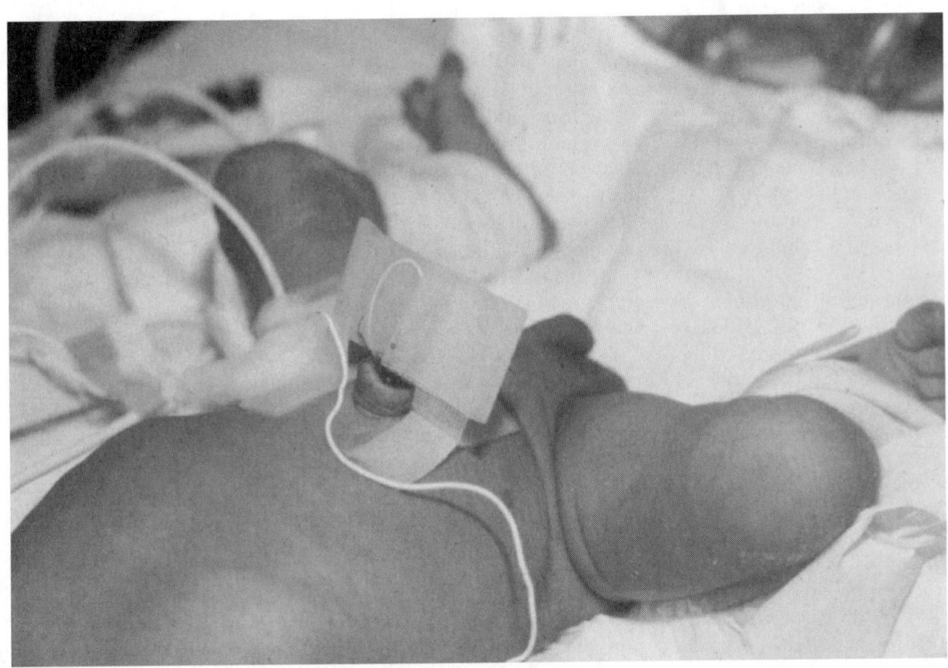

FIGURE 32–18. Hollihesive. (From Kuller, J. [1995]. Skin care management of the low-birthweight infant. In L. Gunderson & C. Kenner [Eds.], *Care of the 24–25 week gestational age infant* (2nd ed.) Petaluma, CA: NICU Ink. Reprinted with permission.)

1994). TEWL is influenced by many factors: ambient humidity, gestational age at birth, postnatal age, ambient temperature, weight, activity, and body temperature (Sedin et al., 1985). Differences in TEWL exist between infants whose weight is appropriate for gestational age and those who are small for gestational age. Infants who are small for gestational age have a lower TEWL in the first day after birth than that of infants whose weight is appropriate for gestational age who are the same gestational age.

In the infant who is 28 to 30 weeks' gestational age, water losses may be as much as 15 times greater than that in a full-term infant on day one after birth. A baby less than 30 weeks' gestation who weighs 0.9 kg, is 1 day old, and is provided nursing care while naked in an incubator loses about 75 ml of water from the skin each day (about 85 ml/kg/day) (Rutter & Hull, 1979). TEWL as high as 200 ml/kg/day has been measured through the skin of the very low birthweight (VLBW) infant. The prevention of hyperosmolarity and its rapid development depend on measures taken to minimize transcutaneous water loss (effective shielding and an optimal thermal environment) and administration of water in sufficient volume to compensate for transepidermal losses (Korones & Bada-Ellzey, 1993). The hyperosmolar state at its worst consists of oliguria, inordinately rapid weight loss, hypernatremia, and hyperkalemia. In its early stages, serum sodium and potassium levels may be increased in the absence of diminished urine output. If inadequately addressed, the dehydration progresses to hypovolemia, shock, renal failure, and death. Experience has shown that administration of large fluid volumes on the day of birth has remarkably diminished the incidence of hyperosmolarity and renal failure in infants weighing less than 800 g (Korones & Bada-Ellzey, 1993).

Evaporative heat loss is the primary source of heat loss in small premature infants. Increased evaporation from the skin surface always means an increase in heat loss as well. Evaporation produces heat loss through the energy used in the conversion of water to its gaseous state. Evaporation of 1 l of water utilizes 600 kcal of heat. Evaporative heat loss may be insensible (from skin and respiration) or sensible (from sweating) (Thomas, 1994).

Because temperature and evaporation are directly related, increases in temperature decrease vapor pressure and increase evaporation. Therefore, warm air temperatures required by the infant are associated with high evaporative loss. However, raising the ambient humidity increases vapor pressure and decreases evaporative loss (Thomas, 1994).

Servocontrol, used with increasing frequency to maintain an infant's temperature within specific ranges, is less effective in immature infants because of their higher evaporative water losses (Loper, 1992). The servocontrol system is based on the assumption that the temperature of the skin reflects that of the surrounding skin. However, attaching the temperature probe to the skin reduces TEWL at that site where the temperature is being monitored. Thus, the temperature probe may record skin temperatures that are higher than the rest of the infant's body and may lead to failure to keep the infant warm (Hey & Scopes, 1987). Increasing humidity may reduce these differences. Hey and Scopes estimated that increasing the humidity of the VLBW infant by 50 percent was similar to increasing the ambient temperature 1.5°C.

Evaporation rate measurements in full-term infants at different ambient humidities revealed a linear relationship between the evaporation rate and the relative humidity: a much higher evaporation rate existed at a lower (20-percent) humidity than at a higher (60-percent) humidity (Sedin et al., 1985). In addition, a linear relationship existed in premature infants, but the TEWL values were much higher in the premature than in the term infant.

Transepidermal water loss in a VLBW infant in an ambient humidity of 85 to 95 percent is only about 10 percent of that in an ambient humidity of 50 percent and is only about 5 percent of that in an ambient humidity of 20 percent. Sedin and colleagues (1985) concluded that the most premature infant (23 to 24 weeks' gestation) may lose as much as 13 percent of his or her body weight as TEWL during the first day of life, even at an ambient humidity of 50 percent. The infant loses much more body weight at a lower level of ambient humidity.

Management of the VLBW infant with high evaporative water losses, with the resulting electrolyte imbalance, high fluid demands, and heat loss, is a nursing challenge. Because the rate of insensible water loss is increased under radiant warmers, the use of double-walled isolettes for the VLBW infant has become commonplace. The incubator not only assists with control of evaporative and convective heat losses, it also serves as a type of barrier between the caregiver and the infant, thus promoting a developmental philosophy of environmental shielding and minimal handling of the infant.

Bell and associates (1980) did measurements of insensible water loss, carbon dioxide production, and oxygen consumption in single-walled incubators and under radiant warmers with and without heat shields. They found that the insensible water loss was greater under radiant warmers than incubators without shields. The addition of the heat shield reduced insensible water loss in the incubator but not under the radiant warmer. Baumgart (1984) found that the use of a plastic blanket under a radiant warmer reduced oxygen consumption, insensible water loss, and radiant warmer demands.

In 1995, Kjartansson and colleagues measured the rate of evaporation from the skin of 12 full-term and 16 preterm infants (gestational age, 25 to 34 weeks), both during incubator care and when cared for under a radiant warmer. They concluded that the evaporative water loss from the skin depends on the ambient water vapor pressure, irrespective of whether the infant is nursed under a radiant warmer or in an incubator. The higher rate of evaporation during care under a radiant warmer is due to the lower ambient water vapor pressure and not to any direct effect of the nonionizing radiation on the skin.

Other measures to reduce TEWL in the VLBW infants that have been used or studied are the topical application of paraffin and semipermeable dressings; an increase in humidity; or the use of a plastic hood, plastic thermal blankets, heat shields, or plastic wraps, such as Glad Wrap, Seal Wrap, and Saran Wrap. These films should never be placed in direct contact with the skin because this could result in maceration of the skin or thermal burns from the direct heating of the wrap by the radiant warmer (LeBlanc, 1991). Mancini and others (1994) studied the effect of a nonadhesive semipermeable dressing on the epidermal barrier of 15 premature infants by measuring TEWL on control and on treated skin. Treated skin showed a significantly decreased TEWL on the treated site; TEWL was measured after temporary dressing removal on days l, 2, 4, and 7. Increased cellular proliferation was documented; this phenomenon is associated with improved epidermal barrier function.

Whether the infant is on a radiant warmer or in an incubator, providing ambient humidity can reduce skin water losses (Sulyok et al., 1972). Humidity has been removed from most incubators over the past decade out of fear of the spread of *Pseudomonas* infection. In a large-scale controlled study performed in the early 1960s by Silverman and others (1957, 1963), infants were studied in varying ambient humidities. These investigators found no increase in the incidence of sepsis in the babies cared for in humidity. It has been shown that *Pseudomonas* will grow in the humidity reservoirs if they are not changed and cleaned frequently. It has never been shown that the growth of these organisms increases the incidence of sickness in the babies themselves (LeBlanc, 1991). LeBlanc has seen extremely high, unpredictable water losses in these infants that necessitated 300 to 600 ml/kg/day to maintain free water balance. Because of clinical experience in managing VLBW infants, LeBlanc (1991) and Harpin and Rutter (1983) suggested that these infants be treated in humid incubators.

One of the easiest ways to deliver a humidified environment is with an incubator that delivers servocontrolled humidity. Two such incubators are currently on the market: the Air Shields C550 LX and the Drager. The Dew-ette II incubator humidification system (Air Shields) uses a water vapor method of controlling humidity. With the incubator set at 36.0°C, the relative humidity set point may be adjusted to any level from 30 to 85 percent or higher. A hygrometer built inside the isolette allows the clinician to monitor the amount of humidity delivered. The LX model of the C550 Quiet Touch has built-in servocontrol for humidity, in addition to improved patterns of air flow and an enhanced air curtain. This servocontrol prevents the temperature from decreasing more than a few degrees when the door is opened for extended periods and decreases the amount of time required to return to the temperature set point after the door is closed. A study was performed at the Children's Hospital of Philadelphia to verify that the design of the Dew-ette allowed incubators to run at increased humidity levels without increasing the risk of infection to the baby (McGowan, 1990). In phase 3 of the study, *Pseudomonas aeroginosa* was placed in the Dew-ette humidity reservoir of three incubators. The incubators were set for 30-percent, 60-percent, and 90-percent humidity. After the fifth day of operation, the reservoir water, the target plates in the incubator, and the inside areas of the hose of the incubator were cultured for signs of infection. Although the reservoir water of the humidifiers set at 30-percent and 60-percent humidity were "swarming" with *Pseudomonas*, no growth was noted on the target culture plates or recovered from the surface cultures inside the incubator. These test results seem to show that the design of the Dew-ette humidifier adequately contains the bacteria that may otherwise have been deposited inside the infant compartment.

The best percentage of humidity for infants of varying gestational ages and weights has not been established. How long the humidity should be left on is another question that has not been studied. Because the maturation of the skin occurs so rapidly during the first 2 weeks of life, some protocols cite 2 weeks as the ideal length of time to leave the humidity on. Hammarlund and Sedin (1979) showed that although TEWL for premature and term infants gradually diminishes with age, at 4 weeks after birth, TEWL is still twice as high for the preterm infant than for the term infant. Close monitoring of fluid requirements gives some indication of the decreasing insensible water losses that occur with skin maturation.

MANAGEMENT OF SKIN CARE PROBLEMS

The stratum corneum can be traumatized by a variety of insults, including epidermal stripping from removal of adhesives; burns from transcutaneous oxygen electrodes; pressure sores; infection; nutritional inadequacies, such as zinc and essential fatty acid deficiency; extravasation of intravenous fluids; and diaper dermatitis. The goal of all skin care for neonates should be the maintenance of skin integrity; however, even with meticulous care, skin breakdown can occur. Strategies to prevent injury and treat skin disruptions after injury are reviewed in the Newborn Skin Care Protocol at the end of the chapter.

Skin Excoriations

When a skin excoriation is noted, the first step is to identify the cause of the injury before determining a treatment strategy. In cases in which no trauma has been known to occur, it is especially important to rule out infectious causes, such as staphylococcal scalded skin syndrome and cutaneous candidiasis, because these conditions may require culturing and either systemic or topical treatment.

If the skin excoriation has a known cause, such as adhesive removal, the care should include cleansing with sterile water and possibly application of some type of antimicrobial ointment or dressing. If an ointment is prescribed, Polysporin or bacitracin ointment is used sparingly over the excoriation and reapplied every 8 to 12 hours. Neosporin is another common topical ointment, but some dermatologists have noted increased sensitization from early uses of this ointment and potential allergy later in life.

Skin excoriations may benefit from some type of dressing. Transparent adhesive dressings, such as Op-Site, Tegaderm, and Bioclusive, have been widely used for many purposes in the

NICU. These dressings are made from a polyurethane film backed with adhesive that is impermeable to water and bacteria but allows air flow so that the skin can "breathe." They adhere well but require a rim of intact skin for attachment. Other uses for transparent adhesive dressings include the securing of intravenous catheters and percutaneous Silastic catheters and as a dressing for central venous lines. Another use is the prevention of skin breakdown, and it can be applied to bony prominences, such as the knees and the sacrum, when the potential for friction burns or pressure sores exists (Fig. 32–19).

Transparent adhesive dressings can also be applied over superficial or deep wounds; they have been shown in adult literature to promote faster, "moist" healing. The one caution is that the wound must be uninfected, or "clean" because bacteria and fungus proliferate under the dressing. When these dressings are used for wound care, a milky white or yellow exudate forms under the dressing; this is often mistaken for pus, but it is actually composed of leukocytes that prevent infection during the process of healing. The dressing should remain in place until healing has occurred or until it falls off because removal may result in further skin excoriation because of the tenacious nature of the adhesive backing.

Another use for transparent adhesive dressings in premature infants that has been reported is reduction of some of the massive transepidermal water losses and evaporative heat losses that result from the immature stratum corneum. Bustamante and Steslow (1989), Knauth and colleagues (1989), and Vernon and associates (1990) all described decreased TEWL and improved thermoregulation when large areas of the skin of premature infants who were younger than 1 week were covered by transparent adhesive dressing (Fig. 32–20). The mechanism of the success of this technique is that the dressings created a "second skin," an additional layer of the stratum corneum that functioned as a mature stratum corneum in preserving fluid and preventing heat loss.

Concerns over the uses of this method include the possibility that infections could occur and proliferate under the dressings and that the normal process of maturation of the stratum corneum would be impaired, although preliminary research indicates that this is not the case: In addition, the infant looks unusual, and skin trauma may occur when the dressings are eventually removed. However, this application is certainly of interest, and future research may address some of the questions about the use of transparent adhesive dressings in the premature infant.

Some of the skin excoriations seen in the patient in the NICU cannot be easily covered with transparent adhesive dressings if no rim of intact skin exists around the site or if it is located in close proximity to other skin that cannot be separated or that folds over the excoriation, such as the neck folds and the groin. Treatment of excoriations includes irrigating with sterile normal saline every 4 to 6 hours and then leaving the area exposed to air. This simple, basic procedure is effective in keeping the excoriation clean, and it promotes healing with little risk of sensitization or infection. Other products used for healing include Vigilon, a gelatinous hydrophilic dressing without an adhesive backing, and DuoDerm, a hydrocolloid dressing with a pectin base; both of these products promote moist healing similar to that seen with transparent adhesive dressings. There is no research that suggests which method is superior; in both types of dressings, it is important that the wound be uninfected.

Large wounds, such as those that occur after surgery, can result in skin disruption when healing fails to progress in the normal fashion. Dehiscence of wounds is occasionally encountered in the neonate, although wound healing is generally less complicated in the NICU if the infant's nutritional status is appropriate and basic precautions against infection are taken. For more information about wound healing in pediatrics, a review article by Garvin (1990) is recommended.

Nutritional Deficiencies

Zinc is an essential trace element—essential because it is crucial for growth and development, and a trace element because it is present in humans in quantities equal to or less than the quantities in which iron is present. Zinc is a cofactor in the reaction of more than 15 enzymes in many areas of metabolism. It is essential for lymphocyte transformation and is important for the metabolism of proteins, nucleic acids, and mucopolysaccharides of the skin and subcutaneous tissues. It is also an essential part of the enzyme structure of alkaline phosphatase (Dixon, 1987). In addition, zinc is required for normal taste, smell, and wound healing.

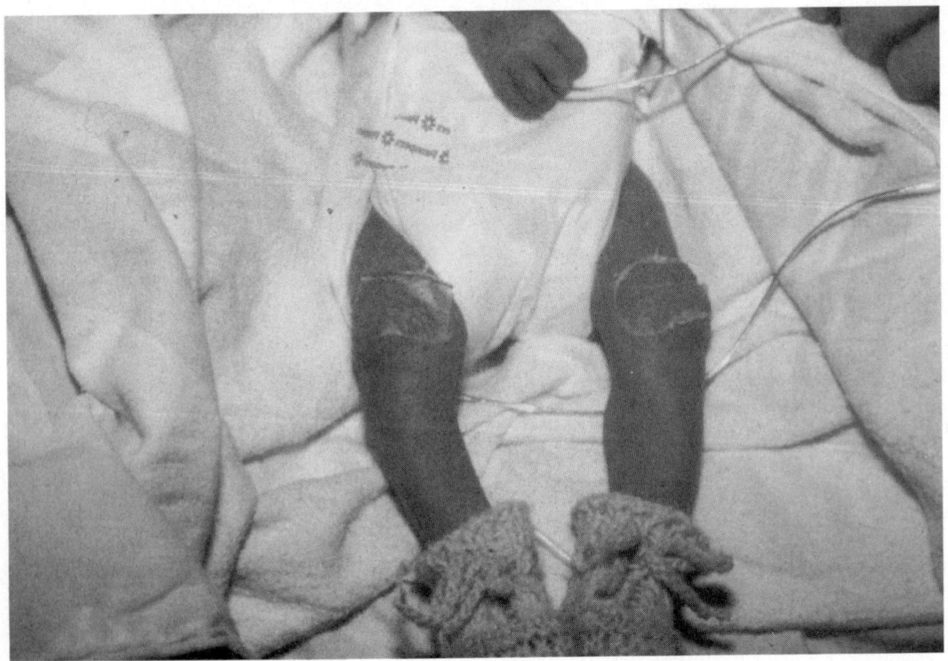

FIGURE 32–19. Knees covered with Op-Site dressing.

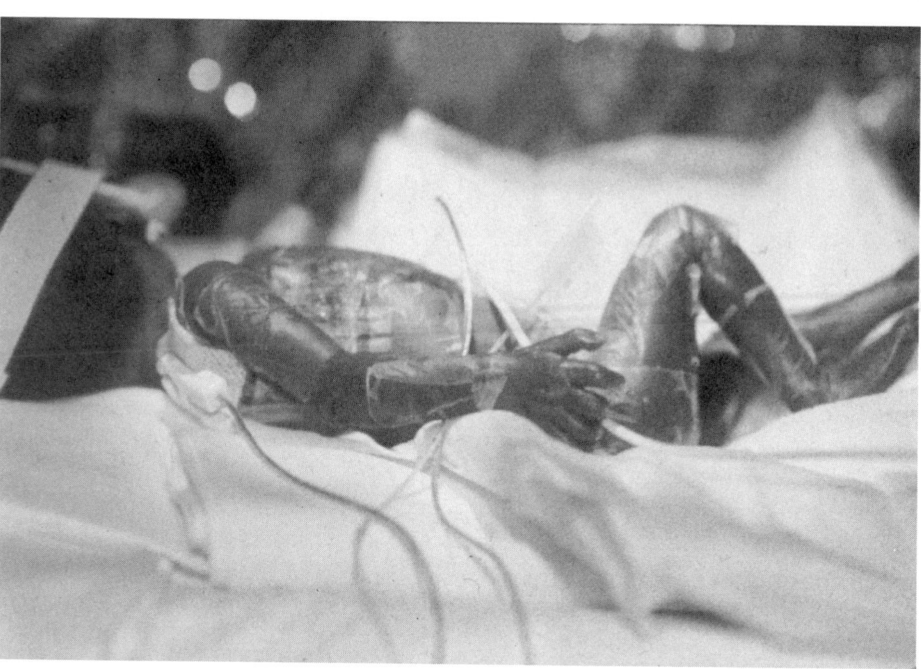

FIGURE 32–20. Body covered with Op-Site dressing.

Total body zinc doubles between 32 and 40 weeks' gestation, with two thirds of the maternal-fetal transport occurring during the last 10 weeks of gestation (Lefrak, 1984). Absorption and excretion of zinc occur primarily through the gastrointestinal tract. Deficiencies are related to abnormal losses of zinc in stool or urine, poor stores, or increased demands, as occur during rapid growth phases or stress. Premature infants are at special risk for developing a zinc deficiency. Because they have trouble absorbing zinc and have not received adequate stores before birth, they may be in negative zinc balance for several weeks after birth. Other infants at risk for zinc deficiency include those with gastrointestinal pathology, chronic diarrhea, short-gut or short-bowel syndrome with jejunoileal bypass, necrotizing enterocolitis, or an ileostomy. Any patient receiving total parenteral nutrition who is not receiving mineral supplements is also at risk (Dixon, 1987).

The clinical manifestations of zinc deficiency include lethargy, growth retardation, skin lesions, alopecia, and diarrhea; the striking sign of zinc deficiency, however, is some form of skin lesions. Common sites of involvement are the groin and perianal area (Fig. 32–21), the neck folds, and the face, particularly the angles of the mouth and the cheeks. Lesions have also been noted at sites of trauma, such as endotracheal and cardiac monitor tape sites (Esterly & Spraker, 1985). The skin lesions are reddened, scaly, and moist. The skin eruption of zinc deficiency strongly resembles acrodermatitis enteropathica in its morphologic features and distribution.

Hair and plasma zinc levels do not accurately reflect tissue zinc levels, making the diagnosis of zinc deficiency difficult. In an infant with clinical symptoms of deficiency, diagnosis is made when the serum zinc levels are low (normal, 68 to 120 μg/ml) and are accompanied by a low alkaline phosphatase level (Zimmerman et al., 1982). Treatment consists of zinc supplementation. For infants receiving total parenteral nutrition, the range is between 150 and 350 μg/kg/day (Zlotkin & Buchanan, 1983). However, the choice of which commercial amino acid should be used in conjunction with the supplementation must be considered when zinc deficiency is being treated or prevented because some deactivate or decrease absorption of zinc (Dixon, 1987). Premature infants in whom a zinc deficiency acrodermatitis develops while they are breastfed exclusively must be given oral zinc supplements with zinc sulfate.

Recovery from zinc deficiency is dramatic once adequate zinc supplementation has begun. In general, skin conditions caused by nutritional deficiencies are often confused with infections and other irritants but do not respond until the deficiency state itself is treated.

Intravenous Extravasations

The extravasation of intravenous fluids and medications can result in skin injury and, in some cases, deep tissue injury to muscle and nerves. The most serious extravasation injuries are iatrogenic complications that can lead to pain, prolonged hospitalization, and increased morbidity, such as infection. Extravasation injuries can also result in increased hospital costs and the potential for legal action. Despite vigilant nursing assessment, intravenous extravasations do occur in about 11 percent of patients in the NICU (Upton et al., 1979). Tissue sloughing occurs in as many as 43.6 percent of these infants (Collinge & Aranda, 1984). Therefore, nursing actions, such as the monitoring of intravenous sites, and other preventive strategies, as well as immediate interventions that can reduce the extent of tissue injury are important considerations for all nurseries that care for newborns with intravenous devices for fluid administration and medications.

Some of the factors identified by Zenk (1981) that increase the risk of tissue injury include

1. The length of exposure after extravasation occurs, especially when the patients are unable to verbalize the discomfort of pain or pressure.
2. The nature of the drug or solution; hypertonic solutions with high concentrations of calcium, potassium, glucose, or amino acids, and medications such as nafcillin have been identified as high risk for causing injury.
3. The mechanical compression caused by electronic infusion pumps.

Another risk factor is compromised perfusion to the skin, as evidenced by the poor capillary refill exhibited by the most critically ill neonates, or by the obstructed venous circulations seen

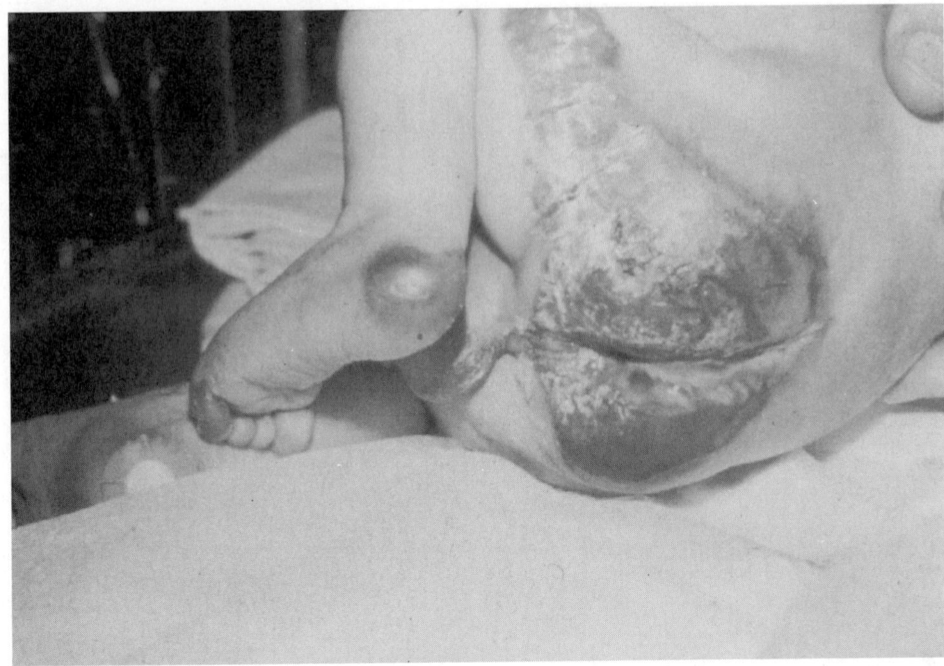

FIGURE 32–21. Infant with zinc deficiency.

with taping methods that constrict the extremities in which the intravenous device is placed.

Prevention of skin injury after infiltration is the first important consideration. Strategies include ensuring that the insertion site is clearly visible by using transparent adhesive dressing or clear tape to secure the device, and observing the site with appropriate documentation every hour. In addition, the tape should be carefully placed on the extremity to avoid obstruction of venous return. Tape placed loosely over a bony prominence, such as the knee or elbow, permits extravasated fluids and medications to disperse over a larger surface area and thus reduce the risk of injury, compared with extravasation that is limited to a small surface area. Avoiding extremities with poor perfusion in favor of better-perfused, scalp veins (except, of course, those on the forehead) may also be prudent; in some cases, the wiser choice may be the placement of central venous lines for access. Nursery policies that limit the glucose (<12.5 percent), amino acid (<2 percent), and calcium (10%) concentrations are also strategies to reduce the risk of tissue injury from the extravasation of intravenous fluids and medications.

Once an intravenous extravasation has been identified, immediate measures to reduce injury are instituted. The device should be carefully removed, and the extremity should be elevated (if it is an arm or leg). Treatment with heat or moisture is not recommended (Brown et al., 1979), because the delicate tissue could be further injured by a burn or the effects of maceration. If tissue damage is visible, the use of a topical antimicrobial ointment (e.g., povidone-iodine, silver sulfadiazine) or saline soaks has been described as having equal efficacy. In the most severe cases of deep tissue necrosis after extravasation injury, a surgical or plastic surgical consultation is necessary, and skin grafts may be needed (Fig. 32–22). In all cases of tissue injury, the open wound should be considered to be a potential portal for infection, and topical or systemic treatment may be required.

Hyaluronidase (Wydase) is an agent that has proved to be highly effective in reducing the incidence of tissue damage that results from intravenous infiltration. Hyaluronidase should be initiated within an hour of injury. It is administered by subcutaneous injections around the periphery of extravasation immediately after the device is removed. (Laurie et al., 1984: Zenk, 1981). Hyaluronidase is an enzyme that temporarily breaks down the normal interstitial barrier, resulting in the rapid diffusion of extravasated fluid over an enlarged surface area. Within 10 minutes of injection, hyaluronidase produces the diffusion of extravasated fluid over an area three to five times larger than an untreated area. The interstitial barrier is regenerated within 24 to 48 hours.

Hyaluronidase was used in the 1950s, when dermolysis (the delivery of fluid subcutaneously) was used for infants with dehydration who were not candidates for intravenous therapy because of a lack of appropriate-sized devices. It is also used in the delivery of dermatologic preparations that require dispersion over a large surface area.

Hyaluronidase is supplied in a vial that is reconstituted with 1 ml of normal saline to 150 U/ml. After reconstitution, 0.1 ml of this solution is withdrawn and added to 0.9 ml of normal saline. The final concentration is 15 U/ml, which is the dose suggested for the treatment of extravasation injuries in neonates. It is administered subcutaneously, in five 0.2-ml injections around the periphery of the site of extravasation. Use of hyaluronidase is contraindicated if the vasoconstriction would become worse if the extravasation were to spread to a larger surface area. Sites that may benefit from treatment with hyaluronidase include those with

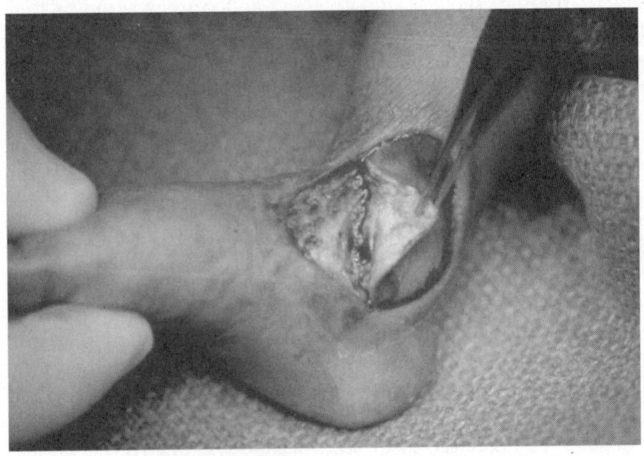

FIGURE 32–22. IV extravasation injury.

evidence of blanching (except alpha-adrenergic agents), discoloration, or blistering, or in any in which hypertonic solutions, such as calcium-containing fluids, are involved. Some injuries may appear relatively minor at first inspection but have the potential for injury, for example, if they contain calcium; treatment with hyaluronidase may prevent deep tissue injury if it is given promptly.

The antidote for extravasation due to alpha-adrenergic agents or those causing vasoconstriction, such as dopamine and norepinephrine, is phentolamine (Regitine). It is delivered in the same manner as hyaluronidase, and the recommended dose is 0.5 mg diluted to 1 ml, delivered around the periphery of the extravasation (Zenk & Sills, 1986). Phentolamine works by causing local vasodilatation, thus increasing blood flow and accelerating the speed of absorption of these caustic substances. Excessive blanching in an area of dopamine infusion, especially associated with extravasation, benefits from the administration of phentolamine. Treatment is effective if it is administered within 12 hours of infiltration but should be given as soon as possible after the diagnosis is made. Small areas of blanching are commonly seen along the vein into which dopamine is infusing. This blanching usually reverses when treatment is discontinued or when the intravenous site is changed.

Another treatment identified as being effective for intravenous infiltrates is the use of glyceryl trinitrate, in the form of a Transderm-Nitro patch. Because of the potentially variable absorption rate, however, these patches are not indicated in neonates younger than 21 days of age or in infants with skin breakdown (Flemmer & Chan, 1993).

Diaper Dermatitis

A common skin disruption that occurs in neonates and infants is diaper dermatitis. This term encompasses a range of processes that affect the perineum, groin, thighs, buttocks, and anal area of infants who are incontinent and wear some covering to collect urine and feces. Diaper dermatitis can be caused by many different mechanisms, but the condition of the skin has a direct role in the progression of skin injury.

The pathogenesis of diaper dermatitis is partly related to the degree of wetness of the skin. Skin that is moist and macerated becomes more permeable (Berg, 1987) and susceptible to injury because wetness increases friction. In addition, moisture-laden skin is more likely to contain microorganisms than dry skin.

Another component in the process of skin injury from diaper dermatitis is the effect of an alkaline pH. The normal skin pH is acidic, ranging between 4.0 and 5.5, but can become alkaline when it is exposed to urine, which generally has a higher pH. It is the resulting increased pH of the skin, and not the effect of ammonia in urine, as previously thought, that increases its vulnerability to injury and penetration by microorganisms (Berg et al., 1986; Leydon et al., 1977). Another problem associated with increased pH of the skin is that it stimulates fecal enzyme activity (Buckingham & Berg, 1986). Specifically, both protease and lipase, which are found in stool, can injure the skin, which is made up of protein and fat components. These enzymes can cause significant injury to the epidermis fairly quickly and are responsible for the contact irritant diaper dermatitis that is commonly seen.

Once the epidermis has been impaired or becomes a less efficient barrier because of one of the aforementioned mechanisms, invasion by bacteria or fungus can occur. Thus, a contact irritant diaper dermatitis can turn into a staphylococcal or fungal rash if this progression occurs.

S. aureus can be found in large numbers on the skin surface, especially if it is inflamed or impaired, and can result in secondary infection. The classic presentation for *S. aureus* is pustule formation at the site of hair follicles.

Fungal rashes, primarily those caused by *C. albicans*, may have different mechanisms of invasion. Many researchers have identified *C. albicans* as a secondary invader of skin that has been injured by other mechanisms, whereas others suggest that *C. albicans* is a primary causative factor in diaper dermatitis (Rasmussen, 1987). This theory is based on the ability of *C. albicans* to penetrate the stratum corneum, especially in a warm and moist environment, such as that found under an occlusive diaper. The resulting intense inflammation is significant and appears as brightly erythematous, sharply marginated dermatitis, involving the inguinal folds as well as the buttocks, thighs, abdomen, and genitalia, characteristically with satellite lesions that may extend the rash over the trunk (Fig. 32–23). The gastrointestinal tract is often the reservoir for *C. albicans*, and it can frequently be recovered in stool. Thus, oral therapy may be indicated, especially if evidence of oral infection, such as thrush, is apparent.

Some diaper dermatitis can be the result of a primary dermatologic condition, such as psoriasis, eczema, and seborrheic dermatitis. Significant family history of these skin conditions may identify infants who are especially vulnerable to developing severe reactions to inflammation in the diaper area.

Collaborative Management

Prevention is the first goal of intervention and is paramount in breaking the cycle of diaper dermatitis. Frequent diaper changes result in skin that is drier with a more normal pH and thus maintain the functional barrier of the skin. Strategies to keep the skin dry also include the use of highly absorbent gelled diapers that act to "wick" moisture away from the skin (Campbell et al., 1987; Davis et al., 1989). Use of talcum powders has been discouraged, owing to the risk of inhalation of silicone particles into the respiratory tract. Cornstarch has been substituted for talc and has recently been shown not to promote yeast growth (Leydon, 1984); however, efficacy of this approach has not been researched.

Once diaper dermatitis occurs—and it is not completely avoidable in most infants—protection of injured skin during healing is the primary goal. Use of a generous layer of protective skin barriers containing zinc oxide prevents further trauma and allows impaired skin to heal. Opening the skin to light and air is not effective if the fecal contents are allowed to have direct contact with already injured areas. Because protective skin barriers tend to adhere well to the skin, it is neither necessary nor desirable to completely remove them during diaper changes before more cream is applied. It is best to generously apply more cream to the site in order to protect the area from further injury.

Treatment of diaper dermatitis that is solely due to invasion with *C. albicans* requires the use of antifungal creams or ointments; sometimes, the addition of a steroid cream reduces in-

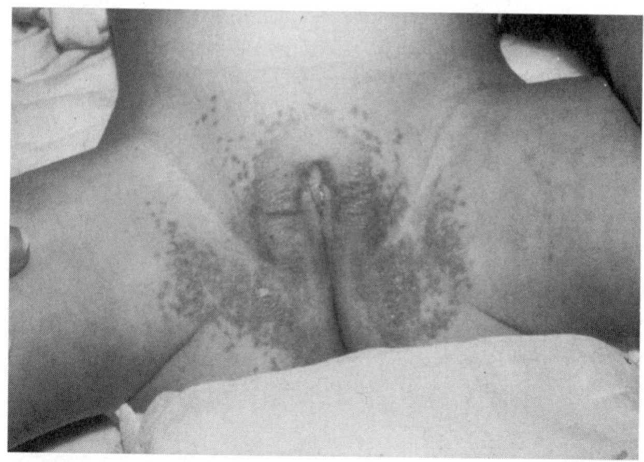

FIGURE 32–23. Diaper dermatitis.

flammation and promotes healing faster. Some of the antifungal preparations include nystatin, miconazole, and clotrimazole. If the diaper dermatitis involves both fungus and a contact irritant component, alternating applications of the topical creams or ointments is effective.

Serious diaper dermatitis is observed in infants with severe malabsorption syndrome secondary to intestinal resection or mucosal injury. In this case, the stool is extremely caustic, containing a higher level of enzyme activity, a lower pH as the result of rapid transit through the intestine, and significant amounts of undigested carbohydrates. In addition, stool frequency is often greatly increased. Although skin disruption frequently becomes the focus of nursing interventions, this symptom may be a significant indication of more serious physiologic concerns. These infants' stools should be carefully monitored by documentation of number, volume, pH, and carbohydrate testing. The infants must be observed for the dehydration caused by extensive water losses in diarrhea. Once dietary manipulations and hydration have stabilized the general physiologic status, a program of skin protection is imperative because some level of chronic diarrhea may be ongoing for many weeks or months. Products such as pectin-based powders or pectin-containing pastes without alcohol may be better barriers to the caustic, constant fecal irritation if traditional zinc oxide creams do not work adequately. If yeast is present, antifungal creams may be applied in conjunction with protective barriers.

CONCLUSION

Neonatal skin management is a complex problem that requires a collaborative approach. Some research has been conducted in this area, but there is still a lot to be done regarding the use of routine NICU equipment and its impact on neonatal skin, the use of skin barriers for protection, and the effect of a consistent approach to skin care on the integrity of neonatal skin. This chapter has outlined the development and structure of the skin. It has addressed differences in the skin based on gestational age variations. Normal physiologic as well as common dermatologic abnormalities have been presented. The chapter concludes with a protocol for newborn skin care.

NEWBORN SKIN CARE PROTOCOL

PURPOSE

Maintenance of skin integrity in the neonatal patient promotes the following skin functions:

1. Protects internal organs
2. Provides a barrier against foreign substances and organisms
3. Provides tactile perception
4. Regulates body temperature
5. Stores fat and discharges electrolytes and water
6. Facilitates initial attachment phase between mother and infant

GOAL	INTERVENTION	RATIONALE
Maintain Skin Integrity		
Provide general skin care	1. An initial bath with mild soap is given once the infant's temperature has stabilized	Use of mild soap reduces surface colonization
	Owing to HIV considerations, *all* infants should receive a soap bath as soon as possible. A mild soap, such as Neutrogena, can be used. Warm water baths are given during the first week of life. Thereafter, use of a low-alkaline soap for bathing should be employed two or three times per week during the first weeks. On other days, water or no bath regimen is followed.	Alkaline soaps affect skin pH and temporarily destroy the acid mantle that provides a bactericidal defense mechanism.
	For the infant weighing 800 g or less, warm sterile water is used for all baths except for the first one; soap may be instituted after 2 weeks.	Premature skin matures within the first 2 weeks of life.
	For the infant older than 2 months, daily soap baths using a low-alkaline soap may be given.	
	2. Avoid the use of creams and emollients unless skin becomes prone to develop cracks or fissures	Creams and emollients change skin pH and are readily absorbed by preterm skin. Cracked skin provides a portal of entry for bacteria.
	If an emollient is necessary, Heb cream is recommended. It should be used sparingly once every 8 hours.	Heb cream is a hydrophilic cream base that moisturizes the skin and allows for evaporation of skin moisture through the cream.
Provide skin preparation	1. Use povidone-iodine solution as a prepping agent prior to invasive procedures. Allow to dry for 60 seconds prior to puncturing the skin.	Povidone-iodine destroys many organisms that may be present on the skin.
	Remove solution with sterile water.	Removing the iodine solution minimizes the absorption of the solution and risk of an adverse reaction to it.
	Isopropyl alcohol may be used to remove povidone-iodine only in older infants.	Alcohol is very drying to the skin, is readily absorbed through the poorly keratinized stratum corneum of immature skin, and can cause skin irritation.
	2. Liberal use of disinfectant agents is not recommended.	Skin protection from chemical irritants is dependent on a mature stratum corneum. Skin irritation and chemical burns can result from use of disinfectant agents on preterm skin.

NEWBORN SKIN CARE PROTOCOL *Continued*

GOAL	INTERVENTION	RATIONALE
Prevent Injury		
Epidermal stripping	1. Limit the amount of adhesive used to secure monitoring and life support devices.	Adhesive removal causes the stripping of the epidermal layer because of the decreased cohesion between epidermal and dermal skin.
	2. Use Hollihesive as a blanket barrier between skin and tape to secure the following devices: endotracheal tube, umbilical arterial catheter, temperature probe, nasal oxygen cannula, nasogastric tube, and urine bag.	Hollihesive is a pectin-based barrier that adheres well to the skin but can be gently removed without causing skin excoriations.
	Do not use Hollihesive over a monilial rash.	
	Apply Hollihesive to clean, dry skin that is free of oil or soap residue.	
	Facilitate adherence of Hollihesive by holding it in place for 30 to 60 seconds.	Hollihesive readily molds to contours of the infant's skin.
	3. Remove cardiorespiratory monitor electrodes only when nonfunctional.	Epidermal stripping occurs with removal of adhesives.
	For the very low birth weight infant one of the following options may be used: limb electrodes, water-activated gel electrodes, electrodes that have been trimmed down and secured with a flexible dressing material (such as Kling or Coban).	
	4. Remove adhesives with water-soaked cotton balls.	Adhesive removers (solvents such as Wisk, Dermasol, and Unisolve) are drying to the skin and are combustible; the effects of absorption are unknown.
	5. BenBenzoin is not recommended for routine use.	Benzoin can provide a stronger bond between tape and epidermis than the cohesion between the epidermis and the dermis in preterm skin. The effects of absorption are unknown.
	6. Avoid the use of plasticized polymers (Skin Gel, Skin Prep, and Bard Protective Film).	The effects of absorption are unknown.
Prevent thermal burns	1. Use the lowest effective temperature for the continuous transcutaneous monitor, and change the site every 3 to 4 hours, or more often with the very low birth weight infant.	Minimizing the time and intensity of heat contact with the skin minimizes the degree of thermal burn caused by the electrode.
	2. Avoid direct contact of a heat source with the infant's skin. Heated mattresses or warm water-filled gloves should be covered with a blanket or pillowcase.	Direct contact between a heat source and an infant's skin, especially preterm skin, can result in a thermal burn.
Prevent pressure necrosis	1. Prevent use of constrictive tape or devices that may interfere with circulation.	Preterm infant is especially at risk because of immaturity of the skin and the initial tendency toward edema.
	2. Change the infant's position every 2 hours.	
	3. Use a waterbed or sheepskin to soften the mattress surface.	
Prevent IV infiltrates	1. Use clear tape to secure IVs.	Clear tape facilitates frequent and effective assessment of catheter site.
	2. Assess IV catheter sites at least hourly, and document in patient's record.	This is a standard nursing practice.
	3. IVs should be removed at the first sign of infiltration.	IV infiltrates can decrease circulation to the affected area and promote tissue damage. Many IV chemical substances are caustic to the tissues if deposited interstitially and can cause tissue necrosis and skin sloughing.
Treat skin disruptions	1. Before determining interventions for skin disruptions, determine the cause. Infection may need to be considered.	Infections, such as staphylococcal scalded skin syndrome and yeast infection, may present with massive areas of denuded skin.
	2. Treat excoriations as follows:	
	Cleansing may be done with quarter-strength hydrogen. Sterile water can also be used to cleanse excoriated areas.	Undiluted hydrogen peroxide can cause tissue damage.
	After cleansing the area, exposure to air is recommended.	
	If an antimicrobial ointment is warranted, the use of Polysporin or bacitracin is preferred.	Neomycin, a commonly used antimicrobial ointment, has been shown to increase sensitization and potential for allergic reaction later in life.
	Use of a transparent dressing (such as Op-Site) to serve as a "second skin" may be preferred.	Op-Site is impermeable to water and bacteria and allows moisture and air to flow freely through the surface.
	Op-Site is contraindicated over a monilial rash.	

Procedure continued on following page

NEWBORN SKIN CARE PROTOCOL *Continued*

GOAL	INTERVENTION	RATIONALE
Treat skin disruptions *Continued*	3. Determine the cause of a diaper rash. Most diaper rashes are direct irritant contact dermatitis. Treatment includes exposing the area to light and air. Once healing is under way, protective ointments (zinc oxide or Desitin) may be used to promote further healing and prevent more extensive skin breakdown.	If bacterial or monilial infection is present, appropriate medication is needed.
Minimize insensible water and heat loss	1. Transfer infant to double-walled incubator with servocontrol as soon as possible.	Radiant warmers increase insensible water loss.
	2. Place infant in a heat shield. A Saran "tent" in close proximity to the infant's skin can be used on a radiant warmer or in an incubator. A plastic shield can be used in an incubator.	Heat shields minimize evaporative and convective heat losses.
	3. Maintain relative humidity in the range of 40 to 60% by providing warm humidified air in the infant's environment.	Humidity decreases insensible water loss and evaporative loss.
	The plastic shield or Saran "tent" should be changed every 1 to 3 days.	A warm humidified environment provides a medium for bacterial growth.
	4. Give priority to interventions that maintain skin integrity.	Denuded skin allows a two- to sixfold increase in insensible water loss.
Protect against absorption of topical substances	Evaluate all substances that come in direct contact with the infant's skin. Question the use and amount of such substances.	Topically applied substances are readily absorbed through the infant's skin. This is especially true for the preterm infant, whose increased surface area–to–body weight ratio puts him or her at risk for toxicity from topically applied substances.

From Kuller, J. (1995). Skin care management of the low-birthweight infant. In L. Gunderson & C. Kenner (Eds.), *Care of the 24–25 week gestational age infant* (2nd ed., pp. 136–139). Petaluma, CA: NICU Ink. Reprinted with permission.

REFERENCES

Ackerman, A. (1985). Structure and function of the skin. In S. Moschella & H. Hurley (Eds.), *Dermatology* (Vol. 2, 2nd ed.). Philadelphia: W. B. Saunders Co.

Adamkin, D. (1977). Is the neonate defenseless? *Contemporary Ob-Gyn, 10*, 73–75.

American Academy of Pediatrics. (1974). Skin care of newborns. *Pediatrics, 54*(6), 682–683.

American Academy of Pediatrics. (1977). *Standards and recommendations for hospital care of newborn infants*. Evanston, IL: Author.

Apfelberg, D., Maser, M., & Lash, H. (1978). Argon laser treatment of cutaneous vascular abnormalities. *American Plastic Surgery, 1*(1), 14.

Arndt, K. (1978). *Manual of dermatologic therapeutics* (2nd ed.). Boston: Little, Brown & Co.

Artnak, K., Moore, L., & Clements, C. (1981). Epidermolysis bullosa: An inherited skin disorder. *American Journal of Nursing, 81*(10), 1837–1840.

Avery, G. B., Fletcher, M. A., & MacDonald, M. G. (Eds.) (1994). *Neonatology: Pathophysiology and management of the newborn* (4th ed.). Philadelphia: J. B. Lippincott Co.

Baley, J., & Silverman, R. (1988). Systemic candidiasis: Cutaneous manifestations in low birth weight infants. *Pediatrics, 82*(2), 211–215.

Baley, J. E., Kliegman, R. M., Boxerbaum, B., & Fanaroff, A. A. (1986). Fungal colonization in the very low birth weight infant. *Pediatrics, 78*(2), 225–232.

Baumgart, S. (1982). Radiant energy and insensible water loss in the premature newborn infant nursed under a radiant warmer. *Clinics in Perinatology, 9*(3), 483–503.

Behrendt, H., & Green, M. (1971). *Patterns of skin pH from birth through adolescence*. Springfield, IL: Charles C Thomas Publishers.

Bell, E. F., Weinstein, M. R., & Oh, W. (1980). Heat balance in premature infants: Comparative effects of convectively heated incubator and radiant warmer with and without plastic shield. *Journal of Pediatrics, 96*(3, Part 1), 460–465.

Berg, R. (1987). Etiologic factors in diaper dermatitis: A model for development of improved diapers. *Pediatrician, 14*(1), 27–33.

Berg, R. W., Buckingham, K. W., & Stewart, R. L. (1986). Etiologic factors in diaper dermatitis: The role of urine. *Pediatric Dermatology, 3*(2), 102–106.

Boyle, R. J., & Oh, W. (1980). Erythema following transcutaneous pO2 monitoring. *Pediatrics, 65*(2), 333–334.

Brice, H., Rutter, N., & Hull, D. (1981). Reduction of skin water loss in the newborn: II. Clinical trial of two methods in very low birth-weight babies. *Archives of Disease in Childhood, 56*(9), 673–675.

Brown, A., Hoelzer, D., & Piercy, S. (1979). Skin necrosis from extravasation of intravenous fluids in children. *Plastic and Reconstructive Surgery, 64*(2), 145–150.

Buckingham, K. W., & Berg, R. W. (1986). Etiologic factors in diaper dermatitis: The role of feces. *Pediatric Dermatology, 3*(2), 107–112.

Bustamante, S., & Steslow, J. (1989). Use of a transparent adhesive dressing in very low birthweight infants. *Journal of Perinatology, 9*(2), 165–169.

Campbell, R. L., Seymour, J. L., Stone, L. C., & Milligan, M. C. (1987). Clinical studies with disposable diapers containing absorbent gelling materials: evaluation on infant skin condition. *Journal of the American Academy of Dermatology, 17*(6), 978–987.

Cartlidge, P. H., & Rutter, N. (1987). Karaya gum electrocardiographic electrodes for preterm infants. *Archives of Disease in Childhood, 62*(12), 1281–1282.

Chabrolle, J., & Rossier, A. (1978). Goiter and hypothyroidism in the newborn after cutaneous absorption of iodine. *Archives of Disease in Childhood, 53*(6), 495–498.

Choudhuri, M., McQueen, R., Inoue, S., & Gordon, R. C. (1990). Efficiency of skin sterilization for a venipuncture with the use of commercially available alcohol or iodine pads. *American Journal of Infection Control, 18*(2), 82–85.

Clark, D. (1986) Perinatal infections. In *Pathology of the neonate slide series* (Vol. I, No. 2). Philadelphia: Wyeth-Ayerst Laboratories.

Clark, D., & Thompson, J. (1986). Dermatology of the newborn. Parts 1 and 2. In *Pathology of the neonate slide series* (Vol. III, Nos. 3 and 4). Philadelphia: Wyeth-Ayerst Laboratories.

Collinge, J. M., & Aranda, J. V. (1984). Nonmetabolic complications of neonatal intravenous therapy: Epidemiologic considerations. *American Journal of Perinatology, 1*(2), 185–189.

Cosman, B. (1980). Experience in the argon laser therapy of port wine stains. *Plastic & Reconstructive Surgery, 65*(2), 119–129.

Cowen, J., Ellis, S., & McAinsh, J. (1979). Absorption of chlorhexidine from the intact skin of newborn infants. *Archives of Disease in Childhood, 54*(5), 379–383.

Cunico, R. L., Maibach, H., Khan, H., & Bloom, E. (1977). Skin barrier properties in the newborn: Transepidermal water loss and carbon dioxide emission rate. *Biology of the Neonate, 32*(3-4), 177–182.

Curley A., Kimbrough R. D., Hawk, R. E., et al. (1971). Dermal absorption of hexachlorophene in infants. *Lancet, 2*(719), 296–297.

D'Angio, C. T., McGowan K. L., Baumgart, S., et al. (1989). Surface colonization with coagulase-negative staphylococci in premature neonates. *Journal of Pediatrics, 114*(6), 1029–1034.

Davies J., Babb J. R., & Ayliffe, G. A. (1977). The effect on the skin flora of bathing with antiseptic solutions. *Journal of Antimicrobial Chemotherapy, 3*(5), 473–481.

Davis, J. A., Leyden, J. J., Grove, G. L., & Raynor, W. J. (1989). Comparison of disposable diapers with fluff absorbent and fluff plus absorbent polymers: Effects on skin hydration, skin pH, and diaper dermatitis. *Pediatric Dermatology, 6*(2), 102–108.

Dietel, K. (1978). Morphological and functional development of the skin. In U. Stave (Ed.), *Perinatal physiology* (pp. 761–773). New York: Plenum Press.

Dixon, A. (1987). Think zinc. *Neonatal Network, 5*(4), 29–33.

Elias, P. M. (1983). Epidermal lipids, barrier function and desquamation. *Journal of Investigative Dermatology, 80*, 44S–49S.

Enjolras, O., Riche, M., Merland, J., & Escade, J. (1990). Management of alarming hemangiomas in infancy: A review of 25 cases. *Pediatrics, 85*, 491–498.

Esterly, N. B., & Solomon, L. M. (1995). The skin. In A. A. Fanaroff & R. J. Martin (Eds.), *Neonatal-perinatal medicine: Diseases of the fetus and infant* (5th ed., pp. 1328–1358). St. Louis: C. V. Mosby Co.

Esterly, N., & Spraker, M. (1985). Neonatal skin problems. In S. Moschella & H. Hurley (Eds.), *Dermatology* (Vol. 2, 2nd ed., pp. 1882–1903). Philadelphia: W. B. Saunders Co.

Evans, N. J., & Rutter, N. (1986a). Development of the epidermis in the newborn. *Biology of the Neonate, 49*(2), 74–80.

Evans, N. J., & Rutter, N. (1986b). Reduction of skin damage from transcutaneous oxygen electrodes using a spray on dressing. *Archives of Disease in Childhood, 61*(9), 881–884.

Evans, N., Rutter, N., Hadgraft, J., & Parr, G. (1985). Percutaneous administration of theophylline in the preterm infant. *Journal of Pediatrics, 107*(2), 307–311.

Ezekowitz, R., Mulliken, J., & Folkman, J. (1992). Interferon alfa-2a therapy for life-threatening hemangiomas of infancy. *New England Journal of Medicine, 326*, 1456–1463.

Fisch, R. O., Berglund, E. D., & Bridge, A. G. (1963). Methemoglobinemia in a hospital nursery: A search for causative factors. *Journal of the American Medical Association, 185*, 760–763.

Flemmer, L., & Chan, J. (1993). A pediatric protocol for management of extravasation injuries. *Pediatric Nursing, 19*(4), 355–358.

Freedman, R., & Baltimore, R. (1990). Fatal *Streptococcus viridans* septicemia and meningitis: Relationship to fetal scalp electrode monitoring. *Journal of Perinatology, 10*(3), 272–274.

Friedman, Z. (1980). Essential fatty acids revisited. [Review]. *American Journal of Diseases of Children, 134*(4), 397–408.

Frosch, P. J., & Kligman, A. M. (1979). The soap chamber test: A new method for assessing the irritancy of soaps. *Journal of American Dermatology, 1*(44), 35–41.

Garvin, G. (1990). Wound healing in pediatrics. *Nursing Clinics of North America, 25*(1), 181–192.

Golden, S. M. (1981). Skin craters: A complication of transcutaneous oxygen monitoring. *Pediatrics, 67*(4), 514–516.

Gordon, M., & Montgomery, L. A. (1996). Minimizing epidermal stripping in the very low birth weight infant: Integrating research and practice to affect infant outcome. *Neonatal Network, 15*(1), 37–44.

Hammarlund, K., & Sedin, G. (1979). Transepidermal water loss in newborn infants: Relation to gestational age. *Acta Paediatrica Scandinavica 68*(6), 759–801.

Harmon, J., & Steele, S. (1975). *Nursing care of the skin: A developmental approach*. New York: Appleton-Century-Crofts.

Harpin, V. A., & Rutter, N. (1983). Barrier properties of the newborn infant's skin. *Journal of Pediatrics, 102*(3), 419–425.

Harpin, V., & Rutter, N. (1982). Percutaneous alcohol absorption and skin necrosis in a preterm infant. *Archives of Disease in Childhood, 57*(6), 477–479.

Hey, E. N., & Katz, G. (1969). Evaporative water loss in the newborn baby. *Journal of Physiology, 200*(3), 605–619.

Hey, E., & Scopes, J. W. (1987). Thermoregulation in the newborn. In G. B. Avery (Ed.), *Neonatology, pathophysiology, and management of the newborn* (pp. 201–211). Philadelphia: J. B. Lippincott Co.

Holbrook, K. A. (1982). A histological comparison of infant and adult skin. In H. I. Maibach & E. K. Boisits (Eds.), *Neonatal skin: Structure and function* (pp. 3–31). New York: Marcel Dekker.

Hutchinson, J. H., Kerr, M. M., William, K. A., & Hopkinson, W. I. (1963). Hyperbaric oxygen in the resuscitation of the newborn. *Lancet, 2*, 1019–1022.

Hymes, D. (1983). Epidermolysis bullosa in the neonate. *Neonatal Network, 1*(4), 36–39.

Jackson, H. J., & Sutherland, R. H. (1981). Effect of povidine- iodine on neonatal thyroid function. *Lancet, 2*(8253), 992.

Jones, K. L. (1988). *Smith's recognizable patterns of human malformations* (4th ed.). Philadelphia: W. B. Saunders Co.

Kjartansson, S., Arsan, S., Hammarlund, K., Sjörs, G., & Sedin, G. (1995). Water loss from the skin of term and preterm infants nursed under a radiant heater. *Pediatric Research, 37*(2), 233–238.

Klaus, M. H., & Fanaroff, A. A. (1987). *Yearbook of perinatal/neonatal medicine*. Chicago: Year Book Medical Publishers.

Knauth, A., Gordin, M., McNelis, W., & Baumgart, S. (1989). Semipermeable polyurethane membrane as an artificial skin for the premature neonate. *Pediatrics, 83*, 945– 950.

Kopelman, A. E. (1973). Cutaneous absorption of hexachlorophene in low-birth weight infants. *Journal of Pediatrics, 82*(6), 972–975.

Korones, S. (1986). *High-risk newborn infants* (4th ed.). St. Louis: C. V. Mosby Co.

Korones, S., & Bada-Ellzey, H. (1993). (pp. 44–45). Maintenance of fluid. In *Neonatal decision making*. St. Louis: B. C. Decker.

Kuller, J. (1990). Assessment and management of integumentary dysfunction. In M. Auvenshine & M. Enriquez (Eds.), *Comprehensive maternity nursing: Perinatal and women's health* (2nd ed.). Boston: Jones & Bartlett Publishers.

Kuller, J. (1995). Skin care management of the low-birthweight infant. In L. P. Gunderson & C. Kenner (Eds.), *Care of the 24–25 week gestational age infant*. (2nd ed.) Petaluma, CA: NICU Ink.

Laurie, S., Wilson, K., Kernahan, D., et al. (1984). Intravenous extravasation injuries: The effectiveness of hyaluronidase in their treatment. *Annals of Plastic Surgery, 13*(3), 191–194.

LeBlanc, H. (1991). Thermoregulation: Incubators, radiant warmers, artificial skins, and body hoods. *Clinics in Perinatology, 18*(3), 403–422.

Lefrak, L. (1984). Nutrition and its effects on the skin. *Neonatal Network, 3*(3), 36–39.

Leydon, J. J., Katz, S., Stewart, R., & Kligman, A. M. (1977). Urinary ammonia and ammonia-producing micro-organisms in infants with and without diaper dermatitis. *Archives of Dermatology, 113*(12), 1678–1680.

Leydon, J. J. (1984). Cornstarch, *Candida albicans* and diaper rash. *Pediatric Dermatology, 1*(4), 322–325.

Lo, J. S., Oriba, H. A., Maibach, H. I., & Bailin, P. L. (1990). Transepidermal potassium ion, chloride ion, and water flux across delipidized and cellophane tape-stripped skin. *Dermatologica, 180*(2), 66–68.

Loper, D. (1992). The integumentary system. In S. Blackburn, & D. Loper (Eds.), *Maternal physiology*, (pp. 491–521). Philadelphia: W. B. Saunders Co.

Lorenz, J. M., Kleinman, L., Kotagal, U. R., & Reller, M. D. (1982). Water balance in very low-birth-weight infants: Relationship to water and sodium intake and effect on outcome. *Journal of Pediatrics, 101*(3), 423–432.

Lund, C., Kuller, J., Tobin, C., & Lefrak, L. (1986). Evaluation of a pectin-based barrier under tape to protect neonatal skin. *Journal of Obstetric, Gynecologic, and Neonatal Nursing, 15*(1), 39–44.

Mancini, A., Sookdeo-Drost, S., Madison, K., et al. (1994). Semipermeable dressings improve epidermal barrier function in premature infants. *Pediatric Research, 36*, 306–314.

Margileth, A. M. (1994). Dermatologic conditions. In G. Avery, M. A. Fletcher, & M. G. MacDonald (Eds.), *Neonatology: Pathophysiology and management of the newborn* (4th ed, pp. 1229–1268). Philadelphia: J. B. Lippincott Co.

McGowan, K. L. (1990). Air shields. *Microbiological Clinical Test Results.* Philadelphia: The Children's Hospital of Philadelphia.

Montagna, W., Van Scott, E., & Stoughton, R. (1972). *Advances in the biology of the skin: Vol. XII. Pharmacology and the skin.* New York: Appleton-Century-Crofts.

Montagu, A. (1971). *Touching: The human significance of skin.* New York: Columbia University Press.

Moore, K. L., & Persaud, T. V. N. (1993). *Before we are born: Basic embryology and birth defects* (5th ed.). Philadelphia: W. B. Saunders Co.

Morad, A. B., McClain, K. L., & Ogden, A. K. (1993). The role of transexamic acid in the treatment of giant hemangiomas in newborns [Review]. *American Journal of Pediatric Hematology-Oncology, 15*(4), 383–385.

Morelli, J. G., & Weston, W. L. (1987). Soaps and shampoos in pediatric practice [Review]. *Pediatrics, 80*(5), 634– 637.

Moschella, S., & Hurley, H. (1985). *Dermatology* (Vol. 2, 2nd ed.). Philadelphia: W. B. Saunders Co.

Nachman, R. L., & Esterly, N. B. (1971). Increased skin permeability in preterm infants. *Journal of Pediatrics, 79*(4), 628–632.

Nasemann, T., Sauerbrey, W., & Burgdorf, W. (1983). *Fundamentals of dermatology.* New York: Springer- Verlag.

National Committee for Clinical Laboratory Standards. (1986). *Procedures for the collection of diagnostic blood specimens by skin puncture* (2nd ed.). Approved standard (NCCLS Publication No. H4-A2). Villanova, PA: Author.

Nonato, L., & Guy, R. (1995). *Light and transmission electron microscopy: Developmental changes in neonatal skin structure.* Unpublished manuscript.

Patrick, C. (1990). Coagulase-negative staphylococci: Pathogens with increasing clinical significance [Review]. *Journal of Pediatrics, 116*(4), 497–507.

Patrick, C. C., Kaplan, S. L., Baker, C. J., et al. (1989). Persistent bacteremia due to coagulase-negative staphylococci in premature neonates. *Pediatrics, 84*(6), 977–985.

Peck, S., & Botwinick, J. (1964). The buffering capacity of infants' skin against an alkaline soap and neutral detergent. *Journal of Mt. Sinai Hospital, 31*, 134–137.

Potts, R. O., Buras, E. M., Jr., & Chrisman, D. A., Jr. (1984). Changes with age in the moisture content of human skin. *Journal of Investigational Dermatology, 82*(1), 97–100.

Pyati, S., Ramamurthy, R., Krauss, M. T., & Pildes, R. (1977). Absorption of iodine in the neonate following topical use of povidone-iodine. *Journal of Pediatrics, 91*(5), 825–828.

Rasmussen, J. (1987). Classification of diaper dermatitis: An overview. *Pediatrician, 14*(1), 6–10.

Rathburn, A. M., Holland, L. A., & Geelhoed, G. N. (1986). Preoperative skin decontamination: A study on efficiency and effect. *AORN Journal, 44*(1), 62–65.

Rosen, T., Lanning M., & Hill, M. (1983). *The nurses' atlas to dermatology.* Boston: Little, Brown & Co.

Rutter, N., & Hull, D. (1979). Water loss from the skin of term and preterm babies. *Archives of Disease in Childhood, 54*(11), 858–868.

Rutter, N., & Hull, D. (1981). Reduction of skin water loss in the newborn: I. Effect of applying topical agents. *Archives of Disease in Childhood, 56*(9), 669–672.

Sarkany, I., & Arnold, L. (1970). The effect of single and repeated applications of hexachlorophene on the bacterial flora of the skin of the newborn. *British Journal of Dermatology, 82*(3), 261–267.

Schick, J. B., & Milstein, J. M. (1981). Burn hazard of isopropyl alcohol in the neonate. *Pediatrics, 68*(4), 587–588.

Sedin, G., Hammarlund, K., Nilsson, G. E., et al. (1985). Measurements of transepidermal water loss in newborn infants. *Clinics in Perinatology, 12*(1), 79–99.

Shalita, A. (1981). *Principles of infant skin care.* Skillman, NJ: Johnson & Johnson Baby Products Company.

Silverman, W. A., Agate, F. J., & Ferwig, J. W. (1963). A sequential trial of the nonthermal effect of atmospheric humidity on survival of human infants of low birth weight. *Pediatrics, 31*, 710–724.

Silverman, W. A. (1957). Effect of humidity on survival of newly born premature infants. *Pediatrics 20*, 447.

Solomon, L., & Esterly, N. (1973). Neonatal dermatology. In A. Schaffer (Ed.), *Major problems in clinical pediatrics* (Vol. IX). Philadelphia: W. B. Saunders Co.

Sulyok, E., Jequier, E., & Ryser, G. (1972). Effect of relative humidity on thermal balance of the newborn infant. *Biologia Neonatorum, 21*, 210–218.

Tagami, H., & Yoshikuni, K. (1985). Interrelationship between water-barrier and reservoir functions of pathologic stratum corneum. *Archives of Dermatology, 121*(5), 642–645.

Tagami, H., Kanamaru, Y., Inoue, K., et al. (1982). Water sorption-desorption test of the skin in vivo for functional assessment of the stratum corneum. *Journal of Investigative Dermatology, 78*(5), 425–428.

Thomas, K. (1994). Thermoregulation in neonates. *Neonatal Network 13*(2), 15–22.

Thune, P., Nilsen, T., Hanstad, K., et al. (1988). The water barrier function of the skin in relation to the water content of stratum corneum, pH and skin lipids: The effect of alkaline soap and syndet on dry skin in elderly, non-atopic patients. *Acta Dermato-Venereologica, 68*(4), 277–283.

Tupker, R. A., Pinnagoda, J., & Nater, J. P. (1990a). The transient and cumulative effect of sodium lauryl sulfate on the epidermal barrier assessed by transepidermal water loss: Inter-individual variation. *Acta Dermato-Venereologica, 70*(1), 1–5.

Tupker, R. A., Pinnagoda, J., Coenraads, P. J., & Nater, J. P. (1990b). Evaluation of detergent-induced irritant skin reactions by visual scoring and transepidermal water loss measurement. *Dermatologic Clinics, 8*(1), 33–35.

Upton, J., Milliken, J., & Murray, J. (1979). Major intravenous extravasation injuries. *American Journal of Surgery, 137*, 497–506.

Vernon, H. J., Lane, A. T., Wischerath, L. J., et al. (1990). Semipermeable dressing and transepidermal water loss in premature infants. *Pediatrics, 86*(3), 357–362.

Walton, R. (1971). Pigmented nevi. *Pediatric Clinics of North America, 18*(3), 897–922.

Watson, W. (1978). Selected genodermatoses. [Review]. *Pediatric Clinics of North America, 25*(2), 263–284.

West, D. P., Worobec, S., & Solomon, L. M. (1981). Pharmacology and toxicology of infant skin. *Journal of Investigative Dermatology, 76*(3), 147–150.

Wester, R., & Maibach, H. (1982). Comparative percutaneous toxicity. In H. I. Maibach & E. K. Boisits (Eds.), *Neonatal skin: Structure and function* (pp. 137–148). New York: Marcel Dekker.

Wheldon, A. E., & Hull, D. (1983). Incubation of very immature infants. *Archives of Disease in Childhood, 58*(7), 504–508.

Wilhelm, K. P., & Maibach, H. I. (1990). Factors predisposing to cutaneous irritation. [Review]. *Dermatologic Clinics, 8*(1), 17–22.

Zenk, K. (1981). Management of intravenous extravasations. *Infusion, 5*(4), 77–79.

Zenk, K., & Sills, J. (1986). Management of dopamine-induced perivascular blanching and extravasation in LBW infants. *Journal of Perinatology, 6*(1), 82.

Ziai, M., Clark, T., & Merritt, T. (1984). *Assessment of the newborn.* Boston: Little, Brown & Co.

Zimmerman, A., Hambidge, K. M., Lepow, M. L., et al. (1982). Acrodermatitis in breast-fed premature infants: Evidence for a defect in mammary gland zinc secretion. *Pediatrics, 69*(2), 176– 183.

Zlotkin, S. H., & Buchanan, B. E. (1983). Meeting zinc and copper intake requirements in the parenterally fed preterm and full-term infant. *Journal of Pediatrics, 103*(13), 441–446.

RESOURCES

ALOPECIA AREATA

National Alopecia Areata Foundation (NAAF)
714 C Street
Suite 216
San Rafael, California 94901
(415) 456-4644
Vicki Kalabokes, Executive Director

CONGENITAL PORT-WINE STAIN

National Congenital Port-Wine Stain Foundation
125 East 63rd Street
New York, New York 10021
(212) 755-3820
Martha Woodhouse, Executive Director

ECTODERMAL DYSPLASIAS

National Foundation for Ectodermal Dysplasias (NFED)
108 North First Street
Suite 311
Mascoutah, Illinois 62558
(618) 566-2020
Mary Kaye Richter, Executive Director
Contact: Beverly Meier

EPIDERMOLYSIS BULLOSA

Dystrophic Epidermolysis Bullosa Research Association of America, Inc. (D.E.B.R.A.)
c/o Kings County Medical Center
451 Clarkson Avenue
Building E-6-101
Sixth Floor
Brooklyn, New York 11203
(718) 774-8700
Arlene Pessar, R.N., Executive Director

ICHTHYOSIS

Foundation for Ichthyosis and Related Skin Types, Inc.
(F.I.R.S.T.)
3640 Grand Avenue
Suite Two
Oakland, California 94610
(415) 763-9839
Charles Elchhorn, Executive Director

SCLERODERMA

United Scleroderma Foundation, Inc. (USF)
P.O. Box 350
Watsonville, California 95077--0350
(800) 722-HOPE
(408) 728-2202
Diana Williams, Executive Director

XERODERMA PIGMENTOSUM

Xeroderma Pigmentosum Registry
UMDNJ–NJ Medical School
Department of Pathology
Medical Science Building
Room C-520
100 Bergen Street
Newark, New Jersey 07103
(201) 456-6255
W. Clark Lambert, MD, Executive Director

CHAPTER 33

Assessment and Management of Auditory Dysfunction

KATHLEEN HAUBRICH

RESEARCH AGENDA

What are the risk factors associated with neonatal hearing loss?

What is the relationship between neonatal hearing loss of any degree and later school behavioral problems?

What is the effect of music in the incubator on heart and respiratory rates?

What is the response to in utero auditory stimuli and neonatal auditory testing?

What factors have an impact on otologic problems in infants with Down syndrome?

VIGNETTE

I first met Kevin when he was only 10 hours old. I had received a call from the clinical specialist on the hospital's family unit. She informed me that a baby had been born the previous day with a bilateral complete cleft lip and palate, and she wanted me to provide the infant's parents with information and support. On the basis of the information in the baby's chart, it appeared that Kevin had an isolated craniofacial defect that was not associated with any syndrome or other systemic problems.

When I arrived at Mrs. T's room, she and her husband were trying to get acquainted with their new baby. Mr. and Mrs. T were initially surprised at a visit from a speech–language pathologist, but I explained that I had been called to answer some of the questions they may have about Kevin's lip and palate.

The pediatrician had provided a basic explanation of the defect, and the nursing staff had already begun instructing the parents in special feeding techniques, but they still had many questions and concerns. In addition to their insecurity about feeding and caring for Kevin, Mrs. T became tearful as she expressed her concern over how Kevin would be accepted by his 2-year-old sister, grandparents, and all other family members and friends. I explained that Kevin would likely undergo the first stage of his lip repair in just a few weeks. I added that we were fortunate to have a multidisciplinary craniofacial anomaly team that would guide them through the long process that lay ahead. The team would provide them with any support services they would need.

Besides their concerns about Kevin's appearance and surgical management, Mr. and Mrs. T questioned how Kevin would learn to talk. We discussed the importance of providing Kevin with the same kind of rich language environment they had given their first child. I explained to them that although Kevin's speech may be delayed or affected by the palatal defect, his language should develop normally. We briefly discussed the otologic problems that are frequently associated with palatal clefts and the need for careful monitoring of his hearing through routine screenings. Although there was no way to anticipate Kevin's individual speech problems at the time, his hearing would be screened through auditory brain stem response testing before he left the hospital. The results of this screening would be shared with both Kevin's parents and his pediatrician.

I gave the parents some literature from the Cleft Palate Foundation and recommended that they use this as a resource in the future. I also encouraged them to contact a speech–language pathologist with questions or for future guidance regarding Kevin's speech and language development.

Robin Roe
Cynthia DeAngelis

Hearing is a prerequisite to cognitive, social, and emotional development. Any impairment of hearing from birth to 18 months can have a profound effect on the auditory stimulation necessary for language development. Sensory deprivation affects the acquisition of communication skills, even though correction of the hearing loss may be accomplished. The effect is approximately proportional to the amount of deprivation and is inversely proportional to the age at which the deprivation occurred; the infant with a total hearing loss is more affected than the adult with a minor loss (Ruben, 1984).

The importance of early identification of hearing impairment in the neonate has been well documented in the literature (Allen & Capute, 1986; Moeller et al., 1986; Osberger, 1986). In a study of childhood language development and academic achievement, Osberger and associates (1986) reported that hearing impairment has a significant impact on the future development of the child. These investigators further substantiated earlier findings by reporting that children with a hearing impairment demonstrated limited speech-production skills. Moeller and associates (1986) and Osberger (1986) looked at another aspect of childhood development—namely, receptive and expressive language skills—and found that children with a hearing impairment demonstrated a significant delay in the development of these skills. Allen and Capute (1986) studied academic achievement in language-related areas, and their findings supported earlier reports that demonstrated reduced academic achievement in hearing-impaired children.

To prevent or minimize the detrimental effects of hearing impairment on social, cognitive, and educational development, hearing impairment must be identified at the earliest possible time. Reliable data on the incidence of hearing loss in infants and young children are difficult to obtain. National statistics indicate that of the approximately 3.76 million children born each year, 7 to 12 percent are at risk for hearing impairment (Mahoney & Eichwald, 1987). Moderate-to-profound hearing impairment is reported to be present in fewer than 2 percent of infants at risk (Mahoney & Eichwald, 1987). Approximately one in 100 infants has been reported to be born deaf at birth (Early Identification of Hearing Impairment in Infants and Young Children, National Institutes of Health Consensus Development Conference, 1993).

In spite of the sequelae of auditory impairment in infants and young children, the average age for identification of hearing impairment in the United States is 3 years, well past the critical age for speech and language development.

The Early Identification of Hearing Impairment in Infants and Young Children, National Institutes of Health Consensus Development Conference (1993) on early identification of hearing impairment in infants and young children concluded that all infants should be screened for hearing impairment. This conclusion is based on two premises, first, advances in technology have led to improved screening methods, and second, current criteria fail to identify 50 to 70 percent of children born with an impairment. Current practice, however, dictates that only infants identified with one or more risk factors be screened for hearing impairment.

Assessment and management of auditory dysfunction present a challenge to nurses committed to the welfare of the neonate. The intent of this chapter is to describe a comprehensive nursing approach that identifies current practice as well as future trends and management of infants at risk for hearing impairment.

AUDITORY DEVELOPMENT AND MECHANISM OF FUNCTION

A basic understanding of the embryologic development of the ear is essential to the early identification and management of hearing loss. By understanding the developmental timetable of the various structures and the relationship of the processes to the final structure, the nurse can apply estimates of developmental deviations and of the association of hearing loss with other disorders that may cluster with an auditory abnormality. For example, if an assessment of a malformation of pinna formation is found, on physical examination of the newborn, then malformation of the ossicles in the middle ear may also be suspected because both structures develop simultaneously. A chronologic timetable of the important events in the development of the ear is given in Table 33–1.

Embryology

The ear is a singular organ that functions in both hearing and equilibrium. In the embryo, the ear develops from three different parts.

Internal Ear

The internal ear is the first area of the ear to develop in the embryo. As early as the fourth week of gestation, a thickening of the surface ectoderm on the sides of the rhombencephalon appears as the otic placodes. Each otic placode invaginates to the underlying mesenchyma of the surface ectoderm, eventually forming an otic pit. The periphery of the otic pit fuses to form the otic vesicle, which is the rudimentary membranous labyrinth.

As the otic vesicle loses its connection with the surface ectoderm, a diverticulum develops from the otic vesicle and lengthens to form the endolymphatic duct. The dorsal portion of the otic vesicle gives rise to the semicircular canals of the utricle and the endolymphatic duct. A ventral component gives rise to the saccule and the cochlear duct.

Diverticula extend from the utricular portion of the membranous labyrinth. Central portions eventually fuse and disappear. Peripheral portions of the diverticula eventually become the semicircular canals.

Ampullae develop at the end of each semicircular duct, with the sensory nerve ending differentiating in the specific regions. Cells of the ampulla form a crest; the crista ampullaris contains cells for the maintenance of equilibrium. Sensory areas of the utricle and the saccule, known as maculae acousticae, develop similarly. Impulses generated from these areas are transmitted to the brain by the eighth cranial nerve.

By the sixth week of gestation, the ventral saccule of the otic vesicle forms an outpouching at its lower end that is known as the cochlear duct, which grows in a spiral fashion to form the cochlea. A narrow pathway remains between the saccule and the cochlea, the ductus reuniens.

Mesenchyma surrounding the cochlear duct differentiates into a cartilaginous shell that gives rise to the formation of vacuoles and two perilymphatic spaces, the scala vestibuli and the scala tympani. Further differentiation within the cochlear duct is then accomplished through separation of the scala vestibuli by the vestibular membrane, and of the scala tympani by the basilar membrane. Lateral walls of the cochlear duct remain attached to the surrounding cartilage by the spiral ligament.

Epithelial cells of the cochlear duct further develop to form two ridges, an inner ridge and an outer ridge. The outer ridge forms hair cells, which are the sensory cells of the auditory system. Hair cells are covered by the tectorial membrane. The sensory cells and tectorial membrane are called the spiral organ of Corti. Impulses are transmitted by the organ of Corti to the spiral ganglion and then to the nervous system by the auditory fibers of the eighth cranial nerve.

By the 20th to 22nd week of gestation, the internal ear reaches its adult size and shape.

Middle Ear

The tympanic cavity is derived from the first pharyngeal pouch. The distal portion of the pouch, the tubotympanic recess, widens to become the primitive tympanic cavity, and the proximal end narrows to form the auditory, or eustachian, tube.

The malleus and the incus develop from the cartilage of the first pharyngeal arch, and the stapes develops from the second arch. During the first half of fetal life, the ossicles are embedded in mesenchyma until the tissue dissolves. Endodermal lining of the tympanic cavity extends into the new developing space. With the ossicles free from the surrounding mesenchyma, the endodermal epithelium connects them to the wall of the cavity. Ligaments that support these ossicles are developed from mesenteries.

The tympanic cavity expands dorsally to form the mastoid antrum by the formation of vacuoles. The mastoid antrum is well developed in the newborn; however, there are no mastoid cells present. Mastoid cells are well developed by 2 years of age and produce projections called mastoid processes.

External Ear

The external ear develops around the first branchial groove. The meatal plug is derived as the ectodermal cells form a funnel-

TABLE 33–1 Embryology Summary of the Ear

Fetal Week	Inner Ear	Middle Ear	External Ear
3rd	Auditory placode; auditory pit	Tubotympanic recess begins to develop	
4th	Auditory vesicle (otocyst); vestibular-cochlear division		Tissue thickenings begin to form
5th			Primary auditory meatus begins
6th	Utricle and saccule present; semicircular canals begin		Six hillocks evident; cartilage begins to form
7th	One cochlear coil present; sensory cells in utricle and saccule		Auricles move dorsolaterally
8th	Ductus reuniens present: sensory cells in semicircular canals	Incus and malleus present in cartilage; lower half of tympanic cavity formed	Outer cartilaginous third of external canal formed
9th		Three tissue layers at tympanic membrane present	
11th	Two and one-half cochlear coils present; nerve VIII attaches to cochlear duct		
12th	Sensory cells in cochlea; membranous labyrinth complete; otic capsule begins to ossify		
15th		Cartilaginous stapes formed	
16th		Ossification of malleus and incus begins	
18th		Stapes begins to ossify	
20th	Maturation of inner ear; inner ear adult size		Auricle in adult shape but continues to grow until age 9
21st		Meatal plug disintegrates, exposing tympanic membrane	
30th		Pneumatization of tympanum	External auditory canal continues to mature until age 7
32nd		Malleus and incus complete ossification	
34th		Mastoid air cells develop	
35th		Antrum is pneumatized	
37th		Epitympanum is pneumatized; stapes continues to develop until adulthood; tympanic membrane changes relative position during first 2 yr of life	

From Northern, J., & Downs, M. (1984). *Hearing in children.* Baltimore: Williams & Wilkins. Reprinted with permission.

shaped tube. Central cells of the meatal plug degenerate to form a cavity known as the external auditory meatus.

The tympanic membrane is derived from the first branchial membrane. As embryonic development continues, the mesenchyma separates two parts of the branchial membrane that later develops into two layers of fiber in the tympanic membrane. The external covering of the tympanic membrane is derived from the surface ectoderm, and the internal lining is derived from the endoderm of the tympanic recess.

The auricle, or pinna, is derived from six mesenchymal swellings known as auricular hillocks around the first branchial groove. Mesenchyma in the hillock is derived from mesoderm in the first and second branchial arches. The lobule of the auricle is the last part to develop.

STRUCTURE OF THE EAR

The ear is the anatomic unit involved in hearing and equilibrium. The ear consists of three parts: the external, the middle, and the inner ear. The external ear is composed of the auricle (pinna) and the external ear canal (Fig. 33–1). A complex cartilage framework gives structure to the auricle. Because of this anatomic position, the auricle is susceptible to trauma from external forces. The external ear canal is curved posterosuperiorly and anteromedially. The shape of the canal is oval, and the long axis is positioned superorinferiorly. Normally, the outer portion of the canal is cartilaginous, and the medial portion is bony. Before 34 weeks' gestation, the pinna is a slightly formed, cartilage-free double thickness of skin. In the newborn, however, most of the canal is cartilaginous and collapsed. But as ear development ensues, the cartilage becomes more firm, making the outer two thirds of the canal more patent. Cerumen glands and tiny hairs are present in the outer portion of the cartilaginous canal. The medial two thirds of the canal lies immediately over a bony area and is referred to as the osseous region. The auditory meatus assumes an irregular path from the concha to the tympanic membrane.

At the termination of the external canal is the eardrum, or tympanic membrane, which forms the boundary between the outer and the middle ear (Fig. 33–2). It is a complicated shape, loosely resembling a flat cone, that moves with changes in air

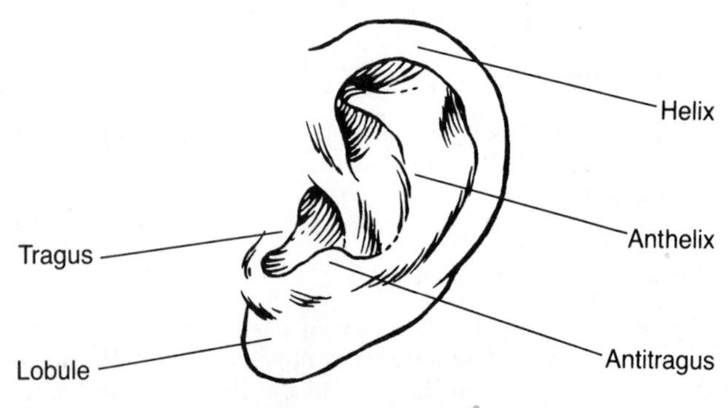

FIGURE 33–1. External ear.

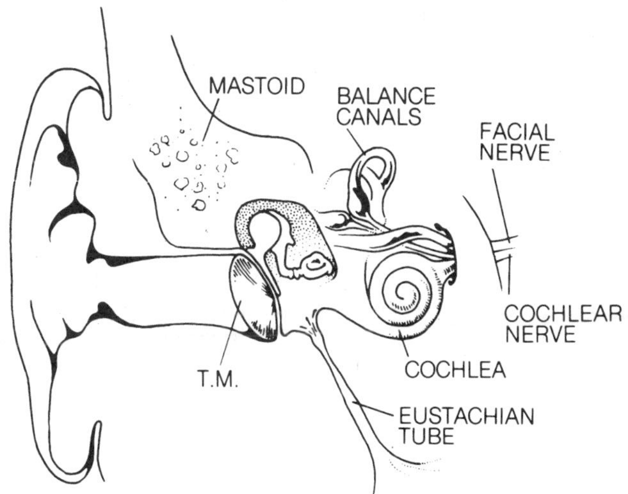

FIGURE 33–2. General framework of the outer, middle, and inner ear. T.M., tympanic membrane. (From Pappas, D. [1985]. *Diagnosis and treatment of hearing impairment in children* [p. 6]. San Diego, CA: College-Hill Press. Reprinted with permission.)

pressure. The tympanic membrane is oval and translucent, so middle ear structure can often be visualized through it. Short and long processes of the malleus are attached to the fibrous layer of the tympanic membrane and are visible on the lateral surface. The middle ear cavity is an air-filled space connected by an air cell system posteriorly to the mastoid and by the eustachian tube anteriorly to the nasopharynx. Neither of these communications is in a dependent position for drainage of fluids. Ciliated columnar cells cover the walls of the tympanic cavity and mastoid air cells. Secretory cells are distributed throughout the middle ear, with the greatest number being present in the eustachian tube. In the middle ear region, the malleus, incus, and stapes occupy the region between the tympanic membrane and the oval window of the middle ear. During otoscopic examination, the long process of the incus can often be seen through the tympanic membrane.

The stapedius and the tensor muscles of the tympanic membrane attach in the middle ear to the malleus and the stapes by tendons. The chorda tympani nerve passes across the posterior surface. The medial wall of the middle ear cavity contains the oval and the round windows. Between the oval and the round windows, the lower portion of the cochlea forms a prominence known as the promontorium tympani on the medial wall of the middle ear.

The inner ear consists of a bony labyrinth composed of three parts: the semicircular canals, the vestibule, and the cochlea. These hollow spaces are surrounded by a dense, bony capsule in the petrous protein of the temporal bone; this capsule contains perilymph and endolymph. Each of the semicircular canals has a dilated portion at the end, referred to as ampullae, which contain the crista ampullaris, a vestibular sense organ. Within the vestibule, the utricle and saccules are formed. The utricle and saccules contain sensory endings for equilibrium.

The cochlea is a tubular structure that has 2½ spirals; the structure closely resembling that of a snail shell, with a base and an apex. The cochlea is divided into the scala vestibuli and the scala tympani. The two tracts connect at the apex. The scala vestibuli begins at the oval window, and the scala tympani terminates at the round window. The basilar membrane side of the duct gives rise to the organ of Corti, the organ of hearing. The organ of Corti includes hair cells and supporting cells; attached to the hair cells is a gelatinous membrane called the tectorial membrane.

The membranous labyrinth of the inner ear is composed of connective tissue filled with endolymph that forms within the bony labyrinth. Hair cells of the cochlea and the vestibular labyrinth are attached by afferent nerve fibers to the neurons of the auditory system, the spiral ganglion, and the Scarpa ganglion in the temporal bone. Efferent nerve fibers from ganglia form the auditory and vestibular division of the eighth nerve and exit the temporal bone on its posterior surface to enter the brain stem.

PHYSIOLOGY OF AUDIOLOGIC FUNCTION

External Ear

The external ear consists of the auricle (pinna) and the external auditory meatus (external canal). The primary function of the external ear is to funnel sound to the tympanic membrane. Absence of the auricle contributes to difficulty in sound localization.

Middle Ear

Advancing sound entering the auditory canal directly strikes the tympanic membrane. The tympanic membrane and the ossicles serve as transmitters from the outer ear to the inner ear. The malleus, which is continuous with the tympanic membrane and is connected with the incus and stapes, moves the ossicles. Ossicles transfer sound energy into the inner ear through the oval window, which holds the stapes by means of an angular ligament.

The middle ear is lined by respiratory mucosa that is composed of ciliated columnar epithelial cells, supporting cells, and secretory cells. Secretory cells secrete mucus that forms a complex mucous layer. Cilia of the middle ear interact with the mucus by transporting mastoid and middle ear secretions through the eustachian tube to the nasopharynx, where they are swallowed. This mechanism is known as the mucociliary transport system. Glycoproteins in the mucus determine the viscosity and elasticity of the middle ear mucus. Mucus that is too thick or too thin impedes effective transport of bacteria and cellular debris from the mastoid and middle ear cleft. This transport has a protective effect against ear infections. In addition to being an exit for secretion into the nasopharynx, the eustachian tube equalizes the pressure between the middle ear and the ambient atmosphere.

Inner Ear

Before this point in the hearing mechanism, all of the sound energy is contained in the air-filled spaces of the external and middle ear. From the stapes onward, the pathway for sound takes place in fluid-filled spaces. When sound is transferred from the tympanic membrane to the inner ear, the stapes creates a fluid wave that is transmitted to the round window. This transmission creates fluid waves that travel from the basal aspect of the cochlea to the apex. As the fluid wave moves, it displaces the basilar membrane. A maximum movement of the basilar membrane exists at the point that is specific to the frequency of sound entering the ear. High-frequency sounds cause minimal disturbance at the basal end of the cochlea, and low-frequency sounds cause minimal disturbance at the apex.

Vibrations within the basilar membrane cause movement of the organ of Corti. This organ contains receptor hair cells that are on the basilar membrane. Vibrations of the hair on the hair cells cause either polarization or depolarization, depending on the direction of the bend. When sufficient depolarization occurs, action potentials are produced that are propagated along the auditory pathway to the auditory cortex. The cochlea provides input by coding information about loudness and frequency in the action potentials that are sent to the cortex, giving meaning to the sound. Hair cells of the spiral organ of Corti are stimulated as they touch the tectorial membrane. Hair cells act as transducers, converting mechanical energy into electrical impulses in the fibers of the spiral ganglion. Axons of these cells become the auditory nerve (vestibulocochlear nerve). Nerve fibers pass to the medulla, the pons, and the midbrain, and finally to the temporal lobes of the cortex, where the impulses are interpreted as sound.

The vestibular system is similar to the auditory system. Fluid moves within the vestibular labyrinth when the head moves. The semicircular canals respond to angular acceleration (rotation), and the utricle and saccule respond to linear acceleration (position). Movement of endolymph places forces on the hairs of the sensory cells of the cristae and the maculae. Depolarization of the sensory cells produces action potentials that are transmitted to the vestibular cortex. The vestibular apparatus functions in conjunction with proprioception and visual orientation to maintain balance.

PERINATAL AUDITORY DEVELOPMENT

There is increasing evidence that the fetus can perceive auditory stimulation and act on it at an early age. This evidence comes from investigation of fetal heart rate responses to sounds and from studies of audition in preterm infants. A study by Johansson et al., (1964), using high-frequency pure tones presented by microphone to the uterus, elicited a fetal heart rate acceleration response in the fetus as early as the 20th week of gestation. Elliot and Elliot (1964) reported that physiologically, the cochlea has normal function by the 20th week of pregnancy. A study by Rotteveel and colleagues (1987) reported that auditory, brain stem, middle latency, and cortical responses emerge at about 25 weeks of conceptual age. Further maturation of the nerve fibers continues well into the first year of life. These reports suggest that the newborn has been hearing sounds within the fluid-filled environment for many months before birth.

Other researchers have attempted to positively correlate fetal response to acoustic stimulation as an indicator of fetal well-being. Goodlin and Schmidt (1972) reported that auditory stimulation evoked various arousal levels in the fetus. Elicitation of auditory arousal levels was used to predict fetal well-being and subsequent fetal outcome. Further studies, by Read and Miller (1977), compared the use of an antepartum surveillance tool, the oxytocin challenge test, to fetal acoustic stimulation. Acoustic stimulation was found to be as reliable an indication of fetal status as the oxytocin challenge test in predicting pregnancies at risk for antepartal distress and fetal demise. Grimwade and associates (1971) reported changes in the fetal heart rate in response to low-frequency stimuli presented via a speaker placed in the birth canal.

Vibroacoustic stimulation by use of an artificial larynx attached to the mother's abdomen has been reported to test well-being in the fetus. Jensen (1984) found that impaired response to stimulation correlated with severity of hypoxia and was of greater predictive value than a nonreactive nonstress test in predicting a compromised fetus.

Although reproducible, the clinical applications of such work are still considered tentative. Lack of uniformity in research methodologies makes it difficult to determine the predictive value that acoustic stimulation has in measuring fetal well-being (Gagnon, 1989).

With implanted microphones in the uterine cavity, Querleu and colleagues (1981) observed seven patients at term. External speech was recorded within the uterus, and 64 percent of the mother's and 57 percent of the father's phonemes were recognizable. Other studies by Querleu and colleagues (1988) demonstrated that the fetus was able to recognize audible speech and acted on it. In the absence of fetal distress, the fetus reacted to voice stimulus by a change in heart rate that was often accompanied by movement. In a review of perinatal behavior, Querleu and coauthors (1989) concluded that despite the relative immaturity of the human fetus, experimental data indicate that some fetal learning does take place. The role of this prenatal experience in the functional development of language has yet to be defined.

DeCasper and Fifer (1980) demonstrated the newborn's unique ability to discriminate and demonstrate a preference for the mother's voice. By sucking on a nonnutritive nipple, a newborn could elicit either its mother's or another female's voice. Findings showed that the infant learned how to produce the mother's voice and produced it more often than the other voice. This study indicated that the newborn is capable of auditory responsiveness with respect to speech at a fairly sophisticated level.

Condon and Sander (1974) reported that the neonate moves in precise movements that are synchronous with the articulated speech structure. Eiman and Tartter (1979) indicated that the neonate is also able to discriminate segmental aspects of speech in a categorical and linguistic manner. Selectivity to the dimensionality of human speech may be connected to other attention-getting responses or may be an early manifestation of linguistic ability. Butterfield (1968) demonstrated a consistent ability to regulate auditory events in the environment in 1-day-old infants. These conclusions were made after the authors observed that the infants in the study made sucking responses to an instrumental pacifier that operated musical selections. Eisenberg's (1976) observations on the responses to sound gives significance to the newborn's ability for higher processing of sound stimuli. Overt reactions cited were arousal, gross body movements, orienting behavior, turning of the head, wide-eyed appearance, pupillary dilation, motor reflexes, facial grimaces, displacement of a single digit, crying or cessation of crying, and acceleration or deceleration of heart rate (Kaminski & Hall, 1996). Preterm infants have also been shown to have changes in heart rate and various types of body movements in response to sound (Graven, 1996; Mencher et al., 1985).

It is important that the auditory centers be highly stimulated and that early vocalization attempts be rewarded in the prelinguistic period. In 1981, Maskarinec and associates studied vocalizations of deaf and normal infants from birth to 32 weeks of age. They concluded that during this time, speech-like sounds increased and non–speech-like sounds decreased in normal infants, whereas speech-like and non–speech-like production both decreased with age in deaf children. The babbling response in both deaf and hearing infants appears to represent an innate preprogrammed linguistic process that is unique to the human infant. Certain critical periods in development exist when the neonate is programmed to receive and use particular types of stimuli for important prelinguistic activities, but once the period has passed, the effective use of this stimuli diminishes. Webster and Webster (1979) reported that environmental sounds have their greatest impact in shaping auditory ability from the time that the inner ear and the eighth cranial nerve become functional to the time of central nervous system (CNS) maturation—from approximately 5 months' gestation to between 18 and 28 months of age. A long period of receiving complex adult auditory language symbols exists, before which speech and language present as a culmination of coding and organizing grammatical structure into the child's language structure.

The results of these studies indicate that early identification and intervention is imperative to an optimal outcome. Auditory development is an area in which neonatal nurses assume important roles in parental teaching, role modeling, and evaluation of the child. Additional research studies are needed in all areas of in utero and early neonatal auditory stimulation. Protocols for supporting parents in meeting this essential need in infancy will need to be developed and tested to ensure positive outcomes. The area of perinatal auditory behavior holds great potential as another surveillance tool for the identification of hearing loss.

The ability of the fetus to respond to auditory stimuli in utero may at some point be added to the risk assessment for the early identification of hearing impairment. Research studies need to be conducted to establish a relationship between multiple variables, including response to in utero auditory stimuli, fetal well-being, postnatal risk assessment, and neonatal auditory testing results.

HEARING IMPAIRMENT

Hearing impairment is defined by the American Speech–Language Hearing Association as "a loss of auditory sensitivity that can be measured at birth and for which intervention strategies are known and available." Hearing impairment represents a spectrum of hearing loss that is classified as mild, moderate, severe, or prolonged (Northern & Downs, 1984). The criterion for measuring bilateral conductive and sensorineural hearing deficit in children is the frequency range that is important for speech recognition, namely 1000 to 4000 Hz.

Types of Hearing Impairment

The types of hearing impairment have been classified according to the location of the problem. Impairments may be one of three types: conductive, sensorineural, or a combination of these. Conditions that affect the outer and the middle ear are categorized as conductive losses. A sensorineural loss results from inner ear disorders. Combination losses result from deviations in both areas of the ear.

A conductive hearing loss exists when dysfunction exists in the outer or middle ear that disrupts the normal sequence of sound localization and vibration. Commonly, occlusion of the external auditory meatus occurs as a result of cerumen (wax), which impedes the transmission of sound. Otitis media, an infection of the middle ear, is the most common cause of conductive hearing loss. In this instance, fluid accumulates in the middle ear, preventing the tympanic membrane and ossicular chain from vibrating normally. Congenital deformities of the outer ear can also have an impact on the neonate's ability to hear. Because the function of the external ear is to funnel sound, variations in the structure and protrusion of the pinna may contribute to conductive hearing loss.

A missing or deformed pinna can result from a malformation of the auricular folds. Atresia of the auditory meatus or abnormal ossicular chain development may result from branchial chain development.

Disorders of conduction can be revealed by auditory pure-tone testing. Individuals with conductive hearing loss have difficulty hearing low-frequency sounds, that is, in the 125- to 500-Hz range. Collaborative management of the neonate with conductive hearing loss is directed toward early observation, detection, and intervention to eliminate the source of infection or to remove the blockage, which results in the restoration of normal hearing.

Sensorineural hearing impairment results from damage to the sensory nerve endings of the cochlea or dysfunction of the auditory nerve (eighth cranial nerve). A typical characteristic of inner ear dysfunction is the inability of the inner ear to interpret fluid changes in the cochlea. With sensorineural loss, hearing is normal at low frequencies. Deficits with sound are evident at frequencies greater than 1000 Hz.

Sensorineural hearing loss may present as a congenital inner ear abnormality, resulting in congenital deafness. Other conditions that may result in sensorineural hearing loss include trauma to the inner ear from injury, effects of certain drugs, prolonged exposure to loud noise, infections, infectious conditions such as measles, and effects of aging.

Collaborative Management

Collaborative management of the neonate with hearing loss is directed toward early identification, detection, and restoration with amplification of sound, if indicated. For some neonates, the hearing deficit may cause a severe distortion of the sound, and amplification of sound is indicated. For other neonates, the hearing deficit may cause a severe distortion of the sound, and amplification would not be an appropriate treatment modality. Rather, early intervention with visual cues offers the greatest potential for the growth and development of the child.

IDENTIFICATION OF THE HEARING-IMPAIRED INFANT

Physical Examination

Physical examinations of the infant should be performed in a quiet, warm, draft-free area to afford adequate surroundings for observation and inspection of auditory function. Observing the infant's behavior before the actual examination of the ear yields valuable baseline assessments. The alert, normal newborn reacts by turning toward the sound of human speech, reacts by turning toward a ringing bell, and startles to the stimulus of a loud noise. Observation of the preterm infant (34 to 38 weeks' gestation) is deferred to a later time, when maturation of behavioral response has occurred (Mencher et al., 1985). This test is a crude estimate of neonatal hearing ability. Neonates that do not respond as expected to sound should be suspected of audiologic dysfunction.

Inspection of the ear begins with the medial and the lateral surfaces of the pinna and the surface of the scalp, face, and neck. Development of the pinna correlates with the gestational age of the infant. At term, the pinna of the newborn is well shaped and contains sufficient cartilage to maintain a normal shape and resistance (Fig. 33–3). Before 34 weeks' gestation, the pinna is a slightly formed double thickness of skin.

When folded, the pinna in the term infant demonstrates instant recoil and remains erect from the head. In contrast, the premature infant exhibits a flat, shapeless pinna that remains folded on inspection. As gestation continues, the pinna develops more cartilage, resulting in better form.

The pinna should be inspected for location as well as for its relationship to other facial structures. Normal attachment is to the side, level with the middle third of the face, and fixed in position to the lateral aspect of the external auditory canal. Major convolutions of the pinna are termed the helix, anthelix, tragus, antitragus, and lobule. The lobule of the external ear contains no cartilage. The angle of the placement is almost vertical. If the angle is more than 10 degrees from normal, it is considered abnormal. The superior helix is located at the outer canthus of the eye, and the tragus is roughly level with the infraorbital rim (Fig. 33–4). A finding of low-set auricles is frequently associated with other abnormalities of the first and second branchial cleft and with abnormalities of the urinary system (Jones, 1988). Other abnormalities that may be noted are skin tags, sinuses, or pits, which are often associated with other auditory or renal malformations. The pinna may often be observed to have bruising from a forceps delivery. Depending on the degree of bruising, the discoloration should subside within the first week of life.

The external auditory meatus should next be observed for patency. Atresia or stenosis of the external meatus may be observed. This abnormality results in a conductive hearing loss because it blocks sound transmissions; it should be noted as part of the physical findings.

The next phase of the examination is directed toward inspection of the middle ear and the tympanic membrane. The depths of the external meatus can be examined with a brightly illumi-

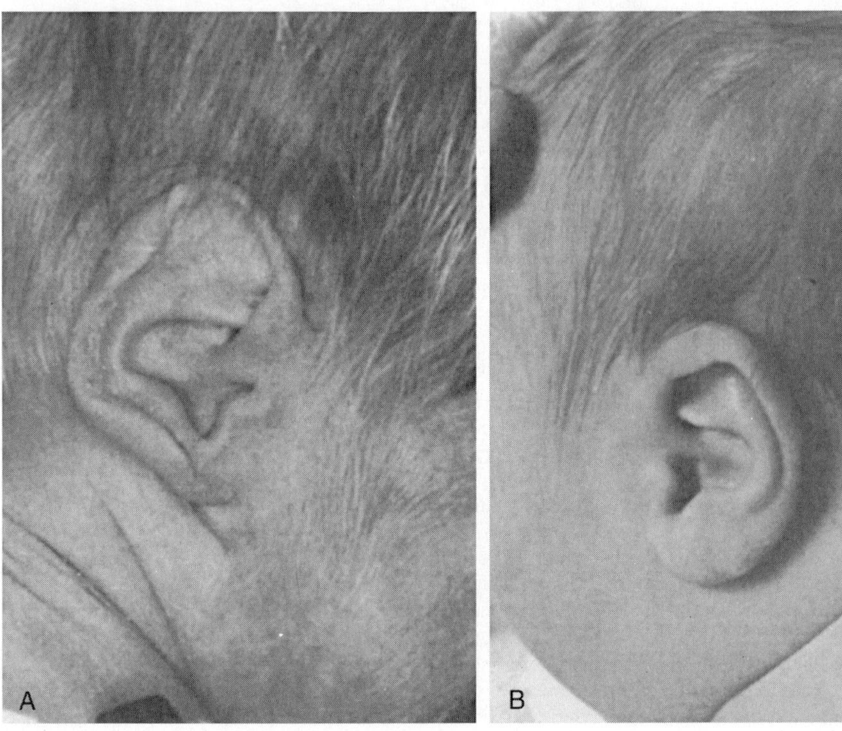

FIGURE 33–3. Premature *(A)* and full-term *(B)* ear. (From Schreiner, R. L., & Bradburn, N. C. [1987]. *Care of the newborn* [2nd ed., p. 35]. New York: Raven Press. Reprinted with permission.)

nated pneumatic otoscope. Vernix caseosa is frequently encountered in the ear canal of the neonate. Introduction of the otoscope into the ear canal is accomplished by gentle traction posterosuperiorly on the auricle. In the neonate, the tympanic membrane lies in a nearly horizontal plane. Visualization of the tympanic membrane through the collapsed neonatal ear is accomplished by gentle dilation of the ear canal with the speculum as the cartilaginous canal is traversed. The tympanic membrane should be examined for thickness, vascularity, and contour. All areas, including the area above the short process of the malleus (pars flaccida), should be visualized for completeness. Normally, the tympanic membrane appears translucent. White shadows of the ossicles can usually be seen through the membrane. Mobility of the tympanic membrane can be assessed by applying intermittent pressure through a bulb or by blowing through a polyethylene tube connected to an otoscope. Otitis media can occur in the first days of life and can be diagnosed by otoscopic examination. Otitis media often presents as a poorly mobile, bulging, yellow, opacified tympanic membrane (Schwartz & Rodriguez, 1981). Complications of otitis media are common. Otitis media with middle ear effusion may cause hearing loss, perforation of the tympanic membrane, and potential intracranial complications, including meningitis, encephalitis, and brain abscess. Shurin (1976) demonstrated that middle ear effusion occurs in both out-patient and in-patient populations of neonates. Balkany and associates (1979) reported that 30 percent of 125 infants randomly selected from the neonatal intensive care unit (NICU) were found to have middle ear effusion. They also found that endotracheal intubation of longer than 7 days contributed to the incidence of middle ear effusion. This finding has implications for the long-term auditory development of the neonate and supports the need for visualization of the middle ear as part of the septic work-up of all neonates. Nursing research is needed in this area to identify risks as well as interventions directed at minimizing the harmful sequelae of prolonged intubation.

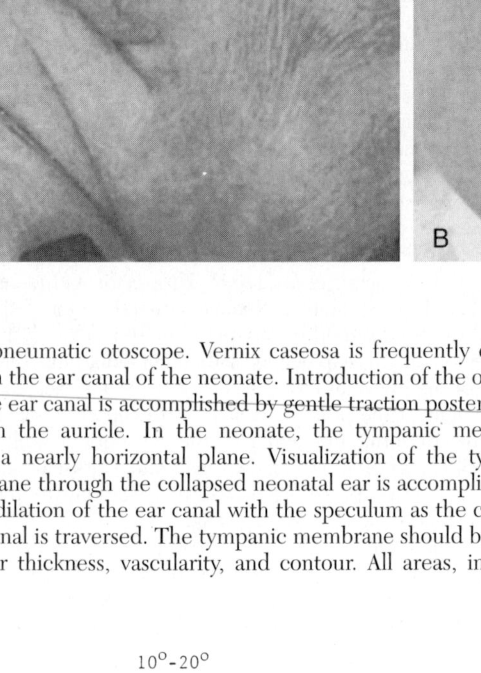

10°-20°

FIGURE 33–4. Pinna in relationship to structures of the face. (From Northern, J., & Downs, M. [1984]. *Hearing in children* [p. 34]. Baltimore: Williams & Wilkins. Reprinted with permission.)

History

The importance of obtaining a comprehensive history for identifying the infant at risk cannot be underestimated. The newborn carries a history extending back to the time of conception and is influenced by perinatal events as well as parental genetic composition. The gathering of data on the infant's history is the first step in identifying infants at risk for hearing impairment. Early identification of hearing-impaired infants aids in minimizing the detrimental effects of reduced auditory input.

In 1974, the Joint Committee on Newborn Hearing developed

a high-risk register, a list of categories that would identify a satisfactory number of infants at risk. Downs and Silver (1972) referred to these categories as the ABCDs of deafness. Further expansion and revision of the 1974 guidelines gave way to the current list developed by the Joint Commission in 1981. The 1981 list of the ABCDs of deafness is a format for screening factors in the perinatal or genetic history that place the neonate at risk for hearing impairment. An abundance of information is available from studies on various aspects of the high-risk register.

Factors are presented to facilitate identification of infants at risk for hearing impairment (American Speech–Language Hearing Association Joint Committee on Hearing, 1990). The only infants screened are those identified with one or more high-risk factors associated with hearing impairment. It is of paramount importance that nurses in the labor and delivery department and the newborn nursery use the high-risk register as an essential part of early screening for all neonates (Table 33–2).

Asphyxia

Asphyxia, or anoxia, a condition in which there is a lack of oxygen with an increase in the carbon dioxide level in the tissue, is particularly damaging to the CNS. The incidence of asphyxia is indirectly related to gestational age and birth weight. MacDonald and associates (1980) reported that the preterm infant is at greater risk for anoxic episodes than the full-term infant. A postulated cause of asphyxia includes hypoxic-ischemic injury to the brain stem. It is essential that an adequate supply of oxygen be available for adequate functioning of the organ of Corti. The incidence of sensorineural hearing loss in children with severe perinatal asphyxia has been reported to be approximately 4 percent (Stein et al., 1983). In the neonate, the anoxia is reflected in the Apgar score assessment taken at 1 minute (Apgar & James, 1962). The 5-minute Apgar assessment is a more accurate index of the likelihood of death or neurologic sequelae (Behrman, Kliegman, & Arvin, 1995).

The clinical definition of asphyxia remains an item of debate among authors. The use of multiple measures in determining clinically significant asphyxia has been suggested. Scheiner (1980) suggested that the following measures be used to determine clinically significant asphyxia: (1) the length and degree of intrapartum asphyxia; (2) the infant's response to the intrapartum asphyxia, as measured by the Apgar score; and (3) the infant's ability to repair the effects of the hypoxic insult, as evidenced by behavioral characteristics during the neonatal period and as monitored by serial electroencephalograms. The hearing loss that is evident in cases of asphyxia is sensorineural, with a steep slope noted, especially in the high-frequency range (Simmons, 1980). Because the type of hearing impairment associated with asphyxia is not progressive, screening can be implemented early in the neonatal period.

TABLE 33–2 Risk Identification Criteria: Neonates (Birth–28 Days)

The risk factors that identify those neonates who are at risk for sensorineural hearing impairment include the following:

1. Family history of congenital or delayed onset childhood sensorineural impairment.
2. Congenital infection known or suspected to be associated with sensorineural hearing impairment, such as toxoplasmosis, syphilis, rubella, cytomegalovirus, and herpes.
3. Craniofacial anomalies, including morphologic abnormalities of the pinna and ear canal, absent philtrum, low hairline, etc.
4. Birth weight less than 1500 g (3.3 lb).
5. Hyperbilirubinemia at a level exceeding indication for exchange transfusion.
6. Ototoxic medications, including but not limited to the aminoglycosides used for more than 5 days (e.g., gentamicin, tobramycin, kanamycin, streptomycin) and loop diuretics used in combination with aminoglycosides.
7. Bacterial meningitis.
8. Severe depression at birth, which may include infants with Apgar scores of 0–3 at 5 minutes or those who fail to initiate spontaneous respiration by 10 minutes or those with hypotonia persisting to 2 hours of age.
9. Prolonged mechanical ventilation for a duration equal to or greater than 10 days (e.g., persistent pulmonary hypertension).
10. Stigmata or other findings associated with a syndrome known to include sensorineural hearing loss (e.g., Waardenburg's or Usher's syndrome).

From Joint Committee on Infant Hearing. (1991, March). Position statement. *ASHA, 28*, 15–17. Reprinted with permission.

Bacterial Meningitis

Bacterial meningitis is a common infection and sequela of bacteria in the neonate. Meningitis, which is a disease of the CNS, presents as an inflammation of the meninges and the cerebrospinal fluid that may extend to adjacent organs, such as the brain and the ear. Meningitis presents in approximately 1 in 2500 live births (Feigin et al., 1992). In the neonate, meningitis may be acquired from a maternal infection transmitted transplacentally or at the time of delivery. The mode of transmission may also be from infant to infant via nursery personnel or contaminated equipment. In most cases, meningitis is acquired after birth and is the most common cause of hearing loss in infants (Pappas, 1985). Paparella and Suguira (1967) proposed that the course of infection passes from the meninges to the inner ear via the cochlear aqueduct and along vessels and nerves from the internal and auditory meatus. Because clinical manifestations of neonatal meningitis are often subtle and deceptive, clinical vigilance and verification by laboratory studies provide the only means of diagnosis in the newborn. The ability of meningitis to cause neurologic damage has been studied by numerous researchers (Ueda et al., 1979). Factors such as host differences, bacterial virulence, age of the infant, time between exposure to the disease and onset of treatment, intensity of treatment, and duration of the disease have been implicated in neurologic damage.

Meningitis may be viral in origin; however, most cases resulting in neurologic deficits are caused by bacterial organisms. Three organisms, *Haemophilus influenzae, Diplococcus pneumoniae*, and *Neisseria meningitidis*, have been identified as the responsible agent in 89 percent of cases studied (Pappas & Mundy, 1982). Of these agents, *H. influenzae*, type B, has been reported to be the most common organism (Northern & Downs, 1984).

Treatment modalities for infants with meningitis are supportive, with antibiotic therapy being an important aspect of the regimen. Antibiotic drugs, such as gentamicin and kanamycin, which are widely used in treatment, are often potential ototoxic agents. Careful monitoring of drug levels is imperative to decrease the risk of hearing loss.

Sensorineural hearing loss has been reported in 7 to 35 percent of patients with bacterial meningitis (Finitzo-Hieber et al., 1981). The hearing loss is generally bilateral and ranges from severe to profound. Reports of mild-to-moderate hearing loss have also been documented. Meningitic hearing loss may be recovered to some degree. Rosenhall and Kankkunen (1980) reported partial or complete recovery in both or one ear in one fourth of postmeningitis patients. Further studies, by Friel-Patti and associates (1982), reported a 35-percent sensorineural hearing loss after meningitis. Bacterial meningitis with subsequent hearing loss is subject to fluctuations and progression. Reports that 50 percent of infants who have had meningitis are subject to unstable hearing loss are important and call for close monitoring to ensure proper identification of at-risk patients (Pappas, 1985). Some investigators recommend performing audiometry immediately after the meningitis and every 3 months until the age of 3 years (Pappas, 1985).

Congenital Perinatal Infection

The occurrence of certain infections during the perinatal period place the fetus at risk for various congenital malformations that affect auditory function. The most common and best-referenced infections are represented by the acronym TORCH, for toxoplasmosis, other infections, rubella, cytomegalovirus (CMV), and herpes. Although "other infections" does not include syphilis, this infection is discussed here in relation to its potential impact on hearing impairment. Stagno and associates (1981) investigated the impact of perinatal infections on the fetus throughout the course of pregnancy. They reported that early in gestation, if the infection is severe, termination of the pregnancy may result. The degree of involvement with late-gestation exposure to infection may range from subclinical to severe multisystem disease.

Lack of symptomatology, which is often associated with the TORCH infections, makes identification difficult in the prenatal period. In general, infants exposed to congenital perinatal infections experience varying degrees of ocular, cardiovascular, and psychoneurologic problems, among which is hearing impairment.

An estimated 1 to 5 percent of all deliveries are infected by the TORCH agents (Nahmias, 1974). According to these estimates, 2000 infants are born yearly with significant sequelae from one of the TORCH infections. The potential impact of the TORCH infections on the viability as well as the long-term outcome of the pregnancy makes this an area of interest for nurses involved with mothers and infants. Collaborative research needs to be conducted on the development of more sensitive tools for identifying mothers at risk for transmitting these infections.

Toxoplasmosis

Toxoplasmosis infection is caused by the parasite *Toxoplasma gondii*. Toxoplasmosis is acquired as an active disease in 2 to 7 per 1000 pregnant women. Of these women, 30 to 40 percent transfer the organism transplacentally to the fetus (Babson, 1980). The route of transmission is transplacental and is thought to be evoked by maternal contact with the organism in uncooked meat or in cat feces. The most severe impact on the fetus results from exposure during the first and second trimesters. Congenital toxoplasmosis is manifested by chorioretinitis, cerebral calcification, psychomotor retardation, hydrocephalus or microcephaly, and convulsions (Feigin et al., 1992).

Although research directly relating toxoplasmosis to hearing disorders is sparse, the disease is similar to cytomegalovirus and therefore may have a similar impact on hearing. Pathologic studies have demonstrated changes in the soft tissue mesenchyma and mucoperiosteum and calcium deposits in the spiral ligament of the inner ear (Keleman, 1958).

More than 70 percent of infants with toxoplasmosis do not manifest clinical signs in the neonatal period (Feigin et al., 1992). Infants who do demonstrate generalized disease are likely to manifest low birth weight, hepatosplenomegaly, icterus, and anemia in the first weeks of life. Findings indicating neurologic disease are convulsions, intracranial calcification, and hydrocephalus or microcephaly and are not seen until 1 month of life in most infants (Feigin et al., 1992). In a 4-year follow-up study of infants that demonstrated the effects of toxoplasmosis in the newborn period, Abrams (1977) found that 17 percent had hearing loss. In another study of 11 children who were asymptomatic as neonates but were later diagnosed with toxoplasmosis, 73 percent had neurologic sequelae (Wilson et al., 1980). These studies indicate the need for follow-up of infants at risk, because of maternal and neonatal history, until 1 year of age. Collaborative studies with larger sample sizes need to be conducted in order to replicate reports currently in the literature.

Syphilis

Syphilis, now thought to be on the increase, continues to pose a threat to the mother and fetus. Syphilis is caused by the *Treponema pallidum* spirochetal organism, which is transmitted in utero to the fetus from an infected mother (Feigin et al., 1992). It was previously thought that before the 18th week of gestation, the Langhans layer of the chorion acted as a barrier to protect transmission of the spirochete to the fetus (Feigin et al., 1992; Stome, 1977). Krugman and Katz (1981) suggested that the infection takes place earlier but that pathologic changes do not occur until the fifth month of gestation, when the fetus becomes immunocompetent and inflammatory cells can be found. Treatment of the disease before 18 weeks of gestation almost always prevents signs of infection in the fetus (Feigin et al., 1992).

Transmission of the spirochete to the fetus occurs in 70 to 100 percent of pregnancies with untreated primary syphilis and approximately 30 percent of pregnancies with latent syphilis (Krugman & Katz, 1981).

Early symptoms of congenital syphilis in the neonate include nasal discharge (snuffles), rash, anemia, jaundice, and osteochondritis. Late symptoms include saddle nose, saber skin, and dental abnormalities (Northern & Downs, 1984). Congenital syphilis has a profound effect on the inner ear. Pathologic changes include osteitis of all three layers of the otic capsule, with inflammatory infiltration of the membranes of the cochlea and the vestibular labyrinth. Hearing impairment may be profound as a result of severe degeneration of the organ of Corti, spiral ganglion, and nerve cells, along with destruction of the membranous labyrinth (Karmody & Schuknecht, 1966; Schuknecht, 1974).

Spirochetes remain visible in the perilymph of the ear despite massive therapy because penicillin does not readily cross the barrier to enter the endolymphatic fluid of the inner ear (Wiet & Milko, 1975).

Congenital syphilis affects hearing in approximately 35 percent of children (Sando & Wood, 1971). Hearing deficit associated with congenital syphilis presents a challenge to health care providers. Some of the complex issues surrounding hearing impairment related to congenital syphilis include the following:

1. Congenital syphilis may be asymptomatic in up to 50 percent of neonatal cases (Stagno et al., 1981).
2. Routine hospital screenings for syphilis through the Venereal Disease Research Laboratory test have high false-positive and false-negative rates and may show a positive reaction in other diseases, such as malaria, infectious hepatitis, infectious mononucleosis, and disseminated lupus erythematosus. In comparison, the fluorescent treponemal antibody absorption test is more sensitive but more expensive (Harner et al., 1968).
3. The progressive pattern of hearing impairment demonstrates variations as to the time of onset and the rapidity of progression (Patterson, 1968).
4. In early childhood, the onset of infantile congenital syphilis is usually between 8 and 20 years of age. Hearing loss is sudden, bilateral, symmetric, and profound, and with no accompanying symptoms (Schuknecht, 1974).
5. Hearing loss as a result of congenital syphilis presents as poor function and limited use of hearing aid devices that results from neural atrophy with poor discrimination (Wilson et al., 1980).
6. Penicillin therapy does not prevent or retard the progressive hearing loss (Patterson, 1968).

Treatment modalities include early identification of infants suspected of having a syphilitic infection and prompt treatment with large doses of penicillin. Steroids are the drugs of choice for the treatment of hearing loss secondary to congenital syphilis. However, not all patients improve with steroid therapy (Abrams et al., 1983).

Because syphilitic hearing impairments pose a grave threat to the future developmental milestones of the infant, early identification, testing, and lengthy follow-up are imperative.

Rubella

Congenital rubella infection is a major threat to the fetus and newborn. In the prevaccine period, before 1969, congenital rubella was the leading cause of deafness in children attending schools for the hearing impaired in the United States (Cooper et al., 1969).

Acquired rubella is a mild disease of children and adults that is transmitted by droplet contact with the virus. The virus is congenitally acquired by the fetus through placental transfer (McCracken, 1963). The critical factor in determining pregnancy outcome is the gestational age of the fetus at the time of exposure. There is a 50-percent prevalence of congenital rubella defects in infants exposed during the first month of pregnancy. The prevalence decreases to 22 percent in infants exposed during the second month of pregnancy, and to 6 to 10 percent in those exposed during the third, fourth, and fifth months (Pumper & Yamashiroya, 1975). Clinically, the infant with congenital rubella may present with a wide range of features. Many present as normal newborns, whereas others display cardiac lesions, low birth weight, eye defects, growth retardation, thrombocytopenia purpura, hepatosplenomegaly, hepatitis, and CNS defects, such as psychomotor retardation (Baley & Goldfarb, 1992). Hearing defects are the most common result of the viral insult. Congenital rubella is manifested as chronic infection in fetal tissues that causes an inhibition of fetal cell multiplication; therefore, it is not a static disease (Baley & Goldfarb, 1992). The degree of pathology caused by the arrest of development varies and reflects the clinical variations demonstrated in hearing loss. Histopathologic studies after rubella infection have revealed a degeneration of the organ of Corti as well as anomalies of the middle ear, such as fixed stapedial footplate (Sando & Wood, 1971; Scholl et al., 1951).

Hearing deficit associated with congenital rubella syndrome is severe-to-profound bilateral sensorineural loss, with an audiometric configuration that depicts the greatest degree of loss in the midrange, from 500 to 2000 Hz (Konigsmark & Gorlin, 1976). Although the incidence of congenital rubella defects is related to the time of onset, no special relationship appears to exist between the degree of loss and the time of the infection (Ueda et al., 1979).

It is difficult to verify rubella exposure during pregnancy because it often presents as a mild, unrecognized disease. Infants with a history of rubella or rubella exposure should be observed with serial audiograms until they are 18 to 24 months of age because of the potential late onset and the progressive nature of congenital rubella syndrome.

Cytomegalovirus

Cytomegalovirus, a virus of the herpes family, is the most common cause of congenital viral infection in humans. An estimated 20 percent of pregnant women carry CMV; 2.5 percent of the infants are infected at birth, and 10 to 20 percent are at risk for later sequelae (Baley & Goldfarb, 1992).

The virus can be transmitted to the fetus transplacentally or at the time of delivery via the cervix. CMV can also be transmitted after birth through infected urine, saliva, breast milk, tears, feces, and blood transfusions (Weller, 1971). Nearly all congenital infections occur in infants whose mothers had the antibody to the virus before conception and represent reactivation of a latent infection. A report by Panjvani and Henshaw (1981) suggested that the risk to the fetus may be related to both the time of infection in utero and the immune status of the mother. During pregnancy, cervical reactivation of the CMV infection is common. Panjvani and Henshaw (1981) reported the risk of infecting the infant to be approximately 40 percent with a reactivated cervical infection.

The effects of CMV range from severe CNS involvement to asymptomatic carrying of the virus. Asymptomatic infants are at risk for late sequelae, manifested as bilateral sensorineural hearing loss that may be mild to profound. This observation is supported by Stagno and associates (1977), who found a 7- to 14-percent hearing loss in infants identified as CMV positive by urine screenings in the first week of life. In 25 percent of these infants, the hearing loss developed or became severe after 1 year of age.

Symptomatic congenital infection, also known as cytomegalic inclusion disease (CID), occurs in only 5 to 10 percent of infected infants and is nearly always associated with maternal infection around the time of conception (Baley & Goldfarb, 1992). Manifestations of CID include enlargement of the liver and spleen, jaundice, petechial rash, chorioretinitis, cerebral calcifications, and microcephaly (Baley & Goldfarb, 1992).

CMV infections of the inner ear cause either partial or total cochlear and labyrinthine end-organ destruction. The damaged cell reaction is clearly manifested among the cells of the organ of Corti and the neurons of the spiral ganglion (Stagno et al., 1977). In a follow-up study of symptomatic infants with CID, 30 percent were found to have severe-to-profound bilateral sensorineural hearing loss (Pass et al., 1980).

The following basic tenets should be considered in the care of the neonate identified at risk for CMV (Northern & Downs, 1984):

1. Excretion of the CMV virus may continue for several years after birth, contributing to degenerative hearing loss. Therefore, follow-up testing should take place at shorter time periods than for nonprogressive disease processes. Audiologic evaluation at 3-month intervals is recommended.
2. In the case of CID, any pattern and degree of hearing loss can occur. Screening of these infants should be performed with electrophysiologic testing, because the opportunity to detect a mild-to-moderate loss is greater with this technique.
3. In the case of asymptomatic viral infection, hearing loss may manifest at a later date. This knowledge may help determine the cause of childhood-onset hearing loss.

Herpes Simplex Virus

Herpes simplex virus (HSV), a member of a group of DNA viruses that cause latent infection characterized by periodic recurrences, poses a threat to the health of both the mother and the neonate. HSV-1 infections generally occur in the oral cavity or above the waist and are most prevalent among children and young adults. Transmission is usually spread via the respiratory route from contact with family members who are asymptomatic. Recurrence of the oral lesions takes place in 20 to 45 percent of individuals with the disease (Baley & Goldfarb, 1992).

Herpes simplex virus–2 infections generally occur in the genital region and are transmitted by sexual contact. Isolation of the virus can be found in sexually active individuals. Most genital infections are asymptomatic. Patients who are symptomatic report local tenderness and burning involving the labia and vaginal mucosa. Both symptomatic and asymptomatic individuals may transmit the infection.

Jenistra (1984) reported that 10 to 35 percent of women are infected with the virus before childbearing. The persistence of the virus and the frequency of infection are both increased during pregnancy (Baley & Goldfarb, 1992). The most common route of HSV to the fetus is during vaginal birth if the mother is actively infected.

The risk of genital herpes infection to the infant during vaginal delivery has not been clearly defined. Baley and Goldfarb (1992) reported that the risk may be as high as 40 to 60 percent with active infections at term. Fewer than 10 percent of infants are infected after birth, either through airborne infection or with direct contact with the virus from labial sores on the mother or open lesions on face, lips, or hands of the father or nursery personnel (Hatherly et al., 1980). An ascending mechanism of infection has also been reported as a mode of transmission, despite the presence of intact membranes (Hain et al., 1980). Transplacental transmission of the virus, although a rare occurrence, may occur during maternal viremia (Gershan, 1981).

Although HSV infections are often asymptomatic in the adult, they are rarely so in the neonate. Vaginally contracted HSV in the neonate does not manifest initially; an incubation period of from 6 to 12 days exists before clinical symptoms appear (Whitley et al., 1980). Neonatal infections are classified as disseminated with or without CNS involvement, or localized. Disseminated infections may involve virtually every organ system. With CNS involvement, most cases result in death; of the survivors, only 4 percent lack sequelae. Without CNS involvement, 12 percent survive without sequelae. Of infants with localized infections, 41 percent suffer from progressive neurologic damage resulting in death; 42 percent of those who survive have severe neurologic sequelae (Whitley et al., 1980).

Specific reports linking HSV to hearing loss have thus far not been made in the literature; however, Ventry et al. (1981), through histopathologic studies, demonstrated that herpes infects the sensory cells of the labyrinth. In light of the similarities of all of the perinatal viral infections, nurses should implement careful follow-up of this at-risk group.

Collaborative research studies need to be conducted in many different areas. First, the incidence of HSV infection during various stages of pregnancy, as well as at the time of delivery, needs to be documented. Longitudinal studies of neonates exposed to HSV need to be conducted to ascertain if the virus contributes to progressive hearing loss.

Defects of the Head and Neck

The anatomy of the head and neck should be assessed for deficits as part of the screening process for all neonates. Ear anomalies associated with head and neck anomalies may occur as a result of a primary regional defect, secondary to a primary defect in an area contiguous to the temporal bone, as part of an inherited defect involving the skeletal system, or as part of a chromosomal disorder. Malformations of the head and neck may be relatively simple or complex. Any neonate presenting with a defect, even if it is minor, should be closely examined for hidden major malformations.

Ear

The relationship of the pinna to the remainder of the structures of the head and face is important in the initial assessment. In normal placement, the helix is located at the level of the outer canthus, and the tragus is roughly level with the intraorbital rim. Low-set auricles are frequently associated with abnormalities of the urinary system (Eavey, 1989). Jaffe (1977) reported unilateral conductive hearing losses in children with normal-sized pinnae and unilateral absence of the superior crus. He also reported hearing losses in patients with a fused, anthelix–helix, thickened, hypertrophied ear lobes, a "cup" ear, as well as a protruding pinna. The pinna may be noted to be abnormally small (microtia) or totally absent (anotia). Atresia (closure of the external auditory canal) may be observed. Atresia is classified as mild severity, indicating a small ear canal; medium severity, indicating a bony atresia plate that replaces the canal with ossicular malformation; or severe, indicating a small or absent ear canal and middle ear space (Naunton & Valvassori, 1968).

Multiple combinations of atresia and microtia may coexist; therefore, all children with these abnormalities should be suspected of having middle ear abnormalities. Naunton and Valvassori (1968) reported that sensorineural hearing loss was found in 12 percent of patients with congenital atresia of the outer ear. Atresia is often observed with cranial, facial, mandibular, or acrofacial dysostoses. Abnormalities of the skeletal system or chromosomal aberration may also present with atresia. Aural atresia may also be associated with facial, labial, or palatal clefts. Infants with atresia often have conductive hearing loss related to the inability of the ear canal to transmit sound.

Preauricular abnormalities, including pits or tags (Fig. 33–5) and branchial fistulas, are often accompanied by external or middle ear malformations. These appendages may present with an otherwise normal-appearing pinna. Preauricular tags or pits usually require only cosmetic surgery or excision if they are draining.

Nose

Examination of the nose should be directed toward identification of suspicious defects, such as unusual broadness with a flat base and a short length (saddle nose), small nostrils, and notched alae. Deformities of the nose often present with other craniofacial abnormalities.

Mouth

Defects in the oral cavity are the most common defects associated with hearing impairment. Babson (1980) reported that cleft lip or palate, or both, occur in every 600 births. The child with cleft lip or palate displays a deficiency in palate musculature that is primarily related to the inability of the tensor muscle of the velum palatinum to dilate the eustachian tube actively during swallowing (Doyle et al., 1980). Helias and colleagues (1988)

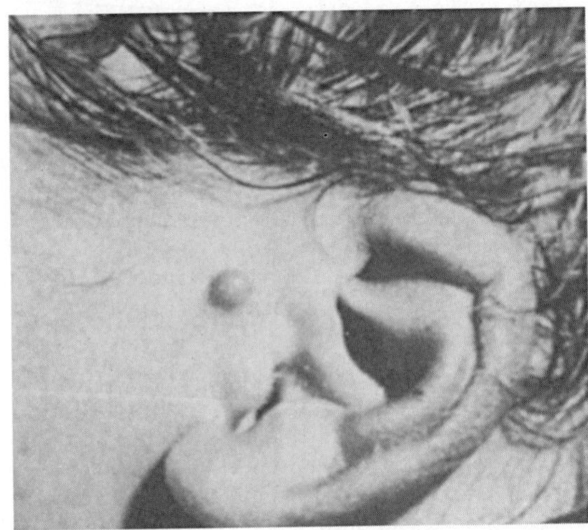

FIGURE 33–5. Preauricular tag. (From Schreiner, R. L., & Bradburn, N. C. [1987]. *Care of the newborn* [2nd ed., p. 21]. New York: Raven Press. Reprinted with permission.)

reported that hearing problems are observed in cleft palate cases, depending on the age of the patient on examination and the means of the exploration.

This condition leaves the child vulnerable to the effusion of fluid and, as a result, to varying degrees of hearing loss. The consequences of effusion of fluid raise the rates of otitis media, for which 50- to 90-percent incidences have been reported (Bluestone & Shurin, 1974; Doyle et al., 1980). The hearing loss associated with cleft lip or palate is generally conductive; however, there have been reports of sensorineural or combination losses, or both (Bergstrom & Hemenway, 1971). Helias and colleagues (1988) studied a group of 23 infants younger than 12 months of age with cleft palate before they underwent surgical repair and found that hearing loss was detectable at an early age in direct relationship to the degree of malformation.

Eyes

Deformities of the eyelids are the most usual abnormalities involving the eyes. A variation in eyelid configuration has been noted in which the upper eyelid forms an almost vertical curve at the level of the medial limit of the cornea and fuses with the lower eyelid. The distance of the two medial angles is increased. These findings are typically noted in Waardenburg's syndrome, an autosomal dominant disorder resulting in mild-to-severe sensorineural hearing loss in 50 percent of patients. The hearing loss may be unilateral or bilateral and progressive (Marcus & Valvassori, 1970; Pantke & Cohen, 1971).

Epicanthal folds, which are true vertical folds extending from the nasal fold into the upper eyelid, are commonly noted in infants with Down syndrome, or trisomy 21. Other physical features presenting in Down syndrome include low-set ears, small pinna, and narrow external ear canal. Infants with this syndrome display a strong tendency for recurrent otitis media and anomalies of the middle ear ossicles. The incidence of hearing loss is high and consists of sensorineural, conductive, or combination types (Balkany et el., 1979).

Hair

Unusual hair texture or hairline should be regarded with suspicion in assessments for abnormalities associated with hearing loss. Twisted hair (pili torti) has been associated with sensorineural hearing loss. The hair may be twisted, dry, brittle, or easily broken. Other observations that may be significant are aberrant scalp-hair patterning.

Neck

Defects of the neck that may be associated with hearing defects are branchial cleft fistulas and mildly webbed or shortened neck (Feingold, 1982). Not all infants with defects of the head or neck also have hearing impairments; many variations may be observed in the normal neonate (Jones, 1988). The presence of such defects does increase the risk of hearing impairment, however, and should be followed up in the long-term interest of the child.

Elevated Bilirubin

Hyperbilirubinemia, also referred to as neonatal jaundice, occurs when an excess amount of bilirubin is present in the blood. The condition can be neurotoxic to the infant at high concentrations. Jaundice is observed in approximately 60 percent of term infants and in 80 percent of preterm infants (Behrman & Kliegman, 1992). Any number of factors that interfere with the transport of bilirubin to the liver or that reduce or prohibit the liver from metabolizing bilirubin can lead to toxic levels of the unconjugated bilirubin. Unconjugated bilirubin has the ability to cross the blood–brain barrier. Kernicterus, a neurologic syndrome, results from the deposit of unconjugated bilirubin in the basal ganglia of the brain, causing motor and sensory deficits, mental deficits, or death (Behrman & Kliegman, 1992). Exchange transfusions are performed in order to lower bilirubin levels on infants at risk for developing kernicterus (Levine, 1979). Simmons (1980) reported that hyperbilirubinemia was the most common sequela of neonatal problems that results in deafness. In a study of 405 infants with hemolytic disease or hyperbilirubinemia, Hyman and associates (1969), found mild-to-profound sensorineural hearing impairment in 4.2 percent, and the highest number occurred in preterm infants.

The Joint Committee on Infant Hearing suggested that infants with a bilirubin level that exceeds indications for an exchange transfusion are at risk for hearing impairments. The Committee of the Fetus and the Newborn of the AAP (1982) suggested that the following birth weights and bilirubin levels be used as guidelines for deciding whether or not an infant should be placed on the high-risk register:

Birth Weight (g)	Bilirubin Level (mg)
<1000	10
1001–1250	10
1251–1500	13
1501–2000	15
2001–2500	17
>2500	18

Family History

More than 50 types of hereditary hearing loss have been described. A significant number of hearing impairments may be classified as genetically based. Hereditary hearing loss must be identified on the basis of a thorough medical and family history, the components of which should include the following:

1. Determination of the cause and circumstances under which the hearing impairment was first noticed. Many different circumstances surrounding the onset of the hearing loss may cause it to be labeled as congenital, or hereditary, or both. An example of hearing loss that is hereditary and not congenital is that in Alport's syndrome, which has an autosomal dominant inheritance resulting in deafness that appears at 8 years of age.
2. A complete family history, including a history of all previous as well as current pregnancies.
3. An extended family history of data relating to hearing impairments of immediate as well as extended family members.
4. A thorough physical examination, with particular inspection of the head and neck region to detect abnormalities.
5. Selective testing procedures for assessing possible causes of sensorineural hearing loss.

A form for identification through query of the mother is shown in Figure 33–6. Although the questions may easily be asked verbally, the questionnaire provides a structured format that can be used by the neonatal nurse to ensure consistency during the interview. The questionnaire should be given to all new mothers to be completed before discharge. This tool provides an excellent opportunity for educating the mother on normal speech and language development.

Hereditary Hearing Loss

Autosomal Dominant

Autosomal dominant inheritance accounts for 10 to 25 percent of cases of hereditary hearing impairment (Fraser, 1976; Nance &

MOTHER'S NAME:________
ROOM NO.:________

1. Do you know any of the baby's relatives who now have a hearing loss which started before the age of five? Think hard about all of your family and the baby's father's family . . . .
   Yes ______ No ______
   A. In no, proceed to question No. 2.
   B. If yes, ask the following:
      (1) Who were they? (relationship to baby)
          (A).______ (B).______ (C).______
      (2) Do you know what caused the loss? . . . .
          Yes ______ No ______
          (A).______ (B).______ (C).______
      (3) What makes you think the onset of the hearing loss was before age five?
          (A).______ (B).______ (C).______
      (4) Did he/she wear a hearing aid before age five? . . (A) ______ (B) ______ (C) ______
          Does he/she still wear an aid? . . . . (A) ______ (B) ______ (C) ______
      (5) Did he/she attend a special school for the deaf? . (A) ______ (B) ______ (C) ______
          Did the person attend public school? . . . . . . (A) ______ (B) ______ (C) ______
      (6) Did he/she have a speech problem? . . . . . . (A) ______ (B) ______ (C) ______
2. During your pregnancy, did you have 3-day measles, German measles, rubella, or a rash with a fever? . . . . Yes______ No______
   WHEN: 1st 3 mo.______ Middle 3 mo.______ Last 3 mo.______
3. During your pregnancy, were you around anyone who had 3-day measles, German measles, rubella, or a rash with fever? . . . . Yes______ No______
   WHEN: 1st 3 mo.______ Middle 3 mo.______ Last 3 mo.______
4. Do you have any reason to be concerned about your baby's hearing? . . . .
   Yes______ No______
   If yes, why?______
5. What pediatrician or clinic will be caring for your baby when he/she leaves the hospital? ______
   Approximate location______
6. Nearest relative or friend: Name:______
   Address:______
   Phone:______

FIGURE 33–6. Mother's interview. (From Northern, J., & Downs, M. [1984]. *Hearing in children* [p. 237]. Baltimore: Williams & Wilkins. Reprinted with permission.)

Sweeney, 1975). The hearing loss may be unilateral or bilateral, and both sexes are affected equally. Autosomal dominant hearing disorders vary in severity ("variable expressivity") and in progression of hearing loss. A typical example of autosomal dominant hearing disorder occurs in Waardenburg's syndrome. In this syndrome, severe-to-profound bilateral sensorineural hearing loss presents with integumentary system involvement. Histopathologic studies indicate the absence of the organ of Corti and atrophy of the spiral ganglion (Marcus & Valvassori, 1970; Pantke & Cohen, 1971).

Another example of autosomal dominant hearing loss with incomplete penetrance and variable expression occurs in Treacher Collins syndrome. Major features include facial anomalies, small displaced or absent external ears, external auditory canal atresia, and poorly developed or malformed tympanic ossicles. Deafness is generally complete and conductive (Linsey, 1971).

Klippel-Feil syndrome, if familial, is another example of autosomal dominance with variable expression. Characteristics of this syndrome include craniofacial disorders, fusion of some or all of the cervical vertebrae, occasionally cleft palate, and severe sensorineural hearing loss (Windle-Taylor et al., 1981). Crouzon's disease is another disease in which hearing loss is attributed to autosomal dominance with variable expression. This disease is characterized by an abnormally shaped head, a beaked nose, and marked bilateral exophthalmos caused by premature closure of the cranial sutures. Hearing loss may be conductive or sensorineural, owing to middle ear deformities (Baldwin, 1968).

Autosomal Recessive

Autosomal recessive inheritance accounts for about 40 percent of childhood deafness (Proctor & Proctor, 1967). An estimated one in eight individuals is a carrier for a recessive form of hearing impairment. The incidence of recessive inheritance is increased in marriages of recent common ancestry. This type of union increases the possibility that each parent will be the carrier of an identical defective gene that may express itself as an abnormal trait. Hearing loss in people with an autosomal recessive gene tends to be more severe than in those with autosomal dominant inheritance. This is because most cases of recessive hearing loss are associated with the Scheibe deformity of the cochlea. In Scheibe's dysplasia, the entire organ of Corti is rudimentary, with hair cells missing and the supporting cells distorted or collapsed. The vestibular membrane is usually collapsed (Konigsmark & Gorlin, 1976). Pendred's syndrome, a condition marked by hearing loss and goiter detected in the first 2 years of life, is an example of an autosomal recessive disorder (Illum et al., 1972).

X-Linked

Approximately 3 percent of hereditary deafness is due to the X-linked mode of transmission (Northern & Downs, 1984). The mutant gene is on the X chromosome, and males transmit only Y chromosomes to their male offspring; thus, only males are affected. The female is the carrier and has the chance to transmit the gene to 50 percent of her sons, who manifest the disease, and 50 percent of her daughters, who carry the abnormality. The hearing loss is characteristically not present at birth but develops in infancy to varying degrees. X-linked hearing losses, with exceptions, are sensorineural, and some retention of hearing in all frequencies often occurs. Recessive, or X-linked, Duchenne's muscular dystrophy is an example of this type of disorder. Characterized by muscle wasting, the severe infantile form of muscular dystrophy is also associated with mild-to-moderate sensorineural hearing loss (Black et al., 1971). (For a complete discussion of genetic inheritance patterns, see Chapter 9, Human Genetics.)

Cytogenetic Disorders

Cytogenetic disorders are caused by structural changes in one or more of the chromosomes or by errors in the distribution of the chromosomes. Down syndrome, the most common chromosomal aberration syndrome, presenting in 1 in 600 to 800 births, is usually caused by an extra chromosome 21 (Nyhan, 1983). Approximately 5 percent of cases of Down syndrome are due to translocation and fusion of part of this chromosome 21 to chromosome 14.

Balkany and associates (1979) reported on the relatively high incidence of hearing loss in children with trisomy 21. Characteristic otologic findings that have an impact on the hearing performance of these children during the early years are (1) a high incidence of stenosis of the external auditory canal; (2) a high incidence of serous otitis media; and (3) a high incidence of cholesteatoma-persistent growth of squamous epithelium from the ear canal into the middle ear or mastoid through a tear in the tympanic membrane (Pappas, 1985).

The ear canal of infants with Down syndrome tends to be stenotic, with an hourglass appearance. The narrowed segment is located at the junction of the cartilaginous and the bony portions of the canal. With increasing age, the canal has been noted to assume a more typical appearance as the thickened tissue recedes.

The degree of hearing loss in these infants varies, but it is rarely ever profound. Balkany (1980) reported that children with Down syndrome had normal-appearing otoscopic examinations; however, on aperture examination, congenital ossicular malformations and destruction caused by inflammations resulting from chronic infection were revealed.

Mental retardation is a clinical condition frequently observed with Down syndrome. The impact of the otologic handicap on the developmental potential of these children is uncertain (Saxon & Witriol, 1976). Because of the high incidence of hearing loss in this group, it becomes imperative that early and frequent monitoring be instituted. Collaborative research studies need to be performed in order to identify factors that have an impact on the otologic problems of infants with Down syndrome and on early strategies to optimize their potential.

Low Birth Weight

Low birth weight (<1500 g), especially when associated with such complications as hyperbilirubinemia and perinatal asphyxia, is widely accepted as a risk factor for congenitally acquired hearing impairment. Numerous reports of frequencies between 4 and 16 percent for hearing loss have been recorded in low birth weight infants (Abramovich et al., 1979; Anagnostakes et al., 1982). Other conditions that have been reported to enhance the risk of neurologic sequelae, including hearing impairment, are acidosis, sepsis, ototoxic drug therapy, sound trauma, and hypoglycemia (Bess et al., 1979; Perlman et al., 1980). Ascertaining the exact cause of hearing loss in neonates with multiple risk factors remains difficult. Any of these factors alone may cause hearing impairment, but when they are associated with immature physiologic status, the risk of hearing impairment increases. The hearing loss most often demonstrated in low birth weight infants is sensorineural, particularly in the high-frequency range (Clark, 1978).

Berman and associates (1978) reported a high correlation between prolonged intubation, otitis media, and hearing loss in low birth weight infants. Halpern and coauthors (1987) examined hearing in 799 infants who had been in the NICU and found that two overall measures of health—length of stay in the NICU and gestational age—predicted hearing loss in this group. The higher incidence of hearing loss in low birth weight infants has been attributed to several factors: (1) premature physiologic status; (2) perinatal complications, such as hyperbilirubinemia, hypoxia, acidosis, and apneic spells, which are likely to produce brain damage in low birth weight infants; (3) constraints of intensive care; and (4) combined effects of the preceding factors (Minoli & Moro, 1985).

"Constraints of intensive care" refers to the iatrogenic factors common in the care of newborns admitted to the NICU that have an impact on the incidence of hearing impairment. These factors include ambient noise and exposure to ototoxic drugs (Minoli & Moro, 1985). (For a complete discussion, see Chapter 44, Iatrogenic Complications of the NICU.)

Galambos and colleagues (1994) presented a retrospective study of hearing loss in level two (n = 1527) and three (n = 4374) graduates. Findings indicated that 1.4 percent of level two and 2.1 percent of level three infants failed two rounds of ABR testing and subsequently required hearing aid devices within the first year of life.

Ototoxic Drugs

The effects of ototoxic drugs commonly used in the care of low birth weight infants, which potentiate damage to the cochlea or the vestibular portion of the inner ear, have been well documented in the literature (Lerner et al., 1981; Pettigrew et al., 1988). Drugs that have been reported to be potentially ototoxic include antibiotics, diuretics, and antimalarial pharmaceuticals (Northern & Downs, 1984). Considerable individual susceptibility appears to exist to these ototoxic drugs, which usually cause bilateral symmetrical hearing loss of varying degrees. Numerous factors may enhance the risk of ototoxicity, including increased drug serum levels, decreased renal function, use of more than one ototoxic drug simultaneously or in increased dose or for an extended period of time, age, health, heredity, and concurrent noise. In a study using perinatal histories of 16 preterm infants, Pettigrew and associates (1988) reported that aminoglycoside therapy of 15 days' duration significantly increased the incidence of moderate-to-profound hearing loss in those infants, as compared with 266 preterm infants who did not receive drug therapy.

Colding and colleagues (1989) reported that there was no indication that continuous 24-hour intravenous infusion of gentamicin causes more hearing impairment than the intermittent intravenous or intramuscular mode of therapy. Specific aminoglycosides reported to have ototoxic potential include amikacin, clindamycin, gentamicin, kanamycin, tobramycin, and vancomycin (Pettigrew et al., 1988). The most recent guidelines (American Speech–Language Hearing Association, 1990) suggested that aminoglycoside therapy administered for more than 5 days in combination with loop diuretics be added to the risk criteria for potential sensorineural hearing loss.

Neonatal nurses are urged to monitor peak and trough serum concentrations of antibiotics and creatinine clearance to avoid high systemic levels in cases of impaired renal function.

Sound Trauma

The potential for noise-induced hearing loss in the neonate has been the subject of numerous reports in the literature (Abramovich et al., 1979; Long et al., 1980). In the NICU, a magnitude of sound sources exist that constantly generate background and alarm sounds. Noise levels within the NICU have been reported to be 20 dB higher than in the well-baby nursery.

Douek and coauthors (1976) demonstrated destruction in the outer cochlear hair cell of the guinea pig when it was exposed to incubator noise. In contrast, according to Abramovich and colleagues (1979) and Anagnostakes and associates (1982), the noise level of incubators per se does not cause sensorineural hearing loss in otherwise healthy preterm infants. NICU sudden noises have been reported to produce hypoxemia in preterm infants, which leads to decreases in transcutaneous oxygen tension and increases in intracranial pressure, heart rate, and respiratory rate (Long et al., 1980).

Nearly all the reported sound pressure levels of incubators are consistently less than the risk levels for adults, being between 60 and 80 dB (Douek et al., 1976; Falk & Farmer, 1973; Thomas, 1989). The damage risk level of 90 dB for adults is based on intermittent exposure to noise, whereas for neonates, exposure is continuous for weeks and months at a time (Brown & Glass, 1979). In a follow-up study of children aged 4 to 6 years treated in incubators for prolonged periods, Winkel and coauthors (1978) reported that no cause of severe sensorineural hearing loss could be established; however, testing suggested minor noise-induced cochlear damage. In an 8-year follow-up study, Kitchen and associates (1979) demonstrated that premature infants who received care in a NICU had a higher incidence of sensorineural deafness than those who were in a routine care unit. Safe noise standards have not been established for NICUs. The NICU Design Standards Task Force has made recommendations that background noise be no greater than 90 dB (White, 1996). However, when background noise is greater than 50 dB, sleep is disturbed (Robertson & Philbin, 1996). The possible potentiating effects of constant noise with other risk factors on the neonate are also not known.

Newborns at risk for hearing impairment may be exposed to hazardous sound levels during transport procedures. In these conditions, noise levels between 90 and 110 dB can be reached in a helicopter (Despland & Galambos, 1982). Use of ear protectors during air transport has been suggested (Minoli & Moro, 1985).

The increased incidence of hearing loss in at-risk newborns indicates the need for further research studies to evaluate the potentiating effects of some of these factors in determining neonatal hearing loss. Accurate follow-up studies of infants in the NICU who are treated in different ways can provide indicators of the potential risks of various treatment modalities.

Conclusion

The high-risk register provides the nurse with a systematic approach for assessing auditory risk in the neonate (Table 33–3). As research in the area continues, further clarifications of the present risk factors and new findings will emerge.

SCREENING METHODS FOR IDENTIFICATION OF HEARING LOSS

Hearing screening is a method of detecting hearing impairment before the deficit becomes obvious in the infant. Within the past 15 years, programs and procedures for screening newborns have been developed, modified, and improved.

The goal of any screening program is to accomplish the task rapidly, accurately, and economically. To date, no current diagnostic screening methods fully meet all criteria.

Screening criteria such as the high-risk register should be the basis for any infant screening program. Infants who demonstrate no risk factors receive no audiologic follow-up unless some factor in the history indicates that delayed onset, degenerative disease, or intrauterine infection may present with progressive or fluctuating hearing loss. In all cases, teaching about the speech and hearing milestones and the identification of community agencies for long-term follow-up should be shared with the parents by the neonatal nurse before discharge. Because the focus of all screening programs is to identify and habilitate hearing-impaired children as early as possible, the Early Identification of Hearing Impairment in Infants and Young Children, National Institutes of Health Consensus Development Conference on the Early Identification of Hearing Impairment in Infants and Young Children (1993) recommended that all neonates be screened for hearing impairment. Only infants who are identified as having one or more high-risk factors are screened, leaving 50 to 70 percent of children with an impairment unidentified.

Infant screening is a collaborative effort involving nurses, physicians, audiologists, and public health agency members. Each play a vital role in the program's potential success.

Infants who present with any item on the high-risk register should undergo audiologic testing in the nursery or shortly after discharge.

Behavioral Measurements of Hearing Function

Early attempts at infant behavioral screening focused on observational assessments of the neonatal behavioral response to sound,

TABLE 33–3 Common Manifestations of Hearing Loss

	Most Common Manifestations of Hearing Loss					
High-Risk Factor	***Conductive***	***Sensorineural***	***Mixed***	***Unilateral***	***Bilateral***	***Degree***
Asphyxia		+			+	Mild–profound
Bacterial meningitis		+			+	Severe–profound
Toxoplasmosis*		+			+	Moderate–profound
Syphilis		+			+	Severe–profound
Rubella*		+			+	Profound
Cytomegalovirus*		+		+	+	Mild–profound
Herpes*		+		?	?	?
Defects of head and neck	+	+	+	+	+	Mild–profound
Elevated bilirubin		+		+	+	Mild–profound
Family history*	+	+	+	+	+	Mild–profound
Low birth weight		+			+	Moderate–severe

*These factors may exhibit progressive hearing loss and should be followed serially.
From Gerkin, K. P. (1984). The high risk register for deafness. *ASHA, 26*, 22. Reprinted with permission.

using noisemakers to obtain orienting responses. A squeeze toy, bell, or rattle was used to test for a behavioral response based on the maturational level of the subject (Fig. 33–7). The expected response at 0 to 4 months included eye widening, eye blink, and arousal from sleep. With this method, the false-positive or false-negative results were found to be unacceptably high. Errors can be minimized by having more than one observer. Even under these conditions, Moneus (1968) reported that trained observers can incorrectly perceive a response in 39 percent of control trials. In response to the high false-negative and false-positive results, Gerber and colleagues (1985) suggested the following protocol be established for observational behavioral testing. Response from auditory stimulation should constitute an eye movement and the movement of at least one limb, both of which should occur within 2.5 seconds of signal onset, and both of which must be observed by two independent observers or one observer subjected to auditory masking. The validity of the test lies partly on the identification of infant state and the control of environmental noise. For testing purposes, a light sleep state is best. This state can be assessed by the clinician's noting a quiver of the eyelid or small body movement when the eyelid is stimulated with a finger or a tongue blade.

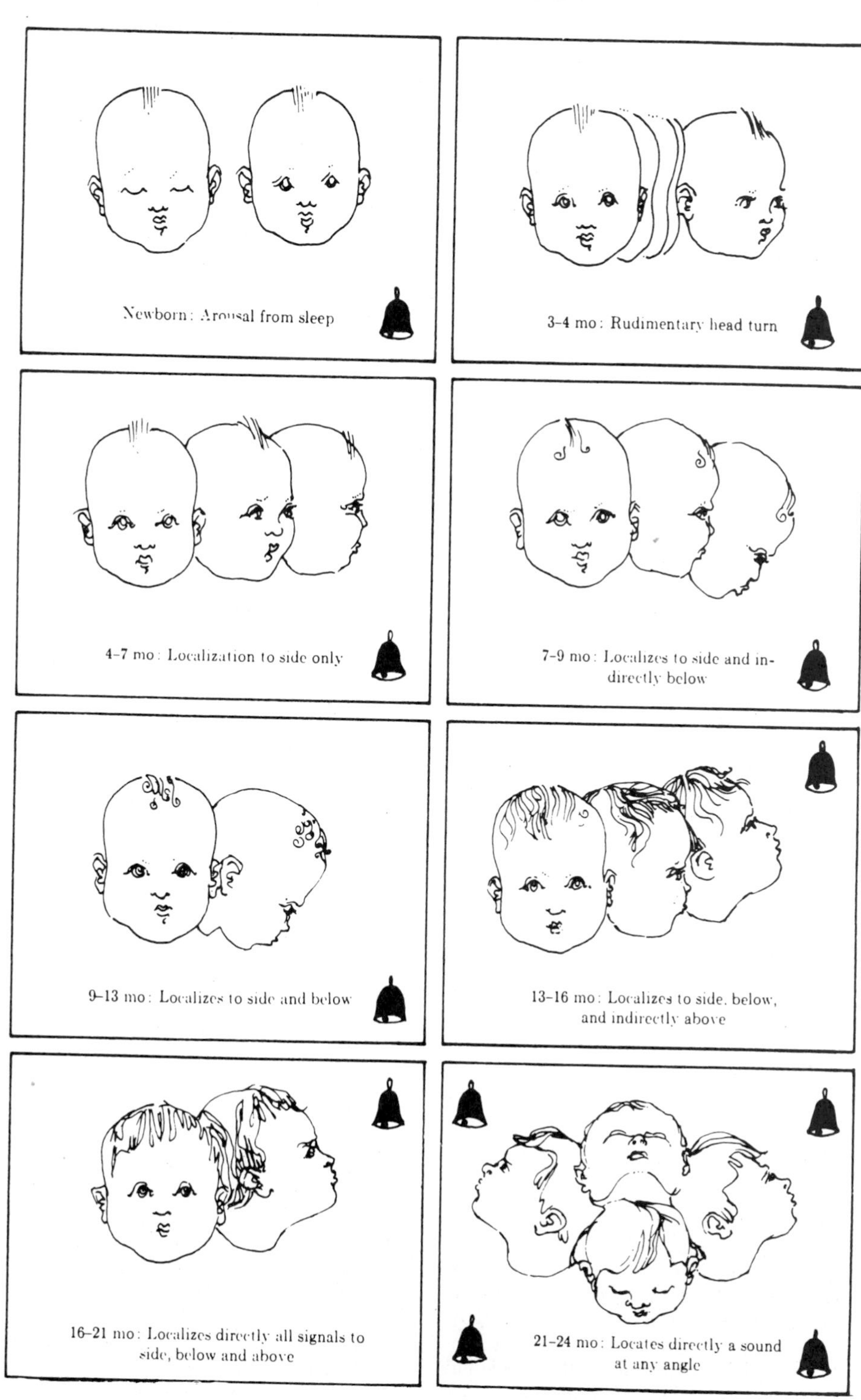
Newborn: Arousal from sleep
3–4 mo: Rudimentary head turn
4–7 mo: Localization to side only
7–9 mo: Localizes to side and indirectly below
9–13 mo: Localizes to side and below
13–16 mo: Localizes to side, below, and indirectly above
16–21 mo: Localizes directly all signals to side, below and above
21–24 mo: Locates directly a sound at any angle

FIGURE 33–7. Maturation of auditory response. (From Northern, J., & Downs, M. [1984]. *Hearing in children* [p. 252]. Baltimore: Williams & Wilkins. Reprinted with permission.)

Automated Screening Devices

Disappointing results from observational screening methods prompted the development of automated instrumentation methods of detecting hearing loss.

Crib-O-Gram

The Crib-O-Gram (Simmons & Russ, 1974) is an ingenious automated system aimed at monitoring behavioral and physiologic responses to auditory stimuli. This test is accomplished by placement of a motion-sensitive transducer under the crib mattress. The infant's state is monitored automatically by measurement of crib movements before and after each sound presentation. The test sound, 92 dB, is presented by an earphone placed in the bassinet. Responses are recorded from 10 seconds before until 3.5 seconds after the stimuli onset until a statistically valid decision is made by a microprocessing unit (Marcellino, 1986).

Auditory Response Cradle

Like the Crib-O-Gram, the Auditory Response Cradle (ARC), which was designed by Bennett and Lawrence (1980), monitors behavioral and physiologic responses to auditory stimuli by an automatic, microprocessor-controlled device. The system is composed of a cradle that houses the electronic components of the device, including the microprocessor. Four response types are monitored during the test: (1) head and trunk movements are monitored by a pressure-sensitive mattress; (2) startle responses are detected by the microprocessor and transducer; (3) body movements are detected by pressure transducers beneath the mattress; and (4) respiratory movements of the chest are monitored by a transducer within a band fixed around the infant's chest or abdomen. Noise stimulus is presented at 85 db through earphones, and the analysis procedure takes into account the number of responses that occur with sound and control trials. The device assesses infant activity in the prestimulus period and defers testing if the subject is restless. Davis and colleagues (1991) reported the mean test time to be 11 minutes for infants at risk. This time is short, compared with the 2- to 3-hour test time reported for the Crib-O-Gram studies.

Screening Studies Using the Behavioral Method

One of the most extensive studies of the behavioral method for infant screening was reported by Feinmesser and Tell (1976). These investigators reported on a group of 17,731 newborns by use of behavioral methods at birth, 6 months, and 3 years: the screening test conducted at birth detected hearing loss in only six of the 23 children who were ultimately diagnosed as having profound hearing loss. A false-positive rate of 75 percent was also reported. Many of these children (17 of 23) would have been identified by a high-risk register assessment. A more recent study, by Marcellino (1986), who used a Crib-O-Gram as the behavioral tool on 1195 babies in the special care unit, indicated a false-positive rate of 14 to 16 percent; no false-negative responses were reported. Initial studies of the ARC looked promising. Bennett and Wade (1981) obtained an initial false-positive rate of 5.3 percent after testing 1899 infants. Tucker (1986) identified 23 infants who had some degree of hearing impairment and seven who had definite hearing loss who originally passed the ARC test. ARC testing of preterm infants (McCormick et al., 1984) was reported to result in a false-positive rate of 19 percent after one test. Before more screening of preterm infants is used, much more research is needed about the development of sensory and response systems and the patterns of attentiveness.

Automated devices have reduced errors introduced by observers; however, more sensitive parameters for assessing physical response to auditory stimuli will need to be collaboratively researched before present devices can be used without hesitation.

Peripheral Measurements of Hearing Function

In assessing the hearing activity of the neonate, recent focus has been directed toward a two-tiered approach, in which a test that measures otoacoustic emissions is initially used, and ABR follow-up is performed for infants whose hearing impairment is detected on the initial screening. Otoacoustic emissions are low-intensity sounds that can be measured by use of a sensitive microphone placed in the ear canal. Hearing screening using otoacoustic emissions is quick, inexpensive, and relatively accurate. If an infant's hearing impairment is detected on the otoacoustic emissions, additional testing by the ABR confirms the validity of the otoacoustic emissions. The ABR test records the electrical potentials that arise from the auditory nerve system. During this measurement, disk electrodes are attached to the vertex and the mastoid areas, and repetitive sounds are then presented to the ear in the form of clicks caused by a direct current pulse. The response recorded is a sequence of waves that represents the action potential of the auditory nerve. The wave latencies in infants at risk tend to show smaller and more prolonged responses. The absolute latency of the ABR waves depends on the intensity of the click stimulus. Thresholds of hearing are identified by decreasing the click stimuli from intensities of 60 dB to 30 to 40 dB. Absence of all waves indicates the presence of a peripheral lesion. An abnormal ABR result may be defined as one in which there is an absence of response at the 40-dB intensity or a wave V latency that exceeds the norm by two standard deviations (Cox et al., 1984). Wave V responses in infants are highly repeatable and reveal little variability in normal-hearing subjects; thus, they are used to determine response abnormality. The ABR appears to be a sensitive method in that no false-negative results have been reported. Considering that any screening method should be quick, inexpensive, and easily administered and should allow easy interpretation of a large number of infants, ABRs are at a disadvantage. Specialized personnel are needed to administer this test, which in most cases takes from 60 minutes to 2 hours to perform. Nevertheless, the ABR can be justified as a neonatal hearing test, especially in preterm or high-risk infants.

In some infants whose initial ABR test results meet risk criteria, ongoing audiologic follow-up and management may be appropriate. These infants include those with risk factors associated with possible progressive or fluctuant loss, such as family history of progressive hearing loss, CMV, and persistent fetal circulation.

Infants who do not demonstrate a repeatable ABR wave V to the signal presented at 40 dB in at least one ear should have a comprehensive hearing evaluation at no later than 6 months of age (National Institutes of Health Consensus Development Conference, 1993). This follow-up includes general physical examination, including examination of the head and neck, otoscopy and otomicroscopy, identification of relevant physical abnormalities, and laboratory tests for perinatal infections. A comprehensive audiologic evaluation may include additional evoked potential evaluation, behavioral testing, and acoustic emittance measures. Although precise data on hearing sensitivity cannot be obtained until the infant can respond to operant conditioning test procedures at approximately 6 months of age, habilitation should not be delayed (Thompson & Wilson, 1984). Modifications of the treatment protocols can be made as additional hearing evaluation data become available. Some institutions are now using ABR and otoacoustic emissions as early as 24 hours of age. The rationale is that the earlier a problem is identified, the quicker a treatment can be started (Ronge, 1997).

Infants can be fitted with hearing aids before 3 months of age. Attention to early identification, amplification, and education does not necessarily ensure but certainly facilitates speech and language acquisition, even in the most profoundly hearing-impaired child (Markides, 1986).

MANAGEMENT OF THE HEARING-IMPAIRED NEONATE

Among the recommendations advanced by the Joint Committee on Infant Hearing is that the hearing of infants who present with any item on the high-risk register should be screened optimally by 3 months but no later than 6 months of age, and that whenever possible, the diagnostic process should be complete and the habilitation begun by 6 months of age (AAP, 1982). An infant with a positive hearing test result should be retested within 6 weeks of the initial screening procedure. Infants who, by virtue of their history, are at risk for late-onset hearing loss should be observed by periodic audiologic testing.

For the infant with a confirmed hearing loss, efforts are directed at treatment. In accordance with Public Law 99, early intervention services are (1) evaluation and assessment and (2) development of an individualized family service plan. The full evaluation plan is to be completed within 45 days of referral. This plan may include various treatment modalities directed at the treatment of serous otitis media, which is a major cause of temporary conductive hearing loss. For the infant with a permanent conductive hearing loss, amplification with a hearing aid may facilitate stimulation in the early critical period. Infants can be fitted with a hearing aid device as soon as the impairment is diagnosed. In addition to amplification, the family should be taught total communication skills that will enhance the interactional process between the sender and the receiver. The basic premise is to use every means to communicate, such as gesturing, touching, and attending to stimuli (Brewster, 1985).

Hearing screening is a task for a team of professionals— pediatricians, otolaryngologists, audiologists, and nurses. Local public health agencies may provide services such as data collection and referral. Many large metropolitan medical centers have speech and hearing centers as part of a broad base of services ranging from diagnosis to rehabilitation. At the national level, the following organizations disseminate information to health professionals and consumers on the diagnosis and treatment of hearing impairments:

American Speech–Language Hearing Association (ASHA)
10801 Rockville Pike
Rockville, MD 20852

Alexander Graham Bell Association for the Deaf
3417 Volta Place, N.W.
Washington, D.C. 20007

The overall goal of any treatment program for the hearing impaired is to optimize the potential communication skills and abilities of the infant. To achieve this goal, a comprehensive evaluation, follow-up, and management system must be implemented. The multidisciplinary, multiservices approach should be instituted only when all components are available to the infant and the family (American Speech–Language Hearing Association, 1988).

In addition to qualified professionals and services, many other factors influence the management and habilitation of the hearing-impaired infant. These factors facilitate or hamper entry into the system, and compliance with the treatment regimen (Northern & Downs, 1984).

Facilitates	Hampers
Parental involvement	Length of waiting list
Expeditious referral arrangements	Poor communication between speech and hearing departments

Outcome measures of the treatment program are early identification and implementation of a comprehensive habilitation plan to maximize communication potential and parental acceptance of the infant's disability.

The infant with severe-to-profound hearing impairment who is not at risk for recurrent otitis media and cannot receive results with a hearing aid is a candidate for cochlear implant (Northern & Downs, 1984). In this procedure, implanted electrodes into the cochlea stimulate the auditory nerves and obtain some hearing where none was before.

For the hearing-impaired infant, multiple referral sources exist in which a multidisciplinary approach optimizes the potential for the infant's future growth and development.

Parental Support

Support for the parents of a hearing-impaired child is based on the foundation of trust and acceptance between the nurse and the family. Notification of a hearing impairment is an extremely traumatic and deeply disturbing situation for the parents and is one that often provokes denial. Often, delays in identification occur because parents cannot admit that something is wrong. Some practices in the diagnostic work-up for hearing impairment seem to favor separation of the parents from the diagnostic process. Otoacoustic emissions and ABR testing may foster denial because the findings are abstract and parents need to have visible, tangible evidence of the impairment. The nurse plays a major role in reiterating, interpreting, and reinforcing the information conveyed by the audiologist. Sensitivity for the parents in their need to grieve the loss of the "perfect child" is important. Facilitating acceptance of the handicap can be aided by enlisting the parents as codiagnosticians. Asking the parents what they think the problem is and making them part of the decision-making process objectifies the diagnoses and aids in future compliance to the habilitative regimen. By listening to the parental feelings of inadequacy and by indirect teaching, nurses can teach more fruitful coping strategies (Luterman, 1985).

The mother–infant relationship is potentially damaged when the infant is hearing impaired. Reciprocal communication that normally occurs between the mother and the infant on an affective and a verbal level has been reported to be diminished with infants who are hearing impaired (Greenstein et al., 1976). The handicapped infant may miss intended signals from parents and may emit signals that are not understood. The parents need to capture their infant's visual attention so that their efforts are effectively stimulating. A potential asynchrony may develop that can retard the ability to acquire language even beyond the limits of the hearing loss itself (Luterman, 1985). The family can be taught total communication skills (gesturing, touching, and attending) to support interaction with the infant.

CONCLUSION

Most nursing research in this area has centered on the effect of noise on infants in NICUs. Further research is needed in the areas of identification of additional risk factors, comparative cost for various screening procedures, strategies to enhance acquisition of early linguistic skills, and the parent–infant relationship. Additional research is also needed in order to identify the cost–benefit ratio of universal screening procedures, as well as the impact of environmental noise on the neonate and the caregiver.

REFERENCES

Abramovich, S. J., Gregory, S., Slemink, M., & Stewart, A. (1979). Hearing loss in very low birth weight infants treated with neonatal intensive care. *Archives of Disease in Childhood, 54*(6), 421–426.

Abrams, D. A., Kerr, A. G., Smyth, G. D., & Cinnamond, M. J. (1983). Congenital syphilitic deafness: A further review. *Journal of Laryngology and Otology, 97*(1), 399–404.

Abrams, I. F. (1977). Nongenetic hearing loss. In B. F. Jaffe (Ed.), *Hearing loss in children*. Baltimore: University Park Press.

Allen, M. C., & Capute, A. J. (1986). Assessment of early auditory and visual abilities of extremely premature infants.

Developmental Medicine and Childhood Neurology, 28(4), 458–466.

American Academy of Pediatrics (AAP). (1982). Joint Committee on Infant Hearing: Position statement. *Pediatrics, 70*(3), 496–497.

American Speech–Language Hearing Association Committee on Infant Hearing (ASHA). (1988). Guidelines for the identification of hearing impairment in at risk infants age birth to six months. *ASHA, 30*(4), 61–64.

American Speech–Language Hearing Association Joint Committee on Hearing. (1990). Position statement. *ASHA, 32*(3), 15–17.

Anagnostakes, D., Petmezakis, J., Papzissis, G., et al. (1982). Hearing loss in low birth weight infants. *American Journal of Diseases in Children, 136*(7), 602.

Apgar, V., & James, L. (1962). Further observation on the newborn scoring system. *American Journal of Diseases of Children, 104*(10), 419–428.

Babson, S. G. (1980). *Diagnosis and management of the fetus and neonate at risk*. St. Louis: C. V. Mosby Co.

Baldwin, J. L. (1968). Dysostosis craniofacialis of Crouzon. *Laryngoscope, 78*(10), 1660–1675.

Baley, J., & Goldfarb. J. (1992). Viral infections. In A. Fanaroff & R. J. Martin (Eds.), *Neonatal perinatal medicine: Diseases of the fetus and infant* (5th ed., pp. 662–682). St. Louis: C. V. Mosby Co.

Balkany, T. J., Downs, M. P., Jafek, B. W., & Krajicek, M. J. (1979). Hearing loss in Down's syndrome: A treatable handicap more common than generally recognized. *Clinical Pediatrics, 18*(2), 116–118.

Balkany, T. J. (1980). Otologic aspects of Down's syndrome. *Seminars in Speech, Language and Hearing, 1*(1), 39.

Behrman, R. E., Kliegman, R. M., & Arvin, A. M. (Eds.) (1995). *Nelson textbook of pediatrics* (15th ed.). Philadelphia: W. B. Saunders Co.

Behrman, R. E., & Kliegman, R. M. (1992). Disturbances of organ systems. In R. E. Behrman (Ed.), *Nelson textbook of pediatrics* (14th ed., pp. 460–493). Philadelphia: W. B. Saunders Co.

Bennett, M. J., & Lawrence, R. J. (1980). Trials with the Auditory Response Cradle: II. The neonatal respiratory response to an auditory stimulus. *British Journal of Audiology, 14*(1), 1–6.

Bennett, J. J., & Wade, H. K. (1981). Computerized hearing test for neonates. *Hearing Aid Journal, 10*, 52–53.

Bergstrom, L., & Hemenway, W. G. (1971). Otologic problems in submucous cleft palate. *Southern Medical Journal, 64*(10), 1172–1177.

Berman, S. A., Balkany, T. J., & Simmons, M. A. (1978). Otitis media in the neonatal intensive care unit. *Pediatrics, 62*(2), 198–201.

Bess, F. H., Peek, B. F., & Chapman, J. J. (1979). Further observations on noise levels in infant incubation. *Pediatrics, 63*(1), 100–106.

Black, F. O., Bergstrom, L., & Downs, M. P. (1971). *Congenital deafness: A new approach to early detection through a high risk register*. Boulder, CO: Associated University Press.

Bluestone, C. D., & Shurin, P. A. (1974). Middle ear disease in children: Pathogenesis, diagnosis and management. *Pediatric Clinics of North America, 21*(2), 379–399.

Brewster, L. C. (1985). Interaction analysis of mother and hearing impaired child. *Ear and Hearing, 6*(1), 54–56.

Brown, A. K., & Glass, L. (1979). Environmental hazards in the newborn nursery. *Pediatric Annals, 8*(1), 698–705.

Butterfield, E. C. (1968). *An extended version of modification of sucking with auditory feedback*. Unpublished manuscript. Topeka: University of Kansas Medical Center, Bureau of Child Research Laboratory, Children Rehabilitation Unit.

Clark, G. M. (1978). Cochlear implant surgery for profound or total hearing loss [Editorial]. *Medical Journal of Australia, 2*(13), 587–588.

Colding, H., Andersen, E. A., Pragtz, S., et al. (1989). Auditory function after continuous infusion of gentamicin to high risk newborns. *Acta Paediatrica Scandinavica, 78*(6), 840–843.

Condon, W. S., & Sander, L. W. (1974). Neonate movement is synchronized with adult speech: Interactional participation and language structure. *Science, 183*(120), 99–101.

Cooper, L. Z., Ziring, P. R., Ockerse, A. B., et al. (1969). Rubella: Clinical manifestations and management. *American Journal of Diseases of Children, 118*(1), 18–29.

Cox, L. C., Hack, M., & Metz, D. A. (1984). Auditory brainstem response abnormalities in the very low birth weight infant: Incidence and risk factors. *Ear and Hearing, 5*(4), 47–51.

Davis, A. C., Wharrad, H. J., Sancho, J., & Marshall, D. H. (1991). Early detection of hearing impairment: What role is there for behavioural methods in the neonatal period? *Acta Oto-Laryngologica. Supplement, 482*, 103–109.

DeCasper, A. J., & Fifer, W. P. (1980). Of human bonding: Newborns prefer their mothers' voices. *Science, 208*(4448), 1174–1176.

Despland, P. A., & Galambos, R. (1982). The brainstem auditory evoked potential is a useful diagnostic tool in evaluating risk factors for hearing loss in neonatology. *Advances in Neurology, 32*, 241–247.

Douek, E., Bannister, L. H., Dodson, H. C., et al. (1976). Effects of incubator noise on the cochlea of the newborn. *Lancet, 2*(7995), 1110–1113.

Downs, M. P., & Silver, H. K. (1972). A.B.C.D.'s to hear: Early identification in the nursery office and clinics of the infant who is deaf. *Clinical Pediatrics, 11*(10), 563–566.

Doyle, W. J., Cantekin, E. I., & Bluestone, C. D. (1980). Eustachian tube function in cleft palate children. *Annals of Otology, Rhinology, and Laryngology, 89*(Suppl. 68), 34–40.

Early Identification of Hearing Impairment in Infants and Young Children, National Institutes of Health and Consensus Development Conference. (1993). *American Journal of Otology, 15*(2), 130–131.

Eavey, R. D. (1989). Management strategies for congenital ear malformations. *Recent Advances in Pediatric Otology, 36*(6), 1521–1540.

Eiman, P. D., & Tartter, V. C. (1979). On the development of speech perception: Mechanisms and analogies. *Advances in Child Development and Behavior, 13*(1), 303.

Eisenberg, R. B. (1976). *Auditory competence in early life*. Baltimore: University Park Press.

Elliot, G. B., & Elliot, K. A. (1964). Some pathological radiological and clinical implications of the precocious development of the human ear. *Laryngoscope, 74*(7), 1160–1171.

Falk, S. A., & Farmer, J. C. (1973). Incubator noise and possible deafness. *Archives of Otolaryngology, 97*(1), 385–387.

Feigin, R. D., Adcock, L., & Miller, D. (1992). Postnatal bacterial infections. In A. Fanaroff & R. J. Martin (Eds.), *Neonatal-perinatal medicine: Diseases of the fetus and infant* (5th ed., pp. 619–661). St. Louis: C. V. Mosby Co.

Feigin, R. D., Adcock, L., & Edwards, M. S. (1992). Fungal and protozoal infections. In A. Fanaroff & R. J. Martin (Eds.), *Neonatal-perinatal medicine: Diseases of the fetus and infant* (5th ed., pp. 683–690). St. Louis: C. V. Mosby Co.

Feingold, M. (1982). Clinical evaluation of a patient with a genetic birth defect syndrome. *Alabama Journal of Medical Science, 19*(2), 151–156.

Feinmesser, M., & Tell, L. (1976). Neonatal screening for detection of deafness. *Archives of Otolaryngology, 102*(5), 297–299.

Finitzo-Hieber, T., Freedman, F. J., Gerling, I. J., et al. (1981). Auditory brainstem response abnormalities in post-meningitic infants and children. *International Journal of Pediatric Otorhinolaryngology, 3*(4), 275–286.

Fraser, G. R. (1976). *The causes of profound deafness in childhood*. Baltimore: Johns Hopkins University Press.

Friel-Patti, S., Finitzo-Hieber, T., Conti, G., & Brown, K. C. (1982). Language delay in infants associated with middle ear disease and mild, fluctuating hearing impairment. *Pediatric Infectious Diseases, 1*(2), 104–109.

Gagnon, R. (1989). Stimulation of human fetuses with sound and vibration. *Seminars in Perinatology, 13*(5), 393–402.

Galambos, R., Wilson, M. J., & Silva, P. (1994). Identifying hearing loss in the intensive care nursery: A 20-year summary. *Journal American Academy of Audiology, 5*(3), 151–162.

Gerber, S. E., Wile, E., & Hamai, N. T. (1985). Central auditory dysfunction in deaf children. *Human Communication Canada, 9*(1), 39–44.

Gershan, A. (1981). Infection of fetus and newborn infants. *Journal Perinatal Medicine, 9*(4), 204–206.

Goodlin, R. C., & Schmidt, W. (1972). Human fetal arousal levels as indicated by heart rate recordings. *American Journal of Obstetrics and Gynecology, 114*(5), 613–621.

Graven, S. N. (1996). Concepts of fetal sensory development. Paper presented at the Physical and Developmental Environment of the High Risk Neonate, January 31, 1996. Clearwater Beach, FL: University of South Florida College of Medicine.

Greenstein, J. M., Greenstein, B. B., McConnville, K., et al. (1976). *Mother-infant communication and language acquisition in deaf infants*. New York: Lexington School for the Deaf.

Grimwade, J. C., Walter, D. W., Bartlet, M., et al. (1971). Human fetal heart rate change and movement in response to sound and vibration. *American Journal of Obstetrics and Gynecology, 109*(1), 90.

Hain, R. J., Doshi, N., & Harger, J. H. (1980). Ascending transcervical herpes simplex infection with intact fetal membranes. *Obstetrics and Gynecology, 56*(1), 106.

Halpern, J., Hosford-Dunn, H., & Malachowski, N. (1987). Four factors that accurately predict hearing loss in "high risk" neonates. *Ear and Hearing, 8*(1), 21–25.

Harner, R. E., Smith, J. L., & Israel, C. W. (1968). The FTA-ABS test in late syphilis: A serological study in 1,985 cases. *Journal of the American Medical Association, 203*(8), 103–106.

Hatherly, L. I., Hayes, K., & Jack, I. (1980). Herpes virus in an obstetric hospital: III. Prevalence of antibodies in patients and staff. *Medical Journal of Australia, 2*(6), 325.

Helias, J., Chobaut, J., Muorot, M., & Lafon, J. (1988). Early detection of hearing loss in children with cleft palate by brain-stem auditory response. *Archives of Otolaryngology—Head and Neck Surgery, 114*(2), 154–156.

Hyman, C. B., Keaster, J., Hanson, V., et al. (1969). CNS abnormalities after neonatal hemolytic disease or hyperbilirubinemia: A prospective study of 405 patients. *American Journal of Diseases of Children, 117*(4), 395–405.

Illum, P., Kiaer, H. W., Hvidberg-Hansen, J., & Sondergaard, G. (1972). Fifteen cases of Pendred's syndrome: Congenital deafness and sporadic goiter. *Archives of Otolaryngology, 96*(4), 297–304.

Jaffe, B. F. (1977). Middle ear and pinna abnormalities. In B. J. Jaffe (Ed.), *Hearing loss in children* (pp. 294–309). Baltimore: University Park Press.

Jenistra, J. A. (1984). Perinatal herpes virus infections. In M. S. Amstey (Ed.), *Virus infection in pregnancy*. Orlando, FL: Grune & Stratton.

Jensen, O. H. (1984). Fetal heart rate response to a controlled sound stimulus as a measure of fetal well-being. *Acta Obstetrica et Gynecologica Scandinavica, 63*(2), 97–101.

Johansson, B., Wadenberg, E., & Westin, B. (1964). Measurement of tone response by the human fetus. *Acta Oto-Laryngologica, 57*, 188–192.

Jones, K. L. (Ed.). (1988). *Smith's recognizable patterns of human malformation* (4th ed.). Philadelphia: W. B. Saunders Co.

Kaminski, J., & Hall, W. (1996). The effect of soothing music on neonatal behavioral states in the hospital newborn nursery. *Neonatal Nursing, 15*(1), 45–54.

Karmody, C. S., & Schuknecht, H. F. (1966). Deafness in congenital syphilis. *Archives of Otolaryngology, 83*(1), 18–27.

Keleman, G. (1958). Toxoplasmosis and congenital deafness. *Archives of Otolaryngology, 68*, 547–561.

Kitchen, W. H., Richards, A., Ryan, M. M., et al. (1979). A longitudinal study of very low-birthweight infants: II. Results of controlled trial of intensive care and incidence of handicaps. *Developmental Medicine and Childhood Neurology, 21*(5), 582– 589.

Konigsmark, B. W., & Gorlin, R. J. (1976). *Genetic and metabolic deafness*. Philadelphia: W. B. Saunders Co.

Krugman, S., & Katz, S. (1981). *Infectious diseases of children*. St. Louis: C. V. Mosby Co.

Lerner, S. A., Mantz, G., & Hawkins, J. (1981). *Aminoglycoside ototoxicity*. Boston: Little, Brown & Co.

Levine, R. L. (1979). Bilirubin: Worked out years ago? *Pediatrics, 64*(3), 380–385.

Linsey, J. R. (1971). Inner ear pathology in congenital deafness. *Otolaryngologic Clinics of North America, 4*(2), 249–290.

Long, J. G., Lucey, J., & Philip, A. (1980). Noise and hypoxemia in the intensive care nursery. *Pediatrics, 65*(1), 143–145.

Luterman, D. M. (1985). The denial mechanism. *Ear and Hearing, 6*(1), 57–58.

MacDonald, H. M., Mulligan, J. C., Allen, A. C., & Taylor, P. M. (1980). Neonatal asphyxia: I. Relationship of obstetric and neonatal complications to neonatal mortality in 38,405 consecutive deliveries. *Journal of Pediatrics, 96*(5), 898–902.

Mahoney, T., & Eichwald, J. (1987). The ups and "Downs" of high risk hearing screening: The Utah statewide program. In K. Gerkin & A. Amochaev (Eds.), *Seminars in Hearing, 8*(2), 155–163.

Marcellino, G. R. (1986). "The Crib-O-Gram" in neonatal hearing screening. In E. T. Swigart (Ed.), *Neonatal hearing screening*. Basel, Switzerland: Karger.

Marcus, R. E., & Valvassori, G. (1970). Cochleo-vestibular apparatus, radiologic studies in hereditary and familial hearing loss. *International Audiology, 9*, 95–102.

Markides, A. (1986). Age at fitting of hearing aids and speech intelligibility. *British Journal of Audiology, 20*(2), 165–167.

Maskarinec, A. S., Cairns, G. F., Jr., Butterfield, E. C., & Weamer, D. K. (1981). Longitudinal observations of individual infant's vocalizations. *Journal of Speech and Hearing Disorders, 46*(3), 267–273.

McCormick, B., Curnock, D. A., & Spavins, F. (1984). Auditory screening of special care neonates using the Auditory Response Cradle. *Archives of Disease in Childhood, 59*(12), 1168–1172.

McCracken, J. S. (1963). Rubella in the newborn. *British Medical Journal, 2*, 420–422.

Mencher, G. T., Mencher, L. S., & Rohland, S. L. (1985). Maturation of behavioral response. *Ear and Hearing, 6*(1), 10–14.

Minoli, I., & Moro, G. (1985). Constraints of intensive care units and follow-up studies in prematures. *Acta Oto-Laryngologica. Supplement, 421*, 62–67.

Moeller, M. P., Osberger, M. J., & Eccarius, M. (1986, March). Language and learning skills of hearing-impaired students: Receptive language skills. *ASHA Monographs*, pp. 41–53.

Moneus, J. P. (1968). Judge reliability in infant testing. *Journal of Speech and Hearing Research, 11*(1), 348–411.

Nance, W. E., & Sweeney, A. (1975). Genetic factors in deafness of early life. *Otolaryngologic Clinics of North America, 8*(1), 19–48.

Naunton, R. J., & Valvassori, G. E. (1968). Inner ear abnormalities: Their associations with atresia. *Laryngoscope, 64*(6), 1041–1049.

Nahmias, A. J. (1974). The TORCH complex. *Hospital Practice, 9*(5) 65–72.

Northern, J. L., & Downs, M. P. (1984). *Hearing in children*. Baltimore: Williams & Wilkins.

Nyhan, W. L. (1983). Cytogenetic diseases. *Clinical Symposia, 35*(1), 1–32.

Osberger, M. J., Moeller, M. P., Eccarius, M., et al. (1986). Expressive language skills. In M. Osberger (Ed.), Language and learning skills of hearing impaired students. *ASHA Monographs, 23*, 54–65.

Panjvani, Z. F., & Henshaw, J. B. (1981). CMV in the perinatal period. *American Journal of Diseases of Children, 135*(1), 56–60.

Pantke, O. A., & Cohen, M. M. (1971). The Waardenburg syndrome. *Birth Defects, 7*(7), 147–152.

Paparella, M., & Suguira, S. (1967). The pathology of suppurative labyrinthus. *Annals of Otology, Rhinology and Laryngology, 76*(3), 554–586.

Pappas, D. G. (1985). *Diagnosis and treatment of hearing impairment in children*. San Diego: College-Hill Press.

Pappas, D. G., & Mundy, M. R. (1982). Sensorineural hearing loss: Infectious agent. *Laryngoscope, 92*(7), 752–754.

Pass, R. F., Stagno, S., Meyers, F. J., & Alford, C. (1980). Outcome of symptomatic congenital cytomegalovirus infection results of long term longitudinal follow up. *Pediatrics, 66*(5), 758–762.

Patterson, M. E. (1968). Congenital luetic hearing impairment. *Archives of Otolaryngology, 87*(4), 378–382.

Perlman, M. A., Gartner, L. M., Lee, K., et al. (1980). The association of kernicterus with bacterial infection in the newborn. *Pediatrics, 65*(1), 26–29.

Pettigrew, A. G., Edwards, D. A., & Henderson-Smart, D. J. (1988). Perinatal risk factors in preterm infants. *Medical Journal of Australia, 148*(4), 174–177.

Proctor, C. A., & Proctor, B. (1967). Understanding hereditary nerve deafness. *Archives of Otolaryngology, 85*(1), 23–40.

Pumper, R. W., & Yamashiroya, H. M. (1975). *Outline of medical virology*. Philadelphia: W. B. Saunders Co.

Querleu, D., Renard, X., Boutteville, C., & Crepin, G. (1989). Hearing by the human fetus. *Seminars in Perinatology, 13*(5), 409–420.

Querleu, D., Renard, X., & Crepin, G. (1981). Perception auditive et ré activité foetale aux stimulations sonores. *Journal de Gynecologie, Obstetrique et Biologie de la Reproduction, 10*(1), 307–314.

Querleu, D., Renard, X., & Versyp, F. (1988). Fetal hearing. *European Journal of Obstetrics, Gynecology, and Reproductive Biology, 29*(1), 191–212.

Read, J. A., & Miller, F. C. (1977). Fetal heart rate acceleration in

response to acoustic stimulation as a measure of fetal well-being. *American Journal of Obstetrics and Gynecology, 129*(5), 512–517.
Robertson, A., & Philbin, M. K. (1996). Studies of sound and auditory development. Paper presented at the Physical and Developmental Environment of the High Risk Neonate, January 31, 1996. Clearwater Beach, FL: University of South Florida College of Medicine.
Ronge, L. J. (1997). Making a sound decision. *AAP News, 13*(4), 10–11.
Rosenhall, U., & Kankkunen, A. (1980). Hearing alterations following meningitis. *Ear and Hearing, 2*(4), 170–176.
Rotteveel, J., DeGraaf, R., Stegema, D. F., et al. (1987). The maturation of the central auditory conduction in preterm infants until 3 months post term: V. The auditory response. *Hearing Research, 27*(1), 95–110.
Ruben, R. J. (1984). Experimental otitis media with effusion: An inquiry into the minimal amount of auditory deprivation which results in a cognitive effect in man. *Acta Oto-Laryngologica. Supplement, 414*, 157–164.
Sando, I., & Wood, R. P. (1971). Congenital middle ear anomalies. *Otolaryngologic Clinics of North America, 4*(2), 291–318.
Saxon, S. A., & Witriol, E. (1976). Down's syndrome and intellectual development. *Journal of Pediatric Psychology, 1*(1), 45–47.
Scheiner, A. P. (1980). Perinatal asphyxia: Factors which predict developmental outcome. *Developmental Medicine and Child Neurology, 22*(1), 102–104.
Scholl, L. A., Lurie, M. H., & Keleman, G. (1951). Embryonic hearing organs after maternal rubella. *Laryngoscope, 61*(2), 99–112.
Schuknecht, H. J. (1974). *Pathology of the ear.* Cambridge, MA: Harvard University Press.
Schwartz, R. H., & Rodriguez, W. J. (1981). Acute otitis media in children eight years old and older: A reappraisal of the role of *Hemophilus influenzae. American Journal of Otolaryngology, 2*(1), 19–21.
Shurin, P. A. (1976). Antibacterial therapy and middle ear effusions. *Annals of Otology, Rhinology, and Laryngology,* 85(2, Suppl. 25, Part 2), 250–253.
Simmons, F. B., & Russ, F. N. (1974). Automated newborn hearing screening "The Crib-O-Gram." *Archives of Otolaryngology, 100*(1), 1–7.
Simmons, F. B. (1980). Patterns of deafness in newborns. *Laryngoscope, 90*(3), 448–453.
Stagno, S., Pass, K., & Alford, C. (1981). Perinatal infections and maldevelopment. *Birth Defects, 17*(1), 31–50.
Stagno, S., Reynolds, D. W., Amos, C. S., et al. (1977). Auditory and visual effects resulting from symptomatic and subclinical congenital cytomegalovirus and toxoplasma infection. *Pediatrics, 59*(5), 669–678.
Stein, L., Ozdamar, O., Kraus, N., & Paton, J. (1983). Follow-up of infants screened by auditory brainstem response in the neonatal intensive care unit. *Journal of Pediatrics, 103*(3), 447–453.
Stome, M. (1977). Sudden and fluctuating hearing losses. In B. F. Jaffe (Ed.), *Hearing loss in children* (pp. 478–479). Baltimore: University Park Press.
Thomas, K. (1989). How the NICU environment sounds to a preterm infant. *MCN, American Journal of Maternal Child Nursing, 14*(4), 249–251.
Thompson G., & Wilson, W. R. (1984). Clinical application of visual reinforcement audiometry. *Seminars in Hearing, 8*(2), 149–154.
Tucker, S. M. (1986). Auditory screening of normal and preterm infants using the auditory response cradle. *Audiology in Practice, 11*(4), 5–7.
Ueda, K., Nishida, Y., Oshima, K., & Shepard, T. H. (1979). Congenital rubella syndrome: Correlation of gestational age at time of maternal rubella with type of defect. *Journal of Pediatrics, 94*(5), 763.
Ventry, R. W., Wilson, W. R., Sprinkle, P. M., et al. (1981). Implications of virus in idiopathic sudden hearing loss: Primary infection of reactivation of latent viruses. *Archives of Otolaryngology—Head and Neck Surgery, 89*(1), 137–141.
Webster, D. B., & Webster, M. (1979). Effects of neonatal conductive hearing loss on brain stem auditory nuclei. *Annals of Otology, Rhinology and Laryngology,* 88(5, Part 1), 684–688.
Weller, T. H. (1971). The cytomegalovirus ubiquitous agents with protein clinical manifestations. *New England Journal of Medicine, 285*(4), 203–214.
White, R. (1996). Neonatal intensive care unit structure and design: Recommended standards. Paper presented at the Physical and Developmental Environment of the High Risk Neonate, January 31, 1996. Clearwater Beach, FL: University of South Florida College of Medicine.
Whitley, R. J., Nahmias, A. J., Bisintine, A. M., et al. (1980). The natural history of H.S.V. infection of mother and newborn. *Pediatrics, 66*(4), 489–494.
Wiet, R. J., & Milko, D. A. (1975). Isolation of the spirochetes in the perilymph despite prior antisyphilitic therapy. *Archives of Otolaryngology, 101*(2), 104–106.
Wilson, W. R., Byl, F. M., & Laird, N. (1980). The efficacy of steroids in the treatment of idiopathic sudden hearing loss: A double-blind clinical study. *Archives of Otolaryngology, 106*(12), 772–776.
Windle-Taylor, P., Emery, P. J., & Phelps, P. D. (1981). Ear deformities associated with Klippel-Feil syndrome. *Annals of Otology, Rhinology and Laryngology, 90*(1), 210–216.
Winkel, S., Bonding, P., Larsen, P. K., & Roosen, J. (1978). Possible effects of kanamycin and incubation in newborn children with low birth weight. *Acta Paediatrica Scandinavica, 67*(6), 709–715.

CHAPTER 34

Assessment and Management of Ophthalmic Dysfunction

FRANCES STRODTBECK

RESEARCH AGENDA

What impact will surfactant treatment have on the incidence and severity of retinopathy of prematurity?

What is the optimal treatment for severe retinopathy of prematurity and at what point should intervention occur?

VIGNETTE

Mrs. K presented to the emergency room in preterm labor with ruptured membranes; she delivered Andrew 2 hours later. He weighed 1180 g and was 12 weeks early. After he was stabilized and transferred to the NICU, I became his primary nurse.

Andrew was a fighter from the first. He received three doses of surfactant during the first 2 days and was weaned from the ventilator to nasal cannula oxygen. He had a fairly unremarkable course, which included mild apnea of prematurity, normal head ultrasounds, and steady weight gain. Andrew was alert and responsive to all who interacted with him. His parents were actively involved in his care and wanted to know and understand everything.

At 6 weeks of age Andrew had his first eye exam to screen for retinopathy of prematurity (ROP). Both of Andrew's eyes were prethreshold for ROP, meaning that they could improve spontaneously or worsen. If they worsened, he would probably need cryotherapy surgery. It was necessary to follow Andrew's eyes closely, and another eye exam was scheduled for the following week. The parents were quite concerned about this news. They spent the week reading and learning all they could about ROP. Mrs. K stated at one point that waiting to see what the next eye exam would show was the longest week of her life.

Both parents were at the bedside for the next exam. On completing the exam, Dr. L (the pediatric ophthalmologist) discussed the findings with them. She explained that the ROP had progressed to the threshold stage and that Andrew needed surgery, but first, she wanted to verify her findings with another ophthalmologist.

The second ophthalmologist confirmed the findings. Together, they spent time explaining the procedure, risks, and benefits to the parents. They also informed the parents that Andrew had a 50 percent chance for success. The parents were naturally upset by the news, and Mrs. K stated, "I thought we were finished with problems; it seems like it never ends." After agreeing to the surgery, the date was set for 2 days later.

My colleagues and I spent the next 2 days answering questions and discussing what to expect during and after the surgery, and that he would most likely be very sensitive to light for several days and we would need to shield his eyes with patches. We also discussed the importance of providing calming sensory stimulation to the other senses, such as rocking, gentle stroking, and talking during the interval the patches were on. We discussed that he would receive frequent eye exams after surgery and that his eyes might need cryotherapy again.

On the day of the surgery, Andrew's parents were there bright and early. He came through the procedure with flying colors. On post-op day 3, Andrew had another eye exam, and everything looked good according to Dr. L. She told the parents that Andrew would need close follow-up because the highest risk of detachment would be in the next 3 months. Andrew's eyes would be rechecked in 2 weeks and in another 2 months to determine whether more laser surgery was needed. If everything proceeded well, exams would be scheduled every 3 months for the first year and then annually. Dr. L also informed the parents that Andrew would be at risk for various eye problems and that he might require corrective glasses as he matured.

Five weeks later, Andrew was discharged home weighing 2600 g. His eye exams remained normal. Six months later, I saw Andrew when he returned to the ophthalmology clinic. According to his mother, everything looked good; he was a happy little boy who smiled and babbled and loved watching his mobile and followed the objects.

Kimberly S. Burton

The eye begins to develop early in gestation, making this body system vulnerable to insults during the growth process. Neonatal visual problems occur as a result of transplacental, congenital, or neonatal infections; congenital or genetic malformation; exposure to drugs; or abnormal adaptation of the developing eye and its vascularity to stimuli such as oxygen. Visual disturbances in the newborn can range from minor refractory problems to complete blindness. Early detection and treatment are essential if the best possible outcome is to be achieved.

This chapter briefly outlines the embryologic development of the eye, reviews the key points of assessment of the newborn's eye, and describes specific ophthalmic dysfunctions. Collaborative management and appropriate nursing care are also discussed.

EMBRYOLOGY

Our understanding of the forces that control and govern the development of the eye is growing but limited. About 2 weeks after fertilization, the embryonic plate elongates, and the primitive streak develops along the dorsal surface. The brain and eye develop from the neuroectoderm anterior to the primitive streak. The optic pits (optic sulci) are formed by the indentation of neuroectoderm. Closing of the neural tube leads to movement of the optic pits laterally and outward, toward the surface ectoderm. This movement results in the formation of the optic vesicles (Moore & Persaud, 1993).

As the optic vesicle approaches the outer wall of the embryo, it stimulates a focal thickening of cells called the lens placode. At the fourth week of gestation, invagination of this tissue occurs, resulting in formation of the optic cup. The inferior portion of the cup is the last to close. The two layers of the optic cup oppose one another to form the retina. At the same time, the lens placode sinks beneath the ectoderm and later becomes the crystalline lens. Mesoderm surrounding the optic cup differentiates to form the sclera, choroid, and a portion of the cornea (Moore & Persaud, 1993).

Mesoderm anterior to the lens develops into the pupillary membrane; the periphery of the pupillary membrane becomes the iris. The center degenerates to form the pupil. Ectoderm that covers the mesodermal folds appears above and below the lens placode to form the eyelids. The eyelids are fused until about 26 weeks of gestation. The lacrimal gland, the lacrimal drainage system, and the eyelashes form from the ectoderm that covers these folds. Tear production does not begin until 2 to 4 months after birth, when the lacrimal system process is complete (Moore & Persaud, 1993).

ASSESSMENT OF THE EYES

History

A thorough history is imperative to determine the presence of risk factors for eye problems. A complete family, medical, pregnancy, and psychosocial history, along with a maternal review of systems, should be obtained. The interviewer should ask questions related to the family history of vision problems, such as strabismus, glaucoma, retinoblastoma, and refractive errors, such as myopia. The maternal history should include questions regarding exposure to infectious diseases, such as gonorrhea, chlamydia, rubella, and cytomegalovirus, which are known to cause significant eye problems in newborns. The perinatal history should include questions on any difficulties that might have resulted in hypoxia or anoxia, conditions that are associated with adverse optical changes. Previous pregnancies that resulted in preterm births can provide important information about prior experience with retinopathy of prematurity (ROP).

Examination

Examination of the eyes of a newborn can be a challenge. Care must be taken during the examination process to protect the newborn from injury and cold stress (Cohen & Byrne, 1989). Infant state is also important to success. Newborns in the quiet alert state are more responsive to visual stimuli.

Most important information about the eye of the newborn can be obtained from inspection and observation. An examination with an ophthalmoscope is usually not indicated unless findings suggestive of serious problems, such as cataracts or glaucoma, exist.

It is easier to examine the newborns eyes when they are spontaneously open. Dimming the lights in the environment, talking to the infant, and holding him or her upright may facilitate natural opening of the eyes. Newborn eyes should be assessed for their shape, symmetry, and size and for the presence of obvious features, such as eyebrows and eyelashes. The eyes should appear clear, unswollen, and without discharge. Occasionally, irritation may result from the prophylactic drops or ointment used to prevent ophthalmia neonatorum. The eyelids should be evaluated for redness or swelling as well as for evidence of colobomas and abnormal tumor masses. Inability to elevate the eyelids or ptosis (drooping) of one or both eyelids may lead to amblyopia or poor visual development. The presence of unusual folds and the slant of the eye should be noted. Pupils should be checked for size, equality, reaction to light, and accommodation. The color and clarity of the red reflex should be checked. The color of the reflex in African-American infants may be pale orange rather than red (Johnson, 1993).

The cornea should be evaluated for clarity and size. A cloudy cornea may be caused by congenital glaucoma, inborn error of metabolism, or congenital corneal dystrophy. Trauma at birth can result in injury to the cornea, which can give the cornea a hazy appearance.

Directly behind the iris is the lens. Cloudiness or opacity in the lens is by definition a cataract. Any cataract found in a newborn should be evaluated by an ophthalmologist as soon as possible to determine if it is visually significant. Surgery should be performed in order to remove vision-threatening cataracts as soon as the infant is able to tolerate the procedure. Early surgery is critical to the prevention of amblyopia (lazy eye) that develops in these eyes when the condition is ignored for a few months.

Leukocoria is the descriptive term for a whitish-appearing pupil. This condition is almost always indicative of a serious eye problem. The differential diagnosis of leukocoria includes cataract, retinoblastoma, persistent hyperplastic primary vitreous, retrolental fibroplasia, toxocariasis, and Coats' disease.

Examination of the posterior pole of the eye (optic nerve, macula, and blood vessels) is performed with a direct ophthalmoscope with the pupil dilated. Newborns often squirm and move their head to avoid the light of the ophthalmoscope. An assistant should be used to stabilize the infant's head and body. It is often helpful to give the infant a bottle or a pacifier as a calming measure. A topical anesthetic, such as 0.5-percent proparacaine, may be instilled to dull the corneal and conjunctival sensitivity. The assistant may separate the eyelids, or a small pediatric eyelid speculum can be used. Care should be taken to avoid causing a corneal abrasion while the speculum is inserted. Normal saline should be used in order to avoid corneal drying (especially under the heat of a radiant warmer).

The infant's ability to see can be assessed by getting the newborn to fix and follow on brightly colored objects. The examiner should hold the object steady about 7 to 9 inches from the eye until the newborn fixes on it (examiner notes the reflection of the object in the middle of the newborn's pupil). Newborns should be able to follow an object about 90 inches either direction from a midline or a central position (Algranati, 1992). Care should be taken to avoid talking or other distractions because infants respond best to the presentation of one stimulus at a time.

Several important measurements should be obtained. The interpupillary distance and palpebral fissure width should be determined; abnormal values may be indicative of an underlying syndrome, such as fetal alcohol syndrome (Algranati, 1992). The interpupillary distance (distance from midpupil to midpupil when the eyes are looking forward) determines whether the eyes are spaced appropriately. Abnormal findings are hypotelorism (eyes too close together) or hypertelorism (eyes too far apart). Palpebral fissure width is the distance from the medial canthus to the lateral canthus of each eye. This measure determines the appropriateness of the opening for the eye. Measurements obtained should be compared with published norms to determine if the value is normal or abnormal (Algranati, 1992).

Determining visual acuity in a newborn is difficult. Several methods are available, including visual preference charts and visual evoked potential. At term, newborn visual acuity ranges from 20/100 to 20/400, depending on the testing method used. This visual acuity improves to 20/80 to 20/200 by 4 months of age, 20/40 to 20/80 by 12 months of age, and 20/20 by 2 years of age (Green, 1992).

Attention should also be directed to an eye motility examination. In the neonate, the position of the eyes varies greatly. Most infants display intermittent outward deviation (exotropia). This deviation usually disappears within the first few months of life. Any constant inward (esotropia) or outward deviation should be evaluated for a possible nerve or muscle palsy. Intermittent nystagmus (rapid movements of the eye) is a common finding in the newborn. Persistent nystagmus is abnormal; patients with this disorder should be referred for further evaluation (Carey, 1993).

Eye Drops

Great care must be taken in the selection of dilating drops for use in newborns. Systemic absorption of the eye drops, although unavoidable to some extent, can cause severe reactions, including death. Cardiovascular consequences, including arterial hypertension, which is a predisposing factor for intracranial hemorrhage, have been reported in premature infants (Rosales et al., 1993). Excess medications that flow out of the eyelids are easily absorbed through the porous skin of the newborn and should be wiped off to prevent systemic absorption. Absorption of the medication from the nasolacrimal system can also occur. This absorption can be minimized by the application of pressure with a fingertip over the nasolacrimal duct for approximately 1 minute after instillation of the drops.

The most commonly used mydriatics are cyclopentolate, phenylephrine, and tropicamide. For maximum dilation and minimal risk of side effects, a combination of drugs is routinely used in most clinical settings. According to Bolt and colleagues (1992), the combination of phenylephrine, 2.5 percent, and tropicamide, 0.5 percent (one drop of each followed by a second drop of tropicamide 20 minutes later), produced a better mydriasis with no systemic side effects than the combination of cyclopentolate and tropicamide. A complete listing of ophthalmic medications commonly used in newborns can be found in Table 34–1.

After the examination, the infant's eyes should be shielded from light until the pupils have returned to their normal size. This shielding can be achieved by covering the eyes with an occlusive eye shield, such as phototherapy shields, or by placing an isolette cover over the baby's incubator. Unshielded, dilated eyes are very sensitive to light. The excessive light entering a dilated pupil can result in intense pain in an infant. Premature infants or those with underlying health problems may react to the pain with systemic responses, such as apnea, bradycardia, cyanosis, and agitation (Blackburn, 1996).

NEONATAL CONJUNCTIVITIS

Any conjunctivitis occurring within the first 28 days of life is classified as neonatal conjunctivitis, according to the World

TABLE 34–1 Commonly Used Eye Medications

Generic Name	Brand Name
Topical Anesthetics	
Proparacaine hydrochloride	Alcaine, Ophthaine, Ophthetic
Tetracaine hydrochloride	Anacel, Pontocaine
Mydriatics (Dilating Drops)	
Atropine sulfate	Atropisol, BufOpto Atropine, Isopto-Atropine
Cyclopentolate hydrochloride	Cyclogyl
Homatropine hydrobromide	Isopto Homatropine
Scopolamine hydrobromide	Isopto Hyoscine
Tropicamide	Mydriacyl
Phenylephrine hydrochloride	Mydfrin, Neo-Synephrine
Anti-Inflammatory Agents	
Dexamethasone	Maxidex Ophthalmic Suspension
Dexamethasone sodium phosphate	Decadron Phosphate
Fluorometholone	FML Liquifilm Ophthalmic
Prednisolone acetate	Econopred, Pred Forte, Pred Mild
Prednisolone sodium phosphate	AK-Pred, Inflamase Forte, Inflamase, Metreton
Anti-Infectives	
Antibacterials	
Bacitracin	
Chloramphenicol	Chloromycetin, Chloroptic, Econochlor
Erythromycin	Ilotycin
Gentamicin sulfate	Garamycin
Polymyxin B sulfate	
Silver nitrate 1%	
Sulfacetamide sodium	Bleph-10, Cetamide, Sodium Sulamyd
Tetracycline hydrochloride	Achromycin
Tobramycin	Tobrex
Antivirals	
Idoxuridine	IDU
Trifluridine	Viroptic
Vidarabine	Vira-A
Miscellaneous	
Timolol maleate	Timoptic (antiglaucoma medication)
Fluorescein sodium	Diagnostic drop for corneal abnormalities

Health Organization. An infection of the conjunctiva with a discharge may develop within the first 24 to 48 hours of life. Because of the various causes of newborn conjunctivitis, laboratory investigations are important in determining the exact cause. Rapid treatment in some cases of conjunctivitis is important for the prevention of vision loss.

Silver Nitrate Conjunctivitis

Most states in the United States require prophylaxis against neonatal conjunctivitis with the instillation of a 1-percent solution of silver nitrate. These drops typically cause an irritative reaction that leads to conjunctival edema, redness, and watery discharge. The reaction starts within a few hours of the instillation of the drops and usually resolves within 48 hours.

Silver nitrate conjunctivitis is self-limiting. Laboratory cultures and smears should be obtained to rule out an infectious cause for the conjunctivitis. Parents should be informed of the benign nature of the inflammation once the proper diagnosis has been made. Any secretions from the eyes should be cleansed frequently to avoid skin irritation.

Silver nitrate is effective against *Neisseria gonorrhea* and most bacteria; however, it is not effective against chlamydia. Some states substitute tetracycline ointment or erythromycin ointment for routine prophylaxis. These antibiotics usually do not cause eye irritation.

Chlamydial Conjunctivitis (Inclusion Conjunctivitis)

In recent years, *Chlamydia trachomatis* has been recognized as the most common cause of conjunctivitis in the newborn. The infection is transmitted from the infected mother to the infant at the time of birth. The conjunctivitis usually arises 4 to 14 days after birth. It may be mild or moderate and resolves within 6 weeks with proper treatment. Clinical symptoms include swollen eyelid or eyelids and mucopurulent discharge. Chronic infection can lead to more serious consequences, such as conjunctival scarring, adhesions of the eyelid, and deposits of connective tissue under the cornea (Weiss, 1993).

Diagnosis is made from laboratory studies. The conjunctiva is scraped with a spatula, and a smear is made for Giemsa staining. This classically reveals a dark-staining cytoplasmic inclusion body. Direct immunofluorescent antibody staining or enzyme immunoassay should be obtained to confirm the diagnosis.

Topical treatment to the eye should consist of sulfacetamide or tetracycline drops or ointment for 3 weeks. Although the eye infection is generally not serious, a chlamydial pneumonitis develops in 11 to 20 percent of infected neonates. Systemic therapy with oral erythromycin estolate or erythromycin ethylsuccinate for 3 weeks is often necessary to eradicate the organism from the respiratory tract (Weiss, 1993).

Gonorrheal Conjunctivitis

Routine prophylaxis of neonates with silver nitrate has greatly reduced the incidence of gonorrheal conjunctivitis. Because of the potential for blindness from this infection, early detection and prompt treatment are critical. Gonorrheal conjunctivitis typically presents as an acute, purulent, bilateral conjunctivitis with eyelid edema. If not treated appropriately, the infection may progress rapidly to corneal ulceration and endophthalmitis. Gram stains and cultures should be performed routinely in all cases of neonatal conjunctivitis. The presence of *N. gonorrhea* confirms the diagnosis. Treatment consists of intravenous or intramuscular antibiotics and topical ointment to the eye. Irrigation of the eye with sterile saline may be necessary to cleanse the eye of drainage.

Staphylococcal Conjunctivitis

This bacterial infection is usually acquired during vaginal delivery or by contact with an infected mother or nursery personnel. Symptoms usually appear 2 to 4 weeks after birth. The conjunctivitis is usually mild with a purulent discharge. It may progress to a corneal ulcer, endophthalmitis, or generalized skin infection. Diagnosis is made with cultures and Gram stain. Staphylococci can be found in the conjunctiva of healthy neonates; therefore, laboratory results should be interpreted cautiously. Treatment involves application of topical bacitracin or erythromycin ointment and cleansing of exudate from the eyelids.

Herpes Simplex Conjunctivitis

Herpes simplex infections at birth may be part of a localized or a systemic disease. The neonate is usually infected during passage through the birth canal. The conjunctivitis presents with eyelid swelling, conjunctival inflammation, corneal opacity, and epithelial dendrites. These dendrites can best be seen by staining the cornea with a fluorescein dye and then examining the cornea under the blue light of a portable slit lamp. The onset of the conjunctivitis is usually 2 to 14 days after birth. The disseminated form of the disease may also lead to cataracts and optic neuritis.

Laboratory diagnosis is based on conjunctival epithelia scrapings for Giemsa staining and tissue cultures. The Giemsa stain should reveal multinucleated giant cells and intranuclear inclusion. Fluorescent antibody techniques are also helpful in the diagnosis. This disease should always be kept in mind when a history of maternal or paternal genital herpes exists. Treatment should be instituted with the topical antiviral trifluridine. Systemic treatment may be helpful in disseminated cases.

LACRIMAL DYSFUNCTION

Obstructed Nasolacrimal Duct

Blockage of the nasolacrimal duct occurs when the duct fails to canalize at the entrance to the nose. This blockage occurs in 2 percent of all newborns and is the most common cause of chronic conjunctivitis in infants. The infant presents after 1 month of age with excessive tearing and pooling in the medial canthal region and signs of infection. Pressure on the lacrimal sac area usually causes pus or mucus to exude from the puncta. Because the problem resolves spontaneously in 50 percent of affected neonates by 6 months of age, conservative treatment of lacrimal massage and topical antibiotics is recommended. Obstruction lasting beyond this point may necessitate lacrimal probing (Weiss, 1993). This problem must be differentiated from congenital glaucoma, a foreign body on the eye, or corneal injury or inflammation.

Mucocele

Mucoceles occur because of the one-way valve effect at the end of the nasolacrimal duct. Mucus accumulates or amniotic fluid is trapped in the nasolacrimal sac. The infant presents with a bluish mass in the inferomedial region of the eyelid. This swelling is most frequently confused with a hemangioma. If simple massage does not decompress the mucocele, probing of the nasolacrimal duct may be necessary.

RETINOPATHY OF PREMATURITY

Retinopathy of prematurity, a disease resulting from proliferation of abnormal blood vessels in the newborn retina, was first described by Terry, in 1942. His description of a fibrous growth behind the lens and retinal detachment in premature infants gave birth to the name retrolental fibroplasia (Weakley & Spencer, 1992). This name was changed to retinopathy of prematurity in 1984 by an international committee to provide a uniform classification system for the disease. The classification system uses a standard description of the location of retinopathy (zone, clock hours), the severity of the disease (stage), the presence of special risk factors (plus disease), and the features of regression (International Committee on Retinopathy of Prematurity, 1984) (Fig. 34–1).

Retinopathy of prematurity was responsible for an epidemic of blindness in young children in the 1940s and early 1950s until the link to supplemental oxygen therapy was made in 1952. Subsequently, the practice of limiting oxygen administration in the care of premature infants led to the near disappearance of RLF (Phelps, 1992). Improvements in neonatal health care in the past 30 years have increased the survival of preterm infants, yet ROP remains the leading cause of blindness in premature infants (Javitt et al., 1993). According to data from the multicenter cryotherapy trial of more than 4000 infants, the greatest risk occurs in premature infants weighing less than 750 g at birth (90 percent) and in those with birth weights of 751 to 1000 g (78 percent) (Phelps, 1992). The overall incidence of ROP is increasing, with current estimates at 25 percent annually (Hunter & Mukai, 1994). Although most of these cases will regress, the incidence of severe disease has reached a plateau of 5 to 10 percent, with over 500 new cases of blind infants reported annually in the United States (Hunter & Mukai, 1994; Vander, 1994).

Pathophysiology

Retinopathy of prematurity is a disease produced by an abnormal adaptation of normal maturational processes in the face of physiologic stress. The disease develops gradually and is divided into five stages of increasing severity, described in Table 34–2. The key factor in the development of ROP, especially in the premature infant, is the developing retinal blood vessels. Mature retinal vasculature is not susceptible to the adverse effects of severe stress. Retinal vascularization begins at the optic nerve at about 16 weeks of gestation. Retinal vascular development proceeds slowly and reaches the retinal periphery (ora serrata retinae) during the ninth month of gestation (Phelps, 1992; Vander, 1994). Exposure of undifferentiated mesenchymal cells, which are critical to the process of capillary development, to severe physiologic stress during this migration can cause cells to die or lose their orientation. The newly developing capillaries become obliterated, resulting in retinal ischemia (Roth, 1977).

TABLE 34–2 Stages of Retinopathy of Prematurity

Stage	Finding
1	Demarcation line at avascular retina
2	Ridge with height and width
3	Ridge with fibrosis extending into vitreous
4	Partial retinal detachment
	A. Without the fovea
	B. With the fovea
5	Complete retinal detachment

From George, D.S., Stephen, S., Fellows, R.R., & Bremer, D.L. (1988). The latest on retinopathy of prematurity. *MCN, American Journal of Maternal Child Nursing, 13*(4), 256. Reprinted with permission.

The ischemia becomes a potent inducer of new vessel growth (neovascularization). As the new blood vessels proliferate, they tend to grow into the vitreous and can result in bleeding and formation of fibrous tissue (Roth, 1977). Mild degrees of ROP are often transient and regress once the abnormal stimuli are removed or corrected. Moderate retinopathy can lead to excessive fibrous tissue formation or scarring in the peripheral retina, which may lead to traction on the macula and reduced vision. In severe cases of ROP, fibrous tissue development may lead to retinal detachment and blindness (Hunter & Mukai, 1994). Severely affected neonates may also present with leukocoria, or glaucoma, or both.

Risk Factors

Retinopathy of prematurity is a multifactorial disease related to conceptual age that occurs primarily in premature infants. Although many risk factors have been identified, prematurity is the single most important factor leading to the development of ROP (Fielder & Levene, 1992; Hunter & Mukai, 1994; Phelps, 1992). Other risk factors include use of supplemental oxygen, low birth weight, intraventricular hemorrhage, sepsis, multiple births, acidosis, and blood transfusions (Cooke et al., 1993; Fielder & Levene, 1992; Hittner, 1981; Phelps, 1992; Todd et al., 1994; Weakley & Spencer, 1992).

For some variables linked to the development of ROP, the

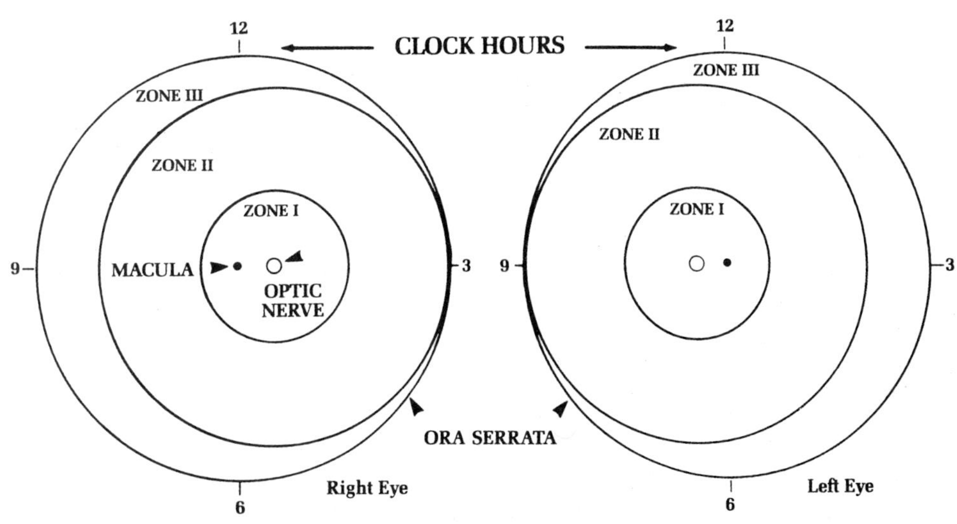

FIGURE 34–1. Diagram for documenting retinal disease. (From George, D. S., Stephen, S., Fellows, R. R., & Bremer, D. L. [1988]. The latest on retinopathy of prematurity. *MCN, American Journal of Maternal Child Nursing, 13*[4], 254–258. Reprinted with permission.)

evidence is less conclusive and there is no direct link to the treatment or management of medically unstable premature infants. Often, these factors are interlinked and include antioxidant deficiencies; administration of beta-adrenergic blockers late in pregnancy for preterm labor; maternal bleeding; apnea of prematurity; use of xanthines, such as caffeine and theophylline; abnormal blood gas findings; number of days on mechanical ventilation; early intubation; ambient lighting; hypotension; necrotizing enterocolitis; and patent ductus arteriosus treated with indomethacin (Arroe & Peitersen, 1994; Fielder & Levene, 1992; Gallo et al., 1993; Muller, 1992; Phelps, 1992; Robinson & Fielder, 1992; Todd, et al., 1994). An association between ROP and glucocorticoid steroid use has not been substantiated (Wright & Wright, 1994); although the use of steroids may increase the chance of surgical intervention for ROP (Todd et al., 1994). The impact of surfactant therapy on ROP is a major concern. Preliminary reports suggest that the incidence and severity of ROP are not altered by surfactant therapy (Holmes et al., 1994; Rankin et al., 1992; Repka et al., 1993; Tubman et al., 1992).

Although most ROP occurs in premature infants, there have been rare case reports of the disease in full-term infants, stillborn infants, infants with hypoxia, and infants who were not given supplemental oxygen (Kushner & Gloeckner, 1984; Naiman et al., 1979; Stefani & Ehalt, 1974). These reports, along with the striking similarity of disease presentation from infant to infant, have led some to conclude a genetic component to ROP may exist (Flynn, 1992). Further research is needed in order to increase our understanding of the cause and the pathophysiology of this disease.

Treatment

Treatment of ROP can be divided into three categories: preventive, interdictive, and corrective (Weakley & Spencer, 1992). Until premature birth can be abolished, the major focus of ROP treatment is early detection and appropriate follow-up of significant disease. Javitt and colleagues (1993) estimated that properly timed screening and treatment for ROP is not only cost saving but may also save approximately 320 infants per year from a lifetime of blindness. Despite the international effort to standardize ROP and the combined efforts of the multicenter, randomized clinical trial known as the Cryotherapy for Retinopathy of Prematurity Study (1988), no universally accepted guidelines exist for the screening of premature infants for ROP. Screening protocols vary from institution to institution. Several widely used, published guidelines are summarized in Table 34–3.

Preventive Treatment

Other preventive strategies that have been used or are under consideration are antioxidant therapy, oxygen monitoring, and modifications of environmental light. High-dose vitamin E, which is an antioxidant, gained popularity in the 1980s as a prophylactic therapy for ROP (Hittner, 1981); however, most clinical studies failed to document a protective effect (Muller, 1992). Significant side effects, such as sepsis, necrotizing enterocolitis, intraventricular hemorrhage, and death, were noted in numerous studies, prompting most nurseries to avoid the use of high-dose vitamin E (Pierce & Mukai, 1994). Preliminary evidence suggests that penicillamine, an antioxidant used in the treatment of hyperbilirubinemia in Hungary, may lower the incidence of ROP; however, the substance has not been tested for this purpose outside of Hungary (Phelps, 1992). Inositol, an antioxidant found in breast milk and other dietary sources, is being investigated for a possible role in decreasing the incidence of chronic lung disease (Hallman et al., 1992). Preliminary data reveal an unexpected decrease in the incidence of ROP in treated infants (Phelps, 1992). Other investigators are exploring whether bilirubin is protective against ROP (Fauchére et al., 1994). Multicenter, randomized, controlled studies are needed before the true value of these antioxidants is known.

Oxygen monitoring has been the major emphasis in the prevention of ROP. Elaborate policies and practices for continuous monitoring of oxygenation have evolved over the years, including invasive (fiberoptic umbilical catheters) and noninvasive (transcutaneous oxygen monitoring, pulse oximetry) technologies. Despite these efforts, few data answer the question of what is a safe level of oxygenation in infants at risk for ROP. Early efforts at restricting oxygen delivery in the 1950s to 1960s traded visual problems for neurologic sequelae (Weakley & Spencer, 1992). Current practice aimed at minimizing oxygen exposure while preserving optimal functioning of vital organs must continue until research determines appropriate strategies.

Environmental lighting in nurseries has been implicated as a contributing factor in the development of ROP (Ackerman et al., 1989; Robinson & Fielder, 1992). Although the clinical studies claiming this relationship have many limitations, some authorities believe that there are sufficient data to warrant concern (Phelps, 1992). Multicenter clinical trials will hopefully shed some light on the subject (Seiberth et al., 1994). Many nurseries have already instituted reduced environmental lighting and shielding of incubators as part of a developmental approach to care (Blackburn, 1996).

Interdictive Treatment

The second strategy for treating ROP focuses on therapies aimed at minimizing or preventing blindness once the disease has

TABLE 34–3 Guidelines for Retinopathy of Prematurity Screening Examinations

Recommending Group	Infant Criteria	Examination Protocol
Cryotherapy for Retinopathy of Prematurity Cooperative Group (1988)	Birth weight <1251 g	First examination, 4–6 weeks after birth; continue every 2 weeks. Increase to weekly examinations if prethreshold disease develops
American Academy of Pediatrics; *Guidelines for Perinatal Care* (1988)	Birth weight <1800 g OR gestational age <35 weeks who require oxygen Birth weight <1300 g OR gestational age <30 weeks	Examine 5–7 weeks after birth or before discharge to home (whichever comes first)
British College of Ophthalmologists and British Association of Perinatal Medicine (Fielder & Levene, 1992)	Birth weight <1500 g OR gestational age <31 weeks	Infants <25 weeks' gestation: first examination, 6–7 weeks after birth; continue every 2 weeks Infants 26–31 weeks' gestation: first examination 6–7 weeks after birth; continue every 2 weeks

developed. Interdictive therapies include cryotherapy and laser photocoagulation.

Cryotherapy, the most widely used technique, was developed in the 1970s in Japan. It gained popularity in the United States in the 1980s after the release of data from the Cryotherapy for Retinopathy of Prematurity study. The study was terminated early, when preliminary analysis revealed a significant benefit in eyes treated with cryotherapy (Phelps, 1992). The improvements noted in study subjects persisted in follow-up studies (Cryotherapy for Retinopathy of Prematurity Cooperative Group [CRPCG], 1988).

Cryotherapy is a surgical procedure that involves the insertion of a probe cooled with liquid nitrogen on the medial aspect of the eye. Confluent spots on the avascular retina are ablated (destroyed by freezing), reducing the release of an angiogenic factor that appears to induce retinal vasoproliferation. Although the exact way in which cryotherapy works remains unknown, substantial evidence indicates that the therapy works and improves the outcome of ROP (CRPCG, 1988; Göbel & Richard, 1993; Javitt et al., 1993; Schulenburg & Acheson, 1992; Trese 1994).

Despite the proven benefits of cryotherapy, it is not a benign procedure. Ocular and other complications can occur. Ocular complications include edema of the eyelid or eyelids, laceration of the conjunctiva, intraocular hemorrhage, and late retinal detachment (Vander, 1994). Other complications reported include apnea, bradycardia, arrhythmias, increased oxygen requirement, seizures, and, rarely, cardiorespiratory arrest (Batton et al., 1992; Brown et al., 1990).

Neonatal nurses and other health care professionals should work closely with the ophthalmologist performing the cryotherapy. Infants undergoing the procedure must have their pupils dilated because of the need for indirect ophthalmoscopy. Although the procedure is usually performed with local or general anesthesia, it can severely stress the infant. The oculocardiac reflex, a vagal nerve–mediated reflex, may be triggered during the procedure, causing bradycardia (Clarke et al., 1985). This reflex can be prevented by the preoperative administration of atropine (Phelps, 1992). It is imperative that cardiorespiratory status be closely monitored throughout the procedure and the immediate postoperative period. Analgesia during and after the procedure is also recommended. Premature infants, especially those with bronchopulmonary dysplasia, often experience increased oxygen requirements and apnea episodes after cryotherapy (Brown et al., 1990). Nasal stuffiness, which is another common side effect of cryotherapy, may be partially responsible for the increase in apnea and/or oxygen requirements after surgery (Phelps, 1992).

Laser photocoagulation, a recent technique used in the treatment of ROP, is showing promise and may eventually replace cryotherapy (Goggin & O'Keefe, 1993; Hunter & Repka, 1993). Argon and infrared diode lasers have been successfully used to ablate the avascular retina in a similar manner to that used in cryotherapy. Evidence to date suggests that laser therapy is as effective as cryotherapy; however, no conclusive evidence indicates that it is better than cryotherapy (Goggin & OKeefe, 1993; Hunter & Repka, 1993; Pierce & Mukai, 1994). Advantages of laser photocoagulation therapy described have included technical ease to perform; usefulness in posterior ROP, which is difficult to treat with cryotherapy; lower stress to the infant receiving the therapy; fewer side effects; and fewer delayed consequences of myopia and retinal detachment (Hunter & Repka, 1993; Preslan, 1993). Some evidence indicates that laser therapy may increase the risk of cataracts in treated infants (Christiansen & Bradford, 1995).

Corrective Treatment

The focus of corrective treatment is surgery for the repair of detached retinas. Scleral buckling, or vitrectomy, or both, with or without lensectomy are the techniques currently available (Trese, 1994). Scleral buckling involves the placement of silicone or plastic band around the globe of the eye. After the band is constricted, the sclera is brought into closer proximity to the retina, and retinal reattachment is facilitated. This procedure is often performed in conjunction with cryotherapy or laser therapy to salvage any remaining vision for the infant (Phelps, 1992).

When retinal detachment progresses beyond the point of a scleral buckle procedure, the ophthalmologist must consider anatomic reattachment of the retina. Vitrectomy involves surgical opening of the eye, removal of the lens, and gentle excision of the proliferative scar tissue. This process allows the retina to lie against the pigmented epithelium and reattach (Hunter & Repka, 1993; Trese, 1994). Despite the skill involved in these procedures, most infants receiving corrective therapy do not experience significant improvement in their vision. Functional success rates range from 3 to 43 percent (Hunter & Repka, 1993).

Nursing Care

Parents often express concern about the development of ROP in their premature infant. Open communication between the neonatal health care team and the parents is crucial for successful coping with the multiple stress of a hospitalized premature infant. The amount of information a parent can handle is important to determine. General information about the relationship of ROP and prematurity can be shared at first. Once the first eye examination is performed, the information can be specific to their baby (Phelps, 1992). The neonatal health care team must work closely with the ophthalmologist in providing a consistent message to the family. Information shared should take into account known cultural differences, such as that the occurrence of severe ROP is approximately 50% less in black infants than in white infants (Palmer et al., 1991). Parent teaching should focus on providing a basic understanding of ROP, the purpose of the screening examinations, and the importance of regular vision testing in their infant after discharge. Explanations of eye examination results may need reinforcing as parents try to assimilate the overwhelming amount of information they are receiving. Misconceptions about the disease and the use of oxygen need to be corrected.

Once ROP is diagnosed in an infant, parents may need more support than usual. Some parents may exhibit denial because they cannot see any physical evidence of a problem. Families of infants who need surgical intervention may experience increased stress from their concern for their infant's vision and the added communication with an ophthalmologist or retinal surgeon. Nursery staff can help parents cope by providing support during discussions about decision making with the eye specialists, by asking questions to clarify information, and by reinforcing information (Phelps, 1992).

Information given to the parents about the prognosis of ROP in their infant must be included in any discharge planning. Parents need to understand that eye problems are more common in premature infants and may develop in infants with regressed ROP (Gallo et al., 1993; King & Cronin, 1993; Quinn et al., 1992; Robinson & O'Keefe, 1992). Myopia (nearsightedness), strabismus (crossed eye), astigmatism, and amblyopia (lazy eye) are common sequelae. Glaucoma and late retinal detachment are common sequelae in infants with severe ROP (Hartnett et al., 1993; Quinn, et al., 1992).

Outcome studies suggest that the incidence of long-term problems has been underestimated (Gallo et al., 1993; Quinn et al., 1992; McGinnity & Bryars, 1992; Schraeder & McEvoy-Shields, 1991). McGinnity and Bryars (1992) compared 200 low-weight infants with a matched group of full-term infants at 9 years of age. They found a significant excess of visual problems, such as strabismus, refractive errors, cicatricial ROP, and optic atrophy.

They also found that 70 percent of children with poor vision needed special resources to succeed in school. Clearly, early detection and referral to programs for visual impairment are essential. Parents need to understand the importance of regular eye examinations by a pediatric ophthalmologist or by an ophthalmologist knowledgeable about ROP and its complications (Blackburn, 1995; Gallo et al., 1993; Schraeder & McEvoy-Shields, 1991). Many families may benefit from referral to community resources, support groups, and special programs for children with visual problems.

CONGENITAL DEFECTS

Aniridia

This condition is a severe ocular abnormality that presents with bilateral absence of the iris. The defect is usually accompanied by cataracts, corneal pannus, macular dysfunction, and glaucoma. Most of the infants have a significant reduction in their visual acuity, to a level of 20/200 or worse. About 20 to 30 percent of children with the noninherited form of aniridia eventually have Wilms' tumor of the kidney.

Persistent Hyperplastic Primary Vitreous

This condition is a unilateral disorder that affects both sexes equally. It results from persistence of the hyoid vessels that connect the optic nerve and the posterior surface of the lens. It should be considered in the differential diagnosis of leukocoria. The involved eye is invariably small, and a mature cataract is often present. Surgery may improve the integrity of the eye; however, useful vision is usually not restored.

Rubella

Congenital rubella is responsible for a wide variety of ocular complications, including pigmentary retinopathy, glaucoma, cataract, and microphthalmos. Newborns classically present with hearing, eye, and cardiac defects; although, a wide spectrum of clinical presentations exists.

Today, the incidence of congenital rubella syndrome is low; however, new information from long-term follow-up studies (Elango et al., 1994; Givens et al., 1993) suggests that the prevalence of ocular problems is nearly twice the previously thought rate (78 percent instead of 43 percent). Several trends have also been noted including an increase in delayed disease and new associations of combination problems. Microphthalmia, cataracts, and glaucoma are more likely to occur in combination than independently. Pigmentary retinopathy produces a characteristic salt-and-pepper appearance and can result in sudden vision loss during adulthood. Poor visual acuity and diabetic retinopathy are also of concern in individuals with congenital rubella syndrome (Givens et al., 1993). Parents of infants with congenital rubella need to understand that vision problems may occur at any time and that they must have their affected children screened on a regular basis.

Capillary Hemangiomas of the Eyelid

Capillary hemangioma of the eyelid, a blood vessel tumor, usually appears before the age of 6 months. It tends to enlarge, stabilize, and then regress by the time the child is 5 years of age. The tumor is usually elevated and reddish purple. Capillary hemangiomas are often referred to as strawberry nevi because of their appearance.

Superficial tumors of the eyelid cause cosmetic and visual problems. Pressure on the globe from the tumor may result in significant astigmatism and subsequently amblyopia. If the tumor is large, it may cover the pupil and prevent normal visual development. Deep tumors in the orbit may present with proptosis. These tumors may be treated with surgical removal, radiation, or steroid injection. Tumors that are exclusively cosmetic should be allowed to regress on their own.

Ptosis

Ptosis refers to a drooping of one or both eyelids as a result of neurologic, muscular, or mechanical factors. If the ptosis is significant enough to cover the pupil, a dense amblyopia may result. If bilateral ptosis is present, the infant may have slowed motor development and delayed ambulation later in life. These problems are caused by the awkward chin-up position the child must maintain in order to see. Mild ptosis that causes a problem with appearance is generally not repaired until the child is 4 or 5 years old because the results are usually better at this age.

A thorough family history should be obtained. Several familial syndromes are associated with ptosis, including blepharophimosis syndrome and double-elevator palsy. Significant birth trauma may result in damage to the cervical ganglion and in an infantile Horner's syndrome. The infant presents with different-colored pupils, miosis, anhidrosis (lack of sweating), and mild ptosis. Direct trauma to the eyelid or a tumor in the eyelid may also cause ptosis. Surgical repair corrects this defect easily.

Congenital Glaucoma

Congenital glaucoma occurs in approximately 1 in 25,000 births. Glaucoma is a disease in which the intraocular pressure is increased to a level sufficient to damage the optic nerve. Because of the blinding potential of this disease, it must be detected early in the infant's life and treated properly. The neonate presents with tearing, light sensitivity, eyelid spasm, and a large cloudy cornea. The disease is slightly more common in males than in females.

It is critical that congenital glaucoma be differentiated from other diseases that present with similar symptoms. Nasolacrimal duct obstruction presents with tearing but does not cause light sensitivity or a cloudy cornea. Difficult labor or forceps injury may damage the cornea and cause temporary clouding, but the intraocular pressure is not increased, which is the hallmark feature of glaucoma. The large eyes of the infant with congenital glaucoma may appear beautiful to the parents, but health professionals should be alert to the possibility of this disease.

The abnormality in congenital glaucoma is a maldevelopment of the filtering system that controls the level of intraocular pressure within the eye. Treatment of congenital glaucoma is surgical. The surgical results are usually good, but parents must be educated regarding the need for continued monitoring of this condition throughout the child's life.

Congenital Cataracts

The causes of significant lens opacities in the newborn are numerous. Cataracts are an important cause of blindness because they may interfere with the process of visual development early in the infant's life. For this reason, visually significant cataracts must be detected and treated before they cause amblyopia, which may be unresponsive to the most persistent treatment.

Heredity is an important cause of congenital cataracts. A thorough family history is critical in determining the cause of the lens opacity. The inheritance pattern may be autosomal dominant, autosomal recessive, or sex linked. A maternal history of diabetes, x-ray exposure, or malnutrition may be an important factor in cataract formation. In premature infants, transient cataracts or insignificant opacities are commonly seen, as a result of remnants of developmental tissues. ROP can also lead to cataracts in premature infants.

Several inborn errors of metabolism, including galactosemia, Alport's syndrome, Fabry's disease, and Lowe's syndrome, cause cataracts. Intrauterine rubella infection is also associated with cataracts in the neonate.

Cataract surgery early in life is critical to the infant's visual rehabilitation. Useful vision is especially difficult to achieve in eyes with monocular cataracts. It is important for nurses to work closely with the infant's parents. The parents' persistence in handling contact lenses and in amblyopia therapy often determines the outcome for their child's vision.

Retinoblastoma

Retinoblastoma is the most common intraocular neoplasm in childhood. The tumor occurs in approximately 1 in 25,000 births. Most cases appear sporadically and occur in infants with no family history of the disease. An autosomal dominant pattern is usually responsible for the 5 to 10 percent of inherited retinoblastomas, most of which are bilateral. A somatic mutation accounts for 80% of unilateral tumors.

Leukocoria is the most common presenting symptom. Most of the tumors are not detected in the neonatal period, except in infants with a positive family history. The tumor is highly malignant and may spread to the bone marrow, the central nervous system, or other organs. Untreated patients rarely survive. The standard treatment for advanced cases of retinoblastoma is enucleation. Less severe cases are treated with radiation, laser photocoagulation, or cryotherapy. Children with this tumor require close follow-up for possible recurrence after treatment. Parents must be educated about the disease so that they are aware of the need for ongoing follow-up for the constant monitoring of their child.

CONCLUSION

Visual disturbances, although sometimes difficult to detect, have a dramatic impact on a newborn's behavioral and psychosocial development. ROP is the most common cause of serious eye disease in children. Although significant advances have been made in the diagnosis, treatment, and follow-up of infants with ROP, the incidence and long-term sequelae continue to increase as smaller neonates survive. Treatment of vision problems requires collaborative efforts between the neonatal health care team, the ophthalmologist, and the families of children with this problem. Clear, consistent communication between health care providers and parents and education of parent are important to quality care, as is good follow-up.

REFERENCES

Ackerman, B., Sherwonit, E., & Williams, J. M. (1989). Reduced incidental light exposure: Effect on the development of retinopathy of prematurity in low birth weight infants. *Pediatrics, 83*(6), 958–962.

Algranati, P. S. (1992). *The pediatric patient: An Approach to history and physical examination* (pp. 22–85). Baltimore: Williams & Wilkins.

American Academy of Pediatrics, American College of Obstetricians and Gynecologists. (1988). *Guidelines for perinatal care* (2nd ed.). Washington, DC: Author.

Arroe, M., & Peitersen, B. (1994). Retinopathy of prematurity: Review of a seven-year period in a Danish neonatal intensive care unit. *Acta Paediatrica, 83*(5), 501–505.

Batton, D. G., Ivery, P., & Trese, M. (1992). Respiratory complications associated with cryotherapy in premature infants. *American Journal of Perinatology, 9*(4), 296–298.

Blackburn, S. (1996). *Studies of light and its application to clinical practice.* Paper presented at the Physical and Developmental Environment of the High-Risk Neonate, January, 1996. Clearwater Beach, FL: University of South Florida College of Medicine.

Blackburn, S. (1995). Problems of premature infants after discharge. *Journal of Gynecologic and Neonatal Nursing, 24*(1), 43–49.

Bolt, B., Benz, B., Koerner, F., & Bossi, E. (1992). A mydriatic eyedrop combination without systemic effects for premature infants: A prospective double-blind study. *Journal of Pediatric Ophthalmology and Strabismus, 29*(3), 157–162.

Brown, G. C., Tasman, W. S., Naidoff, M., et al. (1990). Systemic complications associated with retinal cryoablation for retinopathy of prematurity. *Ophthalmology, 97*(7), 855–858.

Carey, B. (1993). Neurologic assessment. In E. P. Tappero & M. E. Honeyfield (Eds.), *Physical assessment of the newborn* (pp. 121–138). Petaluma, CA: NICU Ink.

Christiansen, S. P., & Bradford, J. D. (1995). Cataract in infants treated with argon laser photocoagulation for threshold retinopathy of prematurity. *American Journal of Ophthalmology, 119*(2), 175–180.

Clarke, W. N., Hodges, E., Noel, L. P., et al. (1985). The oculocardiac reflex during ophthalmoscopy in premature infants. *American Journal of Ophthalmology, 99*(6), 649–651.

Cohen, K. W., & Bryne, S. M. (1989). The role of the nurse in assisting with eye examinations on premature infants. *Neonatal Network, 8*(2), 31–35.

Cooke, R. W., Clark, D., Hickey-Dwyer, M., & Weindling, A. M. (1993). The apparent role of blood transfusions in the development of retinopathy of prematurity. *European Journal of Pediatrics, 152*(10), 833–836.

Cryotherapy for Retinopathy of Prematurity Cooperative Group (CRPCG) (1988). Multicenter trial of cryotherapy for retinopathy of prematurity: Preliminary results. *Archives of Ophthalmology, 106*(4), 471–499.

Elango, S., Reddy, T. N., & Shriwas, S. R. (1994). Other abnormalities in children from a Malaysian school for the deaf. *Annals of Tropical Paediatrics, 14*(2), 149–152.

Fauchére, J., Meier-Gibbons, F. E., Koerner, F., & Bossie, E. (1994). Retinopathy of prematurity and bilirubin: no clinical evidence for a beneficial role of bilirubin as a physiological anti-oxidant. *European Journal of Pediatrics, 153*(5), 358–362.

Fielder, A. R., Levene, M. I. (1992). Screening for retinopathy of prematurity [Review]. *Archives of Diseases in Childhood, 67*(7, Spec. No.), 860–867.

Flynn, J. T. (1992). The premature retina: A model for the in vivo study of molecular genetics? *Eye, 6*(Part 2), 161–165.

Gallo, J. E., Holmstrm, G., Kugelberg, U., et al. (1993). Regressed retinopathy of prematurity in children aged 5-10 years. *Acta Ophthalmologica, 111*(Suppl. 210), 41–43.

Gallo, J. E., Jacobson, L., & Broberger, U. (1993). Perinatal factors associated with retinopathy of prematurity. *Acta Paediatrica, 82*(10), 829–834.

George, D. S., Stephen, S., Fellows, R. R. & Bremer, D. L. (1988). The latest on retinopathy of prematurity. *American Journal of Maternal Child Nursing, 13*(4), 254–258.

Givens, K. T., Lee, D. A., Jones, T., & Ilstrup, D. M. (1993): Congenital rubella syndrome: Ophthalmic manifestations and associated systemic disorders. *British Journal of Ophthalmology, 77*(6), 358–363.

Göbel, W., & Richard, G. (1993). Retinopathy of prematurity: current diagnosis and management [Review]. *European Journal of Pediatrics, 152*(4), 286–290.

Goggin, M., & O'Keefe, M. (1993). Diode laser for retinopathy of prematurity: Early outcome. *British Journal of Ophthalmology, 77*(9), 559–562.

Green, M. (1992). *Pediatric diagnosis* (pp. 16–36). Philadelphia: W. B. Saunders.

Hallman, M., Bry, K., Hoppu, K., et al. (1992). Inositol supplementation in premature infants with respiratory distress syndrome. *New England Journal of Medicine, 326*(19), 1233–1239.

Hartnett, M. E., Gilbert, M. M., Hirose, T., et al. (1993). Glaucoma as a cause of poor vision in severe retinopathy of prematurity. *Graefes Archive for Clinical and Experimental Ophthalmology, 231*(8), 433–438.

Hittner, H. (1981). Retrolental fibroplasia: Efficacy of vitamin E in a double-blind clinical study of preterm infants. *New England Journal of Medicine, 305*, 1365–1371.

Holmes, J. M., Cronin, C. M., Squires, P., & Myers, T. M. (1994). Randomized clinical trial of surfactant prophylaxis in retinopathy of prematurity. *Journal of Pediatric Ophthalmology and Strabismus, 31*(3), 189–191.

Hunter, D. G., & Mukai, S. (1994). Retinopathy of prematurity: Pathogenesis, diagnosis, and treatment. *International Ophthalmology Clinics, 34*(3), 163–184.

Hunter, D. G., & Repka, M. X. (1993). Diode laser photocoagulation for threshold retinopathy or prematurity. *Ophthalmology, 100*(2), 238–244.

International Committee on Retinopathy of Prematurity (ICROP). (1984). An international classification of retinopathy of prematurity. *Pediatrics, 74*(1), 127–133.

Javitt, J., Cas, R. D., & Chiang, Y. (1993). Cost-effectiveness of screening and cryotherapy for threshold retinopathy of prematurity. *Pediatrics, 91*(5), 859–866.

Johnson, C. B. (1993). Head, eyes, ears, nose, threat (HEENT) assessment. In E. P. Tappero & M. E. Honeyfield (Eds.), *Physical assessment of the newborn* (pp. 41–54). Petaluma, CA: NICU Ink.

King, K. M., & Cronin, C. M. (1993). Ocular findings in premature infants with grade IV intraventricular hemorrhage. *Journal of Pediatric Ophthalmology and Strabismus, 30*(2), 84–87.

Kushner, B. J., & Gloeckner, E. (1984). Retrolental fibroplasia in full-term infants without exposure to supplemental oxygen. *American Journal of Ophthalmology, 97,* 148–153.

McGinnity, F. G., & Bryars, J. H. (1992). Controlled study of ocular morbidity in school children born preterm. *British Journal of Ophthalmology, 76*(9), 520–524.

Moore, K., & Persaud, T. V. N. (1993). *Before we are born* (4th ed.). Philadelphia: W. B. Saunders.

Muller, D. P. (1992). Vitamin E therapy in retinopathy of prematurity [Review]. *Eye, 6*(Part 2), 221–225.

Naiman, J., Green W. R., & Patz, A. (1979). Retrolental fibroplasia hypoxic newborn. *American Journal of Ophthalmology, 88*(1), 55–58.

Palmer, E. A, Flynn, J. T., Hardy, R. J., et al. (1991). Incidence and early course of retinopathy of prematurity. *Ophthalmology, 98*(11), 1628–1640.

Phelps, D. L. (1992). Retinopathy of prematurity. *Current Problems in Pediatrics, 22*(8), 349–371.

Pierce, E. A., & Mukai, S. (1994). Controversies in the management of retinopathy of prematurity. *International Ophthalmology Clinics, 34*(3), 121–148.

Preslan, M. W. (1993). Laser therapy for retinopathy of prematurity. *Journal of Pediatric Ophthalmology and Strabismus, 30*(2), 80–83.

Quinn, G. E., Dobson, V, Repka, M. X., et al. (1992). Development of myopia in infants with birth weights less than 1251 grams. *Ophthalmology, 99*(3), 329–340.

Rankin, S. J., Tubman, T. R., Jalliday, H. L., & Johnston, S. S. (1992). Retinopathy of prematurity in surfactant treated infants. *British Journal of Ophthalmology, 76*(4), 202–204.

Repka, M. X., Hardy, R. J., Phelps, D. L., & Summers, C. G. (1993). Surfactant prophylaxis and retinopathy of prematurity. *Archives of Ophthalmology, 111*(5), 618–620.

Robinson, J., & Fielder, A. R. (1992). Light and the immature visual system. *Eye, 6*(5), 166–172.

Robinson, R., & O'Keefe, M. (1992). Follow-up study on premature infants with and without retinopathy of prematurity. *British Journal of Ophthalology, 77*(2), 91–94.

Rosales, T., Isenberg, S., Leake, R., & Everett, S. (1981). Systemic effects of mydriatics in low weight infants. *Journal of Pediatric Ophthalmology and Strabismus, 18*(6), 42–44.

Roth, A. M. (1977). Retinal vascular development in premature infants. *American Journal of Ophthalmology, 84*(5), 636–640.

Schraeder, B. D., & McEvoy-Shields, K. (1991). Visual acuity, binocular vision, and ocular muscle balance in VLBW children. *Pediatric Nursing, 17*(1), 30–33.

Schulenburg, W. E., & Acheson, J. F. (1992). Cryosurgery for acute retinopathy of prematurity: Factors associated with treatment success and failure. *Eye, 6*(Part 2), 215–220.

Seiberth, V., Linderkamp, O., Knorz, M. C., Liesenhoff, H. (1994). A controlled clinical trial of light and retinopathy of prematurity. *American Journal of Ophthalmology, 118*(4), 492–495.

Stefani, F. H., & Ehalt, H. (1974). Non-oxygen induced retinitis proliferans and retinal detachment in full-term infants. *British Journal of Ophthalmology, 58*(5), 490–513.

Todd, D. A., Kennedy, J., Roberts, S., et al. (1994). Retinopathy of prematurity in infants less than 29 weeks gestation at birth. *Australian and New Zealand Journal of Ophthalmology,* 22(1), 19–23.

Trese, M. T. (1994). Surgery for retinopathy of prematurity. *International Ophthalmology Clinics, 34*(3), 105–111.

Tubman, T. R., Rankin, S. J., Halliday, H. L., & Johnston, S. S. (1992). Surfactant replacement therapy and the prevalence of acute retinopathy of prematurity. *Biology of Neonate, 61*(Suppl. 1), 54–58.

Vander, J. F. (1994). Retinopathy of prematurity: Diagnosis and management. *Journal of Ophthalmic Nursing and Technology, 13*(5), 207–212.

Weakley, D. R., Jr., & Spencer, R. (1992). Current concepts in retinopathy of prematurity [Review]. *Early Human Development, 30*(2), 121–138.

Weiss, A. H. (1993). Chronic conjunctivitis in infants and children. *Pediatric Annals, 22*(6), 366–374.

Wright, K., & Wright, P. (1994). Lack of association of glucocorticoid therapy and retinopathy of prematurity. *Archives of Pediatric and Adolescent Medicine, 148*(8), 848–852.

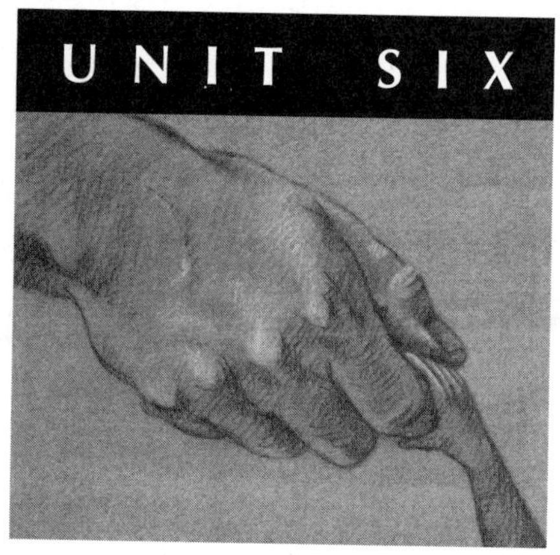

Neonatal Monitoring and Evaluation

Everything seemed so out of proportion in the NICU. The machines were enormous, bulky, and cumbersome. And they were everywhere. The babies were so dwarfed by comparison that they seemed almost to vanish. Above some isolettes, ropes and cords dangled from IV poles like giant wads of spaghetti. The hoses that were hooked up to endotracheal tubes would have looked equally at home watering the lawn, or maybe putting out a fire. Monitors that sat atop many isolettes looked like they might crush the unsuspecting babies beneath them.

Mostly, the NICU was a very noisy place. The machines gurgled and spat and hissed and spewed and roared. The monitors were all connected at alarms. If the preterm child's underdeveloped nervous system forgot to remind the baby to breathe, the apnea monitor would shriek like the siren on a police car. If the baby's heart rate dropped suddenly, a bradycardia alarm bellowed out news of this development. The monitors were so sensitive that sometimes, if the babies moved abruptly or awkwardly, they could activate the sound system. The beepers and buzzers were at once harsh and shrill. They reminded me of movies I had seen of London during the blitz.

ELIZABETH MEHREN
Born Too Soon

CHAPTER 35

Monitoring Neonatal Biophysical Parameters

CAROLE KENNER

RESEARCH AGENDA

What is the effect of gestational age on the accuracy of pulse oximetry?

What factors influence the accuracy of biophysical monitoring in the neonate?

What is a safe and effective temperature of a transcutaneous monitor probe for the very low birth weight infant?

What is the effect of blood flow and limb position on the pulse oximeter values?

What is the effect of skin color on the accuracy of transcutaneous bilirubin measurements?

Do hypoxemic episodes occur in the neonate that are not detected by routine cardiorespiratory monitoring?

Successful management of the patient in the neonatal intensive care unit (NICU) is reliant on the timely assessment of physiologic and biochemical status during the early period of the neonate's adaptation to extrauterine life. It is important to have instantaneous data on the newborn infant because of the highly dynamic changes that occur during this adaptation period. Advances in transduction technology and clinical computer applications have greatly improved the availability of physiologic and biochemical vital signs data at the bedside in the intensive care unit. The transcutaneous oxygen, carbon dioxide, and oxygen saturation monitors, which generate instant responses to changes in vital signs, have had an immense impact on the care of the sick premature infant. The neonate presents numerous transduction problems that make the availability of instantaneous data difficult. The small physical size of the neonate, for example, creates a serious limitation in the area available for mounting sensing electrodes. In general, clinical medicine adapts new technologic techniques from nonmedical areas in which the techniques have been proved accurate and reliable. Measurement in a living biologic system, however, creates some problems that are not encountered elsewhere. Regardless of the signal to be measured and monitored, there are some fundamental principles that should be applied to ensure accuracy and repeatability in the measurement process. This chapter discusses these principles as well as the physics and engineering bases used for their implementation. Examples are given on how these transduction tools are applied clinically to measure specific biophysical phenomena. Potential problems in the use or functioning of the specific techniques that could create erroneous measurements are identified. Significant clinical problems with interfacing the monitors that rely on sensors to contact the infant's skin are discussed. The basic measurement principles and monitoring system configurations are outlined in a general overview because these same basic concepts can be applied to any type of biophysical measurement and monitoring system. This review of transduction and monitoring system principles should assist the clinician in the identification and correction of errors in the use of continuous invasive and noninvasive monitoring systems. New techniques in monitoring that may be used in transport or in the NICU are also outlined.

BIOLOGIC SIGNALS

In intensive care monitoring, it is desirable to measure spontaneous events to provide instant information on the biologic status of the patient, for example, as is done with an electrocardiograph (ECG). In some cases, it is necessary to stimulate the system to generate a transducible signal that can be processed for interpretation, as with the use of a sphygmomanometer to measure blood pressure. The accurate measurement of a biologic signal depends on the ability of the applicable sensing system to detect some transducible property of the signal and convert it to electrical energy, which can then be processed to provide some type of visual presentation of the transduced information. The transducer must be able to distinguish the signal from other biologic signals by having a high degree of specificity and must also filter out extraneous or biologic noise, such as muscle movement artifact. Biologic signals can be categorized based on physical properties described by chemical, electrical, mechanical, electromagnetic, or thermal behavior (Fig. 35–1).

Many biologic processes involve chemical reactions. The actual reaction or the end product of the reaction may provide some detectable difference in chemical state to form a basis for detection and signal generation. In most cases, however, biochemical reactions and associated signals are inaccessible to in vivo transduction with current methods and require the removal of the tissue or fluid for processing and state analysis. Because of its ionic origin, the bioelectrical signal can be considered a special type of biochemical signal. Bioelectrical signals range from low-voltage transmembrane potentials in cells to the medium-voltage ECG of the heart. Bioelectrical signals are the most widely used in clinical medicine because of the relative ease with which they can be transduced and manipulated to provide discernible information to the caretaker using conventional signal processing tools such as the amplifier and the computer.

Blood pressure, flow, and velocity are important biomechanical signals that are easily transduced. Electromagnetic signals are

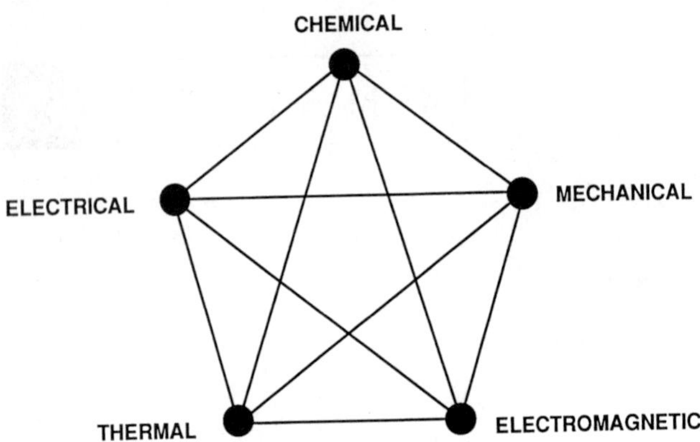

FIGURE 35–1. Biologic signal types. Interconnecting lines represent biologic events that could have a cascade of physical properties.

those that have energies in the wavelength region of non-ionizing radiation. These electromagnetic signals are, in some cases, detectable by a change in energy at some wavelength or by a shift in the wavelength of peak energy emission. Because most biochemical reactions result in the release or consumption of energy, biologic status can be assessed by the transduction of specific thermal properties, for example, by measuring temperature changes or heat released. Temperature is the most widely used biophysical indicator of health status (Table 35–1).

Biopotentials are the most frequently transduced physiologic parameters. The ECG, for example, measures the biopotential that is generated by cardiac tissue, which is detectable even on the surface of the skin. The single cell is the basic unit from which all biologic systems are constructed. It is single-cell membrane potentials that form the basis for all biopotentials. In biologic systems, it is the movement of ions in an electrolyte solution that produces electrical activity. This principle is the same one that generates current flow in the typical lead–acid battery used in automobiles. Biopotentials are also used in biologic systems for communication or stimulation of specific responses. Biopotentials can be converted into electrical voltages, using, for example, ECG electrodes to transduce an electrical response. Although not accessible noninvasively, each cell has its own state of electrical activity, which can characterize its biologic status.

The body is composed of a wide range of physical systems that communicate with each other and are adjusted and controlled to provide a specific response or state. Electrical, mechanical, chemical, and thermal systems are used for both communication and stimulation in living biologic systems. The cardiovascular, respiratory, and nervous systems have been studied in depth using biophysical transduction techniques. The biophysical transducers and monitoring systems for these systems form the basis for the majority of on-line continuous monitoring tools.

The biochemical system that controls the energy for body activity and the messenger system for cellular communication are the most inaccessible to noninvasive transduction. Biophysical transducers have been developed to make indirect measurements on these biochemical systems, for example, in the determination of the oxygen saturation level of hemoglobin using optical techniques. In this application, light pulses are timed to the cardiac pulse wave, and the difference in absorption properties between oxygenated and unoxygenated hemoglobin is detected as changes in the intensity of transmitted optical levels. These light level differences can be correlated with the level of oxygen saturation.

In particular, at the biochemical level, much is unknown with respect to the interaction and interrelationship of both individual cell types and overall systems. This interaction among cell types and higher order physiologic systems makes the detection of parameters in nonisolated intact biologic systems extremely difficult. Hence, there continues to be a great clinical reliance on the analysis of isolated tissue or body fluids for the assessment of biochemical status. As the understanding of the interactions is improved, it is conceivable that noninvasive optical techniques could be developed and applied to expand the use of noninvasive biophysical transduction at the bedside.

TABLE 35–1 Biophysical Parameters and Their Associated Signal Types

Sensor Type	Transduced Parameter
Chemical	Po_2, Pco_2
Electrical	Heart rate, respiration rate
Mechanical	Blood pressure, intracranial pressure
Electromagnetic	Skin temperature, oxygen saturation
Thermal	Temperature, metabolic rate

BIOPHYSICAL MONITORING SYSTEMS

Biophysical monitoring systems can be described as open-loop or closed-loop architecture (Fig. 35–2*A*). The open-loop systems are the simplest and are used to transduce spontaneous events, such as is done in ECG monitoring. Closed-loop systems use a stimulus to the patient and have a feedback signal that is used to adjust the stimulus in response to the level of the transduced signal from the patient. This type of closed-loop system is used in monitoring applications in which a transducible response is not normally present, for example, as in the control of cuff pressure to transduce blood pressure in automated noninvasive blood pressure monitors.

A block diagram of an open-loop biophysical monitoring system is shown in Figure 35–2*B*. The basic components are the same for most types of in vivo monitoring systems. The system consists of three main components: a sensor that is connected to the patient, signal conditioning equipment that conditions and processes the signal, and an output device such as a computer terminal or printer to present the transduced information to the caretaker.

The sensor typically has two main components: the interface and the transducing element. The interface is the part of the sensor that is in contact with the patient, for example, electrically conductive paste on an ECG electrode. The transducing element is designed to be responsive to and recognize the specific parameter of interest and to generate some type of electrical signal, for example, the oxygen electrode used in transcutaneous oxygen measurement. The electrical signal is then sent to the signal conditioning and processing equipment. For certain transduction applications, it is necessary to incorporate a membrane between the patient and the sensor to filter out noise or to allow only a specific anolyte to reach the sensing element. In these cases, the membrane becomes the interface to the patient. This use of membranes increases the specificity of the sensor. The selectivity of a transcutaneous oxygen transducer to oxygen, for example, is controlled by placing a membrane that is permeable to oxygen between the patient and the sensing element. Some biophysical parameters facilitate the use of electronic filters within the transducer to remove noise and to make the sensor more sensitive to signals with a particular frequency response. The disadvantage of this approach is that it can be used only to remove noise in frequency ranges that are higher and lower than the actual physiologic response being measured. These electronic filters are also used when the amplitude of the sensor signal is low and could be subject to interference from ambient radio waves. Additionally, in these low biologic signal power applications, local amplification

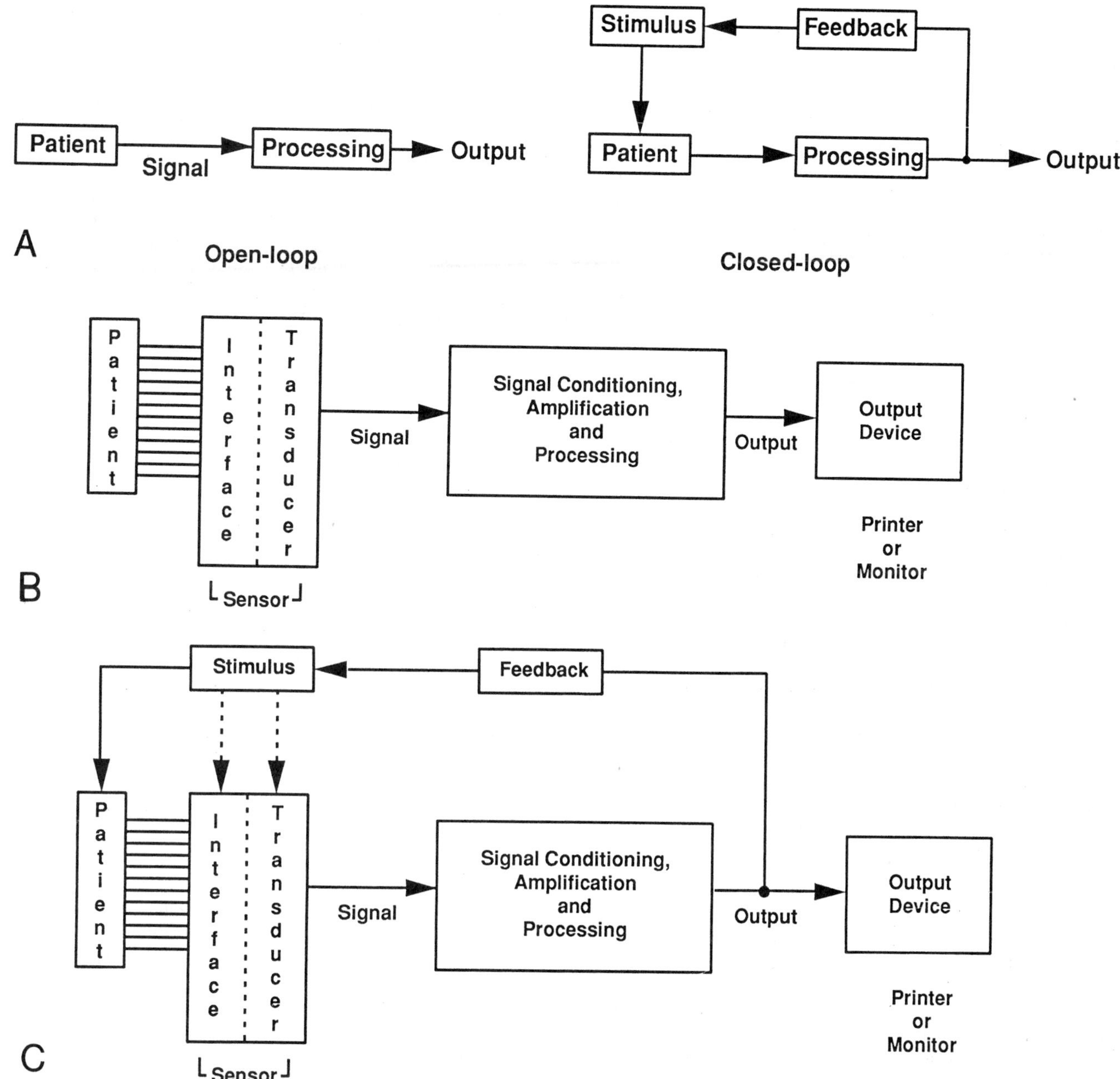

FIGURE 35–2. *A*, Monitoring system architectures. *B*, Open-loop biophysical monitoring system. *C*, Closed-loop biophysical monitoring system.

at the transducer is used to boost the strength of the signal, thereby making it less sensitive to external interferences.

The output from the transducer is always some form of analog signal. The signal is usually carried through wires to the signal conditioning equipment. Although not widely used in neonatal monitoring, telemetry in the radio frequency or optical ranges can be used to send the transduced signal to the conditioning equipment. Telemetry eliminates the need for wires between the transducer and the conditioning or display equipment.

The signal conditioning system processes the signal and converts it into a form that can be displayed on a cathode-ray tube or sent to some other type of output device, for example, a printer or a strip chart recorder. It is in the signal conditioning section of the system that the transduced signal is converted from some type of voltage signal to clinically relevant units (Fig. 35–2*C*); for example, the output from a blood pressure transducer is an analog voltage that is processed to provide a readout in millimeters of mercury to the clinician.

When a biophysical parameter of interest cannot be transduced from spontaneous events, it may be feasible to induce a transducible response through the use of some type of external stimulus, such as with the use of light to produce a visual-evoked response, which is an electrical signal that can be transduced and recorded. In other types of evoked response transduction, it may be desirable or necessary to control the degree of stimulation. This control can be accomplished by modifying the level of stimulation based on the level or strength of the transduced signal. This type of feedback control is used in noninvasive blood pressure monitoring, in which the cuff pressure is progressively increased to occlude blood flow. The occlusion force is patient dependent, and it is the use of closed-loop control of the cuff pressure that makes this type of transduction feasible for automated continuous or intermittent monitoring of blood pressure. In Figure 35–2*C*, the dotted lines to the sensor indicate a feedback system in which the sensor itself is actuated or adjusted in response to the transduced signal.

Components and General Considerations

Biophysical Sensors

The biophysical sensor is the combination of the interface to the patient and the physical element that transduces the biologic response and converts it to some form of electrical energy. These sensors can be as straightforward as the ECG electrode or as complex as the optical transducer used to measure transcutaneous oxygen saturation ($TcSaO_2$). Biophysical sensors are categorized as being invasive or noninvasive. It is always desirable to use a noninvasive sensing system, and all sensors should be electrically isolated from the patient. Insertion of a catheter with a pressure sensor at its tip into an artery to provide continuous recording of pressure waves is highly invasive compared with the use of the noninvasive automated sphygmomanometer to provide intermittent recording of blood pressure. Except for the ECG and other highly electrically active biologic systems, there are few biologic signals that can be easily transduced from the skin. In most cases, the interface of the transducing element of the sensor must be in intimate contact with the tissue or anolyte of interest.

Biophysical monitoring of the neonate also requires that each sensor be physically small to maximize the surface area available for other skin contact sensors and to accommodate invasive applications, because of the small vessels encountered. As shown in Figure 35–3, closed-loop feedback control is sometimes incorporated in the sensor to modify the interface of the sensor to the biologic system. The heater on a transcutaneous oxygen sensor elevates the temperature of the skin to increase the permeation of oxygen through the skin. This heater is servo controlled to maintain the skin temperature at specific levels that have been characterized to promote specific rates of diffusion. In this case, the interface between the sensor and the anolyte of interest is modified to produce oxygen permeation levels that are transducible. Feedback is also used in the $TcSaO_2$ sensor to maintain the level of incident light at the minimal level to detect a cardiac pulse wave. The ideal biophysical sensor requires no direct patient contact or any type of external stimulus to produce a detectable response. Such a sensor is the infrared thermometer, which can transduce skin temperature directly from the emission characteristics of electromagnetic energies from the skin.

Electric Circuits and Patient Insulation

Electricity is a fundamental property of all matter and involves the movement of electrons under a force field in an electric circuit. The electric circuit is a set of components that can conduct electricity. The force field in an electric circuit is the potential difference that exists between conductors. The potential difference unit is the volt (V). The conduction property of electricity is current, and current flows in a circuit when there is a driving force or voltage of sufficient magnitude to overcome the total of all resistances to current flow. An electric circuit can conduct current only when the circuit is closed. The unit of electric current is the ampere (A). The amount of current flowing in a circuit under a particular voltage is also a function of the resistance to current flow in the circuit. The unit of resistance is the ohm. Circuits are usually composed of conducting elements that can be classified as resistors, capacitors, or inductors (Fig. 35–4).

Voltage and current in a circuit can be described as either alternating current (AC) or direct current (DC). AC voltages are cyclic at some frequency and have associated cyclic currents. The AC voltage source that provides electric power to wall outlets is sinusoidal and has a frequency of 60 hertz (Hz). This AC voltage source can be used directly to power appliances or instruments, but, in most cases, it is converted to lower voltage AC or DC. DC voltages and associated currents are produced at constant or steady-state levels. DC voltages can be either positive or negative and are generated from AC by rectifying the AC, that is, converting the voltage to either all positive or all negative voltages (Fig. 35–5). AC current cannot be stored for later use. DC current can be stored in batteries.

Current flow in a DC circuit is described by Ohm's law, where voltage = (current × resistance). For example, current flow in a circuit whose resistance is 20,000 ohms would be 0.0005 A (0.5 mA), but, at a 10-V potential difference, it would increase to 0.005 A (5 mA) at 100 V. In AC circuits, the analysis of current flow can be complex and frequently requires the solution of complex mathematical relationships that describe the interaction of the various components of the circuit. Circuit power, usually expressed in watts, is the product of the voltage and current in a DC circuit. Power calculations in an AC circuit, like current flow calculations, are more complex; voltage, current, and the power factor must be known for the specific circuit. The power factor is a function of the capacitance and inductance of the circuit.

Biophysical sensing instruments are either DC powered (usually by battery) or AC powered. The AC-powered instruments

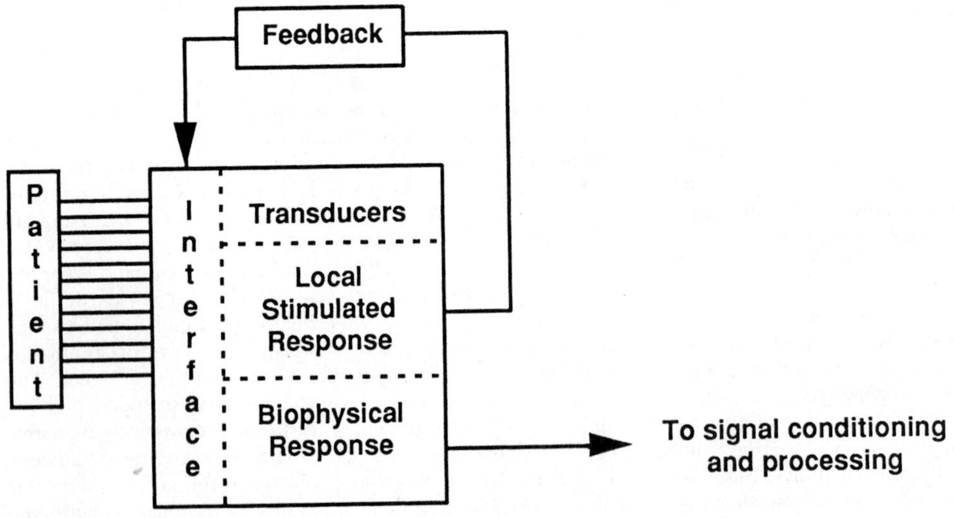

FIGURE 35–3. Block diagram of a complex biophysical transducer.

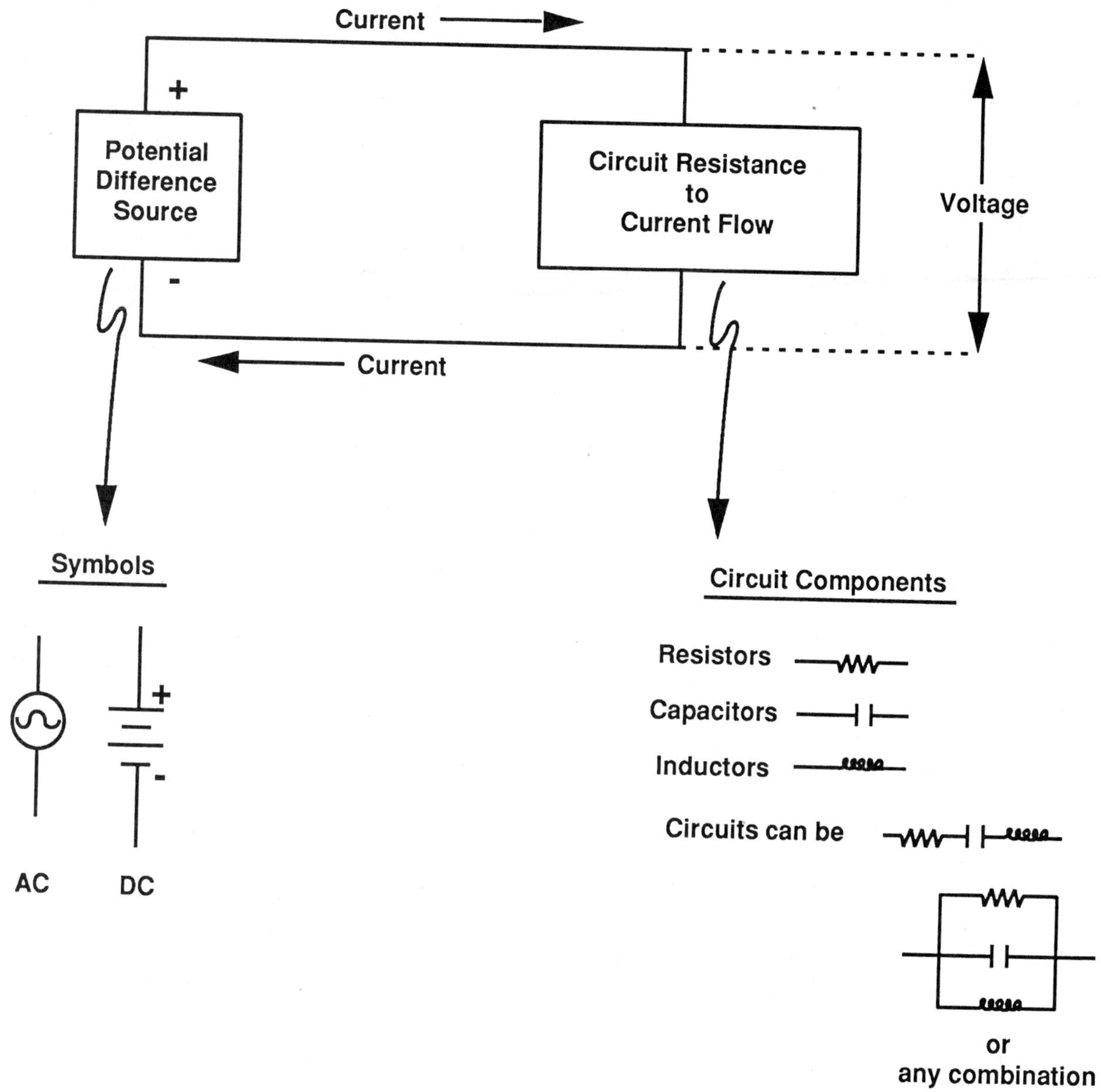

Current
+
Potential Difference Source
-
Current
Circuit Resistance to Current Flow
Voltage
Symbols
AC
DC
+
-
Circuit Components
Resistors
Capacitors
Inductors
Circuits can be
or
any combination

FIGURE 35–4. Basic circuits.

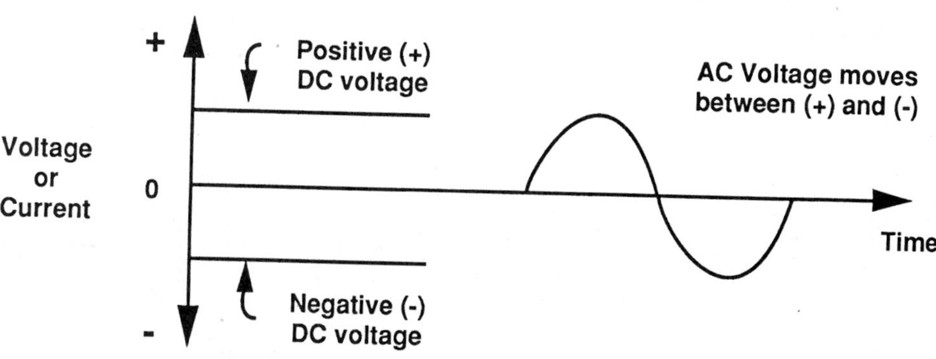

FIGURE 35–5. Classification of voltage and currents as AC or DC. DC voltage and currents can be positive or negative but typically do not change over time. AC voltage and currents can oscillate between positive and negative currents over time.

+
Positive (+)
DC voltage
Voltage
or
Current
0
-
Negative (-)
DC voltage
AC Voltage moves
between (+) and (-)
Time
DC
AC

have a power supply that converts the higher voltage AC from the wall outlet to a lower level AC or DC. When biophysical sensing systems are powered by AC, there is a potential for the caretaker or the patient to come in contact with high-level voltages and to complete circuits such that high currents could flow through the body. Dry skin has a high resistance and normally makes the body a poor conductor. However, voltages could be present that could produce high current flow through the body, particularly if the body forms part of the circuit to the high voltages from a wall outlet.

Electrical power distribution systems in hospitals must have a ground wire at each receptacle, and all modern biophysical instrument systems have a ground wire. The ground wire is physically connected to all exposed conducting surfaces of the instrument and it is intended to provide a low-resistance path for current flow (Fig. 35–6). If the instrument is properly grounded and there is a fault situation in which a high-voltage conductor comes in contact with the conducting surfaces, then the current flows through the ground wire. If there is a break in the continuity of the ground wire and a patient or caretaker touches an exposed conducting surface, then current could flow through the body if contact is made with a grounded object.

In some monitoring systems, redundant insulation (i.e., double insulation) is used to protect the patient and the caretaker, such that even if a high-voltage AC wire comes in contact with conducting surfaces, all the surfaces have been protected with at least two levels of nonconducting material to prevent the flow of current. The use of double insulation does not obviate the need to protect the biophysical transducer from potential fault situations that could result in high-current flow through the body of the patient with whom the transducer may form an electrical connection. A ground wire is not protection from excessive current flow through the body if the patient or the caretaker completes an electrical connection between both conductors of a high-voltage supply line. Current flow through the body is dependent on the voltage source and the resistance of the body.

Current flow is categorized as a microshock if the current is less than 0.001 A (1 mA); currents of more than 1 mA are considered macroshocks. Microshocks are only hazardous when delivered directly to biologic tissue and can cause ventricular fibrillation if delivered directly to the heart. Microshocks on the skin surface are not considered hazardous, because the stratum corneum protective layer of the skin is highly resistive and protects the underlying tissue from current flow. Macroshocks can be hazardous even on the body surface; they can cause pain and can result in the "can't let go" phenomenon, by causing muscle depolarization and tetanic contraction.

All monitoring systems have a fuse or circuit breaker (fuse that can be reused) that ultimately breaks the electrical connection to discontinue current flow. Fuses are the last line of defense, however, and provide no protection against microshock or macroshock hazards. Fuses protect the monitoring system itself and prevent power dissipation in the monitoring system, which generates sufficient heat to pose a fire hazard.

Another type of fuse is the ground fault circuit interrupter (GFCI). The GFCI monitors current flow in the conductors at the wall outlet, and, if an imbalance is detected, both conductors are disconnected, which terminates current flow to the monitoring system. The protection given by the GFCI is based on the assumption that if an imbalance in current flow is detected, some of the current must be flowing through some other circuit or to ground through the ground wire. The GFCI does not protect against the hazard of the patient or caretaker being connected to both conductors of the high-voltage wall outlet.

The opto-isolator is an electronic device that has an internal transmitter and receiver (Fig. 35–7). The transmitter converts electrical energy received at its input to optical energy. This optical energy is then detected at the receiver. The receiver is an optical detector that converts the optical energy back to electrical energy. The distance between the transmitter and receiver determines the degree of protection provided by the isolator against the passage of electric current. Greater distances require larger voltages to initiate current flow. Most opto-isolators provide protection of as much as 5000 V.

The opto-isolator is a safe and effective mechanism to deliver power to a transducer that must contact the patient, while ensuring that under fault conditions, the patient cannot come in direct electrical contact with the main power supply of the monitoring system or the high voltage from the wall outlet. Similarly, transducers in contact with the patient utilize opto-isolators to transmit

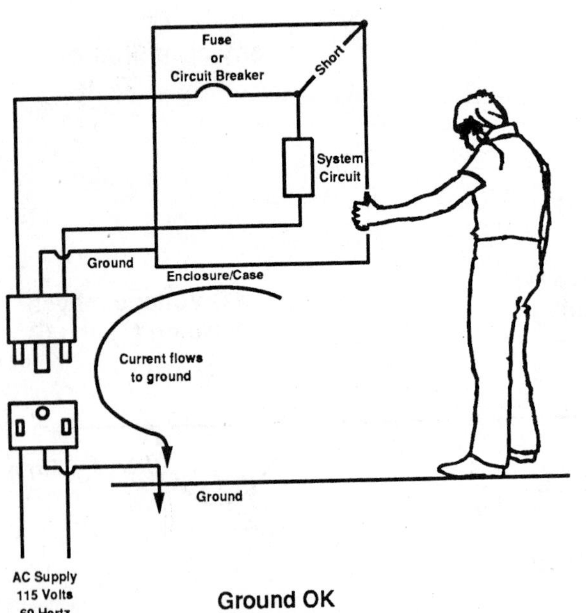

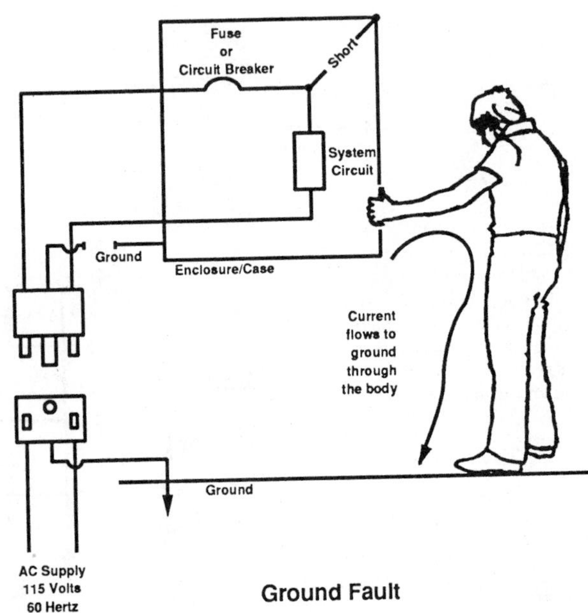

FIGURE 35–6. If a short develops and completes a circuit to the conductive components of a grounded instrument, current flows to ground and the fuse should protect from excessive current flow. When a ground fault or discontinuity occurs, a large current can flow through the body if physical contact is made to the enclosure before the fuse breaks the circuit.

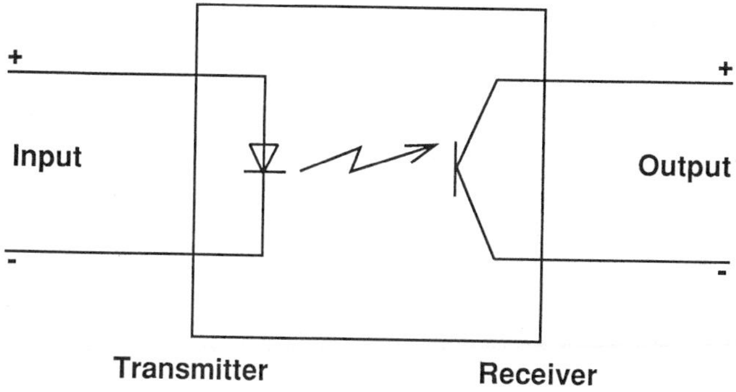

FIGURE 35–7. Opto-isolator.

the transduced signal to the signal conditioning circuits. The conversion of electrical energy to optical energy and the transduction of biologic signals using optics provide degrees of protection and patient safety that cannot be achieved by any other means. The transducer in a $TcSaO_2$ transcutaneous oxygen saturation monitoring system provides total electrical isolation to the patient, because it uses optical energies for stimulation, and the sensing system transduces an optical response that is then converted to electrical energy for processing.

Electromagnetic Radiation

The electromagnetic spectrum includes energies with wavelengths ranging from those of x-ray, to visible light, to radio frequencies (Fig. 35–8). Electromagnetic energy can be classified based on its wavelength or its frequency. Of particular interest in biologic applications are the ultraviolet, visible, and infrared regions of the spectrum. Radiation at these wavelengths is nonionizing. Electromagnetic radiation and its interaction with matter are governed by wave theory and, as such, can be manipulated just like light. All matter radiates energy, and the wavelength of the emitted energy is a function of its temperature. A hotter object emits radiation whose wavelength is shorter than that of a cooler object.

The human body emits electromagnetic energy with wavelengths in the 3- to 50-micrometer (μm) range (Fig. 35–9). Analysis of the transmitted radiation from the skin can be used to determine the temperature of the skin without making physical contact. Clinical infrared thermometers rely on this principle to measure skin or tissue temperature. Also, electromagnetic radiation can be reflected, absorbed, or transmitted at the skin surface. Energies in those wavelengths in which little energy is absorbed by the skin can be used to noninvasively examine underlying tissue or fluids. Electromagnetic energy in the visible region could be directed at the skin, and a detector sensitive to the same range of visible wavelengths could be positioned to measure the level of transmitted radiation. This basic technique is used in the detection of oxygen saturation, in which the quantity of energy absorbed is a function of the degree of oxygenation of hemoglobin. Electromagnetic radiation systems have a transmitter and a receiver that are responsive to specific wavelengths. This specificity can be implemented by optical filters. Optical sensors, even when absorbance and reflectance in living intact biologic systems are used for transduction, are considered to be noninvasive. This categorization as noninvasive is based on the extremely low-level photon energies available in the optical wavelengths from visible to near infrared. The available photon energies in these wavelengths are less than those required for ionization. Ionization can occur at energy levels of 10 electronvolts (eV) (Table 35–2).

Computerized Signal Processing

Biologic signals can be categorized as being analog or digital. Analog signals are those in which the amplitude or frequency changes with time. Digital signals are a specific type of analog signal. Digital signals exhibit on–off types of analog behavior; for example, a digital signal could be considered to be present when a certain voltage level was present continuously and would be considered absent if no voltage was present. This presence or absence of a discrete analog voltage forms the basis for describing digital signals. Digital signals are categorized as ones or zeroes and are mathematically processed in the binary system. This type of representation makes digital signals suitable for a variety of automated processing approaches using computers. An analog signal can be represented as a group of ones and zeroes. The ones and zeroes can then be stored and processed by a computer. The biologic system is of the analog type, in that all systems and processes change amplitude or frequency and periodicity as a function of time (Fig. 35–10). Respiration is an analog behavior and the depth or amplitude of respiration can change independently of the respiration rate or frequency of respiration.

Frequency and periodicity are related mathematically. The pe-

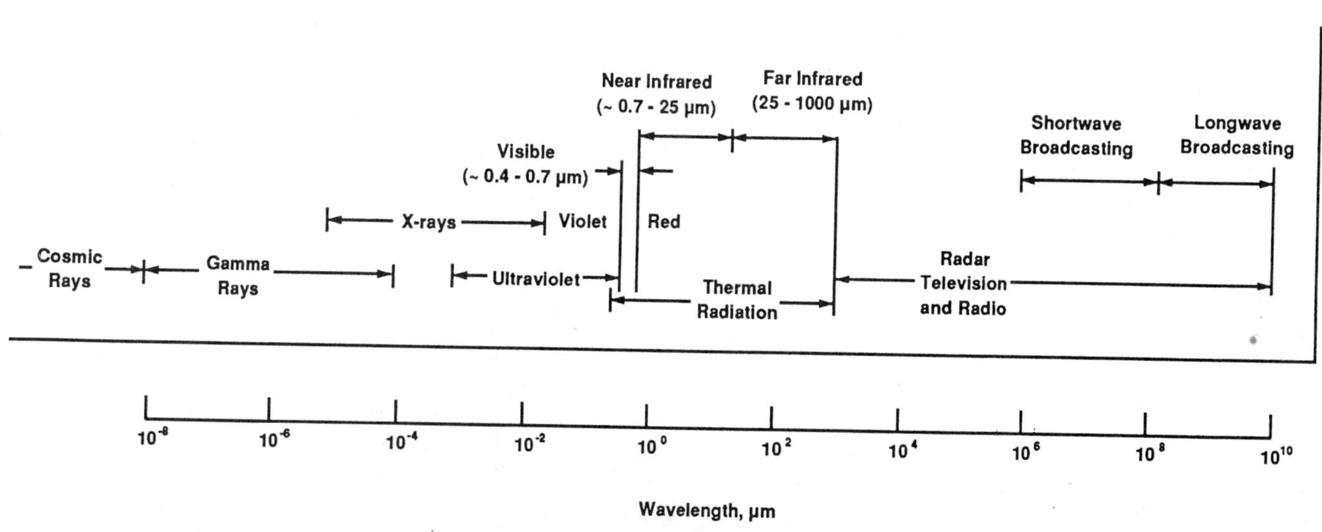

FIGURE 35–8. Electromagnetic spectrum.

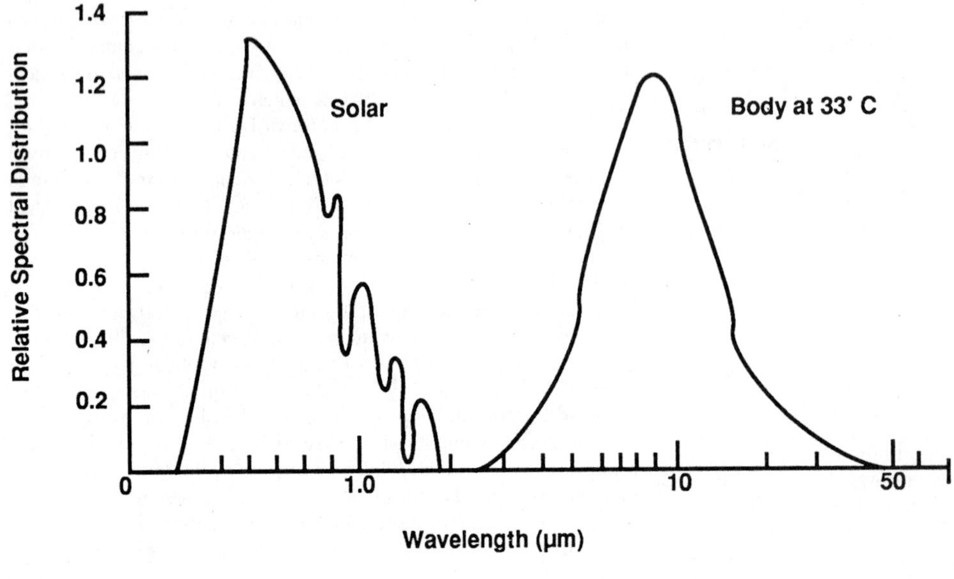

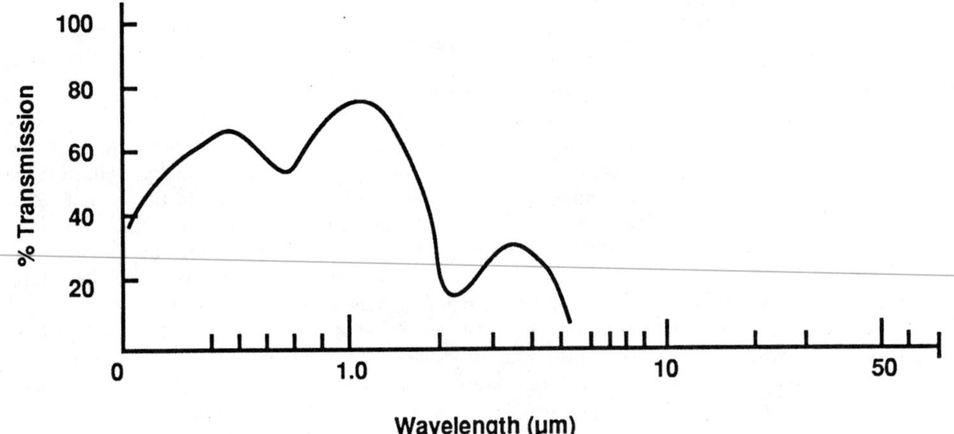

FIGURE 35–9. Relative spectral distribution of energy from the human body and the sun, and the spectral transmission of the skin.

riodicity is the length of time it takes for a specific response to be repeated, and the frequency is the number of times a specific response is repeated per unit of time. Frequency is usually expressed in hertz, which measures cycles per second. Period is expressed in second or minute time units. The period of an analog signal is the inverse of its frequency.

Biologic signals transduced as analog voltages must be conditioned and processed for interpretation to the caretaker. The biophysical transducer may also detect other biologic information that interferes with the primary sensing function. This type of interference would be categorized as artifact. Additionally, the sensor may also respond to energies or noise in the environment.

TABLE 35–2 Photon Energies for Spectrum Segments

Spectrum Segment	Frequency (GHz)	Photon Energy (eV)
Gamma and X radiation	2.3×10^{16}–2.3×10^{7}	10^{11}–10^{2}
Ultraviolet	2.3×10^{7}–10^{6}	10^{2}–4.4
Visible light	10^{6}–3.8×10^{5}	4.4–1.7
Infrared	3.8×10^{5}–300	1.7–1.3×10^{-3}
Microwaves	300–0.3	1.3×10^{-3}–1.3×10^{-6}
Radio waves	0.3–10^{-4}	1.3×10^{-6}–4.4×10^{-10}

To convert the signal to an interpretable format, it is necessary to remove the artifact and noise. This type of processing can be performed on the raw analog signal or on a digital version of the signal. The wide availability of computers makes it more economical and efficient to perform the conditioning and processing of the signal in the digital format. The first step in processing is usually to filter out the noise. Filters that block out noise allow only the analog information in preselected frequency ranges to pass to the next stage of processing. Other types of filters may be used. For example, a filter may remove the 60-Hz noise that results from interference from the 60-Hz AC wall outlet power.

Analog signals are converted to a digital format by an analog-to-digital converter (A/D converter) (Fig. 35–11). The A/D converter samples the signal and generates a set of digital codes to represent the amplitude of the signal. The sampling rate or frequency used must be at least twice the highest frequency of the analog signal and is usually selected to be much higher so that the original analog signal can be accurately reconstructed from the digital information. The precision of the A/D converter is dependent on the number of digital bits used, called the word length. The word length can be 8, 12, 16, or other multiples of 2 bits. An 8-bit converter has 256 (2^8) available combinations of its digital outputs. This, for example, would give the converter a precision of 10/256 V for a 10-V input range. In a similar way, a digital signal can be converted to an analog signal by a device called a digital-to-analog converter.

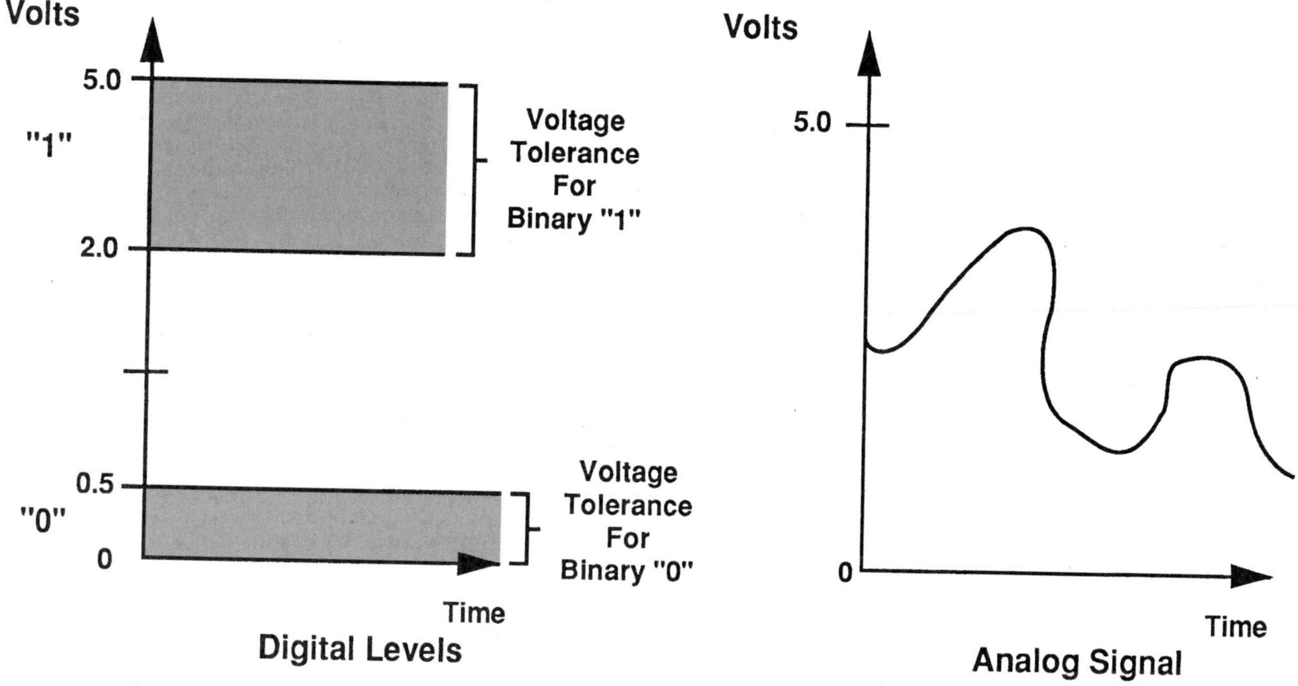

FIGURE 35–10. Analog and digital signals.

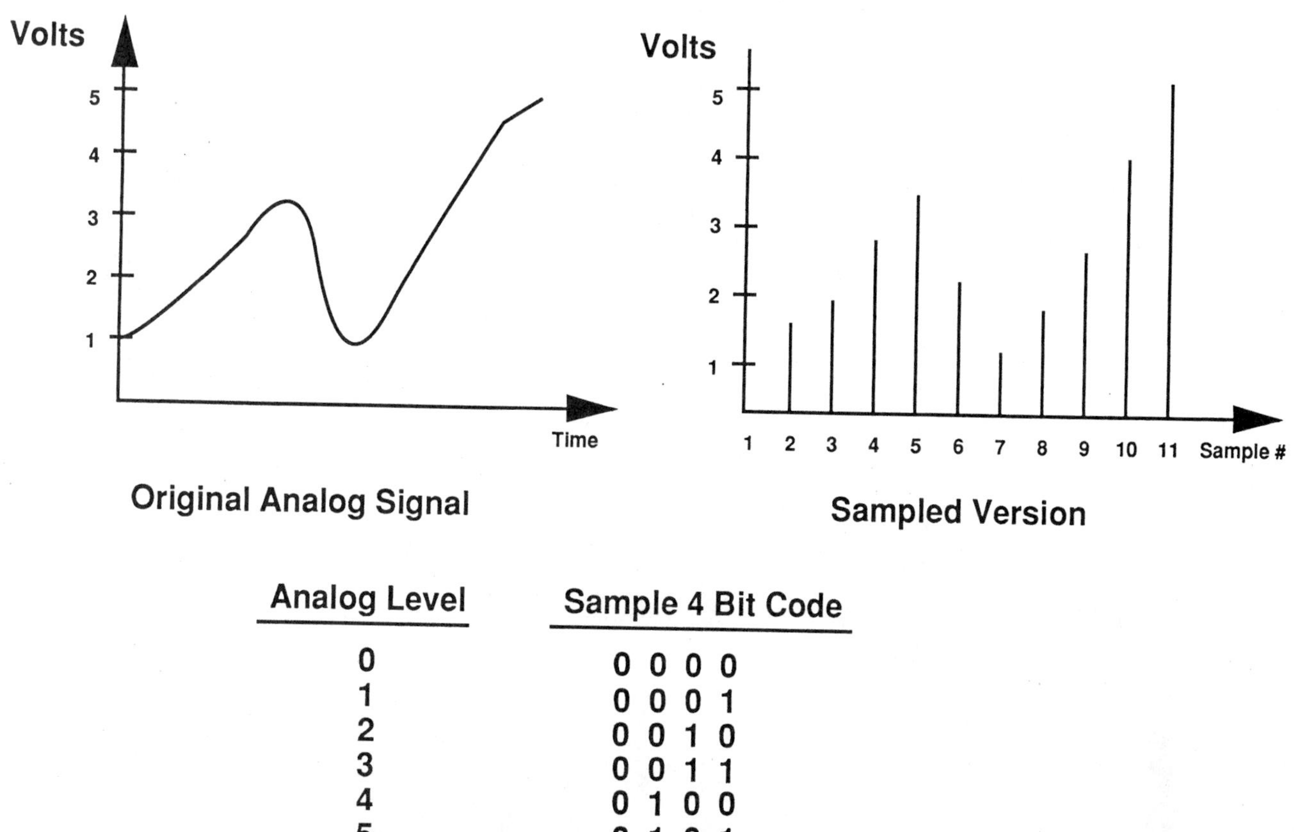

Analog Level	Sample 4 Bit Code
0	0 0 0 0
1	0 0 0 1
2	0 0 1 0
3	0 0 1 1
4	0 1 0 0
5	0 1 0 1

FIGURE 35–11. Analog and digital conversion. The analog signal is sampled, and each sample is assigned a digital code that represents the voltage level of the sample. The digital code system is a 4-bit code.

Computers are composed of hardware and software. The hardware is the physical electronic devices, and the software is the set of instructions that regulate the function of the hardware. A simplified computer has an input and output system (I/O system), a central processing unit (CPU), and a memory system (Fig. 35–12). The interaction of these three components is controlled by the software. The software is the set of instructions that has been developed for the specific task to be performed by the computer. The software is usually stored in the memory. The computer can have multiple layers of memory that are designed for either slow- or high-speed tasks.

It is through the I/O system that the computer communicates with other devices. A digitized biophysical signal would be sent to the input of the computer, and a processed version of this signal could then be sent to the output to be printed or displayed on a video monitor. The CPU manipulates the signal based on the set of processing instructions. The speed of the computer is usually determined by the clock speed. The clock speed is the frequency at which instructions are processed. For example, a clock speed of 10 MHz means that it takes 0.1 microsecond to execute one instruction cycle in the CPU. High-speed computers can take a transduced biophysical signal that has been contaminated with noise and artifact and rapidly filter it, then convert it to a format interpretable by the caretaker. Biophysical data can be stored in the computer memory for later analysis or for the development of patient-specific trends. Most biophysical monitoring systems use some type of computer for signal conditioning and processing. Computers can be used to perform data reduction or transformation tasks on large data sets so that the data can be more readily interpreted by the caretaker. Computers are used to implement pattern recognition algorithms and process control functions that would be extremely time consuming or impossible to implement manually.

Factors That Influence Monitoring Reliability

Computers have greatly influenced biophysical monitoring systems, but the computer processing and manipulation are limited and are ultimately dependent on the quality of the transduced signal. The computer cannot add physiologic information to the transduced biophysical signal or compensate for unforeseen errors in the transduction processes. The effective application of measurement systems to biophysical monitoring is dependent on how error-free the process can be. Errors can occur in the transducer at the site of signal detection, in the conditioning and processing equipment, or in both. The conventional approach to the elimination of errors is to calibrate the system using a known standard. Monitoring system performance is based on the types and magnitude of the errors that may be encountered in the application. Calibration is an effective way to detect and correct for amplitude errors. Errors are usually defined in the manufacturer's specifications for the specific monitoring system.

Because the biologic system primarily generates AC or time-varying complex periodic signals, it is important that the monitoring system architecture accurately reproduce the transduced signals in both amplitude and frequency. The ECG waveform is a complex periodic biologic signal. The primary frequency of this wave is heart rate. However, the basic wave is complex in that the amplitude of the wave changes at different rates over one cycle. If the biophysical transduction or signal conditioning system does not have adequate frequency response, it is possible that the signal will be distorted. The frequency response of the system is defined as that range of frequencies over which there is accurate detection of the amplitude and phase of the biologic signal (Fig. 35–13). The preferred response is for the amplitude ratio of the signal to be constant over the range of frequencies encountered in the signal. The signal is attenuated when the system absorbs more energy at one set of frequencies than at other frequencies. The system can exhibit resonance at some frequencies. Resonance is a type of amplification of the signal that is undesirable. It is therefore important to know the frequency content of the biologic signal being measured and to select a monitoring system that has adequate frequency response or bandwidth.

The important aspect with respect to the bandwidth of a signal is to determine the fastest changing portion of the signal. Analysis of this fast-changing part yields the highest frequency component of the signal. For complex biologic signals, however, spectral analysis tools are used to dissect the signal. This type of spectral analysis process is based on the Fourier theorem, which states that it is always possible to decompose a complex periodic waveform into a series of simple sine waves of varying frequencies. Each of the sinusoids has a contribution to the original signal. These sinusoids are referred to as harmonics, and the contribution of each harmonic to the original signal is weighted as a function of its amplitude. The bandwidth of the signal is defined by the frequency range of the simple sinusoids required to recreate the signal. This type of analysis is widely used and is referred to as spectral or Fourier analysis. Fourier analysis also yields information on the phase angle characteristics of the signal. The phase angle of the signal is a function of the capacitive and inductive components of the signal source. Distortion of the phase angle by the monitoring system can cause shifts in the timing of the signal. In most cases, however, phase angle distortion results only in delaying the signal and does not alter the actual shape of the signal. Table 35–3 provides a listing of some routine physiologic determinations and their associated biophysical systems, with amplitude and frequency ranges of the signals encountered in these systems.

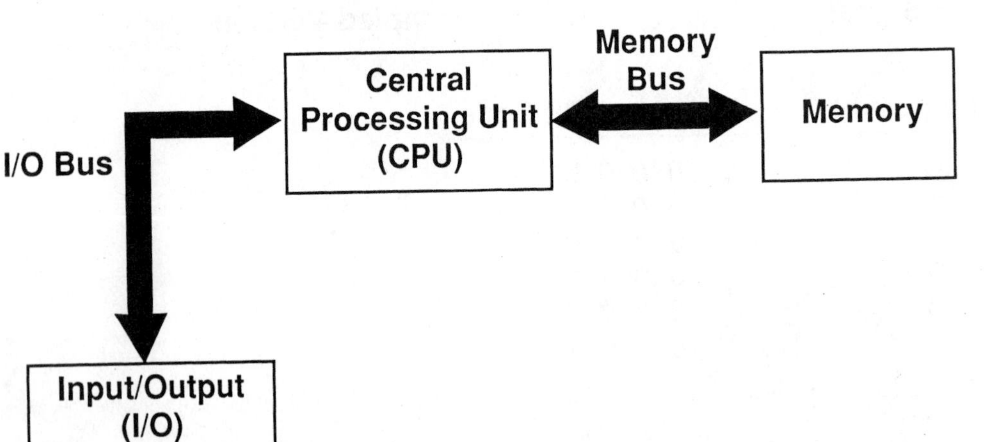

FIGURE 35–12. Block diagram of a simple computer.

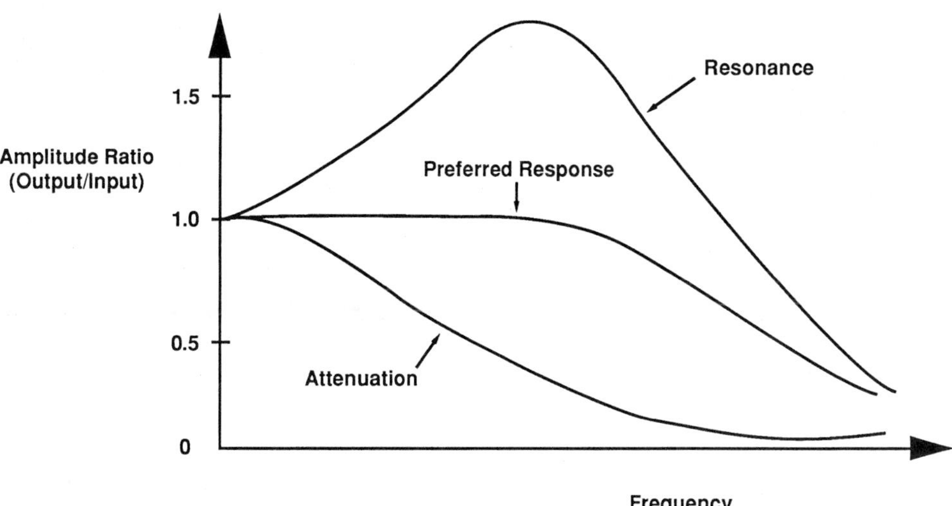

FIGURE 35–13. Influence of frequency response on a signal.

Most monitoring systems can have expected errors that incorrectly represent the amplitude of the signal (Fig. 35–14). Some of these errors occur over time and are referred to as drift errors. Drift can be caused by changes in the transducer properties with time and usually occurs slowly. A drift error usually starts out small and increases gradually with time. These types of errors can increase or decrease the amplitude of the signal but are different from offset errors because the magnitude of the error changes with time. With offset error, the magnitude of error remains constant. Another type of error can occur when there is a change in the degree of error based on the amplitude of the signal. This type of error is categorized as a proportional error.

TABLE 35–3 Amplitude and Frequency Ranges of Frequently Monitored Biophysical Parameters

	Amplitude Range	Frequency Range
Cardiovascular system		
ECG		
Skin surface	0–5 mV	0.05–80 Hz
Direct cardiac	0–20 mV	0.05–80 Hz
Pressure		
Arterial	20–300 mm Hg	0–15 Hz
Ventricular	5–300 mm Hg	0–15 Hz
Blood flow		
Cardiac output	0–1 L/second	0–15 Hz
Velocity	0–5 m/second	0–15 Hz
Respiratory system		
Flow rate	0–1 L/second	0–5 Hz
Blood gases		
Po_2	10–650 mm Hg	0–2 Hz
Pco_2	10–90 mm Hg	0–2 Hz
pH	6.9–7.7	0–2 Hz
Neuromuscular system		
EEG		
Body surface	5–300 mV	0.2–50 Hz
Brain surface	10–5000 μV	0.2–50 Hz
Evoked potentials	0–50 mV	10–500 Hz
Core temperature	30–40°C	DC
Skin temperature	20–42°C	DC
H_2O evaporation rate	0–70 g/m²/h	0–5 Hz

ECG, electrocardiogram; EEG, electroencephalogram.

Proportional errors can also be nonlinear, and this makes them extremely difficult to correct. Hysteresis errors are caused when the current measurement is dependent on the previous measurement level. The error may be different when the signal goes from a low to a higher level, or from a high to a lower level. Most electronic devices are susceptible to hysteresis errors.

Computer processing of the transduced signal can compensate and correct for certain of these errors when they are nonrandom. In some monitoring systems, these errors are small and cannot be corrected or compensated for in the conditioning and processing components of the system. In these cases, the error is used to quantify the accuracy of the system in the form of a tolerance for the output. Tolerances are expressed as a percentage of the range or are assigned limits to the range. For example, the output for a transcutaneous monitor could be specified as being accurate to within ±5 mm Hg.

In the transduction of information from the biologic system, the positioning of the transducer may alter the response and introduce errors. This is the major practical limitation in the transduction of biologic information using transducers that must make physical contact with the living tissue. Another important parameter in the performance of measurement systems is the signal-to-noise ratio. This ratio expresses the level of noise in a system in reference to the level of signal. This ratio should be as high as possible to minimize the effect of noise on the monitoring system. Sometimes, wires used to connect a transducer to the patient act like an antenna and pick up electrical noise from the environment, which could cause interference, for example, in an ECG. Biologic noise may affect the actual transducer if the sensing element cannot be protected from biologic matter that generates characteristics similar to those of the anolyte of interest.

Stability is another important criterion in the assessment of monitoring system performance. Stability can be affected by temperature changes in the operating environment. Additionally, the monitoring system itself may be dependent on its own operating temperature, which may change as a function of the length of time that power is supplied. This operating temperature change is characterized as warm-up time.

In neonatal monitoring, the effect of temperature must be considered for all types of transduction, because nearly all neonates are in beds that have altered environments. In most cases, neonatal bed environments are convectively warmed enclosed incubators or open bassinet infrared radiant heaters. It is also important to consider how high-intensity optical radiation from phototherapy or examination lights may affect the transducers or conditioning and processing devices.

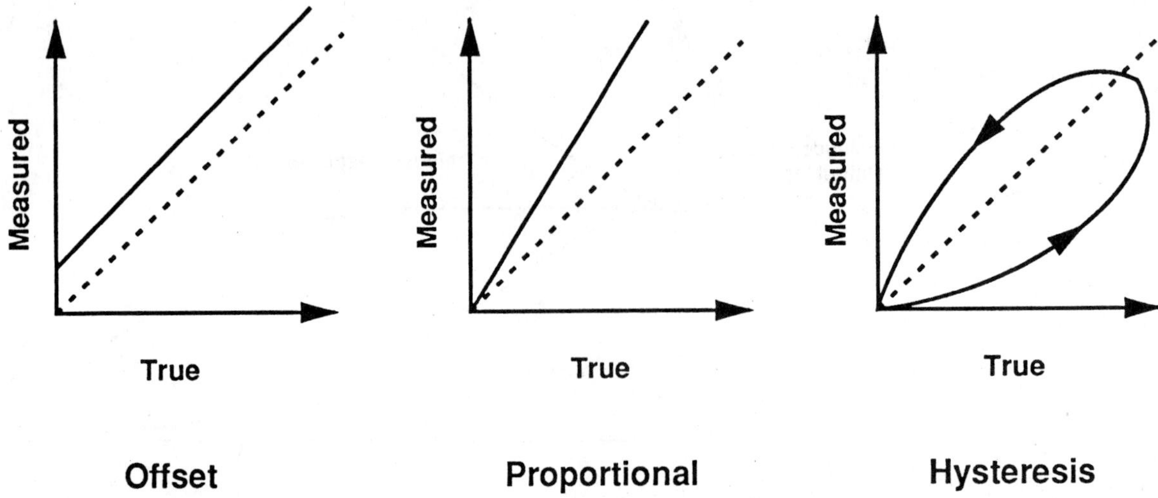

FIGURE 35–14. Amplitude errors. Linear response is shown as dotted line.

Specific Applications

Temperature Measurement

Contact thermometry is the prevalent technique for the routine measurement of body temperature. Neonatal body temperature is assessed by either rectal or skin surface temperature measurement. Rectal temperature is an indicator of core or "deep body" temperature. Skin temperature is widely used because, unlike rectal temperature, it is easily transduced to provide continuous temperature information to the caretaker. In most clinical situations, however, skin temperature alone provides no real quantitative assessment of patient status. Skin temperature, when coupled with core and ambient air or environment temperature, can be an effective indicator of the infant's thermal balance.

Temperature is one of the most important indicators of the health status of newborns. Rectal temperature measurement using mercury-in-glass thermometers is gradually being replaced by electronic thermometers. Temperature measurement by electronic thermometers is an inexpensive technique that can be used to ensure sterility and prevent cross-contamination. Protective plastic sleeves can be used on the sensing element, or, in some cases, the sensing element itself is a single-use disposable item.

A common problem with all types of contact thermometry is that the indicated temperature is a reflection of the entire surface in contact with the sensing element. A large sensing element indicates an average temperature for its entire surface contact area. Also, the temperature sensing device must have adequate time to equilibrate with its environment before a reliable temperature can be measured. This time to an acceptable response is a function of the time constant of the sensor. The time constant is the standard notation for classifying how fast a temperature is sensed and is defined as the time to reach 63 percent of the final value in response to an abrupt change in temperature. The length of time to reach the final temperature is usually multiple time constants. The time constant is primarily a function of the physical size and density of the temperature-sensing element. Temperature measurement devices with large time constants cannot be used for temperature monitoring when rapid temperature changes are expected.

Traditional mercury-in-glass type rectal thermometers, like skin thermometers, have been replaced with electronic devices. Electronic thermometers are based on the principle that most materials exhibit some type of physical change in response to temperature. The thermistor, the platinum resistance temperature device (RTD), and the thermocouple are the most common temperature-sensing elements used in electronic thermometers. The temperature-dependent physical changes in each of these devices are reversible and can be transduced with repeatability and acceptable accuracy for biologic applications.

The thermistor is a thermally sensitive resistor that changes its resistance as a function of its temperature. Thermistors are fabricated from semiconductor materials. Semiconductor materials are usually some form of metal oxide and are similar to the basic materials used to produce the semiconductor components used in electronic instrumentation (e.g., transistors, integrated circuits). The electrical conduction and resistance properties of these materials change exponentially with temperature. This exponential resistance change makes these devices very sensitive to temperature, but the exponential nature of the change makes the resistance curve for the thermistor nonlinear. The nonlinear change in resistance with temperature must be corrected in the signal conditioning and processing component of the monitoring system to provide useful temperature data to the caretaker. When a constant current is passed through a thermistor, changes in resistance due to temperature produce a change in the voltage measured across the thermistor. Thermistors can be made very small and, with laser cutting techniques, can be produced in large quantities with low variability in the resistance temperature response.

Platinum RTDs are based on the resistance change of metal wire with temperature changes. The wire is wound on an insulating core for physical support. The mechanical winding process requires much larger dimensions than those required for thermistors. The resistance change of an RTD is always linear, and it is this linear response to temperature that is the significant advantage of RTDs over thermistors. Because they are much larger than thermistors, however, the RTDs have larger time constants. Also, RTDs cannot be applied to invasive applications as easily as the much smaller thermistors.

The thermocouple, unlike the thermistor or the RTD, does not require an applied voltage or current at the transducing element to measure temperature. The thermocouple is based on the principle that when two dissimilar metals are placed in contact, a voltage difference is created across this metal contact. Because the thermocouple is fabricated from metals, the voltage difference is a function of temperature. This difference in voltage results in current flow through the circuit, which can then be transduced and processed. Thermocouples can be fabricated as small as the available wire diameters. The small physical size gives the thermocouple a faster response time than either the thermistor or the RTD. For biologic in vivo tissue exposure, however, the metals must be protected from oxidation. The protective coating required to achieve this protection can adversely affect the time constant of the thermocouple because of increased thermal mass.

Advances in automated manufacturing have greatly reduced the cost of thermistors, RTDs, and thermocouples, such that these sensing elements can be designed to be single-use and disposable. For example, because the actual resistance of a thermistor is a function of its physical size, automated cutting equipment can adjust the size to meet a very specific resistance range. This type of manufacturing process can ensure that each thermistor produced is virtually the same.

The use of these types of temperature-sensing elements in disposable thermometers can also overcome an inherent problem in that each of these devices deteriorates with age. In particular, the resistance of a thermistor changes over time. This type of failure mode is gradual and can go totally undetected if calibration is not regularly checked. Calibration of equipment using thermistors should be closely monitored if the thermistors are not routinely replaced.

The most common failure mode for thermistors, RTDs, and thermocouples is an open circuit or short circuit. For a thermistor, a short circuit occurs as a very high temperature reading (zero resistance). Most clinical thermometers provide some type of alarm indication when catastrophic failures such as this occur.

The most common problem with temperature measurement is ensuring that the sensor has good contact with the surface being measured. Measuring skin temperature of a newborn in the delivery room is difficult because it is virtually impossible to attach a skin probe to the infant's wet skin. When the sensor is not in intimate contact with the skin surface, the temperature measured is greatly influenced by the temperature of the environment. For example, a poorly adhered skin probe on the skin of an infant in an incubator is highly influenced by the air temperature of the incubator. Also, a skin probe used on an infant under a radiant warmer does not accurately indicate the infant's skin temperature if the temperature sensor is not shielded from the direct radiation of the radiant warmer heating system by a reflective pad. The pad reflects the incident radiation and prevents the absorption of energy, which would heat the sensor and elevate the sensed temperature.

Noncontact infrared thermometers and infrared thermographic cameras can be used to measure temperatures without contact with the surface to be measured. This type of temperature measurement system offers the greatest level of sterility and protections because no physical contact is required to measure temperature. These noncontact thermometers work on the principle that all materials emit radiation. The intensity and the wavelength of the emitted radiation from an object are a function of the temperature of the object. As the temperature increases, so does the intensity or power at a given wavelength. The peak of the energy curve moves toward the shorter wavelengths as the temperature increases (Fig. 35–15).

By measuring the power of the radiation emitted over a range

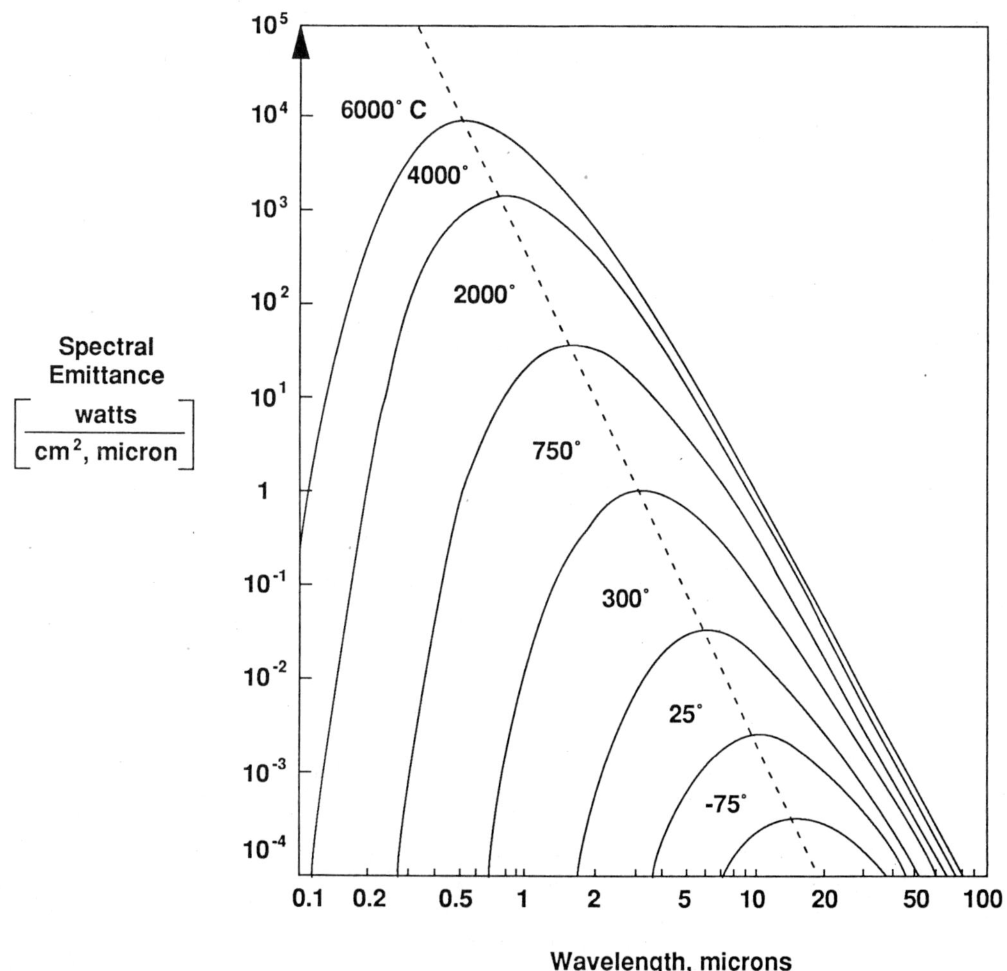

FIGURE 35–15. Blackbody radiation curves. There is an increase in intensity with temperature, and the wavelength of the peak moves toward shorter wavelengths.

of wavelengths, it is possible to determine the temperature of the surface emitting the radiation. For temperatures in the physiologic range, the energy is emitted in the infrared region. A sufficient amount of energy is emitted from objects, such that with sensitive detectors, the energy can be measured even at great distances from the object. The infrared detectors for human body temperature measurement are designed for the 5- to 25-μm wavelengths. These infrared devices can be used for single-point temperature measurements or can be used to provide thermal images for an entire surface. Infrared detectors, like all optical measurement systems, can have interference either from reflections from other objects or from infrared energy that is transmitted through the surface being observed. The total energy received at the detector is a combination of the emitted, reflected, and transmitted energies (Fig. 35–16).

When using infrared thermometers, it is important to ensure that there are no other sources of heat that can interfere with the surface being sensed. Infrared energies are reflected just like visible light. Infrared thermometers are used to measure tympanic membrane temperature. The tympanic membrane has been documented to be a good indicator of core temperature. However, the physical size of the optic head on these temperature monitors makes it difficult to position the thermometer in the ear canal to ensure good alignment with the tympanic membrane, particularly in infants. When not aligned properly, the thermometer may read the temperature of the ear canal rather than the tympanic membrane. This type of temperature measuring device can be affected by the depth of the probe into the ear canal and potentially by the presence of vernix or other debris in the ear. Yet, these potential factors have not been addressed in research. Some NICUs are using tympanic temperature measurements with reportedly good results, but clinical trials have yet to be conducted on premature and term infants under various conditions and gestational ages.

Electrodes for the Electrocardiogram

Bioelectrical potentials are transduced from the skin surface for ECG, electroencephalogram (EEG), and evoked potentials. The potentials on the body range from 1 μV to 1 mV. Body surface electrodes attached to the skin (Fig. 35–17) are used to convert the ionic potentials produced by the ionic current flow in tissue to electronic potentials. The surface electrode uses a metal–electrolyte interface. The electrolyte for biologic transduction can be the fluid around the tissue. Artificial electrolytes in a gel substance are usually incorporated into commercial electrodes. An electrical potential is generated at the metal–electrolyte interface when there is a difference in diffusion rates of ions into and out of the metal. Metallic ions in solution with their associated metals always develop an electrode potential. These electrode potentials are referred to as half-cell potentials. The most common electrode is the silver–silver chloride electrode. Pairs of these electrodes can be coupled to produce a voltage source just like in a battery.

Two electrodes are necessary to measure bioelectrical potentials, and the voltage measured is actually the instantaneous potentials of the two electrodes. If the two electrodes are exactly the same, then the voltage difference is dependent on the biologic ionic difference between the two electrodes. If the two electrodes are different, there is a potential or DC voltage between them. This DC voltage is referred to as electrode offset and affects the transduction of ionic potentials. Offsets like this are sometimes caused by a drying of the electrolyte gel in one of the electrodes. Microelectrodes and needle electrodes that are used to penetrate the skin function on the same basic principle as ECG electrodes. The premature infant has a poorly developed stratum corneum. This immature skin has a low resistance to current flow; therefore, it is easy to obtain a good electrical signal during the early postnatal period. As the stratum corneum develops and the skin

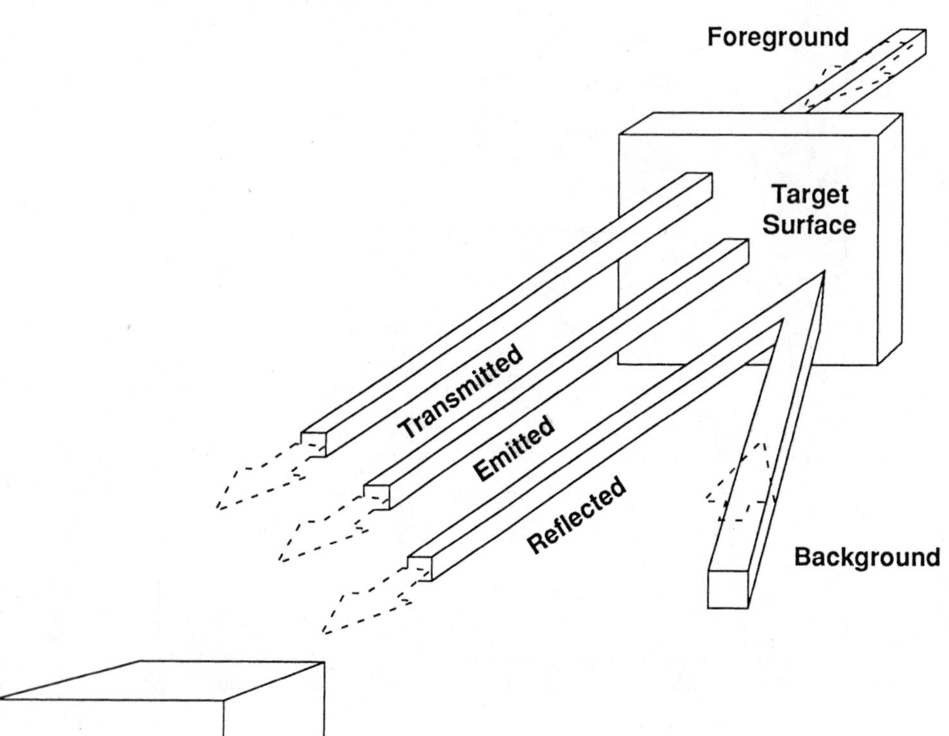

FIGURE 35–16. The total energy received at the detector is a combination of the emitted, reflected, and transmitted energies.

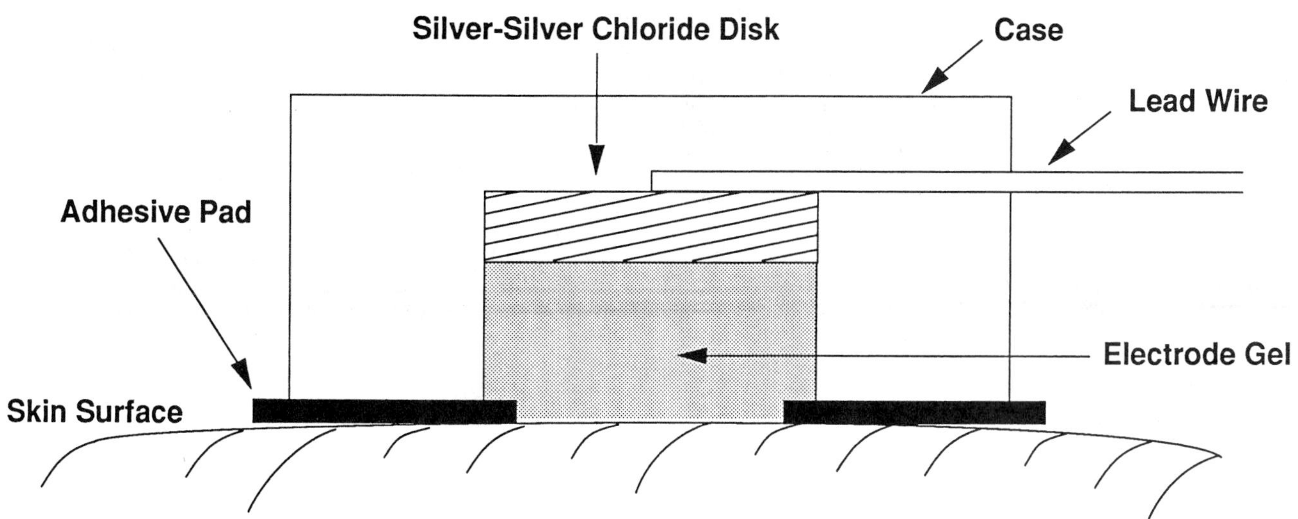

FIGURE 35–17. Diagram of a skin surface electrode.

becomes less moist, however, it is important to check and replace the electrodes to ensure that there is sufficient electrolyte for good electrical conduction. Difficulties with the ECG baseline can usually be attributed to drying of the electrolyte. Also, during the neonate's first week of life, the electrodes are very sensitive to motion artifact and baseline drift.

Impedance Electrodes for Respiration Rate

Impedance electrodes generate an electrical field around tissue. The electrodes are the same type as those used for biopotential transduction such as with the ECG. Measured distortions or changes in the electrical field can then be attributed to specific tissue effects. Impedance electrodes are applied in the form of an impedance bridge, and the electrodes are excited with low-voltage high-frequency AC. There is also no risk of ventricular fibrillation at the high frequencies that are used.

Impedance is the transduction principle used to measure respiration rate and cardiac output. Two electrodes placed at the extremes of the thoracic cavity can be used to detect volume changes caused by respiration (Fig. 35–18). The expansion and contraction of the intervening tissue mass during each respiratory cycle cause detectable changes in the electrical conducting path. This change in the conducting path is referred to as impedance and is transducible if the changes are large enough. In the three-lead ECG configuration, impedance transduction is usually applied to two of the electrodes to determine respiration rate. Because it is the resistance to current flow that is being detected, it is extremely important to have intimate contact with the skin surface. Here also, drying of the electrolyte gel generates impedance changes that can cause baseline drift. This technique for respiration rate monitoring is widely used because it does not require any additional electrodes or connections to the infant other than those required for ECG (heart rate) monitoring.

A recent study by Poets and associates (1995) examined stable premature infants who were on continuous cardiopulmonary monitoring and would not normally have received regular pulse oximeter measurements. They found that of the 96 preterm infants with a median gestation age of 34 weeks and who were

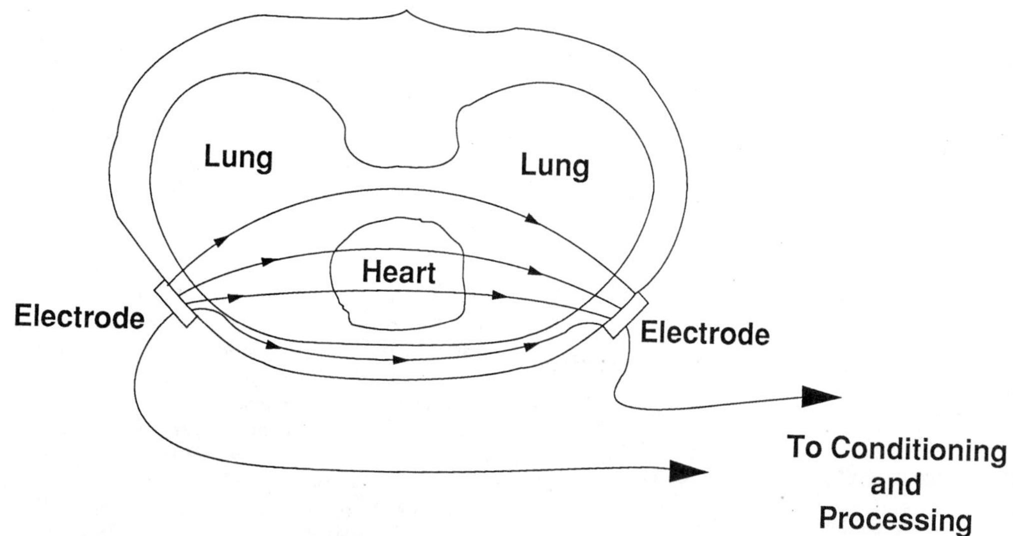

FIGURE 35–18. Electrodes placed on the extremities of the thoracic cavity are sensitive to volume changes caused by respiration. Arrows indicate the current path between the electrodes.

on room air were followed by pulse oximetry, that 88 episodes of oxygen saturation levels less than 80 percent and lasting 20 seconds or longer occurred in 15 infants. These hypoxic episodes did not "set off" the cardiorespiratory monitors. The ramifications are that stable premature infants, at least for a time, probably should be monitored by pulse oximetry in addition to routine cardiorespiratory monitoring.

Pulse Oximetry (Transcutaneous Oxygen Saturation)

Measurement of $TcSaO_2$, referred to as pulse oximetry, is based on the principle of oximetry. Oximetry uses spectrophotometric analysis of light transmitted through or reflected back from light-absorbing substances. Light-absorbing substances have an absorption coefficient for each wavelength. Therefore, the amount of light absorbed at any wavelength is a function of the concentration of the substances that have high absorption coefficients at that wavelength. When the distance that the light travels is kept constant, then it is only the concentration of light-absorbing substances that affects the levels of transmitted or reflected light. Using this basic optical technique, which is based on Lambert-Beers law, the concentration of substances can be determined if there are some unique absorption characteristics at a specific wavelength. Other substances that have similar absorption characteristics must be removed or always be at a constant or known concentration.

Because oxyhemoglobin and deoxyhemoglobin have distinctively different absorption characteristics (Fig. 35–19), it is possible to determine the concentration of each in a sample of blood in vitro. By irradiating the blood sample with light at a wavelength that has different absorption characteristics for oxyhemoglobin and deoxyhemoglobin (approximately 650 nm) and at a wavelength for which the absorption characteristics are the same for oxyhemoglobin and deoxyhemoglobin (805 nm), it is possible to determine the concentrations of each in blood. The percentage of hemoglobin saturated with oxygen can then be calculated from these intensities.

This same principle is used to determine the percent saturation of arterial blood in vivo, using pulse oximetry. As shown in Figure 35–20, the assumption is that changes in the intensity of light transmitted through or reflected from tissue during the inflow phase of the cardiac cycle (systole) are attributable to arterial blood alone. If light intensity is measured during systole and also during the period between heart beats (diastole), then the difference between the light intensities can be attributed to arterial blood alone. Measurements of light intensities at 650 nm and 805 nm are taken for systole and diastole. The light intensities are corrected for tissue variations, and the pulsatile variation can then be attributed to arterial flow only. Consequently, there is no calibration required for the sensor. The ratio of the corrected light intensities gives the beat-to-beat percent saturation.

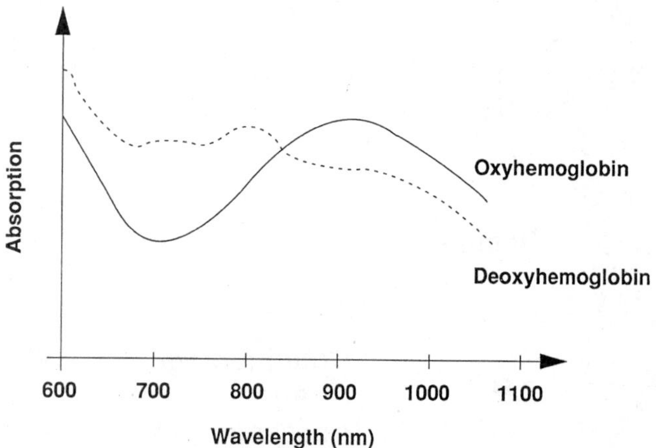

FIGURE 35–19. Absorption characteristics for oxyhemoglobin and deoxyhemoglobin as a function of wavelength.

The first generation of oxygen saturation devices used fiberoptic cables to deliver the light to the sensor tip and another fiberoptic cable to return the transmitted light to the detector. Currently, monochromatic light-emitting diodes and photodetectors are fabricated small enough to encapsulate in self-contained sensors.

Using this optical technique, percent saturation can be influenced by venous pulsatile flow and motion artifact, which can change the effective thickness of the tissue between the light source and the detector. Ambient lights that have high intensities in the levels used for saturation can be detected by the saturation detector if they are not adequately shielded. Also, because the absorption characteristics of fetal hemoglobin are slightly different from those of adult hemoglobin, it is important that saturation monitors used in the early postnatal period be suitably corrected to compensate for these differences. The timing for the activation of the light pulses is critical to the accuracy of the derived percent saturation. The addition of an independent source for the timing of the pulse wave, like an ECG, can improve the accuracy if the triggering of the light pulses is linked to this independent source. To compensate for poor or variable arterial perfusion, the light intensities on the transmitters of most oximeters can be adjusted so that the level of light received at the detector provides an acceptable pulse wave.

Partial Pressure of Oxygen

The partial pressure of oxygen in arterial blood ($TcPO_2$) can be measured using oxygen polarographic techniques. Figure 35–21 shows a general schematic of this technique that is based on the Clark oxygen electrode.

The polarographic cell has a cathode (usually platinum) and an anode (usually silver–silver chloride, or Ag-AgCl), whose surfaces are in contact with an electrolyte, for example, potassium chloride (KCl). The anode and cathode are polarized with 600 mV DC. Oxygen molecules, which can reach and dissolve in the electrolyte, are electrochemically reduced at the cathode. Each O_2 molecule takes four electrons (e^-) from the cathode and combines with two water molecules (H_2O) to form four hydroxyl ions (OH^-). At the anode, silver is oxidized and electrons are liberated. The silver ions combine with chloride ions to form silver chloride. These reactions provide a continuous flow of electrons between the cathode and the anode. Because the supply of electrons to the cathode depends on the supply of oxygen molecules, the PO_2 can be determined. The flow of electrons generates a detectable current, which can be processed to provide its output in mm Hg pressure. A membrane permeable only to oxygen must be used to protect the electrode from all other molecules. A thin membrane of Teflon is used in most commercial devices. The thickness and composition of the membrane, because it affects the flow of oxygen to the electrodes, ultimately determine the response time of the sensor. These oxygen electrodes must be calibrated at two reference levels before use because the build-up of charge on the electrodes over time causes drift.

$TcPO_2$ is based on the concept that it is possible to alter the rate of diffusion of oxygen through the skin by elevating its temperature to more than 40°C. Normally, there is very low or no transport of oxygen through the skin. The skin is usually heated to 43°C to 44°C, at which point there is increased diffusion even through the outer barrier of the skin, the stratum corneum. Because heating also causes vasodilation, there is an increase in

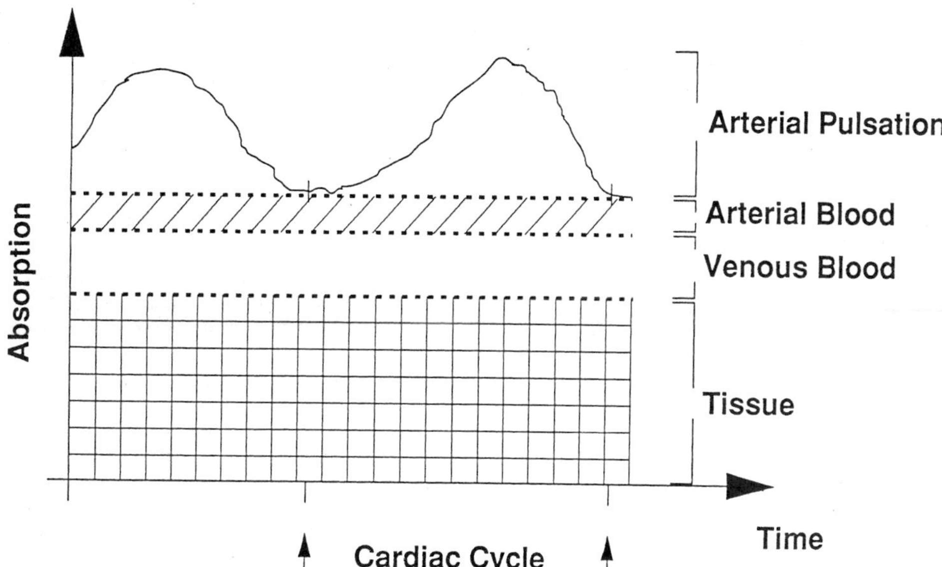

FIGURE 35–20. Changes in the intensity of transmitted or reflected light are a function of the absorption characteristics of the tissue at the measurement site, the absorption caused by venous blood, and the absorption changes that can be accounted for by arterial pulsation.

blood flow to the dermal capillaries, which makes the oxygen tension in these vessels close to the levels of the deeper arterial vessels. To protect the sensor from the effects of oxygen in the air, the probe assembly is attached to the skin with an adhesive that provides a good mechanical air-tight seal. The heating of the skin to promote oxygen diffusion causes mild erythema. This is one monitoring situation in which extreme care must be taken because of the high temperatures used at the surface of the sensor, which is in contact with the very immature skin of the small premature infant. $TcPo_2$ is still not an absolute measurement system and is used primarily as a trending tool in conjunction with absolute gas tensions measured in arterial blood with a laboratory analyzer.

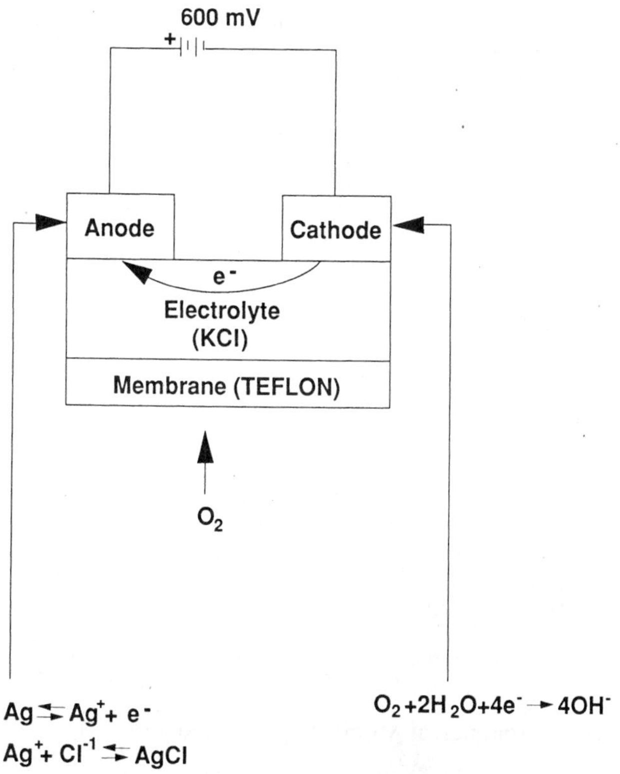

600 mV
Anode
Cathode
e⁻
Electrolyte (KCl)
Membrane (TEFLON)
O_2
$Ag \rightleftharpoons Ag^+ + e^-$
$Ag^+ + Cl^{-1} \rightleftharpoons AgCl$
$O_2 + 2H_2O + 4e^- \rightarrow 4OH^-$

FIGURE 35–21. Schematic of a Po_2 transducer.

Partial Pressure of Carbon Dioxide

The partial pressure of carbon dioxide in arterial blood ($TcPco_2$) can be measured using transduction techniques based on the Severinghaus principle. The Severinghaus principle is based on the measurement of CO_2 using an indirect transduction scheme in which the effect of CO_2 on the pH of a solution is transduced. The resultant pH is measured using standard glass pH electrodes. Figure 35–22 shows a general schematic of this type of transduction.

The CO_2 molecules are absorbed in an electrolyte (HCO_3), forming hydrogen and bicarbonate ions. A potential is generated between the pH electrode and the reference electrode. The potential is proportional to the concentration of CO_2. The CO_2 sensor must be calibrated at two points using reference gases (usually 5 percent and 10 percent CO_2). Heat is also used in the Po_2 sensor to increase the diffusion of CO_2 across the stratum corneum. Because the transduction mechanism is based on the pH glass electrode, the sensor is extremely sensitive to temperature (Fig. 35–23). Both $TcPo_2$ and $TcPco_2$ are highly influenced by skin perfusion. Also, because the response time of the sensors is slow, it is difficult to use data for anything other than gross trending of gas tensions. This slow response is in contrast with the rapid response of transcutaneous oxygen saturation measurement systems.

Another type of carbon dioxide monitoring being tried during transports is a portable infrared end-tidal carbon dioxide monitor. It has been used most widely during pediatric anesthesia and in the transport of critically ill adults. The problem with this type of monitoring in infants is that a 38-mL dead space potentially leads to very small infants rebreathing the air. Biochem International in Waukesha, WI, has devised the Biochem 520 carbon dioxide breath indicator, a side-stream infrared capnometer with only a 2-ml dead space. One reason to use this form of monitoring during transport is to determine whether an endotracheal tube is in proper position for ventilation. Bhende and colleagues (1995) found that when 50 patients aged 1 day to 19 years were identified by this device during transport, 48 of the 50 endotracheal placement positions were verified (sensitivity of 96 percent, specificity of 100 percent). These findings need to be replicated, but

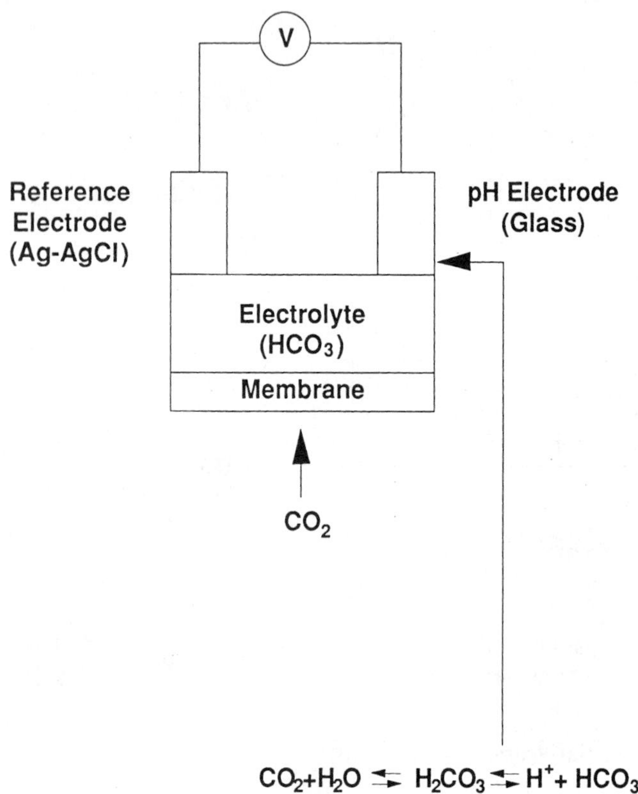

FIGURE 35–22. Schematic of a P_{CO_2} transducer.

they may show that this is a good noninvasive way to monitor the status of neonates during transport.

Serum Bilirubin

Total bilirubin can be measured using a simple optical system (Fig. 35–24). The device is designed to quantify the degree of yellowing of the tissue underlying the skin. Because bilirubin has unique absorption spectra, it is possible to determine the concentration of bilirubin in vivo by analyzing the reflected light from a source directed at the skin. The reflected light is split into two beams using a dichroic mirror. The light is then passed through 460- and 550-mm filters and is converted to electrical energy by photodetectors. The relative energies of the reflected light can be correlated to the concentration of total bilirubin at the measurement site. Measurement accuracy is ultimately dependent on the optical properties of the skin and location of sensor on body.

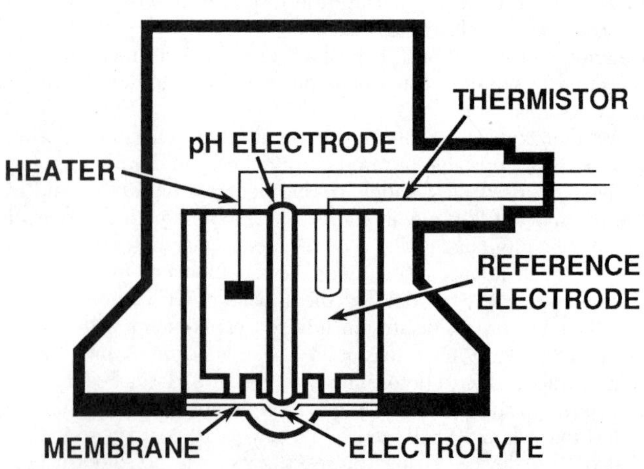

FIGURE 35–23. Cross-sectional diagram of a transcutaneous P_{CO_2} sensor. (Courtesy of Hoffmann-La Roche, Basel, Switzerland.)

Pressure Monitoring

The measurement of pressure is mostly based on strain gauge transduction principles. Strain is the change in length of an object per unit length. The strain gauges are usually constructed of materials that have the ability to detect changes in electrical resistance for small changes in length. The sensitivity of the strain gauge is a function of the force necessary to cause a detectable deflection in the gauge membrane. Attaching an object to the gauge can facilitate the transduction of force. If a fluid exerts force on the active surface of the gauge, then movement of the gauge can be expressed as a pressure. Blood pressure measurement with a catheter is based on this principle. With a sterile saline solution in the catheter, the pressure of the blood for each cardiac cycle is transmitted through this fluid column to the active face of the pressure transducer. The length and the type of material used in the catheter can affect the frequency response in this type of pressure measurement system. Also, the location of the transducer at the same level as the heart helps to avoid pressure offsets.

In all direct pressure measurement systems in which a fluid-filled catheter is used to transmit the pressure wave to the strain gauge, it is important to ensure that the catheter is free of all air bubbles. If there is a significant amount of air in the system, the pressure waveform is distorted because air, unlike saline, can be compressed. The loss of energy because of compression in the catheter can dampen the actual pressure wave. Bubbles can usually be dislodged by gently tapping the pressure transducer manifold.

Semiconductor strain gauges, which can be fabricated to be very small in size, are extremely sensitive and produce measurable outputs with little distortion in the gauge membrane. Displacements as low as a few microns can be detected. Semiconductor-based strain gauges are used in catheters that have the pressure transducer at their tip. In these catheter-tipped pressure transducers, the pressure variations are transduced at the measurement site itself and not through a fluid column.

Indirect blood pressure measurement can be accomplished with an inflatable cuff placed around a major artery. These systems have automated inflation and deflation mechanisms and are designed to measure cuff pressures at the systolic and diastolic end points of the cardiac cycle. With the availability of small sensitive pressure transducers and suitable plastics for the cuff, this technique has gained acceptance as a screening tool for infants. When a timer is incorporated to activate the inflation and deflation pumps at discrete intervals (e.g., every 30 minutes), this technique can be used in a semicontinuous noninvasive way to track pressure. The widespread availability of low-cost sophisticated electronics allows for the incorporation of fail-safe alarm systems to prevent overinflation or continuous inflation of the cuffs. All types of pressure monitoring, direct and indirect, are extremely sensitive to motion artifact and positioning of the pressure transducer. Pressure transducers are usually extremely temperature sensitive because they rely on the detection of small mechanical changes in metals as the transduction mechanism.

New Techniques of Monitoring the Neonate

Cerebral blood flow velocity is an area that, until recently, was followed by researchers rather than clinicians. The equipment

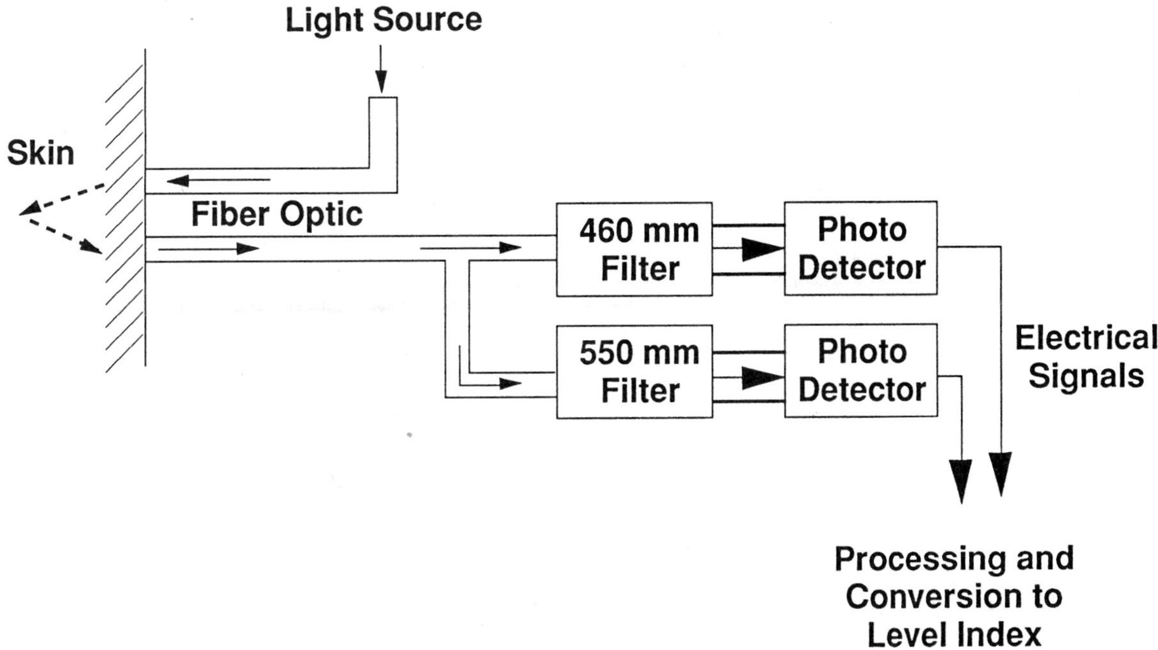

FIGURE 35–24. Block diagram of an optical device for the measurement of bilirubin. Arrows indicate direction of light flow.

necessary to measure this type of blood flow was expensive and not readily available. Yet, cerebral blood flow velocity changes, especially in the very immature neonate, with routine tasks of suctioning, blood draws from arterial lines, flushing of arterial lines, and repositioning of the infant in bed. These changes were observed during surfactant trials, in which considerable increase in cerebral blood flow occurred when the pulmonary and systemic vasculature opened up, potentially leading to intracranial hemorrhages.

Cerebral blood flow can be noninvasively monitored by Doppler flow velocity monitors such as the one by Hewlett Packard Sonos 1000, Waltham, MA. Measurements are usually taken with the neonate in a supine position. A pulsed Doppler flow velocity meter with a 7.5 MHz frequency and continuous multifrequency scanner with a 7.5-MHz shore focus probe is used. Noise from the movement of the blood in the vessel is filtered with a 100-Hz high-pass filter. The probe is positioned transcranially over the temporal bone to "catch" the vessel as it leaves the circle of Willis. Sagittal and coronal measurements are taken "through" the open fontanelle. Audio and visual signals are detectable and projected. Direct measurement can be obtained with an analog output system. These measurements include the systolic velocity, diastolic velocity, and integration of the area under the curve, which is considered to be a close approximation of the blood flow volume (Aziz et al., 1995). Aziz and colleagues used cerebral blood velocity measurements to follow up neurodevelopment in infants whose birth weights were 500 to 1249 g. Their belief was that this form of noninvasive monitoring could detect lesions or changes in cerebral blood flow that might indicate long-term neurodevelopmental difficulties. These types of studies offer new uses for high technology in follow-up outpatient care to identify infants at risk for developmental delays.

Doppler flow monitoring is also being used during infusions of some medications such as indomethacin (Hammerman et al., 1995). If infusion is rapid, indomethacin has the potential of decreasing cerebral blood flow while the patent ductus arteriosus is closed. Hammerman and associates (1995) compared cerebral blood flow changes in infants who received rapid versus continuous infusions of indomethacin. They found that during rapid infusions, cerebral blood flow was diminished, but this was not the case with continuous infusions. For further information on cerebral blood flow monitoring and diagnostic techniques, see Chapter 36, Diagnostic Imaging.

CONCLUSION

Although many different monitoring techniques are used in the management of the neonate, the physiologic basis for these monitors is not widely understood. This chapter has outlined the principles of transduction needed to understand neonatal biophysical monitoring. Because many treatment changes are based on the values obtained from monitoring devices, it is important for the health professional to know which factors may influence monitoring values and how to distinguish between artifact and actual physical changes in the neonate's status. The ability to make this distinction can be critical.

REFERENCES

Aziz, K., Vickar, D. B., Sauve, R. S., et al.(1995). Province-based study of neurologic disability of children weighing 500 through 1249 grams at birth in relation to neonatal cerebral ultrasound findings. *Pediatrics, 95*(6), 837–844.

Bhende, M. S., Karr, V. A., Wiltsie, D. C., & Orr, R. A. (1995). Evaluation of a portable infrared end-tidal carbon dioxide monitor during pediatric interhospital transport. *Pediatrics, 95*(6), 875–878.

Hammerman, C., Glaser, J., Schimmel, M. S., et al. (1995). Continuous versus multiple rapid infusions of indomethacin: Effects on cerebral blood flow velocity. *Pediatrics, 95*(2), 244–248.

Poets, C. F., Stebbens, V. A., Richard, D., & Southall, D. P. (1995). Prolonged episodes of hypoxemia in preterm infants undetectable by cardiorespiratory monitors. *Pediatrics* 95(6), 860–863.

SUGGESTED READINGS

Acree, C. M. (1990). *Comparison of the pulse oximeter to co-oximeter readings in preterm neonates with respiratory distress.* Unpublished master's thesis, University of Cincinnati, Cincinnati, OH.

Bohn, D. J. (1990). Pulse oximetry. In N. Nelson (Ed.), *Current therapy in neonatal-perinatal medicine* (No. 2, pp. 466–472). Philadelphia: B. C. Decker.

Bossi, E., Meister, B., & Pfenninger, J. (1987). Comparison between transcutaneous Po_2 and pulse oximetry for monitoring O_2-treatment in newborns. *Advances in Experimental Medicine and Biology, 20,* 171–176.

Burki, N. K., & Albert, R. K. (1983). Noninvasive monitoring of arterial blood gases. A report of the ACCP section on respiratory pathophysiology. *Chest, 83*(4), 666–670.

Cabel, L. A., Siassi, B., & Hodgmen, J. E. (1992). Neonatal clinical cardiopulmonary monitoring. In A. A. Fanaroff & R. J. Martin (Eds.), *Neonatal-perinatal medicine* (5th ed., pp. 437–455). St. Louis: C. V. Mosby.

Ciba Corning. (1989). *310 Pulse oximeter, technical literature on reflective pulse oximetry: Way ahead of the rest.* Medfield, MA: Ciba Corning Diagnostics Corp.

Comroe, J. H., & Botelho, S. (1947). The unreliability of cyanosis in the recognition of arterial anoxemia. *American Journal of the Medical Sciences, 214,* 1–6.

Coté, C., Goldstein, E. A., Coté, M. A., et al. (1988). A single-blind study of pulse oximetry in children. *Anesthesiology, 68*(2), 184–188.

Dear, P. R. (1987). Monitoring oxygen in the newborn: Saturation or partial pressure? *Archives of Disease in Childhood, 62*(9), 879–881.

Deckardt, R., & Steward, D. J. (1984). Noninvasive arterial hemoglobin oxygen saturation versus transcutaneous oxygen tension monitoring in the preterm infant. *Critical Care Medicine, 12*(11), 935–939.

Durand, M., & Ramanathan, R. (1986). Pulse oximetry for continuous oxygen monitoring in sick newborn infants. *Journal of Pediatrics, 109*(6), 1052–1056.

Fallenstein, F., Baeckert, P., & Huch, R. (1987). Comparison of in-vivo response times between pulse oximetry and transcutaneous Po_2 monitoring. *Advances in Experimental Medicine and Biology, 20,* 191–194.

Gunderson, L. P., & Berns, S. P. (1995). Embryology and development of the infant born at 24–25 weeks of gestation. In L. P. Gunderson & C. Kenner (Eds.), *Care of the 24–25 week gestational age infant: A small baby protocol* (2nd ed., pp. 1–22). Petaluma, CA: NICU Ink.

Gunderson, L. P., & Kenner, C. (1988). Transcutaneous oxygen monitoring: Description and clinical application. *Neonatal Network, 6*(6), 7–14.

Hay, W. W., Jr., Brockway, J., & Eyzaguirre, M. (1987). Application of the Ohmeda Biox 3700 pulse oximeter to neonatal oxygen monitoring. *Advances in Experimental Medicine and Biology, 20,* 151–158.

Hodgson, A., Horbar, J., Sharp, G., Soll, R., & Lucey, J. (1987). The accuracy of the pulse oximeter in neonates. *Advances in Experimental Medicine and Biology, 220,* 177–179.

House, J. T., Schultetus, R. R., & Gravenstein, N. (1987). Continuous neonatal evaluation in the delivery room by pulse oximetry. *Journal of Clinical Monitoring, 3*(2), 96–100.

Jennis, M. S., & Peabody, J. L. (1987). Pulse oximetry: An alternative method for the assessment of oxygenation in newborn infants. *Pediatrics, 79*(4), 524–528.

King, J. D., & Jung, A. L. (1990). Phototherapy. In N. Nelson (Ed.), *Current therapy in neonatal-perinatal medicine* (No. 2, pp. 461–464). Philadelphia: B. C. Decker.

Krauss, A. N., Waldman, S., Frayer, W. W., & Auld, P. A. M. (1978). Noninvasive estimation of arterial oxygenation in newborn infants. *Pediatrics, 93,* 275–278.

Peabody, J. L., & Emery, J. R. (1985). Noninvasive monitoring of blood gases in the newborn. *Clinics in Perinatology, 12*(1), 147–160.

Ramanathan, R., Durand, M., & Larrazabal, L. (1987). Pulse oximetry in very low birth weight infants with acute and chronic lung disease. *Pediatrics, 79*(4), 612–617.

Riedel, K. (1987). Pulse oximetry: A new technology to assess patient oxygen needs in the neonatal intensive care unit. *Journal of Perinatal and Neonatal Nursing, 1*(1), 49–57.

Severinghaus, J. W. (1987). History, status and future of pulse oximetry. *Advances in Experimental Medicine and Biology, 220,* 3–8.

Taeusch, H. W., Ballard, R. A., & Avery, M. E. (1991). *Schaffer & Avery's diseases of the newborn* (6th ed.). Philadelphia: W. B. Saunders.

Tremper, K. K. (1989). Pulse oximetry [Editorial]. *Chest, 95*(4), 713–715.

Vreman, H. J., Ronquillo, R. B., Ariagano, R. L., et al. (1988). Interference of fetal hemoglobin with the spectrophotometric measurement of carboxyhemoglobin. *Clinical Chemistry, 34*(5), 975–977.

Walsh, M. C., Noble, L. M., Carlo, W. A., & Martin, R. J. (1987). Relationship of pulse oximetry to arterial oxygen tension in infants. *Critical Care Medicine, 15*(12), 1102–1105.

CHAPTER 36

Diagnostic Imaging

CATHERINE JURSICH THEORELL

■ **RESEARCH AGENDA**

What are the effects of maternal magnetic resonance imaging done during pregnancy on neonatal hearing?

What are the long-term effects of ionizing radiation from a diagnostic radiograph on the neonate?

What are the effects of iodine-containing salts on neonatal kidneys?

Is there a significant change in a very low birth weight infant's core temperature when placed on the x-ray plate?

Diagnostic imaging has assumed an increasingly important role in neonatal diagnosis and the assessment, evaluation, and follow-up of neonatal care. The technologic advances since the 1970s have resulted in a variety of imaging modalities that demonstrate not only the internal structure but also the function of organ systems in the fetus and neonate. The spectrum of diagnostic imaging modalities includes radionuclide imaging, ultrasonography, and magnetic resonance imaging as well as conventional roentgenologic techniques. These many imaging modalities require complex, problem-oriented decision-making to determine which techniques should be used or omitted in any given clinical situation. In addition, these diagnostic imaging examinations are expensive, with ultrasonography being the least expensive and magnetic resonance imaging the most expensive. As the public, the government, private insurers, and health care providers have become increasingly more cost conscious, pressures have increased to make more efficacious and cost-effective decisions about the use of imaging examinations.

The selection of a particular imaging examination should be based on the inherent patient risks, the likelihood that the examination will establish or refute the diagnosis, the potential benefit to the patient, and the risk of liability if the examination is requested or if the examination is not requested (Haller & Slovis, 1984; Juhl & Crummy, 1993; Kirks, 1991; Squire & Novelline, 1988; Swischuk, 1989, 1995). When selecting an imaging examination, the clinician must carefully consider how much the examination will affect the certainty of the differential diagnosis and whether the information derived from the examination will alter the diagnostic approach or choice of treatment. Diagnostic certainty never reaches 100 percent. Because of the costs, imaging examinations with a low diagnostic yield or examinations that only duplicate information must be omitted. The acceptable level of compromise depends on the specific clinical problem, the type of imaging abnormality, and the experience of the radiologist. To minimize the risks and maximize the diagnostic benefit from any imaging examination, the diagnostic procedure must be tailored to the specific clinical problem under consideration. Thus, diagnostic approaches vary among radiologists and institutions (Gyll & Blake, 1986; Haller & Slovis, 1984; Hilton & Edwards, 1994; Kirks, 1991; Swischuk, 1989, 1995).

The roles of the nurse, neonatologist, nurse practitioner, and radiologist are critically interrelated in diagnostic imaging. It is essential that the history, clinical presentation, physical examination, and laboratory data are understood in order to select the imaging modalities that are indicated for the diagnostic evaluation and subsequent therapy for each neonate. After a diagnostic imaging examination has been ordered by the neonatologist or nurse practitioner, the radiologist evaluates whether the requested examination is indicated, what views should be obtained, what sequence of examinations is necessary, and whether contrast or supplementary examinations are required (Poznanski, 1976; Swischuk, 1989). Nurses should be aware of the rationale for the selection and sequencing of these diagnostic evaluations, the indications for various imaging modalities, the need for patient preparation, and the biophysical principles used in producing the image. The nurse ensures that the correct neonate undergoes the diagnostic imaging procedure, monitoring the neonate during and after the procedure, and reducing alterations to the thermal environment. The nurse may also be responsible for preparing information about the infant that is essential for the interpretation of these examinations. For example, the gestational, postnatal, and corrected gestational ages are important considerations when interpreting bone density, and the perinatal history is an important consideration when interpreting intracranial calcifications or hemorrhages. In addition, the nurse must often act as a liaison between the medical staff and the parents. The relationship that the nurse establishes with the family often provides an opportunity to inform the parents of the benefits and risks of the procedure as well as for the parents to express their questions and concerns. With a thorough understanding of these concepts, the nurse is able to coordinate the acquisition of diagnostic information with minimal disruption to patient care. Knowledge of patient preparation, proper positioning, and potential risks of each procedure is incorporated into the care plans and parent teaching. These plans of care and acknowledgment of risks facilitate the development of unit policies and procedures.

DIAGNOSTIC IMAGING IN INFANTS

The diagnostic imaging used for infants and newborns is unique, differing in several ways from that used for older children and adults. Infants and newborns are not just small adults for

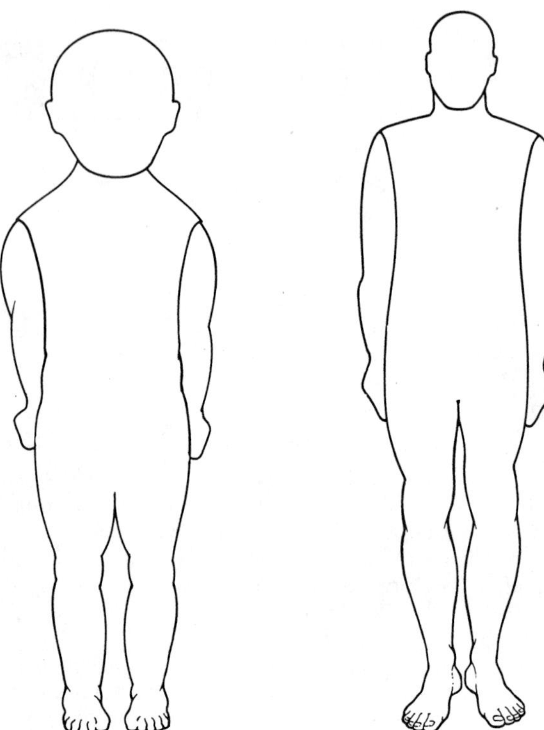

FIGURE 36–1. Proportional anatomic differences between a neonate and an adult.

whom smaller films and less exposure are all that is required. There are significant differences not just in size but also in the origin and imaging appearance of disease entities, anatomic proportions, exposure factors, radiation protection, and methods of immobilization (Gyll & Blake, 1986; Hilton and Edwards, 1994; Swischuk, 1989, 1995).

Conditions Requiring Diagnostic Imaging

Pathologic conditions commonly encountered in adults are often not found in infants, and many abnormal conditions are exclusive to the newborn period. Examples of these pathologic conditions are the congenital abnormalities of the newborn, such as atresias of the gastrointestinal (GI) tract, severe congenital heart defects, surgical causes of respiratory distress, spina bifida, and bilateral choanal atresia. These lesions are lethal if left untreated and are often symptomatic in the first days of life. Medical problems related to premature and postmature birth, intrauterine growth disturbances, nonlethal developmental defects, genetic abnormalities, and perinatal asphyxia are of greatest concern in the newborn period. In addition, malignant tumors, such as neuroblastoma and Wilms' tumor, may appear in the newborn period and up to approximately 4 years of age. Lastly, certain infections, such as cytomegalovirus, toxoplasmosis, and syphilis, have a distinct radiographic and ultrasonic presentation if the exposure occurred in utero rather than in the neonatal period (Fanaroff & Martin, 1997; Gyll & Blake, 1986; Haller & Slovis, 1984; Hilton & Edwards, 1994; Kirks, 1991; Swischuk, 1989, 1995).

Anatomic Proportions

The anatomic proportions of infants are very different from those of the adult, and the younger the infant, the more marked the differences. A thorough knowledge of these proportions is essential for accurate patient positioning for field exposure limitation and interpretation of diagnostic imaging (Gyll & Blake, 1986; Hilton & Edwards, 1994). It is important that only the area in question and the whole of it appear in the imaging field.

Figure 36–1 shows that the neonate's head is large in proportion to the body, and the cranial vault is large in proportion to the area of the face. The neck is short and the diaphragm is high. The kidneys are low, about midway between the diaphragm and symphysis pubis. The abdomen is large because of the relative size of the liver and stomach. The pelvic cavity is very small, and the bladder extends above the symphysis pubis. The chest, pelvis, and limbs are small in proportion to the abdomen (Gyll, 1985; Hilton & Edwards, 1994; Poznanski, 1976; Swischuk, 1989, 1995; Vogler et al., 1986).

In an anteroposterior (AP) projection, the neonate's lungs appear wider than they are long and much higher up in the thoracic cavity than is normally expected (Hilton & Edwards, 1994; Swischuk, 1989, 1995; Vogler et al., 1986; Wesenberg, 1973). The diaphragm is located just below the level of the nipples. On a lateral projection, the posterior aspect of the lungs may extend to twice the depth of the anterior part (Gyll & Blake, 1986; Swischuk, 1989, 1995).

The neonate's abdomen bulges laterally wider than the pelvis,

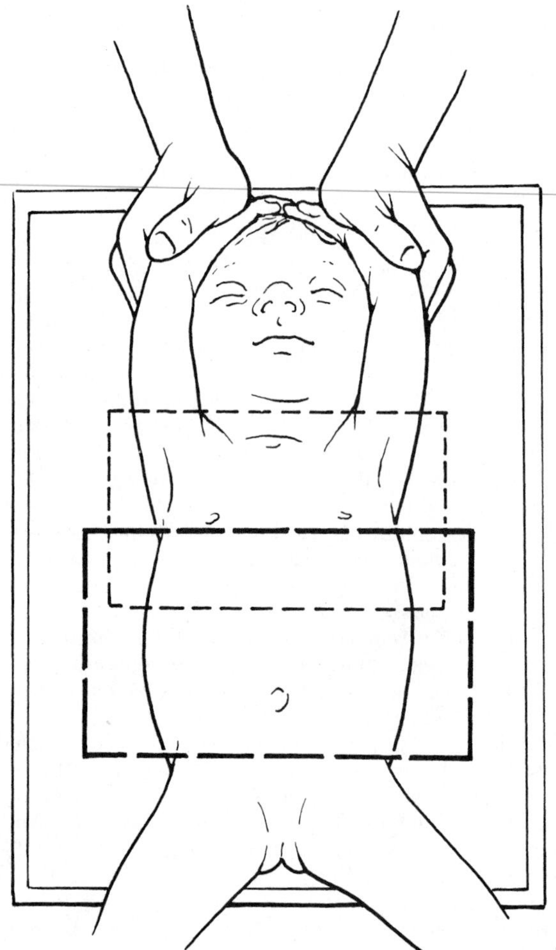

FIGURE 36–2. Neonatal radiographs should be limited to only the area of interest. Total body radiographs should be avoided. The top box (*light dashed lines*) defines the area of interest for an anteroposterior chest radiograph. Bottom box (*heavy dashed lines*) defines the area of interest for an anteroposterior abdominal film. Gonad shield has been omitted for illustrative purposes.

and the bulge contains abdominal organs displaced by the large liver and stomach. Care must be taken to include this area of the abdomen in the imaging field (Gyll, 1985; Hilton & Edwards, 1994; Poznanski, 1976; Swischuk, 1989, 1995). The smallest possible body area should be irradiated, consistent with producing the necessary information. Often, the field is too large, particularly in premature infants and newborns. Arms and legs should not appear on the abdominal film, nor should half the skull and abdomen appear on a chest film (Fig. 36–2) (Fanaroff & Martin, 1997; Gyll & Blake, 1986; Hilton & Edwards, 1994; Kirks, 1991; Swischuk, 1989, 1995).

TYPES OF DIAGNOSTIC IMAGING

Diagnostic imaging methods are limited to the demonstration of pathologic features no smaller than a few millimeters in diameter, whereas biochemical and histologic methods document disease at a molecular or cellular level. It is commonly thought that diagnostic imaging provides only anatomic information; however, a significant amount of physiologic data may be derived from studies such as barium examinations or urography, as well as from dynamic radionuclide and ultrasonographic imaging. There are four major types of diagnostic imaging modalities: x-ray (roentgenologic) imaging, radionuclide imaging, ultrasonographic imaging, and magnetic resonance imaging (Bushong, 1992; Juhl & Crummy, 1993; Horowitz, 1995; Treves, 1995). This chapter discusses each of these imaging modalities in relation to the biophysical principles responsible for producing the image, the potential risks of the procedure, and the nursing care of the neonate undergoing such an examination.

X-Ray Imaging (Roentgenology)

The principles of conventional radiography have not changed since the discovery of x-rays in the late 1800s. However, the equipment and techniques have become far more sophisticated and include tomography, fluoroscopy, computed tomography (CT), and digital radiography.

X-rays are one form of electromagnetic energy that travels at the speed of light (3×10^8 m/second, or 6.7×10^8 miles/hour). Other forms of electromagnetic energy include gamma rays, radio waves, microwaves, and visible light (Fig. 36–3). Only x-rays and gamma rays have enough energy to produce an ion pair by separating an orbital electron from its parent atom (Alpen, 1990; Bushong, 1992; Juhl & Crummy, 1993; Kelsey, 1985; Squire & Novelline, 1988). The amount of radiation present is measured by detecting such ionization. Radiation exposure is measured either in units of coulombs per kilogram (C/kg) or in roentgens (1 R = 258 μC/kg). Although the roentgen is no longer an official scientific unit, it is still widely used in radiology. The amount of radiation absorbed by the body is measured in rads (Alpen, 1990; Bushong, 1992; Gofman, 1983; Juhl & Crummy, 1993; Kelsey, 1985; Noz & Maguire, 1985).

When an x-ray beam is directed toward a part of the body, there is differential absorption of the x-ray photons by different types of

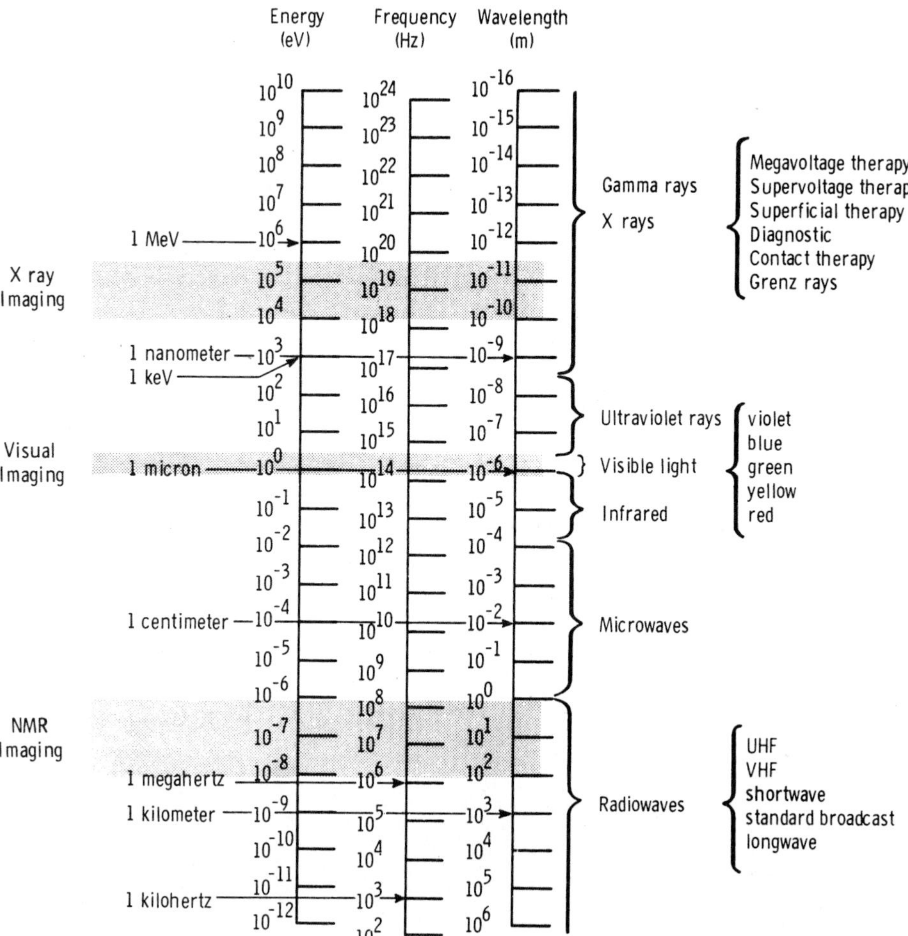

FIGURE 36–3. The electromagnetic spectrum extends over 25 orders of magnitude. This chart illustrates the values of frequency, energy, and wavelength and identifies some common regions of the spectrum. (From Bushong, S. C. [1984]. *Radiologic science for technologists* [3rd ed., p. 58.] St. Louis: C. V. Mosby. Reprinted with permission.)

body tissue. A beam of x-ray photons is variously attenuated as it passes through the body tissues to produce a shadow image that is recorded on photographic film, while the absorbed x-ray photons interact with the tissue, causing ionization within the body (Alpen, 1990; Bushong, 1992; Gofman, 1983; Juhl & Crummy, 1993). Bone and metal fragments absorb x-ray photons and therefore appear white, whereas air-containing structures such as lung and bowel gas absorb few x-ray photons and appear black. Soft tissues and blood vessels appear as intermediate shades of gray.

A radiograph gives a two-dimensional projection of three-dimensional structures. An x-ray tube is positioned to direct the x-ray beam through the part of the neonate to be examined, so as to record different views or projections on the film. Although this type of imaging modality can distinguish between only air, fat, and tissues having densities approximately equal to those of water or metals, this simple technique continues to be enormously valuable and is still the most commonly used diagnostic imaging method in neonatal care.

X-ray photons are generated in the tungsten anode of the tube when it is bombarded by a stream of high-energy electrons emitted from the cathode (Fig. 36–4) (Alpen, 1990; Bushong, 1992; Juhl & Crummy, 1993; Kelsey, 1985). The energy, or penetrating power, of the resulting x-ray photons is a function of the electron energy, which is controlled by the voltage gradient across the cathode–anode gap. In diagnostic radiology, this is usually between 60 and 120 kilovolts (kV) (Hilton & Edwards, 1994; Juhl & Crummy, 1993; Kelsey, 1985; Squire & Novelline, 1988). Low-kilovoltage x-rays have poor penetrating ability, whereas higher kilovoltage x-rays have deeper penetrating ability. Thus, the kilovoltage across the cathode–anode gap controls the penetration of the x-ray beam.

The milliamperage (mA) indicates the amount of current applied to the cathode filament (Alpen, 1990; Bushong, 1992; Kelsey, 1985). The greater the current, the more electrons are produced for transmission across the cathode–anode gap, and the greater the number of x-ray photons generated by the anode in a finite time. The product of the exposure time and the milliamperage given to the cathode filament controls the amount, or dose, of x-rays and is expressed in milliampere-seconds (mAs) (Alpen, 1990; Bushong, 1992; Juhl & Crummy, 1993; Kelsey, 1985; Shapiro, 1990).

Early radiographs required exposure times of as long as 30 minutes to produce a satisfactory image (Bushong, 1992; Gofman, 1983; Juhl & Crummy, 1993). It is not surprising then to find reports of radiation injury in the early days of radiology (Gofman, 1983; Kelsey, 1985). Reports of superficial skin and tissue damage, hair loss, and anemia were common among the patients as well as their physicians because of the prolonged exposure times and the low-energy radiation that was available. The development of an interrupterless transformer by H. C. Snook in 1907 and progressive improvements in the development of the cathode ray tube resulted in a marked decrease in the reports of radiation injury (Gofman, 1983; Kelsey, 1985; Noz & Maguire, 1985). Since that time, continued improvements in film sensitivity and fluorescent screens have further reduced exposure times, so that the average exposure time for a chest radiograph is approximately one twentieth of a second (Alpen, 1990; Juhl & Crummy, 1993; Kelsey, 1985). The short exposure time reduces image blurring caused by involuntary and cardiovascular motion and decreases the radiation exposure to the neonate. It is also important to limit the cross-sectional area of the x-ray beam to the region of interest to reduce unnecessary radiation to adjacent organs (Alpen, 1990; Bushong, 1992; Gofman, 1983; Gyll, 1985; Juhl & Crummy, 1993; Kelsey, 1985; Shapiro, 1990; Squire & Novelline, 1988).

The common method of recording conventional radiographic images is with large-size photographic film that is enclosed within an aluminum or plastic light-proof cassette. The film is compressed between fluorescent screens that emit visible light when exposed to x-rays. It is the fluorescence from the phosphor screens rather than the direct effect of x-ray upon the photo-

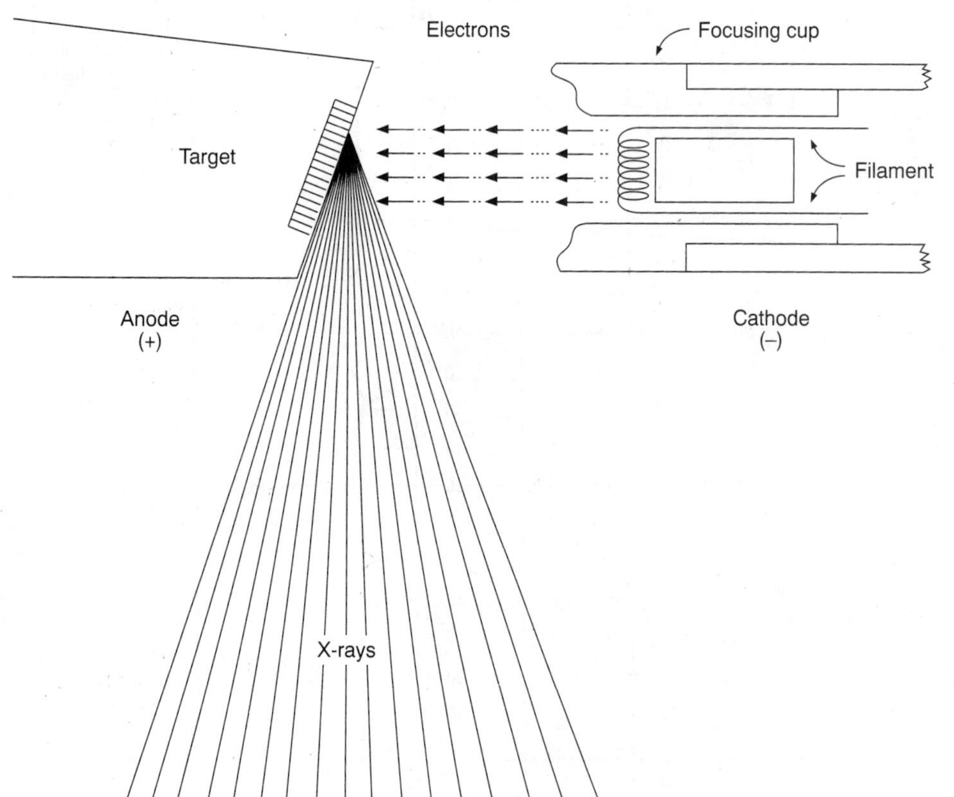

FIGURE 36–4. The generation of x-ray photons in a tungsten anode–cathode tube.

graphic emulsion that produces most of the image on the film (Alpen, 1990; Bushong, 1992; Juhl & Crummy, 1993; Kelsey, 1985). In addition to conventional film radiography, other diagnostic imaging methods use ionizing radiation as well.

Other Radiographic Imaging Techniques

Xeroradiography

Xeroradiography is a radiographic imaging technique used to evaluate soft tissue. In this technique, the electrical charge of a photoconductive plate is altered in proportion to the intensity of the transmitted radiation image (Alpen, 1990; Bushong, 1992; Juhl & Crummy, 1993; Kelsey, 1985). The image is recorded on this plate rather than on x-ray film. This modality provides much better contrast than conventional radiography for soft tissue structures that differ only slightly in density. It also provides an "edge effect" at the margins of discontinuous structures and therefore is indicated for detection of nonmetallic foreign bodies and for evaluation of complex upper airway abnormalities in the neonate (Juhl & Crummy, 1993; Kelsey, 1985; Swischuk, 1995). Despite these benefits, the risks associated with this imaging technique must be considered. The radiation exposure is 6 to 12 times greater than that of conventional radiographs (Alpen, 1990; Juhl & Crummy, 1993; Kelsey, 1985; Kirks, 1991; Poznanski, 1976; Swischuk, 1995; Whalen & Balter, 1984).

Fluoroscopic Imaging

The fluoroscope was developed in 1898 by Thomas Edison (Bushong, 1992). His work focused on the use of fluorescent materials in this new imaging modality. During the period of his investigation, Edison analyzed the fluorescent properties of more than 1800 materials, including zinc cadmium sulfide and calcium tungstate, both of which are still used. Edison halted his research in this area when his assistant and long-time friend, Clarence Dally, suffered severe x-ray burns that required bilateral upper extremity amputation. Clarence Dally's subsequent death in 1904 is considered the first x-ray fatality (Bushong, 1992; Juhl & Crummy, 1993).

Fluoroscopic imaging is a radiologic technique used to evaluate the motion of an organ system. After passing through the patient, the fluoroscopic x-rays interact with the input phosphor of the image-intensifier tube. The input phosphor converts the incident x-rays into visible light, which causes the photocathode to emit electrons (Alpen, 1990; Bushong, 1992; Juhl & Crummy, 1993; Kelsey, 1985; Squire & Novelline, 1988). These electrons are accelerated and focused by electrodes within the image intensifier onto the output phosphor to produce visible light that can be viewed directly through an optical system or by a television system (Bushong, 1992; Kelsey, 1985; Squire & Novelline, 1988). Fluoroscopic images can be recorded either on film or on videotape. Videotape recording of fluoroscopy has become essential. It is easier and safer to rerun a videotape several times to evaluate dysfunction rather than to prolong the radiation exposure from fluoroscopy.

During a fluoroscopic examination, the anatomic structure may be evaluated by obtaining a spot film by photographing the output phosphor on 100-mm or 105-mm film. This type of intensifier optical-coupled spot-film camera decreases the radiation dose to the infant by at least 75 percent when compared with a conventional spot-film device (Juhl & Crummy, 1993; Kelsey, 1985; National Council on Radiation Protection [NCRP], 1993a, 1993b, 1993c; Noz & Maguire, 1985). Videotapes are used to record motions, and spot films are used to document anatomy. Although fluoroscopy has many advantages, the radiation dose of 1 minute of fluoroscopy is equivalent to the dose in more than thirty 105-mm spot films or more than eight conventional radiographs (Aplen, 1990; Gofman, 1983; NCRP, 1993a, 1993b, 1993c; Noz & Maguire, 1985; Shapiro, 1990; Squire & Novelline, 1988; Whalen & Balter, 1984).

Electronic intensification of the faint fluoroscopic image allows fluoroscopy to be performed in subdued lighting. Improved intensifier systems have made invasive catheter studies such as cardiac angiography much easier to perform (Kelsey, 1985; Kirks, 1991; Moss et al., 1984).

Fluoroscopically guided cytologic biopsy of the lung, bone, pancreas, and lymph nodes has become possible with percutaneous needle insertion. Embolization of arteriovenous malformations may be performed, arterial stenoses may be dilated with balloon catheters, and plastic stents can be inserted to provide drainage through biliary strictures under fluoroscopy (Hilton & Edwards, 1994; Moss et al., 1984). Although these surgical-radiologic procedures apply to a relatively small proportion of neonates, all procedures require cooperation between the neonatal, surgical, and radiologic teams to achieve the best results and are dependent on high-quality image intensification.

Conventional X-Ray Tomography

Tomography is a radiologic method of imaging a slice of tissue at a specific level. A coordinated movement of the x-ray tube and film cassette gives a defined image in the two-dimensional plane of interest, whereas the structures in front of or behind this plane are blurred out (Alpen, 1990; Juhl & Crummy, 1993; Kelsey, 1985; Kirks, 1991). Tomography is useful in many circumstances, but its usefulness has been overshadowed by the development of computed tomography (CT).

Computed Tomography

CT was first developed in 1961 by Oldendorf and, by 1973, became a recognized diagnostic imaging tool. CT scanning obtains cross-sectional images rather than the shadow images of conventional radiography. Conventional radiography is based on variable attenuation of the x-ray beam as it passes through tissue. Only the sum total of this attenuation is available for recording on the film, so that conventional radiography can only detect differences of 10 percent attenuation (Juhl & Crummy, 1993; Kelsey, 1985; Moss et al., 1984). Thus, detailed characterization of various soft tissue densities cannot be made by conventional radiographs. The densities that can be visualized on conventional radiographs are air, fat, soft tissue, and bone. CT passes multiple, highly collimated beams through the same cross-sectional slice of tissue at different angles during different intervals of time. In CT scanning, a fan x-ray beam from a source rotating about the infant passes through the body, and the exit transmission of x-ray beam intensity is monitored by a series of detectors (Alpen, 1990; Bushong, 1992; Kelsey, 1985; Kirks, 1991). The x-ray beam "cuts a slice" from 3 to 13 mm thick through the infant. The exit transmission at any angle can be used to calculate the average attenuation coefficient along the length of the x-ray beam. By measuring the exit transmission at a large number of angles around the infant, a complex series of mathematical equations can be solved by computer to calculate and determine the mass attenuation coefficient of small (approximately 0.5 mm × 0.5 mm × 10 mm) volume elements or voxels. The final cross-sectional image is then made up of a display of the gray scale value of every voxel, which can be projected on a cathode-ray tube and recorded photographically (Alpen, 1990; Bushong, 1992; Juhl & Crummy, 1993; Kelsey, 1985; Moss et al., 1984). Bone is the most dense, absorbs the largest amount of x-rays, and appears white; air is the least dense and appears black; soft tissues are displayed as intermediate shades of gray. CT scanning has the ability to separate spatial and contrast resolution and is much more sensitive to tissue densities than conventional radiographs. CT can distinguish differences in attenuation coefficients as small as 0.1 percent, detects changes in density in very small areas of tissue, and permits identification of various components of soft tissue such as subarachnoid space, white matter, gray matter, and ventricles (Alpen, 1990; Bushong, 1992; Juhl & Crummy, 1993; Kelsey, 1985; Moss et al., 1984; Squire & Novelline, 1988). CT of the body is technically more difficult than cranial examination because of cardiac and respiratory motion; however, a modern body scanner can complete a scan in 2 to 4 seconds, which decreases movement artifact. In the neonate, the rapid heart rate and respiratory rate limit the usefulness of this technique for thoracic examination.

In CT, the density, or contrast resolution, depends on radiation dose and scan time (Alpen, 1990; Bushong, 1992; Juhl & Crummy, 1993; Kelsey, 1985). As the radiation dose (i.e., scan time) increases, the number of photons collected in each area increases and the statistical noise decreases, resulting in better contrast resolution. CT demonstrates tissue structure with precise clarity, showing superior anatomic detail as compared with conventional radiographic imaging (Alpen, 1990; Juhl & Crummy, 1993; Kelsey, 1985; Kirks, 1991; Moss et al., 1984). CT permits two-dimensional visualization of entire anatomic sections of tissue to help determine the extent of the disease or malformation. Anatomic and physiologic information can be visualized despite overlying gas and bone. Contrast enhancement can measure blood flow and help define pathologic abnormalities (Moss et al., 1984; Squire & Novelline, 1988; Swischuk, 1989, 1995). Bolus injection of contrast material permits excellent visualization of vascular structures.

As good as CT is as an imaging modality, it is still not a radiologic microscope. CT does have its drawbacks. It also uses ionizing radiation, and, because the computers require a cool room for proper equipment performance, there is a significant alteration in the neonate's environment, which must be considered.

Digital Radiography and Digital Vascular Imaging

Digital radiography is the term used to describe those techniques that use computers to produce projectional images similar to those of conventional radiography (Kelsey, 1985; Kirks, 1991). Although standard CT instruments have been designed to produce two-dimensional images of two-dimensional body slices, they can also be used to project three-dimensional structures into two-dimensional images that are similar to conventional radiographs. These projections do not have the fine detail of conventional radiographs, but, because the pictorial data are stored in the computer, it is possible to manipulate the image and enhance subtle features (Bushong, 1992; Kelsey, 1985; Squire & Novelline, 1988).

Another method of digital radiography converts the image intensifier picture to digital signals that can be stored and manipulated. The most important use of this method is to obtain digital subtraction images of the heart and major arteries from data recorded before and after the injection of angiographic contrast material (Bushong, 1992; Kelsey, 1985; Squire & Novelline, 1988). This method is much less invasive than catheterization, although the technique is new and the equipment is expensive. It has been used on a very limited basis in the neonate.

Radiographic Contrast Agents

Plain radiography can differentiate only four kinds of body tissue: tissue containing gas (lung and bowel), fatty tissue, tissue containing calcium (bone or pathologic calcifications), and tissues of water density (solid organs, muscle, and blood). To demonstrate blood vessels within solid organs or surrounded by muscle or to demonstrate other hollow structures, it is necessary to introduce artificial radiographic contrast agents. The contrast medium may be negative or positive and may be injected, swallowed, or administered as enemas (Gyll & Blake, 1986; Haller & Slovis, 1984; Hilton & Edwards, 1994; Squire & Novelline, 1988; Swischuk, 1989, 1995).

Negative contrast media absorb less radiation than adjacent soft tissues and so cast a darker radiographic image. Gases such as air, oxygen, and carbon dioxide can be used as negative contrast media. The amount of contrast provided by negative media for conventional radiography is limited and is not readily used (Fanaroff & Martin, 1997; Kirks, 1991; Swischuk, 1989, 1995).

Positive contrast media use elements with a high atomic number, which absorb much more radiation than surrounding soft tissues and therefore cast a lighter image. Barium and iodine are the two elements that are currently used. Barium sulfate is a relatively stable, nontoxic compound that is the major contrast agent used for outlining the walls of the GI tract. Iodine-containing salts that are excreted by the kidneys are used for a wide variety of urographic and angiographic studies. Newer non-ionic iodine-containing media are also excreted by the kidneys. These newer agents are less painful than iodine-containing salts when injected into arteries because of their lower osmolality, and they are rapidly being used in place of the older contrast agents (Table 36–1) (Fanaroff & Martin, 1997; Gyll & Blake, 1986; Haller & Slovis, 1984; Hilton & Edwards, 1994; Kirks, 1991; Swischuk, 1989, 1995).

Ionizing Radiation Interactions With Tissue

When an infant undergoes a radiologic procedure, most of the radiation passes through the infant's body and strikes the fluorescent screens encompassing the film. The roentgen (or C/kg) is a measure of how many x-rays were present. For the infant, the more important quantity is the number of x-rays that stop in the body and how much energy is deposited by those x-rays. The radiation dose (rads) is a measure of the energy deposited. X-rays that pass through the infant are attenuated by photoelectric absorption and Compton scattering (Alpen, 1990; Bushong, 1992; Juhl & Crummy, 1993; Kelsey, 1985; Shapiro, 1990).

Photoelectric absorption involves the complete interaction and

TABLE 36–1 Radiopharmaceuticals Used in Neonatal Diagnostic Imaging

Technetium 99m: sulfur or tin colloid
Used for imaging liver, spleen, bone marrow, ventilation, gastrointestinal bleeds
Technetium 99m: albumin microspheres
Used for imaging lung perfusion
Technetium 99m: pyrophosphate, diphosphate
Used for imaging skeletal and myocardial infarcts
Technetium 99m: pertechnetate
Used for imaging thyroid, brain, and gastrointestinal tract
Technetium 99m: DTPA glucoheptonate
Used for imaging kidney and brain
Technetium 99m: HIDA or PG
Used for imaging the biliary system
Iodine 131
Used for imaging thyroid, fibrinogen, clot localization
Xenon 131, Krypton 81m
Used for imaging lung ventilation
Thallium 201
Used to image myocardial perfusion and testicular localization

absorption of the incoming x-ray photon by the atom. The photon energy is transferred to one of the orbital electrons, which is then ejected as a photoelectron (Alpen, 1990; Kelsey, 1985; Shapiro, 1990). The ejected electron leaves a vacancy in one of the inner orbits, and this vacancy is immediately filled by an outer orbit electron. The difference in binding energies between the outer orbit and the inner orbit is released as a characteristic x-ray (Alpen, 1990; Bushong, 1992; Gofman, 1983; Juhl & Crummy, 1993; Kelsey, 1985; Shapiro, 1990; Squire & Novelline, 1988). The attenuation of the photoelectric effect is dependent on the atomic number of the material and the amount of incoming energy. The photoelectric interaction decreases rapidly with increasing energy and increases rapidly with increasing atomic number (Alpen, 1990; Bushong, 1992; Kelsey, 1985; Shapiro, 1990). This is why lead is such an effective shield and why bone has so much more absorption than soft tissue.

In Compton scattering, only part of the energy of the incoming x-ray photon is transferred to the atom, which reduces the energy of the original photon and produces a scattered electron (Kelsey, 1985; Shapiro, 1990). The scattered electron has a range of less than 1 mm in tissue. The reduced-energy x-ray photon can do exactly what the original x-ray photon could do. It can interact with another atom, causing a photoelectric effect and transferring all its energy to set an electron in motion, or it can itself undergo the Compton effect, scattering an electron and creating a new x-ray photon whose energy is still further reduced (Alpen, 1990; Bushong, 1992; Gofman, 1983; Juhl & Crummy, 1993; Kelsey, 1985; Shapiro, 1990; Squire & Novelline, 1988). Through these two processes, all the energy is eventually transferred to electrons to set them into high-velocity motion. At low photon energies (less than 60 kV), photoelectric interactions predominate. At approximately 140 kV, the photoelectric and Compton interactions transfer equal energy to tissue; at more than approximately 200 kV, most of the energy transfer to tissue is through the Compton interaction (Alpen, 1990; Bushong, 1992; Kelsey, 1985; Shapiro, 1990; Swischuk, 1989). Most diagnostic radiographs in the neonate use photon energies between 60 and 100 kV (Fanaroff & Martin, 1997; Gyll & Blake, 1986; Hilton & Edwards, 1994; Kirks, 1984; Poznanski, 1976; Swischuk, 1989, 1995).

X-ray photons with energies greater than 1.02 meV cause both a photoelectric effect and Compton effect and have an additional capability as well. In the vicinity of the atom, the incoming x-ray photons disappear and, in the process, create new matter in the form of one electron and one positron (Alpen, 1990; Bushong, 1992; Kelsey, 1985; Shapiro, 1990; Squire & Novelline, 1988; Whalen & Balter, 1984). A positron is a particle of the same size and mass as an electron, but the positron has one unit of positive charge. To create this pair, exactly 1.02 meV of energy is consumed in the conversion of energy into matter. If the incoming x-ray photon has more energy than 1.02 meV, the residual energy is distributed equally to the electron and the positron in the form of kinetic energy (Alpen, 1990; Gofman, 1983; Shapiro, 1990).

The effects of the electron when placed in high-velocity orbit are the same as previously described for the photoelectric and Compton effects. The positron effects are different. The positron expends some of its energy interacting with atoms of the material in which it has been set in motion. Eventually, it meets an electron, and the two annihilate each other. When this occurs, both the electron and the positron disappear and two gamma rays appear, each with 0.51 meV of energy (Alpen, 1990; Bushong, 1992; Juhl & Crummy, 1993; NCRP, 1993a, 1993b, 1993c; Noz & Maguire, 1985; Shapiro, 1990).

With ionizing radiation, electrons are removed from their atoms and endowed with energies 14 to 20,000 times greater as compared with those in ordinary biochemical reactions (Alpen, 1990; Bushong, 1992; Gofman, 1983; Kelsey, 1985; Noz & Maguire, 1985). As compared with biochemical reactions, such electrons maraud through tissue for some distance and have the capability to break any kind of chemical bond in the body (Gofman, 1983; NCRP, 1993a, 1993b, 1993c; Noz & Maguire, 1985; Shapiro, 1990). In biochemical systems, the reactions are carefully controlled, often by special geometric juxtaposition of the reactants. A high-speed electron is akin to a bull in a china shop—it can break anything, anywhere. Once it has ripped an electron out of an atom in a molecule, the molecule itself is placed at such a high energy level that it can produce all kinds of chemical reactions that would never have been possible without ionizing radiation (Alpen, 1990; Gofman, 1983; NCRP, 1993a, 1993b, 1993c; Shapiro, 1990).

X-rays and gamma rays are identical in nature, except that, in general, x-rays are made in high-voltage machines, whereas gamma rays originate from the nuclei of atoms. Radiations emitted from such naturally unstable atoms as uranium are commonly more energetic per unit than x-ray photons. For example, gamma rays are commonly measured in the millions of eV per photon (meV), whereas x-rays are commonly measured in 50 to 100 keV (50,000 to 100,000 eV) (Gofman, 1983). Gamma rays from unstable nuclei do all of the things that x-rays do, that is, they can undergo photoelectric effect and Compton effect, and they can produce high-energy electrons and positrons.

There are also other radiation decay products that create particulate radiation called alpha and beta rays. Beta rays are not truly rays but high-speed electrons emitted from the nuclei of decay products of uranium (Alpen, 1990; Cowan, 1959). Once emitted from the nuclei, beta particles act identically to any high-speed electron. Alpha rays are also not rays and are unlike beta particles. Alpha particles are emitted from the nuclei of uranium. Alpha particles are the "stripped" nuclei of helium and consist of any two protons. Ultimately, these two protons find two electrons in the environment and become helium gas. Most beta particles have energies in the million eV range, although they are always accompanied by beta particles of lesser energies ranging down to nearly zero. Alpha particles, however, have energies in the 5 million eV range (Alpen, 1990; Gofman, 1983). X-rays and gamma rays, which pass through the body and do not produce effects with tissue, have no biologic effect. However, alpha and beta particles interact at every millimeter along their path through tissue, so that, if they gain access to tissue, biologic harm is guaranteed (Gofman, 1983; NCRP, 1993a, 1993b, 1993c; Noz & Maguire, 1985; Shapiro, 1990).

Biologic damage from ionizing radiation depends on the quantity of energy that is deposited in a particular tissue. X-rays and gamma rays produce harmful effects only to the extent that they place high-speed electrons in motion. If the same number of electrons are placed in motion by gamma rays from plutonium or from deposited radionuclide, or by agents from external x-rays, the biologic effects are the same (NCRP, 1993a, 1993b, 1993c).

Factors Affecting Radiograph Quality

Interpretation of a neonatal radiograph requires a rapid evaluation to determine whether the radiograph is technically satisfactory. There are several factors that determine technical quality of a radiograph, including film exposure, phase of respiration, motion, tube angulation, and infant positioning. If one of these factors is unsatisfactory, there may be misinterpretation of the film. Understanding of these factors by the nurse results in improved technical quality of radiographs.

A reasonable criterion to judge film exposure is satisfactory visualization of the dorsal intervertebral disk spaces through the entire cardiothymic silhouette (Fanaroff & Martin, 1997; Gyll, 1985; Hilton & Edwards, 1994; Kirks, 1991; Poznanski, 1976; Wesenberg, 1973). An underexposed film results in a loss of the dorsal disk spaces and in the lungs and other structures having a homogeneous "whitewashed" appearance. An overexposed film results in a progressive loss of pulmonary vascular markings, until the lungs have a black, "burned out" appearance (Hilton & Edwards, 1994; Swischuk, 1989, 1995; Wesenberg, 1973).

The phase of respiration at the time that the film was obtained has considerable influence on the appearance of the radiograph (Fig. 36–5). An expiratory film may show that the heart appears grossly enlarged and the lung fields appear opaque, which may simulate diffuse atelectasis, and the diaphragm is located above the seventh rib (Gyll, 1985; Hilton & Edwards, 1994; Kirks, 1991; Swischuk, 1995; Wesenberg, 1973).

Inspiratory films show the diaphragm at the eighth rib, normal cardiothymic diameter, and prominent pulmonary vascularity. The right hemidiaphragm is slightly higher than the left. If the right hemidiaphragm is at or above the level of seventh rib, the film is in an expiratory phase or the infant has hypoaeration (Gyll, 1985; Hilton & Edwards, 1994; Kirks, 1991; Swischuk, 1995; Wesenberg, 1973).

If the infant moves just as the radiograph is being made, the resulting film is blurred. Motion causes blurring of the hemidiaphragms, the cardiovascular silhouette, and all fine pulmonary detail (Hilton & Edwards, 1994; Swischuk, 1989, 1995; Wesenberg, 1973). The avoidance of movement blur on diagnostic images is achieved in one of two ways: fast imaging and adequate immobilization.

Speed

Short exposure times are essential for obtaining clear images. This can be achieved by limiting the time of exposure to the energy source and increasing use of computerized imaging.

Immobilization

The nursing staff is primarily responsible for ensuring adequate immobilization during diagnostic imaging. Inadequate immobilization is an important cause for poor quality of neonatal images. Proper immobilization techniques improve image quality, decrease length of the examination, and eliminate the need for repeat studies (Gyll & Blake, 1986; Hilton & Edwards, 1994; Kirks, 1991; Swischuk, 1989, 1995). Proper immobilization may be less traumatic than manual restraint alone. An immobilization board may be required, or tape, foam rubber blocks and wedges, towels, diapers, or clear plastic acetate sheets may be used (Gyll & Blake, 1986).

There are physical risks to neonates associated with immobilization. Trauma may occur as a result of restraint or use of an ill-designed immobilization device. Tape or plastic sheets may cause skin and soft tissue damage if not carefully applied and removed. In addition, there may be thermal stress encountered when placing a neonate on a noninsulated board or film cassette. The nurse should position and immobilize the infant properly so that the technician can center the tube, position the beam, and make the exposure. With the nurse and the technician working together, superior results are achieved with greater speed and less disruption than if they worked separately.

Infants lie still only when they are very ill. Otherwise, they greatly resent being forcibly restrained, especially in an unusual position. There are a number of immobilization devices available, but the best method of immobilization is using a pair of adequately protected adult hands (Gyll, 1985; Haller & Slovis, 1984; Hilton & Edwards, 1994; Kirks, 1991; Swischuk, 1989, 1995).

Another factor that affects radiographic quality is x-ray tube angulation and improper field limitation. Often, neonatal chest films appear mildly lordotic, with the medial clavicular ends projected on or above the dorsal vertebrae. This results in a rather peculiar chest configuration. The preossified anterior arcs of the upper ribs have a position that is superior to the posterior arcs (Fig. 36–6). The lordotic projection tends to increase the apparent transverse cardiac diameter, making it difficult to determine heart size. Lordotic projections result from the x-ray tube being angled cephalad, centering the x-ray beam over the abdomen, or from an irritable infant whose back is arched at the time of the film exposure (Gyll & Blake, 1986; Hilton & Edwards, 1994; Kirks, 1991; Swischuk, 1989, 1995; Wesenberg, 1973). Caudad angulation or centering the x-ray beam over the head results

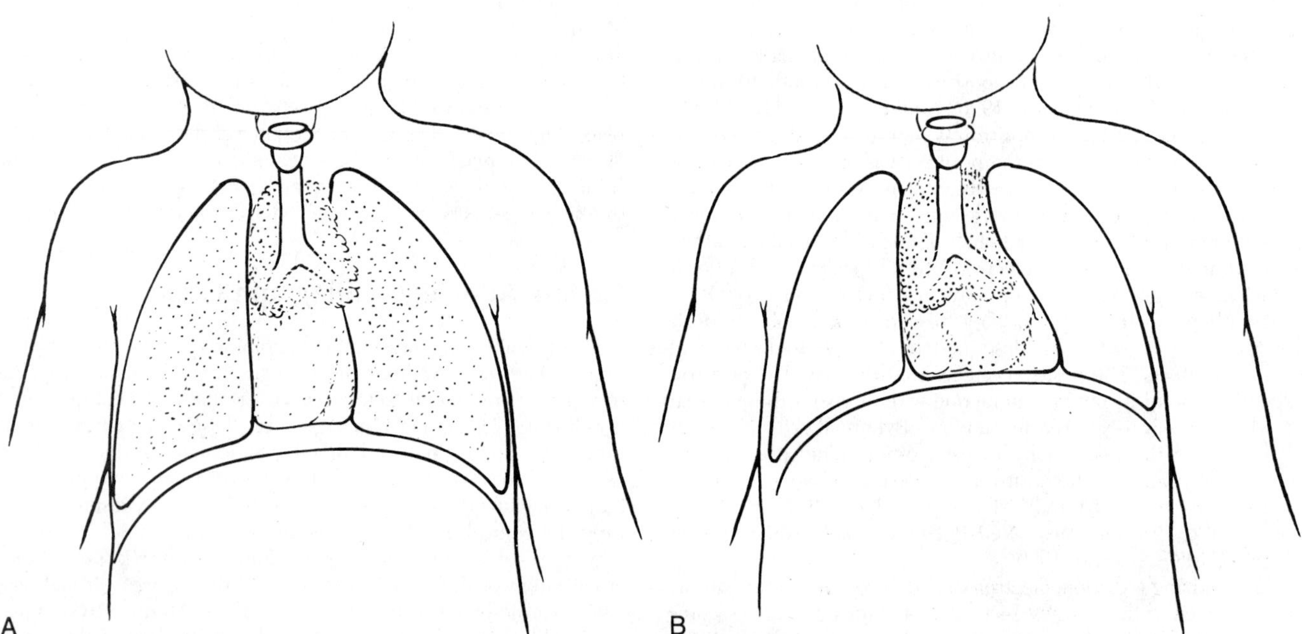

FIGURE 36–5. The differences in appearance between inspiration (*A*) and expiration (*B*) in a neonatal chest radiograph. On full inspiration, the diaphragm is located at the eighth rib, and the lungs appear larger and darker. During expiration, the diaphragm is above the seventh rib, and the lung fields appear smaller and lighter. The heart size may also appear larger on expiratory films.

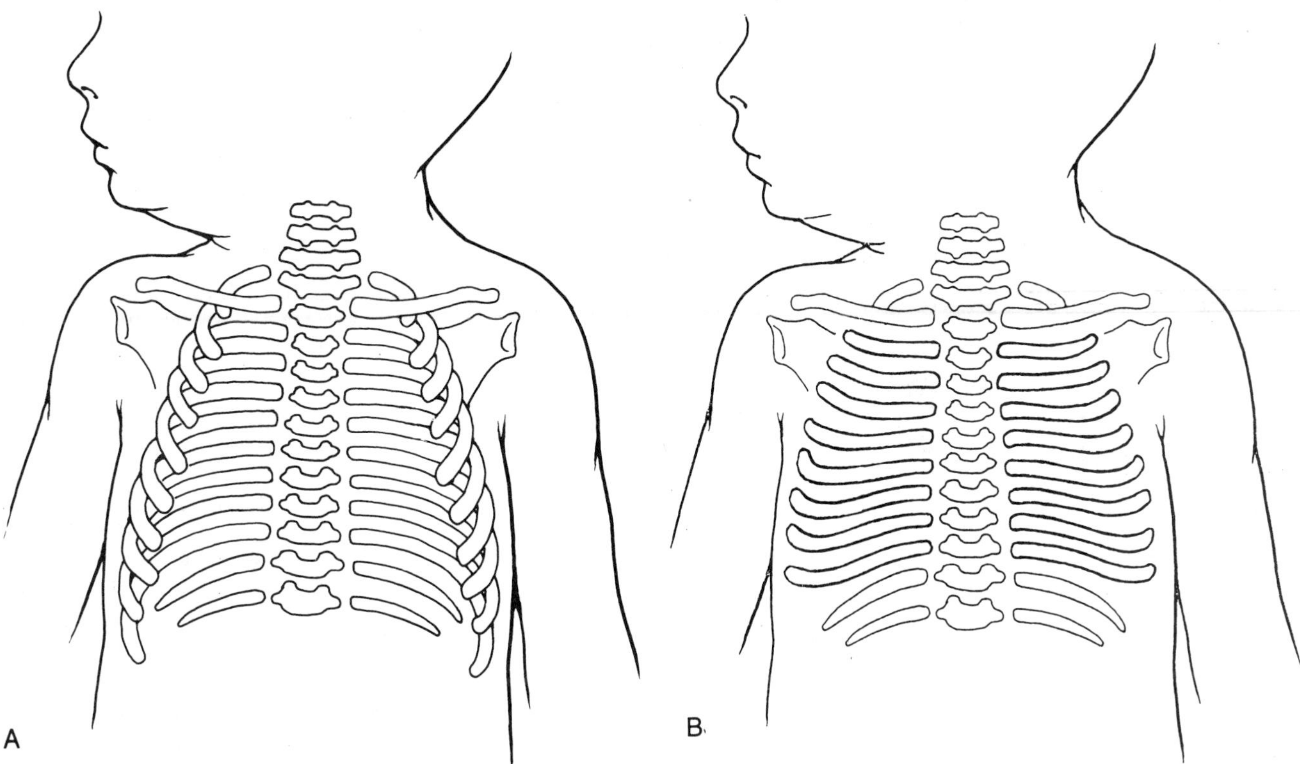

FIGURE 36–6. Skeletal position in a normally positioned radiograph *(A)* and in a film obtained with cephalad positioning of the x-ray tube *(B)*.

in the anterior rib arcs being angulated sharply downward in relation to the posterior arcs (Hilton & Edwards, 1994; Swischuk, 1989, 1995; Wesenberg, 1973).

Proper infant positioning is important in radiographic quality and interpretation. If the infant is rotated, there may be a false impression of a mediastinal shift (Fig. 36–7) (Gyll & Blake, 1986; Hilton & Edwards, 1994; Swischuk, 1989, 1995; Wesenberg, 1973). The direction and degree of rotation can be estimated by comparing the lengths of the posterior arcs of the ribs from the costovertebral junction to the lateral pleural line at a given level. The infant is rotated toward the side with the greatest posterior arc length (Hilton & Edwards, 1994; Kirks, 1991; Swischuk, 1989, 1995; Wesenberg, 1973). Another measurement to determine the degree of rotation is the distance from the medial aspect of the clavicles to the center of the vertebral body at the same level. If the infant is properly positioned, the medial aspects of the clavicles should be equidistant from the center of the vertebral body (Hilton & Edwards, 1994; Poznanski, 1976; Wesenberg, 1973). The measurement is increased on the side toward which the infant is rotated. On a lateral view, rotation can be readily determined by observing the amount of offset between the anterior tips of the right and left sets of ribs.

Prior to interpretation of any chest film, these factors need to be systematically evaluated. Through experience, this evaluation becomes automatic and the film can be rapidly scanned.

Radiologic Projections

Radiologic projections are the geometric views of the radiograph and vary among institutions and radiologists. They can be customized to the specific infant or clinical condition. For example, the skull may require a simple AP film to make the diagnosis of a fracture, or a complete skull series may be necessary in the evaluation of congenital malformations. For the neck and upper airway, a lateral film in inspiration with the infant's head extended may be sufficient in the evaluation of stridor, or a xeroradiograph of the soft tissue structures of the neck may be required. Because the radiation dose of a xeroradiograph is much greater than a plain lateral neck film, the indications for this examination should be clearly present (Gyll, 1985; Kirks, 1991; Poznanski, 1976; Swischuk, 1995).

In the evaluation of the spine, the AP projection is most commonly used. Oblique views of the spine in the infant are usually difficult to obtain because it is difficult to position and immobilize the infant. In addition, diagnostic information gained does not outweigh the risk of the greater radiation required to obtain such views. In the evaluation of congenital hip dysplasia, an AP view of the entire pelvis and both hips is required. Gonadal exposure should be minimized with proper shielding during radiographic examination of the hips. Assessment of skeletal maturation in the infant requires an AP film of the left hemiskeleton, whereas a long bone series requires a film of the upper and lower extremities (Gyll & Blake, 1986; Hilton & Edwards, 1994; Kirks, 1991; Poznanski, 1976; Swischuk, 1989, 1995).

Chest radiographs are the most frequently performed diagnostic imaging procedure in the neonatal intensive care unit (NICU). In most cases, an AP projection from a supine position is satisfactory to evaluate the infant's chest, heart, and lung fields. Lateral projections of the chest are often poorly positioned, have reduced technical quality, and require greater radiation exposure of the infant. For the experienced radiographer, an AP film in the supine position is sufficient in most cases. Rarely, a lateral chest film with esophageal barium contrast may be desired to evaluate the left atrium of the heart (Hilton & Edwards, 1994; Swischuk, 1989, 1995; Wesenberg, 1973).

Abdominal x-ray films are also frequently obtained in the NICU. The most commonly used radiographic projections are the AP and cross-table lateral views (Hilton & Edward, 1994; Kirks, 1991; Poznanski, 1976; Swischuk, 1995; Wesenberg, 1973). Because the infant's abdomen is relatively cylindrical, a lateral

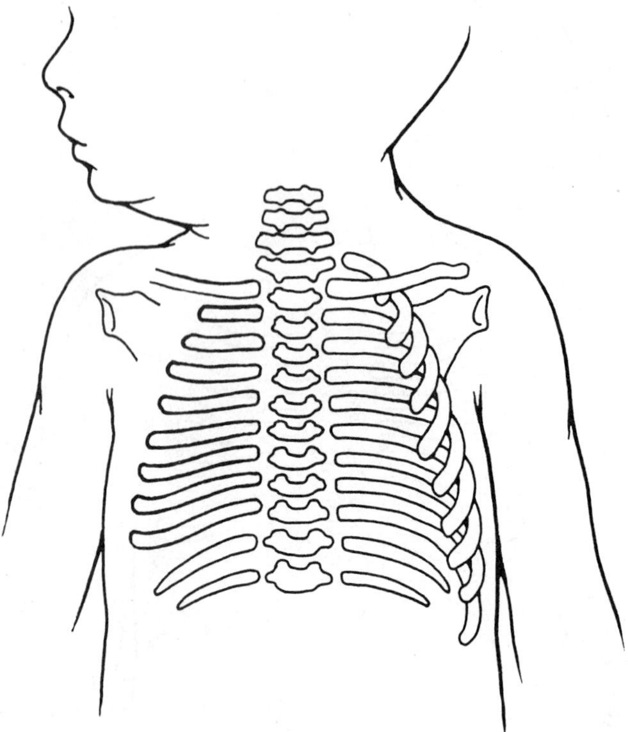

FIGURE 36–7. Skeletal configuration in a film obtained with the infant rotated to the right.

view provides more information than it does in an older child or adult (Gyll, 1985). AP views define the gas pattern, intestinal displacement, some masses, and ascites, whereas the cross-table lateral view is recommended in the diagnosis of intestinal perforation, pneumoperitoneum, and portal venous air (Hilton & Edwards, 1994; Swischuk, 1995).

Exposure Factors in Infancy

There are numerous radiographic variables involved in x-ray exposure. The x-ray machine, films, screens, type of cassettes, processing methods, and radiologist's preference may vary greatly from one department and institution to another. However, a few general principles can be stated. Exposure time should be short to avoid movement blur and limit radiation dose. Radiographic technicians should be knowledgeable of factors and variables that affect exposure to prevent repeating a radiograph obtained using poor technique. The largest dose of unnecessary radiation to an infant is caused by a repeat film (Gyll, 1985; Haller & Slovis, 1984; Hilton & Edwards, 1994; Kirks, 1991; Swischuk, 1989, 1995). Every possible precaution should be taken to ensure that the first attempt produces a film of diagnostic quality. Before repeating a film, the film should be shown to the radiologist or neonatologist who requested it. Although the technical quality of the film may not be ideal, it may provide sufficient information.

Another method of reducing radiation exposure is to use other diagnostic imaging modalities such as ultrasonography and magnetic resonance scans, which do not use ionizing radiation to create an image (Gyll & Blake, 1986; Horowitz, 1995; Kirks, 1991; Swischuk, 1989, 1995). If radiologic imaging is the best diagnostic approach to the infant's condition, then it may be important to "customize" the examinations, limit the area being examined, and reduce the number of follow-up films. The radiologist and technician should be knowledgeable about the rapidly advancing technology related to the film–screen combinations, filtration, projections, and film processing, which helps to produce a film of fine diagnostic quality while minimizing the radiation exposure (Alpen, 1990; Gyll & Blake, 1986; Kirks, 1991; Swischuk, 1989, 1995; Wesenberg, 1973).

Ideally, there are no "routine" radiologic examinations, just problem-oriented approaches. There is, however, a logical approach to radiographic examinations. Plain films should be obtained first. Then, if indicated, a dye contrast study such as an excretory urograph should be performed, because the contrast material is rapidly eliminated from the body. Lastly, barium contrast studies should be obtained (Hilton & Edwards, 1994; Kirks, 1991; Swischuk, 1995). Barium contrast studies are performed after the others because (1) barium interferes with any nuclear scintigraphic scans, body computed tomograms, and ultrasonographic scans, and (2) barium is slowly eliminated from the GI tract, thereby causing a delay in further diagnostic evaluation. The possibility of additional radiation exposure occurs if the barium must be completely eliminated before the next imaging procedure (Gyll & Blake, 1986; Hilton & Edwards, 1994; Swischuk, 1989, 1995).

Adequate patient preparation is another way to reduce radiation exposure (Gyll, 1985; Hilton & Edwards, 1994; Kirks, 1991; Shapiro, 1990; Swischuk, 1995). If GI and genitourinary (GU) imaging are both to be performed, the GU examination should be scheduled first. Although each institution may have its own policies, in preparation for a GU examination such as excretory urography, the infant should be on NPO (nothing by mouth) status for no longer than 3 hours. This is often accomplished by withholding the early morning feeding and scheduling the examination for 8 A.M. No preparation is necessary for excretory urography in infants with abdominal masses, trauma, or GU emergencies. If the infant has impaired renal function, the radiologist and the neonatologist should discuss the condition thoroughly so that the risks of this procedure are minimized. To prepare an infant for a GI contrast study, the infant who has been feeding should be kept on NPO status for no longer than 3 hours before the examination. Generally, if a contrast study of the entire GI tract is desired, the lower GI series is performed before the upper GI series (Gyll, 1985; Hilton & Edwards, 1994; Kirks, 1991; Swischuk, 1989, 1995). This allows time for the barium in the colon to be eliminated and prevents its interfering with the diagnostic quality of the upper GI study. Colon preparation is usually unnecessary in the neonate and should be avoided in neonates with an acute abdomen or in suspected Hirschsprung's disease (Gyll & Blake, 1986; Haller & Slovis, 1984; Kirks, 1991; Swischuk, 1989, 1995).

Collaborative Care

Radiation Protection

Any radiation is considered harmful to the infant, and all efforts must be made to reduce radiation exposure without decreasing diagnostic information. Radiation risks include both genetic and somatic effects (NCRP, 1993a, 1993b, 1993c; Noz & Maguire, 1985; Shapiro, 1990; Whalen & Balter, 1984). Reduction of radiation exposure should be the goal for sites that are sensitive genetically (gonads) and somatically (eye, bone marrow). Although there is no evidence that somatic damage (e.g., carcinogenesis or cataract production) occurs as a result of low-dose diagnostic radiologic procedures, dose reduction should be accomplished for the site examined as well as for the rest of the body (Gofman, 1983, 1990; Noz & Maguire, 1985; Shapiro, 1990; Whalen & Balter, 1984). Methods used to reduce radiation exposure include performing examinations only when they are clinically indicated, selecting the appropriate imaging modality, using the lowest radiation dose that achieves an image of diagnostic quality, avoiding repeat examinations, reducing the number of films obtained, using appropriate projections with tight field limitation, ensuring proper positioning and immobilization, and shielding the gonads (Alpen, 1990; Gofman, 1983, 1990; Hilton & Edwards, 1994; NCRP, 1993a, 1993b, 1993c; Noz & Maguire, 1985; Wesenberg, 1973; Whalen & Balter, 1984).

Gonadal exposure, if the gonads are not within the area of interest, depends on the adequacy of field limitation. The maximum gonadal dose occurs when the gonads are unshielded and exposed to the primary x-ray beam. This dose decreases rapidly as the distance from the gonads to the primary beam increases. Gonadal exposure in an AP film that includes the gonads can be reduced by 95 percent with proper contact shielding (Kirks, 1991; Shapiro, 1990). The gonads should be shielded whenever they are within 5 cm of the primary x-ray beam.

Contact gonadal shields are easy to make from 0.5 mm thick lead rubber sheets and should be sized for sex and age (Fig. 36–8) (Gyll & Blake, 1986; Kirks, 1991; Shapiro, 1990; Swischuk, 1989, 1995). In males, proper positioning of the shield avoids obscuring any bony detail of the pelvis if the upper edge of the shield is placed just below the pubis and the testicles have descended into the scrotum. In a female, the position of the ovaries varies with bladder distention. Because of their anatomic location, the ovaries cannot be shielded without obscuring lower abdominal and pelvic structures. The lower margin of the gonad shield should be placed at the level of the pubis, and the upper margin should cover at least the lower margin of the sacroiliac joints (Gyll & Blake, 1986; Hilton & Edwards, 1994; Kirks, 1991; Swischuk, 1989, 1995; Whalen & Balter, 1984).

Radiation Safety

There are three ways to reduce radiation exposure of personnel: (1) reduce the time of radiation exposure, (2) increase the distance from the radiation source, and (3) provide radiation shielding between the nurse and the radiation source (Alpen, 1990; NCRP, 1993a, 1993b, 1993c; Poznanski et al., 1974; Shapiro, 1990; Whalen & Balter, 1984). Portable radiologic examinations are the most common form of diagnostic imaging routinely performed in the NICUs. During these diagnostic procedures, there is a tendency for all the nurses to leave the room when an exposure is being produced. Thus, other infants may be left unattended for this interval, and this practice has resulted in the expression of parental fears for environmental radiation hazards for their infants.

Poznanski and others studied radiation exposure to personnel in a neonatal nursery (Poznanski et al., 1974). They studied the amount and location of scattered radiation dosage in microroentgens (10^{-6} R) and calculated the radiation exposure at 1-foot intervals away from the x-ray target. They found that the amount of scattered radiation is infinitesimally small. They used a situation of an infant who receives two radiologic examinations per shift and calculated the total dose outside a 1-foot radius of the primary beam as 70 microroentgens (μR). If the staff nurse worked a 250-day work year and held an infant who received two x-ray examinations per shift, this would represent a cumulative dose of 17,500 μR or 18 mrad per year (1000 μR = 1 mrad) (Poznanski et al., 1974). This value is considerably less than background radiation in a building, which is between 100 and 150 mrad per year (Cowan, 1959; Shapiro, 1990).

Other radiologic studies done in the NICU have found that, within 6 feet of the target, an unshielded person receives 100 mrad *per hour* of exposure (Poznanski et al., 1974; Poznanski, 1976; Shapiro, 1990; Whalen & Balter, 1984). Time of exposure is approximately 0.1 second, so radiation dose is 0.003 mrad per exposure. This amount of radiation is far below the safety limit of 500 mrad per year (Shapiro, 1990). At this rate of radiation exposure, a full-time staff nurse would have to be exposed to more than 6000 x-rays each day to reach the radiation safety limit per year (Gofman, 1983 & 1990; NCRP, 1993a, 1993b, 1993c; Noz & Maguire, 1985; Poznanski, 1976; Shapiro, 1990).

It appears that, if certain basic radiation protection precautions are observed, it is unnecessary for nurses and other personnel in a

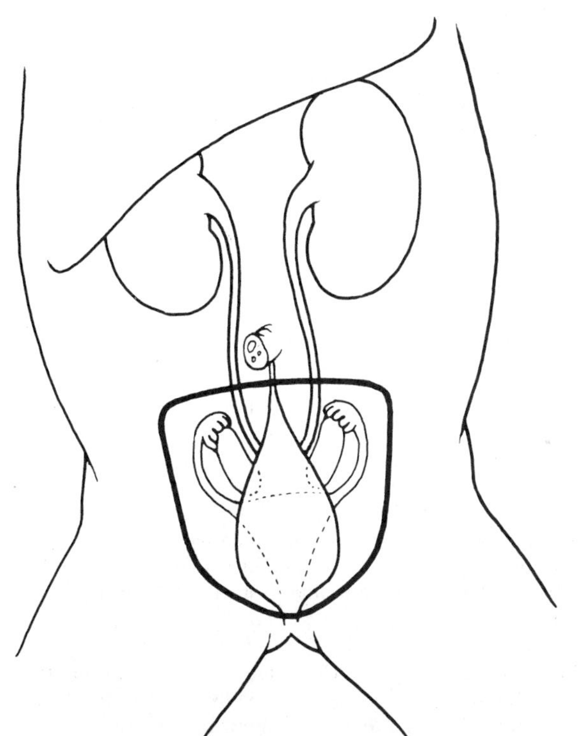

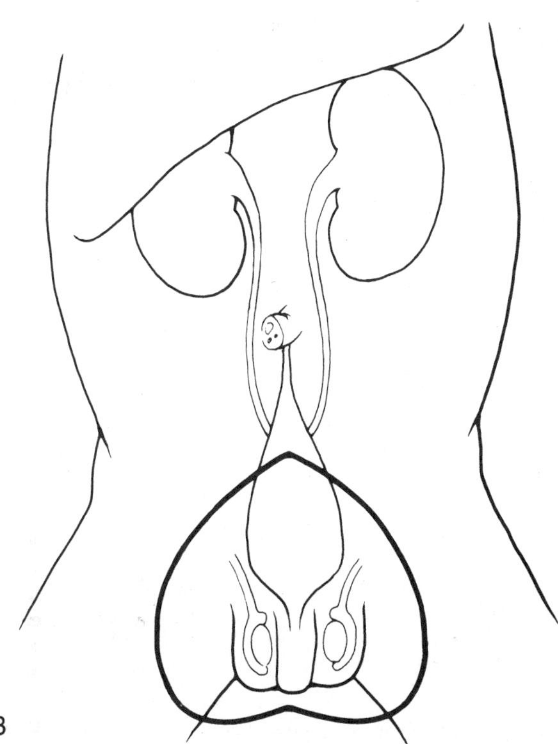

FIGURE 36–8. Anatomic placement of gonad shield for female infants *(A)* and for male infants *(B)*.

NICU to leave the room during x-ray exposures. As a precaution, however, staff members should stay 1 foot or more away from the infant who is being radiographed. Care must be taken to ensure that, if a horizontal beam film is obtained (e.g., in a cross-table lateral projection), no one is in the direct x-ray beam, because the radiation dose in the primary beam is considerably higher than in the scattered dose. When a horizontal beam is used, it should not be directed at any other patient or personnel. If an employee is within 1 foot of the incubator or is holding the infant for the exposure, lead gloves and aprons should be worn (Shapiro, 1990).

The x-ray beam must be confined to within the cassette edges. There is not much scatter from an infant, but an adult's hands can easily come within the field of primary radiation and cause scatter (Gyll, 1985; Kirks, 1991; Shapiro, 1990). It is important to properly position and secure the infant while keeping hands out of the x-ray beam. If correct radiographic technique is used, the dose to the nurse's lead-protected hands is approximately 0.01 mSv. The annual dose limit to the hands of nondesignated personnel is 500 mSv (Gyll, 1985; Shapiro, 1990).

Radionuclide Imaging

The use of radioisotopes has brought a new dimension to diagnostic imaging, because they can be used to trace a wide range of physiologic functions in virtually every organ in the body, thereby complementing conventional radiography and ultrasonographic imaging. Whereas ultrasonographic imaging does not use radiation, the difference between conventional radiology and radionuclide imaging is that, in the former, images are produced by the transmission of radiation, and, in the latter, images are produced by the emission of radiation (gamma rays) previously introduced into the body and recorded on film or in a computer (Fig. 36–9) (Alpen, 1990; Bushong, 1992; Juhl & Crummy, 1993; Kirks, 1991; Siddiqui, 1985; Treves, 1995; Walker & Margouleff, 1984).

Radionuclide studies yield physiologic information as well as anatomic representations of the distribution of radioactivity, dependent upon the selective uptake of radionuclide by different organs of the body (Siddiqui, 1985; Treves, 1995; Walker & Margouleff, 1984). The primary disadvantage of radionuclide imaging is the limited anatomic resolution to diameters greater than 2 cm.

Relatively small amounts of radioactivity are used in radionuclide imaging, and the radiation hazard is significantly smaller than for corresponding conventional radiographic investigations (Gofman, 1983; Noz & Maguire, 1985; Shapiro, 1990; Siddiqui, 1985; Treves, 1995; Whalen & Balter, 1984). The radioactive substance injected is usually distributed throughout the body, and the site of maximum radiation is not always at the site of the same organ that is being investigated (Siddiqui, 1985; Treves, 1995; Whalen & Balter, 1984). For example, the thyroid gland selectively concentrates radioactive iodine even if this compound is being used to study another organ. Thyroid iodine uptake may need to be blocked pharmaceutically in this case. In addition, radioactive phosphonate agents used for skeletal scanning are excreted by the kidneys, and the maximal radiation dose is to the bladder mucosa (Siddiqui, 1985; Treves, 1995; Whalen & Balter, 1984). This dose effect can be reduced by promoting diuresis. Thus, the radiation hazards in radionuclide imaging are affected by the physiologic distribution of the agent and its physical half-life, the dose of radionuclide administered, and the pharmacologic half-life in the body (Kirks, 1984; Shapiro, 1990; Siddiqui, 1985; Squire & Novelline, 1988; Treves, 1995; Whaler & Balter, 1984).

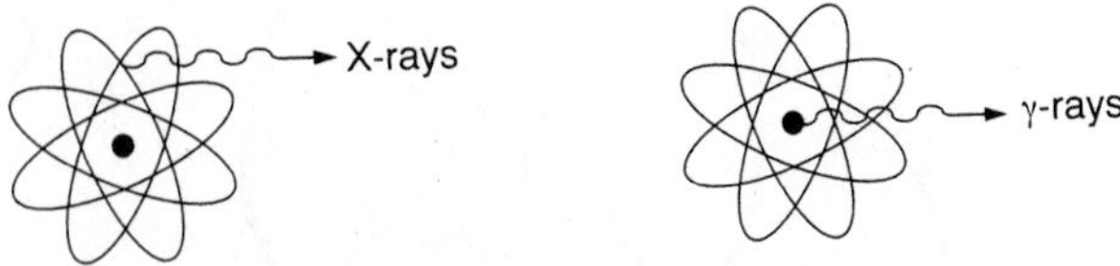

FIGURE 36–9. X-rays are produced outside the nucleus of artificially excited atoms; gamma rays are produced inside the nucleus of radioactive atoms.

In nuclear diagnostic imaging, several factors help determine how much energy is actually deposited in the tissue and may influence the choice of radionuclide. These factors include the following (Gofman, 1983; Shapiro, 1990; Treves, 1995):

- Route of entry
- Fraction of the administered dose that actually reaches the tissue
- Rate of biologic removal of the radionuclide
- Amount of radiation the tissue of interest receives from the portion of the radionuclide deposited in tissues other than the one of interest
- Number of microcuries of radionuclide taken in
- Careful calculation of the average energy of the beta particles emitted, of any ancillary gamma rays emitted, and any loss of radiation out of the specific tissue
- Metabolic or other factors that might alter the distribution of the radionuclide in various tissues of the human population studied

Thus, estimating the true dose of energy delivered to a specific tissue from radionuclide exposure, plutonium contamination, or external x-ray exposure has serious technical problems and requires the efforts of physicists skilled in such measurements.

Nearly all radionuclides used in medicine are artificially produced in nuclear reactors. The most versatile of these compounds is technetium 99m (^{99m}Tc), which has many ideal physical properties (Gofman, 1983; Treves, 1995):

1. It is nontoxic and nonallergenic.
2. It easily bound to other physiologic compounds.
3. It is relatively inexpensive
4. It circulates in the blood and accumulates in small amounts in gastric mucosa, salivary glands, and thyroid tissue.
5. It is excreted in the feces and urine primarily but can also be found in sweat and tears
6. It does not accumulate in the brain (except in the choroid plexus) unless the blood–brain barrier is disrupted
7. It has a short physical half-life (6 hours), which is long enough for tests to be completed while at the same time enabling high initial radioactivities to be administered within an acceptable radiation hazard
8. It emits only gamma photons, which can be detected by the sodium iodide crystals of gamma cameras.

Despite wide use of technetium, not all investigations can be done with it, and a number of alternative isotopes are available (see Table 36–1).

After injection and distribution of the radionuclide, the ideal instrument to detect radiation emission is the gamma camera. With this camera, images are rapidly acquired and dynamic studies are easily performed and quantified. Multiple views from various projections can be obtained. The camera consists of a large crystal of sodium iodide protected by a heavy lead collimator. The shielded crystal is placed over the target organ, and the gamma photons emitted from the body strike it and are converted into light scintillations. The pinhole and converging collimators allow the image to be magnified without loss of resolution. These light scintillations are manipulated electronically to define the distribution and intensity of the radioactivity. The final copy of the image is produced on film or stored on videotapes or magnetic disk (Alpen, 1990; Siddiqui, 1985; Squire & Novelline, 1988; Treves, 1995; Walker & Margouleff, 1984).

Radiopharmaceuticals are rarely organ specific. Therefore, there is always interference from radioactivity outside the organ of interest. Advances in computer processing similar to CT have been developed to eliminate this interfering background data, thereby increasing the accuracy of derived data. Two types of computer-enhanced radionuclide imaging are available: single photon emission computed tomography (SPECT) and positron emission tomography (PET). Both of these modalities have significant advantages over conventional planar radionuclide imaging in that (1) there is much greater sensitivity and qualifications of the distribution and density of radioactivity, (2) three-dimensional imaging is possible with computer reconstruction, (3) the dose of radionuclide is the same, and (4) artifactual lesions can be eliminated (Bushong, 1992; Siddiqui, 1985; Swischuk, 1989, 1995; Treves, 1995; Walker & Margouleff, 1984).

In SPECT, a gamma camera is rotated 360 degrees around the infant, and a series of equally spaced cross-sectional images is obtained and stored in the computer. These images are used to reconstruct a series of cross-sectional slices at right angles to the axis of rotation of the camera. Each cross-sectional slice comprises a series of squares arranged in a matrix. Using a mathematical model, the computer can readily reconstruct these cross-sectional slices in other planes such as lateral or coronal. The image is then viewed directly from the computer screen or formatted on film. This type of computer-enhanced emission tomography scan uses the standard gamma-emitting radionuclides such as technetium, thallium, gallium, or iodine (Bushong, 1992; Siddiqui, 1985; Treves, 1995).

In PET, a different type of radiopharmaceutical called a positron is used. Positrons are the same size and shape as electrons, but they have a positive charge. Typical positrons used in this type of imaging are carbon 11, oxygen 15, and nitrogen 13. By using the metabolic nucleotide from oxygen, carbon, or nitrogen, PET scans create images that depict the "metabolic" function of tissue such as the brain (Bushong, 1992; Kirks, 1991; Siddiqui, 1985; Treves, 1995; Walker & Margouleff, 1984). Whereas SPECT is widely available for general use, PET scanning is only available at large university medical centers with access to a cyclotron, which can produce the short-lived positrons required for this imaging modality. Continued advances in particle physics enhance the development of the technique as a research tool in the study of cerebral blood flow and physiology. The recent substitution of fluorine into the glucose molecule has been very useful in the study of cerebral metabolism in neonates after intracranial hemorrhage (Kirks, 1991; Siddiqui, 1985; Swischuk, 1989, 1995). Although this modality is not used frequently in clinical medicine, the nurse should understand its potential as a research tool.

Collaborative Care

The care of a neonate undergoing a radionuclide scan requires knowledge about the patient's history and clinical manifestations, the type of nuclear scan requested, and the radiopharmaceutical used. In general, the doses of radiopharmaceuticals are based on the infant's body weight, and the total whole body irradiation is considerably less than that of a conventional radiograph. The infant poses no radioactivity hazard for the nursing staff or other neonates. Linen, diapers, and body excreta can be disposed of in the usual manner. The nurses should be aware of the ability of the radionuclide to concentrate in areas other than the organ of interest so that proper thyroid iodine-uptake blocking agents can be administered or diuresis can be promoted.

Ultrasonographic Imaging

Ultrasonography is a form of diagnostic imaging, frequently used in the evaluation and treatment of the neonate, that evaluates internal anatomic structures. Unlike conventional radiography, it emits no ionizing radiation. Instead, sound waves are used to evaluate tissue densities, movement of tissues, and flow of blood (Bushong, 1992; Fanaroff & Martin, 1997; Kirks, 1991; Martin, 1985; Swischuk, 1989, 1995). The images can be recorded on videotape, photographic film, or light-sensitive paper.

By definition, ultrasound is any sound that has a frequency greater than 20,000 cycles per second (Hz), which exceeds the audible range of human hearing (20 to 20,000 Hz) (Bushong, 1992). Ultrasonography, which uses high-frequency (3.5 to 10 MHz) sound waves, is used to evaluate internal anatomic structures. In echocardiography and Doppler studies, ultrasound frequencies range in the millions of cycles per second (Feigenbaum, 1986). The advantages of ultrasonography as a diagnostic tool are as follows (Bushong, 1992; Fanaroff & Martin, 1997; Feigenbaum, 1986; Kirks, 1991; Martin, 1985; Swischuk, 1989, 1995):

1. It emits no ionizing radiation and has no known deleterious somatic or genetic effects; therefore, follow-up examinations may be repeated at will.
2. Ultrasound waves can be directed as a beam.
3. Sound waves obey laws of reflection and refraction.
4. Ultrasound waves are reflected by objects of small size.
5. Ultrasonography can be used in a variety of transverse, longitudinal, sagittal, or oblique planes.
6. Ultrasonography is considerably less costly than either CT or magnetic resonance imaging.
7. Ultrasound equipment is easily portable.
8. The examination is relatively painless and well tolerated.
9. Sedation is rarely required
10. Ultrasonography relies on acoustic impedance of tissue to demonstrate anatomy.
11. Diagnostic ability is accurate.

The principal disadvantages of ultrasonography are as follows (Bushong, 1992; Feigenbaum, 1986; Martin, 1985):

1. The technique is operator dependent.
2. Ultrasonography does not provide information on organ function, as does urography.
3. Ultrasonography has limited value as a screening procedure for "acute abdominal distress," but should be focused on a particular area of interest.
4. CT is superior in demonstrating the extent of the disease, because ultrasonography demonstrates a smaller area of interest and less anatomic detail.
5. Ultrasonography is adversely affected by bone, excessive fat, and gas artifacts.

As a result, certain parts of the body, such as the brain, must be imaged through an ultrasound "window," for example, the anterior fontanelle. In addition, because ultrasonography is poorly propagated through gaseous medium, the transducer must have airless contact with the surface being examined, and it is difficult to examine parts of the body that contain large amounts of air.

High-frequency sound passes through the body tissues at a fairly constant speed of approximately 1500 m/second, or 1.5 mm/microsecond (Bushong, 1992). Using electronic mechanisms, it is possible to time the passage of an ultrasound impulse to within a fraction of a microsecond so that the distance between an ultrasound transducer and a reflecting interface of tissue can be determined to a fraction of a millimeter. The transducer converts electrical energy into ultrasonography energy and acts as both the emitter of the initial impulse and the receiver of the reflected impulse.

The velocity of sound wave transmission is the product of

the sound frequency and the wavelength. How rapidly sound is transmitted varies and depends on the density and compressibility of the medium (Bushong, 1992). The velocity of sound transmission is low in a gaseous medium because of the large compressibility and low density of the substance. Sound does not exist in the vacuum of outer space but is readily transmitted through objects of greater density, such as water or metal. This principle can be readily illustrated with the use of a tuning fork. When struck, the tuning fork vibrates and emits sound that can be easily heard. However, when the vibrating tuning fork is placed against the mastoid bone of the cranium, the sound is transmitted to the ear much more readily and is perceived as being louder.

The frequency and wavelength are inversely proportional in ultrasonography (Bushong, 1992; Kirks, 1991). That is, as ultrasound frequency increases, the wavelength decreases. The ability of ultrasonography to distinguish objects of small size is directly related to the sound wavelength. High-frequency ultrasonography has short wavelengths and results in better image resolution than low-frequency, long-wavelength ultrasonography. This occurs because, as the ultrasound frequency increases, the degree of interaction with the conducting medium increases and absorption of the ultrasound beam is increased. Thus, at higher ultrasound frequencies, there is less tissue penetration. For example, ultrasound examinations of the eye typically use 10-MHz frequencies, whereas an examination of deep structures of the abdomen uses frequencies in the 2.5-MHz range (Moss et al., 1984).

The frequency-dependent characteristic of ultrasonography results in its highly directional and collimated nature, which enhances its imaging ability (Bushong, 1992). As the frequency of sound increases, its dispersion from the source becomes less and its transmission becomes more like that of a collimated beam. This becomes apparent when experimenting with a household stereo. The woofers, which produce low-frequency bass sound, fill the entire room with sound. A person's perception of these low-frequency sounds does not change, no matter where the person stands in the room. However, the higher frequency sound produced by the tweeters does not disperse as well in the room and can best be heard when the person is positioned directly in front of the speakers. In addition, low-frequency sounds seem at times to penetrate and reverberate within the body, whereas this is not true with higher-frequency sounds. These same principles govern ultrasound transmission through tissue. At higher ultrasound frequencies, the beam becomes more collimated in a forward direction. As ultrasound frequency is increased, the ability to distinguish small objects increases, but the penetrability of the beam decreases. Therefore, the highest frequency transducer is chosen to provide the greatest depth for the tissue or organ imaged (Martin, 1985).

In addition, ultrasonography is useful as a diagnostic imaging method because it is reflected at tissue interfaces. A principle called "sonic momentum" describes the velocity of sound transmitted through tissue. Sound transmission through different tissues varies with sound velocity, the freedom of motion of the molecules (density), and the sound waves' compressibility. The nature of how sound travels through a tissue is frequently referred to as the acoustic impedance of that tissue. As a sound wave travels through a homogeneous tissue, it continues in a straight line. When the sound wave reaches an interface between two tissues with different acoustic impedances, it undergoes reflection and refraction (Fig. 36–10) Bushong, 1992; Kirks, 1991). The amount of sound reflected depends on the degree of difference between the two tissues; the greater the disparity, the greater the reflection. Diagnostic ultrasound has little interest in the refracted wave but is primarily interested in the intensity of the reflected

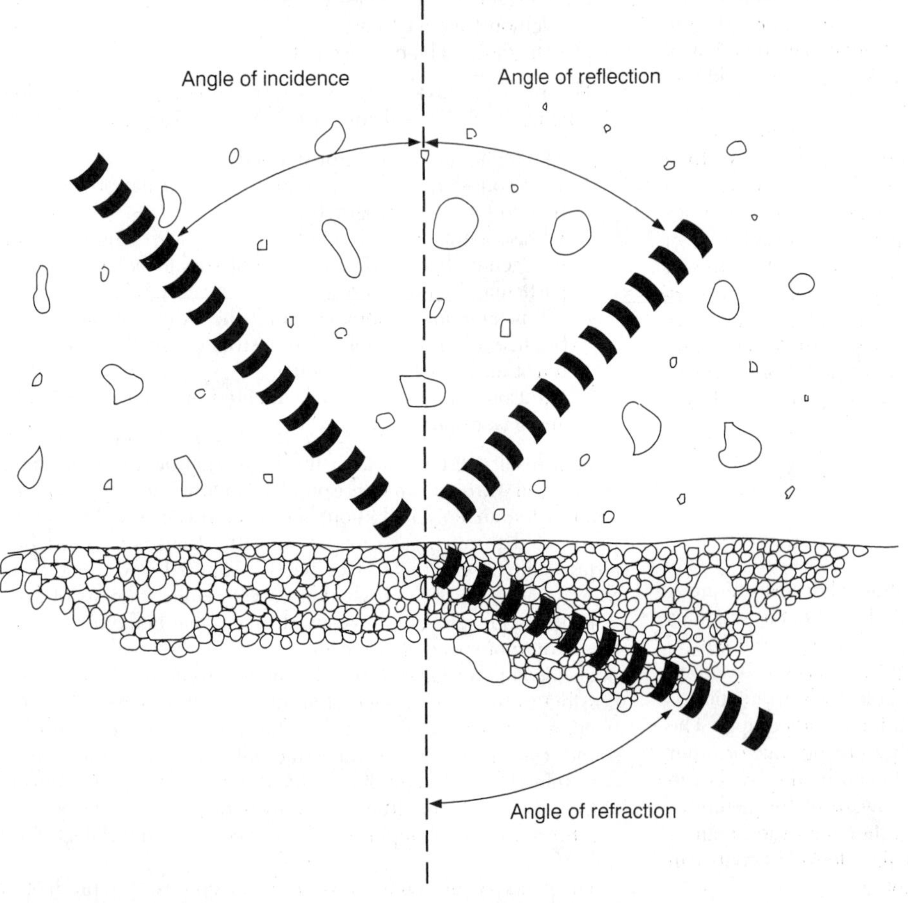

FIGURE 36–10. The reflection and refraction of ultrasound.

beam relative to the original sound wave (Bushong, 1992; Kirks, 1991). The major patterns of ultrasound reflection are anechoic, echoic, and mixed. An anechoic structure is described as sonar lucent and is a structure in which the acoustic medium is homogeneous and the sound waves are unimpeded. An anechoic structure may be fluid filled (bladder), cystic (hydronephrosis), or solid (lymphoma), as long as the tissue is homogeneous. Cystic structures usually have sharp echogenic margins anteriorly and posteriorly. Echoic structures are inhomogeneous and reflect sound waves. These tissues are generally solid with a variety of densities (typical Wilms' tumor) or may be cystic (hemorrhagic Wilms' tumor). A mixed pattern of reflections has the combined qualities of anechoic and echoic tissues. In addition, ribs and calculi may cause imaging artifacts on an ultrasonographic image. These dense structures prevent further penetration of the ultrasound beam and cause a band-like region of decreased sound transmission beyond that point, called acoustic shadowing (Kirks, 1992; Martin, 1985; Vogler et al., 1986).

When applying these principles to clinical practice, it is known that ultrasound is propagated differently in various human tissues and is reflected from each acoustic interface (Feigenbaum, 1986). A stationary interface results in a reflected ultrasound wave that has the same frequency as the transmitted wave. When the tissue interface is moving, for example, the movement of red blood cells in a vessel, the reflected ultrasound wave has a shifted frequency directly proportional to the velocity of the reflecting blood cells, in accordance with a principle called the Doppler effect. If the movement of the blood cells is toward the transducer, the frequency of the reflected wave is higher than the transmitted frequency. Conversely, movement of blood away from the transducer results in a lower frequency of the reflected wave (Feigenbaum, 1986). The difference between the transmitted frequency and the reflected frequency is called the Doppler shift. It is the principle of sound frequency shifts that allows the application of the mathematical relationship between the velocity of the target and the Doppler frequency in order to calculate flow. This is used most commonly in the echocardiographic evaluation of the heart and in cerebral blood flow determinations (Feigenbaum, 1986; Martin, 1985).

Modes of Ultrasonography

There are currently five modes of ultrasonic imaging. There are two static modes (A-mode, B-mode), two dynamic modes (M-mode, real-time), and one Doppler mode. All these modes, except Doppler, use a pulse-echo transducer. A pulse-echo transducer sends ultrasound waves for 0.0001 second, then waits for the reflected sound for 0.999 second. The first reflection of a sound wave occurs at the transducer–patient interface, and this is the most intense. At each succeeding tissue interface, reflection of the sound wave decreases in intensity as the tissue is penetrated. The time required for the pulse to be reflected to the transducer and its returned intensity indicates the position of the interface and is indicated as a blip on the video display screen (Bushong, 1992; Martin, 1985).

In A-mode, ultrasonic images are displayed on the video screen as a series of vertical blips that represent the returning echoes (Fig. 36–11*A*). The distance between these blips is proportional to distances between the tissue interfaces, and the height of each blip is proportional to the intensity of the reflected beam. Thus, distal reflections produce lower blips (Feigenbaum, 1986). The main purpose of A-mode imaging is to measure depths of interfaces and detect their separation accurately. A-mode ultrasonography is primarily used in echoencephalography to determine cranial midline and is also used for ultrasonically guided aspiration techniques such as amniocentesis. The advantages of A-mode are that it relies on axial resolution, is relatively inexpensive, and is easy to use. The primary disadvantage of this mode is that is requires frequent calibration (Bushong, 1992; Martin, 1985).

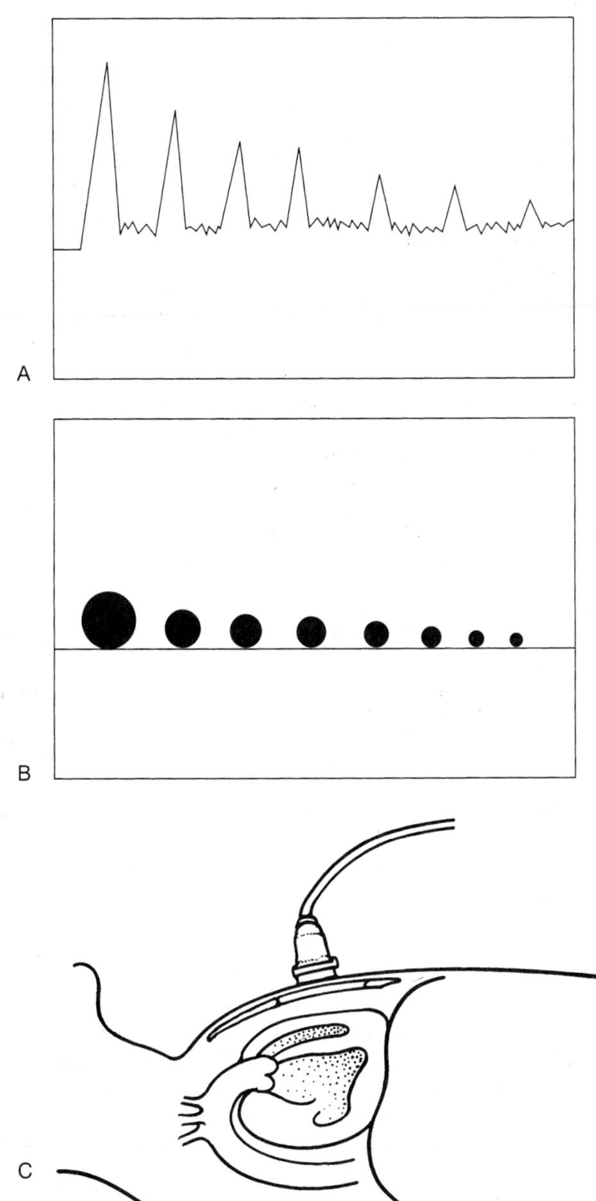

FIGURE 36–11. *A*, A-mode ultrasound display pattern consists of a series of vertical blips that correspond to tissue density and depth. *B*, B-mode ultrasound display pattern consists of a series of dots whose brightness corresponds to the tissue density and depth. *C*, M-mode ultrasound display pattern produces a strip chart for tracing moving tissue interfaces.

B-mode, or brightness mode, ultrasonic imaging displays information as dots, with the brightness of the dot corresponding to the distance of the reflecting interface from the transducer (see Fig. 36–11*B*). Advances in microcomputers and electromechanical coupling have resulted in a compound B-mode image (Bushong, 1992; Martin, 1985). This is achieved when the spatial position and direction of the ultrasound beam is coupled to the video display screen and the B-mode pulses are individually stored while the transducer is moved about the body. Thus, the image that appears on the video display screen is the summation of many individual B-mode lines. The spatial resolution of this type of imaging is highly variable and dependent on transducer characteristics and the electromechanical linkages available commercially. This mode of imaging has become widely used especially for abdominal examinations. The B-mode transducer can be moved linearly to provide a rectangular scan view or it can be angled to provide a sector scan (Bushong, 1992; Martin, 1985).

M-mode, or motion mode, is an imaging process that incorporates pulse-echo ultrasonography to define tissue movement. If an ultrasound transducer is operated in A-mode over the heart, it detects a number of vertical blips from stationary objects, which indicate the motionless interfaces of the tissue. The amplitude of these blips is proportional to the intensity of the echo. The magnitude of the moving objects represents the degree of movement of tissue interface. If this A-mode scan is converted into a B-mode scan, the image is transformed into a number of dots, some of which are fixed and some of which are moving. If this image is driven on the X-axis according to time as in a chart recording, a tracing of the dots results (see Fig. 36–11*C*). The stationary dots trace a regular pattern according to the motion of the tissue interface. The Y-axis is the depth of the tissue plane. This type of imaging is used primarily to monitor heart function and can be synchronized with the electrocardiograph (Bushong, 1992; Martin, 1985).

Real-time ultrasonic imaging is another dynamic form of examining tissues. Real-time is considered the ultrasonic fluoroscope and has several advantages over B-mode imaging, including the following:

1. The cost for real-time ultrasonography units is considerably less than for B-mode units.
2. Real-time images obtained are much less dependent on operator skill.
3. Time required for real-time examinations is less because real-time imaging is relatively easy to use.
4. Portable versions are readily available.

In real-time ultrasonography, the transducer is longer than is required in B-mode, and thus more gel is needed. The transducer is then moved over the surface until the anatomic region of interest is found. The dynamic image is recorded on videotape, and stop action frames are obtained by taking sequential photographs of the display. The disadvantages of real-time ultrasonography are that (1) the ultrasound beam interacts with tissue interfaces from only one direction, whereas B-mode transducers can move while storing the image from many directions, and (2) lateral resolution is superior in B-mode imaging as compared with real-time imaging (Bushong, 1992; Martin, 1985).

The popularity of real-time ultrasonography as an imaging modality has generated three types of real-time transducer devices—mechanical, linear array, and phased array—which have distinct characteristics in their display. The mechanical transducer was the first real-time device developed. In this device, the transducer is motorized so that the ultrasound beam is mechanically swept across the field in an oscillating fashion. Each sweep results in one image frame, and as many as 15 frames per second may be obtained. This transducer can be moved linearly for a rectangular view or in an angulated fashion for a sector view (Bushong, 1992; Martin, 1985). This mechanical transducer device was not popular in the early days of real-time ultrasonography because of the limitation of frame rate per second, restricted field of view, and distortion. In recent years, manufacturers have improved this transducer by increasing the frame rate, expanding the viewing field, and decreasing the distortion.

Linear array is a type of ultrasonographic transducer device that has a line of 32 transducers aligned in a single case. Because each transducer is only 2 mm wide, the overall length of the transducer case is 64 mm. In linear array, each transducer is energized in sequence from 1 to 32. This provides 32 image lines over the pulse of ultrasound and is called sequential linear array. If four or five contiguous transducers are energized simultaneously, each pulse of the ultrasound results in four or five scan image lines called segmental linear array. In a typical system, the transducers are fired in an overlapping pattern so that numbers 1 through 5, then 2 through 6, 3 through 7, and so on are segmentally then sequentially energized (Bushong, 1992; Martin, 1985). This type of transducer device provides for greater image line density and improved image quality over sequential linear array devices. As with the mechanical devices, sequential and segmental linear array devices have poor lateral resolution.

Phased-array real-time ultrasonic imaging is similar to linear array in that it incorporates segmental excitation of the transducer elements. The transducers are segmentally sequenced and have programmable electronic circuity to incorporate delay lines to precisely time the excitation and reception of the ultrasound waves by each element. This delay allows a plane of sound waves from the transducer to be directed or "phased." The result is a sector scan with a maximum sector angle of 90 degrees (Bushong, 1992; Martin, 1985). The scan line rate, frame rate, and depth of scan can be selected. The electronic delay lines on the receiver circuitry allow some depth of focusing by synchronizing the returning reflected pulses. The transducer size is smaller than with linear array, and there is good axial resolution. As with real time imaging, lateral resolution is poor but can be improved with acoustic focusing.

Biologic Effects of Ultrasonography

Ultrasonic imaging was first introduced into obstetrical practice in 1966. Since that time, despite the widespread use of this imaging modality and the use of multiple scans during an individual pregnancy, there has not been any report of manifested injury or late effects that occurred to humans (or fetuses) exposed to diagnostic levels of medical ultrasound (Bushong, 1992; Kirks, 1991; Martin, 1985). In the laboratory, however, it has been shown that much higher levels of ultrasound can produce measurable tissue effects. The levels of ultrasound energy required to produce these effects are approximately 1000 times greater than those used in diagnostic medical ultrasonography. In vitro, the mechanism of action of the ultrasonic effects on tissue is thought to be caused by increased tissue temperature, cavitation, and various viscous stresses on the tissue (Bushong, 1992; Kirks, 1991).

The thermal effects of ultrasonography occur because of the molecular agitation and relaxation processes caused by the passing sound waves (Bushong, 1992). Extremely high levels of ultrasound are required to produce even a measurable increase in tissue temperature. The effects of the elevation in tissue temperature not only occurs with ultrasonography but also occurs with fever or hyperthermia. At the local tissue level, significant changes in tissue temperature regardless of cause result in structural changes in macromolecules and membranes and alter the rate of biochemical reactions. The thermal effects of diagnostic medical ultrasonography do not result in any increase in tissue temperature.

High levels of experimental ultrasound can also result in alteration in the structure and function of macromolecules and cells without an increase in tissue temperature. These changes can result from cavitation, which occurs when tiny bubbles of gas are formed during the molecular relaxation after sound wave agitation (Bushong, 1992). As the cavitation increases, more energy is absorbed from the incident ultrasound beam. This is thought to cause disruption of molecular bonds and the production of free hydrogen and hydroxide radicals produced by the dissociation of water vapor. Cavitation effects have not been observed with the levels of sound used in diagnostic medical ultrasonography.

Every tissue has a specific density, and the density of tissues on either side of an interface may not be equal. As ultrasound waves interact along this tissue interface, the differences in density result in stress exerted on the tissue boundary. This tissue boundary stress results in small-scale fluid motions called microstreaming (Bushong, 1992). It is theoretically possible that such microstreaming can disrupt membranes and cells in the region of the interface. Microstreaming has been observed in vitro only after exposure to extremely high levels of ultrasound.

Experimental evidence has shown that ultrasound in sufficiently high doses is able to degrade macromolecules and may produce chromosomal aberrations and cause cellular death. To induce these effects in living tissue, however, ultrasound intensities of 10 W/cm^2 exposure over considerable periods of time are necessary. The absolute minimum dose level that has been reported to have an observable effect in experimental specimens is 100 mW/cm^2, and then only after many hours of continuous ultrasonographic application (Bushong, 1992). The intensity range of diagnostic ultrasound is from 1 to 10 mW/cm^2, and examinations using this modality frequently require only a few minutes of ultrasound exposure. There are no reports of human chromosomal effects or changes in prenatal or neonatal death rates after exposure to ultrasound. Nor is there evidence that ultrasound induces latent malignant disease. It is for these reasons that ultrasonic imaging has grown in its application in all areas of medicine and is rapidly increasing its application in neonatal care.

Indications for ultrasonography in neonatal intensive care commonly include evaluation of brain parenchyma and ventricular size, myocardial function and structure, cholelithiasis, choledochal cysts, intestinal duplication, renal neoplasms, urinary tract dilation and duplication, pelvic masses, and skeletal anomalies of the spine and hips (Fanaroff & Martin, 1997; Feigenbaum, 1986; Martin, 1985).

Collaborative Care

The care required for a neonate undergoing a diagnostic ultrasound examination is to ensure that any disruption of the infant's microenvironment is minimal. The infant's temperature can be maintained more easily if the ultrasound examination is performed by placing the transducer in the incubator. Although this method is technically more cumbersome for the ultrasonographer, cooperative interchange between the ultrasonographer and the nurse facilitates the procedure. In addition, the transducer gel should be warmed to the same temperature as the infant's incubator to minimize heat loss. A diaper or other pad placed under the imaged area and quick removal of the gel and drying the skin after the scan also decrease heat loss caused by wet blankets or skin.

The nurse's understanding of the imaging examination to be performed helps in more accurately positioning the infant and moving electrodes, tape, or other artifacts that limit the surface area to be scanned. The nurse's assistance in performing an ultrasound examination is important to monitor the infant's tolerance of the procedure and provide information that may be of diagnostic importance to the ultrasonographer. In addition, the nurse's presence at the bedside allows for immediate visual feedback and interpretation of the extent of the pathologic condition that may be present. This knowledge allows better support of the infant's parents during further diagnostic testing and treatment decisions after their discussions with the medical staff. Interaction with the ultrasonographer at the bedside may also help the nurse to anticipate future health care needs of both an immediate and long-term nature.

Magnetic Resonance Imaging

The theoretical basis of magnetic resonance imaging is a development of research conducted since the 1940s for studying atomic nuclear structure, which resulted in the awarding of the Nobel Prize for physics in 1952 to Edward Purcell and Felix Block. In addition to the advances in atomic nuclear research, other developments, such as the development of superconductivity and advances in computer programming, were necessary before this this concept was applied to diagnostic imaging.

As an imaging modality, magnetic resonance imaging has several advantages over CT (Dubowitz & Bydder, 1985; Friedman et al., 1989; Horowitz, 1995; Moss et al., 1984):

1. Magnetic resonance, like ultrasonography, does not use ionizing radiation to produce the image, but rather uses magnetic fields and radio waves.
2. The magnetic resonance image depends on three separate molecular parameters that are sensitive to changes in structure and bioactivity rather than on x-ray photon interaction with tissue electrons, as in CT.
3. The region of the body imaged in magnetic resonance imaging is not limited by the gantry geometry as in CT, but can be controlled electronically, allowing imaging in transverse planes as well as in true sagittal, coronal, and oblique planes.
4. Magnetic resonance images are free of high-intensity artifacts produced in CT scans by sharp, dense bone or metallic surgical clips.

The principal disadvantages of magnetic resonance imaging are its high cost and limited availability and its limited use for clinically unstable infants on life support, because there is interference by the strong magnetic field with monitoring devices and limited access to the infant during the procedure (Horowitz, 1995; Kirks, 1991; Swischuk, 1989, 1995).

Despite the disadvantages of magnetic resonance imaging, its clinical applications are rapidly expanding. The image quality is excellent, with the advances in the use of surface coils, and more sensitive head and body coils allow structures such as cranial nerves and small joints to be evaluated more precisely. The increased use of gating and fast scanning techniques has improved the evaluation of the spinal cord and of vessels and mediastinal pathologic conditions (Dubowitz & Bydder, 1985; Friedman et al., 1989; Horowitz, 1995; Moss et al., 1984; Swischuk, 1989, 1995).

Biophysical Principles

All particles in an atom have either a positive or negative charge and a "spin" like a tiny spinning top. The total spin of the protons and neutrons on the nucleus is the sum of the individual spins. Moving charges create magnetic fields, thus the nucleus of an atom develops north and south magnetic dipoles (Bushong, 1992; Friedman et al., 1989; Horowitz, 1995). In most materials such as soft tissue, these little spinning magnetic dipoles are randomly oriented (Fig. 36–12*A*). This random orientation causes all the spins and magnetic forces to cancel in the material so that the net magnetic force is zero. However, if the material is placed in a strong magnetic field, the magnetic dipoles align themselves, much like a compass needle aligns itself with the Earth's magnetic field. The alignment of these magnetic dipoles produces a net magnetic force or vector that is oriented parallel to the direction of the imposed magnetic field (see Fig. 36–12*B*). Not all magnetic dipoles become aligned; some are in constant thermal motion so that nuclei are being continually knocked out of alignment (Bushong, 1992; Friedman et al., 1989; Horowitz, 1995).

In magnetic resonance imaging, after imposing the strong magnetic field to align the molecular magnetic dipoles, radio frequency pulses are applied. The known specific frequency of these radio waves displaces the net magnetic moment by an amount determined by the strength and duration of the pulse. The frequency is directly proportional to the strength of the magnetic field and is known as the resonant frequency. After the pulse, the

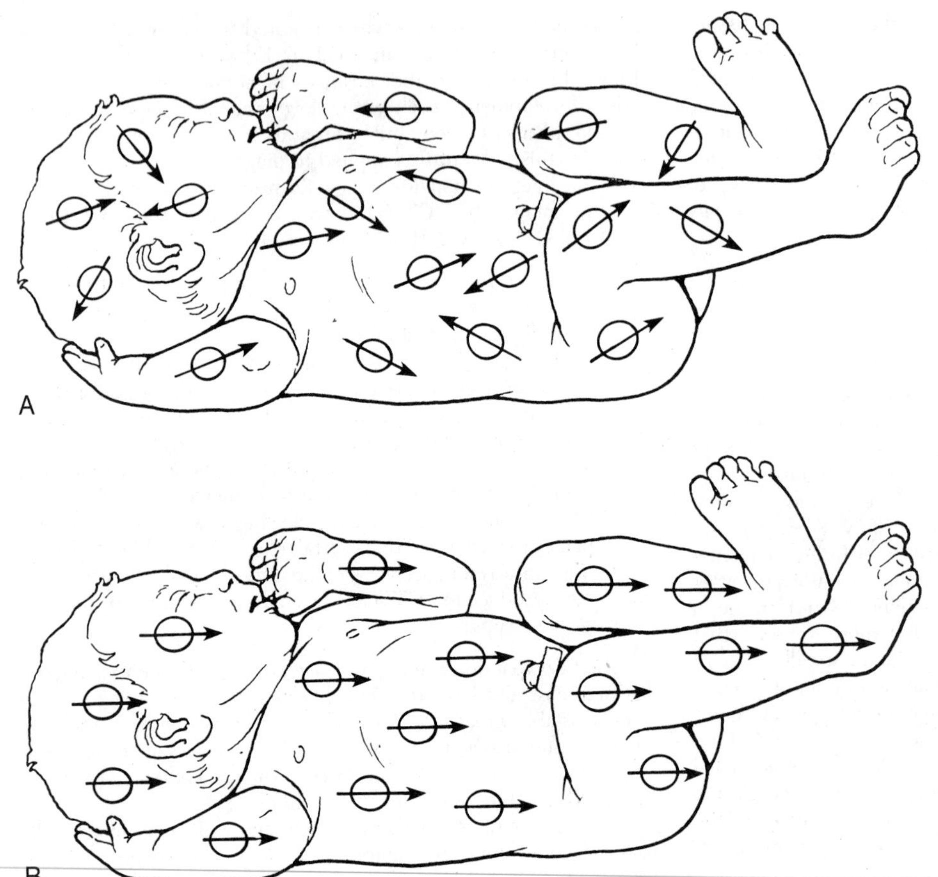

FIGURE 36–12. *A,* All the magnetic moments are randomly oriented in the body so that the net magnetic charge is zero. *B,* Applied radio frequency pulses align the magnetic moments along a predetermined axis. The rate at which the atoms return to their "normal" magnetic moment after the radio frequency is stopped is characteristic for physiologic and pathologic tissues and is responsible for creating the magnetic resonance image.

protons emit radio frequencies as they return to their original orientation. Therefore, the frequency of signals emitted by the protons after the application with radio frequency waves reflects their position in the tissue. Although any stable nuclei can be used in theory, hydrogen is the most abundant and has the strongest resonance (Bushong, 1992; Friedman et al., 1989; Horowitz, 1995).

After placement of protons in a magnetic field, the alignment of protons is not instantaneous but increases exponentially with a time constant characterized by T_1, or spin-lattice relaxation time, which reflects the interaction of the hydrogen nucleus with its molecular environment (Bushong, 1992; Friedman et al., 1989; Horowitz, 1995). T_1 characterizes the return of the net magnetization from its displaced position to its normal vertical position resulting from spin-lattice interactions. To form an image, the radio frequency pulses must be applied repetitively. After each radio frequency pulse, the net magnetic force of the sample is reduced. Therefore, too rapid a radio frequency repetition depletes the magnetization of the tissue and an image cannot be produced. Thus, radio frequency pulses are sequenced with a certain time interval to allow the magnetic force to be reestablished. The longer the time interval, the greater the magnetic force and the longer the imaging time (Friedman et al., 1989; Horowitz, 1995).

After exposure to the radio frequency pulse, the signal emitted from the sample of protons decays exponentially with a time constant referred to as T_2, or spin–spin relaxation time. T_2 reflects the magnetic interactions between protons. T_2 characterizes the exponential loss of signal caused by dephasing or desynchronization of magnetic force, which results from spin–spin interactions (Bushong, 1992; Friedman et al., 1989; Horowitz, 1995). The interval between the application of a radio frequency pulse and the emitted signal depends on the alignment and synchronization of magnetic dipoles. A strong magnetic force results in a long interval for the emitted signal after the pulse. Thus, the contrast between tissues with different values of T_2 changes. T_1 is not equal to T_2, because each nucleus is not located within identical magnetic fields. Each hydrogen nucleus is subject to different local magnetic fields because of the presence or absence of other hydrogen nuclei.

The third parameter that affects image resolution of magnetic resonance imaging is spin density. Spin density refers to the strength of the signal received from the nuclei before any of the decay processes have taken place (Bushong, 1992; Friedman et al., 1989; Horowitz, 1995). This is proportional to the number of nuclei within the detection volume of the scanner. Spin density is an indication of hydrogen concentration in the tissue.

A magnetic resonance image results from the mixture of these three properties (T_1, T_2, and spin density) unique to each tissue. The values of T_1 and T_2 for various tissues have been defined. There is a wide range of values between various types of tissue, and considerable differences have been documented between pathologic tissue and normal tissue (Friedman et al., 1989; Horowitz, 1995; Moss et al., 1984). Each number defined for the relaxation times (T_1 and T_2) for various tissues is dependent upon the primary external magnetic field and thus may vary from scanner to scanner. The visual projection of the magnetic resonance image is similar to that obtained in computed tomography. By controlling the gradient field of radio frequency pulses, a series of projections at uniform angles through the tissue can be collected. The computer can then reconstruct the image and can emphasize the individual T_1, T_2, or spin density parameters to further define detail (Friedman et al., 1989; Horowitz, 1995; Moss et al., 1984).

The spatial resolution of an MRI scan compares favorably to CT. If the object scanned is of high tissue contrast, a lesion as small as 1 mm can be defined. As more data are being collected on this imaging modality, even greater spatial resolution is being obtained. As stronger magnetic fields are used, the emitted signals become stronger, and greater resolution may be possible using even higher radio frequency pulses (Horowitz, 1995; Moss et al., 1984).

MRI has greater ability than CT to detect differences between low-contrast structures. The difference in T_1 and T_2 MRI between biologic tissues is frequently 10 percent or more. For example, in CT scans, the x-ray photon attenuation coefficient between gray and white matter is approximately 0.5 percent, whereas the differences in T_1, T_2, and spin density between gray and white matter are great, allowing for more accurate definition of these two tissues (Horowitz, 1995; Moss et al., 1984). Thus, MRI has become the diagnostic imaging mode of choice for certain neurologic conditions such as multiple sclerosis. Although not readily done in neonatal patients, MRI may be useful in the early diagnosis of periventricular leukomalacia before development of the characteristic cystic lesions (Dubowitz & Bydder, 1985).

Safety of Magnetic Resonance Imaging

MRI scanning uses three kinds of fields associated with the imaging process: (1) a static, moderately strong magnetic field, (2) a switched, weaker magnetic field gradient, and (3) radio frequency waves. The energies associated with the imaging process are approximately 10^{-8} eV/quantum, which are too weak to cause ionization or breakage of chemical bonds (Bushong, 1992; Horowitz, 1995; Moss et al., 1984). Energies associated with body temperature elevations are 10^5 to 10^6 times greater, so temperature effects are far more disruptive to chemical bonds than the energy associated with MRI (Horowitz, 1995; Moss et al., 1984).

In the laboratory, biologic responses on animals, chromosomes, plant seeds, and molecular specimens have shown effects only after extremely high intensities of MRI energy. There is an apparent dose response relationship present, although the biologic threshold is exceedingly high. In humans, tests for genetic damage have proved negative, and studies of workers in particle accelerators exposed to static magnetic fields six to seven times greater than those in MRI have shown no detrimental effect (Bushong, 1992; Friedman et al., 1989; Horowitz, 1995; Shapiro, 1990). Long-term studies of humans exposed to radio frequency waves have not demonstrated any deleterious effect (Bushong, 1984; Friedman et al., 1989; Horowitz, 1995; Moss et al., 1984).

The hazards of MRI relate primarily to any ferromagnetic objects (e.g., tools, oxygen cylinders, watches, bank cards, pens, and paper clips) that are accelerated toward the center of the magnetic field. The magnetic propulsion of these objects can result in projectile damage. Thus, any patient with a pacemaker or an extensive metal prosthesis should be excluded from this imaging technique. In addition, MRI has not been fully tested on pregnant women.

Collaborative Care

The care of a neonate who requires an MRI scan includes the careful preparation and elimination of any ferromagnetic objects brought near the magnetic field. The infant must be clinically stable, because the strong magnetic field affects some monitoring devices and visualization of the neonate is impossible during the scan. Surface respiratory monitors and possibly an esophageal stethoscope may be used. An MRI scan is degraded by motion, so the infant must be positioned comfortably and safely within the magnetic cylinders. Because the infant must remain motionless for a period of minutes, an MRI scan is best done after the infant has been fed and is sleeping. If the infant is unable to remain motionless for the duration of the scan, oral chloral hydrate sedation may be recommended.

CONCLUSION

Marked technical advances over the past 2 decades have produced a variety of imaging methods for use in the diagnosis, treatment, and evaluation of neonates. Great expenditures have been directed toward improving image presentation and quality on the assumption that a trained clinical eye can make diagnostic use of the data provided. Investigations are useful only in so far as they reduce the diagnostic uncertainty. The final product of any radiologic imaging procedure is not a set of photographic pictures, but a diagnostic opinion that should be of benefit to the infant's management. Before initiating any imaging modality, the physician should always consider whether further information is really needed and to select the imaging modality that will give the required information with sufficient reliability and with minimal risk to the patient. The value of any diagnostic imaging examination must be balanced against the potential hazards.

REFERENCES

Alpen, E. L. (1990). *Radiation biophysics*. Englewood Cliffs, NJ: Prentice Hall.

Bushong, S. C. (1992). *Radiologic science for technologists: Physics, biology & protection* (5th ed.). St. Louis: Mosby–Year Book.

Cowan, F. P. (1959). Natural radioactive background. In H. Blatz (Ed.), *Radiation hygiene handbook*. New York: McGraw-Hill.

Dubowitz, L. M. S., & Bydder, G. M. (1985). Nuclear magnetic resonance imaging in the diagnosis and follow-up of neonatal cerebral injury. *Clinics in Perinatology, 12*(1), 243–260.

Fanaroff, A. A., & Martin, R. J. (Eds.). (1997). *Neonatal-perinatal medicine* (6th ed.). St. Louis: C. V. Mosby.

Feigenbaum, H. (1986). *Echocardiography*. Philadelphia: Lea & Febiger.

Friedman, B. R., Jones, J. P., Chaves-Munoz, J., et al. (1989). *Principles of MRI*. New York: McGraw-Hill.

Gofman, J. W. (1983). *Radiation and human health*. New York: Pantheon Books.

Gofman, J. W. (1990). *Radiation-induced cancer from low-dose exposure: An independent analysis*. San Francisco, CA: Committee for Nuclear Responsibility.

Gyll, C. (1985). *A handbook of pediatric radiography* (2nd ed.). Oxford: Blackwell Scientific Publications.

Gyll, C., & Blake, N. (1986). *Pediatric diagnostic imaging*. London: William Heinemann Medical Books.

Haller, J. O., & Slovis, T. L. (1984). *Introduction to radiology in clinical pediatrics*. Chicago: Year Book Medical Publishers.

Hilton, S., & Edwards, D. K. III. (1994). *Practical pediatric radiology* (2nd ed.). Philadelphia: W. B. Saunders.

Horowitz, A. L. (1995). *Magnetic resonance imaging (MRI): Physics for radiologists: A visual approach* (3rd ed.). New York: Springer-Verlag.

Juhl, J. H., & Crummy, A. B. (Eds.). (1993). *Paul and Juhl's essentials of radiologic imaging* (6th ed.). Philadelphia: J. B. Lippincott.

Kelsey, C. A. (1985). *Essentials of radiology physics*. St. Louis: Warren H. Green.

Kirks, D. R. (1991). *Practical pediatric imaging* (2nd ed.). Boston: Little, Brown.

Martin, D. J. (1985). Neonatal disorders diagnosed with ultrasound. *Clinics in Perinatology, 12*(1), 219–242.

Moss, A. A., Ring, E. G., & Higgins, C. B. (Eds.). (1984). *NMR, CT and interventional radiology*. San Francisco: University of California Printing Department.

National Council on Radiation Protection and Measurements. (1993a). *Risk estimates for radiation protection*. NCRP Report Number 115. Bethesda, MD: National Council on Radiation Protection Publication.

National Council on Radiation Protection and Measurements. (1993b). *Research needs for radiation protection*. NCRP Report Number 117. Bethesda, MD: National Council on Radiation Protection Publication.

National Council on Radiation Protection and Measurements. (1993c). *A practical guide to the determination of human exposure to radiofrequency fields.* NCRP Report Number 119. Bethesda, MD: National Council on Radiation Protection Publication.

Noz, M. E., & Maguire, G. Q. (1985). *Radiation protection in the radiologic and health sciences* (2nd ed.). Philadelphia: Lea & Febiger.

Poznanski, A. K. (1976). *Practical approaches to pediatric radiology.* Chicago: Year Book Medical Publishers.

Poznanski, A. K., Kanellitsas, C., Roloff, D. W., & Borer, R. C. (1974). Radiation exposure to personnel in a neonatal nursery. *Pediatrics, 54,* 139–141.

Shapiro, J. (1990). *Radiation protection: A guide for scientists and physicians* (3rd ed.). Cambridge, MA: Harvard University Press.

Siddiqui, A.R. (1985). *Nuclear imaging in pediatrics.* Chicago: Year Book Medical Publishers.

Squire, L. F., & Novelline, R. A. (1988). *Fundamentals of radiology* (4th ed.). Cambridge, MA: Harvard University Press.

Swischuk, L. E. (1995). *Differential diagnosis in pediatric radiology* (2nd ed.). Baltimore: Williams & Wilkins.

Swischuk, L. E. (1989). *Imaging of the newborn, infant, and young child* (3rd ed.). Baltimore: Williams & Wilkins.

Treves, S. T. (Ed.). (1995). *Pediatric nuclear medicine* (2nd ed.). New York: Springer-Verlag.

Vogler, J. B., Helms, C. A., & Collen, P. W. (1986). *Normal variants and pitfalls in imaging.* Philadelphia: W. B. Saunders.

Walker, J. M., & Margouleff, D. (Eds.). (1984). *A clinical manual of nuclear medicine.* Norwalk, CT: Appleton-Century-Crofts.

Wesenberg, R. L. (1973). *The newborn chest.* Hagerstown, MD: Harper & Row.

Whalen, J. P., & Balter, S. (1984). *Radiation risks in medical imaging.* Chicago: Year Book Medical Publishers.

CHAPTER 37

Diagnostic Tests and Laboratory Values

JEANNE HARJO

Care of the neonate can involve numerous diagnostic procedures used to identify dysfunction related to birth, prematurity, or congenital malformations. Although these procedures are usually helpful in developing a medical or surgical diagnosis, many implications for nursing care exist. Appropriate assessment of pre- and postprocedural status is vital in promoting optimal outcomes for an already compromised infant. This chapter highlights some of the more common diagnostic tests and laboratory values. For full discussions of these tests and values, see the appropriate assessment chapters. The values given in this chapter represent the broader normal range, but values in a specific chapter may vary slightly, depending on what the author considers to be within normal limits. Every attempt has been made to provide consistent diagnostic and laboratory values. In addition, this chapter describes the procedures and pre- and postprocedural care considerations.

LABORATORY VALUES

A wide variety of laboratory tests are available for use in both diagnosis and care of the neonate. Although a general range of normal values is established, many hospitals have compiled their own list of acceptable values; specific laboratories should be contacted when evaluating laboratory results (Tables 37–1 to 37–18).

CARDIOLOGY PROCEDURES

Cardiac Catheterization

The use of radiopaque dye allows for clarification of congenital heart defects. A radiopaque catheter is inserted into an arm or leg vessel by percutaneous puncture or cutdown. Under fluoroscopy, the catheter is visualized and passed into the heart. Selected chambers and vessels of the heart can then be evaluated for size and function. Intracardiac pressures and oxygen saturations can also be measured during this procedure.

Immobilization of the neonate and constant monitoring are required during cardiac catheterization. The infant must be restrained to maintain supine positioning. Electrocardiographic electrodes must also be placed to provide constant vital sign monitoring. To maintain proper positioning during the procedure, sedation may be a consideration.

A local anesthetic agent is administered at the insertion site. The catheter is then inserted and guided into the chambers and vessels of the heart. Contrast medium is injected through the catheter in order to visualize the various cardiac structures.

After the desired information is obtained, the catheter is carefully removed. If a cutdown was performed, the vessel is ligated and the skin is sutured. Pressure should be applied over a percutaneous puncture site to enhance clot formation. For continued bleeding problems, pressure dressings may be applied to the insertion site; these must be checked frequently for active bleeding.

Following cardiac catheterization, vital signs should be measured frequently, comparing them with precatheterization baseline vital signs. Evaluation for localized bleeding or signs of hypotension resulting in changes in heart rate and blood pressure is essential. Assessment of the insertion site and affected extremity for bleeding, color, peripheral pulses, temperature, and capillary refill should continue for at least 24 hours after the procedure.

Complications of catheterization may include hypovolemia (as a result of bleeding or fluid loss during the procedure), infection, thrombosis, or tissue necrosis. Peripheral intravenous fluids may be required to compensate for fluid losses. Localized infection of the catheterization site may be demonstrated by redness, swelling, warmth, or drainage. Management usually involves use of antibiotic ointment on the site followed by protection with a dry sterile dressing. Assessments of skin color and temperature, as well as quality and characteristics of bilateral peripheral pulses, are essential after cardiac catheterization.

Echocardiography

Echocardiography is a commonly used noninvasive diagnostic procedure. By means of high-frequency sound waves, vibrations are sent to the heart. Structures within the heart then reflect energy, which is transmitted into a visual image. Single-dimension echocardiography allows for evaluation of anatomic structures, including valves, chambers, and vessels. Two-dimensional echocardiography provides more in-depth information about relationships between the heart and the great vessels (Flanagan & Fyler, 1994).

Echocardiographic examination also allows for evaluation of structural function within the heart. This information can be important not only in preoperative assessment of cardiac defects but also in postoperative evaluation of procedures.

Doppler echocardiography is used in various forms to evaluate characteristics of blood flow through the heart, valves, and great vessels. It can measure not only cardiac output but also flow velocity changes as demonstrated in stenotic lesions. Regurgitation through insufficiently functioning valves can also be identified through Doppler studies. Directional Doppler echocardiography can also be used to identify shunting through a patent ductus arteriosus (Hohn & Stanton, 1995).

Electrocardiography

Electrocardiography is another noninvasive diagnostic tool that is sometimes employed in the neonatal population. It is used in conjunction with other diagnostic measures to evaluate cardiac function—specifically, circulatory demands placed on individual heart chambers. Dysrhythmias may also be diagnosed by the use of electrocardiography (Flanagan & Fyler, 1994).

GENETIC PROCEDURES

Chromosome Analysis

Analysis of chromosome composition can assist in identification of various genetic disorders. A blood specimen is obtained from the infant and used to harvest an actual set of chromosomes. During active cell division, usually during metaphase, the chromosomes are photographed and then arranged in pairs by number. This *karyotype* is then evaluated for the appropriate number of pairs, chromosome size, and structure. Specific genetic disorders can be associated with abnormal numbers of chromosomes, as in trisomy 21, or abnormal structure of chromosomes, as in cri du chat syndrome, which reflects loss of part of the short arm of chromosome 5 (Kuller et al., 1996). Abnormal genes on the chromosomes can also cause genetic disorders, such as Duchenne's muscular dystrophy, an X-linked recessive disorder. Bone marrow cells may be analyzed for chromosomes if a more rapid evaluation is required. Skin fibroblast analysis is required when an infant has been transfused, making lymphocyte analysis inaccurate. In cases such as stillbirth, tissue biopsy specimens can be used for chromosome testing because viable lymphocytes are absent (Jones & Cahill, 1994).

Sweat Chloride

The sweat chloride procedure is an evaluation of sodium and chloride content in sweat. It is a mechanism by which neonates can be evaluated for cystic fibrosis. Sweat, produced by an electrical current, is collected onto a gauze pad or filter paper. The sweat content is then evaluated; a sweat chloride of greater than 60 mEq/L is consistent with cystic fibrosis (Vanderhoof et al., 1994).

GASTROINTESTINAL PROCEDURES

Barium Enema

A barium enema is used to evaluate the structure and function of the large intestine. The diagnosis of disorders such as Hirschsprung's disease and meconium plug syndrome can easily be supported by the use of this procedure.

In the enema procedure, a contrast solution such as barium sulfate is instilled and a series of films are taken under fluoroscopy. The infant must be well restrained, initially starting in the supine position. As the contrast solution is instilled, its flow through the bowel is observed as the infant's position is changed. A series of abdominal x-ray films should be taken once the bowel has been filled with contrast solution. Follow-up films may also be necessary to document evacuation of the contrast solution from the bowel. Evaluation of the bowel is essential following this procedure in order to prevent constipation or obstruction. Assessment of bowel elimination is an important nursing concern following barium enema.

Upper Gastrointestinal Series With Small Bowel Follow-Through

As in the barium enema, barium sulfate or other water-soluble contrast solution is used in this procedure. However, the contrast solution is swallowed in order to examine the upper gastrointestinal tract. Three main areas are examined (Kenner et al., 1988):

1. The esophagus, for size, patency, reflux, and presence of a fistula or swallowing abnormality.
2. The stomach, for anatomic abnormalities, patency, and motility.
3. The small intestine, for structures, patency, and function.

Follow-up x-ray films may be desirable to evaluate the emptying ability of the stomach and intestinal motility as the contrast material moves through the small bowel. Again, care of the infant includes assessment of temperature and cardiac and respiratory status throughout the procedure. The nurse should be alert for reflux or vomiting, which can be accompanied by aspiration. Evacuation of contrast material from the bowel remains a concern after upper gastrointestinal series with small bowel follow-through and should be monitored by the nurse. It is also possible for fluid to be pulled out of the vascular compartment and into the bowel. The side effects are thus fluid loss and hypotension. It is imperative that the health care team assess the infant for signs of these complications.

Rectal Suction Biopsy

Rectal biopsy is a procedure commonly used to evaluate the presence or absence of ganglion cells in the bowel (the latter being seen in Hirschsprung's disease). Prior to a rectal biopsy, it is essential to obtain bleeding times, prothrombin time, partial thromboplastin time, and platelet counts as well as a spun hematocrit to ensure that the infant is not in danger of excessive bleeding.

- The infant is positioned in a supine fashion with legs held toward abdomen.
- Small specimens of rectal tissue from the mucosa and submucosa levels are excised with a suction blade apparatus inserted through the anus into the bowel.
- Specimens are evaluated by the pathology department for the composition of ganglion cells.

Care of the infant following this procedure should focus on assessments for bleeding or intestinal perforation. These assessments should include evaluation of vital signs for increased heart rate or decreased blood pressure, fever, persistent guaiac-positive stools, or frank rectal bleeding (Kenner et al., 1988).

Liver Biopsy

Open or closed liver biopsy may be required in the neonatal population. Open liver biopsy is a surgical procedure that requires general anesthesia, whereas a closed liver biopsy may be done using local anesthetic. As with the rectal biopsy, coagulation studies including bleeding time, platelet count, and spun hematocrit are essential. Preoperative care may include sedation of the infant, requiring frequent monitoring of vital signs. Throughout the procedure, assessment of vital signs remains essential in identifying changes in hemodynamics or respiratory states. Following the procedure, assessment of vital signs for signs and symptoms of hemorrhage is essential. Indications of hemorrhage also include decreases in the hemoglobin and hematocrit, thus making laboratory monitoring an important element of postbiopsy care. The biopsy site must be evaluated for signs of active bleeding, ecchymosis, swelling, or infection.

Abdominal Ultrasonography

Ultrasonography is a mechanism by which sound waves are emitted from a transducer through tissues and then collected by the transducer as they bounce off of structures. These sound waves can then be visualized for evaluation.

Ultrasonography of the abdomen enables the evaluation of structures such as the liver, biliary system, and gallbladder. Space-occupying lesions such as cysts or tumors can also be identified and measured by the use of ultrasonography (Vanderhoof et al., 1994).

GENITOURINARY PROCEDURES

Cystoscopy

Utilization of this procedure provides direct visualization of the urinary structures, including the bladder, urethra, and urethral orifices. This enables the diagnosis of abnormalities in the structure of the bladder and urinary tract.

A cystoscopy is performed under general anesthesia. The urethral opening is prepared with an antiseptic solution followed by sterile draping. The lubricated cystoscope is inserted through the urethra, and visualization of the urinary structures is performed.

As with any postanesthesia patient, postprocedural care includes vital sign assessment. However, particular attention should be paid toward assessing for adequate urinary output and the presence of hematuria (Spitzer et al., 1995).

Excretory Urography and Intravenous Pyelography

Complementary to the evaluation of structures by cystoscopy are excretory urography and intravenous pyelography, which not only evaluate structures but also focus on the function of those structures. Small amounts of contrast media are injected through the intravenous route. As the contrast material is excreted through the urinary system, a sequence of x-ray films is taken. These films reflect the configuration of organs as well as the rate of excretion of the contrast media.

These procedures are relatively safe for use in the neonatal population and should result in no postprocedural complications.

Radioisotope Renal Scan

This procedure includes the intravenous injection of a radioisotope, after which radioactive counters monitor the movement of the radioisotope through the urinary system. Comparison of the kidneys in terms of blood flow, renal tubule function, and excretion is made possible by this procedure. Following injection of the radioisotope, films are taken approximately every 5 minutes for at least 30 minutes. Follow-up films may be desirable if compromised kidney function is suspected.

It must be remembered that the infant's urine is radioactive for 24 hours after injection of the radioisotope. Consequently, gloves should be worn when changing diapers or handling soiled diapers. Also, provisions must be made for linens or trash that is contaminated with radioactive urine.

Voiding Cystourethrogram

The purpose of this procedure is to visualize the lower urinary tract following instillation of contrast media through urethral catheterization. The infant's bladder is emptied after catheterization and then filled with the contrast media. Serial films under fluoroscopy in a variety of positions are taken during voiding. Following voiding, additional films are obtained. Pathologic results of a voiding cystourethrogram demonstrate residual urine in the bladder, as with a neurogenic bladder, posterior valve obstructions, or vesicourethral reflux.

As with the cystoscopy procedure, the infant should be evaluated for hematuria. In addition, symptoms of infection (fever, cloudy or sedimented urine, foul-smelling urine) as a result of contaminated catheterization should be evaluated.

Renal Ultrasonography

Using the same technique as for abdominal ultrasonography, kidney ultrasonography is used to evaluate size and position of kidneys, obstructions in urinary structures, or abnormal accumulation of fluid such as residual urine found in the bladder.

NEUROLOGIC PROCEDURES

Computed Tomography and Magnetic Resonance Imaging

Chapter 36, Diagnostic Imaging, gives an in-depth description of the biophysics of computed tomography and magnetic resonance imaging. They are used in the neonatal population to identify structural defects, atrophy, hydrocephaly, or hemorrhage. They are noninvasive procedures that can be quickly and safely performed (Miller & Murray, 1995).

Electroencephalography

Electroencephalographic examination records the electrical activity of the brain. Numerous electrodes are placed at precise locations on the infant's head in order to record electrical impulses from various parts of the brain. This procedure can be important in diagnosing lesions or tumors, identifying nonfunctional areas of the brain, or pinpointing the focus of seizure activity.

The infant may require sedation during this procedure to prevent crying or movement. As much equipment as is safely possible should be removed in order to decrease electrical interference. Also, calming procedures such as decreasing light stimulation or warming the environment may assist in quieting the infant during electroencephalography. The infant should be closely observed throughout the procedure for any signs of seizure activity.

Radioisotope Brain Scan

As described with radioisotope renal scans, intravenous injection of radioisotope solution and monitoring of uptake in the brain constitute a diagnostic procedure used in neonates. At specified intervals, various views of the brain are taken, showing the presence of the radioisotope in abnormal brain tissue. Tumors or abscesses as well as areas of hematoma or infarct can be identified with this procedure.

Head Ultrasonography

Ultrasonography of the head is a noninvasive procedure commonly used to assess intracranial structures. Ventricular size, intraventricular hemorrhage, or intracranial masses can be detected using ultrasonography. Accumulation of cerebrospinal fluid, as seen in hydrocephalus or shunt malfunction, is easily diagnosed with this procedure (Miller & Murray, 1995).

RESPIRATORY PROCEDURES

Laryngoscopy and Bronchoscopy

These procedures are commonly done in tandem under general anesthesia. Examination of structures by direct visualization provides the opportunity to identify congenital anomalies, obstructions, masses, or mucous plugs and to evaluate stridor or respiratory dysfunction.

Possible complications related to these procedures include bronchospasm, laryngeal spasms, laryngeal edema, or pneumothorax or bradycardia resulting in hypoxia. Close respiratory observation in the immediate postoperative period is essential to maintain a patent airway and promote optimal gas exchange. In addition, bleeding may occur after tissue biopsy, but frank bleeding is abnormal and should be investigated (Nickerson et al., 1995).

REFERENCES

Flanagan, M. F., & Fyler, D. C. (1994). Cardiac disease. In G. B. Avery, M. A. Fletcher, & M. G. MacDonald (Eds.), *Neonatology: Pathophysiology and management of the neonate* (4th ed., pp. 516–559). Philadelphia: J. B. Lippincott.

Hohn, A. R., & Stanton, R. E. (1995). The cardiovascular system. In A. A. Fanaroff & R. J. Martin (Eds.), *Neonatal-perinatal medicine: Diseases of the fetus and infant* (5th ed., pp. 883–940). St. Louis: C. V. Mosby.

Jones, O. W., & Cahill, T. C. (1994). Basic genetics and patterns of inheritance. In R. K. Creasy & R. Resnik (Eds.), *Maternal-fetal medicine* (3rd. ed., pp. 3–60). Philadelphia: W. B. Saunders.

Kenner, C. A., Harjo, J., & Brueggemeyer, A. (1988). *Neonatal surgery: A nursing perspective*. Orlando, FL: Grune & Stratton.

Kuller, J. A., Chescheir, N. C., & Cefalo, R. C. (1996). *Prenatal diagnosis & reproductive genetics*. St. Louis: C. V. Mosby.

Miller, M. J., & Murray, G. S. (1995). Noninvasive diagnostic techniques. In A. A. Fanaroff & R. J. Martin (Eds.), *Neonatal-perinatal medicine: Diseases of the fetus and infant* (5th ed., pp 700–702). St. Louis: C. V. Mosby.

Nickerson, B. G., Barnhart, S. L., & Czervinske, M. P. (1995). Bronchoscopy. In S. L. Barnhart & M. P. Czervinske (Eds.), *Perinatal and pediatric respiratory care* (pp. 103–113). Philadelphia: W. B. Saunders.

Spitzer, A., Bernstein, J., Boichis, H., & Edelmann, C. M., Jr. (1995). Kidney and urinary tract. In A. A. Fanaroff & R. J. Martin (Eds.), *Neonatal-perinatal medicine: Diseases of the fetus and infant* (5th ed., pp. 1293–1327). St. Louis: C. V. Mosby.

Vanderhoof, J. A., Zach, T. L, & Adrian, T. E. (1994). Gastrointestinal disease. In G. B. Avery, M. A. Fletcher, & M. G. MacDonald (Eds.), *Neonatology: Pathophysiology and management of the neonate* (4th ed., pp. 605–629). Philadelphia: J. B. Lippincott.

APPENDIX

TABLE 37–1 Summary of Common Laboratory Values

Test	Normal Value	Test	Normal Value
Complete Blood Count (CBC)		***Serum Electrolytes***	
Red blood cell count (RBC)	5.1 to 5.8 (1,000,000/mm^3)	Sodium (Na)	135 to 145 mEq/L
White blood cell count (WBC)	18,000/mm^3	Potassium (K)	4.5 to 6.8 mEq/L
Hemoglobin (Hgb)	16.8 to 18.4 g/dl	Chloride (Cl)	95 to 110 mEq/L
Hematocrit (Hct)	52% to 58%	Carbon dioxide (CO_2)	20 to 25 mmol/L
Platelets	150,000 to 400,000/mm^3		
Differential		***Serum Chemistries***	
Band neutrophils (Bands)	1600/mm^3 (9%)	Blood urea nitrogen (BUN)	6.0 to 30.0 mg/dl
Segmented neutrophils (Segs)	9400/mm^3 (52%)	Calcium (Ca)	7 to 10 mg/dl
Eosinophils (Eos)	400/mm^3 (2.2%)	Creatinine (Cr)	0.2 to 0.9 mg/dl
Basophils (Baso)	100/mm^3 (0.6%)	Glucose (G)	40 to 97 mg/dl
Lymphocytes (Lymphs)	5500/mm^3 (31%)	Magnesium (Mg)	1.5 to 2.5 mg/dl
Monocytes (Monos)	1050/mm^3 (5.8%)	Phosphorus (P)	5.4 to 10.9 mg/dl

Data from Fanaroff, A., & Martin, R. (1987). *Neonatal-perinatal medicine: Diseases of the fetus and infant* (4th ed.). St. Louis: C. V. Mosby; Cohen, S., Kenner, C., & Hollingsworth, A. (1991). *Maternal, neonatal and women's health nursing*. Springhouse, PA: Springhouse; Kenner, C., Harjo, J., & Brueggemeyer, A. (1988). *Neonatal surgery: A nursing perspective*. Orlando: Grune & Stratton; and Streeter, N. S. (1986). *High risk neonatal care*. Rockville, MD: Aspen Publishers.

TABLE 37–2 Summary of Normal Urine Laboratory Values

Test	Age	Normal Value
Urine Values		
Ammonia	2 to 12 months	4 to 20 μEq/min/m^2
Calcium	1 week	<2 mg/dl
Chloride	Infant	1.7 to 8.5 mEq/24 hours
Creatinine	Newborn	7 to 10 mg/kg/day
Glucose	Preterm	60 to 130 mg/dl
	Full-term	12 to 32 mg/dl
Glucose (renal threshold)	Preterm	2.21 to 2.84 mg/ml
	Full-term	2.20 to 3.68 mg/ml
Magnesium		180 ± 10 mg/1.73 m^2/dl
Osmolality	Infant	50 to 600 mOsm/kg
Potassium		26 to 123 mEq/L
Protein		<100 mg/m^2/dl
Sodium		0.3 to 3.5 mEq/dl (6 to 10 mEq/m^2)
Specific gravity	Newborn	1.006 to 1.008

From Ichikawa, I. (1990). *Pediatric textbook of fluids and electrolytes*. Baltimore: Williams & Wilkins. Reprinted with permission.

TABLE 37–3 Electrocardiographic Data in the Neonate*

Parameter	Age: *0–24 Hours*	*1–7 Days*	*8–30 Days*	*1–3 Months*
Heart rate (beats/min)	119 (94–145)	133 (100–175)	163 (115–190)	154 (124–190)
PR interval (sec)	0.1 (0.07–0.12)	0.09 (0.07–0.12)	0.09 (0.07–0.11)	0.1 (0.07–0.13)
P wave amplitude II	1.5 (0.8–2.3)	1.6 (0.8–2.5)	1.6 (0.08–2.4)	1.6 (0.8–2.4)
QRS duration (sec)	0.065 (0.05–0.08)	0.06 (0.04–0.08)	0.06 (0.04–0.07)	0.06 (0.05–0.08)
QRS axis (degrees)	135 (60–180)	125 (80–160)	110 (60–160)	80 (40–120)
R amplitude V_{4R} (mm)	8.6 (4–14.2)	—	6.3 (3.3–8.5)	5.1 (1.1–10.1)
R amplitude V_1 (mm)	11.9 (4.3–21)	—	11.1 (3.3–18.7)	11.2 (4.5–18)
R amplitude V_5 (mm)	10.2 (4–18)	10.7 (3.4–19)	11.9 (3.5–27)	13.6 (7.3–20.7)
R amplitude V_6 (mm)	3.3 (2.3–7)	5.1 (2.2–13.1)	6.7 (1.7–20.5)	8.4 (3.6–12.9)
S amplitude V_{4R} (mm)	3.8 (0.2–13)	—	1.8 (0.8–4.6)	3.4 (0–9.3)
S amplitude V_1 (mm)	9.7 (1.1–19.1)	—	6.1 (0–15)	7.5 (0.5–17.1)
S amplitude V_5 (mm)	11.9 (0.24)	6.8 (3.6–16.2)	4.8 (2.7–12.3)	4.7 (2–12.7)
S amplitude V_6 (mm)	4.5 (1.6–10.3)	3.3 (0.8–9.9)	2.0 (0.6–9)	2.4 (0.8–5.8)

*Mean (5th to 95th percentile).

From Fanaroff, A., & Martin, R. (1987). *Neonatal-perinatal medicine: Diseases of the fetus and infant* (4th ed., p. 1256). St. Louis: C. V. Mosby. As modified from Liebman, J., & Plonsey, R. (1977). Electrocardiography. In A. J. Moss, F. H. Adams, & G. C. Emmanovillides (Eds.), *Heart disease in infants, children and adolescents* (2nd ed.). Baltimore: Williams & Wilkins. Reprinted with permission.

TABLE 37–4 Time of First Void in 5000 Infants

Hours Since Delivery	395 Full-Term Infants		80 Preterm Infants		25 Postterm Infants	
	No. of Infants	*Cumulative (%)*	*No. of Infants*	*Cumulative (%)*	*No. of Infants*	*Cumulative (%)*
<1	51	12.9	17	21.2	3	12
1–8	151	51.1	50	83.7	4	38
9–16	158	91.1	12	98.7	14	84
17–24	35	100	1	100	4	100
>24	0	—	0	—	0	—

From Clark, D. A. (1977). Times of first void and first stool in 500 newborns. *Pediatrics, 60,* 457–459. Reproduced by permission of *Pediatrics.*

TABLE 37–5 Time of First Stool in 500 Infants

Hours Since Delivery	395 Full-Term Infants		80 Preterm Infants		25 Postterm Infants	
	No. of Infants	*Cumulative (%)*	*No. of Infants*	*Cumulative (%)*	*No. of Infants*	*Cumulative (%)*
<1	66	16.7	4	5	8	32
1–8	169	59.5	22	32.5	9	68
9–16	125	91.1	25	63.8	5	88
17–24	29	98.5	10	76.3	3	100
24–48	6*	100	18†	98.8	0	—
>48	0	—	1‡	100	0	—

*At 25, 26, 27, 28, 33, and 37 hours.
†Five stooled more than 36 hours after birth at 38, 39, 40, 42, and 47 hours.
‡At 59 hours.
From Clark, D. A. (1977). Times of first void and first stool in 500 newborns. *Pediatrics, 60,* 457–459. Reproduced by permission of *Pediatrics.*

TABLE 37–6 Acid–Base Status

Determination	Sample Source	Birth	1 Hour	3 Hours	24 Hours	2 Days	3 Days
Vigorous Term Infants, Vaginal Delivery							
pH	Umbilical artery	7.26					
	Umbilical vein	7.29					
P_{CO_2} (mm Hg)	Arterial	54.5	38.8	38.3	33.6	34	35
	Venous	42.8					
O_2 saturation	Arterial	19.8	93.8	94.7	93		
	Venous	47.6					
pH	Left atrial		7.30	7.34	7.41	7.39	7.38
CO_2 content (mEq/L)	—	—	20.6	21.9	21.4	temporal artery	temporal artery
Premature Infants							
	Capillary (skin puncture)						
pH	<1250 g				7.36	7.35	7.35
P_{CO_2} (mm Hg)					38	44	37
pH	>1250 g				7.39	7.39	7.38
P_{CO_2} (mm Hg)					38	39	38

From Schaffer, A. J. (1971). *Diseases of the newborn* (3rd ed.). Philadelphia: W. B. Saunders. Reprinted with permission.

TABLE 37–7 Selected Chemistry Values in Full-Term and Preterm Infants

Constituent	Preterm	Term	Reference
Ammonia (μg/100 ml)	—	90–150	1
Base, excess (mmol/L)	—	−10 to −2	2
Bicarbonate, standard (mmol/L)	18–26	20–26	2
Bilirubin, total (mg/dl)			
Cord	<2.8	<2.8	2
24 hours	1–6	2–6	
48 hours	6–8	6–7	
3–5 days	10–12	4–6	
≥1 month	<1.5	<1.5	
Bilirubin, direct	<0.5	<0.5	2
Calcium, total (mg/dl), week 1	6.0–10.0	7.0–12.0	3
Calcium, ionized (mg/dl), 72 hours	2.5–5.0	2.5–5.0	4
Ceruloplasmin (mg/dl)	—	20–40	
Creatinine phosphokinase			
Day 1	—	44–1150	5
(arb U) Day 4	—	14–97	
Creatinine (mg/dl)			
Birth	Mother's level	Mother's level	1,6
10 days	1.3 ± 0.07 (mean ± SD)	0.8–1.4	
1 month		—	
	0.6 ± 0.05 (mean ± SD)	14–331	7
Gamma-glutamyl transferase (U/L)			
Glucose (mg/dl)			
<72 hours	20–125	30–125	8
>72 hours	40–125	40–125	
Lactate dehydrogenase (U/L)	—	357–953	7
Magnesium (mg/dl)	—	1.5–2.8	9
Osmolality (mOsm/L)	—	280–295	2
Phosphatase, acid (U/L)	—	7.4–19.4	2
Phosphatase, alkaline (U/L) (mean ± SD)			
26–27 weeks	320 ± 87	164 ± 68	10
28–29	292 ± 87	—	
30–31	281 ± 85	—	
32–33	254 ± 72	—	
34–35	236 ± 62	—	
36	207 ± 60	—	
Phosphorus (mg/dl)			
Birth	5.6–8.0	5.0–7.8	11
Week 1	6.1–11.7	4.9–8.9	
Month 1	6.6–9.4	5.9–9.5	

TABLE 37–7 Selected Chemistry Values in Full-Term and Preterm Infants *Continued*

Constituent	Preterm	Term	Reference
SGOT (aspartate aminotransferase)	—	24–81	7
SGPT (alanine aminotransferase)	—	10–33	7
Urea nitrogen (mg/dl)	—	5–25	2
Uric acid (mg/dl)	—	3.0–7.5	2

[1]Meites, S. (1977). *Pediatric clinical chemistry: A survey of normals.* Washington, DC: American Association of Clinical Chemistry.
[2]Wallach, J. B. (1983). *Interpretation pf pediatric tests.* Boston: Little, Brown.
[3]Meites, S. (1975). *Critical Reviews in Clinical Laboratory Sciences, 6,* 1.
[4]Brown, D. M., Boen, J., & Bernstein, A. (1972). *Pediatrics, 49,* 841.
[5]Drummond, L. M. (1979). *Archives of Disease in Childhood, 54,* 362.
[6]Stonestreet, B. S., & Oh, W. (1978). *Pediatrics, 61,* 788.
[7]Statlan, B. E., & Freer, D. E. (1978). *Clinical Chemistry, 24,* 1010 [abstract].
[8]Cornblath, M., & Schwartz, R. (Eds.). (1976). *Disorders of carbohydrate metabolism* (2nd ed.). Philadelphia: W. B. Saunders.
[9]Tsang, R. C. (1972). *American Journal of Diseases of Children, 124,* 282.
[10]Glass, L., et al. (1982). *Archives of Disease in Childhood, 57,* 373.
[11]O'Brien, D. (1974). Interpretation of biochemical values. In C. H. Kempe & H. K. Silver (Eds.), *Current pediatric diagnosis and treatment* (3rd ed.). Los Altos, CA.: Lange Medical Publications.

From Fanaroff, A., & Martin, R. (1987). *Neonatal-perinatal medicine: Diseases of the fetus and infant* (4th ed., p. 1262). St. Louis: C. V. Mosby. Reprinted with permission.

TABLE 37–8 Serum Total Protein and Electrophoresis Fractions

Fraction	Cord Blood	Age: *Birth*	Age: *1 Week*	Age: *1–3 Months*
Total protein	4.78–8.04	4.6–7.0	4.4–7.6	3.64–7.38
Albumin	2.17–4.04	3.2–4.8	2.9–5.5	2.05–4.46
Alpha-1	0.25–0.66	0.1–0.3	0.09–0.25	0.08–0.43
Alpha-2	0.44–0.94	0.2–0.3	0.30–0.46	0.40–1.13
Beta	0.42–1.56	0.3–0.6	0.16–0.60	0.39–1.14
Gamma	0.81–1.61	0.6–1.2	0.35–1.3	0.25–1.05

From Fanaroff, A., & Martin, R. (1987). *Neonatal-perinatal medicine: Diseases of the fetus and infant* (4th ed., p. 1263). St. Louis: C. V. Mosby. Reprinted with permission.

TABLE 37–9 Heptoglobin Levels in Preterm Infants*

Gestation (weeks)	Days After Birth: *0*	*5*	*10*	*15*	*21*	*28*
<32	10 (3)	—	—	—	—	—
32–34	—	18.5 (2)	51.6 (3)	42.6 (3)	12 (1)	12 (1)
34–36	9.8 (9)	14.9 (11)	11.4 (10)	11.6 (9)	7.1 (7)	16.5 (4)
36–38	13.0 (7)	18.3 (3)	16.6 (5)	16.3 (2)	11 (1)	7.5 (1)
38+	9.3 (8)	28.3 (6)	20.9 (4)	10.1 (5)	9.2 (3)	7.0 (1)
Totals	10.5 (27)	19.6 (22)	19.5 (22)	16.1 (19)	8.3 (12)	13.2 (7)

*Heptoglobin levels are measured as mg/dl metHb binding capacity. Numbers in parentheses indicate number of samples from which mean values were derived.
From Philip, A. G. (1971). Heptoglobins in the newborn. II. Low birth weight babies. *Biology of the Neonate, 19,* 322–328. Reprinted with permission.

TABLE 37–10 Heptoglobin Levels in Full-Term Infants

	Birth	5 days
Heptoglobin (mg/dl Hgb binding capacity)	23.9 (10.6–50)	52.3 (14.8–100)

From Fanaroff, A., & Martin, R. (1987). *Neonatal-perinatal medicine: Diseases off the fetus and infant* (4th ed., p. 1263). St. Louis: C. V. Mosby. Reprinted with permission.

TABLE 37–11 Plasma Immunoglobulin Concentrations in Premature Infants (25–28 Weeks' Gestation)

Age (months)	n	IgG* (mg/dl)†	IgM* (mg/dl)†	IgA* (mg/dl)†
0.25	18	251 (114–552)	7.6 (1.3–43.3)	1.2 (0.07–20.8)
0.5	14	202 (91–446)	14.1 (3.5–56.1)	3.1 (0.09–10.7)
1	10	158 (57–437)	12.7 (3.0–53.3)	4.5 (0.65–30.9)
1.5	14	134 (59–307)	16.2 (4.4–59.2)	4.3 (0.9–20.9)
2	12	89 (58–136)	16 (5.3–48.9)	4.1 (1.5–11.1)
3	13	60 (23–156)	13.8 (5.3–36.1)	3 (0.6–15.6)
4	10	82 (32–210)	22.2 (11.2–43.9)	6.8 (1–47.8)
6	11	159 (56–455)	41.3 (8.3–205)	9.7 (3–31.2)
8–10	6	273 (94–794)	41.8 (31.1–56.1)	9.5 (0.9–98.6)

*Geometric mean.
†The normal ranges in parentheses were determined by taking the antilog of (mean logarithm ± 2 SD of the logarithms).
From Ballow, M., Cates, K. L., Rowe, J. C., et al. (1986). Development of the immune system in very low birth weight (less than 1500 g) premature infants: Concentrations of plasma immunoglobulins and patterns of infections. *Pediatric Research, 20,* 899–904. Reprinted with permission.

TABLE 37–12 Plasma Immunoglobulin Concentrations in Premature Infants (29–32 Weeks' Gestation)

Age (months)	n	IgG* (mg/dl)†	IgM* (mg/dl)†	IgA* (mg/dl)†
0.25	42	368 (186–728)	9.1 (2.1–39.4)	0.6 (0.04–1)
0.5	35	275 (119–637)	13.9 (4.7–41)	0.9 (0.01–7.5)
1	26	209 (97–452)	14.4 (6.3–33)	1.9 (0.3–12)
1.5	22	156 (69–352)	15.4 (5.5–43.2)	2.2 (0.7–6.5)
2	11	123 (64–237)	15.2 (4.9–46.7)	3 (1.1–8.3)
3	14	104 (41–268)	16.3 (7.1–37.2)	3.6 (0.8–15.4)
4	21	128 (39–425)	26.5 (7.7–91.2)	9.8 (2.5–39.3)
6	21	179 (51–634)	29.3 (10.5–81.5)	12.3 (2.7–57.1)
8–10	16	280 (140–561)	34.7 (17–70.8)	20.9 (8.3–53)

*Geometric mean.
†The normal ranges in parentheses were determined by taking the antilog of (mean logarithm ± 2 SD of the logarithms).
From Ballow, M., Cates, K. L., Rowe, J. C., et al. (1986). Development of the immune system in very low birth weight (less than 1500 g) premature infants: Concentrations of plasma immunoglobulins and patterns of infections. *Pediatric Research, 20,* 899–904. Reprinted with permission.

TABLE 37–13 Plasma Amino Acids in Preterm and Full-Term Infants

Amino Acid	Premature, First Day	Newborn, Before First Feeding	16 Days–4 Months
Taurine	105–255	101–181	
OH-proline	0–80	0	
Aspartic acid	0–20	4–12	17–21
Threonine	155–272	196–238	141–213
Serine	195–345	129–197	104–158
Aspartic acid + glutamic acid	655–1155	623–895	
Proline	155–305	155–305	41–245
Glutamic acid	30–100	27–77	
Glycine	185–735	274–412	178–248
Alanine	325–425	274–384	239–345
Valine	80–180	97–175	123–199
Cystine	55–75	49–75	33–51
Methionine	30–40	21–37	15–21
Isoleucine	20–60	31–47	31–47
Leucine	45–95	55–89	56–98
Tyrosine	20–220	53–85	33–75
Phenylalanine	70–110	64–92	45–65
Ornithine	70–110	66–116	37–61
Lysine	130–250	154–246	117–163
Histidine	30–70	61–93	64–92
Arginine	30–70	37–71	53–71
Tryptophan	15–45	15–45	
Citrulline	8.5–23.7	10.8–21.1	
Ethanolamine	13.4–105	23.7–72	
α-Amino-*n*-butyric acid	0–29	8.7–20.4	

From Fanaroff, A., & Martin, R. (1987). *Neonatal-perinatal medicine: Diseases of the fetus and infant* (4th ed., p. 1264). St. Louis: C. V. Mosby. Reprinted with permission.

TABLE 37–14 Urine Amino Acids in Normal Newborns

Amino Acid	μmol/day	Amino Acid	μmol/day
Cysteic acid	Tr–3.32	Methionine	Tr–0.892
Phosphoethanolamine	Tr–8.86	Isoleucine	0–6.11
Taurine	7.59–7.72	Tyrosine	0–1.11
OH-proline	0.0–9.81	Phenylalanine	0–1.66
Aspartic acid	Tr	β-Aminoisobutyric acid	0.264–7.34
Threonine	0.176–7.99	Ethanolamine	Tr–79.9
Serine	Tr–20.7	Ornithine	Tr–0.554
Glutamic acid	0–1.78	Lysine	0.33–9.79
Proline	0–5.17	1-Methylhistidine	Tr–8.64
Glycine	0.175–65.3	3-Methylhistidine	0.11–3.32
Alanine	Tr–8.03	Carnosine	0.044–4.01
α-Amino-*n*-butyric acid	0–0.47	Arginine	0.088–0.918
Valine	0–7.76	Histidine	Tr–7.04
Cystine	0–7.96	Leucine	Tr–0.819

Tr, trace.

From Fanaroff, A., & Martin, R. (1987). *Neonatal-perinatal medicine: Diseases of the fetus and infant* (4th ed., p. 1264). St. Louis: C. V. Mosby. Modified from Meites, S. (ed.) (1977). *Pediatric clinical chemistry: A survey of normals, methods and instruments.* Washington, DC: American Association for Clinical Chemistry. Reprinted with permission.

TABLE 37–15 Cerebrospinal Fluid Values in Healthy Term Newborns*

	Age			
	0–24 Hours	*1 Day*	*7 Days*	*>7 Days*
Color	Clear or xanthochromic	Clear or xanthochromic	Clear or xanthochromic	
Red blood cells/mm^3	9 (0–1070)	23 (6–630)	3 (0–48)	
Polymorphonuclear leukocytes/mm^3	3 (0–70)	7 (0–26)	2 (0–5)	
Lymphocytes/mm^3	2 (0–20)	5 (0–16)	1 (0–4)	
Proteins (mg/dl)	63 (32–240)	73 (40–148)	47 (27–65)	
Glucose (mg/dl)	51 (32–78)	48 (38–64)	55 (48–62)	
Lactate dehydrogenase (IU/L)	22–73	22–73	22–73	0–40

*Values are given as mean, with range in parentheses.

From Fanaroff, A., & Martin, R. (1987). *Neonatal-perinatal medicine: Diseases of the fetus and infant* (4th ed., p. 1265). St. Louis: C. V. Mosby. Reprinted with permission.

TABLE 37–16 Cerebrospinal Fluid Cytology in 46 Low Birth Weight and Term Neonates*

Category	Weight (g)	RBCs/mm^3	WBCs/mm^3	Polymorphonuclear leukocytes (%)	Lymphocytes (%)	Macrophages (%)
Low birth weight (n = 22)	1437 (652–2438)	50 (0–431)	7 (0–28)	16 (0–100)	28 (0–100)	56 (0–100)
Normal birth weight (n = 24)	3240 (2665–3997)	131 (0–478)	11 (1–38)	21 (0–100)	20 (0–100)	59 (0–100)

*Values are given as mean, with range in parentheses.

From Pappu, L. D., Purohir, D. M., Levkoff, A. H., & Kaplan, B. (1982). CSF cytology in the neonate. *American Journal of Diseases of Children, 136,* 297–298. Copyright 1982 American Medical Association. Reprinted with permission.

TABLE 37–17 Colloid Osmotic Pressure (torr) in Infant's Blood

Term, vaginal delivery	19.5 ± 2.1 (SD)
Term, cesarean section	16.1 ± 2.0
Term, vaginal (sick) (sepsis, asphyxia, heart failure, abdominal surgery)	19.5 ± 3.1
Preterm (700–1980 g) (hyaline membrane disease, asphyxia, necrotizing enterocolitis, etc.)	12.5 ± 2.5

From Taeusch, H. W., Ballard, R. A., & Avery, M. E. (Eds.) (1991). *Schaffer and Avery's diseases of the newborn* (6th ed., p. 1078). Philadelphia: W. B. Saunders. Reprinted with permission.

TABLE 37–18 Thyroid Function in Full-Term and Preterm Infants

	Serum T_4 Concentration in Premature and Term Infants					Serum Free T_4 Index in Premature and Term Infants				
	Estimated Gestational Age (wk)					*Estimated Gestational Age (wk)*				
	30–31	***32–33***	***34–35***	***36–37***	***Term***	***30–31***	***32–33***	***34–35***	***36–37***	***Term***
Cord										
Mean	6.5°	7.5	6.7‡	7.5	8.2			5.6	5.6	5.9
SD	1.0	2.1	1.2	2.8	1.8			1.3	2.0	1.1
n	3	8	18	17	37			12	10	14
12–72 hr										
Mean	11.5‡	12.3‡	12.4‡	15.5†	19.0	13.1§	12.9§	15.5‖	17.1	19.7
SD	2.1	3.2	3.1	2.6	2.1	2.4	2.7	3.0	3.5	3.5
n	12	18	17	15	6	12	14	14	14	6
3–10 days										
Mean	7.7‡	8.5‡	10.0‡	12.7†	15.9	8.3§	9.0§	12.0¶	15.1	16.2
SD	1.8	1.9	2.4	2.5	3.0	1.9	1.8	2.3	0.7	3.2
n	7	8	9	9	29	6	9	5	4	11
11–20 days										
Mean	7.5†	8.3‡	10.5	11.2	12.2	8.0°°	9.1¶	11.8	11.3	12.1
SD	1.8	1.6	1.8	2.9	2.0	1.6	1.9	2.7	1.9	2.0
n	5	11	9	9	8	5	8	8	5	8
21–45 days										
Mean	7.8‡	8.0‡	9.3‡	11.4	12.1	8.4°°	9.0¶	10.9		11.1
SD	1.5	1.7	1.3	4.2	1.5	1.4	1.6	2.8		1.4
n	11	17	13	5	5	11	17	5		5
46–90 days			30 to 73 weeks					30 to 35 weeks		
Mean		9.6			10.2	9.4				9.7
SD		1.7			1.9	1.4				1.5
n		16			17	13				10

°$p < .05$
†$p < .005$
‡$p < .001$
§$p = .001$
‖$p = .025$
¶$p = .01$
°°$p = .005$
For comparison of premature vs. term infants (t test).
From Cuestas, R. A. (1982). *Journal of Pediatrics*, 92, 963. Reprinted with permission.

UNIT SEVEN

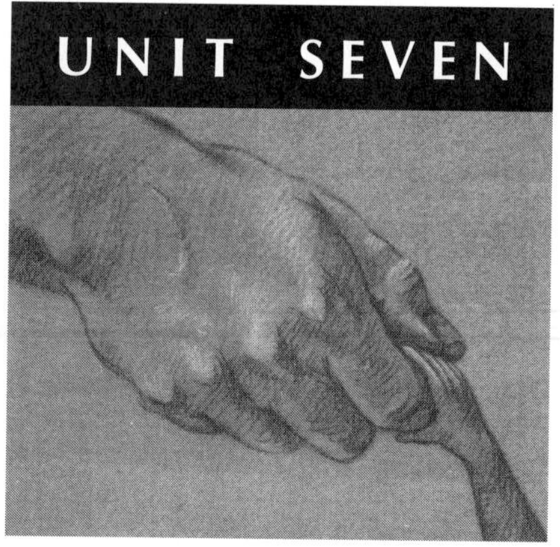

Special Clinical Concerns

Leslie knew how much I wanted to hold Emily. She knew I wanted to clutch her close to my chest, to stroke her, to tell her we loved her, and to thank her for being so brave. So at midmorning, she carefully opened Emily's isolette. All her tubes and devices were still attached, and Emily had more than doubled in size from edema. Her labia had puffed up fiercely. Her head had so increased in size that her hair, a pale golden brown, barely stretched around it. From lying in one position she had a small bedsore on the side of her head. An "owie," one would have said to an older child. I wanted to kiss her and tell her the kiss would make it well. But of course I knew it would not.

ELIZABETH MEHREN
Born Too Soon

CHAPTER 38

Fetal Therapy

KATHY BERGMAN CAROLE KENNER
LORI J. HOWELL JODY FARRELL MARIBETH INTURRISI

RESEARCH AGENDA

What impact do the following factors have on patient and family decision-making when considering maternal and fetal well-being?

Religious values and personal values
Previous experience with the health care system
Education and ability to read and understand medical information
Financial resources
Available support systems

Considering the women's rights issue, what impact will the decision of individual states not to allow physicians to discuss prenatal testing with families have on perinatal and neonatal outcomes?

The *Webster vs Reproductive Health Services* Supreme Court decision turns more of the decision-making power about abortions over to the states. This change from the individual to the government may potentially result in an ethical dilemma. What are the maternal perceptions of this ruling on the woman's own right about the continuation of the pregnancy?

What are the physiologic and psychological risks to the mother from fetal surgery?

Fetal treatment, a recent development that often involves experimental techniques, presents a wide variety of challenges to the nursing profession. The nurse is called on to provide counsel, education, organization, and technical skill to the treatment team and to families, while weighing ethical and moral considerations (Perry et al., 1986). This chapter describes the historical perspective of fetal treatment, including fetal surgery. It describes and defines fetal treatment. Collaborative management is discussed. In addition, future trends for fetal treatment are outlined.

HISTORICAL OVERVIEW

Throughout history, fetal development has been considered a mysterious process. In the past, cultural rituals often centered on protection of the mother from evil spirits so that the fetus would not be harmed. All this changed with the advent of ultrasonography. Suddenly events within the uterus became visible to the human eye. No longer was the fetus considered untouchable, nor was prenatal diagnosis left up to expert hunches.

In the 1950s and 1960s, ultrasonography began to be used in health care. Ian Donald is credited with having developed obstetrical ultrasonography (Lopez, 1989). He developed a scanner that was two-dimensional with capabilities allowing greater accuracy in visualizing the fetus (Donald, 1964). It used a transducer made of barium titanate, which turned vibratory sensations into electrical waves through a chemical process. These waves were transmitted to a cathode ray tube, allowing visualization of a pictorial representation of the waves. This picture was captured and recorded by a camera on film (Donald, 1964). Because the resulting picture is a facsimile of the actual structure being filmed, much is left to the interpreter of the ultrasonogram to make sense of the shadows of light and dark. This interpretation is one of the most critical elements in the accuracy of the diagnostic technique. Interpretation is further complicated by fetal movement and size. Thus, accuracy in achieving a good ultrasonographic picture in the first place is essential.

Erythroblastosis fetalis, a life-threatening fetal and neonatal complication, prompted the first attempt at in utero treatment of a fetal condition. In 1963 in New Zealand, A. W. Liley, guided by fluoroscopy, performed an in utero exchange transfusion on a 32-week fetus by infusing red blood cells into the fetal abdomen, where lymphatics carried the cells into the fetal blood stream. The attempt, let alone the success of the procedure, was heralded as a new dimension of obstetrical and pediatric care (Liley, 1963). This actual in utero medical intervention or correction of a fetal condition is called *fetal treatment.* Today, treatments for erythroblastosis fetalis and other fetal anemias can be accomplished by direct transfusion of O negative irradiated packed red blood cells into fetal umbilical blood vessels under the guidance of ultrasonography (percutaneous umbilical blood sampling) (Laifer & Kuller, 1996). Other forms of fetal treatment used today include genetically engineered antibodies that can be inserted into humans and aerosol gene therapy that introduces genetic matter directly into the lungs, which is being tested in animals (Waldmann, 1991). The implications of the latter work may be in relation to pulmonary immaturity in the neonate.

The use of noninvasive ultrasonography in obstetrical care has become commonplace in many countries. In Europe, routine ultrasonographic examinations are performed at 18 and 32 weeks' gestation to assess the progress of fetal growth (Pringle, 1986). In the United States, it is suggested under certain conditions only; it is still considered controversial in the United States, where the concern lies in the cost:risk:benefit ratio. Colodny (1987) identified the following assessments as indications for prenatal ultrasonography: (1) fetal growth or gestational age, (2) placental site, (3) amniocentesis, (4) fetal lie, (5) certain high-risk conditions of pregnancy, and (6) the cephalopelvic ratio.

Another concern about the use of ultrasonography is the accuracy of the procedure itself. Although the technique is able to differentiate between fluid-filled cavities and solid structures, the exact determination of a potential problem depends on the experience of the technician and the position of the fetus and the mother. Since fetal movements interfere with interpretation of results, real-time films or videotapes are often a useful adjunct to ultrasonography (Lopez, 1989). The position of the pregnant woman's uterus also can alter the interpretation of the ultrasonography results.

Ultrasonography is capable of determining the following: (1) gestational age; (2) fetal growth patterns; (3) certain congenital anomalies, especially structural malformations (when accomplished prior to 24 weeks' gestation); (4) fetal well-being (through the biophysical profile); (5) abnormal levels of amniotic fluid; and (6) abnormal positioning of the placenta. It is the ability to detect congenital structural malformations that links the ultrasonographic procedure to fetal diagnosis and treatment.

Ultrasonography (see Chapter 36, Diagnostic Imaging) has provided an essential adjunct to other prenatal diagnostic procedures such as amniocentesis, chorionic villus sampling, and percutaneous umbilical blood sampling. These techniques, along with ultrasonography, have laid the groundwork for the new frontier of fetal treatment. Once early detection and determination of abnormal fetal conditions could be made, they became amenable to fetal treatment. No longer are the options for management limited to abortion or postnatal treatment.

Table 38–1 describes the malformations that may be amenable to in utero treatment either medically or surgically.

In 1981, Harrison and a multidisciplinary team at the University of California at San Francisco became the first to attempt to correct a urinary obstruction in utero (Harrison et al., 1981; Levine & Imai, 1982). The rationale for selecting this particular problem on which to try their experimental procedure was the knowledge that infants with bilateral congenital hydronephrosis due to an outlet obstruction are often stillborn or die during the neonatal period. These deaths are due to either a failure of the lungs to develop or renal failure (Levine & Imai, 1982). (For a complete discussion of this association, see Chapter 31, Assessment and Management of Genitourinary Dysfunction.) The team performed its first attempt at a closed surgical procedure on a human using local anesthesia. A closed procedure involves the passage of a catheter needle through the maternal abdominal wall into the fetal bladder (Fig. 38–1). An indwelling bladder catheter is secured so that fluid drains from the bladder into the amniotic sac. Bladder decompression is achieved. More important, the amniotic fluid volume is restored. This catheter remains in place until birth (Levine & Imai, 1982). Although the cause of the obstruction is not corrected until the neonatal period, the deleterious effects of the obstruction are averted while the fetus continues to grow and develop.

The success of this intervention led the way for a new frontier in fetal and neonatal medicine. Other physicians started considering the possibilities raised by this type of surgical procedure. Thus, by the early 1980s, it became evident that this new treatment frontier was not just a passing trend. An international group of physicians and scientists met in Santa Ynez, California to discuss the new directions of medical science. Out of this meeting came the formation of the International Fetal Surgery Society, renamed in 1985 the International Fetal Medicine and Surgery Society (Manning, 1986). The society then created the International Fetal Surgery Registry in order to track the number, type, and outcomes of fetal surgical attempts. Since reporting was strictly voluntary, this registry by no means represented all the cases of fetal surgery, but it was a beginning for obtaining more accurate statistics on procedures performed. It is still voluntary today. There are now three registries, all created to collect data

TABLE 38–1 Malformations Amenable to In Utero Treatment

Problem	Intervention
Fetal Therapy: Medical Treatment	
Rh sensitization	Red cell transfusion: into umbilical vessel or intraperitoneal
Pulmonary immaturity	Betamethasone (transplacental)
Vitamin B_{12} deficiency	Vitamin B_{12} (transplacental)
Carboxylase deficiency	Biotin (transplacental)
SVT (supraventricular tachycardia)	Digoxin, flecainide, or similar drug (transplacental)
Heart block	Betamimetics (transplacental)
Hypothyroidism	Thyroxine (transplacental)
Adrenal hyperplasia	Steroids
IUGR (intrauterine growth retardation)	Protein–calories (transamniotic)
SCID (severe combined immunodeficiency) syndrome	Stem cell transplantation into umbilical vessel
Fetal Therapy: Surgical Treatment	
Urinary tract obstructions	Closed procedure:
Hydronephrosis	Percutaneous
Lung hypoplasia	Catheter placement
Renal and respiratory failure	*or*
Diaphragmatic hernia	Open procedure:
Lung hypoplasia	Vesicostomy
Respiratory failure	Open procedure:
	Decompression of chest contents
	Placement of Gore-Tex patch
	Repair of diaphragm
Cystic adenomal formation	Closed procedure:
Lung hypoplasia	Catheter placement to decompress
Respiratory failure	*or*
	Open procedure:
	Correction of malformation

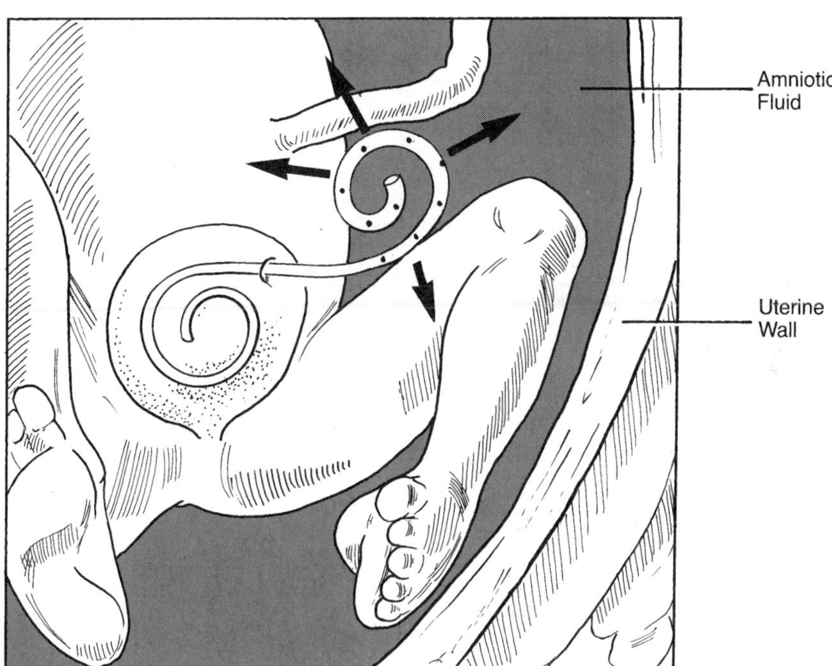

FIGURE 38–1. Posterior urethral valve obstruction. Perforations allow urine to flow outward into amniotic fluid as indicated by arrows. (Courtesy of Dr. Michael R. Harrison, University of California, San Francisco.)

from around the world on many types of fetal problems (Collins, 1994). Several centers offer treatment options and catheter placements, including Denver, Colorado; University of California at San Francisco, San Francisco, California; Harvard University, Boston, Massachussetts; Georgetown University, Washington, DC; Chicago, Illinois; University of Manitoba, Winnipeg, Manitoba; University of Toronto, Toronto, Ontario; Wayne State University, Detroit, Michigan; and University of Montreal, Montreal, Quebec. Fetal surgery is also practiced in Italy, Germany, France, Denmark, England, New Zealand, Australia, Israel, Chile, and Yugoslavia (Michejda et al., 1986). In the United States, the only centers currently performing open procedures that involve a hysterotomy and direct fetal surgery are the fetal treatment center of the University of California at San Francisco and Wayne State University under Dr. Alan Flake.

CRITERIA FOR FETAL SURGERY

Fetal or antenatal surgery is still considered experimental and should be undertaken only under certain circumstances. Also, in light of the potential risk to both the mother and the fetus it is suggested that fetal surgery be carried out only in centers that are committed to research as well as clinical application (Sullivan & Adzick, 1994).

Manning (1986), head of the International Fetal Surgery Registry, suggests that the natural history of the disease process or prognosis is an important consideration. Fetal age and the associated maturity as well as the natural progression of the disease if untreated are other important considerations (Manning, 1986). Above all, Manning cautions that fetal surgery should be undertaken only when the natural progression of the disease will probably result in fetal demise or neonatal death if surgery is not undertaken at this time (Elias & Annas, 1987; Manning, 1986). An overriding concern is maternal health. Maternal morbidity has been associated with fetal therapy and surgery and cannot be ignored when this treatment modality is considered (Pringle, 1986). Also, financial factors cannot be overlooked in today's economic environment. Cost–benefit and cost–effectiveness analyses influence decision-making (Collins, 1994).

When discussing fetal treatment, one must assess the risks to the mother as well as those to the fetus. Closed procedures (percutaneous, catheter placements) carry fewer risks to the mother but may be less beneficial to the fetus. The risks to the mother undergoing a closed procedure include minor discomfort (the procedure is performed under local and intravenous sedation with a narcotic or benzodiazepine); preterm labor (mild to moderate, usually amenable to bed rest or oral tocolytic agents, or both); premature rupture of membranes (infrequent); and chorioamnionitis (infrequent but would require premature delivery). The risks to the fetus include injury to a fetal part (performed under ultrasonographic guidance) or lack of successful placement owing to fetal position or dislodgment of the catheter from the fetal bladder by fetal movement during or after the procedure. Open procedures (hysterotomy) carry greater risks to the mother and fetus, yet if successful result in amelioration of the in utero condition. Maternal risks include those of general anesthesia and cesarean section. In addition, there is the risk of premature rupture of membranes, chorioamnionitis, and preterm labor. The latter is always a result of this procedure and requires a combination of intravenous, subcutaneous, and rectal tocolytics to control it. The risks of tocolytic therapy to the mother and fetus must be considered. Long-term tocolysis and bed rest are required in almost all cases. In addition, the mother has a uterine scar in the fundus of the uterus, requiring repeat cesarean section for all births following this procedure to avoid the risk of uterine rupture near term or during labor. These women are not generally considered good candidates for vaginal deliveries after birth even though that is the trend in other women who undergo cesarean section. The fetal risks include intraoperative death secondary to an inability to repair the lesion, correction of the lesion but unrecognized or disabling fetal abnormalities of another kind or intraventricular hemorrhage in utero, or injury from side effects of the tocolytic agents. Since this surgery is often performed very early in gestation, the fetus is small for such a procedure. Figure 38–2 illustrates just how small the fetus is in relationship to a mother's hand.

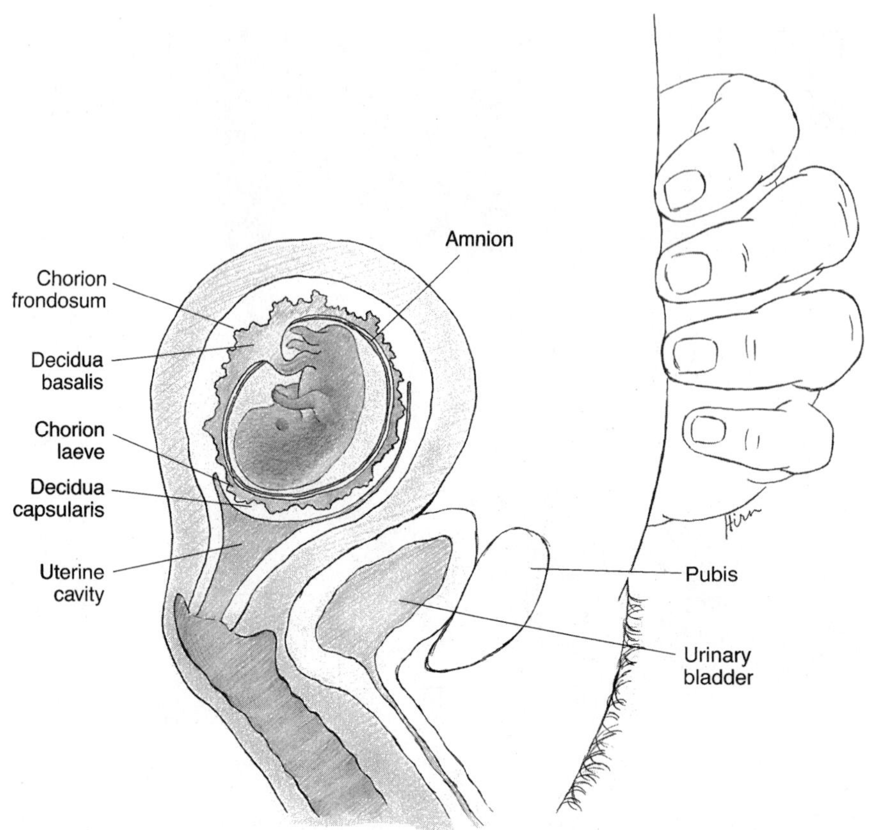

FIGURE 38–2. At 8 weeks, the 1½-inch-long embryo is approximately half as long as its mother's forefinger.

ANESTHESIA

In the event that in utero treatment is necessary, either percutaneously or as an open surgical procedure, anesthesia is used. The anesthesiologist must consider the two patients who are being anesthetized simultaneously for any fetal manipulation.

Anesthetizing pregnant women during major surgery while maintaining the pregnancy requires specially trained anesthesiologists. First and foremost is maternal safety. The particular hazards of anesthesia during pregnancy are related to physiologic changes in the mother and to possible adverse effects on the fetus (Blustein, 1988). The goal is to provide low-level anesthesia and pain management for the maternal-fetal unit with minimal side effects (Collins, 1994). Fetal monitoring is essential because of the effect anesthesia has on the fetus. Radiokinetic devices are attached to the fetus' back to monitor heart rate, respiratory rate, temperature, and intrauterine pressure (Sullivan & Adzick, 1994).

Some of the physiologic differences between healthy pregnant women and healthy adults are (1) a decrease in peripheral vascular resistance (cardiac output increase with no increase in blood pressure, resulting in a decrease in peripheral vascular resistance); (2) a decrease in functional residual capacity and an increase in alveolar ventilation (therefore the rapidity of induction with inhalation anesthetics is increased); (3) an increase of oxygen consumption (a decreased functional residual capacity combined with an increased oxygen consumption makes pregnant women more likely to become hypoxic); and (4) hypotension due to aortocaval compression (by lying supine, a pregnant woman in the second and third trimesters may experience hypotension as the result of aortocaval compression by the gravid uterus). Direct compression of the aorta by the gravid uterus directly decreases uterine blood flow. For displacement of the uterus from the great vessels, lateral tilt of the operating table should be used for all anesthesia procedures to prevent supine hypotension and uterine hypoperfusion. In addition, mechanical vena cava compression is likely to occur during fetal surgery when the fetus is returned to the uterus. This complication is one of the reasons that there is an almost constant exchange of information on the patients' status between the anesthesiologists and surgeons during fetal surgery.

As the pregnant uterus grows, the stomach is displaced cephalad and horizontally, which changes the angle of the gastroesophageal junction and predisposes the mother to passive regurgitation. This, along with the increased gastric acid production, makes her more susceptible to regurgitation and aspiration when anesthetized (Chen et al., 1988; Christ, 1986). To decrease the acidity of the gastric juice, prophylactic administration of an oral antacid is recommended prior to general anesthesia. Pregnant women are also more sensitive to inhalation anesthetics because the endorphin level is elevated; therefore, they are more susceptible to overdosing. Regional anesthetics also require special attention because with the increase in femoral venous and intra-abdominal pressure, the epidural veins are enlarged, which decreases the epidural space, thus decreasing the amount of anesthesia needed.

Fetal oxygenation is dependent on maternal arterial oxygen content. If the mother's partial pressure of arterial oxygen, partial pressure of arterial carbon dioxide, and uterine blood flow are maintained within normal limits, fetal asphyxia does not occur. Elevated maternal oxygen tension, which commonly occurs during anesthesia, is safe for the fetus; however, maternal hyperventilation can cause fetal hypoxia and acidosis. Other causes of fetal asphyxia are maternal hypotension, which causes decreased uterine blood flow, and uterine vasoconstriction caused by anxiety, insufficient anesthesia, or vasoactive drugs.

While the mother is anesthetized for fetal surgery, the fetus also receives anesthesia via placental transfer. It has been shown through animal studies that operating on an unanesthetized fetus results in autonomic nervous system stimulation, increased hormonal activity, and increased motor activity (Colodny, 1987).

Thus, general anesthesia is used for all open procedures to provide both maternal and fetal anesthesia.

Halothane anesthesia has been found to be both safe and effective. Intraoperative halothane anesthesia not only inhibits uterine contractions but also provides the necessary uterine relaxation for surgical exposure through a small hysterotomy incision and for replacement of the fetus back into the uterus when the surgical repair is finished (Connor & Ferguson-Smith, 1987). A newer technique is uterine stapling, which decreases maternal blood loss (Sullivan & Adzick, 1994).

Since fetal surgery is experimental, informed consent and institutional review board approval are necessary prior to performing any procedure. An ethics committee is useful for challenging cases and offers assistance to the fetal treatment team. The determination of the course of action should respect the patient's authority and elicit the preferences of the patient and acknowledge the patient's life values (Chervenak & McCullough, 1993). Each institution has policies outlining the exact steps that must be taken when an experimental treatment is to be used. These institutional guidelines should be consulted.

Once a congenital condition is recognized as potentially correctable with surgery, several other points must be considered. A level II sonogram, a fetal echocardiogram, and chromosomal fetal testing (chorionic villus sampling or amniocentesis) must be performed to determine whether any other congenital anomalies or genetic defects exist that may be incompatible with life. The fetal condition that is identified for surgical intervention might just be a small part of a larger syndrome, such as trisomy 18, that includes urinary or renal problems (Elias & Annas, 1987). Even if these concurrent conditions are not lethal, the surgery may be compromised if, for instance, a congenital cardiac abnormality is also found.

CONDITIONS TREATED WITH FETAL SURGERY

Fetal surgery is performed on the fetus to alter the destructive physiology caused by hydrocephalus, urinary tract obstructions, diaphragmatic hernias, congenital cystic adenomatoid malformations of the lung, and sacral coccygeal teratomas.

Hydrocephalus

Hydrocephalus is the accumulation of fluid within the ventricles of the brain, resulting in an enlargement of the cranial cavity. The condition is due to either an actual defect in the structure of the ventricles themselves (e.g., Arnold-Chiari malformation, communicating hydrocephalus), which affects the movement or absorption of cerebral spinal fluid (CSF), or an obstruction along the circulatory pathway of the CSF, especially at the aqueduct of Sylvius or the fourth ventricle, as in the Dandy-Walker malformation, noncommunicating hydrocephalus. Both these malformations may accompany a meningomyelocele or neural tube defect. Aqueductal stenosis is the usual cause of hydrocephalus (Manning et al., 1986).

The problem is most often detected during the second trimester. Treatment involves relief from any obstruction that may be present and the resumption of CSF circulation and absorption. The first attempts at correction of the condition were carried out at Harvard. Encephalocentesis (the drainage of fluid within the ventricles) was performed, which offered only temporary relief. The fluid returned rapidly because the problem causing the fluid's accumulation was not corrected (Michejda et al., 1986). Guided by ultrasonography, a team at the University of Colorado used percutaneous placement (a closed procedure) of a small polymeric silicone (Silastic) tube. With a one-way silicone valve to prevent backflow of amniotic fluid, one end of the tubing was placed within the brain's ventricles to allow fluid to flow from the cranium (parietal region), and the other end of the tubing was placed in the amniotic fluid (ventriculoamniotic shunt). The excess fluid was excreted by the maternal body. Thus, the circulatory movement of fluid was restored by this Denver shunt, and the enlarged ventricles and cranial vault were reduced. There are variations of this shunt, some with rubber or silicone catheters without the valve (Michejda et al., 1986). Whichever shunt is used, the insertion is similar. It is inserted through a 13-gauge needle guided by a stylet and threaded from the amniotic cavity into the ventricles (Michejda et al., 1986).

The rationale for performing hydrocephalic surgery in utero is to allow the brain to develop normally without pressure from the dilated ventricles, which might ultimately damage delicate brain tissue. Complications from the procedure have led to questions about the actual benefits of this intervention. One argument against the procedure is that the fetal fontanelles are open, thus allowing a great deal of swelling to occur before actual damage is probably done to the fetal brain. Another concern is the trauma that has resulted from the fetal intervention. The surgery itself has resulted in fetal death secondary to chorioamnionitis, prematurity, or multiple coexisting congenital problems not previously detected. Brain damage has occurred in some cases. Most of the cases of hydrocephalus were associated with chromosomal disorders. As of 1986, of the 44 patients reported to the Fetal Registry, 36 survived the treatment; the other 8 died during the treatment or by age 3 months postnatally. Only 12 of the surviving infants were reported to be developing normally; 18 had severe neurologic deficits (Michejda et al., 1986).

The shunt has also posed problems (Michejda et al., 1986). Often, at birth it is noted that the shunt has become dislodged by fetal movement or obstructed by glial tissue. Indications are that the dislodgment or obstruction happened before birth, thus leaving concerns about how effective the surgery really is. Although the newer shunts are less likely to present these problems, they still occur. Survival may improve, but long-term outcomes are questionable (Manning et al., 1986). Thus, such in utero shunt treatments are no longer performed.

A caveat for this type of surgery is that an accurate determination of any coexisting conditions should be made, since hydrocephalus is often just one of many congenital defects present in the same fetus. Other criteria that should be used to determine whether the surgery should be undertaken are (1) gestational age of less than 30 weeks (before a safe delivery is advisable), (2) ventricular dilation and cortical mantle decrease, (3) a multidisciplinary team consultation and discussion with the family that concludes with the family's understanding of their treatment options, and (4) long-term family follow-up (Michejda et al., 1986).

Urinary Obstructions

Urinary obstructions (bladder outlet obstructions, most of which are ureteropelvic junction or posterior urethral valve obstructions, and urethral atresia) offer the most hope for positive outcomes in fetal corrections (Manning, 1987; Perry et al., 1986). The danger of such an obstruction is that the back-up of urine in the fetal bladder leads to hypertrophy of the bladder, loss of abdominal wall strength, hydroureter, hydronephrosis, and renal failure. The resultant oligohydramnios limits fetal movement, resulting in contractures or arthrogryposis and flattening of the facial features. In addition, lung maturation is halted by the lack of amniotic fluid and by the lack of space for lung growth in the chest, which is occupied by the enlarged kidneys (Fig. 38–3). Catheters have been placed in the fetal bladder to decompress this system and allow drainage of fluid into the amniotic sac surrounding the fetus. If the lesion has not been prolonged, renal

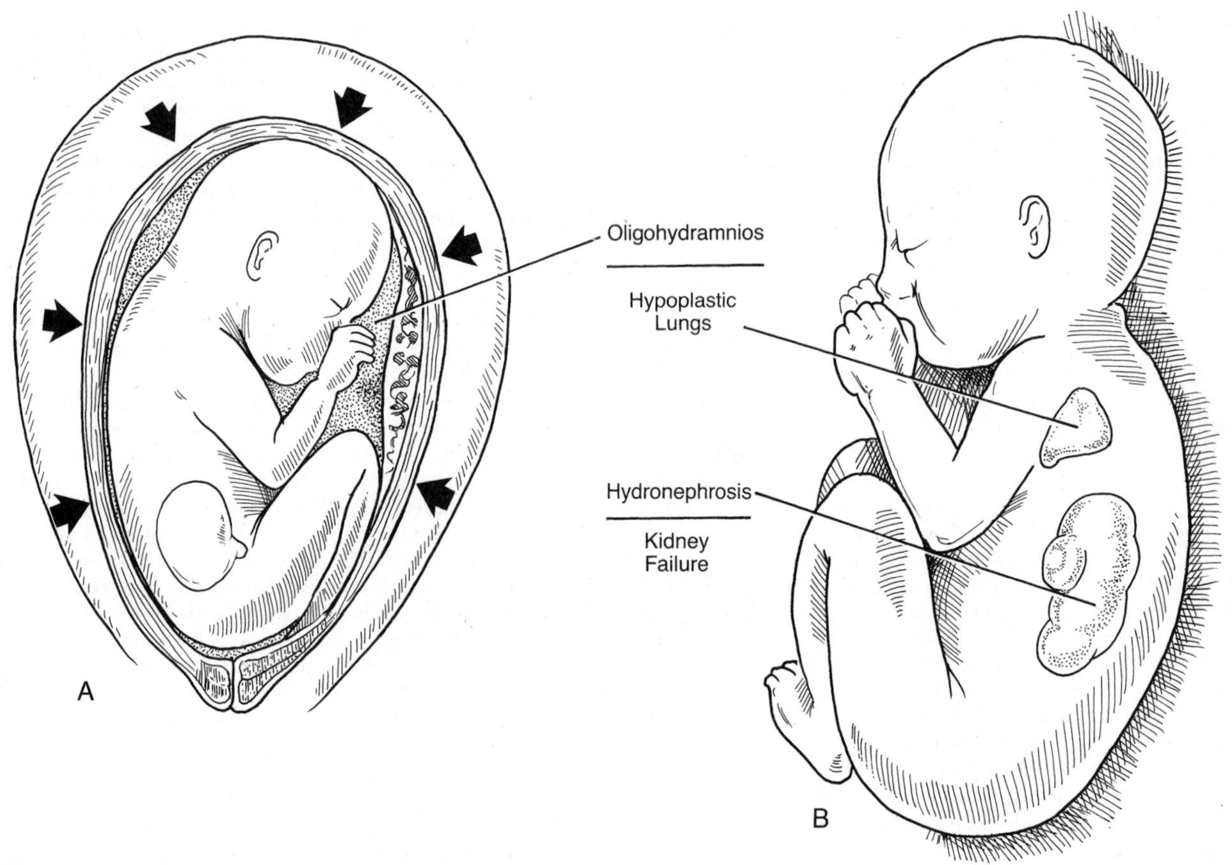

FIGURE 38–3. Urethral obstruction. (Courtesy of Dr. Michael R. Harrison, University of California, San Francisco.)

and lung damage may be minimal, and decompressing the system with catheters can prevent any further damage.

When there is a urinary tract obstruction, the status of kidney function must be determined prior to any decision about fetal surgery. The decision should be made after the fetal bladder has been tapped (a procedure similar to amniocentesis) and fetal urine examined for electrolytes and osmolarity. If the sodium concentration is less than 100 mEq/L, renal function is considered to be good (Harrison et al., 1991).

The glomerular filtration rate is a more accurate parameter for kidney function. Fetal urine osmolarity of less than 210 mOsm predicts good renal function if ultrasonography also shows fairly normal kidney appearance and absence of renal cysts (Harrison et al., 1991).

Fetal surgery is aimed at prevention of long-term renal and pulmonary compromise. The exact mechanism of pulmonary hypoplasia secondary to urinary obstruction is not known. It is hypothesized that it is related to damage to the fetal metanephros, preventing the release of arginase. This substance is needed for the chemical conversion of arginine to ornithine to proline. The latter is believed to induce cellular development of mesenchymal tissue vital to the pulmonary system (Colodny, 1987). Pulmonary hypoplasia has been reported when oligohydramnios is present (Colodny, 1987). However, it may be present even in the absence of oligohydramnios. It is the pulmonary hypoplasia rather than the kidney disease itself that often results in neonatal death. Pulmonary hypoplasia is responsible for approximately 81 percent of fetal and neonatal deaths, even when the renal problem has been treated in utero (Manning, 1987); however, these deaths occurred before it was known which fetuses had adequate renal function left to make more amniotic fluid.

Of the 73 closed procedures (i.e., percutaneous catheter placements) reported to the Fetal Registry, 20 percent of the fetuses were born preterm; 41 percent survived the surgery, and 27 percent of those who survived the procedures died of pulmonary compromise within the first 24 hours after birth (Grupe, 1987; Seeds & Mandell, 1988). The infants' survival rate was ultimately 76.2 percent (Manning, 1987).

Thus the fetus must be viable (no concurrent lethal conditions); the mother must have oligohydramnios that poses a threat to fetal pulmonary development; and there must be positive renal function (not completely compromised, which might suggest irreversible kidney damage). If no oligohydramnios is present and the hydronephrosis is unilateral but renal function is positive, treatment may be properly postponed until the postnatal period. Infants with unilateral disease may not suffer permanent renal damage, since the unaffected kidney maintains adequate kidney function and seems to prevent pulmonary hypoplasia (Newnham et al., 1987).

The corrective renal surgery can be conducted via three major routes: (1) percutaneous needle aspiration or bladder tap to decompress the bladder, (2) shunt placement, and (3) open urinary tract surgery (Colodny, 1987; Grupe, 1987). The first two options are poor because they provide only short-term relief of the obstruction and often require more than one attempt.

The exact surgical procedure varies according to the fetal renal disorder or the surgical team's preference. Posterior urethral valve obstruction may be treated by percutaneous placement of a shunt (catheter) in the fetal bladder to the amniotic sac (closed procedure). This shunt uses a Harrison French double-reversed pigtail catheter (see Fig. 38–1) developed by Harrison and the surgical group at the University of California at San Francisco. The catheter or stent is in the shape of a pigtail, with openings at either end of the catheter. The diameters of the catheter's two ends are dissimilar, a safety feature of the catheter in case it should become dislodged. The larger of the two ends is located in the amniotic cavity so that it is more likely that the catheter would move back into this cavity rather than the fetal bladder.

A polyethylene catheter, which is more rigid and therefore less likely to bend or become kinked, is sometimes used. The catheter is introduced through the maternal abdomen and uterus into the fetal abdomen and bladder via a needle and trocar guidance system, much as angiocatheters are used for intravenous therapy. Once the catheter is in place, one end is in the renal pelvis and the other end is in the amniotic sac, thus providing a way for the amount of amniotic fluid to increase. The guidance system is withdrawn, leaving the tubing in place. More than one insertion attempt may be necessary for successful placement. The fetus must undergo later corrective surgery during the neonatal period, consisting of bladder and abdominal wall repair and relief of the urethral obstruction.

An open technique can be used to correct hydronephrosis in the fetus. When an open procedure is performed, as for the treatment of hydronephrosis, a maternal hysterotomy is carried out under general anesthesia. The uterine cavity is opened under ultrasonographic guidance to avoid the placenta and to guide the incision over the fetal abdomen. The fetal abdomen and thorax are exposed, but the fetus is not removed (Fig. 38–4). A pulse oximeter, to sense fetal heart rate and fetal oxygen, is taped to the hand of the fetus to provide telemetry for the assessment of fetal well-being and uterine activity during the procedure. On completion of the procedure, a device is sewn under the skin of the fetal thorax to provide telemetry for fetal heart and uterine pressure. This device is left in place postoperatively until delivery. A vesicostomy is performed, and a large volume of urine is drained from the fetal bladder. This vesicostomy is used in postnatal life to continue to drain urine from the bladder (Fig. 38–5). The bladder is marsupialized to the fetal abdominal wall, leaving an avenue for urine to flow from the fetal bladder into the amniotic sac. On closure of the uterus, an infusion of lactated Ringer's solution into the amniotic space via a red Robinson catheter returns the amniotic fluid volume to within normal limits, thus correcting the oligohydramnios (Perry et al., 1986). The membranes and uterus are closed by suture and sealed with fibrin glue in an attempt to prevent intra-abdominal leakage of amniotic fluid.

To prevent long-term renal and pulmonary problems, it is essential that early treatment be undertaken. Fetal surgery for posterior urethral valve obstruction has been accomplished as early as 18 weeks and as late as 26 weeks of gestation. The ultimate goal is to prevent irreversible renal damage and pulmonary hypoplasia (Quinlan et al., 1986).

Congenital Diaphragmatic Hernias

Diaphragmatic hernia, occurring once in 2400 to 5000 live births, is the movement of abdominal contents upward into the thoracic cavity through an incomplete area of the diaphragm. (For a complete description, see Chapter 24, Assessment and Management of Gastrointestinal Dysfunction.) The current survival rate is approximately 40 percent (Harrison et al., 1991). With the introduction of extracorporeal membrane oxygenation, survival rates of these neonates may increase even without fetal surgery. With improvement in neonatal survival and improved treatment techniques, the need for fetal surgery is questioned by some authorities. Fetal surgical repair of this type of hernia has been reported for several years. Harrison's group in California has demonstrated in fetal lambs that in utero repair of these hernias improved the overall survival. When diaphragmatic hernias remained untreated in fetal lambs, alveolar tissue failed to grow, but type II cells proliferated and yet were smaller in the left upper lobe. These findings suggest that lung tissue undergoes morphologic changes secondary to the anatomic hernia (Pringle, 1986).

A hysterotomy is performed as described in the section on repair of urinary bladder obstruction. Two subcostal incisions are made in the fetus, and the chest is decompressed by removing the abdominal contents from it. A ventral pocket is created with a piece of lined Gore-Tex and this is attached to the fetus where the subcostal incision was made. The intestines, stomach, and spleen are housed in this "silo" similar to a gastroschisis to help the undersized abdomen accommodate these organs. A Gore-Tex graft is sewn to the edges of the diaphragmatic rim. The uterus and membranes are then closed in the same fashion described in the section on urinary obstructions.

Diaphragmatic hernia can be repaired only by an open procedure. At present the only lesions amenable to repair in utero are

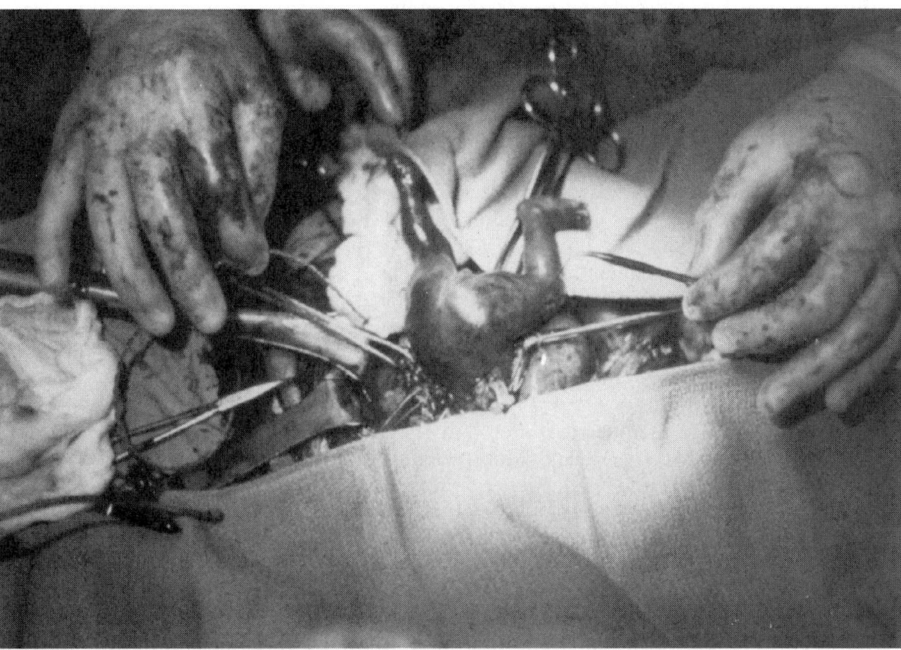

FIGURE 38–4. Exposure of fetus for vesicostomy in posterior urethral valve obstruction. (Courtesy of Dr. Michael R. Harrison, University of California, San Francisco.)

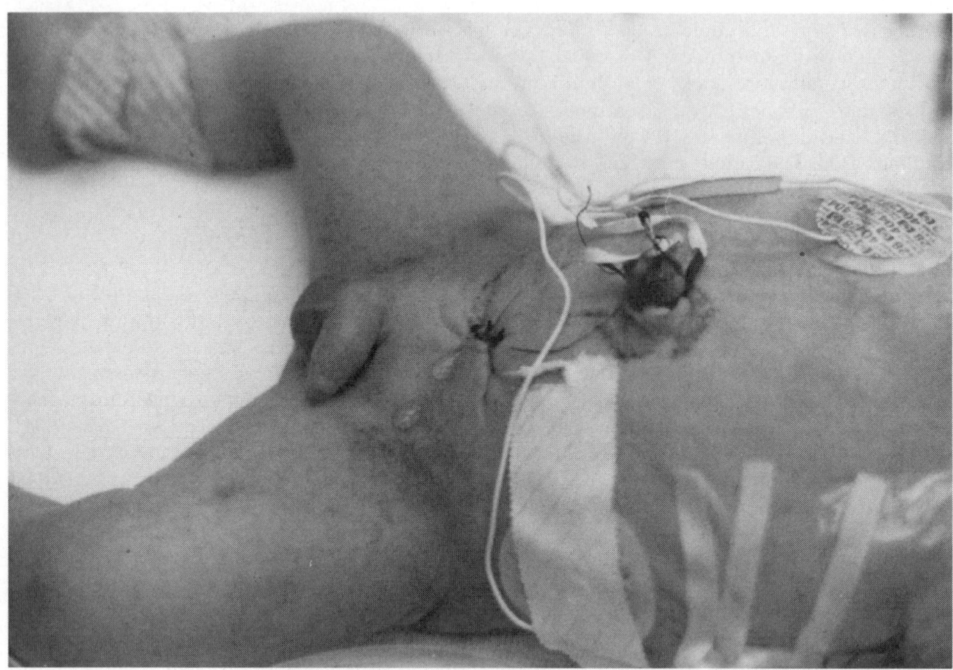

FIGURE 38–5. Newborn voiding through vesicostomy at birth. (Courtesy of Dr. Michael R. Harrison, University of California, San Francisco.)

those in which the liver is below the level of the diaphragm. In all patients with the liver above the defect, death in utero occurs secondary to liver hemorrhage from manipulation or kinking of major fetal vessels or some other unknown cause related to the location and manipulation of the liver. For a step-by-step description of congenital diaphragmatic hernia repair, see Figure 38–6.

Congenital Cystic Adenomatoid Malformation

Congenital cystic adenomatoid malformation (CCAM) is a rare pulmonary malformation that is usually restricted to one part of the lung and includes a wide variety of clinical manifestations. It is often accompanied by maternal polyhydramnios, fetal hydrops, and pulmonary hypoplasia.

There are two categories, based on gross anatomy ultrasonographic findings and prognosis. Macrocystic tumors appear as large cystic tumors; microcystic tumors appear almost solid because there are so many tiny cysts throughout the lesion. Macrocystic lesions are more common, are not associated with hydrops, and have a more favorable outcome. Microcystic lesions lead to hydrops, lung hypoplasia, and neonatal demise.

Macrocystic lesions have been decompressed by the closed percutaneous catheter placement technique, allowing lung growth. Microcystic lesions have been removed by open (hysterotomy) technique, with subsequent resolution of hydrops (Harrison et al., 1991). Hydrops is associated with CCAM. If this condition occurs before 32 weeks' gestation, the fetus can undergo fetal surgery. As previously stated, it may be as simple as a thoracoamniotic catheter shunt to drain the mass and decompress it to allow fetal lung growth (Morin et al., 1994). If the mass is solid, resection is necessary. This surgical procedure has been performed at 21 to 27 weeks' gestation (Morin et al., 1994). This period of gestation is when lung growth is continuing and the air exchange surface becomes more complex and extensive as fetal life continues. Type II cells are producing surfactant, so the infant may tolerate the surgical procedure better than at an earlier stage. This timing allows the lung tissue to resume a normal growth pattern for optimal lung development.

Delivery of this fetus–neonate should take place at a tertiary center because pulmonary hypoplasia is also certain (Morin et al., 1994). Postnatal radiography studies are needed to observe for any residual or return of the CCAM. Some children have been reported to aquire lung masses following prenatal diagnosis of CCAM (Morin et al., 1994).

Sacral Coccygeal Teratoma

Sacral coccygeal teratoma, or sacrococcygeal teratoma, is a neural tube defect. It consists of a tumor growth in the sacral and coccygeal areas of the spinal cord. This condition can be detected by ultrasonography. Once identified, an open fetal surgical procedure can be performed to remove the mass. A hysterotomy is performed, and the buttocks and lower spinal cord are exposed (Harrison & Adzick, 1993). A fetal radiotelemetry device for monitoring is placed on the upper portion of the fetus' spinal cord. The surgery consists of removing the tumor either by resection or stapling. The stapling procedure is accomplished by using a uterine staple machine that was devised for minimizing trauma to the mother's uterus. In the case of the fetus, this stapling is used when the tumor is small. It applies pressure to the highly vascular tissue, cutting off the blood supply and thus killing the tumor. This procedure minimizes fetal blood loss (Harrison & Adzick, 1993). If the tumor is larger than can safely be handled by stapling, umbilical tape can be pulled tightly over the tumor mass. The tape binds the tumor and cuts off the blood supply, allowing the surgeon to remove or resect the tumor with little danger of bleeding. Because these tumors sometimes recur or are not completely removed, there may be a need for further surgery during the neonatal period (Harrison & Adzick, 1993).

CONSIDERATIONS FOR COLLABORATIVE CARE PLANNING

When fetal surgery is contemplated, the individual case may be divided into six distinctive phases: (1) the diagnostic phase, (2) the information and decision-making phase, (3) the surgery and postoperative phase, (4) the home care and follow-up phase, (5) the delivery, and (6) the neonatal period. Each of these phases involves distinct and important nursing input.

Diagnostic Phase

The initial or diagnostic phase generally covers the period from the time of referral for diagnosis through the initial evaluation process. Typically this phase requires the family, often with limited information about the reason for referral, to wait—first for an appointment and then for the potential findings from the evaluation (Matthews et al., 1984). Often families say that this waiting period is most difficult (Costello, 1987). The nurse should help provide appropriate information about the process and use available resources—such as social services, support groups, and counseling services—to cushion the fears inherent in a stressful situation. It is important for the nurse to recognize that the family is undergoing the loss of a normal pregnancy.

Major concerns during the initial phase relate to the diagnosis and cause of the fetus' problem and the couple's sense of responsibility for causing the problem. Families need reassurance that the cause is unknown.

Information and Decision-Making Phase

During the decision-making phase, the differential diagnosis is established by the perinatologist and pediatric surgeon. The family is offered options: termination of the pregnancy if it is early enough, surgical intervention, or simply waiting until term and accepting a high risk of fetal loss at that time. The question of whether invasive therapy is offered and recommended or offered but not recommended is confronted at this point according to Chervenak and McCullough (1993). Such therapy should be offered and recommended only if all of the criteria are met: (1) the therapy is judged to have a high likelihood of being life-saving or of preventing serious, irreversible disease, injury, or disability for the fetus and the child to come and (2) the therapy has a low risk of mortality and a low or manageable risk of disease, injury, or disability to the fetus. Although the risk for the pregnant woman is expected to be low or at least manageable, there is a risk of morbidity and mortality from the surgical procedure (Chervenak & McCullough, 1993).

This time is when the family's worst fears may be confirmed. There is often an increase in the intensity of the feelings of family members as the grief reaction begins. The family must confront the religious, moral, and ethical as well as financial and practical implications of the decisions to be made (Costello, 1987). A particularly graphic example of a possible issue that arises is found in the case of the twin-to-twin transfusion syndrome. In this syndrome there are abnormal placental chorionic vessels that connect the circulation between the twins causing an imbalance in the blood flow (Sullivan & Adzick, 1994). There is a "pump twin" and a "recipient twin" (Crombleholme, 1994). The pump twin is usually structurally normal, but without treatment there is a high probability of death. Several techniques for fetal therapy have been used to correct this problem; however, the issue of risk to both twins, even the one who would most likely be fine during extrauterine life, must be confronted.

The fetal treatment nurse coordinator and the obstetrical nurse specialist from the tertiary center where the fetal surgery is to be performed have a role in assisting with family decision-making. The family is invited to meet the fetal treatment team, consisting of the pediatric surgeon, obstetrical specialist, perinatologist, anesthesiologist, neonatologist, operating room nurse, sonographer, nurse coordinator, nurse specialists, and a social worker. In a team meeting, each member provides detailed information regarding preoperative, intraoperative, and perioperative hospital and home care, and questions are answered. The family meets privately with the perinatal social worker, who makes a psychosocial assessment and evaluates the family's ability to cope with each of the management choices. The evaluation includes an assessment of the marital relationship, the available support systems, coping strategies they have used in previous crisis situations, previous experience of loss, current stress factors in the family (such as concern for care for children at home), recent unemployment or financial constraints, and other health problems. The mother ought to be healthy and a nonsmoker (Sullivan & Adzick, 1994). Thus a good history and assessment is essential. All this information assists the team in assessing how well the family may cope with the present crisis and what resources may be helpful in working with them (Matthews et al., 1984).

Perioperative Phase

Once decisions are made, the nurse, as part of the team, helps prepare the family for the procedure. This third phase is the surgery and perioperative phase. The exact patient management during the preoperative and postoperative periods is outlined in Table 38–2. The nurse provides extensive preoperative teaching and preparation. At this time it may be appropriate to discuss seeing, holding, and naming the infant in case of fetal loss at any point in the perioperative phase (Costello, 1987).

During the 7- to 10-day postoperative period, the nurse provides support, encouragement, education, and confidence during a critical time. The mother and family undergo great uncertainty about whether the fetus will survive the postoperative period or whether preterm labor can be halted. Additionally, with all these uncertainties the mother is under the influence of medications that alter her mental status, postoperative discomfort, and sleep patterns.

Home Follow-Up

The discharge to home can bring about a great deal of anxiety. During this fourth phase, home follow-up, the mother is often restricted to complete bed rest and tocolytic therapy. Nitrous oxide is a powerful vasodilator that promotes uterine relaxation. It is being used experimentally with tocolytic agents as adjunctive therapy to decrease the incidence of preterm labor (Harrison, 1993; Sullivan & Adzick, 1994). There may be constant concern that something she does or fails to do will lead to preterm labor, premature rupture of membranes, or some other harm to the fetus. Home care nursing is generally provided on a once-a-week basis to provide continuing instruction in self-care and management and support.

Patients are encouraged and sometimes required to stay near the medical center with a family member or friend. This enables the mother to visit the medical center once or twice a week for fetal evaluation (nonstress test [NST], amniotic fluid index [AFI], and sonogram [sono]) and signs of preterm labor. Other sources of anxiety are the emotional strain from being separated from friends, family, and young children and the potential financial strain of time away from work and lost income.

Delivery

The fifth phase is the delivery phase, which may occur any time after the surgery but most commonly 4 to 6 weeks after the procedure. During this phase, major concerns include the fears and fantasies involving what the infant will look like and whether he or she will survive. For the congenital diaphragmatic hernia plug procedure, delivery must take place under controlled circumstances. The entire fetal treatment team must be present. The fetus is removed from the uterus, but the umbilical cord is not clamped. The tracheal clip is removed and an endotracheal

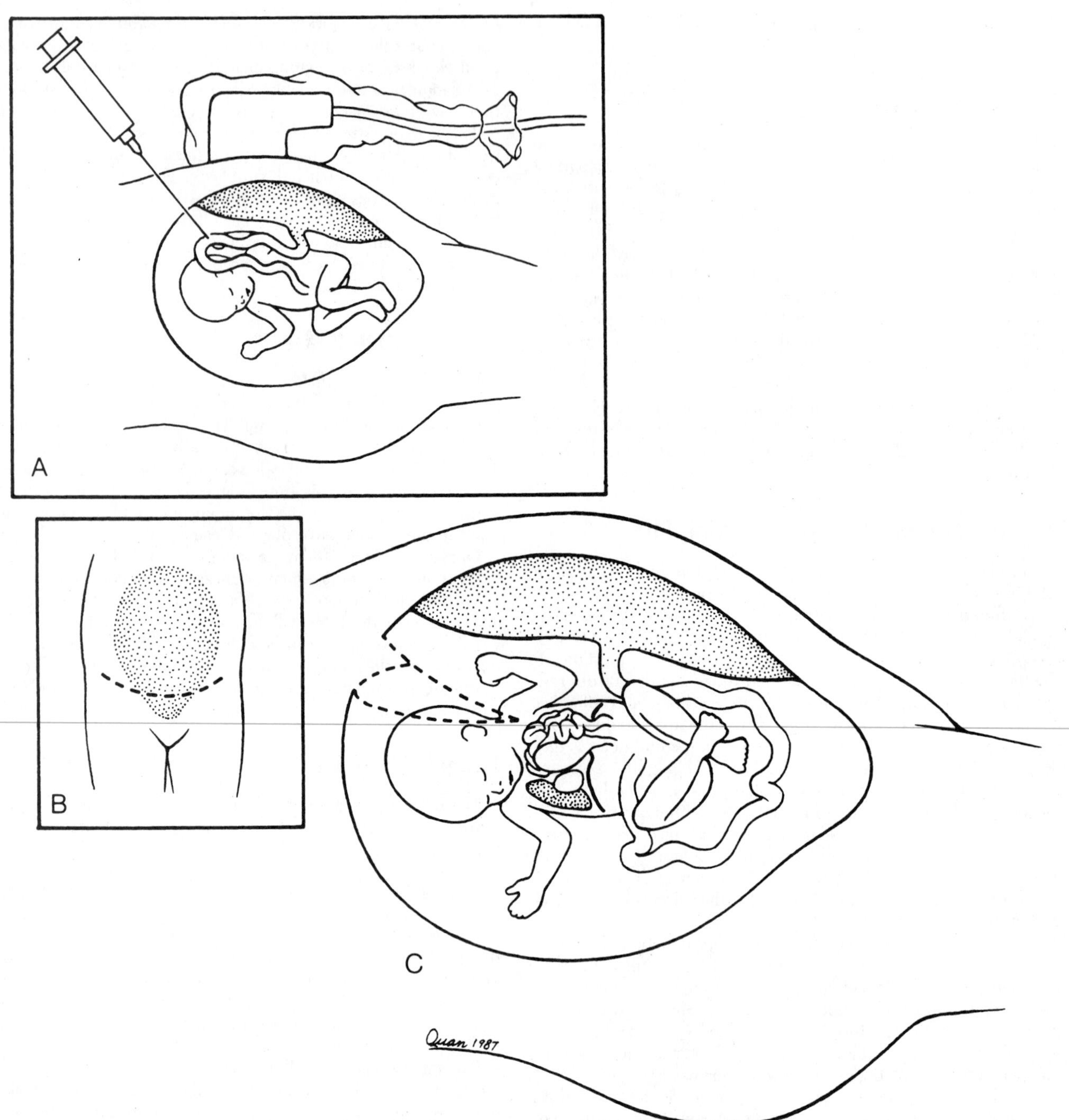

FIGURE 38–6. Steps in fetal repair of congenital diaphragmatic hernia. *A,* Sonogram on mother's stomach shows surgeons the position of fetus. *B,* Incision in the uterus. *C,* Incision is made into the uterus; the fetal intestines and stomach are visible in the left lung cavity.

tube is placed through which surfactant is given. The cord is then clamped and cut and the newborn is resuscitated. This fetal bypass procedure is completed within 20 to 50 minutes.

The parents should have the opportunity to see and touch the infant as soon after birth as possible, regardless of the outcome. If the infant does not survive, parents should be encouraged to hold and view the infant, and pictures should be taken. All these interventions help the parents accept the outcome and experience closure.

If the infant survives, it is equally important for parents to see and touch the infant as soon as possible after birth to provide reassurance. If this is not possible because of the physical conditions of both mother and infant, pictures should be taken and given to the family immediately.

Neonatal Period

The final phase, the neonatal period, requires the team to work closely with the family's long-term health care providers to ensure that there is appropriate management of the case. Even when the infant does not survive, contact should be maintained with the family so that autopsy results and genetic counseling can be provided. Discussions of the various stages of the grief process

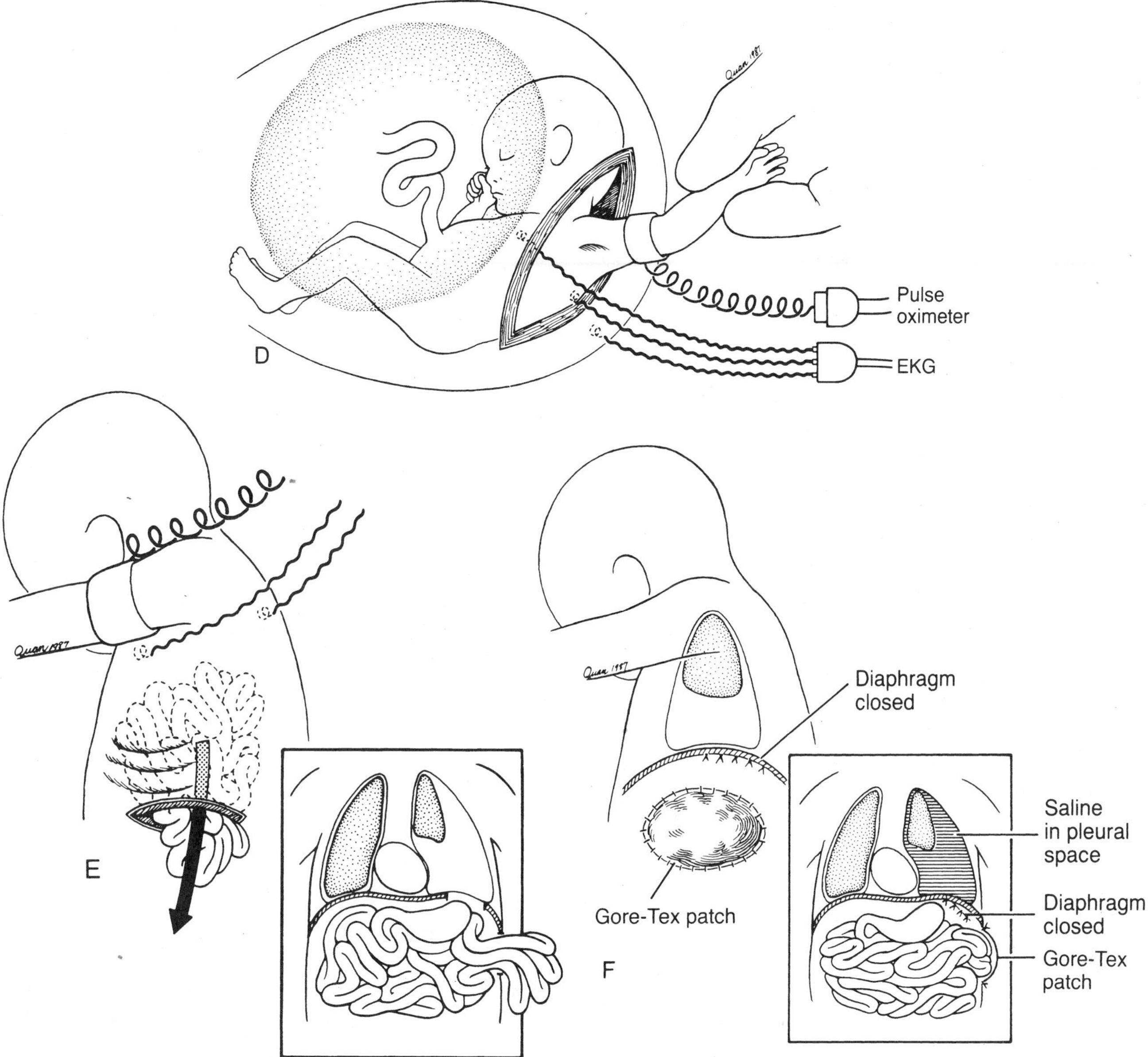

FIGURE 38–6 *Continued D,* Arm and left side of fetal chest are brought out of the uterus so that surgeon can operate. *E,* Moving the intestines and stomach from the lung cavity gives the lung room to grow. *F,* Hole in diaphragm is repaired with a patch. (Used with permission from the University of California, San Francisco.)

with the parents may help alleviate fears of never "getting back to normal." This is also an appropriate time to discuss the reactions of friends and family (Matthews et al., 1984). For the family whose infant has survived, the realization that the infant may require further surgical intervention surfaces during this period. They may even learn that the infant, in spite of the fetal surgery, may not live long. Even when the infant is doing well and has minimal risk of further illness, the family may not readily accept the information given. They may anticipate the infant's death, even though to the health care professionals this is not a realistic concern. They may require significant psychosocial support following the discharge of the mother and the infant to make sure that the transition to home is successful. This can be accomplished through telephone contact, home visits, and clinic visits soon after discharge in order to assess the family's adjustment. Referrals to support groups, psychologists, or professionals of other disciplines should be made immediately if the family appears to have trouble coping with having the infant home.

MULTIDISCIPLINARY COLLABORATIVE APPROACH

The focus of the multidisciplinary collaborative approach is the maternal-fetal unit, which requires continuous monitoring of both patients in the intensive care setting (Harrison, 1993). With the preceding discussion of the complexity of fetal surgery, it should be obvious that there is a need for a multidisciplinary team approach. Fetal surgery requires a collective approach to caregiving. The multidisciplinary team should include the following: perinatologist, neonatologist, pediatric surgeon, sonographer, anesthesiologist, operating room and obstetrical nurses, and social worker. In addition to these team members, a compassionate nurse coordinator should be available as a family liaison (Sullivan & Adzick, 1994).

Time is of the essence in these cases, not only because of the legal time frame dictated by the *Roe vs. Wade* decision regarding

TABLE 38–2 Pathway Used at the University of California, San Francisco

1. All patients who are admitted for intrauterine fetal surgery have preadmission consultation with the following members of the University of California, San Francisco fetal treatment team:
   Perinatologist
   Pediatric surgeon
   Operating room nurse specialist
   Ultrasonographer
   Obstetrical anesthesiologist
   Obstetrical nurse specialist
   Perinatal social worker
2. All patients are admitted the evening before surgery.
3. All patients are placed on tocolysis. The usual regimen is as follows:
   Indomethacin 50 mg PR at 10 P.M. prior to surgery, on call to operating room, then every 6 hours for at least 24–48 hours after procedure.
   Magnesium sulfate 2 g/hour intravenously beginning near the end of the procedure (intraoperatively) and continued until uterine activity is controlled for 48 hours.
   Subcutaneous betamimetics are begun prior to discontinuing magnesium sulfate and continued until delivery.
4. The clinical nurse specialist, the fetal treatment nurse coordinator, and the perinatal social worker provide continuity for issues of coping.
5. All patients undergo general anesthesia for the procedure and have an epidural catheter placed postoperatively for pain management via epidural morphine.
6. Postoperatively patients receive intravenous antibiotics until they are afebrile for 48 hours.
7. Patients receive one-to-one care for 48 to 72 hours.
8. Postoperative fluid management is crucial because the patient has some degree of blood loss requiring fluid replacement *and* receives intravenous tocolysis requiring fluid restriction to prevent pulmonary edema.
9. Pain management includes epidural morphine sulfate for the first 72 hours via continuous drip as ordered by the anesthesiologist. Good pain control is essential not only for the well-being of the patient but also for the fetus.
10. Patients generally remain in the hospital 7 to 10 days and then nearby until delivery with one home visit per week and one to two visits to the medical center for preterm labor evaluation and sonographic follow-up of the effects of fetal surgery and nonstress tests.

Fetal Surgery Preoperative Orders

1. Admit to:
2. Diagnosis:
3. Condition:
4. Vital Signs: Heart rate, respirations, blood pressure on admission and prior to surgery.
5. Fetal-tocolysis monitor strip 20 minutes after admission and prior to surgery. Maintain continuous tocolysis if uterine activity present.
6. Height and weight on admission.
7. Call ______________ perinatologist, beeper No. ______ for:
   A. Abnormal fetal heart rate.
   B. Uterine activity ≥4 uterine contractions per hour, ______________ >20 minutes per hour of uterine activity.
   C. Other.
8. Notify house officer for:
9. Activity: Bed rest, bathroom privileges.
10. Diet: Regular, nothing by mouth after midnight prior to surgery.
11. Laboratory:
    A. Complete blood count; differential.
    B. Sodium, potassium, chloride, carbon dioxide, blood urea nitrogen, creatinine, glucose, aspartate aminotransferase, uric acid, alanine aminotransferase.
    C. Type and crossmatch 2 units packed red blood cells; check specimen.
    D. Clot for quad pack of O negative, cytomegalovirus negative, sickle cell negative, irradiated.
    E. Fibrin glue.
    F. Urinalysis with microtube.
12. Intravenous therapy: D5LR at 100 ml/hour via 16-gauge angiocatheter to begin at 2200.
13. Electrocardiogram.
14. TED hose to thighs in place for surgery.
15. Medications: Allergies: ______________ Ht ______ (cm) Wt ____ (kg):
    A. Preoperative
       1. Indomethacin 50 mg PR at half strength.
       2. Nembutal 100 mg orally at half strength as needed for sleep.
    B. On call to operating room:
       1. Indomethacin 50 mg PR.
       2. Alka Seltzer Gold 2 tablets in 20 ml water
    C. Send to operating room with patient:
       1. Indomethacin 50 mg PR times 2.
       2. Ceftizoxime 2 g.
       3. Magnesium sulfate 50 g/500 ml drip primed on AVI tubing and set at 4-g load.
       4. Terbutaline.
       5. Fetal surgery pack.
    D. Pharmacy to make up nitroglycerin drip in D5NS and send to operating room 6 for intraoperative use. Prepare adequate amount of nitroglycerin to provide 20 μg/kg/minute for 6 hours.

Fetal Surgery Postoperative Orders

1. Admit to:
2. Diagnosis:
3. Condition:
4. Vital parameters: Heart rate, respirations, blood pressure every ______, temperature every ______. Continuous arterial blood oxygen saturation. Daily weight, 1 + intake and output 1 hour. Continuous tocolysis. Continuous fetal electrocardiogram, temperature and contraction monitor via indwelling electrode. Continuous arterial line and central venous pressure monitoring.

TABLE 38–2 Pathway Used at the University of California, San Francisco *(Continued)*

5. Call fetal surgery fellow: ______________ beeper No. ______:
   A. If unable to monitor TOCO/electronic fetal monitor continuously.
   B. Mean arterial pressure <60, pulse >120, respiratory rate >30, urine output <30 ml every hour, fetal bradycardia.
6. Activity: bed rest in lateral position; modified Trendelenburg position.
7. Diet: Nothing by mouth.
8. Nasogastric tube attached to low intermittent suction.
9. Foley catheter to gravity drainage.
10. Diagnostic studies:
    A. Fetal echocardiogram every day and as necessary.
    B. Sonogram every day and as necessary.
    C. Laboratory: Complete blood count, electrolytes, magnesium, calcium phosphate, creatinine, blood urea nitrogen, glucose, methemoglobin, arterial blood gas on arrival, every 6 hours times 24 hours. Accucheck every 6 hours.
    D. Chest film on arrival and every A.M.
11. Intravenous therapy
    A. Total intravenous fluids ____________ ml/hour
    B. Nitroglycerin ____________ μg/kg/minute (100 mg/250 ml D5NS = 400 μg/ml prepared by pharmacy only.
    C. Lactated Ringer's solution at ____________ ml/hour.
12. Oxygen via nasopharyngeal to keep arterial oxygen saturation >95%. Incentive spirometer every 3 to 4 hours while awake.
13. Thigh-high TEDS and Venodyne boots with sequential compression device.
14. Medications: Allergies:
    A. Refer to antimicrobial order sheet.
    B. Tocolysis: Nitroglycerin in D5NS titrate up to 10 μg/kg/minute maximum to keep mean arterial pressure >65.
    C. Indocin:
    D. Begin intravenous insulin drip when glucose >130 mg/dl. Check Accucheck every hour while on drip.

glucose	*units*
<130	0
131–150	2
151–170	4
171–190	6
191–210	8
>210	Notify house officer. Give 10 units.

    E. Pain: Per pain service.

Discharge Teaching

1. Ensure that patient has viewed the videotape "Recognizing Preterm Labor" (or another similar tape). Review signs and symptoms with patient and family.
2. Provide the following handouts and review each with patient and family:
   A. Preterm labor.
   B. Bed rest and diet.
   C. Bed rest and exercises.
3. Review the actions, dosage, frequency, and side effects of oral tocolytics with patient.
4. Assess with patient realities of home care management:
   A. Evaluate support systems and help at home.
   B. Physical layout of home.
   C. Management of meals.
   D. Factors that may interfere with bed rest.
5. Arrange home care as needed.

D5LR, 5% dextrose in lactated Ringer's solution; D5NS, 5% dextrose in normal saline; PR, per rectum.
Courtesy of Fetal Treatment Team, University of California, San Francisco.

women's rights to abortion but also because delays can lead to morbidity and mortality. For maximal potential benefit, candidates for fetal surgery should be identified and referred before 23 weeks' gestation. Early referral allows time for the fetal surgery team to carefully study the situation and perform appropriately timed interventions (Reedy et al., 1984).

Use of the multidisciplinary approach and specific interventions are outlined in Table 38–2 developed by the fetal surgery team at the University of California, San Francisco.

FETAL THERAPY: NEW HORIZONS

As previously mentioned, therapies and treatments for genetic problems are being attempted through fetal therapies. Such problems include treatment for inborn errors of metabolism in which the mother is given medication, vitamins, or the substance noted to be lacking in the infant. This substance passes through the placenta to the fetus for therapy (see Chapter 25, Assessment and Management of Metabolic Dysfunction). Other therapies have aimed at blood incompatibility problems. Exchange transfusions can be performed in utero. One of the newer fetal therapies has exciting potential. This treatment is for severe combined immune deficiency syndrome which carries a high mortality rate. This deficiency in the immune system resulted in infants and children having to live in protected bubbles so that they would not be exposed to infectious agents. Their immune systems are generally dead. Stem cell transplantation has been successful in treating this condition in utero. These stem cells can be obtained from a parent and then transfused through the umbilical cord of the fetus. The cells migrate to the spaces in the fetal bone marrow. There is a lot of space there because the liver is the main hemopoietic organ during gestational development. These cells do not trigger an immune response because a fetus generally does not mount such a reaction. These cells proliferate and replace the fetal stem cells and become differentiated into the various cell types of the immune system (Wiley, 1996). In the neonatal period, tests can be run and the T lymphocytes, in particular, can be identified. They can be tested to determine cell origin. In the successful treatment case in Detroit at Wayne State, the cells were paternal in origin and in sufficient number to suggest a cure for the severe combined immune deficiency syndrome. The infant is doing well (Flake, 1995). If this therapy continues to be successful, the treatment modality may be attempted for all forms of hemoglobinopathies—sickle cell anemia and thalassemia in particular. There is already a national network for cord blood banks to allow families the opportunity to save cord blood for use later in life if an immune problem arises. This movement toward embracing this new therapy is bringing with it ethical considerations that the nurse must remain aware of (McMillan, 1996).

CONCLUSION

This chapter has described fetal treatment and, more specifically, fetal surgery. It has highlighted the state of the art regarding this area of perinatal and neonatal health care. A critical pathway for care for the families undergoing fetal surgery has been included (see Table 38–2). This area of perinatal practice and research is growing. It is reasonable to assume that more neonatal health care professionals are going to be questioned about fetal treatment or surgery. It is important that neonatal nurses have a basic understanding of this newer technology. Community hospital–based nurses need to have some familiarity with this technology because the mother and fetus–neonate are often transferred to another hospital for follow-up care (Collins, 1994).

REFERENCES

Blustein, J. (1988). Mortality and parenting: An ethical framework for decisions about the treatment of imperiled newborns. *Theoretical Medicine, 9*(1), 23–32.

Chen, H., Moore, L. A., & Veghte, A. (1988). *Gene pool.* Dayton, OH: Children's Medical Center.

Chervenak, F. A., & McCullough, L. B. (1993). Ethical issues in recommending and offering fetal therapy. *Fetal Medicine (special issue), West Journal of Medicine, 159*(3), 396–399.

Christ, J. E. (1986). Fetal surgery: A frontier for plastic surgery [Editorial]. *Plastic and Reconstructive Surgery, 77*(4), 645–647.

Collins, J. E. (1994). Fetal surgery: Changing the outcome before birth. *Journal of Obstetric, Gynecologic, and Neonatal Nursing, 23*(2), 166–169.

Colodny, A. H. (1987). Antenatal diagnosis and management of urinary abnormalities. *Pediatric Clinics of North America, 34*(5), 1365–1381.

Connor, J. M., & Ferguson-Smith, M. A. (1987). *Medical genetics* (2nd ed.). Boston: Blackwell/Year Book Medical Publishers.

Costello, A. (1987). Psychosocial management of patients in a fetal medicine and surgery program. *Birth Defects, 23*(6), 62–74.

Crombleholme, T. M. (1994). Invasive fetal therapy: Current status and future directions. *Seminars in Perinatology, 18*(4), 385–397.

Donald, I. (1964). Ultrasonography in two dimensions. *Medical Biological Illustration, 14,* 216–224.

Elias, S., & Annas, G. J. (1987). *Reproductive genetics and the law.* Chicago: Year Book Medical Publishers.

Flake, A. (1995, October). *Fetal surgery.* Presentation at the National Association of Neonatal Nurses Regional Conference From Conception to Kindergarten, Chicago, IL.

Grupe, W. E. (1987). The dilemma of intrauterine diagnosis of congenital renal disease. (Review). *Pediatric Clinics of North America, 34*(3), 629–638.

Harrison, M. R. (1993). Fetal surgery. *Fetal Medicine (special issue), West Journal of Medicine, 159*(3), 341–349.

Harrison, M. R., & Adzick, N. S. (1993). Fetal surgical techniques. *Seminars in Pediatric Surgery, 2*(2), 136–142.

Harrison, M. R., Golbus, M. S., & Filly, R. A. (1981). Management of the fetus with a correctable congenital defect. *Journal of the American Medical Association, 246*(7), 774–777.

Harrison, M. R., Golbus, M. S., & Filly, R. A. (1991). *The unborn patient: Prenatal diagnosis and treatment* (2nd ed.). Philadelphia: W. B. Saunders.

Laifer, S. A., & Kuller, J. A. (1996). Percutaneous umbilical blood sampling. In J. A. Kuller, N. C. Chescheir, & R. C. Cefalo (Eds.), *Prenatal diagnosis and reproductive genetics* (pp. 151–158). St. Louis: C. V. Mosby.

Levine, A. H., & Imai, P. K. (1982). Intrauterine treatment of fetal hydronephrosis. *AORN Journal, 35*(4), 655–662.

Liley, A. W. (1963). Intrauterine transfusion of foetus in haemolytic disease. *British Medical Journal, 5365,* 1107–1109.

Lopez, E. I. (1989). Prenatal diagnosis by ultrasound. *Journal of Perinatal and Neonatal Nursing, 2*(4), 34–42.

Manning, F. A. (1986). International Fetal Surgery Registry: 1985 update. *Clinical Obstetrics and Gynecology, 29*(3), 551–557.

Manning, F. A. (1987). Fetal surgery for obstructive uropathy: Rational considerations. *American Journal of Kidney Diseases, 10*(4), 259–267.

Manning, F. A., Harrison, M. R., & Rodeck, C. (1986). Catheter shunts for fetal hydronephrosis and hydrocephalus. Report of the International Fetal Surgery Registry. *New England Journal of Medicine, 315*(5), 336–340.

Matthews, A. L., Costello, A. J., & Scott, J. A. (1984). The fetus as a patient: Some preliminary data from the first year of a fetal medicine and surgery program. *Birth Defects, 20*(6), 192–196.

McMillan, M. P. (1996). Banking on cord blood. *Journal of Obstetric, Gynecologic, and Neonatal Nursing, 25*(2), 115.

Michejda, M., Queenan, J. T., & McCullough, D. (1986). Present status of intrauterine treatment of hydrocephalus and its future. *American Journal of Obstetrics and Gynecology, 155*(4), 873–882.

Morin, L., Crombleholme, T. M., & Dalton, M. E. (1994). Prenatal diagnosis and management of fetal thoracic lesions. *Seminars in Perinatology, 18*(3), 228–253.

Newnham, J. P., Thomson, M. R., Murphy, A., et al. (1987). Successful placement of a pyeloamniotic shunt catheter for ureteropelvic junctional obstruction in utero. *Medical Journal of Australia, 146*(10), 540–542, 544.

Perry, S. E., Inturrisi, M., & Filly, R. A. (1986). Meeting the challenge of fetal surgery. *Dimensions in Critical Care Nursing, 5*(4), 196–205.

Pringle, K. C. (1986). In utero surgery [Review]. *Advances in Surgery, 19,* 101–138.

Quinlan, R. W., Cruz, A. C., & Huddleston, J. F. (1986). Sonographic detection of fetal urinary anomalies. *Obstetrics and Gynecology, 67*(4), 558–565.

Reedy, N. J., Ford, K. L., & Depp, R. (1984). Intrauterine fetal surgery: A nursing challenge. *Journal of Obstetric, Gynecologic, and Neonatal Nursing, 13*(5), 291–295.

Seeds, J. W., & Mandell, J. (1988). Prenatal diagnosis and management of fetal obstructive uropathies. In L. R. King (Ed.), *Urologic surgery in neonates and young infants* (pp. 41–58). Philadelphia: W. B. Saunders.

Sullivan, K. M., & Adzick, N. S. (1994). Fetal Surgery. *Clinical Obstetrics and Gynecology, 37*(2), 355–371.

Waldmann, T. A. (1991). Monoclonal antibodies in diagnosis and therapy [Review]. *Science, 252*(5013), 1657–1662.

Wiley, J. M. (1996). Stem cell transplantation for the treatment of genetic disease. In J. A. Kuller, N. C. Chescheir, & R. C. Cefalo (Eds.). *Prenatal diagnosis and reproductive genetics.* (pp. 243–269). St. Louis: C. V. Mosby.

CHAPTER 39

The Surgical Neonate

JEANNE HARJO

RESEARCH AGENDA

What is the relationship between the neonate's initial reaction to the stress of surgery and the postoperative acid–base balance?

What factors influence the neonate's ability to tolerate delays in surgical interventions?

What factors put the neonate at risk for surgical complications during the intraoperative period?

Combined with low-dose narcotics, does acetaminophen achieve satisfactory analgesia with minimal complications during the postoperative period?

VIGNETTE

As the ice cream choices in the freezer case absorbed my attention, I was startled to hear someone calling my name. I turned to see a woman in her early 20s with a babbling, tottering toddler at her feet. Why, it was Sarah and her mom! Sarah was smiling, wide-eyed, and full of energy, the picture of a healthy child. But there was a telltale scar in the center of her neck.

Sarah had been born full-term 2 years earlier and transported to the NICU. The left side of her face was much enlarged. An ear, nose, and throat consult diagnosed the presence of cystic hygroma. An airway was placed at her bedside. Sarah was in need of supplemental O_2, so she was placed in a head hood. Capillary O_2 saturation was monitored closely. The cystic hygroma rapidly collected fluid, putting more and more pressure on Sarah's airway. Her respiratory problem became so life-threatening that a tracheostomy was performed.

Sarah was the first child of her young, single mother. Although the father was not involved, her mother did get support from the maternal grandparents. They came and held Sarah daily. Sarah loved her pacifier. Her family and I brought toys for stimulation and a tape cassette of nursery rhymes. Daily explanations were given to the mother about Sarah's condition. However, she was overwhelmed by the number of people who came in contact with her daughter each day. The equipment alone was terrifying—all those tubes! At times, she would come into the nursery in the evening and sit by Sarah's bed and cry. I was her primary nurse, so I would go over and talk with her. Sometimes, there were questions for me to answer; other times, we just sat together and she would share her concerns and hopes.

When the ENTs considered Sarah adequately stable, she was prepared for surgery. Although she was in the OR for only 3 hours, it seemed like days had gone by when they brought Sarah back to the unit. Her color was good, her lips were pink, her eyes were open, and no ventilator was necessary. A little O_2 was blown through her tracheostomy. Sarah began to wiggle and move about in her crib. Her vital signs were within the normal range. Her incisions were minimally dressed. She was to be closely monitored for the next few days. Her mother stayed at her bedside stroking her head. Day by day her condition improved. Her IV fluids were decreased as gavage feedings were started. Sarah's respiratory status improved so much that her tracheostomy was closed. It became difficult to calm Sarah—she wanted her pacifier. Soon, her fluids and medications were discontinued and oral feedings were begun.

Sarah continued to grow and heal. Revision would be done as she grew. Discharge instructions were taught, along with well-baby care. When Sarah was deemed ready to be discharged, I carried her to the grandparents' waiting car. Although her mother was excited and pleased to be taking her daughter home, she verbalized her fear related to the severity of the illness Sarah had experienced and doubts about her ability to care for her.

Vicky Merritt

Care of the surgical neonate is an exciting challenge. To provide complete care and achieve optimal survival, a multidisciplinary team must be involved. This team must include neonatal nurses, neonatologists, pediatric surgeons, radiologists, and anesthesiologists. Members of this team must work together, guided by the knowledge that all of the principles of neonatal care, as well as additional considerations related to surgical care, apply in each case.

In this chapter, the challenges faced by the surgical neonate are discussed. Stressors such as hypoxia, acidosis, hypothermia, and fluid and electrolyte imbalances are poorly tolerated by the neonate, especially when complicated by prematurity. When these stressors are prevented or minimized, however, surgical stress is tolerated remarkably well. This chapter is an overview of the global concerns facing any neonate who is undergoing surgery. The specific care regimens of the surgical problems are discussed in detail in the respective assessment and management chapters of the text.

PREOPERATIVE PERIOD

Stabilization of the neonate in the preoperative period determines the infant's ability to survive the trauma of surgical intervention. The major factors to be considered in effective stabilization include oxygenation, acid–base balance, thermoregulation, fluid and electrolyte balance, and pharmacologic support.

Oxygenation

Adequate tissue oxygenation is necessary to prevent irreversible organ damage resulting from hypoxia. Establishment of effective ventilation is a primary concern in providing optimal air exchange and oxygenation.

Ventilatory insufficiency can occur with various surgical problems. For example, airway obstruction occurs with choanal atresia, whereas an ineffective airway clearance mechanism is experienced with a tracheoesophageal fistula with esophageal atresia. Hypoventilation is encountered with a diaphragmatic hernia as well as with those defects causing increased abdominal pressure on the diaphragm and lungs. Defects that manifest this type of problem include omphalocele or gastroschisis, necrotizing enterocolitis, and bowel obstructions.

It is imperative that the numerous causes of altered neonatal ventilation be considered and properly treated. A surgical neonate is not immune to problems such as prematurity, respiratory distress syndrome, persistent pulmonary hypertension, atelectasis, aspiration pneumonia, or bronchopulmonary dysplasia.

Neonates are obligate nose breathers. With choanal atresia, an oral airway is required to establish adequate ventilation. Intubation, if required, is performed through the orotracheal route.

Diaphragmatic breathing is also characteristic of neonates. Any intra-abdominal pressure changes can lead to respiratory compromise. To minimize this problem, care must be taken to position the infant so as to avoid abdominal pressure from an abdominal wall defect. Placing these infants in the side-lying or semi–side-lying position may relieve diaphragmatic pressure from the defects and enhance ventilator assistance and pulmonary function.

Omphalocele or gastroschisis, necrotizing enterocolitis, and bowel obstructions all cause increased abdominal distention. Gastric decompression is necessary to decrease this source of pressure on the diaphragm and the increasing difficulty in lung expansion. This decompression is achieved through use of an oronasogastric tube to gravity drain or suction. The patency of this tube must be maintained to allow for adequate gastrointestinal decompression. Continued abdominal distention may further compromise respiratory effort. Increased oxygenation or ventilation needs may reflect unresolved abdominal distention and worsening of the disease process. In addition, the ascites encountered in renal defects such as ureteropelvic junction obstructions can cause respiratory difficulty. Mechanical ventilation may be required until surgical intervention relieves the abdominal pressure.

A neonate with a diaphragmatic hernia has special respiratory needs. Mask ventilation must be avoided. This method of oxygenation is contraindicated because air is forced into the gastrointestinal tract, causing the volume to be increased in the chest, thus increasing the respiratory compromise in an infant with already limited lung function. Ventilation must focus on the use of the minimal pressures necessary to oxygenate the infant adequately, thereby avoiding damage to the functional lung. The prevention of persistent pulmonary hypertension must also be a primary concern. To accomplish this, adequate ventilation must be established to avoid hypoxia, hypercarbia, and acidosis, which are known factors in the pathophysiology of pulmonary hypertension.

Mask ventilation is also contraindicated when a tracheoesophageal fistula with esophageal atresia is present. Rupture of the esophageal pouch and overdistention of the stomach may occur. As a result, stomach contents can reflux through the fistula into the trachea, causing pneumonia. Proper positioning of the endotracheal tube, if needed, and the use of minimal ventilator pressure minimize these complications.

The prevention of aspiration pneumonia is a major concern with a tracheoesophageal fistula with an esophageal atresia. If the blind esophageal pouch fills with saliva, overflow occurs into the lungs, causing pneumonia. Maintaining the patency of a double-lumen suction tube to drain the esophageal pouch prevents this complication. If diagnostic testing is necessary to evaluate the esophageal pouch, the contrast fluid must be kept from spilling out of the pouch, which, again, can cause aspiration pneumonia. This danger can be avoided by using a plain anteroposterior chest and abdomen radiograph taken with a radiopaque tube placed in the esophageal pouch. The esophageal pouch is clearly outlined, and visualization of air in the stomach confirms the presence of a tracheoesophageal fistula. Elevating the head of the infant's bed or placing the infant in the prone position minimizes possible reflux of gastric secretions through the tracheoesophageal fistula, preventing aspiration pneumonia.

Maintenance of a patent airway can be of concern with various defects. In some circumstances, intubations may be avoided if proper positioning is used. Extension of the neck may be necessary when a large, obstructing cystic hygroma is present. Hydrocephalus of severe proportions may also require slight extension of the neck and turning of the head to either side.

Regardless of the type of defect present, nursing priorities in regard to oxygenation status include respiratory assessment for the quantity and quality of respiratory effort. Wide changes in the respiratory rate should be investigated. Adequate ventilation can be demonstrated by ease of respirations, absence of retractions or nasal flaring, and appropriate pink color of lips, mucous membranes, or nailbeds.

Acid–Base Balance

Alterations in acid–base balance can be caused by a variety of factors in the surgical neonate. Major areas that can result in acidosis include inadequate respiratory support and fluid or electrolyte imbalances. The effects of sepsis and tissue necrosis are also significant causes of acidosis. Acidosis in the surgical neonate can be respiratory, metabolic, or mixed.

Respiratory acidosis could occur with decreased ventilation, resulting in increased $P\text{CO}_2$ levels and decreased pH. An overproduction of acids may occur with any condition that causes decreased oxygenation or decreased perfusion. Impaired kidney function, such as that which occurs in acute renal failure or renal tubular necrosis, decreases elimination of hydrogen ions, contributing to the development of metabolic acidosis. Bicarbonate losses are increased with severe diarrhea, intestinal fistulas, vomiting, and gastric drainage, resulting in metabolic acidosis.

The neonate with a diaphragmatic hernia is at great risk for development of respiratory acidosis, metabolic acidosis, or both. Such an infant requires aggressive ventilation as well as the administration of a buffering agent (e.g., sodium bicarbonate, tromethamine [Tham]) to prevent acidosis, which could contribute to the development of persistent pulmonary hypertension.

Poor tissue perfusion causes acidosis, as is seen with multiple gastrointestinal anomalies that are accompanied by large fluid losses. These include tracheoesophageal fistula with esophageal atresia, ruptured omphalocele and gastroschisis, bowel obstructions, and necrotizing enterocolitis. Adequately replenishing fluid or blood volume usually corrects this metabolic acidosis. When necrosis or perforation occurs, however, the acidosis may not be correctable until the necrotic bowel is removed and any resulting sepsis is treated.

Thermoregulation

See Chapter 16 for further discussion of neonatal thermoregulation. This discussion offers information concerning the prevention of cold stress in the surgical neonate.

Neonates may have poorly developed mechanisms for thermoregulation. The large body surface area of a neonate coupled with the lack of insulating subcutaneous fat enhances heat loss. Also, oxygen consumption is not decreased with prolonged cooling of a neonate; rather, oxygen consumption increases as the metabolic rate increases to maintain body temperature. This increased metabolic work results in acidosis and tissue hypoxia.

Prevention of hypothermia is imperative to the surgical neonate in the preoperative period. Maintenance of a neutral thermal environment is a constant challenge. In this atmosphere, metabolic activity is minimal as body temperature is kept stable. Oxygen consumption is reduced, and acidosis is prevented. Any prolonged deviations from the neutral thermal environment further stresses the already limited thermoregulation abilities of the neonate.

Heat loss occurs through evaporation, conduction, convection, and radiation. Evaporative heat loss occurs with the exposure of the intestinal contents of a ruptured omphalocele or gastroschisis. In the case of an encephalocele or a myelomeningocele, the unprotected spinal cord may allow heat loss. The exposed bladder mucosa seen in an exstrophy of the bladder also contributes to heat loss. Prevention of this heat loss can be accomplished by applying warm dressings to the defects, then covering these areas with plastic.

Conductive heat loss occurs with direct skin contact on a cold surface, such as cold or wet linens, a weight scale, an examining table, x-ray plates, or an unwarmed bed. To avoid this type of heat loss, linens should be prewarmed as the bed or incubator is warmed. Examining or x-ray tables can be warmed with heat lamps before and during procedures. Linens that become wet should be replaced with dry, warmed linens; x-ray plates and scales should be covered with warmed linens before being placed under the infant.

Heat loss by convection occurs when air blows over the infant. Use of warmed oxygen in head hoods and ventilators can decrease this type of heat loss. Also, it is essential that the incubator door not be open for prolonged periods. Insertion of nasogastric tubes, placement of intravenous lines, x-ray studies, physical examination, and phlebotomy procedures should be performed through the incubator portholes to decrease heat loss. An additional heat source may be placed over the incubator when the door must be open.

Heat loss by radiation is the most difficult to control. This type of heat loss occurs during transportation of the neonate in cold hallways, in cold examining rooms, or in the cold operating room. To prevent this cold stress, the infant should be covered with warmed linens during transport. Examining rooms and operating rooms should be prewarmed to well above the "comfortable" temperature.

Nursing care focusing on the thermoregulation process of the neonate is vitally important in preventing complications related to poor temperature control. Maintenance of a constant temperature, whether inside an incubator or in a radiant warmer bed, is a top priority. It is also beneficial to use warmed solutions for suctioning and dressing changes. Frequent monitoring of the infant's temperature is extremely important. Consistency in the method of measuring temperature and appropriate documentation are also essential. Prevention of cold stress decreases the chance of surgical complications, prompting more neonatal surgeries (e.g., patent ductus arteriosus ligations) to be performed within the neonatal intensive care unit (NICU). The lack of transport of the neonate to the operating room suite avoids subjecting the infant to environmental temperature changes during the move to and from the operating room and in the operating room itself.

Fluid and Electrolyte Balance

Fluid Losses

Adequate fluid volume is required to ensure adequate perfusion of all organ systems. An inadequate vascular volume interferes with the oxygen supply to peripheral tissues, resulting in cellular damage and acidosis.

A neonate with a normally functioning cardiovascular system can tolerate the administration of intravenous fluids and blood products, as long as the delivery of these fluids is precise and appropriate. Precision in fluid management is essential, and there is little margin for error.

All fluid losses must be accurately measured to allow for adequate replacement. Estimation of insensible fluid losses is essential, including those caused by humidification through ventilation, radiant heating, and phototherapy. Unexpected fluid losses and inadequate fluid replacement delay the neonate's preoperative stabilization.

With an esophageal atresia in the neonate, continuous losses of saliva suctioned from the esophageal pouch must be measured and replaced. The large exposed intestinal area seen with a ruptured omphalocele or gastroschisis results in tremendous amounts of fluid losses. Replacement of these losses may involve up to twice the normal maintenance fluids of a neonate. If an omphalocele is protected by a membranous sac, the fluid requirement is less.

Gastrointestinal obstructions cause fluid losses from vomiting and from the suctioning required for gastric decompression. Peritonitis, as occurs with perforations in necrotizing enterocolitis, midgut volvulus, or ruptured meconium ileus, causes third spacing of fluid or fluid shifts into the bowel, necessitating increased fluid replacement.

Infants with open neural tube defects also have increased fluid losses. A leaking myelomeningocele requires increased fluid administration to keep up with the loss of cerebrospinal fluid.

Third spacing of fluids, or capillary leak syndrome, is the result of trauma to the gastrointestinal system. The capillary membrane's permeability is changed. This phenomenon may be due to secretion of natural fibronectin, a glycoprotein secreted by epithelial cells in the pulmonary and gastrointestinal trees. It is secreted in response to stimulation of the immune system to heal a wound. Fibronectin alters capillary permeability, shifting fluid and resulting in a "leaky capillary" and the third spacing of fluid. The body's compensatory response to any gastrointestinal trauma, then, can result in a movement of fluid across this "leaky" membrane. Fluid moves out of the vascular compartment and into the tissues. The infant becomes swollen with generalized edema. Abdominal swelling creates pressure on the thoracic cavity, increasing the work of breathing. Gas exchange and ventilation are compromised as a result of (1) the pressure, (2) the decreased circulation, (3) the increased workload of the heart, which delivers oxygen to the tissues, and (4) the increasing loss of the buffer system through decreased kidney perfusion and gastric losses.

The immediate reaction by inexperienced health professionals is to restrict fluids in this edematous infant, even though the vascular compartment is severely depleted of fluids. The infant is hypotensive, which increases cardiopulmonary compromise. Thus, liberalization of fluids is necessary to avoid total vascular collapse.

The performance of diagnostic enemas with hyperosmolar solutions can have catastrophic results in a neonate who is not properly hydrated. Adequate intravenous access and good hydration are essential. Vascular collapse and even shock can occur rapidly if the fluid is shifted from the vascular bed to the bowel and the fluid is extracted with the enema and not appropriately replaced.

Glucose Level

Fluctuation in the glucose level is a major indication of stress as well as infection. Preoperative hyperglycemia can result from sepsis or excessive intravenous administration of glucose. Hypoglycemia may result from a multitude of problems. For example, reduced glycogen stores are seen in premature infants and in infants with intrauterine growth retardation. Excessive insulin production occurs in the infant of a diabetic mother and with sudden or prolonged cessation of glucose infusions, as may occur with difficult or delayed intravenous line insertions. Abnormalities in glucose metabolism are evident with sepsis, shock, and asphyxia, as well as with various central nervous system abnormalities. Careful titration of glucose infusions is necessary to provide adequate hydration while slowly restoring serum glucose to an acceptable level, avoiding extremes in serum glucose levels.

Electrolyte Imbalances

The numerous conditions affecting the surgical neonate may result in imbalances of serum electrolytes, especially sodium and potassium. Fluid losses as well as inadequate intake result in hypokalemia and hyponatremia.

Hyperkalemia occurs with acidosis, excessive potassium intake, and renal failure. Renal failure may result from genitourinary obstructions or from sepsis and poor perfusion as seen in necrotizing enterocolitis with perforation or peritonitis.

Hypernatremia is generally the result of iatrogenic causes. An excessive intake of sodium occurs with the administration of hypertonic solutions, intravenous flushes with normal saline or heparinized normal saline, or sodium bicarbonate for treatment of acidosis. Therapy with antibiotics such as ampicillin also adds to the potential for hypernatremia.

Return to proper fluid and electrolyte balance is needed to improve the neonate's ability to tolerate any necessary operative procedure and to reduce potential complications.

Pharmacologic Support

Calculations of medication doses must be carefully individualized to the neonate. The neonate's weight is only one factor to be considered in these calculations. An immature renal and hepatic system may result in a decreased ability to metabolize and excrete drugs. To prevent toxicity, serum levels of medications should be closely monitored. (See Chapter 41, Neonatal Pharmacology.)

Preoperative antibiotic therapy may be required for the treatment of sepsis. Untreated sepsis may progress, causing deterioration of the respiratory and cardiovascular systems. Respiratory distress requires increased ventilation. Inotropic drugs may be needed to support the cardiovascular system. In many NICUs, gentamicin sulfate is used in combination with aminoglycoside therapy as treatment for sepsis. This antibiotic increases the sodium intake and must be considered in monitoring electrolyte balance. Clindamycin is an effective agent used in the treatment of anaerobic organisms, which are generally found in gastrointestinal infections.

Surgical problems in the neonate necessitate the use of antibiotic therapy. With suspected gastrointestinal obstructions, antibiotics may be needed to treat peritonitis or enterocolitis. The progression of necrotizing enterocolitis may be slowed with vigorous antibiotic therapy. Omphalocele and gastroschisis treatment should include antibiotics to protect the exposed gastrointestinal contents and to help prevent ischemic injury to the abdominal contents. If pneumonia accompanies an esophageal atresia with tracheoesophageal fistula, aggressive antibiotic treatment should be instituted to clear the pneumonia and promote an optimal surgical repair of the defect. The infant with a myelomeningocele requires antibiotic treatment to prevent meningitis.

Inotropic agents may be necessary to improve cardiac function and thus improve organ perfusion that has been impaired as a result of sepsis and stress. The most frequently used agents are dobutamine and dopamine. Dobutamine achieves organ perfusion by increasing cardiac output. Dopamine, used in low to moderate doses, causes vasodilation with resultant improvement in cardiac, renal, gastrointestinal, and cerebral blood flow. Use of dopamine at high doses, however, causes vasoconstriction of renal and gastrointestinal vessels. This vasoconstriction could worsen a renal system affected by obstruction or poor flow status, as well as the gastrointestinal system already compromised in necrotizing enterocolitis, omphalocele, gastroschisis, or obstructions. Thus, dobutamine and dopamine doses must be carefully calculated and continually titrated to achieve the desired effect. Furthermore, these medications are incompatible with many other drugs. For example, alkaline solutions such as sodium bicarbonate, ampicillin, gentamicin, and furosemide can inactivate dobutamine and dopamine. These inotropic agents are also irritating to vessels, and close monitoring of intravenous sites for infiltration is essential.

A buffering agent may be required to treat the acidosis that may accompany a diaphragmatic hernia, necrotizing enterocolitis, omphalocele, gastroschisis, or obstruction with resulting ischemic injury. Adequate ventilation and tissue perfusion must be established and maintained before medication is used to treat acidotic conditions.

OPERATIVE PERIOD

Timing of the Operation

The proper timing of a surgical procedure is an important factor in minimizing the stress encountered by a surgical neonate. If the infant is hemodynamically stable, then major intervention may be tolerated with surprisingly few complications. However, the infant with untreated sepsis or acidosis may not even survive the induction of anesthesia without severe problems.

A surgical neonate may suffer from a multitude of medical as well as surgical problems. A complete evaluation is needed, as long as the infant can tolerate this delay. A metabolically stable, growing infant is a much better surgical risk than an unstable, acidotic, premature baby.

The emergent nature of any surgical problem takes precedence over minor defects. For example, resection of a perforated bowel requires intervention before the repair of a mild congenital heart defect; however, severe congenital heart disease may be repaired before an uncomplicated intestinal atresia is corrected.

Perforation of the stomach or intestines is one of the few reasons an emergency surgical repair is performed. If such a case is untreated, hypovolemia, acidosis, and shock occur. Delay in treating necrotizing enterocolitis with perforation or midgut volvulus results in further infarction of an already compromised bowel, leading to further shock and death. The physiologic response to perforation is not correctable until the diseased bowel is resected. Even in these emergent situations, hypovolemia must be aggressively treated to attain an optimal surgical outcome.

The treatment of a congenital diaphragmatic hernia is directed toward aggressive stabilization of respiratory status, including extracorporeal membrane oxygenation (ECMO), before the repair of the hernia. The repair is performed when the infant is stable and while the infant is still on ECMO.

An infant with a tracheoesophageal fistula with an esophageal atresia receives a gastrostomy tube as soon as possible to prevent reflux of gastric contents into the lungs through the fistula. The repair of the atresia and fistula can be delayed until the infant is stable and a complete evaluation is performed for other anomalies. The fistula may be ligated and the esophageal anastomosis delayed to allow for better growth and an optimal surgical outcome. Treatment of pneumonia must be done before any surgical procedure is undertaken.

When a neonate is not stable enough for a primary closure of an omphalocele or gastroschisis or the defect is too large, a Silastic pouch, or "silo," may be performed. This pouch helps to prevent infection, alleviate the restriction of venous return to the extremities, and reduce renal compromise. This procedure relieves abdominal pressure, which may cause respiratory compromise by suspending the defect above the abdomen. Slow, daily reduction of this "silo" over 7 to 10 days allows closure with minimal complications.

A myelomeningocele can be protected with sterile normal saline soaked dressings to allow for full evaluation of the infant's neurologic status before repairing the defect. An ultrasound of the head helps determine whether placement of a ventriculoperitoneal shunt is needed. Evaluation by an orthopedist for determination of potential intervention for the lower extremities can be delayed until the back repair is done and is healing.

If the infant with an encephalocele is stable, a full evaluation should be performed to reveal the type of tissue and vascular access involved in the defect. This information is useful to the surgeon who removes the encephalocele and allows for preparation of the family for the infant's postoperative prognosis.

The timing factor is important when a sacrococcygeal teratoma is present. Evaluation of the defect preoperatively is essential to determine the surgical technique and the postoperative outcome. Relevant questions include the following:

Is the spinal cord involved?
Is the defect extremely vascular?
What will be the result if the defect is excised?

A great loss of blood can occur and should be anticipated. Preoperative stabilization of the infant's hematologic status is imperative to optimize surgical outcome.

An infant with an imperforate anus requires radiologic evaluation to identify the location of the rectum. This evaluation determines the surgical procedure, that is, whether an anoplasty or a colostomy is required.

Timing of the operation can also be extremely important to the family. In a stabilized infant, thorough evaluation of a surgical defect is essential. This information, as complete and accurate as time allows, enables the family to truly give informed consent.

Intraoperative Care

The stressors encountered by the surgical neonate during the preoperative period continue to present a challenge for patient management during the intraoperative period. Although the stabilization of the infant remains a major consideration, the effects of anesthesia during the surgical procedure present additional problems. Vascular access must be established in order to rapidly give drugs, fluids, and blood products. Arterial lines may be needed to monitor blood gases and arterial pressures. Critical assessments of vital signs and exact fluid management directly affect the positive or negative outcome of surgical intervention.

Oxygenation

A number of factors can limit gas exchange during anesthesia in the neonate. The gestational age and birth weight of the infant dictate the size of the endotracheal tube used for intubation. Smaller gauge tubes create increased airway resistance and, thus, increased difficulty in ventilation. Specific defects such as diaphragmatic hernia, omphalocele, and gastroschisis cause additional considerations. When the abdominal contents of the defects are replaced in the abdominal cavity, pressure on the diaphragm is increased and ventilation must be adjusted to compensate for this change. Stress and fatigue in the infant also decrease respiratory effort and necessitate prolonged manual or mechanical ventilation.

Anesthetic agents can cause respiratory depression, as can narcotic and sedative medications. The capacity of the neonate to tolerate anesthesia for a prolonged period is limited. Residual effect of anesthesia can delay the recovery of the infant from the surgical procedure, as seen by the infant's decreased respiratory effort or apnea. Oxygenation of the neonate should be directed toward maintenance of a PO_2 in the range of 60 to 80 mm Hg or an O_2 saturation range of 90 to 95 percent.

Acid–Base Balance

Acidosis during surgery remains a challenge for management. As previously discussed, the effects of sepsis and tissue necrosis as well as poor tissue perfusion add to the potential for an acidotic state. Acid–base balance may also continue to be altered as a result of impaired renal function or prolonged fluid imbalances. Monitoring of blood gases and the administration of buffering agents are important aspects of patient care throughout the surgical procedure as discussed for the preoperative period.

Thermoregulation

Concerns related to temperature regulation continue during the intraoperative period. Although it is always helpful to achieve a normal core temperature in the infant before surgery, this is not always possible. The body temperature should be monitored throughout the procedure by use of either a skin or a rectal probe. A radiant warmer should be used during line placement, preparation, draping, and induction of anesthesia. A warming blanket can also be used to achieve constant temperature control. In addition, the room temperature should be increased to assist in compensating for the neonate's inability to stabilize temperature. Another mechanism for improving temperature control is through humidification and warming of anesthetic gases. Slightly warming blood products, irrigation fluids, and intravenous fluids also assists in temperature maintenance. Surgical drapes should be replaced, if possible, when they become wet.

Another challenge in temperature maintenance is encountered during transport of the neonate to and from the operating room. To ensure temperature stability, the infant should be covered with warmed linen during transport. During the operative procedure, the bed should be warmed to allow for some warmth during transport postoperatively.

Fluid and Electrolyte Balance

Constant monitoring of fluid balance should continue throughout the surgical procedure. Early treatment of hypovolemia is essential. Intravenous fluid administration rates must be monitored to prevent fluid boluses, which could compromise fluid and electrolyte balance. Fluid loss from the surgical defect and blood loss during the operative procedure must be monitored and replaced. Metabolic response to surgery may also alter the infant's fluid and electrolyte balance. Hyperglycemia is a common response to surgical stress. Cold stress adds to this metabolic response and consequent fluid needs.

Glucose stability is an additional consideration during surgery. Glucose metabolism is not stable in the neonate; prematurity magnifies this problem. The glucose level should be monitored frequently to maintain a narrow range of normal. As discussed, the infusions of intravenous fluids should be monitored closely to prevent inaccurate rates of administration, resulting in hypoglycemia or hyperglycemia.

Pharmacologic Support

Use of medications during the intraoperative period can be affected by many variables. Irregular patterns of metabolism, immature or compromised renal function, and variations in hepatic blood flow can influence the action and effectiveness of medications. Bradycardia can result from narcotics such as fentanyl and morphine, inhalation anesthetics, and muscle relaxants. The resultant hypoxia must be considered a major problem and must be resolved quickly to ensure successful surgical outcome.

When considering the use of muscle relaxants, it must be remembered that neonates are particularly sensitive to succinylcholine. Bradycardia can be associated with this drug, and a predose of atropine may be given to avoid this complication. Intermediate and long-acting muscle relaxants such as pancuronium are commonly preferred for their ability to achieve or maintain a hemostatic state by increasing the heart rate and blood pressure.

Inhalation anesthetics and intravenous anesthetics can depress the ventilatory response to hypoxemia and hypercarbia. An increased pulmonary uptake of some agents causes high tissue levels and eventual cardiac compromise. However, the successful use of inhalation anesthetics in combination with narcotics has been achieved in the neonatal population (Reyes & Vidyasagar, 1989). However, careful monitoring of fluid status as well as cardiovascular and renal function is essential throughout the surgical procedure.

POSTOPERATIVE PERIOD

The initial postoperative period is a critical time in the recovery of the surgical neonate. Neonatal surgery is done only when it is absolutely necessary; therefore, the infant is already in a compromised situation before the procedure. The skillful assessment and management of the neonate is required to achieve a positive surgical outcome. This requires experience and collaborative care before, during, and after surgery. There are times when, no matter how careful and diligent the care is before surgery, the outcome in terms of morbidity and mortality is not good.

Close monitoring of the neonate includes frequent assessment of core temperature, surface temperature, heart and respiratory rate, blood pressure, perfusion, and oxygen saturation. Ventilatory assistance must also be evaluated frequently for rate, pressure, and oxygen administration. Intravenous infusions should also be assessed for rate to ensure an adequate urine output of at least 1 to 2 cc/kg/hour (Ingelfinger, 1985). Serum glucose levels should be monitored and adjusted appropriately.

Oxygenation

Respiratory care in the postoperative period can present a great challenge to the caregiver. The respiratory tract can be traumatized by intubation, anesthetic gases, and the stress of the procedure. Depression of respiratory drive can also be seen as a residual effect of anesthesia. Airway clearance may also be difficult to maintain. These alterations in respiratory mechanics may lead to respiratory insufficiency and the need for prolonged mechanical support (Leape, 1987). Although specific respiratory needs may vary depending on the surgical procedure, a conservative approach to respiratory care is essential to maintain optimal oxygenation. An aggressive plan of weaning may cause recurring acidosis, hypoxia, or damage to the surgical repair.

In the postoperative neonate with diaphragmatic hernia, care should be geared toward prevention of persistent pulmonary hypertension, caused by pulmonary vasoconstriction, and prevention of damage to the "good lung," resulting from excessive ventilator pressures. Paralysis with pancuronium can be beneficial in the postoperative period to assist in adequate ventilation and oxygenation. Such an infant should be weaned cautiously.

Respiratory support for the postoperative infant with tracheoesophageal fistula may range from humidified mist to endotracheal intubation, depending on the type of repair and the complications encountered in surgery (Kenner et al., 1988). The infant should be suctioned frequently to minimize both endotracheal and oropharyngeal secretions. A measured catheter should be used to avoid damage to the surgical sites. A thoracotomy may also be done to prevent atelectasis or pneumothorax and to promote expansion of the lung.

Respiratory compromise is a common complication following primary closure of an omphalocele or gastroschisis. Excessive pressure on the diaphragm and poor peripheral perfusion related to pressure on the inferior vena cava may require ventilatory support to improve lung expansion and oxygenation status. Paralysis with pancuronium may be helpful with ventilation efforts and to prevent rupture of incisions.

Postoperative care of the neonate with necrotizing enterocolitis includes aggressive ventilation. Many of these infants are small, premature, or have low birth weight with already compromised lung function. The stresses of severe infection and the surgical procedure itself, and the prematurity of the lungs may necessitate a prolonged ventilation with a slow weaning process.

Acid–Base Balance

As in the preoperative and intraoperative periods, acid–base balance continues to present a challenge to the neonate postoperatively. Although the neonate's initial reaction to the stress of surgery influences this balance, the concern over acidosis continues for a significant period of time. Monitoring of blood gases, attention to fluid balance, and delivery of appropriate respiratory support are a large part of postoperative care. As sepsis is resolved, fluid status is stabilized, and urine output is optimized, acid–base balance also stabilizes.

Thermoregulation

Temperature regulation of the neonate can remain a problem in the immediate postoperative period. Use of radiant warmers is a method of choice in maintaining both core and surface temperatures. The premature, small infant may require enclosure in an incubator to maintain consistent temperature control.

The principles of thermoregulation used in the preoperative and intraoperative periods are again useful in the postoperative plan of care for the surgical neonate. Use of warmed linens immediately following transport of the infant may be helpful in maintaining temperature stability. Removal of wet dressing and warming of irrigation fluids also assist in alleviating variations in body temperature.

Fluid and Electrolyte Balance

The goal of postoperative care is to provide fluid and electrolyte balance without overhydration. Hypovolemia is a major cause of hypotension and must be resolved quickly to ensure adequate perfusion to all organ systems and to combat acidosis. However, extreme care must be taken in administering fluids because premature infants are susceptible to third spacing and edema. Neonates are also very easily overloaded with excessive fluids.

Vital signs should be monitored frequently, initially every 15 to 30 minutes. Drastic changes in heart rate or blood pressure could indicate shock or undetected fluid loss for which the body is trying to compensate. Assessment of temperature continues to be an important factor and must be considered when evaluating fluid needs.

Serum electrolyte and glucose levels should be evaluated immediately postoperatively and then every 4 to 6 hours until stable. Sodium losses may continue through wound drainage as well as gastric decompression. Thus, intravenous fluids, both maintenance and replacement, require reevaluation to achieve and maintain electrolyte balance. Glucose metabolism may be altered as a response to surgery. Serum glucose levels should be monitored every 1 to 2 hours after surgery (Kenner et al., 1988).

Attempts to correct glucose or electrolyte problems overzealously can result in a rebound effect. The neonate may change from being hyperglycemic to hypoglycemic without intervention over a period of minutes or hours. The neonate moves from a catabolic to an anabolic state fairly rapidly compared with an older child or adult. These phases may occur over a few days or weeks in the infant instead of over months as in the adult. Thus, it is best to obtain baseline serum electrolyte and glucose levels. These values should be obtained every 1 to 4 hours, depending on how extreme the levels are. When any intervention is needed, the sodium, potassium, or other electrolyte should be increased or decreased slowly and in small increments. These incremental changes should be followed by repeated measurement of serum levels, which must be closely monitored.

Third spacing of fluids causing edema in the first few postoperative days is an additional consideration. The infant's weight, renal function, and nutritional needs must continue to be evaluated. Additionally, nursing care must include measures to maintain skin integrity during this period of edema and fluid mobilization.

Nutritional Needs

Concern during the convalescent period for some surgical neonates goes beyond fluid and electrolyte balance. The nutritional needs of infants with altered function of the gastrointestinal tract present unique problems. A small stomach size with altered emptying ability, as is sometimes seen with diaphragmatic hernia, gastroschisis, omphalocele, and bowel resections may present paramount problems in providing proper nutrition when feedings are started. Use of continuous feedings may help with these problems.

Gastroesophageal reflux may present challenges to feeding. Assessments of vomiting and large gastric aspirates must be made. Treatment of reflux may include positioning the infant prone or in an upright position after feedings and thickening the feeding. Continued reflux without appropriate weight gain is cause for evaluation for surgical intervention such as pyloroplasty or pyloromyotomy.

The neonate with bowel resection following perforation (e.g., in necrotizing enterocolitis) can present a significant challenge. Concerns should center around vomiting, diarrhea, distention, or the presence of glucose or blood in the stool. The infant may not tolerate standard formulas, and an alternative formula such as Pregestimil may be required. (See Chapter 23, Nutrition: Physiologic Basis of Metabolism and Management of Enteral and Parenteral Nutrition.)

Pharmacologic Support

During the postoperative period, antibiotic therapy remains aggressive. Ampicillin sodium and gentamicin sulfate remain the most commonly used combination of drugs. Penicillin G, clindamycin, cefotaxime sodium, and ceftriaxone sodium are also frequently used.

Inotropic agents, dopamine and dobutamine, may be needed postoperatively to maintain organ perfusion and renal function. As fluid balance is achieved and cardiac compromise resolves, monitoring and titration of these drugs remains essential.

Management of pain in the surgical neonate is an ongoing challenge in the postoperative period. Narcotic analgesics have both advantages and disadvantages. Although they are potent and achieve effective analgesia in all age groups, their most adverse effect is the respiratory depression and apnea produced. The sedative effect of narcotics can be advantageous in the immediate postoperative period. When unstable vital signs are present, however, potential bradycardia and hypotension, which can be side effects of a variety of narcotic preparations, must be considered.

Use of acetaminophen is common when concerns about respiratory depression exist. Combined with low-dose narcotics, acetaminophen may achieve satisfactory analgesia with minimal complications. Also, acetaminophen has no significant effect on platelet aggregation, thus causing no risk for increased bleeding (Reyes & Vidyasagar, 1989).

CONCLUSION

Care of the surgical neonate is a multidimensional challenge. The infant possesses many strengths that assist in tolerance of the surgical procedure and promotion of recovery. Rebound from surgery can occur rapidly if the case is properly managed and complications are anticipated. Nursing care requires ongoing assessment and timely interventions to produce optimal outcomes in the surgical neonate.

REFERENCES

Ingelfinger, J. R. (1985). Renal conditions in the newborn period. In J. P. Cloherty & A. R. Stark (Eds.), *Manual of neonatal care* (2nd ed., pp. 377–394). Boston: Little, Brown.

Kenner, C., Harjo, J., & Brueggemeyer, A. (1988). *Neonatal surgery: A nursing perspective.* Orlando: Grune & Stratton.

Leape, L. L. (1987). *Patient care in pediatric surgery.* Boston: Little, Brown.

Reyes, H., & Vidyasagar, D. (1989). Neonatal surgery. Preface. *Clinics in Perinatology, 16*(1), xi–xii.

SUGGESTED READINGS

Avery, G. B., Fletcher, M. A., & MacDonald, M. G. (Eds.). (1994). *Neonatology: Pathophysiology and management of the newborn.* (4th ed.). Philadelphia: J. B. Lippincott.

Bell, S. G. (1989). Vercuronium bromide as an alternative to pancuronium bromide for neuromuscular blockage in mechanically ventilated neonates. *Neonatal Network,* 7(5), 21–25.

Burke, J. F. (1983). *Surgical physiology.* Philadelphia: W. B. Saunders.

Coran, A. G. (1978). *Surgery of the neonate.* Boston: Little, Brown.

Crockett, M., & Tappero, E. (1989). Dopamine, dobutamine: Neonatal indications and implications. *Neonatal Network,* 7(5), 13–19.

Fanaroff, A. A., & Martin, R. J. (Eds.). (1997). *Neonatal-perinatal medicine* (6th ed.). St. Louis: C. V. Mosby.

Filston, H. C., & Izant, R. J. (1985). *The surgical neonate: Evaluation and care* (2nd ed.). Norwalk, CT: Appleton-Century-Crofts.

Freeman, N. V., Burge, D. M., Griffiths, M., & Malone, P. S. J. (Eds.). (1994). *Surgery of the newborn.* New York: Churchill Livingstone.

King, L. R. (1988). *Urologic surgery in neonates and young infants.* Philadelphia: W. B. Saunders.

Noerr, B. (1988). Tolazoline HC1 (Priscoline). *Neonatal Network,* 7(3), 74–75.

Noerr, B. (1989). Sodium bicarbonate. *Neonatal Network,* 7(5), 70–71.

Norton, S. (1988). After-effects of morphine and fentanyl analgesia: A retrospective study. *Neonatal Network,* 7(3), 25–28.

Pawlak, R. P., & Herfert, L. A. T. (1988). *Drug administration in the NICU: A handbook for nurses.* Petaluma, CA: Neonatal Network.

Sethling, L. C. (1982). *Common problems in pediatric anesthesia.* Chicago: Year Book Medical Publishers.

CHAPTER 40

Identification, Management, and Prevention of Pain in the Neonate

LINDA STURLA FRANCK

■ RESEARCH AGENDA

What are the mechanisms of neonatal pain?

What are the behavioral responses to neonatal pain?

What are the long-term consequences of neonatal pain?

How can pain be best evaluated in the critically ill or premature infant?

How do the attitudes, beliefs, and knowledge of nurses, physicians, and parents about opioid analgesics influence the management of neonatal pain?

How do analgesics commonly used in the intensive care nursery (ICN) compare in their efficacy and side effects?

Does frequent, intense pain or pharmacologic pain treatment have long-term consequences for ICN infants?

In comparison to the dramatic advances that have been made in other aspects of neonatal care, there has been a conspicuous lack of progress in the understanding and treatment of neonatal pain. Because of scientific and social influences, however, advances in these areas are beginning to be made. This chapter describes current knowledge regarding neonatal pain, identifies gaps in that knowledge and opportunities for research, and discusses the role and responsibilities of the neonatal nurse in caring for the neonate in pain.

HISTORICAL OVERVIEW

Scientific Study of Pain

The current definition of pain, adopted in 1979 by the International Association for the Study of Pain, holds that "Pain is an unpleasant sensory and emotional experience associated with actual or potential tissue damage, or described in terms of such damage" (Merskey, 1979). This definition recognizes the subjective nature of pain and avoids linking it to a specific stimulus. Current pain theory organizes the experience into sensory-discriminative, cognitive-evaluative, and affective-motivational dimensions (Melzack & Creasy, 1968). Major advances have occurred primarily in understanding the sensory-discriminative dimension of pain. Pain sensation is thought to involve a dynamic process of excitation and inhibition within a constantly shifting pattern of interneuronal communication along ascending nerve tracts. Descending projections inhibit or amplify pain information transmission at multiple spinal and supraspinal levels (Anand & Carr, 1989). Advances in all aspects of adult pain research have been comprehensively reviewed by Price (1988) and by Wall and Melzack (1994).

Before the mid-1970s, infants were believed to be reflexive, decorticate beings who could only experience pain at the level of a semianesthetized adult (Swafford & Allen, 1968). Although behavioral responses of infants to painful stimuli were observed, they were thought to be of no consequence based on a lack of understanding of both pain and infant neurologic development. However, newborn infants possess anatomic substrates to perceive and respond to pain that are similar (if not identical) to those of the adult.

Most significant to the progress of infant pain research, is the refutation of the belief that myelination is necessary for nerve function. Even though the role of myelin has been established as one of insulation, affecting the speed of impulse conduction and not necessary for nerve function (Schulte, 1975), the potential for infants with immature (largely unmyelinated) nervous systems to perceive pain was not recognized and fully appreciated until it was established that up to 80 percent of fibers that transmit pain information in adults remain unmyelinated (Price & Dubner, 1977).

Emergence of an Imperative for Treatment of Infant Pain

Concurrent with developments in pain science, three factors led to the emergence of an imperative for the treatment of infant pain: (1) the advent of neonatal intensive care, (2) the realization of the influence of environment on the developing central nervous system (CNS), and (3) the emergence of an ethical mandate for treatment of infant pain.

First, and most dramatic, were the changes that occurred in the care of newborn infants. Before the advent of neonatal intensive care, most infants did not survive life-threatening illness or medical treatment of the kind that would cause intense pain in adults. Techniques to support all vital functions of the preterm or ill infant created a new population of patients in the intensive care nursery (ICN) who are exposed to frequent noxious stimuli (Barker & Rutter, 1995a, 1995b; Franck, 1987; Gottfried & Gaiter, 1985). Clinicians, who had been practicing under the assumption that infants did not perceive pain or at least would not remember pain, were reluctant to change practice, claiming that the risks and consequences of pain management outweighed any benefit for the physiologically fragile newborn infant (Truog & Anand, 1989).

The discovery of the importance of neural plasticity in CNS development was the second factor contributing to the emergence of an imperative for the study and treatment of infant pain. (For a more complete discussion of plasticity, see Chapter 29, Assessment and Management of Neurologic Dysfunction). In the 1980s, the functional interaction between environmental stimuli and developing brain structures was described. Research revealed that environmental stimuli, particularly during periods of rapid brain growth, had profound and developmentally essential effects (Gollin, 1981). However, this neural plasticity also implies a profound vulnerability to the environment and can result in abnormal structural and functional development (Duffy et al., 1984). A realization has gradually emerged that, in the ICN, pain is one of the most frequent and significant environmental stimuli with potential effects on the infant's developing CNS.

Third, parents of infants receiving intensive care played a significant role in creating the imperative for pain management for infants. They advocated the use of anesthesia for infant surgery, a practice that was not the standard of care even as late as the mid-1980s (Lawson, 1988; Shearer, 1986). This change prompted discussion regarding the ethical aspects of pain management for infants (Butler, 1987, 1989; Campbell, 1989) and the publication of a position statement regarding neonatal anesthesia by the American Academy of Pediatrics (AAP, 1987).

Taken together, these historical developments led to the current conceptualization of the neonatal CNS as an organ system at risk (whether as a result of premature birth or pathologic condition), requiring scientific attention and thoughtful intervention. An imperative has been created for research to better understand the mechanisms and management of neonatal pain.

NEURODEVELOPMENT OF PAIN MECHANISMS

Infants have the neurologic capability to feel pain before birth, even premature birth. The scientific evidence for this statement has been comprehensively reviewed (Fitzgerald & Anand, 1993; Franck, 1991). Briefly, the peripheral, spinal, and central structures necessary for pain information transmission are present and functional early in gestation (between the first and second trimesters). Rapid synaptogenesis begins in the cortex with demonstrated functional maturity by 20 to 24 weeks of gestation. Infants possess a well-developed hypothalamic-pituitary-adrenal axis and can mount a fight-or-flight stress response with release of catecholamines and cortisol. Neuropeptides, which mediate analgesia (inhibit or amplify), are also present and functional before birth. Cortisol and endorphin levels have been shown to increase during intrahepatic transfusion in 23- to 34-week-old fetuses (Giannakoulopoulos et al., 1994), demonstrating an appropriate hormonal response to needling of the abdomen.

PATHOPHYSIOLOGY

There are two major reasons for concern about the effects of pain experienced by critically ill infants. First, pain causes many adverse physiologic consequences. Second, the developing CNS is extremely vulnerable to environmental influences and can be altered by external events. Acute and chronic pain cannot, as yet, be differentiated in the infant. Nor is the clinician able to determine the quality of pain (e.g., stinging, burning) or even the location of pain in infants. Therefore, immediate and potential long-term effects of pain experienced by newborn infants are discussed without distinguishing between acute and chronic pain. Assessment of pain focuses solely on the measurement of pain intensity.

IMMEDIATE EFFECTS

Pain causes adverse physiologic effects in all major organ systems, which can be life-threatening in the acutely ill patient. These effects include reduced tidal volume and vital capacity in the lungs, increased demands of the cardiovascular system, and hypermetabolism resulting in neuroendocrine imbalances (Kehlet, 1986). The increased metabolic demands on the cardiovascular and respiratory systems caused by pain can lead to increased oxygen consumption, hypoxemia, and myocardial ischemia in the patient with compromised cardiovascular and respiratory function (O'Gara, 1988; Phillips & Cousins, 1986).

The newborn infant's immature sympathetic response to pain is less predictable than that of the adult. The mobilization of endocrine and metabolic resources results in changes in blood pressure (which can be either increased or decreased) and changes in skin color and temperature. The immature cerebral vascular bed is particularly vulnerable to injury because there is a lack of autoregulation and any stimuli that increase cerebral vascular congestion or result in hypoxemia (e.g., crying) may increase the risk for intraventricular hemorrhage (Brazy, 1988). Endorphin release may also affect blood pressure and respiration. These changes may be dramatic or subtle depending on the level of maturity of the infant's CNS regulatory mechanisms and the amount and intensity of stress to which the infant is subjected.

Research regarding the stress responses of both full-term and preterm infants to surgical trauma has been succinctly summarized by Anand (1990). The hormonal-metabolic changes seen in full-term infants are greater in magnitude but shorter in duration than in adults undergoing similar surgery. Immature enzyme processes and decreased lipid stores result in an even greater degree of tissue breakdown in preterm infants after surgery (Anand, 1990). It has also been demonstrated that anesthesia can reduce the magnitude of the hormonal-metabolic stress response. Several studies of premature infants undergoing ligation of the patent ductus arteriosus demonstrated substantial and prolonged catabolic reactions as well as circulatory and metabolic complications after surgery when anesthetic agents were not administered or were administered in inadequate doses (Anand & Aynsley-Green, 1988a, 1988b; Anand et al., 1987). These studies also suggest that the use of anesthesia not only decreases the neonate's stress response but also results in decreased postoperative morbidity and mortality, as has been shown in adults (Anand & Carr, 1989; Anand & Hickey, 1992).

Neonates may exhibit acute behavioral and physiologic instability to stimuli that are considered only mildly noxious or nonpainful to the adult or older child. This increased sensitivity of premature neonates to most sensory stimuli has been well documented (Gorski et al., 1983). Excessive light and noise in the ICN elicit dramatic physiologic and behavioral stress responses (Blackburn, 1996; Grauer, 1989; Long et al., 1980; Robertson & Philbin, 1996). In addition, handling and caregiving procedures cause significant physiologic distress to the premature neonate, including blood pressure and heart rate instability as well as hypoxia (Long et al., 1980; Norris et al., 1982; Perry et al., 1990; Porter et al., 1991). The cardiorespiratory effects of handling may result from increased circulating catecholamines, particularly norepinephrine, and cortisol (Gunnar et al., 1989; Lagercrantz et al., 1986). For the premature neonate, social interaction (e.g., the human voice and face) can cause physiologic and behavioral distress similar in magnitude to that occurring with chest physiotherapy (Gorski et al., 1983).

Potential Long-Term Effects

Studies of both animal and human neonates have demonstrated that environmental manipulations can permanently alter behavior, brain function, and even brain structure, particularly when the event occurs during critical periods of development (Duffy et al., 1984). The developing human brain is most vulnerable to environmental influences during periods of rapid growth between 10 to 18 weeks' gestation and again between 30 weeks' gestation and 3 months of postnatal age (Dobbing & Smart, 1974). Although the infant brain undergoes a tremendous period of growth, the process of neuronal competition for synaptic connections (particularly during the third trimester) results in a large amount of cell death and remodeling of the neuronal structure (Volpe, 1987). It is on this process that environmental influences can have the most profound effects. Patterned neuronal activity selects those cell populations that will proliferate from those that will degenerate (Janowsky & Finlay, 1986). The amount and frequency of painful stimuli inflicted on the infant receiving intensive care could possibly result in a reallocation of cortical resources and permanent alterations in cerebral neuroanatomy.

The arousal resulting from a painful event may be overwhelming for the infant who then may attempt to shut out all stimuli and alter interactions with caregivers and sleep patterns (Emde et al., 1971; Marshall et al., 1982). It has been suggested that a mismatch between the environmental demands of the ICN and the infant's neurobehavioral maturity can result in aberrant patterns of social interaction that may persist beyond infancy (Als, 1983).

Animal research suggests that pain and stress in the neonatal period result in altered pain sensitivity, decreased weight gain, decreased ability to learn mazes, body temperature instability, and even immunosuppression in the adult (Anand & Plotsky, 1995; Sandman et al., 1979; Vorhees, 1981). Studies of human neonates have revealed marked differences in cortices of healthy term infants as compared with preterm infants (Duffy, 1985). Two recent studies (Grunau et al., 1994a, 1994b) suggest that pain experience in the ICN may alter the normal course of development of pain behavior in toddlers.

ICN caretakers have been described as "brain shapers" in the care of their preterm patients (Spinelli, 1990). Studies point to the long-term negative effects of noxious stimuli in the ICN on the infant's developing CNS (Field, 1990; Gorski et al., 1990). Modulation of the negative effects with modifications of the ICN environment can improve developmental outcome (Als et al., 1986; Barnard & Bee, 1983).

Premature infants who spend the neonatal period in the ICN are at risk for developmental delays, permanent CNS handicap, and emotional disorders (Sell, 1986). Although the contribution of painful procedures to these risks is unknown, the possibility should not be disregarded. The neonatal CNS must be considered as an organ system at risk, as important as the cardiovascular or pulmonary systems, and protected from adverse environmental events, including pain.

MEASUREMENT OF INFANT PAIN RESPONSES

Assessment of pain in the neonate is challenging, and the appropriateness of treatment depends on an accurate assessment. Most instruments used to assess pain in adults or older children require language skills and are therefore not applicable to the assessment of pain in infants. Reliable physiologic and biochemical markers have not been developed, in part, because of the ethical constraints on inflicting pain on infants who cannot give their consent in a controlled experimental setting. Nevertheless, clinicians must use available information and determine, to the best of their ability, the presence of pain in their neonatal patients. Assessment of pain in infants can be made with information gathered from the following three categories of responses: behavioral, physiologic and autonomic, and neuroendocrine.

Behavioral

Several surveys have shown that nurses still rely primarily on behavioral cues to assess presence of pain in neonates (Franck, 1987; Pigeon et al., 1989; Sparshott, 1989). However, the neonate's ability to demonstrate behavioral responses to painful stressors is strongly influenced by neuromuscular maturation and severity of illness (Coll, 1990; Tronick et al., 1990) and may not be a reliable indicator. Premature neonates demonstrate decreased behavioral responsiveness to painful stressors (Stevens & Johnston, 1994). Behavior becomes more organized and under inhibitory control as the neonate matures and health improves (Als, 1984). Therefore, it may be difficult at times to assess pain in infants from their behavioral responses. Behavioral assessment of infant pain includes evaluation of vocalization (i.e., cry), facial expression, and gross motor movement.

Infant pain cries have been shown to be spectrographically distinct in terms of acoustic frequency and pitch from cries resulting from other stimuli (Fuller, 1991; Levine & Gordon, 1982; Porter et al., 1988a, 1988b). These differences can be detected by adult listeners (Porter et al., 1988a, 1988b). Cry latency has also been used as a measure of pain (Franck, 1986; Grunau and Craig, 1989).

The infant also forms a "cry face" characteristic of pain. The facial expression in response to heelstick is different from that from other tactile stimuli such as rubbing or cleaning the heel, and it has been shown to be a sensitive and reliable measure of pain (Craig & Grunau, 1989; Grunau et al., 1990). Key features of the cry face include brow bulge, eye squeeze, and deepening of the nasolabial folds. While premature neonates have less robust facial expression, these indicators of pain can be accurately and reliably detected and correlated with physiologic signs of pain.

The healthy infant displays vigorous gross motor movement and attempts to withdraw from painful stimuli (Franck, 1986). The critically ill or premature infant, however, may exhibit diffuse, disorganized behavior but quickly becomes limp and flaccid in response to noxious stimuli.

The flexor reflex of the neonate can be evoked by a cutaneous mechanical stimulus to the heel that produces a clear, distinct withdrawal of the leg. The flexor reflex threshold response increases (i.e., the neonate becomes less reactive to cutaneous stimuli) with gestational age (Andrews & Fitzgerald, 1994; Fitzgerald et al., 1988a). Repeated stimulation has been shown to produce sensitization (rhythmic flexion and extension or tonic flexion of the leg) in the premature infant less than 30 weeks' gestation, whereas habituation (i.e., diminished responsivity to repeated stimulation) has been observed in most infants at 32 to 35 weeks' gestation (Andrews & Fitzgerald, 1994; Fitzgerald et al., 1988a). Repeated heelsticks lower the flexor reflex threshold (i.e., greater sensitivity to cutaneous stimuli) in the injured heel as compared with the intact heel (Fitzgerald et al., 1988a, 1989). The hypersensitivity of the injured heel was reversed with application of a topical local anesthetic (Fitzgerald et al., 1989). These data suggest a clear organization of spinal sensory processing and a high level of excitability within the developing spinal cord of the premature neonate.

Absence of Overt Response

The absence of overt responses to painful stimuli does not necessarily indicate lack of pain perception. Whereas behavioral responses are consistently associated with increases in neuroendocrine measures, elevations in neuroendocrine parameters are not always accompanied by increases in behavioral responses. Response to pain stimuli may also be delayed or cumulative. The infant may appear to tolerate several procedures well and then exhibit signs of compromise with increased oxygen requirements in the absence of further stimulation. In the very immature or very stressed infant, there may be no response at all to noxious stimuli. The immature CNS has a limited ability to withstand stress, and the absence of response may only indicate the depletion of response capability and not lack of perception. In such cases, perception of pain must be inferred empirically, based on the likelihood of a pain response in an older child or adult under the same conditions.

Differentiation of Pain From Agitation

Agitation is a term commonly used to describe excessive gross motor behavior and crying. Agitation in the ill neonate can be disruptive to physiologic processes. Because it is difficult to interpret the behavioral language of infants, distinguishing irritable, restless behavior caused by pain from agitation resulting from other causes is one of the most challenging tasks of infant pain management. Excessive gross motor movement and crying occur frequently in ICN infants experiencing respiratory insufficiency and CNS dysfunction. Characteristics of the irritable infant have also been described (Budreau & Craft, 1992). However, because treatment decisions are made based on the suspected cause of the behavior (i.e., pain versus air hunger), every effort must be made to accurately assess the reason for the agitated behavior.

Physiologic and Autonomic

Measurement of neonatal physiologic responses to painful stimuli includes changes in heart rate, respiratory rate, blood pressure, transcutaneous oxygen and carbon dioxide levels, oxygen saturation, intracranial pressure, cardiac vagal tone, and palmar sweat (Harpin & Rutter, 1983; Porter et al., 1988a, 1988b; Rawlings et al., 1980; Schwartz & Jefferies, 1990; Stevens & Johnston, 1994). However, the accuracy and sensitivity of these measures, particularly in the ill or premature infant, have been difficult to establish because of the influence of other nonpainful stimuli (Cabal et al., 1992).

A promising physiologic measure of pain response may be heart rate variability (HRV), which examines the amplitude of beat-to-beat changes in heart rate to estimate the parasympathetic or sympathetic influences on heart rate. One method of determining HRV—vagal tone index (VTI)—appears sensitive to differences in stimulus intensity and may discriminate between pain and nonpain states in neonates. For example, in full-term neonates, decreases in VTI following restraint were smaller than the decreases following circumcision (Porter et al., 1988a, 1988b). In addition, precircumcision VTI was predictive of the magnitude of the change in VTI following the procedure, whereas heart period was not. Neonates with higher baseline VTI values had larger decreases in VTI after circumcision. Thus, in neonates, VTI may provide better specificity and sensitivity in detecting the parasympathetic response to painful stimuli than either heart rate or heart period variability (Porter, 1989). Further research is required to determine whether VTI is a more sensitive measure of the neonatal pain responses than heart rate.

Neuroendocrine

Infants release catecholamines, cortisol, endorphins, and other chemicals with neuroendocrine effects in response to pain (Boix-Ochoa et al., 1987). Although neonates clearly demonstrate catecholamine responsiveness to painful stimuli, there is marked variability in both the baseline values and the degree of change in plasma E and NE levels associated with pain. The sources of the variability in responses have not been identified.

Changes in plasma, urinary, and salivary cortisol levels are also observed in response to painful stressors (Gunnar et al., 1991). The degree of cortisol responsiveness of neonates correlates closely with the intensity of the stressor, increasing only slightly with mild restraint and fourfold during circumcision (Gunnar et al., 1991). Healthy infants habituate to repeated mild stressors (handling) and become more reactive (sensitized) to repeated painful stressors (heelstick), whereas less healthy infants do not habituate or sensitize to stressors (Gunnar et al., 1989; Gunnar et al., 1991). Even though increased cortisol levels are usually seen during behavioral distress, elevated cortisol levels in response to painful stressors are not always accompanied by behavioral signs of distress (Gunnar et al., 1988).

Neuroendocrine measures are difficult to obtain in the clinical setting but, in the future, may prove valuable in assessing the neuroendocrine response to stressors such as pain (Hughes et al., 1987). The development of an assay for salivary cortisol (Gunnar et al., 1991) may provide a clinically useful measure of neuroendocrine stress response to pain.

Variability in Neonatal Responses to Pain

Although specific neonatal data are lacking, factors that influence pain responses in adults (i.e., specificity, magnitude, intensity, and duration of stressors) presumably influence the mode of expression and magnitude of the neonatal nociceptive stress responses. In addition, expression of neonatal stress responses is further modulated by (1) the increased sensitivity of premature neonates to sensory stimuli, (2) the initial behavioral state of the neonate, and (3) the neonate's ability to habituate to stressors. In the healthy neonate, stress responses may diminish with repeated pain stimuli, indicating adaptation to the stressor. These mechanisms are not well developed in the premature neonate, resulting in a relative hypersensitivity of the premature neonate to painful stimuli and normally nonpainful stimuli (Fitzgerald, 1991). Furthermore, lack of stress responses in ill neonates may indicate exhaustion. The inability to reliably distinguish between habituation and exhaustion is a significant challenge in neonatal pain assessment (Stevens et al., 1996).

Behavioral state is a significant factor modulating the observed behavior of infants in response to pain as well as other stimuli. Infants who are awake, inactive but attentive, show the strongest behavioral response to stimuli (Craig & Grunau, 1989).

Some of the intraindividual variability seen in neonatal responses to painful stimuli may be due to differences in baseline behavioral state during the study periods, which may influence the neonate's degree of responsiveness to stimuli. Thus, any evaluation of stress responses requires careful examination of the influence of the individual's baseline state and reactivity, as well as the context of the stressful stimuli (Boyce et al., 1992; Manuck et al., 1990; Porges, 1992).

Neonates often exhibit the same stress responses to painful and nonpainful stimuli. The degree of responsiveness to stressors may also be predictive of later behaviors and health status (Brazelton, 1973; Gunnar et al., 1989; Izard et al., 1991; Lewis, 1992; Porges, 1992). Lewis (1992) suggested that it is a combination of genetic determinants of temperament and environmental conditions that accounts for the differences in responsiveness to stressors among neonates. Porter (1989) believed that the interindividual variability in behavioral responses to nociceptive stressors may indicate the early development of individual coping styles.

CLINICAL ASSESSMENT OF INFANT PAIN

Although advances in understanding and measurement of infant pain responses have been dramatic over the last decade, ideal clinical pain assessment tools remain elusive. Behavioral indices have been combined into a pain scoring instrument (Barrier et al., 1989). Using this scoring tool, the clinician rates the infant's sleep, cry, motor activity, tone, excitability, facial expression, sociability, consolability, and sucking. The tool has been used to assess the effectiveness of analgesia (Mayer et al., 1989) but requires validity and reliability testing before its usefulness can be determined.

Another pain score, the Neonatal Infant Pain Scale (NIPS), was shown to be a valid and reliable measure of infant responses (including facial expression, cry, breathing pattern, arm and leg movement, and behavioral state) to arterial, venous, or capillary needle puncture (Lawrence et al., 1993). Gestational age and 5-minute Apgar scores were positively correlated with NIPS scores, indicating that older, healthier infants were more capable of demonstrating behavioral responses to painful stimuli than younger, sicker infants.

A scoring tool combining both physiologic and behavioral indices (Krechel & Bildner, 1995) demonstrated initial validity and reliability in 32- to 60-week-old infants in assessment of postoperative pain. The simplicity of the scale and inclusion of quantitative physiologic parameters may increase the acceptance and use of pain-scoring tools in the ICN.

Only one pain assessment scoring tool has been developed and validated in premature neonates. The Premature Infant Pain Profile (Stevens et al., 1994) rates changes in heart rate, oxygen saturation, facial action (degree of brow bulge, eye squeeze, and nasolabial furrow) on a 3-point scale. Gestational age and behavioral state are also factored into the pain score. This scoring tool has been used for premature neonates undergoing heelstick, but further validation studies using other pain stimuli are needed.

Despite the need for further research and development of infant pain assessment methods, there is clear evidence from adult studies that implementation of a standardized pain assessment protocol (no matter how imperfect the tool) improves pain management for patients (Au et al., 1994). The importance of routine assessment, using standardized terms, and incorporating discussion of pain issues into medical and nursing rounds makes pain "visible." The importance of having pain assessment protocols and tools has been underscored in the Acute Pain Management Guidelines from the Agency for Health Care Policy and Research (AHCPR, 1992), which requires institutions to develop an organized program to evaluate the effectiveness of pain assessment. Pain assessment has also received greater attention from hospitals since it became a focus for quality improvement activities. Friedrichs and colleagues (1995) provide an excellent example of a successful unit-based multidisciplinary approach to the improvement of neonatal pain assessment and management. Figure 40–1 represents one example of a documentation form for pain assessment.

With regard to pain assessment in neonates, the following advertising slogan seems apropos: "Just do it!"

TABLE 40–1 Minimal Handling Protocol (Children's Hospital, Oakland)

Protect From Light
Shade infant's eyes with blanket over isolette or table, or use cut-out box over infant's head.

Protect From Noise
Do not talk over infant.
Set speakers as low as possible.
Do not allow telephones to ring in the room.
Close isolette doors softly.
Do not set bottles or other objects on top of isolettes.
Remove all sources of loud, jarring noise such as trash receptacles with lids that bang shut.

Protect From Overstimulation
Cluster nursing care activities.
Allow the infant 2- to 3-hour periods of undisturbed rest.
Do not routinely suction or perform postural drainage (perform as needed only).
Contain the infant's limbs (swaddle) during suctioning or other procedures.

Provide Boundaries
Position the infant prone or side-lying.
Cover, wrap, swaddle the infant.

Adapted from VandenBerg, K. A., & Franck, L. S. (1990). Behavioral issues for infants with bronchopulmonary dysplasia. In C. H. Lund (Ed.), *Bronchopulmonary dysplasia: Strategies for total patient care* (p. 126). Petaluma, CA: Neonatal Network. Reprinted with permission

MANAGEMENT OF NEONATAL PAIN

The goals of pain management in infants are (1) to minimize intensity, duration, and physiologic cost of the pain experience and (2) to maximize the infant's ability to cope with and recover from the painful experience.

Nonpharmacologic Management

Noninvasive, nonpharmacologic pain management techniques support the neonate's own coping mechanisms. Many of the noxious stimuli in the ICN result from routine handling and nursing procedures. Therefore, the intensity and duration of pain can often be minimized by gentle handling and quick, efficient, skilled execution of invasive procedures. For example, use of a spring-loaded lancet for heelstick significantly reduces pain responses in neonates compared with local anesthetic cream or nursing comfort measures (McIntosh et al., 1994). Infants must be allowed periods of rest between procedures. Other stressors should be eliminated and a minimal handling protocol initiated (Table 40–1).

Minimizing the physiologic cost of pain can be achieved by providing proper support to the infant during the procedure. This support includes providing containment for the premature infant to limit excessive, immature motor response. Full-term and older infants may be distracted during procedures with oral, visual, auditory, or tactile stimulation. Interventions such as swaddling, assisting the infant with hand-to-mouth contact, or nonnutritive sucking assist the infant in coping with noxious stimuli (Campos, 1989; Field & Goldson, 1984). Pacifiers should be offered to mechanically ventilated neonates to reduce behavioral and physiologic distress during painful procedures (Miller & Anderson, 1993). Recent studies suggest that a pacifier dipped in a sucrose solution reduces behavioral and physiologic signs of distress associated with heelstick to a greater degree than using a pacifier dipped in water (Blass & Hoffmeyer, 1991; Bucher et al., 1995). Animal studies suggest that the effect of sucrose is mediated by endogenous opioid pathways (Blass et al., 1987). Findings from studies using sucrose-dipped pacifiers during circumcision are contradictory, with one study reporting decreased crying (Blass & Hoffmeyer, 1991) and another study showing no difference in crying between neonates who received a sucrose-dipped pacifier and those who received a water-dipped pacifier (Rushforth & Levene, 1993).

In adults, counterirritation (i.e., nonpainful tactile stimulation of the opposite limb) is helpful in blocking pain sensation. In neonates, contralateral tactile stimulation resulted in a significant increase in functional response time (FRT) (decreased sensitivity) in the injured heel following repeated heelstick (Andrews & Fitzgerald, 1994).

In general, nurses should begin with nonpharmacologic inter-

Pain score	Degree of pain	Behavioral Assessment	Pain score	Degree of pain	Behavioral Assessment
0	No apparent pain	Not crying/resting, calm, sleeping/ relaxed body posture/comfortable without intervention	2 (cont.)	Mild pain	Tense muscles/difficult to distract and console
1	Uncomfortable	Intermittent whimpering, cry/ intermittent restlessness, but able to sleep/intermittently tense muscles/comforts–calms self	3	Moderate pain	Sobbing; strong, loud cry/ continuous restlessness, irritability, sleep disruption/tense, rigid body/ only intermittently distractible
2	Mild pain	Whimpering cry, moaning/restless, irritable, but able to sleep	4	Severe/ extreme pain	High pitched scream/thrashing, tremulous/unable to sleep

CHILDREN'S HOSPITAL OAKLAND
INTENSIVE CARE NURSERY
24 HOUR NURSE'S RECORD

INFANT POSITION
R = Right side down S = Supine HOB↑ = Head up HL = Head to left
L = Left side down P = Prone HR = Head to right HM = Head midline

INFANT STATE
I = Deep sleep III = Drowsy V = Active alert P = Paralysis (drug)
II = Light sleep IV = Quiet alert VI = Crying O = Other (described)

BREATH SOUNDS C/D	RESP. RX / PD	SITE	SUCTION AMOUNT / COLOR	LAB WORK DRAWN RESULTS PREVIOUS AMT.: HGB__ CS__	BLOOD OUT AMT / TOT.	X-RAY/ OTHER DIAG. TESTS	POSITION Body / Head	STATE	PAIN SCORE	COMMENTS

FIGURE 40–1. Example of a 24-hour nurse's record. (Courtesy of Children's Hospital, Oakland.)

ventions before progressing to pharmacologic agents. However, nonpharmacologic interventions may not be appropriate for situations in which severe or prolonged pain is assessed. The questions listed in Table 40–2 serve as a guide to the nurse in determining appropriate strategies for relieving pain in the hospitalized infant.

Pharmacologic Management

Pharmacologic agents are often required to alleviate the pain caused by invasive procedures. A reluctance to use drugs to treat infant pain persists among many physicians and nurses despite the safety of analgesic and anesthetic agents and the potential harm caused by unrelieved pain (Yaster & Deshpande, 1988).

Opioids

Opioid analgesics are considered the "gold standard" for pain relief. Opioid analgesia is mediated primarily by mu receptor subtypes mu1 and mu2. Opioid drugs act at these receptors to hyperpolarize the cell membrane and reduce neuronal excitability.

Use of opioids, however, is not without risks or side effects. The neonate's responses to opioids differ from those of the older child or adult. These response variations may be due to differences in the amount and type of mu receptors in the brain and spinal cord. In the neonatal rat, the number of high-affinity mu receptors is associated with the pain relief and the number of low affinity mu receptors is associated with the degree of respiratory depression. In one study, neonatal rats (2 days of age) had fewer high-affinity mu receptors and were less sensitive to morphine's analgesic effects, despite having higher brain concentrations of the drug (Pasternak et al., 1980). These findings suggest that higher concentrations of opioids may be needed to provide adequate analgesia for neonates than for older patients. Data on the kinetics of opioids administered to neonates are limited. Nor are there data on the plasma opioid concentrations associated with analgesia or cardiorespiratory side effects in neonates or on the influence of previous exposure to opioids (e.g., prenatally) on analgesia or cardiorespiratory side effects.

Neonates exhibit increased clearance and decreased half-life of opioids as gestational age increases (Bhat et al., 1994). There is also evidence to suggest rapid maturation of opioid metabolic mechanisms during postnatal life, with clearance levels approaching those of adults by 6 months of age (Lynn & Slattery, 1987). The pharmacokinetics of multiple intermittent opioid dosing in neonates have not been evaluated.

TABLE 40–2 Question Guide to Determining Infant Pain Treatment

Assessment

What behavior is the infant displaying that is actually or potentially harmful? Is there interference with adequate ventilation, circulation, nutrition, sleep–wake cycle, or social development?
Is the infant compromised physiologically?
Can any precipitating factors be identified?
Is ventilation or oxygenation optimized?
  Is the oxygen delivery system functioning adequately?
  Does the infant need to be suctioned?
  Is the infant breathing in synchrony with the ventilator?
Have painful procedures been recently performed?
Will painful procedures be performed frequently?
Does the infant have a painful condition?

Nonpharmacologic Support

Have nonpharmacologic comfort measures been attempted?
  Is the infant's temperature stable?
  Has a wet diaper or bedding been removed?
  Has abdominal distention been relieved?
  Has the infant been repositioned or swaddled?
  Has the infant been offered nonnutritive sucking?
Has a minimal handling protocol been implemented?

Selecting Appropriate Analgesics

What routes are available for delivery of medication?
Is a brief period of analgesia needed for an invasive procedure? Is prolonged analgesia required for a painful condition?
What is the drug half-life?
What are the side effects?
Will blood levels be helpful in assessing efficacy or toxicity?
How many doses will need to be given before the drug reaches steady-state?

Evaluation of Drug Treatment

Did the drug achieve the desired effect?
Was the drug given at an appropriate interval for an appropriate period of time (to achieve steady-state)?
Were there any side effects?
How will weaning from pharmacologic support be achieved?

Adapted from VandenBerg, K. A., & Franck, L. S. (1990). Behavioral issues for infants with bronchopulmonary dysplasia. In C. H. Lund (Ed.), *Bronchopulmonary dysplasia: Strategies for total patient care* (p. 136). Petaluma, CA: Neonatal Network. Reprinted with permission.

Morphine

Mean elimination half-life following single-dose administration of morphine ranges between 2.6 and 14 hours (Bhat et al., 1990, 1994). There are differences in the pharmacokinetics of morphine administered to premature neonates in the first week of life (Bhat et al., 1990). Neonates less than 40 weeks' gestation have longer elimination half lives and delayed clearance than older neonates (Lynn & Slattery, 1987) after bolus administration. In addition, approximately 80 percent of morphine is unbound by plasma proteins in premature neonates. This unbound morphine may account for its increased CNS concentrations (Kupferberg & Way, 1963). When morphine was administered as a continuous infusion, plasma concentrations were three times greater and the elimination half-life was seven times longer in neonates than in older infants and children (Koren et al., 1985). In several patients, morphine plasma concentrations increased after the infusion was discontinued, suggesting that there is enterohepatic recirculation of the drug. Other studies have demonstrated that continuous infusion of morphine is well tolerated and effective in neonates postoperatively (Farrington et al., 1993; Lynn et al., 1984).

Morphine has few effects on the neonatal cardiovascular system in the well-hydrated neonate; however, hypotension commonly occurs in dehydrated patients. Decreased intestinal motility and abdominal distention may also occur.

Meperidine

The pharmacokinetics of meperidine specific to neonates are not known. During the first 2 days of life, more meperidine than normeperidine is excreted. By 3 days of age, the reverse is true, indicating that there is rapid activation of the enzymes responsible for meperidine metabolism after birth. Because normeperidine is an active metabolite, delayed respiratory depression and reduction in seizure threshold can occur with meperidine administration.

Fentanyl

Fentanyl is frequently used to provide anesthesia to neonates during surgical procedures. It is short acting and must be administered as a continuous infusion or as an intravenous bolus every 1 to 2 hours. The mean elimination half-life following single-dose administration of fentanyl ranges between 6 and 32 hours (Collins et al., 1985; Gauntlett et al., 1988; Koehntop et al., 1986). Serum concentrations of fentanyl are lower in neonates than in older infants and children, and the pharmacokinetics of fentanyl in premature and full-term neonates are similar (Koehntop et al., 1986). The elimination half-life and total body clearance are larger in neonates than in adults. The lower initial steady-state plasma levels are due to larger initial volumes of distribution and volumes of distribution at steady-state. The latter prolongs administration of the drug. More than 90 percent of fentanyl is metabolized by the liver (Gauntlett et al., 1988). Increased intra-abdominal pressure can triple the elimination half-life of fentanyl (Koehntop et al., 1986), probably because there is reduced hepatic artery blood flow. Although it has only been demonstrated for fentanyl, increased intra-abdominal pressure probably occurs with other opioids that are metabolized by the liver. Because many neonates have increased intra-abdominal pressure, elimination is an important consideration when administering opioids to neonates. Rarely, fentanyl can significantly reduce chest wall compliance (stiff chest syndrome). This naloxone-reversible side effect can be prevented by slow infusion (as opposed to rapid bolus administration), administration of doses less than 3 μg/kg, or concomitant use of muscle relaxants.

Fentanyl blunts increases in pulmonary vascular resistance and pressure in stressed (but normoxic) neonates (Hickey et al., 1985). This finding led to the use of continuous fentanyl infusion in neonates with pulmonary hypertension or requiring extracorporeal membrane oxygenation (ECMO). A major problem with long-term fentanyl administration is the development of tolerance and physical dependence (Franck & Vilardi, 1995). A morphine infusion can provide similar pain relief, better sedative effects, and less tolerance and physical dependence when long-term use of an opioid is required (Vilardi et al., 1994).

Sufentanil and Alfentanil

Sufentanil is 10 times more potent than fentanyl and is used to provide anesthesia for neonates undergoing cardiac surgery. The volume of distribution of sufentanil is about half as large in infants as it is in older patients. The shorter elimination half-life and smaller volume of distribution shorten the duration of anesthesia. Sufentanil has a mild negative inotropic effect and reduces serum catecholamine concentrations in infants. Sufentanil has been used to premedicate children for surgery. However, the dose required often causes decreased lung compliance, which is a significant risk for the spontaneously breathing infant. More recently, sufentanil was administered to premature neonates in a continuous infusion and was well tolerated with no decrease in heart rate or blood pressure (Seguin et al., 1994).

Alfentanil is also very short acting and is used in older children for brief procedures in which rapid return to consciousness is desired (White et al., 1986). The elimination half-life is approximately 30 percent shorter in neonates than in adults. Alfentanil use during brief painful procedures in neonates has not been reported. Decreased lung compliance may occur in neonates, and clinicians should be prepared to intervene.

Methadone

Methadone is more commonly known for its use in the opioid-dependent pregnant woman. However, its long-acting properties and good oral bioavailablity make it an attractive option to treat postoperative pain in neonates (Berde et al., 1991; Gourlay et al., 1982) and prevent neonatal abstinence syndrome (Maas et al., 1990). One study demonstrated effective relief of pain in neonates for 6 to 10 hours, using 50 to 100 μg/kg of methadone (Franck & Gregory, 1993).

Epidural

Improved catheter design and insertion technique has finally made this effective mode of analgesia administration available to neonates. Morphine or fentanyl administered alone or in combination with local anesthetics can provide good intraoperative anesthesia and postoperative analgesia after abdominal or lower extremity surgery. Use of epidural analgesia may potentially expedite extubation (Valley & Bailey, 1991; Murrel et al., 1993). Because the opioids act directly on the neurons in the spinal cord, lower doses are used for epidural or intrathecal administration and fewer opioid side effects are generally seen. Opioid side effects can still occur and require careful monitoring of the patient for side effects such as respiratory depression, hypotension, or urinary retention. Catheter-related side effects include systemic overdose related to catheter migration or infection. Epidural analgesia should not be used in the septic patient.

Cardiovascular and Respiratory Side Effects of Opioids

In neonates, opioids can depress heart rate and blood pressure (Gregory, 1994a). As with the respiratory effects, cardiovascular effects vary depending on the specific opioid administered as well as on the route and rate of administration. Hydration status is also a key factor in the maintenance of cardiovascular stability, with opioid-induced hypotension more likely to occur in the hypovolemic neonate than in the normovolemic neonate (Gregory, 1994a, 1994b; Yaster & Deshpande, 1988). Therefore, comparison of postopioid measures to baseline parameters for individual neonates provides the most accurate method to evaluate opioid-induced changes in heart rate and blood pressure.

Only one study (Purcell-Jones et al., 1987) documented the incidence of opioid-induced respiratory depression in neonates. This retrospective chart review of 933 neonates during the postoperative period revealed a 13.5 percent incidence of opioid-induced respiratory depression in spontaneously breathing neonates. Four of 83 ventilated neonates (4.5 percent) who received codeine or papaveretum experienced delays in weaning from ventilatory support because of opioid-induced respiratory depression as judged by clearly defined criteria, although none of the 10 neonates who received morphine had delays in weaning. In contrast, two other studies (Koren, et al., 1985; Farrington, et al., 1993) reported no cases of respiratory depression in neonates receiving up to 40 μg/kg/hour of morphine, with serum morphine levels as high as 90 ng/ml.

The respiratory effects of opioids have been directly measured in two studies (Lynn et al., 1993; Way et al., 1965). In the first study (Way et al., 1965), 10 normal full-term neonates demonstrated a 22 percent decrease in responsiveness to carbon dioxide (CO_2) after an intramuscular morphine injection compared with a control group who received an injection of saline. No changes in CO_2 responsiveness were seen after the administration of meperidine in an equianalgesic dose. Administration of both drugs resulted in the loss of a regular sigh that normally occurs as part of the newborn's respiratory pattern.

More recently, Lynn and associates (1993) found steady-state serum morphine levels above 20 ng/ml were associated with a greater occurrence of hypercarbia and depressed CO_2 responsiveness in infants and children receiving continuous morphine infusion after cardiac surgery. There was no correlation between age and morphine serum levels or CO_2 responsiveness. Three neonates with cyanotic heart disease retained CO_2 responsiveness despite high serum morphine levels.

Opioid-induced decreases in heart rate, respiratory rate, and blood pressure may reach statistical significance but be well within normal physiologic limits (Hartley et al., 1993). Provision of analgesia may improve ventilation and cardiovascular status through depressant effects on cardiorespiratory parameters (Elias-Jones et al., 1991; Irazuzta et al., 1993; Robinson & Gregory, 1981; Vacanti et al., 1984). Conversely, failure to adequately relieve pain could lead to hypoventilation. For example, Pokela

(1994) administered 1 mg/kg meperidine or saline to premature neonates before endotracheal suctioning and routine procedures (weighing, bathing, temperature measurement, chest radiograph). Neonates in both groups experienced a similar number of episodes of hypoxemia. However, these episodes were of significantly shorter duration in the neonates who received meperidine before the procedures.

To discriminate between inadequate analgesia and opioid-induced cardiorespiratory side effects, vital signs must be evaluated within the context of the clinical situation and timing of opioid administration.

Local Anesthetics

Local infiltration of anesthetics (e.g., 0.25 to 0.5 ml/kg of 25 percent bupivacaine or 0.5 to 1.0 percent lidocaine) can be used for procedures such as lumbar puncture or intravenous catheter insertion. Some clinicians have argued that the administration of local anesthesia by subcutaneous injection results in more pain than performing the procedure without anesthesia. However, there are no data to support this claim. In contrast, a large study of premature and full-term neonates demonstrated decreased behavioral distress in neonates who received local anesthesia (Pinheiro et al., 1993). There was no difference in the success rate of lumbar puncture between the two groups.

Topical Application of Local Anesthetics

The use of topical anesthetics for procedures such as venipuncture has significantly improved the management of pain in pediatrics (Yaster et al., 1994). The effectiveness of topical local anesthesia for reducing pain in neonates has not been as clearly demonstrated. While use of Emla (eutectic mixture of local anesthetics; Astra Pharmaceuticals) decreased behavioral and physiologic responses to circumcision (Benini et al., 1993), it was not effective for heelstick procedures (Barker & Rutter, 1995a, 1995b). Further studies must be conducted to determine whether topical local anesthesia is useful in decreasing infant pain. Studies must also be conducted to determine the safety of repeated application of topical local anesthetics in premature and full-term neonates.

Nerve Blocks

Peripheral nerve and caudal epidural blocks using local anesthesia (or a combination of local anesthetic and an opioid) can be used to provide intraoperative regional or general anesthesia and postoperative pain relief for neonates (Yaster et al., 1994). Careful monitoring of the patient during the postoperative period is required to assess potential complications including bleeding, compartment syndrome, excessive sensorimotor blockade, and systemic local anesthetic toxicity (Yaster & Maxwell, 1989). In addition to pain assessment, nurses caring for infants receiving local anesthetics via epidural infusion should assess the patient sensorimotor blockade by eliciting withdrawal reflex of the legs every few hours.

Non-Opioid Analgesics

Acetaminophen

Acetaminophen is useful for treating mild to moderate pain in children. The use of acetaminophen in neonates is limited because it can only be administered orally or rectally. Rectal administration is unpredictable (Roberts, 1984). Although acetaminophen is metabolized by the liver, hepatic toxicity should not be a concern in neonates if standard doses are used (Berde et al., 1991).

Use of Adjunctive Drugs

In the ICN, the use of sedatives, alone or in combination with analgesics, is controversial. Although sedatives suppress the behavioral expression of pain, they have no analgesic effects and can even increase pain. Sedatives should only be used when pain has been ruled out (Hartley et al., 1989). Use of sedatives or antianxiety agents in combination with analgesics is common practice in care of the critically ill adult or older child to reduce the fear and anxiety that accompany critical care as well as to minimize some of the psychological side effects of narcotic analgesics. No research has been done to determine the safety or efficacy of combining sedatives and analgesics for the treatment of pain in infants.

Benzodiazepines

Until recently, diazepam was the most commonly used benzodiazepine in neonates. Because of its long half-life (approximately 31 hours), it should not be administered on a fixed schedule, but only as clinical signs indicate.

Midazolam is a short-acting benzodiazepine used to provide sedation for mechanically ventilated neonates. Because it is highly lipid soluble at a physiologic pH, midazolam readily enters the brain, resulting in a rapid onset. Up to 90 percent of midazolam is protein bound. Therefore, the neonate with low serum protein may have increased midazolam entering the CNS with increased sedation and respiratory depression. Midazolam is metabolized in the liver by microsomal oxidation (Laegreid et al., 1992). In normoxic neonates, midazolam is not associated with hypotension. The elimination half-life of midazolam is estimated at 6.5 hours in the critically ill neonate. Midazolam administered in an intravenous bolus can cause hypotension and decreased cerebral blood flow in ill neonates (van Straaten et al., 1992).

Lorazepam is used in neonates to provide sedation and to prevent seizures. It provides effective maintenance sedation for mechanically ventilated infants without affecting heart rate or causing apnea. In patients with renal failure, repeated doses of lorazepam can result in hypotension or apnea, and weaning from mechanical ventilation may be delayed. The dose of benzyl alcohol preservative in lorazepam is below the dose known to cause fatal toxicity in premature neonates (100 to 400 mg/kg/day). However, with frequent dosing, benzyl alcohol toxicity is a potential risk. Given orally, lorazepam is a useful alternative to chloral hydrate for the nonventilated infant with chronic lung disease who requires ongoing or intermittent sedation to prevent respiratory distress associated with activity or agitation.

Chloral Hydrate

Chloral hydrate has been used in single doses to sedate neonates during pulmonary function, radiographic, and other diagnostic testing for which the patient must lie still. Although clinically effective, concern has been raised about the potential carcinogenic and genotoxic effects of chloral hydrate administered to animals (Salmon et al., 1990). Chloral hydrate has also been used in repeated doses to sedate neonates on mechanical ventilation. Alternative sedatives (i.e., benzodiazepines) should be used when possible because chloral hydrate has other gastrointestinal side effects (Roberts, 1984) and may be associated with direct hyperbilirubinemia (Lambert et al., 1990). The extremely long half-life (greater than 72 hours) of chloral hydrate (Mayer et al., 1991) increases the risk of toxicity with repeated administration, which may be manifest as increased agitation (Hartley et al., 1989).

Phenobarbital, Pentobarbital, Secobarbital

Little is known about the pharmacokinetics and clinical effects of phenobarbital, pentobarbital, and secobarbital when used as sedatives. Phenobarbital is commonly given to control seizures in neonates and does have a short-lived sedative effect. Pentobarbital is more commonly used in older children in the pediatric intensive care unit to induce coma. Secobarbital has also been used to provide sedation to mechanically ventilated neonates, but it has been reported to cause prolonged sedation 24 to 96 hours after the last dose (Nahata et al., 1991).

The use of nonanalgesic psychoactive drugs in combination with analgesics has proven effective in reducing pain in adults. It is postulated that these drugs reduce anxiety and muscle tension, which otherwise exacerbate pain. Benzodiazepines such as lorazepam and midazolam are also powerful amnesiacs. Adults and children given these agents in combination with analgesics while in intensive care units often have no memory of the experience, even though they demonstrated responsiveness to painful and other stimuli (Booker et al., 1986). No research has been conducted regarding the efficacy or safety of combining analgesics with sedative or hypnotic agents in the neonatal population. These practices, however, do occur. Care must be taken to assess the use of analgesia as opposed to simple sedation, and prolonged use may potentially impair development because of the amnesiac effects.

Pharmacologic Management of Neonatal Pain for Specific Procedures

Circumcision

Provision of anesthesia and analgesia for circumcision remains controversial. Circumcision is performed on healthy, spontaneously breathing newborn infants, and provision of analgesia is perceived by some clinicians as overly risky. Dorsal penile nerve block is a safe and effective method of providing local anesthesia to infants during circumcision. Numerous studies have demonstrated safety and efficacy, with a reduction in physiologic and behavioral distress, with the use of dorsal penile nerve block (Dixon et al., 1984; Stang et al., 1988). However, many physicians remain reluctant to use the technique. Infants who received comfort measures such as music, intrauterine sounds, or pacifier exhibited the same degree of behavioral distress as did control infants who received no intervention during circumcision (Benini et al., 1993). Acetaminophen has also been shown to have no effect in reducing distress during and after circumcision. In one study, provision of a sucrose-dipped pacifier or topical local anesthesia decreased distress in infants undergoing circumcision compared with infants who received no treatment at all (Benini et al., 1993). However, these methods provide only brief analgesia and have not been compared with dorsal penile nerve block in controlled trials.

Preprocedure Anesthesia and Analgesia

Local anesthesia is used to prevent pain for other procedures performed in the ICN such as chest tube insertion (Franck, 1987) and lumbar puncture (Porter et al., 1988a, 1988b). Use of topically applied local anesthesia for heelstick has recently been reported (Fitzgerald et al., 1989). Further exploration of topical administration of analgesic agents is warranted.

Local anesthesia may not be sufficient for procedures that affect deeper tissue, such as chest tube insertion or surgical cutdown of vessels. Central analgesia is then required to prevent pain. For the nonventilated patient, in whom there is concern for the respiratory depressant effects of opioids, one half the standard dose may be administered. The infant's respiratory status and responsiveness to pain stimuli can then be assessed before further drug administration. For the infant who is receiving opioid analgesics on a regular basis, a higher dose may be required to provide adequate analgesia during an invasive procedure.

Anesthesia for Surgical Procedures

Anesthesia is required for prolonged surgical procedures involving deep tissue. In 1987, the AAP published a position statement validating the use of anesthesia in infants and discounting infant age or perceived degree of cortical maturation as reasons for withholding anesthesia (AAP, 1987). The AAP recommended that the usual guidelines for safe administration of anesthetics to high-risk, potentially unstable adult patients be applied to critically ill infants as well. Nurses should assist physicians and parents in weighing the risks and benefits and understanding the need for anesthesia in infants undergoing surgery.

Overall, the results of these studies support the use of opioids for both preterm and full-term neonates during surgery and suggest that opioids are efficacious in attenuating hemodynamic, hormonal, and metabolic effects of surgical stress. Based on these data, some clinicians advocate use of 50 to 100 μg/kg of fentanyl anesthesia and continuation of a 10- to 15-μg/kg fentanyl infusion during the early postoperative period to prevent neuroendocrine stress responses and hemodynamic instability in infants undergoing cardiac surgery (Wessel, 1993).

Postoperative Analgesia

Adequate analgesia is important during the immediate postoperative period for the optimal recovery of the patient. Concern is often expressed by physicians and nurses that infants may not be easily weaned from ventilation with the use of narcotic analgesics. However, unrelieved pain can also interfere with ventilation and delay weaning. Use of low-dose continuous infusion of narcotic analgesics has been proven effective in the care of the postoperative adult patients and is gaining wider acceptance in pediatric and neonatal care. This delivery method can provide more constant, effective pain relief with less medication (Truog & Anand, 1989).

Mechanical Ventilation

Opioids are frequently used to sedate, promote respiratory synchrony, improve ventilation, and relieve pain or discomfort in neonates (Bell & Ellis, 1987; Koren & Maurice, 1989). Results of the studies to date (Goldstein & Brazy, 1991; Irazuzta et al., 1993; Quinn et al., 1992; Seguin et al., 1994; Vacanti et al., 1984) suggest that opioids can be used to improve the cardiac and respiratory status of mechanically ventilated neonates. Measurement of comfort level and sedative effects of the opioids in mechanically ventilated neonates has not been well described. Further research is needed to evaluate the relative risks and benefits of using opioids as analgesics to attenuate the stress responses related to pain, particularly in critically ill neonates.

Extracorporeal Membrane Oxygenation

ECMO is one of the most prolonged invasive therapies experienced by neonates in the ICN. Most ECMO patients are given an anesthetic dose of an opioid (usually fentanyl) for cannulation and then are kept sedated with a continuous fentanyl drip. Often, benzodiazepines are also used (lorazepam or midazolam) and additional injections of morphine are given. Rapid tolerance to fentanyl has been reported as has severe withdrawal following decannulation and weaning of drug (Arnold & Truog, 1990). Continuous morphine infusion may provide better sedation than fentanyl and reduce the incidence of post-ECMO opioid withdrawal symptoms (Vilardi et al., 1994).

Prevention of Withdrawal Symptoms

Over time (as little as several hours with some agents), physical dependence to psychoactive drugs (e.g., opioids and benzodiazepines) develops in infants, as it does in adults. Opioid analgesics, sedatives, or antianxiety agents given around the clock should never be discontinued abruptly (Maguire & Maloney, 1988). To prevent withdrawal symptoms, the infant should be weaned from opioid and sedative drugs. Abstinence scoring methods commonly used in the care of the infant with prenatal drug exposure must be used in assessing the infant during the opioid weaning (Franck & Vilardi, 1995).

PARENTS

Nurses caring for the infant in pain must care for the infant's family as well. Parents have many concerns and fears about their infant's pain and about the drugs used in treatment of pain (Lawson, 1988). Parents may fear the effects of pain on their child's development. They may also fear that their infant may become "addicted" to the analgesics. Nurses must be prepared to respond to questions from parents and encourage parent participation in providing nonpharmacologic comfort measures to their infant. Parents must be reassured that they are expected to ask questions about their infant's pain management (American Association of Critical-Care Nurses, 1987).

Attitudes of Health Care Professionals as a Barrier to Optimal Neonatal Pain Management

The attitudes and beliefs of health care professionals have played a major factor in the undertreatment of pain in both adults and children, despite emerging scientific evidence. Fear of addiction and disproportionate concern for side effects have resulted in severe underutilization of narcotic analgesics for acute postoperative pain (Schechter, 1989). Patients often suffer needlessly because of the nurse's or physician's unfounded fears of addiction or misinformation about analgesics.

Research has shown that pain management is strongly influenced by a nurse's biases, personal experience with pain (Burokas, 1985), and area of specialization (Page & Halvorson, 1991). Nurses must examine closely their own beliefs and attitudes about pain, explore the impact that their attitudes might have on their patient care, and challenge their beliefs to determine whether they are based on science or tradition.

NEONATAL NURSE'S ROLE AND RESPONSIBILITIES

Providing comfort and relieving pain are two central care goals. Neonatal nurses must prevent pain when possible, assess pain in their neonatal patients who cannot verbalize their subjective experience of pain, provide relief or reduction of pain, and assist the infant in coping when pain cannot be prevented (Table 40–3). The nurse is also obligated to find effective methods to communicate the assessments and recommendations to maximize the collaboration for an effective pain management.

TABLE 40–3 Strategies to Prevent or Minimize Pain in the Critically Ill or Premature Infant

Group blood draws to minimize the number of venipunctures per day
Use noninvasive monitoring devices when possible
Establish central vessel access to minimize vein and artery punctures
Have only expert staff attempt intravenous access on the most unstable patients
Use minimal amount of tape and remove tape gently
Ensure proper premedication before invasive procedures

From *OGN nursing practice resource: Prevention, recognition and management of neonatal pain* (pp. 3–4) (1991). Washington, DC: NAACOG. Reprinted with permission.

Much remains to be done to develop valid and reliable pain assessment tools for use in the clinical setting. In the absence of such instruments, it is imperative that each infant's pain assessment and treatment be systematically approached. The effective management of infant pain requires nurses to collaborate with each other, with physicians, and with the infant's parents. Neonatal nurses must remain informed about new research and scientific developments regarding pain management and be able to communicate assessments and recommendations in an objective, concise manner. Evaluation of pain treatment is the most important but most often neglected aspect of pain management. When the nurse intervenes with the infant in pain, the nurse must be continually evaluating the effect of treatment and modifying the treatment plan accordingly. A sample of protocol for pain management is in this chapter's Appendix.

CONCLUSION

Current understanding of pain experienced by infants is relatively limited, and much research remains to be done. It is clear, however, that caring for infants in pain requires attention not only to the immediate effects but also to the long-term developmental consequences of pain and pain treatment. Through objective assessment, effective collaboration, and systematic application of treatment plans, nurses will achieve greater comfort for individual patients and add to the body of knowledge in this rapidly evolving field.

APPENDIX
CHILDREN'S HOSPITAL OAKLAND DEPARTMENT OF NURSING NEONATAL PAIN MANAGEMENT PROTOCOL

Purpose:

To outline the nursing management of the neonate in pain

Level:

Interdependent (requires physician's order for dependent functions)

Supportive Data:

Neonates, even extremely premature neonates, are capable of perceiving and responding to pain. Pain can cause physiologic compromise in the ill infant. However, it can be difficult to distinguish instability caused by pain from that resulting from medical condition or immature neurologic development. Pain should be presumed in neonates in all situations that are usually painful for adults and children, even (or especially) in the absence of behavioral or physiologic signs. In addition, the risks of the pain treatment must be balanced against the risks of the pain.

Assessment:

1. *Identify* actual and potential sources of pain for the neonate:
   Invasive or surgical procedures
   Fractures, edema
   Noxious environment (e.g., noise, light, handling)
2. *Assess* the patient's vital signs and compare with baseline:
   Infants may respond to pain stimuli with either decreases or increases in heart rate and blood pressure and decrease in O_2 saturation.
3. *Observe* and score pain behaviors using the Children's Hospital of Ontario behavioral scoring system (0–4).
4. *Identify* physiologic behavior compromise resulting from pain:
   Decrease in oxygen saturation
   Hypertension and hypotension, tachycardia and bradycardia
   Inability to sleep or feed
5. *Evaluate* above parameters (1–4) at regular intervals:
   Every shift (minimum); every 4 hours if pain source is identified or suspected
   Every 4 to 72 hours postoperatively and after each intervention to relieve pain

Pain Management:

6. *Implement* noninvasive comfort measures:
   Positioning, swaddling, pacifier
   Reduction of stressors in the environment (e.g., light, noise, handling)
7. *Evaluate* efficacy of comfort measures by assessing change in physiologic and behavioral parameters.
8. *Implement* pharmacologic comfort measures:
   A. Administer opioids as ordered:
      Obtain one-time order of either fentanyl or morphine before invasive procedures.
      Suggest scheduled or continuous drip morphine for frequent or continuous pain.
      Avoid giving PRN orders.
      Use fentanyl drip only when hemodynamic instability is a concern.
      Suggest continuous morphine drip for prolonged and continuous analgesia and sedation needs
   B. Administer adjunctive drugs as ordered:
      Use choral hydrate for one-time sedation only, if ordered.
      Reevaluate sedation needs if giving more than three doses per day.
      Use lorazepam to produce sedation, not as a substitute for analgesia.
9. *Evaluate* efficacy of pharmacologic measures by comparing pretreatment and posttreatment assessment.
10. *Monitor* for side effects (e.g., respiratory depression, decreased gastrointestinal motility)
11. *Wean* from opiates as patient tolerates using opiate-weaning protocol and flowsheet.

Reportable Conditions:

12. *Notify physician* of assessment of behavioral or physiologic signs of pain unrelieved by noninvasive comfort measures or pharmacologic measures.
    Notify physician of sources of pain requiring analgesia (e.g., surgical procedures).
13. *Notify physician* of any side effects from pharmacologic measures.

Discontinue:

14. *Discontinue protocol* if no invasive procedures are performed, there is no painful medical condition, and the patient is free from signs or pain for 48 hours.

Safety:

15. *Directly observe* patient during periods of pain-induced hemodynamic instability and during administration of opioids and sedatives.
16. *Double-check* opiate and sedative doses per ICN Policy.

Psychosocial:

17. *Provide* infant with opportunities for human interaction that do not involve painful procedures.

Parent Instruction:

18. *Instruct* parent on need for analgesia and infant signs.
19. *Instruct* parent on nonpharmacologic comfort measures and encourage use.

Documentation:

20. *Record* all assessment data on nursing process record (NPR) every shift and with each occurrence (see 24-hour nurse's record).
21. *Record* medication as given on NPR, including patient response.
22. *Document* the effectiveness of this protocol in the NPR, including the following:
    Behavioral pain score and vital signs assessments before and after interventions
    Environmental conditions that reduce or exacerbate pain responses
    Side effects of treatments
    Parent involvement and understanding of their infant's pain management

REFERENCES

Agency for Health Care Policy and Research. (1992). *Acute pain management guidelines*. Rockville, MD: Author.

Als, H. (1984). Newborn behavioral assessment. In W. J. Burns & J. V. Lavigne (Eds.), *Progress in Pediatric Psychology* (pp. 1–46). New York: Grune & Stratton.

Als, H. (1983). Infant individuality: Assessing patterns of very early development. In J. Calls, E. Galenson, & R. Tuson (Eds.), *Frontiers of infant psychiatry* (pp. 363–378). New York: Basic Books.

Als, H., Lawhon, G., Brown, E., et al. (1986). Individualized behavioral and environmental care for very low birth weight preterm infants at high risk for bronchopulmonary dysplasia: Neonatal intensive care unit and developmental outcome. *Pediatrics, 78*(6), 1123–1132.

American Academy of Pediatrics. (1987). Neonatal anesthesia. *Pediatrics, 80*(3), 446.

American Association of Critical-Care Nurses. (1987). *It is critical that you know...what you should do when your baby is in the neonatal intensive care unit* [Pamphlet]. Newport Beach, CA: Author.

Anand, K. J. (1990). The biology of pain perception in newborn infants. In D. C. Tyler & E. C. Krane (Eds.), *Advances in pain research and therapy: Pediatric pain* (Vol. 15, pp. 113–122). New York: Raven Press.

Anand, K. J., & Aynsley-Green, A. (1988a). Does the newborn infant require potent anesthesia during surgery? Answers from a randomized trial of halothane anesthesia. In R. Dubner, G. F. Gebhart, & M. R. Bond (Eds.), *Proceedings of the 5th World Congress on Pain* (pp. 329–335). New York: Elsevier.

Anand, K. J., & Aynsley-Green, A. (1988b). Measuring the severity of surgical stress in newborn infants. *Journal of Pediatric Surgery, 23*(4), 297–305.

Anand, K. J., & Carr, D. B. (1989). The neuroanatomy, neurophysiology, and neurochemistry of pain, stress, and analgesia in newborns and children [Review]. *Pediatric Clinics of North American, 36*(4), 795–822.

Anand, K. J., & Hickey, P. R. (1992). Halothane-morphine compared with high dose sufentanil for anesthesia and post-operative analgesia in neonatal cardiac surgery. *New England Journal of Medicine, 326*(1), 1–9.

Anand, K. J. S., & Plotsky, P. M. (1995). Repetitive neonatal pain alters weight gain and pain threshold during development in infant rats. *Critical Care Medicine, 23*(Suppl.), A22.

Anand, K. J. S., Sippell, W. G., & Aynsley-Green, A. (1987). Randomized trial of fentanyl anaesthesia in preterm babies undergoing surgery: Effects on the stress response. *Lancet, 1*(8526), 234.

Andrews, K., & Fitzgerald, M. (1994). The cutaneous withdrawal reflex in human neonates: Sensitization, receptive fields, and the effects of contralateral stimulation. *Pain, 56*(1), 95–101.

Arnold, J. H., & Truog, R. D. (1990). *For infants undergoing extracorporeal membrane oxygenation* [Abstract]. Presented at ECMO Conference.

Au, E., Loprinzi, C. L., Dhodapkar, M., et al. (1994). Regular use of a verbal pain scale improves the understanding of oncology inpatient pain intensity. *Journal of Clinical Oncology, 12*(12), 2751–2755.

Barker, D. P., & Rutter, N. (1995a). Exposure to invasive procedures in neonatal intensive care unit admissions. *Archives of Disease in Childhood, 72*(1), F47–F48.

Barker, D. P., & Rutter, N. (1995b). Lignocaine ointment and local anaesthesia in preterm infants. *Archives of Disease in Childhood, 72*(3), F203–F204.

Barnard, K. E., & Bee, H. L. (1983). The impact of temporally patterned stimulation on the development of preterm infants. *Child Development, 54*(5), 1156–1167.

Barrier, G., Attia, J., Mayer, N. M., et al. (1989). Measurement of postoperative pain and narcotic administration in infants using a new clinical scoring system. *Intensive Care Medicine, 15*(Suppl. 1), 537–539.

Bell, S. G., & Ellis, L. J. (1987). Use of fentanyl for sedation of mechanically ventilated neonates. *Neonatal Network, 6*(2), 27–31.

Benini, F., Johnston, C. C., Faucher, D., & Aranda, J. V. (1993). Topical anesthesia during circumcision in newborn infants. *JAMA, 270*(7), 850–853.

Berde, C. B., Beyer, J. E., Bournaki, M. C., et al. (1991). Comparison of methadone and morphine for prevention of postoperative pain in 3–7 year old children. *Journal of Pediatrics, 119*(1, Part 1), 136–141.

Bhat, R., Chari, G., Gulati, A., et al. (1990). Pharmacokinetics of a single dose of morphine in preterm infants during the first week of life. *Journal of Pediatrics, 117*(3), 477–481.

Bhat, R., Chari, G., & Iver, R. (1994). Postconceptual age influences pharmacokinetics and metabolism of morphine in sick neonates. *Pediatric Research, 35*(4, Part 2), 81A.

Blackburn, S. (1996). *Studies of light and its application to clinical practice.* Paper presented at The Physical and Developmental Environment of the High Risk Neonate. Clearwater Beach, FL: University of South Florida College of Medicine.

Blass, E. M., & Hoffmeyer, L. B. (1991). Sucrose as an analgesic for newborn infants. *Pediatrics, 87*(2), 215–218.

Blass, E., Fitzgerald, E., & Kehoe, P. (1987). Interactions between sucrose, pain and isolation distress. *Pharmacology, Biochemistry & Behavior, 26*(3), 483–489.

Boix-Ochoa, J., Ibanez, V. M., Potau, N., & Lloret, J. (1987). Cortisol response to surgical stress in neonates. *Pediatric Surgery, 2,* 267–270.

Booker, P. D., Beechey, A., & Lloyd-Thomas, A. R. (1986). Sedation of children requiring artificial ventilation using an infusion of midazolam. *British Journal of Anaesthesia, 58,* 1104–1108.

Boyce, W. T., Barr, R. G., & Zeltzer, L. K. (1992). Temperament and the psychobiology of childhood stress. *Pediatrics, 90*(3), 483–486.

Brazelton, T. B. (1973). Neonatal behavioral assessment scale. *Clinics in developmental medicine, No. 50.* Philadelphia: J. B. Lippincott.

Brazy, J. E. (1988). Effects of crying on cerebral blood flow and cytochrome aa3. *Journal of Pediatrics, 112*(2), 457–461.

Bucher, H., Moser, T., von Siebenthal, K., et al. (1995). Sucrose reduces pain reaction to heel lancing in preterm infants: A placebo-controlled, randomized and masked study. *Pediatric Research, 38,* 332–335.

Budreau, G., & Craft, M. (1992). The Budreau infant irritability scale. *Childrens Health Care, 21*(3), 184–189.

Burokas, L. (1985). Factors affecting nurses' decisions to medicate pediatric patients after surgery. *Heart & Lung: Journal of Critical Care, 14*(4), 373–379.

Butler, N. C. (1987). The ethical issues involved in the practice of surgery on unanesthetized infants. *AORN Journal, 46*(6), 1136–1142.

Butler, N. C. (1989). Infants, pain and what health care professionals should want to know: An issue of epistemology and ethics. *Bioethics, 3,* 181–199.

Cabal, L. A., Siassi, B., & Hodgman, J. E. (1992). Neonatal clinical cardiopulmonary monitoring. In A. A. Fanaroff & R. J. Martin (Eds.), *Neonatal-perinatal medicine: Diseases of the fetus and infant* (pp. 437–455). St. Louis: C. V. Mosby.

Campbell, N. (1989). Infants, pain and what health care professionals should want to know: A response to Cunningham Butler. *Bioethics, 3,* 200–225.

Campos, R. G. (1989). Soothing pain-elicited distress in infants with swaddling and pacifiers. *Child Development, 60*(4), 781–792.

Coll, C. G. (1990). Behavioral responsivity in preterm infants. *Clinics in Perinatology, 17*(1), 113–123.

Collins, C., Koren, G., Crean, P., et al. (1985). Fentanyl pharmacokinetics and hemodynamic effects in preterm infants during ligation of patent ductus arteriosus. *Anesthesia and Analgesia, 64*(11), 1078–1080.

Craig, K. D., & Grunau, R. V. E. (1989). Neonatal pain perception and behavioral measurement. In K. J. S. Anand & P. J. McGrath (Eds.), *Neonatal pain and distress.* Amsterdam: Elsevier.

Dixon, S., Snyder, J., Holve, R., & Bromberger, P. (1984). Behavioral effects of circumcision with and without anesthesia. *Development and Behavioral Pediatrics, 5*(5), 246–250.

Dobbing, J., & Smart, J. L. (1974). Vulnerability of developing brain and behaviour. *British Medical Bulletin, 30*(2), 164–168.

Duffy, F. H. (1985). *Evidence for hemispheric differences between fullterms and preterms by electrophysiologic measures* [Abstract]. Presented at Patterns of Brain Function in the Premature Infant Symposium.

Duffy, F. H., Mower, G., Jensen, F., & Als, H. (1984). Neural plasticity: A new frontier for infant development. In H. E. Fitzgerald, B. M. Lester, & M. W. Yogman (Eds.), *Theory and research in behavioral pediatrics* (Vol. 2, pp. 67–96). New York: Plenum Press.

Elias-Jones, A. C., Barrett, D. A., Rutter, N., et al. (1991). Diamorphine infusion in the preterm neonate. *Archives of Disease in Childhood, 66*(10, Spec. No.), 1155–1157.

Emde, R. N., Harmon, R. J., Metcalf, D., et al. (1971). Stress and neonatal sleep. *Psychosomatic Medicine, 33*(6), 491–497.

Farrington, E. A., McGuinness, G. A., Johnson, G. F., et al. (1993). Continuous intravenous morphine infusion in postoperative newborn infants. *American Journal of Perinatology, 10*(1), 84–87.

Field, T. (1990). Alleviating stress in newborn infants in the intensive care unit. [Review]. *Clinics in Perinatology, 17*(1), 1–10.

Field, T., & Goldson, E. (1984). Pacifying effects of nonnutritive sucking on term and preterm neonates during heelstick procedures. *Pediatrics, 74*(6), 1012–1015.

Fitzgerald, M. (1991). The developmental neurobiology of pain. In M. R. Bond, J. E. Charlton, & C. J. Woolf (Eds.), *Proceedings of the 5th World Congress on Pain* (pp. 253–261). New York: Elsevier.

Fitzgerald, M., & Anand, K. J. S. (1993). Developmental neuroanatomy and neurophysiology of pain. In N. L. Schechter, C. B. Berde, & M. Yaster (Eds.), *Pain in infants, children, and adolescents* (pp. 11–31). Baltimore: Williams & Wilkins.

Fitzgerald, M., Millard, C., & McIntosh, N. (1989). Cutaneous hypersensitivity following peripheral tissue damage in newborn infants and its reversal with topical anaesthesia. *Pain, 39*(1), 31–36.

Fitzgerald, M., Shaw, A., & McIntosh, N. (1988). Postnatal development of the cutaneous flexor reflex: Comparative study of preterm infants and newborn rat pups. *Developmental Medicine and Child Neurology, 30*(4), 520–526.

Franck, L. S. (1986). A new method to quantitatively describe pain behavior in infants. *Nursing Research, 35*(1), 28–31.

Franck, L. S. (1987). A national survey of the assessment of pain and agitation in the national intensive care unit. *Journal of Obstetric, Gynecologic, and Neonatal Nursing, 16*(6), 387–393.

Franck, L. S. (1991). *Pain control in critical care.* Rockville, MD: Aspen Publishers.

Franck, L. S., & Gregory, G. A. (1993). Clinical evaluation and treatment of infant pain in the neonatal intensive care unit. In N. L. Schechter, C. B. Berde, & M. Yaster (Eds.), *Pain in infants, children, and adolescents* (pp. 519–535). Baltimore: Williams & Wilkins.

Franck, L., & Vilardi, J. (1995). Assessment and management of opioid withdrawal in ill neonates. *Neonatal Network, 14*(2), 39–48.

Friedrichs, J. B., Young, S. H., Gallagher, D., et al. (1995). Where does it hurt? An interdisciplinary approach to improving the quality of pain assessment and management in the neonatal intensive care unit. *Nursing Clinics of North America, 30*(1), 143–159.

Fuller, B. F. (1991). Acoustic discrimination of three types of infant cries. *Nursing Research, 40*(3), 156–160.

Gauntlett, I. S., Fisher, D. M., Hertzka, R. E., et al. (1988). Pharmacokinetics of fentanyl in neonatal humans and lambs: Effects of age. *Anesthesiology, 69*(5), 683–687.

Giannakoulopoulos, X., Sepulveda, W., Kourtis, P., et al. (1994). Fetal plasma cortisol and β-endorphin response to intrauterine needling. *Lancet, 344*(8915), 77–81.

Goldstein, R. F., & Brazy, J. E. (1991). Narcotic sedation stabilizes arterial blood pressure fluctuations in sick premature infants. *Journal of Perinatology, 11*(4), 365–371.

Gollin, E. S. (Ed.). (1981). *Developmental plasticity: Behavioral and biological aspects of variations in development*. New York: Academic Press.

Gorski, P. A., Hole, W. T., Leonard, C. H., & Martin, J. A. (1983). Direct computer recording of premature infants and nursery care: Distress following two interventions. *Pediatrics, 72*(2), 198–202.

Gorski, P. A., Huntington, L., & Lewkowicz, D. J. (1990). Handling preterm infants in hospitals: Stimulating controversy about timing of stimulation. *Clinics in Perinatology, 17*(1), 103–112.

Gottfried, A. W., & Gaiter, J. L. (1985). *Infants under intensive care: Environmental neonatology*. Baltimore: University Park Press.

Gourlay, G. K., Wilson, P. R., & Glynn, J. C. (1982). Pharmacodynamics and pharmacokinetics of methadone during the postoperative period. *Anesthesiology, 57*(6), 458–467.

Grauer, T. T. (1989). Environmental lighting, behavioral state, and hormonal response in the newborn. *Scholarly Inquiry for Nursing Practice, 3*(1), 53–66.

Gregory, G. A. (1994a). Pharmacology. In G. A. Gregory (Ed.), *Pediatric anesthesia* (3rd ed., pp. 13–45). New York: Churchill Livingstone.

Gregory, G. A. (1994b). Anesthesia for premature infants. In G. A. Gregory (Ed.). *Pediatric anesthesia* (3rd ed., pp. 351–373), New York: Churchill Livingstone.

Grunau, C., & Craig, K. D. (1989). Facial and cry responses to invasive and non-invasive procedures in neonates [Abstract]. *Journal of Pain and Symptom Management, 4*(4), S4, 9.

Grunau, R. V., Johnston, C. C., & Craig, K. D. (1990). Neonatal facial and cry responses to invasive and non-invasive procedures. *Pain, 42*(3), 295–305.

Grunau, R. V., Whitfield, M. F. & Petrie, J. H. (1994a). Pain sensitivity and temperament in extremely low-birth-weight premature toddlers and preterm and full-term controls. *Pain, 58*(3), 341–346.

Grunau, R. V. E., Whitfield, M. F., Petrie, J. H., & Fryer, E. L. (1994b). Early pain experience, child and family factors, as precursors of somatization: a prospective study of extremely premature and fullterm children. *Pain, 56*(3), 353–359

Gunnar, M. R., Connors, J., & Isensee, J. (1989). Lack of stability in neonatal adrenocortical reactivity because of rapid habituation of the adrenocortical response. *Developmental Psychobiology, 22*(3), 221–233.

Gunnar, M. R ., Connors, J., Isensee, J., & Wall, L. (1988). Adrenocortical activity and behavioral distress in human newborns. *Developmental Psychobiology, 21*(4), 297–310.

Gunnar, M. R., Hertsgaard, L., Larson, M., & Rigatuso, J. (1991). Cortisol and behavioral responses to repeated stressors in the human newborn. *Developmental Psychobiology, 24*(7), 487–505.

Harpin, V. A., & Rutter, N. (1983). Making heel pricks less painful. *Archives of Disease in Childhood, 58*(3), 226–228.

Hartley, S., Franck, L. S., & Lundergan, F. (1989). Maintenance sedation of agitated infants in the NICU with chloral hydrate: New concerns. *Journal of Perinatology, 9*(2), 162–164.

Hartley, R., Green, M., Quinn, M., & Levene, M. I. (1993). Pharmacokinetics of morphine infusion in premature neonates. *Archives of Disease in Childhood*, 69(1, Spec. No.), 55–58.

Hickey, P. R., Hansen, D. D., Wessel, D., et al. (1985). Pulmonary and systemic hemodynamic responses to fentanyl in infants. *Anesthesia and Analgesia, 64*(5), 483–486.

Hughes, D., Murphy, J. F., Dyas, J., et al. (1987). Blood spot glucocorticoid concentrations in ill preterm infants. *Archives of Disease in Childhood, 62*(10), 1014–1018.

Irazuzta, J., Pascucci, R., Perlman, N., & Wessel, O. (1993). Effects of fentanyl administration on respiratory system compliance in infants. *Critical Care Medicine, 21*(7), 1001–1004.

Izard, C. E., Porges, S. W., Simmons, R. F., et al. (1991). Infant cardiac reactivity: Developmental changes and reactions with attachment. *Developmental Psychobiology*, 27(3), 432–439.

Janowsky, J. S., & Finlay, B. L. (1986). The outcome of perinatal damage: The role of normal neuron loss and axon retraction [Review]. *Developmental Medicine and Child Neurology, 28*(3), 375–389.

Kehlet, H. (1986). Pain relief and modification of the stress response. In M. F. Cousins & G. D. Phillips (Eds.), *Acute pain management* (pp. 49–76). New York: Churchill Livingstone.

Koehntop, D. E., Rodman, J. H., Brundage, D. M., et al. (1986). Pharmacokinetics of fentanyl in neonates. *Anesthesia & Analgesia, 65*(3), 227–232.

Koren, G., & Maurice, L. (1989). Pediatric uses of opioids. *Pediatric Clinics of North America, 36*(5), 1141–1156.

Koren, G., Butt, W., Chinyanga, H., et al. (1985). Post-operative morphine infusion in newborn infants: Assessment of disposition characteristics and safety. *Journal of Pediatrics, 107*(6), 963–967.

Krechel, S. W., & Bildner, J. (1995). Cries: A new neonatal postoperative pain measurement score. Initial testing of validity and reliability. *Pediatric Anaesthesia*, 5, 53–61.

Kupferberg, H. J., & Way, E. L. (1963). Pharmacologic basis for the increased sensitivity of the newborn rat to morphine. *Journal of Pharmacology and Experimental Therapy, 141*, 105–112.

Lagercrantz, H., Nilsson, E., Redham, I., & Hjemdahl, P. (1986). Plasma catecholamines following nursing procedures in a neonatal ward. *Early Human Development, 14*(1), 61–65.

Laegreid, L., Hagberg, G., & Lundberg, A. (1992). The effect of benzodiazepines on the fetus and the newborn. *Neuropediatrics, 23*(1), 18–23.

Lambert, G. H., Muraskas, J., Anderson, C. L., & Myers, T. (1990). Direct hyperbilirubinemia associated with chloral hydrate administration in the newborn. *Pediatrics, 86*(2), 277–281.

Lawrence, J., Alcock, D., McGrath, P., et al. (1993). The development of a tool to assess neonatal pain. *Neonatal Network, 12*(6), 59–66.

Lawson, J. R. (1988). Pain in the neonate and fetus [Letter]. *New England Journal of Medicine, 318*(27), 1398–1399.

Levine, J. D., & Gordon, N. C. (1982). Pain in prelingual children and its evaluation by pain-induced vocalization. *Pain, 14*, 85–93.

Lewis, M. (1992). Individual differences in responses to stress. *Pediatrics, 90*(3), 487–490.

Long, J. G., Lucey, J. F., & Philip, A. G. (1980). Noise and hypoxemia in the intensive care nursery. *Pediatrics, 65*(1), 143–145.

Lynn, A. M., Nespeca, M. K., Opheim, K. E., & Slattery, J. T. (1993). Respiratory effects of intravenous morphine infusions in neonates, infants, and children after cardiac surgery. *Anesthesia and Analgesia, 77*(4), 695–701.

Lynn, A. M., Opheim, K. E., & Tyler, D. C. (1984). Morphine infusion after pediatric cardiac surgery. *Critical Care Medicine, 12*(10), 863–866.

Lynn, A. M., & Slattery, J. T. (1987). Morphine pharmacokinetics in early infancy. *Anesthesiology, 66*(2), 136–139.

Maguire, D. P., & Maloney, P. (1988). A comparison of fentanyl and morphine use in neonates. *Neonatal Network, 7*(1), 27–32.

Manuck, S. B., Kasprowicz, A. L., & Muldoon, M. F. (1990). Behaviorally-evoked cardiovascular reactivity and hypertension: Conceptual issues and potential associations. *Annals of Behavioral Medicine*, 12(1), 17–29.

Marshall, R. E., Porter, F. L., Rogers, A. G., et al. (1982). Circumcision: II. Effects upon mother–infant interaction. *Early Human Development, 7*(4), 367–374.

Maas, U., Kattner, E., Weingart-Jesse, B., et al. (1990). Infrequent neonatal opiate withdrawal following maternal detoxification during pregnancy. *Journal of Pediatric Medicine, 18*(2), 111–118.

Mayer, D. J., Hindmarsh, K. W., Sankaran, K., et al. (1991). Chloral hydrate disposition following single-dose administration to critically ill neonates and children. *Developmental Pharmacology and Therapeutics, 16*(2), 71–77.

Mayer, M. N., Attia, J., Amiel-Tison, C., et al. (1989). Measurement of post-operative pain in infants after general versus regional anesthesia (Abstract). *Journal of Pain and Symptom Management, 4*(4), S7.

McIntosh, N., van Veen, L., & Brameyer, H. (1994). Alleviation of the pain of heel prick in preterm infants. *Archives of Disease in Childhood, 70*(3), F177–F181.

Melzack, R., & Creasy, K. L. (1968). Sensory, motivational and central control determinants of pain: A new conceptual model. In D. Kenshalo (Ed.), *The skin senses* (pp. 423–443). Springfield, IL: Charles C Thomas.

Merskey, H. (1979). Pain terms: A list with definitions and notes on usage. Recommended by the IASP Subcommittee on Taxonomy. *Pain, 6*(3), 249–252.

Miller, H. D., & Anderson, G. C. (1993). Nonnutritive sucking: Effects on crying and heart rate in intubated infants requiring assisted mechanical ventilation. *Nursing Research, 42*(5), 305–307.

Murrell, D., Gibson, P. R., & Cohen, R. C. (1993). Continuous epidural analgesia in newborn infants undergoing major surgery. *Journal of Pediatric Surgery, 28*(4), 548–553.

Nahata, M. C., Starling, S., & Edwards, R. C. (1991). Prolonged sedation associated with secobarbital in newborn infants receiving ventilatory support. *American Journal of Perinatology, 8*(1), 35–36.

Norris, S., Campbell, L. A., & Brenkert, S. (1982). Nursing procedures and alterations in transcutaneous oxygen tension in premature infants. *Nursing Research, 31*(6), 330–336.

O'Gara, P. T. (1988). The hemodynamic consequences of pain and its management. *Journal of Intensive Care Medicine, 3,* 3–5.

Page, G. G., & Halvorson, M. (1991). Pediatric nurses: The assessment and control of pain in preverbal infants. *Journal of Pediatric Nursing, 6*(2), 99–106.

Pasternak, G. W., Zhang, A., & Tecott, L. (1980). Developmental differences between high and low affinity opiate binding sites: Their relationship to analgesia and respiratory depression. *Life Sciences, 27*(13), 1185–1190.

Perry, E. H., Bada, H. S., Ray, J. D., et al. (1990). Blood pressure increases, birth weight-dependent stability boundary, and intraventricular hemorrhage. *Pediatrics, 85*(5), 727–733.

Phillips, G. D., & Cousins, M. F. (1986). Neurological mechanisms of pain and the relationship to pain, anxiety, and sleep. In M. F. Cousins & G. D. Phillips (Eds.), *Acute pain management* (pp. 21–48). New York: Churchill Livingstone.

Pigeon, H. M., McGrath, P. J., Lawrence, J., & Brock-MacMurray, S. (1989). Nurses' perceptions of pain in the neonatal intensive care unit. *Journal of Pain and Symptom Management, 4*(4), 179–183.

Pinheiro, J. M. B., Furdon, S., & Ochoa, L. F. (1993). Role of local anesthesia during lumbar puncture in neonates. *Pediatrics, 91*(2), 379–382.

Pokela, M. (1994). Pain relief can reduce hypoxemia in distressed neonates during routine treatment procedures. *Pediatrics, 93*(3), 379–383.

Porges, S. W. (1992). Vagal tone: A physiological marker of stress vulnerability. *Pediatrics, 90*(3), 498–504.

Porter, F. L. (1989). Pain in the newborn. *Clinics in Perinatology, 16*(2), 549–564.

Porter, F. L., Miller, J. P., Cole, F. S., & Marshall, R. E. (1991). A controlled clinical trial of local anesthetic for lumbar punctures in newborns. *Pediatrics, 88*(4), 663–669.

Porter, F. L., Miller, J. P., & Marshall, R. E. (1988a). Local anesthesia for painful medical procedures in sick newborns. *Pediatric Research, 26,* 374A.

Porter, F. L., Porges, S., & Marshall, R. E. (1988b). Newborn pain cries and vagal tone: Parallel changes in response to circumcision. *Child Development, 59*(2), 495–505.

Price, D. D. (1988). *Psychological and neural mechanisms of pain.* New York: Raven Press.

Price, D. D., & Dubner, R. (1977). Neurons that subserve the sensory-discriminative aspects of pain [Review]. *Pain, 3*(4), 307–338.

Purcell-Jones, G., Dormon, F., & Sumner, E. (1987). The use of opioids in neonates: A retrospective study of 933 cases. *Anaesthesia, 42*(12), 1316–1320.

Quinn, M. W., Otoo, F., Rushforth, J. A., et al. (1992). Effect of morphine and pancuronium on the stress response in ventilated preterm infants. *Early Human Development, 30*(3), 241–248.

Rawlings, D. J., Miller, P. A., & Engel, R. R. (1980). The effect of circumcision on transcutaneous Po_2 in term infants. *American Journal of Diseases of Children, 134*(7), 676–678.

Roberts, R. J. (1984). *Drug therapy in infants: Pharmacologic principles and clinical experience.* Philadelphia: W. B. Saunders.

Robertson, A., & Philbin, M. K. (1996). *Studies of sound and auditory development.* Paper presented at The Physical and Developmental Environment of the High Risk Neonate. Clearwater Beach, FL: University of South Florida College of Medicine.

Robinson, S., & Gregory, G. A. (1981). Fentanyl-air-oxygen anesthesia for ligation of patent ductus arteriosus in preterm infants. *Anesthesia and Analgesia, 60*(5), 331–334.

Rushforth, J. A., & Levene, M. I. (1993). Effect of sucrose on crying in response to heel stab. *Archives of Disease in Childhood, 69*(3), 388–389.

Salmon, A. G., Zeise, L., Jackson, R. J., & Book, S. (1990). *Hazards from pediatric uses of chloral hydrate.* Unpublished report, Health Hazards Assessment Division, California Department of Health Services, Berkeley, CA.

Sandman, C. A., McGivern, R. F., Berka, C., et al. (1979). Neonatal administration of beta-endorphin produces "chronic" insensitivity to thermal stimuli. *Life Sciences, 25*(20), 1755–1760.

Schechter, N. L. (1989). The undertreatment of pain in children: An overview [Review]. *Pediatric Clinics of North America, 36*(4), 781–794.

Schulte, F. J. (1975). Neurophysiological aspects of brain development. *Mead-Johnson Symposia on Perinatal Development, 6,* 34–47.

Schwartz, M. E., & Jefferies, I. P. (1990). Neonatal pain assessment: Physiological responses to heel lancing. *International Pediatrics, 5*(4), 344-349.

Seguin, J. N., Erenberg, A., & Leff, R. D. (1994). Safety and efficacy of sufentanil therapy in ventilated infant. *Neonatal Network, 13*(4), 37–40.

Sell, E. J. (1986). Outcome of very very low birth weight infants. *Clinics in Perinatology, 13*(1), 451–459.

Shearer, M. H. (1986). Surgery on the paralyzed, unanesthetized newborn. *Birth, 13*(2), 36–38.

Sparshott, M. (1989). Minimizing discomfort of sick newborns. *Nursing Times, 85*(43), 39–42.

Spinelli, D. N. (1990). Plasticity triggering experiences, natures, and the dual genesis of brain structure and function. *Clinics in Perinatology, 17*(1), 77–82.

Stang, H. J., Gunnar, M. R., Snellman, L., et al. (1988). Local anesthesia for neonatal circumcision: Effects on distress and cortisol response. *Journal of the American Medical Association, 259,* 1507–1511.

Stevens, B. J., & Johnston, C. C. (1994). Physiological responses of premature infants to a painful stimulus. *Nursing Research, 43*(4), 226–231.

Stevens, B., Johnston, C. C., Petryshen, P., Taddio, A. (1994). *The development and validation of a measure to assess pain in premature infants.* Paper presented at the 3rd International Symposium on Pediatric Pain, Philadelphia, PA, June 6–9.

Stevens, B., Johnston, C., Petryshan, P., & Taddio, A. (1996). Premature infant pain profile: Development and initial validation. *Clinical Journal of Pain, 12,* 13–22.

Swafford, L. I., & Allen, D. (1968). Pain relief in the pediatric patient. *Medical Clinics of North America, 52,* 131–136.

Tronick, E. Z., Scanlon, K. B., & Scanlon, J. W. (1990). Protective apathy, a hypothesis about the behavioral organization and its regulation to clinical and physiological status of the preterm infant during the newborn period. *Clinics in Perinatology, 17*(1), 125–154.

Truog, R., & Anand, K. J. S. (1989). Management of pain in the postoperative neonate [Review]. *Clinics in Perinatology, 16*(1), 61–78.

Vacanti, J. P., Crone, R. K., Murphy, J. D., et al. (1984). The pulmonary hemodynamic response to perioperative anesthesia in the treatment of high-risk infants with congenital diaphragmatic hernia. *Journal of Pediatric Surgery, 19*(6), 672–679.

Valley, R. D., & Bailey, A. G. (1991). Caudal morphine for postoperative analgesia in infants and children: A report of 138 cases. *Anesthesia and Analgesia, 72*(1), 120–124.

van Straaten, H. L., Rademaker, C. M., & de Vries, L. S. (1992). Comparison of the effect of midazolam or vercuronium on blood pressure and cerebral blood flow velocity in the premature newborn. *Developmental Pharmacology Therapeutics, 19*(4), 191–195.

Vilardi, J., Franck, L. S., & Powers, R. J. (1994). Morphine sulfate versus fentanyl infusion for sedation and analgesia in neonates on ECMO. *Pediatric Research* 25(4, Part 2), 83A.

Volpe, J. J. (1987). Neuronal proliferation, migration, organization and myelination. In J. J. Volpe (Ed.), *Neurology of the newborn* (2nd ed., pp. 33–68). Philadelphia: W. B. Saunders.

Vorhees, C. V. (1981). Effects of prenatal naloxone exposure on postnatal behavior development of rats. *Neurobehavioral Toxicology and Teratology, 3*(3), 295–301.

Wall, P. D., & Melzack, R. (1994). *Textbook of pain* (3rd ed.). New York: Churchill Livingstone.

Way, W. L., Costley, E. C., & Way, E. L. (1965). Respiratory sensitivity of the newborn infant to meperidine and morphine. *Clinical Pharmacology and Therapeutics, 6*(4), 454–461.

Wessel, D. L. (1993). Hemodynamic responses to perioperative pain and stress in infants. *Critical Care Medicine, 21*(9, Suppl.), S361–S362.

White, P. F., Coe, V., Shafer, V., & Sung, M. C. (1986). Comparison of alfentanil with fentanyl for outpatient anesthesia. *Anesthesiology, 64*(1), 99–106.

Yaster, M., & Deshpande, J. K. (1988). Management of pediatric pain with opioid analgesics. *Journal of Pediatrics, 113*(3), 421–429.

Yaster, M. & Maxwell, L. G. (1989). Pediatric regional anesthesia. *Anesthesiology, 70*(2), 324–338.

Yaster, M., Tobin, J. R., Fisher, Q. A., & Maxwell, L. G. (1994). Local anesthetics in the management of acute pain in children. *The Journal of Pediatrics, 124*(2), 165–176.

CHAPTER 41

Principles of Neonatal Drug Therapy

LINDA TIMM WAGNER CHARLOTTE A. KENREIGH

RESEARCH AGENDA

Which administration method is better for neonatal drugs: syringe pump or continuous infusion?

Can standardized nursing procedures for administration of drugs, such as gentamicin, and sampling blood concentrations lead to better attainment of safe and effective drug levels?

What are the pharmacokinetic parameters of medications used in ECMO patients?

The principles that govern the use of medications in the neonatal population are no different from those in other age groups. However, the neonate is significantly different physiologically from other populations, and this difference affects how the neonate responds to medication therapy.

Approaches to neonatal drug therapy are influenced by several factors. Literature on the use of medications in the neonatal population remains sparse, and few drugs have been evaluated in a well-controlled manner in this population of patients. Often, health care practitioners are required to review data available in other populations, such as adults, and extrapolate that information to the neonatal patient on the basis of knowledge of neonatal physiology. The available literature on neonatal drug use includes case reports and small sample size studies, making extrapolations to the entire neonatal population difficult. Within the practice of medicine, neonatology is a relatively young field. Advances in medical care have provided for the survival of infants as young as 24 weeks' gestation, resulting in an even more pharmacologically challenging patient. The health care practitioner caring for the neonate receiving medications has to be aware of these factors when interpreting a neonate's response to a medication regimen.

GENERAL PRINCIPLES OF DRUG THERAPY

One of the most important considerations in prescribing or administering medications to any patient is the understanding of what is expected from the administration of the drug. A definite outcome should be determined for each medication and a monitoring plan established for evaluation of achievement of that outcome. It is important to design a monitoring plan that establishes the limits of toxicity that will be tolerated as well as the expected therapeutic benefit of the drug regimen. How a patient will respond to therapy is influenced by characteristics such as the patient's age, size, and development; concomitant administration of other medications; concurrent disease states; and organ function.

Drug-related morbidity and mortality are common problems in health care (Manasse, 1989). The prevention of drug-related morbidity and mortality is the responsibility of all patient care providers. Drug-related problems can be divided into eight situations (Hepler & Strand, 1989) in which the patient (1) has a medical problem that requires drug therapy but is not receiving a drug for that indication; (2) has a drug indication but is taking the wrong drug; (3) has a medical problem that is being treated with a subtherapeutic dose of the right drug; (4) has a medical problem that is the result of the patient's not receiving the drug (e.g., formulation or drug delivery problems); (5) has a medical problem that is being treated with too much of the right drug; (6) has a medical problem that is a result of an adverse drug reaction or side effect; (7) has a medical problem that is the result of a drug–drug, drug–food, or drug–laboratory interaction; or (8) has received a medication for no medically valid indication.

Health care providers should evaluate medication regimens and ensure that a drug-related problem does not exist. Tools such as laboratory tests and other diagnostic aids should be incorporated into the overall plan for the patient's medication regimen.

ADVERSE DRUG REACTIONS

An adverse drug reaction (ADR) is defined as any effect or response from a drug that is noxious and unintended when the drug is given in appropriate dosages (Fincham, 1992). An ADR may be caused either by the active drug or by an inert component of the drug such as a filler or preservative. ADRs may be considered either bothersome events that do not hinder continuation of therapy or toxic events that necessitate discontinuation of therapy. ADRs are designated as either of these categories on the basis of several factors: temporal relationship of administration of drug to occurrence of adverse event; improvement of symptoms with discontinuation of medication (dechallenge); reappearance of adverse reactions when the medication is restarted (rechallenge); and absence of concomitant medications or disease states that could possibly be responsible for development of an ADR.

ADRs are a common reason for hospitalization of patients and also a major reason for delay in discharge of hospitalized patients (Manasse, 1989). Recognizing and reporting of ADRs are the responsibility of all health care providers (Faich, 1986). Neonatology is an especially important area for reporting of ADRs. Because most drugs are not initially studied in the neonatal population and are frequently used before significant numbers of infants have been exposed, little is known about the ADRs that may be more common in this population. Each hospital has its own system for monitoring and evaluating ADRs. The Food and Drug Administration (FDA) has also established a MedWatch program for reporting of ADRs nationally (U.S. Department of Health and Human Services, 1993). Information compiled by this program is collated and evaluated to note trends associate with the use of specific medications.

DRUG INTERACTIONS

Understanding drug interactions, not only with other medications but also with food and other laboratory tests, is important. Many drug interactions are so common that almost all health care providers are aware of them (e.g., erythromycin–theophylline). There are also many uncommon but no less important drug interactions. Therefore, whenever a patient's response to a prescribed regimen is different than expected or laboratory values are inconsistent with clinical findings, it is important to consider a drug interaction. The potential for a drug interaction should be evaluated in any patient receiving multiple drugs.

Drug interactions may take many forms (Hansten & Horn, 1993). It is important to consider the expected time course of the drug interaction in evaluating a potential interaction. Not all interactions occur immediately when two drugs are administered to the same patient. Each interaction has a time course of maximal risk. For example, in adults, the risk of the erythromycin–theophylline interaction is maximum on about day 5 of combined therapy. If the crossover of drug therapies is for only 1 or 2 days, it may be acceptable to combine the two drugs (Hansten & Horn, 1993).

Drug–drug interactions may be grouped into several categories. Certain drugs may interfere with the absorption of other medications from the gastrointestinal tract. This interference can be from altered motility, altered gastrointestinal pH, alterations in gastrointestinal flora, or actual drug binding within the gut lumen. Antacids not only alter the gastric pH but may also bind to medications within the gastrointestinal tract, resulting in inactivation of medications. The prokinetic agents cisapride and metoclopramide may decrease gastrointestinal transit time and therefore reduce the time available for absorption of other medications.

Drug–drug interactions can also occur because of altered plasma or tissue protein binding. One drug may interfere with the metabolism or excretion of another medication, thereby increasing or decreasing effectiveness, creating toxicity, or producing subtherapeutic levels. Certain medications that may be administered to the neonate may result in increased activity of liver enzymes and an increased metabolism of drugs. Rifampin and phenobarbital are classic examples of medications that increase liver enzymes (Hansten & Horn, 1993). Medications such as cimetidine reduce enzyme activity and result in a decreased clearance of certain other medications.

Drug activity may also be interfered with by concurrent disease states. Congestive heart failure results in alterations in blood flow to the liver, thereby decreasing the metabolism of medications that require hepatic biotransformation (Rowland & Tozer, 1989). Interferences such as these are referred to as drug–disease state interactions.

MEDICATION ADMINISTRATION

Oral Formulations

Most medications have not been approved by the FDA for use in the pediatric or neonatal population. The drug approval process is complicated, and the numbers of patients that would be required in order to obtain FDA approval would be difficult to achieve. Many of the medications that are used orally are available only as tablets or capsules. Therefore, oral medications administered for the neonatal population are often extemporaneously prepared in the pharmacy. These preparations are usually formulated from available literature on in vitro stability. However, little is usually known about the bioavailability of the product—that is, the extent to which the active ingredient is absorbed and the time at which a maximum serum concentration is achieved. Some ingredients necessary for the preparation of these medications may not be readily available and therefore make acquisition of the drugs difficult after discharge from the hospital.

With drugs that are commercially available as suspensions and oral solutions, the volume of medication is often not appropriate for the neonate. The product may be concentrated in such a way that accurate measuring for a neonatal dose is difficult. These preparations may also contain silent or inert ingredients such as preservatives that are harmless in adults but may, when administered frequently to neonates, result in toxicity.

Osmolality must also be considered in providing neonatal enteral medications. High-osmolality substances administered to the neonate have been associated with many adverse effects, including the development of necrotizing enterocolitis and decreased transit time (Ernst et al., 1983). Many enteral medications add a significant osmolar load to formula or breast milk (White & Harkavy, 1982). It is important to stagger neonatal enteral medication administration to avoid simultaneous administration of highly osmolar medications.

Intravenous Administration

Accurate neonatal medication delivery is critical to the interpretation of the efficacy or toxicity of a prescribed regimen. Much has been written about neonatal drug administration with regard to accurate monitoring of the serum drug concentration. The majority of medications administered are evaluated clinically without use of serum drug concentration monitoring. Regardless of whether serum drug concentrations will be obtained, it is important to keep in mind the following principles when administering any medication, because the interpretation of the effectiveness of the therapy may be affected.

Factors that may affect the rate and completeness of drug administration include the site of injection, rate of intravenous (IV) fluid administration, medication dosage and fluid volume, administration of multiple medications, and properties of the drug solution such as specific gravity, osmolality, and pH (Gould & Roberts, 1979). Interpretation of pharmacokinetic parameters can be difficult because of the multitude of factors influencing the delivery and timing of the administration. Incomplete medication administration may occur secondarily to the low flow of IV fluids that these patients often receive, and peak serum concentrations may be reached several hours after what is expected because of these confounding variables. Several techniques are currently used to administer neonatal medications (Fig. 41–1).

In the antegrade system, medications are administered at a port (Y-site, flashball) and are assumed to flow to the patient from that site (Roberts, 1981). In this system, the time to peak effect and the total drug delivery are dependent on the volume of medication administered, the rate of administration of the IV fluid, and the site of injection. It is often difficult to predict the time to peak effect with this method. If the injection site is distal to the patient, clinical interpretation of the effectiveness of a medication and its side effects may be difficult. For this reason, many clinicians suggest avoiding medication administration at distal ports of entry unless absolutely necessary.

Another technique, first started in the early 1970s, that is in use today is the retrograde system (Benzing & Loggie, 1973). In this system, two three-way stopcocks are used, separated by ex-

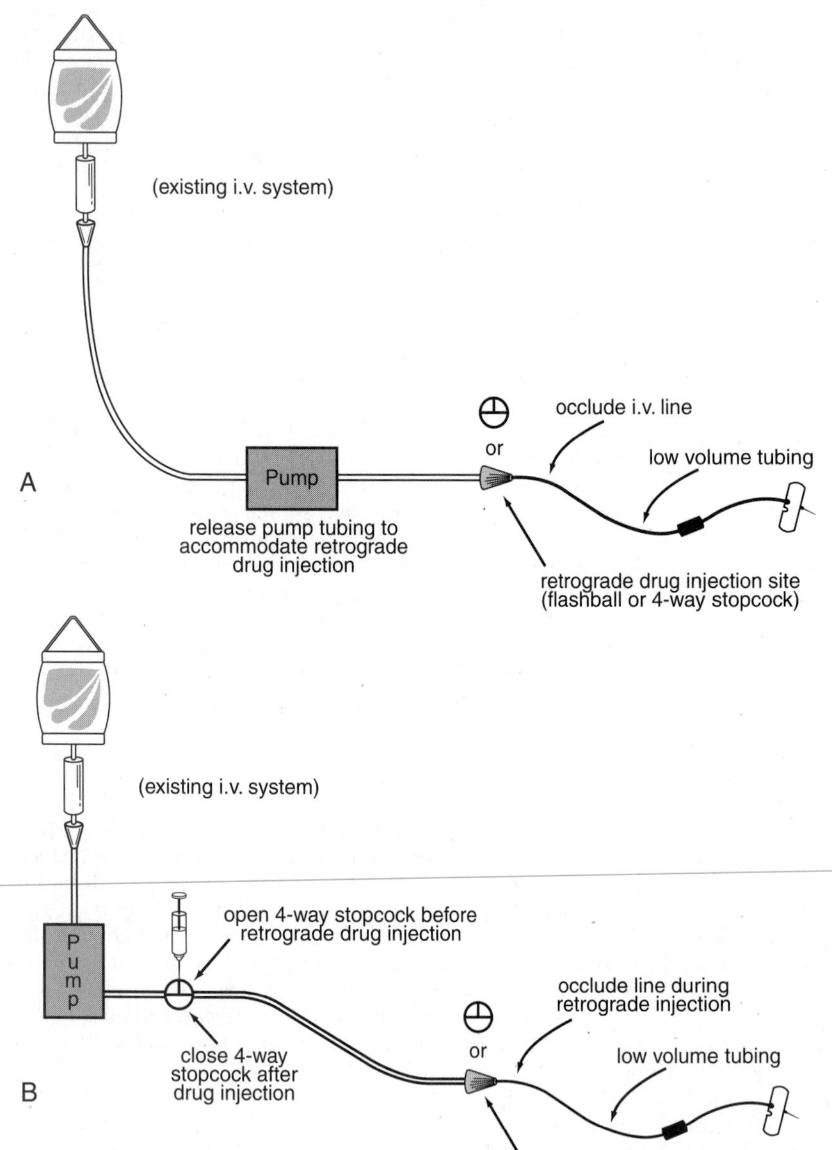

FIGURE 41–1. Intravenous drug administration. *A*, Construction of IV system for manual retrograde injection. An injection site (flashball or stopcock) and low-volume extension tubing are located at the distal end of the existing IV setup. *B*, Construction of IV system for retrograde injection modified for a volume infusion pump device unable to accept retrograde injections. System consists of existing IV to which is attached an extension set with a proximal four-way stopcock and distal flashball injection site. A large-volume syringe is attached to the four-way stopcock and acts as an overflow reservoir for the IV fluid displaced by the dosage volume. (Redrawn from Leff, R. D., & Roberts, R. J. [1981]. Methods for intravenous drug administration in the pediatric patient. *Journal of Pediatrics*, 98[4], 631–635.)

tension tubing that becomes part of the maintenance infusion line. The medication is infused at the most proximal port, and the dose is injected away from the patient and displaces fluid in the tubing up into a syringe on the distal stopcock. Then both stopcocks are opened to the patient and the IV line, resulting in delivery of medication to the patient. This method is more reliable than the anterograde method but is still influenced by drug dosage volumes, the IV fluid rate, and the tubing diameter. Commercially manufactured retrograde systems are available.

Many practitioners have begun using syringe pumps to administer medications to neonatal patients. Syringe pumps provide a rate of medication delivery that is independent of the rate of IV fluid and dosage volume. Studies of medication administration via syringe pump have demonstrated that this method yields reproducible and consistent results (Leff & Roberts, 1981). Complicated medication regimens in which there is a lot of tubing between the syringe pump and the patient is still influenced by factors such as drug volume and IV fluid rate.

Syringe pumps have provided neonatal health care providers with a more consistent method for administration of intermittent dosages of medications to their patients. Many medications are currently administered as continuous infusions. Because daily fluid requirements for many neonatal patients are somewhat restricted, the continuous infusion rate is frequently less than 1 ml/hour. In an effort to be cost conscious, there has been a movement to use syringe pumps to administer continuous infusions. However, several authors have questioned the accuracy of this method of drug delivery to the neonatal patient (Carl et al., 1995; Rooke & Bowdle, 1994).

Many of the same problems that plague the commercially available medications for oral administration to the neonate also can be found in available products for IV administration. Many of the available IV medications are provided in concentrations that prohibit accurate measurement and administration of neonatal doses. This can affect the interpretation of the infant's response to the therapy. Another important consideration is the concentration of fluid that the infant is receiving through an IV line; many medications may be hyperosmolar and cause irritation at the site of infusion. Intermittent administration of other medications into a line that is dedicated to a continuous infusion of a medication may result in an inadvertent bolus of the initial medication, which could potentially be harmful to the patient. This is particularly troublesome with vasoactive medications, sedatives, and narcotics. Sudden changes in drug delivery may also occur when medication lines are changed.

Extravasation and *infiltration* are terms used interchangeably in the literature; both terms reflect a misdirection of IV fluid or medication into tissue surrounding the IV site (MacCara, 1983). The extent of damage that follows such an event depends on the extravasated substance and the volume of the fluid that has leaked into the interstitium. Many of the medications (potassium, calcium, parenteral nutrition, dopamine, epinephrine, and nafcillin) incorporated into the drug regimens of patients in the neonatal intensive care unit are capable of causing tissue damage if extravasation occurs. Unless absolutely necessary, the use of small or superficial venous access sites should be avoided for administration of these agents. The best prevention is close attention to the IV site where the medication is infusing. Extravasation of medications with alpha-adrenergic activity (epinephrine, dopamine) may be treated with the alpha-adrenergic blocking agent phentolamine. Hyaluronidase, an enzyme that destroys tissue cement, may be useful for the treatment of other extravasations (Table 41–1).

Aerosolized Medication Administration

Aerosolized medications are becoming a more common addition to the medication regimen of the neonate. Delivery of medications to the lung appears to be optimal, inasmuch as this is the desired site of action of many therapies prescribed in the neonatal population. Targeting the therapy to the site of action and minimizing the systemic effects are appealing concepts leading to the increased use of aerosolized medications (Newman & Clarke, 1983). Most of the available literature on the effectiveness of various aerosolized medications and dosing confirms that the airways of a neonate are much smaller than the airways of an adult or older pediatric patient. The particle size produced by various inhalers and nebulized solutions may be much larger than the airway diameter itself. These limitations may prevent the premature infant from receiving the most benefit from a medication administered via inhalation, because the larger particles of the drug may become deposited in the airway before reaching the intended site of activity.

PHARMACOKINETICS

Pharmacokinetics is the study of the movement of a substance through the various body compartments (Levy, 1992). It reflects a time-dependent relationship between a drug dosage and the resulting measurable concentration of medication, usually in the serum or plasma. Measurement of blood levels is usually much simpler than measurement of tissue levels. Pharmacodynamics is the study of how that substance affects the body and the clinical effect that is desired when a medication is administered (Lalonde, 1992). Pharmacodynamic studies are difficult to conduct; most of

TABLE 41–1 Extravasations

Extravasated Drug/ Fluid	Treatment
Calcium	Hyaluronidase
Dopamine	Phentolamine
Dextrose	Hyaluronidase
Norepinephrine	Phentolamine
Parenteral nutrition	Hyaluronidase
Potassium	Hyaluronidase

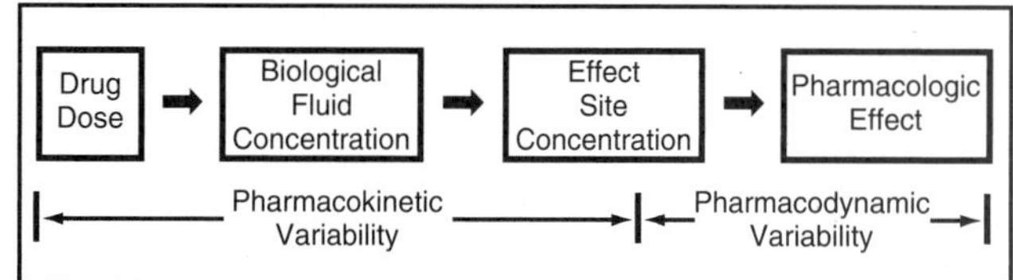

FIGURE 41–2. Pharmacokinetics and pharmacodynamics as determinants of the dose–effect relationship. (Redrawn by permission from *Applied Pharmacokinetics: Principles of Therapeutic Drug Monitoring,* third edition, edited by William E. Evans, Jerome J. Schentag and William J. Jusko, published by Applied Therapeutics, Inc., Vancouver, Washington, © 1992.)

the information that is available on neonatal response to medications is based on pharmacokinetic and not pharmacodynamic data (Fig. 41–2).

It is important to understand some terminology involved in pharmacokinetics. These terms are referred to frequently in this chapter and throughout the available literature on the use of medications in the neonatal population.

Volume of distribution (Vd) refers to an imaginary space into which a medication is distributed once it reaches the blood stream and assumes an equal distribution of drug throughout all body compartments (Rowland & Tozer, 1989). It is the mathematical relationship between the dose administered and the serum concentration of the medication. A volume of distribution for a medication is dependent on the chemical properties of the drug itself and the physiologic status of the patient. Factors such as extent of plasma and tissue binding, lipid solubility, an increased volume of distribution for medications that distribute into body water, increases in a patient's intravascular and extravascular fluid, changes in protein concentration and binding capacity, and changes in fat content can alter a volume of distribution.

Half-life ($t_{1/2}$) refers to the time it takes for the serum concentration of a medication to decrease to half of its original concentration (Winter, 1988). Half-life may be influenced by other medications, tissue perfusion, and organ function.

Steady state refers to the time at which for each dosing interval the patient is receiving the same amount of drug that is being excreted by the body; rate of drug administration equals the rate of drug elimination. Steady state does not imply a steady serum concentration; rather, it implies that the changes that occur over a dosing interval are the same with each dosing interval. In clinical practice, steady state is considered to be achieved after about four to five half-lives of the drug have passed (Shargel & Yu, 1985).

Clearance (Cl) refers to the amount of drug cleared from the blood stream per unit of time (Rowland & Tozer, 1989). This rate of elimination encompasses all routes in relation to the concentration of drug in the biologic fluid. Clearance of a medication depends on many factors, including the volume of distribution, the half-life, the physiologic status of the patient, blood flow to the organs, organ function, and the properties of the medication itself. Patients with altered organ function, as in renal or hepatic failure, may have impaired clearance of certain medications and require dosage adjustments.

Clearance may be of several types. In clinical practice, clearance is generally referred to as linear (first order) or nonlinear (zero order). For a drug whose clearance follows linear pharmacokinetics, an increase in the dose proportionately and predictably increases the serum proportional to the concentration of drug achieved at steady state. The majority of medications used in neonates (aminoglycosides, vancomycin, phenobarbital, caffeine, and catecholamines) follow this type of elimination. Theophylline is also eliminated on a linear basis when concentrations are in the normally accepted therapeutic range. However, when concen-

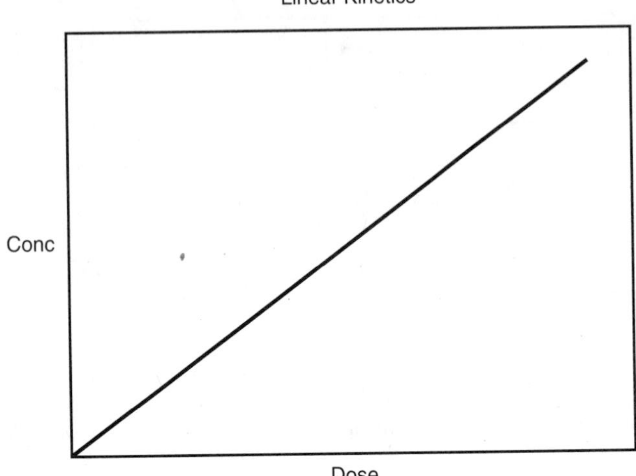

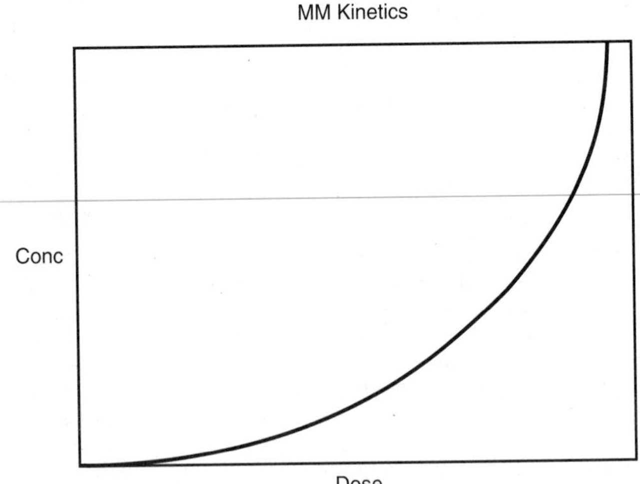

FIGURE 41–3. Linear versus nonlinear clearance.

trations above the therapeutic range are exceeded, theophylline deviates from linear elimination.

For a drug that follows nonlinear pharmacokinetics, there may be a rapid rise in serum concentration in response to a small increase in dose. This unpredictable dose response is a result of enzyme saturation in the liver. Elimination now becomes dose-dependent. All medications cleared hepatically follow nonlinear pharmacokinetics; however, elimination may appear linear over the therapeutic range and change to nonlinear elimination when levels exceed the therapeutic range. An increase in dose yields a predictable increase in serum concentration unless the serum concentration exceeds what is normally considered therapeutic. At these elevated serum concentrations, the nonlinear pharmacokinetic parameters are observed. Phenytoin is a classic example of a medication with nonlinear kinetics; once the enzymes responsible for the elimination of phenytoin are saturated, elimination can no longer occur at the rate of drug administration. A proportional increase in clearance is not seen with a dosage increase; rather, serum concentrations become excessively elevated with small dosage increases. Elimination of medication through this saturable enzyme process is often referred to as Michaelis-Menton kinetics (Rowland & Tozer, 1989) (Fig. 41–3).

Loading Doses

Medications gradually accumulate in the body over a period of time if the body cannot totally eliminate a drug in the time between dosing intervals. This occurs mainly with drugs that have longer half-lives and the doses of which must be scheduled to maintain serum concentrations in order to produce a desired effect. As a scheduled medication is given, the concentration of drug in the body slowly approaches the desired steady-state concentration. When there is an immediate need to achieve a desired therapeutic concentration in order to elicit an effect, and when accumulation of drug is expected, a loading dose of medication may be necessary. This is true of medications such as antiarrhythmics, phenobarbital, caffeine, gentamicin, and theophylline. If a loading dose is not given, it may take hours to days to achieve the desired therapeutic concentration.

Therapeutic Drug Monitoring

Pharmacokinetics is frequently associated with the monitoring of medications for which a therapeutic range has been identified. A therapeutic range is a definable range of drug concentrations in which the drug is expected to exert the desired effect with little or low toxicity. This range can be applied to therapy considerations for the majority of patients; however, some patients respond at serum concentrations outside this range, and others experience toxic effects within or below the defined therapeutic range. Therapeutic drug monitoring requires availability of an assay to measure serum concentrations as part of the daily monitoring of drug therapy. It is important to understand what is measured when serum drug concentrations are evaluated. For some medications (aminoglycosides) it is important to evaluate both peak and trough serum concentrations. In general, elevation of trough concentrations reflects an inability of the body to eliminate a medication, and the dosing interval should be extended. Conversely, if the trough concentration is below a desired level, the dosage interval must be shortened. Subtherapeutic or elevated peak levels necessitate actual dosage adjustment instead of interval changes. For other medications (antiepileptics, cardiac medications, theophylline, caffeine), it is most important to be able to determine that the serum drug concentration remains within the therapeutic range throughout the dosing interval. In such cases, an evaluation of a trough concentration provides the most benefit. For these medications, peak concentrations are evaluated only if the patient exhibits signs of toxicity.

When the clinician decides whether and when serum concentrations should be evaluated, the pharmacokinetic parameters of the drug should be identified (Table 41–2). Obtaining levels once

TABLE 41–2 Common Pharmacokinetic Equations

$$\text{Volume of distribution (Vd)} = \frac{\text{dose (mg/kg)}}{\text{peak conc (mg/L)}}$$

$$\text{Half-life } (t_{1/2}) = \frac{0.693}{k_e}$$

$$\text{Clearance (Cl)} = \frac{0.693 \times \text{Vd}}{t_{1/2}}$$

$$\text{Elimination rate constant } (k_e) = \frac{\ln \text{conc}_a - \ln \text{conc}_b}{\Delta t}$$

Conc, concentration.

a patient achieves steady-state concentrations usually provides the health care provider with the most accurate information concerning how the patient may handle the medication on a long-term basis. Patients with altered organ function or rapidly changing clinical status may require closer monitoring of serum concentrations than do other patients. Because obtaining serum concentrations may require obtaining significant volumes of blood in a neonate, assessing the patient's clinical status may provide more useful information than obtaining serial serum concentrations of drugs.

Certain medications are highly protein bound. For these medications, two types of assays may be available: total and free serum concentrations. Free levels indicate the amount of free, unbound drug that is available to exert its effects on target tissues. Phenytoin, for example, should be monitored by evaluating free levels in the neonate because it is highly bound to plasma proteins and its pharmacokinetic parameters are significantly altered in this age group. If free phenytoin serum assays are not available, caution must be used in the interpretation of total serum concentrations. Levels may be falsely interpreted as low when the actual amount of active drug is adequate or toxic.

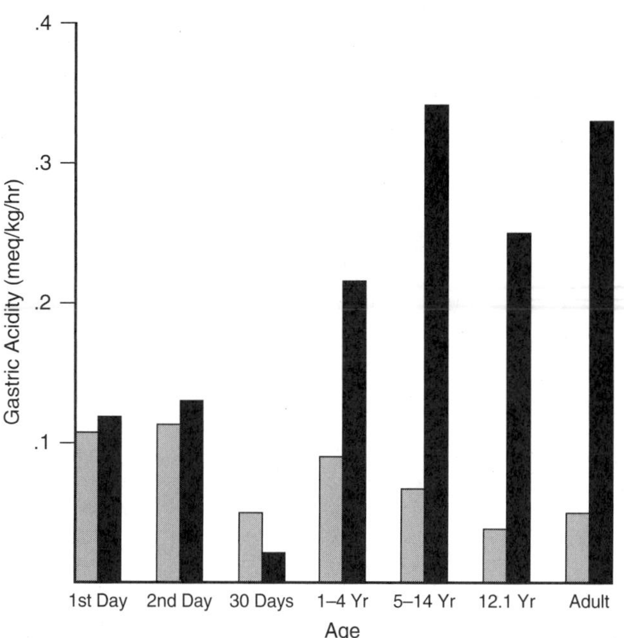

FIGURE 41–4. Ontogeny of gastric pH. Basal (□) and stimulated (■) gastric acid secretion from the first day of life to adulthood. (Originally published in Stewart, C. F., & Hampton, E. M. [1987]. Effect of maturation on drug disposition in pediatric patients. *Clinical Pharmacy*, 6[7], 550.)

FACTORS UNIQUE TO THE NEONATE

Absorption

Medications may be administered via many routes. No absorption phase is required for IV or intra-arterial administration of medications. Other routes of administration such as intramuscular (IM), oral, topical, rectal, and subcutaneous require absorption of the medication from the site of administration in order for drug to be recovered from the blood stream.

Absorption of a medication from an IM injection is influenced by muscle tone, muscle mass, and regional blood flow to the area (Stewart & Hampton, 1987). Neonates, especially premature infants, may have significantly decreased muscle mass and decreased tone. Blood flow to the muscle tissue itself can be compromised by hypoxemia, sepsis, shock, and congestive heart failure. IM injections of some medications may result in a delay in therapy because of poor or erratic absorption. A longer duration of action and a delay in the time to peak serum concentration may occur with IM administration of medications to neonates, and this route should be avoided unless absolutely necessary for the patient to receive the drug therapy.

Absorption from the gastrointestinal tract is dependent on many variables, including gastrointestinal pH, gastric emptying time, microbial colonization of the gastrointestinal tract, intestinal transit time, pancreatic enzyme activity, biliary function, and the clinical status of the infant (Morselli et al., 1980). The gastric pH in neonates differs significantly from that in adults. The gastric pH at birth is about 6 to 8. Gastric acid production is initiated soon after birth and then decreases over the first 30 days of life. An infant's gastric pH does not approach adult values until about 1 year of age (Stewart & Hampton, 1987). This difference in pH affects the absorption of many medications. Medications that are weak acids (phenobarbital, phenytoin, acetaminophen) are more poorly absorbed in neonates than in adults and older pediatric patients. Medications such as penicillin that are weak bases are absorbed to a much greater extent in the neonate than in either adults or pediatric patients. This difference in absorption may result in either a lack of drug absorption or excess absorption compared with that of medications administered intravenously but usually results in a longer duration of action. This may or may not be clinically significant (Fig. 41–4).

Absorption and time to peak serum concentration are influenced by the contact time of the medication with the absorptive surface. Gastric emptying time is delayed in the neonatal patient, especially in the premature infant (Morselli et al., 1980). This delay can enhance the absorption of medications that are absorbed in the stomach. Most medications are absorbed, not in the stomach, but in the small intestine. The slow intestinal transit time may influence the timing and peak effect of medications absorbed in the small intestine.

Concurrent disease states and some medications may produce alterations in transit time that affect drug absorption and peak serum concentration. The presence of diarrhea increases the gastrointestinal motility, resulting in less absorption of drug. Patients receiving narcotics usually develop a prolonged transit time that may result in increased absorption of other medications the patient is receiving.

Neonates have a state of relative pancreatic insufficiency; pancreatic activity reaches adult values by 9 months of age (Reed & Besunder, 1989). Pancreatic enzymes are required for the breakdown of nutrients. They are also required for the intraluminal hydrolysis of some medications (chloramphenicol, clindamycin).

Biliary function and the bile acid pool increase over the first month after birth (Watkins et al., 1973). The relative state of bile acid depletion affects medications administered with food. Bile acids are required for absorption of fat-soluble vitamins; patients with poor biliary function may have difficulty absorbing these nutrients.

The rate and composition of the colonization of the gastrointestinal tract are variable with time. The colonization may be affected by diet and by early exposure to antibiotics. The microbial colonization in the gut facilitates the breakdown of some medications and is involved in the enterohepatic recirculation of some medications. Changes in the gut flora may influence the metabolism of some drugs and some drug–drug interactions.

The absorption of medications through the skin depends on the skin integrity, blood flow to the skin, and the amount of subcutaneous fat (Stewart & Hampton, 1987). The ratio of skin to body surface area of premature infants is three times that of an adult. Because of smaller amounts of subcutaneous fat and an

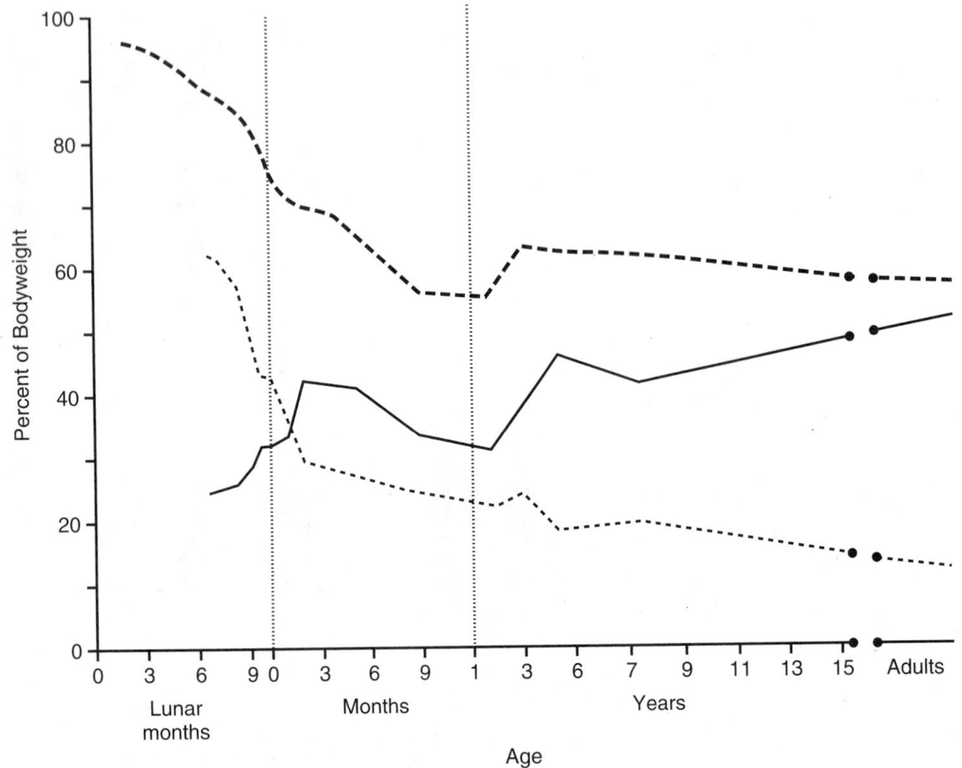

FIGURE 41–5. Distribution of body water. Percent of total water *(bold dashed line),* extracellular water *(solid line),* and intracellular water *(dashed line)* as a function of age. (Redrawn from Friis-Hansen, B. [1983]. Water distribution in the foetus and newborn infant. *Acta Paediatrica Scandinavica, 305*[Suppl.], 7–11.)

overall decreased skin barrier, agents applied topically can be absorbed to a significant degree. For example, application of hydrocortisone cream or ointment may result in therapeutic serum concentrations (Rutter, 1987). This enhanced absorption of topically applied medications can lead to toxicity, but it can also be exploited therapeutically. Use of the topical route of administration has been proposed for theophylline administration to premature infants (Micali et al., 1993).

Rectal administration of medications may be a valuable alternative for the administration of certain medications (e.g., aspirin, acetaminophen, diazepam, and sodium polystyrene sulfonate [Kayexalate]) when other routes of administration are not available. Rectal absorption is dependent on blood flow, retention of the drug in the rectum, and chemical properties of the drug and its formation.

Distribution

Once the medication has reached the blood stream, the next step is its distribution to other body compartments. This distribution phase is affected by the binding to tissue or plasma proteins, the nature and size of available body compartments, and the chemical properties of the drug itself. Most medications that are protein bound bind to serum albumin. Serum albumin and serum total proteins are decreased during infancy and rise slowly over the first year of life to adult values (Brodersen & Honore, 1989). Newborns also have a higher serum concentration of substances (maternal estrogens and bilirubin) that compete with medications for binding sites on albumin. Only the amount of medication that is biologically active is the free or unbound fraction. Decreased available sites for protein binding and increased displacement may influence therapeutic efficacy and toxicity at lower measured serum concentrations than would be evident in an adult. Patients with hepatic dysfunction or renal failure have alterations in protein binding and will also have increased amounts of free or unbound drug (Besunder et al., 1988). Trimethoprim-sulfamethoxazole and phenytoin are examples of highly protein bound medications that may result in the availability of increased free drug, depending on the age of the patient and on organ function.

Total body water and its distribution in the intracellular and extracellular spaces vary with the gestational age of the infant (Stewart & Hampton, 1987). A fetus of less than 3 months' gestation is 92 percent water, the majority of which is extracellular fluid. As the fetus matures, total body water decreases to a total of 75 percent at term, only about half of which is extracellular fluid (Fig. 41–5).

The central nervous system of neonates is immature and does not fully develop until the child reaches approximately 8 years of age (Levin, 1988). The formation of the blood–brain barrier is also incomplete, resulting in an increased accessibility of drugs to the central nervous system. Increased sensitivity to many drugs, especially those with sedative and central nervous system effects, may occur in the neonatal period.

Knowledge of the changing body composition of the developing fetus is important and is combined with knowledge of the chemical properties of a drug to predict how the distribution of a medication may be different in the neonate in comparison to published data in adults or older pediatric patients. Medications that are hydrophilic have a much higher volume of distribution in neonates than in adults; therefore, neonatal dosing is higher on a per kilogram basis. Likewise, medications that are lipophilic have a much smaller distribution volume in a neonate than in an adult, because less of a neonate's body mass is composed of adipose tissue. Neonatal dosing of medications that are lipophilic is probably lower on a per kilogram basis than is the adult dosing.

Metabolism

Many drugs undergo metabolism before they are eliminated from the body. The process of biotransformation occurs mainly in the liver, although other tissues may also be involved (Reed & Besunder, 1989). Many pathways are available for the metabolism of drugs, and each pathway matures at a different rate. For medications that are metabolized, this step is frequently the rate-limiting factor for elimination from the body.

At birth, concentrations of drug-oxidizing enzymes in the fetal liver are similar to those of an adult (Besunder et al., 1988). The activity of these enzymes may be markedly reduced. Enzymatic pathways, including methylation, reduction, and sulfation, appear to be well developed at birth. Other pathways such as demethylation, hydroxylation, glucuronidation, and conjugation do not develop until later in postnatal life. The delay in maturation of these pathways affects how the neonate metabolizes many medications and thereby affects the neonate's response to medication. For example, morphine is glucuronidated to a morphine-6-glucuronide compound in the adult. This glucuronidated morphine product is much more potent an analgesic than the parent morphine. Because glucuronidation is limited in neonates, they may require more of the parent drug per weight to produce adequate analgesia (Chay et al., 1992).

The maturation of these processes begins at birth and is independent of the length of gestation. Consideration must also be given to medications that the mother might have taken during her pregnancy. During intrauterine life, the fetus depends on both the mother's liver and its own liver to detoxify compounds. There is some evidence that prenatal exposure to drugs that have the capacity to induce hepatic enzymes may affect neonatal metabolism (Rudd & Brazy, 1988).

Excretion

The primary route of elimination of medications from the body is via the kidney. The neonatal kidney is significantly different from the adult kidney in that it has a high resistance to blood flow, has incomplete glomerular and tubular development, has a short and incompletely differentiated loop of Henle, and receives a low fraction of the cardiac output (Prandota, 1985). The glomerular filtration rate is lower in infants than in adults and significantly lower in premature infants than in those born at term. The first increase in the glomerular filtration rate is seen at 34 weeks of postconceptional age. Tubular reabsorption and secretion are also decreased in the neonate. Therefore, drugs excreted primarily via the renal route must have extended dosing intervals in comparison to the adult dosing. The kidney reaches adult capacity by 1 year of age. Prolonged excretion of some drugs in the neonate requires extension of dosing intervals. Gentamicin is administered only once or sometimes twice a day in most neonates, in comparison with the adult dosing of three times a day.

SPECIAL NEONATAL POPULATION

Extracorporeal membrane oxygenation (ECMO) has become a more frequently used mode of medical management for certain neonatal patients, including those with persistent pulmonary hypertension, meconium aspiration, sepsis, and congenital diaphragmatic hernia; it is also used as a bridge to heart transplant. Patients undergoing ECMO are often treated with numerous medications, including antibiotics, sedatives, analgesics, inotropes, diuretics, and antiepileptics. Medications may be administered to ECMO patients either into the ECMO circuit or directly to the patient. Varying pharmacokinetics may be observed, depending on the actual site of injection (Hoie et al., 1993).

Medications delivered into the ECMO circuit may be injected directly into the venous reservoir either before the filter or after the filter. The effects of the pump may cause an incomplete admixture of the medication, depending on the site of injection. Distribution and delivery of medication are more consistent when drugs are injected after the filter. Administration into this site places the patient at risk for development of air emboli, and

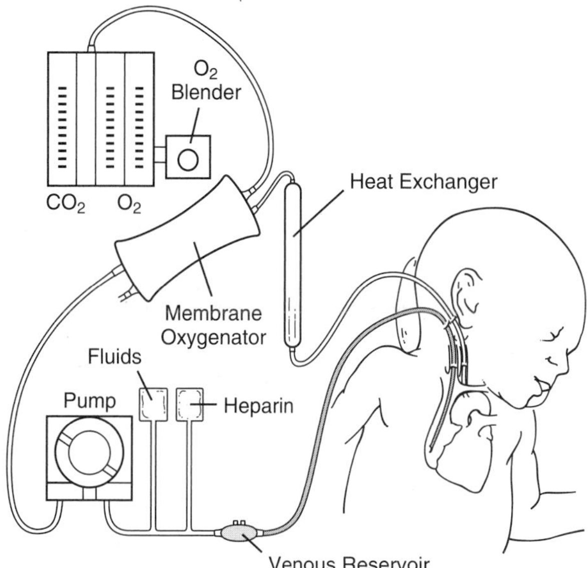

FIGURE 41–6. ECMO diagram. Venoarterial ECMO circuit with cannulation of the right common carotid artery and right internal jugular vein. (From Lotze, L., Short, B. L., & Taylor, G. A. [1987]. Lung compliance as a measure of lung function in newborns with respiratory failure requiring extracorporeal membrane oxygenation. *Critical Care Medicine, 15*[3], 226–229.)

administration of medications here should be done with great caution. Medications injected directly into the reservoir or before the filter usually result in a prolonged time of actual drug delivery to the patient and incomplete drug administration. Interpretation of pharmacokinetic parameters in this type of patient is often difficult because of the influences of the site of injection, flow rate of the ECMO circuit, and clinical status and organ function of the patient. There is often a delay in peak effect for these patients, resulting in false interpretation of serum peak levels for aminoglycoside antibiotics (Fig. 41–6).

In addition to the pharmacokinetic influences of ECMO, drugs such as heparin and fentanyl bind to the ECMO circuit, resulting in a reduced amount of bioavailable drug for the patient (Hynynen, 1987). Once the circuit becomes saturated with these medications, the medications reach the infant's circulation. Therefore, increased doses may be required initially when these medications are used or when the circuit is changed during ECMO therapy.

Patients placed on ECMO often have underlying hepatic and renal dysfunction secondary to hypoxic insults. The physiologic effects of ECMO further compound this dysfunction. Frequently, renal function continues to deteriorate during ECMO. Dosing adjustments need to be made for any medications cleared renally (Southgate et al., 1989).

Pharmacokinetic parameters have been established for few medications used in ECMO patients. Studies have noted an increased volume of distribution, which has been attributed to the volume of the ECMO circuit. Some of the observed increased in volume of distribution may have resulted from concurrent disease states. Increased volume of distribution should not be assumed for all medications. Dosing should be individualized on the basis of the medications and clinical status.

FETAL AND INFANT EXPOSURE TO MATERNAL MEDICATIONS

Fetal Exposure

Virtually any medication or substance given to the mother, either intentionally or inadvertently, can cross the placental mem-

TABLE 41–3 Pregnancy Risk Categories

Pregnancy Risk Categories	Definition*
Category A:	Controlled studies fail to demonstrate a risk to the fetus when exposed in the first trimester; possibility of fetal harm appears remote.
Category B:	Either animal-reproduction studies have not demonstrated a fetal risk but there are no controlled studies in pregnant women, or animal-reproduction studies have shown an adverse effect that was not confirmed in controlled studies in women in the first trimester.
Category C:	No controlled studies in women or animals available, or studies in animals have revealed adverse effects on the fetus. Drugs should be given only if the benefit outweighs the risk.
Category D:	Positive evidence of human fetal risk; benefits of use in pregnant women may outweigh risk because of life-threatening or serious disease state.
Category X:	Studies in animals or human beings have demonstrated fetal abnormalities, or there is evidence of fetal risk based on human experience; risk outweighs any potential benefit.

*Definitions used by the U.S. Food and Drug Administration, adapted from *Federal Register* (1980), *44*, 3734–3767.

brane. The consequence of fetal exposure to a substance may result in deleterious effects on the exposed fetus or may result in minimal or no adverse outcome. The effects seen are dependent on the agent, the amount of the substance, and the stage of gestation at which the fetal exposure occurs. Since the 1980s, there has been an increase in the amount of both prescription and over-the-counter drug use in women during pregnancy (Yaffe, 1994).

The amount of drug that passes into the fetal circulation is dependent on several factors, including molecular weight of the substance, protein binding, lipid solubility, ionization of drug, maternal serum concentrations, and integrity of the placental barrier. The FDA (1980) published definitions indicating pregnancy risk categories for certain medications. Drug companies have been required since 1983 to assign each medication a risk category (Table 41–3).

Unfortunately, medications passed through the placenta to the fetus are not efficiently cleared by the fetus. The effects on the fetus may be magnified. Medications given to expectant mothers close to delivery that affect liver enzymes by activation or inhibition will potentially affect the neonate's ability to clear medications that are hepatically metabolized. Sedation from maternal narcotic administration just before delivery may also result in some sedative effects in the newborn infant.

Lactation Exposure

An often overlooked source of exposure of a neonate or infant to medications is via transfer from the maternal circulation into breast milk. A nursing mother may produce up to 600 ml/day of milk (Anderson, 1991). The milk contains sufficient amounts of carbohydrate, protein, and fat to meet the daily nutritional requirements of the infant. Drugs may reach the breast milk after binding to fat or protein or by the passage of lipid-soluble drugs into the milk. Protein binding, degree of ionization, and concentration of drug in the maternal circulation also contribute to the amount of drug that reaches the milk supply. Considerations in determining the amount of medication the infant will receive also include the time the medication is taken in relation to the period of nursing, the amount or dose of medication, the length of nursing, and the amount of milk ingested.

The American Academy of Pediatrics Committee on Drugs (1994) published guidelines regarding the transfer of drugs and chemicals into human milk. These guidelines include a list of medications and chemicals for which there are available data concerning the transfer of a substance into the mother's milk and the subsequent effects to expect in the nursing infant. The list does not contain information on every available drug, because for some drugs there may not be any information available in the literature. If a breastfed infant develops any adverse effects from a medication prescribed to the mother, this information should be documented.

REFERENCES

American Academy of Pediatrics Committee on Drugs. (1994). The transfer of drugs and other chemicals into human milk. *Pediatrics, 93*(1), 137–150.

Anderson, P. O. (1991). Drug use in breast-feeding [Review]. *Clinical Pharmacy, 10*(8), 594–624.

Benzing, G., III, & Loggie, J. (1973). A new retrograde method for administering drugs intravenously. *Pediatrics, 52*(3), 420–425.

Besunder, J. B., Reed, M. D., & Blumer, J. C. (1988). Principles of drug biodisposition in the neonate: Part I [Review]. *Clinical Pharmacokinetics, 14*(4), 261–286.

Brodersen, R., & Honore, B. (1989). Drug binding properties of neonatal albumin. *Acta Paediatrica Scandinavica, 78*(3), 342–346.

Carl, J., Erstad, B., Murphey, J., & Slack, M. (1995). Fluid delivery from infusion-pump syringes. *American Journal of Health-System Pharmacy, 52*, 1428–1432.

Chay, P. C., Duffy, B. J., & Walker, J. S. (1992). Pharmacokinetic-pharmacodynamic relationships of morphine in neonates. *Clinical Pharmacology and Therapeutics, 51*(3), 334–342.

Ernst, J., Williams, J., Glick, M., & Lemons, J. (1983). Osmolality of substances used in the intensive care nursery. *Pediatrics, 72*(3), 347–352.

Faich, G. (1986). Adverse-drug-reaction monitoring. *New England Journal of Medicine, 314*(24), 1589–1592.

Fincham, J. (1992). Monitoring and managing adverse drug reactions. *American Pharmacy, 32*(2), 74–81.

Gould, T., & Roberts, R. (1979). Therapeutic problems arising from the use of the intravenous route for drug administration. *Journal of Pediatrics, 95*(3), 456–471.

Hansten, P., & Horn, J. (1993). *Drug interactions & updates quarterly* (pp. 1–25, 95–99, 119–124). Vancouver, WA: Applied Therapeutics.

Hepler, C., & Strand, L. (1989). Opportunities and responsibilities in pharmaceutical care. *American Journal of Pharmaceutical Education*, Winter suppl., p. 7s.

Hoie, E. B., Hall, M. C., & Schasf, L. J. (1993). Effects of injection site and flow rate on the distribution of injected solutions in an extracorporeal membrane oxygenation circuit. *American Journal of Hospital Pharmacy, 50*(9), 1902–1906.

Hynynen, M. (1987). Binding of fentanyl and alfentanil to the extracorporeal circuit. *Acta Anaesthesiologica Scandinavica, 31*(8), 706–710.

Lalonde, R. (1992). Pharmacodynamics. In W. E. Evans, J. J. Schentag, & W. J. Jusko (Eds.), *Applied pharmacokinetics: Principles of therapeutic drug monitoring* (pp. 1–31). Vancouver, WA: Applied Therapeutics.

Leff, R., & Roberts, R. (1981). Methods for intravenous drug administration in the pediatric patient. *Journal of Pediatrics, 98*(4), 631–635.

Levin, R. (1988). Pediatric and neonatal therapy. In E. T. Herfindal, D. R. Gourley, & L. L. Hart (Eds.), *Clinical pharmacy and therapeutics* (pp. 1011–1029). Baltimore: Williams & Wilkins.

Levy, G. (1992). Applied pharmacokinetics—A prospectus. In W. E. Evans, J. J. Schentag, & W. J. Jusko (Eds.), *Applied pharmacokinetics: Principles of therapeutic drug monitoring* (pp. 1–8). Vancouver, WA: Applied Therapeutics.

MacCara, M. (1983). Extravasation: A hazard of intravenous therapy. *Drug Intelligence and Clinical Pharmacy, 17*(10), 713–717.

Manasse, H., Jr. (1989). Medication use in an imperfect world: Drug misadventuring as an issue of public policy: Part I. *American Journal of Hospital Pharmacy, 46*(5), 929–944.

Micali, G., Bhatt, R. H., Distefano, G., et al. (1993). Evaluation of transdermal theophylline pharmacokinetics in neonates. *Pharmacotherapy, 13*(4), 386–390.

Morselli, P., Franco-Morselli, R., & Bossi, L. (1980). Clinical pharmacokinetics in newborns and infants. Age-related differences and therapeutic implications [Review]. *Clinical Pharmacokinetics, 5*(6), 485–527.

Newman, S. P., & Clarke, S. W. (1983). Therapeutic aerosols 1—Physical and practical considerations [Review]. *Thorax, 38*(12), 881–886.

Prandota, J. (1985). Clinical pharmacokinetics of changes in drug elimination in children. *Developmental Pharmacology and Therapeutics, 8*(5), 311–328.

Reed, M., & Besunder, J. (1989). Developmental pharmacology: Ontogenic basis of drug disposition. *Pediatric Clinics of North America, 36*(5), 1053–1074.

Roberts, R. (1981). Intravenous administration of medication in pediatric patients: Problems and solutions. *Pediatric Clinics of North America, 28*(1), 23–34.

Rooke, G., & Bowdle, T. (1994). Syringe pumps for infusion of vasoactive drugs: Mechanical idiosyncrasies and recommended operating procedures. *Anesthesia and Analgesia, 78*(1), 150–156.

Rowland, M., & Tozer, T. N. (1989). *Clinical pharmacokinetics: Concepts and applications* (2nd ed., pp. 17–31, 156–158, 182–187). Philadelphia: Lea & Febiger.

Rudd, C., & Brazy, J. (1988). Drugs in the perinatal period: Implications for the preterm infant. *Comprehensive Therapy, 14*(12), 30–37.

Rutter, N. (1987). Percutaneous drug absorption in the newborn: Hazards and uses. *Clinics in Perinatology, 14*(4), 911–930.

Shargel, L., & Yu, A. (1985). *Applied biopharmaceutics and pharmacokinetics* (2nd ed., pp. 214). Norwalk, CT: Appleton-Century-Crofts.

Southgate, W. M., DiPiro, J. T., & Robertson, A. F. (1989). Pharmacokinetics of gentamicin in neonates on extracorporeal membrane oxygenation. *Antimicrobial Agents and Chemotherapy, 33*(6), 817–819.

Stewart, C. F., & Hampton, E. M. (1987). Effect of maturation on drug disposition in pediatric patients [Review]. *Clinical Pharmacy, 6*(7), 548–564.

U.S. Department of Health and Human Services. (1993). MedWatch Reporting Program. *FDA Medical Bulletin, 23*(2), insert.

U.S. Food and Drug Administration. (1980). Drug use in pregnancy risk categories. *Federal Register, 44,* 3734–3767.

Watkins, J. B., Ingall, D., Szczepanek, P., et al. (1973). Bile salt metabolism in the newborn: Measurement of pool size and synthesis by stable isotope technic. *New England Journal of Medicine, 288*(9), 431–434.

White, K., & Harkavy, K. (1982). Hypertonic formula resulting from added oral medications. *American Journal of Diseases of Children, 136*(10), 931–933.

Winter, M. (1988). *Basic clinical pharmacokinetics* (2nd ed., pp. 7–63). Vancouver, WA: Applied Therapeutics.

Yaffe, S. (1994). Introduction. In G. E. Briggs, R. K., Freeman, & S. J. Yaffe (Eds.), *Drugs in pregnancy and lactation* (4th ed., pp. 11–17). Baltimore: Williams & Wilkins.

CHAPTER 42

Neonatal Acquired Immunodeficiency Syndrome: Human Immunodeficiency Virus

CAROLE KENNER

RESEARCH AGENDA

What subtle signs and symptoms does a neonate or infant display before being diagnosed as having human immunodeficiency virus (HIV) or undergoing seroconversion?

What factors influence the shorter incubation period of HIV in the neonate and infant as compared with that in an older child or adult?

What effect does the parental diagnosis of HIV have on the health professional's care of the neonate?

What impact does being HIV-positive have on maternal and fetal outcomes during and following pregnancy?

What effect does prenatal administration of certain HIV medications have on the seropositive mother and her fetus?

What effect does prenatal use of zidovudine (azidothymidine [AZT]) have on vertical HIV transmission to the fetus or neonate?

Does preconceptional teaching about HIV have an impact on perinatal and neonatal HIV infection rates?

What impact does a boarder baby have on the care and neurobehavioral development of the infant with HIV?

Evaluate strategies that are meant to help increase the adherence to therapeutic regimens of persons with HIV infection.

Examine the relationship of psychosocial variables such as social support to patient and family adaptation to HIV infection.

Evaluate the long-term effects of death and dying and the grief process on personnel providing care to persons with HIV infection.

Test strategies to promote the use of universal precautions by health care personnel.

VIGNETTE

"It's a boy!" the doctor announced as the baby was born. Tears spilled down LuAnn's face as she gazed at the tiny newborn on her abdomen. She gently touched the baby and said, "You're my little Bobby Joe." I wondered what thoughts were going through her mind as I congratulated her. She watched intently as the neonatologist and I assessed her baby and provided the initial resuscitation. It had only been 6 weeks since LuAnn had been diagnosed HIV-positive.

As Dr. James and I quickly dried the baby and cleared his airway, we took care to use universal precautions. As I held the oxygen mask near his face, I noted how tiny Bobby Joe's head looked when compared with his body. He looked small, even for a 36-week baby. We began to assess for the distinctive facial features found in neonates who have contracted HIV in utero. Dr. James commented about the eyes. "He has the features of an HIV baby. Look at the increased inner and outer canthal distance and the prominent triangular philtrum," he said in a hushed voiced.

LuAnn continued to watch us closely. "How's he doing?" she asked. "He's pretty small, but he's breathing well and looks good," Dr. James replied. By this time, I had slowly withdrawn the oxygen, and Bobby Joe remained pink. After weighing him and wrapping him in warm blankets, I took Bobby Joe to LuAnn to see and hold her newborn son.

"Since he's stable, he can stay with you for awhile before we take him to the nursery," Dr. James told an anxious LuAnn. He had already palpated the baby's abdomen and noted hepatosplenomegaly. He left orders for me to send a cord blood specimen for maternal HIV antibodies.

I dimmed the lights to facilitate their bonding, and the baby responded by opening his distinctive eyes. LuAnn's mother had been her support person through the labor and delivery. She exclaimed, "My first grandson! He's so beautiful!" I agreed and pointed out that he had light hair, like LuAnn's.

As the three of them continued to bond, I thought back over the prenatal history I had read and the feelings LuAnn had shared with me while she was in labor. She had lived with her boyfriend for 2 years. When his intravenous drug habit became too much for her to tolerate, this 20-year-old

For further information on HIV Clinical Trials call AIDS Clinical Trials Information Service at 1-800-TRIALS-A.

high school graduate moved home with her mother. She soon discovered she was pregnant. Her mother was supportive of her decision to keep the baby. She accompanied LuAnn on her prenatal visits. LuAnn ignored the symptoms of fatigue and night sweats in the early months of her pregnancy, thinking it was hormonal changes. She lost weight during her first trimester because of constant nausea and poor appetite but had attributed it to "morning sickness." At her 16-week visit, LuAnn had a fever and continued poor weight gain. That morning, the OB clinic received a call from the public health department, reporting a positive HIV III antibody test for her former boyfriend. An enzyme-linked immunosorbent assay (ELISA) was performed on LuAnn that day and returned positive. Both a repeat ELISA and subsequent Western blot test showed positive results. LuAnn described her emotional turmoil, fear, and confusion to me. She immediately inquired about the danger to her unborn baby. When told there was a 20 to 30 percent chance that she would transmit the disease to her baby, she requested an abortion but was refused because of advanced gestation. LuAnn verbalized fear and guilt about her baby's possible HIV status. She also verbalized anger at her boyfriend for passing the deadly infection to both of them.

Her doctor had explained much about acquired immunodeficiency syndrome (AIDS) to her: that the progress of the disease is unpredictable and possibly fatal, that research is ongoing to identify medications and treatments, that not all HIV-positive persons progress to AIDS, and that the course of the infection appears to be unaffected by pregnancy. The OB clinic nurse gave LuAnn and her mother support and educational pamphlets on HIV and explained the importance of adequate rest, nutrition, and avoiding infection. She referred her to several support groups for AIDS patients and their families. LuAnn and her mother found a group near their home and attended regularly.

Bobby Joe was about 45 minutes old, so I gently told the new mother and grandmother that he needed to go to the nursery to be examined. The two women kissed the baby before giving him to me.

As I reported mother's history and baby's stability to the nursery nurse, the smile faded from her face. She immediately put on gloves and cover gown. I reported Dr. James's findings on initial examination and his request to be notified when Bobby Joe arrived in the nursery.

I returned after LuAnn's recovery period and transfer to her room to find Dr. James finishing his admission note on the baby. On further examination, he had noted other facial abnormalities of HIV babies: boxy forehead; flat, broad nasal bridge; and spreading lips. The tiny newborn was breathing well; his color was pink and vital signs stable as he sucked vigorously on his fist. Dr. James sighed as he told the nursery nurse further signs to watch for with the baby in the next few days: oral candidiasis and respiratory distress indicative of interstitial pneumonitis.

I did not see LuAnn again, since they were discharged before I returned to work. As I left the hospital that morning, I felt sad and wondered if their family would get the support they desperately needed and deserved from other nurses and physicians. The social stigma, chronic and debilitating illness, pain, and strong possibility of death require committed intervention on the part of all health care team members.

Judi Hostiuck

The number of infants exposed to HIV is an increasing problem in many areas of the United States (Ellerbrock & Rogers, 1990). Neonatal nurses need to be familiar with HIV: its mode of transmission, tests to detect it, signs and symptoms, assessment, and physical findings. They must be aware that in most instances infants who are infected perinatally progress to AIDS and die before the age of 5 years (Chin, 1994). Chin (1994) estimated that by the year 2000, there will be 320,000 HIV-positive women in North America and western Europe with 25,000 HIV-positive infants, 20,000 pediatric AIDS patients, and 25,000 orphans less than 5 years of age and 120,000 less than 15 years of age from the same geographic area. It is the single largest cause of pediatric death due to infectious agents in the United States (Chin, 1994). Additionally, nurses need to be aware of ways to provide both physical and developmental support to the infant who has been exposed to HIV and the infant's family. Once aware of the factors related to HIV, the neonatal nurse is better prepared to deal with the growing number of infants who have been exposed to or infected with HIV. Neonatal nurses are also drawn into the ethical and legal discussions about whether or not there should be mandatory HIV screening for newborns (Rhodes, 1995). These controversies are dealt with in Chapters 3, Ethical Aspects of Perinatal Care, and 4, Legal Aspects of Perinatal Care.

The purpose of this chapter is to define HIV and discuss its pathophysiology, signs and symptoms, and mode of transmission, as well as the testing and management of the infant who has been infected. In addition, nursing diagnoses for both the asymptomatic and symptomatic infant with HIV infection are presented. Methods for prevention as well as issues for health care workers are addressed. Finally, the problem of boarder babies, especially those with HIV, is discussed.

HUMAN IMMUNODEFICIENCY VIRUS INFECTION AND ACQUIRED IMMUNODEFICIENCY SYNDROME

AIDS is an impairment of the body's immune system. It is a relatively new disease. The origin of the AIDS retrovirus is thought to be Africa, with the first cases occurring in the mid-1970s (Viscarello, 1990). However, it was not until the 1980s that full attention became focused on HIV. Although still relatively uncommon in the general population, the incidence of HIV and AIDS has increased dramatically over the past decade. Unfortunately, the sharp rise in the number of HIV and AIDS cases has not excluded the infant population.

In the literature, the virus is known by three names: (1) HIV, human immunodeficiency virus; (2) LAV, lymphadenopathy-associated virus; and (3) HTLV-III, human T-cell lymphotropic virus type III. The term *AIDS* is a generic label referring to individuals who may be infected but are asymptomatic or individuals who are symptomatic. Therefore, owing to the generic use of the label, it is more appropriate to use the term *HIV infection*, which covers the entire range from asymptomatic to the terminally ill individual.

Definition of Human Immunodeficiency Syndrome

The Centers for Disease Control and Prevention (CDC) case definition for AIDS is as follows: "AIDS is a disabling or life threatening illness caused by human immunodeficiency virus (HIV) characterized by HIV encephalopathy, HIV wasting syndrome, or certain diseases due to immunodeficiency in a person with laboratory evidence for HIV infection or without certain other causes of immunodeficiency" (CDC, 1987a).

In contrast, the CDC case definition for pediatric AIDS is presented in Table 42–1. The pediatric definition includes anyone 13 years of age or younger. Individuals older than 13 years of age are reported in the adult statistics. In addition to the definition,

TABLE 42–1 Centers for Disease Control Case Definition for Pediatric AIDS

1. Without laboratory evidence of HIV infection (tests not done or inconclusive), a patient with AIDS:
   A. Does not have another cause of immunodeficiency, such as the following:
      1. High-dose or long-term systemic corticosteroid therapy or other immunosuppressive-cytotoxic therapy ≤3 months before the onset of the indicator disease
      2. Hodgkin's disease, non-Hodgkin's lymphoma (other than primary brain lymphoma), lymphocytic leukemia, multiple myeloma, other cancer of lymphoreticular-histocytic tissue, angioimmunoblastic lymphadenopathy ≤3 months after diagnosis of the indicator disease
      3. A genetic (congenital) immunodeficiency syndrome or an acquired immunodeficiency syndrome atypical of HIV infection (such as one with hypogammaglobulinemia)

   AND

   B. Has had one of the following AIDS indicator diseases definitively diagnosed:
      1. Candidiasis of the esophagus, trachea, bronchi, or lungs
      2. Extrapulmonary cryptococcosis
      3. Cryptosporidiosis with diarrhea persisting >1 month
      4. Cytomegalovirus disease of an organ other than liver, spleen, or lymph nodes in a patient >1 month
      5. Herpes simplex virus infection causing a mucocutaneous ulcer persisting >1 month, or bronchitis, pneumonitis, or esophagitis in a patient >1 month of age
      6. Primary lymphoma of the brain in a patient <60 years of age
      7. Kaposi's sarcoma in a patient <60 years of age
      8. Lymphoid interstitial pneumonia or pulmonary lymphoid hyperplasia in a child <13 years of age
      9. *Mycobacterium avium* complex of *Mycobacterium kansasii* disease disseminated to site other than lungs, skin, or cervical or hilar lymph nodes
      10. *Pneumocystis carinii* pneumonia
      11. Progressive multifocal leukoencephalopathy
      12. Toxoplasmosis of the brain in a patient >1 month of age
2. With laboratory evidence of HIV infection, a patient with AIDS:
   A. Has had one of the already-listed AIDS indicators or diseases definitively diagnosed or one of the following AIDS indicator diseases definitively diagnosed:
      1. Multiple or recurrent bacterial infections (at least two within 2 years) in a child <13 years of age, including septicemia, pneumonia, meningitis, bone or joint infection, abscess of internal organ body cavity (except otitis media or superficial skin or mucosal abscesses)
      2. Coccidioidomycosis disseminated to a site other than lungs or cervical or hilar lymph nodes
      3. HIV encephalopathy
      4. Histoplasmosis disseminated to a site other than lungs or cervical or hilar lymph nodes
      5. Isosporiasis with diarrhea persisting >1 month
      6. Kaposi's sarcoma
      7. Primary lymphoma of brain
      8. Other non-Hodgkin's lymphoma of B-cell or unknown immunologic phenotype (small, noncleaved Burkitt's or non-Burkitt's lymphoma or immunoblastic sarcoma)
      9. Disseminated nontubercular mycobacterial disease involving a site other than lungs, skin, or cervical or hilar lymph nodes
      10. Tuberculosis involving at least one site other than lungs
      11. Recurrent nontyphoid *Salmonella* bacteremia
      12. HIV wasting syndrome

   OR

   B. One of the following AIDS indicator diseases diagnosed presumptively:
      1. Esophageal candidiasis
      2. Cytomegalovirus retinitis with loss of vision
      3. Kaposi's sarcoma
      4. Lymphoid interstitial pneumonia or pulmonary lymphoid hyperplasia in a child <13 years of age
      5. Acid-fast infection (species not identified) disseminated to a site other than lungs, skin, or cervical or hilar lymph nodes
      6. *Pneumocystis carinii* pneumonia
      7. Toxoplasmosis of the brain in a patient >1 month of age

   AND

   Has had *Pneumocystis carinii* pneumonia definitively diagnosed

   OR

   C. Has had a definitive diagnosis of one of the AIDS indicator diseases listed in section 1, plus a T-helper (T4) lymphocyte count <400/mm^3

AIDS, acquired immunodeficiency syndrome; HIV, human immunodeficiency virus.

From Centers for Disease Control. (1987). Classification system for human immunodeficiency virus (HIV) infection in children under 13 years of age. *MMWR Morbidity and Mortality Weekly Report, 36*, 225–230.

TABLE 42–2 Summary of the Classification of HIV Infection in Children Younger Than 13 Years of Age

Class P-0 Indeterminate Infection

Class P-1 Asymptomatic Infection

Subclass A. Normal immune function
Subclass B. Abnormal immune function
Subclass C. Immune function not tested

Class P-2 Symptomatic Infection

Subclass A. Nonspecific findings
Subclass B. Progressive neurologic disease
Subclass C. Lymphoid interstitial pneumonitis
Subclass D. Secondary infectious disease
Category D-1. Specified secondary infectious diseases listed in the CDC surveillance definitions for AIDS
Category D-2. Recurrent serious bacterial infections
Category D-3. Other specified secondary infectious diseases
Subclass E. Secondary cancers
Category E-1. Specified secondary cancers listed in the CDC surveillance definition for AIDS
Category E-2. Other cancers possibly secondary to HIV infection
Subclass F. Other diseases possibly due to HIV infection such as hepatitis, cardiopathy, nephropathy, hematologic (anemia, thrombocytopenia), dermatologic diseases

HIV, human immunodeficiency virus; CDC, Centers for Disease Control and Prevention; AIDS, acquired immunodeficiency syndrome.
From Centers for Disease Control. (1987). Classification system for human immunodeficiency virus (HIV) infection in children under 13 years of age. *MMWR Morbidity and Mortality Weekly Report, 36,* 225–230.

the CDC has developed a classification system. The CDC recommends that physical assessment data should be gathered with the classification system in mind (Table 42–2). To meet the classification system, physical examination findings must be multiple and present for at least 2 months before they can be related to HIV (Mendez & Jule, 1990). Table 42–3 summarizes the definition of HIV for infants and children. The information and data presented from the CDC in these three tables formulate the foundation on which a diagnosis of pediatric HIV infection is established.

Incidence

For the pediatric and adult population, it is estimated that between 1 and 1.5 million persons in the United States have been infected by HIV (CDC, 1991). Many of the individuals infected by HIV may not be aware that they harbor the virus and are classified in the asymptomatic category. These individuals may have no visible signs of illness and are able to transmit the virus throughout their lifetime. Even though these individuals are infected with the virus, that does not necessarily mean that they will contract AIDS as classified by the CDC.

Some of these individuals may get AIDS-related complex (ARC). ARC was previously used to describe certain clusters of symptoms. The term *ARC* is no longer used, owing to the confusion that surrounds it from a public health perspective (Institute of Medicine/National Academy of Sciences, 1988). A more appropriate label is *HIV-positive.* This term distinguishes between individuals who are seropositive and do not meet the 1987 CDC definition but who manifest some of the signs and symptoms associated with AIDS and those who are seropositive and meet the 1987 CDC definition for having AIDS (CDC, 1987a, 1987b).

In 1979, AIDS was first recognized as a syndrome (CDC, 1982). It was not until 1984 that the HIV virus was discovered as the infectious cause of AIDS. The first cases in the early 1980s were associated with homosexual or bisexual males (CDC, 1982). As more data and information on HIV was obtained, the HIV virus has been associated with certain patterns or lifestyles (CDC, 1982). The current high-risk groups in the United States include homosexual or bisexual men, intravenous drug users, recent African immigrants, heterosexual partners of persons with HIV, hemophiliacs and other persons receiving blood or blood products, and infants born to HIV-positive mothers (Edmondson, 1988). Most recently it has been recognized that the heterosexual population is at increasing risk if multiple partners are involved and safe sexual practices are not followed. Table 42–4 lists the three major categories of groups at high risk for possible HIV exposure.

In Africa and developing countries, the pattern and mode of transmission are different from those in the United States (Viscarello, 1990). In other areas of the world, transmission of HIV is primarily through heterosexual contact. The remainder of this chapter focuses on HIV in the United States.

TABLE 42–3 Summary of the Definition of HIV Infection in Children

Infants and Children Younger than 15 Months of Age with Perinatal Infection

1. Virus in blood or tissues
or
2. HIV antibody present
and
Evidence of both cellular and humoral immune deficiency
and
One or more categories in class P-2
3. Symptoms meeting CDC case definitions for AIDS

Older Children with Perinatal Infection and Children with HIV Infection Acquired Through Other Modes of Transmission

1. Virus in blood or tissues
or
2. HIV antibody
or
3. Symptoms meeting CDC case definition for AIDS

HIV, human immunodeficiency virus; CDC, Centers for Disease Control and Prevention; AIDS, acquired immunodeficiency virus.
From Centers for Disease Control. (1987). Classification system for human immunodeficiency virus (HIV) infection in children under 13 years of age. *MMWR Morbidity and Mortality Weekly Report, 36,* 225–230.

Human Immunodeficiency Virus in the United States

In 1982, the first case of perinatal transmission was described by the CDC (CDC, 1982; Rogers et al., 1987). By 1986, there had been 20,000 cases of HIV reported in the United States. Of those 20,000 cases, 307 of the HIV cases were in infants and children (Rogers et al., 1987). In 1987, the number of HIV cases doubled from the previous year to 40,532, with approximately 1 percent of the total cases being in infants and children younger than 13 years of age (Rogers et al., 1987). The CDC predicted

TABLE 42–4 Three Major Categories of Risk Factors for HIV Infection

Perinatal

During pregnancy
Intrapartum
Postpartum
Breastfeeding

Exposure to Blood

Mother or father intravenous drug user
Parent has had blood transfusion
Infant received contaminated blood transfusion

Sexual

Bisexual father
Mother having sexual relations with high-risk individuals

that by the end of 1991 there would be 2900 pediatric cases in the United States alone (CDC, 1991).

When dealing with the actual number of HIV cases, it is difficult to quote the latest statistics because of the ever-changing numbers. Until the mid-1990s, fewer than 1 percent of individuals with HIV were infants; unfortunately this figure is rapidly changing. The overall trend through 1991 was for increasing numbers of maternal and infant cases. Unfortunately the trend has not changed to date. The pattern of increasing pediatric cases is presented in Table 42–5. The prognosis and clinical course for these infants are more grim and shorter than those of the adult with HIV (American Academy of Pediatrics, 1988). The average age for survival is 8 to 9 years (Yoder & Polin, 1997).

The pattern and number of individuals infected with HIV vary by geographic region and proximity to large metropolitan areas. In the United States, HIV has been reported in women in all 50 states (Ellerbrock & Rogers, 1990). The largest numbers of cases are reported along the northeastern coast, in the South, and in western coastal regions. More specifically, these states are New Jersey; New York; Washington, DC; Connecticut; Maryland; Rhode Island; Massachusetts; Florida; South Carolina; Georgia; California; and Delaware.

More than 40 states are testing neonatal blood collected for other screening purposes, such as phenylketonuria testing, to look for the presence of HIV. These samples, representing 90 percent of all newborns in the areas being screened, were devoid of all identifying factors. Dondero and associates (1988) and Hoff and colleagues (1988) reported the seroprevalence of HIV in women experiencing live births. From these investigations, it was estimated that there were eight HIV-infected women per 10,000 live births (range 2 to 66). These data were calculated based on neonatal blood samples.

In women, a predominance (one third) of the diagnosed cases is found in the childbearing ages between 20 and 29 years (Ellerbrock & Rogers, 1990). When the incubation period and time to the manifestation of symptoms are taken into consideration, most of these women were likely infected in their teenage years (Ellerbrock & Rogers, 1990). Eighty-five percent of the women infected with HIV are between the ages of 15 and 44 years (Ellerbrock & Rogers, 1990). Culturally, a majority (85 percent) of the HIV cases among women are reported in the black and Hispanic populations (Harrison, 1990).

Etiology and Pathophysiology

HIV-1 is part of the lentivirus subfamily of human retroviruses and requires a cell surface receptor for attachment and penetration into the cell. The current theory is that HIV is an RNA virus that has a gp120 surface molecule that attaches to the CD4+ receptor sites on the cell's surface. The gp120 surface molecule acts as a key to open the lock on the surface of the CD4+ (T-helper cell), thus allowing the HIV to move inside the cell easily. In older HIV literature, the CD4+ cells were referred to as T-helper lymphocytes or T4 cells (CDC, 1991; Fahrner, 1992). The term *retrovirus* refers to the ability of the virus to enter the target cell via the receptor site; then during cell division, the virus's RNA material is copied into the DNA. By using the enzyme reverse transcriptase, the new cell continues to replicate the virus throughout the infected individual's life (American Academy of Pediatrics, 1988). Other cells that have CD4+ receptor sites include B lymphocytes, monocytes, macrophages, and glial cells of the brain (Levy, 1989). Any of these cells may also become infected with the retrovirus using the process previously described for the CD4+ cells (Fahrner, 1992), thus explaining the variety of symptoms a person infected with HIV may manifest. In addition, HIV may also attack other cells that do not have the CD4+ receptor sites that are readily detectable on the surface membrane (Fahrner, 1992). Therefore, other receptor sites in certain cells, such as those of the central nervous system, may allow the lock-and-key mechanism with the HIV gp120 on the cell's surface. Once HIV has entered a cell, it results in immunodeficiency that renders the cell incapable of combating infections (Fahrner, 1992). The reason is that the CD4+ cells that normally assist in an immune response are rendered useless. At this point, not only does the HIV infection result in immunodeficiency but the infected cells can also readily pass into the peripheral and central nervous system, gastrointestinal (GI) tract, heart, lungs, and kidney of the infected individual (Fahrner, 1992).

The premature or term infant has an immature immune system (Polin & Fox, 1992). The T-cell or cell-mediated immune system is mature. However, the B-cell or humoral system is physiologically immature (Polin & Fox, 1992). The B cells are involved in the formation of functional antibodies. T cells are differentiated into CD4+ cells (previously referred to as T-helper cells) and CD8+ cells (previously referred to as T-suppressor cells). In the noninfected infant, CD4+ cells enhance an immune response to infection, and CD8+ cells dampen a response. In the case of HIV in the adult, the ratio of CD4+ cells to CD8+ cells is reversed, thus leaving the individual vulnerable to bacterial and opportunistic infections (Fahrner, 1992). It is unclear whether the CD4+:CD8+ ratio in the infant follows the same pattern as in the adult (Fahrner, 1992).

Therefore, infants exposed to HIV may manifest signs and symptoms at an earlier stage owing to the inability of the humoral system to manufacture antibodies (Fahrner, 1992). Hence, bacterial infections and other types of opportunistic infections are more likely to occur in the infant infected with HIV than in the adult infected with HIV, in whom a mature immune system exists.

TABLE 42–5 Number of Reported Infant and Pediatric HIV Cases in the United States from 1982 to 1991

Year	Number of Cases
1982	16
1983	35
1984	48
1985	132
1986	410
1987	525
1988	839
1989	977
1990	1600
1991	2900

HIV, human immunodeficiency virus.

Data from Centers for Disease Control. (1991, March). *Centers for Disease Control HIV/AIDS surveillance report*. Washington, DC: US Government Printing Office.

Transmission

Another concept addressed in the literature is the degree of infectiousness. The infectiousness increases as HIV progresses (Ellerbrock & Rogers, 1990). The degree of infectiousness may correlate with CD4+ cell counts. Thus, the longer an individual has been seropositive for HIV, and the lower the CD4+ cell counts, the more correlation there is with the risk of transmission. Therefore, there is an increased frequency of the viremia and secretion of HIV (Ellerbrock & Rogers, 1990).

Isolation of Human Immunodeficiency Virus

HIV has been isolated from the blood, brain tissue, saliva, tears, semen, vaginal secretions, amniotic fluid, breast milk, and organs of infected individuals (Fahrner, 1992; Mundy et al., 1987). However, HIV cannot reproduce outside a living cell. The majority of infants who have become infected with HIV are born to mothers who have AIDS or who are in high-risk groups (i.e., intravenous drug users, those with multiple sexual partners, sexual partners of men infected with HIV) (see Table 42–4).

Transplacental Transmission

Neonates and infants younger than 15 months of age most likely contract HIV via vertical or transplacental transmission, although some cases may be contracted via maternal blood, vaginal secretions, or breast milk. The CDC states that 80 percent of all pediatric cases are reported in infants younger than 15 months of age. In the past, the remaining 20 percent of pediatric HIV patients contracted the disease from infected blood products (most commonly used for the treatment of hemophilia and sickle cell anemia). However, this pattern is changing as the result of better screening of the nation's blood supply. The risk and rate of infection are dramatically decreasing for the population with hemophilia and sickle cell anemia, although such infection is still present.

For the adolescent population, the mode of transmission is similar to that for the adult. The problem with the adolescent population is that they are of childbearing age and are delivering more and more infants, thus increasing the possibility of placing the infant at risk if any of the high-risk behaviors for HIV are present in the mother or father.

In addition to the noted routes of possible exposure or transmission, individuals have become exposed via artificial insemination, tissue transplantation, and occupational contact (Marcus and the CDC Cooperative Needlestick Surveillance Group, 1989). Occupational exposure is discussed at the end of this chapter in the section discussing HIV and the health care worker.

Exposure Through Artificial Insemination

In Australia, Stewart and coworkers (1985) reported that eight women were artificially inseminated with cryopreserved semen from an asymptomatic HIV-infected donor. Four of the eight women tested positive for the HIV antibody. Additionally, another individual exhibited symptoms of lymphadenopathy. Chiasson and colleagues (1990) reported one case of HIV infection in the United States resulting from artificial insemination with fresh semen.

Effect of Pregnancy on Progression of Human Immunodeficiency Virus

Becoming or being pregnant does not appear to aggravate the course of HIV infection in asymptomatic women. However, other sources state that evidence exists that a pregnant woman infected with HIV is more apt to become HIV-positive or acquire AIDS than is a nonpregnant women with HIV (Ellerbrock & Rogers, 1990). In addition, there is some evidence that pregnancy may aggravate the course of the disease in a woman who is in the advanced stages of HIV infection (Ellerbrock & Rogers, 1990). Regardless of the findings, the long-term impact of being pregnant and infected with HIV is unknown (Selwyn et al., 1989). Therefore, further research in the area of HIV during pregnancy needs to be carried out.

PERINATAL EXPOSURE OF INFANTS OF INFECTED MOTHERS

The transmission of HIV infection from mother to infant predominantly occurs over one of the following routes: (1) in utero via transplacental passage of the virus, (2) during labor and delivery through exposure to infected blood and vaginal secretions, or (3) postpartally through breastfeeding (Ellerbrock & Rogers, 1990). In addition, other modes of transmission may occur, as previously discussed.

Rate of Mother-to-Infant Transmission

It is difficult to determine the actual rate of transmission of the HIV virus from mother to infant. Ellerbrock and Rogers (1990) noted that there may be an underestimation of the rate of transmission because most of the women are asymptomatic during pregnancy. Therefore, if the mother–infant dyad were followed for a longer period, the rate of 25 to 35 percent may prove to be an underestimation of the actual number of cases (Ellerbrock & Rogers, 1990).

Maternal factors that may be related to an increased rate of transmission include (1) immunologically compromised seropositive mothers, (2) seropositive mothers with CD4+ counts greater than 400/mm^3, and (3) maternal age and elevated maternal IgA levels (Ellerbrock & Rogers, 1990). The exact physiologic mechanism for those associations and linkages is not fully understood (Hutto et al., 1989).

Effect of Human Immunodeficiency Virus Infection on Pregnancy Outcomes and Obstetrical Complications

Current evidence has not established an increased risk of adverse perinatal outcomes for the pregnant woman (Ellerbrock & Rogers, 1990). Selwyn and associates (1989) found no differences in the frequency of spontaneous abortion, ectopic pregnancy, preterm delivery, stillbirth, or low birth weight infants between a group of seropositive women and a group of seronegative women. In their investigation, they found a slightly increased rate of bacterial pneumonia during pregnancy as well as breech presentation (Selwyn et al., 1989). In the investigation, there were no differences between the seropositive and seronegative women regarding the occurrence of antepartal, intrapartal, or neonatal complications.

Tovo and associates (1994) found that the more rapidly the infection progressed maternally, the more rapidly it would progress in the infant. Thus this research, if substantiated in further studies, would suggest that prevention of vertical transmission must be aimed at slowing maternal progression of the disease. It also suggests that there may be genetic linkages that need to be examined. Ahmad and associates (1995) found that genetic markers that have to do with the HIV-1 sequences found proximal to the first cysteine in the DNA protein in a mother are similar in her infected infant. Similar genotypes between the mother–infant dyad may help with preventive vertical transmission strategies.

To minimize the risk of transmission from the HIV-infected mother to the fetus, invasive procedures involving the passage of needles and instruments through the skin or tissue of the infected mother to the fetus should be avoided whenever possible (Mendez & Jule, 1990). The risks and benefits should be carefully weighed before performing amniocentesis and chorionic villus sampling.

Ways to Minimize Vertical Transmission

Clinical trials are exploring the possibility of ways to stop or minimize vertical transmission from the mother to the infant during pregnancy or before delivery (Minkoff, 1990). These trials may include the use of zidovudine, Soluble CD4+ (rs CD4+), CD4+ immunoadhesion, dideoxyinosine (ddI), and HIV immunoglobulin (Viscarello, 1990). These drugs have been shown in animal models to reach the fetus about as easily as a mother's natural proteins do. Hopefully, these drugs may be able to block perinatal transmission of HIV. Further investigation examining the benefit and safety of prenatal administration of medication needs to be conducted. However, blocking or decreasing the risk of transmission is possible only in individuals who have been identified as HIV-positive. Unfortunately, many of the infants exposed to HIV are delivered to mothers who have no knowledge regarding their HIV status.

Newer techniques include the prenatal-intrapartal use of zidovudine such as studied in the Research Project AIDS Clinical Trial Group or ACTG 076 (Baker, 1994; Craven et al., 1994). This clinical trial enrolled HIV-infected pregnant women who were between 14 and 34 weeks pregnant. They were randomized to either a zidovudine (100 mg orally five times per day) or a placebo group. During the intrapartal period, these women were given 2 mg/kg intravenously for 1 hour and then 1 mg/kg/hour until delivery. The newborn received the drug at 2 mg/kg orally every 6 hours for 6 weeks. Results from those 477 women enrolled between April 1991 and December 1993 showed a 67.5 percent relative reduction in the risk of vertical transmission between the treatment and control groups at 18 months of age (Connor et al., 1994). When this medication is given in the premature infant, a prolonged clearance and potential effect on bilirubin levels should be considered. This trial shows great promise for neonates. One area in need of further research that this study does not address is the long-term effects of this treatment on infected and noninfected infants (Health Resources & Services Administration, 1995).

Another study is examining the use of a recombinant human antibody that will encase the gp120 glycoprotein that houses CD4 binding sites (Burton et al., 1994). If effective, this monoclonal antibody could neutralize the HIV-1 virus. This research is in the preliminary stages. Researchers are also looking at maternal vitamin A levels and transmission. Women who have higher vitamin A levels appear to transmit less virus to the fetus. The reason for this is not known and further research is needed, but it is probably linked to the vitamin's role in mucosal integrity and cell-mediated immunity (Bridbord & Willoughby, 1994). Another effective method of decreasing transmission is avoiding the use of invasive procedures prenatally.

Intrapartally, the spread of the HIV infection from an HIV-positive mother to her fetus is discouraged by avoiding any procedures that would disrupt the integrity of the fetus's skin. Therefore, cordocentesis, internal scalp monitoring and fetal scalp pH sampling, internal uterine pressure monitoring, and vaginal examinations following the rupture of membranes should be avoided if possible (Mendez & Jule, 1990; Minkoff, 1990). There does not seem to be an elevated risk factor for vaginal delivery over cesarean section (Blanche et al., 1989; European Collaborative Study, 1988; Italian Multicentre Study, 1988).

Fetal Outcome

Fetal outcome appears to deteriorate in women who have had increased progression in the stage of AIDS illness. Koonin and associates (1989) found that symptomatic women had a poor prognosis regarding fetal outcome when compared with asymptomatic women. In their investigation, the gestational age ranged from 24 to 35 weeks, with a mean of 29 weeks. In addition, the health history often included premature birth, low birth weight, or small for gestational age infants. More controversial is the aspect of dysmorphic features, including growth retardation; microcephaly; box-like forehead; hypertelorism; short, flat nose; wide palpebral fissures; blue sclerae; and short philtrum (Laurence, 1987). The controversy surrounding the dysmorphic features is that they may be associated with substance abuse, for example, alcohol, rather than with HIV itself (Minkoff, 1990). The problem is, too, that many known HIV-positive neonates do not display these characteristics. These dysmorphic features and their tie to HIV are in need of further research.

Care of the Neonate in the Delivery Room

In the delivery room, newborns who have been exposed to HIV do not differ from those who have not. The maternal histories, mode of delivery, rate of obstetrical complications, Apgar scores, and initial physical examination findings are similar for both groups (Blanche et al., 1989; Johnson et al. 1989; Mendez et al., 1987). The recommendations for the management of the exposed neonate are the same as those for all neonates (Mendez & Jule, 1990).

Airway Management

When suctioning is required to clear the nares, oropharynx, and hypopharynx, either a bulb syringe or a mechanical device should be used. The amount of negative pressure for the mechanical device should be low to avoid tissue trauma breaking the integrity of the skin. The traditional DeLee trap, requiring mouth suctioning, should be avoided. Newer devices are now on the market that have modified the DeLee trap to prevent secretions from inadvertently entering the care provider's mouth. The advantages of the modified DeLee trap as compared with a mechanical device need to be explored.

Thermoregulation

The recommendations for maintaining body temperature are those found in the *Guidelines for Perinatal Care* (American Academy of Pediatrics and American College of Obstetricians and Gynecologists, 1993). The infant should be placed under a warmer and either toweled off or put in plastic and bundled. Both methods are designed to reduce the amount of evaporative heat loss. It should be noted that nurses and other health care professionals should wear gloves to avoid exposure to potentially infectious material on the skin of the infant.

Resuscitation and Stabilization

Regardless of whether the infant has been exposed to HIV or not, all infants should be treated and handled identically. As with the previous interventions, gloves should be worn when resuscitating and stabilizing the infant. In addition, a suction apparatus, manual resuscitation bag with appropriate neonatal-sized airways, and endotracheal tubes should be present for all deliveries. Mendez and Jule (1990) recommend that any volume-expanding agents or drugs should be given through the umbilical vein. Before placing the umbilical vessel catheter, care should be taken to cleanse the site with antiseptic solutions to avoid the introduction of any microorganisms that may be present. Albumin or Ringer's lactate solution is recommended instead of administering filtered, heparinized placental blood (Mendez & Jule, 1990). It is crucial that gloves, eye protection, and gowns or aprons be worn throughout the entire resuscitation and stabilization period.

COLLABORATIVE CARE OF THE INFANT EXPOSED TO THE HUMAN IMMUNODEFICIENCY VIRUS

Care of the Neonate in the Nursery

Once the neonate has been stabilized in the delivery room, he or she is transferred to either the regular nursery or intensive care nursery. In the nursery, routine neonatal care can be implemented, depending on the infant's gestational age, Apgar score, and current physical status.

Thermoregulation is of utmost importance. However, once the neonate's temperature has stabilized, many normal newborn nurseries bathe the infant. A warm water bath with soap may help minimize the risk of infection (Mendez & Jule, 1990).

Cord care should involve the use of antimicrobial agents such as triple dye or bacitracin. Following the prophylactic treatment against ophthalmia neonatorum, the next step is vitamin K administration. The skin should be thoroughly cleansed before the parenteral administration of vitamin K to prevent the introduction of microorganisms.

As with the procedure in the delivery room, nursing personnel and other health care providers should wear gloves for the bath, cord care, eye care, and vitamin K administration. Following completion of these procedures, gloves are no longer necessary (Mendez & Jule, 1990). Routine procedures such as weighing, dressing, cleansing, and feeding the newborn do not require gloves. However, gloves are recommended for diaper changes or any procedures that place nursing and other health care providers in contact with body secretions.

If a neonate's condition deteriorates and invasive procedures are required, such as heelsticks; venous or arterial punctures; insertion, flushing of, or drawing blood from the umbilical line; lumbar punctures; chest tube insertion; or any procedure that involves actual or potential contact with blood or body fluids, universal precautions should be followed (CDC, 1988). In addition to the precautions taken by the nursing staff and other health care providers, the skin should be cleansed with antiseptic solutions before any invasive procedure to prevent the potential entry of materials from the skin (Mendez & Jule, 1990).

Isolation

Isolation is not necessary for the neonate who has been exposed to HIV. If, however, enteritis, draining wounds, congenital syphilis, cytomegalovirus, herpes, rubella, or other viral infections are present, the neonate should be placed in isolation for these disease entities, not the HIV itself.

If none of the reasons to isolate the infant is present, the nursing staff should promote early contact between the neonate and the mother. Nursing staff should instruct the mother to wash her hands and change soiled gowns and linen before handling her infant. During this period, the mother or care provider should be educated regarding signs and symptoms of infections and ways to minimize them (Mendez & Jule, 1990).

Transmission Through Breastfeeding

Oxtoby (1988) noted that there is an increasing body of knowledge and evidence linking breastfeeding and the transmission of HIV. The first reports that the transmission of HIV through breast milk was possible began appearing in the medical literature in late 1984 and early 1985 (Thiry et al., 1985; Zeigler et al., 1984; Zeigler et al., 1988). Since then, the virus has been isolated in both the cellular portion and the liquid portion of breast milk (Ellerbrock & Rogers, 1990). The exact risk of HIV transmission from seropositive mother to infant via breastfeeding is unknown. The rate of risk found in the literature is conflicting (Ellerbrock & Rogers, 1990). Some investigators have reported neonatal patients who have acquired HIV from being breastfed by HIV-positive mothers (Colebunders et al., 1988; Lepage et al., 1987; Oxtoby, 1988; Stanbacket et al., 1988; Weinbreck et al., 1988; Zeigler et al., 1984; Zeigler et al., 1988). However, one must interpret the findings with caution because of the fact that many of the early investigations included women who had received blood transfusions of contaminated blood during or following delivery. Thus, in essence these women had become HIV-positive after delivery. In investigations in which mothers who were HIV-positive before delivery and breastfed their infants were compared with HIV-positive mothers who bottle fed their infants, the investigators found no differences in the incidence of HIV for either group (Minkoff, 1990).

Clinically, what does this all mean when it comes to a decision about breastfeeding? The recommendation by the American Academy of Pediatrics and the CDC for mothers who are HIV-positive is not to breastfeed. In the United States, there are alternative commercial formulas that are readily available (Mendez & Jule, 1990). However, in other geographic areas where ready-made formula is not as easily available and the water supplies are contaminated, the advantages of breastfeeding far outweigh the disadvantages of bottle feeding.

In Africa, for example, where HIV is prevalent, the danger of either contaminated water or formula as well as the problem of malnutrition or necrotizing enterocolitis, resulting in death, is greater than the danger of acquisition of HIV through breast milk. Breastfeeding in Africa is not discouraged (Anderson & Kliegman, 1991).

Neonatal Discharge

Many infants who have been exposed to HIV do not go home with their mothers. Some of the infants are placed in foster care, and others become boarder babies, a concept discussed in further detail at the end of this chapter. If foster care is to be used, the foster family needs to be aware of the mother's serostatus, if it is known. Being knowledgeable about the mother's HIV status is important so that the family or care provider can be educated regarding what it means to be exposed to HIV and also to detect signs and symptoms of an infection at the earliest possible time. The foster family or care provider should learn about providing care for the neonate, including when they need to follow universal precautions for certain aspects of infant care.

Regardless of where and to whom the neonate is discharged, the pediatrician or nurse practitioner responsible for follow-up should be apprised of the mother's serostatus (Mendez & Jule, 1990). Being aware of the mother's serostatus, if possible, will help the follow-up care provider devise a plan of care that is focused on possible signs and symptoms indicative of HIV infection and take appropriate measures in other aspects of care provision. Additionally, the mother, foster family, or other care provider should be counseled and educated by the follow-up provider regarding the frequency and possible content of the infant's follow-up visits (Mendez & Jule, 1990).

It is important that throughout the neonatal and infancy period immunizations be given and methods to enhance or boost the immune system such as the use of immunoglobulins be encouraged when there is a risk of infection. An infected neonate or infant should receive zidovudine and immunoglobulins (Craven et al., 1994).

Latency Period

During the nursery stay, most infants are found to be asymptomatic. Signs and symptoms of HIV infection are not usually detected in the nursery but instead are seen several months up to a year after delivery if the infant is going to undergo seroconversion (Goedert et al., 1989; Johnson et al., 1989) (Table 42–6).

The period of latency is different for the infant than for the adult. The latency period for the infant is much shorter than the 6 months to 10 years for the adult (De Wolf et al., 1987; Fahrner, 1992; Pizzo, 1990). Rubinstein and Bernstein (1986) reported that 6 months was the average time between exposure to HIV

TABLE 42–6 Incubation Period for Infants Converting to HIV Seropositive

Approximately one third of the infants born to HIV seropositive mothers will go on to seroconvert and become HIV infected.

The incubation period for these infants is as follows:

Less than 1 year:	60%
Less than 1½ years:	39.5%
Longer than 5 years:	1.5%

Currently, 85% of all infants will die within 1 year of diagnosis.

HIV, human immunodeficiency virus.

From Harrison, C. J. (1990). *Pediatric AIDS*. Pediatric Grand Rounds, March 8, 1990. Cincinnati, OH: Children's Hospital Medical Center. Reprinted with permission.

and the development of HIV symptoms in the infant. The latency period ranges from 6 weeks to 23 months for the infant exposed in utero according to Mendez and Jule (1990). The median age for the appearance of opportunistic infections is 9 months after birth (Rogers et al., 1989). The reason for the shortened time span may be the immature humoral immune system of the neonate as compared with that of the older child or adult. However, not every infant exposed to HIV becomes infected with HIV; only about one third of these infants become HIV-positive (see Table 42–6). There are some children who are now between 9 and 16 years of age who acquired HIV perinatally and yet are asymptomatic, but this is not the norm (Grubman et al., 1995).

Progression to Acquired Immunodeficiency Syndrome

It is impossible to pinpoint when the infant will acquire AIDS after exposure to HIV infection. HIV, once it has entered a cell, may remain latent until it is activated by certain factors, which may include (1) a decreased number of CD4+ cells, (2) an increased number of CD8+ cells, (3) a reduced level of HIV antibodies, and (4) an increased level of cytomegalovirus antibody (Polk et al., 1987). The progression of HIV may also be linked to (1) age, (2) physiologic stress, and (3) poor nutritional status (Viscarello, 1990).

Infant Follow-Up

Infants who have been exposed to HIV require close and careful periodic medical, developmental, and psychosocial evaluation (Mendez & Jule, 1990). In addition, specific interventions are necessary. Mendez and Jule (1990) have noted that many of the infants, regardless of their serostatus, are born to mothers who may have used drugs while pregnant and also may have other environmental factors that may have an impact on the mother–infant relationship. Whether or not an infant is seropositive, an infant born to such a mother requires routine screening for developmental delays and referral when indicated.

Routine Infant Care

An infant born to a seropositive mother needs to be followed in a tertiary center, in a clinic, or by an individual knowledgeable about HIV exposure and possible subsequent HIV infection. Mendez and Jule (1990) found that the case management model, in which a pediatrician and nurse followed a given infant, was beneficial in the delivery of routine care and follow-up.

Following discharge from the nursery, follow-up visits should occur monthly for the first 6 months, unless the infant was exposed to drugs in utero. In that case, the infant should be seen on a biweekly basis (Chasnoff, 1986). After 6 months, the visits should occur every 2 to 3 months until 1 year of life. From 1 to 2 years of age, the follow-up visits should occur quarterly (Mendez & Jule, 1990).

At 1 month of age, the initial follow-up visit to the physician or nurse practitioner should occur. Data to be gathered should include antenatal, intrapartal, and postpartal histories. For the infant, a neonatal history regarding possible exposure to hepatitis B, syphilis, and other sexually transmitted diseases and drugs should be obtained at this time.

Physical Examination

The physical examination should incorporate the normal steps used in assessing an infant. The CDC (1987a, 1987b) recommends that physical assessment findings be gathered in relation to the pediatric classification system (see Table 42–2). However, as mentioned earlier, the physical findings must be multiple, present for at least 2 months, and not related to any other disease state before the infant can be classified as having AIDS.

In addition, the assessment includes reviewing the following three areas: (1) pertinent history including growth and development, (2) physical findings, and (3) psychosocial concerns (discussed later).

Pertinent History

In the infant, Rubinstein (1986) noted that there might be a link between HIV and the occurrence of small for gestational age development. However, a variety of factors may be related to the small for gestational age diagnosis. In addition to the pertinent history, a thorough assessment of growth and development must be conducted. The growth history, which includes plotting weight, height, and head circumference on a grid, must be conducted at each visit if they occur on an outpatient basis. There may be no difference in birth weight or length of gestation among HIV-infected and noninfected neonates (Spinillo et al., 1994).

In the older infant and young toddler, there are a number of signs that may be indicative of HIV infection. The signs include failure to thrive, chronic diarrhea, persistent respiratory infections, fever, malaise, night sweats, fatigue, muscle and joint weakness, history of blood product transfusions (although this is not as much of a problem as it was in years past), and prenatal or postnatal exposure to a infected parent infected with HIV (Tables 42–7 and 42–8).

Physical Findings

A summary of physical assessment findings that may be related to HIV is presented in Table 42–9. On the physical examination,

TABLE 42–7 Medical History that May Indicate HIV Infection

Recurrent fever	Lymphadenopathy
Bacterial (systemic) infection	Parotitis
Recurrent otitis media	Failure to thrive
Recurrent and/or chronic thrush	Poor feeding
Recurrent and/or chronic diarrhea	Microcephaly
Monilial diaper rash	Developmental delay

HIV, human immunodeficiency virus.

Data from Boland, M., & Conviser, R. (1992). Nursing care of the child. In J. H. Flaskerud & P. J. Ungvarski (Eds.), *HIV/AIDS: A guide to nursing care* (2nd ed., pp. 199–238). Philadelphia: W. B. Saunders; and Husson, R. N., Comeau, A. M., & Hoff, R. (1990). Diagnosis of human immunodeficiency virus infection in infants and children. *Pediatrics, 86,* 1–10.

TABLE 42–8 Major Clinical Manifestations of HIV in Infants and Children

Failure to thrive	Hypergammaglobulinemia
Lymphoid interstitial pneumonia	Persistent oral candidiasis
Opportunistic infections	Generalized lymphadenopathy
Chronic otitis media	Hepatosplenomegaly
Recurrent bacterial sepsis	Encephalopathy
Recurrent or persistent diarrhea	Cardiomyopathy
Salivary gland enlargement	Hepatitis
Encephalopathy	Renal disease (nephrotic syndrome)
Thrombocytopenia	

HIV, human immunodeficiency virus.

Data from Centers for Disease Control. (1988). Universal precautions for prevention of transmission of human immunodeficiency virus, hepatitis B virus, and other bloodborne pathogens in healthcare settings. *MMWR Morbidity and Mortality Weekly Report, 37,* 377.

findings may be vague or nonspecific, depending on the infant's age and the progress of the disease state. Characteristic findings include lymphadenopathy, hepatosplenomegaly, bacterial sepsis, herpetic lesions, anemia, candidiasis (thrush), encephalopathy, lymphoid interstitial pneumonia, lymphopenia (specifically with a positive HIV culture), normal or increased immunoglobulin levels, laboratory and physical findings consistent with specific opportunistic infections, and neurologic alterations (American Academy of Pediatrics, 1988).

Early signs and symptoms in the infant include recurrent bacterial infections with sepsis, candidiasis (thrush), and failure to thrive. As the disease progresses, later manifestations include lymphadenopathy, hepatosplenomegaly, chronic or recurrent diarrhea, and enlarged salivary glands. As the HIV progresses, the infant may manifest failure to thrive, developmental delays, neurologic disease, and thrombocytopenia. The exact cause of the thrombocytopenia—a reduced number of platelets—is not clearly understood.

Other aspects of the initial visit include evaluating the growth, nutritional intake, and development; effects of perinatal drug exposure; and the quality of the mother–infant interaction (Mendez & Jule, 1990).

Mendez and Jule (1990) caution the physician or practitioner to discuss the findings with the mother, foster family, or care provider, stressing the need for continual follow-up. The diagnosis of AIDS should not be arrived at prematurely. Careful examination and exploration of the findings should occur to rule out other diseases and possibilities.

TABLE 42–9 Physical Assessment Findings Possibly Linked with HIV*

Failure to thrive (as evidenced by failure to maintain height, weight, and head circumference curves)	Hepatomegaly
Dermatitis	Splenomegaly
Monilial diaper rash	Clubbing
Candida or seborrhea	Failure to maintain and/or loss of developmental milestones
Otitis media	Neurologic abnormalities
Rhinitis	Interstitial pneumonia
Parotitis	Chronic diarrhea
Generalized lymphadenopathy	Microcephaly
Cervical	
Axillary	
Inguinal	

* None of these findings are diagnostic without a positive HIV culture or antigen test.

Differential Diagnosis

Careful screening to rule out any immunodeficiency disorders must be conducted to determine if there are other possible causes for the presenting signs and symptoms. The following diseases and clusters of disorders should be ruled out:

1. *X-linked agammaglobulinemia.* This is a B-cell deficiency that is characterized by recurrent bacterial sinopulmonary infections, diarrhea, and otitis media. The cluster of symptoms may be similar to those of HIV.
2. *Wiskott-Aldrich syndrome* (chronic granulomatous disease). This is a T-cell deficiency characterized by severe eczema and thrombocytopenia with platelets of reduced size and function. In addition, the infant or child presents with recurrent infections with encapsulated bacteria.
3. *Ataxia-telangiectasia.* This is a T-cell deficiency characterized by telangiectasis (a dilation of capillaries and small blood vessels), ataxia, recurrent sinopulmonary infection, and malignancy.
4. *DiGeorge's syndrome.* This is another T-cell deficiency, which is characterized by hypertelorism ear anomalies; abnormalities of the aortic arch and neonatal tetany and candidiasis are not uncommon.
5. *Severe combined immunodeficiency.* This consists of T- and B-cell deficiency characterized by low immunoglobulin levels and by absent antibody responses with recurrent or chronic bacterial, fungal, viral, and protozoan infections.

When any of these five disorders are suspected, the follow-up care provider should order a blood test for HIV.

Human Immunodeficiency Virus Signs and Symptoms

In the infant, the manifestations of the signs and symptoms of HIV can range from subclinical to mild, moderate, and severe. Symptoms usually do not present as a single entity; instead, manifestations of HIV involve multiple organ systems. The multiple organ involvement leads to progressive clinical deterioration and eventually to immune dysfunction, opportunistic infections, and secondary cancers (Mendez & Jule, 1990). Infants with HIV infection most often present with chronic parotitis, lymphocytic interstitial pneumonitis, and serious recurrent bacterial infections. The latter may include meningitis, pneumonia, osteomyelitis, septic arthritis, and septicemia (Mendez & Jule, 1990; Nesheim et al., 1994).

The medical provider needs to review the infant's medical history closely, looking for symptoms that may be related to HIV (see Table 42–7). Factors that may indicate a deteriorating immune system are listed in Table 42–8. Laboratory tests, including markers that may predict the progression to AIDS, are also part of the evaluation procedure. Laboratory findings that might be linked to HIV infections in infants and children are presented in Table 42–10. The entire picture of presenting symptoms is not complete without a thorough medical history. Physical assessment findings that may indicate possible HIV infection are found in Table 42–9.

Serologic Evaluation

Managing the infant with HIV includes monitoring the hemoglobin, hematocrit, prothrombin time, partial thromboplastin time, platelet counts, gamma globulin levels, CD4+ counts, and other serologic parameters. The hemoglobin and hematocrit should be carefully evaluated for anemia. The frequency of serologic testing should be every 6 months to correspond with other laboratory studies (Mendez & Jule, 1990). Bruising and bleeding

TABLE 42–10 Laboratory Findings Possibly Linked with HIV*

Anemia	Low CD4+ count
Elevated liver function panels	Viral culture
Hypergammaglobulinemia	Mitogen unresponsive
Hyperproteinemia	Reversed CD4+ : CD8+ ratio
Leukopenia	Lymphopenia
Thrombocytopenia	Hypoglobulinemia (3%)
p24 antigen	

* None of these findings are diagnostic without a positive HIV culture or antigen test.

HIV, human immunodeficiency virus.

Data from Boland, M., & Conviser, R. (1992). Nursing care of the child. In J. H. Flaskerud & P. J. Ungvarski (Eds.), *HIV/AIDS: A guide to nursing care* (2nd ed., pp. 199–238). Philadelphia: W. B. Saunders; Harrison, C. J. (1990). *Pediatric AIDS.* Pediatric Grand Rounds, March 8, 1990. Cincinnati, OH: Children's Hospital Medical Center; and Husson, R. N., Corneau, A. M., & Hoff, R. (1990). Diagnosis of human immunodeficiency virus infection in infants and children. *Pediatrics, 86,* 1–10.

problems have also been noted in infants infected with HIV. Occult bleeding in gastric secretions, stool, and urine should be assessed. If the laboratory evidence indicates that an infant is experiencing bleeding problems, a replacement transfusion may be necessary. The frequency of the testing may have to be modified and the infant monitored more closely when he or she begins to show symptoms of HIV infection (Mendez & Jule, 1990).

Infants born to seropositive mothers are seropositive at birth and during the early stages of follow-up (Mendez et al., 1987). These infants have maternal antibodies that were passed transplacentally. Approximately one third of the infants born to women infected with HIV go on to seroconversion (Mendez & Jule, 1990).

At birth and immediately after, it is difficult to make the laboratory diagnosis of HIV. The reason for this difficulty is that the serologic and virologic techniques that are currently available for clinical use have significant limitations for identifying infant antibodies (Andiman, 1989).

Antibodies

The antibody status of the neonate represents the infection status of the mother. While in utero, the infant passively acquires maternal antibodies. In the case of a mother infected with HIV, the fetus may acquire HIV antibodies. If the infant is then tested, the maternal antibodies will be detected in testing (Ellerbrock & Rogers, 1990). Therefore, all newborns born to HIV-positive mothers have maternal antibodies at birth and thus test positive. Approximately 25 to 30 percent (range 30 to 80 percent) of these infants acquire HIV if born to a mother infected with the virus (Nanda, 1990). The number of HIV cases and the number of infants born to mothers infected with HIV vary from one area to the next.

Testing

Before discussing the various tests, the terms *specificity* and *sensitivity* need to be defined. Specificity refers to a test's ability to detect a given organism, whereas sensitivity deals with the test's ability to detect the organism when it is present in a sample.

Infants exposed to HIV can be identified at birth if the mother has been tested during her pregnancy. The recommendations of many public health officials focus on voluntary, confidential testing of all pregnant individuals or those individuals contemplating pregnancy (Boland & Conviser, 1992). After delivery and before testing the infant, the need for HIV testing should be discussed with the parent or legal guardian and informed consent should be obtained.

Another important issue to be considered when HIV testing is to be implemented is the need for counseling of the parents or primary care providers. Counseling, along with access to medical treatment and possible clinical trials for drugs and treatment protocols, is a vital aspect of the testing process (Husson et al., 1990).

For the adult, routine screening for HIV is carried out with the enzyme-linked immunosorbent assay (ELISA). If the ELISA indicates that antibodies for HIV are present, a second test, the Western blot (also known as the immunoblot), may be used as a more definitive test. HIV infection can be detected with a high degree of sensitivity and specificity with the ELISA and the Western blot test (National Center for Nursing Research, 1990).

For the infant, the ELISA and Western blot may not be useful in detecting the presence of HIV owing to the fact that maternal antibodies for HIV (IgG) cross the placenta and may be found in the infant's serum for up to 15 months after birth (Husson et al., 1990). The maternal antibodies may give a false-positive test result rather than an actual indicator of how the infant's immune system is responding to the HIV infection. In theory, all infants with a confirmed HIV-positive mother may test seropositive. However, only one third of these infants actually go on to become seropositive themselves (American Academy of Pediatrics, 1988).

Mendez and associates (1989) found that infants and children with reactive ELISA and immunoblot (Western blot) results over time show the following pattern: (1) increasing reactivities of previously existing bands, (2) fading and reappearance of bands, and (3) appearance of new bands. A record of immunoblot reactivities for comparison to the latest test results must be kept in the record of each infant (Mendez & Jule, 1990).

Approximately one third of the infants born to women with HIV infection will go on to seroconversion. In these infants, the ELISA test result becomes nonreactive. Most of the test results are nonreactive by a median age of 12 months, with a range of 3 to 15 months (Mendez & Jule, 1990). For the Western blot test, reactivities show a steady disappearance of all bands. Most immunoblot results are negative by 15 months of age. In some cases, the p24 may show bands, but they too eventually disappear. Since the results of the ELISA and Western blot may not be beneficial in the early stages of follow-up, if the p24 antigen is positive after 1 month of age, the infant is considered positive (Kellinger, 1994). Other types of testing and cultures may need to be explored. One that appears to hold promise for infants older than 6 months of age is the HIV IgA immunoblot test. It is a diagnostic test with a reported sensitivity and specificity greater than 75 percent and is especially useful in the diagnosis of pediatric HIV in developing countries because it is easy and requires frozen sera samples (Deluchi et al., 1994).

Antigen Testing

The purpose of antigen testing is to look specifically at the p24 HIV antigen. The HIV p24 antigen, or p24 core protein of HIV, has been isolated from an adult population in the acute stage of HIV infection as well as during the late stages of AIDS. Therefore, when detectable levels of p24 antigen are present, there is an increased association for the development of AIDS (Allain et al., 1987; De Wolf et al., 1987; Goudsmit et al., 1986; Pedersen et al., 1987).

The level of p24 is variable in the initial, asymptomatic stage of HIV in infected infants. Detection of the p24 antigen in the neonatal population might be used to help predict the onset or impending development of AIDS. However, this test may not be the first choice for making a definitive diagnosis.

Viral Culture

The viral culture is a way of allowing the HIV infection, if present, to grow in a sample. Again, as with antigen testing, the goal is to measure the p24 antigen or reverse transcriptase enzyme activity. The culture is specific in identifying HIV when it is present. However, the sensitivity (i.e., the actual detection of HIV when it is present), is only approximately 90 percent. In approximately 10 percent of cases, HIV is not detected when it is present (Boland & Conviser, 1992).

Since the antigen testing and viral culture are not always sensitive in detecting HIV when it is present, other modes of testing are necessary.

Antibody Detection

IgG antibodies readily pass through the placenta from the infected mother to the infant. The M and A antibodies, however, do not cross the placenta. Therefore, any IgM or IgA antibodies found in the infant's blood may be indicative of HIV infection.

One drawback to the detection of IgM or IgA is that they may be present in minute quantities, therefore making early detection difficult. One way to overcome this limitation is to perform serial testing over time to see if enough IgM or IgA is found in increasing quantities. A negative, one-time antibody detection test does not necessarily mean that the infant is seronegative (Husson et al., 1990). A negative test result or culture and the absence of HIV antigens *does not* rule out the possibility of infection. It may be that the individual has not had time to undergo seroconversion and therefore is in the initial phases before detection.

Polymerase Chain Reaction

Newer biologic and chemical techniques such as the polymerase chain reaction (PCR) may be more diagnostically valid (National Center for Nursing Research, 1990). The PCR is less expensive and less time-consuming than performing a culture for the HIV virus (Rogers et al., 1989).

The PCR looks specifically for the presence of HIV antigen as well as proviral deoxyribonucleic acid. When both are found to be present, the test result is considered positive.

Through PCR, the nucleic acid sequence specific to HIV as written in the cell's DNA is amplified for easier detection. The PCR has shown greater promise with adults than it has with infants and children (Husson, et al., 1990). However, that does not negate the test's usefulness. The sensitivity of PCR in the first few months after birth is affected by the low levels of HIV present. In addition, Husson and associates (1990) noted that there is a relatively high false-negative rate, or low sensitivity, associated with PCR. Although problematic, PCR is still useful when the results are triangulated with other diagnostic tests and the complete clinical physical assessment and laboratory findings for the infant.

CD4+ Count

One of the predictors used to help quantify the progression of HIV is the CD4+ lymphocyte count. This count entails a quantification of CD4+ cells present in a sample. The CD4+ cells show a general progression or decline from the initial infection with HIV to the actual conversion to AIDS. One of the benefits of the CD4+ test is that it can be ordered readily in a variety of settings, from hospital to community-based follow-up care providers.

The results of the CD4+ counts in the infant population differ greatly from those in the adult population (Boland & Conviser, 1992). Moss and coworkers (1988) noted that in the adult, the normal CD4+ values range from 900 to 1000/mm^3. For the uninfected newborn, the level is 3500/mm^3, declining to 1500 to 2000/mm^3 by 1 to 2 years of age. An infant is considered immunocompromised when the level is 1500/mm^3 or less. The infant is considered at risk when the level is less than 1000/mm^3 by 1 to 2 years of age (Connor et al., 1991; Leibovitz et al., 1990). The CD4+ count for the neonate is much lower owing to the immaturity of the immune system. However, the overall pattern in decline is similar for both the infant and the adult. The time frame in which the pattern occurs is compressed for the infant when compared with that for the adult. For the neonate who undergoes seroconversion after birth, the pattern occurs over months versus years as in the adult (Moss, 1989).

CD4+:CD8+ Ratio

HIV infects the CD4+ cells, leading to a defective cell-mediated immunity response and thus the potential for opportunistic infections. According to Lane and Fauci (1985), the effect that HIV has on the CD4+ cells is both quantitative and qualitative. In the early stages of infection, the number of CD4+ cells and CD8+ cells is normal. As the disease progresses, there appears to be a low CD4+ count and a high CD8+ count, leading to a low CD4+:CD8+ ratio (Oleske et al., 1983; Pahwa et al., 1986; Rubinstein, 1986; Scott et al., 1984).

The CD4+:CD8+ ratio, formerly known as the T4-helper:T8-suppressor ratio, is approximately 2:1 in adults. A ratio of less than 1 may indicate immune dysfunction (Fahrner, 1992). The exact ratio seems to fluctuate more in the infant than in the adult in part owing to the infant's immature humoral immune system (Fahrner, 1992). However, the variable ratio for the infant may not be as helpful in establishing the diagnosis of HIV infection (Fahrner, 1992).

Neopterin

Another marker that is possibly linked with the conversion to AIDS following seropositivity is neopterin. This is a by-product associated with macrophage activity and is considered a possible indicator of cell-mediated immunity activation. A rise in the neopterin level, as measured in the urine, is generally inversely proportional to the number of CD4+ lymphocytes (Fuchs et al., 1988).

Other Tests in the Clinical Trial Phase

On June 18, 1991, Dr. Thomas C. Quinn, from the National Institutes of Health and Johns Hopkins University, announced from Florence, Italy, the development of a rapid new test that can detect HIV reliably in infants as young as 3 to 6 months of age. The new, faster test detects the IgA protein. This protein is formed only when an infant is infected with HIV and does not pass from mother to infant in utero, as previously discussed. Earlier diagnosis and treatment of HIV-infected infants may potentially increase their life expectancy. The cost of the new test is much less than that of previous tests. However, tests for earlier detection, as soon after birth as possible, still need to be developed.

Any or all of the tests just discussed may be used in the future to document the progression of disease in both infants and adults. Early detection holds the promise of earlier intervention and therapy, thus possibly attempting to slow the progression of the disease.

When one suspects that an infant may be HIV-positive, one of the best approaches to the diagnosis of HIV is frequent follow-up visits and repeated laboratory testing (Husson et al., 1990).

Husson and colleagues (1990) recommend the following approach for testing the infant: (1) serial antibody testing through 15 months of age (ELISA and Western blot [immunoblot]), (2) serial p24 antigen testing, (3) HIV culture, and (4) one or more methods such as PCR or IgM detection.

The testing intervals for infants born to HIV-infected women are outlined by Mendez and Jule (1990). These children should be tested at the initial follow-up (1 month) and at 6, 12, 18, and 24 months of age. In addition, Mendez and Jule (1990) recommend that sera be saved and properly labeled and placed in storage at −20°C to −70°C for future reference.

If the result is positive, appropriate referrals should include local HIV service groups, social workers for planning of physical and financial assistance, mental health personnel, and support groups for infants with HIV.

Resources include many local as well as national organizations. With the increasing number of individuals diagnosed with HIV, there are more and more local support groups within the community. However, national organizations may be helpful in linking the family to appropriate resources. In addition, the Department of Health for each state or community is able to provide information regarding a variety of resources. Several HIV resource groups and foundations at the national level are listed in Table 42–11.

Infection

Passive immunity in the form of IgG affects the infant's ability to mount a response to infections such as HIV. An infant who has been exposed to HIV is vulnerable owing to the attack by HIV on the CD4+ cells that are present. The neonate and infant with HIV are left immunocompromised and require care that is focused on protection against secondary sources of infection (see Chapter 27, Assessment and Management of Immunologic Dysfunction, for further details on the immune system.)

One of the major goals in caring for an infant who has been infected with HIV is preventing opportunistic infection. HIV destroys the infant's ability to build antibodies against bacterial, viral, and fungal infections. No matter how careful the nurse and family are, opportunistic infections occur. Such infections most often strike the skin, lungs, and GI tract. These infections can be oral thrush, diaper rash, and other infections of the skin, pulmonary system, and GI tract (see Table 42–9).

Infected infants who survive are faced with repeated illness that may become chronic, lasting for the months or years of their limited lives.

TABLE 42–11 National HIV Resources

AIDS Action Council
1875 Connecticut Avenue, N.W.
Washington, DC 20009
(202) 986–1300

National AIDS Fund
1400 I Street, N.W.
Washington, DC 20005
(202) 408–4848

CDC National AIDS Hotline
(800) 342–AIDS

CDC National AIDS Information Clearinghouse
P.O. Box 6003
Rockville, MD 20850
(800) 458–5231

NIAID Intramural Trials for HIV Infection and AIDS
(800) AIDS-NIH [(800) 243–7644]

HIV, human immunodeficiency virus.

It is not uncommon for infants with HIV infection to experience multiple oral candidiasis (thrush) infections. These infants may suffer from chronic thrush outbreaks. Managing such episodes involves the administration of nystatin suspension. Careful monitoring for the spread to and through the GI tract may be necessary. Many times it is beneficial to use a nystatin ointment on the diaper area for prophylactic prevention of skin breakdown and possible infection.

If the infant has a gastrostomy tube, central line, or peripheral intravenous lines, a careful nursing assessment of the insertion site for signs and symptoms of rashes, skin breakdown, or infection is critical. Aseptic techniques must be employed by both the nurse and the care provider when the lines and dressings are changed.

Respiratory Infections

Respiratory infections are the most common type of infection contracted by the infant with HIV infection (Harrison, 1990). The nurse can look for changes in pulmonary status. Additionally, he or she can teach the family or care providers to look for fever, increased pulse, increased respirations, adventitious breath sounds, retractions, cough, and other indicators of compromised pulmonary status.

Pneumocystis carinii pneumonia (PCP) is the most frequent opportunistic infection according to Ammann (1992). In more than half of the infants who acquired PCP, it was often the initial clinical sign of HIV infection: Before the development of PCP, these infants were not recognized as being infected with HIV. The March 5, 1991, *Morbidity and Mortality Weekly Report* published guidelines for prophylactic prevention of PCP, which the CDC believes must begin in the first few months of the infant's life. The report describes several chemoprophylactic regimens that have been used for similar disease. However, the FDA has not approved the various regimens for PCP prophylaxis recommended by the CDC. In addition, the doses of the various regimens have not been examined in infants and children infected with HIV. The exact approach for PCP management and treatment in infants and children is still being examined. The American Academy of Pediatrics has not made any new recommendations regarding the CDC's recommendation (Lang, 1991). Zidovudine for 6 weeks following birth is used by some pediatricians as prophylactic treatment against secondary infections (Yoder & Polin, 1997). Some physicians also recommend prophylactic treatment against PCP with trimethoprim/sulfamethoxazole 75 mg/m^2 twice daily, 3 days per week for the first year of life or until HIV is ruled out. This treatment is begun at about 6 weeks of age (Yoder & Polin, 1997).

As soon as a respiratory infection is suspected, rapid evaluation and diagnosis must follow. Antibiotic therapy must begin immediately to prevent overwhelming sepsis. It is vital that the entire prescribed amount of the drug be taken at specific intervals. If an antibiotic course is incomplete, the infant can experience a relapse and even more severe complications.

If the infant's respiratory status is such that hospitalization is necessary, a careful nursing assessment of the need for supplemental oxygen or respiratory support may have to be implemented. The key role for the nurse is ongoing clinical assessment, regardless of an inpatient or outpatient setting, to detect any changes in respiratory status.

Pharmacologic Management

There is no known cure for HIV. Opportunistic infections can be treated with appropriate therapy, although they may not respond positively in all cases. More than 200 investigational drugs have been tried, but none has effectively halted or reversed the immunodeficiency process. In the coming years, there may be new drugs developed that can inhibit HIV from invading healthy cells (Lo et al., 1991; Merluzzi et al., 1990). Current work at the cellular level suggests that there may be a specific receptor site on CD4+ that may be used by HIV to enter healthy cells (Murphy et al., 1990). If this work shows promise, drugs can be developed that may be able to block the receptor site, thus preventing HIV from entering the cell.

Current drug therapy for the infant and pediatric population centers primarily on gamma globulin therapy and zidovudine. The latter works by blocking the virus from reproducing in the newly infected cells. One of the main problems associated with zidovudine therapy in infants and children is bone marrow suppression, primarily in the form of anemia and neutropenia (Pizzo et al., 1988).

Another drug that has been considered for critically ill adults is ddI. On October 9, 1991, the Food and Drug Administration (FDA) approved the antiviral drug to be used by patients who are not helped by zidovudine. The approval of ddI by the FDA was highly criticized because the approval was based on less scientific data than is normally required by the FDA for approval of a new drug. In addition, ddI is currently being tested in the infant and pediatric populations in controlled, experimental clinical trials.

Vaccines

Dr. Wayne C. Koff, chief of the AIDS vaccine research and development branch of the National Institute of Allergy and Infectious Disease, noted on May 6, 1990, that there are at least nine different experimental HIV vaccines undergoing clinical trials in humans (Cohen, 1991). The initial studies have focused on the safety of the vaccines and their capacity to evoke an immune response (Cohen, 1991). Currently, most of the HIV vaccines in human trials are made from parts of HIV that are incapable of causing the disease. However, none of the clinical trials has been a real-time test of effectiveness (Cohen, 1991). Future clinical trials need to explore whether the vaccine is capable of building immunity against HIV (Cohen, 1991). One active trial that is beginning to show promise is at the Chicago Community Programs For Clinical Research Center, which is part of a 16-site National Institutes of Health study (Zurlinden & Verheggen, 1994). In this study, a therapeutic vaccine is given to nonpregnant adults who are known to be infected with HIV in the hope of at least decreasing transmission to others and at best controlling the virus in infected persons.

The National Institutes of Health has given HIV vaccine research high priority because the development of new drugs to combat the disease has not been as successful as previously hoped. The main difficulty in developing a vaccine is attempting to overcome HIV's ability to mutate constantly, thereby constantly changing the vaccine's target. HIV is skilled at evading a major part of the immune system by hiding in the immune system cells.

To overcome the ability of HIV to mutate rapidly, vaccines are being developed that contain key proteins from a variety of virus strains. If this type of vaccine is successful, it could work like the influenza vaccine; the influenza vaccine is updated on a regular basis by adding different strains of the flu virus as they mutate with each new flu season. A similar approach might be used with an HIV vaccine.

Vaccines for the treatment of AIDS are in the developmental stages (Sabin, 1991). Most of the work with vaccines has been conducted on animal models, namely, chimpanzees and monkeys. The success with the vaccine in monkeys has been achieved with the whole, killed simian immunodeficiency virus, a close cousin of HIV (Cohen, 1991). To date, the preparations have protected more than 150 monkeys in challenge experiments (Cohen, 1991).

Researchers favor a genetically engineered HIV vaccine based on subunits of the whole virus because they pose far less risk than whole, killed virus preparations (Cohen, 1991). The FDA, in 1990, approved testing in California for an experimental AIDS vaccine developed by Dr. Jonas Salk. Current testing is being conducted on individuals who are already infected with HIV, rather than as a method of preventive treatment. The current clinical trial is designed to find out whether the inactivated virus causes the body to produce specific cells (T cells) that destroy other cells infected with virus. A second purpose of the investigation is to find out if the vaccine stimulates the individual's immune system to respond to the HIV infection. It is hoped that the vaccine might halt or reverse the spread of the virus in asymptomatic, seropositive individuals.

Although work looks promising with a vaccine developed for monkeys, it is more than 5 years away for use in the infant and adult populations if the vaccine is to follow normal channels for approval through the FDA. However, if the vaccine work is highly successful in the animal model, the approval process may be shortened or abbreviated, as with the approval process for ddI. Even with current testing, the efficacy of the vaccine will not be known for quite some time (Cohen, 1991). Additionally, vaccines to protect infection-free infants, children, and adults from the general population will take longer to develop than vaccines used for treatment of HIV-infected individuals. The reason for the longer developmental time is that researchers need to rule out any possibility that an HIV vaccine might accidentally cause HIV infection.

Experimental Therapy

Other modes of treatment are currently in the experimental stages. On June 9, 1990, Edward A. Berger, a senior scientist at the National Institute of Allergic and Infectious Disease, announced the development of a two-staged therapy for the treatment of HIV. The process uses a genetically engineered molecule CD4-PE40. The molecule CD4-PE40 finds and destroys the CD4+ cells that are producing HIV. CD4-PE40 works in the following manner:

1. CD4-PE40 has two component parts: CD4, which is a copy of a receptor found on the CD4+ cell surface, and PE40, a small fatal substance that researchers attach to the CD4 receptor.
2. The CD4-PE40 attaches to the CD4+ cells that are infected with HIV through a lock-and-key mechanism involving CD4 and gp120.
3. The CD4-PE40 then binds to the cell, and the PE40 enters the cell and kills it.

The reason healthy CD4 cells are not killed is that uninfected cells lack gp120 proteins; thus, the lock-and-key mechanism cannot occur. Therefore, CD4-PE40 cannot bind to the cell surface and the healthy cells are spared. The second step in the experimental treatment process is the administration of zidovudine. This agent blocks the virus from reproducing in newly infected cells. The two-step treatment process is not a cure but possibly is an effective way of managing and actually treating HIV-infected individuals.

Genetically engineered molecules similar to CD4-PE40 are being examined. One such molecule is CPF. It seems to use a mechanism similar to that described for CD4-PE40. Further work must be conducted on the two-step method and other genetically engineered molecules before widespread use in humans. Even in the late 1990s, these genetically engineered molecules are still being tested.

Immunizations

Infants and children should be immunized according to the American Academy of Pediatrics recommendations (American

Academy of Pediatrics, 1988). The American Academy of Pediatrics recommends that diphtheria, tetanus, and pertussis vaccine; inactivated polio vaccine (IPV); measles, mumps, rubella (MMR) vaccine; and *Haemophilus influenzae* B vaccine be administered to infants and children who are known to be either asymptomatic or symptomatic. In addition, immunizations should be given at the recommended intervals, regardless of the mother's serostatus (Yoder & Polin, 1997). The only exception is the oral polio vaccine (live). This vaccine should be replaced with the IPV. Additionally, the American Academy of Pediatrics recommends that the IPV be administered to all other infants and children in the household.

The MMR vaccine is a live virus that has thus far caused no serious complications when given to an infant infected with HIV. More risk is involved in the potential for allowing the infant to acquire these childhood diseases at a later time when the immune system may be compromised (Kellinger, 1994).

Infants and children with HIV infections lose vaccine-associated antibodies as the disease progresses (Mendez et al., 1988). Many of the infants may present with vaccine-preventable diseases, even if they have been previously immunized (Adamson et al., 1989). In such cases, infants with HIV infection who are symptomatic should receive postexposure prophylaxis, regardless of previous immunization (Mendez & Jule, 1990).

Currently, it is debatable whether infants and children who are asymptomatic should be treated prophylactically following exposure to infections (Mendez & Jule, 1990). However, both asymptomatic and symptomatic infants should be treated prophylactically following exposure to measles and varicella zoster. The treatment involves the use of serum immunoglobulin and varicella zoster immunoglobulin, respectively (Mendez & Jule, 1990). It is too early to tell whether or not the varicella vaccine will be advocated by most pediatricians. It is a live virus, so it may be more of a risk to give it than to risk the disease itself. At present, if an infant or child who is infected with HIV is exposed to varicella there is a 72-hour window of opportunity in which to give varicella zoster immune globulin to prevent infection. If varicella is acquired, a 10-day course of acyclovir (Zovirax) is sometimes prescribed (Kellinger, 1994).

The only other issue facing the primary care provider is whether to use antibiotic therapy prophylactically to prevent PCP, pneumococcal infections, and *Haemeophilus influenzae* type B sepsis. Currently, there are no clear guidelines regarding prophylactic antibiotic use (Mendez & Jule, 1990). There are concerns about the use of prophylactic antibiotic therapy and the development of resistant strains of bacteria or secondary fungal infections, so even for infants at risk, the costs versus long-term benefits must be weighed.

Subsequent Follow-up Visits

At each follow-up visit, a review of systems and an assessment of growth, nutritional intake, development, and the quality of mother–infant interaction should take place. Additionally, age-appropriate anticipatory guidance and screening should be conducted according to the American Academy of Pediatrics guidelines for problems such as iron deficiency, lead poisoning, tuberculosis, and renal disease.

Nutrition

Fluid and Electrolyte Balance

Fluid and electrolyte balance is necessary in the infant infected with HIV. Even before any reported history of diarrhea, these infants may manifest imbalances. One way to monitor the status is to carefully assess the weight and skin turgor on an outpatient basis. The nurse can teach the care provider signs and symptoms associated with altered fluid intake and dehydration. Any change in fluid intake should be reported to the primary care provider, especially during the warm months when insensible water loss may be greater and the infant's intake may not match the output.

When the infant is in an acute phase and hospitalized, the nurse should carefully monitor intake and output and electrolyte balance (Edmondson, 1988). Daily measurements of urine specific gravity as well as urine dipstick tests should be conducted. In addition, serum electrolytes should be monitored closely in the infant with HIV infection who is in an acute phase of illness (Edmondson, 1988).

Caloric Balance

One of the classic signs of HIV is failure to thrive. Rubinstein (1986) and Rubinstein and Bernstein (1986) found that failure to thrive was not always related to chronic diarrhea. It appears that some other, yet unidentified, mechanism may be involved in the chronic growth problem.

HIV can have a devastating effect on the GI tract. Chronic diarrhea is one of the common problems experienced by the infant with HIV infection. In some cases, the infant is unable to absorb enough calories as the result of the increased transitory time in the GI tract, leading to diarrhea. Therefore, a central line may be needed to meet the infant's nutritional, caloric, and growth needs.

There are no special dietary recommendations or restrictions for infants and children who are infected with HIV (Fahrner, 1992). The actual type of nutritional intake depends on the infant's age at the time of diagnosis. In the young infant, a high-calorie formula should be used in an attempt to maintain adequate calories to meet growth needs and to promote healing.

Nutritional monitoring on the part of the nurse includes age-appropriate weight and height measurements. If the weight begins to decline, and difficulty in feeding and maintaining nutritional status ensues, gastrostomy tube feedings and intravenous alimentation via central lines may need to be initiated.

If the infant is unable to take formula or food by mouth because of anorexia, vomiting, or diarrhea, a nasogastric tube may be necessary (Fahrner, 1992). Infants may need nutritional supplementation. In some cases, gastrostomy tubes are necessary when prolonged nutritional support is required.

Encephalopathy

One of the classic signs of HIV is developmental delays. Failure to meet developmental milestones may be linked to neurologic damage that has been documented on computed tomography scans during the first weeks of life (Rubinstein, 1986). Rubinstein (1986) suggested that the HIV virus may lead to brain damage in utero, thus leading to encephalopathy.

Because HIV is able to enter the glial cells—a major supporting cell in the nervous system—complications and alterations in central nervous system function can occur. Many infants and children do not manifest signs and symptoms of encephalopathy in the early stages of infection (Fahrner, 1992). Other causes for the encephalopathy have been associated with HIV, such as cytomegalovirus, herpes simplex, varicella zoster, Epstein-Barr virus, meningitis, and retinitis (Boland & Conviser, 1992). Whatever the reason for the encephalopathy, it is not until the disease process is advancing that signs and symptoms begin to be noticed.

The pattern of encephalopathy is one marked with plateaus of relatively stable neurologic function and behavior punctuated by episodes of deterioration of neurologic function and behavior. Any possible combination of motor skills, cognitive function, and behavioral problems may be manifested with the growing infant or child. Fahrner (1992) noted that the periods of stability followed by the episodic periods of deterioration in neurologic function closely parallel the degree of immunodeficiency. The more marked the immunodeficiency, the grimmer the prognosis and the higher the incidence of encephalopathy (Epstein et al., 1988).

The progression of motor deficits in the infant with HIV infection depends on the infant's age and developmental abilities. The degree and type of delay or regression in neuromuscular and neurobehavioral development may be associated with or compounded by a maternal history of substance abuse, premature birth, and the current social and environmental living conditions (Boland & Conviser, 1992; Fahrner, 1992; Wishon & Gee, 1988).

Falloon and associates (1989) reported that acquired microcephaly is frequently found in the infant and child infected with HIV. The reason for the microcephaly may be related to diffuse cortical atrophy and calcifications found in the basal ganglia.

Regardless of the presence or absence of microcephaly, an analysis of the cerebrospinal fluid obtained by a spinal tap in infants infected with HIV shows normal protein and glucose levels and cell counts (Fahrner, 1992). However, Boland and Conviser (1992) reported that there may be an elevated protein level and mild pleocytosis.

Role of the Nurse in Managing the Infant Infected With the Human Immunodeficiency Virus

The role of the nurse in caring for the infant with HIV infection is multidimensional. Families and care providers need a variety of nursing services that may include home care, hospice care, respite care, counseling, and educational programs. Nurses may also be able to assist in and direct the families and care providers to services focused on housing, transportation, financial, and legal issues.

In the inpatient or outpatient setting, the nursing process can be applied to the management of the infant on an ongoing basis. The major emphasis is placed on the area of assessment and documentation of findings so that early intervention and treatment can be carried out.

Psychosocial Concerns: Developmental Factors

Fear and anxiety may be one of the major problems in dealing with infants or pediatric patients because of their cognitive inability to understand what is happening to them. The major burden, therefore, is placed on the parent or care provider to deal with the diagnosis and complications of HIV. The parents or care providers go through a period of anxiety and denial following the diagnosis. The steps for acceptance of the diagnosis of HIV for the infected mother or father are similar to Elisabeth Kubler-Ross's five steps in the grief process for an individual who is dying (see Chapter 8, Bereavement: A State of Having Suffered a Loss.)

Usually, following the diagnosis the parents or care providers need time before teaching or educational activities are of any benefit. Following the period of denial is a period in which the parents or care providers seek out any available material regarding the disease process and its cause, prognosis, and treatment. It is at this time that the nurse working collaboratively with the health care team provides the family with accurate information.

MANAGEMENT

The overall goal in providing care to the infant who has been infected with HIV is to promote an optimal level of wellness regardless of the severity of the signs and symptoms. The level of wellness depends on the infant's disease state and course of the progression of HIV. The provision of care focuses on routine medical care, including immunization, nutrition, and developmental interventions. One of the major problems in working with the infant and child with HIV infection is the developmental regression that appears to be one of the classic signs and symptoms (American Academy of Pediatrics, 1988).

At each visit, baseline respirations, respiratory effort, skin color, presence or absence of cough, sputum production, and presence of dyspnea with activity should be assessed. If warranted, a pulmonary function test might be of benefit. Other baseline data, including heart rate and temperature, are obtained at each visit or on a daily basis if the infant is hospitalized. The child's pattern of elimination and hydration status need to be observed and recorded so that any subtle changes can be recognized and treatment implemented as soon as possible. Usually during the examination, parents verbalize concerns regarding their child's nutritional status or other problems that may be worrying them.

In addition to the clinical management of the infant, the developmental needs should be closely followed and documented. The nurse must document the infant's developmental abilities as well as deficits. Once these are documented, the care providers need to learn about appropriate developmental interventions to stimulate the infant's visual, kinesthetic, auditory, and tactile senses (Fahrner, 1992).

Family Unit

Knowledge about HIV has been presented to the public through a variety of print and television media. However, a majority of the information in the past has focused on the adult with HIV. Many individuals lack information regarding HIV in the infant or pediatric client. Even with adequate information, many care providers are not ready to accept the diagnosis. Many families and care providers go through a period of denial during which additional information or teaching is not absorbed. Parents and care providers must be ready, willing, and able to work through the process.

Maternal Considerations

To date there is no evidence that casual contact or providing routine infant care such as bathing, bottle feeding, diapering, and playing increases the likelihood of spreading the HIV infection from mother to infant (Nanda, 1990). Therefore, there should be no restrictions placed on a mother with HIV infection in regard to providing care for her infant.

Emergency Department Management

The infant presenting in the emergency room deserves special attention and consideration according to Mendez and Jule (1990). Parents and foster families should be encouraged to disclose the serostatus of their infants in emergency situations or when coming into contact with alternative care providers. Mendez and Jule (1990) recommend immediate medical attention on arrival in the triage area for any symptomatic infant. One of the steps in emergency care is to perform an HIV-oriented physical examination to evaluate the HIV status and the possible presence of an opportunistic infection. In contrast, Mendez and Jule (1990) recommend no special treatment for asymptomatic infants who have been exposed to HIV. The emergency team should provide standard pediatric care. Following discharge of either an asymptomatic or symptomatic infant, the primary health care provider must be notified. Such notification is imperative so that close supervision and follow-up of any treatment begun in the emergency department can be carried out.

Mortality

Minkoff (1990) reported that in some regions and cities in the United States, HIV is endemic and more infants will die of HIV than of any other cause. Oleske and colleagues (1988) reported that HIV in infants is rapidly becoming the number two cause of death in infants.

The causes of death following HIV infection are as follows: (1) 50 percent of infants die of PCP, (2) 10 to 15 percent die of *Mycobacterium avium-intracellulare* (atypical tuberculosis) infection, (3) 10 percent die of fulminate bacterial infection, and (4) 10 percent die of neurologically related causes (Harrison, 1990).

Currently, 100 percent of individuals diagnosed with AIDS are expected to die from the disease (CDC, 1991). The mean survival time for infants and children is 19.7 months after birth, much shorter than the survival times for adults. Eighty percent of the infants and children diagnosed with AIDS die within the first 2 years after diagnosis (Edmondson, 1988).

Nursing Diagnoses

The primary focus for the nurse caring for a seropositive HIV infant or an infant with AIDS is to alleviate existing symptoms and prevent further complications (Edmondson, 1988). Using the nursing model, there are several nursing diagnoses that are applicable to developing a plan of care for the infant who has HIV infection. The nursing plan of care should have both an infant- and family-centered focus. The term *family* is used to encompass both biologic and extended families, as well as alternative care providers. Possible nursing diagnoses that may be modified for either the asymptomatic or symptomatic infant with HIV are presented in Table 42–12.

Three "Cs" of Care

When providing care to the HIV patient, three "Cs" can be applied to the situation: comprehensive, consistent, and compassionate. Comprehensive care includes an alliance of mental health and medical professionals to provide both emotional and physical supportive care. Consistent care refers to building a sense of trust and rapport between parents and care providers. Lastly, compassionate care refers to supportive education, stressing the importance of empathy, including human touch, when dealing with the individual with HIV.

Closely aligned to the three Cs of care are the basic principles of nursing care. Four important points must be kept in mind to provide high-quality comprehensive care to newborns infected with HIV. The first point is that the infant and family are the unit of treatment, not the disease itself. To carry out this principle, the aspects of infant development and psychosocial concerns need to be taken into consideration. The second principle is that care should be community-based and family-centered. Every effort should be made to devise and support outpatient and family-centered treatment. One of the primary reasons is that community-based care is less costly than in-hospital care. In addition, community-based care attempts to improve the quality of life of the infant and family (Ross Laboratories, 1989).

Third, culturally appropriate and sensitive questions must be asked to determine the psychosocial dimensions of the illness and the milieu in which it occurs. The health care providers need to be nonjudgmental of the parents, who may be from culturally diverse backgrounds or have a history that may involve prior or current drug abuse. These are just two examples of modifying ways that nursing care needs to be culturally appropriate.

Lastly, another factor to take into consideration is the quality of the infant's and family's life and the family's right to a dignified death. Dignity in all stages of care and impending death must be an underlying theme in the care of an infant or child infected with HIV. The fact that HIV is currently fatal does not lessen the infant's and family's need for love, physical intimacy, and social and cognitive stimulation.

TABLE 42–12 Possible Nursing Diagnoses That May Be Modified for the Asymptomatic or Symptomatic HIV-Infected Infant

1. Potential for infection related to immunosuppression
2. Impaired gas exchange related to viscous secretions, ineffective cough, and fatigue
3. Ineffective breathing pattern related to hepatosplenomegaly
4. Alteration in oral mucous membranes related to immunosuppression
5. Alteration in nutrition; less than body requirements related to anorexia, altered oral mucous membranes, and so on
6. Alteration in bowel elimination; diarrhea related to impaired intestinal lining
7. Alteration in fluid volume related to nutritional intake and diarrhea
8. Alteration in skin integrity related to immunosuppression
9. High risk for ineffective family coping related to perception or reaction to HIV diagnosis
10. Alteration in growth and development related to neurologic changes associated with HIV
11. High risk for injury related to neurologic changes associated with HIV
12. High risk for knowledge deficit related to implications of diagnosis

Diagnoses derived from material from American Academy of Pediatrics. (1988). *Report of the Committee on Infectious Disease* (21st ed., pp. 91–115). Elk Grove, IL: Author; and Gee, G., & Moran, T. A. (1988). *AIDS: Concepts in nursing practice.* Baltimore: Williams & Wilkins.

Educational Principles

Prevention of HIV in the adult population decreases the number of cases in infants and children. Ways to prevent the spread of HIV include practicing "safe sex"; decreasing intravenous drug use, especially in childbearing women; abortion; and avoidance of pregnancy in high-risk women. This form of education ideally should be preconceptional teaching (Lindberg, 1995).

A second goal of the free-standing clinics is to offer programs that outline options for limiting the transmission of the disease to the infant and child. Such programs might focus on birth control, abortion (where cultural and government regulations allow), and sterilization. In addition to reaching childbearing women, attempts to reach sexual partners should be carried out. Individuals should be counseled not to donate blood, plasma, sperm, organs, or breast milk (American Academy of Pediatrics, 1988).

Another way to minimize the spread or to work on prevention of HIV is to provide heath care to the underserved populations, which include a large number of inner city women in high-risk areas. The care could be provided in the form of free-standing clinics for prenatal care and outreach for both infants and children. Counseling, including AIDS education, and ways to minimize the spread of HIV for the diagnosed individual should also be readily available to underserved individuals. The American Academy of Pediatrics (1988) recommends that counseling be ongoing. The provision of education should focus on HIV and its transmission. An emphasis should be placed on outlining precautions to be taken within the household and the community to prevent the spread of HIV. Counseling should be directed toward women of childbearing age and pregnant women. Women of childbearing age who are infected with HIV need to be aware of the risks of having an infected infant if they become pregnant. Factors to take into consideration in counseling include culturally appropriate approaches and using language and terminology that is familiar to the individuals being addressed.

A perinatal HIV counseling checklist has been reported by Holman and associates (1989). The checklist covers the major areas of education concerning the woman's own health and her role as a care provider for her infant. Included on the checklist are specific areas for follow-up counseling appointments and for questions and concerns that the woman may have.

The general public still needs to be educated regarding the methods and likelihood of transmission of HIV. The programs should be targeted to all childbearing populations that may be exposing an unborn child to HIV. Providing information or educational programs to teenagers and childbearing populations is not enough. The childbearing population must be empowered to use the information. Knowing is not doing! Authorities on HIV recommend that the education should focus on two major areas (Ross Laboratories, 1989):

- Learning about HIV in a structured setting with consistent, factual information
- Learning about HIV from parents

Educational strategies need to include programs that discuss precautions in day care and nursery schools to protect all those who are participating and providing care to infants and children.

In addition, educational programs should focus on the provision of needed medical and social services for infants, children, and families with HIV.

Health care providers, parents, and extended family members should be aware that infants and children with HIV should not receive live virus vaccines, with the exception of MMR. Therefore, follow-up care providers need to ask specific questions regarding HIV before administering immunizations to any child.

When infants or children with HIV have cutaneous eruptions or draining lesions that cannot be covered, they should not attend day care or school until the lesions can be covered or have healed (American Academy of Pediatrics, 1988). Infants and children who have inappropriate behaviors, such as biting, and the infant or child with incontinence or uncontrolled diarrhea should not be in a day care setting or attending school until the problem is resolved. Teachers and parents should be counseled that an infant or child with HIV infection should not be attending day care or school during outbreaks of chickenpox or other communicable diseases because infants or children with HIV have weakened immune systems, thus making them more susceptible to infections. The infections may not be easily combated and may carry added risk or negative outcomes for the infant or child infected with HIV (American Academy of Pediatrics, 1988). Noninfected infants and children pose a greater threat to the health of an HIV-positive infant or child than the converse.

HUMAN IMMUNODEFICIENCY VIRUS AND THE HEALTH CARE WORKER

In the United States, there are approximately 6.8 million health care workers. Of these workers, 1875 individuals have been found to be seropositive for HIV. Ninety-five percent of the 1875 individuals have exhibited high-risk behaviors (CDC, 1991). The remaining 5 percent have been exposed in the work setting via needlesticks or breaks in universal blood and body fluid precautions. The CDC (1987c) published "Recommendations for Prevention of HIV Transmission in Health Care Settings." In the document, the CDC recommended that blood and body fluid precautions be observed for all patients regardless of diagnosis or HIV status. Thus, the recommendations by the CDC in August 1987 have come to be known as the *universal blood and body fluid precautions.* Table 42–13 lists the guidelines for caring for the infant regardless of serostatus.

TABLE 42–13 Guidelines for Caring for Infants Regardless of Seropositivity

Use universal blood and body fluid precautions when providing direct patient care.
Maintain confidentiality in the communication of the diagnosis for the infant with HIV infection. (Avoid engendering anxiety among families of other patients on the units.)
Maintain scrupulous attention to disposal of needles and other sharp instruments; place contaminated needles and other "sharps" into designated containers *without* recapping.
Label specimens and laboratory slips with "biohazard" or other approved designation to prevent injury to laboratory personnel or transporters of specimens.
Avoid contamination when drawing blood or collecting other specimens; dispose of diapers and linens as dictated by hospital protocols.
Supervise patient environment during emergency situations so that unwary personnel responding to crisis are not inadvertently contaminated.

HIV, human immunodeficiency virus.

Universal precautions are recommended by the CDC for all health care workers. The use of the precautions applies to both the nurse in the delivery room and the nursery nurse (Table 42–14).

In the delivery room, the use of appropriate barrier precautions to prevent exposure of the skin and mucous membranes to blood or other body fluids from any patient has been recommended by the CDC (1987a, 1987b, 1987c, 1988). More specifically, precautions specify the following:

- Gloves: to be worn to avoid direct contact with blood and potentially infectious body fluids

TABLE 42–14 Health Care Workers' Protection Against HIV

1. Intact skin is an effective barrier against HIV; health care workers with exudative dermatitis or lesions should not provide direct patient care.
2. Hands should be washed carefully and thoroughly before and after each patient contact and after any contact with body fluids.

Universal Blood and Body Fluid Precautions:

1. Gloves should be used for any contact with body fluids (blood, vomitus, feces, urine); the gloves should be discarded and the hands washed after contact.
2. Gloves should be worn by all dental health personnel.
3. Body spills should be disinfected with bleach (1 part bleach to 9 parts water); this solution should be prepared daily.
4. Use chlorine bleach in laundry for items soiled with blood, urine, feces, or vomitus.
5. Health care workers should be careful to avoid accidental puncture by lancets, needles, and other sharp objects.
6. All used needles, lancets, and other sharp objects should be disposed of in puncture-proof containers.
7. Disposable diapers, dressings, syringes, gloves, and so on should be placed in plastic bags, which should be tied securely.
8. Disposable Ambu bags should be used for mouth-to-mouth resuscitation.
9. Use masks for indirect, sustained contact with patients who are coughing.
10. Protective eye wear (i.e., goggles) should be worn if splattering of body fluids is anticipated.
11. Gowns are necessary only if soiling of clothing with body fluids is anticipated.

HIV, human immunodeficiency virus.

Data from Gee, G., & Moran, T. A. (1988). *AIDS: Concepts in nursing practice.* Baltimore: Williams & Wilkins; and American Academy of Pediatrics. (1988). *Report of the Committee on Infectious Disease* (21st ed., pp. 91–115). Elk Grove, IL: Author.

- Masks, protective eyewear or face shields, and gowns or aprons: to protect against dispersion of blood or other body fluid and splashes of these fluids during procedures

All personnel in the delivery room should wear gloves. This includes all nursing personnel. Gloves must also be worn during venipuncture and other modes of vascular access. Additionally, proper resuscitative equipment, including masks, manual resuscitation bags, and oral airways, should be available in various newborn and infant sizes for each and every delivery.

Universal precautions and infection control guidelines should be employed by every nurse and health care provider regardless of the mother's serostatus. All individuals should be approached using the universal precautions as outlined by the CDC.

The CDC has been collecting data since 1983 on more than 300 institutions in the United States to determine the risk of acquiring HIV infection after exposure to blood from patients infected with HIV (Marcus and the CDC Cooperative Needlestick Group, 1989). Of those individuals stuck with needles or cut by sharp objects, 4 of 982 had a seropositive status (0.41 percent). Three of the four experienced seroconversion after being stuck. The remaining individual had no baseline data available to determine seroconversion (Marcus and the CDC Cooperative Needlestick Surveillance Group, 1989). The CDC (1986) notes that occupational transmission of HIV may occur in rare instances. The transmission is generally related to contamination of mucous membranes or nonintact skin or from prolonged and extensive skin contact with contaminated blood and body fluids.

The media have been focusing a great deal of attention on HIV and health care professionals. The current debate is whether health care professionals should be routinely tested for HIV. In addition, there is a great deal of controversy surrounding the issue of mandatory versus voluntary testing. To date, the major medical and nursing organizations do not support mandatory testing. On June 30, 1991, the American Nurses' Association passed a resolution opposing mandatory testing. In 1991, the American Nurses' Association President Lucille Joel said "Compulsory universal testing isn't reliable, and it is extremely expensive." The CDC's (1991) position on mandatory testing of medical, dental, and health workers is that it is not justified because the risk of HIV transmission by health care workers to their patients is too small. However, the CDC is currently trying to identify invasive medical, surgical, and dental procedures that if performed by a health care provider who is infected with HIV should require notification of the patient. Several of the major medical and nursing organizations are opposed to such regulations. There is no compelling evidence that such testing would control AIDS (Rhodes, 1995).

OTHER ISSUES SURROUNDING THE DIAGNOSIS OF HUMAN IMMUNODEFICIENCY VIRUS

An issue that has not received a great deal of media attention is the fact that many of these infants may become orphaned or experience the death of a parent or sibling in their short life span. The onset and progression of HIV in the neonate are generally more rapid owing to the immaturity of the immune system, coupled with the inability to acquire an adequate supply of antibodies to overcome opportunistic infections (Oleske et al., 1988). This rapid disease progression coupled with fear has led to the "boarder baby" phenomenon.

Boarder Babies

Despite all the protection and education, there is an inherent fear about the spread of AIDS. Some parents are so ill themselves that by the time of the infant's birth they are no longer able to care for him or her. Other family members may be afraid to care for such an infant if the parents are known to be HIV-positive. This is also true when it comes to foster care or adoption of the infant. Therefore, another important aspect of HIV is the social issue of *boarder babies.* This term is used not only for HIV-positive neonates or infants but also for those who are exposed to drugs and potentially at risk for the later development of HIV. It is estimated that significantly more infants who have been exposed to drugs than infants who have not become boarder babies. It has been estimated that more than 50 percent of infants who have been exposed to cocaine in utero are at risk of becoming boarder babies (Barton et al., 1995). Of these infants, more than half will eventually be placed in foster care (Marcenko et al., 1992). Marcenko and associates (1992) found in a study of 20 boarder babies from an eastern city in the United States that the total number of days they required boarding was 195 with a cost in 1992 of $117,000. The cost of such infants has significantly increased since 1993. In another study, Marcenko and Spence (1994) found that when foster care was not possible, home visits for women infected with HIV and their infants was a good and safe alternative. Boarder or abandoned infants is a growing problem. The exact definition of boarder babies varies across the United States.

Boarder babies is a term used to describe infants who live in the hospital without medical necessity; they simply do not have a safe place to go home to. Other labels attached to these children are *children in limbo, hard-to-place, abandoned infants,* and *long-stay newborns.*

The first documented report about boarder babies was published in 1946 by the Citizens Committee for Children of New York, Inc. They reported at least 100 healthy children living in New York hospital wards (New York Citizens' Committee for Children, 1971). Historically, reasons for boarder babies have included parental neglect, illness, substance abuse, and imprisonment. Poverty and teenaged pregnancy are risk factors, as are chronic illness or mental retardation of the infant (Dahl-Regis & Oyefara, 1990). Having a mother who abuses drugs or one who is infected with HIV are newer risk factors.

Inner city hospitals that treat mothers with many of these risk factors seem to have the most boarder babies. A study at Howard University Hospital, Washington, DC, 1988–1989, was designed to identify variables that predicted abandonment (Dahl-Regis & Oyefara, 1990). Of the 968 babies delivered, 28 (or 2.9 percent) became boarder babies for varying lengths of time. During the same period, boarder babies constituted 4.6 percent of all pediatric admissions. Mothers of boarder babies were determined to be single and primarily of low socioeconomic status. The authors postulate that mothers with limited resources, particularly those who live on the streets, are simply not able to care for a child with special health needs.

The recent surge in the drug epidemic, thought to be related to ready availability of "crack" cocaine, has compounded the problem. Many drug-abusing mothers are unable to handle more than one dependency at a time. Infants withdrawing from drug exposure are often irritable, have a stiff posture, and do not tolerate eye contact, making bonding difficult. As previously indicated, women addicted to drugs often have other high-risk factors that may influence their inability to care for their newborns. The ability of the extended family to care for the infant continues to change; fewer grandparents are in a position to rear and support grandchildren than in years past. Foster families are difficult to find, mostly because of fear, ignorance, and prejudice. This is particularly true if the infant has a medically or developmentally disabling condition that requires "special foster care."

AIDS is also a new risk factor. Whether or not an infant is HIV-positive, one or both parents may have AIDS and be too ill to care for the child. In many cases, the woman with AIDS is a single parent (AIDS women, boarder babies: Complex discharge problems, 1991). A generational effect may occur if the infant's grandmother has to choose between caring for her daughter with AIDS and providing a home for her grandchildren, who may or may not be infected with HIV. A mother who receives Aid to Families with Dependent Children monies loses her benefits if her child is placed in a foster family. Such families may be afraid to care for an HIV-positive infant. All these issues compound the boarder baby dilemma. A study at Harlem Hospital Center, New York, between 1981 and 1986 found that boarder babies with AIDS had an average length of stay nearly four times longer than AIDS infants with homes (Hegarty et al., 1988).

Caring for Boarder Babies

It is not always obvious at birth or on admission that infants will become boarder babies. Mothers are sometimes involved in their child's care at the onset: visiting, kissing, and cuddling, and promising to take them home. It may be in retrospect that a nurse will realize it has been several days since the parent has been in to see the baby. A parent may be difficult to reach by phone and when contacted may give legitimate reasons for not being more involved. The parent is given the benefit of the doubt for as long as possible. When the parent does not comply with visiting requirements set forth by the social worker, and it is apparent that the child will not go home with the parent, the court system is involved to grant custody to the state, and foster care is pursued.

Boarder babies present different challenges for nurses. They do not usually require intensive medical care, and the focus shifts to normalizing their environment and fostering growth and development. Some of the problems boarder babies encounter in the hospital are nosocomial infections with resistant organisms, fresh air deprivation, inappropriate developmental stimulation, and inappropriate housing (environmental light, sounds, and smells). Perhaps the major challenge for nurses is finding time during the shift to address these issues. These infants are at risk of being neglected in a hospital environment because they are not acutely sick. It is important for the hospital administration first to recognize that these infants have different needs and that their nursing care, although different from acute care, is just as important for optimal healthy outcomes.

These children benefit by having child life specialists (individuals with a college degree in child development who are employed by hospitals to normalize the environment and daily activities as much as possible) or nurses specializing in chronic care involved in planning their nursing care. "Baby holders"—volunteers from the community who give their time to cuddle and rock abandoned infants—are becoming a popular and valued asset to nurseries. Some boarder babies with medically complex conditions, such as those on ventilators, become boarder children, particularly if no specialty foster homes are found and the area nursing homes do not accept small children. The longer a child stays on a hospital unit, the more intricate the issue may become. Having nurses take the infants on pass for the weekend, power struggles between nurses who become surrogate mothers, possible on-again, off-again involvement of the birth parents, toilet training and behavioral modification programs, and eventually transportation to day care or preschool all present milestones to be dealt with.

Alternatives for Boarder Babies

The 1988 Congress Act P.L. 100-505, entitled the Abandoned Infants Assistance Act, has helped institutions develop multidisciplinary programs to meet the needs of these infants (Marceko et al., 1992). Once such program is in Florida. The Social Work Department at Jackson Memorial Hospital, Miami, Florida, has responded to the crisis of inadequate numbers of foster homes (Boarder babies: Winning the battle, 1991). In March 1989, they had 36 boarder babies. By working with a national child advocacy organization, the news media, and the state's protective service system, their average discharge delay was reduced to 1½ days, with an average of two boarder babies on any given day. Other hospitals with large numbers of boarder babies are working with community and state groups to expand the available pool of specialty foster homes. For-profit hospitals are particularly concerned about the cost of infants staying in the hospital without medical necessity, and some are involved in negotiating with state bureaucracies to make provisions for these children.

Some hospitals have made arrangements with "shelter homes," which are group homes for children, where care is provided until a family is found for the infant. Another organization, Children with AIDS Project of America, was started in 1989 by a nurse in Phoenix, Arizona, to provide permanent, loving homes for children with AIDS (Jenkins, 1990). They also support the child's birth, adoptive, and foster parents. Their toll-free number is 1-800-866-2437. In Arizona, the number is 1-602-843-8654.

Allegheny–Hahnemann University Hospital in Philadelphia also started a program in 1989 to respond to the growing problem of boarder babies. It was funded by Robert Wood Johnson (Gentry, 1993). Their special caretakers program resulted in a reduction in unreimbursable hospital days from 257 to 77. It used foster care recruitees from their own employees. These employees were screened via community foster agencies. Once the screening was completed, normal state procedures were followed for foster placements. Other funding for the program was found from formula companies and through donations.

Project CONNECT in New York State serves prenatal and postpartum women who are at risk and their infants (Randolph & Sherman, 1993). It provides a partnership with health delivery services and human support services with the goal of keeping families together as much as possible. The success rate has been good in its 5 years. It is another alternative to boarder babies.

In 1989, Incarnation Children's Center in New York started a temporary home for boarder babies (Clark & Byrne, 1993). It worked with a community foster care agency and city and state child welfare agencies to recruit foster parents. At present, the need for the center has changed. Because of the increasing numbers of foster parents, the center now provides respite care for natural or foster parents and enhanced care for the children who need professional care but are not sick enough for hospitalization.

The problem of boarder babies will be a reality as long as the family and the environmental risk factors exist. Although there are no quick cures or wonderful solutions in the offing, nurses and the caring they give fill the gap for these infants who need what every child needs—love and a sense of security.

CONCLUSION

The literature on HIV and AIDS infection is rapidly changing. It is impossible to create a chapter that is up to date with the latest facts and figures. As soon as the material is gathered, it rapidly becomes obsolete. Statistics focusing on the incidence and prevalence of HIV in the infant and pediatric population are always changing. A great deal of effort and federal dollars are being allocated from the National Institutes of Health for the explicit purpose of focusing on HIV research. Based on the findings from these investigations, new treatment protocols are and will be continually emerging.

For now, the medical and nursing profession must rely on the existing drugs, including zidovudine and ddI, and aggressive treatment of opportunistic infections. Even with treatment protocols, there is a continued need for educational programs for nurses, other health care professionals, and the lay population. Currently, the prognosis for the HIV-infected infant is grim at best. However, the future holds promise and hope as new treatment protocols and the possibility of a vaccine are currently being examined in both human and animal models.

REFERENCES

Adamson, P. C., Wu, R. C., Meade, B. D., et al. (1989). Pertussis in a previously immunized child with human immunodeficiency virus infection. *Journal of Pediatrics, 115*(4), 589–592.

Ahmad, N., Baroudy, B. M., Baker, R. C., & Chappey, C. (1995). Genetic analysis of human immunodeficiency virus type 1 envelope V3 region isolates from others and infants after perinatal transmission. *Journal of Virology, 69*(2), 1001–1012.

AIDS women, boarder babies: Complex discharge problems. (1991, January–February). *Discharge Planning Update, 1,* 16–17.

Allain, J. P., Laurian, Y., Paul, D. A., et al. (1987). Long-term evaluation of HIV antigen and antibodies to p24 and gp41 in patients with hemophilia. Potential clinical importance. *New England Journal of Medicine, 317*(18), 1114–1122.

American Academy of Pediatrics. (1988). *Report of the Committee on Infectious Disease* (21st ed., pp. 91–115). Elk Grove, IL: Author.

American Academy of Pediatrics and American College of Obstetricians and Gynecologists. (1993). *Guidelines for perinatal care* (3rd ed.). Elk Grove, IL: American Academy of Pediatrics.

Ammann, A. J. (1992). Pediatric acquired immunodeficiency syndrome. In R. D. Feigin & J. D. Cherry (Eds.), *Textbook of Pediatric Infectious Diseases* (3rd ed., pp. 1044–1049). Philadelphia: W. B. Saunders.

Anderson, D. M., & Kliegman, R. M. (1991). Relationship of neonatal alimentation practices to the occurrence of endemic necrotizing enterocolitis. *American Journal of Perinatology, 8*(1), 62–67.

Andiman, W. (1989). Virologic and serologic aspects of human immunodeficiency virus infection in infants and children. *Seminars in Perinatology, 13*(1), 16–26.

Baker, D. A. (1994). Management of the female HIV-infected patient. *AIDS Research and Human Retroviruses, 10*(8), 935–938.

Barton, S. H., Harrigan, R., & Tse, A. M. (1995). Prenatal cocaine exposure: Implications for practice, policy development, and needs for future research. *Journal of Perinatology, 15*(1), 10–22.

Blanche, S., Rouzioux, C., Moscato, M. L., et al. (1989). A prospective study of infants born to women seropositive for human immunodeficiency virus type 1. *New England Journal of Medicine, 320*(25), 1643–1648.

Boarder babies: Winning the battle. (1991, January–February), *Discharge Planning Update, 1,* 15.

Boland, M., & Conviser, R. (1992). Nursing care of the child. In J. H. Flaskerud & P. J. Ungvarski (Eds.), *HIV/AIDS: A guide to nursing care* (2nd ed., pp. 199–238). Philadelphia: W. B. Saunders.

Bridbord, K., & Willoughby, A. (1994). Vitamin A and mother-to-child HIV-1 transmission [Commentary]. *Lancet, 343*(8913), 1585–1586.

Burton, D. R., Pyati, J., Koduri, R., et al. (1994). Efficient neutralization of primary isolates of HIV-1 by a recombinant human monoclonal antibody. *Science, 266*(5187), 1024–1027.

Centers for Disease Control. (1982). CDC: Update on acquired immunodeficiency syndrome (AIDS)–United States. *MMWR Morbidity and Mortality Weekly Report, 31*(37), 507–514.

Centers for Disease Control. (1986). Recommendations for preventing transmission of infection with human T-lymphotrophic virus type II/lymphadenopathy associated virus during invasive procedures. *MMWR Morbidity and Mortality Weekly Report, 35*(14), 221–223.

Centers for Disease Control. (1987a). Classification system for human immunodeficiency virus (HIV) infection in children under 13 years of age. *MMWR Morbidity and Mortality Weekly Report, 36,* 225–230.

Centers for Disease Control. (1987b). Revision of the CDC surveillance case definition for acquired immunodeficiency syndrome. *MMWR Morbidity and Mortality Weekly Report, 36*(Suppl. 1), 35–55.

Centers for Disease Control. (1987c). Recommendations for prevention of HIV transmission in health care settings. *MMWR Morbidity and Mortality Weekly Report, 36*(Suppl. 2), 1–18.

Centers for Disease Control. (1988). Universal precautions for prevention of transmission of human immunodeficiency virus, hepatitis B virus, and other bloodborne pathogens in health-care settings. *MMWR Morbidity and Mortality Weekly Report, 37,* 377.

Centers for Disease Control. (1991, March). *Centers for Disease Control HIV/AIDS surveillance report.* Washington, DC: U.S. Government Printing Office.

Chasnoff, I. J. (1986). *Drug use in pregnancy: Mother and child.* Norwell, MA: MTP Press.

Chiasson, M. A., Stoneburner, R. L., & Joseph, S. C. (1990). Human immunodeficiency virus transmission through artificial insemination. *Journal of Acquired Immune Deficiency Syndromes, 3*(1), 69–72.

Chin, J. (1994). The growing impact of the HIV/AIDS pandemic on children born to HIV-infected women. *Clinics in Perinatology, 21*(1), 1–14.

Clark, P. J., & Byrne, M. W. (1993). A step up from home: Enhanced care for medically complex HIV infected children. Part 1. *MCN, American Journal of Maternal/Child Nursing, 18*(2), 1–4, 6.

Cohen, J. (1991). AIDS vaccine meeting: International trials soon. *Science, 254*(5032), 647.

Colebunders, R., Kapita, B., Nekwei, W., et al. (1988). Breast-feeding and transmission of HIV. *Lancet, 2*(8626–8627), 1487.

Connor, E., Bagorzzi, M., McSherry, G., et al. (1991). Clinical and laboratory correlates of *Pnenumocysis carinii* pneumonia in children infected with HIV. *Journal of the American Medical Association, 265*(13), 1693–1697.

Connor, E. M., Sperling, R. S., Gelber, R., et al., for the Pediatric AIDS Clinical Trials Group Protocol 076 Study Group. (1994). Reduction of maternal-infant transmission of human immunodeficiency virus type 1 with zidovudine treatment. *New England Journal of Medicine, 331*(18), 1173–1180.

Craven, D. E., Steger, K. A., & Jarek, C. (1994). Human immunodeficiency virus infection in pregnancy: Epidemiology and prevention of vertical transmission. *Infection Control & Hospital Epidemiology, 15*(1), 36–47.

Dahl-Regis, M. M., & Oyefara, B. I. (1990). Boarder babies: Children with special health needs. *Journal of the National Medical Association, 82*(7), 473–477.

Deluchi, G., Canizal, A. M., Zarwanitzer, S., et al. (1994). HIV IgA immunoblot as a diagnostic tool in pediatrics [Abstract PBO447]. *International Conference on AIDS. 10*(1), 254.

De Wolf, F., Goudsmit, J., Paul, D. A., et al. (1987). Risk of ARC and AIDS in homosexual men with persistent HIV antigenaemia. *British Medical Journal, 295*(6598), 569–572.

Dondero, T. J., Jr., Pappaioanou, M., & Curran, J. W. (1988). Monitoring the levels and trends of HIV infection: The Public Health Service's HIV surveillance program. *Public Health Report, 103*(3), 213–220.

Edmondson, K. S. (1988). Acquired immune deficiency syndrome in the neonate. *Neonatal Network, 6*(4), 7–12.

Ellerbrock, R. V., & Rogers, M. F. (1990). Epidemiology of human immunodeficiency virus infection in women in the United States. *Obstetrics and Gynecology Clinics of North America, 17*(3), 523–544.

Epstein, L. G., Sharer, L. R., & Goudsmit, J. (1988). Neurologic and neuropathologic features of human immunodeficiency virus infection in children. *Annals of Neurology Journal, 23*(Suppl.), S19–S23.

European Collaborative Study. (1988). Mother-to-child transmission of HIV infection. *Lancet, 2*(8619), 1039-1043.

Fahrner, R. (1992). Pediatric HIV infection and AIDS. In P. L. Jackson & J. A. Vessery (Eds.), *Primary care of the child with a chronic condition* (pp. 408–425). St. Louis: C. V. Mosby.

Falloon, J., Eddy, J., Wiener, L., & Pizzo, P. A. (1989). Human immunodeficiency virus: Infection in children. *Journal of Pediatrics, 114*(1), 1–30.

Fuchs, D., Hausen, A., & Reibnegger, G. (1988). Neopterin as a marker of activated cell-mediated immunity. *Immunology Today, 9,* 150–155.

Gentry, L. R. (1993). Practice forum: The special caretakers program: A hospital's solution to the boarder baby problem. *Health & Social Work, 18*(1), 75–77.

Goedert, J. J., Mendez, H., Drummond, J. E., et al. (1989). Mother to infant transmission of human immunodeficiency virus type 1: Association with prematurity or low anti-gp120. *Lancet, 2*(8676), 1351–1354.

Goudsmit, J., Paul, D. A., Lang, J. M. A., et al. (1986). Expression of human immunodeficiency virus antigen (HIV-Ag) in serum and cerebrospinal fluid during acute and chronic infection. *Lancet, 2*(8500), 177–180.

Grubman, S., Gross, E., Lerner-Weiss, N., et al. (1995). Older children and adolescents living with perinatally acquired human immunodeficiency virus infection. *Pediatrics, 95*(5), 657–663.

Harrison, C. J. (1990). *Pediatric AIDS.* Pediatric Grand Rounds, March 8, 1990. Cincinnati, OH: Children's Hospital Medical Center.

Health Resources & Services Administration. (1995). *Draft: Program advisory: ZDV therapy for reducing perinatal HIV: Implementation in HRSA-Funded Programs*, pp. 1–28. Washington, DC: U.S. Government Printing Office.

Hegarty, J. D., Abrams, E. J., Hutchinson, V. E., et al. (1988). The medical care costs of human immunodeficiency virus–infected children in Harlem. *Journal of the American Medical Association, 260*(13), 1901–1905.

Hoff, R., Berardi, V. P., Weiblen, B. J., et al. (1988). Seroprevalence of human immunodeficiency virus among childbearing women. *New England Journal of Medicine, 318*(9), 525–530.

Holman, S., Berthaud, M., Sunderland, A., et al. (1989). Women infected with human immunodeficiency virus: Counseling and testing during pregnancy. *Seminars in Perinatology, 13*(1), 7–15.

Husson, R. N., Corneau, A. M., & Hoff, R. (1990). Diagnosis of human immunodeficiency virus infection in infants and children [Review]. *Pediatrics, 86*(1), 1–10.

Hutto, C., Scott, G. B., & Mitchell, C. (1989). Maternal risk factors for perinatal transmission of human immunodeficiency virus–1 (HIV–1). *Abstracts of the Fifth International Conference on AIDS* (p. 71, No. ThAO 8). Montreal: International Development Research Center.

Institute of Medicine/National Academy of Sciences. (1988). Confronting AIDS: Update: 1988. *Journal of Acquired Immune Deficiency Syndromes, 1*(2), 173–186.

Italian Multicentre Study. (1988). Epidemiology, clinical features, and prognostic factors of paediatric HIV infection. *Lancet, 2*(8619), 1043–1046.

Jenkins, J. E. (1990). Caring for boarder babies [Letter to the Editor]. *Nursing 90, 20*(9), 4.

Johnson, J. P., Nair, P., Hines, S. E., et al. (1989). Natural history and serologic diagnosis of infants born to human immunodeficiency virus–infected women. *American Journal of Diseases of Children, 143*(10), 1147–1153.

Kellinger, K. G. (1994). Providing primary care to the HIV-at-risk and infected child. *Nurse Practitioner: American Journal of Primary Health Care, 19*(8), 48–52.

Koonin, L. M., Ellerbrock, R. V., Atrash, H. K., et al. (1989). Pregnancy-associated deaths due to AIDS in the United States. *Journal of the American Medical Association, 261*(9), 1306–1309.

Lane, H. C., & Fauci, A. S. (1985). Immunologic abnormalities in the acquired immunodeficiency syndrome. *Annual Review of Immunology, 3*, 477–500.

Lang, R. (1991). CDC issues guidelines for HIV-infected infants. *American Academy of Pediatrics News, 7*(10), 3.

Laurence, J. (1987). HIV infections in infants and children. *Infectious Medicine, 4*, 44–56.

Leibovitz, E., Rigaud, M., Pollack, H., et al. (1990). *Pneumocystis carinii* pneumonia in infants infected with the human immunodeficiency virus with more than 450 CD4+ lymphocytes per cubic millimeter. *New England Journal of Medicine, 323*(8), 531–533.

Lepage, P., Van de Perre, P., Carael, M., et al. (1987). Postnatal transmission of HIV from mother to child [Letter]. *Lancet, 2*(8555), 400.

Levy, J. A. (1989). Human immunodeficiency viruses and the pathogenesis of AIDS [Review]. *Journal of the American Medical Association, 261*(26), 2997–3006.

Lindberg, C. E. (1995). Perinatal transmission of HIV: How to counsel women. *MCN, American Journal of Maternal/Child Nursing 20*(4), 207–212.

Lo, S. C., Tsai, S., Benish, J. R., et al. (1991). Enhancement of HIV–1 cytocidal effects in CD4+ lymphocytes by the AIDS-associated mycoplasma. *Science, 251*(4997), 1074–1076.

Marcenko, M. O., & Spence, M. (1994). Home visitation services for at-risk pregnant and postpartum women: A randomized trial. *American Journal of Orthopsychiatry, 64*(3), 468–478.

Marcenko, M. O., Seraydarian, L., Huang, K., & Rohweder, C. (1992). Hospital boarder babies and their families: An exploratory study. *Social Work in Health Care, 17*(2), 73–85.

Marcus, R., & the CDC Cooperative Needlestick Surveillance Group. (1989). Health-care workers exposed to patients infected with human immunodeficiency virus (HIV). United States. *Abstracts of the Fifth International Conference on AIDS* (p. 63, No. WAO 1). Montreal: International Development Research Center.

Mendez, H., & Jule, J. E. (1990). Care of the infant born exposed to human immunodeficiency virus. *Obstetrics and Gynecology Clinics of North America, 17*(3), 637–649.

Mendez, H., Fikrig, S., & DeForest, A. (1988). Response to childhood immunizations in children with human immunodeficiency virus infection [Abstract]. *Proceedings of the Fourth International Conference on AIDS*. Stockholm: Swedish Ministry of Health and Social Affairs.

Mendez, H., Holman, S., & Stevens, R. (1989). HIV ELISA (E) and Western blot (WB) patterns in infants born to seropositive (SP) women [Abstract]. *Pediatric Research, 25*, 166A.

Mendez, H., Willoughby, A., & Hittelman, J. (1987). Human immunodeficiency virus (HIV) infection in pregnant women and their offspring [Abstract]. *Pediatric Research, 21*, 418A.

Merluzzi, V. J., Hargrave, K. D., Labadia, M., et al. (1990). Inhibition of HIV–1 replication by a nonnucleoside reverse transcriptase inhibitor. *Science, 250*(4986), 1411–1413.

Minkoff, H. L. (Ed.). (1990). HIV disease in pregnancy. *Obstetrics and Gynecology Clinics of North America, 17*(3).

Moss, A. R. (1989). Predicting who will progress to AIDS. *British Medical Journal, 297*(6656), 1067–1068.

Moss, A. R., Bachetti, P., Osmond, D., et al. (1988). Seropositivity of HIV and the development of AIDS or ARC: Three year follow-up of the San Francisco General Cohort. *British Medical Journal Clinical Research Education, 296*(6624), 745–750.

Mundy, D. C., Schinazi, R. F., Gerber, A. R., et al. (1987). Human immunodeficiency virus isolated from amniotic fluid. *Lancet, 2*(8556), 459–460.

Murphy, K. M., Heimberger, A. B., & Loh, D. Y. (1990). Induction by antigen of intrathymic apoptosis of CD4+ CD8+ TCR10 thymocytes in vivo. *Science, 250*(4988), 1720–1723.

Nanda, D. (1990). Human immunodeficiency virus infection in pregnancy. *Obstetrics and Gynecology Clinics of North America, 17*(3), 617–626.

National Center for Nursing Research. (1990). HIV infection: Prevention and care. Bethesda, MD: Author.

Nesheim, S. R., Lindsay, M., Sawyer, M. K., et al. (1994). *AIDS, 8*(9), 1293–1298.

New York Citizens' Committee for Children. (1971). *A dream deferred—child welfare in New York City* (p. 2). New York: Author.

Oleske, J., Minnerfor, A., Cooper, R., Jr., et al. (1983). Immune deficiency syndrome in children. *Journal of the American Medical Association, 249(17)*, 2345–2349.

Oleske, J. M., Connor, E. M., & Boland, M. G. (1988). A perspective on pediatric AIDS. *Pediatric Annals, 17*(5), 319–321.

Oxtoby, M. J. (1988). Human immunodeficiency virus and other viruses in human milk: Placing the issue in broader perspective [Review]. *Pediatric Infectious Disease Journal, 7*(12), 825–835.

Pahwa, S., Kaplan, M., Fikrig, S., et al. (1986). Spectrum of human T-cell lymphotropic virus type III infection in children: Recognition of symptomatic, asymptomatic and seronegative patients. *Journal of the American Medical Association, 255*(17), 2299–2305.

Pedersen, C., Nielsen, C. M., Vestergaard, B. F., et al. (1987). Temporal relation of antigenaemia and loss of antibodies to core antigens to development of clinical disease in HIV infection. *British Medical Journal Clinical Research Education, 295*(6598), 567–569.

Pediatric AIDS. (1989). Columbus, OH: Ross Laboratories.

Pizzo, P. A. (1990). Pediatric AIDS: Problems within problems. *Journal of Infectious Disease, 161*(2), 316–325.

Pizzo, P. A., Eddy, J., Falloon, J., et al. (1988). Effect of continuous intravenous infusion of zidovudine (AZT) in children with symptomatic HIV infection. *New England Journal of Medicine, 319*(14), 889–896.

Polin, R. A., & Fox, W. W. (1992). *Fetal and neonatal physiology*. Philadelphia: W. B. Saunders.

Polk, B. F., Fox, R., Brookmeyer, R, et al. (1987). Predictors of the acquired immunodeficiency syndrome developing in a cohort of seropositive homosexual men. *New England Journal of Medicine, 316*(2), 61–66.

Randolph, L. A., & Sherman, B. R. (1993). Project CONNECT: An interagency partnership to confront new challenges facing at-risk women and children in New York City. *Journal of Community Health, 18*(2), 73–81.

Rhodes, A. M. (1995). Can mandatory HIV testing be justified? *MCN, American Journal of Maternal/Child Nursing, 20*(4), 231.

Rogers, M. F., Ou, C. Y., Rayfield, M., et al. (1989). Use of the polymerase chain reaction for early detection of the proviral sequences of human immunodeficiency virus in infants born to seropositive mothers. *New England Journal of Medicine, 320*(25), 1649–1654.

Rogers, M. F., Thomas, P. A., Starcher, E. T., et al. (1987). Acquired immunodeficiency syndrome in children: Report of the Centers for

Disease Control National Surveillance, 1983 to 1985. *Pediatrics, 79*(6), 1008–1014.

Rubinstein, A. (1986). Pediatric AIDS. *Current Problems in Pediatrics, 16*(7), 367–409.

Rubinstein, A., & Bernstein, L. (1986). The epidemiology of pediatric acquired immunodeficiency syndrome [Review]. *Clinical Immunology and Immunopathology, 40*(1), 115–121.

Sabin, A. B. (1991). Effectiveness of AIDS vaccines [Letter]. *Science, 251*(4998) 1161.

Scott, G. B., Buck, B. E., Leterman, J. G., et al. (1984). Acquired immunodeficiency syndrome in infants. *New England Journal of Medicine, 310*(2), 76–81.

Selwyn, P. A., Schoenbaum, E. E., Davenny, K., et al. (1989). Prospective study of human immunodeficiency virus infection and pregnancy outcomes in intravenous drug users. *Journal of the American Medical Association, 261*(9), 1289–1294.

Spinillo, A., Iasci, A., Dal Maso, J., et al., for the SIGO study group of HIV infection in pregnancy. (1994). *European Journal of Obstetrics & Gynecology and Reproductive Biology, 57*(1), 13–17.

Stanbacket, M., Pape, J. W., & Verdier, R. (1988). Breastfeeding and HIV transmission in Haitian children. *Abstracts of the Fourth International Conference on AIDS* (No. 5101). Stockholm: Swedish Ministry of Health and Social Affairs.

Stewart, G. J., Tyler, J. P., Cunningham, A. L., et al. (1985). Transmission of human T-cell lymphotropic virus type III (HTLV-III) by artificial insemination by donor. *Lancet, 2*(8455), 581–585.

Thiry, L., Sprecher-Goldberg, S., Jonckheer, T., et al. (1985). Isolation of AIDS virus from cell free breast milk of three healthy virus carriers [Letter]. *Lancet, 2*(8460), 891–892.

Tovo, P. A., de Martino, M., Gabiano, C., et al. (1994). AIDS appearance in children is associated with the velocity of disease progression in their mothers. *Journal of Infectious Diseases, 170*(4), 1000–1002.

Viscarello, R. R. (1990). AIDS: Natural history and prognosis [Review]. *Obstetrics and Gynecology Clinics of North America, 17*(3), 545–555.

Weinbreck, P., Loustaud, V., & Denis, F. (1988). Postnatal transmission of HIV infection [Letter]. *Lancet, 1*, 482.

Wishon, S. L., & Gee, G. (1988). Children and HIV Infection. In G. Gee & T. A. Moran (Eds.), *AIDS: Concepts in nursing practice* (pp. 41–61). Baltimore: Williams & Wilkins.

Yoder, M. C., & Polin, R. A. (1997). The immune system (pp. 685–811). In A. A. Fanaroff & R. J. Martin (Eds.), *Neonatal-Perinatal Medicine* (6th ed.). St. Louis: Mosby–Year Book.

Zeigler, J. B., Cooper, D. A., Johnson, R. O., & Gold, J. (1984). Postnatal transmission of AIDS-associated retrovirus from mother to infant. *Lancet, 1*(8434), 896–898.

Zeigler, J. B., Stewart, G. J., & Penney, R. (1988). Breast-feeding and transmission of HIV from mother to infant. *Abstracts of the Fourth Annual International Conference on AIDS* (No. 5100). Stockholm: Swedish Ministry of Health and Social Affairs.

Zurlinden, J. & Verheggen, R. (1994). HIV vaccines: A report from the front. *RN*, 57(1), 36–40.

CHAPTER 43

Hepatic and Renal Transplantation in Infants and Children

FREDERICK C. RYCKMAN SUSAN PEDERSEN-RYCKMAN

RESEARCH AGENDA

What impact does transplantation have on family function?

What are the perinatal and neonatal risk factors that result in the need for infant organ transplantation?

What are the ethical considerations regarding organ transplantation in the neonate?

How does organ transplantation affect parent–infant interaction?

In the past decade, few areas of medicine have experienced the expansion in technology and pharmacology that has occurred in the field of organ transplantation. Procedures that were once experimental and rarely led to long-term survival are routinely undertaken in severely ill infants and children with tremendous success. As a consequence of continued improvements in donor maintenance, organ preservation surgical implantation, and immunosuppressive management, solid organ transplantation is becoming a safe and reliable option for the treatment of end-stage organ failure in the smallest infants and children. This chapter outlines the present status of liver and kidney transplantation in infants and children as a basis for the study of future progress.

HEPATIC TRANSPLANTATION IN INFANTS AND CHILDREN

Transplantation of the liver in infants and children has been recognized for many years to be a possible solution to many inherited metabolic diseases and primary abnormalities of liver function. Although the first attempts at clinical transplantation were failures, in 1967, the prolonged survival of a child who received a transplant following hepatoma resection was reported. With improving survival, indications for transplantation have broadened, and transplant volume has increased. Following the introduction of cyclosporine in 1980, the number of liver transplants greatly increased because of the improved survival of recipients. A graphic example of the increase in overall transplant volume and pediatric liver transplantation is shown in Figure 43–1 (Annual Report on the U. S. Scientific Registry for Organ Transplantation and the Organ Procurement and Transplantation Network, 1988–89, 1989). At present, liver transplantation is offered to all children with progressive liver failure, regardless of age or weight.

Etiology

The disease entities leading to liver transplantation in infants and children at Children's Hospital Medical Center, Cincinnati, are summarized in Table 43–1. The table lists the most common conditions requiring transplantation.

Biliary Atresia

Infants with biliary atresia account for the majority of patients requiring pediatric liver transplantation (Ryckman et al., 1991a; Starzl et al., 1986). Within the first 60 days of life, most infants have a constellation of progressive jaundice and acholic stools. A percutaneous liver biopsy demonstrates bile duct obliteration, and ultrasonographic examination does not visualize a gallbladder. The primary use of hepatic portoenterostomy (Kasai procedure) is indicated in patients who are diagnosed in infancy. Long-term correction of liver function is achieved in approximately one third of all cases, and, although the patients require careful follow-up, transplantation may not be necessary. In the remaining children, progressive cirrhosis, portal hypertension, and nutritional failure develop, requiring liver transplantation. Vigorous institution of nutritional support is essential to maintain growth and development while sufficient hepatic function exists. Transplantation should be undertaken when growth failure develops, portal hypertensive complications occur, or the synthetic function of the liver deteriorates. Transplantation in these infants is technically more difficult because of their small size, intra-abdominal adhesions from previous operations, and frequently associated anomalies of the portal vein, hepatic artery, and inferior vena cava. In addition, malrotation or abdominal situs inversus can complicate organ placement. (See Chapter 24, Assessment and Management of Gastrointestinal Dysfunction.)

TABLE 43–1 Indications for Orthotopic Liver Transplantation in 107 Infants and Children at Children's Hospital Medical Center, Cincinnati

Diagnosis	Reduced-Sized Allografts	Whole Organ Allografts
Biliary atresia (50%)	33	20
Metabolic disease (23%)	25	0
Fulminant hepatic failure (12%)	3	9
Cirrhosis (7%)	2	6
Hepatitis (6%)	3	3
Cholestatic syndromes (3%)	1	2

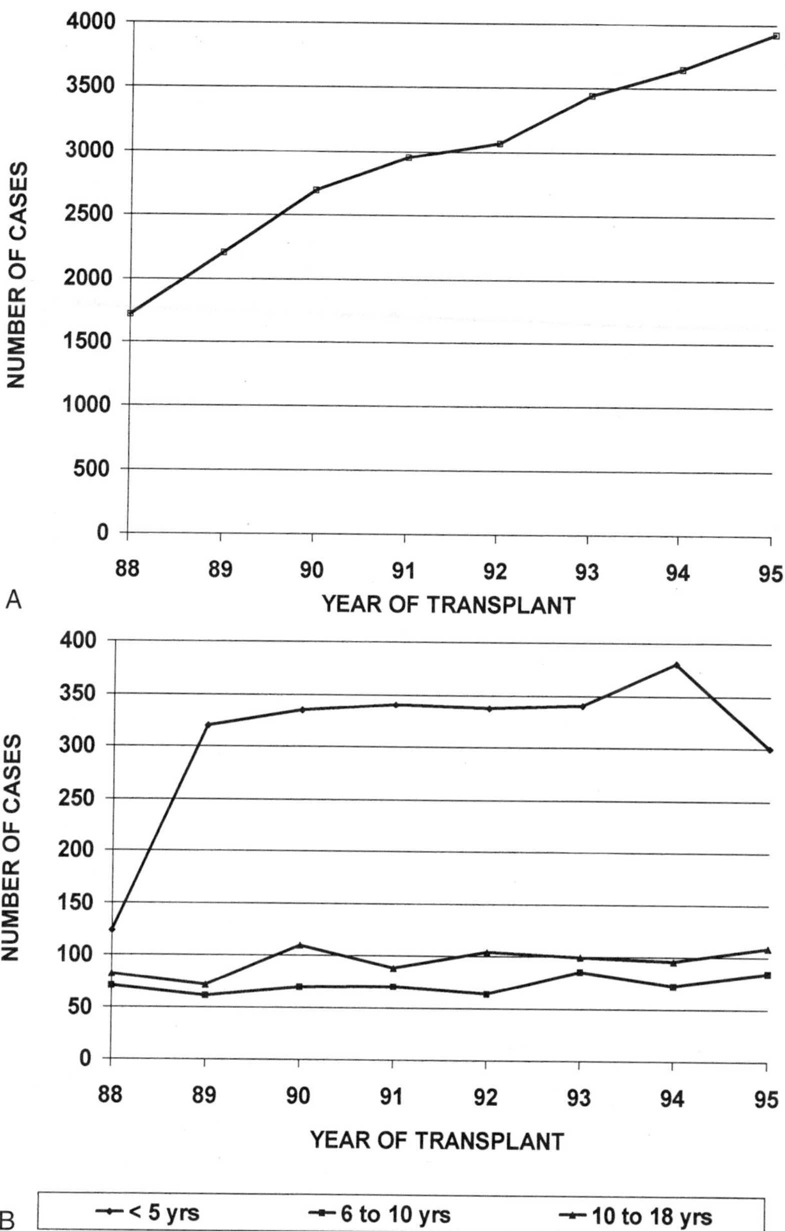

FIGURE 43–1. *A*, Overall liver transplant cases, 1988–1995. *B*, Pediatric liver transplant cases, 1988–1995.

Inborn Errors of Metabolism

Many inborn errors of metabolism have been addressed by liver transplantation. Although these errors are often diagnosed in infancy, the need for transplantation during this period is rare. α_1-Antitrypsin deficiency, Wilson's disease, tyrosinemia, glycogen storage disease, and familial hypercholesterolemia have all been significantly improved or cured by liver replacement. (See Chapter 25, Assessment and Management of Metabolic Dysfunction.) Appropriate genetic counseling is indicated when the diagnosis is made. The prognosis for these patients is good, owing to the predictability of transplantation and the patients' larger size. Inherited urea cycle abnormalities, such as ornithine transcarbamoylase deficiency, can also be cured by liver transplantation. However, careful dietary intervention to prevent irreversible central nervous system injury secondary to hyperammonemia is required in infancy. (See Chapter 26, Assessment and Management of Endocrine Dysfunction.)

Acute Hepatic Failure

Liver replacement in acute fulminant liver failure is performed more frequently in children than in infants. The primary cause may range from viral hepatitis to unrecognized metabolic disturbances. The prognosis is directly related to the primary disease and the severity of the neurologic impairment at the time of transplantation. The rapidity of hepatic failure in these patients makes pretransplant diagnosis uncommon, and their prognosis is impaired by the rapidity of disease progression and their common neurologic abnormalities.

Other Diagnoses

Familial cholestasis, chronic active hepatitis, biliary hypoplasia, cryptogenic cirrhosis, and hepatic tumors represent other indications for hepatic replacement in selected infants and children.

Pretransplant Management

The pretransplant management of infants and children with progressive end-stage liver disease is paramount in achieving later success with liver transplantation.

Selection of Candidates for Transplantation

In general, indications for transplantation in children include (1) progressive end-stage liver disease, (2) stable liver disease with a known lethality, (3) fatal hepatic-based metabolic disease, (4) metabolic disease correctable by liver cell replacement, and (5) social invalidism, or inability to participate in any social or extracurricular activities (A-Kader et al., 1991). Although specific size and age limitations do not exist, complications and technical difficulties with transplantation increase greatly in small donors and recipients. At present, transplantation is limited to infants of term gestation without other life-threatening abnormalities.

The selection of candidates for transplantation and the most appropriate allocation of available organs have been difficult issues in pediatric transplantation. Standard liver function tests do not quantitate hepatic reserve or progression. Several attempts at quantitating and stratifying infants and children have been undertaken. Malatack and associates (1987) developed a scoring system by retrospective review of 70 variables, 23 of which had prognostic significance. Patients were stratified into one of three risk groups—high, medium, or low—according to their overall score. This score was complex and, although helpful, assessed the severity of hepatic disease and its complications rather then the degree of potential hepatic reserve. Further attempts to quantitate hepatic functional reserve and predict patient deterioration using a quantitative assessment of lidocaine metabolism have been undertaken in pediatric candidates (A-Kader et al., 1989; Gremse et al., 1987; Oellereich et al., 1987; Schroeder et al., 1989). The formation of monoethylglycinexylidide (MEGX), a product of lidocaine metabolism in the liver, is decreased in proportion to the severity of the liver disease. MEGX has been shown to be predictive of hepatic function, not only in potential recipients but also in transplant donors (Schroeder et al., 1989). This test is simpler to administer and correlates well with the more complex Malatack score (Gremse et al., 1987). Quantitative stratification of the severity of liver disease in the potential recipient should allow earlier referral of patients with deteriorating hepatic status before they reach the point at which transplantation is not practical and survival is not possible. Although each of these tests is helpful in assessment of potential recipients, no single test reliably predicts hepatic reserve or impending failure.

Nutritional Support

Attention to nutritional assessment and support is particularly important. Initial assessment, height, weight, anthropometric data, and growth velocity properly establish a nutritional data base. Chronic intake and oxygen consumption measurement allows nutritional goals to be set. The goal of nutritional management should be the acquisition of positive nitrogen balance and progressive weight gain. Management of complications of liver failure, such as ascites, coagulopathy, and increased infection risks, requires meticulous coordination of fluid and dietary intake. Fat-soluble vitamins (A, D, E, and K) are administered. Early institution of nocturnal supplemental nasogastric or nasojejunal feedings is often necessary to achieve adequate caloric intake. Periodic reassessment is essential to ensure timely adjustment of the feeding schedule (Balistreri et al., 1995).

Portal Hypertension

Regardless of the primary diagnosis, the common complications of portal hypertension develop in most patients with progressive cirrhosis. These include esophageal varices, gastrointestinal hemorrhage, and hypersplenism. Esophageal varices complicated by hemorrhage are the most common manifestations of this process. Endoscopic assessment with sclerotherapy of the varices is used to treat both acute and chronic bleeding. Sequential reevaluation and repeat sclerotherapy can prevent recurrent hemorrhage while attempts at donor organ acquisition occur. Pharmacologic management of acute hemorrhage includes the administration of vasopressin and octreotide (somatostatin). The use of a Sengstaken-Blakemore tube to achieve direct balloon tamponade of bleeding varices, or transthoracic ligation of the bleeding varices, is rarely necessary. Portal azygos venous disconnection (Segura procedure) is an accepted long-term alternative when transplantation is not immediately required. Portacaval shunting should be avoided when possible in transplant candidates.

Other complications of portal hypertension such as hypersplenism and ascites can also occur. Splenic sequestration of blood components can be recognized by leukopenia, thrombocytopenia, or anemia. Most instances resolve with transplantation and resolution of the portal hypertension. When severe leukopenia (white blood cell count less than 3000) or thrombocytopenia (platelet count less than 50,000) occurs, splenectomy may be necessary at the time of transplantation. This splenectomy is rarely, if ever, necessary in infants and small children because there is an increased risk of sepsis and a likelihood of resolution following transplantation. Dietary salt restriction, caloric support, and occasional albumin supplementation in association with diuretics are used to control ascites.

Infection

Patients with end-stage liver disease are especially prone to both normal infections seen in infants and children (e.g., meningitis, otitis media, pneumonia) and infections from unique sources. Any fever or physical examination suggestive of infection requires vigorous investigation. Identification of specific organisms by blood, urine, sputum, nasal wash, or spinal fluid cultures allows directed antibiotic treatment. Paracentesis to exclude peritonitis is essential in patients with increased or newly recognized ascites, as well as in those with chronic ascites. Cholangitis is particularly common in patients with biliary tract abnormalities or biliary atresia. Direct bile cultures are rarely available, but percutaneous liver biopsy cultures often identify specific organisms in refractory cases.

Antibiotic treatment should be instituted empirically and modified according to culture and sensitivity results. The potential for rapid clinical progression in these patients necessitates hospital admission for the initiation of treatment in most cases. Antibiotic coverage to include *Staphylococcus epidermidis*, enterococcus, and gram-negative enteric organisms should be administered until culture evidence is available. Use of long-term prophylactic antibiotics promotes the development of resistant organisms and is not recommended. Prophylactic administration of hepatitis B vaccine should be undertaken. Older infants and children should receive all scheduled immunizations and polio vaccine before transplant evaluation when possible. Influenza immunizations are administered to older children but not to neonates.

Education and Psychosocial Concerns

The child and family facing liver transplantation need to acquire a significant amount of knowledge related to their disease and the transplant process, as well as integration into a complex health care system (Simon & Smith, 1992). This acquisition of knowledge is most appropriately facilitated by the efforts of a multidisciplinary transplant team, composed of medical, surgical, nursing, social service, nutritional, and hospital administrative services. Preparation of the patient and the family for transplantation optimally begins at the time of initial diagnosis and progresses throughout the transplant process. A variety of media can be used for family and age-appropriate patient education, including written materials, play therapy, and frequent, direct communication with members of the multidisciplinary transplant team. Liver transplantation disrupts the family's lifestyle and expectations and has profound financial ramifications. Therefore, anticipatory emotional, spiritual, and financial assessment of the family unit is critical and continues throughout the transplant process.

Psychiatric assessment and support of the entire family unit is highly beneficial, if not critical. Travel and extended-stay accommodation arrangements should be made in advance to minimize confusion and anxiety at the time of transplantation. Because extended preoperative hospitalization is often required in addition to the transplant procedure, financial counseling and support assistance is necessary for all patients.

Operative Procedure

The adequate preoperative preparation for liver transplantation includes provisions for significant perioperative life support. Blood bank resources, including packed red blood cells, platelets, fresh-frozen plasma, and cryoprecipitate to replace two patient blood volumes, should be available. Upper-extremity large-bore intravenous lines, central venous access, and an arterial catheter for blood gas and blood pressure measurement are necessary. An underpatient warming blanket, as well as blood and intravenous fluid warmers, assists in the difficult temperature management of small recipients. Provisions for inotropic support using dopamine, dobutamine, and epinephrine should be made. As in all complex operative procedures, extensive preoperative and intraoperative communication among the surgical, nursing, and anesthesia team is invaluable.

Critical junctures in the operative procedure occur at several intervals. Blood loss must be carefully avoided; all losses should be replaced, especially when the native diseased liver is being removed. Prior operative procedures and concurrent portal hypertension complicate this goal. When the native diseased liver is removed, hemodynamic stability often decreases because of diminished venous blood return from the lower extremities of the portal system resulting from the divided intrahepatic inferior vena cava and portal vein. This problem persists throughout the anhepatic phase (phase without the liver). Careful and extensive flushing of the transplant liver to remove hyperkalemic preservation solutions is necessary to avoid cardiac arrhythmias when circulation to the allograft is restored. After implantation, temperature must be returned to normal by vigorous warming and coagulation function reestablished by judicious administration of coagulation factors. The overall operative procedure may require 6 to 18 hours of diligent monitoring and care by the operative team. However, careful operative and anesthetic coordination allows the operative procedure to proceed without difficulty in most circumstances.

Surgical Techniques

Successful transplantation requires not only meticulous surgical technique but also appropriate donor selection and postoperative care. The surgical options available include (1) whole organ transplantation, (2) reduced-sized liver transplantation, (3) auxiliary transplantation, and (4) living related donor transplantation.

Whole Organ Transplantation

Replacement of the diseased liver with a size-matched allograft is the standard procedure for older children and adults. In infant recipients, however, an insufficient number of size-matched organs for anatomic replacement is available. Reliance on size-matched livers for transplantation led to a pretransplant waiting list mortality rate of 25 to 50 percent in many pediatric transplant centers (Broelsch et al., 1988; Ryckman et al., 1991a). When organs are available from infant donors, the long-term quality and survival of these allografts are still poor (Tan et al., 1988). When suitable size-matched donors are available, however, successful transplantation is technically possible (Fig. 43–2). Whole organ transplantation involves anatomic replacement of the liver with direct vascular reconstruction. Biliary continuity is reestablished using a Roux-en-Y hepaticojejunostomy, with an internal biliary Silastic stent being placed because of the small size or absence of the extrahepatic biliary tree in small children (Fig. 43–3). Reliance on whole organ replacement techniques does not appear to be feasible for all potential pediatric recipients because there is not a sufficient supply of adequate infant donor organs.

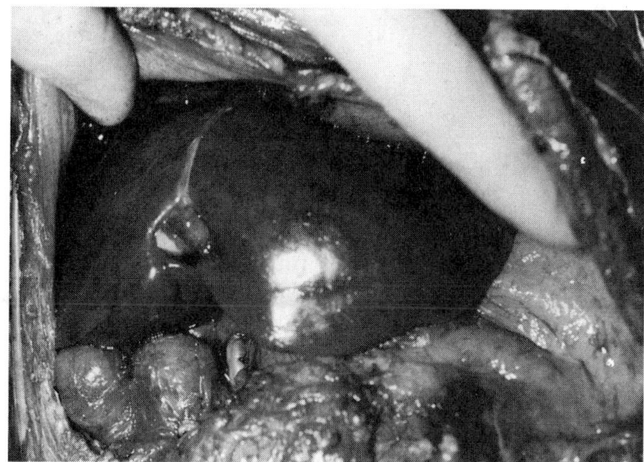

FIGURE 43–2. Five-day-old infant donor liver transplanted into a 5-kg recipient.

Reduced-Sized Liver Transplantation

Segmentation of the liver into fully functional but reduced-sized allografts has allowed liver transplantation into the smallest recipients (Bismuth & Houssin, 1984; Broelsch et al., 1988; Emond et al., 1989; Kalayoglu et al., 1989; Otte et al., 1990b; Ryckman et al., 1991a). Division along the known anatomic planes

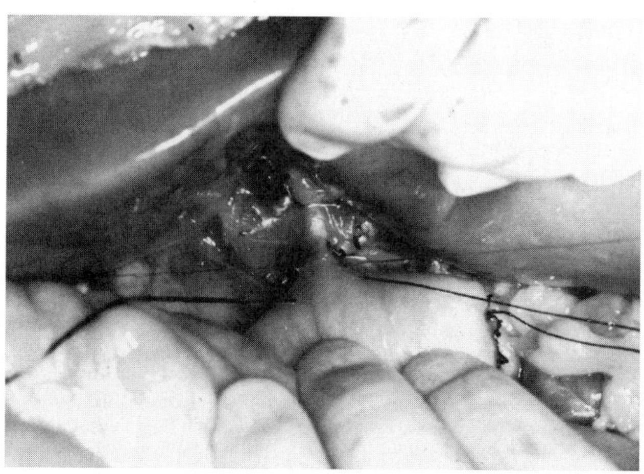

FIGURE 43–3. Placement of an internal biliary Silastic stent.

within the hepatic parenchyma allows the preparation of various-sized liver allografts from larger donor livers (Figs. 43–4 and 43–5). Donor-to-recipient weight ratios of 4:1 are possible with left lobe (segments 1 to 4) reduced-sized grafts, and 10:1 ratios are possible using the left lateral segment (segments 2 and 3). Right lobe allografts (segments 5 to 8) are less commonly used in children because there is increased thickness of the right hepatic lobe. Survival in infants receiving reduced-sized allografts is significantly improved over those receiving whole organ transplants (Ryckman et al., 1991a). This improved survival is a consequence of fewer life-threatening complications in the postoperative period, including a lower incidence of vascular thrombosis, and no increased risk of primary nonfunction or biliary complications.

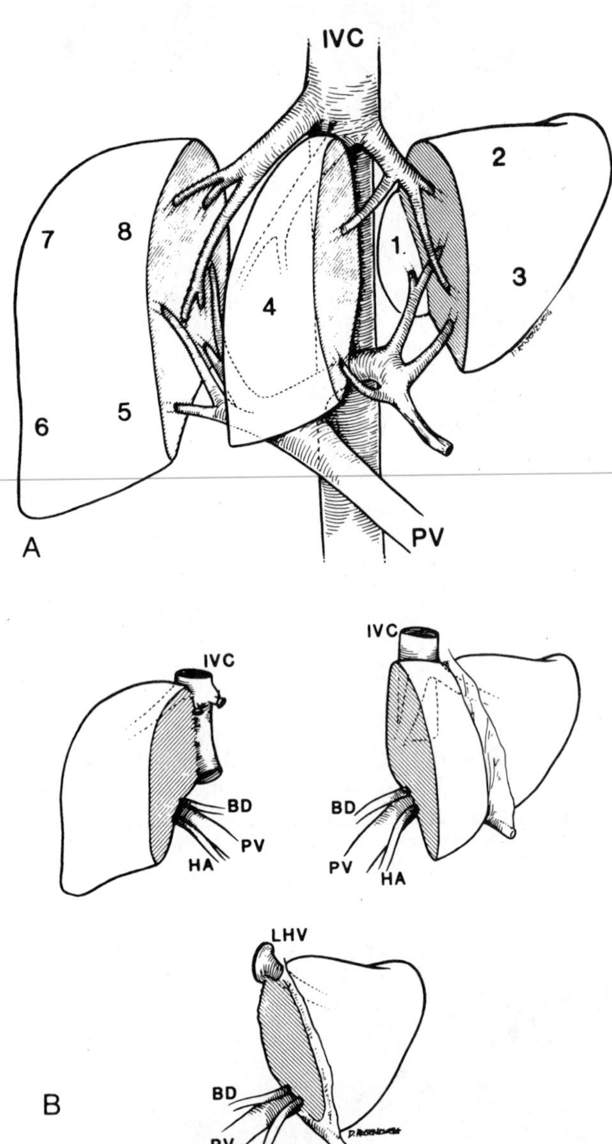

FIGURE 43–4. Segmental anatomy of the human liver. *A*, Functional allografts can be constructed from segments that have discrete vascular supply and bile drainage. *B*, In practice, the right lobe graft *(upper left)* consists of segments 5 to 8, the left lobe graft *(upper right)* of segments 1 to 4, and the left-lateral segment graft *(lower)* of segments 1 to 3. IVC, inferior vena cava; PV, portal vein; HA, hepatic artery; LHV, left hepatic vein, BD, bile duct. (From Emond, J. C., Whitington, P. F., Thistlethwaite, R., et al. [1989]. Reduced size orthotopic liver transplantation: Use in the management of children with chronic liver disease. *Hepatology, 10*[5], 867–872. Reprinted with permission.)

Split Liver Transplantation

Division of a single donor liver into two usable reduced-sized allografts has also been undertaken (Fig. 43–6) (Emond et al., 1990; Otte et al., 1990a). The results of this procedure, known as split liver grafting, are not as successful as reduced-sized allografts, but they are nearly equivalent to whole organ transplantation with respect to survival and complication rates.

Living Related Donor Transplantation

The use of living related donors for small children has also become a primary mode of transplantation for children (Fig. 43–7) (Broelsch et al., 1990). Organ and patient survival results are equivalent to those of reduced-sized transplantation. The immunologic advantages of living related donor liver transplants may decrease the overall incidence of rejection, although this is not apparent in the initial patient series. Morbidity to the donor is minimal but not absent; death of the donor is rare but possible after the donor hepatectomy.

These options are designed to increase the donor pool to meet the needs of an increasing transplant population. These innovative techniques need continued reevaluation in light of the donor-to-recipient mismatch seen in pediatrics and the progressively increasing need for donor organs.

Auxiliary Liver Transplantation

The placement of a second liver in an auxiliary position within the abdomen has been used as an option for the treatment of metabolic diseases or acute hepatic failure (Terpstra et al., 1988). In infants and small children, the lack of available intra-abdominal space to accommodate the transplanted liver mass limits this option. In older children, replacement of the left lobe of the liver using a left lateral segment allograft has successfully corrected metabolic disease without requiring total removal of the recipient's native liver (Broelsch et al., 1990). In acute hepatic failure, recovery of the native liver has been reported while function was supported by the auxiliary graft (Gubernatis et al., 1991). Further uses of this technique need to be evaluated. The use of isolated hepatocytes as cellular transplants is also currently under laboratory investigation (Hoofnagle et al., 1995; Balladur et al., 1995).

Postoperative Care

The postoperative care of the liver transplant patient does not differ from that of patients having other extensive operative procedures. Particular attention to temperature management often requires the use of overhead radiant warmers and heating blankets. Intravenous fluid support to maintain central venous pressures of 8 to 10 cm H_2O should ensure adequate perfusion. The hematocrit should be maintained at 35 percent, and a urine output of 1 to 2 ml/kg/hour is expected. Prophylactic antibiotics directed against *S. epidermidis*, enterococcus, and enteric organisms are administered preoperatively, intraoperatively, and for several postoperative doses. Antifungal and antiherpesvirus prophylaxis is also administered. Ventilatory assistance should be discontinued when adequate blood gases are maintained, organ function is documented, and fluid balance is adequate.

The function of the transplanted organ is best assessed by monitoring coagulation parameters. An increasing Factor VII level establishes hepatocellular recovery. Rapid and accurate daily

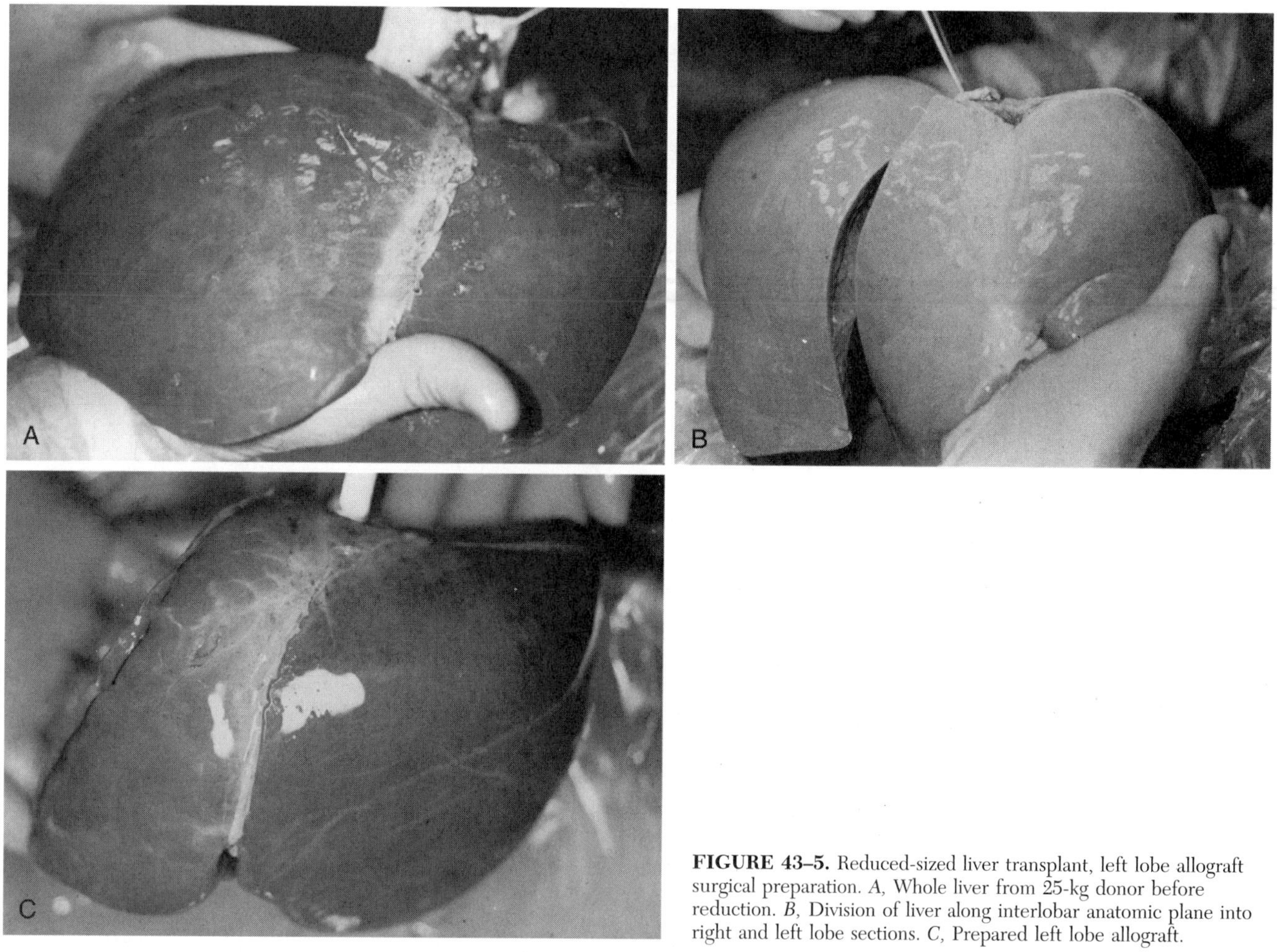

FIGURE 43–5. Reduced-sized liver transplant, left lobe allograft surgical preparation. *A*, Whole liver from 25-kg donor before reduction. *B*, Division of liver along interlobar anatomic plane into right and left lobe sections. *C*, Prepared left lobe allograft.

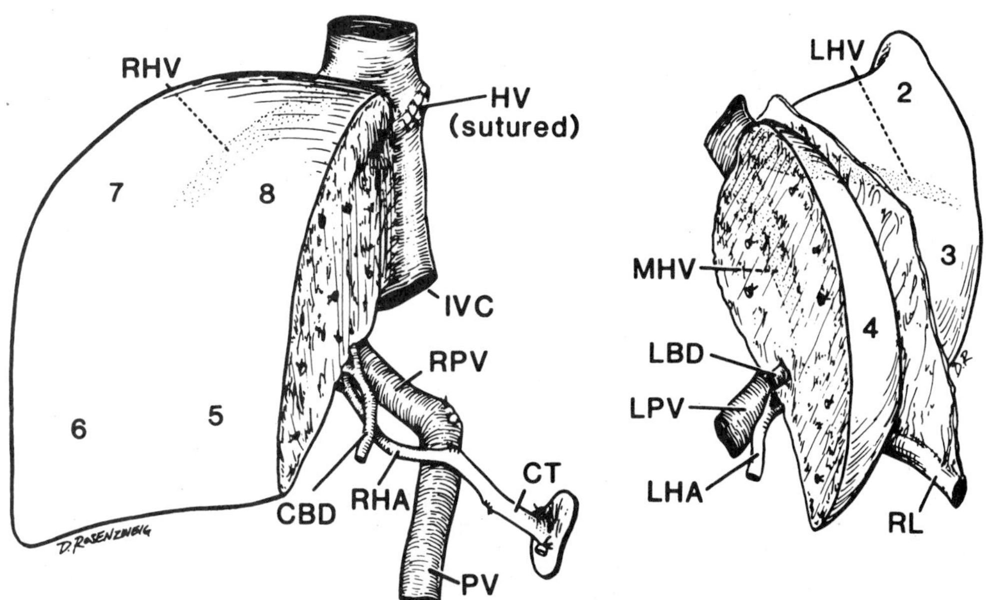

FIGURE 43–6. Diagram of two grafts after preparation from one donor liver. All the main vascular and biliary structures remain attached to the right lobe and the left lobe is supplied by lobar pedicles. IVC, inferior vena cava; PV, portal vein; CT, celiac trunk; CBD, common bile duct; HV, hepatic vein; RPV, right portal branch; RHA, right branch of the hepatic artery; RHV, right hepatic vein; RL, right lobe; LHA, left branch of the hepatic artery; LPV, left portal branch; LBD, left bile duct; LHV, left hepatic vein; MHV, middle hepatic vein. Numbers indicate hepatic segments according to Couinaud. (From Emond, J. C., Whitington, P. F., Thistlethwaite, J. R., et al. [1990]. Transplantation of two patients with one liver. Analysis of a preliminary experience with "split-liver" grafting. *Annals of Surgery, 212*[1], 14–22. Reprinted with permission.)

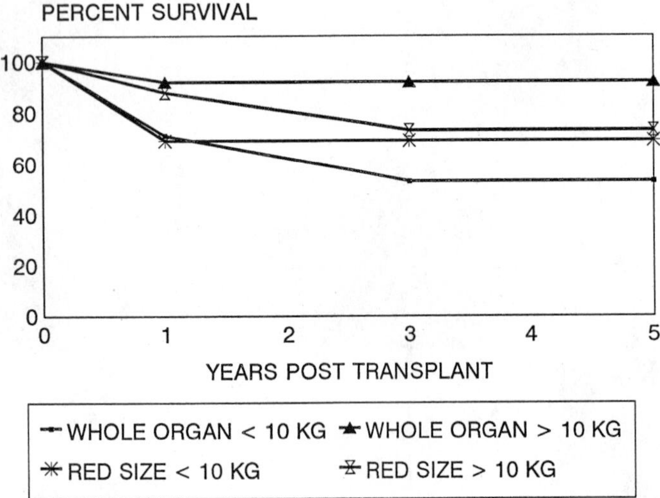

FIGURE 43–7. Liver transplant patient survival comparing whole versus reduced-sized allografts by recipient weight.

assessment of allograft blood flow can be undertaken using real-time ultrasonography at the bedside. Episodes of hypotension, acidosis, fever, or deterioration of hepatocellular enzyme or coagulation profiles require immediate and vigorous investigation.

Immunosuppressive Management

In addition to prednisone, primary immunosuppressive management in infants and children includes cyclosporine or tacrolimus. Azathioprine is used in some centers as part of a cyclosporine-based initial immunotherapy program. It is usually discontinued early in the posttransplant period. Rejection is treated with steroid pulses, steroid recycling, or the monoclonal anti–T-cell antibody muromonab-CD3 (Orthoclone OKT3). Daily monitoring of immunosuppressive medications is necessary for proper dose adjustment in infants and children in whom intestinal absorption is variable (Ryckman et al., 1991b, Starzl & Demetris, 1990; Todo et al., 1990).

Postoperative Complications

Many complications following liver transplantation are heralded by an increase in hepatocellular enzymes, often associated with malaise, fever, leukocytosis, and jaundice. This clinical picture defines hepatic allograft dysfunction, but it does not separate allograft rejection from other allograft complications such as primary nonfunction, bile duct abnormalities, hepatic artery thrombosis, or allograft infection. The use of real-time ultrasonography to assess hepatic vasculature and the use of computed tomography to assess allograft structure are often necessary. Allograft biopsy is definitive when the cause of the graft abnormality is rejection; it can strongly support the diagnosis of viral infection or cholangitis when the characteristic histologic markers and microscopic appearance occur. Definitive diagnosis of the cause of the allograft dysfunction should precede immunologic manipulation. Selected complications unique to liver transplantation are outlined in the following sections.

Primary Nonfunction

Primary nonfunction is defined as a failure of the transplant allograft to recover function despite successful operative implantation. Careful evaluation of the donor allograft, using frozen section biopsy, can assist in identifying failures associated with primary nonfunction such as allograft stenosis (Markin et al., 1993; Strasberg et al., 1994). Since the introduction of University of Wisconsin preservation solution, initial nonfunction of the transplanted allograft is uncommon. In our experience, initial nonfunction occurs in 2 percent of cases, regardless of allograft type. Hepatic allograft preservation for up to 24 hours can be accomplished; however, preservation times of less than 12 hours are associated with excellent organ function following reperfusion. When primary nonfunction occurs, rapidly increasing hepatocellular enzymes and bilirubin are accompanied by a failure of functional recovery, manifested by an uncorrectable coagulopathy. Treatment with prostaglandin E_2 has been helpful in restoring hepatocellular function in nonrandomized trials in primary nonfunction, although controlled trials to support its use have not been undertaken (Todo et al., 1990). Retransplantation is required if no functional improvement is recognized within 48 hours.

Rejection

Acute cellular rejection occurs in up to 95 percent of patients treated by conventional immunosuppressive protocols using prednisone, cyclosporine, and azathioprine (Ryckman et al., 1991b). In our experience, when sequential induction immunotherapy using Orthoclone OKT3, prednisone, and azathioprine is combined with the delayed introduction of cyclosporine, the incidence of rejection is decreased to 46 percent (Ryckman et al., 1991b; Starzl & Demetris, 1990). Rejection episodes are treated aggressively with methylprednisolone or Orthoclone OKT3 and are reversible in 95 percent of cases. Individuals failing medical therapy for rejection require retransplantation.

Bile Duct Complications

Biliary leak or stricture formation at the site of the surgical anastomosis or within the liver parenchyma can result from prolonged or incomplete ischemia preservation or from viral infection; however, these complications most often occur following hepatic artery thrombosis. Treatment is individualized and includes anastomotic revision, percutaneous dilation and internal stent placement, or retransplantation. Bile duct disruption with intrahepatic biloma formation can also occur. Adequate drainage using percutaneous techniques is necessary at the time of diagnosis to prevent the formation of an intrahepatic abscess. Resolution may occur with prolonged drainage, although allograft replacement is often required because of the extensive bile duct injury. Associated infection complications are common with all bile duct abnormalities, most often with a combination of enteral bacteria and fungal organisms. Vigorous antimicrobial treatment must accompany restoration of unobstructed bile flow (Peclet et al., 1994).

Hepatic Artery Thrombosis

Clotting within the arterial circulation of the transplanted liver occurs in approximately 15 percent of all patients, with the incidence inversely proportional to the recipient's size at the time of transplantation and the age of the liver donor (Tan et al., 1988). Early thrombosis presents with signs of fulminant hepatic failure, biliary leak or stricture, or systemic sepsis. Immediate thrombectomy is occasionally successful. When ischemia allograft damage has occurred, retransplantation is nearly always required (Langnas et al., 1991). Late thrombosis can present similarly or be silent. The incidence of arterial thrombosis is decreased in reduced-sized allografts, possibly because of the improved stability of the donor, the larger size of the arterial vasculature in these older donors, or direct implantation of the hepatic artery into the infrarenal aorta (Ryckman, et al., 1991b).

Retransplantation

In all cases of irreversible liver failure following transplantation, retransplantation is the only option allowing survival. The use of reduced-sized liver allografts has greatly improved the likelihood of a replacement allograft being located within the abbreviated time frame imposed by allograft failure. Retransplant rates of 15 percent are common in pediatric series involving small infant recipients (Ryckman et al., 1991b). Survival following retransplantation is similar to survival after primary transplantation and is directly related to the severity of illness of the recipient before operation.

Long-Term Survival of Transplantation

Survival following liver transplantation is directly related to the severity of the patient's illness before undergoing surgical therapy (Shaw et al., 1989). Despite the often serious complications regularly encountered in these individuals, the overall survival rate is rewarding. The present overall survival rate for pediatric transplantation is 67 to 88 percent (Broelsch et al., 1990; Kalayoglu et al., 1989; Ryckman et al., 1991a; Starzl et al., 1986). Improvements in immunosuppressive therapy, anesthetic and perioperative management, and innovative surgical procedures such as reduced-sized or living related liver transplantation have all improved patient survival (Broelsch et al., 1990; Emond et al., 1989; Kalayoglu et al., 1989; Ryckman et al., 1991a, 1991b). Survival has historically been diminished by the following factors: (1) small patient size and weight, (2) previous extensive operative procedures, and (3) the disease severity of the recipient at the time of transplantation (see Fig. 43–7). Improved preoperative care, careful donor selection, the use of innovative technical procedures, and evolving immunosuppressive management promise further increases in recipient survival.

Improved survival of infants and children following transplantation has allowed health care professionals to focus on the overall goals of complete rehabilitation with appropriate growth and development, social reintegration, enhanced self-esteem, and improved quality of life (Stewart et al., 1989). Recent advances in posttransplant management have been directed at minimizing complications related to immunosuppression, enhancing growth velocity, and promoting normalcy and lifestyle improvement (Sokal, 1995). Increased energy and motor dexterity, decreased number of medications and hospitalizations, success in school, and attainment of satisfying peer relationships have been seen in our pediatric liver transplant population, as well as in other centers, and these attributes have contributed to the perception of an improved quality of life (Chin et al., 1991).

After transplantation, establishment of a satisfactory lifestyle should remain as important a goal as patient survival. At present, all of our surviving recipients have returned to a normal lifestyle for their age and have shown satisfactory developmental progress consistent with their age and developmental status before transplantation. This experience has been seen in other centers as well (Zitelli et al., 1987).

RENAL TRANSPLANTATION IN INFANTS AND CHILDREN

From the vast strides achieved through extensive experience with older children and adults, renal transplantation in infants and children has become an increasing reality. Recent advances in the techniques of dialysis and the management of end-stage renal disease (ESRD) in infants have allowed many patients with complex urologic or hereditary abnormalities to reach the age and size at which transplantation is possible. These advances have allowed the implementation of renal transplantation along with dialysis as a complementary treatment modality in the care of infants with irreversible renal dysfunction.

Etiology

Acute renal failure in infants is most often the consequence of hemodynamic instability, hypoxia, or malperfusion, resulting in acute tubular necrosis. Most of these infants either recover sufficient function for normal long-term survival or die of multisystem failure. Chronic renal failure is also uncommon in infants, with the estimate of infants with ESRD at 0.2 per million total population for infants younger than 1 year of age (Fine, 1984; Potter et al., 1980). Congenital nephrosis, dysplasia–hypoplasia, and other anatomic abnormalities associated with complex urogenital malformations are the most common causes of ESRD in infants. In children younger than 5 years of age with glomerulonephritis, 46 percent have a congenital cause for ESRD. Lupus nephritis and recurrent pyelonephritis, which are more common in older patients, are uncommon causes of ESRD in the infant. Hereditary causes of renal failure are important to identify to plan appropriate overall treatment strategy; evaluating other family members and providing genetic counseling when needed must also be considered. Appropriate identification of the cause of the ESRD also allows assessment of the potential for recurrence within a transplant allograft and consideration of living related donor transplantation.

Pretransplant Management

The present management of infants with renal failure has improved significantly with an increased understanding of fluid and electrolyte management and the introduction of dialysis techniques suitable for the small infant. These advances, coupled with improvements in infant nutritional support and medical management, allow extended survival for the infant with ESRD.

Dialysis

Dialysis is indicated in infants, as in older children, if complications of medical management of ESRD occur, namely, hyperkalemia, volume overload, acidosis, intractable hypertension, and uremic symptoms such as vomiting. In addition, dialysis may be necessary to allow the administration of adequate protein as part of an extensive nutritional resuscitation plan. However, there is no requirement that dialysis be undertaken before transplantation in infants or children. In the North American Pediatric Renal Transplant Cooperative Study (NAPRTCS), 22 percent of children underwent transplantation without previous dialysis (McEnery et al., 1992). If dialysis is undertaken, the use of peritoneal dialysis is preferred for the following reasons: (1) it avoids multiple transfusions associated with hemodialysis, (2) it allows smoother gradual correction of electrolyte abnormalities, preventing cerebral disequilibrium syndrome in small infants, and (3) its administration is easier. Hemodialysis can be used in infants with an unsuitable peritoneal cavity or with peritoneal infections; however, the construction and maintenance of adequate vascular access in small infants and children are difficult. Use of centralized venous catheters rather than arteriovenous fistulas is our preferred mode for hemodialysis access in small children, although infection and vascular clotting difficulties complicate this therapy.

Nutritional Support

The need for vigorous nutritional support of the infant with uremia has been supported by the well-documented growth retardation seen in infants and children with ESRD. The cause of growth disturbance is multifactorial, including both protein and calorie insufficiency, renal osteodystrophy, aluminum toxicity, acidosis, impaired somatomedin activity, and insulin resistance. Because the most intense period of growth occurs during the first 2 years of life, careful nutritional support during that time is essential. Despite extensive nutritional efforts, the mean height for all patients at the time of transplantation was 2.2 standard deviations (SD) below the appropriate age- and sex-adjusted mean for normal children in the recent NAPRTCS study. This growth deficit was greater (−2.8 SD) in children younger than 5 years of age. Transplantation afforded a +0.8 SD increase in growth over the first posttransplant year; however, this accelerated growth then reached a stable plateau. After 2 to 3 years, the mean weight values were comparable to those in normal children (McEnery et al., 1992). If epiphyseal closure has occurred, additional bone growth (bone age older than 12 years) is often not achieved (Fine, 1984; Grushkin & Fine, 1973). Normalization of growth rarely occurs with the introduction of either hemodialysis or peritoneal dialysis.

The importance of efforts to normalize nutritional parameters is emphasized by the adverse impact of uremia on the developing nervous system in the infant. The significance of the problem was emphasized in the study by Rotundo and colleagues (1982), in which progressive encephalopathy, developmental delay, microcephaly, hypotonia, seizures, and dyskinesia developed in 20 of 23 children younger than 1 year of age with ESRD. All of these patients had significant growth impairment. Monitoring of the head circumference has been suggested to identify the infant at risk, with the intent to initiate dialysis, nutritional support, or transplantation if this parameter deviates from the normal curve (Fine, 1984).

Transplant Management

Preoperative Evaluation

In addition to the nutritional parameters described, an extensive evaluation of the urinary tract and immunologic status of the patient is necessary before transplantation.

The increased frequency of urinary tract abnormalities as the primary cause of ESRD in infants and children necessitates the investigation of the urinary tract for sites of obstruction, the presence of ureteral reflux, and the functional state and capacity of the urinary bladder (Najarian et al., 1986). This investigation is best accomplished by obtaining an intravenous pyelogram or ultrasonogram to evaluate the upper urinary tract, and a voiding cystourethrogram to assess bladder and reflux parameters. Any questions related to bladder function or structure require cystometry and cystoscopy. In infants with long-standing oliguric ESRD, the bladder capacity may appear very small. In the absence of abnormal obstructive or neuromuscular bladder pathology, adequate enlargement of the bladder in the face of normal urinary production is to be expected. Any surgical correction of urethral obstruction or augmentation of bladder size should be undertaken far in advance of undertaking transplantation. Preoperative sterilization of the urinary tract and development of unobstructed urinary outflow should be the ultimate goals of evaluation and reconstruction. Although complex anomalies of the urogenital tract often require many extensive operative procedures to augment, reconstruct, or create an acceptable lower urinary tract, virtually all children with such anomalies can undergo successful reconstruction with continent urinary reservoirs without the use of intestinal conduits (Sheldon et al., 1994).

Immunologic assessment includes tissue typing and panel reactive antibody analysis. Patients should be monitored periodically for the development of a positive crossmatch to their potential donor or the development of positive cytotoxic antibody to a panel of random donors to assess immunologic reactivity. In addition, reactivity to cytomegalovirus, Epstein-Barr virus, herpes simplex virus, and hepatitis should be investigated. Childhood immunizations should be current, and immunization against the hepatitis B virus should be instituted when indicated. Any immunizations with live virus vaccines should be given well in advance of transplantation, because their use is contraindicated in the early posttransplant period.

Selection of the appropriate donor source for transplantation is a decision for the transplant team and family to consider together. A living related donor kidney from an immediate family member has the advantage of a low incidence of postoperative acute tubular necrosis; improved histologic matching, leading to fewer rejection episodes and the need for less immunosuppression; and the possibility of extended organ function. In addition, the operative procedures required for preparation, as well as the transplant procedure, can be scheduled around the needs of the patient, simplifying preoperative care and potentially avoiding the complications of dialysis. Parents form the majority of donors; siblings younger than 18 years of age are not considered. At present, 43 percent of children receive a living related donor kidney. Cadaveric kidneys are successfully transplanted in infants and children, with improved results when sequential immunotherapy and cyclosporine or tacrolimus is used (Najarian et al., 1990). The unpredictability of donor organ availability and the need to establish a negative antibody crossmatch for cadaver transplantation make surgical planning more difficult. The size of the allograft, cadaveric or living related, is of importance. Adult kidneys from small-sized donors can be transplanted into infants weighing as little as 5 kg with good technical success (Turcotte et al., 1988). Cadaveric organs from pediatric donors older than 4 years of age are most appropriate and should be preferentially used in pediatric recipients when possible. However, a progressive decrease in 1-year graft survival has been observed when kidneys from donors younger than 3 years of age have been used (Ildstad et al., 1990). This decrease in graft and patient survival is related to the donor organ source, because infants and children younger than 5 years old who receive organs from older children and adults enjoy similar survival to the overall pediatric population using living related donors (Kim et al., 1991; McEnery et al., 1992). Caution should be exercised when using donors younger than 3 years of age until the factors responsible for this decreased graft survival are defined. The decision to use a cadaveric donor is often strengthened by the likelihood of disease recurrence within the transplanted kidney. In small infants, a cadaveric kidney may be recommended for short-term improvement, with the use of a living related donor reserved for the later expected growth needs of the developing child, when the larger kidney can be more easily implanted.

Operative Procedure

Preparation for transplantation should include the placement of adequate large-bore intravenous lines and the largest Foley catheter possible. Central venous lines are used in all infants and children to ensure vascular access and a route for postoperative immunosuppressive delivery. Perioperative prophylactic antibiotics are administered.

Transplantation in infants and small children can be undertaken through a generous retroperitoneal approach or transabdominal placing of the allograft within the peritoneal cavity posterior to the right or left colon. Retroperitoneal placement allows the maintenance of postoperative peritoneal dialysis and should be strongly considered with cadaveric allografts when size permits. The arterial anastomosis should be to the distal aorta using a Carrel patch, and venous outflow of the allograft should be to the inferior vena cava or common iliac vein (Fig. 43–8). Ureteral implantation using the Lich external ureteroneocystostomy avoids the presence of a cystotomy and minimizes postoperative blood clots within the bladder, which may obstruct the Foley catheter.

Anesthetic management of the infant and small child during both liver and kidney transplantation is complex. Intravascular blood volume must be augmented during allograft implantation to allow restoration of flow to the kidney without sudden sequestration of blood in the allograft, precipitating hypotension. In addition, blood sequestered in the lower extremities during caval and aortic occlusion is acidotic and hyperkalemic. Efforts to remove the hyperkalemic graft preservation solution before implantation are necessary to avoid massive potassium infusion with reconstitution of allograft perfusion. Blood volume loading to a central venous pressure of 13 to 15 cm H_2O and administration of bicarbonate, calcium, and insulin–glucose mixtures can be necessary. Vasopressors (dopamine, dobutamine, epinephrine) should be immediately available in the operating room.

Postoperative Management

Fluid and electrolyte monitoring every 15 to 30 minutes is necessary immediately after transplantation, because adult kidneys can excrete the equivalent of the infant's blood volume within a single hour. Careful attention to serum concentrations of calcium, phosphorus, and magnesium in addition to electrolytes is necessary. Glucose-free urine replacement fluids minimize hyperglycemia and attendant osmotic diuresis in the recipient. Maintenance of catheter patency is essential, and any episode of decreased urinary output should be rapidly investigated to exclude Foley catheter occlusion and bladder distention.

Immunosuppression

Many immunosuppressive regimens are available and all share similar strategy (Turcotte et al., 1988). Our present preference is sequential immunotherapy using antilymphocyte globulin, azathioprine, and steroids at the time of transplantation, with the introduction of cyclosporine following demonstration of stable renal function. Maintenance immunotherapy uses cyclosporine, azathioprine, and steroids. By using multiple agents, it is hoped that steroid dosing can be minimized and growth parameters maximized in infants and children. Overall, half of all transplant recipients have a bout of rejection within 2 months of transplantation. Factors that increase the likelihood of rejection or long-term graft loss include the use of cadaveric donors rather than living related donors, receiving a kidney from a donor younger than 5 years of age, allowing the kidney to be more than 24 hours in cold storage, black race, and delayed graft function from acute tubular necrosis. Overall, 54 percent of rejection episodes were reversed, 38 percent were partially reversed, and 8 percent ended in graft failure. Success in treating rejection declines with each successive rejection episode (McEnery et al., 1992). Rejection episodes are treated with steroid administration or monoclonal anti–T-cell agents such as Orthoclone OKT3. As with liver transplantation, tacrolimus can be used in place of cyclosporine, and in conjunction with steroids.

Posttransplant Management

Posttransplant management requires careful screening for rejection and recurrence of the primary renal disease, as well

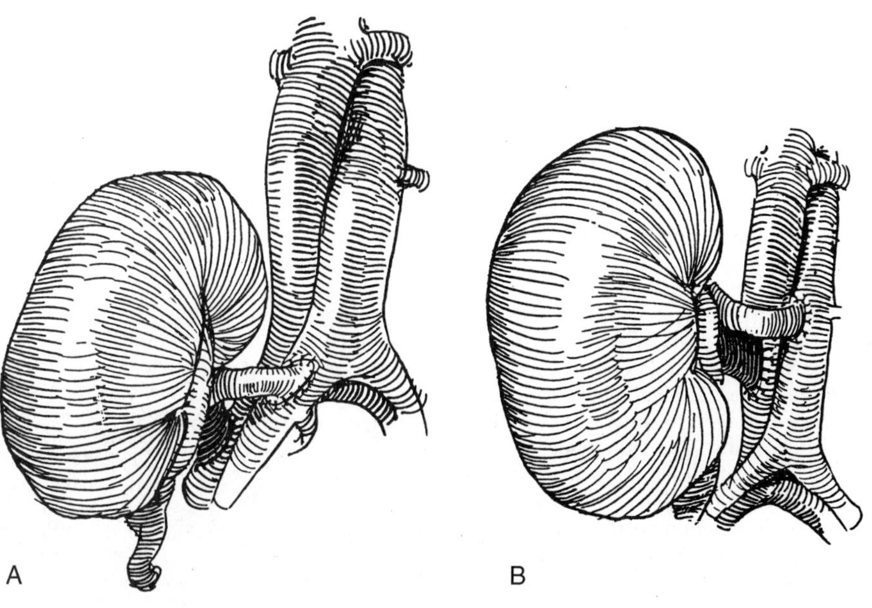

FIGURE 43–8. Renal transplant anatomy in pediatric recipients. *A*, Renal artery and vein implanted into the recipient's iliac vessels. *B*, Renal artery and vein implanted into the recipient's aorta and vena cava. (Modified from Flye, M. W. [1995]. *Atlas of Organ Transplantation* [p. 113]. Philadelphia: W. B. Saunders.)

as prevention of immunosuppression-related complications. Any preexisting hypertension is augmented by the immunosuppressive drugs cyclosporine, tacrolimus, and prednisone. Careful attention to the pretransplant control of hypertension and dietary management improves posttransplant management. Antihypertensive control is especially important to preserve all possible renal function when using small allografts in infants. Development of hypertension more than 3 months after transplantation suggests the possibility of renal artery stenosis and warrants ultrasonographic Doppler flow studies and arteriography in questionable cases. Transluminal angioplasty has been successful in managing most of these cases when recognized; surgical correction is reserved for angioplasty failures.

Most long-term complications are related to infection and occur within the first 6 posttransplant months. During this time, immunosuppression is greater and susceptibility to life-threatening infection is increased. The use of organs from donors who have had prior exposure to cytomegalovirus and Epstein-Barr virus in infants and children who are seronegative enhances the risk of these specific infections. Expanded use of antiviral prophylaxis using ganciclovir and acyclovir has decreased the intensity of these infections as well as their associated morbidity or mortality. Trimethoprim-sulfamethoxazole is used for *Pneumocystis carinii* pneumonia prophylaxis as well.

Chronic steroid toxicity presenting as posterior subcapsular cataracts, excessive weight gain, hyperlipidemia, or aseptic necrosis of the bone must be carefully sought and treated.

Results of Renal Transplantation

The overall results of renal transplantation in children are similar to those in adults. Overall, 1-year transplant graft survival rates of 88 to 100 percent have been reported for living related allografts, with results for cadaveric allografts being 50 to 72 percent (Fine, 1984; Flye, 1989; Ildstad et al., 1989; Turcotte et al., 1988). In the recent NAPRTCS report, 1- and 3-year survival rates were 74 and 62, respectively, with cadaveric donors and 89 and 80 percent, respectively, with living related donors. In the living related donor recipient who was younger than 1 year of age at transplantation, a 71 percent 2-year graft survival rate was achieved (McEnery et al., 1992). These optimistic results further strengthen the need for rapid transplantation in children with ESRD to avoid the secondary growth and developmental consequences.

ORGAN PROCUREMENT

A problem common to all types of transplantation is donor organ availability. This problem is intensified in small pediatric recipients by a relative maldistribution of donors and recipients, with the most common pediatric organ donor being in midchildhood to teenage years. This problem is most significant in liver, heart, and lung transplant recipients for whom the donor organ must be a special size, that is, matched to the size of the removed diseased organ.

Organ procurement and distribution are monitored and managed through the United Network for Organ Sharing (UNOS), a congressionally mandated organization. Computer-generated scoring systems take into account tissue or blood type matching, organ size, disease severity, and donor location to direct distribution of allografts. Ultimate donor organ selection and acceptance are the responsibilities of the transplant team.

Operative removal of the donor organ is undertaken by a surgical team composed of specialists in multiple organ harvest and preservation. Multiple organs, including heart, lung, liver, pancreas, kidneys, and intestine, can all be sequentially harvested from a single donor using hypothermic preservation techniques. Other tissue grafts, such as cornea, skin, bone, heart valves, and tendons, can be removed after the solid perfused organs are successfully removed. Organs are preserved using simple hypothermic sterile packaging for transport to the recipient's transplant center. Preservation times have been significantly prolonged by the University of Wisconsin preservation solution, with cold ischemic preservation times exceeding 48 hours for kidney allografts, 18 hours for liver allografts, and 24 hours for pancreas allografts. Heart and heart–lung preservation times remain limited to 4 to 6 hours.

The present success of transplantation has led to a vast discrepancy between donor organ availability and the rapidly increasing recipient waiting lists. Only through increased donor organ acquisition, achieved by creative surgical options and improved professional and community education, can the goals and success of pediatric transplantation be offered to all needy potential recipients.

CONCLUSION

Transplantation offers the possibility of relief from the complications of end-stage liver and renal failure in infants and small children. However, these procedures treat the primary disease only at the cost of the potential complications of long-term immunosuppressive treatment. Only through the development of new and innovative transplant techniques and through further research in the mechanisms of transplant tolerance can the hope for safe and successful transplantation become reality for all patients with end-stage organ failure.

REFERENCES

A-Kader, H. H., Ryckman, F. C., & Balistreri, W. F. (1991). Liver transplantation in the pediatric population: Indications and monitoring. *Clinical Transplant, 5,* 161.

A-Kader, H. H., Schroeder, T. J., & Balistreri, W. F. (1989). Lidocaine metabolism: A quantitative liver function test in children. *Hepatology, 10,* 616.

Annual Report on the U. S. Scientific Registry for Organ Transplantation and the Organ Procurement and Transplantation Network (1988–89). (1989). Richmond, VA: United Network for Organ Sharing.

Balistreri, W. F., Bucuvalas, J. C., & Ryckman, F. C. (1995). *The effect of immunosuppression on growth and development.* Presented at the American Association for the Study of Liver Disease, Chicago, IL, November, 1995.

Balladur, P., Crema, E., Honiger, J., et al. (1995). Transplantation of allogenic hepatocytes without immunosuppression: Long-term survival. *Surgery, 117*(2), 189–194.

Bismuth, H., & Houssin, D. (1984). Reduced sized orthotopic liver graft in hepatic transplantation in children. *Surgery, 95*(3), 367–370.

Broelsch, C. E., Emond, J. C., Thistlethwaite, J. R., et al. (1988). Liver transplantation, including the concept of reduced-size liver transplants in children. *Annals of Surgery, 208*(4), 410–420.

Broelsch, C. E., Emond, J. C., Whitington, P. F., et al. (1990). Application of reduced-size liver transplants as split grafts, auxiliary orthotopic grafts, and living related segmental transplants. *Annals of Surgery, 212*(3), 368–377.

Chin, S. E., Shepherd, R. W., Cleghorn, G. J., et al. (1991). Survival growth and quality of life in children after liver transplantation: A 5 year experience. *Journal of Pediatrics and Child Health, 27*(6), 300–305.

Emond, J. C., Whitington, P. F., Thistlethwaite, J. R., et al. (1989). Reduced size orthotopic liver transplantation: Use in the management of children with chronic liver disease. *Hepatology, 10*(5), 867–872.

Emond, J. C., Whitington, P. F., Thistlethwaite, J. R., et al. (1990). Transplantation of two patients with one liver. Analysis of a preliminary experience with "split-liver" grafting. *Annals of Surgery, 212*(1), 14–22.

Fine, R. N. (1984). Renal transplantation in children. In P. J. Morris (Ed.), *Kidney transplantation: Principles and practice* (2nd ed., pp. 509–546). Orlando, FL: Grune & Stratton.

Flye, M. W. (1989). Renal transplantation. In E. Wickland (Ed.), *Principles of organ transplantation* (pp. 264–293). Philadelphia: W. B. Saunders.

Gremse, D. A., Schroeder, T. J., & Balistreri, W. F. (1987). Lidocaine metabolism: A quantitative assessment of liver function in children. *Pediatric Research, 25,* 114.

Grushkin, C. M., & Fine, R. N. (1973). Growth in children following renal transplantation. *American Journal of Diseases of Children, 125*(4), 514–516.

Gubernatis, G., Pichlmayr, R., Kemnitz, J., & Gratz, K. (1991). Auxiliary partial orthotopic liver transplantation (APOLT) for fulminant hepatic failure: First successful case history. *World Journal of Surgery, 15*(5), 660–666.

Hoofnagle, J. H., Carithers, R. J., Jr., Shapiro, C., & Ascher, N. (1995). Fulminant hepatic failure: Summary of a workshop [Review]. *Hepatology, 21*(1), *240–252.*

Ildstad, S. T., Tollerud, D. J., Noseworthy, J., et al. (1990). The influence of donor age on graft survival in renal transplantation. *Journal of Pediatric Surgery, 25*(1), 134–139.

Ildstad, S. T., Tollerud, D. J., Noseworthy, J., et al. (1989). Renal transplantation in pediatric recipients. *Transplant Proceedings, 21*(1, Part 2), 1936–1937.

Kalayoglu, M., Stratta, R. J., Sollinger, H. W., et al. (1989). Liver transplantation in infants and children. *Journal of Pediatric Surgery, 24*(1), 70–76.

Kim, M. S., Jabs, K., & Harmon, W. E. (1991). Long-term patient survival in a pediatric renal transplantation program. *Transplantation, 51,* 413–417.

Langnas, A. N., Marujo, W., Stratta, R. J., Wood, et al. (1991). Hepatic allograft rescue following arterial thrombosis. Role of urgent revascularization. *Transplantation, 51*(1), 86–90.

Malatack, J. J., Schaid, D. J., Urbach, A. H., et al. (1987). Choosing a pediatric recipient for orthotopic liver transplantation. *Journal of Pediatrics, 111*(4), 479–489.

Markin, R. S., Wisecarver, J. L., Radio, S. J., et al. (1993). Frozen section evaluation of donor livers before transplantation. *Transplantation, 56*(6), 1403–1409.

McEnery, P. T., Stablein, D. M., Arbus, G., & Tejani, A. (1992). Renal transplantation in children: A report of the North American Pediatric Renal Transplant Cooperative Study. *The New England Journal of Medicine, 326*(26), 1727–1732.

Najarian, J. S., Ascher, N. L., & Mauer, S. M. (1986). Kidney transplantation. In K. J. Welch, J. G. Randolph, M. M. Ravitch, et al. (Eds.), *Pediatric surgery* (4th ed., pp. 360–373). Chicago: Year Book Medical Publishers.

Najarian, J. S., Frey, D. J., Matas, A. J., et al. (1990). Annual Meeting of the American Surgical Association, Washington, DC.

Oellereich, M., Raude, E., Burdelski, M., et al. (1987). Monoethylglycinexylidide formation kinetics: A novel approach to assessment of liver function. *Journal of Clinical Chemistry and Clinical Biochemistry, 25*(12), 845–853.

Otte, J. B., de Ville de Goyet, J., Alberti, D., et al. (1990a). The concept and technique of the split liver in clinical transplantation. *Surgery, 107*(6), 605–612.

Otte, J. B., de Ville de Goyet, J., Sokal, E., et al. (1990b). Size reduction of the donor liver is a safe way to alleviate the shortage of size-matched organs in pediatric liver transplantation. *Annals of Surgery, 211*(2), 146–157.

Peclet, M. H., Ryckman, F. C., Pedersen, S. H., et al. (1994). The spectrum of bile duct complications in pediatric liver transplantation. *Journal of Pediatric Surgery, 29*(2), 214–220.

Potter, D. E., Holliday, M. A., Piel, C. F., et al. (1980). Treatment of end-stage renal disease in children: A 15 year experience. *Kidney International, 18*(1), 103–109.

Rotundo, A., Nevins, T. E., Lipton, M., et al. (1982). Progressive encephalopathy in children with chronic renal insufficiency in infancy. *Kidney International, 21*(3), 486–491.

Ryckman, F. C., Flake, A. W., Fisher, R. A., et al. (1991a). Segmental orthotopic hepatic transplantation as a means to improve patient survival and diminish waiting list mortality. *Journal of Pediatric Surgery, 26*(4), 422–428.

Ryckman, F. C., Schroeder, T. J., Pedersen, S. H., et al. (1991b). The use of monoclonal immunosuppressive therapy in pediatric renal and liver transplantation. *Clinical Transplantation, 5,* 189.

Schroeder, T. J., Gremse, D. A., Mansour, M. E., et al. (1989). Lidocaine metabolism as an indicator of liver function in hepatic transplant donors and recipients. *Transplant Proceedings, 21*(1, Part 2), 2299–2301.

Shaw, B. W., Starzl, T. E., Iwatsuki, S., & Gordon, R. D. (1989). An overview of orthotopic transplantation of the liver. In E. Wickland (Ed.), *Principles of organ transplantation* (pp. 347–363). Philadelphia: W. B. Saunders.

Sheldon, C. A., Gonzalez, R., Burns, M. W., et al. (1994). Renal transplantation into the dysfunctional bladder: The role of adjunctive bladder reconstruction. *Journal of Urology, 152*(3), 972–975.

Simon, N. B., & Smith, D. (1992). Living with chronic pediatric liver disease: The parents' experience. *Pediatric Nursing, 18*(5), 453–458.

Sokal, E. M. (1995). Quality of life after orthotopic liver transplantation in children. An overview of physical, psychological and social outcome [Review]. *European Journal of Pediatrics, 154*(3), 171–175.

Starzl, T. E., & Demetris, A. J. (1990). Liver transplantation. A 31-year perspective: Part III. In S. A. Wells, Jr. (Ed.), *Current problems in surgery* (pp. 183–240). Chicago: Year Book Medical Publishers.

Starzl, T. E., Iwatsuki, S., & Shaw, B. W. (1986). Liver transplantation. In K. J. Welch, J. G. Randolph, M. Ravitch, et al. (Eds.), *Pediatric surgery* (4th ed., pp. 373–382). Chicago: Year Book Medical Publishers.

Stewart, S. M., Uauy, R., Waller, D. A., et al. (1989). Mental and motor development, social competence, and growth one year after successful pediatric liver transplantation. *Journal of Pediatrics, 114*(3), 547–581.

Strasberg, S. M., Howard, T. K., Molmenti, E. P., & Herti, M. (1994). Selecting the donor liver: Risk factors for poor function after orthotopic liver transplantation [Review]. *Hepatology, 20*(4, Part 1), 829–838.

Tan, K. C., Yandza, T., de Hemptinne, B., et al. (1988). Hepatic artery thrombosis in pediatric liver transplantation. *Journal of Pediatric Surgery, 23*(10), 927–930.

Terpstra, O. T., Schalm, S. W., Weimar, W., et al. (1988). Auxiliary partial liver transplantation for end-stage chronic liver disease. *New England Journal of Medicine, 319*(23), 1507–1511.

Todo, S., Fung, J. J., Starzl, T. E., et al. (1990). Liver, kidney, and thoracic organ transplantation under FK 506. *Annals of Surgery, 212*(3), 295–307.

Turcotte, J. G., Campbell, D. A., Dafoe, D. C., et al. (1988). Pediatric renal transplantation. In G. J. Cerilli (Ed.), *Organ transplantation and replacement* (pp. 349–360). Philadelphia: J. B. Lippincott.

Zitelli, B. J., Gartner, J. C., Malatack, J. J., et al. (1987). Pediatric liver transplantation: Patient evaluation and selection, infections, complications, and life style after transplantation. *Transplant Proceedings, 19*(4), 3309–3316.

CHAPTER 44

Iatrogenic Complications of the Neonatal Intensive Care Unit

LINDA LEFRAK

The word *iatrogenic* is derived from the Greek words *iatros*, meaning physician, and *genesis*, meaning origin. The current definition of this word has been broadened to include complications related to therapeutic treatments and routine care interventions. This chapter takes this definition a step further and addresses the role of nursing in the arena of iatrogenic complications.

The neonatal intensive care unit (NICU) provides a close and unique collaboration between medicine and nursing, thus placing the nurse in a position to contribute to the complications of diagnostic and therapeutic interventions as well as to detect and prevent them. This chapter reviews iatrogenic events in the history of newborn care and reviews the nursing practices and techniques that most contribute to iatrogenic complications of newborn care. It also presents a program for reduction and prevention of iatrogenic error as it relates to the delivery of medical orders and nursing care.

HISTORICAL PERSPECTIVE

The historical complications of care are grouped into six categories: (1) false assumptions, (2) long-term consequences, (3) "if a little is good, a lot is better," (4) equipment–therapy interactions, (5) social-environmental issues, and (6) limited clinical trials. Many of the present-day iatrogenic complications can be categorized in the same way, which may guide the clinician in the evaluation of new therapies and practices.

False Assumptions

Two classic examples of practice based on false assumptions include the management of fluids in preterm infants in the 1950s and the use of castor oil in the delivery room during the same period. The first assumption made was that infants born prematurely were puffy and therefore had too much total body fluid. The treatment at the time of birth was to withhold all fluids to reduce the edema. This led to dehydration and hypoglycemia, the latter of which most likely was undiagnosed. The second practice involved the administration of 1 teaspoon of castor oil by mouth in the delivery room. It helped evacuate meconium from the bowel rapidly, which was assumed to be advantageous to the infant. Aspiration of the castor oil was a risk.

To some extent, assumptions continue to guide practice and should be acknowledged as such. Practice based on assumption should receive close monitoring, and, if complications occur, the practice should be systematically reviewed using the continuous quality assurance/continuous quality improvement (CQA/CQI) process.

Long-Term Consequences of Care

Long-term consequences of care are seen in the practice of irradiation of the thymus gland in the 1930s and 1940s. This practice was almost routine in some newborn nurseries and was thought to reduce the incidence of sudden infant death syndrome. In many of these infants, cancer of the thyroid gland developed in adult life as a consequence of the newborn therapy. Concern over long-term complications has greatly affected the introduction of all new therapies in the NICU during the past 30 years and has pushed the clinician to design long-term follow-up studies. Phototherapy, diagnostic ultrasonography, total parenteral nutrition, and postnatal steroid use were all approached cautiously because of concern over long-term consequences. In some cases, these therapies were not used because of widespread questions about future complications.

If a Little Is Good, a Lot Is Better

If a little is good, a lot is better is a premise that has plagued the field of neonatal care. The classic example occurred in the 1940s, when the use of vitamin K to prevent hemorrhagic disease of the newborn was modified from a small dose to a dose 10 times larger. The higher dose, 10 mg, led to red blood cell destruction, resulting in hemolysis, hyperbilirubinemia, and, in some cases, kernicterus.

Equipment–Therapy Interactions

A classic example of equipment–therapy interactions occurred with the introduction of better-constructed incubators in the 1950s and 1960s. The reduction of leaks in incubators allowed a higher oxygen concentration to be achieved via the back of the unit. Although this may have improved outcome in some infants with respiratory distress syndrome, it led to an increase in the incidence of retinopathy of prematurity (ROP). The introduction of new equipment and supplies into the NICU setting continues to bring about unforeseen complications.

Social-Environmental Issues

One of the first complications related to a social policy occurred as a result of visitation rules in most nurseries before the mid-1970s. NICUs and premature nurseries prohibited parental visitation until immediately before the infant's discharge. This practice was thought to reduce the risk of hospital-acquired infection in the neonate. The complications of this practice included absent or inadequate parent–infant attachment and subsequent failure to thrive, abuse, and neglect. This practice took a swing in the 1980s, when unlimited visitation by parents and grandparents, as well as sibling visitation, became the standard in many NICUs. With this acknowledgment of the need to address the family unit during a time of crisis came the adverse exposure of the neonate to viral and bacterial infections from visitors. Most recently, the resurgence of chicken pox, measles, and tuberculosis has led to the need for isolation of exposed infants and, hence, the complications of another social change that was not readily anticipated.

The NICU environment—namely, noise, light, and social interaction—has also been cited in many recent studies as a cause of neonatal complications (Long et al., 1980; Rushton, 1986). Problems ranging from intermittent hypoxia to hearing loss are being reported as they directly relate to the properties of the NICU environment.

Limited Clinical Trials

The limited clinical trials category includes complications resulting from practices that have been tested on a limited number of infants and then reported to be successful. The issues of safety and potential risk of the practice are often not addressed in the published research. More commonly, the complications become evident only in the hands of the clinician when the practice is instituted. Complications then become evident in a particular unit when the practice gains widespread use. As the saying goes, "If you haven't seen complications yet, then you haven't done enough." One recent example of this category was the introduction in the late 1970s of a specialized formula for low birth weight infants. After the formula had been used for a period, reports began to surface about the formation of lactobezoars in these infants. The lactobezoar formed in the gastrointestinal tract of premature infants and created large, hard curds that, in serious cases, had to be surgically removed. When formula manufacturers changed to whey-predominant premature formula, the problem of lactobezoars was essentially eliminated (Tsang & Nichols, 1988). This bezoar formation was a direct result of intolerance to the formula ingredients by some premature infants.

The introduction of a specialized formula for the low birth weight infant is routinely preceded by clinical trials by the manufacturer. The number of infants in these clinical trials varies, but, until the 1980s, was limited to as few as 20 physiologically stable premature infants. Although complications may not occur in the 20 infants, when the formula is marketed, widespread use can uncover problems not anticipated by the manufacturer or clinician. Some of the complications are directly related to the immaturity and illness of the infant. The infants used in most clinical trials are physiologically stable and tend to be approximately 32 weeks' gestation or greater. The safe use in a sick infant of 26 weeks' gestation is not established. The issue of complications related to infant formulas is not a new one and will most likely continue until formulas are tested and approved as drugs instead of as nutritional products. Although formulas are indeed nutritional products, their potential for serious adverse effects in infants is unquestionable (Jelliffe, 1977).

A second example of limited clinical trials occurred when physicians began to use vancomycin in the early 1980s. Several authors published articles on the pharmacology of the drug and its efficacy against resistant organisms. Schaad and colleagues (1980), in particular, presented data on the pharmacokinetics of vancomycin in the pediatric population. This article clearly stated the ages and weights of the infants in the study and the dosing regimen based on age and gestation. Because of the serious problems with oxacillin-resistant *Staphylococcus epidermidis* infection in the NICU, clinicians were forced to use these suggested doses even in infants much smaller and more premature. Although these doses may have been a logical starting point, the subsequent reports on morbidity related to the use of vancomycin clearly illustrated that they were excessive, and, in fact, the dosing and monitoring of this drug in the NICU are still in a state of flux. The ethical constraints and serious limitations of extensive clinical trials on premature and term infants leave the clinician in a role of weighing the risks and benefits of most new therapies. It also places a burden on nurses and physicians because any new therapy used after limited clinical trials has the potential to cause great harm in some infants.

Summary

In summary, it is essential that the nurse practicing in the NICU be aware of historical aspects of neonatal care. This information should be incorporated into the core curriculum of newly hired nursing staff. The history of failures can only assist in the evaluation of new therapy. It is also essential that nurses consider themselves to be as responsible for therapy evaluation as physicians. Because nurses administer the therapy in many cases and are the constant attendants at the bedside, they are uniquely capable of recognizing unexpected outcomes. It is naive to assume that what nurses do as ordered by physicians is safe. As a professional team member, a nurse must be alert to unintended adverse outcomes in all care delivery.

CURRENT ISSUES IN NEONATAL INTENSIVE CARE

The issues discussed in this section include therapy and practice, equipment evaluation and use, supply evaluation and use, medication administration, and infection control.

Therapy and Practice

The technical and scientific advances that have occurred in the past 30 years have not only improved survival and outcome for infants born prematurely and sick but also placed clinicians, both nurses and physicians, in a role that they could not have anticipated. The potential adverse side effects of advances can readily be appreciated from the great number of MEDLINE citations for iatrogenic disease. As reported by McClead and Menke (1987), 4000 articles have been published since 1966 on iatrogenic disease in all categories. The numbers have been steadily increasing. A search of the literature on newborn iatrogenic complications reveals hundreds of articles (McClead & Menke, 1987). The reports are categorized into five basic areas: (1) medical progress, (2) "new" or "quasi-experimental" modalities, (3) unproven or not fully tested therapies, (4) iatrogenesis imperfecta, and (5) simple human error (McClead & Menke, 1987). The following are therapy and practice categories that more directly relate to the practice of nursing:

1. Nursing practice based on tradition or routine
2. Bandwagon approach
3. Knee-jerk reaction to isolated or rare morbidity
4. Staff and systems problems, including staff skill and knowledge, systems problems, workload and staffing, and human error

Nursing Practice Based on Tradition or Routine

Nursing practice based on tradition or routine involves the complications of a practice that is routine owing to years of tradition and comfort but that is not necessarily backed by scientifically conducted evaluation. The typical defense of routine is,

"We ought not to be overanxious to encourage innovation, in cases of doubtful improvement, for an old system must ever have two advantages over a new one: it is established and it is understood" (Colton in McClead & Menke, 1987). If nurses are systematically going to reduce errors related to their practice, those practices over which they have the most domain must be evaluated. The process involves listing all routine therapy and practice that nurses control or influence and deciding on a priority for evaluation. Evaluation varies based on the practice that is being examined and should include a review of all unusual incidents that have some relation to the practice. For example, if nurses secure central venous catheters in a particular manner and the catheters become dislodged through no fault of the patient, then the securing routine should be questioned.

If no such reports are normally generated, a specific form or audit mechanism should be developed and tested. An example of such an evaluation mechanism is a device security routine, such as for securing central venous lines or endotracheal tubes (ETTs). In many units, nurses are solely responsible for the initial taping and stabilization of the ETT as well as for its ongoing maintenance. If accidental extubation is not considered an unusual incident, then reviewing reports are not helpful. Evaluation requires a form. Evaluation is ideally preceded by literature review and by computer or telephone survey to determine what is published about the practice and to gain as much information as possible. The evaluation may be labor intensive, but groundwork helps determine whether there are data to support a particular practice before another is evaluated. Other examples of nursing routines that could be evaluated for iatrogenic complications include the following:

- All methods of device security, including securing intravenous lines, chest tubes, feeding tubes, and oxygen cannulas
- Skin care practices, including bathing practices, wound management, and application of all topical agents that nurses use without a physician's order
- Intravenous line insertion
- Suctioning procedures
- Medication delivery
- Feeding techniques
- Sample (body fluid) collection
- Positioning

The National Center for Nursing Research (1989) has declared some of these areas a priority for nursing investigation in the care of the low birth weight infant. The potential studies of complications related to these nursing practice topics are numerous and should be as much a priority as the control trials of medical therapy modalities. There is a need, however, for nurses to continue to work on the evaluation of their own practice and not to use all of their resources for the evaluation of medical practice. A sample evaluation form is shown in Figure 44–1; it was developed to look at variables related to securing and monitoring peripheral intravenous devices. This form can be used as a before-and-after tool to assist in problem identification or to look at any change in practice. It can be used randomly, as with an audit, or as a follow-up to a problem, such as after Wydase therapy for an infiltrate. The CQA/CQI literature should be used to assist in the development of methods to evaluate nursing practice. There are many ways to address problem identification and resolution, the key ingredients being that problem reporting is simple and, if necessary, solicited and that review is timely and, in most cases, intradisciplinary. For samples of such programs, refer to *Quality Assurance, A Complete Guite to Effective Programs* (Meisenheimer, 1985).

Bandwagon Approach

Complications of the "bandwagon approach" occur when a practice is rapidly introduced in a new setting. It is most commonly seen when a reputable medical or nursing journal reports what is believed to be a dramatic therapeutic breakthrough. The published study rarely includes any discussion of the technical complications encountered by nursing in the unit where it was studied. An example occurred when the *New England Journal of Medicine* published the study by Hittner and colleagues (1981) showing a reduction of ROP in premature infants who received an oral dose of vitamin E. This practice was hurriedly introduced in many NICUs. Nurses began to observe the limitations of the therapy: sick, very immature infants often did not tolerate the oral solution of vitamin E. The medication often stayed in the stomach or was vomited. Some infants demonstrated complications after vomiting the medication.

To reduce the complications from rapidly introduced therapy, nurses must take an active role. Nurses need to ask pertinent questions related to nursing practice and seek nursing information from units where the practice was initially researched or the practice has existed for a period of time. Telephone communication is often invaluable, and such networking must be encouraged and continued. If there is no information about the nursing implications of the therapy, a prospective approach must be undertaken. This should include communication with staff about the practice, an interpretation of research findings, and a critique of results. The critique should include a discussion of the number and type of patients that the therapy was tried on, the outcome, and the unanswered questions. The introduction of the therapy should be preceded by a stated concern that this is a new therapy and that complications may occur. Many new or inexperienced staff nurses assume that if they encounter a problem during the delivery of care that it is due to their own lack of knowledge or experience and not the fault of the therapy. They must be encouraged to report all complications and must be given a mechanism to facilitate reporting. At my institution's nursery, the use of electronic mail (E-mail) has dramatically improved reporting of complications. Nurses who previously did not generate a hard copy of an incident find it easier to send a rapid one- to two-sentence report encouraging an in-depth investigation of a particular problem.

Reaction to Isolated Morbidity (Knee-Jerk Response)

The third category of complications occurs when nursing practice is restricted because there was an event of isolated morbidity; for example, nurses may not be allowed to pass nasogastric tubes because of a historical event in which there was a serious complication. The "knee-jerk" reaction was to take the practice out of the nursing arena. Yet, if physicians are not available to pass a nasogastric tube on a distended infant, there is potential for vomiting and aspiration, or, if the infant has necrotizing enterocolitis, perforation could occur while waiting for the tube to be passed. In some units, nurses are not allowed to give certain medications by intravenous push because of actual or potential concerns about iatrogenic effects of the therapy. If the medication is not given in a timely manner because no physician is available, then the practice leads to repeated adverse outcomes in the name of reducing adverse outcomes.

All nursing units should look at their written or unwritten rules about what nurses can and cannot do. It should be determined whether the practice is considered standard nursing practice and is supported by the state Nurse Practice Act. Nurses should then openly discuss which of these rules may cause more complications than they were meant to avoid. Even though some of these rules were written by the nursing professionals, they may be so outdated that current evaluation is essential.

IV INFILTRATES

DRAFT #3

DATE ________ PATIENT NAME ________________________ MR#________

WEIGHT ________________ GESTATION ________________________

TYPE OF DEVICE ____

LOCATION IN PATIENT ____

TYPE OF INFUSATE (INCLUDE ADDITIVES) ____

____

RATE OF IV ____

WAS DEVICE SECURED PER PROTOCOL? ________________ IF NO, WHY? AND HOW? ________________

INCLUDE DRAWING IF HELPFUL:

MD/RN NOTIFIED OF OCCURRENCE

TIME NOTIFIED ____

WAS WYDASE USED? ____

LIST ALL OTHER PERTINENT FACTORS: MEDICATION, INFUSING, BLOOD, PRODUCT INFUSING, ETC. ________________

____

____

____

NAME OF PERSON COMPLETING AUDIT ____

PATIENT OUTCOME ____

____

FOLLOW-UP ____

____

____

____

COST OF OCCURRENCE ____

FIGURE 44–1. CQA/CQI audit problem identification form.

Staff and Systems Problems

The staff and systems problems category includes several factors that can be grouped together as errors that result in complications owing to actual nursing practice. These errors result from the following:

- Lack of skill
- Lack of knowledge
- Workload and staffing problems
- Systems problems
- Simple human error

Unusual occurrence reports can be reviewed with these categories in mind and, ideally, classified by incident to allow for systematic review, evaluation, and resolution. Errors that fall into the categories of skill and knowledge deficits should be aggressively addressed by the educators in the clinical area. Addressing the deficit may require an addition to the core curriculum for newly hired nurses, an in-service education offering, or, in some cases, a program for an individual nurse. Other skill and knowledge errors need to be addressed by improving resources for the nurses. This might be as simple as making available a user's manual with a new piece of equipment. Using the concept of competencies in nursing practice has improved management's ability to focus on particular staff practices (Britton et al., 1995).

All factors that contribute to an error must be considered to ensure that the solution is complete and comprehensive. The nurses reviewing the monthly or weekly unusual incident reports may have differing opinions about what is a serious error, and a definition should be written to help assist in the prioritization of review. The factors that contribute to unusual incidents may not be obvious, and the nurse reviewer may need to seek out the consultation of others, including those immediately involved, to assess accurately all of the factors that led to the complication. An example of such an evaluation follows.

A report was filed by a nurse about a 10-fold overdose of oral furosemide (Lasix) solution. The error met the definition of *serious* because of the consequence to the patient and cost of laboratory tests to follow up the electrolyte replacement therapy. The factor of nursing practice that contributed to the event was knowledge deficit—the nurse did not know the safe dose when questioned. The systems factors were the following:

1. The pharmacy was sending two dilutions of oral furosemide to allow for various doses to be given in small volumes.
2. There was no available reference in the clinical area for the nurse to look up the safe dose.

Human error is probably the most difficult to reduce. Human or careless errors can be made by staff at every level (Folli et al., 1987). Senior, experienced nurses are not exempt from making errors of this nature. One way to assist in the reduction of human error is to inform staff about mistakes that have been made by others. To accomplish this, managers and CQA/CQI committee members must share information about errors. This process educates and alerts staff about the prevalence and the range of errors that can occur. This requires sensitivity to the individuals involved. Staff members should be told that part of the CQA/CQI process is to keep staff informed about complications related to the delivery of nursing care. This philosophy should be presented during orientation to the clinical setting. With each occurrence, nurses should be told about the plan to communicate the information to the staff and they should be assured of their confidentiality beforehand. Nurses need to know that other nurses make mistakes and that experience does not exempt one from making errors. Sharing experiences of human error can often prevent similar errors from being made. An example of how this can work follows.

In a systematic review of unusual incidents in a particular NICU, it was determined that one to two times a month an infant had an iatrogenic blood loss because of a disconnected portion of an intravenous infusion system. When nurses reviewed the type of devices that led to this complication, they learned how to practice in a preventive manner. The review showed that the majority of blood loss occurred on peripheral intravenous lines. It was also noted in the review that in each case the disconnect had occurred at a junction where the connection was not made with a Luer-Lok. The nursing practice at the time required Luer-Lok only on arterial lines and central venous catheters. However, infants can lose significant amounts of blood from peripheral intravenous lines, and routine Luer-Lok connections are always preferred. This systematic review, coupled with a staff notification program, reduced this category of complication in the months following the notification process. The results came about through a change in practice after a problem identification.

The Joint Commission on Accreditation of Healthcare Organizations (JCAHO) standards support and require this type of process in all clinical areas. Through systematic problem review, "the loop" of CQA/CQI can be closed and errors of a similar nature can be dramatically reduced.

Equipment Evaluation and Use

According to Golonka (1986), "the traditional expectation about nursing practice] is that the nurse cares for the psychological and physiologic needs of the patient." Nurses must also regulate and monitor the equipment within the patient's environment, record the effects of devices on the patient, recognize and report equipment malfunction, and often do initial trouble-shooting if a device is not performing correctly (Golonka, 1986). Although these duties are evident in the NICU, there is little formal education provided for nurses on the use of either simple or sophisticated biomedical equipment. Many nurses consider the bedside equipment as a necessary evil to contend with instead of as a potential contributor to adverse patient outcome if not operated or interpreted properly. The lack of education for nurses in this area is compounded by several factors, including (1) inadequate on-the-job instruction, (2) inadequate in-service time for newly introduced equipment, (3) lack of input in the evaluation process for equipment purchases, (4) proliferation of medical device companies with a short and often poor track record for quality control, (5) variable biomedical engineering support, and (6) no systematic recall mechanism for defective devices. On the basis of these factors, nurses should take an active role in the area of equipment use. If a product evaluation committee exists, nurses should be represented in this forum, and at least one nurse representative should attend from the NICU. Once a piece of equipment has been selected for evaluation, nurses should again take an active role in the development of an evaluation tool, determining the amount of time needed for evaluation, the number of devices in need of evaluation, and the in-service requirement for the initial evaluation time. At my institution, one person is responsible for soliciting evaluations from staff. These are needed in adequate numbers for problems to be identified during the trial phase. We have also expanded trial phases to span several months if an item is not used daily, to allow for enough experience by which to decide.

In November 1991, the Safe Medical Devices Act became law. This law requires health care facilities to report information that "reasonably suggests" the probability that a medical device caused or contributed to the death, serious injury, or serious illness of a patient in that facility. At my institution, we view this law in a broad sense, making such reports when there has been patient harm related to small supplies, such as a stopcock, as well as those that occur related to large equipment, such as a pulse oximeter. The nurse is responsible for completing the Unusual Occurrence Report, including device number, serial number, or lot number, and the remainder of the report is completed by biomedical engineering personnel. The facility has 10 working days to complete the report. All nursing units should familiarize themselves with their own reporting mechanism related to this law. While viewed as burdensome by some practitioners, others are relieved to not have to shoulder the burden of direct complaints to the product manufacturer who may not respond in a timely or appropriate manner. The law also provides a mechanism to look at user problems throughout the country and to identify product problems that may not be evident in an individual nursery. The information is only as good as that which is received, however, and reports should include all information that assists in review at a federal level.

If nurses have sole responsibility for the introduction of certain kinds of equipment, two steps can smooth the process of evaluation. The first step is to ask a series of standard questions of all sales representatives before deciding on a device to evaluate. The second step is to create a "critical function" list for any device before evaluation. The standard questions should include the following:

1. How long has your company been in business?
2. How long have you been manufacturing this product?
3. Who currently uses the product? Please provide names and telephone numbers.
4. Are all of the instructional materials currently available for the product?
5. Is all of the clinical trial information available, including what is in print and what was done for product testing?
6. What kind of technical assistance comes with the purchase?
7. How much time can you make available for staff education on the use of the product?

Reputable medical device companies have answers to these questions and should be able to supply potential users with all of this information. The manufacturer should also provide printed information on clinical trials and names of professionals involved in those evaluations. If the manufacturer is vague or has minimal printed materials and is hesitant to supply more, the nurse should strongly consider looking at another product. Vague references to equipment used in "large East Coast hospitals" should be ignored without hard evidence that this is indeed the case. Once these questions have been satisfactorily answered, an evaluation form should be developed. The form should take into consideration all of the information that the staff have determined is critical to the function of the device. Such a form may exist, or there may be another form that can be adapted for a specific equipment evaluation. The development of an evaluation form is best done in collaboration with the medical staff, biomedical engineering personnel, and the bedside nurse. Nurses are often the most capable of stating the essential components for the form based on desired operation of the device and the patient needs. If the device is used by members of another discipline, such as respiratory therapists, their input is also essential. An example of how the process works follows.

A unit determines a need to purchase a new intravenous infusion pump. The nursing staff is asked to assist in evaluation after a product has been selected for trial. The manufacturer of the infusion pump has answered the initial screening questions in a satisfactory manner. A core group of staff members is then selected to develop an evaluation tool based on a list of the essential components they need to infuse intravenous solutions safely. Staff members should be asked to choose and list essential components for the functioning and safety of any new piece of equipment before equipment evaluation. This step saves time and money. It is a learning experience, in that essential functions of medical devices may not be clear to all staff members, and it is a method of obtaining consensus on the function of a piece of equipment. Infusion pump criteria selected for an evaluation might include the following:

- Ability to detect air
- Continuous flow capability
- Ability to deliver from 0.1 to 100 ml/hour
- Inclusion of occlusion alarms
- Measurement and display of pounds per square inch required for infusion
- Presence of a bottle-empty alarm
- Presence of a keep-open mode
- Inclusion of a mechanism to infuse a preset volume over a period of time
- Provision of a cumulative reading of volume infused

If the criteria are established before meeting with the sales representative, then selection time is reduced. When the evaluation tool is complete, it accompanies each device into the unit for evaluation. A product evaluation coordinator collects the evaluation tools and collates the pertinent information. When a problem occurs, the product evaluation coordinator arranges a meeting with the sales representative. If the problem is serious, the product should be pulled from the clinical area until a resolution occurs.

Equipment evaluations are difficult because the device must be interfaced with as many clinical situations and users as possible in a defined period of time. If as many users as possible handle the equipment, its sturdiness is tested and user error that may need future attention during staff education is identified. Most busy NICUs are hard on equipment, and, if an item breaks or is damaged during a relatively short evaluation period, it most likely will not withstand months of continuous use.

Evaluation tests require time, and any major purchase should have a trial period of 1 to 3 months or more when possible. Whereas most busy NICUs with a large staff provide the ultimate test of a product's durability and its vulnerability to user error, smaller units should ask for a longer evaluation time. If this is not possible, they should solicit information from other users to assist in their evaluations. Too short an evaluation period may lead to the purchase of a product that does not perform in a safe and reliable way over time.

Once a piece of equipment is determined to be satisfactory, a final consultation with biomedical engineering staff should precede the purchase. At this time, the preventive maintenance and repair options must be determined and the user manuals should be reviewed for completeness of instruction. The formal introduction into the unit needs to include a mechanism of instruction for all personnel and a written policy and procedure on how to use the device.

Many new medical devices are purchased and placed in the clinical setting with little or no information on their safe use. For example, when pulse oximetry devices were introduced into NICUs several years ago, many nurses and physicians had little or no working knowledge of how to respond to oxygen saturation changes in monitored infants. Policy and procedures related to this instrument would have reduced user error, but they often were not put into place until months or years after product introduction. Although all of the procedural needs related to a piece of equipment may not be clear at the time of introduction, it is essential that they be considered by nursing and medical staff before purchase. Using other professional users as a resource can often assist in this process, and the individual unit can modify the procedure as necessary after firsthand experience. As clinical experience improves the safe use of the product, it should be incorporated into written equipment procedures and revised at least annually. A compilation of user manuals left in a central location is helpful as a supplement to nursing procedures.

Problem Reporting

Problem reporting for equipment failures or malfunctions should be a clear process in all NICUs. Nurses must have a form that is easy to use. Managers should work with biomedical engineering personnel to review equipment malfunction reports to ensure that they are filled out completely. Forms that say "doesn't work" should be discouraged, and the staff should provide complete documentation on the nature of the malfunction to assist in the repair.

Nurses should be taught that marketed equipment is subject to malfunction or failure and that, as responsible clinicians, they must be alert to this possibility. Although nurses may lack the knowledge to sort through all of the technical issues of an equipment failure, they must ensure that when a piece of equipment is malfunctioning, it is sent to the biomedical engineering department for immediate review. This procedure, which should be written by nurses, should be clearly outlined and include the following:

- How to generate a report when equipment malfunctions or fails
- Where to place the equipment so that it is not returned to the patient care area
- How to provide information to the nurse if user error was involved
- How to arrange for equipment rental until repair can be accomplished

The removal and tracking of malfunctioning equipment need not be done by a nurse, but the original report must be completed by a nurse to provide the repair department with as much clinical information as possible to expedite the process. Nurses who fail to complete this information or to facilitate removal of a piece of malfunctioning equipment are potentially contributing to adverse patient outcome. Again, the Safe Medical Devices Act requires that this be done, and the use of E-mail can facilitate the process of information review both to the biomedical engineering department and to the rest of the NICU staff.

The Safe Medical Devices Act of 1990 requires users to report medical device problems that may have contributed to patient injury. The law requires hospitals to report problems to: Food and Drug Administration, Center for Devices and Radiological Health, MDR User Report, P. O. Box 3002, Rockville, MD, 20847-3002.

Reviews of medical equipment failure by Bassen (1986) show that malfunctions of devices are primarily caused by the following: design flaws, defective production processes, user error caused by misuse on the patient, and user error caused by improper maintenance or calibration. Bassen also points out that environmental factors can lead to malfunction and adverse patient reaction. Bassen's review can be used as a reference for those who need a systematic approach to these technologic problems.

In some cases, it is not always clear why equipment fails or malfunctions. When thorough investigation does not uncover the cause, other action must be taken. Interdisciplinary meetings may be held to discuss all of the potential causes of the problem, and similar devices may need to be removed from the area until additional information can be obtained. An alert to nurses and physicians should be posted to inform them of the potential problem and directing them to observe for similar incidents with similar equipment. This process is time-consuming. A protocol should be worked out by a unit-based CQA/CQI committee and not be left to chance. The responsible individuals should be identified and given the time to pursue the matter to completion. Such an investment of time is needed to reduce the potential for serious patient injury and institutional liability.

A recent example of such a process is when an intravenous infusion pump overinfused a solution. The pump was immediately removed from the clinical setting, and an equipment malfunction form was completed by the bedside nurse that included all of the details about how the pump was set to infuse. The pump was examined by the biomedical engineering department and found to be in perfect working condition. It was returned to the unit, but an alert to nurses was posted. Within 1 week, four more incidents occurred, triggering a meeting of staff to discuss other causes. After some time, it was discovered that the manufacturer of the syringes used in the pumps had recently changed the mold for a certain size syringe. The new mold produced a syringe that behaved in a way that was no longer compatible with the infusion pump. The pump was not the problem; the syringes were the problem. Until the mold problem could be solved, an alternate syringe had to be purchased and the pumps reprogrammed to accommodate the new syringe. If prompt action had not been taken and additional overinfusions had occurred, the users would have been found negligent. It was also clear from this incident that the level of expertise needed to sort through the issues was beyond the scope of most hospitals; therefore, it is essential that NICU staff know what resources are available for this type of incident. During such incidents, it is also helpful to note the response of the manufacturer. Companies that do not immediately send a representative to assist fully in the process of discovery should not be considered in future equipment purchases. Responsible manufacturers have a record of cooperation in product investigation and recall.

Finally, it is essential that clinicians be alerted to the possible adverse interaction of new devices in their individual environments. Any new device has the potential to interact adversely with another piece of equipment in an unexpected way and lead to an adverse reaction. Noise, light, humidity, and electrical properties are all areas that may adversely interact. An example of the potential for unexpected interaction includes the effect of intense light on certain ventilator disconnect alarms. Although the alarms work dependably most of the time, they can be triggered when under direct light. Nurses and respiratory therapists prevent the false alarm by protecting that part of the ventilator from direct light when it is needed at the patient bedside. Another example includes the electrical interference with cardiorespiratory monitors by certain types of recordings brought in by families for infants' bedsides. It is best to keep a high index of suspicion when a new medical device or other less technical device is introduced, not only for problems not detected during the evaluation period, but also for unusual and unexpected interactions with other devices or a particular physical environment.

Supply Evaluation and Use

Although equipment purchases are usually preceded by a systematic evaluation, many items costing less than $200 are introduced in the NICU with little or no evaluation. In some cases, they are supplies that materials management personnel substitute for established products if they are less expensive or if the original supply is back ordered. The complications related to the use of medical supplies can be as serious as those related to equipment malfunction in the NICU.

Supplies that warrant a critical evaluation should include all devices that enter the body or connect to the body, such as the following:

- Intravenous catheters
- Intravenous tubing
- Stopcocks
- T-connectors
- Adhesives
- ETTs
- Suction catheters
- Feeding tubes
- Chest tubes

These items are manufactured by dozens of medical supply companies, many of which lack experience in the field. Owing to the large number of manufacturers, quality control, technologic back-up, and clinical trials may be inadequate and lack depth. Businesses have also been forced in the past decade to cut production costs, and many nurses report a general decline in the grade of plastic used and an increase in the number of defective devices found at the time the order is received. Evaluation and ongoing inspection of these products should be similar to the process used for equipment purchases. A committee or group of individuals representing the various disciplines should regularly meet to discuss new products or changes in manufacturers. There should be a predetermined process by which any supply is selected and subsequently evaluated. Changes in the product can also occur when companies change hands or there is some other "transparent" change in the manufacturing. A factor insignificant to the company may lead to patient harm in the hand of the user. Materials management personnel should be involved in this process and should know that substitution cannot be made without clearance by key individuals on the medical team or the entire committee. Evaluation forms should exist or be modified for all new supplies; a lengthy evaluation period is essential to detect as many problems as possible.

It is also helpful to have the users determine the critical qualities that the product must meet before an evaluation is begun. For example, when evaluating a supply item such as a stopcock, basic essential functions and properties should be listed to eliminate time spent evaluating a product that does not meet minimum standards. A list of standards for a stopcock would include properties such as (1) high-grade plastic to reduce the likelihood of cracking and leaking, (2) good visibility to allow for examination for bubbles, (3) ease of movement in turning the device to prevent torque on the intravenous line, (4) Luer-Lok with stationary and swivel adapter, and (5) ability to withstand the use of intravenous fats. Such a list is not all inclusive, but, if the list is made by nurse and physician users before evaluation, it saves time for the product evaluation team and materials management personnel. Many times, the critical properties of a supply item are not clear and surface only during an evaluation period. An index of doubt about the suitability of a new product should be high in staff nurses and physicians evaluating the product. Those staff members responsible for bringing in new supplies should ask the same questions of their sales representatives as are asked for equipment purchases.

If the product lacks testing and there are no known product users in the area, an evaluation may not be justified, because, in reality, such an evaluation provides the manufacturer with a clinical trial site. This service should be approached with caution; it involves planning and arrangements for reimbursement. For example, a device was recently introduced to locate the tip of an ETT without a radiograph. At the time the device was being introduced in the NICU, the published clinical trials included data only on infants larger than 2.4 kg. However, in most NICUs, critical tube placement is problematic in infants weighing less than 1500 g, for whom no data were available. The use of a supply that is new to the NICU is experimental and should be treated as such.

Complications related to the use of supplies can be just as

costly to the patient as those caused by faulty equipment. An example is the use of a cracked stopcock that allows a Broviac catheter to go uninfused. The leak can lead to blood loss, intravenous fluid loss, subsequent hypoglycemia or loss of drug effect, and permanent occlusion of the catheter. The cost in dollars, lengthened hospital stay, and morbidity to the patient must be made clear to personnel who assist in purchasing supplies. Unusual incident reports should accompany all supply failures affecting a patient. Members of the nurse management team or CQA/CQI committee should then talk with materials managers and risk managers to help them understand how the product adversely affected the patient. Although the adverse effect may be clear to clinicians, it may be vague to personnel from another department.

Nurses should be encouraged to save all packaging from each supply item until after the item has been examined and used on the patient for a short period of time. If a defect becomes evident, the lot number can be located and the packaging can be returned to materials management personnel to determine whether there is a bad lot or it is an isolated event. Too often, the nurse assumes that the defect is an isolated event and discards the item with no further notification of personnel. This delays the detection of serious problems and increases the likelihood of adverse patient outcomes. To facilitate the return process, a central location should exist for nurses to leave defective supplies with the package attached and a note identifying the problem. Nurses at the bedside do not have the time to follow up such problems, and the analysis and reporting should be done by managers or unit-based CQA/CQI committees.

Finally, a protocol should be developed by the NICU and the materials management department that provides a standard reporting mechanism for all defective supplies. At my institution, we have chosen to use the Safe Medical Devices Act for such reporting. If the product is defective or a large number of the items fail, the manufacturer should be notified immediately and asked to remedy the problem. Until then, a safe equivalent product must be found. Alternative product lists and suppliers should be maintained for such occasions as well as for supply delays caused by back ordering or unexpected recall. During the recent floods in the midwestern United States, all but one suction catheter manufacturer lost production time. The result was a serious shortage in neonatal suction catheters, and the need to rapidly find a safe alternative highlighted the need to keep this information readily available.

Medication Administration

For many reasons, the most common iatrogenic complications in the NICU are related to medication administration. The first major area of concern involves the limited clinical trials in the neonatal population and the fact that most of the drugs administered in the NICU are not recommended for children younger than 6 years of age. Thus, premature and term infants cannot even be addressed in the dosing or side effect information. The small number of clinical trials that do exist are almost always on term infants or stable premature infants. NICU nurses find themselves in the position of giving a drug that may lead to serious adverse patient reaction. As discussed, one example is the introduction of vancomycin into most NICUs in the late 1980s. As new drugs are introduced, nurses in the NICU must maintain a high index of suspicion related to dosing, side effects, and toxicity.

Side effect identification is difficult in infants because of their inability to communicate and their vulnerability resulting from organ immaturity. Many symptoms of adverse drug reaction are similar to those of other disease states, such as infection. Drug circulars and formularies often list side effects such as nausea or dizziness, which are practically impossible to detect in an infant. It is therefore essential that all medication introduction into the NICU be preceded by a meeting that includes clinical pharmacy, medical, and nursing staff. The meeting should include discussion of the potential adverse effects, properties of the drug (including half-life, clearance, known toxicity in adults), plan for monitoring levels, appropriate method of administration, appropriate dilution, and interactions and compatibilities with other drugs. These issues should be communicated to the staff and included in a readily available reference manual that is modified as new information becomes available. If a particular unit cannot develop its own, such manuals are available commercially, such as *Neofax*, published by Ross Laboratories (Young & Mangum, 1997). At my institution, the most recent edition of *The NICU Medication Reference Manual* will be placed within the Hospital Information System so that, from any unit-based computer terminal, a copy of the medication information can be printed for reference.

Labeling and packaging are additional problems related to medication errors. Manufacturers do not usually consult users about label changes or label similarities that may lead to error. Drugs that come in similarly colored or labeled vials or solutions are frequently cited as contributing to error. The pharmacy department should be solicited to assist the clinicians in this area. All concentrations of oral medications should be standardized by consensus as soon as possible. In other words, oral furosemide should not be dispensed in more than one concentration. All vials and unit doses of drugs that are dispensed to the NICU should also be of like concentrations when possible. If a concentration changes because of a manufacturing changes or changes in suppliers, the NICU should receive adequate notification and a system of alert should be put into place during the introduction of the new concentration. Bright-colored "Nurse Alert" stickers are inexpensive and effective. This agreement with the pharmacy department should be in writing and the process clearly defined. Nurses should also alert pharmacy personnel if the labeling on the vial is misleading or unclear. If these problems cause reconstituting or dosing problems, the manufacturer should be notified and given a suggestion on how to reduce the potential for error through a labeling change. Such reports should be made through the Food and Drug Administration MedWatch problem reporting program. Information and forms can be obtained by calling 1-800-FDA-1088. This program coordinates the reports of units throughout the country and can work directly with the manufacturer to achieve changes that improve the safety of the product, label, and administration instructions. Nurses and pharmacists should use these centralized reporting mechanisms to assist in their own practice as well as contribute to a data base that can lead to product modification in a timely manner.

Preservatives and compatibilities are additional problems. The preservatives used in some medication preparations may be safe in adults but fatal or toxic to infants. Benzyl alcohol is an example (Benda et al., 1986). Many times, the effect of the preservative is unknown in the infant population, and clinical pharmacy personnel need to research the known information and collaborate with medical and nursing personnel to make decisions about the safety or lack of acceptability of the preparation. At my institution recently, we were unable to purchase the usual supply of parenteral morphine sulfate. An alternate manufacturer listed phenol and formaldehyde as the preservatives used in its preparation. Printed information on the safe amounts of phenol and formaldehyde was minimal and vague. An exhaustive search was unable to determine whether this new preparation was safe, and the alternate product was rejected. Because of frequent back ordering and supply problems, it is beneficial to find a second safe supplier of a drug and have this information on file. If an alternate supplier cannot be found, the pharmacy should find a hospital in the area that is willing to sell its supply of the medication when an emergency arises.

The issues related to technical delivery of medication are perhaps those with which nurses are most familiar. Orientation and preceptor programs often have curricula aimed at the special considerations related to administering medications to premature and term infants. However, such administration remains a skill that requires reevaluation based on the medication, the infusion system, and the properties of the medication, and, even then, there is the potential for adverse effects (Bechtel et al., 1993; Gould & Roberts, 1979; Leff & Roberts, 1981; Roberts, 1981). Annual staff surveys that ask for recall of knowledge and that present problems to assess skill (competency) can assist in the planning of staff education needs. Issues that must be addressed systematically include (1) drug dilution recommendations, (2) time to deliver the drug, (3) volume of the administration device (tubing), (4) potential loss of drug in the delivery system, and (5) potential for inadvertent overdose. Continuous drug infusions involve other technical difficulties, in that, depending on the volume of the drug to be infused, the concentration of all other intravenous components can be altered to the ill effect of the patient. Standards must be developed that include how to prime tubing for critical drug drips such as prostaglandin E_1 or dopamine to reduce the risk of bolus administration or delay in infusion. These technical problems must be addressed systematically, usually by nurses, because nurses are most aware of the delivery problems, and in consultation with pharmacy and medical staff when questions cannot be clearly answered. Technical delivery protocols must be included in all orientation of new staff and, ideally, printed in a centrally located reference manual. At my institution, this competency has been added to our annual "skills workshop" because of the high-risk nature of the medications delivered by continuous drip. It is risky to assume that all staff members follow the same procedure for dilution, preparation, and administration when many options exist. For an infant who has only an umbilical artery line, there are many options for drawing up and administering an intravenous dose of digoxin that is less than 0.1 ml of drug. One nurse may draw up the drug directly from the vial and administer it via the umbilical artery line through a stopcock. Then, in the process of aspirating for air from the line, the nurse could administer some of the hub volume of the syringe and overdose the patient. A second nurse could use a 1:10 dilution to increase the volume of the drug and push it through a scalp-vein needle inserted for the drug administration but may not remember to clear the tubing volume in the needle and therefore underdose the patient. To assess staff practices, a survey format is again helpful. Such a survey gives hypothetical information and asks the nurse to list the steps of preparation and administration in detail and to include all math used in the calculation. Once practice can be determined, the units can address issues comprehensively and reduce the technical obstacles to safe delivery of medications.

We have also found it beneficial to study certain technical aspects of medication delivery to determine whether "best practice" does exist. In a recent laboratory assay of 1:10 dilutions of digoxin solutions using two different techniques, we determined that neither technique led to the desired concentration of drug. The use of 0.1 ml of drug and 0.9 ml of diluent was no less accurate than 1 ml of drug and 9 ml of diluent. In each assay, there was less drug in the diluted samples than expected and the concentrations were similar. When the drug is expensive, the former method is preferred. Other technical aspects of administration are more difficult to study in individual practice settings.

Medication administration involves skill and knowledge. Pharmacology, although a standard in all nursing curriculums, is a weak point for most nurses. Adequate clinical pharmacist support, as well as pertinent available references, is essential in any busy NICU. Several articles have looked at medication error rates in NICUs, the types of errors made, and who made them (Folli et al., 1987; Koren et al., 1986; Lesko et al., 1990; Vincer et al., 1989). Folli and colleagues demonstrated a significant impact on the reduction of errors when systematic error review occurred and a pharmacist was involved in routine medication order review. Other researchers have qualified error rates with the use of unit dosage and satellite pharmacies that deal with the subspecialty of pediatrics, specifically neonates. Many have shown that error rates can be positively affected with such services and support. An article by Raju and associates (1989) described a systematic approach for reviewing and reducing medication errors in the neonatal and pediatric intensive care units. The project is labor intensive initially, but the cost of errors both in patient outcome and in potential liability can easily justify the time and personnel expense. Although many units tabulate the number of errors made in a time period and may list the type of error, there is also a tabulation of the total number of medications given so that a percent of error rate can be reviewed over time and in light of specific interventions. It is therefore essential to find a method of obtaining a denominator from which to calculate a medication error rate. Methods to accomplish this include using computer data from the pharmacy department to quantify the number of medications dispensed for a particular time period. If medication errors are reviewed on a monthly basis, looking at the number of drugs given in a month allows the CQA/CQI committee to calculate a reported error rate. If such data do not exist, error rate can be calculated by using patient days as the denominator. This system is crude, however, and does not account for acuity changes that may be associated with a much higher volume of medication administration.

It is also important that other factors be considered when looking at the number of errors. If nurses become more aware of how to recognize errors and they improve their reporting frequency, then an increase in error rate is seen. This is actually an increase in reporting and may not reflect a change in errors made. Most important, there must be a system for collecting data, reviewing data, and developing solutions that can then be evaluated. Several articles put forth a systematic method of error review (Cobb, 1986; Raju et al., 1989; Rasic et al., 1989). JCAHO requires that each patient care unit evaluate iatrogenic errors and assess them against a standard. Without a systematic approach, error tabulation and description may be of little value.

In some units, knowledge is regularly assessed through survey or audit to plan in-service needs related to medication administration. Survey information can also be used to plan the type of reference manuals needed for the unit. Many nurses state that if the information was readily available, the error rate would be less. If nurses have to make telephone calls or search for the *Physicians' Desk Reference (PDR)*, medications may be administered without sufficient information so that they are given on time. The *PDR* is a poor source of information in such cases because it does not recommend that the listed drugs be given to children and therefore does not address the issues of dilution, delivery, compatibility, or side effects in infants. Furthermore, when pharmacists are part of a large general hospital, their knowledge may be limited in the field of pediatrics; therefore, in-unit reference materials must be thorough.

The patient impact of a particular medication error is helpful in focusing intradisciplinary review. Table 44–1 is a tool used at my institution for the past 5 years that scores the error based on type of error, route of administration, drug classification, discovery time, and patient impact. This tool, which is an adaptation of the tool developed by Martha Cobb, is completed by the nurse manager/advanced practice nurse who receives the unusual occurrence report. The weight of the error determines whether it is reviewed by the larger Medication Error Task Force at a monthly meeting. Errors scoring a total of 16 points or more require such a review. All errors are tracked, and any error may be reviewed based on individual request. The patient impact column allows for a value of 5 to be added to the total of the previous four columns, even if there was no effect on the patient but the

TABLE 44–1 Medication Error Tool (to be completed by nurse manager)

A. Type of Error	B. Route of Administration (Actual)	C. Classification of Drug/ IV Solution	D. Error/Discovery Time	E. Patient Impact
.10 Wrong time .... 1 Human error (e.g., forgot) Transcription .11 Wrong route .... 3 Given via wrong IV line Human error Ordered wrong Transcription error IF PO, given IV +2 .12 Wrong dose .... 5 Dispensed wrong Human error (e.g., miscalculated, incorrectly drawn up, mislabeled) Ordered wrong Transcription error Safe dose not checked Wrong IV rate IV pump failure .13 Wrong medication .... 5 Dispensed wrong Human error (e.g., vials looked similar) Ordered wrong Transcription error .14 Unordered medication .... 5 Order expired Order not written Wrong patient (human error) Wrong patient (clerical error; e.g., wrong stamp on order sheet) .15 Administration error.... 3 Drug incompatibility Medication expired Drug omitted Given more frequently than ordered Other........ 1 Medication unavailable Medication not given	IV .... 7 (intraosseous) IM/SC .... 5 PO (NG/GT) .... 3 Others .... 1 (Ear, eye, irrigation, rectal)	Aminoglycosides .... 5 Amphotericin .... 5 Antacids........ 1 Antianxiety agents........ 5 Antibiotics/anti-infectives .... 5 Anticoagulant/ thrombolytic agents...... 7 Anticonvulsants........ 5 Antidepressants........ 3 Antipsychotics .... 3 Antidiarrheals........ 1 Antiemetics .... 3 Antihistamines/ histamines .... 1 Antipyretics .... 2 Barbiturates........ 5 Blood and blood components........ 3 Bronchodilators........ 3 Cardiovascular drugs: antidysrhythmic, inotropics, antihypertensives, vasoactives/ vasodilators........ 7 Cathartics/laxatives .... 1 Chemotherapeutic and antineoplastic agents .... 7 Diuretics........ 3 Electrolytes/mineral bolus .... 5 Expectorant/anti-tussives .... 1 GI drugs (ranitidine)........ 3 Amino acids/enzymes....... 4 Insulin .... 7 IV with electrolytes/ vitamins/minerals........ 3 Muscle relaxants........ 5 Narcotic analgesics........ 7 Narcotic antagonists........ 3 Nonbarbiturate sedatives/ hypnotics .... 3 Nonnarcotic analgesics..... 2 Nonsteroidal anti-inflammatory agents ..... 2 Oral antidiabetic agents .... 3 Oral contraceptives........ 1 Oral vitamins/minerals/ desferol (IV) .... 1 Steroids........ 4 Stock IV solution .... 2 Total parenteral nutrition/ lipids .... 4 Vancomycin........ 5 Other 1	Repeat of error due to delay in discovery........ 5	No clinical change noted, no or minimal financial impact, or no additional lab work/tests ordered (incidental error with little or no risk to patient)........ 0.5 Lab work ordered; side effects noted; adverse change in clinical condition; increase nursing observation required for side effects........ 1.0 Multiple lab test ordered for follow-up; additional medications or treatments required; decreased level of consciousness; vital signs changed; length of stay increased due to side effects........ 1.25 Transferred to higher level of care; cardiac changes required intervention; bleeding (e.g., hematuria); lab values changed from normal to critical levels........ 1.50 Unplanned surgical procedure; placed on respirator; Code Blue; residual physical impairment; critical lab values became more critical........ 1.75 Death 2.00

Key: 1, No impact (0–9); 2, Significant (10–15); 3, Serious (16–21); 4, Patient morbidity (22+).
Total: A____ B____ C____ D____ E____ A+B+C+D+E____ × Impact ____ + Code ____ = ____
For *potential* impact, multiply by 0.5, then add 5 points

potential existed. For example, if an infant received 10 times the dose of an antihypertensive, there would be a score of 5 from column A, 7 from column B, 7 from column C, and, if found immediately, no score from column D, for a total of 19. If there were no clinical changes in the patient and no additional nursing observations, the total score is then multiplied by 0.5 for a total of 9.5. The 5 points is then added for the potential impact for a total of 14.5. The error is weighted as significant on the scale.

Pediatrics has the second highest rate of lawsuits related to medication errors, second only to internal medicine (Folli et al.,

1987). Therefore, it is easy to justify the time needed for CQA/CQI measures related to medication administration.

Infection Control

Hospital-acquired, or nosocomial, infections can occur as a result of an avoidable event and therefore should be considered an area of routine nursing attention in the prevention and reduction of complications. A member of the NICU staff should be on the hospital infection control committee, and a mechanism should exist to review and discuss all nosocomial infections with the nursing and medical leadership monthly. Although it is clear that patients in the NICU are at extreme risk for infection because of their immaturity, their immune incompetence, and the number of invasive tubes and procedures they require, there are some infections that can be avoided through practice changes, education, and systems changes.

A hospital's monthly nosocomial infections are typically reviewed in committee. When an infection appears to have been avoidable, such as the transmission of a resistant organism from one infant to another, the infection control committee usually refers the issue back to the unit of origin. The NICU nurse member of that committee then reports the information back to the NICU nursing leadership group. The nurses, working with the infection control and medical departments, should develop a plan to reduce the potential for additional infections from the same cause. For example, if a particularly resistant strain of *Pseudomonas* is found in the ETTs of three infants who are side by side in the unit, and pneumonia develops in two of the three, it may be ruled that one patient was admitted with the organism but that the other two acquired the organism by hand-to-infant transmission. The review of the infection highlights the need to (1) inform the staff about the presence of the organism, (2) educate the staff about the mode of transmission, (3) develop a method of identifying the infants with the organism to inform ancillary personnel, and (4) instruct staff on how to reduce spread to other infants. Many times, the major focus of the effort is notification and education. If dramatic systems problems are uncovered, the issue is often referred to an interdisciplinary CQA/CQI committee for problem solving. For example, if the infection control department identifies the problem as being related to a cleaning solution or to air filtering within an isolation room, more personnel than nurses are required to facilitate a solution. It is essential that nurses be involved at the committee level in the discussion of infection control, because, without their knowledge and representation, they may end up being told how to change practice with no input in the decision-making process. Nursing is frequently the target of infection control practices, but it is only one of many disciplines in contact with the patient and the patient's equipment and environment.

If a nurse cannot be on the infection control committee, then a formal relationship with the hospital's infection control officer must be stronger than usual. This relationship should include a standard mechanism for informing a member of the NICU nursing staff of which infections are occurring and which ones are seen as unusual or excessive and therefore possibly warrant an evaluation by the nursing CQA/CQI committee. Nurse managers and the staff will find that time spent reviewing hospital-acquired infections is valuable. Such review reassures staff members what practice is appropriate or identifies a need for change. This step is far superior to waiting to be told what to do to reduce infection after a serious problem is identified. The solutions for infection reduction may have little to do with how often disposable supplies are changed and more to do with the overall way that infants are cared for within a particular unit. To address the infections in any nursery, nursing practice must address skin care, nutritional support, and all invasive procedures such as suctioning and intravenous access. These issues have a direct and powerful impact on barriers to infection and immune function.

MONITORING, CONTINUOUS QUALITY ASSURANCE/CONTINUOUS QUALITY IMPROVEMENT, AND RISK MANAGEMENT

As discussed, there are many strategies for reducing the adverse effects of care in the NICU. In units that do not currently have these systems in place, the following summary may be beneficial.

Several groups should be in place to meet the monitoring and CQA/CQI demands of most NICUs. A nursing CQA/CQI committee that is unit based is essential. The committee should include staff members for all shifts, management, and consultation from the hospital-based committee of clinical nurse specialists, where available. Members of this group need to spend some initial time educating themselves in the process of CQA/CQI. In an article by Jain and Vidyasagar (1989), the role of the CQA/CQI committee is defined as one that (1) identifies the major iatrogenic problems, (2) collects data with specifically adapted forms, (3) analyzes collected data, (4) identifies the underlying problem, (5) discusses the possible methods to reduce or eliminate the problem, (6) proposes guidelines to the staff, (7) reviews the outcome of the solutions, and (8) resolves the problems. This is not a simple or straightforward process. Nursing committees may need to begin with a clearly defined problem and use it as an example before they tackle multifactorial problems such as accidental extubation. For example, it may be known by nurse managers that the emergency carts do not get checked every 8 hours as mandated by policy. Although the solution may not be simple, at least the problem is defined. Once the committee has finished the process on a previously defined problem, they can move into problem identification. Membership in such a committee should be consistent because experience is essential to effectiveness. Uninterested staff members should not be solicited because the time and energy commitment is high. Such staff members can be effectively used to perform audits. When given a clear form and told how to proceed with the audit, staff nurses can learn a great deal about the process without being on the committee. Many texts and manuals exist to assist in new committee organization, but there is no substitution for experience in this field. Once the group is educated, it needs to decide on annual goals and to set in motion some audit mechanisms. Forms can be used from other nursing departments or can be developed and piloted by the committee. Many times, an audit may need to be completely reorganized after an initial period, either because the information is not useful or because the practice being audited is not seen as important by the members or staff nurse. The audit process must stay dynamic. The following is an example of one such audit.

If the standard to be evaluated is timely antibiotic administration, and if the outcome is to have antibiotics administered within 30 minutes of the physician's order, the audit is fairly straightforward. The form to be developed must guide the CQA/CQI member on where to obtain the information and what information to retrieve. If the nurse must look for time of the order and time of medication administration, all pertinent data needed to evaluate the chosen outcome must be included on the form. Another such example is an audit to determine whether nurses maintain saturation monitor alarms within predetermined ranges for infants of varying gestation and postnatal age. The form guides the staff member who collects the data, and tabulations and interpretations can be done in the larger forum. With current financial constraints, these audits should be designed so they can be completed on duty time.

Many audits are handed down from a hospital-wide committee. If these are not seen as essential in the NICU, the time spent on the audit is viewed as wasted and the quality of the audit is usually poor. At this juncture, the chairperson of the committee should meet with the hospital-based chairperson and negotiate an alternate audit that is in compliance with the original intent of the higher committee. For example, if a general nursing committee has asked that a specific discharge form be audited and the NICU staff shows consistent low compliance, a problem exists. This form may not be used for the same purpose in the NICU and therefore may not be valued. Unit-based committees must assist the hospital-based committee in developing audits that analyze practice issues that are important and pertinent. Many nurses avoid participation in CQA/CQI programs owing to their lack of pertinence to practice. It is the role of the unit committee to create pertinence; the subsequent interest of the staff will follow.

Once the standard is pertinence to practice, audits can be done in many ways. Effectiveness is improved when (1) the form used to collect the data yields the desired information, (2) the random selection of charts is set up to avoid bias, (3) the auditors are staff members who know how to find the desired information, and (4) after the initial audits, there is a meeting to determine whether the process yielded desired and pertinent information. The results of the audit require critical evaluation. If the reasons for the poor compliance are unclear, consultation is essential. Nurses themselves may be the most important source of information. Many opinions should be solicited to cover all of the possible factors leading to the problem. These factors should then be dealt with one by one. Audits must be shared with the staff in a professional way and the standard redefined if unclear. When the audit reveals that an individual nurse has not complied with the stated standard (policy, protocol, or procedure), individual discussion must take place with that nurse. Nurse managers must meet with individual staff members to identify why that nurse did not act in accordance with written standards. Managers remain an essential component in the total process because their daily attention to standards and compliance is essential to the ultimate solution.

Once the issues have been stated, problem-solving is difficult. Apparent solutions may prove totally unsuccessful in subsequent audits, and the entire process must be repeated. This is not uncommon. Changing practice is one of the most difficult tasks in any work arena. If repeated solutions also fail, the standard needs to be critically evaluated. Perhaps it is a standard in name only and not valued by staff. If the standard has an impact on patient outcome and is not understood or appreciated by staff, managers and nursing CQA/CQI committee members must focus their attention on acceptance of the standard in order to work toward a solution of compliance. If the standard has no apparent bearing on patient outcome but has stayed in the audit process for lack of evaluation or thought, the audit of that standard should probably be dropped after thorough discussion and agreement that the standard is no longer pertinent to quality care. For example, one standard nursing audit was used to check tubing labels to ensure that tubing was changed every 24 hours as mandated. Many nurses found this type of audit a waste because they were unable to link it to any patient outcome. Since practice has shown that such tubing changes can safely be done every 72 hours, the perception has been validated.

In summary, the following issues should be dealt with to improve the success of a unit-based CQA/CQI committee:

1. Select a chairperson with time to devote to the committee and the knowledge to head others in the CQA/CQI process.
2. Select members who are interested and committed to the role of the committee.
3. Set goals.
4. Meet often to work on group education and group process.
5. Begin working on problems that have been clearly identified.
6. Begin with problems that fall completely within the practice of nursing.
7. Develop audit forms that are clear, pilot them, and revise them as needed.
8. Develop a method to evaluate each solution.
9. When solutions fail, look again for underlying problems and the methods chosen to decrease them.
10. Develop a professional and consistent method to inform staff members about their failure to meet an audit standard and to keep a record.
11. Keep the committee members stable to reduce educational needs over time.
12. Develop strong ties with the members of the medical and nursing leadership team (clinical nurse specialist, managers, educators, and advanced practice nurses) to assist in all committee efforts, including daily attention to practice standards to complement infrequent audits.

Unusual Incident Reporting

Nurses have traditionally had somewhat of an aversion to and misunderstanding of the process of completing incident reports. Although it is rare that they are misused in the hands of the nurse manager, nurses often view the form as a "black mark" in their employee personnel file. The unusual incident form is, in fact, an ideal mechanism to track iatrogenic complications ranging from environmental hazards for visitors to malfunctioning equipment. It is traditionally completed when an unexpected occurrence leads to adverse patient effect. It is also completed for all unusual events that could lead to a lawsuit. For both circumstances, the pertinent information surrounding the incident is needed. When the report is filed in a timely and complete manner, it assists nurse managers to identify problems. By tabulating incidents in various areas, the manager and CQA/CQI committee can plan as well as evaluate previous solutions. For example, if the unusual incident reports are tabulated monthly for the category "overdose of medication," once the CQA/CQI committee has put a solution into place to reduce that type of error, the category can be looked at each subsequent month for improvement. Ideally, the nursing CQA/CQI committee should review the current form and its routing process to evaluate its effectiveness. It is not uncommon that the form is developed with no input from nurses. If the form is not clear or easy to use, a meeting should be held with the hospital CQA/CQI department to discuss the possibility of a revision. It is also essential that the NICU staff understand what is done with the information on the form by the hospital CQA/CQI department. The routing of such forms must provide information to and from the sources able to act on the problem. If the forms go to any source and nothing more is heard, then reporting decreases or ceases altogether. It should not be assumed that persons in the department where the report is sent completely understand what happened in the incident or know who else should review the information. NICU staff members should provide a liaison to the hospital CQA/CQI department for consultation, and nurse managers should talk directly with the CQA/CQI department members to recommend how the incident be handled. Often a written addendum or E-mail message helps a centralized department know where to route the report. There is no substitute for direct and timely communication with the individuals or departments directly involved in the error.

For example, if an incident report states that a patient who was ordered to receive a normal saline infusion through an umbilical line actually received a 20 percent glucose solution, the nurse manager reviewing the incident should communicate clearly to the professionals involved in the incident the actual or potential patient effects. If it was a result of labeling error, the incident should be reported to the director of the pharmacy in a confidential manner. The physician should be notified immediately upon discovering the error so that he or she can examine the infant and intervene to correct the hyperglycemia or other side effects. The nursing staff should receive immediate communication about what happened, how it was discovered, how the solution was analyzed, and how the patient was treated for adverse consequences. The more time spent informing members of the treatment team or making a timely diagnosis of the problem, the more likely it is that the staff can avoid similar incidents. The nurse manager should also indicate which departments need to review the incident and where intervention should most likely occur.

The incident form itself, and the process by which the form is handled, should be reviewed for the following to decide whether revision or modification is required:

1. Does the form have a mechanism to quantitate the effect on the patient, and, therefore, when it is sent to the hospital CQA/CQI department, does it receive proper priority?
2. Does the form allow the nurse to record what happened easily, what it meant to the patient, and who else was involved?
3. Is the form easy to fill out?
4. Does the form provide space for the pertinent information related to the incident?
5. Does the staff know what type of occurrence should be documented on the form?
6. Does the staff know who should fill out the form and where it should go after completion?
7. Is the form readily available to the staff?
8. Is the nurse manager's role in form completion and routing clear?
9. Is the routing sequence clear?
10. How is information processed once it reaches its destination?
11. How does feedback occur?

If this process breaks down at any point, the form loses some effectiveness and credibility, and part of the CQA/CQI monitoring benefit is lost. If the form is used appropriately, it can be used to tabulate error rates, total errors, and error types and to assist in the planning of the CQA/CQI committee activities as well as those that require systems changes or in-service education. The use of E-mail to alert nurse managers or advanced practice nurses to a problem should also be encouraged if the individual on duty at the time of the occurrence has not had the time to complete the written report.

Reports can be used by the unit-based CQA/CQI committee to assist in problem identification or to quantitate problems. It can also initiate or trigger further investigation into certain events such as cardiopulmonary resuscitation. The incident report in this case is filled out because the event is unusual, and then the CQA/CQI committee reviews the entire event to audit for compliance with a standard related to aspects of the event.

Risk Managers

Many institutions have employed individuals with varying backgrounds to take on the role of risk manager. Although the role varies from institution to institution, it is generally designed to assist clinicians and administrators in day-to-day issues that have been judged to carry some liability or risk to the institution. In current health care delivery systems, those issues are many, ranging from how to proceed with a court order for care on an infant with absent or incompetent parents to the legalities involved with limiting visitation from a hostile family member. Risk managers have a variety of backgrounds, ranging from law to nursing to hospital administration. Most new positions, however, require a law degree.

The unit manager, physicians, social workers, and CQA/CQI committee should prearrange when to consult with the risk manager. The risk manager is usually a member of the hospital CQA/CQI committee but may have only a consulting role with unit-based committees. It is also beneficial to have the risk manager involved in some portion of orientation of new staff and ongoing staff nurse education. The role of the risk manager in the unusual incident report loop usually involves interviews with key individuals and review of documentation in incidents that are judged to be areas for potential lawsuits. However, there is no substitute for unit-based "risk managers" who are members of the nursing leadership group and unit-based CQA/CQI committee. Members of the NICU staff should take the advice given and discuss it as they would any consultant's advice about patient care. Decisions are best made by the treatment team within the nursery setting after the consultation has been obtained.

If an event is identified by the unit-based staff as serious, the risk manager should be notified by telephone. It is not reasonable to assume that the written report will be correctly interpreted by the risk manager. Because of their clinical expertise, unit-based staff members are the most aware of which events are serious. The immediate telephone call also provides a timely gathering of facts. Fact gathering at this initial stage is far more productive than fact gathering months or years later, when signatures are not legible, nurses have taken other jobs, and notations in the medical record are not clear. If an institution does not have a risk manager, administrators should be asked to identify the individual in the institution who should be contacted for such questions. The role may be delegated to an administrator or legal counsel employed as a consultant to the institution. In any case, such a consultation should be available to staff members who find themselves with ever-increasing legal questions related to the delivery of highly technical care to patients who cannot speak for themselves.

Nurses should not defer to the risk manager's advice routinely if the advice creates concern. Risk managers rely on information from clinicians and on candid feedback about their recommendations. If the advice from the risk manager is evaluated as harmful or inadequate or in any other way not appropriate, the nursing leadership group should speak openly with the risk manager and reopen the discussion about a particular case. It is also of value for the unit to create a list of common occurrences in which legal issues arise and to sort these out before a crisis. An example of such an occurrence is the need to transfuse an infant born to parents who are Jehovah's Witnesses. The steps to follow should be in writing as set forth by risk management and the NICU team; nurses, physicians, and social workers in the nursery should know the steps or how to immediately access the information.

Other Monitoring

Other systems that are valuable in the detection and prevention of iatrogenic complications include an interdisciplinary CQA/CQI committee. This group includes members of nursing, medical, pharmacy, and respiratory therapy departments, as well as a member of the hospital CQA/CQI committee. This group can audit and monitor complications and standards that come under joint practice more effectively than can the nursing CQA/CQI committee. The role, purpose, and education of the committee are similar to those of the nursing CQA/CQI group and vary only in the scope and focus of problem-solving.

Some complications require this multidisciplinary approach. Examples are thermal injury cases, vascular access complications, review of morbidities such as intestinal perforations, and intraoperative complications. Nurses, physicians, pharmacists, and respiratory therapists are all involved in these problems. The solutions to problems are best reached by all disciplines using the CQA/CQI process. These committees are unit based and often structurally placed under the protection of a medical staff committee to ensure confidentiality. The committee's role is often critical to problems that were partially solved when they were addressed by only one department. An interdisciplinary committee receives reports from the other unit-based CQA/CQI committees (such as from nursing, transport, and extracorporeal membrane oxygenation programs) and then addresses those issues that require an interdisciplinary team approach to be successfully managed. It is essential that all unit CQA/CQI functions be coordinated to complement and not duplicate one another. The departments of nursing, pharmacy, respiratory therapy, and medicine must work together closely with ancillary support staff to determine what CQA/CQI programs exist. Staff members need to share audits that are pertinent to other disciplines and work together on projects when appropriate.

CONCLUSION

Newborn intensive care has made many therapeutic and technologic strides in the past decades. It is essential that the same technology that has advanced the field so dramatically be critically evaluated to reduce as many complications as possible. The consequences of therapies must be assessed more carefully before their introduction into practice, and practice routines must also be scrutinized. A healthy skepticism should exist in all nurses about the safety and benefit of all they do to their tiny patients. Nurses must stay alert to potential dangers of all therapies, ranging from positioning infants to using high-frequency ventilators, and they must assume an active role with medicine in monitoring for complications, evaluating the data, and determining the ultimate solutions. McClead and Menke (1987) point out that two principles should guide the prevention of iatrogenic complications: (1) remembering the past so as not to repeat it and (2) controlling the eagerness to embark upon new therapies. They quote a sign in a fireworks factory, "It is better to curse the darkness than to light the wrong candle." The definition of *iatrogenic* clearly must include all nursing practice. In the next decade, one of the major tasks must be the reduction of harm from nursing practice.

Finally, it is clear that, with health care reform, the attention to complications will require more creativity. The leadership of each intensive care nursery must find ways to continue all efforts to report, analyze, and reduce care delivery complications. Complications will not "go away." The burden of their impact has tremendous cost to the infant and family as well as to the institution. Keeping practice safe is an ethical mandate and a professional responsibility. It also helps reduce the cost of care for each infant.

REFERENCES

Bassen, H. I. (1986). From problem reporting to technological solutions. *Medical Instrumentation, 20*(1), 17–26.

Bechtel, G. A., Vertrees, J. L., & Swartzberg, B. (1993). A continuous quality improvement approach to medications administration. *Journal of Nursing Care Quality, 7*(3), 28–34.

Benda, G. I., Hiller, J. L., & Reynolds, J. W. (1986). Benzyl alcohol toxicity: Impact on neurologic handicaps among surviving very low birth weight infants. *Pediatrics, 77*(4), 507–512.

Britton B. P., Raper, J. T., & Walden, C. M. (1995). From development to evaluation: making a competency plan work. *Journal of Nursing Staff Development, 11*(4), 210–214.

Cobb, M. D. (1986). Evaluating medication errors. *Journal of Nursing Administration, 16*(4), 41–44.

Folli, H. L., Poole, R. L., Benitz, W. E., & Russo, J. C. (1987). Medication error prevention by clinical pharmacists in two children's hospitals. *Pediatrics, 79*(5), 718–722.

Golonka, L. (1986). Trends in health care and use of technology by nurses. *Medical Instrumentation, 20*(1), 8–10.

Gould, T., & Roberts, R. J. (1979). Therapeutic problems arising from the use of the intravenous route for drug administration. *Journal of Pediatrics, 95*(3), 465–471.

Hittner, H. M., Godio, L. B., Rudolph, A. J., et al. (1981). Retrolental fibroplasia: Efficacy of vitamin E in a double-blind clinical study of preterm infants. *New England Journal of Medicine, 305*(23), 1365–1371.

Jain, L., & Vidyasagar, D. (1989). Iatrogenic disorders in modern neonatology. [Review]. *Clinics in Perinatology, 16*(1), 255–273.

Jelliffe, E. F. (1977). Infant feeding practices: Associated iatrogenic and commerciogenic diseases. [Review]. *Pediatric Clinics of North America, 24*(1) 49–61.

Koren, G., Barzilay, Z., & Greenwald, M. (1986). Tenfold errors in administration of drug doses: A neglected iatrogenic disease in pediatrics. *Pediatrics, 77*(6), 848–849.

Leff, R. D., & Roberts, R. J. (1981). Methods for intravenous drug administration in the pediatric patient. *Journal of Pediatrics, 98*(4), 631–635.

Lesko, S. M., Epstein, M. F., & Mitchell, A. A. (1990). Recent patterns of drug use in newborn intensive care. *Journal of Pediatrics, 116*(6), 985–990.

Long, J. G., Lucey, J. F., & Philip, A. G. (1980). Noise and hypoxemia in the intensive care nursery. *Pediatrics, 65*(1), 143–145.

McClead, R. E., Jr., & Menke, J. A. (1987). Neonatal iatrogenesis. [Review]. *Advances in Pediatrics, 34*, 335–356.

Meisenheimer, C. G. (Ed.). (1985). *Quality Assurance, A Complete Guide to Effective Programs.* Rockville, MD: Aspen Publications.

National Center for Nursing Research. (1989). *Neonatal nursing care of low birthweight infants, 18*(45), 10–12.

Raju, T. N., Kecskes, S., Thornton, J. P., et al. (1989). Medication errors in neonatal and paediatric intensive-care units. *Lancet, 2*(8659), 374–376.

Rasic, E., Boedicker, M., & Lyon, M. (1989). A new system for managing medication errors. *Nursing Management, 20*(5), 102–112.

Roberts, R. J. (1981). Intravenous administration of medication in pediatric patients: Problems and solutions. *Pediatric Clinics of North America, 28*(1), 23–34.

Rushton, C. H. (1986). Promoting Normal Growth and Development in the Hospital Environment. *Neonatal Network, 4*(6), 21–30.

Schaad, U. B., McCracken, G. H., Jr., & Nelson, J. D. (1980). Clinical pharmacology and efficacy of vancomycin in pediatric patients. *Journal of Pediatrics, 96*(1) 119–126.

Tsang, R. C., & Nichols, B. L. (1988). *Nutrition during infancy.* St. Louis: C. V. Mosby.

Young, T. E., & Mangum, O. B. (1997). *Neofax, a manual of drugs used in neonatal care* (10th ed.). Columbus, OH: Ross Laboratories.

Vincer, M. J., Murray, J. M., Yuill, A., et al. (1989). Drug errors and incidents in a neonatal intensive care unit. *American Journal of Diseases of Children, 143*(6), 737–740.

CHAPTER 45

The Drug-Exposed Neonate

ANN APPLEWHITE FLANDERMEYER

RESEARCH AGENDA

Determine the long-term consequences of passive in utero drug exposure.

Evaluate various approaches to maternal drug rehabilitation treatment programs.

Examine the effectiveness of nursing home follow-up on the achievement of developmental milestones in the infant who has been exposed to drugs in utero.

Develop or find an assessment tool to identify pregnant women at risk for substance abuse.

VIGNETTE

A 23-year-old woman presented in the ER with no prenatal care. She was a gravida 4 with three living children. She stated she had been bleeding the past few hours and was "about 7 months pregnant." She was pale, diaphoretic, and tachycardiac and complained of moderate abdominal pain. It was determined by ultrasound that a partial abruption had occurred in this twin pregnancy. It also showed two fetuses. The decision was made to perform a C-section. The NICU was notified. A pediatrician and a NICU nurse were present for each infant.

Both infants were admitted to the NICU after initial delivery room stabilization. Infant A, a male, weighed 1140 g with Apgars of 1, 2, and 5. He was intubated in the delivery room because of no respiratory effort. Over the next 40 hours, this infant remained unstable. Umbilical arterial and venous catheters were placed. Medical management consisted of plasma protein fraction (Plasmanate), tromethamine (Tham), dopamine, dobutamine, and an infusion of packed red blood cells. He continued to have ventilator assistance with 100% oxygen. Chest compressions and epinephrine were given several times during the last couple of hours. Despite resuscitative efforts, the infant expired. Autopsy was not performed. The only apparent anomaly was a two-vessel cord.

Infant B, a female, weighed 1208 g with Apgars of 6, 8, and 9. She was given 100% blow-by oxygen in the delivery room and during transport to the NICU. She was put in a head hood and weaned to 60% oxygen, maintaining saturations greater than 93%. A gestational age assessment at 12 hours of age showed her to be 33 weeks' gestation. Her length was 39 cm, and her head circumference was 27.5 cm. She was determined to be SGA.

On further evaluation, the mother admitted to cocaine use, dosing up as recently as when the abdominal cramping started "to help the pain." She said she smoked about a pack of cigarettes a day. She was vague about her drinking habit, stating that she had a few drinks a week. She also stated that the twins' father was not to be involved in their care. Her three other children were removed from her care 2 months previously because of neglect. She defended herself, saying she had been "feeling sick a lot" during the pregnancy. She said she was going to take the twins home and be a good mother to them. She named the twins David and Sara. Social Services was notified and became involved with the case.

The day after the twins were born, the mother visited the bedsides of both infants. She was very quiet. She sat in her wheelchair at David's incubator and stared at the lines and equipment as the nurse explained them. The doctor was honest and considerate in discussing David's status. Her only question was, "How much does he weigh?" Later, when David's death was inevitable, she was notified and encouraged to hold him. She refused. A NICU nurse volunteered to hold David in his last few minutes.

At Sara's incubator, the mother was encouraged to stroke and talk to the infant. She asked appropriate questions about Sara's weight, her monitors, and her chances of survival. However, her attention would wander to other infants in the unit.

Sara remained in the head hood for a few more days and was gradually weaned to room air. She was NPO during this time, being maintained on IV fluids and electrolytes. Phototherapy was started for hyperbilirubinemia, and this resolved. Sara was jittery and irritable, sleeping for short periods. She took her pacifier vigorously. Meconium and urine were sent for a drug toxicology screen. Results were positive for nicotine and cocaine.

Over the next few weeks, Sara remained irritable and was easily stimulated. Feedings were attempted with orogastric tubes when she was 3 days old, but she frequently regurgitated and could not tolerate full feeds and so was maintained on IV fluids for an additional week while feeds were gradually increased. She liked her pacifier during the orogastric feeds. When attempts were made to nipple feed, she had a difficult time coordinating sucking with swallowing and breathing. She had a vigorous suck and sometimes she'd cough and choke. Other times she'd suck and swallow but forget to breathe, initiating a bradycardiac episode. Eventually, she got the hang of it. She gained weight slowly and was weaned from the incubator to a crib. Sara's sleeping pattern was still irregular, with short periods of deep sleep and long periods of irritability. Nursing care and lab work were done when she was awake to avoid disturbing her much needed sleep. Rocking and holding her did not provide comfort but made her more irritable. She would become rigid and cry. She found comfort in three things: being bundled, boundaries with blanket rolls, and her pacifier.

When Sara's mother was released from the hospital, she came in to visit one time during the next week. Several unsuccessful attempts were made to contact her by Social Services and Sara's nurses. When Sara was more than 5 lb, steadily gaining weight, and tolerating feeds, she was released into foster care.

Kathleen Spiering

Drug abuse by young women of childbearing age is on the rise among all strata of society, so there is an increased number of pregnancies being complicated by substance abuse. This chapter discusses the effects of prenatal exposure to tobacco, cocaine, heroin, and alcohol. The effects of each substance are considered separately. However, the reader should be aware that multiple substances are often abused simultaneously, which makes it difficult to ascertain which effect is caused by which substance. This determination may be complicated further by an interactive effect of two or more drugs or adulterants, or both, used to dilute illicit drugs.

Interest and discussion of specific drugs within the literature parallels the popularity of drugs of choice among pregnant women. During the 1960s and 1970s, the focus was on examining the effects of alcohol and heroin on the fetus. Attention then shifted to tobacco. In the late 1980s and early 1990s, researchers studied cocaine and polysubstance abuse. Currently, interest in tobacco and alcohol has resurged. Overall, whatever the substance abuse trends, society at large has become acutely aware of the ill effects on the fetus. The average cost for one infant who is undergoing neonatal withdrawal in a neonatal intensive care unit (NICU) has been estimated at $28,000 (Lewis, 1991). Physical, psychosocial, and financial concerns related to substance abuse do not end with birth but continue throughout childhood. Through long-term prospective studies, the health care community has become knowledgeable about the deleterious perinatal effects of substance abuse. It is now the responsibility of health care professionals to educate the public about these consequences.

DEFINITIONS

The following definitions are used in this chapter:

Low birth weight (LBW): 2500 g or less (Gunderson & Kenner, 1995)

Preterm: 37 weeks' gestation or less (Arias, 1984)

Small for gestational age (SGA): "Infant with somatic development below the 10th percentile of the normal variation for gestational age as determined by neonatal examination. The SGA infant may be preterm, term or postterm" (Arias, 1984, p. 39)

NURSING CONSIDERATIONS

Nurses are in a pivotal position to effect change through dissemination of health-related information to the diverse individuals with whom they work. Nursing education includes a liberal base of interview techniques, active listening and, of course, the nursing process. Nurses are able to polish these skills daily through working with their clients.

Epidemic proportions of substance abuse have necessitated that all nurses be taught interviewing strategies to enhance self-reporting of tobacco, alcohol, and drug use. When such interviewing is conducted with all clients, nurses become adept at detecting subtle cues or inferences that may be explored with further questioning. However, even with the best interviewing strategies, tobacco use is underreported (Bardy et al., 1993), so more negatively sanctioned substances such as alcohol and street drugs are prone to be underreported with greater frequency. Underreporting is often due to the woman not wanting to receive health teaching on the merits of stopping use and the socially unacceptable nature of substance use during pregnancy. She may also fear loss of her infant because of child protection laws. Although underreporting is a problem, if women are not asked about substance use, they do not spontaneously divulge the information. Therefore, until there is a better way to screen for substance use, a thorough history is still the best available tool.

Prenatal education regarding substance abuse is essential. Preconception programs need to be offered, such as health classes in high school or during routine gynecologic examinations. The overall emphasis should be on promoting a healthier lifestyle for young women of childbearing age. This strategy could ameliorate the problem of fetal damage occurring from drug exposure during the first 8 weeks of pregnancy. It is during this period that birth defects can occur, yet women may not yet realize that they are pregnant. Therefore, educational programs should focus on young, nonpregnant women who are sexually active. Education should emphasize that all substances of abuse (including tobacco and alcohol) should be avoided during the sexually active years when conception can take place. Once women are pregnant and receiving prenatal care, the importance of abstinence from substance use can be reinforced. Women should be informed that use may be harmful to the fetus during all trimesters of pregnancy. For example, alcohol or cocaine consumption may cause disruption in organogenesis during the first trimester, increase the risk of spontaneous abortion during the second trimester, and exert a potential for intrauterine growth retardation as well as interference with brain maturation during the third trimester. Therefore, there is no safe time to ingest alcohol or cocaine during pregnancy. For these reasons, nurses can and should launch their own personal anti–substance abuse campaign.

Prevention is truly the key to turning the tide in drug-affected infants. Programs to achieve this goal are varied. Admittedly, the "just say no" slogan was a simplistic view of the drug problem. However, a drug prevention program targeted at young children can be influential in forming attitudes that may dissuade future substance use. If such use is negatively sanctioned by society (e.g., smoke-free buildings, mandatory prison time for driving under the influence, and the "three strikes and you're out" policy for repeat offenders), individuals may be less likely to use such substances. Unlike other disease processes, drug-induced anomalies are irreversible. For example, once a child is born impaired with fetal alcohol syndrome (FAS) or fetal alcohol effects (FAE), there is no cure. The damage is lifelong. Other substances, such as cocaine, heroin, and tobacco, have not been correlated with as predictable a pattern of aberrant behavior and appearance as that associated with alcohol. However, cocaine, heroin, and tobacco have been associated with significant fetal harm (e.g., learning delays, irritability, and intrauterine growth retardation) that persists into later life.

TOBACCO

History

Cigarette smoking remains common, even with the broad-based antismoking information and the proliferation of smoke-free environments. As a consequence of the public's increased awareness of the hazards of smoking, the number of adult smokers declined from 50 to 30 percent during the years 1965 to 1980 (U.S. Department of Health and Human Services, 1983). Although the numbers of smokers decreased, there was an increase among young women of low socioeconomic status. The most frequently cited reason for the altered demographics of smokers is that as men gave up tobacco, advertising campaigns targeted a new population: young women. Advertisements have portrayed smoking as romantic, sophisticated, and a reflection of the new emancipated woman. The consequence of these messages is that approximately one third of all women enter their pregnancies as smokers (Nowicki et al., 1984) and 25 percent of these women continue to smoke. Typically, those who continue smoking during pregnancy are young, poor, black, unemployed, and unmarried (U.S. Department of Health and Human Services, 1990).

Smoking includes a psychological addiction or "habit" as well as a physiologic addiction to nicotine. In addition, most smokers also report a true enjoyment of tobacco (McKool, 1987). Enjoyment is associated with a sense of relaxation during stress and arousal, especially with the first cigarette of the day (Benowitz, 1989).

To overcome the strong addictive properties of nicotine, the pregnant woman must be motivated and supported during her attempts to quit. First she needs to be educated about the risks of smoking on her pregnancy, such as the association between tobacco and LBW, prematurity, and placental abruption. Practical implications such as the myriad complications of prematurity, ranging from mild learning disabilities to death, must be explained.

Health is a prime motivating force for the cessation of smoking (McCool, 1987), so maintenance of a healthy pregnancy may be the driving force behind such cessation. Women may quit out of concern for their unborn child when they may not quit to promote their own well-being. Women may have tried to stop unsuccessfully in the past but should be reassured that more individuals succeed in achieving cessation in subsequent attempts than in initial attempts (U.S. Department of Health and Human Services, 1983).

Few individuals recognize cigarette smoking's vast array of pregnancy-related dangers. Tobacco-induced hazards are discussed in the following section as they relate to various stages in the developing child's life (fetus, infancy, and childhood).

Risk Factors

In addition to the perinatal complications smoking causes, it also places women at risk for infertility before pregnancy is achieved. Women who smoke are at risk for tubal infertility (Lincoln, 1986; McGarry, 1983). Lincoln (1986) discussed Campbell's research conclusion that the underlying cause of ectopic pregnancies was thought to be related to altered tubal motility in association with cigarette smoking. Tobacco smoke has also been found to have antiestrogen effects that cause smokers to enter menopause at an earlier age, thus reducing the number of reproductive years (Baron, 1984). Baron also found that the antiestrogen effects are reversed after smoking cessation.

Smokers have an increased incidence of spontaneous abortion. Kline and associates (1977) controlled for confounding variables and found that among women who had miscarried, there was a twofold increase in the incidence among smokers. Himmelberger and associates (1978) reported similar findings. Heavy smokers in their populations were found to have 1.7 times more spontaneous abortions. The study used a survey to examine the rates of miscarriage and congenital anomalies among professional women who worked in the operating room. The study controlled for other extraneous variables that could affect the pregnancy (e.g., maternal age, exposure to trace anesthesia gases, and history).

Unexplained vaginal bleeding, abruptio placentae, and placenta previa are more common among smokers (Meyer et al., 1976; Naeye, 1980; Naeye et al., 1977). Placenta previa and abruptio placentae contribute to the increased rate of stillborn infants among smokers (U.S. Department of Health and Human Services, 1980). Naeye (1980) also found that among smokers who quit, the risk of these placental abnormalities was almost as low as among women who had never smoked.

A finding that was associated with abruptio placentae was "decidual necrosis at the margin of the placenta" (Naeye, 1980, p. 764). This decidual necrosis was not present in the placentas of nonsmokers or in women who had stopped smoking. Meyer and colleagues (1976) also found an increased incidence of perinatal mortality associated with abruptio placentae or placenta previa among smokers. They concluded that "the striking regularity with which both of these complications increase with maternal smoking makes it highly convincing that this is one avenue through which maternal smoking increases perinatal loss" (Meyer et al., 1976, p. 473).

There is some controversy regarding tobacco as a teratogen. Himmelberger and colleagues (1978) found smoking mothers to have a risk 2.3 times greater than nonsmokers of having an anomalous child, whereas Evans and associates (1979) found no evidence that smoking was teratogenic except with regard "to neural tube defects where the effect is at most modest" (p. 171). Golding and Butler (1983) found no increase in the incidence of anencephaly among their population after they controlled for social class. Tobacco in and of itself is not considered a teratogen (U.S. Department of Health and Human Services, 1980). However, smokers are known to have low levels of vitamin C, implying that the tobacco itself might not be a direct teratogen but creates a vitamin deficiency, including that of folic acid, which may be responsible for an increased number of neural tube birth defects.

Fetal Hazards

Low Birth Weight

Maternal smoking has been documented as responsible for reduced birth weight among term infants (Chomitz et al., 1995; Crosby et al., 1977; Curet et al., 1983; Luke et al., 1993; Meyer et al., 1976) and has also been correlated with an increased incidence of prematurity (U.S. Department of Health and Human Services, 1980). With reduced birth weight being found among infants of comparable gestation, an underlying mechanism other than prematurity was felt to be responsible. The report on smoking by the U.S. Department of Health and Human Services (1980) found that the average weight differential between infants of smokers and those of nonsmokers was 200 g. They further reported a dose-related response, with birth weight reduced in relation to the number of cigarettes smoked. The infants also had smaller crown-to-heel lengths and smaller head, chest, and shoulder circumferences. The report estimated that smoking during pregnancy is responsible for 14 percent of all LBW infants.

Luke and colleagues (1993) stated that maternal smoking doubled the risk of having a LBW infant and tripled the incidence of neurologic sequelae. de Jong-Pley and associates (1994) found that smoking adversely influenced the infant's condition at birth by correlating with a birth weight that was an average of 350 g less, a lower umbilical venous pH, and a lower neurologic score than was seen in controls.

Effects of tobacco on fetal weight gain can be avoided by maternal cessation of smoking. Butler and Goldstein (1973) found that when mothers stopped smoking early in pregnancy, their infants weighed the same as their nonsmoking counterparts, thus documenting the importance of encouraging women to stop smoking once they become pregnant.

Morbidity and mortality associated with smoking may be

masked by the method of reporting. Fetal deaths are not listed under "smoking." Instead, they are reported by presenting symptoms such as anoxia, prematurity, or respiratory distress.

Fetal Heart Rate Variability

Other fetal hazards are related to the direct effect of smoking on the fetus in utero. Fetal well-being has been commonly assessed by fetal heart rate (FHR) variability (the ability of the fetal heart to increase or decrease in rate within a range of 5 to 10 beats per minute in response to fetal activity). Forss and colleagues (1983) found an acute decrease in FHR variability after the mother had smoked a standard filtered cigarette. They concluded that tobacco had both a narcotic and a hypoxic effect on the fetus during the third trimester. These workers also investigated the effects of maternal smoking on FHR variability during the second trimester (22 to 26 weeks' gestation). They found that smoking had a narcotic but not a hypoxic effect. They believe that further investigation is needed to explain the difference in action of tobacco use on the fetus in different stages of gestation. Goodman and associates (1984) studied 10 pregnant women between 37 and 40 weeks' gestation. They measured the effects of smoking two low-tar filtered cigarettes on fetal movement and FHR variability. They found that "there was a significant reduction in the percentage of time the fetus spent moving during the first 16 minutes of smoking" (p. 657). They also found "significant reductions in the number of accelerations in beat to beat variation and in heart rate variation around the basal value within the smoking period" (p. 658). These findings uphold the belief that tobacco use directly affects fetal homeostasis (see Chapter 14, The Effects of Labor on the Fetus and Neonate).

Placental Effects

Visible differences are also seen in the placental structures of women smokers (Christianson, 1979; Wingerd et al., 1976). Christianson (1979) studied 7651 placentas and found that smokers had an "increased prevalence of calcification and patchy subchorionic fibrin" (p. 179). This increase in fibrin and calcium has been associated with longer gestation. Thus, if women who smoked had longer gestation than nonsmokers, this would be a consistent finding. However, the smokers had a shorter mean gestational age than did the nonsmokers (Christianson, 1979). Therefore, the patchy fibrin and calcification occur earlier in gestation when mothers smoke. Smoking hastens the placenta's aging process, making the uterine environment less favorable for fetal habitation. Smoking also hastens the skin's aging, resulting in excess wrinkles (Daniell, 1971).

Another smoke-related finding is the ratio of placental weight to birth weight increases (Christianson, 1979). This relatively large placental ratio is especially significant considering that the average birth weight of infants of smokers is less than nonsmokers (Christianson, 1979). Therefore, the larger placenta is a compensatory mechanism that facilitates fetal oxygenation. A large placental ratio is also seen in studies of infants born in high altitudes.

Jouppila and colleagues (1983) studied the effects of smoking on blood flow in 19 fetuses. They found that smoking one cigarette "did not produce immediate alterations in the blood flow in the fetal thoracic aorta or in the umbilical vein" (p. 7). However, although there were no sudden changes in fetal blood flow associated with smoking, the infants were smaller, probably secondary to chronic intrauterine hypoxia.

Causes of Intrauterine Hazards

Cigarette smoke has been associated with between 2000 and 4000 chemicals. Recognized constituents of cigarette smoke include nitrosamines, nicotine, carbon monoxide (Enkin, 1984), and cyanide (Lehtovirta et al., 1983). All these elements readily cross the placenta. An additional element is cadmium, which is entrapped by the placenta (Kuhner et al., 1982).

Nitrosamines. These agents are known carcinogens (Enkin, 1984). They are linked with the increased cancer incidence among smokers. Therefore, it is hypothesized that prenatal exposure to nitrosamines may place the fetus at risk for the development of cancer later in life.

Carbon Monoxide. Cigarette smoke contains carbon monoxide. Maternal carbon monoxide levels rise in relation to the quantity of cigarettes smoked (Bureau et al., 1982). Therefore, a woman smoking one pack of cigarettes per day would not have as high a carbon monoxide level as a woman smoking two packs per day. Carbon monoxide readily diffuses across the placenta. Once in fetal circulation, carbon monoxide competes with oxygen for the binding sites on hemoglobin, forming carboxyhemoglobin (Guyton, 1996). When carboxyhemoglobin is formed, the oxygen molecules are displaced, thus lowering the fetal oxygen partial pressure and impairing tissue oxygenation (Longo, 1976). Therefore, the fetus experiences intrauterine hypoxia. Normal fetal Po_2 is already only 20 to 30 mm Hg, compared with an adult norm of 100 mm Hg (Longo, 1976).

A fetal response to this state of hypoxemia (lower than normal range) is to produce more red blood cells (polycythemia), thus increasing available oxygen binding sites. The result is a 30 percent increase in fetal blood viscosity (Buchan, 1983). The viscosity further reduces blood flow and increases the hypoxia (Buchan, 1983). Polycythemia also predisposes the neonate to a multitude of potential problems, including, but not limited to, the development of venous thrombi or hyperbilirubinemia, or both.

Curet and associates (1983) observed that infants of smokers had a reduced incidence of respiratory distress syndrome (RDS). They attributed this to either a direct effect of smoking on the fetal lungs or an indirect effect of inducing chronic hypoxia from vasoconstriction of the placental vessels. Chronic hypoxia is believed to stimulate the fetal stress response, hastening the fetal secretion of glucocorticoids, which facilitates surfactant production. Surfactant, in turn, stabilizes the alveolar membrane, which reduces the incidence of RDS.

Nicotine. Cigarette smoke contains nicotine, which readily crosses the placenta. In the adult, "nicotine reduces pain and anxiety and produces a pleasurable, euphoric state that can be as addictive as narcotics" (McKool, 1987, p. 29). Nicotine reaches the brain within seconds of inhalation, producing a period of alertness followed by euphoria and relaxation (Pomerleau et al., 1983). Nicotine is physiologically addictive, as withdrawal accompanies smoking cessation (McKool, 1987).

Nicotine has the same vasoconstrictive properties as carbon monoxide. It reduces the uteroplacental blood flow and consequently fetal-placental exchange (Buchan, 1983; Bureau et al., 1982; Longo, 1976).

Cadmium. This is another substance that becomes more prevalent in the body after smoking. Kuhner and associates (1982) found that cadmium levels were highest in the placenta, followed by maternal serum and then by fetal cord blood. A normal dietary intake of cadmium may be 50 mg/day. This level is increased by as much as 20 mg/day in heavy smokers (Kuhner et al., 1982). In later gestation, the placenta seems to entrap cadmium, preventing it from reaching the fetus. However, it is uncertain if the placenta possesses similar capabilities during early gestation because the rudimentary placenta is a fairly ineffective protective barrier. The effect of elevated cadmium levels on the human fetus is uncertain. However, since it can and does accumulate in the placenta (at higher rates among smokers), Kuhner and associates (1982) concluded that pregnant women should avoid exposure to cadmium because it has been shown to alter placental function in animals. Cadmium has no known biologic function.

Cyanide. Cigarette smoke also contains small amounts of cyanide, which readily crosses the placenta. The U.S. Department of Health and Human Services (1980) stated that cyanide is suspected to "contribute to retarded infant growth and increased perinatal mortality" (p. 234). Cyanide inhibits cellular respiration and, in sufficient doses, can readily induce death.

Risk Factors in Infancy

Neonatal Thyroid Enlargement

Maternal smoking has been associated with an increased neonatal thyroid volume as documented by cord levels of thiocyanate, a metabolite of tobacco smoke (Chanoine et al., 1991). The lighter birth weight compared with the larger thyroid volume resulted in a significant birth weight to thyroid volume ratio. The study population was derived from 82 randomly selected mothers in Brussels who had no history of thyroid disease or iodine deficiency. The neonates were asymptomatic; however, the correlation of maternal smoking and enlarged thyroid to body weight was significant and adds another potential complicating influence of tobacco. The long-term effects are as yet unknown.

Strabismus

Maternal prenatal smoking possibly is linked to strabismus (Chew et al., 1994; Hakin & Tielsch, 1992). Two types of strabismus, which is an abnormal gaze deviation, include exotropia (eyes diverge) and esotropia (eyes converge). Untreated strabismus may lead to amblyopia or blindness in the weak eye. Although the cause of strabismus is unknown, it may be from a defect in central nervous system (CNS) control over the oculomotor system (Chew et al., 1994). The risk of strabismus increases with heavy smoking during the third trimester—the period of rapid brain growth and myelinization of the optic nerve tracts as well as development of oculomotor and sensorimotor tracts of the eye (Hakin & Tielsch, 1992)

Maternal smoking continues to place infants at risk for morbidity and mortality. Rhead (1977) found an increased incidence of sudden infant death syndrome (SIDS) among infants of smoking pregnant women.

These infants also experience more frequent upper respiratory infections and otitis media than do their nonsmoking counterparts. This increased illness rate results in more physician's office visits and hospital admissions during the first year of life (Rantakallio, 1983).

There is some controversy regarding whether these ill effects are caused by the actual fetal exposure to smoking during pregnancy or to passive smoking after birth. The latter refers to exposure to the smoke emitted from the burning end of the cigarette (sidestream smoke). This smoke consists of the "smoke emitted from the burning cigarette [and] includes more toxins and carcinogens than mainstream smoke" (McKool, 1987, p. 28).

To document the effects of passive smoking on infants, Greenberg and colleagues (1984) examined the saliva and urine of infants of smokers for cotinine, a by-product of nicotine. The presence of nicotine excretion in the saliva and urine reflects recent exposure, whereas cotinine is indicative of chronic exposure to tobacco (Greenberg et al., 1984). They suggested "that a dose response relationship can be established between the intensity of passive exposure to tobacco smoke and urinary excretion of cotinine, the major metabolite of nicotine, and to a lesser extent excretion of nicotine itself" (p. 1078). They were able to document, by the presence of nicotine and cotinine in the infants' excreta, that infants exposed to passive smoking were inhaling nicotine.

Nicotine has also been found in breast milk of lactating women who smoke (Luck & Nau, 1984). However, much less nicotine and cotinine was found in the urine of infants who were nursed than in the fetal blood, amniotic fluid, and placental tissue (Luck & Nau, 1984). Their conclusion was that intrauterine nicotine exposure was more significant than that from breastfeeding or passive smoking.

The nurse needs to support the pregnant woman's decision to stop smoking. The nurse should recognize smoking as a true addiction. Counseling should provide information on adverse perinatal effects. Also, the nurse should act as an appropriate role model by not smoking. If the woman is unable to quit, she should be encouraged to reduce the number of cigarettes smoked.

Residual Effects of In Utero Exposure to Tobacco

The long-term effects of maternal smoking on offspring have been questioned. As a result, the growth and development of infants born to smoking mothers has been followed throughout childhood. Their cognitive and developmental achievements have been compared with those of their nonsmoking counterparts (a control group). However, even with a well-controlled study design, it is difficult to determine if the observed differences in outcome are from intra- or extrauterine exposure to tobacco. Women who smoke are more often married to men who smoke, doubling the infants exposure (Rantakallio, 1983). Smoking women have poorer health and are often in less stable marital situations (Rantakallio, 1983). These variables make it intrinsically more difficult for these mothers to care for their children.

Rantakallio (1983) conducted a follow-up study of 1819 Finnish children whose mothers smoked during pregnancy as compared with a control group of children born to nonsmoking women. The children were examined at 14 years of age with regard to height and school performance. Children of women who smoked during pregnancy were shorter, even though the mothers were slightly taller than the nonsmoking women. The children of smokers had poorer school performance. After the variables of the mother's height and age, father's social class, number of older and younger siblings, and sex of the child were controlled for, the children's height deficit remained significant. When the same variables were controlled with regard to school performance, the effect of smoking was "less marked" (p. 749).

Naeye and Peters (1984) conducted a large prospective study consisting of more than 50,000 pregnant women who smoked. They followed the effects of smoking on the children's development. The researchers controlled for extraneous variables (e.g., heredity, lifestyle, and socioeconomic status) by studying the children of women who smoked during one pregnancy and comparing those data with those from siblings born when these women did not smoke. By following the development of the siblings, they were confident that maternal smoking during pregnancy was the independent variable. The results were that "hyperactivity, short attention span and lower scores on spelling and reading tests were more frequent for children whose mothers had smoked throughout pregnancy" (p. 601). After this correlation had been made, the researchers reviewed past medical records and discovered a correlation between children with behavioral abnormalities and high fetal hemoglobin levels.

Butler and Goldstein (1973) conducted a British longitudinal study examining the effect of maternal smoking on the children's subsequent development. "At ages 7 and 11 years physical and mental retardation due to smoking in pregnancy (p. 573) was found."

Common Attributes of Women Who Smoke

A common debate focuses around whether the childhood effects of maternal smoking are directly related to the actual smoking or more to the type of woman who smokes. Women who choose to smoke are inherently at risk for poorer fetal outcome on the basis of their socioeconomic status, educational level, age, and race. Consistent attributes included belonging to a lower socioeconomic class and being urban, tall, thin, less likely to use family planning, and more likely to also drink coffee, beer, and whiskey than the nonsmoker. She also had less frequent prenatal and postpartum care (Cardozo et al., 1982; Enkin, 1984).

Yerushalmy (1971) found that smoking women had a lower age of menarche; were less likely to have used contraceptives or to plan the pregnancy; consumed more coffee, beer, and whiskey; and were also more often extreme in their behavior than were nonsmokers.

COCAINE

History

Cocaine is a CNS stimulant first synthesized in 1858 from the *Erythroxylon coca* leaves (Fig. 45–1) (Stimmel, 1979). Previously, South American natives chewed coca leaves to experience mood-altering effects and to forestall hunger in times of famine (Bingol et al., 1987). Once cocaine was synthesized, it was proclaimed as a cure-all. Use became so widespread that it was a major ingredient in the original Coca-Cola. Soon after cocaine's ill effects were recognized, legal production was halted (Stimmel, 1979). Historically, cocaine was so expensive, use was restricted to the wealthy, and it was known as the "champagne of drugs." In recent years, cocaine has become more available, purer, and less expensive. As a consequence, recreational use has rapidly proliferated among all social classes (Pollin, 1985; Smith, 1988).

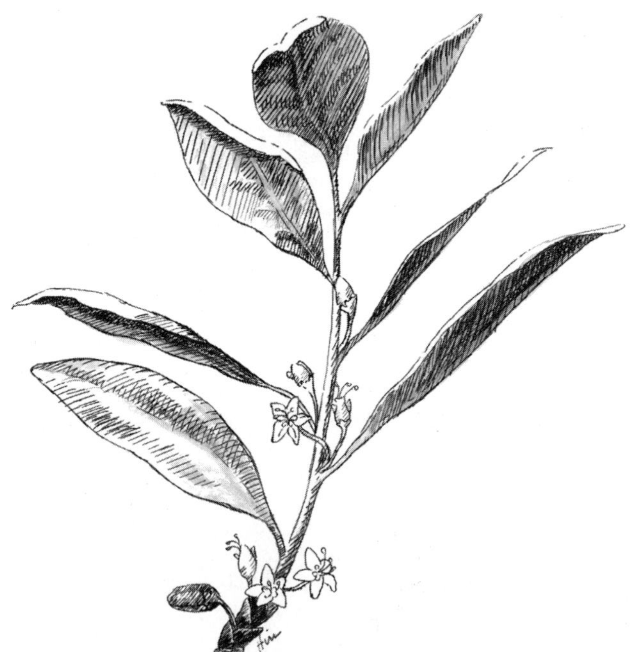

FIGURE 45–1. Coca branch.

Mechanism of Action

In 1884, cocaine was first used as a topical anesthetic (Cregler & Mark, 1985). Its anesthetic properties are produced by the inhibition of peripheral nerve conduction and the prevention of norepinephrine uptake (Smith & Asch, 1987). Norepinephrine accumulates, creating vasoconstriction, tachycardia, and hypertension (Smith & Asch, 1987; Smith & Deitch, 1987). Local vasoconstriction is an asset during minor surgery. These same vasoconstrictive properties are the basis for many of the complications of cocaine use, such as hypertensive episodes, tachycardia, and local nasal septum tissue necrosis with repeated "snorting."

Route of Administration

Cocaine can be administered intranasally, by smoking, by injection, or even intravaginally (Lewis, 1991). Traditionally, cocaine hydrochloride was snorted via intranasal application. More recently, a much purer form of cocaine, cocaine alkaloid or "crack," has come into vogue. The term *crack* evolved owing to the cracking or popping sound heard when it is smoked (Atkins, 1988). Heating does not destroy crack but rather delivers the drug efficiently to the pulmonary vasculature, where it is absorbed within 30 seconds (Atkins, 1988; Cregler & Mark, 1986). The rapid onset is similar to that achieved by the intravenous route of administration (Cherukuri et al., 1988). The mood-altering effects experienced with smoked crack and intravenously injected cocaine are intensified over a briefer time as compared with the somewhat longer duration of euphoria associated with intranasal consumption (Resnick et al., 1977). Crack use is accompanied by intense drug craving and is sustained in "runs" until supply has been exhausted (Cregler & Mark, 1985, 1986; LeBlanc et al., 1987). Crack is also highly purified and less expensive than cocaine. Atkins (1988) reported "street" cocaine as being 20 to 30 percent pure, whereas crack can be as much as 80 percent pure. However, crack is so highly addictive that the user consumes large quantities of the drug, leading to a more expensive addiction than with cocaine hydrochloride. When snorted, cocaine is of lower concentration and is associated with local vasoconstriction of the tissues within the nasal septum. Thus, there is a self-limited effect. Euphoria is followed by dysphoria that is characterized by anxiety, depression, fatigue, and cravings for more cocaine (Resnick et al., 1977).

Metabolism

Cocaine is metabolized by the esterase enzymes, which are produced within the liver and are present in the plasma. The rate of individual metabolism varies according to the level of cholinesterase activity (Bingol et al., 1987). For example, pregnant women and their fetuses are slower to metabolize cocaine as a consequence of a lower level of plasma cholinesterase activity (Pritchard, 1955). This has practical implications when considering screening newly delivered mothers and their infants for cocaine metabolites. According to Chasnoff and colleagues (1987), if a woman has ingested cocaine 2 to 3 days prior to delivery, her urine contains metabolites for 24 hours and the neonate's urine continues to test positive for 4 to 7 days. However, the more immature the fetal liver, the longer the cocaine metabolites may linger in the fetal system (Udell, 1989).

There may be circumstances in which the mother tests positive and the child tests negative, or vice versa. Udell (1989) reported that the timing of maternal cocaine ingestion influences whether the metabolites are present and in which system, maternal or fetal. If a woman has taken cocaine with the onset of labor, she tests positive but the infant may not, the rationale being that sufficient time may not have elapsed for the metabolites to cross the placenta, since cocaine induces vasoconstriction and precipitous deliveries. Udell (1989) suggested that a converse scenario may also be true. Cocaine's metabolites may be absent in the woman's system after birth, although the infant may continue to excrete metabolites for a longer period. Cocaine metabolites may persist for 2 weeks in a very premature infant (Udell, 1989).

Hazards of Cocaine Addiction

Cocaine is felt to be the most dangerous of all illicit drugs (Smith, 1988), and its use has become more prevalent than that of heroin. Personal and social deterioration are commonplace among cocaine users, and severe and sometimes fatal cardiovascular complications have been documented (Bates, 1988; Cregler & Mark, 1985, 1986; Lichtenfeld et al., 1984). Bozarth and Wise (1985) were able to document the overall impact of cocaine use by studying the animal model. Their study compared and contrasted drug-seeking behavior among heroin- and cocaine-addicted rats. Two similar but mutually exclusive groups of rats were allowed unlimited access to heroin or cocaine. The rats addicted to cocaine exhibited more intense levels of abuse, with erratic patterns of administration, exaggerated deterioration of health, and dramatic weight loss. After 30 days, 90 percent of the rats addicted to cocaine had died of drug use. By comparison, the rats addicted to heroin suffered less deterioration of health and less weight loss. By the end of the same 30-day period, 36 percent of the heroin-abusing rats had died.

If these data could be generalized to humans, they would uphold the belief that cocaine is more dangerous than heroin. Human patterns of drug consumption seem to parallel the animal patterns in the report by Bozarth and Wise (1985). Humans use cocaine sporadically but with frequent episodes of consumption. Cocaine is known to cause anorexic effects, with weight loss among chronic users (Bingol et al., 1987); social deterioration related to drug-seeking behavior; and death related to its direct effects (e.g., stroke and myocardial infarction). Perhaps the fatal consequences of cocaine addiction have not been as profound in humans as in the animal model because cocaine has rarely been available in unlimited quantities.

Euphoria generated by cocaine is caused by blocking the reuptake of neurotransmitters such as dopamine and norepinephrine, which prolong contact with the postsynaptic receptor. Continued cocaine use depletes the body's supply of neurotransmitters and results in depression and other symptoms of withdrawal (Tronick & Beeghly, 1992). It is as if cocaine accelerates the consumption of a finite supply of biochemical sources of joy (e.g., neurotransmitters), until the individual experiences chronic depression and sadness.

Heroin is also a dangerous drug; however, the human usage patterns are somewhat predictable given an adequate drug supply. If heroin is consistently of a stable dose and if needles and other drug paraphernalia are sterile, deaths are fewer than those associated with cocaine use. Heroin-related deaths are generally due to an overdose from unexpectedly pure heroin, infections (e.g., hepatitis and acquired immunodeficiency syndrome [AIDS]), or unknown agents used to dilute the drug (adulterants) (Stimmel, 1979).

Risk Factors Associated With Cocaine Abuse

Current widespread cocaine abuse is in part the result of the past public myth that cocaine is a benign, nonaddicting drug (Howard et al., 1985), whereas, in fact, cocaine is highly addictive (MacGregor et al., 1987; Pollin, 1985). Cocaine use is on the increase among young women of childbearing age (Atkins, 1988), with more and more pregnancies being complicated by such use. An estimated 11 percent of all pregnant women have used cocaine sometime during their pregnancy (Tronick & Beeghly, 1992), with an estimated 25 million individuals having used cocaine sometime in their life (Udell, 1989). Cocaine use cuts across socioeconomic lines. The picture of the "typical" drug addict is no longer valid. Women who use cocaine are often from middle to upper socioeconomic classes and lack the classic needle track marks. Chasnoff (1989) exemplified this new concept by his report of the results of blinded urine toxicology studies among pregnant women of various populations within the health care system. Urine was screened for cocaine, opiates, marijuana, and alcohol. Women obtaining prenatal care from a private practice had positive urine toxicology screen results of 13.7 percent, and clinic patients had a positive rate of 16.3 percent. These results demonstrate that fetal cocaine exposure is prevalent among varied socioeconomic classes.

General Health Risks

This section discusses the reported ill effects of cocaine on the woman, the condition of her pregnancy, and fetal well-being. Adverse effects associated with all routes of cocaine ingestion include myocardial infarctions in otherwise healthy individuals (Bates, 1988; Cregler & Mark, 1985; Howard et al., 1985), subarachnoid hemorrhage and cardiac dysrhythmias (Lichtenfeld et al., 1984), tachycardia and hypertension (Finnegan, 1988), and hyperpyrexia (Bingol et al., 1987). Death generally results from direct cardiovascular effects or from an accident that was incurred while the individual was under the influence of cocaine.

Pregnancy-Associated Risks

Potential complications specific to pregnancy are spontaneous abortion (Chasnoff et al., 1985); an increased rate of placental abruption, which is associated with stillbirths (Acker et al., 1983; Chasnoff et al., 1987; Townsend et al., 1988); and an elevated incidence of prematurity (MacGregor et al., 1987; Oro & Dixon, 1987). The initial reporting of these cocaine-induced pregnancy-related problems heightened awareness among health care professionals. As a consequence, there has been much recent documentation relating spontaneous abortion, placental abruption, and prematurity to maternal cocaine ingestion. The association has become so strong that in some institutions, placental abruption and unexplained premature labor are often a signal of suspected drug use, and a drug screen may be ordered. The underlying mechanism of action of cocaine that is responsible for precipitating spontaneous abortion is thought to be placental vasoconstriction and increased uterine irritability (Chasnoff et al., 1985). These physiologic changes can induce miscarriage; however, this is a potential adverse reaction to cocaine and is not a primary mechanism of action.

The news media have discussed the attempts of self-induced abortion by cocaine ingestion (Beck et al., 1989). This publicity is worrisome, as it may influence a vulnerable population: young pregnant women. Using cocaine to induce abortion subjects the woman and the fetus not only to cocaine's ill effects but also to potential addiction. Furthermore, the pregnancy may not abort; the cocaine may instead inflict irreparable fetal harm (e.g., congenital anomaly and cardiovascular accident) or a premature infant.

Cocaine has been implicated in inducing placental abruption owing to its cardiovascular effects. Acker and colleagues (1983) hypothesized that placental vasoconstriction associated with an abrupt hypertensive episode precipitated placental separation from the uterine lining. Once this occurs, there is a significant incidence of associated fetal death, thus contributing to the reported number of stillbirths.

Woods and associates (1987) investigated the effects of maternal cocaine ingestion on placental blood flow in the pregnant ewe. Their findings were consistent with the hypothesis of Acker and coworkers (1983). Cocaine was found to induce placental vasoconstriction, thereby reducing uterine blood flow and inhibiting oxygen transfer to the fetus (Woods et al., 1987).

Fetal Hazards

Cocaine readily diffuses across the placenta because it is of low molecular weight and is lipophilic (Bingol et al., 1987; Cregler & Mark, 1986). Therefore, cocaine is easily transported transplacentally to the fetus, with a mimicking of maternal effects (e.g., tachycardia and hypertension). The resulting infant is often referred to as a *drug-exposed neonate* or a *prenatally drug-exposed infant* (Lewis, 1991).

Maternal cocaine abuse has been associated with preterm labor and delivery of LBW and SGA infants, abnormalities of fetal monitoring, and fetal meconium staining (Chasnoff et al., 1987; MacGregor et al., 1987). The mechanism of preterm labor is thought to be cocaine-induced uterine irritability (Chasnoff et al., 1985). The characteristics of LBW and SGA are caused by cocaine-induced placental vasoconstriction. It is believed that when the placental vessels are constricted, there is a reduction in uteroplacental exchange; therefore, fetal nutrition is diminished. As with any reduction in nutrition, fetal growth is hampered, thus resulting in LBW infants. Often infants have symmetrical growth retardation because of early or prolonged cocaine use during pregnancy. Symmetrical growth retardation is more serious than asymmetrical, or brain-sparing, growth retardation because all organs, including the brain, are malnourished (Tronick & Beeghly, 1992).

One positive effect of this placental vasoconstriction is a reduction in the amount of cocaine that reaches the fetus. This was demonstrated by Moore and coworkers (1986), who found that after cocaine was ingested by the pregnant ewe, fetal cocaine levels were "about {1/8} of those observed in the mother" (p. 888). Although fetal cocaine levels are not as high, clearance is slower owing to the immature metabolic capabilities of the fetal liver. As a consequence, fetal cocaine exposure is prolonged. Another pathway of fetal clearance of cocaine is via the maternal system. Once the maternal system has metabolized its cocaine, the concentration gradient is reversed and unmetabolized fetal cocaine can diffuse back into the maternal system. Once again, there is a time lag that is responsible for prolonging fetal exposure to cocaine.

Placental vasoconstriction also hampers fetal oxygenation and nutrition. Therefore, intrauterine hypoxic episodes may coincide with maternal cocaine ingestion. The total complement of associated ill effects from these hypoxic episodes has yet to be documented. Chasnoff and associates (1986) reported "an infant who developed cerebral infarction after delivery at term to a woman who had used a large amount of cocaine in the 72 hours before delivery" (p. 456). Similar occurrences have been reported in the adult population (Lichtenfeld et al., 1984). It is logical to think that since the cardiovascular effects of cocaine are similar in the fetus and the mother, cocaine could have been responsible for the fetal "stroke" in utero that was reported by Chasnoff and associates (1986). Cocaine has also been associated with FHR arrhythmias that may persist into the neonatal period, which for some children resulted in congestive heart failure, arrest, and death (Frassica et al., 1994).

Vasoconstriction also occurs within the fetal vascular system that supplies the gut. As a result, there is a correlation between cocaine exposure and necrotizing enterocolitis and anomalies of the viscera, including gastroschisis (Udell, 1989; Torfs et al., 1994). There has been a case report of a term infant with necrotizing enterocolitis (Telsey et al., 1988) and a case report of intrauterine fetal death (Critchley et al., 1988) associated with maternal cocaine use. Since 1988, when these observations were first made, practitioners have continued to observe a propensity toward gastrointestinal (GI) manifestations among infants exposed to cocaine, ranging from difficulty stooling and feeding to severe anomalies of the GI system. The correlation between increased fetal mortality (e.g., in utero stroke and prematurity) and cocaine exposure has become undeniable.

Cocaine as a Teratogen

Cocaine has been implicated as a potential teratogen when ingested during early pregnancy (Bingol et al., 1987; Chasnoff et al., 1988). It is difficult to document this definitively owing to the human fetus being exposed to multiple environmental and hereditary variables. It is unethical to perform fetal experimentation. Retrospective documentation is often the method of data collection. This form of investigation requires large samples and relies on the historian's accuracy. Many women use more than one substance, do not take consistent dosages, ingest cocaine at erratic times of gestation, and may not remember exact dates, dosages, or frequency of cocaine use. However, as health care workers are more aware of the large-scale cocaine use among pregnant women, they are diagnosing the abuse more frequently and noting correlations between drug exposure and vasoconstrictive anomalies.

Madden and colleagues (1986) reported no significant birth anomalies among eight infants of cocaine-abusing mothers. However, one child had a sacral exostosis and a capillary hemangioma, and a second child had a capillary hemangioma and a subgaleal hematoma.

Bingol and associates (1987) studied infants of three groups of women. These groups consisted of women who were abusing only cocaine (n = 50), women who were using multiple or polydrugs (n = 110), and women who were drug-free (control group n = 340). Birth anomalies were more prevalent among the infants who were exposed to cocaine. Five of the 50 infants exposed to cocaine had significant anomalies, which included two infants with congenital heart disease and three with skull anomalies. Seven of the 340 members of the control group manifested anomalies. Therefore, the rate of anomalies in the infants exposed to cocaine was five times that of the control group.

Chasnoff and colleagues (1988) compared the rate of anomalies of infants born to women addicted to cocaine with that in infants born to women abusing multiple drugs, excluding cocaine. All women had the benefit of prenatal care and counseling. Nine of 50 infants exposed to cocaine had major birth anomalies. Two infants had ileal atresia, and seven had malformations of the genitourinary tract. One infant with myelomeningocele was born to a cocaine-using mother but was excluded from the sample because the woman received no prenatal care. These genitourinary findings are often refuted by other researchers, such as those cited in this section, the belief being that other variables are more responsible for these anomalies than is cocaine.

When considering cocaine as a teratogen, a significant extraneous variable to be considered relates to the adulterants used to "cut" the cocaine. Common fillers are lactose, mannitol, lidocaine, and procaine (Bingol et al., 1987). These are foreign substances whose influence on fetal development is unknown.

The cause of cocaine's suspected teratogenesis may be related to its vasoconstrictive properties. If the fetal blood supply is compromised by cocaine-induced vasoconstriction during a critical period of organogenesis, impaired oxygenation and nutrition of fetal tissue may result (Bingol et al., 1987; Chasnoff et al., 1988). This impaired nutrition during a critical time in organ formation restricts the growth and development of sensitive developing cells, with the resultant disruption or absence of growth of particular fetal tissue. Thus, an anomaly is seen after delivery. Cocaine-induced hyperpyrexia may also be a cause of birth anomalies (Bingol et al., 1987). A function of the amniotic fluid is to buffer temperature changes. However, if maternal temperature is persistently elevated, the homeostatic function of the amniotic fluid is overwhelmed. The fetal tissue is then exposed to elevations in temperature, and alterations in cell division may occur. This hypothesis seems reasonable in light of the observation that infants born to women who soaked in hot tubs on a regular basis had an increased incidence of anomalies.

Risks Associated With the Neonatal Period

Irritability

There has yet to be a readily identifiable withdrawal pattern among infants born to women who abuse cocaine. However, by observing increasing numbers of these infants, commonalities of behavior have emerged. The infants are often irritable and difficult to handle (Schneider & Chasnoff, 1987). When these infants were assessed using the Brazelton behavioral scale, it was found that they "had significant depression of interactive behavior and a poor organizational response to environmental stimuli (state organization)" (Chasnoff et al., 1985, p. 666). These infants were part of the Northwestern Hospital study, in which all mothers had prenatal care. By comparison, Cherukuri and colleagues (1988) studied the effects of intrauterine exposure to crack on the neonate in cases in which only 40 percent of the women had prenatal care. Their findings were consistent in that 38 percent of the infants had symptoms consisting of "tremulousness, irritability, and muscular rigidity [that] were usually mild and self limiting" (p. 150). These infants are therefore difficult to console, which is frustrating for the caregiver.

Doberczak and colleagues (1988) studied electroencephalograms (EEGs) of 39 infants exposed to cocaine. The EEGs of 34 infants indicated CNS irritability. However, all EEGs (with one pending) reverted to normal by 12 months of age. The researchers concluded that the effects of cocaine were self-limiting as opposed to being a permanent manifestation of cocaine exposure. This provides some optimism that infants can "outgrow" these nervous system alterations.

Residual Effects of In Utero Cocaine Exposure

Infancy

Schneider and Chasnoff (1987) tracked the growth and development of infants exposed to cocaine in utero. They were found to be "irritable, hypertonic infants who are easily overstimulated" (p. 62). This complicates mothering, as the infants are difficult to hold owing to hyperextension and posturing and are easily overloaded by sensory stimulation. "Normal" attempts at interaction by the mother may be poorly tolerated by the infant. As a result of stimulation, the infant may "shut down" into a deep sleep or begin incessant crying (Schneider & Chasnoff, 1987). This also makes caretaking difficult for the nurse. Eisen and associates (1991) found that infants exposed to cocaine exhibit more stress behaviors according to the Brazelton behavioral scale. This change in behavior or stress response may be related to an increased catecholamine level, which has been demonstrated in pilot work by Mirochnick and coworkers (1991). These neurologic changes have implications for the collaborative management of these infants (nursing care is discussed later).

Another risk is that of living in an environment in which cocaine or crack is used. Infants and toddlers may attain a high from passive inhalation of crack cocaine (Bateman & Heagarty, 1989). Children who are crawling may find and eat pieces of crack from the floors of their home (Udell, 1989). Furthermore, cocaine may be passed to the infant via breast milk (Chasnoff et al., 1987). Therefore, infants with a history of prenatal drug exposure need to be carefully followed throughout childhood. Parents need to be cautioned about mechanisms of unplanned cocaine ingestion.

Early Childhood

As more infants who were exposed to cocaine in utero have been followed into early childhood, data are becoming available as to the drug's long-term effects. Children seem to be fulfilling the projected poor outcome scenarios and are manifesting more permanent disabilities, such as attention deficits, difficulties in concentration, abnormal play patterns, and flat, apathetic moods (Hurt, 1989). What is frightening is that the more that becomes known, the more serious and tenacious the effects of in utero cocaine exposure appear to be. However, to avoid a self-fulfilling prophecy, these children should not be labeled *cocaine babies.* This type of labeling is counterproductive for the children and for their families.

HEROIN

History

Heroin is a derivative of the opium poppy. The poppy's presence has been traced to times of antiquity, with evidence of poppy seeds and capsules being present during the Stone Age. Organized cultivation of the poppy existed among the Sumerians of Mesopotamia in 4000 to 3000 B.C. (Stimmel, 1979). It seems evident that the Sumerians experienced the mood-altering effects of the poppy, as its name, *gil,* meant happiness or joy (Stimmel, 1979). From this point in history, the organized cultivation and trade of the poppy spread extensively. In the early 1800s, a German named Serturner produced morphine from opium. Wright followed in 1874 to synthesize heroin from morphine (Stimmel, 1979).

Action

Heroin is a CNS depressant that is six times as potent as morphine; it is highly addictive, and serves no medical purpose (Malseed & Harrigan, 1989). In current times, heroin is illegal and is used solely for the mood-altering effects that it generates. It is not used for therapeutic intentions such as pain relief, for which other narcotics, such as morphine, are prescribed instead. Narcotics induce vasoconstriction of the placental blood vessels and reduce uteroplacental exchange (Eriksson et al., 1973). Narcotics may also depress respirations by interfering with the body's response to elevated P_{CO_2} levels.

Routes of Administration

Heroin is self-administered by sniffing, swallowing, smoking, or injecting subcutaneously or intravenously (Kroll, 1986). "Mainlining" (intravenous injection) is the most common route to achieve the maximal level of euphoria. Heroin is rapidly absorbed, producing a brief but orgasmic high followed by a drowsy, detached, peaceful period of several hours that is followed by an intense craving for more drug (Flandermeyer, 1987; Kroll, 1986). This craving leads to a regular pattern of administration every 3 to 4 hours to sustain the drug's effects. Regular use leads to tolerance, and increasing doses are required to attain a high. If administration is stopped, symptoms of withdrawal ensue. Users soon fall prey to the cycle of addiction. Women addicts often resort to prostitution, stealing, or selling illegal drugs to support their habits.

A difficulty in studying the effects of maternal addiction on the fetus is in estimating the extent and type of drug usage. Heroin's level of purity on the street varies considerably (Flandermeyer, 1987). A common method of conceptualizing the dose is by determining the number of "bags" used per day or the money spent to purchase the drug. However, even if the heroin dose is known, there are unknown agents used to adulterate the drug. Kroll (1986) quoted the 1971 Misuse of Drugs Act as citing "talc, starch, quinine, or scouring powder" as frequently used heroin adulterants. Since purity and dose are so variable, the user may experience withdrawal when the dose received is unexpectedly low or nonexistent. Accidental overdose may also occur when purity is higher than expected. This wide variance of purity was substantiated when Louria and colleagues (1967) analyzed bags of street heroin and found that some contained no drug. The addict may be purchasing anything from pure heroin to pure adulterants.

General Risk Factors Associated With Heroin Abuse

Women addicted to heroin generally live in substandard conditions. They typify the general conceptualization of a drug addict. This stereotyping includes a transient, perhaps homeless, lifestyle whereby food is scarce or perhaps not a priority. The result is a poorly nourished woman with a lack of adequate prenatal care and poor personal hygiene who is at risk for contracting an infectious disease. As previously discussed, this picture does not apply to all substance-abusing women. Most research and documentation pertaining to heroin addiction is from the 1960s and 1970s. The substance-abusing woman of the 1990s seems to be less obvious than previously thought.

As already stated, heroin addicts have often resorted to prostitution to finance their addiction (Connaughton et al., 1975). As a consequence of multiple sexual partners, they are exposed to many sexually transmitted diseases (STDs), which can adversely affect the health of the parturient dyad. Rates of STDs among women who use drugs are double those of the general population (Tronick & Beeghly, 1992). Among the common STDs are herpes, syphilis, gonorrhea, and AIDS.

Another lifestyle risk is associated with multiple unsterile injections or the sharing of hypodermic needles with acquaintances. These practices place the woman at risk for contracting a variety of infectious diseases and communicating these to her fetus. Naeye and colleagues (1973) reported that more than 50 percent of the infants in their study who were born to heroin addicts had been infected with hepatitis. The actual extent of AIDS among this population is difficult to ascertain; however, it is becoming increasingly more prevalent. Tetanus and infectious endocarditis are other serious causes of maternal morbidity and mortality (Stimmel, 1979) (see Chapter 42, Neonatal Acquired Immunodeficiency Syndrome).

Heroin has also been documented as being responsible for anovulation and associated amenorrhea. Therefore, when the addicted woman has stopped menstruating, she feels no need to use birth control or to question if she has become pregnant. However, ovulation can occur in times of irregular heroin supply, and thus impregnation is possible. The woman may be pregnant and not realize it because erratic or absent menses is commonplace. The woman's cognitive abilities are also clouded by heroin, with judgment and problem-solving abilities impaired. Most methods of birth control require forethought and planning, as does the procurement of an abortion. Therefore, the woman finds herself pregnant with no way out. Hopeless and out of control, many may continue drug use as a way of coping. Others may acknowledge the effects of heroin on the fetus and become motivated to seek a drug rehabilitation program. Unfortunately, there is a paucity of such programs, as many exclude pregnant women.

Effects of In Utero Exposure

Fetal Low Birth Weight

Infants who are exposed to heroin weigh significantly less than do infants who are not (Naeye et al., 1973; Reddy et al., 1971; Zelson et al., 1971, 1973). Morbidity and mortality are disproportionately high among LBW infants (Boobis & Sullivan, 1986; Connaughton et al., 1977). The exact mechanism for this decreased intrauterine growth is debatable. Is it from the direct effects of heroin or from the associated lifestyle (e.g., prostitution and poor maternal nutrition)? This does not seem to be the only factor (Abrams & Laros, 1986).

Connaughton and associates (1975) compared two groups of pregnant women who received no prenatal care. One group was addicted to heroin, whereas the other group was not using illegal substances. Of the addicted group, 48.2 percent delivered LBW infants, whereas of the nonaddicted group, 16 percent delivered LBW infants. These findings imply that there was an exogenous variable that affected birth weight other than maternal nutritional status and prenatal care. Heroin readily crosses the placenta, as it is of low molecular weight and is lipid soluble (Kroll, 1986; Smith & Asch, 1987). Heroin may have directly depressed fetal growth.

Naeye and coworkers (1973) also felt that maternal malnutrition was not the only variable involved in LBW infants who had been exposed to heroin in utero. When the growth patterns of these infants were examined, it was found that their organs were smaller owing to a reduction in the number of cells, which is typical of malnourished infants (Naeye et al., 1973). "A reduction in the growth hormone and uteroplacental blood flow may be responsible, but fetal growth retardation in other uteroplacental disorders is different from that observed in the offspring of heroin addicts" (Naeye et al., 1973, p. 1060).

Fetal Distress

During pregnancy, maternal heroin ingestion creates a passive fetal addiction. When the mother's heroin supply is erratic, or if she tries to "kick the habit," the fetus mirrors the mother's withdrawal response. Withdrawal symptoms in an adult consist of irritability, anxiety, tremulousness, and abdominal cramping. The fetus also becomes agitated, which expends energy and increases oxygen demands. However, during this time of enhanced metabolic needs, there is an actual reduction in uteroplacental exchange secondary to uterine cramping (Ostrea & Chavez, 1979). This results in fetal hypoxia, which, in turn, induces deep breathing movements and fetal straining. During straining, meconium may be passed and subsequently aspirated (Ostrea & Chavez, 1979). In utero withdrawal has also been associated with fetal demise. Maternal detoxification is not recommended during the last trimester of pregnancy because of the likelihood of these complications. Generally, the pregnant addict is placed on methadone maintenance and given prenatal care, nutritional assistance, and counseling. Once the child is delivered, detoxification may be attempted (Connaughton et al., 1977).

Another complicating factor in the delivery process is that infants who have been exposed to heroin have an increased incidence of LBW related to prematurity and SGA status (Boobis & Sullivan, 1986). Early studies failed to differentiate LBW infants from those who were SGA. However, with more reliable estimation of gestational age by examination, studies since the late 1960s began to differentiate among babies who were premature, LBW, and SGA (Wilson, 1975). There is also an increased incidence of breech presentation among infants who have been exposed to heroin, which is believed to be from heightened fetal activity during episodes of hypoxia (Connaughton et al., 1975).

Heroin as a Teratogen

It is generally accepted that opiates, heroin, and methadone are not teratogenic (Boobis & Sullivan, 1986). Therefore, the pregnant woman is maintained on methadone until delivery. There is a cross-dependence between heroin and methadone, so fetal withdrawal is prevented. The benefit of methadone over heroin is that methadone can be prescribed by exact dose, can be given orally, and does not exert the mood-altering effects of heroin. The methadone level can be maintained at a more constant level; thus, in utero fetal withdrawal is avoided. Unknown adulterants are also avoided, and the psychological addiction to needles can be overcome. Women in methadone programs are provided with support services such as counseling, prenatal care, and assistance for food and shelter.

Residual Effects in the Neonatal Period

Neonatal Abstinence Syndrome. The majority of infants born to women addicted to heroin undergo withdrawal (Naeye et al., 1973; Reddy et al., 1971; Zelson et al., 1971). It is unclear why all infants do not display withdrawal symptoms. Perhaps in some infants, the symptoms are subtle and go unrecognized. The onset of withdrawal can occur up to day 6 of life (Reddy et al., 1971), and symptoms last for 8 to 16 weeks (Philips, 1986). The term *neonatal abstinence syndrome* (NAS) was coined because of the consistent pattern of symptoms (Fig. 45–2). The findings in infants exposed to heroin in utero include CNS and GI symptoms, and these infants are SGA. Infants who are poorly nourished in utero have already been discussed. CNS symptoms are the first to appear and include behaviors such as hyperactivity, irritability, tremors (Reddy et al., 1971), high-pitched cry, hypertonicity, and convulsions (Zelson et al., 1971).

Symptoms related to the GI tract appear later. Reddy and colleagues (1971) found these symptoms to appear on day 4 to day 6 of life and to include regurgitation, poor feeding, vomiting, and diarrhea. Incessant crying associated with withdrawal often makes the caretaker think that the infant is hungry. This may lead to overfeeding or caretaker frustration when the infant continues to cry instead of sucking from the bottle. Less frequent symptoms are hyperpyrexia, nasal congestion, tachypnea (Reddy et al., 1972), yawning, and sweating (Zelson et al., 1971). All these symptoms are similarly seen in adult drug addicts during withdrawal.

Physiologic jaundice was less frequent among infants of addicted women than among infants of nonaddicted women. Zelson and associates (1971) hypothesized that the heroin, or a substance used to adulterate the heroin, prematurely induces microenzymes in the liver. Glucuronosyltransferase was present earlier in the neonatal period in infants who were exposed to heroin. This early induction of glucuronosyltransferase facilitated the clearance of bilirubin, thus lowering the incidence of hyperbilirubinemia. Signs and symptoms of withdrawal can be categorized and scored (Tables 45–1 and 45–2).

There is no precise predictive correlational pattern between maternal addiction and infant withdrawal. However, a general pattern is that infants of mothers who have long-standing, heavy patterns of abuse are most likely to experience withdrawal (Zelson et al., 1971). Also, NAS has been reported to last longer in infants born to mothers who were maintained on methadone than in those whose mothers were taking heroin (Kaltenbach, 1992). Soepatmi (1994) followed the development of 144 children who were exposed to heroin or methadone in utero. Of the 144 who were eligible, 91 participated in the follow-up study. NAS was evident in all infants exposed to heroin or methadone. Thirty-five percent of the exposed infants experienced a resurgence of withdrawal symptoms or subacute abstinence symptoms after discharge.

Incidence of Respiratory Distress. The incidence of RDS among infants addicted to heroin is less than would be expected when compared with infants of similar size and gestation who were not exposed to heroin (Glass et al., 1971). A possible mechanism to explain this lower rate of RDS relates to the fetal stress response being repeatedly stimulated by periodic episodes of in utero withdrawal and associated hypoxia. This hastens lung maturity by stimulating the fetal adrenal gland to produce glucocorticoids, which, in turn, facilitate the production of surfactant within the lung. Another possible mechanism is that heroin may exert a direct action on the fetal lung to enhance pulmonary surfactant production (Glass & Evans, 1977).

Infants addicted to heroin do have a greater incidence of meconium aspiration and aspiration pneumonia. The underlying mechanism relates to the intermittent episodes of intrauterine hypoxia that are associated with maternal withdrawal in times of sparse drug supply (Philips, 1986). If the fetal P_{CO_2} increases to sufficient levels, the fetus may begin deep respiratory movements that predispose to aspiration of amniotic fluid either in utero or during delivery. If meconium has been passed in utero as a result of heroin-induced hypermotility of the intestines and stress, meconium aspiration results (Flandermeyer, 1987; Philips, 1986).

Risks Associated With Infancy and Early Childhood

Infancy

Infants of addicted mothers often have abnormal sleep patterns. Pinto and coworkers (1988) found that these infants spend less time in quiet sleep. They are also more easily aroused, as they have heightened auditory awareness. Overall, these infants are irritable, difficult to console, and easily aroused (Philips, 1986). Caretakers refer to infants who have been exposed to heroin in utero as being "uncuddly," in that they lack many reciprocal attachment behaviors such as maintaining eye contact, cuddling by conforming to the caretaker's chest, and being easily calmed. Instead they cry, posture, and lack the ability to interact with the caretaker. This behavior reduces caretaker satisfaction, making care difficult.

SIDS has been reported as being 5 to 10 times more common among infants who have been exposed to opiates in utero (Ward et al., 1986). The cause is obscure; however, abnormal ventilatory patterns are hypothesized as being a predisposing factor to SIDS. Ward and associates (1986) recorded overnight pneumograms on infants exposed to opiates, phencyclidine hydrochloride (PCP), and cocaine. The inclusion of all three types of drugs reflects the trend toward polydrug use. They found a higher prevalence of abnormal ventilatory patterns (32 percent) when compared with the control group (9.3 percent). Among the differences were "longer total sleep time, greater durations of apnea, a higher total duration of apneas, more periodic breathing, a higher mean respiratory rate, and a lower mean heart rate" (Ward et al., 1986). At the time this study was performed, data were beginning to be gathered regarding the association of maternal cocaine use and SIDS. However, in more recent studies, it has become clear that SIDS is more prevalent among infants exposed to cocaine when compared with those exposed to methadone (Chasnoff et al., 1987).

NEONATAL ABSTINENCE SCORING SYSTEM

SYSTEM	SIGNS AND SYMPTOMS	SCORE	AM	PM	COMMENTS
CENTRAL NERVOUS SYSTEM DISTURBANCES	Excessive High Pitched (Or other) Cry Continuous High Pitched (Or other) Cry	2 3			Daily Weight:
	Sleeps < 1 Hour After Feeding Sleeps < 2 Hours After Feeding Sleeps < 3 Hours After Feeding	3 2 1			
	Hyperactive Moro Reflex Markedly Hyperactive Moro Reflex	2 3			
	Mild Tremors Disturbed Moderate-Severe Tremors Disturbed	1 2			
	Mild Tremors Undisturbed Moderate-Severe Tremors Undisturbed	3 4			
	Increased Muscle Tone	2			
	Excoriation (Specific Area)	1			
	Myoclonic Jerks	3			
	Generalized Convulsions	5			
METABOLIC/VASOMOTOR/RESPIRATORY DISTURBANCES	Sweating	1			
	Fever<101 (99-100.8 F./37.2-38.2C.) Fever>101 (38.4C. and Higher)	1 2			
	Frequent Yawning (> 3-4 Times/Interval)	1			
	Mottling	1			
	Nasal Stuffiness	1			
	Sneezing (> 3-4 Times/Interval)	1			
	Nasal Flaring	2			
	Respiratory Rate > 60/min Respiratory Rate > 60/min with Retractions	1 2			
GASTRO-INTESTIONAL DISTURBANCES	Excessive Sucking	1			
	Poor Feeding	2			
	Regurgitation Projectile Vomiting	2 3			
	Loose Stools Watery Stools	2 3			
	TOTAL SCORE				
	INITIALS OF SCORER				

FIGURE 45–2. Neonatal abstinence scoring system. (From Finnegan, L. P. [1986]. Neonatal abstinence syndrome: Assessment and pharmacotherapy. In F. F. Rubaltelli & B. Granati [Eds.], *Neonatal therapy: An update*. New York: Excerpta Medica. Reprinted with permission.)

Early Childhood

There is conflicting documentation as to the lingering effects of in utero heroin exposure on growth and development during early childhood. A review of the following longitudinal studies demonstrates this lack of consensus on the impact of heroin on later cognitive and behavioral development. Lifschnitz and colleagues (1983) examined the growth of 3-year-old children who had been exposed to heroin (group 1) and methadone (group 2) and those who were drug-free but of similar socioeconomic status (control group). When environmental factors were controlled, there was not a significant drug-imposed effect on later growth. Lifestyle patterns were felt to be the main variable in growth patterns. Strauss and associates (1976) followed the motor and mental development of infants exposed to opiates in utero during the first year of life and found that they were within normal limits. Wilson and associates (1979) followed the growth and behavior of 3-year-old children exposed to heroin in utero as compared with children in two control groups. One control group consisted of women who were peripherally involved in the drug culture without actively using heroin themselves. Some of these women were married to drug-using men or began using drugs after they delivered. The other control group included mothers of similar socioeconomic status who were not involved in the

TABLE 45–1 Neonatal Abstinence Syndrome: Clinical Manifestations

Birth Weight	Gastrointestional	Central Nervous System	Other
Small for gestational age	Regurgitation	First to appear	Hyperpyrexia
	Poor feeding	Hyperactivity	Nasal congestion
	Vomiting	Irritability	Tachypnea
	Diarrhea	Tremors	Yawning
		High-pitched cry	Sweating
		Hypertonicity	
		Convulsions	
		Incessant crying	

drug culture. The latter group's pregnancies and deliveries were routine. Wilson and coworkers (1979) reported that children exposed to heroin in utero exhibited aberrant behavior. These children were described as having an "uncontrollable temper, impulsiveness and difficulty making and keeping friends" (p. 139). The mental performance of the infants exposed to heroin was within normal limits; however, it was consistently lower than that of the other groups.

Researchers in the Netherlands conducted a longitudinal, prospective study of a group of children who had been exposed to a combination of methadone, heroin, and cocaine in utero (van Barr et al., 1994). The purpose of the study was to evaluate the children's development as compared with a control group of children who were not exposed to drugs. Cognitive delays, especially around early language development, were detected by the Bayley Scales of Infant Development (mental scale) by 2 years of age. When the children were re-evaluated between their fourth and fifth birthdays, half of the scores of the children who were exposed to drugs were markedly lower (e.g., one standard deviation below the average). Results of evaluation of the children at 5 years demonstrated developmental and behavioral problems, as well as cognitive difficulties. Behavioral problems included aggression, depression, and difficulties involving interactions with peers and adults. Another observation was that half of the children who had been exposed to drugs in utero lived with a parent substitute by the age of 5 years. It is difficult to ascertain causality between living with an alternate caregiver and more impaired behavior. Did the disruption of being placed in foster care contribute to the behavioral-cognitive difficulties or were the more affected children removed from the home because their parents could not adequately handle the behavioral and cognitive problems? On the positive side, the children's physical development was normal and they appeared healthy. Neurologic development also was normal as evaluated by the Bayley Scales of Infant Development (motor scale) and the Bruininks-Oseretsky test of motor proficiency.

Soepatmi (1994) reported the developmental outcomes of infants who had been exposed to heroin or methadone in utero. Exposed children were smaller at birth and continued to be small for their age. Subjects were born during 1974 to 1983 and were 3½ to 12 years of age at the time of developmental evaluation. The children had an increased incidence of school problems, IQ scores less than 85, and an increased incidence of behavioral problems as defined by a score of greater than 90 on the Total Social Competence Scale. Another finding was that children faired better when they lived with their biologic parents. However, children in early foster placement had fewer behavioral problems than did children removed from the home at an older age.

Kaltenbach (1992) reviewed the literature and found six longitudinal studies that evaluated the developmental outcome of infants exposed to methadone as measured by the Bayley Scales of Infant Development. There were mixed findings, with three studies reporting that the infants exposed to methadone scored lower than the infants who were not exposed, and the other three studies finding no significant differences.

Inconsistencies in the literature regarding the developmental outcomes of infants who are exposed to heroin or methadone in utero may be attributed to the following:

1. Children may not be followed for a sufficient period to detect differences. Long-term follow-up of this population is difficult because of the transient lifestyle, missed clinic appointments, lack of phone service, and adeptness at "disappearing" resulting from the mother's continued use of illegal drugs.
2. Methodologic issues such as self-selection may not include those infants who were most affected by drug exposure. Children who maintained enrollment in studies have a parent or parents who are more motivated to provide their child with services to enhance outcome.
3. Individual variations in the dose of the drug and variance with respect to the timing of drug use during pregnancy influence the impact on the child.
4. Women may have used multiple substances and reported only one, for example, receiving methadone but also taking cocaine.
5. Raising the child in a drug culture in which parents are more concerned with seeking their next "fix" than in meeting their child's needs hampers development.
6. The impact of exposure to infectious diseases (e.g., hepatitis, HIV) in utero and their parents' deteriorated health status also has a negative impact on the child's development.

TABLE 45–2 Dysmorphic Characteristics of Fetal Alcohol Syndrome

Facial anomalies	Low nasal bridge
Narrow receding forehead	Minor ear anomalies
Microcephaly	Short upturned nose
Short palpebral fissures	Micrognathia
Flat midface	Ptosis
Indistinct philtrum	Myopia
Thin upper lip	Strabismus
Epicanthal folds	

PROFILE OF THE DRUG-ADDICTED WOMAN

The woman who is addicted to drugs generally was abusing drugs before her pregnancy. Therefore, when a pregnant addict seeks prenatal care, she requires more than actual drug treatment. She often has an underlying personality disorder that requires in-depth psychotherapy (Atkins, 1988). The woman has often turned to drugs to dispel anxiety or depression. Drugs are also a mechanism of escape from poverty, personal problems, and hopelessness. The poverty level may be perceived to be so impermeable and so inescapable that drugs are the only way out. Likewise, depression may be so intense that cocaine provides temporary relief. However, as larger amounts of cocaine are taken, happiness and joy seem more elusive. Depression during the "postcoke blues" may trigger the use of other drugs such as heroin to ease the pain of "coming down."

Drug-abusing women were often raised in dysfunctional families, being victims of abuse and rape. Therefore, a void exists with respect to what is entailed in a healthy parent–child relationship. Individuals tend to parent as they were parented; thus, a dysfunctional parent–child relationship may ensue without systematic intervention throughout early childhood. Individuals may become socially isolated as a consequence of their addiction. The woman's acquaintances within the drug community may have no more emotional reserve for coping and problem-solving than she has. Therefore, intervention must come from outside her immediate social network.

In addition to a lack of social support and low self-esteem, the addicted woman is poorly equipped to earn a living for herself and her child (Daghestani, 1988). To further complicate the parenting scenario, the addict often has unrealistic expectations of her infant. She may look to the infant to meet her needs rather than seeing herself as the infant's caretaker. She may think the infant is capable of giving her love and approval and is sadly disappointed when this is not possible. The reality of the situation is that there is an isolated, insecure woman trying to care for a very irritable infant. Instead of gaining satisfaction from the relationship, she may become angry or perhaps guilty, as she may interpret the infant's behavior as a "punishment" or outcry against her for her addiction. This, coupled with the fact that most women return to drug abuse after delivery, sets the stage for poor or abusive parenting. Drug-seeking behavior interferes with the individual's ability to function in society, including the ability to parent. As previously discussed, when an infant is presented to the drug-addicted woman, her deficient coping mechanisms are readily depleted and, without assistance, she may pattern her parenting after that which she received, leading to child neglect or abuse.

ALCOHOL

The consumption of alcohol is easily traced to Biblical times. It is debatable at what point in history the ill effects of alcohol on the fetus were recognized. Some authors have interpreted the Biblical verse "Behold, thou shalt conceive and bear a son; and now drink no wine or strong drink" (Judges 13:7) as cautioning women to abstain from alcohol during times that they can conceive. Others believe that the relationship between maternal alcohol consumption and deleterious effects on the fetus was unknown until 18th-century England. During that time, gin consumption soared to epidemic proportions owing to a cheap, available supply. Men and women alike drank excessively. As a consequence of pregnant women drinking, their offspring were described as being born "feeble and dull witted" (Abel, 1984). Today, excessive maternal perinatal alcohol consumption is associated with infant and child cognitive delays. Lipson (1988) made the statement that "alcohol abuse during pregnancy is the most frequent teratogenic cause of mental retardation in the western world" (p. 385). FAS is the number one cause of mental retardation and is completely preventable (Phelps & Grabowski, 1992). The reported rate of FAS was six times higher in 1993 than in 1979 (AWHONN, 1995). It is not clear if this reflects increased awareness and reporting or simply increased drinking among pregnant women.

Although regular drinking during pregnancy has historically been ill advised, until recently no researchers had systematically examined the offspring of alcoholics to identify a predictable pattern of external malformations. Any association between alcohol and its effects was made retrospectively. The cluster of anomalies termed *FAS* was not identified until 1973. At that time, Jones and Smith (1973) observed the external characteristics of 11 infants born to women with chronic alcoholism, and distinct patterns of anomalies emerged. Their observations were the first clues that alcohol might be a teratogen producing a specific pattern of anomalies. Unknown to Jones and Smith (1973), an earlier French paper (Lemoine et al., 1968) had been published with similar findings. Since these reports, hundreds of studies have been conducted investigating the effects of alcohol on the fetus. Subsequent publications discussed similar anomalous patterns. Alcohol-induced aberrations fall on a continuum, ranging from mild to severe, with some children manifesting all or more characteristics and others exhibiting few or none. In fact, two classifications of alcohol-related effects exist. FAS is on the severe end of the continuum, and FAE refers to mild symptoms (see Table 45–2).

The diagnosis of FAS is not always made easily or immediately based solely on external characteristics. Little and associates (1990) argued that FAS is 100 percent underdiagnosed during the neonatal period unless the mother is admitted in labor while intoxicated or if the amniotic fluid smells of alcohol, or both. There is no definitive test for FAS, so diagnosis is based on a positive drinking history during pregnancy, and the triad of findings (dysmorphic characteristics, CNS dysfunction, and growth deficiency). However, most women are hesitant to disclose drinking during pregnancy, and FAS often goes undiagnosed until preschool or early school years. A high percentage of children exposed to alcohol in utero are in foster or adoptive care, which further obscures the diagnosis, as the maternal drinking history is missing. Failure to thrive, persistent behavioral problems, or academic failure, or a combination of these factors, provide the impetus for a medical investigation. Parents are often told that if they had greater patience, were more consistent with discipline, or were in essence better parents, their child would respond more appropriately. In fact, the symptoms are rooted in organic damage caused by the alcohol consumption. Foster or adoptive parents respond to the diagnosis differently than do biologic parents. Foster or adoptive parents may feel anger toward the biologic parent, while experiencing some relief about knowing what is responsible for their child's symptoms. Biologic parents who are caring for their children need to cope with the guilt from the realization of how they harmed their child through prenatal drinking, receive treatment to achieve and maintain sobriety, cope with emotional issues underpinning their addiction, and learn consistent parenting strategies.

Mechanism of Action

The active ingredient of alcohol is ethanol. Ethanol and its metabolite, acetaldehyde, are of low molecular weight and fat soluble and thus easily cross the placenta (Abel, 1984). Ethanol is a CNS depressant. It is unknown whether the teratogenic effects are a result of ethanol or its metabolite. Once maternal ingestion occurs, alcohol is absorbed via the length of the GI tract by diffusing into the blood stream. Different blood ethanol levels may be achieved from the same maternal dose owing to individual variables. Factors that influence alcohol absorption include the presence of food in the stomach, a high-protein maternal diet, and individual metabolic variations (Abel, 1984). Alcoholic women often eat little and have a protein-poor diet, which enhances ethanol absorption. Alcohol is distributed equally throughout the body fluid. Since women have less body water than do men, ethanol is concentrated in less fluid, producing higher blood ethanol levels (Abel, 1984; Neri et al., 1988). The activity of gastric alcohol dehydrogenase is reduced in women (Frezza et al., 1990). Therefore, the initial gastric metabolism of alcohol is reduced. For these reasons, women achieve higher levels of intoxication than do men, given the same dose of alcohol. Maternal ethanol diffuses to the fetus and is deposited at highest levels in the fetal liver, pancreas, kidney, lung, thymus, heart, and brain (Abel, 1984). Fetal ethanol metabolism is half that of the adult. As a consequence, a major pathway for fetal ethanol clearance is back diffusion to the maternal system. A consequence of this metabolic lag is that the fetus is bathed in ethanol-rich amniotic fluid (Tranmer, 1985). The infant born with high ethanol levels may appear intoxicated until the immature fetal liver can complete metabolism.

Risk Factors Associated With Alcohol Abuse

General Health Risks

As previously discussed, women who drink heavily often smoke and are poorly nourished (Little, 1977; Wright, 1986). These factors make it difficult to ascertain if the fetal effects are inflicted from a single agent or from the interactive effect of alcohol and smoking. Limitations to many studies are that the "drinking" group consists of alcoholics and not just social to moderate drinkers. Data are reliant on accurate self-reporting of alcohol consumption during pregnancy. Drinking is often underreported by users in an attempt to minimize their addiction or perhaps as a result of impaired recall secondary to intoxication. Also, women who are alcoholics often have other associated health problems (e.g., cirrhosis or poor nutritional status).

Pregnancy-Associated Risks

Spontaneous Abortion

Alcohol has been associated with an increased incidence of spontaneous abortion. Harlap and Shiono (1980) found regular maternal alcohol consumption of one or more drinks daily to result in a higher rate of miscarriage during the second trimester. They were careful to state that although miscarriage rates were not elevated during early pregnancy among their subjects, this did not mean that it was safe to drink during pregnancy. Harlap and Shiono (1980) also compared the impact of drinking versus smoking on spontaneous abortion and found that maternal alcohol consumption exerted a much greater effect on the rate of miscarriage.

A positive correlation was found between a minimal maternal alcohol consumption of two drinks (2 oz absolute alcohol) per week and an elevated rate of spontaneous abortion (Kline et al., 1980). A serving of alcohol was defined as 1 oz of absolute alcohol. This form of reporting standardizes the alcoholic content when all forms of alcoholic beverages are considered (i.e., liquor, beer, and wine). The researchers conjectured that ethanol's mechanism of action on termination of the pregnancy is acute fetal poisoning. Although low thresholds of alcohol consumption are being explored, there is no known safe level during pregnancy.

Fetal Hazards

Infant Weight

Infants of women who drink during pregnancy are of lower birth weight than the general population and do not tend to catch up during postnatal months (Chasnoff, 1986a). Little and associates (1980) sought out the effects of past alcoholism on fetal weight gain in cases in which sobriety was maintained during pregnancy. Three groups were followed: (1) abstaining alcoholics, (2) drinking alcoholics, and (3) a control group. By comparing alcoholic women who were maintaining sobriety (abstaining alcoholics) with actively drinking alcoholics, general health issues were controlled. Variables such as maternal smoking, height, age, parity, gestational age, and sex of the child were controlled. The variable that was left to exert an influence on fetal weight was alcohol. Little and colleagues (1980) found that the infants of drinking alcoholics weighed 493 g less than those of the control group, whereas the infants of abstaining alcoholics weighed 258 g less than those of the control group. The results between the groups were statistically significant. It was revealing that past alcoholism affected the mean birth weight in the absence of current drinking. These researchers suggested that an underlying alteration in the woman's health status existed that interfered with optimal fetal weight gain. The women's diets were reported to be adequate during pregnancy. A possible rationale was preexisting compromised maternal health as a result of "fatty liver, hypertension, anemia, peptic ulcer or obesity" (Little et al., 1980, p. 976).

Little (1977) conducted a prospective study of 263 women. She found that maternal consumption of 1 oz of absolute alcohol per day during the last trimester was correlated with infant birth weight being 160 g less than average. Again, significant variables such as maternal smoking, age, height, parity, and the gestational age and sex of the child were controlled. Observations made by Little regarding the subjects in her middle-class health maintenance organization population were that 60 percent of the women did not drink once they became pregnant and those that drank reduced their consumption during pregnancy.

Numerous studies with consistent reports from other investigations document reduced infant birth weight among infants exposed to alcohol in utero. There is also a consistent dose response in that as maternal alcohol consumption increases, infant birth weight decreases (Ernhart et al., 1987; Mills et al., 1984). This finding would validate alcohol as being the causative agent of lower birth weight.

Alcohol as a Teratogen

Ernhart and coworkers (1987) found that a "critical period for alcohol teratogenicity was confirmed to be around the time of conception" (p. 33). A critical period refers to a time during fetal development when developing tissue is highly vulnerable to a teratogen. Typically, this occurs when cells are rapidly dividing and differentiating. Other investigators (Hanson et al., 1978; Warren & Bast, 1988) observed a consistent pattern between alcohol consumption shortly after conception and an increased incidence of FAS. Kronick (1976) found similar patterns of malformations that occurred when ethanol was given to mice during periods of organogenesis in very early pregnancy. Ernhart and coworkers (1987) found a teratogenic maternal ethanol dose to be more than six drinks per day (i.e., more than 3 oz of absolute alcohol), whereas Wright (1986) found the teratogenic dose of ethanol to be 80 g of alcohol, or about eight large glasses of wine per day both before and during pregnancy. It is important to note that absolute alcohol is equally detrimental be it derived from beer, wine, or liquor (Lewis, 1983).

There is no agreement within the literature as to the exact dose of ethanol required to induce FAS or FAE. Therefore, the minimal threshold of ethanol ingestion responsible for producing ill effects in the fetus is unknown (Chasnoff, 1986a). The rationale is that humans are multifaceted, with many variables affecting each individual. It is also unethical to perform fetal experimentation. Commonly identified variables that are thought to affect fetal response to maternal alcohol ingestion are (1) maternal health, (2) ethanol dose, (3) timing with respect to organogenesis, and (4) fetal tolerance to alcohol (Chasnoff, 1986a; Schnoll, 1986; Streissguth & LaDue, 1985). A discussion of each of these four variables follows.

Maternal health affects the developing fetus. The health status of the dyad is influenced by maternal age, nutritional status, exposure to infectious agents, and socioeconomic status (Schnoll, 1986). Other variables that commonly influence the alcoholic's life are the associated manifestations of alcoholism (e.g., cirrhosis of the liver).

Ethanol dose is a critical component of teratogenicity. For anomalies to occur, a "threshold level" must be present in the maternal system (Schnoll, 1986)—that is, a particular dose must be attained before disruption in organogenesis occurs. It is felt that peak levels of ethanol play a more significant role in teratogenesis than do chronic low levels (Chasnoff, 1986a). Clarren and colleagues (1985) also stated that the higher the amount of maternal alcohol consumption, the greater the risk of the development of FAS. For example, chronic alcoholics have a higher rate of infants with FAS than do women who drink socially. However, there is no known safe level of maternal alcohol consumption during pregnancy.

Timing of ingestion with regard to period of susceptibility (i.e., organogenesis) is a variable in teratogenesis (Chasnoff, 1986a). Organogenesis during early pregnancy is a time when aberrations in organ formation can occur. Therefore, a drug may cause an anomaly if consumed on a particular day when a specific organ system is forming. The same drug consumed later in pregnancy may not exert the same effect (see Chapter 10, Fetal Development: Environmental Influences and Critical Periods).

The fourth variable is the difference in individual fetal tolerance to a particular drug. This conclusion is based on the different responses between twins. Dizygotic twins have reportedly been born to alcoholic mothers with different expressions of teratogenicity (Christoffel & Salafsky, 1975; Chasnoff, 1986b).

Fetal Alcohol Syndrome

FAS is diagnosed by reported maternal alcohol consumption during pregnancy as well as characteristic neonatal features. These findings revolve around three areas: (1) prenatal and postnatal growth deficiency, (2) dysmorphic characteristics, and (3) CNS dysfunction (Jones & Smith, 1973; Jones et al., 1973; Lipson, 1988; Streissguth et al., 1985, Streissguth & LaDue, 1985).

Children diagnosed with FAS are smaller at birth and fail to demonstrate catch-up growth. They are often diagnosed later in infancy, when they present with failure to thrive in spite of adequate calorie intake (Jones et al., 1973; Streissguth et al., 1985) or exhibit learning or developmental difficulties during early childhood (Phelps & Grabowski, 1992). Head growth as measured by head circumference is often below the tenth percentile, as is weight for height. Streissguth and colleagues (1985) followed the original 11 children who were the basis of defining FAS. The males remained extremely thin. The females were short but gained weight during the transition into puberty.

Dysmorphic characteristics of FAS include a series of facial anomalies, abnormal palmar creases, and congenital heart disease. Facial anomalies include microcephaly, short palpebral fissures, flat midface, indistinct philtrum, thin upper lip, epicanthal folds, low nasal bridge, minor ear anomalies, short nose, and micrognathia (Baraitser & Winter, 1996; Streissguth et al., 1985). Other findings related to facial abnormalities are ptosis, myopia, strabismus, narrow receding forehead, and short upturned nose (Plant, 1985). As the children enter adolescence, the facial features change, with the nose becoming prominent, with a distinctive nasal bridge (Wekselman et al., 1995). The preponderance of facial anomalies affect the midface (Fig. 45–3). A hypothesis is that if the internal structures that lie within the same plane as the midface were also deficient or absent, it would explain the cognitive deficiencies among FAS children when considered with other findings.

Diagnosis is based on a cluster of anomalies, not just one isolated finding. Neri and coworkers (1988) felt this was reasonable, as "facial anomalies of the FAS are the expression of a midline defect originating from the disruption of the ordered development of midline mesoderm cells during early embryogenesis" (p. 477). Abnormal palmar creases are useful as a diagnostic tool (Jones et al., 1973). Congenital heart disease mainly involves septal defects (Jones & Smith, 1973; Jones et al., 1973), with many of these closing spontaneously. However, more serious cardiac anomalies have been reported (Steeg & Woolf, 1979). Infants with FAS have a variety of phenotypical expressions. They also have a varying degree of cognitive and CNS impairment, which has a negative impact on the child's functioning within the family and society. At birth, these infants are irritable and tremulous, have a poor sucking reflex, and are easily disturbed by sensory stimulation (Clarren et al., 1985; Warren & Bast, 1988). Older children are generally hypotonic and have increased minor motor movements that interfere with learning (Clarren et al., 1985) (Figs. 45–4 and 45–5). Children with FAS also have been reported as hyperactive. Dorris (1989) discussed the difficulties that his adoptive son endured as a result of fetal alcohol exposure. He described at length his son's inability to learn from past experiences or to assimilate, retain, or use data.

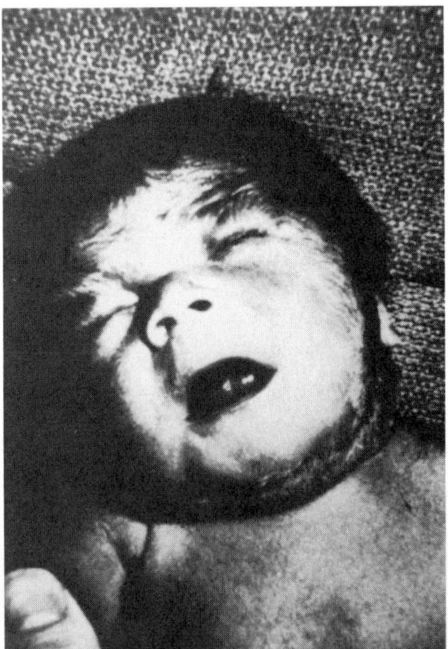
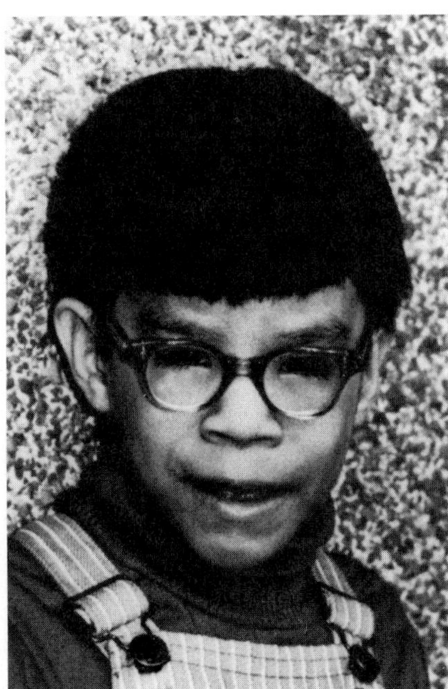
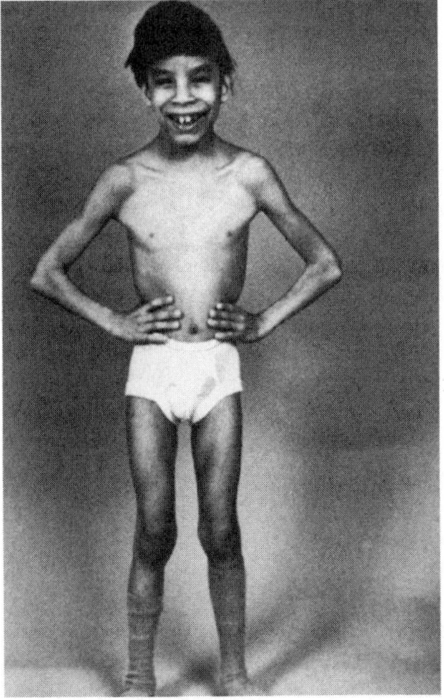

FIGURE 45–3. Fetal alcohol syndrome (FAS). (From Streissguth, A. P., Clarren, S. K., & Jones, K. L. [1985]. Natural history of the fetal alcohol syndrome: A 10-year follow-up of eleven patients. *Lancet,* 2[8446], 85–91. Reprinted with permission.)

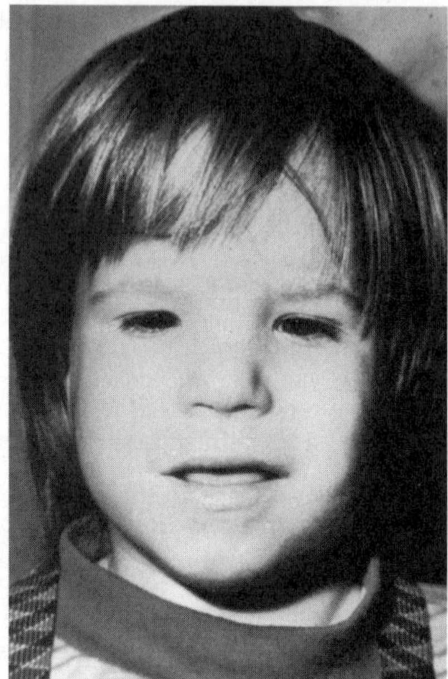
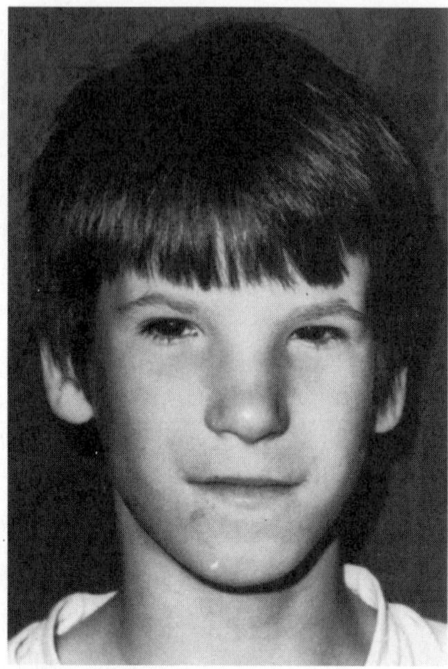
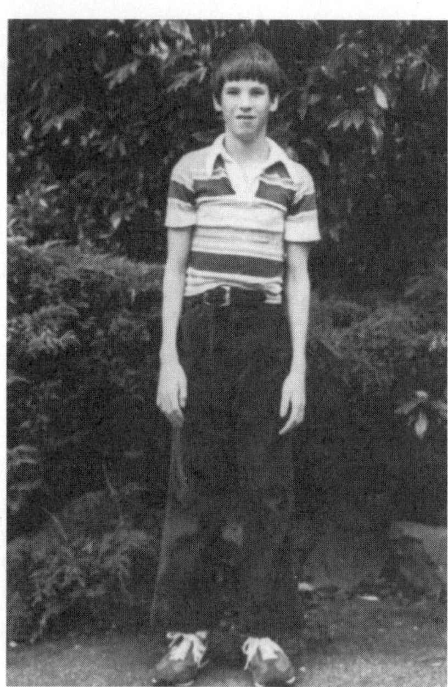

FIGURE 45–4. FAS in older child. (From Streissguth, A. P., Clarren, S. K., & Jones, K. L. [1985]. Natural history of the fetal alcohol syndrome: A 10-year follow-up of eleven patients. *Lancet*, 2[8446], 85–91. Reprinted with permission.)

Behavioral Manifestations. Infants who have been exposed to alcohol in utero often display a predictable set of behaviors after birth. Some researchers refer to these as alcohol related birth defects (ARBD). Characteristic behaviors include irritability, tremors, poor feeding, and hypersensitivity to external stimuli (Clarren et al., 1985; Hanson et al., 1976; LeFrancois, 1984). Infants often have difficulty coordinating their sucking with swallowing and breathing. This difficulty creates feeding problems. Infants who have been exposed to alcohol in utero are easily hyperstimulated by noise, light, and tactile stimulation. This low threshold of stimulation can interfere with the formation of a reciprocal attachment relationship between caretaker and infant by disrupting the normal patterns of early interactions. The clinical picture is similar to that for infants who have been exposed to drugs in utero, with much of the nursing care being the same (nursing care is discussed later).

During preschool years, these children remain hyperactive and fidgety or restless. Learning disabilities emerge secondary to hyperactivity and attention deficit disorder (ADD) (Streissguth et al., 1978). In spite of the prevailing ADD, the children are friendly and outgoing. This gregariousness may mask deficient learning abilities (Streissguth et al., 1985). However, during primary grades, cognitive deficits and learning disabilities become evident. School-aged children with FAS or FAE continue to exhibit similar difficulties with cognition, poor impulse control, and socially acceptable behavior. The children reach an academic

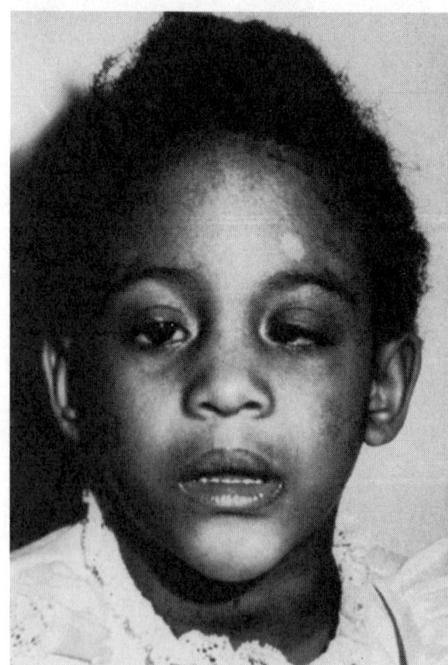
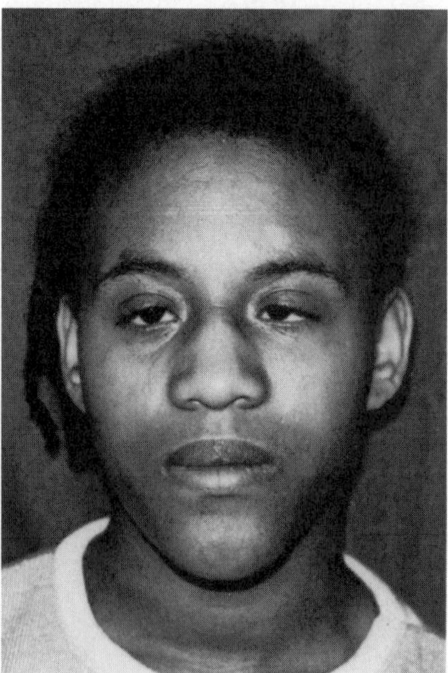
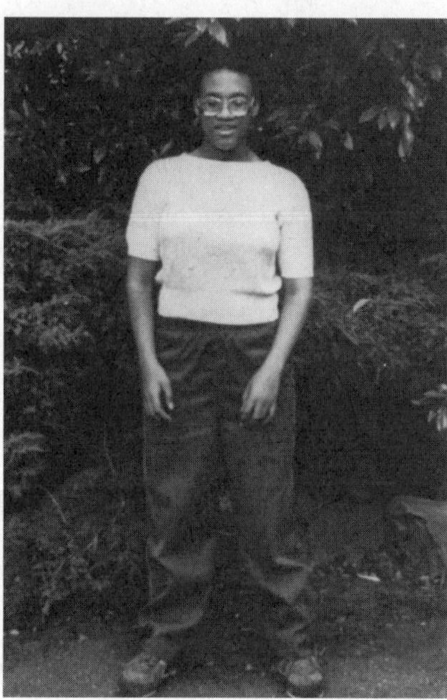

FIGURE 45–5. Adult FAS. (From Streissguth, A. P., Clarren, S. K., & Jones, K. L. [1985]. Natural history of the fetal alcohol syndrome: A 10-year follow-up of eleven patients. *Lancet*, 2[8446], 85–91. Reprinted with permission.)

ceiling by sixth to eighth grade (Wekselman et al., 1995), and behaviors that were accepted as a preschooler (e.g., overly friendly and affectionate) are no longer socially acceptable as an older child.

The most profound effect of FAS is CNS dysfunction. Hyperactivity is pervasive among children with FAS or FAE and is attributed to aberration of the CNS induced by ethanol (Phelps & Grabowski, 1992). As children become school age and enter high school, the hyperactivity is manifested as impulsiveness, not completing tasks, being uncooperative, and being unable to detect social cues that regulate appropriate behavior. Young adults are not able to live independently because of poor judgment, an inability to hold down a job, and a lack of self-discipline. There is a correlation between the extent of overt external manifestations of FAS and the degree of cognitive impairment. When a child displays severe physical dysmorphosis associated with FAS, significant mental retardation is often present (Streissguth et al., 1978). However, the converse is not true. Children with a normal appearance can be affected cognitively owing to alcohol's influence on fetal brain structure and function (Clarren et al., 1985). The level of cognitive impairment may be readily apparent or subtly expressed in the form of learning disabilities and ADD. The IQ of children born to alcoholic mothers has been found to be within normal limits (82 to 113). In spite of this, these children have been seen to experience "persistent academic failure" (Shaywitz et al., 1980, p. 978). This problem demonstrates that the effects of maternal alcohol ingestion cannot be readily detected at birth. Cognitive delays may not be evident until children are challenged with more complex cognitive tasks.

The causative factor seems to be the direct effect of ethanol or its primary metabolite acetaldehyde. Hanson and associates (1976) found a direct correlation between high maternal ethanol levels and expression of FAS. Furthermore, foster care did not improve the child's subsequent development. Hence, the cause of cognitive delays was more than environmental, and the damage was irreversible. Educational enrichment programs can help individuals realize their potential but cannot cure them by restoring cognitive functioning.

Incidence and Classification. Harwood and Napolitano (1985) examined the incidence of FAS. They cited a conservative estimate of 1 in 1000 live births, with a more realistic figure being 1 in 600 live births. The Nurses Association of the American College of Obstetrics and Gynecology (NAACOG) (1988) estimated the incidence as being between 1 and 3 in 1000 live births. The absolute estimates vary, but the ranges are similar. All estimates imply that FAS is far more common than is generally thought by the general population.

A quantifiable result of FAS is cognitive impairment. Such impairment can be categorized as (1) minimally brain damaged, (2) mildly to moderately retarded, and (3) severely to profoundly retarded (Harwood & Napolitano, 1985). Harwood and Napolitano (1985) compared these classifications to incidence. They found that of the children diagnosed with FAS, 52.5 percent were minimally brain-damaged, 45 percent were mildly to moderately retarded, and 2.5 percent were severely to profoundly retarded. The cost to society is immense in terms of lost worker productivity, direct health costs, ongoing educational expenditures, sheltered living and, in some cases, institutionalization (Harwood & Napolitano, 1985).

In early 1996, there were reports in the media (national television news and wire services) of a potential linkage between fetal exposure to alcohol during the second and third trimesters of pregnancy and childhood leukemia. The incidence rate may be increased more than 100 to 200 percent that of the average population. To determine the validity of these reports, long-term research studies must be performed. However, these reports certainly raise questions regarding genetic linkages or possible damage to the immune system by a direct action of the alcohol on the developing fetus.

Children who suffer from FAS or FAE have a devastatingly bleak prognosis. Early diagnosis and intervention can maximize potential, but often damage is so severe that independence cannot be attained. Prevention programs such as those sponsored by the National Organization of Fetal Alcohol Syndrome (NOFAS) have made significant inroads in heightening public awareness of the effects of alcohol on the fetus. Prevention is the only known way to combat FAS for future generations of unborn children.

ASSESSMENT

With abbreviated hospital stays, part of the admission protocol for all women should include a systematic routine assessment for substance use and abuse. The foundation for this form of intervention should be a staff of well-trained nurses. In-services and continuing education programs could be a vehicle to augment the staff's expertise in detecting signs of abuse. Nurses also need to undergo a period of self-examination with respect to their feelings toward addiction. Nonjudgmental therapeutic relationships with drug-abusing clients are impossible until the nurse's own feelings have been identified, contemplated, and resolved.

Nurses gather data through all their senses. They need to observe and interview all women entering the health care system systematically for signs of substance abuse, such as track marks on the arms from injections, an inflamed nasal septum from cocaine, alcohol on the breath, and tobacco stains on the fingers. Beyond observational data comes interview data. Women, especially pregnant women, underreport smoking, drinking, and drug use. However, self-reporting is the best method available to date and without asking about their use, no information will be elicited. In order to increase self-reporting, the nurse needs to create a comfortable atmosphere that encourages the women to disclose sensitive information. This atmosphere can be created through applying the following principles. Interviews should be conducted in a private office and should start with generic questions regarding factual information (e.g., name, address), progressing to the most sensitive information at the end of the interview (e.g, substance use). Questions should be open-ended and phrased in a manner to permit discussion. The interviewer should expect the woman to be open and honest. This attitude is subtly conveyed to the woman and becomes a self-fulfilling prophecy. The tobacco, alcohol, and drug use patterns of a woman resembles those of her partner, and past use parallels current practices. The ordering of questions is important and should begin with questions regarding the partner's use, the woman's past use and, last, the woman's current use. The following includes sample questions.

The interview should begin by the nurse saying that the following questions are asked of everyone.

"I would like to begin by asking a few questions about your partner's habits."

- "How many packs/day of cigarettes does your partner smoke?"
- "How often does your partner drink beer, wine coolers, malt liquor, or hard liquor?"

(Note: Several alcoholic beverages are itemized, as many individuals do not realize that wine coolers and beer contain enough alcohol to harm the fetus.)

- "How many drinks does your partner have at one time?"
- "Does he party?"

If yes, ask

- "Does he ever do pot, crack/cocaine or other drugs when he's out with his friends?"

If yes, ask

- "What do you do when he is partying?"

If no to the party question, ask

- "When was the last time he used pot, crack/cocaine, or other drugs?"

(Note: Women whose partners use are more likely to use themselves. Questions about partner's behaviors should be explored to identify women at risk for substance use.)

- "Considering the last six months before you knew you were pregnant could you answer the following questions?"

(Note: If women admit to use prior to pregnancy, then they may have continued use before they realized they were pregnant or may still be using but not disclosing.)

- "How many packs of cigarettes/day do you smoke?"

(Note: The interviewer should pay particular attention to the woman's smoking status, as smokers are 10 times more likely to use marijuana, 22 times more likely to use cocaine, and 21 times more likely to use amphetamines than nonsmoking women [Vega et al., 1993].)

- "How often do you drink beer, wine cooler, whiskey or other drinks containing alcohol?"
- "Do you have 3 or 4 drinks at a time?"

(Note: By asking about large amounts of drinking, the woman may feel comfortable disclosing that she has one or two drinks per night.)

- "When was the last time you used pot, crack/cocaine, or other drugs?"

These questions are more likely to elicit accurate information than the question "Do you drink?" or "You don't drink, do you?" The recommended questions are nonjudgmental and give the woman permission to report drinking. If the woman is drinking two drinks per day and she is asked if she drinks three or four, then she will feel more comfortable self-reporting drinking. It is also phrased so that the answer will be more than yes or no and prompt some discussion. If the woman responds to any of the questions with ambiguous answers such as "I'm a social drinker" or "I use crack for recreation," the responses need to be clarified with respect to amount and frequency of use (Weiner et al., 1985).

If a woman becomes angry about the questions or refuses to answer, it may be because the questions hit too close to home and she is not willing to discuss her use. She may also react out of shock at being questioned. Her response should be noted and evaluated by the nurse. If the nurse feels that she is perhaps using substances and not disclosing it, the subject can be brought up again later in the course of her prenatal care.

Once substance abuse has been identified, the nurse can begin counseling by exploring with the client the risks of continuing the addiction. Scare tactics and threats are counterproductive in that they heighten maternal anxiety and may exacerbate the abuse. Therefore, the clinician should avoid dwelling on what damage may have already been sustained and instead focus on the potential good that could occur from detoxification or, in the case of heroin, transference to methadone.

One intervention being used in a Centers for Disease Control Perinatal Alcohol Study in Cincinnati, Ohio is the brief intervention model or BIM (Kenner & Hetteberg, 1997). This type of motivational interviewing was adapted to the perinatal client by Dr. Narra Cox from the University of Wisconsin. It is a form of intervention being tried with perinatal women who disclose drinking prior to the 28th week of pregnancy. The brief intervention model requires 10 minutes in which the registered nurse case manager works with the woman to determine her current level of drinking and what triggered her drinking since the last clinic visit. It requires a partnership with the woman to set goals for decreasing or abstaining from drinking. The overall goal is to prevent as much damage to the fetus as possible and to set a lifelong pattern of abstinence to prevent future FAS. One of the difficulties with using this intervention and any other is the inability to predict what complications may evolve from perinatal drinking during each pregnancy. Trying to do so discredits the staff if the outcome does not match the prediction. The woman may also know someone who used alcohol during pregnancy and had, in her estimation, a healthy baby. Often the perception is that if the infant was born with 10 fingers and 10 toes, the infant was "normal." Subtle findings and those with delayed detection may not be associated with substance use (e.g., loss of several IQ points, learning disabilities, poor impulse control) until much later.

A less direct form of data gathering is by looking for high-risk patterns of behaviors. Women addicted to drugs often receive little or no prenatal care, showing up in the emergency room in active labor. These women often "dose up" before arriving at the hospital, so they would obviously appear to be under the influence of an exogenous substance. Maternal behavioral manifestations are related to the substance of abuse and to the last dose of the drug. For example, alcohol may be present on their breath. Their affect may be distorted, judgment impaired, and behavior overly subdued or agitated. Alcohol induces an unsteady gait and slurred speech. Among chronic users of alcohol, a pattern of withdrawal may occur. Manifestations of maternal withdrawal vary according to the extent of the alcoholism. Nurses should assess the mothers for nervousness, nausea, vomiting, and tremors (Powell & Minick, 1988). Other, more profound symptoms of alcohol withdrawal are hallucinations, delusions, agitation, and seizures. Acute withdrawal symptoms can be treated with benzodiazepines such as chlordiazepoxide (Librium), diazepam (Valium), and lorazepam (Ativan) (Powell & Minick, 1988).

Behavioral manifestations of cocaine are different from those of alcohol. Immediately after cocaine ingestion, there is a brief period of euphoria with tachycardia and elevated blood pressure. Once metabolism occurs, depression or "postcoke blues" ensue. Nasal mucosa may be irritated with ulcerations or necrosis from snorting. This ulceration occurs secondary to the vasoconstrictive properties of cocaine.

Unlike cocaine and its stimulant effects, heroin is a CNS depressant. Symptoms include a detached, drowsy period of euphoria, often referred to as a "nod." Since the most common route of administration is intravenous, needle or track marks can be found along blood vessels. There may be scars or sclerosed areas from localized areas of inflammation associated with self-injection. Since the heroin supply is interrupted during hospitalization, the woman may demand narcotics for pain. Owing to the heroin addict's cross-dependence to morphine and meperidine, the usual doses of these painkillers given to laboring or postpartum women are insufficient. Signs and symptoms of maternal withdrawal are nausea and vomiting, watery eyes, runny nose, and agitation. Assessment also includes observing for the drug or its paraphernalia. Cocaine or crack is a white crystalline powder that is stored in glass vials and smoked in a glass pipe. Razor blades and syringes are also used in the preparation and administration of cocaine. Heroin is a white powder that is generally stored in miniature plastic bags. Spoons, needles, and syringes are commonly used in heroin preparation (National Association for Perinatal Addiction Research and Education, 1989).

Once they have delivered their infants, these women may leave the hospital against medical advice (Keith et al., 1988). They may fear exposure of their addiction, with associated legal implications, or worry about insufficient drug or alcohol supply. Early discharge is a true threat to the newborn's well-being, as the infant's onset of withdrawal may be somewhat delayed. This would hamper diagnosis and treatment.

The presence of certain infectious conditions could also raise suspicion of drug use. Such conditions include STDs (e.g., syphilis or gonorrhea), bloodborne illnesses such as hepatitis, and an overall picture of self-neglect (e.g., malnutrition or poor hygiene). A transient lifestyle and a lack of a consistent partner are also consistent with drug abuse. The indicators of potential substance abuse are poor compliance with prenatal visits, initial prenatal care after 20 weeks' gestation, unexplained preterm labor, placental abruption, intrauterine growth retardation, intrauterine fetal demise, history of family violence, other children in foster care, and psychiatric history (Children's Hospital Medical Center of Northern California, 1990; Kaiser Foundation Hospital, 1989). If any of these factors are present, a urine toxicology screen can be ordered. However, this does not definitively document maternal drug use. There are confounding variables, such as narcotics given during labor and the timing of the drug screen with respect to the last dose of drug. If suspicions are raised for substance abuse, a urine sample should be collected. Alcohol is quickly metabolized, so it is difficult to document by this method. Urinary excretion of heroin is accomplished in 24 hours, with cocaine metabolites lingering for 4 to 7 days (Flandermeyer, 1987).

Some substance-abusing women may be harder to detect. Their addiction may be shrouded in a middle- to upper-class home, with care being given by a private physician. Until recently, this patient population was considered exempt from substance abuse. However, a recent study was designed to ascertain the incidence of drug use among pregnant women of various socioeconomic groups. Over a 6-month period, urine samples from pregnant women from five public health clinics (n = 380) and 12 private obstetrical practices (n = 335) were screened for alcohol, cannabinoids, cocaine, and opiates (Chasnoff et al., 1990). Positive result rates were 16.3 percent among public health clinic patients and 13.1 percent among private practice patients. In addition, Chasnoff and associates (1990) stated that even though drug abuse in their study was similar among whites and blacks, black women traditionally have been reported 10 times more often. This adds credence to the suspicion that substance abuse cuts across all socioeconomic lines.

NURSING INTERVENTIONS FOR INFANTS BORN TO SUBSTANCE-ABUSING MOTHERS

Care Related to Central Nervous System Manifestations

Neonatal intervention is largely supportive and dependent on the type of substance the mother has abused (Table 45–3). Infants born to women who abuse various substances are irritable and easily excited by sensory stimuli. Therefore, the environment of these infants should be regulated by the caregiver to reduce the quantity and variety of sensory input (Fig. 45–6). Methods of accomplishing this are dimming the nursery lights and reducing

TABLE 45–3 Summary of the Effects of Maternal Substance Abuse on Pregnancy and the Neonate

	Tobacco	Cocaine	Heroin	Alcohol
Pregnancy-Associated Risks	Placental vasoconstriction Placenta previs Large placental to fetal ratio	Placental vasoconstriction Spontaneous abortion Placental abruption Maternal hyperthermia Implicated as possible mechanism of teratogenesis	Placental vasoconstriction Depresses respiration Unsterile injections Hepatitis AIDS	Spontaneous abortion
Direct Fetal Hazards	Prematurity Decreased FHR variability Decreased fetal movement Exposure to carcinogens Increased polycythemia Reduced birth weight (dose response)	Prematurity Increased stillbirths Increased HR; increased BP Intrauterine hypoxia Meconium staining Cerebral infarction Other vasoconstrictive accidents NEC GU anomalies Ileal atresia Teratogenic	Decreased birth weight SGA LBW Intermittent hypoxia from periodic withdrawal Increased aspiration, pneumonia, and meconium aspiration Stillbirth Increased breech presentation	LBW Teratogenic
Infant Hazards	Increased SIDS Increased frequency of URI and physician's office visits Decreased RDS	CNS irritability Hypertonic Easily overstimulated Hyperextension Posturing Incessant crying	Neonatal abstinence syndrome SGA; CNS, GI manifestations Decreased physiologic jaundice Decreased RDS	FAS-FAE Postnatal growth deficiency Cognitive impairment Dysmorphic characteristics FAS facies Cardiac anomalies Abnormal palmar creases CNS dysfunction Irritability Tremors Poor feeding Easily overstimulated
Hazards Persisting into Childhood	Decreased stature Decreased school performance	Attention deficit disorder Abnormal play patterns Flat, apathetic moods Difficulty in concentration	Effects of drug culture difficult to control for Uncontrolled temper Impulsiveness Difficulty making friends	Attention deficit disorder Learning disorders Cognitive impairment Hypotonic Inability to learn from past experiences

AIDS, acquired immunodeficiency syndrome; FHR, fetal heart rate; HR, heart rate; BP, blood pressure; NEC, necrotizing enterocolitis; GU, genitourinary; SGA, small for gestational age; LBW, low birth weight; SIDS, sudden infant death syndrome; URI, upper respiratory infection; RDS, respiratory distress syndrome; CNS, central nervous system; GI, gastrointestinal; FAS-FAE, fetal alcohol syndrome–fetal alcohol effects.

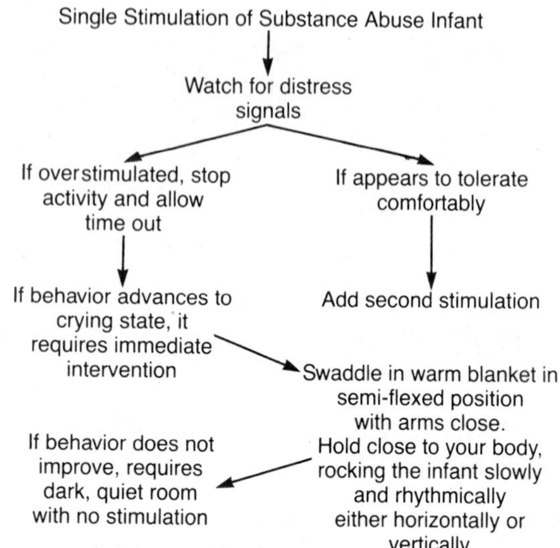
Single Stimulation of Substance Abuse Infant
Watch for distress signals
If overstimulated, stop activity and allow time out
If appears to tolerate comfortably
If behavior advances to crying state, it requires immediate intervention
Add second stimulation
Swaddle in warm blanket in semi-flexed position with arms close. Hold close to your body, rocking the infant slowly and rhythmically either horizontally or vertically
If behavior does not improve, requires dark, quiet room with no stimulation

FIGURE 45–6. Flow chart for stimulation of the infant who was exposed to substances in utero.

noise. If the nursery lights cannot be altered, a blanket can be placed over the infant's incubator. Many noises can be eliminated—for example, by not talking loudly at the bedside, keeping radios and intercom volumes low, silencing alarms after responding, and closing incubator doors quietly. Infants exposed to drugs in utero profit from a private, or isolation, room or a quieter area of the nursery.

The frequency of nursing intervention should be minimized by grouping care to the level of infant tolerance and by using electronic monitoring capabilities for routine vital signs. Unnecessary handling should be avoided. Routine laboratory work should be assessed individually and discontinued if unnecessary. Nurses can use infant behavioral cues as a basis for directing the amount of stimulation to be given. Infants have their own unique personalities; thus, the caregiver learns each infant's signals.

Infants have six wake–sleep states: deep or quiet sleep, active sleep, drowsy, quiet alert, fussy, and crying. Typically, infants possess the capability to modulate their perception of incoming stimuli by altering their level of wakefulness. This ability is termed *state control.* When infants are in the quiet alert phase, they are most in tune to their environment. This is also the ideal phase for mother–infant attachment to occur. The infant is content, alert, and interacts with the caregiver, with the interaction being mutually satisfying. As the infant tires or becomes overly stimulated, "time-out" cues are given to the caregiver. Examples of such cues are gaze aversion, yawning, hiccups, sneezing, and increased movement (Sweeney, 1989). If the caregiver receives such cues from the infant, the interaction must be altered to prevent the infant from either falling asleep or crying. Generally speaking, infants are capable of state transition to regulate their own stimulation. State transition involves transcending from one level of wakefulness to another in response to the perception of environmental stimuli.

In the case of an infant who has been exposed to drugs in utero, the caregiver needs to be more in tune to such subtle behavioral signals. The caregiver can circumvent a prolonged crying episode by minimizing external stressors. For example, if the nurse is rocking, feeding, and speaking to an infant, and the infant begins to avert his or her gaze and increases movement, the caregiver can be still and silent and can position the child facing outward toward the room. Each sensory mode (visual, tactile, auditory, kinesthetic, gustatory) should be evaluated. When the infant's level of tolerance to that stimulus has been determined, plans for further stimulation can be made. Tasks involving complex or multiple sensory interaction may need to be divided into subsets so that infant tolerance to progressive interaction can be assessed. For example, if the infant needs to be fed, the nurse can first stand at the bedside and touch the infant's back, after which the infant can be swaddled in a flexed position with his or her hands crossing at the midline. The infant is then ready to be picked up and fed. The amount of visual, auditory, and kinesthetic stimulation should be individually tailored to meet the infant's needs. The infant must be able to set the pace and tone of the interaction. An understanding of the infant's behavioral cues must be shared with the parents so that they can understand the basis for their child's behavior. This understanding can then influence their caregiving so that they are more responsive to their infant's needs.

Care Related to Gastrointestinal Manifestations

Infants who have been exposed to substances in utero are often of LBW and have a poorly coordinated suck–swallow reflex. Infants who have been exposed to heroin may experience abdominal cramping with diarrhea. Intense crying is often misinterpreted as hunger, with overfeeding creating abdominal distention, vomiting, and diarrhea.

In these situations, infants should be fed smaller quantities more frequently. Three-hour feeds are often tolerated well; however, this can be assessed individually. Since adequate nutrition is essential, accurate intake and output should be recorded. An indwelling, small-diameter (e.g., 5 French) nasogastric (NG) feeding tube is often helpful. Although bolus feedings are desirable because of their physiologic nature, the infant may be unable to finish his or her bottle. Therefore, the remaining milk can be instilled via NG tube. Feeding assisted by gavage reduces expenditure of calories and allows calories to be used for growth. An indwelling NG tube may also be used for the infant's benefit if a feeding is needed during nighttime sleep. Rest can then be maintained while nutrition is provided. Caution should be taken to do what is best for the infant, not what is most convenient for the caretaker; feeding tubes should not be used indiscriminately. Sucking needs can be met via pacifier or hand sucking during gavage feedings.

Feeding requires special consideration with respect to infant state and readiness. As previously discussed, the infant needs to set the pace for the interaction with the caregiver. If the infant is fragile with respect to state control, the caregiver may need to initiate contact slowly. Tactile and kinesthetic stimulation could be used first. For example, in order to feed the infant, the nurse could place a hand on the infant's back. When this has been tolerated, the infant can be picked up, facing out toward the room. This position eliminates visual stimulation. Silence should be used initially. The bottle can then be given. Jaw support may be necessary to encourage the sucking reflex. Also, these infants tend to display an overly extended position of their extremities and have difficulty establishing midline orientation (Schneider & Chasnoff, 1987). Thus, the infant should be swaddled in a warm blanket. Swaddling and warmth decrease motor activity and self-stimulation (Schneider & Chasnoff, 1987). Holding the infant in a flexed position, with the infant's hands past midline, is also helpful. Other soothing techniques include hand holding, vertical rocking, and use of a pacifier (Griffith, 1988).

Daily measurements of weight and head circumference should be obtained to track growth. Weights are most accurate when performed at the same time each day and with the same scale. Infants should be weighed nude and before feeding. Head circumference should be measured over the largest occipitofrontal area. A small ink mark may be placed over the desired area to reduce measurement error.

Drug screens should be performed on breast milk specimens, as cocaine, heroin, and alcohol cross into human milk. Mothers should be informed of this crossover, and, unless abstinence has been achieved, bottle feeding should be encouraged.

Pharmacologic Intervention

Infants who are withdrawing from opiates or who are manifesting NAS may need pharmacologic intervention during withdrawal. Signs and symptoms include fever, vomiting, diarrhea, high-pitched cry, sweating, sneezing, agitation, tremors, and seizures (Chasnoff, 1988).

Pharmacologic intervention is indicated if there has been (1) weight loss from GI symptoms or hyperactivity associated with withdrawal, or both; (2) inability of the infant to rest; (3) fever unrelated to infection; or (4) seizures (Chasnoff, 1988). Paregoric is the drug of choice, as it improves sucking ability and is correlated with weight gain. Paregoric is an opiate and provides direct relief by its cross-dependence with heroin. It also exerts a direct effect on the GI system to reduce diarrhea. Another drug that may help is diazepam. However, diazepam depresses sucking, heart rate, and respirations and is contraindicated in an infant who is jaundiced. Late-onset seizures after the discontinuance of diazepam have been reported (Chasnoff, 1988). Phenobarbital (5 to 12 mg/kg in three divided doses) has also been recommended to ease the symptoms associated with NAS (van Baar et al., 1994). Pharmacologic intervention must be assessed on an individual basis and the dose tapered over time to gradually break the cycle of withdrawal.

Care Related to Risk for Infection

Infants born to substance-abusing women are at risk for the development of an infection as a result of exposure to maternal pathogens. These infants are often poorly nourished in utero and are more susceptible to infectious processes. Care should be taken to maintain universal isolation precautions, as there is an increased incidence of hepatitis and AIDS among these women and their infants. Common signs and symptoms suggestive of sepsis are temperature instability, hypotonicity, color changes (pale or mottled), feeding intolerance, episodes of apnea, and bradycardia (see Chapter 27, Assessment and Management of Immunologic Dysfunction).

Skin excoriations from episodes of crying and flailing may result from rubbing the nose, knees, and elbows against bed linens. The infant should be positioned so that these areas are not contacted and the infant should be comforted consistently. A soft sheepskin may be soothing. Excoriations also need to be kept clean and dry and be assessed periodically for infection. Tegaderm or its equivalent can be used to protect excoriated areas on knees and elbows from further breakdown. The position of choice is prone or side-lying. The supine position should be avoided. Again, swaddling with arms crossing the midline and positioning in a flexed position is most beneficial (Schneider & Chasnoff, 1987).

Care Related to Facilitating Mother–Child Attachment

Attachment is a reciprocal response between the caregiver and the child (Lancaster, 1986). The infant begins interactions with the caretaker by signaling for attention (e.g., crying). Once the caretaker is within close proximity to the infant, the dyad can interact through means such as eye-to-eye contact, smiling, and nuzzling. These behaviors serve to maintain this interaction and promote bonds of affection. However, when the infant continues to be rigid, irritable, and difficult to hold and console, the caretaker becomes frustrated and may stop attempts to calm the child. Maternal apathy toward her infant undermines the reciprocal relationship and impedes attachment. If an early mother–infant relationship is not established, it may be detrimental to their later relationship. It may also be a predisposing factor for future child neglect or physical abuse (Schneider & Chasnoff, 1987). Chasnoff and associates (1982) describe this as a "vicious cycle of infant passivity and maternal rejection" (p. 213). This downward spiraling ensues without appropriate intervention.

Appropriate nursing intervention includes educating parents regarding the expected behavioral manifestations in the infant. It should be explained matter of factly that the infant also experiences drug withdrawal. The nurse can then "interpret" the infant's behavior for the parents. For example, subtle infant cues indicating anxiety (e.g., grimacing) should be pointed out and their significance explained. The mother should also be shown when the infant appears receptive to interaction. An essential comment should be that her infant lacks the cognitive abilities to "dislike" her. These women may misinterpret infant irritability as dislike. In reality, when the infant is irritable, he or she needs extra patience and understanding versus avoidance or resentment. Significant others need to be involved in the infant's care in order to lend assistance to both the mother and the infant. These women have frail coping reserves and need help to care adequately for their infants. A trusting nurse–patient relationship can help immensely. Discharge should be interdisciplinary and include follow-up care. Referrals should be made to a drug rehabilitation program and other appropriate community resources (e.g., the Women, Infants and Children [WIC] program). A new concept of a "resource mom" has been piloted by Children's Hospital of Buffalo (Conway-Orgel, 1990). The resource mom is a volunteer who is specially trained in the special needs of an infant who has been exposed to cocaine in utero. These women serve as big sisters to drug-addicted mothers. The resource mom keeps in close contact with the drug-addicted mother and provides support, information, and troubleshooting when problems arise. The new mother learns parenting skills and has someone to turn to in time of need, with the overall goal being to enable the new mother to be better able to care for her infant.

The nurse should realize that a long pattern of maladaptive behavior is not going to be cured overnight. However, early detection and intervention are the keys to good outcome for the mother and child. If parents understand the dynamics of their infant's behavior and are supported through periods of crisis, perhaps devastating behaviors such as child abuse can be circumvented.

LEGAL AND ETHICAL ISSUES

Currently, throughout the United States, when infants are born to women with behavior suspect of drug abuse, a urine toxicology screen can be ordered and collected. If a positive result on such a screen is found, the results are reported to the state's division of children and family services, a social service consult is initiated, and a family investigation is performed. In order for the infant to be discharged to the mother, she must comply with the recommendations of the division of family services. This generally includes enrolling in a drug rehabilitation program and remaining in close contact with her assigned case worker. The process varies from state to state, with larger urban areas such as New York, Chicago, and San Francisco being more aggressive in identifying neonatal drug exposure. Many smaller midwestern cities seem to perceive the drug problem as less prevalent and are less willing or perhaps less able to deal with the consequences of identifying maternal drug abuse. Therefore, neonatal drug exposure is often underreported. It is unlikely in the near future that widespread routine drug screens will be used because of concern about confidentiality, ethical considerations, and costs.

If the mother chooses not to comply with a drug rehabilitation program or other stipulations, the issue of continued custody arises. The dilemma is an old one. Is it best to have the child remain with the biologic mother or be placed in foster care? A common compromise seems to be to award guardianship to a family member who is living drug-free and who has a stable lifestyle. This approach enables the child to be among family and to have the benefit of a continuous attachment figure. A series of foster homes interferes with the attachment process and is not in the child's best interest. Family custody also eliminates the issue of *boarder babies.* This term refers to infants who are retained by hospitals until suitable homes can be found or until litigation for custody is completed. The boarder baby phenomenon is detrimental to the growth and development of the infant and places a terrific financial burden on the hospital (Saylor et al., 1991) (see Chapter 42, Neonatal Acquired Immunodeficiency Syndrome).

Another related issue is cost. Health care in the United States is often based on crisis. Infants born prematurely or those who are of LBW are readily placed in a NICU at the cost of $1500 to $2000 per day. Lewit and associates (1995) estimate that $11 billion dollars per year is spent on pediatric health care, with $4 billion (35%) of this spent on LBW infants.

Health care dollars could be more efficiently spent on prenatal care and drug rehabilitation programs for the pregnant drug user. There are no easy solutions, and society seems ill equipped to deal with such large-scale issues. However, the economics of the situation may force more attention to be focused on such legal, ethical, and economic issues.

Another legal issue is that relating to the prosecution of drug-abusing women. Should these women be prosecuted not only for drug use but also for in utero child abuse? Many feel that punitive treatment only hurts the infant further, as women will be frightened and thus hide their addiction and not seek prenatal care. A complete lack of pregnancy-related care is detrimental to the mother and infant. Home births could be lethal. The health care team should be perceived as a friend rather than a foe, and help rather than punishment should be offered. Perhaps early intervention before pregnancy could be the goal of the health care network. The official statement on substance abuse in women by NAACOG (1990) is that drug and alcohol addiction are diseases and that punitive approaches to treatment or rehabilitation are not in the woman's best interest and are counterproductive to the role of the health care professional.

VALUE CONFLICT FOR HEALTH PROFESSIONALS

Recognition and discussion of the difficulties faced by professionals who treat infants who have been exposed to drugs in utero are critical to the delivery of quality care (Adams et al., 1990). In a recent unpublished study cited in Adams and associates (1990), a survey was taken to identify some of the issues and feelings nurses had about substance-abusing mothers. Most stated that they felt anger toward these mothers. The NICU nurse caring for infants who have been exposed to drugs in utero must be aware of these feelings and prejudices. The nurse must acknowledge them before working with the mother in an empathetic, nonjudgmental manner. This is a crucial first step toward forming and implementing a treatment plan with the family (Adams et al., 1990).

Support groups and training sessions are forums that can be used by nurses to talk about their feelings. Anger is a primary feeling that generates the energy that can mobilize individuals to take action to deal with and correct a situation. Therefore, the anger felt by the majority of nurses can be a powerful tool in effecting a change in the substance-abusing mother. However, nurses must not lose sight of the fact that they probably cannot cure the substance-abusing mother. Substance abusers, especially those who abuse cocaine, have been labeled "untreatable" by many because of their number of relapses and a lack of motivation to change their lifestyle. Nurses who are accustomed to being successful in their work may feel incompetent and discouraged when they realize that they are not being effective in curing the mother (Adams et al., 1990). Nurses must approach the parent as a holistic being and not just as a substance-abusing parent of a sick infant. They must be nonjudgmental, honest, and empathetic and must look at and integrate good points about the abuser. Showing genuine interest and concern can go a long way toward building a trusting relationship. This can be difficult because manipulative behavior is part of the "survival" techniques of a substance abuser. These mothers go through a phase of testing nurses to discover their views about drug abuse, so honesty is essential at all times. The nurse must remember that abusers have a different set of beliefs and values and that these must be respected as long as they are not harmful to the health of either the mother or the neonate (Adams et al., 1990).

CONCLUSION

For the neonatal nurse, infants who have been exposed to substances in utero present a challenge and require accurate assessments if one is to anticipate the potential problems that may occur. More and more is being learned about these neonates, but many of the long-term risks are still unknown. The complexity of care is increased owing to the pattern of maternal polydrug use; thus, each neonate may present with slightly different clinical manifestations. The basic management outlined in this chapter provides a sound basis for care no matter what combination of maternal drugs the neonate has been exposed to.

PROTOCOL FOR MANAGEMENT OF THE DRUG-EXPOSED NEONATE

GOAL	INTERVENTION	RATIONALE
Motor Dysfunction		
To recognize abnormal motor patterns and provide interventions to promote more normal patterns.	1. Place the infant in a side-lying position with the spine and head flexed.	The side-lying position overcomes both the increased tone and the effects of gravity, as well as brings the infant away from the hyperextended position.
RATIONALE: Intervention is necessary to allow the infant to interact both physically and behaviorally.	2. Position the infant with upper extremities protracted at the shoulder girdle and flex the lower extremities somewhat.	The infant's extensor tone as well as that of the pelvis will be broken up, and midline orientation will be encouraged.

PROTOCOL FOR MANAGEMENT OF THE DRUG-EXPOSED NEONATE *(Continued)*		
GOAL	**INTERVENTION**	**RATIONALE**
Motor Dysfunction *Continued*		
	3. Place rolled-up pads or cloth diapers between the legs and along the spine.	This will help maintain the posture while allowing the infant freedom to move.
	4. Position the awake and alert infant in a prone position with stimulating toys near.	This will help develop antigravity extensor strength by lifting of the head and supporting of the limbs while encouraging pivoting of the trunk.
	5. To carry the infant, position in a more flexed position by setting the infant on the caregiver's hip with an arm under the thighs, keeping arms forward.	This position controls the extensor tone while facilitating head and trunk control as well as promoting the hands coming to midline.
State Control		
To recognize the four common patterns of state control in a drug-exposed infant and to differentiate them from the pattern of a normal infant. *RATIONALE:* Nurses must be knowledgeable about these abnormal patterns so that they can intervene appropriately to promote maximum state control.	1. The normal infant will move through each of the states of arousal with a relatively smooth transition. Each state achieved will be appropriate for the type of stimulation the infant is encountering.	A normal infant is well organized and fully functioning and can move through the states of arousal in a smooth manner.
	2. In the first pattern, the infants pull down into a deep sleep in response to the first stimulation received and remain asleep throughout the rest of the stimulation. The more attempts that are made to wake them, the deeper asleep they become. They awaken only after being swaddled and placed in a dark, quiet room. They may open their eyes and look around, but will shut down again as soon as any type of stimulation is applied.	These infants seem to be aware that deep sleep is their only and best defense against being overstimulated and losing control of themselves.
	3. In the second pattern, the infant cannot or will not wake up during stimulation. In response to stimuli presented, these infants will startle, whimper, change colors, or breathe irregularly, but never awaken.	
	4. Infants displaying the third pattern of state control vacillate between sleep states and cry states, moving abruptly from sleeping to agitated crying. As soon as the stimulation is terminated, they pull back into their sleep shelter.	These infants do not achieve any attention to or responsiveness to visual or auditory stimuli.
	5. The fourth and most common pattern for substance abuse infants is one in which they tend to use both sleeping and crying to shut themselves off from excessive stimulation. However, if managed carefully, they are able to achieve very brief periods of alert responsiveness.	These infants have very low thresholds for overstimulation. The caregiver must be alert to the infant's cues in order to reach responsive states.
Decreased Interactive Abilities		
To recognize signs of depressed interactive abilities of the substance abuse infant and to differentiate them from the behavior of a normal infant. *RATIONALE:* The substance abuse infant may be incapable of responding appropriately to the caregiver.	1. The substance abuse infant will be extremely irritable with a high-pitched, shrill cry and will be very difficult to console.	At delivery, the drug is withdrawn from the drug-dependent infant, who will soon begin to show signs of withdrawal.
	2. The infant will display tremors of the hands, arms, legs, chin, and tongue.	Tremors will occur in infants exposed prenatally to drugs.
	3. The infant will be unable to focus on a caregiver's face and listen to her or his voice at the same time, and will signal this overload by gaze aversion and/or crying.	The substance abuse infant is unable to process complex combinations of stimulation.
	4. The infant will display signals of distress such as yawning, sneezing, hiccups, restless arms and legs, color changes, frowning, gaze aversion, finger splaying, and arching when becoming stressed.	By displaying these distress signals, these infants are protecting themselves from more stimulation than they can handle.

Protocol continued on following page

PROTOCOL FOR MANAGEMENT OF THE DRUG-EXPOSED NEONATE *(Continued)*

GOAL	INTERVENTION	RATIONALE
Optimal Environment		
To control the environment to help the substance abuse infant improve state control and motor patterns, thus improving the infant's ability to interact actively with the outside world by attending to and responding to visual and auditory stimuli. *RATIONALE:* Using caregiver-induced controls will help decrease the infant's level of excitement and disorganization, and the infant may be able to respond to stimuli for brief periods.	1. Swaddle the infant in a warm blanket in a semiflexed position.	The warmth from the blanket causes inhibition of motor behavior, and the flexed position breaks up the extensor tone, decreases tremors, and facilitates hand-to-mouth activity.
	2. Stimuli can be introduced when the infant is in a quiet alert state to work on responsiveness. Present only one type of stimulus at a time, either auditory or visual.	Substance abuse infants have difficulty processing complex combinations.
	3. Each time the caregiver interacts with the substance abuse infant, attempt to gradually increase the time the stimulation is presented. Watch closely for distress signals. Use comforting techniques only as needed, and begin to withdraw them as soon as possible.	As tolerance for stimulation increases and comforting techniques are withdrawn, the infant learns to gain control over his or her state.
	4. Watch the infant closely for early distress signals of overstimulation such as yawns, sneezes, hiccups, and grimaces. Respond by stopping the activity with the infant, allowing a time-out period. Place the infant in a quiet, dimmed environment, swaddled in a warm blanket.	Decreasing stimulation at the first signs of distress may help avoid a crying episode.
	5. A substance abuse infant who reaches a state of crying requires immediate intervention. Swaddle the infant in a warm blanket in a flexed position with arms close to the body and hold the infant close to your body. Rock the infant slowly and rhythmically either horizontally or with the head supported vertically, whichever best soothes.	The earlier in a crying episode intervention is begun, the more quickly the infant will calm down. Vestibular proprioceptive stimulation will immediately arrest crying, decrease irritability, and bring the infant to a visually alert state.
	6. Neonatal hydrotherapy can be utilized for an irritable, crying infant. Place the infant in a small tub filled with water 99 to 101°F, massaging the infant with a firm, calm touch during the bath.	Hydrotherapy is effective in improving posture, muscle tone, and behavioral state in substance abuse infants.
	7. A substance abuse infant who continues to be irritable after the above interventions have been tried must be placed in a quiet, darkened room with no outside stimulation.	This has been proven to work with both pre- and full-term infants exposed prenatally to drugs.
	8. When a substance abuse infant is calm, the caregiver should hold the infant in the en face (face-to-face) position and move her or his face slowly back and forth across the infant's visual field. Watch closely for distress signals of sensory overload. If the infant is able to fix his eyes on the caregiver comfortably, add another stimulus by attempting to talk to the infant in a quiet, rhythmic voice.	The en face position will encourage visual tracking, vocalization, and playful interaction with the caregiver.
Nursing Values and Conflicts		
The NICU nurse will be aware of her or his feelings and prejudices about drug-abusing mothers. *RATIONALE:* The nurse must first identify and acknowledge her or his own feelings and prejudices about drug-abusing mothers.	1. Nurses must talk about their anger toward drug-abusing parents through peer groups and training sessions.	Anger is a primary feeling that generates the energy that can mobilize people to take action to deal with and correct a situation.
	2. Nurses must be aware that they will probably not be able to cure the substance-abusing mother, leading to feelings of incompetence and discouragement.	
	3. Nurses must approach the parent as a holistic being and not just the substance-abusing mother of a sick infant. They must be nonjudgmental, honest, and empathetic and must look at and integrate good points about the abuser.	Showing genuine interest and concern can go a long way toward building a trusting relationship.

REFERENCES

Abel, E. (1984). *Fetal alcohol syndrome and fetal alcohol effects*. New York: Plenum Press.

Abrams, B. F., & Laros, R. K., Jr. (1986). Prepregnancy weight, weight gain, and birth weight. *American Journal of Obstetrics and Gynecology, 154*(3), 503–509.

Acker, D., Sachs, B. P., Tracey, K. J., & Wise, W. E. (1983). Abruptio placentae associated with cocaine use. *American Journal of Obstetrics and Gynecology, 146*(2), 220–221.

Adams, C., Eyler, F. D., & Behnke, M. (1990). Nursing intervention with mothers who are substance abusers. *Journal of Perinatal and Neonatal Nursing, 3*(4), 43–52.

Arias, F. (1984). Preterm labor. In F. Arias (Ed.), *High risk pregnancy and delivery* (pp. 37–62). St. Louis: C. V. Mosby.

Atkins, W. (1988). Cocaine: The drug of choice. In I. Chasnoff (Ed.), *Drugs, alcohol, pregnancy and parenting* (pp. 91–96). Hingham, MA: Kluwer Academic Publishers.

AWHONN [Association of Women's Health, Obstetric, and Neonatal Nurses]. (1995). FAS rises in U.S. *AWHONN Voice, 3*(6), 2.

Baraitser, M., & Winter, R. M. (1996). *Color atlas of congenital malformation syndromes.* St. Louis: Mosby-Wolfe.

Bardy, A. H., Seppala, T., Lillsunde, P., et al. (1993). Objectively measured tobacco and exposure during pregnancy: Neonatal effects and relation to maternal smoking. *British Journal of Obstetrics and Gynaecology, 100*(8), 721–726.

Baron, J. (1984). Smoking and estrogen-related disease [Review]. *American Journal of Epidemiology, 119(1),* 9–22.

Bateman, D. A., & Heagarty, M. C. (1989). Passive free-base cocaine ("crack") inhalation by infants and toddlers. *American Journal of Diseases of Children, 143*(1), 25–27.

Bates, C. K. (1988). Medical risks of cocaine use [Review]. *Western Journal of Medicine, 148*(4), 440–444.

Beck, M., Springen, K., Hager, M., et al. (1989, July 17). Do-it-yourself abortion is hazardous to your health. *Newsweek*, p. 25.

Benowitz, N. (1989). Human pharmacology of nicotine. In H. Cappell, F. Glaser, Y. Israel, et al. (Eds.), *Research advances in alcohol and drug problems* (Vol. 9, pp. 1–52). New York: Plenum Press.

Bingol, N., Fuchs, M., Diaz, V., et al. (1987). Teratogenicity of cocaine in humans. *Journal of Pediatrics, 110*(3), 93–96.

Boobis, S., & Sullivan, F. (1986). Effects of life-style on reproduction. In S. Fabro & A. Scialli (Eds.), *Drug and chemical action in pregnancy: Pharmacologic and toxicologic principles* (pp. 373–425). New York: Marcel Dekker.

Bozarth, M., & Wise, R. (1985). Toxicity associated with long term intravenous heroin and cocaine self-administration in the rat. *Journal of the American Medical Association, 254*(1), 81–83.

Buchan, P. C. (1983). Cigarette smoking in pregnancy and fetal hyperviscosity. *British Medical Journal Clinical Research Edition, 286*(6374), 1315.

Bureau, M. A., Monette, J., Shapcott, D., et al. (1982). Carboxyhemoglobin concentration in fetal cord blood and in blood of mothers who smoked during labor. *Pediatrics, 69*(3), 371–373.

Butler, N., & Goldstein, H. (1973). Smoking in pregnancy and subsequent child development. *British Medical Journal, 4*(892), 573–575.

Cardozo, L. D., Gibb, D. M., Studd, J. W., & Cooper, D. J. (1982). Social and obstetric features associated with smoking in pregnancy. *British Journal of Obstetrics and Gynaecology, 89*(8), 622–627.

Chanoine, J. P., Toppet, V., Bourdoux, P., et al. (1991). Smoking during pregnancy: A significant cause of neonatal thyroid enlargement. *British Journal of Obstetrics and Gynaecology, 98*(1), 65–68.

Chasnoff, I. (1989). The incidence of cocaine use. In I. Chasnoff (Ed.), *Special currents: Cocaine babies* (p. 1). Columbus, OH: Ross Laboratories.

Chasnoff, I. J. (1986a). Alcohol use in pregnancy. In I. Chasnoff (Ed.), *Drug use in pregnancy: Mother and child* (pp. 75–79). Norwell, MA: M. T. P. Press.

Chasnoff, I. J. (1986b). Fetal alcohol syndrome in twin pregnancy. *Acta Geneticae Medicae et Gemellologiae, 34*(3–4), 229–232.

Chasnoff, I. J. (1988). Newborn infants with drug withdrawal symptoms [Review]. *Pediatrics in Review, 9*(9), 273–277.

Chasnoff, I. J., Burns, K. A., & Burns, W. J. (1987). Cocaine use in pregnancy: Perinatal morbidity and mortality. *Neurotoxicology and Teratology, 9*(4), 291–293.

Chasnoff, I. J., Burns, W. J., Schnoll, S. H., & Burns, K. A. (1985). Cocaine use in pregnancy. *New England Journal of Medicine, 313*(11), 666–669.

Chasnoff, I. J., Bussey, M. E., Savich, R., & Stack, C. M. (1986). Perinatal cerebral infarction and maternal cocaine use. *Journal of Pediatrics, 108*(3), 456–459.

Chasnoff, I. J., Chisum, G. M., & Kaplan, W. E. (1988). Maternal cocaine use and genitourinary tract malformations. *Teratology, 37*(3), 201–204.

Chasnoff, I. J., Hatcher, R., & Burns, W. (1982). Polydrug- and methadone-addicted newborns: A continuum of impairment? *Pediatrics, 70*(2), 210–213.

Chasnoff, I. J., Landress, H. J., & Barrett, M. E. (1990). The prevalence of illicit-drug or alcohol use during pregnancy and discrepancies in mandatory reporting in Pinellas County, Florida. *New England Journal of Medicine, 322*(17), 1202–1206.

Chasnoff, I. J., Lewis, D. E., & Squires, L. (1987). Cocaine intoxication in a breast-fed infant. *Pediatrics, 80*(6), 836–838.

Cherukuri, R., Minkoff, H., Feldman, J., et al. (1988). A cohort study of alkaloidal cocaine "crack" in pregnancy. *Obstetrics and Gynecology, 72*(2), 147–151.

Chew, E., Remaley, N., Tamboli, A., et al. (1994). Risk factors for esotropia and extropia. *Archives in Ophthalmology, 112*(10), 1349–1355.

Children's Hospital Medical Center of Northern California. (1990). *Toxicology screening protocol.* San Francisco: Children's Hospital Publisher of Northern California.

Chomitz, V. R., Cheung, L. W., & Lieberman, E. (1995). The role of lifestyle in preventing low birth weight (pp. 121–138). In R. E. Behrman (Ed.), *The future of children: Low birth weight, 5*(1), Los Altos, CA: The Center for the Future of Children, The David and Lucille Packard Foundation.

Christianson, R. E. (1979). Gross differences observed in the placentas of smokers and nonsmokers. *American Journal of Epidemiology, 110*(2), 178–187.

Christoffel, K., & Salafsky, I. (1975). Fetal alcohol syndrome in dizygotic twins. *Journal of Pediatrics, 87*(6, Part 1), 963–967.

Clarren, S., Bowden, D., & Astley, S. (1985). The brain in the fetal alcohol syndrome: Observation in human and nonhuman primates. *Alcohol Health and Research World, 10,* 20–25.

Connaughton, J. F, Jr., Finnegan, L., Schut, J., & Emich, J. P. (1975). Current concepts in the management of the pregnant opiate addict. *Addictive Diseases: An International Journal, 2*(1–2), 21–35.

Connaughton, J. F., Reeser, D., Schut, J., & Finnegan, L. P. (1977). Perinatal addiction: Outcome and management. *American Journal of Obstetrics and Gynecology, 129*(6), 679–686.

Conway-Orgel, M. (1990). Better outcomes for infants of drug addicted mothers. *SIG Newsletter, 6*(1), 2.

Cregler, L. L., & Mark, H. (1985). Relation of acute myocardial infarction to cocaine abuse. *American Journal of Cardiology, 56*(2), 794.

Cregler, L. L., & Mark, H. (1986). Cardiovascular dangers of cocaine abuse: Part 2. *American Journal of Cardiology, 57*(13), 1185–1186.

Critchley, H. O., Woods, S. M., Barson, A. J., et al. (1988). Fetal death in utero and cocaine abuse: Case report. *British Journal of Obstetrics and Gynecology, 95*(2), 195–196.

Crosby, W. M., Metcoff, J., Costiloe, J. P., et al. (1977). Fetal malnutrition: An appraisal of correlated factors. *American Journal of Obstetrics and Gynecology, 128*(1), 22–31.

Curet, L., Rao, A. V., Zachman, R., et al., & the Collaborative Group on Antenatal Steroid Therapy. (1983). Maternal smoking and respiratory distress syndrome. *American Journal of Obstetrics and Gynecology, 147*(4), 446–450.

Daghestani, A. (1988). Psychosocial characteristics of pregnant women addicts in treatment. In I. Chasnoff (Ed.), *Drugs, alcohol, pregnancy, and parenting* (pp. 7–16). Hingham, MA: Kluwer Academic Publishers.

Daniell, H. W. (1971). Smokers wrinkles: A study in the epidemiology of "crow's feet." *Annals of Internal Medicine, 75*(6), 873–880.

de Jong-Pley, E. A., Wouters, E. J., de Jong, P. A., et al. (1994). Effects of maternal smoking on neonatal morbidity. *Journal of Perinatal Medicine, 22*(2), 93–101.

Doberczak, T., Shanzer, S., Senie, R., & Kandell, S. (1988). Neonatal neurologic and electroencephalographic effects of intrauterine cocaine exposure. *Journal of Pediatrics, 113*(2), 354–358.

Dorris, M. (1989). *The broken cord.* New York: Harper & Row.

Eisen, L. N., Field, T. M., Bandstra, E. S., et al. (1991). Perinatal cocaine effects on neonatal stress behavior and performance on the Brazelton scale. *Pediatrics, 88*(3), 477–480.

Enkin, M. W. (1984). Smoking and pregnancy—a new look. *Birth, 11*(4), 225–229.

Eriksson, M., Catz, C. S., & Yaffe, S. J. (1973). Drugs and pregnancy [Review]. *Clinical Obstetrics and Gynecology, 16*(1), 199–224.

Ernhart, C. B., Sokol, R. J., Martier, S., et al. (1987). Alcohol teratogenicity in the human: A detailed assessment of specificity, critical period, and threshold. *American Journal of Obstetrics and Gynecology, 156*(1), 33–39.

Evans, D. R., Newcombe, R. G., & Campbell, H. (1979). Maternal smoking habits and congenital malformations: A population study. *British Medical Journal, 2*(6183), 171–173.

Finnegan, L. (1988). The dilemma of cocaine exposure in the perinatal period. *National Institute of Drug Abuse Research: Monograph Series, 81,* 379.

Flandermeyer, A. (1987). A comparison of the effects of heroin and cocaine abuse upon the neonate. *Neonatal Network, 6*(3), 42–48.

Forss, M., Lehtovirta, P., Rauramo, I., & Kariniemi, V. (1983). Midtrimester fetal heart rate variability and maternal hemodynamics in association with smoking. *American Journal of Obstetrics and Gynecology, 146*(6), 693–695.

Frassica, J. J., Orav, E. J., Walsh, E. P., & Lipshultz, S. E. (1994). Arrhythmias in children prenatally exposed to cocaine. *Archives of Pediatric and Adolescent Medicine, 148*(11), 1163–1169.

Frezza, M., di Padova, C., Pozzato, G., et al. (1990). High blood alcohol levels in women: The role of decreased gastric alcohol dehydrogenase activity and first-pass metabolism. *New England Journal of Medicine, 322*(2), 95–99.

Glass L., & Evans, H. (1977). Physiological effects of intrauterine exposure to narcotics. In J. L. Rementeria (Ed.), *Drug abuse in pregnancy and neonatal effects* (pp. 108–115). St. Louis: C. V. Mosby.

Glass, L., Rajegowda, B., & Evans, H. E. (1971). Absence of respiratory distress syndrome in the premature infants of heroin-addicted mothers. *Lancet, 2*(726), 685–686.

Golding, J., & Butler, N. R. (1983). Maternal smoking and anencephaly. *British Medical Journal Clinical Research Edition, 287*(6391), 533–534.

Goodman, J. D., Visser, F. G., & Dawes, G. S. (1984). Effects of maternal cigarette smoking on fetal trunk movements, fetal breathing movements and the fetal heart rate. *British Journal of Obstetrics and Gynaecology, 91*(7), 657–661.

Greenberg, R. A., Haley, N. J., Etzel, R. A., & Loda, F. A. (1984). Measuring the exposure of infants to tobacco smoke. Nicotine and cotinine in urine and saliva. *New England Journal of Medicine, 310*(17), 1075–1078.

Griffith, D. (1988). The effects of perinatal cocaine exposure on infant neurobehavior and early mother–infant interactions. In I. Chasnoff (Ed.), *Drugs, alcohol, pregnancy, and parenting* (pp. 105–113). Hingham, MA: Kluwer Academic Publishers.

Gunderson, L., & Kenner, C. (Eds.). (1995). *Care of the 24–25 week gestational age infant: Small baby protocol* (2nd ed.). Petaluma, CA: NICU Ink.

Guyton, A. (1996). *Textbook of medical physiology* (9th ed.). Philadelphia: W. B. Saunders.

Hakin, R. B., & Tielsch, J. M. (1992). Maternal cigarette smoking during pregnancy: A risk factor for childhood strabismus. *Archives of Ophthalmology, 110*(10), 1459–1462.

Hanson, J. W., Jones, K. L., & Smith, D. W. (1976). Fetal alcohol syndrome: Experience with 41 patients. *Journal of the American Medical Association, 235*(14), 1458–1460.

Hanson, J. W., Streissguth, A. P., & Smith, D. W. (1978). The effects of moderate alcohol consumption during pregnancy on fetal growth and morphogenesis. *Journal of Pediatrics, 92*(3), 457–460.

Harlap, S., & Shiono, P. (1980). Alcohol, smoking, and incidence of spontaneous abortions in the first and second trimester. *Lancet, 2*(8187), 173–176.

Harwood, H., & Napolitano, D. (1985). Economic implications of the fetal alcohol syndrome. *Alcohol Health and Research World, 10,* 38–43.

Himmelberger, D. U., Brown, B. W. Jr., & Cohen, E. N. (1978). Cigarette smoking during pregnancy and the occurrence of spontaneous abortion and congenital abnormality. *American Journal of Epidemiology, 108*(6), 470–479.

Howard, R. E., Hueter, D. C., & Davis, G. J. (1985). Acute myocardial infarction following cocaine abuse in a young woman with normal coronary arteries. *Journal of the American Medical Association, 254*(1), 95–96.

Hurt, H. (1989). Medical controversies in evaluation and management of cocaine exposed infants. In I. Chasnoff (Ed.), *Special currents: Cocaine babies* (pp. 3–4). Columbus, OH: Ross Laboratories.

Jones, K. L., & Smith, D. W. (1973). Recognition of the fetal alcohol syndrome in early infancy. *Lancet, 2*(836), 999–1001.

Jones, K. L., Smith, D. W., Ulleland, C. N., & Streissguth, P. (1973). Pattern of malformation in offspring of chronic alcoholic mothers. *Lancet, 1*(815), 1267–1271.

Jouppila, P., Kirkinen, P., & Eik-Nes, S. (1983). Acute effect of maternal smoking on the human fetal blood flow. *British Journal of Obstetrics and Gynaecology, 90*(1), 7–10.

Kaiser Foundation Hospital. (1989). *Perinatal substance abuse protocol.* San Francisco, CA: Author.

Kaltenbach, K. A. (1992). Prenatal opiate exposure: Developmental effects in infancy and early childhood [OSAP Prevention Monograph-11]. In *Identifying the needs of drug-affected children: Public policy issues* (pp. 49–58). Washington, DC: Office of Substance Abuse Prevention.

Keith, L., MacGregor, S., & Sciarra, J. (1988). Drug abuse in pregnancy. In I. Chasnoff (Ed.), *Drugs, alcohol, pregnancy, and parenting* (pp. 17–45). Hingham, MA: Kluwer Academic Publishers.

Kenner, C., & Hetteberg, C., for the FAS Team. (1997). *Perinatal alcohol users: Identification and intervention.* Centers for Disease Control Study: U84/CCU508718-01. Cincinnati, OH: University of Cincinnati College of Nursing and Health.

Kline, J., Stein, Z., Susser, M., & Warburton, D. (1977). Smoking: A risk factor for spontaneous abortion. *New England Journal of Medicine, 297*(15), 793–796.

Kline, J., Zhrout, P., Stein, Z., et al. (1980). Drinking during pregnancy and spontaneous abortion. *Lancet, 2*(8187), 176–180.

Kroll, D. (1986). Heroin addiction in pregnancy. *Midwives Chronicle, 99*(1182), 153–156.

Kronick, J. B. (1976). Teratogenic effects of ethyl alcohol administered to pregnant mice. *American Journal of Obstetrics and Gynecology, 124*(7), 676–680.

Kuhner, P. M., Kuhner, B. R., Bottoms, S. F., & Erhard, P. (1982). Cadmium levels in maternal blood, fetal cord blood, and placental tissues of pregnant women who smoke. *American Journal of Obstetrics and Gynecology, 142*(8), 1021–1025.

Lancaster, J. (1986). Impact of intensive care on the parent–infant relationship. In S. Korones (Ed.), *High-risk newborn infants* (pp. 407–418). St. Louis: C. V. Mosby.

LeBlanc, P. E., Parekh, A. J., Nso, B., & Glass, L. (1987). Effect of intrauterine exposure to alkaloidal cocaine ("crack") [Letter]. *American Journal of Diseases of Children, 141*(9), 937–938.

LeFrancois, C. (1984, April). Maternal alcohol ingestion: Serious consequences for the fetus. *Vermont Registered Nurse,* pp. 3–5.

Lehtovirta, P., Forss, M., Kariniemi, V., & Rauramo, I. (1983). Acute effects of smoking on fetal heart-rate variability. *British Journal of Obstetrics and Gynaecology, 90*(1), 3–6.

Lemoine, P., Harrousseau, H., Borteyru, J., & Menuet, J. C. (1968). Les enfants de parents alcooliques: Anomalies observees: A propos de 127 cas. *Ouest Médicine, 25,* 477–482.

Lewis, D. D. (1983). Alcohol and pregnancy outcome. *Midwives Chronicle and Nursing Notes, 96*(1151), 420–423.

Lewis, K. D. (1991). Pathophysiology of prenatal drug-exposure: In utero, in the newborn, in childhood, and in agencies. *Journal of Pediatric Nursing, 6*(3), 185–190.

Lewit, E. M., Baker, L. S., Corman, H., & Shiono, P. H. (1995). The direct cost of low birth weight (pp. 35–56). In R. E. Behrman (Ed.), *The future of children: Low birth weight, 5*(1). Los Altos, CA: The Center for the Future of Children, The David and Lucille Packard Foundation.

Lichtenfeld, P. J., Rubin, D. B., & Feldman, R. S. (1984). Subarachnoid hemorrhage precipitated by cocaine snorting. *Archives of Neurology, 41*(2), 223–224.

Lifschnitz, M. H., Wilson, G. S., Smith, E. O., & Desmond, M. M. (1983). Fetal and postnatal growth of children born to narcotic-dependent women. *Journal of Pediatrics, 102*(5), 686–689.

Lincoln, R. (1986). Smoking and reproduction [Review]. *Family Planning Perspectives, 18*(2), 79–84.

Lipson, T. (1988). Fetal alcohol syndrome [Review]. *Australian Family Physician, 17*(5), 385–386.

Little, B. B., Snell, L. M., Rosenfeld, C. R., & Gilstrap, L. C. III (1990). Failure to recognize fetal alcohol syndrome in newborn infants. *American Journal of Diseases in Children, 144*(10), 1142–1146.

Little, R. (1977). Moderate alcohol use during pregnancy and decreased infant birth weight. *American Journal of Public Health, 67*(12), 1154–1156.

Little, R. E., Streissguth, A. P., Barr, H. M., & Herman, C. S. (1980). Decreased birth weight in infants of alcoholic women who abstained during pregnancy. *Journal of Pediatrics, 96*(5), 974–977.

Longo, L. D. (1976). Carbon monoxide: Effects on oxygenation of the fetus in utero. *Science, 194*(4264), 523–525.

Louria, D. B., Hensle, T., & Rose, J. (1967). Major medical complications of heroin addiction [Review]. *Annals of Internal Medicine, 67*(1), 1–22.

Luck, W., & Nau, H. (1984). Exposure of the fetus, neonate, and nursed infant to nicotine and cotinine from maternal smoking. *New England Journal of Medicine, 311*(10), 672.

Luke, B., Williams, C., Minogue, J., & Keith, L. (1993). The changing pattern of infant mortality in the U.S.: The role of prenatal factors and their obstetrical implications. *International Journal of Gynecology and Obstetrics, 40*(3), 199–212.

MacGregor, S. N., Keith, L. G., Chasnoff, I. J., et al. (1987). Cocaine use during pregnancy: Adverse perinatal outcome. *American Journal of Obstetrics and Gynecology, 157*(3), 686–690.

Madden, J. D., Payne, T. F., & Miller, S. (1986). Maternal cocaine abuse and effect on the newborn. *Pediatrics, 72*(2), 209–211.

Malseed, R., & Harrigan, G. (1989). *Textbook of pharmacology & nursing care: Using the nursing process.* Philadelphia: J. B. Lippincott.

McGarry, J. (1983). Smoking in pregnancy—A 25-year survey. *Midwives Chronicle and Nursing Notes, 96*(1141), 51–55.

McKool, K. (1987). Facilitating smoking cessation. *Journal of Cardiovascular Nursing, 1*(4), 28–41.

Meyer, M. B., Jonas, B. S., & Tonascia, J. A. (1976). Perinatal events associated with maternal smoking during pregnancy. *American Journal of Epidemiology, 103*(15), 464–476.

Mills, J. L., Graubard, B. I., Harley, E. E., et al. (1984). Maternal alcohol consumption and birth weight: How much drinking during pregnancy is safe? *Journal of the American Medical Association, 252*(14), 1875–1879.

Mirochnick, M., Meyer, J., Cole, J., et al. (1991). Circulating catecholamine concentrations in cocaine-exposed neonates: A pilot study. *Pediatrics, 88*(3), 481–485.

Moore, T. R., Sorg, J., Miller, L., et al. (1986). Hemodynamic effects of intravenous cocaine on the pregnant ewe and fetus. *American Journal of Obstetrics and Gynecology, 155*(4), 883–888.

NAACOG [Nurses Association of the American College of Obstetrics and Gynecology]. (1988). Pregnancy and alcohol: A hazardous mix. *NAACOG Newsletter, 15*(3), 1, 4–8.

NAACOG. (1990, May). *Substance abuse in women* [official statement].

Naeye, R., Harkness, W., & Utts, J. (1977). Abruptio placentae and perinatal death: A prospective study. *American Journal of Obstetrics and Gynecology, 128*(7), 740–746.

Naeye, R. L. (1980). Abruptio placentae and placenta previa: Frequency, perinatal mortality and cigarette smoking. *Obstetrics and Gynecology, 55*(6), 701–704.

Naeye, R. L., & Peters, E. C. (1984). Mental development of children whose mothers smoked during pregnancy. *Obstetrics and Gynecology, 64*(5), 601–607.

Naeye, R. L., Blanc, W., LeBlanc, W., & Khatamee, M. A. (1973). Fetal complications of maternal heroin addiction: Abnormal growth, infections, and episodes of stress. *Journal of Pediatrics, 83*(6), 1055–1061.

National Association for Perinatal Addiction Research and Education. (1989). *Drug information guide.* Chicago: Author.

Neri, G., Sammito, V., Romano, C., et al. (1988). Facial midline defect in the fetal alcohol syndrome: Embryogenetic considerations in two clinical cases. *American Journal of Medical Genetics, 29*(3), 477–482.

Nowicki, P., Gintzig, L., Hebel, J. R., et al. (1984). Effective smoking intervention during pregnancy. *Birth, 11*(4), 217–224.

Oro, A. A., & Dixon, S. D. (1987). Perinatal cocaine and methamphetamine exposure: Maternal and neonatal correlates. *Journal of Pediatrics, 111*(4), 571–578.

Ostrea, E. M., & Chavez, C. J. (1979). Perinatal problems (excluding neonatal withdrawal) in maternal drug addiction: A study of 830 cases. *Journal of Pediatrics, 94*(2), 292–295.

Phelps, L., & Grabowski, J. (1992). Fetal alcohol syndrome: Diagnostic features and psychoeducational risk factors. *School Psychology Quarterly, 7*(2), 112–128.

Philips, K. (1986). Neonatal drug addicts. *Nursing Times, 82*(12), 36–38.

Pinto, F., Torrioli, M., Casella, G., et al. (1988). Sleep in babies born to chronically heroin addicted mothers: A follow-up study. *Drug and Alcohol Dependence, 21*(1), 43–47.

Plant, M. (1985). Fetal alcohol syndrome: An overview. *Midwifery, 1*(4), 225–231.

Pollin, W. (1985). The danger of cocaine [Editorial]. *Journal of the American Medical Association, 254*(1), 98.

Pomerleau, O. F., Fertig, J. B., Seyler, L. E., & Jaffe, J. (1983). Neuroendocrine reactivity to nicotine in smokers. *Psychopharmacology, 81*(1), 61–67.

Powell, A. H., & Minick, M. P. (1988). Alcohol withdrawal syndrome. *American Journal of Nursing, 88*(3), 312–315.

Pritchard, J. (1955). Plasma cholinesterase activity in normal pregnancy and in eclamptogenic toxemia. *South American Journal of Obstetrics Gynecology, 70,* 1083.

Rantakallio, P. (1983). A follow-up study up to the age 14 of children whose mothers smoked during pregnancy. *Acta Paediatrica Scandinavica, 72*(5), 747–753.

Reddy, A. M., Harper, R. G., & Stern, G. (1971). Observations on heroin and methadone withdrawal in the newborn. *Pediatrics, 48*(3), 353–358.

Resnick, R. B., Kestenbaum, R. S., & Schwartz, L. K. (1977). Acute systemic effects of cocaine in man: A controlled study by intranasal and intravenous routes. *Science, 195*(4279), 696–698.

Rhead, W. J. (1977). Smoking and SIDS [Letter to the editor]. *Pediatrics, 59*(5), 791–792.

Saylor, C., Lippa, B., & Lee, G. (1991). Drug-exposed infants at home: Strategies and supports. *Public Health Nursing, 8*(1), 33–38.

Schneider, J. W., & Chasnoff, I. J. (1987). Cocaine abuse during pregnancy: Its effects on infant motor development—A clinical perspective. *Topics in Acute Care, Trauma, & Rehabilitation, 2*(1), 59–69.

Schnoll, S. (1986). Pharmacologic basis of perinatal addiction. In I. Chasnoff (Ed.), *Drug use in pregnancy: Mother and child* (pp. 7–15). Norwell, MA: M. T. P. Press.

Shaywitz, S. E., Cohen, D. J., & Shaywitz, B. A. (1980). Behavior and learning difficulties in children of normal intelligence born to alcoholic mothers. *Journal of Pediatrics, 96*(6), 978–982.

Smith, C. G., & Asch, R. H. (1987). Drug abuse and reproduction. *Fertility and Sterility, 48*(3), 355–373.

Smith, J. (1988). The dangers of prenatal cocaine use. *American Journal of Maternal Child Nursing, 13*(3), 174–179.

Smith, J. E., & Deitch, K. V. (1987). Cocaine: A maternal, fetal, and neonatal risk. *Journal of Pediatric Health Care, 1*(3), 120–124.

Soepatmi, S. (1994). Developmental outcomes of children of mothers dependent on heroin or heroin/methadone during pregnancy. *Acta Paediatrics Supplement, 404,* 36-9.

Steeg, C., & Woolf, P. (1979). Cardiovascular malformations in the fetal alcohol syndrome. *American Heart Journal, 98*(5), 635–637.

Stimmel, B. (1979). *Cardiovascular effects of mood altering drugs.* New York: Raven Press.

Strauss, M. E., Starr, R. H., Ostrea, E. M., et al. (1976). Behavioral concomitants of prenatal addiction to narcotics. *Journal of Pediatrics, 89*(5), 842–846.

Streissguth, A., & LaDue, R. (1985, Fall). Psychological and behavioral effects in children prenatally exposed to alcohol. *Alcohol Health and Research World, 10,* 6–12.

Streissguth, A. P., Clarren, S. K., & Jones, K. L. (1985). Natural history of the fetal alcohol syndrome: A 10-year follow-up of eleven patients. *Lancet, 2*(8446), 85–91.

Streissguth, A. P., Herman, C. S., & Smith, D. W. (1978). Intelligence, behavior, and dysmorphogenesis in the fetal alcohol syndrome: A report on 20 patients. *Journal of Pediatrics, 92*(3), 363–367.

Sweeney, L. (1989). Cocaine babies: The latest management dilemma. *NCAST National News, 5*(3), 1–2.

Telsey, A. M., Merrit, T. A., & Dixon, S. D. (1988). Cocaine exposure in a term neonate: Necrotizing enterocolitis as a complication. *Clinical Pediatrics, 27*(11), 547–550.

Torfs, C. P., Velie, E. M., Oechsli, F. W., et al. (1994). A population-based study of gastroschisis: Demographic, pregnancy, and lifestyle risk factors. *Teratology, 50*(1), 44–53.

Townsend, R. R., Laing, F. C., & Jeffrey, R. B., Jr. (1988). Placental abruption associated with cocaine abuse. *American Journal of Roentgenology, 150*(6), 1339–1340.

Tranmer, J. E. (1985). Disposition of ethanol in maternal venous blood and the amniotic fluid. *Journal of Obstetric, Gynecologic, and Neonatal Nursing, 14*(6), 484–490.

Tronick, E. Z., & Beeghly, M. (1992). Effects of prenatal exposure to cocaine on newborn behavior and development: A critical review [OSAP Prevention Monograph-11]. *Identifying the needs of drug-affected children: Public policy issues* (pp. 25–48). Washington, DC: Office of Substance Abuse Prevention (OSAP).

Udell, B. (1989). Crack cocaine. In I. Chasnoff (Ed.), *Special currents: Cocaine babies* (pp. 5–8). Columbus, OH: Ross Laboratories.

U.S. Department of Health and Human Services. (1980). *The health consequences of smoking for women*. Washington, DC: Public Health Service, Office on Smoking and Health.

U.S. Department of Health and Human Services. (1983). *The health consequences of smoking: Cardiovascular disease* (PHS Pub. 84-50204). Washington, DC: Public Health Service, Office on Smoking and Health.

U.S. Department of Health and Human Services (1990). *Alcohol, tobacco, and other drugs may harm the unborn* (PHS Pub. ADM 90-1711). Washington, DC: Office for Substance Abuse Prevention.

van Baar, A. L., Soepatmi, S., Gunning, W. B., & Akkerhuis, G. W. (1994). Development after prenatal exposure to cocaine, heroin and methadone. *Acta Paediatrics Supplement, 404*, 40–46.

Ward, S., Schuetz, S., Krishna, V., et al. (1986). Abnormal sleeping ventilatory pattern in infants of substance-abusing mothers. *American Journal of Diseases of Children, 140*(10), 1015–1020.

Warren, K. R., & Bast, R. J. (1988). Alcohol-related birth defects: An update [Review]. *Public Health Reports, 103*(6), 638–642.

Weiner, L., Rosett, H., & Mason, E. (1985). Training professionals to identify and treat pregnant women who drink heavily. *Alcohol Health and Research World, 10*, 32–35.

Wekselman, K., Spiering, K., Hetteberg, C., et al. (1995). Fetal alcohol syndrome from infancy through childhood: A review of literature. *Journal of Pediatric Nursing, 10*(5), 296–303.

Wilson, G. (1975). Somatic growth effects of perinatal addiction. In R. Harbison (Ed.), *Perinatal addiction* (pp. 333–345). New York: Spectrum.

Wilson, G. S., McCreary, R., Kean, J., & Baxter, C. (1979). The development of preschool children of heroin-addicted mothers: A controlled study. *Pediatrics, 63*(1), 135–141.

Wingerd, J., Christianson, R., Lovitt, W. V., & Schoen, E. J. (1976). Placental ratio in white and black women: Relation to smoking and anemia. *American Journal of Obstetrics and Gynecology, 124*(7), 671–675.

Woods, J. R., Jr., Plessinger, M. A., & Clark, K. E. (1987). Effect of cocaine on uterine blood flow and fetal oxygenation. *Journal of the American Medical Association, 257*(7), 957–961.

Wright, J. (1986). Fetal alcohol syndrome. *Nursing Times, 82*(13), 34–35.

Yerushalmy, J. (1971). The relationship of parents' cigarette smoking to outcome of pregnancy—Implications as to the problem of inferring causation from observed associations. *American Journal of Epidemiology, 93*(6), 443–456.

Zelson, C., Lee, S. J., & Casalino, M. (1973). Neonatal narcotic addiction. Comparative effects of maternal intake of heroin and methadone. *New England Journal of Medicine, 289*(23), 1216–1220.

Zelson, C., Rubio, E., & Wasserman, E. (1971). Neonatal narcotic addiction: 10 year observation. *Pediatrics, 48*(2), 178–189.

CHAPTER 46

Computer Technology Use in Neonatal Nursing

ELIZABETH ELDER WEINER LINDA STURLA FRANCK

RESEARCH AGENDA

What is the impact of computer technology on neonatal nursing practice?

What variables and relationships best describe the knowledge base of neonatal nursing?

Can computer applications be used effectively to educate students, staff, and families?

What role does increased access to information have in the self-care of patients and families?

How can increased access to various databases contribute to the knowledge base of nursing?

Gathering data and managing information is a key nursing function. As early as 1860, Florence Nightingale described the rationale for this activity by the following:

> In dwelling upon the vital importance of *sound* observation, it must never be lost sight of what observation is for. The collection of data is not for the sake of piling up miscellaneous or curious facts, but for the sake of saving life and increasing health and comfort.
>
> (Nightingale, 1860, p. 125).

For us to give the activity of data collection high priority, data must become meaningful to patient care. Computer technology is fast becoming the major modality for the gathering and transforming of data into information for nurses. Nurses working in neonatal settings rely heavily on monitoring devices, information systems, and communications systems to provide up-to-date care efficiently. However, the technology must make care more efficient and effective rather than providing more machines to "nurse."

The complexity of patient care in the neonatal intensive care unit (NICU) presents some of the greatest challenges as well as the greatest potential benefits for using computers. This chapter provides an overview of the major clinical, administrative, educational, and research applications of computer technology for neonatal nursing, discusses the impact of computer technology use in nursing practice and nursing informatics, and provides a resource for nurses seeking to develop or use computer technology in the NICU setting. Lastly, this chapter describes the process and strategies for finding current information.

NURSING INFORMATICS

The importance of computer technology is perhaps clearest as it relates to its role in nursing informatics. The term *nursing informatics* was introduced in the mid-1980s. Nursing informatics is best defined by Graves and Corcoran (1989) in their classic article as "the combination of nursing science, information science, and computer science." The authors describe the transformation of data into information and then into knowledge as three aspects of a phenomenon that is generically called "information."

Information is an essential phenomenon of study for an information-based discipline such as nursing. Computers and other monitoring systems, by their design, contribute greatly to the input and evaluation of the data into information. However, the study of the management and processing of nursing data, information, and knowledge—that is, nursing informatics—is considered an integral part of the science of nursing and not just an application of computer or information science to nursing.

The understanding of nursing decision-making is critical in the generation of nursing knowledge. Knowledge about nursing decision-making has suffered from a focus on "knowledge about nurses" rather than "knowledge about nursing" (Graves & Corcoran, 1989). The challenge for nursing informatics thus becomes the development of tools to understand the process of nursing knowledge by recording and analyzing relationships between and among variables studied. A prototype system that conceptually maps the relationship of variables discovered in nursing research has been developed by Judith Graves (personal communication and software demonstration, August 8, 1995). She has named the system ARKS (A Research Knowledge System), and, although work began on such a system more than 10 years ago, she hopes to gain insight into possible design features to use in a full-featured knowledge registry soon.

The growing importance of informatics to nursing became apparent when a Priority Expert Panel on Nursing Informatics was established by the National Center for Nursing Research (now the National Institute for Nursing Research) to contribute to nursing's research agenda (National Center for Nursing Research, 1993). In addition, the American Nurses' Association (ANA) recently announced that certification in nursing informatics as a specialty area will soon become available. The ANA also published a scope of practice for nursing informatics in 1994. The establishment of nursing informatics masters' programs in both Maryland and Utah have done much to expand opportunities for nurses interested in nursing informatics. Anderson (1992) provides an excellent overview of job opportunities for nurses interested in entering the computer field to design systems for patient care. Furthermore, the National League for Nursing (NLN) has published its recommendations for informatics competencies for nurses in a variety of roles (NLN, 1990).

Nursing competencies are being developed in the areas of informatics while many applications in the clinical areas are appearing. One of these is bedside information systems.

Bedside Information Systems

A further level of sophistication in data processing brings the data gathering, documentation, communication, and analysis functions to the bedside or point of care (Hughes, 1988). (Point-of-care technology is discussed in subsequent paragraphs.) Storage and retrieval of bedside information has proven to be complex and expensive. Less than 2 percent of hospitals made investments in these areas by 1990 (Gardner, 1990), and, whereas more hospitals had acquired these systems by 5 years later, many others had not. Once the systems are in place, there is tremendous potential for redesign and reengineering of nursing work flow and priorities (Simpson, 1991). Early studies of computerized nursing documentation demonstrate savings in time, paperwork, telephone calls, and other clerical functions as well as reduction in transcription and medication errors (Halford et al., 1989; Hendrickson & Kovner, 1989; Hughes, 1988; Yero, 1988). Cost, lack of flexibility and reliability, perceived difficulty of use, and space limitations remain significant obstacles (Gardner, 1990). Well-designed prospective studies are required to substantiate these preliminary findings. See Table 46–1 for key considerations in developing a bedside information system.

Expert Systems

A significant clinical application of informatics is the expert system. The idea behind expert systems is to make available algorithms (or decision trees) used by experts in the field as a resource to guide patient care decisions of clinicians. Data on any patient can then be fit into the model to determine appropriate actions with an established accuracy level. Instead of having a consultation with one faculty member, the user has the experienced information from as many expert clinicians as are entered into the data base. The software Iliad is one example of a medical-based diagnostic program that evolved from the analysis of thousands of patient cases (Warner et al., 1988).

Expert systems are incomplete in their development, however. One difficulty in developing these expert systems is that the programmers must include all factors considered by the clinician, and these complex problem-solving skills are sometimes difficult to capture for analytical purposes, particularly in the complex NICU environment. The work of Benner (1984) clearly describes the advancing problem-solving skills that grow with greater nursing experience. The decision-making processes and expert knowledge of the NICU nurse have yet to be defined and objectified such that algorithms can be defined.

TABLE 46–1 Considerations in Developing a Bedside Computer System

Implement bedside terminals in one unit initially—ideally in an intensive care unit where large volumes of data are generated and are available in electronic form from monitoring devices.
Install one terminal per bedside—sharing terminals between bedsides has not been effective.
Test system for reliability—staff members will not support a system that has even occasional periods of downtime.
Work with physicians to enter orders and notes directly via computer to realize maximal nursing efficiency.

Adapted from Gardner, E. (1990, July 16). Hospitals not in a hurry to plug in computers by the bedside. *Modern Healthcare*, pp. 31–54. Reprinted with permission from *Modern Healthcare*, copyright Crain Communications, Inc., 740 N. Rush Street, Chicago, IL 60611.

TECHNOLOGY IN CLINICAL PRACTICE

Just as computer hardware has changed rapidly, so have the software applications designed to help organize clinical data. Early attempts to design hospital information systems began in the 1960s and were primarily aimed at streamlining tasks such as registration, billing, and scheduling, which could more easily be programmed into the mainframe hospital computer. In the 1980s, more attention was paid to the support of clinical practice. One of the earliest advocates of organized nursing data was Harriet Werley (1987), who pioneered the development of the Nursing Minimum Data Set. From her early work stem four other data bases that are under development. They are (1) The North American Nursing Diagnosis Association (NANDA) Taxonomy of Nursing Diagnosis, (2) the Omaha System Development by the Visiting Nurse Association of Omaha, (3) the Georgetown University Home Health Care Classification Nursing Diagnoses and Interventions (Saba System), and (4) the University of Iowa Intervention Projects Nursing Interventions Classification (NIC). These have been delineated and compared in a recent report by the ANA (1995), whose publication was supported by W. K. Kellogg Foundation and HBO and Company. Since the late 1980s, many institutions have implemented systems for entering orders, reporting results, and planning care. In addition, vendors began to recognize the technologic possibilities for connectivity between input and output patient devices in critical care settings, particularly in the NICU where a high degree of accuracy is required. A recent article in *Neonatal Intensive Care* (1994) provides an overview of the latest in monitoring products for neonatology and perinatology. Represented by a number of different vendors, the products range from apnea monitors to oximeters to complete bedside systems. Vendor contact numbers are included; however, resource lists such as these must be updated frequently because computer hardware and software markets change rapidly.

The vendor selection process itself has become complicated, with many people involved in the commitment that is usually hospital wide and sometimes regional in scope. The essential criteria for selection of computer applications are time efficiency, ease of use, flexibility, reliability, integration, and completeness of final output.

In some cases, specialized vendors are selected for software applications that are unique to specific areas of practice, such as obstetrical and neonatal areas. For example, Quantitative Sentinel/Perinatal (QS/Perinatal) was developed specifically for the perinatal environment (Quantitative Medicine, Inc., 1995). The system has four main application components: surveillance, archival, chalkboard, and charting. The surveillance automatically configures to display active fetal monitors, with strips that maintain the proper aspect ratio. Upon patient discharge, the patient's record is archived automatically on a per pregnancy basis. The chalkboard shows patient status on a unit-wide basis, much like the information boards on the typical labor and delivery unit. Charting can be completed with a defined set of charts, forms, and reports, or the user can create a customized version. The server can be accessed from a variety of locations, including the prenatal clinic, the patient room, labor and delivery, NICU, or even remote access with appropriate hardware.

QS/Perinatal was first developed more than 20 years ago and is in its fourth revision, providing automated support designed specifically for the NICU environment (Quantitative Medicine, Inc., 1995). Vital signs trending, flowsheets, drug dosage calculations, including hyperalimentation and interfaces to equipment such as ventilators, incubators, and intravenous infusion pumps, contribute to a complete patient profile. The patient record is located at or near the bedside, and patient data are automatically placed in the appropriate flow sheet, thereby minimizing transcription errors. The mother's labor and delivery record is also available to provide information for new admissions. There is also a data export feature that allows for clinical information to be put into spreadsheet format for further analysis at the microcomputer level.

There is great interest currently in the use of point-of-care systems for use within neonatal intensive care. The goals of a clinical information system are (1) to provide real-time acquisition of data from monitors and other patient devices (e.g., ventilators, intravenous pumps), (2) to provide for verification of data and direct documentation of patient care delivered (i.e., the paperless chart), (3) to provide multiple, simultaneous user access to the information being recorded from both local and remote sites (and on multiple patients) and to integrate patient data from other sources (e.g., laboratory, radiology departments) and other professionals to create one (paperless) electronic medical record, (4) to provide data for qualitative improvement analysis, and (5) to provide methods for safety checks, notification of abnormal values, protocol guidelines, and clinical algorithms.

In addition to automated patient data collection, the systems have interfaces to a host of peripheral biomedical devices that rely heavily on graphic displays. The result is a costly workstation (Andrew, 1993a, 1993c).

Although there is growing evidence of the clinical and cost effectiveness of these systems, the initial expenditure for hardware and software (approximately $20,000 per bedside station) and staff time to configure and port the system (1 to 2 full-time employees) make clinical information systems cost-prohibitive to implement in many NICUs. Not all NICU facilities have the budget to afford such an elaborate system. The growth of microcomputers and their increased computing capabilities have allowed other programmers to develop data base systems that function on a smaller scale to produce patient documents such as progress notes or provide a patient data base for use on a local level. At the very least, many units are recognizing the need for computer-based patient records.

In a series of articles, Andrew and Dick (1995) describe the computer-based patient record (CPR) as essential for health care. They report trends for each of the Institute of Medicine's (IOM) CPR attributes for 25 emerging CPR systems. The authors report that, although some growth has taken place in CPR systems development, there continue to be the following needs: adequately defined outcome-based patient care, documentation of clinical rationale for decisions, effective linkages (especially if a single vendor system is not used), high-level security, mirrored clinical data bases in case there is downtime of the primary system, support for simultaneous multiuser views, integration of expert systems, and quick access to other clinical resources. The ideal workstation that allows for clinical data entry and analysis coupled with immediate access to information resources is not yet available, but the funding initiative known as Integrated Academic Information Management Systems (IAIMS) from the National Library of Medicine has done much to encourage academic health centers to develop and implement such models (NCNR Priority Expert Panel on Nursing Informatics, 1993). Andrew (1993b) further cautions that, even though critical care environments have been quick to implement aspects of bedside and point-of-care systems, change may be required in current systems because they cannot address the new IOM requirements for integrated clinical data base functionality.

COMPUTER TECHNOLOGY IN ADMINISTRATION

Finance

Perhaps because of the fiscal implications, computers are a common tool for nursing management. Data bases have been constructed to track and analyze all aspects of personnel management from recruitment to turnover. The computer programs need not be part of the mainframe system of the hospital. A multitude of business programs are available for personal computers and can be used by NICU nurse managers to analyze and forecast budget needs, develop proposals for new programs, and perform "what if" analyses to assess the financial impact of any new program or staffing change before implementation (Fowler, 1989; Lange & Detmer, 1989).

Supervision

Many hospitals use computers to assist in the scheduling of nursing staff as well as for meeting reporting requirements for prospective payment (Mowry & Korpman, 1987). However, staffing programs are often not flexible enough to automate the complex and varied schedules of NICU nurses, and manual entry or manipulation of the computerized schedule is required. Some hospitals use programs that compute the number of staff members needed by category (e.g., registered nurses, licensed practical nurses, and nonlicensed staff) based on patient classification. Productivity analyses and trending are made easier by using computer programs (Marks, 1984). The supervision process can also be made more efficient by use of computer data bases (Frayer, 1985). It is too soon to say whether the use of computers in performance monitoring will be perceived as less intrusive or more like "Big Brother" (Sinclair, 1990). Reference information and the communication of policies and procedural changes as well as other routine communication are facilitated by use of the computer. NICU nurse managers are often frustrated by the difficulty in communicating with a larger and increasingly part-time nursing staff. Use of computer applications (e.g., electronic mail, on-line reference information, remote access from home) can improve communication and ensure that all staff receive information and have the opportunity to participate in unit planning and decision-making.

Interdepartmental Relations

Use of computers in hospitals affects the social and political dynamics of the institution. It results in altered communication patterns, job functions, accountabilities, and departmental boundaries (Sinclair, 1990). The redesign of work results in interdepartmental problems as well as opportunities (Aydin & Ischar, 1989). NICU nurse managers must be particularly cognizant of the implications of computerization on interdepartmental communication and work flow because of the dependence of the NICU on support services such as those of the laboratory and pharmacy.

A number of other management functions benefit from computerization, including using electronic mail and word processing to enhance communication. Many nurse administrators publish newsletters and other correspondence in-house, with significant cost savings. Market share and other data necessary for strategic planning are also enhanced through the use of computers (Barhyte, 1987). Billing and inventory programs can help control costs and provide information for forecasting needs (Spohn & Sponseller, 1988).

CONTINUOUS QUALITY ASSURANCE AND CONTINUOUS QUALITY IMPROVEMENT

Automating patient data used for continuous quality assurance (CQA)/continuous quality improvement (CQI) monitoring offers a number of advantages to NICU nurses and allows for more time to be spent in analysis and follow-up as opposed to data collection (Galante & Woodling, 1987). Many applications exist

(*Journal of Nursing Quality Assurance*, 1987), although NICU special applications are rare (Donn et al., 1991). The potential for data gathering is infinite, and nurses participating in CQA/CQI monitoring must ensure that the data represent important aspects of patient care outcome and are meaningful to the practice of nursing (Greer & Hexum, 1987; Joint Commission on Accreditation of Healthcare Organizations [JCAHO], 1990). In addition, the ability to track the documentation of an individual nurse carries the potential for increased use of CQA/CQI data for the reward and punishment of individuals. Although the computer remains neutral, nurses involved in CQA/CQI are advised to consider all ramifications of their computerized data gathering. Barhyte (1987) recommends leaving the evaluation of data that pertain to individual nurse performance to the management personnel responsible for performance appraisal; CQA/CQI should look at the quality of care delivered on a unit-, division-, or hospital-wide level.

COMPUTER TECHNOLOGY IN CLINICAL EDUCATION

Since the proliferation of microcomputers during the 1980s, the use of computers in nursing education also emerged. With the help of the Helene Fuld Foundation and other funding sources, many undergraduate nursing programs began to expand their learning resources to include those that were computerized.

To trim costs and increase accessibility, regional and state libraries began to link their resources electronically with various charging mechanisms. Ohio Link, Ohio's statewide automated information system involving all publicly state-supported universities (Kohl et al., 1993) is an example of this linking that has increased access to holdings across the state while offering more electronic resources. In addition to the usual software for word processing, spread sheets, and data bases, students have access to on-line searching services to find appropriate resources and software to download selected reference material. These tools are becoming as essential to undergraduate and graduate education as the hand-held calculator once was.

Besides exposure to advanced clinical devices, students are exposed to a multitude of clinical simulations for a variety of reasons. Early simulations were developed to help prepare students for the more complex patient situations that they would later encounter on the nursing units. Most of these simulations were text based with minimal graphics. To make simulations more effective, video was added to the computer in the form of interactive videodisc (IVD) during the mid to late 1980s.

Rizzolo (1994) thoroughly describes the use of IVDs in nursing. The *American Journal of Nursing* (AJN), the Health Sciences Consortium, and the Helene Fuld Foundation were instrumental in offering IVD titles for sale to various nursing programs.

Managing the Experience of Labor and Delivery (Gilman et al., 1990) has become a popular IVD program used in the obstetrical environment. Based on the normal labor and delivery experience for one family, the simulation allows the user to make independent decisions based on each hour of labor. The delivery is followed by the initial newborn assessment. In evaluating this program, the authors found that students who had used the IVD program in conjunction with their clinical experience exhibited much more clinical confidence than did those with clinical experience alone (Weiner et al., 1993). One reason for the popularity of this program is that it filled a curricular void in nursing, that is, sometimes there are no patients in labor during an assigned clinical time and, other times, there are too many patients in labor to process the decision-making.

Video that was originally presented via videodisc can be converted to digital form, which can be read directly by the computer. The quality of the digitized video is improving with each generation of new technology, but, currently, the screens are not full sized. With the incorporation of video, sound, text, and graphics files comes the ability to more easily assemble and deliver multimedia packages. The file sizes become quite large, especially with digitized video, so either large servers are used to deliver the programs or the programs are pressed into CD-ROM, another delivery mechanism that is growing in popularity. The changing role of CD-ROM technology should have an impact on more training possibilities for students, staff, and families. Gleydura and associates (1995) provide an excellent overview of multimedia training in nursing education.

A recent example of a CD-ROM program that can be used by both families and students is the *Nine Month Miracle* (A.D.A.M. Software, Inc., 1995). This program is an interactive study of birth from conception to delivery, utilizing stunning still-photography (from Lennart Nillson's *A Child Is Born*), video segments from the PBS documentary *Nine Months,* and creative animation depicting every stage of the birth process. There are three areas of study: "Anatomy," "The Family Album," and "A Child's View of Pregnancy." The anatomy section allows for both female and male versions (with fig-leaf options available to parents, along with four skin colors). Using various tools, the user is able to view the human body layer by layer, with microscopic and labeling features.

The teaching resources available to nurses continue to grow, and those nursing programs and continuing education facilities that do not take advantage of the technologies will receive considerable criticism. Modern graduates take their licensure examination by computer, thereby streamlining the testing procedures by matching responses with algorithms in problem solving (*Nursing and the NCLEX*, 1995).

COMPUTER TECHNOLOGY IN RESEARCH

Two recent electronic advances represent progressive applications of computer technology to nursing research. The first is the establishment of Sigma Theta Tau's Virginia Henderson International Nursing Library (VHINL), which was announced in the fall of 1993 (Gibbons, 1994; Weiner, 1994). The purpose of the VHINL is to provide electronic data bases of research both completed and in progress (without duplicating current university nursing resources), to provide access to "fugitive" literature (not published anywhere else), to describe other information resources in the health care field, and to provide communication links among researchers internationally. This library can be accessed either by direct dial using a computer or modem or through other Internet access. Table 46–2 shows two records in the current VHINL data base that were obtained when searching "neonatal nursing." At the time this search was conducted, these results were not published in any other journal. Information regarding the researcher can be useful to other potential researchers in the field who wish to contact the researcher for more information.

The second, *The Online Journal of Knowledge Synthesis for Nursing*, was developed to promote research-based practice (Barnsteiner, 1994). This on-line journal is sponsored by Sigma Theta Tau. Knowledge synthesis is the gathering of research studies on a topic, assessment of the validity of the findings, and assertion of implications for practice from the valid findings. Given the huge volume of information available, this task could be helpful to a large number of practicing nurses. Many of the articles are authored by clinician and researcher teams to ensure comprehensive synthesis of the research and relevance to clinical practice. Articles generally appear 48 hours after final acceptance by peer review as compared with 6 to 12 months for traditional printed journals.

TABLE 46–2 Sample Records Found in "Neonatal Nursing" Search via the Virginia Henderson International Nursing Library, August 1995

Document 2 of 3

Name:	Carlson Karen Lou
Project:	The relationship of maternal self-concept, depressive symptoms, and social support to the perception of maternal role attainment and premature infant health outcomes
Yr Comp:	1991
Report in Jrnl:	N
Ages:	Newborn infant, adult
Subjects:	Female, male, caregivers, clients/patients, groups/ethnic groups, employed, unemployed, nuclear families, minority groups
Funding:	NIH, internal academic institution, Sigma Theta Tau chapter
Sites:	Homes, hospitals, intensive care unit/critical care unit
Rsch Type:	Applied, descriptive
Design:	Comparative, longitudinal, quantitative
Data Coll:	Chart audit, interview, physiologic measurements, psychological measurements, questionnaire, scales
Data Analy:	Causal models, correlation, factor analysis, regression analysis
Proj Type:	Individual investigator
Descriptors:	Neonatal developmental stage, attachment/involvement, growth and development, depression, self-concept, social support, mother–child relationships, nurturing, theory construction/model building

Abstract

The relationship of maternal self-concept, depressive symptoms, and social support to the perception of maternal role attainment and premature infant health outcomes

Karen L. Carlson

Sixty-two mothers of prematurely born infants were studied to determine the relative contributions of maternal self-concept, depressive symptoms, and perceived social support to subjective feelings of maternal role attainment and infant health outcomes (weight gain, length gain, head circumference gain, number of rehospitalizations, number of unscheduled visits to acute care) at 1 month post discharge from neonatal intensive care.

The mothers were 40.3 percent primiparous, 59.7 percent multiparous, English speaking, 16 years of age or older, predominantly white (54.8 percent) and Hispanic (35.5 percent), married (72.6 percent), and from the lower three socioeconomic stratifications (72.6 percent) as classified by Hollingshead (1977) and lived within a 75-mile radius of the metropolitan area. Their infants were singleton births, of 37 weeks' gestational age or less ($M = 33.4$ weeks), with birth weights of >1000 g and <2500 g ($M = 1857$ g), a history of grade II or less intraventricular hemorrhage, and no known physical or neurologic congenital defects and did not require any high-technology home care upon discharge from the hospital.

Measurement of the predictor variables used the Tennessee Self-Concept Scale (alpha = .93), the Center for Epidemiological Studies Depression Scale (alpha = .89), and the Arizona Social Support Interview Schedule (alpha = .85). At the postdischarge home visits, mothers completed the Gratification in the Mothering Role Scale (alpha = .70), the Maternal Self-Report Inventory (alpha = .81), and a questionnaire about the number of infant rehospitalizations and the number of unscheduled acute care visits. Infants were also weighed and measured during the home visit.

Ten mothers (16.1 percent) had self-concept scores below those of the majority of the population. Forty-two mothers (67.7 percent) demonstrated high depressive symptoms (scores > 16). Perceived number of social support persons ranged from 2 to 20.

Self-concept contributed to 28 percent of the variance in feelings of maternal role attainment as measured by the Maternal Self-Report Inventory ($R^2 = .28$, $F = 24.60$, $p = .0001$). The other relationships of maternal characteristics to feelings of maternal role attainment or infant health outcomes were statistically nonsignificant ($p < .05$).

Peer Reviewed Abstract

Document 3 of 3

Name:	Davis Megan Murphy
Project:	A history of neonatal ethical dilemmas from 1966 to 1985
Yr Comp:	1994
Report in Jrnl:	N

Abstract

A history of neonatal ethical dilemmas from 1966 to 1985

Megan Murphy Davis

The purpose of this research was to analyze critically the impact of technology and social trends on ethical dilemmas involving hospitalized neonates from 1966 to 1985. A historical methodology was employed, using existing bibliographies, the library card catalog, and computer data bases. The study data were classified by content analysis and analyzed according to eight perinatal categories: ethical dilemma, technology, legislation, professional roles, parental roles, ethics committees, psychological issues, and economic issues. In addition, a focused interview was performed with parents and professionals involved in the care of hospitalized neonates between 1966 and 1985. A total of 400 monographs and 20 interviews were obtained.

A histogram of the frequency of monographs allowed a visual interpretation of the growth of literature over time. A chi-square test determined that the presence of the perinatal categories in the sample went significantly beyond random chance. All eight perinatal categories were discussed in light of their changing representation over the years of the study.

The major ethical dilemma was identified as treatment decisions involving premature or handicapped infants. With the rapid advance of medical technology over the past three decades, very small infants who would have died are now kept alive, although not always benefiting from medical techniques. This study showed that the ability to perform technologic feats, moreover, has not been accompanied by a parallel development in making ethical decisions about the lives of these infants.

The major conclusions of this study were that (1) private decisions involving moral dilemmas in the nursery at the beginning of the study became public fare by the study's end, (2) the decision to treat an infant did not remain completely within the domain of medicine or the family, and (3) the ethical evaluation of medical technology quickly accelerated over the time span of the study.

An exhaustive bibliography on ethical dilemmas involving neonates was compiled for the years 1966 to 1985. Recommendations are made for ethics education and research in nursing.

Peer Reviewed Abstract: N

The journal is available through subscription, and neonatal nurses are encouraged to submit topics relevant to their various practice challenges. Searching in August 1995 resulted in synthesized articles relating to early subnutritional feedings (Buus-Frank & Adams, 1994) and tactile stimulation on preterm infants (Harrison & Bodin, 1994).

Computer technology for searching and downloading of citations is as useful to the nurse researcher as it is to the student. The transformation of powerful statistical packages to more user-friendly microcomputer environments has also aided nurse researchers. Graphics presentation packages have also become easier to use and produce either slide or computer presentations of research findings for dissemination.

INTERNET USE

The growth of microcomputers in the 1980s led to networking of resources in the 1990s to promote sharing of data and information. The explosion of these networks led to a need to coordinate them in some way. Many individual campus, state, regional, and national networks were thus linked together into one single network, all sharing a common address scheme, and became the Internet.

World Wide Web, also called WWW, the web, or W3, is the preeminent Internet tool of the mid-1990s (Tomaiuolo, 1995). The WWW is a hypertext interface to the Internet that requires web browsing software such as Netscape. The WWW began in 1989, arising from large collaborations of physics, engineering, and information specialists (Dern, 1994). Documents are prepared and may contain electronic links to other text, audio, image, or video media. Recent growth in WWW servers has overtaken the gopher servers, which are primarily text-based menu driven interfaces to the Internet (Table 46–3).

Internet resources differ substantially from print resources for a number of reasons. First, the sources of information change minute by minute. Whereas this allows for the most current information possible, the user must frequently access sites for updates. Not all sites note the last information update, but certainly should begin to do so. In addition, persons responsible for "linking" to other sites must ensure that the addresses are current so that users do not become frustrated with dead-end links that cannot find the server. Second, anyone who has an account with access to the Internet can build a site and post information there. It is up to the user to determine the credibility of the information provider and thus the believability of the data. Third, there are several different search engines under development to search the web by identified search terms. Because these engines themselves are in a constant state of development, there is no assurance that any one of them is comprehensive in nature. It remains up to the user to again determine the scope and selection of resources. The final and fourth problem remains that of access. The user must still have access to the Internet with either a commercial account (e.g., America OnLine, CompuServe, or Prodigy) or through university, commercial, or government accounts. Access to the web for Macintosh users is still somewhat limited. Web browsers through most commercial systems have been slow to develop for the Macintosh. Many commercial on-line networks have been adapted from the IBM for the Macintosh, leading to many glitches for Macintosh users.

The speed of transfer of the data relates to how long it takes a screen to fill with the selected pictures (graphic images), sound, and video. The more complex the file, the longer the transfer takes. Other factors slowing this process include the speed of the modem on the computer as well as the bandwidth of the fiber carrying the signal. In addition, in this age of multimedia, end users must decide whether they need to hear the sounds and view the advanced graphics because additional hardware and software may be necessary to do so.

TABLE 46–3 Internet Terms

Archie—helps you locate files available by FTP
Backbone—a high-speed connection within a network that connects shorter, usually slower circuits and serves as the major "highway" for an installed system network.
Cyberspace—a term coined by William Gibson in his fantasy novel *Neuromancer* to describe the "world" of computers and the society that gathers around them
DNS (Domain name system)—the method used to convert Internet names to their corresponding Internet numbers
E-mail address—the domain-based address at which one receives electronic mail. E-mail address for author is Betsy.Weiner@UC.EDU.
Ethernet—a 10-million bit per second networking scheme originally developed by Xerox Corporation. Ethernet has grown in popularity because it can network a wide variety of computers.
File transfer protocol (FTP)—software and standards used to send and receive files between computers
Gopher—organizes information into a hierarchy of menus so it is easier to find
Hypertext interface—hypertext is a format in which the text or message is put into a network; the interface is the connection between computers. An example of a hypertext interface is the World Wide Web. It uses hypertext and markup language (HTML).
Internet—connection of many individual TCP/IP campus, state, regional, and national networks (such as NSFnet, ARPAnet, and Milnet) into one single logical network all sharing a common addressing scheme
Internet protocol address—the mutually exclusive address, which is a series of numbers, assigned to a certain system. The IP for the author at which she is available for video-conferencing is 129.137.194.118.
Network—a group of machines connected together so they can transmit information to one another. Networks are usually considered local or remote.
Resolve—translation of an Internet name into its equivalent IP address
SMTP (simple mail transfer protocol)—the Internet standard protocol for transferring electronic mail messages from one computer to another. SMTP instructs two mail systems to interact and format the exchanged messages
Search engines—alternative methods for searching or finding "things" or information on the web. They will be driven by use of search terms, much like Medline or Cinhal literature searches are now
Telnet—logs into a distant computer to execute programs and look at files
Transmission control protocol/Internet protocol (TCP/IP)—a common language that holds the Internet together
Twisted pair—cable made up of a pair of insulated copper wires wrapped around each other to cancel the effects of electrical noise
Uniform resource locator (URL)—the address used to access a web site
Veronica and Jughead—help find Gopher menus
Web home page—the cyberspace office at which a person can be reached on the Internet. The web home page address for the author is HTTP://WWW.UC.EDU/~WEINERBE.
World Wide Web (WWW)—a method of jumping around the Internet with hypertext while using a multimedia browser
World Wide Web (WWW) browser—a method or searching the web for information
World Wide Web (WWW) servers—web browsers that are not usually text-based menu-driven like the older version of the gopher systems. The gopher server is a type of WWW server.

Regardless of the controversy surrounding the use of the web, there exists meaningful information that could be useful to the neonatal nurse. Table 46–4 lists potential electronic sites with their addresses as of August 1995. Some of the sites are addresses on the web, with their listed universal resource locator (URL) addresses. Others are considered "list serves," which require the user to request being added to the "electronic mail list" for a selected topic and then receiving all the mail sent by users who

TABLE 46–4 Electronic Resources of Interest to Neonatal Nurses, August, 1995

Site	How to Access	Address
PEDINFO—pediatrics web server that includes subspecialties of neonatology and perinatology	Internet—WWW	URL:http://www.lhl.uab.edu:80/pedinfo/index.html
NICU-NET—list serve on neonatal intensive care issues for health care professionals	Electronic mail list serve	E-Mail to: Listproc@u.washington.edu Containing message: SUBSCRIBE NICU-NET Your name Your title
Better Health and Medicine Forum—electronic bulletin board for neonatology on America OnLine	Electronic bulletin board	Subscribers to America OnLine
NeoNet—on-line discussion of neonatal topics on America OnLine	Electronic mail	E-Mail to: TACohen@aol.com or BarryBloom@aol.com for information on how to subscribe. Open to America OnLine clients; others can request hard copies of forum discussions via the two E-mail addresses listed.
NICU-WEB—web site from the University of Washington Children's Hospital Medical Center	Internet—WWW	URL:http://weber.u.washington.edu/~pth/WEB/main.html
PRENATAL DIAGNOSTICS—mailing list that mirrors Prenatal Newsgroup	Electronic mail	E-mail to: biosci-server@net.bio.net or MXT@dl.ac.uk. Containing message: subscribe prenatal or SUB bionet-news.bionet.diagnostics.prenatal
PRENAT-L—perinatal discussion list run by State University of New York	Electronic mail	E-mail to listserv@health.state.ny.us. Containing message: subscribe PRENAT-L
NEONATOLOGY/PEDIATRIC—web site from University of Kansas Medical Center	Internet—WWW	http://www.kumc.edu/instruction/medicine/pedcard/neonatology/neonatology.html
NEONATOLOGY—Extracorporeal Life Support Organization (ELSO), home page web site from University of Michigan Medical Center	Internet—WWW	http://www.med.umich.edu/elso/elsotop.html
NEONATOLOGY—Vermont Oxford Neonatal Network, web site from University of Vermont	Internet—WWW	http://www.vtmednet.org/neonate/vtoxford.ntm. For information contact: Jeffrey D. Horbar, MD, University of Vermont. E-mail to horbar@salus.med.uvm.edu
NEONATOLOGY—web site from Baylor College of Medicine	Internet—WWW	http://1.neo.tch.tmc.edu/neo.html
Birth, pregnancy, and midwifery resources	Internet—WWW	http://www.efn.org/~djz/birth/resources.html
Internet midwifery resources	Internet—WWW	http://www.missouri.edu/~nurswalk/internet.html
Virtual Children's Hospital—presented by the Electric Differential Multimedia Laboratory, Department of Radiology, University of Iowa (pediatric multimedia textbooks, information for parents and families, pediatric patient simulations)	Internet—WWW	http://indy.radiology.uiowa.edu/VirtualChildHosp/VCHHomePage.html
General Sites		
HyperDoc—home page of the National Library of Medicine	Internet—WWW	http://www.nlm.nih.gov
Medical Matrix—Guide to Internet Medical Resources (Project of Internet Working Group of American Medical Informatics Association)	Internet—WWW	http://www.kuhttp.cc.ukans.edu/cwis/units/medcntr/Lee/HOMEPAGE.HTML
Nursing and the NCLEX—web site that is home page for information about the nursing licensure examination	Internet—WWW	http://www.Kaplan.com/etc/nclex/nclex_index.html
NRSING-L Nursing Informatics	Electronic mail list serve	E-mail to listproc@lists.umass.edu
OJKSN—Online *Journal of Knowledge Synthesis for Nursing*—Sigma Theta Tau electronic journal that requests synthesized articles	Dial in modem with Guidon software (subscription required) or WWW access (subscription required)	http://www.ref.oclc.org:2000
OVCHIN—Ohio Valley Community Health Information Network, example of client-oriented electronic health system for public access	Internet—WWW	http://www.ovchin.uc.edu
VHINL—Virginia Henderson International Nursing Library—Sigma Theta Tau electronic library	Internet—Telnet (subscription required but can access by typing "guest" to view demonstration)	telnet stti-sun.iupui.edu With modem, call 317-687-2271
Virtual Nursing Center—collection of various nursing resources	Internet—WWW	http://www-sci.lib.uci.edu/HSG/Nursing.html
Virtual Nursing College	Internet—WWW	ftp://ftp.langara.bc.ca/pub/nursing/vnc.htm

belong to the group. This discussion is topic related, sometimes generated by the "systems operator" of the group or sometimes generated by the users themselves. The web sites have identified "web masters" who are responsible for maintaining and updating the information contained at their location. Identifying information for web masters is generally found on the first page, or "home page," of the site.

For example, one of the most active Internet resources for neonatology is the NICU-NET, started in January 1995, which allows on-line discussions and postings of clinical questions. The NICU-NET is grant supported at the University of Washington. It has 957 health care provider users (70 percent are physicians, 10 percent nurses, 6 percent nurse practitioners, 6 percent respiratory therapists, 3 percent doctors of philosphy, 2 percent pharmacists, and 3 percent ethicists, researchers, and bioengineers). Seventy percent of these users are in academic centers accessing the service through a university system with the remaining 30 percent contacting it through commercial accounts (Tarczy-Hornoch, 1995). Twenty-one countries are represented on this network, lending support to the notion of a global community of professionals concerned about neonatal issues.

USE OF COMPUTERS IN PATIENT CARE: ETHICAL AND LEGAL ISSUES

Confidentiality

The use of computers in patient care does not raise new issues regarding confidentiality, but rather highlights the potential problems of current practice regarding the uses of medical records (Melia, 1989). Patient information is generally accessible to a wide variety of personnel within the hospital setting. Computerization of medical records can make access even easier. The use of physical and operational security measures such as restrictive passwords can prevent unauthorized access at bedside terminals. Issues related to patient and family access must always be addressed (Romano, 1987). Use of the information for purposes other than that which serves the interest of the patient is an ethical concern that remains a human problem with or without the computer.

Standardization of Patient Care

Nurses have also expressed concern regarding the potential for computers to promote routine or depersonalized patient care (Melia, 1989; Sinclair, 1988). The use of expert systems and templates for the assessment and documentation of patient care may discourage individualization of such care, which is a central value of the profession of nursing. Again, the use of computers does not create this dilemma, but rather only increases the potential, particularly in the critical care setting, where extensive technology tends to promote the notion of humans as machines. Alternatively, computers can be viewed as an extension of the nurse in delivering holistic, humanistic care (Ryan, 1985).

Legal Liability

The use of computers in patient care carries additional responsibilities and accountability for nurses, who have an obligation to maximize benefits of technology without sacrificing the interests of nurses and patients (Sinclair, 1990). For example, legal liability is often incurred in critical care settings when available technology that may have benefited a patient is not used. The use of computers to gather and display even more information provides the nurse with the potential for liability if the data are not acted upon. It is not simply a case of more is better. Uses of computers in the NICU must be accompanied by careful training and a clear understanding about the use of the data and the responsibility for ensuring accuracy of monitoring equipment (Sinclair, 1988).

CONCLUSION

It is clear that the nurse who is employed in neonatal settings cannot function without dependence on computer technology. The challenge comes in knowing how to use the technology in an efficient, effective manner to facilitate nursing care. Whether practicing in a clinical, administrative, educational or research setting, there are ever-increasing tools to aid the practicing nurse in finding the best and most current information. The job of nurses thus becomes the integration of this information into their knowledge base.

The challenge of the 1990s is the integration of thorough clinical data systems that effectively interface with other information resources in a timely manner. Nurses must be active participants in this process to learn more about nursing knowledge while contributing to effective technologic solutions.

REFERENCES

A.D.A.M. Software, Inc. (1995). *Nine month miracle* [CD-ROM, Mac and Windows]. Atlanta, GA: Author.

American Nurses' Association. (1994). *Scope of practice for nursing informatics*. Washington, DC: American Nurses Publishing.

American Nurses' Association. (1995). *Nursing data systems: The emerging framework*. Washington, DC: American Nurses Publishing.

Anderson, B. L. (1992). Nursing informatics: Career opportunities inside and out. *Computers in Nursing, 10*(4), 165–170.

Andrew, W. F. (1993a). Bedside/point-of-care technology: This issue's featured vendors. *Computers in Nursing, 11*(1), 42–44.

Andrew, W. F. (1993b). Bedside/point-of-care technology: The window into the integrated clinical database. *Computers in Nursing, 11*(1), 17–19.

Andrew, W. F. (1993c). *Guide to bedside/point-of-care information systems, 1993 edition.* Winter Haven, FL: William F. Andrew & Associates, Inc.

Andrew, W. F., & Dick, R. S. (1995). Applied information technology: A clinical perspective. Feature focus: The computer-based patient record. *Computers in Nursing, 13*(4, Part 3), 176–181.

Aydin, C. E., & Ischar, R. (1989). The effects of computerized order entry on communication between pharmacy and nursing. In L. Kingsland (Ed.), *Proceedings, Thirteenth Annual Symposium on Computer Applications in Medical Care* (pp. 796–801). Washington, DC: IEEE Computer Society Press.

Barhyte, D. Y. (1987). Computer-generated quality assurance: Nontraditional uses of the data. *Journal of Nursing Quality Assurance, 1*(4), 43–49.

Barnsteiner, J. H. (1994). The online journal of knowledge synthesis for nursing. *Reflections, 20*(2), 10–11.

Benner, P. (1984). *From novice to expert: Excellence and power in clinical nursing practice*. Menlo Park, CA: Addison-Wesley.

Buus-Frank, M. E., & Adams, E. (August 23, 1994). Early sub-nutritional feedings [74 paragraphs]. *Online Journal of Knowledge Synthesis for Nursing, 1.* (Online serial, available as Doc. No. 8 via WWW and subscription: http://www.ref.oclc.org:2000)

Dern, D. P. (1994). *The Internet guide for new users*. New York: McGraw-Hill.

Donn, S. M., Gates, M. R., & Kiska, D. J. (1991). User friendly computerized quality assurance program for regionalized neonatal care. *Journal of Perinatology, 13*(3), 190–196.

Fowler, L. M. (1989). Computer-assisted occurrence report analysis. In L. Kingsland (Ed.), *Proceedings, Thirteenth Annual Symposium on Computer Applications in Medical Care* (pp. 991–992). Washington, DC: IEEE Computer Society Press.

Frayer, W. W. (1985). Information management systems in neonatal intensive care: A case report. *Mount Sinai Journal of Medicine, 52*(2), 82–86.

Galante, C. M., & Woodling, C. B. (1987). Using computers to evaluate nursing process documentation. *Journal of Nursing Quality Assurance, 1*(4), 50–60.

Gardner, E. (1990). Hospitals not in a hurry to plug in computers by the bedside. *Modern Healthcare, 20*(28), 31–44.

Gibbons, B. J. (1994). Venture into nursing cyberspace with the Virginia Henderson International Nursing Library. *Reflections, 20*(2), 14.

Gilman, B., Weiner, E., & Gordon, J. (1990). *Managing the experience of labor and delivery* [computer program, interactive videodisc]. Cincinnati, OH: University of Cincinnati. (Video production funded by the College of Nursing and Health, University of Cincinnati; project marketed by Health Sciences Consortium, Raleigh, NC).

Gleydura, A. J., Michelman, J. E., & Wilson, C. N. (1995). Multimedia training in nursing education. *Computers in Nursing 13*(4), 169–175.

Graves, J.R., & Corcoran, S. (1989). The study of nursing informatics. *Image: Journal of Nursing Scholarship, 21*(4), 227–231.

Greer, J., & Hexum, J. (1987). Dimensions of computerized quality assurance systems. *Journal of Nursing Quality Assurance, 1*(4), 9–14.

Halford, G., Burkes, M., & Pryor, T. A. (1989). Measuring the impact of bedside terminals. *Nursing Management, 20*(7), 41–44.

Harrison, L. L., & Bodin, M. B. (March 9, 1994). Tactile stimulation on preterm infants [67 paragraphs]. *Online Journal of Knowledge Synthesis for Nursing, 1.* (Online serial, available as Doc. No. 6 via WWW and subscription: http://www.ref.oclc.org:2000)

Hendrickson, G., & Kovner, C. T. (1989). Effect of various components of computer systems on nurses. In L. Kingsland (Ed.), *Proceedings, Thirteenth Annual Symposium on Computer Applications in Medical Care* (pp. 827–833). Washington, DC: IEEE Computer Society Press.

Hughes, S. (1988). Bedside information systems: State of the art. In M. J. Ball, K. J. Hannah, U. Gerdin-Jelger, & H. Peterson (Eds.), *Nursing informatics: Where care and technology meet* (pp. 260–266). New York: Springer-Verlag.

Joint Commission on Accreditation of Healthcare Organizations. (1990). *Accreditation manual for hospitals.* Chicago, IL: Author.

Kohl, D. F., Sanville, T., Steger, J., & Walters, E. G. (1993). *Creating the virtual library in Ohio: New partnerships, new politics, new money.* Paper presented at the meeting of EDUCOM '93, Cincinnati, Ohio: Crafting New Communities.

Lange, L. L., & Detmer, S. (1989). Developing a unit-level nursing productivity model using spreadsheets and database management systems. In L. Kingsland (Ed.), *Proceedings, Thirteenth Annual Symposium on computer Applications In Medical Care* (pp. 989–990). Washington, DC: IEEE Computer Society Press.

Marks, F. E. (1984). Computer graphics for nursing management. *Nursing Management, 15*(7), 19–26.

Melia, K. (1989). Computer ethics. *Nursing Times, 85*(29), 62–63.

Mowry, M. M., & Korpman, R. A. (1987). Evaluating automated information systems. *Nursing Economics, 5*(1), 7–12.

National League for Nursing (NLN). (1990). *Discussions and recommendations: Informatics competencies for four nursing roles.* New York: Author.

NCNR Priority Expert Panel on Nursing Informatics. (1993). *Nursing informatics: Enhancing patient care* (NIH Publication No. 93-2419). (On-line document, available WWW: gopher://gopher.nlm.nih.gov:70/00/extramural/nurseinfo)

Nightingale, F. (1860). *Notes on nursing: What it is and what it is not.* New York: D. Appleton & Co.

Nursing and the NCLEX. (1995). (On-line document, available via WWW: http://www.Kaplan.com/etc/nclex/nclex_Eindex.html)

Quantitative Medicine, Inc. (Division of Marquette). (1995). *Quantitative Sentinel/Perinatal: Meeting all of the needs for obstetrical and neonatal areas* [Brochure]. San Juan Capistrano, CA: Author.

Romano, C. A. (1987). Privacy, confidentiality and security of computerized systems. *Computers in Nursing, 5*(3), 99–104.

Ryan, L. (1985). Decision: Humanism. *Computers in Nursing, 3*(2), 65–67.

Rizzolo, M. A. (Ed.). (1994). *Interactive video: Expanding horizons in nursing.* New York, NY: American Journal of Nursing Company.

Simpson, R. L. (1991). Adopting a nursing minimum data set. *Nursing Management, 22*(2), 20–21.

Sinclair, V. (1988). High technology in critical care: Implications for nursing's role and practice. *Focus on Critical Care, 15*(4), 36–41.

Sinclair, V. G. (1990). The impact of computer support on social and political dynamics in health care organizations. *Nursing Administration Quarterly, 14*(3), 66–73.

Spohn, D. M., & Sponseller, M. J. (1988). Computers and nursing: Supply requisitions and inventory control. *Today's OR Nurse, 10*(7), 10–15.

Tarczy-Hornoch, P. (1995). Neonatology on-line. *AAP Perinatal Section News, 20*(2), 10.

The latest in monitoring products for neonatology/perinatology. (1994). *Neonatal Intensive Care, 7*(4), 36–41.

Tomaiuolo, N. L. (1995). Accessing nursing resources on the internet. *Computers in Nursing, 13*(4), 159–168.

Warner, H. R., Haug, P., Bouhaddou, O., & Lincoln, M. (1988). ILIAD as an expert consultant to teach differential diagnosis. In R. A. Greenes (Ed.), *Proceedings of the Twelfth Annual Symposium on Computer Applications in Medical Care* (pp. 371–376). Los Angeles, CA: IEEE Computer Society.

Weiner, B. (1994). Frequently asked questions regarding the Virginia Henderson International Nursing Library and the online journal of knowledge synthesis for nursing. *Reflections, 20*(2), 12–13.

Weiner, E., Gordon, J., & Gilman, B. (1993). Evaluation of a labor and delivery interactive videodisc simulation. *Computers in Nursing, 11*(4), 191–196.

Werley, H. (1987). The nursing minimum data set: Status and implications. In K. J. Hannah & M. Reimer (Eds.), *Clinical judgment and decision making: The future with nursing diagnosis* (pp. 540–555). New York: John Wiley & Sons.

Yero, M. (1988). St. Francis goes bedside and beyond: High tech with high touch. *The Bedside Story, 2*(1).

UNIT EIGHT

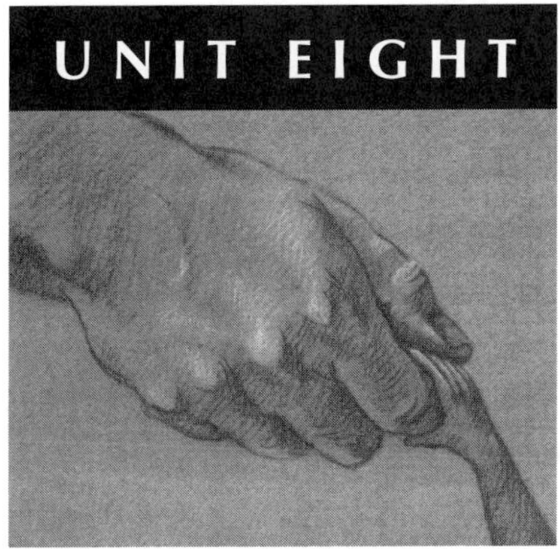

Long-Term Development of the Neonate

Robin's gesture was yet another example of how the nurses seemed to hold this whole place together. The doctors gave the orders, the administrators took care of business, but the nurses kept things human. They were the buffers and the barometers, riding the balance between the parents' panic and the doctors' detachment. In the process, they managed to keep the kids as their primary objects of attention—and often their affections, as well.

One morning, early on, I was in the NICU at about seven o'clock when Eleanor, another nurse who had put in twenty-plus years there, was making her report on the night's activities to the nurse who would succeed her on the day shift.

"They're all my babies while they're up there," she said. "My babies and God's."

ELIZABETH MEHREN
Born Too Soon

CHAPTER 47

Systematic Assessment and Home Follow-Up: A Basis for Monitoring the Neonate's Integration Into the Family Unit

NIA JOHNSON-CROWLEY

RESEARCH AGENDA

What effect does the environment have on neonatal development?

What are the risk factors for poor parent–infant interaction?

What is the relationship between systematic assessment of maternal–infant interaction in the home and compliance with well child follow-up care?

Is infant temperament affected by interaction with the caregiver?

Going home. For parents invested in the day-to-day struggles of their preterm infant within the neonatal intensive care unit (NICU), those two words are guaranteed to make them sit up and take notice. Comments such as "Finally"; "You mean we really can take her home . . . with us?"; "I can't believe this!"; "You're sure it's OK . . . you're really sure?"; "I don't believe I'm ready for this." All reflect the joy, disbelief, anxiety, and ambivalence that many of these parents feel. After days, weeks, and possibly months in the NICU, an important goal is finally reached: Their child is coming home with them.

During their infant's stay in the hospital, parents come to depend on the supportive environment of the NICU to understand and cope with the behavior and care of their infant. Doctors, nurses, nutritionists, and other hospital personnel have been on hand to ensure that their preterm infant not only survived but survived in the best possible condition, setting the stage for as normal a developmental outcome as possible. Knowledge that they must now assume the responsibility that heretofore the hospital personnel assumed for the care of their baby can undermine even the most stalwart person's confidence in his or her parenting ability (Harrison & Kositsky, 1987; Kenner & Lott, 1990; NICHCY, 1988; Sammons & Lewis, 1985). Parents need continued availability of support during the transition between hospital and home and in the ongoing weeks and months as they begin to integrate the new infant into the family unit (Murphy, 1989). Parents need this support not just for their own confidence but because research has shown that no matter how easy or traumatic the infant's stay in the NICU, the home environment has the greatest influence on how well a given preterm infant develops and thrives (Cohen et al., 1986; Gottfried, 1984; Greenberg & Crnic, 1988; Leonard et al., 1990; Sameroff, 1981).

This chapter explores the importance of home follow-up for preterm infants after hospital discharge. Areas discussed include the preterm infant's vulnerability for developing problems that affect later positive outcomes, how parents want and need further monitoring and support when their infant comes home, and the value of nurses in providing this follow-up. The importance of systematic assessment and the use of intervention programs that include the needs of the parents are discussed. Finally, examples of assessments and an intervention program found to be successful with this population are presented.

NEED FOR HOME FOLLOW-UP OF PRETERM INFANTS

It has long been known that disabling neurodevelopmental conditions are prevalent among infants of low birth weight (Bennett, 1984; Blackburn, 1995; Field & Sostek, 1983). However, research has shown that perinatal and neonatal complications do not account alone for these neurodevelopmental conditions (Astbury et al., 1983; Beckwith & Cohen, 1984; Escalona, 1982; Greenberg & Crnic, 1988; Hunt, 1981; Sameroff, 1981). Sameroff (1981), in a review of longitudinal studies, found that 20 to 50 percent of low birth weight infants demonstrate developmental problems in later years. In addition, he found that the variables that most strongly predicted these outcomes were measures of the infant's home environment (Sameroff, 1981). Research studies have provided strong correlations between cognitive development and the quality of a child's overall environment, for both full-term and preterm infants (Cohen et al., 1986; Gottfried, 1984).

Preterm infants are especially vulnerable because of both their biologic status (i.e., being preterm) and environmental factors that interact to put them at high risk for later problems (Barnard et al., 1984; Barnard & Eyres, 1977; Barnard et al., 1985; Beckwith & Cohen, 1980; Bee et al., 1982; Blackman et al., 1987; Crnic et al., 1986; Escalona, 1982; Mitchell et al., 1985; Ramey et al., 1979; Sameroff, 1986). In fact, Greenberg and Crnic (1988) noted that the preterm infants in their study were more strongly influenced by their environment in terms of positive outcomes than were the full-term infants. These studies suggest that ensuring positive environmental conditions after discharge is especially important for the promotion of normal development for preterm infants.

Within the home environment, the parent–infant interaction was found to be the best predictive factor for later positive development in preterm infants (Barnard et al., 1989; Barrera et al., 1986; Bendersky & Lewis, 1986; Crnic & Greenberg, 1987; Field, 1987; Greenberg & Crnic, 1988; Ramey et al., 1979;

Schraeder et al., 1987). Barnard and associates (1989), in their investigation of several research programs studying these interactive qualities for both full-term and preterm infants, stated that "In general, high-quality interactions during the first years of life tend to be positively linked to the infant's subsequent cognitive and linguistic competence and to more secure attachments to major caregivers" (p. 40). Many of these studies identified certain behavioral characteristics that may account for parent–infant interaction difficulties seen in preterm infants and in their parents, resulting in less desirable development outcomes. The next section explores these characteristics and their effect on parenting.

PRETERM INFANT CHARACTERISTICS AND THEIR EFFECT ON CAREGIVER INTERACTION

Studies comparing full-term and preterm infants found preterm infants to be different from their full-term counterparts in several ways: ways that have a tremendous influence on the parent–infant interaction. First, preterm infants as a group were found to be less neurologically mature than full-term infants. As a result of this lack of maturity, preterm infants are less regulatory (organized) in their behavior, which makes it harder to understand and predict how they will behave. This lack of neurologic maturity is directly related to how premature they are: The younger the preterm infant gestationally, the less mature and the more disorganized the infant's behavior. Second, preterm infants as a group exhibited a lower level of behavioral social responsiveness, were less persistent and adaptable, and tended to respond to stimuli in more negative ways than did full-term infants (Anders & Keener, 1985; Barnard, 1980; Barnard & Bee, 1981; Bennett, 1984; Schwartz et al., 1984; Tekolste & Bennett, 1987; Telzrow et al., 1982).

As a result of these characteristics, such infants give hard-to-read cues, making it difficult for their parents to know when to feed them, when to soothe them, when to leave them alone, and when to play with them. Preterm infants, sensitive to stimuli and limited in energy reserves, respond to their parents' attempt to interact by turning away, dropping off to sleep, or crying inconsolably; parents see such behavior as negative and difficult to cope with and understand. If parent–infant interaction is seen as a sort of "dance" in which each participant (parent and infant) must give clear and readable cues that can be read by the partner, must be motorically and neurologically alert to respond quickly and positively to the partner's cues, and must retain enough energy to keep the dance going in a smooth and rhythmic way, it is easy to see why interacting (dancing) with a preterm infant may not be the positive experience that most parents expect it to be. Because parents often expect their preterm infant to behave like a full-term infant, they become confused when this does not occur. In essence, parents are dancing with a partner who does not hold up his or her side of the dance duo, which results in dyssynchrony and discord. Even the most positive mothers and fathers can lose confidence in their ability to parent.

These characteristics of giving unclear cues and being more negative and less socially responsive may also account for the report by parents of preterm infants that they are harder to care for and have a more difficult temperament than full-term infants. Several researchers have studied the temperament of preterm infants. In general, their findings suggest that the older (born at 34 to 37 weeks' gestation), heavier (weight, >1200 g), and healthier preterm infants show no differences in temperament from full-term infants by parent report, whereas the younger (born at less than 34 weeks' gestation), lighter (weight, <1200 g), and sicker preterm infants are described by parents as being more difficult in temperament than those in reports by parents of full-term infants (Barrera et al., 1984; Garcia Coll, 1990; Goldstein & Bracey, 1988; Graham et al., 1973; Medoff-Cooper, 1986; Prior et al., 1989; Riese, 1988; Ross, 1984; Schraeder & Medoff-Cooper, 1983; Schraeder & Tobey, 1989; Thomas, 1981; Washington et al., 1986). Patteson and Barnard (1990), after reviewing several of these studies, concluded that there was some basis for the report of preterm infants' having a more difficult temperament, especially as it related to the lower birth weight infants and those with health problems, specifically respiratory problems.

Riese (1988), Schraeder and Tobey (1989), and Washington and associates (1986) also studied how stable the preterm infant temperament characteristics were over time. Infants in all three studies averaged 1200 g and were essentially healthy, growing preterm infants. Findings from Riese (1988) and Washington and associates (1986) suggested that temperament characteristics are less stable for preterm infants than for full-term infants over the first year of life. Riese reported that by 18 to 24 months, preterm infants were as stable in temperament as the full-term infants (Riese, 1988; Washington et al., 1986). Schraeder and Tobey's (1989) findings differed; they found preterm infants to be rated as more difficult in temperament characteristics up to 4 years of age. However, this was related to conditions of the home environment. The more optimal and positive the home environment, the less difficult the preterm infant was rated by the parent (Schraeder & Tobey, 1989).

Washington and associates (1986) found temperament ratings to be related to the sensitivity of the parent. Ratings of preterm infants as a group varied throughout the year (i.e., they were less stable); however, the more sensitive the caretaker was toward the infant, the less difficult the preterm infant was rated by 12 months of age. Washington and associates (1986) questioned whether altering the environment (i.e., the behavior of the caretaker) changed the caretaker's perception of the infant or whether the infant changed (i.e., became less irritable, more responsive) because the caretaker became more sensitive. Their conclusion was "that temperament, at least early on in life, is not a fixed construct but a reflection both of the changing transactions between caretakers and infants accompanying growth and development, and the discontinuities of the infant's biobehavioral organization" (Washington et al., 1986, p. 501).

In a later study, Zahr (1991) supported earlier work finding a link between temperament and characteristics of the parent–infant interaction. Studying a set of preterm infant–mother dyads (n = 49) from low socioeconomic backgrounds, Zahr reported that the more positive the mother–infant interaction, the less likely that the child's temperament would be perceived as difficult at 4 and 8 months of age and the more social support the mother had. Although birth weight and length of hospitalization also correlated with the positiveness of mother–infant interaction at 4 months of age, only temperament and social support correlated with how well the infant and mother interacted at 8 months of age (Zahr, 1991).

Thomas and Chess (1977) earlier described this mix of infant characteristics and environmental conditions, such as a sensitive caregiver, a "goodness of fit" between the child and the parent. Schraeder and Tobey suggested enhancing this goodness of fit by having nurses help parents assess and understand their preterm infant's "style" of behavior so that parents could better adapt their own behavior and environmental conditions to help the infant adapt and respond better, thus creating a more optimal parent–infant interaction (Schraeder & Tobey, 1989).

More recent studies specifically aimed at determining whether preterm children as a group do differ greatly in temperament and behavior from full-term infants have resulted in conflicting findings. For instance, Gennaro and associates (1992) used secondary analysis of common variables among three cohort study groups to analyze the effects of perinatal factors and NICU influences on infant temperament. Although, as a group, preterm infants in each cohort sample were "significantly more difficult [in temperament] that the comparison groups of full-term infants" (p. 376), by parent report at 6 months, perinatal variables (mechanical ventilation, length of hospital stay, infant birth weight, and gestational age) did not predict well which infants would be perceived as having a difficult temperament. They found that "infants who were the smallest, sickest, and exposed longest to the multiple, often noxious stimuli in neonatal intensive care nurseries in each cohort were not necessarily the infants who had the most difficult temperaments" (p. 376). They concluded that parents could now be assured that "no particular perinatal or neonatal event contributes to this behavioral style" (Gennaro et al., 1992, p. 376).

Oberklaid and associates (1991), however, in their longitudinal study of a group of infants found little difference in temperament between preterm and full-term infants up to age 6 years. Over all the five time periods in which temperament data were gathered (4 and 8 months in infancy and as young toddlers, older toddlers, preschoolers, and early school age children), "the only difference in any temperament rating was in the young toddler age group, when preterm subjects had a tendency to be less intense than control [full-term] subjects . . . [and] significantly more likely to be rated as having an easy temperament" (Oberklaid et al., 1991, p. 857).

Researchers of these most recent studies acknowledge that while preterm infants may be described as more difficult in temperament initially, over time this perception moderates. When problems attributed to a more difficult temperament persist, other factors such as maternal depression, stress, infant illness, medical complications, inadequate support systems, and/or dysfunctional parent–child relationships have been identified as possible correlates. However, how the infant's temperament is influenced by or influences these factors has not been determined and is a matter for further research (Gennaro et al., 1992; Oberklaid et al., 1991; Zahr, 1991).

In conclusion, studies comparing preterm and full-term infants do provide evidence that preterm infants have some characteristics, such as harder-to-read behavioral cues, low responsiveness, and less predictability, that may make them seem more difficult in temperament and make it harder for their parents to care for them, especially during the early weeks and months at home. In addition, these characteristics seem to strongly affect the adaptation between these infants and their caregivers. However, parents who are aware, understand, and adapt to the behavioral and temperament characteristics of their preterm infant report that their preterm infants are easier to care for and more enjoyable to be around at later ages. Unfortunately, not all parents are able to adapt. The next section describes four conditions in which parents do not adapt and that may occur more often in families with preterm infants than in families with full-term infants.

PARENTAL RESPONSE TO THEIR PRETERM INFANT'S BEHAVIOR

Parental burnout, super parent syndrome, vulnerable child syndrome, and higher potential for child abuse are four phenomena described in the literature as maladaptive responses by parents possibly related to the behaviors of preterm infants. Beckwith and Cohen (1980) first described parental burnout in their follow-up study of preterm infants. They found that the level of maternal responsiveness changes over time and is related to the infant's behavior. In general, in normal full-term infants, the more responsive the infant, the more responsive the mother. However, they found that the mothers of preterm infants who had more health problems and who were more premature tended to become less socially responsive over the first year of life. The authors concluded that some reinforcement from the infant was needed to keep the mother responding to her infant's behavior in a positive way. If this reinforcement did not occur, the mother responded less and less over time. Furthermore, they found that there is a limit to how long parents will respond without any reinforcement. If no reinforcement is forthcoming, parents become exhausted trying and eventually "burn out" (Beckwith and Cohen, 1980).

Two other studies have replicated these findings (Barrera et al., 1984; Brandt, 1984). Holditch-Davis and Thoman (1988) reported similar findings in their study, but they concluded that the early lack of responsiveness and low stimulation by the parent was not maladaptive but appropriate, in view of the preterm infant's low tolerance for stimulation. They cautioned, however, that if this parental behavior continued and did not change as the infant grew older, the infant would suffer developmentally (Holditch-Davis & Thoman, 1988). It is possible that Beckwith and Cohen's phenomenon of burnout may be the result of the parents' not adapting their behavior to the infant as he or she grew older, as suggested by Holditch-Davis and Thoman. Whatever the reason, these studies suggest the need for monitoring of the interaction between the parent and preterm infant.

Maygary (1987), in discussing Beckwith and Cohen's "burnout," described how some parents, when confronted with this low social responsiveness in their infant, become "hyperactive" in their interactions; that is, in compensating for the lower level of social responsiveness of the preterm infant, the parent tries harder and harder to get the infant to respond. As the parent heightens his or her response, the infant withdraws further, becoming less and less responsive in an attempt to deal with the increased stimulation. This "super parent syndrome," as Maygary described it, leads to the parental burnout described by Beckwith and Cohen, in which the parent eventually gives up when the responsiveness needed by the infant does not occur. When maladaptation between the infant and the caregiver occurs, as in the case of parental burnout and the super parent syndrome, the positive integration of the infant into the family unit suffers.

Studies show that parents can be taught to be more sensitive to their infants, thus preventing many later problems. For instance, when parents are taught about their infant's sleep–wake organization and appropriate ways of responding to their easily overstimulated infant, they provide more sensitive caregiving to their infant, and disturbances in the parent–infant interaction such as burnout and super parent syndrome do not occur (Barnard et al., 1987; Fuhrmann, 1984; Kang et al., 1995).

Vulnerable child syndrome (VCS), a term first coined by Green and Solnit in 1964, has been associated with preterm infants (Culley et al., 1989; Macey et al., 1987; McCormick et al., 1982; Perrin et al., 1989). In this phenomenon, parents continue to see their infant as vulnerable (susceptibility to a negative outcome) despite evidence to the contrary—that the infant is physically and developmentally normal. This results in maladaptive behavior on the part of both the parent (usually the mother) and the infant. Reported parental behaviors include overprotectiveness (i.e., less willingness to leave infant alone, discouragement of infant exploration), skewed perception of the infant's capabilities, and frequent visits to the hospital or clinic. Behaviors reported in infants and children include less exploration, infantilization, separation anxiety, and psychosocial problems such as somatic complaints and problems in school (Bidder et al., 1974; Forsyth & Canny, 1985; Jeffcoate et al., 1979; Levy, 1984; Macey et al., 1987; McCormick et al., 1982).

However, Scheiner and associates (1985) found no greater degree of overprotectiveness in mothers of preterm infants than they did in mothers of full-term infants, which led them to suggest that VCS is most likely related to certain personality characteristics of the parent or family and other situational events rather than an infant's prematurity per se. A later study by Culley and colleagues (1989) supported the work of Scheiner and associates (1985), concluding that "illness or prematurity in itself does not lead to the [vulnerable child] syndrome" but that "graduates of the NICU had more concerns about their children's health status than did parents of children born at term." In addition, mothers who had a positive supportive relationship reported less of a sense of vulnerability of their preterm infant (Culley et al., 1989).

Work by Schraeder and associates (1992) investigating caregivers' perception of vulnerability, parental subjective stress, and child temperament in 39 very low birth weight [VLBW] and 30 normal birth weight [NBW] children at 7 years of age found "caregivers of healthy normal school-aged VLBW children did not view their children as more vulnerable than parents of NBW children" (Schraeder et al., 1992, p. 163). However, caregivers who viewed their children as vulnerable, whether they were VLBW or NBW, perceived their children as more negative in temperament and reported themselves as having higher levels of subjective stress. In addition, there was no significant correlation between those caregivers who reported more vulnerability in their children and the number of reports of visits and telephone calls to the doctor (Schraeder et al., 1992).

Schraeder and associates concluded that "Temperament dimensions made significant contributions to parental perceptions of child vulnerability over and above birth weight status, supporting the hypothesis that child temperament is a factor in parental perceptions of child vulnerability" (p. 165), but that further research was needed to determine whether child temperament or parental perception was the antecedent construct. They also surmised from their findings that "It is possible that both parental perceptions of child vulnerability and medical-care-seeking behaviors by parents who express fears for the child's health and well-being are responses to stress" (p. 165) and that more research into parental (maternal) depression and anxiety related to stress was needed (Schraeder et al., 1992). Other studies have also reported a link between high levels of stress in families and cognitive and behavioral outcomes of preterm infants (Future of Children, 1993; Oberklaid et al., 1991).

Another phenomenon reported to be associated with preterm infants is child abuse. As with the other three phenomena discussed, reasons for the increase risk of abuse seem to be the combination of infant behavioral characteristics (irritability, lack of clear cues, and low social responsiveness) and certain parental experiences and characteristics (lack of social support, history of violence as a child or with a spouse, insensitivity to the child, annoyance or anger when the infant cries). However, rather than reacting with a lack of responsiveness to the infant (parental burnout), an increase in infant stimulation (super parent syndrome), or overprotectiveness (vulnerable child syndrome), the parent instead abuses the child (Beckwith, 1990; Clark, 1989; Elmer & Gregg, 1967; Klein & Stern, 1979; Ricciuti, 1983; Schmitt & Kempe, 1975).

THE NEED FOR HOME FOLLOW-UP PROGRAMS

There is much evidence in support of providing prevention and intervention programs for families with preterm infants. Patteson and Barnard (1990), in a comprehensive review of intervention programs, found 16 of the 19 studies identified had positive outcomes. Elements believed to be effective in producing these positive results included the use of both hospital and home contacts or home contacts alone and the enlistment and involvement of the parent in the intervention and in interaction with the child. Urging further research in the area of infant intervention, Patteson and Barnard (1990) stated that continued focus should be on "testing ways to help parents cope with the emotional crises of having a low birth weight infant, enhancing positive interactions with their infant, and increasing their knowledge of infant developmental and care needs" (p. 53).

Many researchers studying preterm infants and their families have supported the findings of Patteson and Barnard for continued monitoring and follow-up for these families after discharge. Several of these researchers themselves have been involved in home intervention studies and demonstrated significant results in the cognitive and behavioral outcomes for preterm infants when the needs of the family and infant are met (Bakewell-Sachs & Porth, 1995; Brooks-Bunn et al., 1992; Brown et al., 1989; Heery, 1991; Infant Health and Development Program, 1990; Jones Jessop & Stein, 1991; Kang et al., 1995; Olds & Kitzman, 1993; Ramey et al., 1992; Ryburn Starn, 1992; Zahr, 1994; Zelle, 1995). Their findings suggest the need for follow-up and assessment of the home environment to identify any characteristics or situations that might lead to the maladaptive behaviors previously described. For this to occur, agencies and health care providers must be helped in seeing the need for follow-up and assessment in the home. Once assessment has been completed, intervention strategies can be identified to assist families in recognizing and understanding the behavior of their infant and in meeting the needs of both the infant and the family. The question becomes: "Are parents interested in follow-up, and if so, what kind do they want and need?" This next section explores that question.

NEEDS OF PARENTS WITH A PRETERM INFANT: WHAT DO THEY WANT AND NEED? WHAT ARE THEY GETTING?

The birth of an infant is a major event in the life of a family. Researchers have documented that the parenting role begins in pregnancy (Kemp & Page, 1987; Rubin, 1984) and evolves throughout the first weeks and months at home (Mercer, 1981; Walker et al., 1986). The first year of life has been shown to be a critical time for the adaptation of a new infant into the family milieu (Affonso, 1987; Barnard, 1976; Fein, 1976; Russell, 1974). This adaptation requires enormous amounts of energy and adjustment on the part of the parents and does not always occur smoothly. As discussed previously, preterm infants seem especially vulnerable to this adaptation process because of the conditions of birth and certain characteristics that affect the caregiving they receive. Parental caregiving characteristics have a significant impact on the positive development of their children, either full-term or preterm (Gottfried, 1984). Parental perception and support play a critical role in determining the effectiveness of the caregiving provided infants (Barnard & Eyres, 1977). Therefore, it is important to examine what parents of preterm infants encounter during the first few weeks and months at home, what they need to provide growth-fostering care to their infant, and what they feel they actually are receiving.

Sammons and Lewis (1985) described how the birth and ultimate parenting of a preterm infant are different from those of a full-term infant. Rather than a time of joy, the birth of a preterm baby is one of fear and anxiety. Rather than a process of parental role development, it is a process of grief, dominated by feelings of loss, anger, and resentment. Although hope emerges as the infant survives, these fragile threads can be broken and destroyed should a setback occur. While parents anxiously await the first feelings of attachment to their infant, other feelings such as shame and guilt may emerge from their lack of affective responses to the "little stranger" in the NICU. Rather than a responsive, alert infant, parents are faced with an infant whose response to parental touch and voice is one of withdrawal and bodily system overload. As lights flash, bells ring, buzzers go off, and hospital personnel rush to intervene with the infant's decreased heart rate and lack of breathing, parents learn firsthand what they subconsciously believe: that they do not belong there and their infant does not want them (Sammons & Lewis, 1985).

Faced with a dramatically different birth process and infant than expected, parents form a wall of detachment to deal with the dichotomy of reality versus fantasy. Above all else, although parents of preterm infants worry about their own adaptability to parenthood in much the same way as parents of full-term infants, it is the intensity of the situation that clearly delineates the parents of preterm infants from their counterpart parents of full-term infants. Their feelings regarding whether their infant will survive, whether they will have confidence and competence to deal with the normal everyday responsibilities of parenting, and whether they have the ability to cope with even the slightest changes and challenges (stresses) that occur are extremely intense (Sammons & Lewis, 1985).

As already stated, parents of preterm infants can learn to adapt and deal with all these issues if they have the support and help consistent with their needs and those of the infant. Although most of this adaptation occurs over the weeks and months at home, the positive relationship between parent and child can get a significant boost from measures instituted in the hospital setting (Future of Children, 1993; Kang et al., 1995; Merritt & Vaucher, 1985). Chapter 49 describes ways in which the NICU setting can enhance the development of the infant and support the parenting role. It describes how the NICU environment aids the development of parent and child when it is flexible enough to adjust its procedures and interventions to the biologic development and rhythms of the infant and to the needs and schedules of the parents and other supportive family members. For instance, spacing intrusive (and exhausting) procedures to allow for the infant's recovery, varying levels of light and dark to promote normal levels of infant sleep and awake times, and timing awake times so that they coincide with parent visits all combine to promote normal infant development and positive parent–infant interactions.

Chapter 50, Assessment and Management of the Transition to Home, describes the importance of support for parents to help them cope and manage the stress of the NICU environment, preventing "learned helplessness" that so often occurs. Giving time and attention to really listen to parents, communicating clearly, and teaching effectively all are factors that parents see as important. When support is given and stress is reduced, parents become confident in their ability to care for the infant and are more likely to become actively involved in his or her care—one step toward a positive parent–infant interaction and optimal infant development. Promotion of normal infant development and positive parent–infant interaction are the two key elements that form a basis for the infant's appropriate development and set the stage for coping with the transition from hospital to home and later integration into the family unit.

All parents faced with taking their new infants home have questions and concerns about the care that they should provide. Parents of preterm infants are no different in this regard. Where they differ is in what kinds of concerns and questions they have and the need for an earlier and longer period of continued monitoring and support to ensure the healthy development of the preterm infant (Brooten et al., 1989; Kavanaugh et al., 1995; Rivers et al., 1987; Slater et al., 1987; Swanson & Berseth, 1987). Several studies have documented these differences:

Koral (1987), in a study of gestational age and parents' perception, found that parents with preterm infants differed significantly from those with full-term infants in their ability to respond to or recognize cues involving four behaviors—crying, feeding, spitting, and sleeping. There was no correlation with parents' age, educational level, and income. Koral concluded that members of the health care team needed to work together to provide guidance and special teaching to parents of preterm infants, especially in the area of feeding, with which parents had the most difficulties. The nurse has a pivotal role in this process.

Kenner (1990), in qualitative research involving interviews after hospital discharge with parents of preterm and full-term infants, identified five major issues surrounding the parents' transition from hospital to home: (1) parent–child development, which involved parental and child role expectations, separation of parent and child, and the transition into parenthood; (2) anticipatory grief, related to concern for the infant's health and fear of infant death; (3) stress and coping, related to the parents' ability to deal with the stresses of having a preterm infant; (4) social support, involving parents' perception of whether sources of support were positive or negative; and (5) informational needs, regarding the care and development of the infant to cope with the transition from hospital to home. This information was viewed as important by the parents in their ability to cope with the stresses of a preterm birth.

Kenner (1990) concluded that parents must be viewed as individuals by professionals, that their concerns during and after hospital discharge need to be determined, and that care related to those concerns should be provided. Follow-up visits after hospital discharge were recommended as one way to address parental concerns and provide the information they needed (Kenner et al., 1996).

McKim (1993) also examined mothers' perception, related to information needed and information received, as well as support available and support received. She found that parents of preterm infants perceived the need for, but did not receive, information related to crying and spitting up—a finding similar to Koral's (1987). In addition, reports from both primiparous and multiparous mothers in the sample identified the areas of noisy breathing, infant behavior, infant illness, and prematurity in general for which they needed information and did not receive it, which is similar to Kenner's (1990) findings. McKim found that the mothers who needed support but did not receive it were more anxious and less confident about their caregiving. Multiparous mothers stated they needed less information than primiparous mothers early on, but later they requested a need for more information. This may relate to multiparous mothers' receiving less support at home because they are seen as experienced and not needing information. Finally, in regard to support from health professionals, many mothers reported an increase in confidence and a decrease in anxiety when they received a visit from the public health nurse during the first week after discharge (McKim, 1993).

Baker (1989), using qualitative research similar to Kenner's, involving parent interviews before and after hospital discharge, addressed six specific research questions. The questions involved parental expectations, concerns, feeding, and the general characteristics of the transition period. As in Kenner's study, Baker found several underlying themes that characterized the parents' concerns in one degree or another. They included ambivalence before discharge, impact of the infant on the family, issues of parental competence, infant vulnerability, feeding issues, continued pervasiveness of problems related to the infant's prematurity, and recognition of the possible positive outcomes of the birth of a preterm infant (e.g., stronger marital ties, increased belief in self, and ability to cope).

In addition, several issues discussed previously in this chapter were also mentioned by the parents in Baker's study, such as their preterm infant's being difficult to care for and their own failure to anticipate the emotional and physical toll resulting from having the infant at home. Parents said that their needs for information and support to cope after discharge were significant, yet they judged the teaching and professional support received before discharge to be inconsistent. Those who did establish a supportive relationship with the staff reported being less anxious. Once again, the nurses were noted to be key factors in this regard. In addition, parents reported that when they had a chance to participate more fully in their infant's care, they felt more competent in caring for their infant and less anxious about the infant's forthcoming discharge (Baker, 1989).

The studies of both Brooten and associates (1989) and Kavanaugh and associates (1995) found that there were greater concerns for parents of preterm infants around the area of feedings. Specifically, questions of "getting enough" (milk), increasing "weight gain," and reading "infant cues" were among some of the most frequent areas of concerns addressed in this population. Although mothers of full-term infants have addressed similar concerns as well, these two studies found that the frequency and intensity of concern were greater for the mothers of preterm infants.

Finally, parents are not the only ones to experience difficulty coping and adjusting to the birth of a premature infant. Whereas the birth of a full-term infant in most cases is a positive event during which network members rally to support the family, the birth of a preterm infant causes confusion and ambivalence in network members, leaving them unsure of their roles and how to respond. This may result in an increase in maternal distress rather than the buffering effects usually seen (Zarling et al., 1988). Grandparents report reactions similar to those of parents with regard to the birth of a preterm infant. But although parents received most of their information about the preterm infants directly from nurses, doctors, and support groups, grandparents relied on the parents to keep them informed. This puts an added stress on the already overstressed parents to provide information (Blackburn & Lowen, 1986). Blackburn and Lowen (1986) believe that grandparents, when given access to current accurate information by hospital personnel or through group support, can help reduce their anxiety and enhance their ability to support the infant's parents. Although this may be true, Blackburn and Lowen do not address the issue of legality and hospital policies in being able to provide this information to persons other than the parents or legal guardians. Research needs to be done to study the feasibility of Blackburn and Lowen's recommendations as one way to reduce parental stress. What is clear from all these studies is that parents of preterm infants desire follow-up from the NICU environment, that they have questions and concerns that currently are not being met, and that they look to health professionals to provide these services, especially nursing staff, who have 24-hour contact with the infant (Wereszczak et al., 1997).

IMPORTANCE OF NURSE FOLLOW-UP

Nurses are in key positions to make a difference for parents of preterm infants. In many of the previous studies cited, nurses in the NICU were identified as important sources of information and support in the early weeks after the preterm birth. These studies emphasized the need for nurses to help parents cope with the stress in the hospital environment and make the transition home easier (Hampson, 1989; Kenner, 1990; Krywanio & Jones, 1988; Olds et al., 1993; Ryburn Starn, 1992; Walker, 1992).

Nursing has been synonymous with skill and caring. In the NICU environment, this caring is delivered in a stressful, technical, yet hopeful world (Swanson, 1990). Parents of preterm infants have many concerns, problems, and needs. They have identified the nurse as a key person to help them deal with these issues. They want and need the caring provided by nursing. This is not surprising in view of the fact that the nurse is usually the first person with whom parents come in contact in the NICU environment and is there when they see their child for the first time. Throughout their infant's hospital stay, parents develop a close and often intense relationship with the nurse who provides the primary care for their child. When they leave the hospital, they want and need this relationship to continue.

There are other reasons why nurses may be best suited to provide the follow-up to the family after the preterm infant is discharged. First, studies have documented that nursing intervention makes a difference. Olds and colleagues (1988) found that prenatal and postpartum home visitation by nurses promoted the health and development in a group of socially disadvantaged mothers and their infants. The best outcome measures were obtained on mothers and infants who had nursing visits both prenatally and postnatally through the first 2 years of the infant's life. The investigators concluded that community health nurses could play a key role in reducing unfavorable outcomes of childbearing by socially disadvantaged women, provided they had reasonable caseloads, focused efforts, and augmented training (Olds et al., 1988).

Another major study tested nursing intervention protocols with socially and medically high-risk families. This model of newborn nursing intervention demonstrated that nursing intervention during the first 3 months of life improved parent–infant interaction (Barnard et al., 1983a, 1983b). A reanalysis of this study, comparing full-term and preterm infants, demonstrated that preterm infants and their mothers involved in the nursing intervention study did better than the full-term infants and mothers, although both benefited. They also did better in a previously reported comparison of full-term and preterm infants without nursing follow-up (Barnard et al., 1984). What was interesting in this study was that the preterm infants did not seem healthier than their full-term counterparts during the 3 months of nursing intervention. However, at the 10-month evaluation, there were no parent–infant interaction differences, and the preterm infants scored higher on the Bayley Psychomotor Index. These results led the investigators to conclude that the nursing intervention helped to "sustain" the preterm infants and their mothers, as well as improve the parents' interaction and stimulation over the first year (Barnard et al., 1984). This positive "delay effect" of improved parent–infant interaction was also reported in another intervention home follow-up program (Rauh et al., 1988).

Further support for nursing follow-up came from a study by Ross (1984), in which public health nurses made home visits to low-income families with premature infants. Nursing interventions involved emotional support, instruction on the care and development of preterm infants, and a physical examination. In addition, a pediatric therapist visited monthly to advise the family on feeding and stimulation of the infant. The results showed that infants who received the home intervention had significantly higher scores on the Bayley Mental Scales and on the Home Observation for Measurement of the Environment (HOME) inventory (a measurement of the animate and inanimate home environment) than did a matched set of control infants (Ross, 1984).

A second reason why nurses may be best suited for follow-up was given in a study by Brooten and associates (1986) that demonstrated that nursing intervention could be excellent and cost effective. Brooten and associates implemented an intensive hospital teaching program delivered by nurses with master's degrees who were specially trained to work with preterm infants and their families. Their study included stable, healthy preterm infants and involved teaching parents about health concerns, caregiving activities, and behavioral characteristics of infants born preterm. Follow-up after early hospital discharge included close telephone contact and some home visiting. Brooten and associates demonstrated that stable, healthy preterm infants who were discharged early and monitored by nurses knowledgeable in the special needs of preterm infants fared as well as a set of matched infants not discharged early, with a documented savings of $18,560 per infant for the early-discharge group (Brooten et al., 1986).

More recently, support for earlier discharges of preterm infants is growing as studies demonstrate the benefits to the preterm infants and their families as well as the savings in cost to the community (Ladden, 1990; Shapiro, 1995). This movement toward earlier discharge will only continue to grow as new studies are demonstrating that transitional procedures for preterm infants, such as moving from an isolette to an open crib, can be done safely at lower weights, thereby setting the stage for preterm babies to go home sooner (Medoff-Cooper, 1994).

Another comprehensive home intervention study that demonstrated cost effectiveness, but was not tied to early discharge, was reported by Olds and his colleagues. They also used trained registered nurses who followed up a group of poor, unmarried, teenaged primiparous women (n = 400) from pregnancy until the infants were 2 years of age. Some of the infants were preterm. The nurses in the study "systematically addressed the health, behavioral and psycho-social conditions that lead to poor maternal and child outcomes" (Olds et al., 1993, p. 167). This study demonstrated a savings of $801 per family for government costs, determined by such factors as reduction in later pregnancies and treatment of child abuse. They also demonstrated that their intervention program "saved the most money when it was delivered to women in the lowest social classes" (Olds et al., 1993, p. 166).

A word of caution—all the studies demonstrating improved family outcomes and cost savings had in place an organized home intervention program that followed preterm infants and their families beyond the infants' first year of life (Ladden, 1990; Future of Children, 1993; Shapiro, 1995). Although cost effectiveness should never be the primary reason for providing service delivery, in this age of rising health care costs, the fact that an intervention service can give quality care, improve family outcomes, and be cost effective can only add to its attractiveness and feasibility. The fact that in a review of successful home intervention studies involving pregnant women and young children "programs which employ professionals (especially nurses) and are based on more comprehensive service models stand a greater chance of influencing qualities of parental caregiving and the child's intellectual functioning than do narrowly focused programs staffed by paraprofessionals" (Olds & Kitzman, 1993, p. 79) should make us as nurses stand up, take notice, and demand further support for a service we apparently do so well.

Nurse home follow-up is not a new phenomenon. Most states have in place some form of community health nursing services. Most of these nursing services give priority to high-risk groups. However, in a survey of infants discharged from the NICU in one metropolitan city, fewer than half the preterm infants have any record of public health nurse follow-up. Of those who received visits, the average number of visits was two (Johnson-Crowley & Sumner, 1987a). From the reports of parents and researchers studying preterm infant outcome, two visits would not be enough in a majority of the cases (Future of Children, 1993). Most community health nurses would probably agree to a more intensive follow-up for preterm infants and their families, provided that this follow-up does not increase an already overloaded system.

In addition, nurses involved in home intervention need to do a better job of reporting and evaluating systematically the population they serve and the services they perform. In a research review of intervention programs involving preterm infants from disadvantaged backgrounds, "programs that provide home intervention by nurses through public or private agencies [were excluded because they] do not have an evaluation component and are difficult to quantify" (Zahr, 1994, p. 91). Clearly, if we as nurses wish to influence public, private, and governmental opinion to gain support for nursing home intervention for preterm infants, or for that matter, for all populations, we definitely must start documenting, evaluating, and publicizing our activities along standardized research lines.

Conversations with community health nurses across the nation provide general agreement that they may have little knowledge of the NICU environment from which preterm infants come and are unaware of new research findings that would tailor their services to those needed by preterm infants and their families (Johnson-Crowley & Sumner, 1987a). Many of the researchers cited here would agree that nursing intervention and follow-up of high-risk groups, either socially disadvantaged or preterm, require nurses specially trained to follow those groups (Barnard et al., 1987; Brooten et al., 1986; Future of Children, 1993; Ladden, 1990; Olds et al., 1988, 1993; Shapiro, 1995; Zahr, 1994).

Nurses in the NICU environment may seem to be the logical choice to fulfill this role. As mentioned, parents eagerly want and expect these nurses to provide services to help them understand and cope with their preterm infants. Most NICU nurses, however, would agree that they have little knowledge of community-based follow-up and would feel ill prepared to perform home visitation without additional training. Because both NICU nurses and community health nurses possess knowledge and skill to help families with preterm infants, a collaborative model that blends the knowledge of both these nurses would be ideal, thereby ensuring that consistent information and support are given as the parents move from the hospital environment to the home environment. Such a collaborative model has been implemented successfully between hospital and community nurses (Zelle, 1995).

Research continues to demonstrate the need for home follow-up of preterm infants and their families that is feasible and cost effective. Nurses supported by a large body of research findings now have a great opportunity to see that this service is provided. Throughout this book, collaboration among nurses within the hospital setting is advocated. This collaboration must extend into the community. Hospital nurses and community nurses must work together to promote an early, smooth, and continued transition from hospital to home for preterm infants and their families. Additionally, hospital and community nurses need to collaborate with nurse researchers in their fields to ensure that populations served and services given are documented systematically and effectively. This documentation will allow for comparisons within and among home intervention programs so that services may be individualized for infants and their families and we provide the appropriate "nurse dose" (Brooten & Naylor, 1995)—what they need, when they need, and how they need services. This then will allow us to further refine what important components are necessary for any given home follow-up program. The following section describes what we know are important components for any successful home intervention program.

SYSTEMATIC ASSESSMENTS

An important component of any follow-up with families is the use of systematic assessment. Systematic assessment is the use of validated measures in order to organize the collection of information that can be used to promote strengths, identify concerns, and suggest areas for further evaluation or referral (Barnard et al., 1983a). Bailey and Simeonsson (1988) identified the home environment and parent–infant interaction as important areas to include in any family assessment related to early intervention. Hardy-Brown and colleagues (1987) also advocated assessing the home environment because "assessment of the infant's actual living situation (in contrast to hospital evaluation alone) can permit the most pertinent interventions to be recognized and administered quickly" (p. 8). Barnard and Douglas (1974) identified child rearing and nurturing as two areas in which nursing could make the biggest contributions to families—areas that heretofore were largely neglected but in which parents and professionals identified a need for information and help.

Tekolste and Bennett (1987) supported the findings of Barnard and Douglas (1974) by identifying areas in which nurses can make a difference in home follow-up care with preterm infants and their families. Areas included (1) monitoring and providing support, instructions, and problem solving in the areas of feeding, weight gain and growth, sleeping, and developmental and behavioral concerns, and (2) the concept of the nurse as a complementary liaison with the primary care physician (Tekolste & Bennett, 1987). On the basis of these findings, it seems logical to use measures that assess those areas needed and not being universally monitored, such as sleep–wake organization, parent–infant interaction, and conditions of the home environment.

Nursing Child Assessment Satellite Training Scales

An important aspect of any assessment measure is that it be married to the realities of the health care system; that is, the measure should be easy to use, complement current practice, provide information (for both professional and client), and assess factors found through research to be predictive of a child's later development. In addition, measures should address areas of parent concern to ensure the interest and motivation of the parent in incorporating whatever recommendations are warranted from the assessment (Delerian, 1988). The Nursing Child Assessment Satellite Training (NCAST) Scales are examples of assessment measures that fit these criteria. Developed under the direction of Dr. Kathryn Barnard, a nurse, they are a result of her examinations of characteristics present in families early on that predicted later child outcomes. In addition to assessing the areas of sleep–wake organization, feeding, parent–infant interaction, and the home environment, these scales are useful as a clinical tool to (1) provide information and support to the parent; (2) document the infant's and parent's current behavior; and (3) provide information about predictability of behavior over time, support for positive behavior, and improvement in problem areas when repeated measurements of the same assessment are used (Barnard et al., 1989; Bee et al., 1982; Censullo, 1986; Johnson-Crowley & Sumner, 1987a; Ruff, 1987).

Another advantage is that assessments completed over time generate a picture of the child's changing behavior in a realistic way. This cuts down on exaggeration or understatement of the infant's problems and helps produce a more realistic perception of the infant for the parents.

Professionals find these assessments clinically useful because they help organize the home visit and give them a baseline from which to identify the following (Johnson-Crowley & Sumner, 1987a, 1987b):

1. The developing sleep–wake patterns.
2. The appropriateness of the amount and type of infant feedings.
3. Areas of strength to build the parents' confidence in the care of their infant.
4. Problem areas and relay areas of concern to the parent.
5. When and where further assessments need to be performed.
6. Documented evidence of the behavior of the parent and the child.

Studies using these scales have found correlations with later cognitive performance and behavioral outcomes (Barnard & Eyres, 1977, 1979; Barnard et al., 1983a, 1983b; Eyres et al., 1979; Gottfried, 1984; Hammond et al., 1983; Slater et al., 1987; Zahr, 1991). Thus the NCAST scales are valuable tools for identifying and preventing problems before they occur. Although these assessments were originally designed from observations of a population of full-term infants, they have been validated and found extremely useful with preterm infants and their families (Barnard, 1985; Barnard et al., 1987; Farel et al., 1991; Johnson-Crowley, 1988; Johnson-Crowley & Sumner, 1987a; Slater et al., 1987). The four NCAST assessments are described in the following sections.

Nursing Child Assessment Sleep–Activity Record

The Nursing Child Assessment Sleep–Activity (NCASA) record is a 24-hour record that requires the parent (or caregiver) to keep an hour-by-hour record of the infant's sleep and activity for 1 week (Barnard, 1980, 1989). The record is set up in graph form in which each square represents 60 minutes. Caregivers record sleep; awake times when the child is content and when the child is fussy or crying; feeding; play times; and any other activity for which the parent or nurse identifies a need. An advantage of this record is that symbols are used to represent the activities recorded (Fig. 47–1). The use of symbols has made it useful for parents and caregivers who have low education, difficulty reading, or are non–English speaking (Johnson-Crowley, 1988).

Because the NCASA record is completed over 24 hours and can be filled out week after week, it generates a picture of the child's "increasing temporal integration of activities" (Barnard, 1989). This means that over time the neuromaturational behavior of the infant—a relative decrease in the amount of feedings and night awakenings in infants as they grow and mature—is recorded. With this decrease comes an increase in the amount of time spent awake and more time for play and parent–infant interaction. Parents have found using the NCASA record useful in organizing their activities and providing an ongoing view of their infant's changing behavior, which is an important process for parents of preterm infants, in whom developmental strides may be slow and seemingly nonexistent at times (Johnson-Crowley, 1986).

Nursing Child Assessment Feeding Scale

Whereas the NCASA scale gives a picture of the amount and frequency of feedings the infant is getting, the Nursing Child Assessment Feeding Scale (NCAFS) assesses certain tasks that the parent and the child have for ensuring a positive interactional relationship during feeding, so that the feeding is set in as positive an atmosphere as possible for both parent and child (Barnard & Kelly, 1990). For preterm infants and their families, who may experience feeding as a long, arduous, and often negative process, this scale can provide a very important way to change conditions so that the feeding is a more positive experience. If parents realize that during the early months of life the feeding episode may provide the only times the preterm infant is awake and one of the only times the parent and infant are together and interacting for any length of time, it becomes additionally important that this be as pleasant a time as possible (especially for the parent), because it may set the stage for later interactions (Johnson-Crowley & Sumner, 1987a).

Areas of assessment include the infant's ability to provide clear cues to the parent and respond appropriately and positively to the parent's attempt to interact. For the parents, their ability during the feeding to be sensitive to the infant's cues, respond sympathetically to any distress the infant might experience, provide social and emotional activities that are affectionate and social in nature, and present activities that enhance the infant's cognitive development is assessed as well.

The NCAFS works well as a follow-up to the use of the NCASA record should any feeding difficulties be identified. For instance, if a review of the NCASA record reveals that a breastfeeding preterm infant is getting fewer than the recommended number of feedings per day and discussions with the parent reveal difficulties in getting the infant to eat, the use of the NCAFS may reveal areas in the parent–infant interaction that may be affecting this, such as the parent's inability to read the infant cues (Johnson-Crowley & Sumner, 1987a, 1987b). The use of the NCAFS after discussion of the NCASA record is an example of how assessment measures can complement and build on one another, providing information related to a similar topic

NURSING CHILD ASSESSMENT SLEEP/ACTIVITY RECORD

CAREGIVERS USUAL BEDTIME 8:30 pm
CAREGIVERS USUAL AWAKENING 10 a.m.

CHILD'S NAME ______ (LAST NAME) Jeffrey (FIRST NAME)
BIRTH DATE 12-10-90
DATE OF RECORDING 12-29-90 (38 wks g.a.)

24-HR. SUMMARY

Date	12 Noon	1	2	3	4	5	6	7	8	9	10	11	12 Mid.	1	2	3	4	5	6	7	8	9	10	11	# Feeds	Total # Hrs Sleep	Avg. Nite Sleep	Avg. Day Sleep
12/29															1½ oz										6	14	8	6
12/30						mom's day rest																	at Doctors		8	13	8	5
12/31	Doctors																								8	15	10.5	4.5
1/1	Part of 11 AM feeding										same feeding														7	12.5	8.5	4
1/2								Bye Bye car ride																	6	14	9	5
1/3			Bye Bye																						7	14	10.5	3.5
1/4																									8	12	9	3
Totals																									50	94	63.5	31

SYMBOLS

- [BF] Breastfeeding
- [oz] # ounces Bottle
- — sleep
- eee awake
- MM fussy
- * waken to feed
- ○ mom's rest period

SUMMARY

- avg. 7 feedings/24 hrs.
- one supplemental fdg. in one week
- avg. 13.4 hrs./24 hrs.
- longest awake = 4 hrs.
- had 5 fussy periods during H.S.
- awaken to feed × 1 in week
- one rest period/day for the week

NURSING CHILD ASSESSMENT SATELLITE TRAINING
University of Washington, CDMRC, WJ-10
Seattle, WA 98195 (206) 543-8528

FIGURE 47–1. Nursing Child Assessment Sleep–Activity (NCASA) record completed by mother of a preterm infant. (Courtesy of Kathryn E. Barnard.)

(in this case, feeding) but in different areas. In this way a more comprehensive view of the parent, infant, and the situation is obtained by using multiple assessment measures, which makes assessment, intervention, and evaluation easier and more complete.

Nursing Child Assessment Teaching Scale

The Nursing Child Assessment Teaching Scale (NCATS) assesses the interaction between parent and child while the parent is teaching the child a simple task (Barnard & Kelly, 1990). Although the tasks are chosen by the observer, the parent chooses how he or she wishes to present and teach the task. The areas assessed are similar to those in the NCAFS scale just described, but around a different topic, teaching instead of feeding. Both the NCAFS and NCATS have been shown to be reliable and valid measurements of the parent–infant interaction. Although both assessments measure parent–infant interaction, analysis of the assessments has shown that they offer different and important glimpses of the parent–infant interaction (Barnard et al., 1989; Farel et al., 1991; Gross et al., 1993).

There are other differences as well. First, the NCAFS (feeding) assessment takes as long as a feeding lasts, possibly 15 minutes to more than an hour; the NCATS (teaching) assessment is brief, usually lasting between 1 and 5 minutes. The NCAFS is validated for use up to 12 months of an infant's life, whereas the NCATS can be performed up to 36 months (Barnard et al., 1989). The investigators point out that the feeding situation, because it occurs six times a day, 7 days a week, may be a more familiar, well-rehearsed situation that places few demands on the parent–child pair. The teaching situation, in contrast, set up by the observer, is more novel in approach and places some stress on the parent–child interaction, possibly resulting in more restrictive behavior on the part of the parent (Barnard & Kelly, 1990; Barnard et al., 1989). Barnard and colleagues (1989) stated that "Added together, the two scales give us a richer look at the interactive patterns than either taken separately, but each can be used independently when the situation calls for or allows only one" (p. 47). In addition, the NCAFS (feeding) is useful for measuring parent–infant interaction only as long as the infant and parent are involved in the feeding situation. When the infant is older (older than 1 year), most parents allow infants to feed themselves while parents are engaged in other activities. At this time, the NCATS may be useful to get a more accurate picture of the parent–infant interaction, especially related to cognitive development (Gross et al., 1993).

Home Observation for Measurement of the Environment (HOME)

The HOME is no longer a part of the NCAST assessment package. However, it is a reliable and valid adjunct to NCAST. This instrument, designed by Caldwell, Bradley, and their colleagues, measures "the quality and quantity of support for cognitive, social and emotional development available to the child in the home environment" (Bradley & Caldwell, 1988, p. 97). This assessment is administered using a combination of interview and observation. Both the animate (i.e., people) and the inanimate (e.g., toys) aspects of the home environment are assessed (Caldwell & Snyder, 1978). A review of several studies using the HOME assessment measure has demonstrated that the HOME is a powerful predictor of later cognitive skills both in full-term and preterm infants (Gottfried, 1984). Its ease of use, broad perspective, and extensive use in research make it a popular assessment measure in clinical practice.

Used together in any home follow-up program, the NCASA, NCAFS, NCATS, and HOME assessments offer a way for the health care professional to monitor the ongoing integration of the preterm infant into the family unit by identifying strengths that increase a parent's confidence and competence, assessing systematically those areas found problematic for this population, providing organization to clinical practice, planning individual intervention, measuring outcomes, and most important, providing a way to give support and direction to the parents in relation to caregiving for their child.

HOME-BASED PROTOCOLS OF CARE FOR PRETERM INFANTS AND THEIR FAMILIES

In home follow-up of preterm infants and their families, the assessment component must be attached to a plan of prevention and intervention. This plan should entail a predesigned set of protocols outlining strategies of care. Protocols set up plans of care that are based on the population being served but allow flexibility for individual, cultural, and familial differences. For instance, in the case of the preterm infant, these protocols of care would involve instructions for monitoring weight and growth parameters. Feeding issues and sleep–wake organization would also be included. It is critical that any set of protocols be based on the needs and wants of preterm infants and their families, but they should also include components important to the growth and development of any infant. Protocols have been found to be extremely useful in organizing nursing practice and creating satisfaction in providing care and increasing optimal parenting (Barnard, 1985). In a report on five nurse entrepreneurs, four of the five described the use of nursing protocols as an aid to their practice (Hartman, 1988).

Nursing Systems Toward Effective Parenting—Preterm

Nursing Systems Toward Effective Parenting—Preterm (NSTEP-P) is an example of one type of parent-focused home follow-up intervention program designed specifically to address the problems of parenting a preterm infant. A component of this program is specific protocols of care that help the nurse get organized, allowing her to meet the needs of the family in a way that is comfortable, thorough, supportive, and efficient, thereby increasing nurse satisfaction. The original NSTEP-P program was developed in 1984 through a Continuing Education Grant from Maternal-Child Health Service (Grant #MCJ-009035-01-0), the University of Washington, Department of Parent and Child Nursing, under the direction of Dr. Kathryn Barnard, to test the efficacy of providing nursing services to preterm infants and their families. The nursing protocol that was an integral part of the program was based on research of preterm infants, parenting, and "ecology" of infants and families previously discussed in this chapter (Barnard, 1985).

This home follow-up program was tested in six sites across the nation, involving 23 public health nurses, making eight home visits at specific times. Evaluation data for 76 mothers and their preterm infants were collected and analyzed. The results from this research indicated that the program was successful. Nurses reported that it was helpful to their practice. In addition, measures used to assess parent–infant interaction (NCAFS and NCATS) demonstrated that the techniques used to modulate the infant's sleep–wake state had significantly improved the parent–child interaction. Additional measures of family function, perceived support, and child growth and development were all positive. Follow-up of a subset of these children revealed higher scores on the NCATS, NCAFS, and HOME measurements at 24 months of chronologic age than there were at 5 months of corrected age. Denver Developmental Screening Test (DDST) scores revealed that 95 percent of the children tested normal at

24 months of chronologic age in the area of fine motor, gross motor, and personal-social development. In the area of language, 100 percent of the children were normal (Johnson-Crowley, 1987).

A more recent multi-site field experiment involving NSTEP-P with a group of low-education mothers and their preterm infants was also found to be a "potent intervention to improve the interactive competence of less well-educated mothers to complement the improved social responsiveness of preterm infants and to establish synchronized growth fostering interaction" (Kant et al., 1995).

The following section describes the organization and content of the current NSTEP-P program as an example of what a successful intervention program for preterm infants and their families might include.

Overview

The NSTEP-P protocols of care were developed by nurse researchers and nurse clinicians on the basis of the need to assist parents in learning how to manage their preterm infants after hospital discharge. The overall framework for the NSTEP-P program is the therapeutic relationship in which the nurse structures the interaction to be sensitive to the parents' need while at the same time providing information that will help them learn parenting techniques for the preterm infant who has difficulty feeding, whose state regulation is not well organized, and who tends not to be responsive to the caregiver (Johnson-Crowley & Sumner, 1987b).

The protocols designed as part of the NSTEP-P program are intended to complement a health agency's current strategy of care. Nurses are encouraged to use their agency's routines as well as to incorporate any existing preterm follow-up programs in the community. Although comprehensive in scope, the NSTEP-P program is not designed to take the place of visits to the physician. In fact, an important part of this program is to monitor families to make sure that they continue to see their physicians for well child checkups or for specific health concerns (Johnson-Crowley, 1988).

Content

The content of the program is built on the established characteristics and problems of the preterm infant reported in research and focuses on two main areas.

Content for the Family

Health-related concerns: These issues relate to feeding and nutrition, safety and temperature, illness and infection control, and growth and development. Special health problems more common to the preterm infant, such as anemia, hernias, and vision and hearing problems, are also included.

State modulation: This involves infant state organization, alertness, maintaining state arousal, and stimulation related to the state of the infant.

Parent–infant interaction: This covers behavioral cues, behavioral differences, importance in developing social competence in children, and the preterm infant's effect on his or her caregiver.

Infant's environment: This includes stimulation as provided by the animate and inanimate environment, elements of parent involvement, the important roles of fathers and siblings, stimulation of the preterm infant, and the importance of playing with and enjoying the infant.

Parental coping and support: This involves parental support (family and professional networks), problem-solving, stress appraisal, parental coping, and the challenges of parenting a preterm infant.

As might be expected, issues involving health and state modulation (especially in relation to feeding) take priority early in the program; less time is spent discussing the other content areas. Later, as the problems and concerns in health and state modulation resolve, the content areas of parent–infant interaction and the infant's environment become more paramount. Parental coping and support continues to be a focus throughout the entire home visit program.

Content for the Health Professional

Therapeutic process: This involves contract setting, therapeutic relationships, and closure (termination) with families.

Intervention strategies: These involve the use of systematic assessments, prescriptions of care, and integrated handouts.

Structured protocols: These involve the organization of practice, step-by-step home visiting instructions, and detailed record keeping.

Systematic assessments are given special emphasis because they are critical to the delivery and evaluation of the NSTEP-P program. During delivery of the program, assessments (infant health, parent–infant interaction, parental support, and the home environment) identify potential problems before they develop and delineate when intervention would be most effective. During evaluation, systematic assessments document accomplishment of program goals and promote professional accountability. Assessments found to be important to the success of the NSTEP-P program are anthropometric measures, including height, weight, and head circumference, as well as measures of developmental assessment; the NCAST assessment measures, including the NCASA, NCAFS, NCATS, and HOME; and the network survey, a measurement of the family's support network, including a section assessing support from family, friends, and coworkers and a section assessing support from health agencies and health professionals.

Structure

The NSTEP-P program involves a series of home visits starting from hospital discharge to 5 months of corrected age. One visit is designed to be made before the infant's discharge from the hospital to aid in the transition to home, and "check-in" visits can be scheduled between 9 and 12 months of corrected age to monitor the progress of the family. More visits are made in the beginning, when the parents are most anxious and desirous of contact. As the infant matures and parental confidence increases, the visits are spaced further apart. More visits may occur during the home visit program and after the program has concluded, depending on the needs and wants of the family. This allows for flexibility and takes into account the individual differences and needs of each family.

Format

Presentation of the content information is formulated around a structured format that is consistent from visit to visit. This format, which includes a brief introduction, review of previous content, presentation of new content, summary of the visit, anticipatory guidance, nursing prescriptions, and termination, provides structure for the NSTEP-P families during a period of family disorganization and disequilibrium. This structure and consistency allow nurses and parents to know what to expect with each visit, which reduces the possibility of ambiguity, confusion, and miscommunication. Having clearly defined role expectations helps lessen the parent's need to mobilize additional energy for the

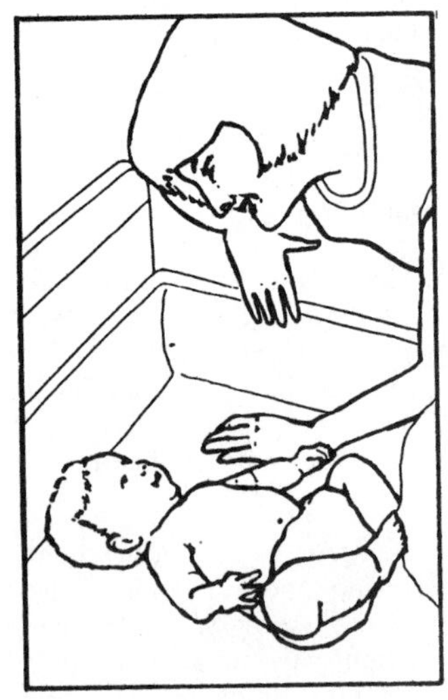

Your baby uses eye contact and his winning smile to reach out to you.

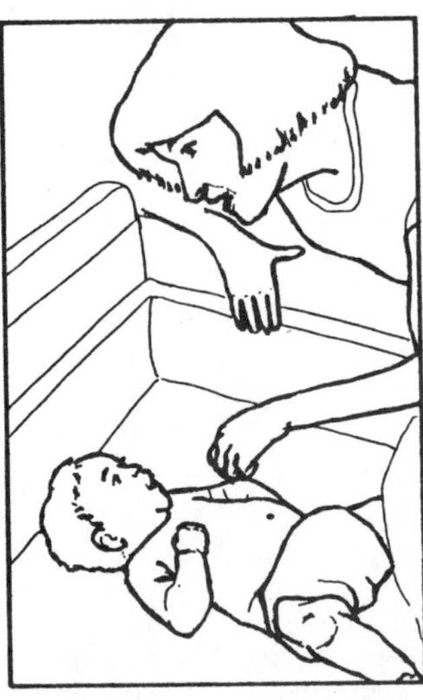

Baby's excitement builds quickly. He smiles and waves his arms and legs.

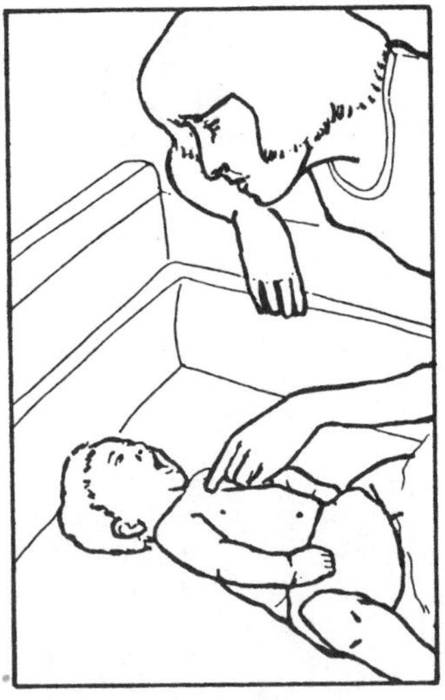

He shows more excitement by making noises, bringing his hands to his mouth, sucking, or clasping his hands.

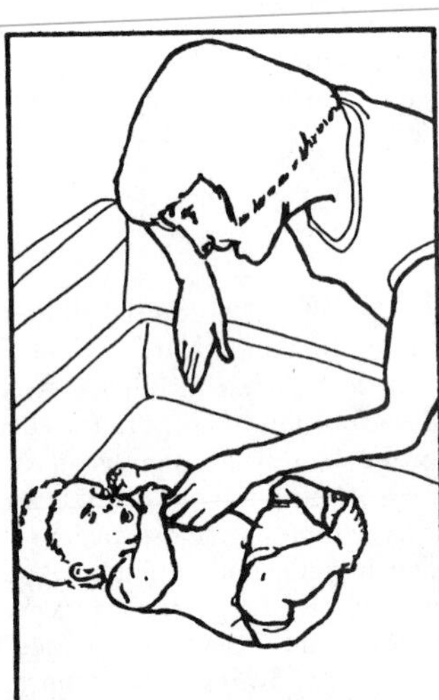

As he gets overwhelmed and needs a break from the interaction.

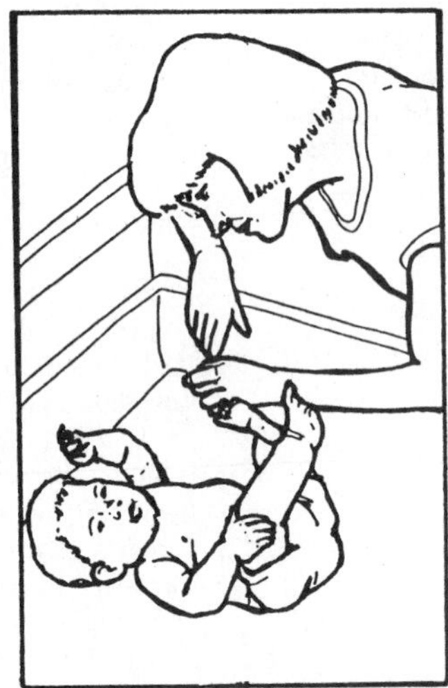

He turns away. You notice his need for a break and stop talking and touching. You look and wait.

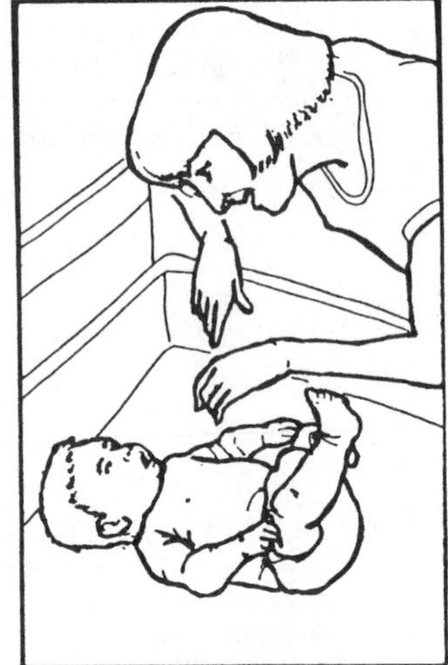

He makes contact again with you to begin the whole cycle again.

FIGURE 47–2. Cues baby uses during interaction. (From Johnson-Crowley, N., & Sumner, G. [1987]. *Protocol manual: Nursing systems toward effective parenting—Preterm.* Seattle: NCAST Publications. Reprinted with permission.)

nurse's visits. However, built-in flexibility allows for the content of the program to be arranged visit-to-visit according to the needs and wants of each family.

Parent Handouts

Handouts are an important source of information for parents. When designed well (a key point), handouts present much of the information—some of it complex—in a format that is easy to read and geared to the interest and education level of the parent. Whenever possible, pictures rather than words are used to convey the information. This is critical, because parents who might be exhausted and overburdened do not need pages of materials to read, when important information can be presented simply, visually, and attractively. Figure 47–2 presents an example of one handout, *Cues Baby Uses During Interaction*, which conveys information about the give and take (synchrony) that occurs during the interaction between the parent and infant.

Designed for parents with an eighth grade education, these handouts would be a problem for parents who cannot read at an eighth grade level or for those who do not read English. However, because the protocol requires that the content of the handouts be explained fully, most professionals have found them applicable for those with less than an eighth grade education. Parents who do not read English often have found another family member to translate the information if they see the value in that information.

Most handouts present information related to the content, but handouts can be used in additional ways, such as (1) an avenue for assessment of the infant by the nurse or parent; (2) a means for the nurse to model appropriate behavior for the parent; (3) a way to transmit information to other members of the family or support network; and (4) a record for the parent and nurse of the home visit. In the NSTEP-P program all five of these functions—providing information, assessing the infant, modeling behavior, relaying information to other family members, and recording the visit—are promoted in a positive and supportive way through handouts. They are an important part of the NSTEP-P protocols of care (Johnson-Crowley, 1988b).

The NSTEP-P program is an example of what should be included in any quality parent-focused follow-up program for preterm infants and their families. Important components to keep in mind for any follow-up program of this population include

- Home visiting to monitor and provide support.
- Measures for systematically assessing the infant and family for identification of problem areas, providing intervention, and evaluating outcomes.
- Protocols of care that are structured, flexible, and consistent from visit to visit.
- Parent involvement in all aspects of care, including assessment, intervention, and evaluation.
- Content encompassing important areas for normal growth and development, yet specific to the needs and problems of preterm infants.
- Research based and supported.

Those programs that include these important components help ensure not only that their NICU graduates survive but also that they develop optimally and as normally as possible—one of the most important considerations for all health professionals, parents, and families.

CONCLUSION

The birth of a preterm infant is a dramatic and frightening event. Before parents really begin to cope with the trauma of their infant's birth and survival, they must bring their infant home. Because of their vulnerability, preterm infants need further monitoring and support to ensure positive developmental outcomes. Nurses have been shown to make a difference when providing home intervention with families who have a high-risk infant. Any intervention program should include parent involvement, systematic assessment, and protocols of care as part of the intervention. Both systematic assessment measures and intervention programs designed with the needs and problems of preterm infants and their families have proved to be a valuable resource in the provision of home follow-up with this population to ensure optimal developmental outcomes. Parents and their preterm infants deserve help and support as they make the transition from hospital to home and integrate their new infant into the family unit. Nurses can play a key role in this process.

For information about the NCAST Assessments and the NSTEP-P program, contact Anita Spietz, NCAST, WJ-10, University of Washington, Seattle, WA 98195, 206-543-8528, fax: 206-685-3284.

REFERENCES

Affonso, D. (1987). Assessment of maternal postpartum adaptation. *Public Health Nursing, 4*(1), 9–20.

Anders, T. F., & Keener, F. (1985). Developmental course of nighttime sleep–wake patterns in full-term and premature infants during the first year of life. *Sleep, 8*, 173–192.

Astbury, J., Orgill, A. A., Bajuk, B., & Yu, V. Y. H. (1983). Determinants of developmental performance of very low birthweight survivors at one and two years of age. *Developmental Medicine and Child Neurology, 25*, 709–716.

Bailey, D. B., & Simeonsson, R. J. (1988). *Family assessment in early intervention*. Columbus, OH: Merrill.

Baker, A. L. (1989). *The transition home for preterm infants: Parents' perceptions*. Unpublished master's thesis, Yale University School of Nursing, New Haven, CT.

Bakewell-Sachs, S., & Porth, S. (1995). Discharge planning and home care of the technology-dependent infant. *Journal of Obstetric, Gynecologic, and Neonatal Nursing, 24*(1), 77–83.

Barnard, D. E. (1976). *A perspective on where we are in early intervention programs*. Adapted from a keynote address at a conference on The Nursing Role in Early Intervention Programs for Developing Disabled Children, University of Utah College of Nursing and Utah State Division of Health, Denver, CO.

Barnard, K. E. (1980). Sleep organization and motor development in prematures. In E. J. Sell (Ed.), *Follow-up of the high-risk newborn: A practical approach*. Springfield, IL: Charles C Thomas.

Barnard, K. E. (1985). *Nursing systems toward effective parenting—Preterm*. Final report supported by Maternal and Child Health Training, Grant #MCH-009035, Bureau of HCDA, HRSA, PHS, and DHHS, Washington, DC.

Barnard, K. E. (1989, May). *State modulation*. Presented at the NCAST Nursing Systems Toward Effective Parenting—Preterm Training Workshop, Seattle.

Barnard, K. E., & Bee, H. L. (1981). *Premature infant refocus project*. Seattle: School of Nursing and the Child Development and Mental Retardation Center, University of Washington.

Barnard, K. E., Bee, H. L., & Hammond, M. A. (1984). Developmental changes in maternal interactions with term and preterm infants. *Infant Behavior and Development, 7*, 101–113.

Barnard, K. E., Booth, C. L., Mitchell, A., & Telzrow, R. (1983a). *Final report: Newborn nursing models* (Grant #RO1 NU-00719-03). Seattle: NCAST Publications.

Barnard, K. E., & Douglas, H. B. (1974). *Child health assessment, part 1: A literature review*. Seattle: NCAST Publications.

Barnard, K. E., & Eyres, S. J. (1977). *Nursing child assessment project final report: The first 12 months of life*. Final report to the Division of Nursing, BHRD, PHS, HRA, and DHEW, Washington, DC.

Barnard, K. E., & Eyres, S. J. (Eds.). (1979). *Child health assessment, part 2: The first year of life*. DHEW Publication No. (HRA) 79–25. Seattle: NCAST Publications.

Barnard, K. E., Eyres, S. J., Lobo, M., & Snyder, D. (1983b). An ecological paradigm for assessment and intervention. In T. B. Brazelton & B.

M. Lester (Eds.), *New approach to developmental screening of infants.* New York: Academic Press.

Barnard, K. E., Hammond, M., Booth, C. L., et al. (1989). Measurement and meaning of parent-child interaction. In F. Morrison, C. Lord, & D. Keating (Eds.), *Applied developmental psychology* (Vol. III, pp. 39–80). New York: Academic Press.

Barnard, K. E., Hammond, M., Mitchell, S. K., et al. (1985). Caring for high-risk infants and their families. In M. Green (Ed.), *The psychosocial aspects of the family.* Lexington, MA: D. C. Heath.

Barnard, K. E., Hammond, M., Sumner, G. A., et al. (1987). Helping parents with preterm infants: Field test of a protocol. *Early Child Development and Care, 27,* 255–290.

Barnard, K. E., & Kelly, J. F. (1990). Assessment of parent-infant interaction. In S. J. Meisels & J. P. Shonkoff (Eds.), *Handbook of early childhood intervention.* Cambridge, UK: Cambridge University Press.

Barrera, M. E., Bronte, B., & Vella, D. (1984). *Behavior patterns of sick and healthy preterm and full term mother–infant dyads.* In abstracts of papers presented at the Fourth International Conference on Infant Studies. *Infant Behavior and Development,* p. 7.

Barrera, M. E., Rosenbaum, P. L., & Cunningham, C. E. (1986). Early home intervention with low birth weight infants and their parents. *Child Development, 57*(1), 20–33.

Beckwith, L. (1990). Adaptive and maladaptive parenting—Implications for intervention. In S. J. Meisels & J. P. Shonkoff (Eds.), *Handbook of early childhood intervention.* Cambridge, UK: Cambridge University Press.

Beckwith, L., & Cohen, S. E. (1980). Interactions of preterm infants with their caregivers and test performance at age 2. In T. M. Field, S. Goldberg, D. Stern, & A. Sostek (Eds.), *High-risk infants and children: Adult and peer interactions.* New York: Academic Press.

Beckwith, L., & Cohen, S. E. (1984). Home environment and cognitive competence in preterm children during the first 5 years. In A. W. Gottfried (Ed.), *Home environment and cognitive development.* New York: Academic Press.

Bee, H. L., Barnard, K. E., Eyres, S. J., et al. (1982). Prediction of IQ and language skill from perinatal status, child performance, family characteristics, and mother-infant interaction. *Child Development, 53,* 1134–1156.

Bendersky, M., & Lewis, M. (1986). The impact of birth order on mother–infant interactions in preterm and sick infants. *Developmental and Behavioral Pediatrics, 7*(4), 242–246.

Bennett, F. C. (1984). Neurodevelopmental outcome of low birth weight infants. In V. C. Kelby (Ed.), *Practice of pediatrics* (Vol. 2). New York: Harper & Row.

Bidder, R. T., Crowe, E. A., & Gray, O. P. (1974). Mothers' attitudes to preterm infants. *Archives of Diseases in Childhood, 49,* 776–777.

Blackburn, S. (1995). Problems of preterm infants after discharge. *Journal of Obstetric, Gynecologic, and Neonatal Nursing, 24*(1), 43–49.

Blackburn, S., & Lowen, L. (1986). Impact of an infant's premature birth on the grandparents and parents. *Journal of Obstetric, Gynecologic, and Neonatal Nursing, 15*(2), 173–178.

Blackman, J. A., Lindgren, S. D., Hein, H. A., & Harper, D. C. (1987). Long-term surveillance of high-risk children. *American Journal of Diseases of Children, 141,* 1293–1299.

Bradley, R. H., & Caldwell, B. M. (1988). Using the HOME inventory to assess the family environment. *Pediatric Nursing, 14*(2), 97–102.

Brandt, L. (1984). *Effects of prematurity, illness and maternal occupation on the mother-infant interaction at 12 months of age.* In abstracts of papers presented at the Fourth International Conference on Infant Studies. *Infant Behavior and Development,* p. 7.

Brooks-Gunn, J., Gross, R. T., Kraemer, H. S., et al. (1992). Enhancing the cognitive outcomes of low birth weight, premature infants: For whom is the intervention most effective? *Pediatrics, 89*(6), 1209–1215.

Brooten, D., Gennaro, S., Knapp, H., et al. (July-August, 1989). Clinical specialist pre- and postdischarge teaching of parents of very low birth weight infants. *Journal of Obstetric, Gynecologic, and Neonatal Nursing,* 316–322.

Brooten, D., Kumar, S., Brown, L., et al. (1986). A randomized clinical trial of early hospital discharge and home follow-up of very-low-birth-weight infants. *New England Journal of Medicine, 315,* 934–939.

Brooten, D., & Naylor, M. D. (1995). Nurses' effect on changing patient outcomes. *Image, 27*(2), 95–99.

Brown, L. P., Brooten, D., Kumar, S., et al. (1989). A sociodemographic profile of families of low birthweight infants. *Western Journal of Nursing Research, 11*(5), 520–532.

Caldwell, B. M., & Snyder, C. (1978). *HOME–Home observation for measurement of the environment.* Seattle: NCAST Publications.

Censullo, M. (1986). Home care of the high-risk newborn. *Journal of Obstetric, Gynecologic, and Neonatal Nursing, 15*(2), 146–153.

Clark, M. C. (1989). In what ways, if any, are child abusers different from other parents? *Health Visit, 62*(9), 268–270.

Cohen, S. E., Parmelee, A. H., Beckwith, L., & Sigman, M. (1986). Cognitive development in preterm infants: Birth to 8 years. *Developmental and Behavioral Pediatrics, 7*(2), 102–110.

Crnic, K. A., & Greenberg, M. T. (1987). Transactional relationships between perceived family style, risk status and mother–child interaction in two-year-olds. *Journal of Pediatric Psychology, 12*(3), 343–362.

Crnic, K. A., Greenberg, M. T., & Slough, M. M. (1986). Early stress and social support influences on mothers' and high risk infants' functioning in late infancy. *Infant Mental Health Journal, 7*(1), 19–33.

Culley, B. S., Perrin, E. C., & Chaberski, M. J. (1989). Parental perception of vulnerability of formerly premature infants. *Journal of Pediatric Health Care, 3,* 237–245.

Delerian, D. (1988). *Focus on patient education.* Seminar presented by The Continuing Education Project, Seattle, WA.

Elmer, E., & Gregg, G. (1967). Developmental characteristics of abused children. *Pediatrics, 40,* 596–602.

Escalona, S. K. (1982). Babies at double hazard: Early development of infants at biologic and social risk. *Pediatrics, 70,* 670–676.

Eyres, S. J., Barnard, K. E., & Gray, C. A. (1979). *Child health assessment, part 3: 2–4 years* (Final report, Grant #RO2-NU-00559). Seattle: NCAST Publications.

Farel, A. N., Freeman, V. A., Keenan, N. L., & Huber, C. J. (1991). Interaction between high-risk infants and their mothers: The NCAST as an assessment tool. *Research in Nursing and Health, 14,* 109–118.

Fein, R. (1976). The first weeks of fathering: The importance of choices and supports for the new parents. *Birth and Family Journal, 3*(2), 53–58.

Field, T. M. (1987). Interaction and attachment in normal and atypical infants. *Journal of Consulting and Clinical Psychology, 55*(6), 853–859.

Field, T. M., & Sostek, A. (Eds.). (1983). *Infants born at risk: Physiological, perceptual and cognitive processes.* Orlando, FL: Grune & Stratton.

Forsyth, B. W., & Canny, P. (1985, May). *Long-term implications of problems of feeding and crying behavior in early infancy: A 3½ year follow-up.* Presented at the annual meeting of the Ambulatory Pediatric Association, Washington, DC.

Fuhrmann, P. J. (1984). *The effect of preterm infant state regulation on parent–child interaction.* Unpublished master's thesis. University of Washington, Seattle.

The Future of Children: Home Visiting, 3(3) (Winter, 1993). Los Altos, CA: Center for the Future of Children, The David and Lucile Packard Foundation.

Garcia Coll, C. (1990). Behavioral responsivity in preterm infants. *Clinics in Perinatology, 17*(1), 113–123.

Gennaro, S., Medoff-Cooper, B., & Lotas, M. (1992). Perinatal factors and infant temperament: A collaborative approach. *Nursing Research, 41*(6), 375–377.

Goldstein, D. J., & Bracey, R. J. (1988). Temperament characteristics of toddlers born prematurely. *Child Care Health and Development, 14*(2), 105–109.

Gottfried, A. (1984). *Home environment and early cognitive development.* New York: Academic Press.

Graham, P., Rutter, M., & George, S. (1973). Temperamental characteristics as predictors of behavior disorders in children. *American Journal of Orthopsychiatry, 43*(3), 328–339.

Green, M., & Solnit, A. J. (1964). Reactions to the threatened loss of a child: A vulnerable child syndrome. *Pediatrics, 34,* 58–66.

Greenberg, M. T., & Crnic, K. A. (1988). Longitudinal predictors of developmental status and social interaction in premature and full-term infants at age two. *Child Development, 59,* 554–570.

Gross, D., Conrad, B., Fogg, L., et al. (1993). What does the NCATS measure? *Nursing Research, 42*(5), 260–265.

Hammond, M. A., Bee, H. L., Barnard, K. E., & Eyres, S. J. (1983). *Child health assessment, part 4: Follow-up of second grade* (Final report of project, Grant #RO1 NU 00816). Seattle: NCAST Publications.

Hampson, S. (1989). Nursing intervention for the first three postpartum months. *Journal of Obstetric, Gynecologic, and Neonatal Nursing, 18*(2), 116–122.

Hardy-Brown, K., Miller, B., Dean, J., et al. (1987). Home based intervention: Catalyst and challenge to the therapeutic relationship. *Zero to Three, 8,* 8–12.

Harrison, H., & Kositsky, A. (1987). *The premature baby book*. New York: St. Martin's Press.

Hartman, K. (Ed.). (1988). Nurses offer home health-care alternatives—Part II. *NAACOG Newsletter, 15*(5), 4–8.

Heery, K. (June, 1991). Getting high-risk infants out of the hospital. *RN,* 58–63.

Holditch-Davis, D., & Thoman, E. B. (1988). The early social environment of premature and fullterm infants. *Early Human Development, 17*(2–3), 221–232.

Hunt, J. V. (1981). Predicting intellectual disorder in childhood for preterm infants with birthweights below 1501 grams. In S. L. Friedman & M. Sigman (Eds.), *Preterm birth and psychological development*. New York: Academic Press.

The Infant Health and Development Program. (1990). Enhancing the outcomes of low-birth-weight premature infants—a multisite, randomized trial. *JAMA, 263*(22), 3035–3042.

Jeffcoate, J. A., Humphrey, M. E., & Lloyd, J. K. (1979). Disturbance in parent–child relationship following preterm delivery. *Developmental Medicine and Child Neurology, 21*(3), 344–352.

Johnson-Crowley, N. (1986). Guidelines for nursing intervention NCASA record with prematures. *NCAST National News, II*(2), 2–4.

Johnson-Crowley, N. (1987). *NSTEP-P: A home visit program for preterm infants and their families.* Poster session presented at the Fifth Biennial National Training Institute for National Center for Clinical Infant Programs, Washington, DC.

Johnson-Crowley, N. (1988). *NSTEP-P: A Home visit program for preterm infants and their families.* Presentation at the Annual Pediatric Nursing Conference, Chicago.

Johnson-Crowley, N., & Sumner, G. A. (1987a). *Concept manual: Nursing systems toward effective parenting—Preterm.* Seattle: NCAST Publications.

Johnson-Crowley, N., & Sumner, G. A. (1987b). *Protocol manual: Nursing systems toward effective parenting—Preterm.* Seattle: NCAST Publications.

Jones Jessop, D., & Stein, R. E. K. (1991). Who benefits from a pediatric home care program? *Pediatrics, 88*(3), 497–505.

Kang, R., Barnard, K., Hammond, M., & Oshio, S. (June, 1995). Preterm infant follow-up project: A multi-site field experiment of hospital and home intervention programs for mothers and preterm infants. *Public Health Nursing, 12,* 171–180.

Kavanaugh, K., Mead L., Meier, P., & Mangurten, H. H. (1995). Getting enough: Mothers' concerns about breastfeeding a preterm infant after discharge. *Journal of Obstetric, Gynecologic, and Neonatal Nursing, 24*(1), 23–32.

Kemp, V. H., & Page, C. K. (1987). Maternal prenatal attachment in normal and high-risk pregnancies. *Journal of Obstetric, Gynecologic, and Neonatal Nursing, 16*(3), 179–184.

Kenner, C. (1990). Caring for the NICU parent. *Journal of Perinatal and Neonatal Nursing, 4*(3), 78–87.

Kenner, C., Flandermeyer, A., & Thornburg, P. (1996). Parenting in the NICU (pp. 93–108). In J. Zaichkin (Ed.), *Newborn intensive care: What every parent needs to know.* Petaluma, CA: NICU Ink.

Kenner, C., & Lott, J. W. (1990). Parent transition after discharge from the NICU. *Neonatal Network, 9*(2), 31–37.

Klein, M., & Stern, L. (1979). Low birthweight and the battered child syndrome. *American Journal of Diseases of Children, 122*(1), 15–18.

Koral, P. A. (1987). *Parents' perceptions of the premature infant.* Unpublished master's thesis, University of Cincinnati College of Nursing and Health, Cincinnati, OH.

Krywanio, M. L., & Jones, L. C. (1988). Developing an early intervention program for infants at risk. *Journal of Pediatric Nursing, 3*(6), 375–382.

Ladden, M. (1990). The impact of preterm birth on the family and society. Part 2: Transition to home. *Pediatric Nursing, 16*(6), 620–626.

Leonard, C. H., Clyman, R. I., Piecuch, R. E., et al. (1990). Effect of medical and social risk factors on outcome of prematurity and very low birth weight. *Journal of Pediatrics, 116,* 620–626.

Levy, J. C. (1984). Vulnerable children: Parents' perceptions and the use of medical care. *Pediatrics, 65,* 956–963.

Macey, T. J., Harmon, R. J., & Easterbrooks, M. A. (1987). Impact of premature birth on the development of the infant in the family. *Journal of Consulting and Clinical Psychology, 55*(6), 846–852.

Maygary, D. (1987). Parent–infant interaction. In N. Johnson-Crowley & G. A. Sumner (Eds.), *Nursing systems toward effective parenting—Preterm.* Seattle: NCAST Publications.

McCormick, M. C., Shapiro, S., & Starfield, B. (1982). Factors associated with maternal opinion of infant development—Clues to the vulnerable child? *Pediatrics, 69,* 537–543.

McKim, E. (1993). The information and support needs of mothers of premature infants. *Journal of Pediatric Nursing, 8*(4), 233–244.

Medoff-Cooper, B. (1986). Temperament in very low birth weight. *Nursing Research, 35,* 139–143.

Medoff-Cooper, B. (1994). Transition of the preterm infant to an open crib. *Journal of Obstetric, Gynecologic, and Neonatal Nursing, 23*(4), 329–335.

Mercer, R. (1981). A theoretical framework for studying factors that impact on the maternal role. *Nursing Research, 30*(2), 73–77.

Merritt, T. A., & Vaucher, Y. E. (1985). Infant follow-up programs: Their impact on infants and families. *Developmental and Behavioral Pediatrics, 8*(5), 285–286.

Mitchell, S. K., Bee, H. L., Hammond, M. A., & Barnard, K. E. (1985). Prediction of school and behavior problems in children followed from birth to age eight. In W. K. Frankenburg (Ed.), *Early identification of children at risk.* New York: Plenum.

Murphy, M. A. (1989). What price success: Can we afford "saved" babies? *Journal of Pediatric Health Care, 3*(6), 285–286.

NICHCY—National Information Center for Children and Youth with Handicaps. (1988). Early intervention for children birth through two. *News Digest,* #10.

Oberklaid, F., Sewell, J., Sanson, A., & Prior, M. (1991). Temperament and behavior of preterm infants: A six-year follow-up. *Pediatrics, 87*(6), 854–861.

Olds, D. L., Henderson, C. R., Phelps, C., et al. (1993). Effect of prenatal and infancy nurse home visitation on government spending. *Medical Care, 31*(2), 155–174.

Olds, D. L., Henderson, C. R., Tatelbaum, R., & Chamberlin, R. (1988). Improving the life-course development of socially disadvantaged mothers: A randomized trial of nurse home visitation. *American Journal of Public Health, 78,* 1436–1445.

Olds, D. L., & Kitzman, H. K. (1993). Review of research on home visiting for pregnant women and parents of young children. In *The Future of Children: Home Visiting, 3*(3) (Winter, 1993). Los Altos, CA: Center for the Future of Children, The David and Lucile Packard Foundation.

Patteson, D. M., & Barnard, K. E. (1990, Spring). Parenting of low-birthweight infants: A review of issues and interventions. *Infant Mental Health Journal,* 37–56.

Perrin, E. C., West, P. S., & Culley, B. S. (1989). Is my child normal yet? Correlates of vulnerability. *Pediatrics, 83,* 355–363.

Prior, M. R., Sanson, A. V., & Oberklaid, F. (1989). The Australian temperament project. In J. E. Kohnstamm, & M. K. Rothbart (Eds.), *Temperament in childhood.* London: John Wiley & Sons.

Ramey, C. T., Bryant, D. M., Wasik, B. H., et al. (1992). Infant health and development program for low birth weight, premature infants: Program elements, family participation and child intelligence. *Pediatrics, 3*(3), 454–465.

Ramey, C. T., Farram, D. C., & Campbell, F. A. (1979). Predicting IQ from mother–infant interactions. *Child Development, 50,* 804–814.

Rauh, V. A., Achenbach, T. M., Nurcombe, B., et al. (1988). Minimizing adverse effects of low birthweight: Four-year results of an early intervention program. *Child Development, 59*(3), 544–553.

Ricciuti, H. N. (1983). Interaction of multiple factors contributing to high-risk parenting. In V. J. Sasserath (Ed.), *Minimizing high-risk parenting—Pediatric Round Table: 7.* Skillman, NJ: Johnson & Johnson Baby Products.

Riese, M. (1988). Temperament in full-term and preterm infants: Stability over ages 6 to 24 months. *Journal of Developmental and Behavioral Pediatrics, 9*(1), 6–11.

Rivers, A., Caron, B., & Hack, M. (1987). Experience of families with very low birthweight children with neurologic sequelae. *Clinical Pediatrics, 26*(5), 223–230.

Ross, G. (1984). Home intervention of premature infants of low-income families. *American Journal of Orthopsychiatry, 54*(2), 263–270.

Rubin, R. (1984). *Maternal identity and the maternal experience.* New York: Springer.

Ruff, C. C. (1987). How well do adolescents mother? *MCN; Journal of Maternal Child Nursing, 12,* 249–253.

Russell, C. (1974). Transition to parenthood: Problems and gratifications. *Journal of Marriage and Family, 36,* 294–302.

Ryburn Starn, J. (1992). Community health nursing visits for at-risk women and infants. *Journal of Community Health Nursing, 9*(2), 103–110.

Sameroff, A. J. (1981). Longitudinal studies of preterm infants. In S. Friedman & M. Sigman (Eds.), *Preterm birth and psychological development.* New York: Academic Press.

Sameroff, A. J. (1986). Environmental context of child development. *Journal of Pediatrics, 109,* 192–200.

Sammons, W. A. H., & Lewis, J. M. (1985). *Premature babies: A different beginning.* St. Louis: C. V. Mosby.

Scheiner, A., Sexton, M., Rockwood, J., et al. (1985). The vulnerable child syndrome: Fact and theory. *Developmental and Behavioral Pediatrics, 6*(5), 298–301.

Schmitt, B., & Kempe, H. (1975). Neglect and abuse of children. In V. Vaughan & R. McKay (Eds.), *Nelson textbook of pediatrics* (pp. 108–111). Philadelphia: W. B. Saunders.

Schraeder, B. D., Heverly, M. A., O'Brien, C., & McEvoy-Shields, K. (1992). Vulnerability and temperament in very low birth weight school-aged children. *Nursing Research, 41*(3), 161–165.

Schraeder, B. D., & Medoff-Cooper, B. (1983). Development and temperament in very low birth weight infants—The second year. *Nursing Research, 32*(6), 331–335.

Schraeder, B. D., Rappaport, J., & Courtwright, L. (1987). Preschool development of very low birthweight infants. *IMAGE: Journal of Nursing Scholarship, 19*(4), 174–177.

Schraeder, B. D., & Tobey, G. Y. (1989). Preschool temperament of very-low-birth-weight infants. *Journal of Pediatric Nursing, 4*(2), 119–126.

Schwartz, S. F., Horowitz, F. D., & Mitchell, D. W. (1984). *A comparison of the behaviors of preterm and full term infants: Implications for mother-infant interaction.* In abstracts of papers presented at the Fourth International Conference on Infant Studies. *Infant Behavior and Development,* p. 7.

Shapiro, C. (1995). Shortened hospital stay for low-birth-weight infants: Nuts and bolts of a nursing intervention project. *Journal of Obstetric, Gynecologic, and Neonatal Nursing, 24*(1), 56–62.

Slater, M. A., Naqvi, M., Andrew, L., & Haynes, K. (1987). Neurodevelopment of monitored versus non-monitored very low birth weight infants: The importance of family influences. *Developmental and Behavioral Pediatrics, 8*(5), 278–285.

Swanson, J. A., & Berseth, C. L. (1987). Continuing care for the preterm infant after dismissal from the neonatal intensive care unit. *Mayo Clinic Proceedings, 62,* 613–622.

Swanson, K. K. (1990). Providing care in the NICU: Sometimes an act of love. *Advances in Nursing Sciences, 13*(1), 60–73.

Tekolste, K. A., & Bennett, F. C. (1987). State of the art, the high risk infant: Transitions in health, development, and family during the first years of life. *Journal of Perinatology, 7*(4), 368–377.

Telzrow, R. W., Kang, R., Mitchell, S. K., et al. (1982). An assessment of the behavior of the premature infant of 40 weeks conceptional age. In L. P. Lipsitt & T. M. Field (Eds.), *Perinatal risk and newborn behavior.* Norwood, NJ: Ablex.

Thomas, A. (1981). Current trends in developmental theory. *American Journal of Orthopsychiatry, 51,* 580–609.

Thomas, A., & Chess, S. (1977). *Temperament and development.* New York: Brunner/Mazel.

Walker, L. O. (1992). *Parent-infant nursing science: Paradigms, phenomena, methods.* Philadelphia: F.A. Davis Company.

Walker, L. O., Crain, H., & Thompson, E. (1986). Mothering behavior and maternal role attainment during the postpartum period. *Nursing Research, 35*(6), 352–355.

Washington, J., Minde, K., & Goldberg, S. (1986). Temperament in preterm infants: Style and stability. *Journal of the American Academy of Child Psychiatry, 25*(4), 493–502.

Wereszczak, J., Miles, M. S., & Holditch-Davis, D. (1997). Maternal recall of neonatal intensive care unit. *Neonatal Network, 16*(4), 33–40.

Zahr, L. (1991). Correlates of mother–infant interaction in premature infants from low socioeconomic backgrounds. *Pediatric Nursing, 17*(3), 259–264.

Zahr, L. (1994). An integrative research review of intervention studies with premature infants from disadvantaged backgrounds. *Maternal-Child Nursing Journal, 22*(3), 90–101.

Zarling, C. L., Hirsch, B. J., & Landry, S. (1988). Maternal social networks and mother-infant interactions in full-term and very low birthweight, preterm infants. *Child Development, 59,* 178–185.

Zelle, R. S. (1995). Follow-up of at-risk infants in the home setting: Consultation model. *Journal of Obstetric, Gynecologic, and Neonatal Nursing, 24*(1), 51–55.

CHAPTER 48

Neonatal Sleep–Wake States

DIANE HOLDITCH-DAVIS

RESEARCH AGENDA

How can practicing neonatal nurses use changes in sleeping and waking state patterns and physiologic measures to more effectively detect medical complications in high-risk infants?

How can the neonatal intensive care unit (NICU) environment and nursing care patterns be modified to promote appropriate development of sleeping and waking in high-risk infants?

To what extent can sleeping and waking state patterns be used clinically to identify infants with neurologic problems or at risk for poor developmental outcome?

How do the sleeping and waking states of individual high-risk infants indicate their needs for specific nursing interventions?

What aspects of sleeping and waking behaviors are practicing neonatal nurses already using as part of their assessments of high-risk infants?

Neonatal nurses are very familiar with interpreting the physiologic status of infants and basing their interventions on physiologic changes. Nurses have placed increased emphasis on the importance of understanding the behaviors of infants under their care because behavior is the only way infants can communicate their needs and their responses to nursing interventions (Als, 1986; Catlett & Holditch-Davis, 1990). However, two factors make this understanding difficult. First, newborn infants have very limited behavioral repertoires. The same behavior may have different meanings in different situations, but busy neonatal nurses may not have the time necessary to correctly interpret infants' behaviors by comprehensively assessing both the infants' actions and the environmental stimulation. Second, the behavior of critically ill infants is even more difficult to interpret because they lack the energy to display characteristic behavioral responses. Thus, neonatal nurses can never rely totally on infants' behaviors to determine infants' needs, but in combination with physiologic parameters, understanding infant behavior enriches both nursing assessment and the evaluation of nursing interventions. This chapter reviews what is known about one major type of newborn infant behavior—sleeping and waking states—and its relevance for neonatal nursing.

SLEEP–WAKE STATES

Sleeping and waking states are clusters of behaviors that tend to occur together and represent the level of arousal of the individual, the individual's responsivity to external stimulation, and the underlying activation of the central nervous system (Ashton, 1973). Three states have been identified in adults: wakefulness, non-REM (rapid eye movement) sleep, and REM sleep. In infants, it is also possible to identify states within waking and states that are transitional between waking and sleeping because infants are less able to make rapid changes between states than are adults. Infants also have more difficulty sustaining alertness when awake. Because the electrophysiologic patterns associated with sleeping and waking states in infants are somewhat different from those in adults (Anders et al., 1971), the sleep states are usually designated active and quiet sleep, rather than REM and non-REM sleep.

Neonatal nurses need to be aware of the infant's present sleep–wake state and typical sleep–wake patterns when making assessments because infant behavior and physiology is affected by state. The functioning of cardiovascular, respiratory, neurologic, endocrine, and gastrointestinal systems differ in different states (Orem & Barnes, 1980). Moreover, sleeping and waking states affect the infant's ability to respond to stimulation (Ariagno, 1996; Columbo & Horowitz, 1987; Korner, 1972). Thus, infant responses to nursing interventions and to parental interactions depend to a great deal on the state the infant is in when the stimulation is begun (Oehler et al., 1988). Timing routine interventions to occur when the infant is most responsive is an important aspect of some current systems of individualized nursing care (Als et al., 1986; Becker et al., 1991). Finally, studies have indicated that sleeping and waking patterns are closely related to neurologic status (Thoman, 1982). Thus, aberrant sleep–wake patterns could potentially be used to identify infants at risk for neurologic complications or poor developmental outcome.

STATE SCORING SYSTEMS

In adults, sleeping and waking are usually scored by electroencephalography (EEG). However, because of the neurologic immaturity of infants, EEG is less reliable and needs to be combined with observation. When EEG and behavioral scoring of states in preterm infants are compared, there is a high degree of agreement (Sahni et al., 1995). Thus, sleeping and waking states in newborn infants, whether full-term or preterm, can be validly scored by directly observing the infant and identifying global categories that are made up of a number of specific behaviors that tend to occur together and reflect a similar level of arousal and responsiveness to the environment. Nurse researchers are currently using four standardized systems for scoring behavioral observations of sleep–wake states. The systems were developed by Brazelton (1984), Thoman (1990), Als (Als et al., 1982), and Anderson (Gill et al., 1988). These systems define states in very similar ways and are probably equally useful for clinical purposes. Figure 48–1 presents a comparison of the state definitions used in these systems.

Clinicians and researchers differ in the ways they use these scoring systems. Neonatal nurses spend a lot of time observing infants and alter their care based on infant behavioral changes. Experienced clinicians are undoubtedly already familiar with the characteristics of sleeping and waking states in these infants even though they may be unable to name specific states. Thus, all they need to do to include judgments of sleeping and waking states clinically is to use the state definitions of any standardized scoring system to systematize their clinical impressions.

For research, however, it is essential that the investigator receive training in the use of a particular scale so that the investigator is using it reliably. It is also important that clinicians reading research understand the differences among the scoring systems so that they can better interpret the findings and understand reports using different names for the same sleep–wake state. Therefore, this chapter briefly examines the characteristics of the various state scoring systems.

Early State Scoring Systems

Sleeping and waking scoring systems for infants have their origins in the work of neurologists, pediatricians, and behaviorists in the 1960s. The neurologists needed a way to systematize the observations they made along with EEG studies, and behaviorists and pediatricians were particularly interested in the waking states and the effect of state on responsiveness to stimulation. Wolff (1959, 1966), a pediatrician, conducted extensive observations of newborn infants in the hospital and at home. As the result of his observations, he proposed a seven-state system. Prechtl and Beintema (1968), pediatric neurologists, proposed a simple five-state system that could be used either to score observations made along with EEG or to ensure that motor reflexes were elicited under optimal conditions. Finally, a team of pediatricians and neurologists at the University of California at Los Angeles

Brazelton	Thoman	Als	Anderson
6. Crying	Cry	6B. Lusty crying	12. Hard crying
		6A. Crying	11. Crying
5. Considerable motor activity	Fuss	5B. Considerable activity	10. Fussing
	Non-alert waking activity	5A. Active	9. Very restless awake 8. Restless awake
4. Alert	Alert	4B. Bright Alert	6. Alert inactivity
		4AH. Hyperalert	
		4AL. Awake and quiet	7. Quiet awake
3. Drowsy	Daze		
	Drowse	3B. Drowsy 3A. Drowsy with more activity	5. Drowsy
	Sleep–wake transition		4. Very restless sleep
2. Light sleep	Active sleep	2A. "Noisy" light sleep	3. Restless sleep
	Active–quiet transitional sleep	2B. Light sleep	2. Quiet sleep: irregular respiration
1. Deep sleep		1A. Deep sleep	
	Quiet sleep	1B. Very still deep sleep	1. Very quiet sleep

FIGURE 48–1. Approximate equivalence of the four major sleep–wake state scoring systems. (Because the criteria used by these systems differ and they are based on different conceptual frameworks, exact equivalence among them is not possible. Isolated instances of infant behavior may be scored quite differently than suggested by this table.)

(UCLA) developed a manual to define the behavioral and EEG criteria for sleeping and waking (Anders et al., 1971). Each of the state scoring systems currently in use is a refinement of these earlier systems.

Brazelton's State Scoring System

T. Berry Brazelton is a pediatrician from Harvard University in Cambridge, Massachusetts. He and his colleagues developed a state scoring system to be used as part of a behavioral evaluation of newborn infants, the Neonatal Behavioral Assessment Scale or NBAS (Brazelton, 1984). The purpose of this tool was to assess the individuality of the infant within the interactional process. This state scale was derived both from Dr. Brazelton's clinical experiences and from the existing state systems of Prechtl and Beintema (1968) and Thoman (1975a). Brazelton's state scoring system consists of six states: deep sleep, light sleep, drowsy, alert, considerable motor activity, and crying. During the administration of the NBAS, this scoring system is used to identify predominant states, state transitions, and the quality of the alertness. However, it can also be used for scoring sleep–wake states during other situations. As of 1983, more than 100 papers had been published using the NBAS and Brazelton's state scale (Brazelton, 1984), and many more have been published since then.

Brazelton's state scoring system has a number of advantages that make it the scoring system of choice for clinicians and also useful for researchers. This state system is easy to learn because the differences between the states are fairly obvious and there are only six states. Because of the widespread use of Brazelton's state scoring system, individuals experienced with this scale are located in virtually every part of the United States. In addition, there are six reliability training centers located throughout the country for those who want to use the entire NBAS or plan to use the state scoring system in research. Thus, obtaining training in this scoring system is relatively easy. Finally, most researchers and experienced clinicians are familiar with the state definitions from this scale so that findings of sleeping and waking observations made with this scoring system are readily understood.

On the other hand, this state scoring system does have some limitations for use in research. First, because of the small number of states, it is not always sensitive enough to identify differences between normal full-term infants and infants with perinatal complications. Moreover, the NBAS state scoring system is appropriate for use only with infants between 36 and 44 weeks' gestational age (GA). The sleeping and waking states of infants born before 36 weeks' gestation and those born after 44 weeks' gestation will not be completely captured with this system. For example, older infants frequently are motorically active and alert during play, but in Brazelton's system, alertness is scored only when the infant is motorically quiet. Young preterm infants are frequently unable to make much sound when crying; thus, their cry periods would be scored as considerable motor activity.

Thoman's State Scoring System

Evelyn B. Thoman is a psychobiologist working at the University of Connecticut. Although trained as an experimental psychologist to work with animals, she became interested in the interactions between human infants and their mothers when she went to work with Dr. Anneliese Korner at Stanford University in 1969 and has been studying them ever since. She developed her first state scoring system in 1975 (Thoman, 1975a) based on the work of Wolff (1966) and Korner (1972). Although some researchers continue to use this system today, it has undergone considerable revision (Thoman, 1990). The Thoman state scoring system consists of 10 sleeping and waking states: alert, nonalert waking activity, fuss, cry, daze, drowse, sleep–wake transition, active sleep, active-quiet transitional sleep, and quiet sleep. Dr. Thoman and others have shown that both acceptable interrater reliability and test–retest reliability can be obtained with her system (Acebo, 1987; Becker & Thoman, 1982b; Holditch-Davis, 1990a; Holditch-Davis & Edwards, 1995a; Holditch-Davis & Thoman, 1987; Thoman, 1975b, 1985; Thoman et al., 1976, 1979, 1987). Predictive validity is demonstrated by evidence that early sleeping and waking behaviors scored on Thoman's scale are related to later developmental outcome (Becker & Thoman, 1981; Thoman et al., 1981).

Thoman's state scoring system has a number of advantages. The documented reliability and validity of this system is of value to researchers. The sleeping and waking states are differentiated enough that they can be used with infants with perinatal complications (Holditch-Davis & Thoman, 1987; Thoman & Becker, 1979; Thoman et al., 1977; Thoman et al., 1985, 1988). This system has been used with preterm infants (Holditch-Davis, 1990a) and with infants older than one month after term (Acebo, 1987). The states in this system can also be combined when an investigator does not need such fine discriminations.

This scoring system has two disadvantages. First, a 10-state system is somewhat more difficult to learn than a 6-state system because it requires more subtle discriminations. However, individuals experienced in using a 6-state system, such as Brazelton's, can readily learn this system. Also, because this state scoring system is not used as generally as Brazelton's, it is more difficult to obtain training in its use.

Als' State Scoring System

Heidelise Als is a psychologist working at Harvard Medical School with Dr. Brazelton and his colleagues. For a number of years, she has worked with these colleagues to modify the NBAS (Brazelton, 1984) to make it more appropriate for use with premature infants. The Assessment of Preterm Infants' Behavior (APIB) is administered in much the same way as the NBAS, but the infant's behavior is scored in much greater detail so as to quantify not only the infant's skills but also the infant's reactivity and stress in response to environmental stimulation (Als et al., 1982). Like the NBAS, the APIB is best administered to infants between 36 and 44 weeks' GA, but the observational portion of the tool can be used with younger preterm infants (Als, 1986). The state scale from the NBAS has been expanded into a 13-state system by subdividing each of the 6 states so that the immature and unclear sleeping and waking states of premature infants can be more adequately described. These 13 states are very still deep sleep, deep sleep, light sleep, "noisy" light sleep, drowsy with more activity, drowsy, awake and quiet, hyperalert, bright alert, active, considerable activity, crying, and lusty crying. The state subscale of the APIB has been shown to differentiate between premature and full-term infants after term (Als & Brazelton, 1981; Als et al., 1988) and to correlate with electrophysiologic measures of brain activity (Duffy et al., 1990). In addition, the APIB and the state subscale are used to provide assessments that are the basis for planning individualized interventions as part of the Neonatal Individualized Developmental Care and Assessment Program (NIDCAP) (Als, 1986; Als et al., 1986) (see Chapter 49, Assessment and Management of Neonatal Neurobehavioral Development, for a detailed description of the NIDCAP system).

The Als' state scoring system has a number of advantages and disadvantages for clinicians and researchers. First, a 13-state system is more difficult to learn than a 6-state system such as Brazelton's (1984). However, inasmuch as the Als system was developed from the Brazelton states, individuals familiar with the Brazelton system should have no difficulty learning it, and when the complexity of the 13 states is not needed they can be collapsed to the 6 states from the NBAS. Second, inasmuch as the APIB, like the NBAS, was never intended for use with infants older than 1 month after term, the state scale may not adequately capture the states of older infants. Finally, because the APIB is a new scale, only a few research reports have been published using this state scoring system separately from the APIB (e.g., Van Cleve et al., 1995). The amounts of individual states exhibited by different groups of infants and developmental changes in each state have not been reported. Thus, it is not yet clear how useful the Als scoring system is describing the sleeping and waking patterns of infants.

Anderson's State Scoring System

Gene Cranston Anderson is a doctorally prepared nurse researcher working at Case Western Reserve University in Cleveland, Ohio. She has long been interested in interventions that keep mother and infant together after birth, reduce infant crying, and promote feeding. She developed a 12-state scoring system, the Anderson Behavioral State Scale (ABSS), to be used with preterm infants based on her own observations of these infants and on the work of Parmelee and Stern (1972). Parmelee was one of the contributors to the UCLA state manual (Anders et al., 1971). The ABSS consists of very quiet sleep, quiet sleep with irregular respirations, restless sleep, very restless sleep, drowsy, quiet awake, alert inactivity, restless awake, very restless awake, fussing, crying, and hard crying (Gill et al., 1988). The states are arranged so that there is a linear relationship between the states and heart rate and energy consumption (Ludington, 1990; McNeely, 1987), with the states with the lowest numbers having the lowest mean heart rates. The ABSS has been used to show the effects of prefeeding nonnutritive sucking (Gill et al., 1988) and kangaroo care (Ludington, 1990) on preterm infant state patterns.

As with the other scoring systems, the ABSS has a number of advantages and disadvantages for clinicians and researchers. As the newest state scoring scale, it has had only limited use outside of nursing. Thus, the reliability and validity of this scale are not well established. Because the ABSS was designed for use with preterm infants, the utility of this scale for full-term infants and older infants is unknown although its similarity to other state scoring systems suggests that it should be applicable for healthy full-term infants. The ABSS may also be difficult to learn because of the complexity of 12 states. As Figure 48–1 illustrates, the sleep states in this system differ markedly from the sleep states defined in other state scoring systems, so this is not a good scoring system to use if one is primarily interested in studying sleep states and wants to compare findings with other studies. Finally, the linear relationship between the states in this system and heart rate may make it the ideal choice for researchers who are primarily interested in studying the energy consumption of infants. However, this feature means the ABSS has a very different theoretical basis than the other state scales. The other state scoring systems differentiate among states based on qualitatively different aspects of the infant's behavior, but the ABSS emphasizes quantitative differences among the states, although Anderson has recently emphasized qualitative differences between states.

DESCRIPTIONS OF INDIVIDUAL STATES

Because the definitions of sleep–wake states are so similar among these scoring systems (see Fig. 48–1), it is possible to describe in general the sleeping and waking states displayed by infants. For clarity's sake, generic state names will be used in all further descriptions. When they are not available, the state names from the Thoman system will be used. Each sleeping and waking state is made up a different constellation of behaviors and serves a different function for the infant. Physiologic functioning is also different in each of these states.

Infants are most responsive to the environment when in the waking states, and, in particular, when alert. When the infant is alert, the eyes are open and scanning. Motor activity is typically low, particularly in full-term newborns, but premature infants and infants older than 1 month after term may be motorically active. Alertness is the state in which the infant exhibits focused attention on sources of stimulation (Brazelton, 1984). Thus, this is the best state in which to test reflexes (Prechtl & Beintema, 1968) and take measures of attention (Colombo & Horowitz, 1987; Hack et al., 1981). Alertness has been suggested to be the optimal state for feeding (Gill et al., 1988). This state is also the one in which infants are most receptive to interactions with their parents and other adults. Yet alertness rarely occurs in the preterm period (Holditch-Davis, 1990a; Holditch-Davis & Edwards, 1995a) and occurs relatively infrequently during the first month after term, only about 10 to 15 percent of the total day (Colombo & Horowitz, 1987).

Crying, another waking state, serves a communication function. However, the meaning of cries differs in different situations and may depend on their intensity (Hopkins et al., 1987; Thoman et al., 1983). Although crying that occurs when the infant is alone may elicit parental attention, crying that occurs during social exchanges may actually disrupt the parent–infant relationship. In full-term infants, crying during social interactions is related to the overall amount of maternal stimulation (Acebo, 1987) and to consistency in the patterning of maternal activities over weeks (Thoman et al., 1983). In both studies, infants exhibiting the highest amounts of social crying received less appropriate maternal stimulation. Crying in ill infants can have even more ominous implications. Studies have indicated that the intensity of crying, ranging from mild fussing to hard crying, is directly related to the heart rate of the infant (Ludington, 1990; McNeely, 1987), and the higher the heart rate the greater the energy consumption of the infant (Woodson et al., 1983). Thus, the infant who spends a lot of time crying will need more calories to grow. In addition, this state is associated with decreased oxygenation in the blood stream (Huch & Huch, 1981) and brain (Brazy, 1988).

The final waking state, nonalert waking activity, is characterized by periods when the infant is motorically active but not alert or crying. Usually the infant's eyes are open. One study of nonalert activity found that excess amounts of this state in full-term infants is associated with inconsistency in the patterning of states over weeks (Becker & Thoman, 1982b), and, in turn, inconsistency in state patterning is related to poor developmental outcome (Thoman et al., 1981). Premature infants, after term, exhibit elevated levels of this state (Holditch-Davis & Thoman, 1987) and are known to be at increased risk of poor developmental outcome (Aylward et al., 1989; Eilers et al., 1986; Hack et al., 1992; Kitchen et al., 1990). However, whether there is a relationship between these findings is unknown.

The states transitional between sleeping and waking have rarely been studied. In fact, the Prechtl scoring system omits them altogether on the grounds that they are not true states but just transitions between states (Prechtl & Beintema, 1968). However, newborn infants, both term and preterm, actually spend significant amounts of time in them, ranging from about 6 percent of the day at 29 weeks' GA to 14 percent in the first month after term (Holditch-Davis, 1990a; Holditch-Davis & Thoman, 1987). Thoman (1985) describes three states transitional between waking and sleeping: drowse, when the infant is quiet and appears sleepy with eyes opening and closing slowly; daze, when the infant is quiet with eyes that are open but dazed in appearance; and sleep–wake transition, when the infant exhibits mixed signals of waking and sleeping, is motorically active, and may appear to be waking up. Drowse and daze typically occur in the midst of periods of waking or as the infant is falling asleep. Sleep–wake transition typically occurs at the end of sleeping as the infant is awakening but may also occur in the middle of sleep particularly in premature infants. Drowse, daze, and sleep–wake transition are often combined in research reports. However, studies have indicated that these states have different patterns of correlations with other states (Thoman et al., 1987). During the first month after term, premature infants have been found to spend significantly more time in sleep–wake transition and less time in drowse or daze than full-term infants (Holditch-Davis & Thoman, 1987). If these three states had been combined, these differences would have been missed. In addition, hospitalized preterm infants spend more time in sleep–wake transition when they are with nurses, rather than parents, but do not differ in the amount of drowsiness occurring with these different caregivers (Miller & Holditch-Davis, 1992).

There are two major sleep states—active sleep and quiet sleep—although some state systems define a transitional state between them. In active sleep, the infant's respiration is uneven and primarily costal in nature. Sporadic motor movements occur, but muscle tone is low between these movements. The most distinct characteristic of this state is rapid eye movements that occur intermittently.

Active sleep is the most common state from birth throughout infancy, but it occurs only during about 20 percent of sleep in adults (Roffwarg et al., 1966). Because of this dramatic developmental decrease and the frequent movements seen in infants during active sleep, many clinicians think of active sleep as a disorganized and primitive state. Surprisingly, this state has relatively recent phylogenetic origins, occurring only in birds and mammals (Roffwarg et al., 1966). Thus, it has been hypothesized to be necessary for brain development (Roffwarg et al., 1966). This hypothesis has received support from a recent study of full-term infants (Denenberg & Thoman, 1981). In animal studies, prolonged deprivation of active sleep in infancy permanently altered brain functioning and resulted in hyperactivity, distractibility, and altered sexual performance (Mirmiran, 1986). Inasmuch as respiratory patterns are relatively unstable in active sleep (Haddad et al., 1987) and transcutaneous oxygen values are lower and more variable (Gabriel et al., 1980; Martin et al., 1979), the large amount of active sleep seen in young preterm infants (Holditch-Davis, 1990a; Holditch-Davis & Edwards, 1995a) may contribute to their respiratory difficulties.

The other sleep state, quiet sleep, is characterized by a lack of body movements and the presence of regular respiration. A tonic level of motor tone is maintained in this state. The major purpose of quiet sleep seems to be rest and restoration (Adam, 1980). This state has been hypothesized to be necessary for healing (Adam & Oswald, 1984). Quiet sleep may also be needed for growth because it is in this state that growth hormone is secreted in adults (Chuman, 1983). However, a study of full-term infants did not find any relationship between growth hormone secretion and quiet sleep (Shaywitz et al., 1971). Oxygenation is higher during this sleep state; thus, quiet sleep may be beneficial for infants with respiratory problems (Norris et al., 1982).

The amount of quiet sleep is also very sensitive to the environment. Infant stimulation studies, for example, have found that quiet sleep is the state most likely to be increased by vestibular and kinesthetic interventions (Cordero et al., 1986; Ingersoll & Thoman, 1994; Korner et al., 1982; Thoman & Graham, 1986). The stimulation provided by routine nursing care, on the other hand, results in significantly reduced amounts of quiet sleep as compared with times when the preterm infant is undisturbed (Holditch-Davis, 1990b), and the amount of this state is further reduced when the infant experiences painful or uncomfortable procedures (Holditch-Davis & Calhoun, 1989). Thus, this is the state most likely to be affected by the neonatal intensive care unit (NICU) environment.

EFFECT OF PHYSIOLOGIC PARAMETERS ON STATE

As previously mentioned, physiologic functioning varies in different states. In turn, abnormalities in physiologic functioning can alter the sleeping and waking states of infants. This discussion focuses on the interrelationship of sleeping and waking and four areas of physiologic functioning of interest to neonatal nurses—perinatal illness, the central nervous system, circulatory system, and respiration.

Perinatal Illness

The state patterns of infants who experienced perinatal complications may differ markedly from the state patterns of healthy full-term infants (Clausen et al., 1977; Prechtl et al., 1973; Thoman & Becker, 1979; Watt & Strongman, 1985). Small for gestational age full-term infants, for example, have more disorganized sleep as evidenced by more active sleep without rapid eye movements than healthy full-term infants (Watt & Strongman, 1985) and more quiet sleep with ocular movements (Bhatia et al., 1980). They also exhibited poorer responsiveness during alertness as measured by the NBAS (Als et al., 1976; Lester et al., 1986).

The sleep of premature infants after term is known to differ from that of full-term infants of the same corrected ages, in that there is a decreased total amount of sleep, longer episodes of quiet sleep, more body movements, more frequent REM episodes, and somewhat lower correlation among the various behavioral criteria of the sleep states (Booth et al., 1980; Dreyfus-Brisac, 1975; Ellingson & Peters, 1980; Holditch-Davis & Thoman, 1987; Parmelee et al., 1967; Watt & Strongman, 1985). Premature infants show day–night differentiation in their sleeping and waking patterns at the same or an earlier postconceptional age than full-term infants (McMillen et al., 1991; Shimada et al., 1993). In addition, their EEG patterns differ from those of full-term infants. Premature infants display longer bursts during trace alternans, earlier sleep spindle appearance, more immature EEG patterns, and poorer phase stability for EEG frequencies (Ellingson & Peters, 1980; Karch et al., 1982). Premature and full-term infants also differ on architectural, phasic, continuity, spectral, and autonomic measures (Curzi-Dascalova et al., 1988; Scher et al., 1992b, 1994b, 1994c).

The ways that the waking states differ between full-term and premature infants are less well established. The results of studies using relatively brief assessments have been contradictory: Premature infants have been found to be less, more, or equally alert and less, more, or equally irritable than full-term infants (Aylward, 1982; DiVitto & Goldberg, 1979; Friedman et al., 1982; Howard et al., 1976; Lester et al., 1976; McGehee & Eckerman, 1983; Palmer et al., 1982; Telzrow et al., 1982). However, over prolonged observation periods, premature infants exhibited more alertness and nonalert waking activity and less drowsiness than full-term infants (Holditch-Davis & Thoman, 1987).

The severity of illness that the infant experiences during the perinatal period has relatively small additional effects on sleeping and waking. In general, critical illness has immediate effects on sleeping and waking patterns, but these effects disappear after the infant recovers as long as there are no neurologic complications and as long as infants are observed at same ages corrected for GA at birth. Karch and colleagues (1982) studied healthy and ill preterm infants at comparable ages and found that ill infants exhibited more quiet sleep, more indeterminate sleep, and less wakefulness. The ill infants in this study were examined while on mechanical ventilation. Thus, the state differences reflect the immediate influence of critical illness and mechanical ventilation. Preterm infants ill with respiratory distress syndrome have been found to exhibit delayed state development but show state patterns comparable to healthy preterm infants' once they recover (Holmes et al., 1979). Holditch-Davis and Hudson (1995) used changes in sleep–wake to identify a wide variety of acute medical complications in preterm infants, including hydrocephalus, sepsis, and cold stress. Infant medical complications also affected the scores of infants on standardized neurobehavioral assessments but only on items requiring vigorous responses (such as vigor of crying, irritability, and motor development) but not on other state items, including alertness and percent sleeping (Korner et al., 1994).

Studies of infants who have recovered from their illnesses have found fewer differences. High and Gorski (1985) did not find any differences in the sleeping and waking patterns of convalescent premature infants differing in the severity of their previous illness. Likewise, Holditch-Davis (1990a) found that the only difference in the development of sleeping and waking states in convalescent preterm infants was that more severely ill infants showed less fussing and somewhat poorer organization of quiet sleep. Als and colleagues (1988) found no difference in the state organization of premature infants born at less than 33 weeks' GA and premature infants born between 33 and 37 weeks' GA when state organization was measured two weeks after term. In addition, scores on the NBAS state scale did not differ significantly between sick and healthy full-term infants at the time of hospital discharge (Holmes et al., 1982).

Infants with chronic lung disease are more likely than other premature infants to have oxygen desaturations when sleeping (Zinman et al., 1992). Yet it is unclear whether this illness has any effect on sleeping and waking patterns. Holditch-Davis and Lee (1993) compared high-risk preterm infants with and without chronic lung disease from 32 to 36 weeks' postconceptional age on sleep–wake states and sleep organization exhibited over 4-hour observations in the intermediate care unit. The only difference between the infants with and without chronic lung disease was that infants with chronic lung disease had more irregular respiration in quiet sleep. Despite the fact that many clinicians believe that infants with chronic lung disease are more sensitive to stimulation, there were also no differences in sleeping and waking when the infants with and without chronic lung disease were with caregivers (Holditch-Davis, 1995). However, at term age, premature infants with chronic lung disease had less active sleep, more frequent arousals, and more frequent body movements in sleep than premature infants who never experienced any respiratory illnesses (Holditch-Davis, 1995; Scher et al., 1992c) and performed more poorly on the interactive and motor clusters of the NBAS (Myers et al., 1992).

Neurologic System

Because sleeping and waking states are assumed to reflect the underlying activation of the central nervous system (CNS), it is not surprising that there is a close relationship between sleep–wake states and CNS functioning. Four factors illustrate this interrelationship. First, sleeping and waking exhibit a large amount of development in the first year of life, the time of the most rapid CNS development. Sleeping and waking state affect neurologic responses. Infants with neurologic abnormalities exhibit abnormal sleeping and waking patterns. Finally, sleeping and waking states can be used to predict developmental outcome.

Development of Sleeping and Waking State

Infants exhibit definite developmental changes in their sleeping and waking state patterns throughout the first year of life. The age at which sleep–wake states first appear is unknown. The earliest study of sleeping and waking in preterm infants younger than 30 weeks' GA found that these infants had only a single active sleep-like state (Dreyfus-Brisac, 1968), but these findings are questionable because all of the infants in this study were dying at the time of the state recordings. More recent studies of preterm infants have found that by 24 weeks' GA, cycling between waking and sleeping can be identified by EEG in some preterm infants (Hellstrom-Westas et al., 1991). By 28 weeks' GA (the earliest age studied), infants exhibit distinct waking and sleeping states (Curzi-Dascalova et al., 1988; High & Gorski, 1985; Holditch-Davis, 1990a; Holditch-Davis & Edwards, 1995a; Stefanski et al., 1984). However, prior to 30 weeks' GA, the various behaviors associated with sleep and waking—eye movements, body movements, respiration, and muscle tone—are not well coordinated; and not until at least 36 weeks' GA do preterm infants exhibit the same degree of correlation between these parameters as do full-term infants (Aylward, 1981; Curzi-Dascalova et al., 1988; Dreyfus-Brisac, 1970, 1975; Parmelee & Stern, 1972; Petre-Quadens, 1974; Prechtl et al., 1979). Studies of sleeping and waking states in fetuses, conducted using observations made during ultrasound examinations, have had similar findings (Arduini et al., 1986; Nijhuis, 1986; Nijhuis et al., 1982; Swartjes et al., 1990; Visser et al., 1987).

Infants exhibit greater amounts of active sleep and indeterminate states during the preterm period and lower amounts of waking states than after term (Dreyfus-Brisac, 1975; High & Gorski, 1985; Holditch-Davis, 1990a; Holditch-Davis & Edwards, 1995a; Holmes et al., 1984; Parmelee et al., 1967). Active sleep occupies as much as 60 to 70 percent of the day for young preterm infants (High & Gorski, 1985; Holditch-Davis, 1990a; Holditch-Davis & Edwards, 1995a) and is further increased during acute illness (Holmes et al., 1979). The major developmental change during the preterm period is a decrease in the amount of active sleep (High & Gorski, 1985; Holditch-Davis, 1990a; Holditch-Davis & Edwards, 1995a). In addition, quiet sleep and waking states, especially crying, increase (Aylward, 1981; High & Gorski, 1985; Holditch-Davis, 1990a; Holditch-Davis & Edwards, 1995a; Korner et al., 1988; Vles et al., 1992). The organization of the sleep states, as measured by the percentages of the state with typical state criteria or by the correlation between criteria, also increases throughout the preterm period (Curzi-Dascalova et al., 1988; Dreyfus-Brisac, 1970; Holditch-Davis, 1990a; Holditch-Davis & Edwards, 1995a; Prechtl et al., 1979). The mean duration and frequency of episodes of each state also changes over the preterm period: quiet waking, active waking, and sleep–wake transition episodes occurred more frequently, and active waking and quiet sleep bout length increased over age (Ariagno, 1996; Fajardo et al., 1990; Holditch-Davis & Edwards, 1995b).

The sleeping and waking states of infants in the first month after term differ dramatically from those of preterm infants. Healthy full-term neonates spend approximately 40 percent of the daytime in active sleep and 20 percent in quiet sleep (Holditch-Davis & Thoman, 1987). Slightly higher amounts of sleep states occur at night (Hoppenbrouwers et al., 1988; Thoman & Whitney, 1989). Waking states make up the rest of the day, with alertness (14 percent) and drowsiness (13 percent) being the most common (Holditch-Davis & Thoman, 1987).

The major developmental trends exhibited by full-term infants in the first month are a decrease in active sleep and an increase in the amount of alertness (Denenberg & Thoman, 1981; Kohyama & Iwakawa, 1990). Moreover, the mean lengths of episodes of the sleep states change, with active sleep decreasing and quiet sleep increasing (Thoman & Whitney, 1989). Similar trends occur for premature infants during this period (High & Gorski, 1985; Holditch-Davis & Thoman, 1987).

Sleeping and waking states continue to develop throughout the first year. Waking periods become longer and more consolidated

(Coons & Guilleminault, 1982; Meier-Koll et al., 1978). The infant spends an increasing proportion of wakefulness in the alert state and gains the ability to remain alert while crying (Acebo, 1987). The amount of time spent crying decreases (Michelsson et al., 1990). In addition, total sleep time decreases, with almost all of this decrease due to a decrease in active sleep time (Hoppenbrouwers et al., 1988; Kohyama & Iwakawa, 1990). The amount of quiet sleep remains the same or increases from term age on; thus, by about 6 months of age, the amount of quiet sleep exceeds the amount of active sleep (Anders & Keener, 1985; Coons & Guilleminault, 1982; Emde & Walker, 1976; Hoppenbrouwers et al., 1988). The nature of these changes depends somewhat on feeding type, as breast-fed infants exhibit longer sleep latency, more non-REM sleep, and shorter duration of REM sleep than formula-fed infants (Butte et al., 1992). In addition, the number of sleep episodes decreases and becomes consolidated primarily into nighttime (Anders & Keener, 1985; Bamford et al., 1990; Coons & Guilleminault, 1982, 1984; Hoppenbrouwers et al., 1988), although the majority of infants continue to exhibit some amount of night waking (Scher, 1991). By 1 year, the infant is taking about two daytime naps (Weissbluth, 1995) and sleeping about 10 to 12 hours through the night, although prematurely born infants may display shorter night sleep and more night wakenings than full-term infants (Ju et al., 1991).

Other developmental changes during the first year affect the organization of sleep. The cycling between active and quiet becomes more consistent over the first few months, and by 4 months of age, the complete sleep cycle first exhibits a standard length of about 1 hour (Harper et al., 1981). The sleep states also develop the EEG patterns typical of adults (Parmelee et al., 1968). By 3 months of age, the EEG stages within quiet sleep can be identified, and this sleep state can now be called non-REM sleep (Coons & Guilleminault, 1982; Ellingson & Peters, 1980).

Neurologic Responses

Infants exhibit different neurologic responses in different sleeping and waking states. The magnitude of neurologic reflexes is known to differ greatly in different states (Prechtl & Beintema, 1968). Therefore, standardized infant assessments and neurologic examinations specify which states are optimal for testing each reflex (Brazelton, 1984; Prechtl & Beintema, 1968). The amplitude, wave form, and latency of visual evoked potentials are different in different sleeping and waking states with the greatest differences being between sleep and waking (Apkarian et al., 1991).

Neurologic Problems

The state patterns of infants with neurologic insults differ markedly from those of healthy infants (Prechtl et al., 1969b). Infants with Down syndrome have been found to spend more time awake and to have abnormally long periods of quiet sleep (Goldie et al., 1968; Prechtl et al., 1973). At term, premature infants with intraventricular hemorrhage have been found to have lower arousal using the NBAS than healthy full-term infants (Anderson et al., 1989). Full-term infants with hyperbilirubinemia show decreased amounts of wakefulness (Prechtl et al., 1973). As compared with full-term infants with only mild bilirubin elevations, infants with moderately elevated bilirubin values exhibit significantly lower scores in state regulation and range on the NBAS and exhibit minor neurologic abnormalities as evidenced by increased latency of brain stem auditory evoked potentials (Vohr et al., 1990). Infants who eventually died from sudden infant death syndrome (SIDS) moved less during sleep, had more REM in the newborn period, and showed less waking in the early morning hours than control infants (Kahn et al., 1992; Schechtman et al., 1992), and male infants at high risk for SIDS fail to show an increase in wakefulness with age (Cornwell, 1993). Abnormal cry patterns have been found in infants with neurologic injuries, with hyperbilirubinemia, or at risk for SIDS (Golub & Corwin, 1982; Prechtl et al., 1969a; Vohr et al., 1989). Milder insults, such as slight hyperbilirubinemia not requiring phototherapy, have not been found to affect infant sleeping and waking (Paludetto et al., 1986).

In addition, infants exposed prenatally to drugs or alcohol exhibit abnormalities in their state patterns possibly as the result of neurologic insults caused by the drugs (Dixon & Bejar, 1989). For example, alcohol-exposed infants exhibit sleep disruptions (Scher et al., 1988). Infants exposed to marijuana have shorter, higher cries with more variation in frequency (Lester & Dreher, 1989) and exhibit a decrease in quiet sleep time (Scher et al., 1988). Methadone-exposed infants exhibit abnormal cries with short first expirations (Huntington et al., 1990). They are more irritable and less able to sustain a high-quality alert state (Jeremy & Hans, 1985; Strauss et al., 1975). Newborn infants of mothers who smoked during pregnancy spend less time in active and quiet sleep and less time awake than did infants whose mothers did not smoke (Kotzer, 1994). Black and associates (1993) found that infants exposed to cocaine prenatally score less positively on NBAS orientation, state regulation, and autonomic regulation clusters than drug-free infants and that these differences decreased with increasing age. On the other hand, Woods and colleagues (1993) did not find any differences on the NBAS between cocaine-exposed and drug-free infants.

Prediction of Developmental Outcome

Finally, the organization of sleeping and waking, as indicated by individual state criteria or the overall patterning of states, can be used to predict the developmental outcome of infants. In healthy preterm infants, lower spectral EEG energies predicted lower neurodevelopmental performance at 12 and 24 months (Scher et al., 1994a). Low levels of trace alternans, an EEG pattern seen during quiet sleep in neonates, is predictive of lower intelligence quotients (IQs) in premature infants (Beckwith & Parmelee, 1986), and delayed maturity of EEG patterns of preterm infants was found to be associated with poor neurologic outcome (Ferrari et al., 1992; Hahn & Tharp, 1990). Elevated amounts of intense bursts of rapid eye movements are associated with later developmental problems in full-term infants (Becker & Thoman, 1981, 1982a). Acoustic characteristics of infant cries have been used to predict developmental outcome in preterm infants and infants exposed to drugs prenatally (Huntington et al., 1990; Lester, 1987). Measures of sleep–wake states during the preterm period—including the amount of crying during gavage feedings and the overall quality of state organization as compared with other infants—have been found to predict Bayley scores during the first year (DiPietro & Porges, 1991; Fajardo et al., 1992), and measures at term have been shown to relate to developmental outcome at age 8 (Cohen et al., 1986). The development of particular sleep behaviors during the first year after term was related to the outcome of premature infants (Anders et al., 1985; Whitney & Thoman, 1993). In apparently normal full-term infants, the stability of state patterns in the first month has been found to predict developmental outcome (Thoman et al., 1981). This finding has been replicated using EEG measures of state (Lombroso & Matsumiya, 1985), in groups of hospitalized preterm infants (Tynan, 1986), in premature infants after term (Whitney & Thoman, 1993), and in siblings of infants who died from SIDS (Thoman et al., 1988).

Circulatory System

Sleeping and waking states affect the infant's circulatory system. Overall, heart rate is higher in waking than sleeping states, and particularly during crying (Ludington, 1990; van Ravenswaaij-Arts et al., 1989). Mean heart rates in the two sleep states are very similar, but heart rate is more variable in active sleep (Junge, 1979; Visser et al., 1982). This difference in variability is large enough that it is possible to differentiate between the two sleep states on the basis of heart rate variability (DeHaan et al., 1977). Thus, neonatal nurses need to be aware of the infant's state when determining heart rate, and routine vital signs probably should not be obtained while the infant is crying.

Sleeping and waking states also affect the infant's circulation. Cerebral blood flow is highest in waking (Greisen et al., 1985). It is significantly higher in active sleep than in quiet sleep in full-term infants (Milligan, 1979) but not in infants less than term age (Greisen et al., 1985). Variability in cerebral blood flow velocity is lowest in quiet sleep, whereas marked fluctuations occur in active waking (fussing and nonalert waking activity) (Ramaekers et al., 1989). Minor variations in cerebral blood flow velocity occur in active sleep. Blood pressure is slightly higher when the infant is awake than when asleep (van Ravenswaaij-Arts et al., 1989).

Respiration

The effect of sleeping and waking states on the respiratory system is even greater than on the circulatory system. The nervous system controls of breathing are different in different states (Phillipson, 1978). During wakefulness, breathing is regulated by metabolic controls, general stimulation from the reticular activating system, and voluntary activities. In quiet sleep, metabolic controls predominate, and maintaining acid–base and oxygen homeostasis is the primary stimulus for breathing. Medullary respiratory center activity varies during active asleep depending on whether the infant is experiencing rapid eye movements and motor activity (phasic active sleep) or not (tonic active sleep) (Orem, 1980), indicating that these two types of active sleep include different controls on breathing (Phillipson, 1978). During phasic active sleep, behavioral controls, similar to the voluntary controls in waking, predominate. In tonic active sleep, the major respiratory control results from direct stimulation of the state in a manner similar to the reticular stimulation of respiration during wakefulness. As a result of these different controls, infants exhibit higher respiratory rates and lower tidal volumes in phasic active sleep than in tonic active sleep (Haddad et al., 1982).

Respiratory activity responds differently to chemical stimulation in different states. Baseline arterial oxygen and carbon dioxide levels are lower in active sleep than in either waking or quiet sleep (Gabriel et al., 1980; Hanson & Okken, 1980; Martin et al., 1979; Martin et al., 1981; Mok et al., 1988), possibly because of hypoventilation or ventilation–perfusion inequalities in this state. Ventilation is increased in response to hypoxia in all states (Phillipson, 1978; Rigatto et al., 1982), but this hyperventilation is not maintained in active sleep (Rigatto, 1982). In addition, arousal in response to hypoxia is slower in active sleep (Fewell & Baker, 1987; Phillipson & Sullivan, 1978). Response to hypercapnia is also different in different states. There is a shift to the right in the carbon dioxide response curve in quiet sleep as compared to waking (Cohen et al., 1991; Phillipson, 1978). This response is further reduced in tonic active sleep and absent in phasic active sleep (Bryan & Bryan, 1978; Phillipson & Sullivan, 1978; Sullivan, 1980).

As a result of these differing neurologic controls on breathing, a number of respiratory variables in both full-term and preterm infants are influenced by sleep and waking states. Respiration rates are higher and more variable in active sleep (Adamson et al., 1981a; Curzi-Dascalova et al., 1981, 1983; Haddad et al., 1987; Hoppenbrouwers et al., 1978; Thoman et al., 1977). Active sleep has also been shown to result in hypoventilation in preterm infants because of central inhibition of spinal motoneurons (Schulte et al., 1977) and poor coordination between chest and abdominal muscles (Gaultier, 1990). Thus, paradoxic movements of the chest wall and abdominal muscles during breathing are common during active sleep in preterm infants (Carlo et al., 1983; Moriette et al., 1983). However, it is not clear whether lung volume is (Henderson-Smart & Read, 1979) or is not (Beardsmore et al., 1989) decreased in active sleep in full-term infants. Expiratory volumes and flow rates are larger in waking than in sleeping infants (Lodrup et al., 1992).

The frequency of central apnea is also different in different sleep states. Central apnea rarely occurs during waking. Most studies indicate that brief apneic pauses of less than 20 seconds in length occur more frequently in active sleep than quiet sleep in both full-term and preterm infants (Adamson et al., 1981b; Bentele et al., 1985; Booth et al., 1983; Curzi-Dascalova & Christova-Gueorguieva, 1983; Dittrichova & Paul, 1989; Ellingson et al., 1982; Gabriel et al., 1976; Holditch-Davis et al., 1994; Lee et al., 1987; Waite & Thoman, 1981, 1982). The effects of sleep state on the frequency of periodic respiration (cyclic breathing alternating with brief apneic pauses) is less clear: Some studies found that periodic respiration occurs more frequently in active sleep (Booth et al., 1983; Waite & Thoman, 1982), whereas others found no difference in periodic respiration frequency in the two sleep states (Barrington et al., 1987; Holditch-Davis et al., 1994). The mean length of apneic pauses is longer in quiet sleep (Adamson et al., 1981b; Booth et al., 1983; Holditch-Davis et al., 1994; Waite & Thoman, 1981), apparently because of a lower incidence of apneas less than 6 seconds in length in quiet sleep, rather than because of an increased incidence of longer apneas (Flores-Guevara et. al, 1982; Hoppenbrouwers et al., 1980; Waite & Thoman, 1981). In addition, a variety of stresses, including an increase in body temperature and sleep deprivation, have been shown to increase apnea frequency, primarily in active sleep (Gaultier, 1994).

However, it cannot be concluded from these studies that pathologic apneas (apneic episodes longer than 20 seconds and usually associated with bradycardia and hypoxemia) are more common in active sleep because these studies rarely included episodes of pathologic apnea. Infants in these studies were usually older than 36 weeks' GA, even though the peak age for pathologic apnea is less than 32 weeks' GA (Henderson-Smart, 1981). Even when infants of the correct ages are studied, pathologic apnea is often too rare to permit statistical analyses comparing states (Holditch-Davis et al., 1994). One study of older infants being treated for prolonged apnea did not find any difference in the rate of brief respiratory pauses in the two sleep states, nor did the frequency of brief pauses differ from that found in healthy infants (Orr et al., 1985). Yet there may be some association between active sleep and pathologic apnea inasmuch as the methylxanthines, caffeine and theophylline, used to treat this condition are known to increase the amount of wakefulness and decrease the amount of active sleep in addition to their direct effects on respiration (Demarquez et al., 1978; Dietrich et al., 1978; Thoman et al., 1985).

EFFECT OF NURSING INTERVENTIONS ON STATE

Sleeping and waking states are also affected by the types and timing of stimulation that the infant receives from the environment. Thus, nursing interventions have the potential to either promote state organization or to disrupt it. The effects of four common nursing interventions—routine NICU care, painful procedures, social interaction, and infant stimulation—on infant sleeping and waking are examined in this section.

Effect of Environmental Stimulation

Investigators have suggested that the hospital provides stimulation that is inappropriate for the development of premature infants and likely to result in disorganized sleeping and waking patterns (Cornell & Gottfried, 1976). The NICU provides infants with an extremely bright and noisy environment with little diurnal variation and frequent interventions for technical procedures but little positive handling (Barnard & Blackburn, 1985; Blackburn & Barnard, 1985; Duxbury et al., 1984; Gaiter, 1985; Gottfried, 1985; Gottfried et al., 1981; Lawson, 1977; Thomas, 1989; Zahr & Balian, 1995). The sickest infants actually receive the most handling (Duxbury et al., 1984; High & Gorski, 1985; Zahr & Balian, 1995) even though they lack the physiologic reserves to cope with it. These infants become hypoxic in response to virtually any form of stimulation: noise (Long et al., 1980), technical procedures (Long et al., 1980; Norris et al., 1982; Speidel, 1978), and social touches (Gorski et al., 1983; Sehring et al., 1985). Several researchers have suggested that these reductions in oxygenation in response to handling may actually be the result of changes in sleeping and waking states (Gottfried, 1985; Speidel, 1978). Convalescent infants receive less handling than ill infants but do experience social interactions as a greater proportion of their care (High & Gorski, 1985).

Several of the aspects of routine NICU care are known to contribute to disruption of infant sleeping and waking patterns. Nursing and medical interventions frequently result in state changes. The frequency of these interventions in the NICU have been found to be as high as five times per hour (Duxbury et al., 1984). Preterm infants change their sleep–wake states about 6 times per hour, and 78 percent of these changes are associated with either nursing interventions or NICU noise (Zahr & Balian, 1995). Preterm infants are rarely able to sustain quiet sleep during nursing interventions (Holditch-Davis, 1990b) and usually awaken with each intervention. Inasmuch as infants fall asleep in active sleep (Anders & Keener, 1985), frequent nursing interventions are particularly likely to reduce the amount of quiet sleep that the infant experiences. These sleep disruptions result in increased waking and, in particular, crying time. Preterm infants normally spend only a small percentage of their time in waking states (High & Gorski, 1985; Holditch-Davis, 1990a), but this percentage increases significantly when they are with nurses (Holditch-Davis, 1990b).

In addition, neonatal nurses and physicians seldom consider infant sleep–wake states and other infant cues when choosing the time for routine interventions. Although two studies found relationships between nursing care and sleeping and waking for groups of preterm infants (Barnard & Blackburn, 1985; Lawson et al., 1985), it is likely that these results represent infant reactions to nursing care or infants conditioned to anticipate regular nursing procedures, rather than nurses responding to infant states. Infant activity has been found to be decreased after nursing interventions (Blackburn & Barnard, 1985). Gottfried (1985) found that nurses responded to fewer than half the cries of convalescent premature infants. Then too, meeting infant social needs is not a nursing priority. Linn and associates (1985) found no relation between staff–patient ratio and the amount of positive handling infants received. Yet a lack of responsiveness to infant cues may serve to slow the development of stable diurnal patterns of sleeping and waking that several investigators have suggested is the first task of infancy (Barnard & Blackburn, 1985; Sander et al., 1979). Full-term infants receiving responsive care develop day–night differentiation in their sleeping and waking in 5 to 7 days, whereas this differentiation is delayed when the care is not responsive (Sander et al., 1970).

Finally, the lighting of the NICU contributes to sleeping and waking problems in infants. Lighting in most NICUs is continuous, high level, and fluorescent. The American Academy of Pediatrics (AAP) guidelines recommend 100-footcandle intensity at the level of the infant 24 hours a day in NICUs for adequate visualization (Peabody & Lewis, 1985). However, researchers have hypothesized that continuous light can result in endocrine changes, changes in biologic rhythms, and sleep deprivation during the NICU stay (Blackburn, 1996; Gottfried, 1985; Halberg, 1969). The frequency of eye opening and waking states is related to the level of illumination in the NICU, with less eye opening occurring when the lights are brightest (Moseley et al., 1988; Robinson et al., 1989). Sudden decreases in lighting result in increased eye opening (Moseley et al., 1988), providing support for the common nursing and parental intervention of shading infant eyes with one's hand to elicit alertness. In addition, infants exposed to NICUs that vary the intensity of lighting on a diurnal pattern open their eyes significantly more than those exposed to continuous illumination (Robinson et al., 1989).

In view of these problems with routine NICU care, it is not surprising that several researchers have attempted to alter this environment to promote better sleeping and waking patterns in infants. When Gabriel and associates (1981) consolidated nursing care so that convalescent premature infants were disturbed less often, the infants were awake less and had longer sleep episodes. Als and colleagues (1986) developed a system of individualized interventions for preterm infants that included sensitivity to infant cues and careful avoidance of sleep disruptions. Their experimental infants did not exhibit different state patterns than the control infants, but the experimental infants did have fewer medical complications and improved performance on the APIB. Using a modification of Als' intervention system, Becker and associates (1991a, 1991b) also found improvements in infant morbidity but did not find differences in state behaviors on the NBAS at the time of hospital discharge; however, the experimental infants showed higher oxygen saturations, fewer disorganized movements, and more alertness during nursing care than did controls (Becker et al., 1993). Fajardo and coworkers (1990) cared for premature infants in a quiet, private room with a day–night cycle, demand feedings, and social interactions by the nurses. These babies showed an increase in the mean length of active sleep and an increase in the organization of sleep states as evidenced by a decreased number of state changes and increased number of enduring state episodes.

A number of researchers altered NICU lighting patterns. Mann and others (1986) cared for preterm infants in a nursery in which light and noise intensities were reduced between 7 P.M. and 7 A.M. As compared with infants from a control nursery, the experimental infants were found to sleep more but not until after hospital discharge. Blackburn and Patteson (1991) compared preterm infants cared for in a nursery with continuous lighting with infants in a nursery with lighting that was dimmed at night. Infants in cycled light exhibited less motor activity during the night and lower heart rates over the entire day than the control infants. When preterm infants in the intermediate care unit were given four $1\frac{1}{2}$-hour nap periods a day during which their incubators were covered and they received no nursing or medical procedures, they exhibited less quiet waking and longer uninterrupted sleep bouts than preterm infants without naps (Holditch-Davis et al., 1995), and they experienced a more rapid decline in apnea and more rapid weight gain (Torres et al., 1995). Altogether, these findings suggest that neonatal nurses need to examine their routine practices to see if changes could be made to better promote stable sleeping and waking patterns in infants.

Painful Procedures

Infants in intensive care inevitably experience painful procedures. Neonatal nurses need to be alert to the effects of these procedures on infant sleeping and waking states. During painful procedures, infants are more likely to be awake and less likely to be in quiet sleep than during routine nursing care (Field & Goldson, 1984; Holditch-Davis & Calhoun, 1989; Van Cleve et al., 1995). All but the youngest and sickest preterm infants are likely to cry (Field & Goldson, 1984; Dale, 1986; Van Cleve et al., 1995), although the length of time until the cry begins depends on the sleeping and waking state the infant is in at the beginning of the procedure (Grunau & Craig, 1987). Healthy full-term infants have the longest latency to cry when in quiet sleep (Grunau & Craig, 1987), but whether preterm infants would show a similar pattern is unknown. Immediately after the painful procedure, the full-term infant is likely to remain awake (Anders & Chalemian, 1974). However, in preterm infants, this tendency is not any greater than the tendency to stay awake after routine handling (Holditch-Davis & Calhoun, 1989). At times longer than a hour after the procedure, full-term infants who experienced the severe pain of circumcision have been found to exhibit more quiet sleep (Emde et al., 1971), possibly in an effort to shut out the pain.

Nursing comfort measures have the potential to minimize some of these state effects. Yet it is not clear how frequently practicing nurses actually use them inasmuch as in one study nurses were not found to use positive touches or talking any more frequently during painful procedures than during routine care (Holditch-Davis & Calhoun, 1989). Franck (1987) identified nine different comfort measures that nurses report using to soothe infants receiving painful procedures. (See Chapter 40, Identification, Management, and Prevention of Pain in the Neonate.) To date only a few of them have studied. Tactile stimulation, music, and intrauterine sounds were found to be ineffective for both preterm and full-term infants when given during the painful procedure (Beaver, 1987; Marchette et al., 1989). However, pacifiers were found to reduce crying and arousal in full-term and preterm infants when given during and after the procedure (Campos, 1989; Field & Goldson, 1984). A sucrose-flavored pacifier was found to be even more effective than a plain pacifier in reducing the amount of crying done by full-term infants during blood drawing and circumcision (Blass & Hoffmeyer, 1991). Swaddling has also been shown to be effective with full-term infants but less so than pacifiers, and the infants were more likely to be alert if given pacifiers (Campos, 1989). Thus, there is evidence that use of pacifiers or swaddling can help reduce the sleeping and waking changes caused by painful procedures. However, additional research is needed to determine the effects of other comfort measures and of combining different comfort measures.

Social Interaction

Sleeping and waking states are known to influence the interactions between full-term infants and their mothers, and in turn maternal interactions alter infant sleep–wake patterns (Thoman & Becker, 1979). For example, infant crying may lead the mother to pick up the infant. At another time, a mother may awaken a sleeping infant for a feeding, thereby altering the infant's sleeping and waking patterns. Mothers have been found to exhibit different patterns of interactions when infants are in different states (Rosenthal, 1983). Aspects of the infant's state organization, including the degree to which he or she shows different patterns of crying and alertness in different situations, are related to the overall quality of the mother–infant interaction (Acebo, 1987). A responsive style of mothering results in infants developing day–night differentiation in their sleeping and waking patterns sooner (Sander et al., 1970). In addition, maternal emotional stress has been found to relate to the amount of night sleeping that full-term infants exhibit at 4 and 12 months (Becker et al., 1991a, 1991b).

Less is known about the effect of social interaction in the hospital on infant sleeping and waking states. Minde and colleagues (1983) found that ill preterm infants exhibited less eye opening, and thus probably less waking, when interacting with their mothers than did healthier preterm infants. Mothers report being aware of the sleeping and waking behaviors of their preterm infants—especially eye movements, orientation, and body movements—when they attempt to interact; they also report having used specific infant responses as guides to increase or decrease their interactive activity (Oehler et al., 1993). Waking, eye opening, increased body movements, positive facial expressions, and calming encouraged increased interaction; body movements, negative facial expressions and withdrawing discouraged maternal interaction. However, preterm infants exhibit the positive interactive behaviors rather small portions of the time with their mothers (Oehler, 1995).

Moreover, social stimulation affects the physiologic status of preterm infants. The variation in infant oxygen saturation during parent touching was related to behavioral state and GA, such that infants who were more aroused and awake at the beginning of touch and had younger GAs at birth showed greater variation in their oxygen saturations (Harrison et al., 1991). Using a standardized protocol of social stimulation, Eckerman and colleagues (1994) found that preterm infants of at least 33 weeks' postconceptional age responded to talking by eye opening and arousal, but when touching was added to the talking, the infants showed increased periods of eyes closed and negative facial expressions. Infants with more neurologic insults showed even greater negative responses to touching. This finding suggests that preterm infants are responsive to social stimulation of low intensity, but if the intensity of social stimulation is increased, they are no longer able to cope with it and that medical complications further decrease infants' ability to cope with moderate-intensity social stimulation.

Preterm infants have also been found to respond differently to nurses and parents. In one study, preterm infants opened their eyes more when interacting with parents than when interacting with nurses (Minde et al., 1975). In another study with sicker infants, preterm infants spent more time in active sleep and less time in sleep–wake transition when with their parents than when with nurses (Miller & Holditch-Davis, 1992). In both of these studies, parents and nurses behaved differently toward infants, with nurses more likely to engage in routine nursing and medical procedures and parents more likely to hold infants and provide positive social stimulation. These findings suggest that preterm infants respond to the less active, more social stimulation provided by parents at first by sleeping and then, as they mature, by awakening to engage in interaction. The early sleeping may serve to conserve energy consumption and promote growth.

Kangaroo care, a recent nursing intervention to promote mothers' holding their preterm infants in skin-to-skin contact, has been found, by some researchers, to increase amount of quiet sleep as compared with periods when the infant is alone in the incubator (Ludington, 1990; Ludington et al., 1992). Other researchers, however, have not found any changes in state patterns during kangaroo care (de Leeuw et al., 1991) or have found a decrease in active sleep and an increase in transitional sleep but no change in quiet sleep (Bosque et al., 1995).

Infant Stimulation

A number of the stimulation interventions used with infants are known to affect sleeping and waking states. In some cases, the goal of the intervention is to alter sleeping and waking states either to lower the infant's arousal so as to provide more energy for growth or to promote more mature state patterns. In other cases, the state effects are side effects of interventions that were designed to alter other aspects of the infant's functioning. This section examines the effects of several different types of infant stimulation interventions currently in use in NICUs.

Nonnutritive sucking is an intervention that has been variously used to soothe irritable infants and to promote feedings and growth (Burroughs et al., 1978; Schwartz et al., 1987). It is known to decrease restlessness and increase sleep time in full-term and preterm infants (Neeley, 1979; Woodson et al., 1985). However, these effects only last while it is being used. The BNAS state scores were not altered in preterm infants offered regular nonnutritive sucking during tube feedings as compared to control infants (Field et al., 1982). Nonnutritive sucking is effective in reducing crying after painful procedures and promoting either alertness or sleeping (Campos, 1989; Field & Goldson, 1984). When given to preterm infants just prior to feedings, nonnutritive sucking helps them to arouse into a quiet, waking state, in which they are most likely to feed effectively (Gill et al., 1988; McCain, 1992). Nonnutritive sucking is more effective in this arousal than stroking (McCain, 1992). Other researchers did not find a change of state with nonnutritive sucking but did find that preterm infants receiving nonnutritive sucking before feedings had higher feeding performance scores and more sleep after feedings (Pickler et al., 1993).

Waterbeds are another common infant stimulation intervention known to affect the sleeping and waking states of preterm infants. The purpose of this intervention is to provide compensatory vestibular-proprioceptive stimulation for preterm infants who are largely deprived of this form of stimulation in the NICU. Infants on waterbeds exhibit increased amounts of active and quiet sleep, less irritability, fewer state changes, and decreased crying (Deiriggi, 1990; Korner et al., 1990). These effects are enhanced if the waterbed oscillates (Korner et al., 1990), but even infants on plain waterbeds exhibit more sleep than they do on regular incubator mattresses (Deiriggi, 1990). When infants have been on waterbeds for prolonged periods of time, state effects continue even during periods when the infant is off the waterbed, as evidenced by decreased irritability and increased alertness during a standardized assessment of preterm infant behavior (Korner et al., 1983). It has also been suggested that waterbeds reduce apnea (Korner et al., 1975; Korner et al., 1978). However, it is unlikely that this effect has clinical significance. When infants treated with theophylline for apnea of prematurity were placed on waterbeds, they showed the same state effects as found in infants without this complication, but they did not exhibit decreased apnea (Korner et al., 1982).

Infant massage is another common infant stimulation technique. It provides both tactile and kinesthetic stimulation because it is necessary to move the infant to provide tactile stimulation to different parts of the body. The purpose of this type of stimulation is primarily to promote growth and augment development, but it also affects infant sleeping and waking states. White-Traut and Pate (1987) used the Rice Infant Sensomotor Stimulation, a 10-minute structured massage of the infant's entire body that is done from head to toe, to provide extra stimulation for growing preterm infants. They found that during massage infants were more alert, but it is not clear that this effect was due to the massage. In this study, infants were taken out of the incubator for the massage, so the state changes might be the result of changes in the thermal environment. In another study, the intervention protocol was altered to be more contingent to infant cues (White-Traut et al., 1993). Again, the experimental infants showed increased alertness during the intervention and continued to be alert for 30 minutes afterwards.

In other studies, stroking of the infant's body followed by passive flexion and extension of the extremities for 15 minutes 3 times a day for 10 days was shown to result in increased weight gain in preterm infants (Scafidi et al., 1986; Scafidi et al., 1990). During the massage treatments, infants exhibited more active sleep (Scafidi et al., 1990), but it is questionable whether any state effects persisted after the treatment period. In one study, massage-treated infants exhibited better scores on the NBAS and spent more time awake and active (Scafidi et al., 1986), whereas in the replication, no differences in the state organization of treated and control infants were found (Scafidi et al., 1990).

Rocking is a form of infant stimulation usually performed in order to soothe the infant. It has been administered either directly while holding the infant or by placing the infant in special cribs or incubators modified to rock at specific speeds. The immediate effects of rocking are reduced crying (Byrne & Horowitz, 1981; Van den Daele, 1970). However, the rhythm and direction of rocking are important in determining which of the other states the infant was most likely to exhibit (Byrne & Horowitz, 1981). Exposing preterm infants to rocking over a 2-week period had longer-lasting results (Cordero et al., 1986). They exhibited increased quiet sleep and decreased active sleep.

In yet another study, preterm infants were placed in a nonrigid reclining chair twice a day for 3 hours from about 30 weeks' postconceptional age until hospital discharge (Provasi & Lequien, 1993). Sleeping and waking states were observed for a 2-hour period for control infants and two 2-hour periods for the experimental infants (once in their beds and once in the infant seat) shortly before discharge. Experimental infants spent more time in quiet sleep and active sleep and less time in quiet and agitated waking than the control infants, but there were no differences in the state patterns of the experimental infants when in their beds and in the infant seat.

In a final type of infant stimulation, Thoman and Graham (1986) placed a "breathing" stuffed bear in the incubator with a preterm infant. The goal of this intervention was to provide a form of rhythmic stimulation that would help the infant organize his or her sleeping and waking patterns. In addition, this form of stimulation was voluntary. Because the bear took up only a small part of the incubator and babies were usually put to sleep in positions in which they were not in physical contact with the bear, infants could choose whether or not to remain in contact with the bear whenever their random movements brought them into contact with it. As compared with controls, experimental infants spent a much greater percentage of time in contact with the area of the incubator with the bear. By the end of the intervention period, experimental infants exhibited significantly increased quiet sleep time. This study has been replicated with two additional samples, and both have shown increased contact with the breathing bear as well as more quiet sleep and less active sleep than infants given a nonbreathing bear (Ingersoll & Thoman, 1994; Thoman et al., 1991).

USEFULNESS OF NEONATAL SLEEP–WAKE STATES FOR ASSESSMENT

Sleeping and waking states are ubiquitous characteristics of neonates. The infant's behavioral and physiologic responses are filtered through neural controls mediated by the sleeping and waking states. Although it is certainly possible to give competent nursing care to high-risk infants without considering their sleep–wake states, recognizing specific states will enable the nurse to better interpret both physiologic and behavioral changes. By observing sleeping and waking, the nurse will be able to determine whether physiologic parameters are consistent with those expected in a particular state. Changes in sleeping and waking patterns can be used to help the nurse identify the need for interventions and to aid the evaluation of these interventions. But most of all, by observing sleeping and waking behaviors, the nurse will come to know each infant better and, thus, be better able to provide individualized care. This knowledge of individual infants can then be shared with parents to help them develop positive interactions with their babies.

CONCLUSION

This chapter has outlined the current research on sleep–wake cycles and the clinical application of the findings. Nurses can and do play a big role in controlling sleep in the NICU environment. It is important that parents are included in these efforts to promote positive sleep–wake patterns in the NICU and once the infant is home.

REFERENCES

Acebo, C. (1987). Naturalistic observations of mothers and infants: Descriptions of mother and infant responsiveness and sleep–wake development. *Dissertation Abstracts International, 48,* 2134B (University Microfilms No. DA8722598).

Adam, K. (1980). Sleep as a restorative process and a theory to explain why [Review]. *Progressive Brain Research, 53,* 289–305.

Adam, K., & Oswald, I. (1984). Sleep helps healing [Editorial]. *British Medical Journal Clinical Research Edition, 289*(6456), 1400–1401.

Adamson, T. M., Cranage, S., Maloney, J. E., et al. (1981a). The maturation of respiratory patterns in normal full term infants during the first six postnatal months. I: Sleep states and respiratory variability. *Australian Paediatric Journal, 17*(4), 250–256.

Adamson, T. M., Cranage, S., Maloney, J. E., et al. (1981b). The maturation of respiratory patterns in normal full term infants during the first six postnatal months. II: Sleep states and apnoea. *Australian Paediatric Journal, 17*(4), 257–261.

Als, H. (1986). A synactive model of neonatal behavioral organization: Framework for assessment of neurobehavioral development in the premature infant and for support of infants and parents in the neonatal intensive care environment. Part 1: Theoretical framework. *Physical and Occupational Therapy in Pediatrics, 6*(3–4), 3–53.

Als, H., & Brazelton, T. B. (1981). A new model of assessing the behavioral organization in preterm and fullterm infants: Two case studies. *Journal of the American Academy of Child Psychiatry, 20*(2), 239–263.

Als, H., Duffy, F. H., & McAnulty, G. B. (1988). Behavioral differences between preterm and fullterm newborns as measured on the APIB System scores. *Infant Behavior and Development, 11*(3), 305–318.

Als, H., Lawhon, G., Brown, E., et al. (1986). Individualized behavioral and environmental care for the very low birth weight preterm infant at high risk for bronchopulmonary dysplasia: Neonatal intensive care unit and developmental outcome. *Pediatrics, 78*(6), 1123–1132.

Als, H., Lester, B. M., Tronick, E. C., & Brazelton, T. B. (1982). Manual for the assessment of preterm infants' behavior (APIB). In H. E. Fitzgerald, B. M. Lester, & M. W. Yogman (Eds.), *Theory and research in behavioral pediatrics* (Vol. 1, pp. 65–132). New York: Plenum.

Als, H., Tronick, E., Adamson, L., & Brazelton, T. B. (1976). The behavior of the fullterm but underweight newborn infant. *Developmental Medicine and Child Neurology, 18*(5), 590–602.

Anders, T. F., & Chalemian, R. J. (1974). The effects of circumcision on sleep–wake states in human neonates. *Psychosomatic Medicine, 36*(2), 174–179.

Anders, T., Emde, R., & Parmelee, A. (Eds.). (1971). *A manual of standardized terminology, techniques and criteria for scoring of states of sleep and wakefulness in newborn infants.* Los Angeles: UCLA Brain Information Service/BRI Publications Office.

Anders, T. F., & Keener, M. (1985). Developmental course of nighttime sleep–wake patterns in full-term and premature infants during the first year of life. I. *Sleep, 8*(3), 173–192.

Anders, T. F., Keener, M. A., & Kraemer, H. (1985). Sleep–wake organization, neonatal assessment and development in premature infants during the first year of life. II. *Sleep, 8*(3), 193–206.

Anderson, L. T., Garcia-Coll, C., Vohr, B. R., et al. (1989). Behavioral characteristics and early temperament of premature infants with intracranial hemorrhage. *Early Human Development, 18*(4), 273–283.

Apkarian, P., Mirmiran, M., & Tijssen, R. (1991). Effects of behavioural state on visual processing in neonates. *Neuropediatrics, 22*(2), 85–91.

Arduini, D., Rizzo, G., Giorlandino, C., et al. (1986). The development of fetal behavioural states: A longitudinal study. *Prenatal Diagnosis, 6*(2), 117–124.

Ariagno, R. (1996, January). *Sleep, sleep cycles, and sleep deprivation.* Paper presented at The Physical and Developmental Environment of the High Risk Neonate. Clearwater Beach, FL: University of South Florida College of Medicine.

Ashton, R. (1973). The state variable in neonatal research: A review. *Merrill Palmer Quarterly, 19,* 3–20.

Aylward, G. P. (1981). The developmental course of behavioral states in preterm infants: A descriptive study. *Child Development, 52*(2), 564–568.

Aylward, G. P. (1982). Forty-week full-term and preterm neurologic differences. In L. P. Lipsitt & T. M. Field (Eds.), *Infant behavior and development: Perinatal risk and newborn behavior* (pp. 67–83). Norwood, NJ: Ablex.

Aylward, G. P., Pfeiffer, S. I., Wright, A. & Verhulst, S. T. (1989). Outcome studies of low birth weight infants published in the last decade: A metaanalysis. *The Journal of Pediatrics, 115*(4), 515–520.

Bamford, F. N., Bannister, R. P., Benjamin, C. M., et al. (1990). Sleep in the first year of life. *Developmental Medicine and Child Neurology, 32*(8), 718–724.

Barnard, K. E., & Blackburn, S. (1985). Making a case for studying the ecological niche of the newborn. In B. S. Raff & N. W. Paul (Eds.), *NAACOG Invitational Research Conference. Birth Defects: Original Article Series, 21*(3), 71–88.

Barrington, K. J., Finer, N. N., & Wilkinson, M. H. (1987). Progressive shortening of the periodic breathing cycle duration in normal infants. *Pediatric Research, 21*(3), 247–251.

Beardsmore, C. S., MacFadyen, U. M., Moosavi, S. S., et al. (1989). Measurement of lung volumes during active and quiet sleep in infants. *Pediatric Pulmonology, 7*(2), 71–77.

Beaver, P. K. (1987). Premature infants' response to touch and pain: Can nurses make a difference? *Neonatal Network, 6*(3), 13–17.

Becker, P. T., Chang, A., Kameshima, S., & Bloch, M. (1991a). Correlates of diurnal sleep patterns in infants of adolescent and adult single mothers. *Research in Nursing and Health, 14*(2), 97–108.

Becker, P. T., Grunwald, P. C., Moorman, J., & Stuhr, S. (1991b). Outcomes of developmentally supportive nursing care for very low birth weight infants. *Nursing Research, 40*(3), 150–155.

Becker, P. T., Grunwald, P. C., Moorman, J., & Stuhr, S. (1993). Effects of developmental care on behavioral organization in very-low-birth-weight infants. *Nursing Research, 42*(4), 214–220.

Becker, P. T., & Thoman, E. B. (1981). Rapid eye movement storms in infants: Rate of occurrence at 6 months predicts mental development at one year. *Science, 212*(4501), 1415–1416.

Becker, P. T., & Thoman, E. B. (1982a). Intense rapid eye movements during active sleep: An index of neurobehavioral instability. *Developmental Psychobiology, 15*(3), 203–210.

Becker, P. T., & Thoman, E. B. (1982b). Waking activity: The neglected state of infancy. *Brain Research, 256*(4), 395–400.

Beckwith, L., & Parmelee, A. H., Jr. (1986). EEG patterns of preterm infants, home environment, and later IQ. *Child Development, 57*(3), 777–789.

Bentele, K. H., Albani, M., Budde, C., & Schulte, F. J. (1985). Sleep apnoea profile in preterm infants recovering from respiratory distress syndrome. *Archives of Disease in Childhood, 60*(6), 547–554.

Bhatia, V. P., Katiyar, G. P., Agarwal, K. N., et al. (1980). Sleep cycle studies in babies of undernourished mothers. *Archives of Disease in Childhood, 55*(2), 134–138.

Black, M., Schuler, M., & Nair, P. (1993). Prenatal drug exposure: Neurodevelopmental outcome and parenting environment. *Journal of Pediatric Psychology, 18*(5), 605–620.

Blackburn, S. (1996, January). *Studies of light and its application to clinical practice.* Paper presented at The Physical and Developmental Environment of the High Risk Neonate. Clearwater Beach, FL: University of South Florida College of Medicine.

Blackburn, S., & Patteson, D. (1991). Effects of cycled light on activity state and cardiorespiratory function in preterm infants. *Journal of Perinatal and Neonatal Nursing, 4*(4), 47–54.

Blackburn, S. T., & Barnard, K. E. (1985). Analysis of caregiving events relating to preterm infants in the special care unit. In A. W. Gottfried & J. L. Gaiter (Eds.), *Infant stress under intensive care: Environmental neonatology* (pp. 113–129). Baltimore: University Park Press.

Blass, E. M., & Hoffmeyer, L. B. (1991). Sucrose as an analgesic for newborn infants. *Pediatrics, 87*(2), 215–218.

Booth, C. L., Leonard, H. L., & Thoman, E. B. (1980). Sleep states and behavior patterns in preterm and fullterm infants. *Neuropediatrics, 11*(4), 354–364.

Booth, C. L., Morin, V. N., Waite, S. P., & Thoman, E. B. (1983). Periodic and nonperiodic sleep apnea in premature and fullterm infants. *Developmental Medicine and Child Neurology, 25*(3), 283–296.

Bosque, E. M., Brady, J. P., Affonso, D. D., & Wahlberg, V. (1995). Physiologic measures of kangaroo versus incubator care in a tertiary-level nursery. *Journal of Obstetric, Gynecologic and Neonatal Nursing, 24*(3), 219–226.

Brazelton, T. B. (1984). *Neonatal behavioral assessment scale* (2nd ed.). Spastics International Medical Publications, in association with William Heinemann Medical Books Ltd., London, and J. B. Lippincott Co., Philadelphia.

Brazy, J. E. (1988). Effect of crying on cerebral volume and cytochrome aa_3. *Journal of Pediatrics, 112*(3), 457–461.

Bryan, A. C., & Bryan, M. H. (1978). Control of respiration in the newborn. *Clinics in Perinatology, 5*(2), 269–281.

Burroughs, A. K., Asonye, U. O., Anderson-Shanklin, G. C., & Vidyasagar, D. (1978). The effect of nonnutritive sucking on transcutaneous oxygen tension in noncrying, preterm infants. *Research in Nursing and Health, 1*(2), 69–75.

Butte, N. F., Jensen, C. L., Moon, J. K., et al. (1992). Sleep organization and energy expenditure of breast-fed and formula-fed infants. *Pediatric Research, 32*(5), 514–519.

Byrne, J. M., & Horowitz, F. D. (1981). Rocking as a soothing intervention: The influence of direction and type of movement. *Infant Behavior and Development, 4*(2), 207–218.

Campos, R. G. (1989). Soothing pain-elicited distress in infants with swaddling and pacifiers. *Child Development, 60*(4), 781–792.

Carlo, W. A., Martin, R. J., Abboud, E. F., et al. (1983). Effect of sleep state and hypercapnia on alae nasi and diaphragm EMGs in preterm infants. *Journal of Applied Physiology: Respiratory, Environment and Exercise Physiology, 54*(6), 1590–1596.

Catlett, A. T., & Holditch-Davis, D. (1990). Environmental stimulation of the acutely ill preterm infant: Physiological effects and nursing implications. *Neonatal Network, 8*(6), 19–26.

Chuman, M. A. (1983). The neurological basis of sleep. *Heart and Lung, 12*(2), 177–182.

Clausen, J., Sersen, E. A., & Lidsky, A. (1977). Sleep patterns in mental retardation: Down's syndrome. *Electroencephalography and Clinical Neurophysiology, 43*(2), 183–191.

Cohen, G., Xu, C., & Henderson-Smart, D. (1991). Ventilatory response of sleeping newborn to CO_2 during normoxic rebreathing. *Journal of Applied Physiology, 71*(1), 168–174.

Cohen S. E., Parmelee, A. H., Beckwith, L., & Sigman, M. (1986). Cognitive development in preterm infants: Birth to 8 years. *Journal of Developmental and Behavioral Pediatrics, 7*(2), 102–110.

Colombo, J., & Horowitz, F. D. (1987). Behavioral state as a lead variable in neonatal research. *Merrill-Palmer Quarterly, 33*(4), 423–437.

Coons, S., & Guilleminault, C. (1982). Development of sleep–wake patterns and non-rapid eye movement sleep stages during the first six months of life in normal infants. *Pediatrics, 69*(6), 793–798.

Coons, S., & Guilleminault, C. (1984). Development of consolidated sleep and wakeful periods in relation to the day/night cycle in infancy. *Developmental Medicine and Child Neurology, 26*(2), 169–176.

Cordero, L., Clark, D. L., & Schott, L. (1986). Effects of vestibular stimulation on sleep states in premature infants. *American Journal of Perinatology, 3*(4), 319–324.

Cornell, E. H., & Gottfried, A. W. (1976). Intervention with premature human infants. *Child Development, 47*(1), 32–39.

Cornwell, A. C. (1993). Sex differences in the maturation of sleep/wake patterns in high risk for SIDS infants. *Neuropediatrics, 24*(1), 8–14.

Curzi-Dascalova, L., & Christova-Gueorguieva, E. (1983). Respiratory pauses in normal prematurely born infants: A comparison with full-term newborns. *Biology of the Neonate, 44,* 325-332.

Curzi-Dascalova, L., Gaudebout, C., & Dreyfus-Brisac, C. (1981). Respiratory frequencies of sleeping infants during the first months of life: Correlations between values in different sleep states. *Early Human Development, 5*(1), 39–54.

Curzi-Dascalova, L., Peirano, P., & Morel-Kahn, F. (1988). Development of sleep states in normal premature and fullterm newborns. *Developmental Psychobiology, 21*(5), 431–444.

Dale, J. C. (1986). A multidimensional study of infants' responses to painful stimuli. *Pediatric Nursing, 12*(1), 27–31.

DeHaan, R., Patrick, J., Chess, G. F., & Jaco, N. T. (1977). Definition of sleep state in the newborn infant by heart rate analysis. *American Journal of Obstetrics and Gynecology, 127*(7), 753–758.

Deiriggi, P. M. (1990). Effects of waterbed flotation on indicators of energy expenditure in preterm infants. *Nursing Research, 39*(3), 140–146.

Demarquez, J. L., Brachet-Lierman, A., Paty, J., et al. (1978). Traitement preventif des apnees du premature par la theophylline: Etude clinique, pharmacocinetique, neurophysiologique [Preventive treatment with theophylline of apnea in premature infants: Clinical, pharmacokinetic and neurophysiological study]. *Archives Francaises de Pediatrie, 35*(7), 793–805.

Denenberg, V. H., & Thoman, E. B. (1981). Evidence for a functional role for active (REM) sleep in infancy. *Sleep, 4*(2), 185–191.

Dietrich, J., Krauss, A. N., Reidenberg, M., et al. (1978). Alterations in state in apneic pre-term infants receiving theophylline. *Clinical Pharmacology and Therapeutics, 24*(4), 474–478.

DiPietro, J. A., & Porges, S. W. (1991). Relations between neonatal states and 8-month developmental outcome in preterm infants. *Infant Behavior and Development, 14*(4), 441–450.

Dittrichova, J., & Paul, K. (1989). Respiratory patterns during sleep states in preterm infants. *Activitas Nervosa Superior, 31*(3), 213–214.

DiVitto, B., & Goldberg, S. (1979). The effects of newborn medical status on early parent-infant interaction. In T. M. Field, A. M. Sostek, S. Goldberg, & H. H. Shuman (Eds.), *Infants born at risk: Behavior and development* (pp. 311–332). New York: SP Medical & Scientific Books.

Dixon, S. D., & Bejar, R. (1989). Echoencephalographic findings in neonates associated with maternal cocaine and methamphetamine use: Incidence and clinical correlates. *Journal of Pediatrics, 115*(5, Part 1), 770–778.

Dreyfus-Brisac, C. (1968). Sleep ontogenesis in early human prematurity from 24 to 27 weeks of conceptional age. *Developmental Psychobiology, 1,* 162–169.

Dreyfus-Brisac, C. (1970). Ontogenesis of sleep in human prematures after 32 weeks of conceptional age. *Developmental Psychobiology, 3*(2), 91–121.

Dreyfus-Brisac, C. (1975). Neurophysiological studies in human prematures after 32 weeks of conceptional age. *Biological Psychiatry, 10*(5), 485–496.

Duffy, F. H., Als, H., & McAnulty, G. B. (1990). Behavioral and electrophysiological evidence for gestational age effects in healthy preterm and fullterm infants studied two weeks after expected due date. *Child Development, 61*(4), 271–286.

Duxbury, M. L., Henly, S. J., Broz, L. J., et al. (1984). Caregiver disruptions and sleep of high-risk infants. *Heart and Lung, 13*(2), 141–147.

Eckerman, C. O., Oehler, J. M., Medvin, M. B., & Hannan, T. E. (1994). Premature newborns as social partners before term age. *Infant Behavior and Development, 17*(1), 55–70.

Eilers, B. L., Desai, N. S., Wilson, M. A., & Cunningham, M. D. (1986). Classroom performance and social factors of children with birth weights of 1,250 grams or less: Follow-up at 5 to 8 years of age. *Pediatrics, 77*(2), 203–208.

Ellingson, R. J., & Peters, J. F. (1980). Development of EEG and daytime sleep patterns in low risk premature infants during the first year of life: Longitudinal observations. *Electroencephalography and Clinical Neurophysiology, 50*(1–2), 165–171.

Ellingson, R. J., Peters, J. F., & Nelson, B. (1982). Respiratory pauses and apnea during daytime sleep in normal infants during the first year of life: Longitudinal observations. *Electroencephalography and Clinical Neurophysiology, 53*(1), 48–59.

Emde, R. N., Harmon, R. J., Metcalf, D., et al. (1971). Stress and neonatal sleep. *Psychosomatic Medicine, 33*(6), 491–496.

Emde, R. N., & Walker, S. (1976). Longitudinal study of infant sleep: Results of 14 subjects studied at monthly intervals. *Psychophysiology, 13*(5), 456–461.

Fajardo, B., Browning, M., Fisher, D., & Paton, J. (1990). Effect of nursery environment on state regulation in very-low-birth-weight premature infants. *Infant Behavior and Development, 13*(3), 287–303.

Fajardo, B., Browning, M., Fisher, D., & Paton, J. (1992). Early state organization and follow-up over one year. *Journal of Developmental and Behavioral Pediatrics, 13*(2), 83–88.

Ferrari, F., Torricelli, A., Giustardi, A., et al. (1992). Bioelectric maturation in fullterm infants and in healthy and pathological preterm infants at term post-menstrual age. *Early Human Development, 28*(1), 37–63.

Fewell, J. E., & Baker, S. B. (1987). Arousal from sleep during rapidly developing hypoxemia in lambs. *Pediatric Research, 22*(4), 471–477.

Field, T., & Goldson, E. (1984). Pacifying effects of nonnutritive sucking on term and preterm neonates during heelstick procedures. *Pediatrics, 74*(6), 1012–1015.

Field, T., Ignatoff, E., Stringer, S., et al. (1982). Nonnutritive sucking during tube feedings: Effects on preterm neonates in an intensive care unit. *Pediatrics, 70*(3), 381–384.

Flores-Guevara, R., Plouin, P., Curzi-Dascalova, L., et al. (1982). Sleep apneas in normal neonates and infants during the first 3 months of life. *Neuropediatrics, 13*(Suppl.), 21–28.

Franck, L. S. (1987). A national survey of the assessment and treatment of pain and agitation in the neonatal intensive care unit. *Journal of Obstetric, Gynecologic, and Neonatal Nursing, 16*(6), 387–393.

Friedman, S. L., Jacobs, B. S., & Werthmann, M. W., Jr. (1982). Preterms of low medical risk: Spontaneous behaviors and soothability at expected date of birth. *Infant Behavior and Development, 5*(1), 3–10.

Gabriel, M., Albani, M., & Schulte, F. J. (1976). Apneic spells and sleep states in preterm infants. *Pediatrics, 57*(1), 142–147.

Gabriel, M., Grote, B., & Jonas, M. (1981). Sleep–wake pattern in preterm infants under two different care schedules during four-day polygraphic recording. *Neuropediatrics, 12*(4), 366–373.

Gabriel, M., Helmin, U., & Albani, M. (1980). Sleep induced pO_2 changes in preterm infants. *European Journal of Pediatrics, 134*(2), 153–154.

Gaiter, J. L. (1985). Nursery environments: The behavior and caregiving experiences of full-term and preterm newborns. In A. W. Gottfried & J. L. Gaiter (Eds.), *Infant stress under intensive care: Environmental neonatology* (pp. 55–81). Baltimore: University Park Press.

Gaultier, C. (1990). Respiratory adaptation during sleep in infants [Review]. *Lung, 168*(Suppl.), 905–911.

Gaultier, C. L. (1994). Apnea and sleep state in newborns and infants [Review]. *Biology of the Neonate, 65*(3-4), 231–234.

Gill, N. E., Behnke, M., Conlon, M., et al. (1988). Effect of nonnutritive sucking on behavioral state in preterm infants before feeding. *Nursing Research, 37*(6), 347–350.

Goldie, L., Curtis, J. A. H., Svendsen, U., & Roberton, N. R. C. (1968). Abnormal sleep rhythms in Mongol babies. *Lancet, 1*(7536), 229–230.

Golub, H. L., & Corwin, M. J. (1982). Infant cry: A clue to diagnosis. *Pediatrics, 69*(2), 197–201.

Gorski, P. A., Hole, W. T., Leonard, C. H., & Martin, J. A. (1983). Direct computer recording of premature infants and nursery care: Distress following two interventions. *Pediatrics, 72*(2), 198–202.

Gottfried, A. W. (1985). Environment of newborn infants in special care units. In A. W. Gottfried & J. L. Gaiter (Eds.), *Infant stress under intensive care: Environmental neonatology* (pp. 23–54). Baltimore: University Park Press.

Gottfried, A. W., Wallace-Lande, P., Sherman-Brown, S., et al. (1981). Physical and social environment of newborn infants in special care units. *Science, 214*(4521), 673–657.

Greisen, G., Hellstrom-Vestas, L., Lou, H., et al. (1985). Sleep-waking shifts and cerebral blood flow in stable preterm infants. *Pediatric Research, 19*(11), 1156–1159.

Grunau, R. V., & Craig, K. D. (1987). Pain expression in neonates: Facial action and cry. *Pain, 28*(3), 395–410.

Hack, M. M., Breslau, N., Aram, D., et al. (1992). The effect of very low birth weight and social risk on neurocognitive abilities at school age. *Journal of Developmental and Behavioral Pediatrics, 13*(6), 412–420.

Hack, M., Muszynski, S. Y., & Miranda, S. B. (1981). State of awakeness during visual fixation in preterm infants. *Pediatrics, 68*(1), 87–92.

Haddad, G. G., Jeng, H. J., Lai, T. L., & Mellins, R. B. (1987). Determination of sleep state in infants using respiratory variability. *Pediatric Research, 21*(6), 556–562.

Haddad, G. G., Lai, T. L., & Mellins, R. B. (1982). Determination of ventilatory pattern in REM sleep in normal infants. *Journal of Applied Physiology: Respiratory, Environmental and Exercise Physiology, 53*(1), 52–56.

Hahn, J. S., & Tharp, B. R. (1990). The dysmature EEG pattern in infants with bronchopulmonary dysplasia and its prognostic implications. *Electroencephalography and Clinical Neurophysiology, 76*(2), 106–113.

Halberg, F. (1969). Chronobiology. *Annual Review of Physiology, 31*, 675–725.

Hanson, N., & Okken, A. (1980). Transcutaneous oxygen tension of newborn infants in different behavioral states. *Pediatric Research, 14*(8), 911–915.

Harper, R. M., Leake, B., Miyahara, L., et al. (1981). Temporal sequencing in sleep and waking states during the first 6 months of life. *Experimental Neurology, 72*(2), 294–307.

Harrison, L. L., Leeper, J., & Yoon, M. (1991). Preterm infants' physiologic responses to early parent touch. *Western Journal of Nursing Research, 13*(6), 698–713.

Hellstrom-Westas, L., Rosen, I., & Svenningsen, N. W. (1991). Cerebral function monitoring during the first week of life in extremely small low birthweight (ESLBW) infants. *Neuropediatrics, 22*(1), 27–32.

Henderson-Smart, D. J. (1981). The effect of gestational age on the incidence and duration of recurrent apnoea in newborn babies. *Australian Paediatric Journal, 17*(4), 273–276.

Henderson-Smart, D. J., & Read, D. J. (1979). Reduced lung volume during behavioral active sleep in the newborn. *Journal of Applied Physiology: Respiratory, Environmental and Exercise Physiology, 46*(6), 1081–1085.

High, P. C., & Gorski, P. A. (1985). Recording environmental influences on infant development in the intensive care nursery: Womb for improvement. In A. W. Gottfried & J. L. Gaiter (Eds.), *Infant stress under intensive care: Environmental neonatology* (pp. 131–155). Baltimore: University Park Press.

Holditch-Davis, D. (1990a). The development of sleeping and waking states in high-risk preterm infants. *Infant Behavior and Development, 13*(4), 513–531.

Holditch-Davis, D. (1990b). The effect of hospital caregiving on preterm infants' sleeping and waking states. In S. G. Funk, E. M. Tornquist, M. T. Champagne, et al. (Eds.), *Key aspects of recovery: Improving nutrition, rest, and mobility* (pp. 110–122). New York: Springer.

Holditch-Davis, D. (1995). Behaviors of preterm infants with and without chronic lung disease when alone and when with nurses. *Neonatal Network, 14*(7), 51–57.

Holditch-Davis, D., Barham, L. N., O'Hale, A., & Tucker, B. (1995). The effect of standardized rest periods on convalescent preterm infants. *Journal of Obstetric, Gynecologic and Neonatal Nursing, 24*(5), 424–432.

Holditch-Davis, D., & Calhoun, M. (1989). Do preterm infants show behavioral responses to painful procedures? In S. G. Funk, E. M. Tornquist, M. T. Champagne, et al. (Eds.), *Key aspects of comfort: Management of pain, fatigue, and nausea* (pp. 35–43). New York: Springer.

Holditch-Davis, D., & Edwards, L. (1995a). *Modelling the development of sleep–wake states: Part 2. Results from two cohorts of high-risk preterm infants.* Manuscript under review.

Holditch-Davis, D., & Edwards, L. (1995b). *Temporal organization of sleep–wake states in preterm infants.* Manuscript under review.

Holditch-Davis, D., Edwards, L. J., & Wigger, M. C. (1994). Pathologic apnea and brief respiratory pauses in preterm infants: Relation to sleep state. *Nursing Research, 43*(5), 293–300.

Holditch-Davis, D., & Hudson, D. C. (1995). Using preterm infant behaviors to identify acute medical complications. In S. G. Funk, E. M. Tornquist, M. T. Champagne, & R. A. Wiese (Eds.), *Key aspects of caring for the acutely ill: Technological aspects, patient education, and quality of life* (pp. 95–120). New York: Springer.

Holditch-Davis, D. & Lee, D. A. (1993). The behaviors and nursing care of preterm infants with chronic lung disease. In S. G. Funk, E. M. Tornquist, M. T. Champagne, & R. A. Wiese (Eds.), *Key aspects of caring for the chronically ill: Hospital and home* (pp. 250–270). New York: Springer.

Holditch-Davis, D., & Thoman, E. B. (1987). Behavioral states of premature infants: Implications for neural and behavioral development. *Developmental Psychobiology, 20*(1), 25–38.

Holmes, D. L., Nagy, J. N., Slaymaker, F., et al. (1982). Early influences of prematurity, illness, and prolonged hospitalization on infant behavior. *Developmental Psychology, 18*(5), 744–750.

Holmes, D. L., Reich, J. N., & Pasternak, J. F. (1984). *The development of infants born at risk.* Hillsdale, NJ: Lawrence Erlbaum.

Holmes, G. L., Logan, W. J., Kirkpatrick, B. V., & Meyers, E. C. (1979). Central nervous system maturation in the stressed premature. *Annals of Neurology, 6*(6), 518–522.

Hopkins, B., & von Wulfften, Palthe, T. (1987). The development of the crying state during early infancy. *Developmental Psychobiology, 20*(2), 165–175.

Hoppenbrouwers, T., Harper, R. M., Hodgman, J. E., et al. (1978). Polygraphic studies of normal infants during the first six months of life: II. Respiratory rate and variability as a function of state. *Pediatric Research, 12*(2), 120–125.

Hoppenbrouwers, T., Hodgman, J. E., Arakawa, K., et al. (1980). Respiration during the first six months of life in normal infants: III. Computer identification of breathing pauses. *Pediatric Research, 14*(11), 1230–1233.

Hoppenbrouwers, T., Hodgman, J., Arakawa, K., et al. (1988). Sleep and waking states in infancy: Normative studies. *Sleep, 11*(4), 387–401.

Howard, J., Parmelee, A. H., Jr., Kopp, C. B., & Littman, B. (1976). A neurologic comparison of pre-term and full-term infants at term conceptional age. *The Journal of Pediatrics, 88*(6), 995–1002.

Huch, R., & Huch, A. (1981). Continuous pO_2 and pCO_2 monitoring in the neonate. *Journal of Perinatal Medicine, 9*(4), 200–203.

Huntington, L., Hans, S., & Zeskind, P. S. (1990). The relations among cry characteristics, demographic variables, and developmental test scores in infants prenatally exposed to methadone. *Infant Behavior and Development, 13,* 533–538.

Ingersoll, E. W., & Thoman, E. B. (1994). The breathing bear: Effects on respiration in premature infants. *Physiology and Behavior, 56*(5), 855–859.

Jeremy, R. J., & Hans, S. L. (1985). Behavior of neonates exposed in utero to methadone as assessed on the Brazelton Scale. *Infant Behavior and Development, 8*(3), 323–336.

Ju, S.-H., Lester, B., Garcia-Coll, C., et al. (1991). Maternal perceptions of the sleep patterns of premature infants at seven months corrected age compared to full-term infants. *Infant Mental Health Journal, 12*(4), 338–346.

Junge, H. D. (1979). Behavioral states and state related heart rate and motor activity patterns in the newborn infant and fetus ante partum: A comparative study. II. Computer analysis of state related heart rate baseline and macrofluctuation patterns. *Journal of Perinatal Medicine,* 7(3), 134–148.

Kahn, A., Groswasser, J., Rebuffat, E., et al. (1992). Sleep and cardiorespiratory characteristics of infant victims of sudden death: A prospective case-control study. *Sleep, 15*(4), 287–292.

Karch, D., Rothe, R., Jurisch, R., et al. (1982). Behavioural changes and bioelectric brain maturation of preterm and fullterm newborn infants: A polygraphic study. *Developmental Medicine and Child Neurology, 24*(1), 30–47.

Kitchen, W. H., Ford, G. W., Doyle, L. W., et al. (1990). Health and hospital readmissions of very-low-birth-weight and normal-birth-weight children. *American Journal of Diseases in Children, 144*(2), 213–218.

Kohyama, J., & Iwakawa, Y. (1990). Developmental changes in phasic sleep parameters as reflections of the brain-stem maturation: Polysomnographical examinations of infants, including premature neonates. *Electroencephalography and Clinical Neurophysiology, 76*(4), 325–330.

Korner, A. F. (1972). State as variable, obstacle, and as mediator of stimulation in infant research. *Merrill-Palmer Quarterly, 18*(2), 77–94.

Korner, A. F., Brown, B. W., Jr., Reade, E. P., et al. (1988). State behavior of preterm infants as a function of development, individual and sex differences. *Infant Behavior and Development, 11*(1), 111–124.

Korner, A. F., Guilleminault, C., Van den Hoed, J., & Baldwin, R. B. (1978). Reduction of sleep apnea and bradycardia in preterm infants on oscillating water beds: A controlled polygraphic study. *Pediatrics, 61*(4), 528–533.

Korner, A. F., Kraemer, H. C., Haffner, M. E., & Cosper, L. M. (1975). Effects of waterbed flotation on premature infants: A pilot study. *Pediatrics, 56*(3), 361–367.

Korner, A. F., Lane, N. M., Berry, K. L., et al. (1990). Sleep enhanced and irritability reduced in preterm infants: Differential efficacy of three types of waterbeds. *Journal of Behavioral and Developmental Pediatrics, 11*(5), 240–246.

Korner, A. F., Ruppel, E. M., & Rho, J. M. (1982). Effects of water beds on the sleep and motility of theophylline-treated preterm infants. *Pediatrics, 70*(6), 864–869.

Korner, A. F., Schneider, P., & Forrest, T. (1983). Effects of vestibular-proprioceptive stimulation on the neurobehavioral development of preterm infants: A pilot study. *Neuropediatrics, 14*(3), 170–175.

Korner, A. F., Stevenson, D. K., Forrest, T., et al. (1994). Preterm medical complications differentially affect neurobehavioral functions: Results from a new neonatal medical index. *Infant Behavior and Development, 17*(1), 37–43.

Kotzer, A. M. (1994). Maternal smoking and infant sleep behavior. *Neonatal Network, 13*(1), 65.

Lawson, K. (1977). Environmental characteristics of a neonatal intensive care unit. *Child Development, 48*(4), 1633–1639.

Lawson, K. R., Turkewitz, G., Platt, M., & McCarton, C. (1985). Infant state in relation to its environmental context. *Infant Behavior and Development, 8*(3), 269–281.

Lee, D., Caces, R., Kwiatkowski, K., et al. (1987). A developmental study on types and frequency distribution of short apneas (3 to 15 seconds) in term and preterm infants. *Pediatric Research, 22*(3), 344–349.

de Leeuw, R., Colin, E. M., Dunnebier, E. A., & Mirmiran, M. (1991). Physiological effects of kangaroo care in very small preterm infants. *Biology of Neonate, 59*(3), 149–155.

Lester, B. M. (1987). Developmental outcome prediction from acoustic cry analysis in term and preterm infants. *Pediatrics, 80*(4), 529–534.

Lester, B. M., & Dreher, M. (1989). Effects of marijuana use during pregnancy on newborn cry. *Child Development, 60*(4), 765–771.

Lester, B. M., Emory, E. K., & Hoffman, S. L. (1976). A multivariate study of the effects of high-risk factors on performance on the Brazelton Neonatal Assessment Scale. *Child Development, 47*(2), 515–517.

Lester, B. M., Garcia-Coll, C., Valcarcel, M., et al. (1986). Effects of atypical patterns of fetal growth on newborn (NBAS) behavior. *Child Development, 57*(1), 11–19.

Linn, P. L., Horowitz, F. D., Buddin, B. J., et al. (1985). An ecological description of a neonatal intensive care unit. In A. W. Gottfried & J. L. Gaiter (Eds.), *Infant stress under intensive care: Environmental neonatology* (pp. 83–111). Baltimore: University Park Press.

Lodrup, K. C., Mowinckel, P., & Carlsen, K. H. (1992). Lung function measurements in awake compared to sleeping newborn infants. *Pediatric Pulmonology, 12*(2), 99–104.

Lombroso, C. T., & Matsumiya, Y. (1985). Stability in waking-sleep states in neonates as a predictor of long-term neurologic outcome. *Pediatrics, 76*(1), 52–63.

Long, J. G., Lucey, J. F., & Philip, A. G. S. (1980). Noise and hypoxemia in the intensive care nursery. *Pediatrics, 65*(2), 143–145.

Long, J. G., Philip, A. G., & Lucey, J. F. (1980). Excessive handling as a cause of hypoxemia. *Pediatrics, 65*(2), 203–207.

Ludington, S. M. (1990). Energy conservation during skin-to-skin contact between premature infants and their mothers. *Heart and Lung, 19*(5, Part 1), 445–451.

Ludington, S. M., Thompson, C., & Swinth, J. (1992). Efficacy of kangaroo care with preterm infants in open-air cribs. *Neonatal Network, 11*(6), 101.

Mann, N. P., Haddow, R., Stokes, L., Goodley, S., & Rutter, N. (1986). Effect of night and day on preterm infants in a newborn nursery: Randomised trial. *British Medical Journal: Clinical Research Edition, 293*(6557), 1265–1267.

Marchette, L., Main, R., & Redick, E. (1989). Pain reduction during neonatal circumcision. *Pediatric Nursing, 15*(2), 207–210.

Martin, R., Okken, A., & Rubin, D. (1979). Changes in arterial oxygen tension during quiet and active sleep in the neonate. *Birth Defects: Original Article Series, 15*(4), 493-494.

Martin, R. J., Herrell, N., & Pultusker, M. (1981). Transcutaneous measurement of carbon dioxide tension: Effect of sleep state in term infants. *Pediatrics, 67*(5), 622–625.

McCain, G. C. (1992). Facilitating inactive awake states in preterm infants: A study of three interventions. *Nursing Research, 41*(3), 157–160.

McGehee, L. J., & Eckerman, C. O. (1983). The preterm infant as a social partner: Responsive but unreadable. *Infant Behavior and Development, 6*(4), 461–470.

McMillen, I. C., Kok, J. S., Adamson, T. M., et al. (1991). Development of circadian sleep–wake rhythms in preterm and full-term infants. *Pediatric Research, 29*(4, Part 1), 381–384.

McNeely, J. B. (1987). *Preterm heart rate in twelve behavioral states.* Unpublished master's thesis, University of Florida, Gainesville.

Meier-Koll, A., Hall, U., Hellwig, U., et al. (1978). A biological oscillator system and the development of sleep-waking behavior during early infancy. *Chronobiologia, 5*(4), 425–440.

Michelsson, K., Rinne, A., & Paajanen, S. (1990). Crying, feeding and sleeping patterns in 1 to 12-month-old infants. *Child: Care, Health and Development, 16*(2), 99–111.

Miller, D. B., & Holditch-Davis, D. (1992). Interactions of parents and nurses with high-risk preterm infants. *Research in Nursing and Health, 15*(3), 187–197.

Milligan, D. W. A. (1979). Cerebral blood flow and sleep state in the normal newborn infant. *Early Human Development, 3*(4), 321–328.

Minde, K., Ford, L., Celhoffer, L., & Boukydis, C. (1975). Interactions of mothers and nurses with premature infants. *Canadian Medical Association Journal, 113*(8), 741–745.

Minde, K., Whitelaw, A., Brown, J., & Fitzhardinge, P. (1983). Effect of neonatal complications in premature infants on early parent–infant interactions. *Developmental Medicine and Child Neurology, 25*(6), 763–777.

Mirmiran, M. (1986). The importance of fetal/neonatal REM sleep. *European Journal of Obstetrics, Gynecology, and Reproductive Biology, 21*(5-6), 283–291.

Mok, J. Y., Hak, H., McLaughlin, F. J., et al. (1988). Effect of age and state of wakefulness on transcutaneous oxygen values in preterm infants: A longitudinal study. *The Journal of Pediatrics, 113*(4), 706–709.

Moriette, G., Chaussain, M., Radvanyi-Bouvet, M. F., et al. (1983). Functional residual capacity and sleep states in the premature newborn. *Biology of the Neonate, 43*(3–4), 125–133.

Moseley, M. J., Thompson, J. R., Levene, M. I., & Fielder, A. R. (1988). Effects of nursery illumination on frequency of eyelid opening and state in preterm infants. *Early Human Development, 18*(1), 13–26.

Myers, B. J., Jarvis, P. A., Creasey, G. L., et al. (1992). Prematurity and respiratory illness: Brazelton Scale (NBAS) performance of preterm infants with bronchopulmonary displasia (BPD), respiratory distress syndrome (RDS), or no respiratory illness. *Infant Behavior and Development, 15*(1), 27–42.

Neeley, C. A. (1979). Effects of nonnutritive sucking upon the behavioral arousal of the newborn. *Birth Defects: Original Article Series, 15*(7), 173–200.

Nijhuis, J. G. (1986). Behavioural states: Concomitants, clinical implications and the assessment of the condition of the nervous system. *European Journal of Obstetrics, Gynecology, and Reproductive Biology, 21*(5-6), 301–308.

Nijhuis, J. G., Prechtl, H. F., Martin, C. B., Jr., & Bots, R. S. (1982). Are there behavioural states in the human fetus? *Early Human Development, 6*(2), 177–195.

Norris, S., Campbell, L. A., & Brenkert, S. (1982). Nursing procedures and alterations in transcutaneous oxygen tension in premature infants. *Nursing Research, 31*(6), 330–336.

Oehler, J. M. (1995) Development of mother-child interaction in very low birth weight infants. In S. G. Funk, E. M. Tornquist, M. T. Champagne, & R. A. Wiese (Eds.), *Key aspects of caring for the acutely ill: Technological aspects, patient education, and quality of life* (pp. 120–133). New York: Springer.

Oehler, J. M., Eckerman, C. O., & Wilson, W. H. (1988). Social stimulation and the regulation of premature infants' state prior to term age. *Infant Behavior and Development, 11*(3), 333–351.

Oehler, J. M., Hannan, T., & Catlett, A. (1993). Maternal views of preterm infants' responsiveness to social interaction. *Neonatal Network, 12*(6), 67–74.

Orem, J. (1980). Medullary respiratory neuron activity: Relationship to tonic and phasic REM sleep. *Journal of Applied Physiology: Respiratory, Environmental and Exercise Physiology, 48*(1), 54–65.

Orem, J., & Barnes, C. D. (1980). *Physiology in sleep*. New York: Academic.

Orr, W. C., Stahl, M. L., Duke, J., et al. (1985). Effect of sleep state and position on the incidence of obstructive and central apnea in infants. *Pediatrics, 75*(5), 832–835.

Palmer, P. G., Dubowitz, L. M., Verghote, M., & Dubowitz, V. (1982). Neurological and neurobehavioural differences between preterm infants at term and full-term newborn infants. *Neuropediatrics, 13*(4), 183–189.

Paludetto, R., Mansi, G., Rinaldi, P., et al. (1986). Moderate hyperbilirubinemia does not influence the behavior of jaundiced infants. *Biology of the Neonate, 50*(1), 43–47.

Parmelee, A. H., Jr., Schulte, F. J., Akiyama, Y., et al. (1968). Maturation of EEG activity during sleep in premature infants. *Electroencephalography and Clinical Neurophysiology, 24*(4), 319–329.

Parmelee, A. H., Jr., & Stern, E. (1972). Development of states in infants. In C. D. Clemente, D. P. Purpura, & F. E. Mayer (Eds.), *Sleep and the maturing nervous system* (pp. 200–215). New York: Academic Press.

Parmelee, A. H., Jr., Wenner, W. H., Akiyama, Y., et al. (1967). Sleep states in premature infants. *Developmental Medicine and Child Neurology, 9*(1), 70–77.

Peabody, J. L., & Lewis, K. (1985). Consequences of newborn intensive care. In A. W. Gottfried & J. L. Gaiter (Eds.), *Infant stress under intensive care: Environmental neonatology* (pp. 199–226). Baltimore: University Park Press.

Petre-Quadens, O. (1974). Sleep in the human newborn. In O. Petre-Quadens & J. D. Schlag (Eds.), *Basic sleep mechanisms* (pp. 355–376). New York: Academic Press.

Phillipson, E. A. (1978). Control of breathing during sleep. *American Review of Respiratory Disease, 118*(5), 909–939.

Phillipson, E. A., & Sullivan, C. E. (1978). Respiratory control mechanisms during NREM and REM sleep. In C. Guilleminault & W. C. Dement (Eds.), *Sleep apnea syndromes* (pp. 47–64). New York: Alan R. Liss.

Pickler, R. H., Higgins, K. E., Crummette, B. D. (1993). The effect of nonnutritive sucking on bottle-feeding stress in preterm infants. *Journal of Obstetric, Gynecologic and Neonatal Nursing, 22*(3), 230–234.

Prechtl, H. F. R., & Beintema, J. (1968). *The neurological examination of the full-term newborn infant*. Spastics International Medical Publications, in association with William Heinemann Medical Books, Ltd., London, and J. B. Lippincott Co., Philadelphia.

Prechtl, H. F. R., Fargel, J. W., Weinmann, H. M., & Bakker, H. H. (1979). Postures, motility and respiration of low-risk pre-term infants. *Developmental Medicine and Child Neurology, 21*, 3–27.

Prechtl, H. F., Theorell, K., & Blair, A. W. (1973). Behavioural state cycles in abnormal infants. *Developmental Medicine and Child Neurology, 15*(5), 606–615.

Prechtl, H. F., Theorell, K., Gramsbergen, A., & Lind, J. (1969a). A statistical analysis of cry patterns in normal and abnormal newborn infants. *Developmental Medicine and Child Neurology, 11*(2), 142–152.

Prechtl, H. F., Weinmann, H., & Akiyama, Y. (1969b). Organization of physiological parameters in normal and neurologically abnormal infants. *Neuropadiatrie, 1*(1), 101–129.

Provasi, J., & Lequien, P. (1993). Effects of nonrigid reclining infant seat on preterm behavioral states and motor activity. *Early Human Development, 35*(2), 129–140.

Ramaekers, V. T., Casaer, P., Daniels, H., et al. (1989). The influence of behavioural states on cerebral blood flow velocity patterns in stable preterm infants. *Early Human Development, 20*(3-4), 229–246.

Rigatto, H. (1982). Apnea. *Pediatric Clinics of North America, 29*(5), 1105–1116.

Rigatto, H., Kalapesi, Z., Leahy, F. N., et al. (1982). Ventilatory response to 100% and 15% O_2 during wakefulness and sleep in preterm infants. *Early Human Development, 7*(1), 1–10.

Robinson, J., Moseley, M. J., Thompson, J. R., & Fielder, A. R. (1989). Eyelid opening in preterm neonates. *Archives of Disease in Childhood, 64*(7, Spec. No.), 943–948.

Roffwarg, H. P., Muzio, J. N., & Dement, W. C. (1966). Ontogenetic development of the human sleep-dream cycle. *Science, 152*, 604–619.

Rosenthal, M. K. (1983). State variations in the newborn and mother-infant interaction during breast feeding: Some sex differences. *Developmental Psychology, 19*(5), 740–745.

Sahni, R., Schulze, K. F., Stefanski, M., et al. (1995). Methodological issues in coding sleep states in immature infants. *Developmental Psychobiology, 28*(2), 85–101.

Sander, L. W., Stechler, G., Burns, S., & Julia, H. (1970). Early mother–infant interaction and 24-hour patterns of activity and sleep. *Journal of American Academy of Child Psychiatry, 9*(1), 103–123.

Sander, L. W., Stechler, G., Burns, P., & Lee, A. (1979). Changes in infant and caregiver variables over the first two months of life: Regulation and adaptation in the organization of the infant–caregiver system. In E. B. Thoman (Ed.), *Origins of the infant's social responsiveness* (pp. 349–407). Hillsdale, NJ: Lawrence Erlbaum.

Scafidi, F. A., Field, T. M., Schanberg, S. M., et al. (1990). Massage stimulates growth in preterm infants: A replication. *Infant Behavior and Development, 13*, 167–168.

Scafidi, F. A., Field, T. M., Schanberg, S. M., et al. (1986). Effects of tactile/kinesthetic stimulation on the clinical course and sleep/wake behavior of preterm neonates. *Infant Behavior and Development, 9*(1), 91–105.

Schechtman, V. L., Harper, R. M., Wilson, A. J., & Southall, D. P. (1992). Sleep state organization in normal infants and victims of the sudden infant death syndrome. *Pediatrics, 89*(5), 865–870.

Scher, A. (1991). A longitudinal study of night waking in the first year. *Child: Care, Health and Development, 17*(5), 295–302.

Scher, M. S., Richardson, G. A., Coble, P. A., et al. (1988). The effects of prenatal alcohol and marijuana exposure: Disturbances in neonatal sleep cycling and arousal. *Pediatric Research, 24*(1), 101–105.

Scher, M. S., Richardson, G., Salerno, D. G., & Guthrie, R. D. (1992a). Sleep architecture and continuity measures in neonates with chronic lung disease. *Sleep, 15*(3), 195–201.

Scher, M. S., Steppe, D. A., & Banks, D. L. (1994a). Lower neurodevelopmental performance at 2 years in healthy preterm neonates. *Pediatric Neurology, 11*, 121.

Scher, M. S., Steppe, D. A., Dahl, R. E., et al. (1992b) Comparisons of

EEG-sleep measures in healthy full-term and preterm infants of matched conceptual ages. *Sleep 15*(5), 442–448.

Scher, M. S., Sun, M., Steppe, D. A., et al. (1994b). Comparisons of EEG sleep state specific spectral values between healthy full-term and preterm infants at comparable postconceptional ages. *Sleep, 17*(1), 47–51.

Scher, M. S., Sun, M., Steppe, D. A., et al. (1994c). Comparisons of EEG spectral and correlation measures between healthy term and preterm infants. *Pediatric Neurology, 10*(2), 104–108.

Schulte, F. J., Busse, C., & Eichhorn, W. (1977). Rapid eye movement sleep, motoneurone inhibition, and apneic spells in preterm infants. *Pediatric Research, 11*(6), 709–713.

Schwartz, R., Moody, L., Yarandi, H., & Anderson, G. C. (1987). A meta-analysis of critical outcome variables in nonnutritive sucking in preterm infants. *Nursing Research, 36*(5), 292–295.

Sehring, S., Gorski, P., Sweet, D., et al. (1985, April). Bradycardia in preterm infants. One response to caregiver touch. In T. Field (Chair), *Supplemental stimulation of ICU neonates*. Symposium presented at the biennial meeting of the Society for Research in Child Development, Toronto.

Shaywitz, B. A., Finkelstein, J., Hellman, L., & Weitzman, E. D. (1971). Growth hormone in newborn infants during sleep–wake periods. *Pediatrics, 48*(1), 103–109.

Shimada, M., Segawa, M., Higurashi, M.,& Akamatsu, H. (1993). Development of the sleep and wakefulness rhythm in preterm infants discharged from a neonatal intensive care unit. *Pediatric Research, 33*(2), 159–163.

Speidel, B. D. (1978). Adverse effects of routine procedures on preterm infants. *Lancet, 1*(8069), 864–865.

Stefanski, M., Schulze, K., Bateman, D., et al. (1984). A scoring system for states of sleep and wakefulness in term and preterm infants. *Pediatric Research, 18*(1), 58–62.

Strauss, M. E., Lessen-Firestone, J. K., Starr, R. H., Jr., & Ostrea, E. M., Jr. (1975). Behavior of narcotics-addicted newborns. *Child Development, 46*(4), 887–893.

Sullivan, C. E. (1980). Breathing in sleep. In J. Orem & C. D. Barnes (Eds.), *Physiology in sleep* (pp. 213–272). New York: Academic Press.

Swartjes, J. M., van Geijn, H. P., Mantel, R., et al. (1990). Coincidence of behavioral state parameters in the human fetus at three gestational ages. *Early Human Development, 2*(2), 75–83.

Telzrow, R. W., Kang, R. R., Mitchell, S. K., et al. (1982). An assessment of the behavior of the preterm infant at 40 weeks conceptional age. In L. P. Lipsitt & T. M. Field (Eds.), *Infant behavior and development: Perinatal risk and newborn behavior* (pp. 85–96). Norwood, NJ: Ablex.

Thoman, E. B. (1975a). Early development of sleeping behaviors in infants. In N. R. Ellis (Ed.), *Aberrant development in infancy: Human and animal studies* (pp. 122–138). New York: John Wiley & Sons.

Thoman, E. B. (1975b). Sleep and wake behaviors in neonates: Consistencies and consequences. *Merrill-Palmer Quarterly, 21*(4), 295–314.

Thoman, E. B. (1982). A biological perspective and a behavioral model for assessment of premature infants. In L. A. Bond & J. M. Joffee (Eds.), *Primary prevention of psychopathology: Facilitating infant and early childhood development* (Vol. 6, pp. 159–179). Hanover, NH: University Press of New England.

Thoman, E. B. (1985). *Sleep and waking states of the neonate* (rev. ed.). (Unpublished manuscript, available from E. B. Thoman, Box U-154, Graduate Program in Biobehavioral Sciences, 3107 Horsebarn Hill Road, University of Connecticut, Storrs, CT 06268.)

Thoman, E. B. (1990). Sleeping and waking states in infancy: A functional perspective. *Neuroscience and Biobehavioral Reviews, 14*(1), 93–107.

Thoman, E. B., Acebo, C., & Becker, P. T. (1983). Infant crying and stability in the mother-infant relationship: A systems analysis. *Child Development, 54*(3), 653–659.

Thoman, E. B., Acebo, C., Dreyer, C. A., Becker, P. T., & Freese, M. P. (1979). Individuality in the interactive process. In E. B. Thoman (Ed.), *Origins of the infant's social responsiveness* (pp. 305–338). Hillsdale, NJ: Lawrence Erlbaum.

Thoman, E. B., & Becker, P. T. (1979). Issues in assessment and prediction for the infant born at risk. In T. Field, A. Sostek, S. Goldberg, & H. H. Shuman (Eds.), *Infants born at risk: Behavior and development* (pp. 461–483). New York: SP Medical and Scientific Books.

Thoman, E. B., Denenberg, V. H., Sieval, J., et al. (1981). State organization in neonates: Developmental inconsistency indicates risk for developmental dysfunction. *Neuropediatrics, 12*(1), 45–54.

Thoman, E. B., & Graham, S. E. (1986). Self-regulation of stimulation by premature infants. *Pediatrics, 78*(5), 855–860.

Thoman, E. B., Holditch-Davis, D., & Denenberg, V. H. (1987). The sleeping and waking states of infants: Correlations across time and person. *Physiology and Behavior, 41*(6), 531–537.

Thoman, E. B., Holditch-Davis, D., Graham, S. E., et al. (1988). Infants at risk for sudden infant death syndrome (SIDS): Differential prediction for three siblings of SIDS infants. *Journal of Behavioral Medicine, 11*(6), 565-583.

Thoman, E. B., Holditch-Davis, D., Raye, J. R., et al. (1985). Theophylline affects sleep–wake state development in premature infants. *Neuropediatrics, 16*(1), 13–18.

Thoman, E. B., Ingersoll, E. W., & Acebo, C. (1991). Premature infants seek rhythmic stimulation, and the experience facilitates neurobehavioral development. *Journal of Behavioral and Developmental Pediatrics, 12*(1), 11–18.

Thoman, E. B., Korner, A. F., & Kraemer, H. C. (1976). Individual consistency in behavioral states in neonates. *Developmental Psychobiology, 9*(3), 271–283.

Thoman, E. B., Miano, V. N., & Freese, M. P. (1977). The role of respiratory instability in the Sudden Infant Death Syndrome. *Developmental Medicine and Child Neurology, 19*, 729–738.

Thoman, E. B., & Whitney, M. P. (1989). Sleep states of infants monitored in the home: Individual differences, developmental trends, and origins of diurnal cyclicity. *Infant Behavior and Development, 12*(1), 59–75.

Thomas, K. A. (1989). How the NICU environment sounds to a preterm infant. *MCN; American Journal of Maternal/Child Nursing, 14*, 249–251.

Torres, C., Holditch-Davis, D., O'Hale, A., & Tucker, B. (in press). *Effect of standardized rest periods on apnea and weight gain of convalescent preterm infants. Neonatal Network.*

Tynan, W.D. (1986). Behavioral stability predicts morbidity and mortality in infants from a neonatal intensive care unit. *Infant Behavior and Development, 9*, 71–79.

Van Cleve, L., Johnson, L., Andrews, S., et al. (1995). Pain responses of hospitalized neonates to venipuncture. *Neonatal Network, 14*(6), 31–36.

Van den Daele, L. D. (1970). The modification of infant state by treatment in a rockerbox. *Journal of Psychology, 74*(2), 161–165.

van Ravenswaaij-Arts, C. M., Hopman, J. C., & Kollee, L. A. (1989). Influence of behavioural state on blood pressure in preterm infants during the first 5 days of life. *Acta Paediatrica Scandinavica, 78*(3), 358–363.

Visser, G. H., Carse, E. A., Goodman, J. D., & Johnson, P. (1982). A comparison of episodic heart-rate patterns in the fetus and newborn. *British Journal of Obstetrics and Gynecology, 89*(1), 50–55.

Visser, G. H., Poelmann-Weesjes, G., Cohen, T. M., & Bekedam, D. J. (1987). Fetal behavior at 30 to 32 weeks of gestation. *Pediatric Research, 22*(6), 655–658.

Vles, J. S., van Oostenbrugge, R. J., Hasaart, T. H., et al. (1992). State profile in low-risk pre-term infants: A longitudinal study of 7 infants from 32–36 weeks of postmenstrual age. *Brain and Development, 14*(1), 12–17.

Vohr, B. R., Karp, D., O'Dea, C., et al. (1990). Behavioral changes correlated with brain-stem auditory evoked responses in term infants with moderate hyperbilirubinemia. *The Journal of Pediatrics, 117*(2, Part 1), 288–291.

Vohr, B. R., Lester, B., Rapisardi, G., et al. (1989). Abnormal brain-stem function (brain-stem auditory evoked response) correlates with acoustic features in term infants with hyperbilirubinemia. *The Journal of Pediatrics, 115*(2), 303–308.

Waite, S. P., & Thoman, E. B. (1981). Brief apneas and reliable assessment of respiratory instability. *Sleep, 4*(1), 61–69.

Waite, S. P., & Thoman, E. B. (1982). Periodic apnea in the full-term infant: Individual consistency, sex differences, and state specificity. *Pediatrics, 70*(1), 79–86.

Watt, J. E., & Strongman, K. T. (1985). The organization and stability of sleep states in fullterm, preterm, and small-for-gestational-age infants: A comparative study. *Developmental Psychobiology, 18*(2), 151–162.

Weissbluth, M. (1995). Naps in children: 6 months–7 years. *Sleep, 18*(2), 82–87.

White-Traut, R. C., Nelson, M. N., Silvestri, J. M., et al. (1993). Patterns of physiologic and behavioral response of intermediate care preterm infants to intervention. *Pediatric Nursing, 1*(6), 625–629.

White-Traut, R. C., & Pate, C. M. (1987). Modulating infant state in premature infants. *Journal of Pediatric Nursing, 2*(2), 96–101.

Whitney, M. P., & Thoman, E. B. (1993). Early sleep patterns of premature infants are differentially related to later developmental disabilities. *Journal of Developmental and Behavioral Pediatrics, 14*(2), 71–80.

Wolff, P. H. (1959). Observations on newborn infants. *Psychosomatic Medicine, 21,* 110–118.

Wolff, P. H. (1966). The causes, controls, and organization of behavior in the neonate. *Psychological Issues, 5*(1), 1–105.

Woods, N. S., Eyler, F. D., Behnke, M., & Conlon, M. (1993). Cocaine use during pregnancy: Maternal depressive symptoms and infant neurobehavior over the first month. *Infant Behavior and Development, 16*(1), 83–98.

Woodson, R., Drinkwin, J., & Hamilton, C. (1985). Effects of nonnutritive sucking on state and activity: Term-preterm comparisons. *Infant Behavior and Development, 8*(4), 435–441.

Woodson, R., Field, T., & Greenberg, R. (1983). Estimating neonatal oxygen consumption from heart rate. *Psychophysiology, 20*(5), 558–561.

Zahr, L. K., & Balian, S. (1995). Responses of premature infants to routine nursing interventions and noise in the NICU. *Nursing Research, 44*(3), 179–185.

Zinman, R., Blanchard, P. W., & Vachon, F. (1992). Oxygen saturation during sleep in patients with bronchopulmonary dysplasia. *Biology of the Neonate, 61*(2), 69–75.

CHAPTER 49

Assessment and Management of Neonatal Neurobehavioral Development

SUSAN TUCKER BLACKBURN KATHLEEN A. VANDENBERG

RESEARCH AGENDA

What are the effects of specific developmental intervention strategies (such as reduction of sound and light levels, cycled lighting, containment, and kangaroo care) on infant physiologic function and neurobehavioral organization?

What are the long-term effects of developmental care on the extremely low birth weight infant's neurologic development in early childhood?

What are the long-term effects of developmental care on the drug-exposed infant's developmental progress through the first 2 years of life?

The care of high-risk infants, both those born prematurely and those with medical, surgical, or developmental problems, has long been a major focus of health care concern. Efforts to increase the understanding of the pathophysiologic problems encountered by these infants, along with new management strategies and technologies, have markedly improved the outcome of these infants. Much of the focus of the neonatal intensive care unit (NICU) has been on meeting the physiologic needs of these infants, with less attention, until recently, on the social interactive consequences of this environment. Thus, the advances in neonatal care have been accompanied by increasing concerns and documentation regarding the impact of the NICU environment on the infant's physiologic and neurobehavioral functioning, the lack of sensory input geared to meet the individual infant's needs and current level of developmental function, and the effects of stress and overstimulation.

Although tremendous progress has been made in reducing mortality and morbidity in high-risk infants, these infants, especially those born prematurely, are still vulnerable to a wide variety of neurodevelopmental problems. These problems have been referred to as the "new morbidities of low birth weight infants" and include behavioral disorganization, attention deficit disorders, hyperexcitability, language problems, sensory/perceptual and higher-order cognitive problems, and school dysfunction (Blackburn, 1995). Adverse outcomes of high-risk infants may be related to a variety of factors, including immaturity, perinatal trauma, the early NICU environment, the home environment in which the child is raised, and parent–child interactional considerations. The development of many of these infants is characterized by an unevenness that can lead to later difficulties. This unevenness may be as much the result of the impact of the early environment and its incongruences as the effects of perinatal stress.

The immature infant differs in two important ways from the healthy full-term infant. First, these infants are born early and therefore must deal with and adapt to the extrauterine environment with bodily systems, including a central nervous system (CNS), that are not yet mature. Second, this interruption of intrauterine life significantly modifies the environment of the infant (Blackburn & Barnard, 1985). Thus, the preterm infant spends the last weeks or months of gestation in an environment—the NICU—that is much different from that of the uterus or that of a healthy full-term infant. The NICU environment has similar implications for the more mature, although still vulnerable, ill full-term infant. For these infants, this environment is also abnormal and quite different from that experienced by healthy infants who go home with their parents soon after birth. In considering the vulnerabilities of ill and immature infants, it is useful to examine the implications of each of these areas: the state of CNS development, neonatal neurobehavioral development, and the NICU environment.

FETAL AND NEONATAL CENTRAL NERVOUS SYSTEM DEVELOPMENT

As noted in Chapter 29, Assessment and Management of Neurologic Dysfunction, the development of the CNS can be divided into six overlapping stages (see Table 29–1). These stages are important to consider in examining the effects of the NICU environment because the stage of development influences the effect of any insult. In addition, several areas of the CNS continue to undergo significant changes during the period when preterm infants are in the NICU, increasing their vulnerability to insult. The stage of development is also reflected by the behaviors characteristic of immature infants (Table 49–1). The first three stages of CNS development (dorsal induction, ventral induction, and neuronagenesis) are completed before the fourth month of gestation. However, the last three stages (neuron migration, synaptogenesis and arborization, and myelinization) continue during the time many infants are in the NICU (Volpe, 1995). Myelinization, although vulnerable to perinatal insults, is a process that continues for many years. Therefore, unless insults are severe or prolonged, their effects may be mitigated.

Areas of development during the last part of gestation that are particularly critical in considering neurobehavioral vulnerabilities of ill or immature infants include: (1) autonomic homeostatic control; (2) alterations in the germinal matrix; (3) pattern of

TABLE 49–1 Neurodevelopmental Limitations of the Very Low Birth Weight Infant and Related Behavioral Manifestations

Limitations in Neurologic Function	
Sparse myelin	Slow nerve conduction
Lung refractory period	Slow synaptic potential
Weak transmission	Unable to sustain high firing rates
Decreased inhibitory potential	Incomplete cell differentiation
Decreased functional validation (ability to utilize various systems)	Decreased synaptogenesis and dendritic arborization
Behaviors of Immature Infants	
Irregular state regulation	Jerky movements
Increased and decreased tone	Low arousal, inability to sustain an alert state
Alterations in primitive reflexes	Poor coordination
Easily exhausted	Altered autonomic regulation
Irritable, difficult to soothe	Asymmetrical, uncoordinated posture and movement
Inability to inhibit	

dendritic connections; and (4) growth of the cerebellum. From about 28 to 32 weeks' gestational age, preterm infants begin to achieve some degree of physiologic homeostasis, with increasing control of the sympathetic system over their autonomic functioning, at least at the subcortical level. With increasing autonomic control, the infant develops greater autonomic stability. This autonomic stability can be seen, for example, in the decreasing incidence of apnea and bradycardia. As these infants move to greater cortical control over the next months, their development is characterized by periods of temporary organization followed by periods of disorganization as new levels of maturation and control are achieved. These periods of disorganization are reflected in the infant's sleep–wake patterns, proportion of transitional or indeterminate sleep, and fragmented behavioral responses and reflexes (Nelson, 1987; Sarnat, 1984).

The germinal matrix in the periventricular area is a site of origin for neuronal and glial cells, which migrate from this area to their eventual loci within the CNS. Until 32 to 34 weeks' gestational age, the fragile, poorly supported blood vessels in this area receive a significant proportion of cerebral blood flow (Volpe, 1995). Insults to this area before this period may lead to periventricular and intraventricular hemorrhage (see Chapter 29, Assessment and Management of Neurologic Dysfunction).

The pattern of dendritic connections between neurons is a critical growth process that begins during the sixth month of gestation and may be particularly vulnerable to insults from the effects of the NICU environment. The interconnections between individual neurons constitute the "wiring" of the brain. Dendritic connections, or arborization, are critical for processing of impulses and for cell-to-cell communication. Lack of connections can result in hypersensitivity, poorly modulated behaviors, and all-or-nothing responses, which can often be observed in preterm infants in the NICU (see Table 49–1). Similar behavior patterns can also be seen in some children in later infancy and childhood.

The cerebellum is also vulnerable to insults from the early environment. The cerebellum is primarily concerned with control of muscles and coordination of movements; it undergoes a critical growth spurt at 30 to 32 weeks' gestation. This spurt includes an increase in dendritic arborization, which is complete earlier than many other areas of the brain. Insults may lead to the altered sequences of motor development seen in some preterm infants (Nelson, 1987).

NEONATAL NEUROBEHAVIORAL DEVELOPMENT

To provide developmentally supportive care for high-risk infants in the NICU, the nurse must have an understanding of their behavioral capabilities and responses. A model for understanding the organization of neurobehavioral capabilities in the development of the fetus, infant, and young child, developed by Als (1982, 1986), describes emerging behavioral organizational abilities of the neonate (Fig. 49–1). This model is based on the assumption that infants actively communicate via their behavior, which becomes an important route for understanding thresholds of stress or stability. Behavior of the infant not only is the main route of communication but also provides the basis for the structure of developmental assessment and provision of developmentally appropriate care (Als, 1986).

This synactive theory of development (Als, 1982) provides a model through which one can specify the degree of differentiation of behavior and the ability of infants to organize and control their behavior. The focus is not on assessment of skills, but on the unique way each individual infant deals with the world around her or him. The synactive theory of development specifies the range of neonatal behavior as the infant matures as well as the ability of the infant to regulate behavior. This model is based on the assumption that the infant's primary route of communicating both functional stability and the limits for stress is through behavior (Als, 1986). For example, infants who extend their limbs after being turned to supine to have their diaper changed may be communicating that they cannot control their limbs and movement in that position. Containing the limbs of these infants helps them to develop control and reduces stress over the loss of control.

Infants are seen as being in continual interaction with their environment via five subsystems: autonomic/physiologic; motor; state/organizational; attentional/interactive; and self-regulatory. These subsystems mature sequentially, and within each subsystem a developmental sequence can be observed. Thus, at each stage of development, new tasks and organizations are learned against the backdrop of previous development. The subsystems are interdependent and interrelated. For example, physiologic stability provides the foundation for motor and state control; the infant cannot respond socially to caregivers until motor and state control is achieved. The loss of integrity in one subsystem can influence the organization of other subsystems in response to environmental demands. In the preterm, less organized infant, the systems interplay, continuously influencing each other. In the full-term infant, these systems are synchronized and function smoothly. Thus full-term infants can regulate their autonomic, motor, state, and attentional systems with ease and without apparent stress. However, less mature infants tend to be able to tolerate only one activity at a time and may easily lose control if required to do more.

Instability in the autonomic system can be seen in the pattern of respiration (pauses, tachypnea), color changes (red, pale, dusky, mottled), and various visceral signs (regurgitation, twitching, stooling). Organization of the motor system is assessed by observing the infant's tone and posture (flexed, extended, hyperflexed, flaccid); specific movement patterns of the extremities, head, trunk and face; and level of activity. The development of motor responses is closely linked to state organization (Als, 1986, 1996). The organization of neuromotor responses moves from minimal capacity for response, to a phase of obligatory, autonomic (all-or-nothing) response, to development of smoother, more organized responses with more individual variation (Sammons & Lewis, 1985).

The state system is understood by noting the available range of states of consciousness (sleep to arousal, awake to alert, crying); how well-defined each state is (in terms of behavioral and physiologic parameters); transitions between states; and the quality of organization of these states (see Chapter 48, Neonatal Sleep–Wake States). States may be poorly defined at first, especially in the immature infant. For example, jerky body twitches and fussing may accompany sleep and wake states. In addition, the imma-

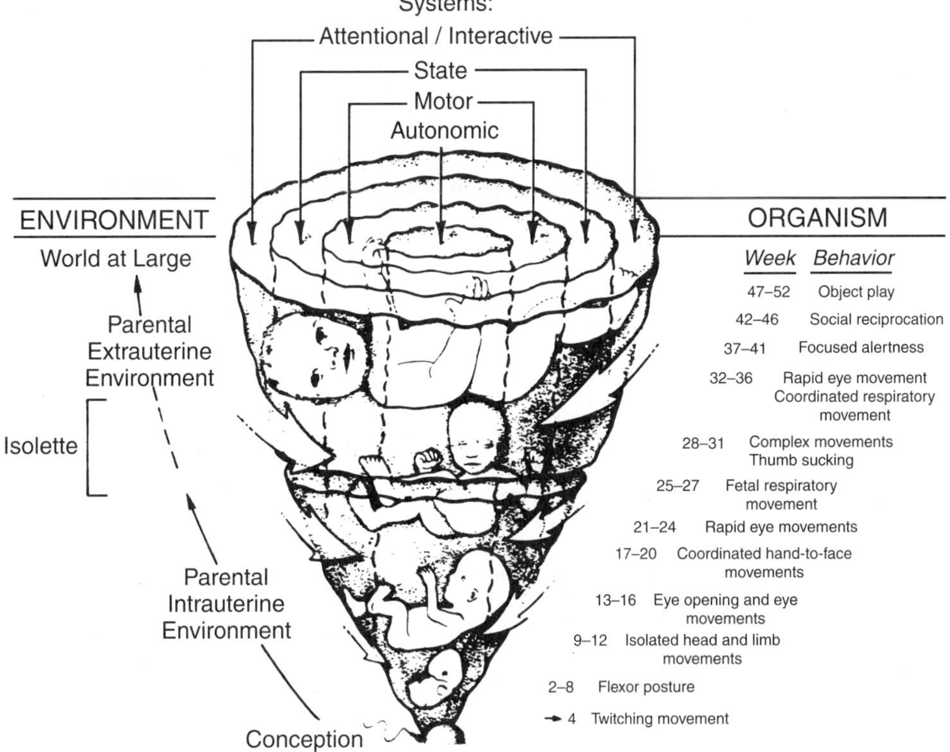

FIGURE 49–1. Model of the synactive organization of behavioral development. (From Als, H. [1982]. Toward a synactive theory of development: Promise for the assessment and support of infant individuality. *Infant Mental Health Journal, 3*[4], 229–243. Reprinted with permission.)

ture infant may not be able to achieve clearly defined states as seen in the mature infant (Ariagno et al., 1996a, 1996b).

Initially, preterm infants tend to be unstable and fragile, with sudden changes in their autonomic, motor, and state systems. These infants often have all-or-nothing responses, that is, they may have minimal response to handling or other sensory input until a threshold is reached, then quickly develop a cascade of responses, ending in several color changes, flaccidity, bradycardia, and apnea. As the infant matures, the responses are more variable and the infant is less likely to totally decompensate (Als, 1986, 1996). Changes within the autonomic, motor, and state systems at all stages of development are not just reactions to stress and overstimulation, but are warning signs. By recognizing these signs early, the nurse can intervene to prevent severe decompensation.

The attentional/interactive system involves the infant's ability to orient and focus on sensory stimuli, such as faces, sounds, or objects—the external environment. This system also includes the range of abilities in states of consciousness: how well-defined periods of alertness are and how transitions into and out of alertness are handled. At first, this alertness may be very brief with a dull look or glassy-eyed stare. As this system matures, the infant is able to interact with greater ease and for longer periods. Social responsiveness requires that the infant has enough state control to sustain some awake and alert states (Als, 1986; Sammons & Lewis, 1985).

The self-regulatory system includes behaviors the infant uses to maintain the integrity and balance of the other subsystems, to integrate the other systems, and to move smoothly between states. For example, some infants can tuck their limbs close to their body in an effort to gain control when stressed, whereas others seem to relax if they can brace a foot against the side of the crib.

In summary, "the process of development appears to be that of stabilization and integration of some subsystems, which allows the differentiation and emergence of others which in turn feed back on the integrated system. In this process the whole system is reopened and transformed to a new level of more differentiated integration from which the next newly emerging subsystem can further differentiate and press to actualization and realization" (Als, 1982, 1996). By observing and assessing the infant's responses to the caregiver and other aspects of the environment across these five subsystems of behavioral functioning, one can develop and implement a plan of care to support the infant's emerging neurodevelopmental organization and reduce stress.

Assessment of Neonatal Neurobehavioral Development

Developmental assessment of newborn functioning emerged with the awareness of the amazing capabilities of neonates. The newborn infant, for years was thought to be nonreactive and incapable of social participation, is now seen as an active participant in social interaction and capable of self-regulation (Als, 1984, 1996; Brazelton, 1984). Even with a greater understanding of newborn capabilities, researchers and clinicians have been unable to accurately predict the future course of an infant's development from early neurologic or behavioral assessments.

Historically, two types of neonatal assessments have evolved, the neurologic examination and the behavioral examination. The neurologic examination assesses the function of the CNS and typically includes assessment of motor tone and reflex behaviors within the context of infant state. The behavioral examination complements and elaborates on the neurologic assessment (Gorski et al., 1987). An assumption underlying the behavioral examination is that the observable behavior of an infant is a reflection of her or his underlying neurologic status. The behavioral examination seeks to describe the quality of behavioral performance (Als, 1984). More recently, these two forms of assessment have been combined into the neurodevelopmental or neurobehavioral assessment.

The neurodevelopmental examination is important because it yields a large pool of early observable behavior, including information about the infant's neurologic status and abilities to cope and interact with the environment. In addition, data from this examination can assist the clinician in estimating maturity and in identifying and evaluating problems that could be precursors to later developmental problems. Because the neurodevelopmental examination provides an immediate basis for determining the status of the infant's development, the results can be used for planning intervention strategies as well as for screening for infants in need of further diagnostic assessments.

Who Needs To Be Assessed?

All neonates and their caregivers can benefit from ongoing neurobehavioral assessment. These assessments provide information on the infant's behavioral capabilities, interactive qualities, and adaptations to the extrauterine environment. This information can be used in planning care, developing individualized intervention strategies, modifying care as the infant matures, and parent teaching and other activities to promote parent–infant interaction. However, for some infants, neurodevelopmental assessment is critical for documentation of neurodevelopmental status, screening, and early case finding.

Certain groups of infants are at increased risk for developmental disabilities and later cognitive impairment (Leonard et al., 1990). Infants that fall into the highest risk category include very low birth weight (VLBW) infants and those with significant intracranial hemorrhages. Preterm infants with known sensory impairment and chronic illness are also at risk for later cognitive dysfunction. Infants with respiratory distress syndrome (RDS) are at greater risk if they also develop chronic lung disease. Severe bronchopulmonary dysplasia (BPD) is generally associated with a prolonged and complicated hospital course, increasing the risk for later neurodevelopmental problems (Ariagno et al., 1996b; Bull & Dodge, 1996).

Neurobehavioral Assessment in the Neonatal Intensive Care Unit

Neurobehavioral assessment can be performed at several different levels and is an essential part of comprehensive care of the high-risk infant in the NICU. Individuals such as Brazelton, Als, and their colleagues have sought to assess preterm and full-term newborn behavior and adaptations. Their work is based on an understanding of newborns as competent individuals with emerging developmental processes who are engaged in dynamic interactions and negotiations with their environment. As a result, several tools have been developed to describe and quantify neurobehavioral organization of both preterm and full-term newborns. The tools that are described here are the Brazelton Neonatal Behavioral Assessment Scale (NBAS) (Brazelton, 1984) and the Assessment of Preterm Infant Behavior (APIB) (Als et al., 1982), which is a component of the neonatal individualized development care and assessment program (NIDCAP) (Als, 1984).

Brazelton Neonatal Behavioral Assessment Scale

The NBAS is a comprehensive behavioral assessment of the healthy full-term neonate. The NBAS combines evaluation of basic reflex responses with the integration of motor capacity, state regulation, and interactive abilities (Brazelton, 1984). Infants are followed through the various states of sleep, arousal, and wakefulness and assessed on their ability to self-regulate in the face of increasingly vigorous activity. A primary focus is observation of the infant's individual and unique ability to respond to outside stimulation while regulating responses to and coping with pleasurable or stressful situations. The infant's best performance is scored. The results are an assessment of the infant's ability to (1) organize states; (2) habituate to external stimulation; (3) regulate motoric activity in the face of increasing sensory input; (4) respond to reflex testing; (5) alert and orient to visual and auditory stimuli; (6) interact with a caregiver; and (7) self-console. Individuals planning to use the NBAS for clinical or research purposes must establish reliability with a recognized trainer. Training in the use of the NBAS is provided in various locations throughout the United States.

The NBAS has been used in numerous studies of neonatal behavior, including investigations of cross-cultural differences, characteristics of drug-addicted infants, effects of obstetric medication, and aspects of maternal-infant interaction (Brazelton, 1984, 1990; Eisen et al., 1991; Gorski et al., 1987). An especially valuable use of the NBAS for nurses and other clinicians is as an intervention. For example, by performing an NBAS in front of the infant's parents, the parents become increasingly aware of and amazed at the remarkable abilities of their infant. An understanding of their newborn's capacity to interact visually, turn to their voices, regulate state and motor activity, and self-console expands the parent's perception of the infant as a unique, competent individual and enhances parent–infant interaction (Als, 1984; Blackburn & Kang, 1991; Brazelton, 1990).

In response to a need to identify the preterm infant's neurobehavioral repertoire, the NBAS was expanded and modified for use with low birth weight infants. Items were added to the original scale, including difficulty of elicitation of alerting, degree of facilitation necessary to support the infant, control over stimulation, robustness, endurance, degree of exhaustion, quality of alertness, and balance of tone (Brazelton, 1984; Kang & Barnard, 1979). These subscales are also useful in describing at-risk full-term infants such as drug-exposed infants.

Assessment of Preterm Infant Behavior

The APIB was developed to respond to the need for a more discrete assessment of preterm infant functioning. Als (1984) felt that the additional items on the NBAS encompassed only the range of behavior close to that of the full-term infant and did not provide a comprehensive description of the subtler differences seen in less mature neonates. The APIB is based on the synactive theory of development, which describes the early behavioral organization and development of the neonate. The APIB is particularly useful for the preterm and full-term high-risk infant from birth to 44 weeks' postconceptional age. The purpose of this assessment is to determine organization of the CNS and how infants cope with the intense environment of the NICU. The focus of the APIB is not only on assessment of skill performance or specific responses to various stimuli, but on the unique way each individual infant deals and interacts with the world around her or him. As described previously, infants are seen as being in continual interaction with their environment and as communicating their responsiveness via five subsystems (autonomic, motor, state, attentional, and self-regulatory) (Als, 1986).

The APIB consists of six packages or sets of maneuvers adapted from the NBAS. The packages are organized to provide increasing input with which the infant must deal, starting with stimulation while the infant is asleep to assess habituation. Subsequent packages move through maneuvers ranging from low and medium tactile manipulations to high tactile and vestibular handling. Throughout the assessment, the infant is continually observed for responses related to each of the five subsystems. Thus, the infant is observed and scored on each of the five subsystems and for examiner facilitation (ability to use support) before, during, and after administration of the items in each package. These responses are called the system scores and range on a 9-point scale from organized (1) to disorganized (9).

The APIB has been used for research and clinical purposes. As a research tool, it has been used to describe and identify neonatal behavioral organization in preterm and other high-risk infants (Als, 1986). Clinically, the APIB has been used by psychologists, neonatologists, neurologists, nurses, developmental specialists, and therapists in providing consultation in the NICU regarding developmental interventions for specific infants. The APIB is useful in determining an infant's degree of fragility and ability to tolerate different caregiving parameters. By measuring maturity of the five subsystems, one can determine maturity of each system and tolerance for handling as well as generate developmental care plans specific to each infant at that stage of development. The APIB is also useful in assessing infant readiness for changes in caregiving routines and in the physical and social environment. Assessing the degree of fragility and tolerance for activities can provide an invaluable piece of information about the infant's functional level and assist staff in making decisions about whether to protect the infant or to advance to the next level of care, as illustrated in the following case:

A 28-week preterm infant had just been extubated and graduated to oxygen by nasal cannula and moved from the open bed to the incubator. An APIB revealed a responsive infant, but one who was working extremely hard to regulate his system amidst two major changes: extubation and change of physical environment. Although successful regulation was noted, it was also apparent that the infant was at maximal capacity in organizing himself. He showed efforts to tuck and maintain hand to mouth; however, he could not maintain these postures for long without help. It was apparent that the infant's threshold had been reached and that any more change or stress would have caused a loss of control in his system's integrity. Immediately after the assessment, nipple feedings once a day were ordered by the neonatologists. With this new demand, the examiner felt that this infant would exceed his threshold and be unable to regulate himself. The developmental specialist recommended waiting 1 week for the infant to stabilize and integrate his new experiences before taking on any new demands. This recommendation was not followed, and feeding continued. Two days later, the developmental specialist returned and noted that the infant had a trial of nippling. He had desaturated, become bradycardic, required bag-and-mouth ventilation, and was considered to have "flunked" nippling. The order was terminated, with the plan to try again in a week. When feeding was reordered a week later, the infant tolerated it well.

Training in the APIB is extensive and requires knowledge of the NICU, including care practices and routines, staffing patterns, and typical infant experiences in that setting as well as physiologic limitations and medical problems.

Neonatal Individualized Development Care and Assessment Program

The NIDCAP incorporates several levels of developmental training in assessment techniques and intervention planning for high-risk preterm and full-term infants. Included in this program is an observation tool (level 1 NIDCAP—naturalistic behavioral observation), which is extremely useful for the NICU nurse. This assessment involves an observation of the infant before, during, and after a routine caregiving episode. It provides the NICU nurse with information on the infant's individual cues for both stress and stable, organized function. The nurse can then structure the infant's experiences, including caregiving interventions and the physical and social environment, to support the infant at the current level of tolerance. This support includes an awareness of the timing of caregiving events, sequencing events and interventions to prevent or reduce stress as well as to enhance stable behavior. Support for parents in understanding their infant's unique behavior and needs is also provided. An example of an assessment and recommended interventions is provided in Table 49–2.

Training in this assessment involves a one-day didactic session and clinical demonstration of the observational tool, after which the trainee completes a specified number of observations on infants of different gestational age, postbirth age, and health status. This observation period is followed by an assessment of reliability for certification by the trainer.

Assessment Beyond Neonatal Development in the NICU

As the infant matures, moves out of the neonatal period, and becomes a "long termer" in the NICU with chronic respiratory or other problems, neurodevelopmental assessments continue to provide important information. For the infant who requires prolonged hospitalization, a developmental assessment at the bedside can provide information on how the infant interacts with objects and people, organizes behavior, and copes with the environment, as well as on the infant's neurologic status. No formal developmental assessments have been standardized for these NICU populations. Most developmental psychologists or specialists adapt items from other examinations such as the Bayley Scales of Infant Development (Bayley, 1969).

Owing to the nature and severity of their illness, these infants may not be able to tolerate a complete examination at one session. To learn about the infant's behavioral capabilities and coping abilities adequately, the examiner must consider events that occurred for several hours preceding the assessment and be aware of the environment in which the infant normally lives and her or his usual types of sensory experiences. Important areas of assessment include (1) availability of alerting; (2) ability to use interventions for consoling or developmental activities; (3) self-soothing capacity; (4) motor activities and strengths; (5) tolerance for handling (how long? with whom?); (6) degree of fragility; (7) degree of distractibility; (8) hand use; (9) parts of body available for use; and (10) respiratory capacity and tolerance.

NEONATAL INTENSIVE CARE UNIT ENVIRONMENT

The high-risk infant in a NICU is living in a highly unusual environment that provides markedly different experiences than the home environment of the healthy full-term neonate. The full-term healthy infant generally has access to a consistent nurturing caregiver and an appropriate variety of stimulation. The full-term infant with 40 weeks of intrauterine development is ready for a variety of sensory experiences, including visual, tactile, auditory, kinesthetic, proprioceptive, olfactory, and gustatory. When these competencies to process sensory information interplay with experience, appropriate patterns of adaptation, cognitive learning, and motor control are formed. The impact of illness on an immature CNS, with accompanying restriction of movement, exposure to high levels of inappropriately patterned sensory input, and loss of a consistent primary caregiver, can alter adaptation patterns and lead to distortions in functioning (Bull & Dodge, 1996; Gorski et al., 1980).

To better understand the possible contributions of early environmental factors to the developmental problems associated with prematurity and other high-risk events and to the development of attachment between high-risk infants and their parents, it is

TABLE 49–2 NIDCAP Behavioral Observation

Peter N. was observed in the NICU from 10:00 AM to 10:32 AM at ABC Hospital in the Intensive Care Nursery on 5/5/95.

Environment

The room is one of 4 rooms in the NICU with 8 beds in it, 4 on each wall. Two large floor-to-ceiling windows behind a partial wall are letting in a flood of light from the outside. Without the overheads on, this is filtered light, and in the corner where Peter is, the light is dim. At the end of the room are two separate isolation rooms with alcoves to each. Overall the room is moderately noisy with staff talking and occasional overhead announcements. There is an ambiance of moderately hectic activity.

Bedding and Bedspace

Peter is bedded on a mattress with sheepskin on it and positioning aid on top of that. His Isolette is covered with a thick printed crib cover which lets in very little light and seems to also block noise. The front flaps can be lifted to let in measured amounts of light as needed. Peter has recently graduated to CPAP and has prongs with long plastic tubing attached to his face, with a hat to hold it all in place. He is wearing only a diaper and has monitor leads taped to his chest. Peter rests in his nest with the wraps of the nest tucked securely over his body to hold his feet and arms in place.

Behavior During Baseline Observation

Peter was lying on his side with his head in midline and was in an active sleep with his legs extended into the soft pillows of the nest at the end of his bed. His arms were flexed with his hands close to his face.

The following cycle of activity was noted repeatedly during this part of the observation. His respirations became irregular and as he became active, he began to squirm, with his respirations becoming even more irregular. He alternated between pausing in respirations, accompanied by squirms, to actively stretching and moving his arms, legs and trunk. He appeared to struggle to regain control of his breathing after long pausing. His respirations were in the 50s, but with squirming episodes, they dropped into the 30s, and then into the 70s after pauses. His color remained pink throughout, but his body tremored, startled, and twitched several times. Peter appeared uncomfortable, with his oxygen level remaining in high 90s when he breathed regularly, but when he paused, his oxygen level dipped into the low 90s with good recovery on his own. Peter completed several of these active uncomfortable cycles as his nurse came to the bedside.

Behavior During Caregiving

Peter immediately settled into a quieter, more regular sleep with more regular respirations as his nurse announced her arrival by putting her hands on his limbs. His breathing stayed in the 60s with improved pink color. He moved into a stable, calm sleep with arms and legs quiet. As vitals were finished, she removed her hands, and his oxygen level dipped into the low 80s, respirations became faster and heart rate was in the 160s with increasing pale color. As she put her hands on him again to change his diaper, his breathing once again became more regular and oxygen levels increased to high 90s, with breathing in 50s. He was able to maintain a stable active sleep state with arms and legs still and very quiet with only an occasional grimace while extending one leg to brace into the nest. As she moved very gently and slowly, Peter responded well, maintaining breathing, heart rate and oxygen levels with slightly improved color, but still fast breathing. As he was rotated to his side, he braced his feet together and grimaced with his hands close but not to his face. He became drowsy and attempted to open his eyes, but frowned and averted his gaze, returning to sleep. His nurse rewrapped the nest wraps around his shoulder and feet, keeping his feet and hands flexed and supported. He remained in light sleep, with pale color; heart rate in 160s and breathing regular but fast in 60s and oxygen levels in 90s.

Behavior Following Caregiving

After his nurse left the bedside, Peter remained with his legs and feet braced into the bottom of the nest and his arms together while in a partial sidelying position. His arms were flexed, but not near his face. He remained sleepy, became drowsy with pale color, and breathing remained fast in 60–70s range with oxygen levels in 72–98 range and heart rate in 150–170s.

Summary of Behavioral Observation

Peter is demonstrating that he has several competent behaviors available to use to stabilize himself such as maintaining his flexed postures and strategies such as leg bracing, hand to mouth, and tucking. When he is uncomfortable (as it appears he is from the CPAP apparatus), he is not able to call these behaviors into play to regulate himself, unless the caregiver helps actively. Peter demonstrates his sensitivity to position changes and handling with variations in his breathing, which becomes irregular and fast, along with pale color and dips in oxygen levels. When his caregiver is available to him, supports him with gentle pacing of care, and protects him from light and noise, Peter responds well and is tolerant of handling.

Peter's Current Goals

Peter apparently seems to be working towards:

1. becoming increasingly effective at maintaining stable regular breathing and oxygen levels, heart rate, and color during caregiving and when on his own.
2. becoming increasingly effective at maintaining flexed postures with hands and feet together.
3. becoming increasingly effective in achieving restful deep sleep and calm awake times during caregiving.

Recommendations

A. *Environment at Large*

1. Consider maintaining quiet around his bedside so that he can achieve deep sleep in between handling.
2. Consider and discuss the possibility of turning off overhead lights and drawing drapes when light is bright.
3. Consider, discuss, and review the alternatives to the loudspeaker system.

B. *Bedspace and Bedding*

1. Consider use of bunting, soft one-piece suit to support flexion and balanced movement in arms and legs.
2. If nest is used, consider use of flaps to keep feet and hands together and near the surrounding softness.
3. Position nest so his feet can brace against it and touch (consider use of diaper in ways that more of softness from nest can be felt).
4. Maintain use of crib cover, considering one that is totally dark for nighttime sleeping and using one with filtered light for day support.

C. *Direct Caregiving*

1. Continue to maintain hands on support before, during, and after caregiving events such as diapering (this is an especially helpful intervention for Peter).
2. Consider the possibility of turning Peter slowly and carefully with hands holding all limbs to allow him to recover from each event before moving on.
3. Consider the possibility of positioning Peter with hands to mouth and together.
4. Before caregiving, consider Peter's readiness for touch. Review lighting and positioning, and anticipate Peter's reaction to being moved.
5. Plan ahead to avoid increased activity and stress for Peter.

NIDCAP, Neonatal Individualized Development Care and Assessment Program; NICU, neonatal intensive care unit.

essential to examine the environment in which these infants spend the critical period of their development. White-Traut and colleagues (1994) noted that although the last two sensory systems to become functional are the visual and auditory systems, these two systems commonly receive the most, and often random, stimulation in the NICU environment. Thus the NICU environment is inconsistent with the preterm infant's level of development and quite different from the intrauterine one.

Intrauterine Environment

The intrauterine environment, with few exceptions, is recognized as the optimal environment to foster the growth and development of the fetus. This environment provides a variety of stimuli to the fetus while modifying the intensity and nature of the sensory input. Characteristics of the intrauterine milieu include (1) auditory input such as the maternal heartbeat, bowel sounds, and muffled sounds from the extrauterine environment; (2) vestibular, tactile, and kinesthetic stimuli from maternal and fetal movements; and (3) rhythmic and cyclic recurrent stimuli such as the maternal heartbeat, maternal sleep and activity patterns, and neurohormonal cycles (Blackburn & Barnard, 1985; Graven, 1996).

NICU Environment: Overview

Birth represents an obligatory change of environments. For high-risk infants, this new environment is the NICU. The infant is thrust into a world of bright lights, sudden and loud noises, and rapid temperature changes, an environment without the containment and movement of the uterus. The infant is exposed to painful and aversive experiences. There is often an irregular pattern of handling and an absence of handling in response to the infant's emerging behavioral organization. Immaturity and health status make the high-risk infant both dependent on and vulnerable to this environment to maintain vital functions, promote growth and development, and provide opportunities for the development and organization of the infant's state and behavior (Blackburn & Barnard, 1985).

Views of the NICU Environment

Three views have been conceptualized regarding the NICU environment (Cornell & Gottfried, 1976). The first is that this environment lacks adequate tactile, kinesthetic, vestibular, and auditory stimuli. This may lead to a state of sensory deprivation, which may contribute to some of the later impairments seen in high-risk infants. Clinical and animal data suggest that a dearth of early stimulation may affect a wide range of behaviors. This is a view held by many who believe in the infant stimulation approach. The second view is that the infant is not sensorially deprived per se, but that there is a lack of appropriate stimulation. In this view, the critical component is the presence or lack of patterned or variable sensory input. The third view is that the NICU environment is too complex and creates a state of sensory overload, overstimulation, and maladaptation. Growing evidence supports this perspective, which underlies the developmental intervention approach (Als et al., 1986, 1994; Becker et al., 1991; Blackburn, 1996; Deiriggi, 1996; Robertson & Philbin, 1996).

Characteristics of the NICU Environment

In examining the environment of the high-risk neonate, one must consider the inanimate (physical) environment and the animate (social) environment (Yarrow, 1968). Interactions between the infant and environment are influenced by infant physiologic, maturational, and behavioral differences and by caregiver factors such as timing, sensitivity to infant cues, and contingency of caregiver actions. Korner (1973) suggested that, ideally, the early environment of preterm infants should create a situation in which infant maturation can take place with a minimum of interference. The more intact the infant is at discharge, the more capable the infant will be of coping with the home environment and responding appropriately to parents.

Potential adverse effects of the physical aspects, social experiences, and hazards associated with neonatal intensive care and the NICU environment are numerous. Every treatment and every characteristic present in the NICU has the potential to be detrimental as well as beneficial to the infant (Peabody & Lewis, 1985). Environmental stimuli in the NICU may be an important factor contributing to the developmental problems associated with prematurity. Recent interest in the NICU environment has yielded documentation of the stresses and hazards existing in today's NICUs and their impact on the high-risk infant. Additional research is needed to further define effects of this environment.

Unfortunately, the medical and nursing management of sick neonates often becomes a source of excessive and disjunctive stimulation at a time when the neonate needs an organizing influence to promote neurobehavioral organization. Environmental conditions also affect the infant's physiologic status. Studies have shown that infants respond to events in the NICU with both behavioral and physiologic responses. The earliest may be a sudden or abrupt fluctuation in heart rate, respiratory rate, or oxygenation in response to specific environmental or caregiving events such as door slamming, suctioning, bathing, or even too close presentation of a caregiver's face (Evans, 1991; Gottfried & Gaiter, 1985; Peters, 1992). Frequently no efforts are made to include modifications in patterns of physical and social stimuli in caregiving routines. NICU patients, staff, and parents are often exposed to an ongoing intense and bizarre onslaught of unpatterned sensory stimuli that has important implications for the physiologic and developmental outcome of infants requiring NICU care.

Inanimate Environment

Sound

Sound and noise levels in the NICU are of concern for two reasons: (1) potential damage to the cochlea with hearing loss; and (2) arousal (Douek et al., 1976; Thomas, 1989). Arousal is a particular concern with immature infants who are unable to inhibit responses. In addition, arousal may deplete the infant's physiologic resources and energy reserves and waste calories over time. Noise interferes with sleep and causes fatigue in adults, and older infants. It increases heart rate, blood pressure, leads to vasoconstriction and alters respiratory patterns and endocrine function (Ariagno, 1996; Peabody & Lewis, 1985; Raymond, 1991). Vasoconstriction of blood vessels in the ear may lead to ischemia and hearing loss (Ciesielski et al., 1980) Sudden loud noises are associated with agitation, crying, irritability, increased intracranial pressure, and decreased oxygenation (Long et al., 1980a; Peabody & Lewis, 1985). Desaturation episodes correlated with peak noise bursts (Satish & Doll-Speck, 1993). Concerns have also been raised about the possible additive effects of drugs and environmental noise. It has been suggested that use of aminoglycosides may increase susceptibility to hearing loss from environmental noise (Bess et al., 1979; Falk, 1974; Peabody & Lewis, 1985).

Loudness of sound is measured in decibels (dB). Ambient sound levels in the NICU have been documented at 50 to 90 dB, which is higher than in the average office or home (Thomas, 1989). Normal adult speech in conversation is usually recorded at a loudness of 45 to 50 dB (Table 49–3). Sound levels inside

TABLE 49–3 Sound Levels and Potential Effects

Source	Sound Level (dB)	Potential Effects (in Adults)
Airplane engine	130	Pain
Rock music	120	
Heavy traffic	90–80	
	80	Potential for hearing damage in adults
Placing bottle on incubator	84	
Closing incubator portholes	80	
Factory	80	
	80	
NICU (general)	70–60	
Closing incubator cabinet	70	Annoying
Adult ICU or recovery room	68–50	
Incubator alarm or opening a plastic sleeve	67	
NICU radio	62–60	
Bubbling water in ventilator tubing	62	
Normal conversation	50–45	
Light traffic	50	
	40	Ambient background noise
Whisper	30	

dB, decibels; NICU, neonatal intensive care unit; ICU, intensive care unit.

Compiled from Baker, C. F. (1984). Sensory overload and noise in the ICU: Sources of environmental stress. *Critical Care Quarterly*, 66–80; Gottfried, A., & Gaiter, J. (1985). *Infant stress under intensive care*. Baltimore, MD: University Park Press; Hilton, B. A. (1985). Noise in acute patient areas. *Research Nursing & Health*, *8*, 283–292; and Thomas, K. (1989). How the NICU environment sounds to a preterm infant. *American Journal of Maternal Child Nursing, 14*, 249–251.

infant incubators have been reported to range from 50 to 80 dB (Agnagnostakis et al., 1980; Bess et al., 1979; Robertson & Philbin, 1996). In adults, levels above 80 to 85 dB have been associated with hearing loss in some individuals. Decibel levels are even higher inside incubators of infants with ventilatory support equipment. However, the incubator does muffle external sounds, an advantage that is not experienced by infants in open radiant warmers.

Transported infants are exposed to both high noise levels and vibration. Rotary wing aircraft have the most vibration and noise, often exceeding 90 dB, followed by fixed wing air and ground transport (Campbell et al., 1984). Infants on high-frequency ventilation are also exposed to vibration and noise. Specific effects of these conditions on infants are not known; however, noise and vibration may have a synergistic effect on hearing loss (Hamernik et al., 1989)

Sound levels in NICUs have two characteristic patterns. There is the relatively loud and continuous pattern of background noise (50 to 90 dB), which has little diurnal rhythm. Interposed with this constant background noise are peak noises, which can significantly increase the decibel level (Bess et al., 1979; Thomas, 1989). These noises are generated by activities such as monitor alarms, telephones, radios, hitting or setting items on the Plexiglas top of the incubator, intercoms, staff calling across the room, equipment dropping, or banging the doors of the incubator cabinet. Reports of peak noise levels as heard by infants inside standard hospital incubators noted that some of the highest levels were associated with events such as dropping the head of the mattress, closing portholes with a snap, tapping fingers or placing a bottle on the Plexiglas top of the incubator or bedside table, banging trash can lids, and closing cabinet doors (Robertson & Philbin, 1996; DePaul & Chambers, 1995; Thomas, 1989). What is striking is that the noise from all of these activities is easily preventable.

Light

Exposure of infants in NICUs to high-intensity, continuous light has also been of considerable concern. If the light intensity is seldom changed, as is the case in many NICUs, the infants never experience diurnal rhythmic patterns necessary for development. Another concern is that intense stimuli, whether light or noise, have a potentially arousing effect on the CNS. This effect may be especially problematic for neonates, who cannot regulate incoming stimuli, leading to wasted energy and sensory overload.

The effects of intense, ambient, cool white fluorescent lights on neonates are unknown. Exposure of animals, older children, and adults has been reported to lead to biochemical and physiologic effects such as alterations in endocrine function, hypocalcemia, cellular transformations, immature gonad development, and chromosomal breakage (Peabody & Lewis, 1985; Wurtman & Cardinali, 1974). Concerns related to phototherapy lights are discussed in Chapter 26, Assessment and Management of Endocrine Dysfunction.

Environmental lighting has been suggested as a factor increasing risks of retinopathy of prematurity (ROP) in VLBW infants, although current studies are inconclusive with many methodologic problems (Ackerman et al., 1989; Glass et al., 1985; Seiberth et al., 1994). In describing the potential additive role between light exposure and oxygen in development of ROP, Marshall (1991) noted the following paradox: "Oxygen is essential for life, but toxic, and light is essential for vision, but toxic. The retina has one of the highest metabolic demands of tissues in the body, thus the combination of light and oxygen greatly enhances the probability of deleterious reactions within its component cells."

Preterm infants are more vulnerable to retinal light damage. Factors influencing the amount of light reaching the retina include lens translucency (increased in preterm infants), amount of time the eye is open (increased in VLBW infant), pupil reactivity (decreased <30 weeks' gestational age), density of optic media (less dense in preterms), macular pigment (immature retinal structures and vascularity) as well as infant position (e.g., facing artificial light sources or windows) and bed position in relation to windows (Blackburn, 1996; Glotzbach et al., 1993; Robinson & Fielder, 1990, 1992; Robinson et al., 1989, 1991).

Common measurements used in describing light environments are irradiance ("what kind of light") or the amount of radiant energy (w/cm^2) emitted over specific wavelength bands, and illuminance ("how much light") in lux (lumens/m^2) or footcandles (ftc). Lux divided by 10 is roughly equivalent to footcandles. Light intensity in the NICU ranges from 192 to 1488 lux (approximately 19 to 148 ftc), with greater intensity during day than night hours (Glotzbach et al., 1993; Landry et al., 1985; MacLeod & Stern, 1972; Robinson et al., 1990). Treatment lights and warming lamps used in the NICU average 200 to 350 ftc (or higher), and bilirubin lights may be as high as 10,000 ftc (Glass, 1990; Glass et al., 1985)

For many years, NICU lighting was bright and continuous throughout the 24-hour day. This lack of diurnal rhythmicity may interfere with the development of natural rhythms. More recently, many nurseries have instituted some dimming of lights at night. The studies done to date have reported that infants experiencing reduced light levels for a portion of the 24-hour period had reduced heart rate, decreased activity, enhanced biologic rhythms, increased sleep, and improved feeding and weight gain. (Blackburn, 1996; Blackburn & Patteson, 1991; Lotus, 1992; Mann et al., 1986; Miller et al., 1995; Shiroiwa et al., 1986; Tenreiro et al., 1991). Thus, reducing light levels may facilitate rest and subsequent energy conservation and promote organization and growth.

Safe levels of light and sound in NICUs have not been established and warrant additional study. Until such data are available, baseline levels should be monitored in units and staff should be informed as to what is currently known about patterns of intense stimuli exposure and the effects on newborn animals and on adults (Catlett & Holditch-Davis, 1990; Messner, 1978). Working to decrease light and sound in NICUs is an important part of providing developmental supportive and safe care (White, 1996).

Animate Environment

For the high-risk infant, the major early caregiver is usually the nurse in the NICU. For any infant, the caregivers, whether parent, nurse, or other individual, have major influences on the amount and variety of sensory input the infant receives. The caregiver selects the specific sensory input to which the infant is exposed, thus helping to shape the sensory environment. In addition to carrying out specific infant care techniques, the caregiver functions by increasing and decreasing sensory thresholds, modulating arousal, and fostering attentional and alerting behaviors (Blackburn, 1979). Initial adaptation of the infant to the extrauterine environment is enhanced by synchrony between infant behaviors and caregiver action.

The majority of caregiving experienced by infants in NICUs involves medical or other caregiving interventions associated with high levels of sensory input. In comparison with healthy full-term infants, these infants experience less adult speech directed toward them, spend more time alone, and are more often asleep during "social" interactions. Most studies have reported that, on average, infants in intensive or intermediate care nurseries are handled for anywhere from 11 to 23 percent of the 24-hour day, although there are wide variations for individual infants (Blackburn, 1979, 1989; Gottfried & Gaiter, 1985). In most cases, this is probably less than that received by the full-term infant at home. What characterizes NICU caregiving is that infants in these settings are handled more frequently with fewer periods for uninterrupted rest and sleep (Ariagno, 1996).

Caregiver–infant interactions often have an all-or-nothing form, ranging from no contact to repeated, frequent, stressful, and often painful interventions. Social interaction with the caregiver may be stressful for the immature or ill infant. For these infants, the critical factor is whether the infant can tolerate the level of sensory input, regardless of whether that input is supposed to be positive or is painful.

Gorski and associates (1983, 1985) found that after completing an intervention, nurses spent a mean of 85 seconds in the immediate infant care area for ill infants and a mean of 45 seconds for intermediate care or growing infants. Signs of distress (such as cyanosis, alterations in respiration and oxygenation, bradycardia, and gastrointestinal upset) in response to caregiving tended to occur within 5 minutes of the nursing intervention, often after the nurse had left the bedside. In addition, many sudden physiologic crises seemed preventable if the caregiver had recognized and responded to stress responses and provided interventions to allow infant recovery and reorganization. Others have noted that more than three fourths of recorded episodes of hypoxemia were associated with handling (Long et al., 1980b; Murdoch & Darlow, 1984; Norris et al., 1982).

Patterns of caregiving in the NICU can profoundly affect the development of infant state organization and biologic rhythms (Blackburn, 1989; Gottfried & Gaiter, 1985). Infants entrain their physical and physiologic activities to regularly recurring endogenous (hunger, secretion of hormones, respiration, elimination) and exogenous (patterns of light, sound, caretaking activities) events. The patterns of care can either enhance or interfere with the infant's neurobehavioral organization. These organizations will be enhanced by caregiving that is based on infant cues.

An important component of the infant's animate environment is the opportunity for contingent caregiving, that is, care in which the experiences and caregiver responses are dependent on the infant's behavior. In this way, infants begin to learn that their behavior influences their environment and vice versa (Blackburn, 1983; Blackburn & Barnard, 1985). Contingent interaction between the infant and caregiver is dependent on three characteristics: (1) readability or clarity of behaviors and cues; (2) predictability of the other in anticipating behavior from immediately preceding behaviors; and (3) responsiveness or reactions of the other with appropriate behaviors within a short latency period (Sammons & Lewis, 1985). These characteristics are inherent in both the infant and the environment, including caregivers. The more readable, predictable, and responsive the infant, the physical environment, and the caregivers, the smoother and more rewarding their interactions. However, as Sammons and Lewis (1985) noted, the NICU environment is far from being easily readable, is often unresponsive, and is highly unpredictable. At the same time, the NICU infant, due to immaturity or illness, is also not easily readable, is unpredictable, and appears unresponsive. The first step in rectifying this situation is for caregivers to learn to recognize infant cues and respond appropriately to provide a more readable, predictable, and responsive environment for the infant.

CHANGING PERSPECTIVES

Historical Overview

In looking back on the care of high-risk infants, especially preterm infants, one finds that, until the early 1960s, these infants were viewed as too fragile to handle. Minimal stimulation was recommended. This approach changed with literature on the effects of maternal deprivation in animal and human infants, along with concerns that the hospital incubator was a sensory deprivation chamber. As a result, there was an increased emphasis on providing stimulation that, in many cases, took on a "more is better" approach to overcoming the effects of the NICU environment. During the 1960s and early to middle 1970s, a variety of approaches to modifying the NICU environment using additional stimulation were suggested and tested (Lott, 1989).

During the 1980s, there was an increasing recognition and validation that what is important is not just sensory input per se, but the pattern of input and timing in relation to the infant's cycles, cues, and maturity. In addition, with increasing technology and its impact on the infant and the infant's environment, along with growing numbers of smaller and sicker infants, there has been increasing concern regarding issues of infant stress and overstimulation. As a result, an alternative approach toward viewing and modifying the NICU environment has been developed. This approach involves specific clinical strategies to modify the NICU environment and to direct caregiving interventions and interactions. These strategies constitute the *developmental intervention* approach, which is much different from the previous *infant stimulation* approach.

Infant Stimulation Approach

The infant stimulation approach derives from early deprivation research with humans and animals. This approach is based on the assumption that infants in the NICU are sensorially deprived. It seeks to reduce the negative effects of the NICU by increasing the infant's sensory experiences. The focus is on providing sensory enrichment, ameliorating developmental delays, and achieving specific developmental milestones. Usually, a similar program is used for a group of infants. The infant stimulation approach has been effective in promoting development of handicapped infants, but is questionable for meeting the needs of very ill and immature neonates in the NICU.

Analysis of Stimulation Studies

Concerns regarding the NICU environment have led to a variety of studies using additional stimulation for high-risk infants, particularly preterm infants. Cornell and Gottfried (1976), Field (1980), Harrison (1985), Masi (1979), and Schaefer and associates (1980) have reviewed many of these intervention studies, including their assumptions, types of interventions used, methodologies, findings, and limitations. The aim of these studies has been to ascertain the effects of environmental manipulations on the behavior and development of the preterm infant. The general assumptions are that:

1. Preterm infants are at high risk for biologic and psychological disabilities.
2. The present nature of care for the preterm infant does not include adequate stimulation.

Types of Interventions

The types of interventions that have been employed fall into two general areas:

1. Use of different types of stimuli characteristic of the experiences of full-term neonates. These include tape recordings of the mother's voice, additional handling or stroking, and programs using mobiles, handling, massage, and rocking (Cornell & Gottfried, 1976; Deiriggi, 1996; White & Labarba, 1976; White-Traut & Nelson, 1988).
2. Attempts to simulate the sensory experiences of the uterus. This involves interventions such as a rockerbed heartbeat program to simulate movement and patterned sound of the uterus; a hammock apparatus, which allows a fetal posture and provides rotation and rhythmic activity similar to that in the uterus; and water beds, which provide vestibular-proprioceptive stimuli similar to that experienced by an infant floating in amniotic fluid (Barnard & Bee, 1983; Burns et al., 1983; Cornell & Gottfried, 1976; Deiriggi, 1990; Korner, 1986; Korner et al., 1975; Neal, 1977).

Methodologies

These studies have differed in their use of a single sensory modality (that is, auditory, visual, tactile, vestibular, or proprioceptive) or use of multimodal stimulation combining modalities such as auditory and kinesthetic or auditory, vestibular, and proprioceptive). The variables used to measure the effects of the interventions have differed, including measures of (1) growth (weight, length, head circumference); (2) gastrointestinal function (feeding, stooling); (3) cardiorespiratory function (heart rate, respiratory rate, apnea); (4) state (patterns, alertness, crying); (5) maternal attitudes and attachment; and (6) performance on behavioral and developmental assessments (Cornell & Gottfried, 1976; Field, 1980; Masi, 1979).

Other differences in components of the various intervention studies include timing and duration of the intervention. Most studies have not incorporated contingency of stimulation. Contingency gives the infant control over the intervention so that sensory input can be individualized to each infant's needs. Minimally, interventions need to be contingent on the infant's state and behavior signals, especially stress and distress cues (Blackburn, 1983; Burns et al., 1994). These differing components point out areas that need to be evaluated when reading and comparing studies.

Findings

The reported results have been as various as the methodologies used. However, as noted by Field (1980), despite considerable differences in both methodology and results, most of the supplemental stimulation studies have cited some benefits for stimulated infants, irrespective of the stimulus modality and the use of unimodal or multimodal stimulation.

General findings include (1) altered weight gain (although there is some evidence on follow-up that the increased weight gain was only temporary); (2) altered activity and crying with both increases and decreases reported; (3) more consistent and better performance on behavioral assessment scales; and (4) more consistent and longer-term increases on motor scales (Cornell & Gottfried, 1976; Field, 1980).

Limitations

Many of the intervention studies have small samples, and few studies have been replicated. Although there have been positive outcomes for groups as a whole, individual infants in experimental groups have been reported to have adverse effects. Most studies have involved relatively stable preterm infants greater than 30 weeks' gestation. There are little data regarding sensory stimulation interventions with those infants who compose the largest populations in many NICUs, that is, infants less than 28 weeks' gestation, ill preterm and full-term infants, and infants with chronic health problems. In addition, studies have varied in the age at which interventions have been initiated. The impact of experience, that is, the infant's postbirth age, is also unknown.

Sleep and wake states have potent effects on infant physiologic and neurobehavioral functioning. Since infants respond differently in different states, this parameter may influence and interact with both the infant's response to stimuli and the measurement of outcome behaviors. In addition, there have been few reports regarding immediate effects of intervention regimens on physiologic and neurobehavioral parameters. Finally, most intervention studies have not examined the existing environment. The baseline stimulation received by the infant, such as ambient sound and light levels and the type and patterns of handling for caregiving, may influence the effectiveness of supplemental sensory input (Blackburn, 1983; Field, 1980; Masi, 1979).

Issues and Questions

Although additional stimulation appears to benefit the preterm and possibly other high-risk infants, questions and concerns regarding early intervention exist. The exact mechanism by which stimulation achieves its results is unclear. Hebb (1949) theorized that brain tissue is activated or established by sensory input and experiences. Schaefer and associates (1980) suggested that "stimulation" takes place through the activation of any sensory modality, which may be why similar findings are reported regardless of the type of stimulation used, and achieves its beneficial effects either by arousing or alerting or by soothing and quieting. Stimulation that arouses or alerts brings the infant into more direct contact with, and focuses the infant's attention on, the environment. Soothing or quieting helps infants to decrease their responsivity to, and the impact of, the environment. Arousing and soothing are state modulation activities that can be utilized by nurses and parents to promote infant adaptation and organization.

Several questions need to be addressed if care for high-risk infants is to be optimized. What is the appropriate type and amount of sensory input to best enhance maturation and development for infants of different gestational ages, postbirth ages, and health status? How does this change over time and with experience? Are there periods when input that arouses is more appropriate, and others when interventions that induce quiescence are more appropriate? For the VLBW or ill infant, the best intervention may be no intervention per se, but rather protection of the infant from the environment. What forms and amount of sensory input are appropriate at each gestational age? What is stressful to the infant? Is single or multimodal stimulation more appropriate, and, if so, for which infants? An infant may respond to sensory input or caregiving activities, but only at significant costs in terms of physiologic status or energy utilization. As more is learned about neurobehavioral development, the need to individualize interventions for each infant and to carefully assess infant responses to caregiving activities and provision of sensory input becomes evident.

As noted above, it is unclear how the NICU environment interacts with provision of supplemental sensory input. It is also unclear how effects of hospital-based interventions are affected by the infant's home environment and experiences. Many studies either have not followed infants long term or have found few effects. Sustained effects have been most clearly demonstrated in studies that continued the intervention after discharge to the home (Cornell & Gottfried, 1976; Field, 1980; Masi, 1979).

TABLE 49–4 Neonatal Auditory and Visual Behavioral Capabilities

Auditory
Anatomic maturation by 20 weeks' gestation
Sounds in extrauterine environment audible to fetus
Auditory evoked potentials recorded as early as 25 weeks' gestation
Active response to sound observed in preterm infants by about 25 to 28 weeks' gestation
Preterm infants respond to sound by autonomic, attentional, and alerting responses
Hearing threshold decreases with gestation from about 40 dB at 28 to 34 weeks' gestation to 20 dB at term
Term neonates can hear and discriminate sounds with acuity best in low- and mid-range frequencies
Neonates differentiate between sounds by attending to sounds of interest and showing aversion to noxious sounds
Neonates can distinguish their mothers' voices and show a preference for high intonations and rhythmic vocalizations
Visual
Layers of retina form by 22 weeks, rods and cones form by 23 weeks, and myelinization of optic nerve begins at 24 weeks' gestation
Neurons forming visual cortex in place by 26 weeks, with rapid development of visual neuronal connections between 28 and 34 weeks' gestation
Visual evoked potentials can be recorded by 25 to 30 weeks' gestation
Visual attention observed in preterm infants by 30 to 32 weeks' gestation
Preterm infants demonstrate pupillary light responses and blinking to a bright light by 29 to 30 weeks, fixate on simple patterns by 30 weeks, and demonstrate pattern preference by 31 to 32 weeks' gestation
Visual scanning by cessation of sucking begins by 30 weeks and is active after 36 weeks' gestation
Preterm infants take longer to fixate, are less visually responsive, and have poorer visual acuity and ability to accommodate than term infants
Neonates have limited accommodation ability, which decreases their ability to focus on objects that are extremely close to or far from their face
Term infants can best perceive objects about 19 cm from their eyes that have high contrast or contour
Neonates can follow movement of an object with their eyes and often with head movement

Derived from Thomas, K. A., & Blackburn, S. T. (1992). The neuromuscular and sensory systems. In S. T. Blackburn & D. L. Loper (Eds.), *Maternal, fetal and neonatal physiology: A clinical perspective* (pp. 522–580). Philadelphia: W. B. Saunders.

Developmental Intervention Approach

The developmental intervention approach is based on the synactive theory (Als, 1982) and focuses on fostering neurobehavioral and physiologic organization. Intervention strategies are individualized for each infant and based on ongoing assessment of that infant. An assumption underlying this approach is that the high-risk infant is vulnerable to sensory overload and overstimulation and demonstrates this via a variety of physiologic, state, motoric, and attentional cues. Therefore, the goal is not to focus on achievement of developmental milestones or to offer stimulation to foster specific skills, but rather to help the infant stabilize at each stage of maturation and to support the infant's emerging behaviors and organization while reducing stress.

The developmental intervention approach does not mean that sensory input is never provided. Sensory input is an important and critical parameter in fostering CNS development. However, sensory input is provided only when appropriate to the infant's physiologic and neurobehavioral status and is individualized to the needs and abilities of the infant at that time. There is also recognition that for the ill, unstable, or fragile infant, the best form of sensory input may be no input. In addition, infants are assessed for early signs of sensory overload so appropriate interventions can be initiated to avoid overstimulation.

Cue-Based Care

Caregiving based on infant cues is an important parameter of providing developmentally appropriate care. These cues provide communications about an infant's needs and status at any given time. Both full-term and preterm infants provide us with specific cues that can be used in planning care. These cues include infant state (see Chapter 48, Neonatal Sleep–Wake States) and behavioral capabilities (Table 49–4) as well as signs of stress, overstimulation, and stability. Caregiving based on infant cues involves attention to messages from the infant that may indicate timing for interventions, such as when to provide care, or opportunities for sensory input and interaction. These cues also indicate how the infant handles stimuli, signals sensory overload, and tolerates stimulation. Thus, information is available as to when the infant cannot tolerate additional handling or stimuli and needs time out to regroup and reorganize.

Behavioral Cues: Stress and Stability

The NICU staff, and especially nurses, play a significant role in shaping the environment and making caregiving more responsive to infants. This requires careful observation and documentation of infant behavior as are done for physiologic status and development of an individualized plan of care. Infant responses to the environment will be influenced by factors such as (1) state; (2) basic needs (for example, hunger); (3) sensory threshold; (4) parameters of the inanimate and animate environment, including readability, predictability, and responsivity; and (5) infant health status and neurobehavioral maturity (Blackburn, 1983). Infant behavioral responses include specific autonomic, motoric, and state cues, which indicate stress and the need for immediate intervention, and stability cues, which indicate that the infant is coping positively. Tables 49–5 and 49–6 summarize infant stability and stress cues. Examples of selected cues are illustrated in Figures 49–2 and 49–3.

Guidelines for Providing Developmental Support

An understanding of behavioral cues and attention to signs of stress are only the first steps in providing developmentally appropriate interventions. Strategies to ameliorate stress and behavioral disorganization must be individualized and appropriate to the infant's level of developmental and health status. Applying

TABLE 49–5 Infant Stability Signals

Autonomic System
Able to regulate color and respiration
Reduction of tremors, twitches, visceral signals
Motoric System
Smooth, well-modulated posture and tone
Synchronous smooth movements with
Hand/foot clasping
Grasping
Hand-to-mouth activity
Suck/suck searching
Hand holding
Tucking
State System
Clear, robust sleep states
Rhythmic, robust crying
Active self-quieting/consoling
Focused, shiny-eyed alertness with intent or animated facial expression
"Ooh" face
Cooing
Attentional smiling

Adapted from Als, H. (1982). Toward a synactive theory of development: Promise for the assessment and support of infant individuality. *Infant Mental Health Journal,* 3(4), 229–243; and Als, H., Lester, B. M., Tronick, E. Z., & Brazelton, T. B. (1982). Assessment of preterm infant behavior (APIB). In H. E. Fitzgerald & M. Yogman (Eds.), *Theory and research in behavioral pediatrics* (Vol. 1, pp. 64–133). New York: Plenum Press.

developmental interventions in this manner may increase the infant's tolerance for stimulation and reduce stressful events that are costly in terms of energy expenditure, caloric utilization, and physiologic homeostasis (Fig. 49–4). This approach may also reduce the need for pharmacologic interventions, including sedatives (VandenBerg & Franck, 1990) and promote adaptation and organization (Als, 1996; D'Apolito, 1991).

As infants become better able to self-regulate through appropriately planned handling and reduction of stressful events, their behavior will reflect a pattern of emerging competency in responding to and interacting with their environment, of which their parents are a critical part. Goals of developmental interventions are to (1) promote an understanding with the parents of their infant's behavior, including manifestations of stress and stability; (2) facilitate neurobehavioral organization based on individualized assessment of the infant's capacity; (3) enhance infant recovery; (4) promote CNS organization; (5) facilitate self-regulatory capabilities; (6) preserve energy and promote growth; (7) reduce stress and prevent agitation; and (8) normalize the environment to the extent that medical care permits (VandenBerg, 1985, 1995).

Because infants in NICUs face challenges to their survival and do not have fully functional biologic systems, the goal is to support these infants and stabilize each of their subsystems, described by Als (1982), as they mature. This requires that a behavioral assessment describing the infant's current level of organization, the infant's individual coping mechanisms, and the impact of the infant's illness on neurodevelopmental functioning be completed before interventions are offered.

Once the infant's current level of organization has been documented, a plan of care can be developed that delineates the degree and kind of environmental support necessary to promote organization and development. This plan should be based on the following guidelines (VandenBerg, 1985):

1. Interventions must seek to normalize or modify the NICU environment to the extent that medical care permits.
2. Interventions must be consistent with the infant's level of maturity and gestational age.
3. Interventions must be appropriately timed in terms of the infant's state, physiologic status, and behavioral responses.
4. Interventions must be individualized to a given infant and be altered with changes in the infant's health status and neurobehavioral maturation.
5. Interventions must be sensitive to the infant's cues.
6. Interventions must take into account how much stimuli each infant can tolerate.

Research supporting the individualized developmental care approach has been published (Als et al., 1994; Becker et al., 1991; Fleisher et al., 1995). Two studies have been conducted by Als and her colleagues at the Brigham and Woman's Hospital in Boston (Als, 1986; Als et al., 1994). Focusing on an understanding of behavioral cues and on documenting the infant's current level of functioning, these studies demonstrated the usefulness of ongoing behavioral management of the high-risk neonate in the NICU. Planned, consistent interventions were carried out by parents and primary care nurses and focused on environmental modifications, handling, positioning, and, in general, reducing stress and enhancing stable functioning. Outcomes of these studies have showed significant reduction in length of stay on the respirator, reduced number of days on supplemental oxygen, reduced number of days to complete gavage feeding, reduction of severity of chronic lung disease, reduction of the incidence of intraventricular hemorrhage and in length of overall hospital stay, as well as reduction in hospital cost. It should be noted that this work was pioneered in the NICU at the Brigham and Women's Hospital and these studies are the result of many years of training and implementation by staff. However, Becker and colleagues (1991) also reported improvement in medical and growth outcomes and in

TABLE 49–6 Infant Stress Signals

Autonomic System
Respiratory pauses, tachypnea, gasping
Color changes (dusky, pale, mottled, cyanotic)
Tremors, startles, twitches
Yawning
Gagging, spitting up
Hiccoughing
Straining
Sneezing, coughing
Sighing
Motoric System
Flaccidity (trunk, extremities, face)
Hypertonicity with hyperextension of legs, arms, trunk
Finger splays
Facial grimace
Hand on face, fisting
Fetal tuck
Frantic diffuse activity
State System
Diffuse sleep–wake states
Fussing or irritability
Staring or gaze averting
Panic or worried alertness
Glassy-eyed alertness
Rapid state oscillation
Irritability
Diffuse arousal

Adapted from Als, H. (1982). Toward a synactive theory of development: Promise for the assessment and support of infant individuality. *Infant Mental Health Journal,* 3(4), 229–243; and Als, H., Lester, B. M., Tronick, E. Z., & Brazelton, T. B. (1982). Assessment of preterm infant behavior (APIB). In H. E. Fitzgerald & M. Yogman (Eds.), *Theory and research in behavioral pediatrics* (Vol. 1, pp. 64–133). New York: Plenum Press.

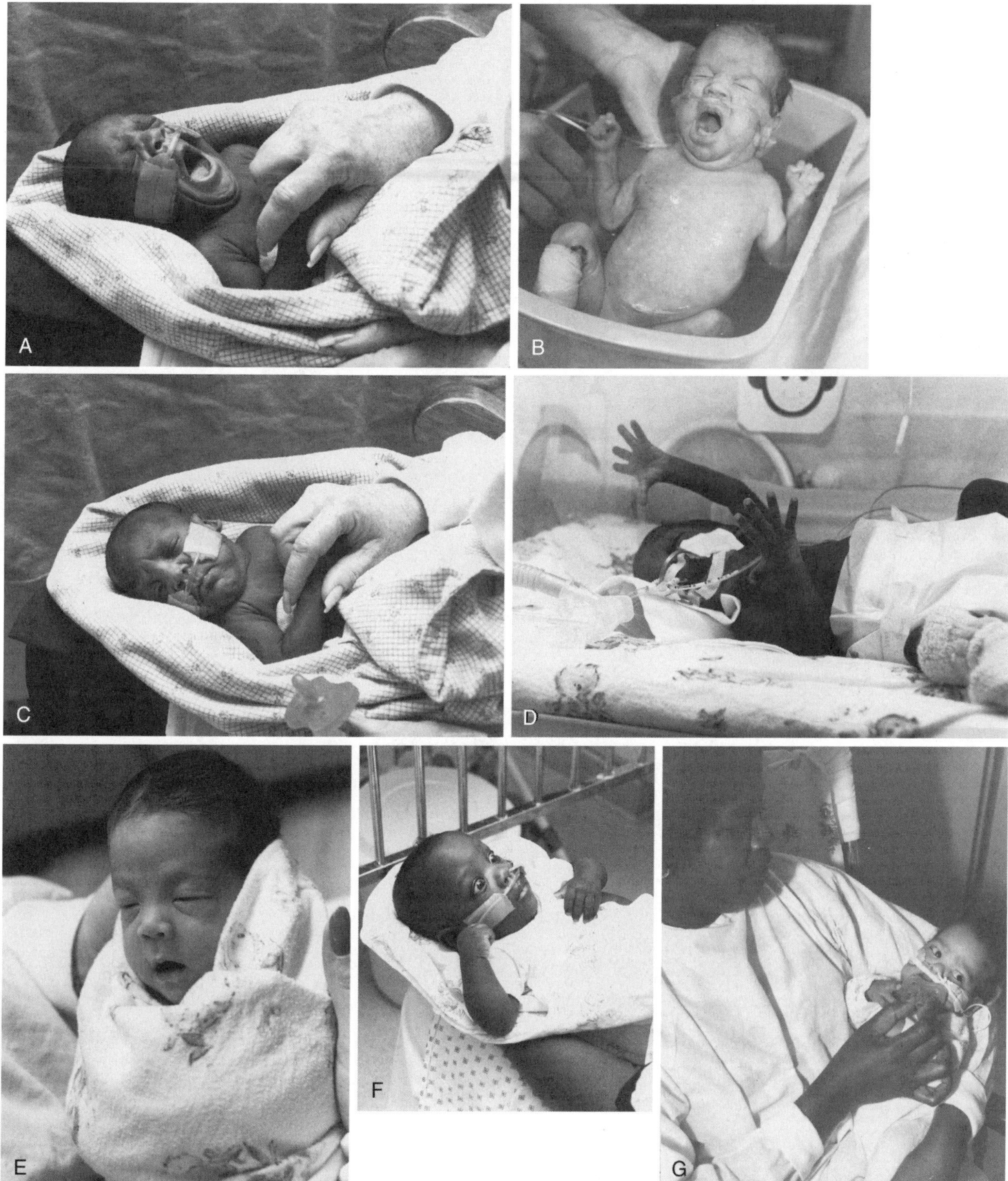

FIGURE 49–2. Examples of selected instability and stress cues. From the autonomic system: *A*, yawning; *B*, mottling. From the motor system: *C*, straining; *D*, finger splay; *E*, facial hypotonia. From the state system: *F*, glassy-eyed, hyperalertness; *G*, gaze aversion; *B*, fussing. (Courtesy of Children's Hospital, Oakland, CA.)

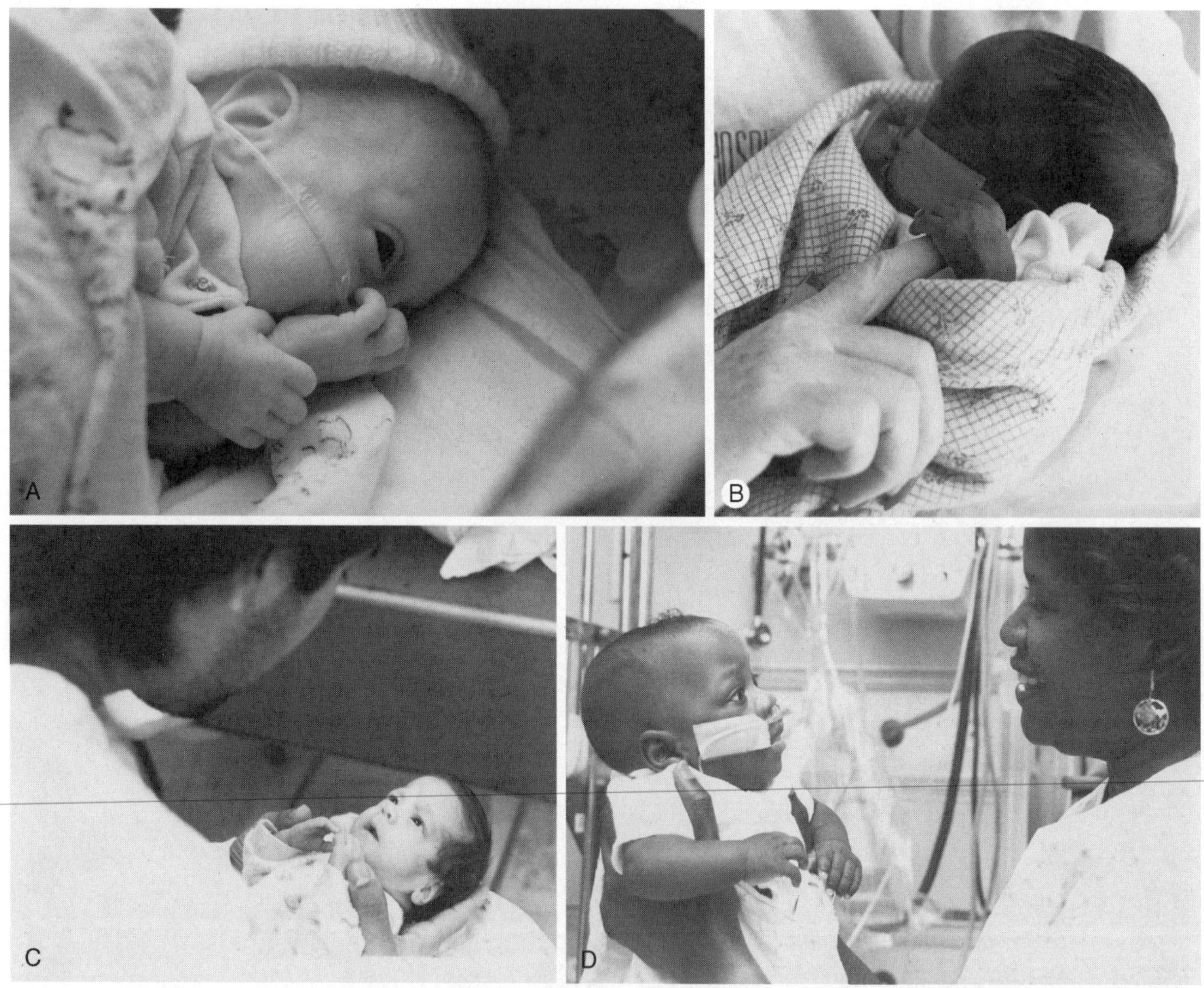

FIGURE 49–3. Examples of selected stability cues. From the motor system: *A,* hand clasp and hand to mouth activity; *B,* grasping; *C,* hands together at midline. From the state system: *A,* active self-quieting; *C* and *D,* focused, shiny-eyed alertness. (Courtesy of Children's Hospital, Oakland, CA.)

motor and behavioral state organization in infants who experienced developmentally supportive care.

A similar study was completed at Lucile Packard Children's Hospital at Stanford (Fleisher et al., 1995). This study was conducted in the postsurfactant era and was carried out in a nursery that had developmental services arranged by consultation. The individualized developmental care approach was introduced and implemented in the first 24 hours for study subjects and carried out consistently until discharge. Experimental infants once again demonstrated fewer days on positive pressure, fewer days in the hospital, and significantly reduced hospital costs ($128,000 per experimental × 17 = $2.18 million saved in hospital charges). Moreover once again one third of the control infants went home several months after the experimental infants, indicating a reduction in chronicity in the experimental group. This study demonstrated that these results could be obtained even when a developmental care program was new to the staff. A National Collaborative Research Institute was funded to test this methodology in three NICUs across the United States, varying in the parameters of primary versus conventional nursing and transport

ENERGY IN +	PHYSIOLOGIC ENERGY OUT +	BEHAVIORAL ENERGY OUT =	GROWTH ENERGY RETAINED
Food calories	Thermocontrol Respiration Cardiovascular system Digestion Other processes	Recycling Stress Overload	Weight gain Growth Formation of new tissues: muscle, fat, dendrites Development and organization of subsystems

FIGURE 49–4. Energy conservation model. (Adapted with permission from Sammons, W. A. H., & Lewis, J. M. [1985]. *Premature babies: A different beginning.* St. Louis: C. V. Mosby.)

versus inborn nurseries. Preliminary results confirm the positive findings of the initial studies (Als & Gilkerson, personal communication, 1995).

These studies demonstrate that an individualized behaviorally based developmental and family-focused care approach stabilizes the infant, reduces stress during NICU hospitalization, and improves neurodevelopmental and medical outcome following premature birth. While continuing to validate this approach, future studies also need to focus on long-term outcome of infants who have been cared for using this model.

Intervention Strategies

Environmental Manipulations

Auditory Environment: Reducing Noise Levels

Sound levels vary in different NICUs and over time within a unit. These levels should be monitored regularly so that problem areas can be identified and modified. Sound levels can be reduced by attending to events that increase both background and peak noise. Increased noise levels result from not closing incubator portholes or cabinet doors gently, and using plastic sleeves. Removing water bubbling in oxygen and ventilator tubing will decrease background noise, as will eliminating radios. Peak noises can also be reduced if staff avoid tapping or banging tops of incubators.

Location of the infant's bed in relation to equipment (including monitors) and to surrounding traffic and activity also needs to be evaluated. By determining from which point on the equipment sounds and alarms emanate, the infant can be repositioned to modify this component of the auditory environment. Noise from equipment belonging to both the infant being cared for and surrounding infants must be considered. For example, depending on how infant beds and equipment are positioned, one infant may be exposed to sounds primarily from equipment from other infants or to sounds from tube systems or pipes in walls. Similar evaluations and modifications can be implemented for telephones, intercoms, and other unit equipment. The effect of a loud overhead speaker system can be reduced by providing staff with pagers that vibrate.

Other sources of noise that should be condensed are the volume of music boxes, tape recorders, and musical toys. The volume can be kept low or muffled with a blanket as needed. These should not be used with infants who are easily disorganized. Audible telephone ringers can be replaced with light signals. Staff should quietly close garbage cans, linen hampers, and equipment carts, and place felt stripping on this equipment and drawers to reduce sound levels. Placing thick, soundproof blankets or other materials around incubators, warmers, and cribs reduces both sound and light. In addition, bottles and other equipment can be placed on blankets or pads rather than directly on the incubator hood. Examples of interventions to reduce noise levels are in Figure 49–5.

Sound levels can also be reduced by eliminating the use of radios, by talking and walking softly, and by avoiding shouting. Some units have instituted the concept of a daily quiet hour. Guidelines for quiet hours are in Table 49–7.

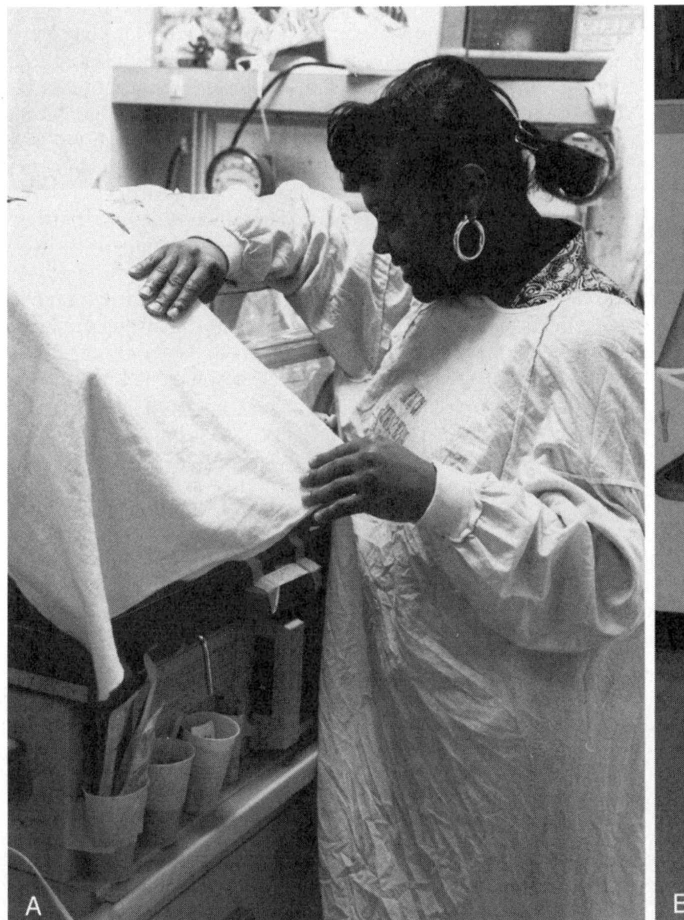

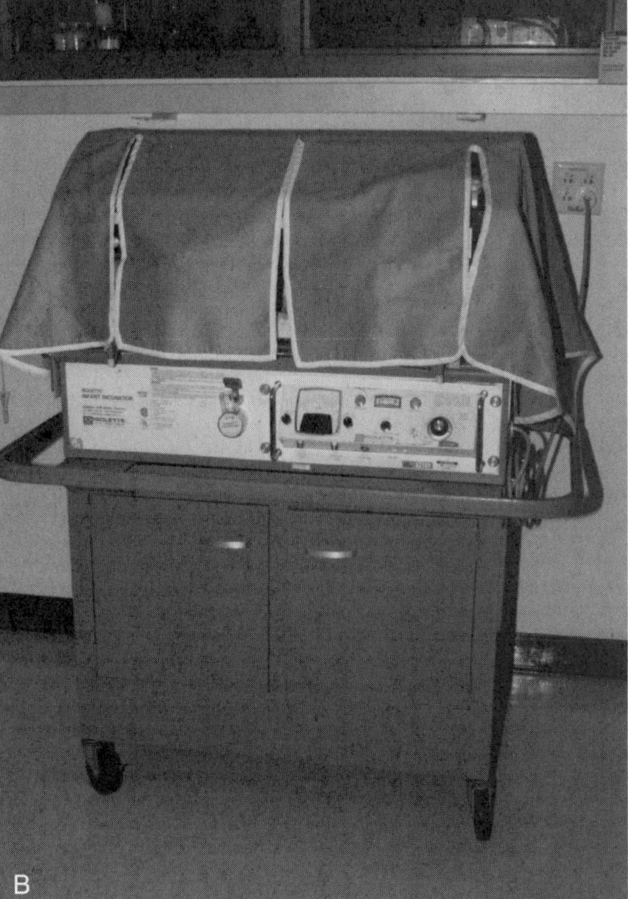

FIGURE 49–5. Examples of environmental modifications to reduce sound and light levels in the NICU. *A,* Reducing light levels with blanket over the incubator; *B,* using a crib cover to reduce light and sound levels. (Courtesy of Children's Hospital, Oakland, CA.)

TABLE 49–7 Protocol for the Implementation of Quiet Hour in the NICU

1. Plan 1 hour per shift to be set aside for quiet hour.
2. Plan elements or protocol and elicit cooperation of medical staff and other health care professionals and departments (e.g., physical, occupational, and respiratory therapists, x-ray and lab technicians, other consultants) who come to the NICU.
3. Plan a research protocol to collect data before and after implementation to evaluate the impact of this change on the infants, family, and staff.
4. Plan quiet hour for a trial run of several weeks and evaluate. Conduct survey (interview or questionnaire) of staff and parents to determine effectiveness and reactions. Modify protocol as needed.
5. During quiet hour, implement the following:
   a. reduce unnecessary tasking at the bedside and talk in a whisper when talking is necessary
   b. do not bring large equipment into the unit
   c. turn down alarms
   d. do not activate loudspeaker
   e. make a special effort not to slam unit doors, drawers, trash cans, or incubator doors
   f. do not perform elective procedures
   g. do not do rounds
6. Parenteral visiting is maintained during this time, with parents encouraged to participate in the activities listed above.
7. Emergency quiet time: Create a feedback system to alert staff when the decibel level in the unit exceeds 60 dB at any time. (For example, a light could be attached to a sound meter that is activated when a reading of greater than 60 dB occurs.) The charge nurse could then implement an emergency quiet time for 5 to 10 minutes to lower the noise level to below 60 dB.

NICU, neonatal intensive care unit.

Visual Environment: Reducing Light Levels

Individually controlled lights at each bedside allow the nurse to control lighting for each infant. Indirect full-spectrum light, which does not have the side effects of cool white light, can be used at the bedside (Peabody & Lewis, 1985). Covering incubators, radiant warmers, and cribs reduces infant exposure to bright overhead lights or daylight. Complete covering can be used for sleep periods, with partial covering during awake times. Dimmer switches, window shades and curtains increase staff control over the light environment. Dimming lights at night may promote development of diurnal cycles. Adjusting lighting levels during other periods fosters state transition and periods of alertness or sleep. Infants who are having brief, predictable alert periods need dim light until they are ready to maintain longer periods of alertness.

The entire visual environment of the infant needs to be evaluated regularly and simplified. Infants in the NICU can accumulate an amazing clutter of toys, pictures, and other equipment. The visual environment is easy to modify. For example, one simple picture can be placed within the infant's visual range on the wall of the incubator or crib. For an older infant, one stuffed animal or toy can be selected at a time for the infant to view. Inasmuch as these toys and pictures have often been brought in by parents, siblings, or other family members, they can become actively involved in planning and arranging their infant's visual environment. Examples of interventions to reduce light levels are in Figure 49–5.

Congestion and Traffic Patterns

Disorganization increases arousal and stress in older children and adults. Much of the data regarding the responses of neonates to congestion and rounds in the NICU is anecdotal. However, these observations suggest that for some infants, these events may lead to physiologic and motoric disorganization, apnea, and bradycardia. Infants need to be assessed and monitored to identify environmental events such as change of shift report and nursing or medical rounds that are disruptive. Infants for whom these events are a problem can be moved out of unit traffic patterns, and reports and rounds moved away from the bedside.

Altering Patterns of Care

As the infant's primary caregiver in the NICU, the nurse has a predominant role in controlling patterns of care. Caregiving patterns can be altered to respond more appropriately to an infant by evaluating the need for routine orders and caregiving interventions (Lawhon, 1986). The need for specific nonemergency interventions must be evaluated for their urgency and the potential impact on the infant. Most NICU infants are being monitored for a variety of physiologic parameters with sophisticated equipment. The data from this equipment can be used to decrease disruption of the infants by routine activities such as monitoring of vital signs. Nonemergency interventions, including monitoring of vital signs, feeding, bathing, diapering, and administration of routine medications, can be done in states other than quiet sleep (infants do not stay in quiet sleep periods for long; often <5 to 10 minutes). Inasmuch as infants spend very little time in the quiet alert state, aversive procedures should be avoided during this state. Duxbury and coworkers (1984) found that infants who received care (except for emergency procedures) only after beginning to awaken spontaneously had improved growth and physiologic function and a significantly decreased length of hospital stay.

Caregiving interventions can also be grouped or clustered to provide longer uninterrupted rest periods. Caregiving involves a significant amount of sensory input and energy utilization. Although some infants do well with clustering of care, others become exhausted and overloaded. Some infants tolerate having aversive interventions (such as blood drawing, injections, suctioning) clustered; others do not. Some infants tolerate clustering of these procedures with infant care interventions (feedings, diapering, and so on); others do not. The amount of time between clusters must be monitored to provide adequate time for recovery and rest (Evans, 1994). Time of interventions within a cluster is also an important consideration, not only in terms of potential side effects, but also in terms of avoiding exhausting an infant before feeding her or him (Gorski, 1985; VandenBerg, 1990). Therefore, clustering of care must be accompanied by ongoing individualized assessment of the infant's responses and may not be appropriate for the VLBW or very fragile infant. In addition, all infants must be observed carefully for signs of stress during caregiving and provided with recovery time as needed. Interventions such as containment can assist the infant in tolerating necessary caregiving interventions.

Interventions With Overstimulated or Stressed Infants

All infants in a NICU will have periods when they cannot deal with environmental stressors and caregiving interventions and will demonstrate signs of sensory overload (see Table 49–6). For the immature or fragile infant, any handling may be stressful, even handling that staff or parents perceive as positive, such as holding, stroking, or talking to the infant. When an infant becomes overloaded, interventions can be implemented to help the infant recover and reorganize. These interventions are illustrated in Figure 49–6. Interventions with overstimulated infants include time out with no or minimal handling or sensory input, containment or swaddling the infant with one's hands or a blanket, holding the infant quietly and providing no other sensory input (e.g., do not talk to, stroke, or jiggle the infant), placing blanket

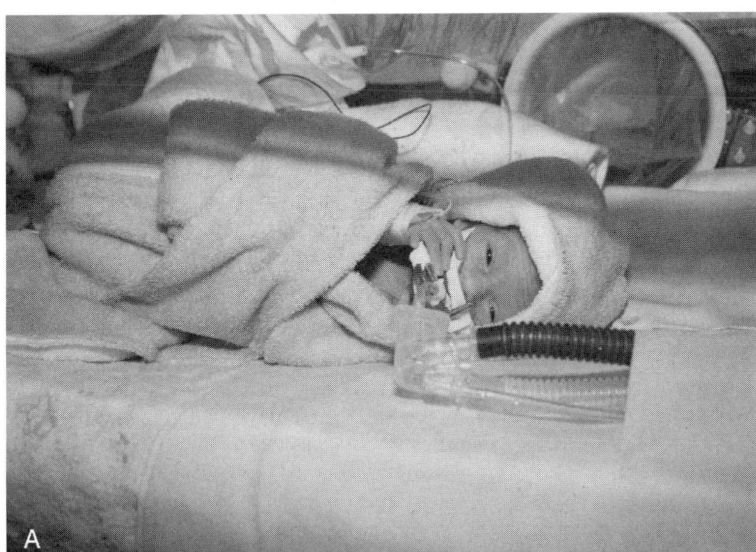
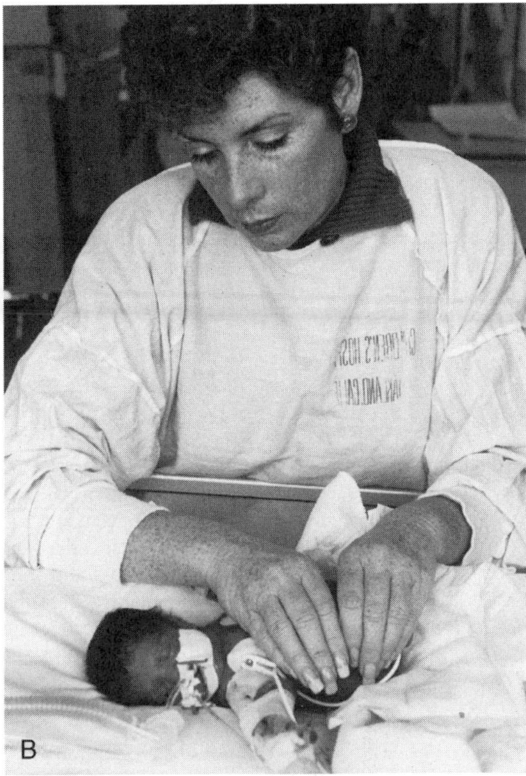

FIGURE 49–6. Interventions with overstimulated, stressed, or irritable infants. *A,* Providing time out in the incubator and swaddling with bunting (available from Terry Co.); *B,* containment with hands. (Courtesy of Children's Hospital, Oakland, CA.)

rolls at the infant's back and feet, or placing one's hands on the soles of the infant's feet.

Positioning

Positioning has been studied in relation to physiologic variables such as arterial oxygen tension, respiratory rate, lung compliance, oxygenation, physical activity, and energy expenditure (Martin et al., 1979; Masterson et al., 1987; Wagaman et al., 1979). To improve the mechanics of breathing, these studies recommend the prone position as the preferred position for low birth weight infants in the NICU. Prone positioning has also been associated with more organized state control, enhancing quiet sleep, and reducing wake states and crying (Masterson et al., 1987).

Positioning of the sick or immature infant includes consideration of the effects of gravity along with neuromuscular characteristics such as variable weak muscle tone and decreased flexion in the limbs, trunk, and pelvis. These infants are at risk for positioning disorders such as widely abducted hips (frog-leg position); retracted and abducted shoulders; ankle and foot eversion; increased neck extension with a right-sided head preference; and increased trunk extension with arching of the neck and back. These positioning disorders affect later development because of their impact on the ability of the child to bear weight, bring the shoulders forward and hands to midline, and rotate the head (Updike et al., 1986). Therefore, in addition to improved physiologic status, developmental goals of positioning include enhancement of flexion in the limbs and trunk, extensor balance, and facilitation of midline skills (Deiriggi, 1996).

These goals are superseded, however, by the importance of stress reduction and enhancement of organized motor system function. This means prevention of ongoing frantic activity (flailing) and frequent recurrent extensions of the extremities and neck. These responses are very costly to the infant in terms of energy expenditure, respiratory function, and oxygenation.

Thus, the immature or sick neonate requires support from caregivers to facilitate and maintain postures that enhance motor control and physiologic functioning and reduce stress. Most infants can be routinely placed in side-lying and prone positions and rotated every 2 to 3 hours. Supine positions are generally avoided. Infants who must be placed supine should be positioned to promote flexion and proper alignment.

Covering, swaddling, and placing blanket rolls around the infant help her or him maintain the desired posture and prevent loss of control of the flexed position. The use of these rolls provides containment and boundaries for the infant, promoting feelings of security, quiescence, and energy conservation. Many infants will seek out boundaries by moving around in their incubator until they rest against its sides, foot, or head. Infants who do so and are resting or sleeping should be left undisturbed in these positions, unless unsafe, until the next caregiving period. At that time, the infant can be repositioned and provided with boundaries or nested with blanket rolls along her or his side and at the feet and head. Nesting is often an effective way of reducing agitation (Lawhon, 1986). Placing rolls at the infant's feet also provides her or him with something to brace against during stressful interventions (Als, 1986, 1996; Lawhon, 1986; Lawhon & Melzar, 1988).

When infants need to be moved and or repositioned, either to provide an alternate position or for caregiving procedures or holding, the infant should be unwrapped and repositioned slowly with containment of the limbs and support of the head and neck. Stress responses are avoided by maintenance of the posture. When repositioning the infant, ensure that the infant is covered or swaddled if possible; if covering is not possible for medical reasons, partial wrapping is encouraged. Swaddling with blankets or containment with the caregiver's hands also reduces stress during procedures. Several investigations have suggested that the use of containment with preterm infants during procedures such as endotracheal suctioning may modify the procedure's physiologic and behavioral consequences by reducing the decrease in arterial blood pressure, heart rate, and oxygenation, promoting more stable intracranial pressure and decreasing behavioral stress cues (Taquino & Blackburn, 1994; Carlos, 1991). Swaddling is also appropriate before and after procedures to minimize motor and physiologic changes.

Infants can also be placed on soft foam, sheepskin or lambskin, waterbeds, or in slings. Sheepskin or lambskin promotes flexion, provides tactile input, and reduces skin abrasion. Waterbeds and slings also promote flexion. In addition, waterbeds provide contingent stimuli (movement in response to the infant's movement) and kinesthetic input. Positioning interventions are illustrated in Figure 49–7.

Handling

Intervention strategies related to handling must be based on two critical components: individualization and timing. The *individualization* of caregiving for each infant includes flexibility and willingness on the part of the caregiver to adapt handling to specific infant needs in order to reduce stress and prevent agitation. The caregiver must also recognize that infant's needs change, so that what may be a well-chosen, appropriate intervention during one shift may not work at all during the next.

Appropriate *timing* of handling is also essential to avoid overtiring, overstimulating infants, or increasing stress. Infants can improve their abilities to regulate their own movements, states, and autonomic function when caregiving activities are offered in sequence and with sensitivity to the infant's degree of tolerance. Examples of timing include stopping and letting the infant gain control of her or his physiologic or motoric status before completing an assessment or procedure or pacing the infant by removing the nipple during oral feeding when respiratory rate exceeds usual limits.

Infants in a NICU, no matter how sick or how small, are experiencing and reacting to every aspect of care and the surrounding environment. A goal of neonatal care is to avoid costly stress in these infants. Slow, sensitive handling for medical procedures and routine caregiving is required to accomplish this goal. Sensitive handling is based on an understanding of infant state and cues (see Tables 49–5 and 49–6). Before gently touching an infant, the caregiver should talk softly. This reduces startling, tremors, or other stress responses from the infant's suddenly being moved by "hands out of nowhere." Minimal handling protocols are necessary for immature, fragile infants (Lawhon, 1986; VandenBerg & Franck, 1990). These protocols involve reduction of environmental stimuli, positioning techniques, and pacing caregiving routines to allow for up to 3 hours of undisturbed rest (Table 49–8). Minimal handling protocols allow infants to have

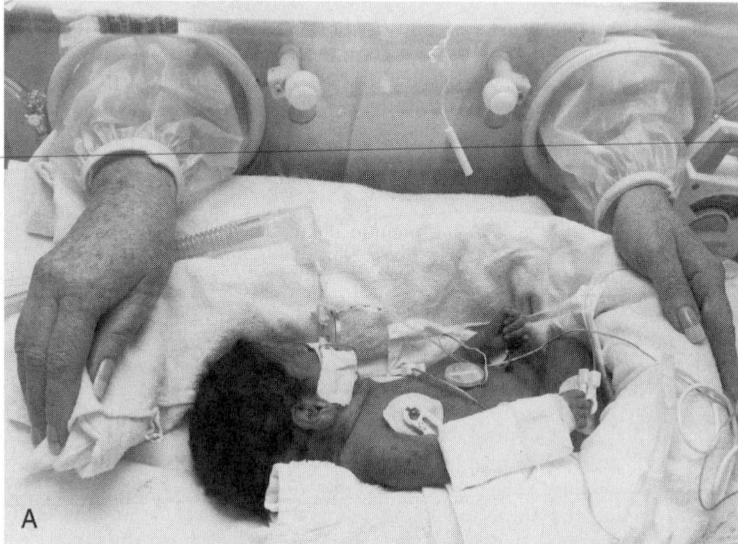

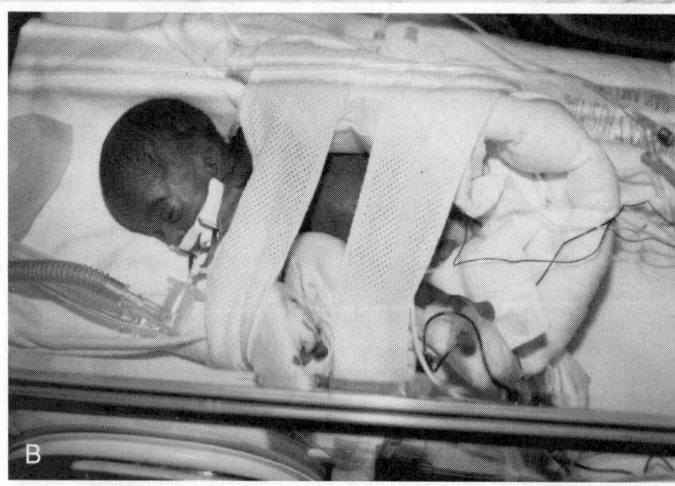

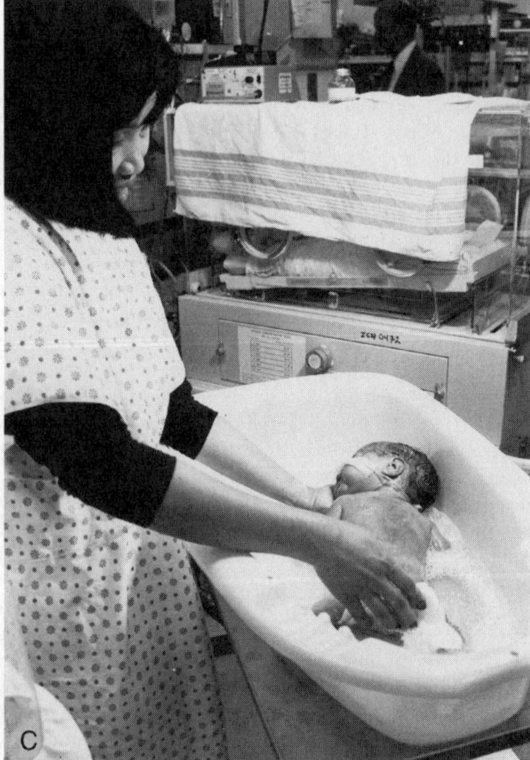

FIGURE 49–7. Handling and positioning of infants in the NICU. *A*, Creating a nest using blankets; *B*, nesting using Snuggle-Up (available from Children's Medical Ventures, Boston, MA); *C*, positioning during a bath. (Courtesy of Children's Hospital, Oakland, CA.)

TABLE 49–8 Minimal Handling Protocol

Protect From Light
Shade infant's eyes (with blanket tent or cutout box)
Cover incubator with blankets
Cover crib with blankets
Protect From Noise
Give shift report away from the bedside
Ensure that telephones do not ring in nursery rooms
Pad all trash receptacles
Close incubator doors gently
Set speakers as low as possible
Close doors softly
Remove sources of loud, jarring noise
Avoid tearing paper near infant
Protect From Overstimulation
Cluster nursing care activities
Allow 2- to 3-hour periods of undisturbed rest.
No routine postural drainage (PRN only)
No routine suctioning (PRN only)
Contain limbs during suctioning (swaddle or have another person help)
Note: Allow for recovery after each intervention
Provide Boundaries
Position prone or side lying
Cover/wrap/swaddle
Use blanket rolls to tuck around sides/back/feet, even at head
Provide objects for suck, grasp

From VandenBerg, K. A. (1990). Behaviorally supportive care for the extremely premature infant. In L. P. Gunderson & C. Kenner (Eds.), *Care of the 24–25 week gestational age infant (small baby protocol)* (p. 151). Petaluma, CA: Neonatal Network. Reprinted with permission.

extended sleep periods, which facilitate autonomic and state control.

State Modulation

One of the primary functions of the caregiver during early life is modulation of levels of arousal in the infant. Lack of interactions organized around soothing or attempts to decrease arousal may contribute to impairment of the high-risk infant's ability to modulate her or his state organization, resulting in an infant who presents fewer or less clear cues to her or his parents.

Initially, state modulation efforts are directed toward protecting the infant from environmental stressors and aversive sensory input by reducing arousal through implementing time-out maneuvers. These early interventions are directed toward protecting the infant from disorganization and decompensation. Infants cannot truly maintain mature states until they achieve control over their autonomic and motoric systems (Als, 1986).

Interventions to organize state include helping these infants to organize their sleep, alerting, and crying. To promote sleep, the caregiver can modify the environment to reduce light, noise, and traffic around the infant's bed. Use of boundaries, prone positioning, minimal handling, and support of flexion, along with predictable routines, will also facilitate sleep organization. Interventions to prevent irritability and crying include predictable routines, reducing environmental stress, timing procedures or other caregiving according to infant cues, and soothing infants when they become stressed. Periods of irritability can be minimized if signs of stress and sensory overload are recognized early and appropriate interventions initiated. Soothing interventions for the immature or ill infant include containment and swaddling, providing time out for recovery, reducing stimulation, holding the infant's hands or feet, prone positioning, and providing sucking opportunities (Als, 1986; Lawhon, 1986; VandenBerg, 1990, 1995).

Immature infants will initially spend very little time in alert states. When they do achieve an alert state, these states are transient and easily disrupted. Caregivers need to approach infants who have reached a quiet alert state carefully. It is often an exciting event when an infant finally opens her or his eyes and reaches a quiet alert state. Unfortunately, caregivers often try to capitalize on this time by providing input and reinforcement that is "too much, too soon." A more appropriate response to interacting with these infants is to allow the infant to initiate and control the interaction. This can be done by slowly approaching the infant with low-keyed input, using one mode of stimuli at a time, then gradually increasing the input based on the infant's cues. If the infant begins to show signs of stress, provide time out, and, after the infant recovers, begin the interaction again. Alert states can be facilitated by shielding the infant's eyes from overhead lights.

As infants mature and their health status improves, they will be able to handle more mature interactions with their parents, nurses, and other caregivers. State modulation activities can then be introduced around caregiving events such as feeding. Fuhrman (1984) studied the effects of a parent-initiated state modulation intervention in which parents were taught to arouse their preterm infants before feeding and to soothe the infants after feeding. These infants were all stable and ready for discharge home. She found that at follow-up 4 weeks after discharge, infants who received this intervention were significantly more alert before feeding, had shorter feeding times, and had higher scores on the Nurse Child Assessment Feeding Scale for both infant and parent subscales.

Alerting activities with healthy full-term or more mature, stable preterm infants include talking to the infant, varying the pitch and intensity of one's voice; unwrapping the infant, even if only the upper extremities; providing a drowsy infant with visual or auditory stimuli; putting the infant in an upright position such as up on one's shoulder; and eliciting the rooting or sucking reflexes. Activities to soothe include talking in a slow, steady monotone; swaddling the infant with hands or blanket; providing a pacifier or helping the infant get her or his fingers or hand into the mouth; and placing one's hands against the soles of the infant's feet (Blackburn & Kang, 1991). As with the more fragile infants, these infants should also be observed for their stress and stability cues in response to each intervention.

Provision of Sensory Input

As the preterm infant matures and the ill preterm or full-term infant recovers and stabilizes, provision of sensory input becomes an important parameter to foster neurologic development. Provision of sensory input is not just providing additional stimulation; careful thought needs to be given to the *appropriate* types of sensory input based on the infant's state, health status, maturity, developmental level, and cues.

Caregivers must be cautious when providing sensory input and must be sensitive to infant responses and abilities to tolerate stimuli. Inasmuch as optimal levels, amount, complexity, and type of sensory input have not yet been established, efforts to stimulate the high-risk infant can quickly result in overstimulation with physiologic, motoric, and behavioral decompensation. The old adage "if a little is good, more must be better" must be avoided to protect the infant from stimulus bombardment (Blackburn, 1983). As noted earlier, for the immature or fragile infant, the best form of additional stimulation is none.

Specific considerations for providing sensory input to high-risk infants include (1) the infant is vulnerable to sensory overload; (2) the infant will benefit from positive experiences; (3) the infant will recover best when sensory input is minimized or when left alone; (4) the infant will take longer to inhibit responses; (5) the infant can deal only with a small amount of stimuli at a time and at a slower rate; and (6) the infant may be able to handle only unimodal rather than multimodal stimuli. If the infant demonstrates signs of stress when presented with sensory input, it should be eliminated and tried again at a later date. Table 49–9 presents examples of types of sensory input for each modality that can be utilized with *stable* high-risk infants.

Feeding

The NICU patient encounters many factors that are likely to jeopardize the development of normal healthy feeding patterns. Treatment factors include prolonged use of endotracheal tubes and gavage feeding and tape placed on the face to hold tubing. These procedures contribute to noxious oral sensations and may lead to oral defensive behaviors such as hypersensitivity to touch (Harris, 1986). Other factors related to the environment and caregiving routines affect the development of feeding skills. These include inconsistent caregivers, intense stimuli, and varied patterns of handling, which disorganize sensory experience. Intense environmental stimuli may overstimulate the infant and interfere with the infant's ability to organize motor activity for efficient sucking.

In addition, owing to the severity of their illness or immaturity, many neonates will not have the energy for feeding. Feeding is a very demanding task, often exceeding what has been asked of an infant up to that point in her or his care. If the infant is preterm, she or he has an immature CNS with weak movement patterns, disorganized states, and oral structures that do not function as those of a full-term neonate. Tongue and jaw movements are affected by immature development, leading to poorer control of suck, swallow, and breathing patterns (Morris & Klein, 1987). Behavioral patterns include weak, poorly sustained sucking and inadequate state control during feeding. This interferes with coordination of suck and swallow with breathing. Nippling even small amounts can lead to exhaustion and flaccidity with disruption of respiratory control. Compounding the problem is staff and parental anxiety over weight gain and growth.

Usually, these infants can suck and swallow a small amount adequately. They then lose control, developing poor coordination of sucking and swallowing with breathing, an inability to sustain sucking, poor suck and swallow rhythm, respiratory irregularities, or exhaustion. This pattern of behavior has been termed the *disorganized feeder*, as opposed to the *dysfunctional feeder* (VandenBerg, 1990).

The dysfunctional feeder is the neurologically abnormal feeder with abnormal jaw and tongue movements during nutritive sucking (Braun & Palmer, 1982). This pattern does not spontaneously improve over time and requires intense therapeutic intervention. Dysfunctional feeders should be assessed by a specialist trained in feeding neonates. This specialist is usually an occupational, physical, or speech therapist or an infant educator. Abnormal oral muscle tone and reflexes are frequently present in this group of infants; professional intervention is required for improvement.

The disorganized feeder pattern usually improves as the infant recovers from neonatal illness and does not require specific therapeutic intervention (Braun & Palmer, 1982; VandenBerg, 1990). However, these infants do require sensitive pacing and accurate reading of their behavioral cues for signs of stress or stability to facilitate adequate nippling (Cagan, 1996).

The goal for the disorganized feeder is to learn self-regulation of autonomic, motoric, and state systems in order to eventually nipple adequately. To do this, the infant must be able to *simultaneously* (1) coordinate suck and swallow with respirations while maintaining heart rate and color; (2) coordinate movement patterns, posture, and tone; and (3) remain in a calm, organized state. In order to help the infant achieve this level of functioning, the caregiver needs to respect the infant's neurobehavioral functional level and not push feeding beyond the infant's capabilities. Fostering state control, timing the feeding, pacing the feeding, positioning the infant, modifying the environment, and respecting the infant's energy level are all part of the neurodevelopmental approach to feeding infants in the NICU (Cagan, 1996; VandenBerg, 1990). Environmental modifications include a quiet setting with indirect lighting and minimal congestion and traffic. Position to facilitate feeding includes promoting generalized body flexion to reduce hypertonia and to assist with swallowing, maintaining the head in midline with hands close to face, providing hip flexion, and swaddling. Other techniques for promoting feeding are described in Chapter 23, Nutrition: Physiologic Basis of Metabolism and Management of Enteral and Parenteral Nutrition. Feeding disorganization is a temporary problem that caregivers can easily facilitate with adequate awareness of the appropriate interventions.

Nonnutritive Sucking

Sucking is one of the earliest coordinated behaviors of the fetus. Sucking is necessary for biologic survival and is an important parameter of caregiver–infant interaction, self-gratification, and soothing (Sammons & Lewis, 1985). Human infants demonstrate two modes of sucking—nutritive and nonnutritive—each with a specific pattern of organization (Medoff-Cooper, 1991). Nonnutritive sucking has a pattern of short, alternating bursts of sucking and rest in contrast to the longer, continuous, rhythmic patterns characteristic of nutritive sucking (Medoff-Cooper et al., 1989). Nonnutritive sucking is present in the fetus as early as 4½ months of gestation (Dubignon & Campbell, 1968). Nonnutritive sucking is seen in VLBW infants. The presence of nonnutritive sucking in these infants does not mean that they have the ability to coordinate and maintain nutritive sucking. The ability to maintain, regulate, and organize the pattern and rhythm of nutritive and nonnutritive sucking is affected by the infant's maturity, illness, and experience.

Nonnutritive sucking is induced by placing a nipple in the infant's mouth without presentation of food. Nonnutritive sucking and rhythmic mouthing (seen in quiet sleep) have similar temporal organization, with regularity of the sucking–pause pattern. Nonnutritive sucking is a state modulation and organizing activity that is used during gavage feeding and interfeeding intervals. It has been associated with improved oxygenation; decreased, more stable intracranial pressure; increased quiet sleep; decreased ac-

TABLE 49–9 Examples of Types of Sensory Input for Stable High-Risk Infants*

Modality	Examples
Tactile/kinesthetic	Sheepskin, lambskin Containment, nesting with blankets Swaddling with blankets or hands Waterbeds, slings, hammocks Kangaroo care
Auditory	Reduction of environmental (background) noise Soft radio, music box, or tape (may need to be muffled) Talking softly within infant's visual range
Visual	Human face within infant's visual range (not closer and do not pursue infant if gaze averts) Single visual stimulus placed within infant's visual range on side of incubator Single stuffed animal or other toy placed in infant's visual range Time visual input to coincide with alert periods, moving slowly so as not to overwhelm infant Mobile (when infant can handle multimodal input)

*Each infant must be assessed regularly to determine her or his ability to tolerate both individual forms of sensory input and unimodal versus multimodal input.

tivity and crying; increased alertness; increased readiness for nipple feeding; better weight gain; and shorter hospital stays (Anderson et al., 1983; Burroughs et al., 1978; Field & Goldson, 1984; Field et al., 1982).

As noted earlier, infants who spend their first months after birth in a NICU or special care nursery experience many factors that may interfere with the acquisition of normal oral functioning and thus condition the infant to respond defensively to any oral stimuli. Nonnutritive sucking can be used to provide the infant with a source of self-consolation and self-regulation and to provide pleasant oral sensation that will serve as a basis for a positive introduction to nutritive sucking and feeding.

Strategies to facilitate development of nonnutritive sucking in intubated infants include (1) using nasal rather than oral intubation; (2) minimizing touch and stress to the oral musculature (and, when necessary, using gentle, slow touch); (3) placing in side-lying position with hands together; (4) positioning with hands tucked under chin or so that hands touch parts of face; and (5) providing pacifiers. After extubation, infants can be positioned with their hands together at the mouth or hands touching their face. In addition, pacifiers can be provided during nasogastric feedings and between feedings.

Kangaroo Care

Kangaroo care is a form of maternal caregiving that grew out of a crisis in the newborn intensive care nursery in Bogotá, Colombia. This type of care was pioneered by two pediatricians working in a large, understaffed, poorly equipped hospital where mortality of low birth weight infants was high. Along with the economic problems, cross-infection was rampant. Infants were often abandoned in the hospital by their mothers. Kangaroo care was developed to be carried out by mothers with stable preterm neonates. This type of care has become, in a modified form, a standard of care in Sweden, England, Germany, and Italy (Affonso et al., 1989; Anderson, 1989; Anderson et al., 1986; Whitelaw et al., 1988).

The kangaroo method of care involves placing a stable full-term or preterm newborn, who requires no assistance with breathing, skin-to-skin in a vertical position between the mother's breasts. The warmth of the skin-to-skin contact and other sensations foster close contact between mother and infant. The infant usually wears only a diaper. The mother wears a loose blouse, dress, or gown that opens in the front and that can be easily wrapped around the infant once placed on the mother's chest (Fig. 49–8). The infant is kept warm by the heat generated by the mother's body and is covered by her clothing, so heat loss is avoided. In fact, most nurses report that close monitoring of the infant's temperature is important during kangaroo care so as to avoid overheating rather than underheating. Infants weighing as little as 1000 g and who are stable have been placed with their mothers kangaroo style.

In Bogotá, infants were discharged home when stable, regardless of weight, with only breast milk supplemented by guava juice. Of the 539 infants who entered the kangaroo program from 1979 to 1981, 72 percent of those under 1000 g survived, significantly decreasing the number of neonatal deaths. In addition, the number of abandoned infants decreased (Anderson et al., 1986).

To determine if the kangaroo method is safe in a tertiary-level NICU, Bosgue and coworkers (1988) conducted a study of six mother–infant pairs, recording physiologic parameters such as heart rate, respiratory rate, temperature, and oxygen saturation, along with maternal and infant behavior on a regular basis in incubator and kangaroo positions, over a 3-week period. Results indicated that for this sample, the kangaroo method was safe and potentially advantageous to both mother and infant. During kangaroo care, infants had a mean skin temperature associated with minimal oxygen consumption. There were no negative effects on physiologic function. Infants receiving this type of care were discharged sooner. DeLeeuw and associates (1991) reported similar findings regarding stability of physiologic parameters in VLBW infants during kangaroo care. Others have also demonstrated positive effects of kangaroo care in preterm infants (Gale et al., 1993; Ludington, 1990; Ludington-Hoe et al., 1991). Kangaroo care also has a positive effect on maternal feelings (Affonso et al., 1989). Other studies have been reported in the United States, Europe, Africa, and Central America (Anderson, personal communication, 1990).

Several variations of kangaroo care allow the procedure to be adapted to the infant, parent, and unit (Table 49–10). Mothers and fathers can both participate in kangaroo care if desired. Infants can receive kangaroo care for extended periods of the 24-hour day or periodically, depending on parental visiting patterns. Table 49–11 describes preparation of infant and parent for kangaroo care.

Interventions with Parents

The ability of the high-risk infant to organize physiologic responses and neurobehavioral activity after birth is crucial (1) in allowing the infant to respond more appropriately to her or his environment, of which the parents are an important part; (2) in providing the parents with a better understanding of their infant's unique rhythms; and (3) in supporting the infant's emerging organization and integration, making her or him more capable of coping with the home environment. Thus, interventions with parents can help not only to enhance the infant's neurobehavioral organization and development but also to promote parent–infant interaction. To intervene with an infant without involving the parents ignores a major component of the infant's environment and developmental care. In the long run, infants spend more time with their parents than with NICU staff. In many studies, the best predictors of later infant outcomes are not the NICU environment per se or the infant's health status, but parental variables and the home environment.

Interventions with parents (Blackburn, 1983; Blackburn & Kang, 1991) include:

1. Discussing discrepancies between the parents' expectations of their infant's appearance and behavior and reality.
2. Encouraging approaches appropriate to the infant's status and maturity.
3. Placing parents in situations in which they will succeed in interacting positively with their infants.
4. Avoiding remarks that unfavorably compare infant responses to parents with infant responses to other caregivers.
5. Involving parents in identifying effective techniques for interacting with their infants.
6. Identifying infant behavioral responses, including subtle signs of attention and response to the parent's touch or voice (i.e., decreased activity, more regular respirations, or increased oxygenation).
7. Teaching parents (a) to recognize and use infant states and stress and stability cues in interacting with their infants and (b) techniques for alerting and consoling their infant that are appropriate to the infant's maturity and health status.
8. Providing anticipatory guidance as the infant matures.

Interventions for working with parents after discharge are discussed in Chapter 47, Systematic Assessment and Home Follow-Up: A Basis for Monitoring the Neonate's Integration Into the Family.

Applications of Intervention Strategies to Specific Situations

The preceding section describes a variety of intervention strategies that can be used with individual infants according to their

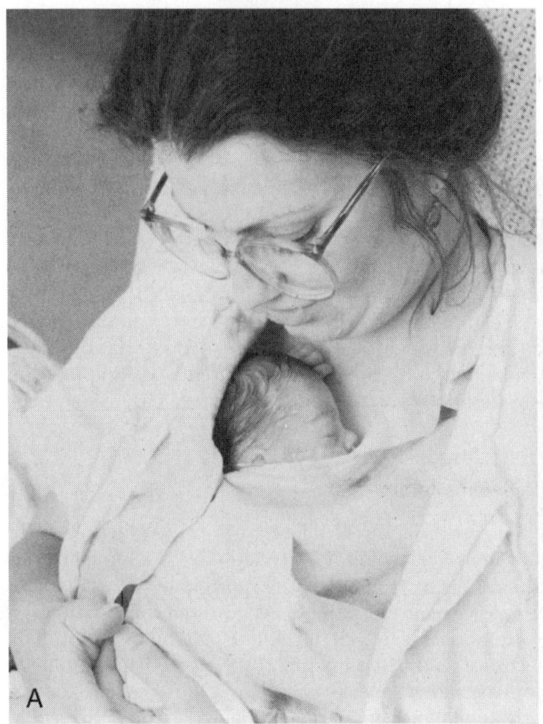

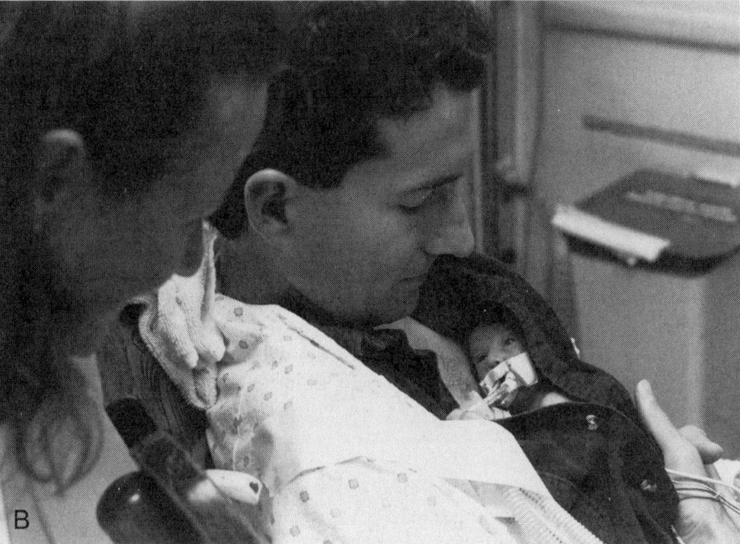

FIGURE 49–8. Skin-to-skin "kangaroo" method of holding preterm infants by mother *(A)* and by father *(B)*. (Courtesy of Children's Hospital, Oakland, CA.)

level of neurobehavioral development and health status. This section examines developmental interventions that the nurse might consider in planning care for infants that fall within specific groups: extremely preterm (VLBW), growing preterm, and ill full-term infants; infants with BPD or requiring prolonged or repeated hospitalization; or infants born to mothers with a history of perinatal substance abuse. These areas are only for consideration because, as emphasized earlier in the chapter, each infant needs to be assessed on an ongoing basis so that the plan of developmental care is individualized to that infant's unique needs, level of developmental function, and ability to tolerate environmental stimuli and other sensory input. Developmental interventions are also an important component in the management of infants experiencing pain. (See the section on nonpharmacologic management of pain in Chapter 40, Identification, Management, and Prevention of Pain in the Neonate.)

TABLE 49–10 Levels of Kangaroo Care

Level	Description
Late K	Begins after the infant has survived the intensive care phase, has stable respirations, and is breathing room air. This can be days or weeks postbirth. This method is being studied experimentally in the United States and Europe.
Intermediate K	Begins after the infant has survived early intensive care, usually about a week postbirth. These infants often still require oxygen and may have periods of apnea and bradycardia. This method is being studied anecdotally and experimentally in Europe and the United States.
Early K	Begins as soon as the infant is stable postbirth, usually during the first day and often the first hours after birth. This is the method used in Bogotá, Colombia.
Very early K	Used with stable infants with Apgars above 6 who are returned to their mothers during the first minutes following birth. If the mothers are lying down, the infants are placed prone on their abdomens. These infants then stay with their mothers thereafter. This is being used by a few obstetricians.

From Anderson, G. C. (1987). Personal communication. Used with permission.

Extremely Preterm Infants

The traumatic and abrupt early transition from intrauterine to extrauterine life places the underdeveloped fetus in a situation

TABLE 49–11 Example of a Protocol for Kangaroo Holding

1. Explain the procedure to the parent so that she or he understands kangaroo holding before starting. Confirm that this is an activity that the parent wants to participate in. Prepare a chair and area where the parent can relax in privacy.
2. To prepare the infant:
   a. remove the infant's clothing except for a diaper
   b. place the infant vertically on the mother or father's chest between the breasts
   c. close the parent's gown around the baby and place a blanket over the infant
3. To prepare the parent:
   a. have the parent wear a scrub gown open in front with no other clothing over the chest
   b. assist infant to position head comfortably once placed on the parent's chest
4. Monitor axillary temperatures of the infant every 15 minutes. Remove the blanket if the infant's temperature is >37.3° (99.2°F). Do not use heat lamps. Most infants will stay very warm next to their parent's skin.

that is incongruent and stressful (Als, 1982). In utero, this infant experienced a warm, comfortable, dimly lit, fluid-filled, gently oscillating environment where basic physiologic, sensory, and motor needs were met. The extrauterine experience, in sharp contrast, provides a noisy, nonadaptive environment that the fetus is unprepared for, but yet must depend on for survival. In utero, functioning in an environment for which she or he is well adapted, the fetus is quite competent. However, a preterm infant in a NICU must cope with a continuous bombardment of inappropriate stimuli. Thus, neonates who are born early must struggle to develop and maintain their autonomic, motor, and sensory systems in organized patterns of functioning in the midst of inappropriate, overwhelming stimuli. If the autonomic system is extremely immature, the infant is often overwhelmed just by the tasks of stabilizing this system, much less by achieving organization or recovering from illness.

The CNS of the preterm infant is well adapted for the intrauterine world at a time when the infant is forced to deal with the extrauterine environment. This leads to an environmental mismatch that influences brain development. The infant brain is undergoing major development and organization during this period. The brain of the immature infant has been described by Als (1986) as overly sensitive and at the mercy of sensory information, unable to buffer input because of the lack of inhibitory controls. Therefore, the extrauterine environment has a strong influence on the development of the immature infant. Experiences such as repeated hypoxic events secondary to handling or environmental stimuli may negatively affect the infant's vulnerable brain, leading to permanent insults (Als et al., 1986; Long et al., 1980b).

Inasmuch as the possibility of CNS dysfunction increases when the environment of the nursery provides overwhelming or inappropriate stimuli to an immature organism, caregivers must be aware of and seek to modify these experiences in relation to stressors from the physical environment (light, sound), caregiving activities and routines, and medical procedures. VLBW infants must first stabilize physiologically, and their behaviors are directed toward this end. Conservation of energy is of utmost importance in accomplishing this task and achieving homeostasis (Tronick et al., 1987). If the tiny amounts of energy available are consumed in coping with overwhelming stimuli and handling, the infant will operate at a deficiency with no reserve. It becomes essential that caregivers interpret the infant's cues for stress and instability and work to protect the infant from the environment and the effects of caregiving interventions. Thus, the primary goal in intervening to promote developmental competence in the VLBW infant is to alter the environment and caregiving events that cause stress and interfere with physiologic homeostasis (VandenBerg & Franck, 1990).

This alteration can be accomplished by identifying the behaviors in the infant that indicate stress and disorganization and the events in the physical environment or associated with caregiving that trigger these behaviors. Interventions can then be provided that reduce the incidence of these stressful behaviors. This approach seeks to support the emergence of developmental maturation, energy conservation, and eventual recovery from acute illness. A primary area of intervention is to work with the parents to promote understanding of the infant's behavior and needs. Parents also need a participatory role in caregiving and in planning and carrying out the developmental protections. Specific intervention strategies for the VLBW neonate are summarized in Table 49–12.

Growing Preterm Infants

As preterm infants recover from their initial health problems and develop increasing neurobehavioral organization, their developmental needs change. Although these infants still need protection from aversive aspects of the environment, they also need increasing opportunities for positive interaction with that environment. Environmental interventions for these infants are directed at modifications to approximate the home environment, including diurnal cycling of light and sound.

By approximately 32 weeks' postconceptional age, infants have achieved enough autonomic regulation and homeostasis to begin to interact more actively with specific aspects of the environment, including caregivers. A primary focus during this period is promotion of state organization. Specific techniques are described in the previous section on state modulation. These infants will also benefit from opportunities for nonnutritive sucking and kangaroo care, both of which also influence state organization.

Interaction with caregivers and the physical environment can be facilitated by opportunities for increasing sensory input (see Table 49–9). Initially, this input must be unimodal, low-keyed, brief, and matched to the infant's behavioral capabilities and ability to tolerate. Social interaction and provision of sensory input should be matched with the appropriate state and should proceed in a graded fashion. Infants should be continuously observed for signs of sensory overload and, if these occur, the stimuli should be reduced or removed (Als, 1996).

Parents and other caregivers must recognize that even when these infants are ready for discharge in terms of their physiologic status, they are still immature neurobehaviorally. Therefore, it is critical that before discharge, parents learn to recognize how their infant indicates that she or he is stressed or sensorially overloaded, what circumstances and events tend to stress the infant, and what interventions are most effective to help the infant deal with stressful situations and reorganize. Table 49–13 provides suggestions for parents in providing routine care for their infant.

Full-Term Ill Infant

Full-term infants have an advantage over preterm infants in that they are better organized, having a more mature CNS. As a result, the full-term infant is better able to deal with the extrauterine environment and is ready for active social interaction. If this infant is critically ill, he or she may not be able to tolerate and interact with the environment in ways similar to a healthy infant. The major focus of developmental care for the ill full-term infant is on conservation of energy and reduction of stress so as not to further compromise physiologic stability and recovery processes, while meeting the infant's developmental needs in a manner that is appropriate to the infant's health status.

Environmental stressors from light, noise, traffic, and congestion must be reduced. Energy conservation and stress reduction can be facilitated by prone or side-lying positioning of the infant to maintain flexion, use of boundaries, and swaddling. Full-term infants are often irritable and frequently cry. Soothing interventions include containing and swaddling, reducing stimulation, holding the infant's hands and/or feet, positioning prone, and providing sucking opportunities. These infants may need minimal handling and sensory input during the period in which they are critically ill. The above recommendations are also appropriate for infants with cardiac problems.

As the infant recovers, she or he will be ready for more active interaction with caregivers and able to tolerate increased sensory input. Considerations in providing sensory input and in facilitating social responsiveness during the recovery period are similar to those for the growing preterm infant. Intervention strategies for the full-term neonate are summarized in Table 49–14.

Infants With Bronchopulmonary Dysplasia

The diagnosis of BPD has significant serious consequences for the parents and staff as well as the infant. BPD is a disorder associated with a prolonged and complicated hospital course. Although BPD can develop in full-term infants, it is seen most frequently in preterm and low birth weight infants. Prolonged hospitalization jeopardizes developmental progress, as infants ex-

TABLE 49–12 A Guide for Prevention and Management of Stress in Very Low Birth Weight Infants

Problem	Goal	Method
Environmental		
Immature, vulnerable CNS	Infant will be protected from environmental stimulation	Reduce light Cover all bedsides, tablebeds, cribs, etc., with dark cloths or covers Reduce noise Implement quiet hour and post signs at bedside to remind staff; pad trash cans, doors, drawers; pad loudspeakers at bedside
Handling		
Easily stressed by all/any procedures	Infant will be prepared to tolerate and recover from procedures with minimal stress as expressed in autonomic/motoric reactions	Before procedure Carry out procedure in stages if possible, allowing recovery and return to appropriate heart and respiratory rates or $TcPo_2$ after each step. Cluster care only as appropriate for individual infants. Some may need slow, continuous, gently efficient carrying out of all procedures, followed by rest. Place according to individual cues. After procedure Continue positioning and containment up to 10 minutes or until infant is stable again, with heart and respiratory rates or $TcPo_2$ back to baseline, and has recovered tone.
Positioning		
Extended flaccid unsupported limbs Abducted hips Retracted shoulder Poor and variable muscle tone (from flaccid to hypertonicity)	Infant's limbs will be flexed; infant will be positioned in postures that permit flexion and minimize flailing, arching, and squirming	Minimal handling protocol Position prone/side lying—never supine Support with blanket rolls Swaddle, wrap to maintain flexion
State Regulation		
Frequent agitation Erratic sleep Exhaustion/excessive fatigue	Infant's sleep will be organized, agitation prevented, and energy and calories preserved for growth, not stress	Modify environment to reduce stimulation Position Provide boundaries Swaddle, contain Handle slowly and gently Cluster care and leave protected/undisturbed for 2- to 3-hour intervals (see minimal handling protocol) Avoid unnecessary stimulation

CNS, central nervous system.
From VandenBerg, K. A. (1990). Behaviorally supportive care for the extremely premature infant. In L. P. Gunderson & C. Kenner (Eds.), *Care of the 24–25 week gestational age infant (small baby protocol).* Petaluma, CA: Neonatal Network. Reprinted with permission.

perience daily exposure to high levels of inappropriate patterns of sensory input from the hospital environment (Blackburn, 1989; Gottfried & Gaiter, 1985; Lawson, 1977). This is compounded by restriction of movement from prolonged ventilation or need for supplemental oxygen and the loss of a consistent primary caregiver. These factors contribute to the higher incidence of developmental problems seen in these infants (Sell & Vaucher, 1988).

Infants with BPD demonstrate many complex behavioral difficulties, often in relation to signs of physiologic compromise. Agitation and stressful episodes are frequently identified by these infants' caregivers as areas of major concern. Other problems include excessive energy expenditure, overreactivity to stimuli, poor self-regulation, repetitive motor behaviors, motor abnormalities, defensive behaviors, frantic activity, and poor feeding (VandenBerg & Franck, 1990).

Because of these behavioral difficulties, the infant with BPD presents several challenges to the NICU nurse. These infants are often unable to provide easily readable cues to signal the onset of severe stress, which often leads to physiologic compromise. The infant with BPD often has an all-or-nothing response to care. These infants may become quickly overstimulated, even from the most benign, routine handling. Instead of a gradual arousal to crying, the infant will abruptly become hypoxic and dusky, requiring immediate physiologic support. These infants do not typically demonstrate a gradual build-up of irritability or other signs of stress. It is extremely difficult to plan or organize care for such an unpredictable patient. State transitions are often unpredictable as well, frustrating the caregiver, who must try to provide care while dealing with an infant who is calm one minute and severely stressed the next. Moreover, the usual soothing techniques of rocking, holding, and talking are not only ineffective, they often exacerbate the infant's stress (VandenBerg & Franck, 1990).

The preterm infant with BPD must also cope with an immature, vulnerable CNS. These infants may be behaviorally disorganized and thus overreact to their environment, unable to shut out stimuli effectively. This may occur at great physiologic cost to their systems and manifest in poor respiratory control, frequent desaturation, and/or a period of duskiness and cyanosis. The infant with BPD also has other physiologic stressors. The contribution of hypoxia, pain, bronchospasm, gastroesophageal reflux, and pharmacologic therapies such as diuretics and xanthine to the agitated state and behavioral disorganization must also be considered.

The complex associations between the infant's behavior and

TABLE 49–13 Guidelines for Incorporating Developmental Principles into Daily Care for the Stable Growing Infant

Caregiving	Easily Stressed Infant	Well-Organized Infant
Waking	Enter room slowly, turn on light, and open curtains or pull up shades slowly	No special adjustment is required
	Avoid arousing if in sleep	Proceed slowly, noting stress and stability cues and helping infant maintain equilibrium
	Vocalize softly	
	Uncover or unwrap gently	
	Avoid overstimulating, even if infant is difficult to arouse	
Changing	Adjust room temperature	As above
	Avoid sudden changes in position	
	Contain limbs while shifting position	
	Keep tactile stimulation mild	
	Frequent consoling may be necessary, but allow infant to use own self-quieting mechanisms	
	Stop changing if infant demonstrates signs of instability	
Feeding	Attend to unique demands for feeding	As above
	Time feeding to coincide with spontaneous alert periods	
	Avoid unessential noise	
	Inhibit disorganized motor activity by wrapping or holding infant close to body	
	Adjust distance from caregiver to suit infant	
Bathing	As above, proceed slowly, watching for signs of exhaustion and disorganization (stress cues)	As above
	Ventral openness may be disruptive	
	Ventral body surface inhibition may be needed, bracing hands or feet against hand or bedside	
	Cover body parts not being bathed	
	Offer support as needed in the form of a finger or pacifier	
	Allow frequent rests	
	Allow infant to organize self when possible	

Adapted from Rauh, V. A., Nurcombe, B., Achenbach, T., & Howell, C. (1990). The mother–infant transactional program: The content and implications of an intervention for the mothers of low-birthweight infants. *Clinics in Perinatology, 17,* 31–45. Reprinted with permission.

physiologic compromise are not yet fully understood. According to a survey by Franck (1987), medication is widely used to manage the agitation of infants with chronic lung disease. The long-term implications of this type of management are unknown. Developmental care for the infant with BPD is essential for preventing and managing agitation in these infants. Applying behavioral and environmental interventions before pharmacologic interventions can, in many cases, prevent stress and eliminate or reduce the need for medication (VandenBerg & Franck, 1990).

TABLE 49–14 Developmental Care for Full-Term Ill Neonates

Type of Strategy	Examples of Interventions
Minimize environment stress	Reduce noise levels
	Reduce light levels
	Reduce congestion
Energy conservation	Minimize environmental stress (see above)
	Individualize handling and use with appropriate timing
	Position infant to foster physiologic stability and state control and prevent agitation
	Provide opportunities for nonnutritive sucking
	Reduce pain (see Chapter 40, Identification, Management, and Prevention of Pain in the Neonate)
Promote neurobehavioral organization	Incorporate developmental care principles into routine care activities (see Table 49–13)
	Promote state organization and state modulation
	Provide sensory experiences appropriate to infant's health status
	Involve parents in planning and implementing care

The goals of developmental care for the infant with BPD include fostering self-regulation, which will help reduce agitation, preserving energy to promote growth, and supporting CNS organization and recovery. Specific strategies for working with these infants are listed in Table 49–15. An essential component of care of these infants is promoting understanding by parents of their infant's behavioral needs and providing opportunities for positive parent–infant interaction.

Infants Requiring Prolonged or Repeated Hospitalization

The infant with BPD or the extremely low birth weight ill infant (<800 g) will frequently have a lengthy hospital course that is often complicated by developmental delays. These infants must recover and achieve physiologic intactness before adequate developmental progress can be expected. Even after discharge, repeated hospitalizations accompanied by disruptions in feeding and recurring infections and other illness will certainly have an impact on a child's overall development and level of functioning. These delays are often transient, but they need careful and ongoing evaluation. As these infants recover, developmental progress usually escalates. Developmental care focuses on continued amelioration and resolution of the stresses of the family as well as promoting CNS organization in the infant.

Developmental interventions for these infants and their parents do not require the aggressive high-level approach necessary with the developmentally disabled infant who needs therapeutic enrichment. This population needs an approach that seeks to facilitate the normal acquisition of developmental skills while taking into account the individual coping behaviors and capacities of the recovering infant.

TABLE 49–15 Developmental Care for Infants With Bronchopulmonary Dysplasia

Type of Strategy	Examples of Interventions
Strategies for behavioral management	Modify environment (light, noise, etc.) Time handling to avoid overtiring and overstimulating Time daily events with appropriate infant states Adapt caregiving routines to individual infant's needs Read infant's subtle cues and provide prompt responses to prevent escalation of stress Minimize handling
Soothing strategies	Reduce activity around bedside Allow 2 to 3 hours of undisturbed rest between caregiving routines Plan nursing care activities around infant states Minimize stressful routines (i.e., suction PRN rather than per a schedule) Reduce activity at first subtle sign of stress (if holding, put back in bed prone; if playing with toys, hold quietly) Swaddle prone or side-lying with pacifier Make a ring of blanket rolls around baby and tuck in Provide sucking opportunities Provide opportunities for grasping

Adapted from VandenBerg, K. A., & Franck, L. (1990). Behavioral issues for infants with BPD. In C. Lund (Ed.), *BPD: Strategies for total patient care*. Petaluma, CA: Neonatal Network. Reprinted with permission.

Developmental care of infants requiring prolonged or repeated hospitalization during infancy presents special challenges to caregivers in dealing with both physiologic and growth and developmental needs. Goldberger (1990) suggests that the goals of stimulation programs for these infants should be to modify the environment to provide adequate and appropriate developmental opportunities and maximized comfort and to enhance the parent's sense of competence and control. Interventions include (1) limiting the number of caregivers; (2) encouraging internal and external rhythmicity and development of diurnal cycles; (3) responding appropriately, rapidly, and consistently to infant crying and other cues; (4) reducing fragmented sensory events such as stomach filling by tube feeding without opportunity for sucking and being held; (5) providing opportunities for coordinated multisensory events such as establishing eye contact with the infant while talking to her or him or reducing the use of radios to provide stimulation, when in actuality this becomes just white background noise; (6) providing predictability in routines and people and providing opportunities for learning cause and effect; (7) providing opportunity for variety, change, and novel situations; (8) respecting the infant's personal space; and (9) providing age-appropriate play materials and opportunities for exploration (Goldberger, 1990).

Drug-Exposed Infants

With the dramatic increase in the incidence of substance abuse among childbearing women, most neonatal units are seeing a dramatic rise in the number of infants who have been exposed prenatally to substances such as heroin, PCP, marijuana, cocaine, and crack. In many cases, women are using multiple drugs and are also using alcohol and tobacco. This problem and its implications are discussed in Chapter 45, The Drug-Exposed Neonate.

The effects of these drugs on the fetus and neonate include increased mortality, dysmorphology, alterations in physiologic function, risk of pathologic problems, and subtle behavioral difficulties (Howard, 1989). Many of these substances markedly alter fetal and neonatal behavioral and neurobehavioral capabilities, increasing the risk for later developmental problems. Specific patterns of behavior described for this population include hyperexcitable states, erratic state behaviors, frantic and disorganized behavior, poor visual processing, and increased startles and tremors (Chasnoff, 1989; Dixon, 1989; Eisen et al., 1991; Howard, 1989). Environmental, physical, and social factors, along with variations in the frequency of use, potency, and mix of drugs, can alter the effects of perinatal substance abuse on infants. As a result, all infants may not be affected in the same way or to the same degree.

In the NICU, the nurse must deal with the neurobehavioral effects not only of drug exposure, but also of illness, low birth weight, and prematurity. The behavioral patterns of many infants exposed to drugs during the prenatal period are similar to those of a sick preterm infant. Therefore, nursing assessment and intervention strategies that are appropriate for a sick, disorganized preterm infant (see Table 49–13) will be beneficial for the disorganized drug-exposed infant. Interventions that are especially useful include protection from overstimulation, environmental modifications, minimal handling, and positioning techniques. Swaddling and providing boundaries with diaper rolls are particularly helpful for drug-exposed infants because their states are usually more erratic.

The staff of the Special Start Program at Children's Hospital in Oakland, California, a federally funded research program and intervention program for drug-exposed neonates, has found that holding these infants reduced agitation and facilitated better state control. They have trained a group of volunteers to hold drug-exposed infants. The time of holding is gradually increased, as tolerated by the infant, to up to 3 hours daily. These infants are held only as long as the infant's autonomic system is regulated. If there is any sudden increase in heart or respiratory rate, oxygen desaturation, or color change, the infant experiences an immediate reduction in handling (Sweet, 1991).

Supportive care for the family is essential, particularly since many women who are substance abusers also have low self-esteem. Nonjudgmental facilitation of parental understanding of the infant's needs and behavior is of primary importance. The mother may be afraid to enter the nursery, may feel guilty about her infant's requiring hospitalization, and may not see herself as an adequate parent. She may view her infant as fragile and be afraid of touching her or him and exacerbating the disorder. Interventions focus on providing these mothers with successful and positive interactions with their infants, such as being able to respond appropriately to their infant's behavioral disorganization. The kangaroo method of holding may be an especially positive experience for these mother–infant pairs. Other intervention strategies for the drug-exposed infant include (1) providing an appropriate environment, including a quiet, darkened room; (2) swaddling; (3) protecting from overstimulation and excessive handling with use of minimal handling protocols; (4) preventing and managing agitation to enhance tolerance for handling as the infant matures and recovers; (5) encouraging visual attention and organization as the infant recovers and alerting emerges; and (6) facilitating caregiver–infant interaction.

COLLABORATIVE CARE

Both the assessment and the management of neurobehavioral development involve a multidisciplinary, collaborative approach. Although the nurse is the primary early caregiver who will usually, along with parents, provide most of the hands-on care, she or he practices in consultation with members of other disciplines who can provide assessments, recommend interventions, or recommend specific therapies. Other professionals involved may include physical therapists, occupational therapists, infant educators, developmental specialists, neonatologists, and developmental psychologists. In addition, provision of consistent and individualized developmental care and modification of the NICU environment require the support, understanding, and cooperation of all individuals in the nursery, including those who have direct (physicians, nurses, therapists, laboratory, and x-ray technicians) and indirect (unit secretaries, cleaners) patient contact.

To provide developmentally appropriate care, the NICU environment, caregiving practices, and caregiving routines must be evaluated on a regular basis. Barriers to providing this type of care can be identified and strategies developed for changes. In most settings, it is unrealistic to expect to institute major changes all at once. Priorities for changes in the environment and care practices, along with their advantages to the institution, staff, patients, and families, need to be identified. It is often best to start with those practices that are likely to be the easiest to change, will generate the least resistance, and will lead to success. The initial proposal for changes in developmental care can begin with a small group of committed nurses and other professionals. This group will need to assess and work with the formal and informal power structures within the unit. However, changes in developmental care can often begin with a few nurses altering the way they care for infants assigned to them. Role modeling, mentoring, and positive reinforcement along with regular educational opportunities and case discussions are useful strategies (McGrath & Valenzuela, 1994). Various models for implementing developmental supportive care programs have been described (Als, 1986; Cole et al., 1990; Grunwald & Becker, 1990; McGrath & Valenzuela, 1994; Tribotti & Stein, 1992).

CONCLUSION

High-risk infants are both dependent on and vulnerable to their early environment—the NICU and intermediate nursery—to maintain their physiologic function, to promote growth and development, and to provide opportunities for the organization of state, behavioral, and social responsiveness. The immaturity and physiologic and neurobehavioral instability of these infants make them particularly vulnerable to environments that do not support their emerging organization and patterns or that do not attend to their cues and respond appropriately.

In summary, the goals in addressing the neurobehavioral needs of high-risk infants are to:

1. Provide an environment that enhances and supports the infant's developing capabilities.
2. Protect the infant from sensory overload and minimize stressors.
3. Assist parents in understanding their infant's unique abilities.
4. Help parents interact with their infant in ways appropriate to the infant's health status, state, and level of maturity.
5. Use the infant's needs and capabilities to foster more positive parent–infant interaction.

REFERENCES

Ackerman, B., Sherwonit, E., & Williams, J. (1989). Reduced incidental light exposure: Effect on the development of retinopathy of prematurity in low birthweight infants. *Pediatrics, 83*(6), 956–962.

Affonso, D., Wahlberg, V., & Persson, B. (1989). Exploration of mother's reactions to the kangaroo method of prematurity care. *Neonatal Network, 7*(6), 43–51.

Agnagnostakis, D., Petmezakis, J., Messaritakis, J., & Matsaniotis, N. (1980). Noise pollution in neonatal units: A potential health hazard. *Acta Paediatrica Scandinavica, 69*(6), 771–773.

Als, H. (1982). Toward a synactive theory of development: Promise for the assessment and support of infant individuality. *Infant Mental Health Journal, 3*(4), 229–243.

Als, H. (1984). Newborn behavioral assessment. In W. J. Burns & J. V. Lavigne (Eds.), *Progress in pediatric psychology*. New York: Grune & Stratton.

Als, H. (1986). A synactive model of neonatal behavioral organization: Framework for the assessment of neurobehavioral development in the premature infant and for the support of infants and parents in the neonatal intensive care environment. *Physical and Occupational Therapy in Pediatrics, 6*(3–4), 3–53.

Als, H. (1996). *The very immature infant—Environmental and care issues.* Paper presented at The Physical and Developmental Environment of the High Risk Neonate. Clearwater Beach, FL: University of South Florida College of Medicine.

Als, H., Lawhon, G., Brown, E., et al. (1986). Individualized behavioral and environmental care for the very low birth weight preterm infant at high risk for bronchopulmonary dysplasia: Neonatal intensive care unit and developmental outcome. *Pediatrics, 78*(6), 1123–1132.

Als, H., Lawhon, G., Duffy, F. H., et al. (1994). Individualized developmental care for the very low birthweight preterm infants: Medical and neurofunctional effects. *Journal of the American Medical Association, 272*(11), 853–858.

Als, H., Lester, B. M., Tronick, E. Z., & Brazelton, T. B. (1982). Assessment of preterm infant behavior (APIB). In H. E. Fitzgerald & M. Yogman (Eds.), *Theory and research in behavioral pediatrics* (Vol. 1, pp. 64–133). New York: Plenum Press.

Anderson, G. C. (1989). Skin to skin care: Kangaroo care in Western Europe. *American Journal of Nursing, 89*(5), 662–666.

Anderson, G. C., Burroughs, A. K., & Measel, C. P. (1983). Nonnutritive sucking opportunities: A safe and effective treatment for preterm neonates. In T. M. Field & A. K. Sostek (Eds.), *Infants born at risk: Physiological, perceptual and cognitive processes* (pp. 129–146). New York: Grune & Stratton.

Anderson, G. C., Marks, E. A., & Wahlberg, V. (1986). Kangaroo care for premature infants. *American Journal of Nursing, 86*(7), 807–809.

Ariagno, R. (1996). *Sleep, sleep cycles, and sleep deprivation.* Paper presented at The Physical and Developmental Environment of the High Risk Neonate. Clearwater Beach, FL: University of South Florida College of Medicine.

Ariagno, R., Fleisher, B., Kugener, B., et al. (1996a). *Individualized developmental care for very low birth weight infants improved state system control without advanced development in sleep measures using the motility monitoring system.* Paper presented at The Physical and Developmental Environment of the High Risk Neonate. Clearwater Beach, FL: University of South Florida College of Medicine.

Ariagno, R., Kugener, B., Thoman, E., et al. (1996b). *A comparison of polysomnographic vs. motility monitoring system sleep state determination during naps in infants.* Paper presented at The Physical and Developmental Environment of the High Risk Neonate. Clearwater Beach, FL: University of South Florida College of Medicine.

Barnard, K. E., & Bee, H. L. (1983). The impact of temporally patterned stimulation on the development of preterm infants. *Child Development, 54*(5), 1156–1167.

Bayley, N. (1969). *Bayley scales of infant development.* New York: The Psychological Corporation.

Becker, P. T., Grunwald, P. C., Moorman, J., & Stuhr, S. (1991). Outcomes of developmentally supportive nursing care for very low birthweight infants. *Nursing Research, 40*(3), 150–155.

Bess, F. H., Peek, B. F., & Chapman, J. J. (1979). Further observations of noise levels in infant incubators. *Pediatrics, 63*(1), 100–106.

Blackburn, S. (1979). *The effects of caregiving activities in the neonatal intensive care unit on the behavior and development of premature infants.* Doctoral dissertation, University of Washington, Seattle.

Blackburn, S. (1983). Fostering behavioral development of high risk neonates. *Journal of Obstetric, Gynecologic, and Neonatal Nursing, 12*(3 Suppl.), 76s–86s.

Blackburn, S. (1989). *NICU caregiving: Impact on preterm infant behavior and function* (Final Report, Grant #R23 NR01260). Bethesda, MD: National Center for Nursing Research.

Blackburn, S. (1995). Problems of preterm infants after discharge. *Journal of Obstetric, Gynecologic, and Neonatal Nursing, 24*(1), 43–49.

Blackburn, S. (1996, January). *Studies of light and its application to clinical practice.* Paper presented at The Physical and Developmental

Environment of the High Risk Neonate. Clearwater Beach, FL: University of South Florida College of Medicine.
Blackburn, S., & Barnard, K. E. (1985). Analysis of caregiving events in preterm infants in the special care unit. In A. Gottfried & J. Gaiter (Eds.), *Infants under stress: Environmental neonatology* (pp. 113–129). Baltimore: University Park Press.
Blackburn, S., & Kang, R. E. (1991). *Early parent–infant relationships* (2nd ed.). White Plains, NY: March of Dimes Birth Defects Foundation.
Blackburn, S., & Patteson, D. (1991). Effects of cycled lighting on activity state and cardiorespiratory function in preterm infants. *Journal of Perinatal and Neonatal Nursing, 4*(4), 47–54.
Bosgue, E. M., Brady, J. P., Affonso, D. D., & Wahlberg, V. (1988). Continuous physiologic measurement of kangaroo vs incubator care in a tertiary level nursery. *Pediatric Research, 23*, 402A.
Braun, M., & Palmer, M. (1982). *Early detection and treatment of infants and young children with neuromuscular disorders*. New York: Therapeutic Media.
Brazelton, T. B. (1984). *Neonatal behavioral assessment scale* (2nd ed.). Philadelphia: J. B. Lippincott.
Brazelton, T. B. (1990). Saving the bath water. *Child Development, 61*(6), 1661–1671.
Bull, M. J., & Dodge, N. N. (1996). *Physical and developmental environment of high-risk infants requiring prolonged hospitalization*. Paper presented at The Physical and Developmental Environment of the High Risk Neonate. Clearwater Beach, FL: University of South Florida College of Medicine.
Burns, K., Cunningham, N., White-Traut, R. C., et al. (1994). Infant stimulation: Modification of an intervention based on physiologic and behavioral cues. *Journal of Obstetric, Gynecologic, and Neonatal Nursing, 23*(7), 581–589.
Burns, K. A., Deddish, R. B., Burns, W. J., & Hatcher, R. P. (1983). Use of oscillating waterbeds and rhythmic sounds for premature infant stimulation. *Developmental Psychology, 19*(5), 746–752.
Burroughs, A. K., Asonye, U. O., Anderson-Shanklin, G. C., & Vidyasagar, D. (1978). The effect of nonnutritive sucking on transcutaneous oxygen tension in noncrying preterm neonates. *Research in Nursing and Health, 1*(2), 69–75.
Cagan, J. B. (1996). *Feeding readiness behavior in preterm infants.* Paper presented at The Physical and Developmental Environment of the High Risk Neonate. Clearwater Beach, FL: University of South Florida College of Medicine.
Campbell, A. N., Lightstone, A. D., Smith, J. M., et al. (1984). Mechanical vibration and sound levels experienced in neonatal transport. *American Journal of Diseases of Children, 138*(10), 967–970.
Carlos, S. A. (1991). *The effects of positioning on nursing care activities in preterm infants: Suctioning.* Unpublished master's thesis, University of Washington, Seattle.
Catlett, A. T., & Holditch-Davis, D. (1990). Environmental stimulation of the acutely ill premature infant. *Neonatal Network, 8*(6), 19–26.
Chasnoff, I. J. (1989). Cocaine and pregnancy—Implications for the child (Editorial). *Western Journal of Medicine, 150*(4), 456–458.
Ciesielski, S., Kopka, J. & Kidawa, B. (1980). Incubator noise and vibration—possible iatrogenic influence on the neonate. *International Journal of Pediatric Otorhinolaryngology, 1*(4), 309–316.
Cole, J. G., Begish-Duddy, A., Judas, M. L., & Jorgensen, K. M. (1990). Changing the NICU environment: The Boston City Hospital model. *Neonatal Network, 9*(2), 15–23.
Cornell, E. H., & Gottfried, A. W. (1976). Intervention with premature human infants. *Child Development, 47*(1), 32–39.
D'Apolito, K. (1991). What is an organized infant? *Neonatal Network, 10*(1), 23–29.
Deiriggi, P. (1996). *The role of position and movement.* Paper presented at The Physical and Developmental Environment of the High Risk Neonate. Clearwater Beach, FL: University of South Florida College of Medicine.
Deiriggi, P. M. (1990). The effects of waterbed flotation on indicators of energy expenditure in preterm infants. *Nursing Research, 39*(3), 140–146.
deLeeuw, R., Colin, E. M., Dunnebier, E. A., & Mirmiran, M. (1991). Physiological effects of kangaroo care in very small preterm infants. *Biology of the Neonate, 59*(3), 149–155.
DePaul, D., & Chambers, S. E. (1995). Environmental noise in the neonatal intensive care unit: Implications for nursing practice. *Journal of Perinatal and Neonatal Nursing, 8*(4), 71–78.
Dixon, S. D. (1989). Effects of transplacental exposure to cocaine and methamphetamine on the neonate. *Western Journal of Medicine, 150*(4), 436–442.
Douek, E., Dodson, H. C., Bannister, L. H., et al. (1976). Effects of incubator noise on the cochlea of the newborn. *Lancet, 2*(7995), 1110–1113.
Dubignon, J., & Campbell, D. (1968). The relationship between laboratory measures of sucking, food intake, and perinatal factors during the newborn period. *Child Development, 40*, 1107–1120.
Duxbury, M. L., Henly, S. J., Broz, L. J., et al. (1984). Caregiver disruptions and sleep of high risk infants. *Heart and Lung, 13*(2), 141–147.
Eisen, L. N., Field, T. M., Bandstra, E. S., et al. (1991). Prenatal cocaine effects on neonatal stress behavior and performance on the Brazelton scale. *Pediatrics, 88*(3), 477–480.
Evans, J. C. (1991). Incidence of hypoxemia associated with caregiving in premature infants. *Neonatal Network, 10*(2), 17–24.
Evans, J. C. (1994). Comparison of two NICU patterns of caregiving over 24-hours for preterm infants. *Neonatal Network, 13*(5), 87.
Falk, S. A. (1974). Combined effects of noise and ototoxic drugs. *Environmental Health Perspectives, 2*, 5–22.
Field, T. (1980). Supplemental stimulation of preterm neonates [Review]. *Early Human Development, 4*(3), 301–314.
Field, T., & Goldson, E. (1984). Pacifying effects of nonnutritive sucking on term and preterm neonates during heelstick procedures. *Pediatrics, 74*(6), 1012–1015.
Field, T. M., Ignatoff, E., Stringer, S., et al. (1982). Nonnutritive sucking during tube feedings: Effects on preterm neonates in an intensive care unit. *Pediatrics, 70*(3), 381–384.
Fleisher, R. F., VandenBerg, K. A., Constantinou, J., et al. (1995). Individualized developmental care for very low birth weight premature infants. *Clinical Pediatrics, 34*(10), 523–529.
Franck, L. S. (1987). A national survey of the assessment and treatment of pain and agitation in the neonatal intensive care unit. *Journal of Obstetric, Gynecologic, and Neonatal Nursing, 16*(6), 387–393.
Fuhrman, P. (1984). *The effect of preterm infant state regulation on parent–child interaction*. Unpublished master's thesis, University of Washington, Seattle.
Gale, G., Franck, L., & Lund, C. (1993). Skin-to-skin (kangaroo care) holding of the intubated premature infant. Neonatal Network, 12(6), 49–57.
Glass, P. (1990). *Environmental manipulations in the NICU: Innovations in practice.* Paper presented at Conference on Developmental Interventions in Neonatal Care, Contemporary Forums, Washington, DC.
Glass, P., Avery, G. B., Subramanian, K. N., et al. (1985). Effect of bright light in the hospital nursery on the incidence of retinopathy of prematurity. *New England Journal of Medicine, 313*(7), 401–404.
Glotzbach, S. F., Rowlett, E. A., Edgar, D. M., et al. (1993). Light variability in the modern neonatal nursery: Chronobiological issues. *Medical Hypotheses 41*(3), 217–224.
Goldberger, J. (1990). Lengthy or repeated hospitalization in infancy: Issues in stimulation and intervention [Review]. *Clinics in Perinatology, 17*(1), 197–206.
Gorski, P. A., Hole, W. T., Leonard, C. H., & Martin, J. A. (1983). Direct computer recording of premature infants and nursery care: Distress following two interventions. *Pediatrics*, 72(2), 198–203.
Gorski, P. A. (1985). Behavioral and environmental care: New frontiers in neonatal nursing. *Neonatal Network, 10*(4), 8–11.
Gorski, P. A., Davison, M. F., & Brazelton, T. B. (1980). Stages of behavioral organization in the high-risk neonate: Theoretical and clinical considerations. In P. M. Taylor (Ed.), *Parent–infant relationships* (pp. 269–290). New York: Grune & Stratton.
Gorski, P. A., Lewkowicz, D. J., & Huntington, L. (1987). Advances in neonatal and infant behavioral assessment: Toward a comprehensive evaluation of early patterns of development [Review]. *Journal of Developmental and Behavioral Pediatrics, 8*(1), 39–50.
Gottfried, A., & Gaiter, J. (1985). *Infant stress under intensive care.* Baltimore: University Park Press.
Graven, S. N. (1996, January). *Concepts of fetal sensory development.* Paper presented at The Physical and Developmental Environment of the High Risk Neonate. Clearwater Beach, FL: University of South Florida College of Medicine.
Grunwald, P. C., & Becker, P. T. (1990). Developmental enhancement: Implementing a program for the NICU. *Neonatal Network*, 9(6), 29–30, 39–45.

Hamernik, R. P., Ahrooon, W. A., Davis, R. I., & Axelsson, A. (1989). Noise and vibration interactions: Effects on hearing. *Journal of Acoustic Society of America, 86*(6), 2129–2137.

Harris, M. B. (1986). Oral–motor management of the high-risk neonate. *Physical and Occupational Therapy in Pediatrics, 6*, 231–253.

Harrison, L. (1985). Effects of early supplemental stimulation programs for premature infants: Review of the literature. *American Journal of Maternal Child Nursing, 14*(2), 69–90.

Hebb, D. O. (1949). *The organization of behavior.* New York: John Wiley & Sons.

Howard, J. (1989). Cocaine and its effects on the newborn [Review]. *Developmental Medicine and Child Neurology, 31*(2), 255–257.

Kang, R., & Barnard, K. (1979). Using the Neonatal Behavioral Assessment Scale to evaluate premature infants. *Birth Defects Original Article Series, 15*(7), 119–144.

Korner, A. F. (1973). Early stimulation and maternal care as related to infant capabilities and individual differences. *Early Child Development and Care, 2*(3), 307–327.

Korner, A. F. (1986). The use of waterbeds in the care of preterm infants. *Journal of Perinatology, 6*(2), 142–147.

Korner, A. F., Kraemer, H. C., Haffner, E., & Cosper, L. M. (1975). Effects of waterbed flotation on premature infants: A preliminary study. *Pediatrics, 56*(3), 361–367.

Landry, R. J., Scheidt, P. C., & Hammond, R. W. (1985). Ambient light and phototherapy conditions of eight neonatal care units: A summary report. *Pediatrics 75*(2, Part 2), 434–436.

Lawhon, G. (1986). Management of stress in premature infants. In D. J. Angelini, C. M. Knapp, & R. M. Gibes (Eds.), *Perinatal/neonatal nursing: A clinical handbook* (pp. 319–328). Boston: Blackwell Scientific Publications.

Lawhon, G., & Melzar, A. (1988). Developmental care of the very low birth weight infant. *Journal of Perinatal and Neonatal Nursing, 2*(1), 56–65.

Lawson, K. (1977). Environmental characteristics of a neonatal intensive care unit. *Child Development, 48*(4), 1633–1639.

Leonard, C. H., Clyman, R. I., Piecuch, R. E., et al. Effect of medical and social risk factors on the outcome of premature and very low birthweight infants. *Pediatrics, 116*(4), 620–626.

Long, J. G., Lucey, J. F., & Philips, A. G. (1980a). Noise and hypoxemia in the intensive care nursery. *Pediatrics, 65*(1), 143–145.

Long, J. G., Philips, A. G., & Lucey, J. F. (1980b). Excessive handling as a cause of hypoxemia. *Pediatrics, 65*(2), 203–207.

Lott, J. W. (1989). Developmental care of the preterm infant. *Neonatal Network, 7*(4), 21–28.

Lotus, M. J. (1992). Effects of light and sound in the neonatal intensive care unit environment on the low-birth-weight infants. *NAACOG's Clinical Issues in Perinatal and Women's Health Nursing, 3*(1), 34–44.

Ludington, S. M. (1990). Energy conservation during skin-to-skin contact between premature infants and their mothers. *Heart and Lung, 19*(5, Part 1), 445–451.

Ludington-Hoe, S. M., Hadeed, A. J., & Anderson, G. C. (1991). Physiologic responses to skin-to-skin contact in hospitalized premature infants. *Journal of Perinatology, 11*(1), 19–24.

MacLeod, P., & Stern, L. (1972). Natural variations in environmental illumination in a newborn nursery. *Pediatrics 50*(1), 131–133.

Mann, N. P., Haddow, R., Stokes, L., et al. (1986). Effect of night and day on preterm infants in a newborn nursery: Randomized trial. *British Medical Journal Clinical Research Edition, 293*(6557), 1265–1267.

Marshall, J. (1991). *The susceptible visual apparatus.* Boca Raton, FL: CRC Press.

Martin, R. J., Herrell, N., Rubin, D., & Fanaroff, A. (1979). Effect of supine and prone positions on arterial oxygen tension in the preterm neonate. *Pediatrics, 63*(4), 528–531.

Masi, W. (1979). Supplemental stimulation of the premature infant. In T. M. Field, A. M. Sostek, S. Goldberg, & H. H. Shuman (Eds.), *Infants born at risk* (pp. 367–387). New York: Spectrum Publications.

Masterson, J., Zucker, C., & Schulze, K. (1987). Prone and supine positioning effects on energy expenditure and behavior of low birth weight neonates. *Pediatrics, 80*(5), 689–692.

McGrath, J. M., & Valenzuela, G. (1994). Integrating developmentally supportive caregiving into practice through education. *Journal of Perinatal and Neonatal Nursing, 8*(3), 46–57.

Medoff-Cooper, B. (1991). Changes in nutritive sucking patterns with increasing gestational age. *Nursing Research, 40*(4), 245–247.

Medoff-Cooper, B., Weininger, S., & Zukowsky, K. (1989). Neonatal sucking as a clinical assessment tool: Preliminary findings. *Nursing Research, 38*(3), 162–165.

Messner, K. H. (1978). Light toxicity to the newborn retina. *Pediatric Research, 12*, 530.

Miller, C. L., White, R., Whitman, T. L., et al. (1995). The effects of cycled and noncycled lighting on growth and development in preterm infants. *Infant Behavior and Development, 18*(1), 87–95.

Morris, S. E., & Klein, D. K. (1987). *Prefeeding skills.* Tucson: Therapy Skills Builders.

Murdoch, D. R., & Darlow, B. A. (1984). Handling during neonatal intensive care. *Archives of Disease in Childhood, 59*(10), 957–961.

Neal, M. V. (1977). Vestibular stimulation and development of the small premature infant. *Communicating Nursing Research, 8*, 291–302.

Nelson, M. (1987). *Development of the newborn.* Presented at the Conference on Developmental Interventions in Neonatal Care, Chicago.

Norris, S., Campbell, L., & Brenkert, S. (1982). Nursing procedures and alterations in transcutaneous oxygen tension in premature infants. *Nursing Research, 31*(6), 330–336.

Peabody, J. L., & Lewis, K. (1985). Consequences of neonatal intensive care. In A. Gottfried & J. Gaiter (Eds.), *Infants under stress: Environmental neonatology* (pp. 199–226). Baltimore: University Park Press.

Peters, K. L. (1992). Does routine nursing care complicate the physiologic stability of the premature neonate with respiratory distress syndrome? *Journal of Perinatal and Neonatal Nursing, 6*(2), 67–84.

Raymond, L. W. (1991). Neuroendocrine, immunologic, and gastrointestinal effects of noise. In T. H. Fay (Ed.), *Noise and health* (pp. 27–40). New York: New York Academy of Medicine.

Robertson, A., & Philbin, M. K. (1996). *Studies of sound and auditory development.* Paper presented at The Physical and Developmental Environment of the High Risk Neonate. Clearwater Beach, FL: University of South Florida College of Medicine.

Robinson, J., Bayliss, S. C., & Fielder, A. R. (1991). Transmission of light across the adult and neonatal eyelid in vivo. *Vision Research 31*(10), 1837–1840.

Robinson, J., & Fielder, A. R. (1990). Pupillary diameter and reaction to light in preterm neonates. *Archives of Diseases in Childhood, 65*(1, Spec. No.), 35–38.

Robinson, J., & Fielder, A. R. (1992). Light and the immature visual system [Review]. *Eye, 6*(Part 2), 166–172.

Robinson, J., Moseley, M. J., & Fielder, A. R. (1990). Illuminance of neonatal units. *Archives of Diseases of Childhood 65*(7, Spec. No.), 679–682.

Robinson, J., Moseley, M. J., Thompson, J. R., & Fielder, A. R. (1989). Eyelid opening in preterm neonates. *Archives of Diseases in Childhood, 64*(7, Spec. No.), 943–948.

Sammons, W. A. H., & Lewis, J. M. (1985). *Premature babies: A different beginning.* St. Louis: C. V. Mosby.

Sarnat, H. B. (1984). Anatomic and physiologic correlates of neurologic development in prematurity. *Topics in neonatal neurology* (pp. 1–25). New York: Grune & Stratton.

Satish, M., & Doll-Speck, L. (1993). *Elevated sound levels increase desaturation episodes in sick preterm infants.* Paper presented at the Annual Meeting, American Academy of Pediatrics, Washington, DC.

Schaefer, M., Hatcher, R. P., & Barglow, P. D. (1980). Prematurity and infant stimulation: A review of research. *Child Psychiatry and Human Development, 10*(4), 199–212.

Seiberth, V., Linderkamp, O., Knorz, M. C., & Liesinhoff, H. (1994). A controlled trial of light and retinopathy of prematurity. *American Journal of Ophthalmology 118*(4), 492–495.

Sell, E. J., & Vaucher, Y. E. (1988). Growth and neurobehavioral outcome of infants who had bronchopulmonary dysplasia. In T. A. Merritt, W. H. Northway, & B. R. Boynton (Eds.), *Bronchopulmonary dysplasia* (pp. 403–420). Boston: Blackwell Scientific Publications.

Shiroiwa, Y., Kamiya, V., Uchibori, S., et al. (1986). Activity, cardiac and respiratory responses of blindfold preterm infants in a neonatal intensive care unit. *Early Human Development, 14*(3–4), 259–265.

Sweet, N. (1991). *The Special Start Project* [Final Report]. Oakland, CA: Office of Education, Children's Hospital.

Taquino, L., & Blackburn, S. (1994). The effects of containment during heelstick and suctioning on the physiologic and behavioral responses of preterm infants. *Neonatal Network, 13*(7), 55.

Tenreiro, S., Dowse, H. B., D'Souza, S., et al. (1991). The development of ultradian and circadian rhythms in premature babies maintained in constant conditions. *Early Human Development, 27*(1–2), 33–152.

Thomas, K. A. (1989). How the NICU environment sounds to a preterm infant. *American Journal of Maternal Child Nursing (MCN), 14*(4), 249–251.

Tribotti, S. J., & Stein, M. (1992). From research to clinical practice: Implementing the NIDCAP. *Neonatal Network, 11*(2), 35–40.

Tronick, E., Scanlon, K. B., & Scanlon, J. W. (1987). Behavioral organization of the newborn preterm infant: Apathetic organization may not be abnormal. In *Infant stimulation: For whom, what kind, when and how much? Johnson & Johnson Pediatrics Round Table* (No. 13, pp. 71–81). Skillman, NJ: Johnson & Johnson Company.

Updike, C., Schmidt, R. E., Macke, C., et al. (1986). Positional support for premature infants. *American Journal of Occupational Therapy, 40*(10), 712–715.

VandenBerg, K. A. (1985). Revising the traditional model: An individualized approach to developmental interventions in the intensive care nursery. *Neonatal Network, 3*(5), 32–38.

VandenBerg, K. (1990). The management of oral nippling in the sick neonate: The disorganized feeder. *Neonatal Network, 9*(1), 9–16.

VandenBerg, K. A. (1995). Behaviorally supportive care for the extremely premature infant. In L. P. Gunderson & C. Kenner (Eds.), *Care of the 24–25 week gestational age infant (small baby protocol)* (2nd ed., pp. 145–170). Petaluma, CA: NICU Ink.

VandenBerg, K. A., & Franck, L. (1990). Behavioral issues for infants with BPD. In C. Lund (Ed.), *BPD: Strategies for total patient care.* Petaluma, CA: Neonatal Network.

Volpe, J. J. (1995). *Neurology of the newborn.* Philadelphia: W. B. Saunders.

Wagaman, M. J., Shutack, J. G., Moomjian, A. S., et al. (1979). Improved oxygenation and lung compliance with prone positioning of neonates. *Journal of Pediatrics, 94*(5), 787–791.

White, J. L., & Labarba, R. C. (1976). The effects of tactile and kinesthetic stimulation on neonatal development in the premature infants. *Developmental Psychobiology, 9*(6), 569–577.

White, R. (1996, January). *Neonatal intensive care unit structure and design: Recommended standards.* Paper presented at The Physical and Developmental Environment of the High Risk Neonate. Clearwater Beach, FL: University of South Florida College of Medicine.

Whitelaw, A., Heisterkamp, G., Sleath, K., et al. (1988). Skin to skin contact in the care of very low birth weight babies. *Archives of Disease in Childhood, 63*(11), 1377–1381.

White-Traut, R. C., & Nelson, M. N. (1988). Maternally administered tactile, auditory, visual, and vestibular stimulation: Relationship to later interactions between mothers and premature infants. *Research in Nursing and Health, 11*(1), 31–39.

White-Traut, R. C., Nelson, M. N., Burns, K., & Cunningham, N. (1994). Environmental influences on the developing premature infants: Theoretical issues and applications to practice [Review]. *Journal of Obstetric, Gynecologic, and Neonatal Nursing, 23*(5), 393–401.

Wurtman, R. J., & Cardinali, D. P. (1974). The effects of light on man. In D. Bergsma & S. H. J. Blondheim (Eds.), *Bilirubin metabolism in man* (Vol. 2). New York: Elsevier.

Yarrow, L. (1968). Conceptualizing the early environment. In L. Dittman (Ed.), *Early childhood care* (pp. 15–27). New York: Atherton Press.

BOOKS/BOOKLETS FOR PARENTS

Cole, J. G. *The competent preemie: A guide for parents.* Boston: Children's Hospital and Wheelock College. (Project WELCOME, Wheelock College, 200 The Riverway, Boston, MA 02215, 617-734-5200, ext. 160.)

Flushman, B. L., & VandenBerg, K. A. (1984). *Developmental steps: A guide for parents on infant development in the intensive care nursery.* Oakland, CA: Children's Hospital Medical Center. (Distributed by Educational Programs Associates, Inc., 1 West Campbell Avenue, Bldg. C, Campbell, CA 95008, 408-374-1210.)

Hatcher, D., & Lehman, K. (1985). *Baby talk: For parents who are getting to know their special care baby.* Omaha: Centering Corporation (Box 3367, Omaha, NE 68103).

Sammons, W. A. H., & Lewis, J. M. (1985). *Premature babies: A different beginning.* St. Louis: C. V. Mosby.

VandenBerg, K. A., & Hanson, M. J. (1993). *Homecoming for babies after the neonatal intensive care nursery: A guide for parents in supporting their babies early development.* Austin: Pro-Ed; and a companion guide for professionals: *Homecoming for babies after the neonatal intensive care nursery: A guide for professionals in supporting families and infants' early development.* (Pro-Ed, Inc., 8700 Shoal Creek Blvd., Austin, TX 78758, 512-451-3246.)

AUDIOVISUAL MATERIALS

Behavior of the premature infant [Videotape or Film]. Cleveland: Case Western Reserve, University Care Video Productions.

Infant behavior: The premature baby [Videotape]. Timonium, MD: Milner-Fenwick, Inc. (1-800-432-8433).

Newborn state and behavior [Videotape]. White Plains, NY: March of Dimes Birth Defects Foundation.

Prematurely Yours [Tape/Slide or Videotape]. Boston: Polymorph Films.

Special delivery [Tape/Slide]. Campbell, CA: Educational Program Associates (1 West Campbell Avenue, Bldg. C, Campbell, CA 95008, 408-374-1210).

CHAPTER 50

Assessment and Management of the Transition to Home

CAROLE KENNER GAIL A. BAGWELL

RESEARCH AGENDA

What are parents' perceptions of the transition to home across three levels of care (levels I, II, and III)?

Are there common concerns in taking an infant home from the hospital that are experienced by parents of well and sick neonates?

How do parents' perceptions of the transition to home change over time?

What are the risk factors for faulty parent–infant interactions when a family receives no follow-up care?

Does an individualized, structured home follow-up teaching session make a difference in the ease of the transition to home and subsequent parent–infant interaction?

Does the transition model (information needs; grief; parent–child development; stress and coping; and social supports) represent a taxonomy of transitional care follow-up?

In the United States, in 1992, 406,501 infants were born with some degree of prematurity. Of these infants, approximately 10 percent were very small infants, weighing less than 1360 g (Ventura et al., 1994). Approximately a quarter million infants are born each year with some degree of prematurity. Of these, 20 percent are very small infants weighing less than 1360 g (Harrison & Kositsky, 1983, p. xi). Modern health care and technology have improved the survival rates of the micropremie within the range of 750 to 999 g from 50 percent in 1982 to 82 percent in 1988 (Cowett, 1990). However, the technology necessary to support these infants requires complex equipment and professional skill. The result is survival and finally discharge after a prolonged hospitalization. The neonatal intensive care unit (NICU) contains not only premature infants, however. The multiple neonatal problems that bring an infant to a NICU have been described, in depth, throughout the preceding chapters. The one common factor when caring for these infants is the parent. Parents also require complex care during and following the infant's discharge. This chapter focuses on the parent and the transition to home for the family unit. Although the NICU label is used throughout the chapter, it actually refers to either a level II or a level III unit, because the authors have found that, for parents, the transition to home from a NICU or special care unit is similar.

THE NEONATAL INTENSIVE CARE UNIT EXPERIENCE

Try to remember the first time you walked into the NICU. What were your thoughts and feelings? We know what ours were: An overwhelming urge to flee. Time seemed to be running. There were people rushing and people talking loudly, alarms buzzing, intercoms blaring, and doors slamming. We suddenly felt tense, on edge, and fearful of our ability to survive in such an environment. We were almost immobilized, and yet we recognized some of the ventilators, intravenous pumps, and monitors. Surely, with this passing acquaintance, we could learn to work in this environment and actually care for the critically ill infant. Then we walked over to an incubator and peered in at a premature infant, born at 28 weeks' gestation and weighing less than 1000 g, who looked as though she had been through a war. Scratches and cuts were visible. Tape cut into the infant's face to hold an endotracheal tube in place. The right arm was pinned to the bed to hold an intravenous line in place, and the legs were restrained to prevent dislodgment of an umbilical arterial line that was being used for blood gas sampling. Our hearts sank. We could never be responsible for providing care to this type of infant. We tried to summon the courage to walk, if not run, out of there.

If we, as beginning professionals, could not at first face the unit or the responsibility of care, what must parents feel? They have the additional fear of the death of a family member. For the most part, they lack the knowledge about the medical diagnosis, equipment, treatments, and routines necessary to support neonates. The mothers must, in addition, make a physiologic and psychological postpartum adjustment. They are also in need of care, yet most express the need to put aside their own time for healing to focus on their infants. For the fathers, the need to run between two units (the postpartum and the NICU) is an added stress even if these units are in the same institution. The parents' concern for their partners and their children often forces them between the two. For the family with other children at home, the stress becomes even greater. Who can take charge of the children? How long will it be necessary for another person to help out with family responsibilities? Is someone who can or will step in to help even available? These are very real family concerns. Along with these concerns comes the assumption of the new parental role. This role adjustment occurs for both first-time and experienced parents. It requires a change from a previous functional pattern to a new one. This change marks a developmental passage or transition.

PARENTAL TRANSITION

Transition involves change—leaving behind the familiar and trying something new. Throughout life, events necessitate change.

Mercer and associates (1989) viewed transitions as means of continued psychosocial development; they are turning points. Taking on a new role requires energy, commitment, and most of all a change in the pattern of functioning—thus a transition. A new role requires an adjustment, a setting of new priorities, and an examination of new expectations. This transition can be negative or positive, depending on the perceptions of the person involved in the transition. The role of parent is a good example of the transition process.

Once a pregnancy is confirmed, the mother and father begin the task of examining their individual roles. For first-time parents, this means considering what it will be like to be a mother or father to a dependent infant. For parents with other children, the new infant will bring a unique personality and another dimension to the already formed family unit. This infant, too, will require role adjustment on the part of the parents (Mercer & Ferketich, 1990).

Maternal Role

Rubin (1973) examined the development of the maternal role. She referred to pregnancy as having a cognitive style, because it is during pregnancy that women question their personal identity. She suggested that women develop their maternal identity in relationship to the developing fetus and newborn (Rubin, 1984). It is the infant's identity that really brings this maternal identity to fruition (Rubin, 1984). If an infant is premature or sick and does not fit the image of the robust full-term infant, women lose their normal frames of reference for the development of their own role expectations and the expectations of their infant as well.

According to Rubin (1973), the first trimester is devoted to the development of the feminine identity, when the only confirmation of the maternal role is that of amenorrhea. The second trimester is the time of beginning the binding-in or attachment process (Kemp & Page, 1987; Rubin, 1973). It is during this period that the first fetal movement is felt or, often, that the infant is visualized via ultrasonography. Thus the abstractness of pregnancy and the fetus is transformed to a more concrete level for both parents. Fetal growth, coupled with the changes in the woman's outward appearance, reinforces the internal changes. The woman begins to model society's expectations and attitudes toward the pregnancy state (Rubin, 1984). If birth occurs during this time, the woman may continue to model the expectations of pregnancy rather than the expectations of motherhood because the "ideal" full-term infant has not developed.

The third trimester completes the binding-in process. Bonding is a natural outgrowth of this process. During the postpartum period, mothers continue to embellish their maternal identity in relationship to their growing infant. Rubin (1984) called this the claiming process. Claiming happens as the mother looks for familial characteristics in her infant. She examines the infant's behavior and appearance in order to tie the image of this infant with the family unit. When the infant lacks common familial characteristics, owing either to prematurity or to illness, the task of claiming is made difficult. If the infant has been transferred to a distant NICU, the lack of spatial proximity to and repeated contacts with the infant add further to the potential for a difficult adjustment. It is through learning about the infant's routine and unique characteristics that the image moves away from the fantasy child created during the gestation and into the realm of reality of the actual infant (Rubin, 1984).

Another facet to be considered for the mother of a premature infant is the prematurity of motherhood itself. Not only are the binding-in and claiming processes affected, but the mother herself is a "premie." She has reached termination of the pregnancy before her own needs are fulfilled. Again, this is the time when society's expectations and rituals help socialize mothers into their impending role. Baby showers, parenting classes, and the purchase of birth announcements all help the parents realize that new responsibilities are forthcoming. When the infant's birth is premature or the infant is sick, some or all of these rituals may be forgotten. Friends and family who would normally be happy to help celebrate the joyous occasion of birth with the exuberant parents may feel uncomfortable and helpless around them. Their support may not be offered, leaving the parents more alone and isolated. Thus the transition to a new role becomes more difficult.

Role Theory

Mercer (1981) used Rubin's concepts of social and cognitive learning coupled with role theory to examine facts that affected the maternal role. She developed a theoretical framework for studying role acquisition. On the basis of her research, Mercer described role acquisition as a staged process that occurs gradually over the infant's first year of life (Mercer, 1981, 1986). The variables that affect this process are (1) maternal age; (2) maternal perceptions of the birth experience; (3) early maternal–infant separation; (4) support system; (5) maternal self-concept; (6) maternal personality traits; (7) maternal illness; (8) childrearing attitudes; (9) infant temperament; (10) infant illness; (11) cultural influences; and (12) socioeconomic level. Stern and Hildebrandt (1986) reported similar findings with regard to maternal perceptions of infants and maternal role expectations. They found that the mothers of premature newborns expected their infants to be different from full-term infants and that they actually shaped their maternal responses to their infants on the basis more of their expectations of them than of the infants' actual behavior.

In part, this discrepancy between the infant's actual behavior and the infant's expected behavior may arise from the lack of experience on the part of the mothers. If one does not know what to expect, it is difficult to plan or respond in less than an anticipatory or contrived manner. Role models may be missing, and so the normal process of change that transpires with a new role is not perceived as normal at all. Sims-Jones (1986) referred to this as normative change, which is greater for mothers of premature or sick infants because norms of reference are lacking. The ease of transition is clearly affected by the maternal expectations of the event whether these expectations are accurate or not (Sheehan, 1981; Sims-Jones, 1986).

Whenever change occurs—leaving the familiar and moving toward an uncharted path—feelings of lower self-esteem, decreased confidence, and decreased ability to cope are expected, even for events that are not tied to an illness or a problem, such as marriage or a new career. When there is an illness or a problem, it is reasonable to assume that these negative feelings may be even more intensely felt. For parents of a NICU infant, the transition may have two phases: one associated with becoming parents at the time of birth, and the other occurring at the time of discharge.

Although the time of NICU discharge is the overriding goal for the health care professional and the family, the actual transition to home can be a time of crisis for the family. The actual assumption of the new parental role can be quite overwhelming. Some researchers and clinicians view this transition as a crisis rather than just a developmental passage to a new functional level.

Transition as a Crisis

Baird (1986) described a crisis as a state of upset and disequilibrium. It is also a time when an individual or a family has the opportunity to grow, mature, and become better able to handle future life problems (Baird, 1986; Mercer et al., 1989). The idea that a crisis is a state of disequilibrium is based on the postulate that humans strive for homeostasis by constantly using coping mechanisms to maintain equilibrium. When a situation that upsets the equilibrium arises, a person employs the usual coping mechanisms to solve the problem. When the usual coping methods do not return the person to a state of equilibrium, a crisis evolves.

A crisis situation is characterized by (1) the event itself, (2) the meaning of the event to the family, and (3) the family's resources in dealing with the event (Baird, 1986). The outcome of the crisis is dependent on these three variables as well as on the help or the hindrance from friends, neighbors, and professionals during the time of disequilibrium (Baird, 1986). These three factors can be present even when a healthy newborn is brought into a family. But for premature or sick infants, the meaning to the family usually is viewed as a crisis. Benner and Wrubel (1989) postulated that caring is the prerequisite to coping. Because caring is the essence of nursing, nurses can make a decided difference for families preparing for discharge.

A crisis usually lasts 4 to 6 weeks, and crisis intervention is most effective when used during this period. When intervention is applied as close to the time of the crisis as possible, it becomes even more effective (Baird, 1986). The aim of crisis intervention is not to restructure a person's personality but to help the person deal with the present problem, relying on history only as it pertains to the present situation. Many things can initiate a crisis in a family. Bringing home a premature infant or a full-term infant who has been in the NICU is seen by parents as a crisis situation for families. Contemplating taking home a medically fragile infant or one that is technology-dependent may create a crisis situation for a parent (Scholtes et al., 1994).

Censullo (1986) stated that the discharge of premature infants renews the crisis for parents. The stress of premature birth becomes compounded by the realization that at home the parents alone must care for the infant. In making the difficult transition between hospital and home care, parents often report feelings of fear, loss, inadequacy, and anger. This period has been documented as a time of a situational crisis. Parents must face their unique situation without the benefit of preparation or experience and with a limited repertoire of responses, because the premature birth has cut short the time to prepare for parenting. The parents often feel overserved in the hospital and then abandoned after discharge, when the need for support and education may be the most intense (Censullo, 1986; McCain, 1990).

Bidder and associates (1974) studied a group of parents whose infants had required intensive care. Parents said they were most anxious about their infant at birth and at the time of discharge from the NICU. Caplan and colleagues (1977) and Trause and Kramer (1983) found that the period after birth, the period before hospital discharge, and the early postdischarge period are the most stressful for parents of premature infants. The crisis that occurs at the time of the infant's discharge is believed to happen because less thought is given to the support available to or needed by a family at that time than when the infant is in the NICU (Noga, 1982).

Other reasons for this crisis, according to Kersten (1984), are that parents of an undersized infant have a great deal of concern about the infant's chances of survival and about understanding information and guidance offered by the physicians and nurses. Kersten also stated that the parental anxiety level is often so high that little or none of the information is remembered. Another factor is the premature infant's behavior. The infant may sleep more than its full-term counterpart. The premature infant is less likely to respond positively to parental interventions at first, thus leaving the parent, especially the mother, with feelings of failure. Adaptation to the new family member is related to the mother's stress level, the social support that is received, and the mother's understanding of the infant's behavior pattern (Zimpelmann, 1990).

Simone (1986) stated that several interrelated factors put parents in a new crisis at the time of discharge: (1) Parents have been totally dependent on other people to care for their infant, and so they are totally unfamiliar with parenting roles, especially parenting roles associated with premature or sick infants; (2) families have often deferred many of their early responses to the preterm or problematic birth because the NICU demanded their attention, and, once home, these feelings and responses reemerge; (3) friends and family believe that the crisis is over once the infant has arrived home, and thus they are less available to the parents for support; (4) parents often become overwhelmed by the demands and dependence of their infant; and (5) the infant often continues to have fluctuations in progress and may even regress, thus affecting the parents' ability to cope. These feelings hold true for any NICU family and not just those of premature infants. These factors and the fact that they put families in a crisis have many implications for neonatal nurses.

For neonatal nurses, it is very important to know when a family is in crisis and what is the cause. Once an impending or a true crisis is recognized, neonatal nurses can implement interventions that will help prevent or alleviate it. Part of crisis intervention involves (1) recognizing and assessing the crisis, (2) planning the intervention, (3) implementing the intervention, (4) resolving the crisis, and (5) anticipatory planning for future crisis situations (Baird, 1986). Anticipatory planning for future crises involves reviewing with the family their coping strategies and how they handled the crisis.

Studies have shown that when people are better prepared to handle a situation, they are less likely to reach a crisis. According to Lazarus and Folkman (1984), "psychological stress is a particular relationship between the person and the environment that is appraised by the person as taxing or exceeding his or her resources and endangering his or her well-being" (p. 19). The meaning that is assigned to an event is done through an evaluative process called *cognitive appraisal* (Lazarus & Folkman, 1984). Coping, then, is the process by which an individual regulates stress. An outcome of coping is usually either control over the stress or being taken over by the stress, as in learned helplessness.

For many parents, the NICU reinforces learned helplessness. Parents express the need to understand their role and what is expected of them in relationship to their infant's care needs, and yet they feel that they are in the way and unable or incapable of caring for their infant. Thus they learn to be helpless. However, at the time of discharge, the picture changes. The parents are told, "Now it is your turn" (Fig. 50–1). It is no wonder that this discharge can be cognitively appraised as being a stress. Nor is it unusual that parents feel helpless and hopeless when it comes to accepting total responsibility for their infant.

According to Lazarus and Folkman's (1984) model, there are two types of coping: *problem-focused coping* and *emotion-focused coping*. Problem-focused coping centers on the need to do something to change the situation. Although parents cannot change the fact of their infant's need for intensive care, they can change the threat (Cobiella et al., 1990). Emotion-focused coping involves regulation of the emotions that result from the perceived stress. Cobiella and coworkers (1990) found that interventions that involved emotion-focused coping strategies effectively decreased parents' stress. These interventions included teaching parents how to recognize anxiety, how to use relaxation techniques, and how these tools could be used in the NICU (Cobiella et al., 1990). Their problem-focused interventions, showing a videotape about the NICU environment and equipment and how the parents could bring clothes for the infant to the unit, were also used. The problem-focused interventions received mixed results with parents. Part of this may be attributable to the inability to interact with a tape versus a person. Parents are very vocal about their feelings regarding their NICU care and preparation for discharge when given the opportunity to discuss their concerns.

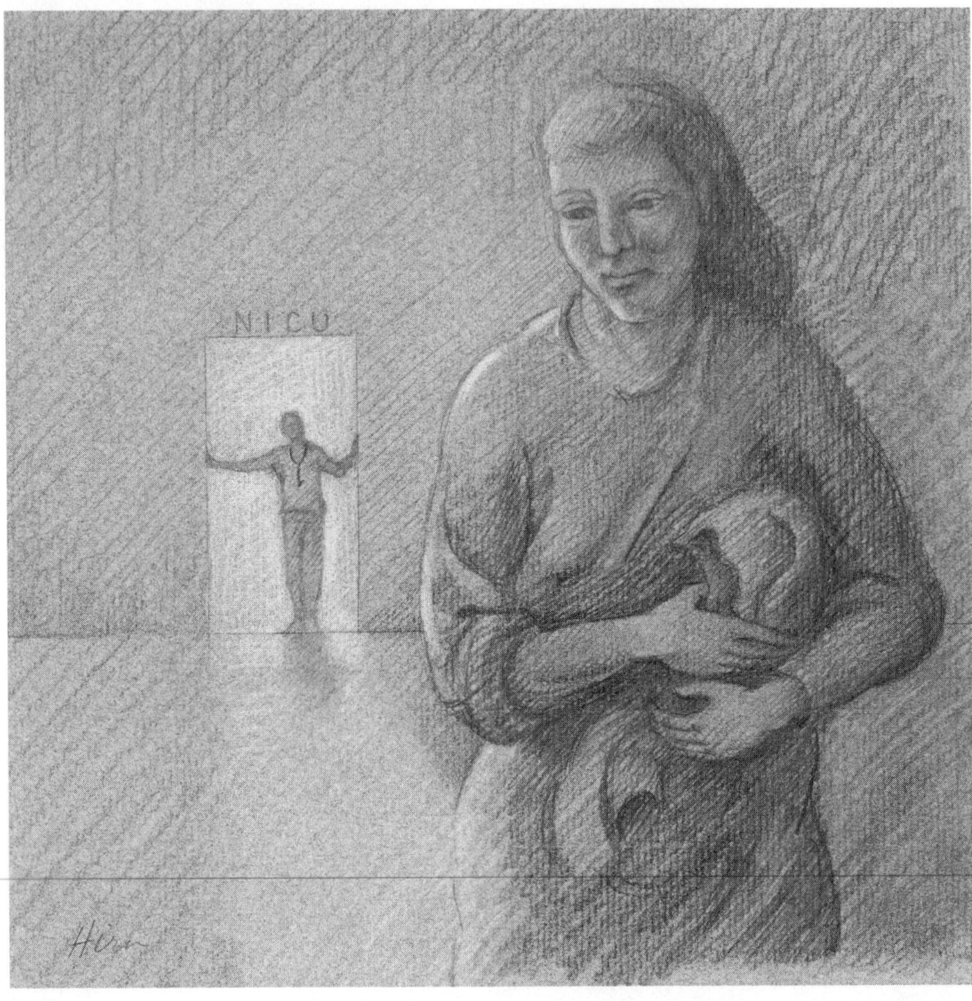

FIGURE 50–1. Leaving the neonatal intensive care unit (NICU).

Another way to meet the needs of those who are problem-focused copers is to present them with transition programs such as one case management–home care program in Utah called Welcome Home (Scholtes et al., 1994). This program was specifically designed to enable parents of medically fragile infants in the NICU to learn how to take care of their child before discharge. After discharge, community resources that were known to the parents before the discharge was completed were made available to the parents. Parents who went through this program felt less of a crisis upon discharge than did parents who had no support.

Parental Concerns

Kenner (1988) and Bagwell and associates (1990) found that parents from level II and III units had similar concerns. (For a more complete description of these and other studies, see Chapter 47, Systematic Assessment and Home Follow-Up: A Basis for the Neonate's Integration Into the Family.) Their concerns fell into five categories: (1) informational needs, (2) grief, (3) parent–child development, (4) stress and coping, and (5) social support.

Informational Needs

The informational needs of parents include how to provide routine newborn care; how to recognize normal newborn characteristics, both physical and behavioral; how to keep the infant healthy after discharge; their own responsibilities about how to provide care; the equipment used on their infant while in the NICU; and a complete explanation of the medical diagnosis and the expected prognosis (McKim, 1993a).

Parents want to feel that they are important enough to know what is really wrong with their infant (Kenner, 1988; Kenner et al., 1996). One family stated, "The only time that the physicians really asked us our opinion or told us about the baby's condition was when they were obligated to get informed consent for an experimental treatment." Another family said, "We would ask the nurses about the baby's apnea but they said they had to check with the physicians and they would have to talk to us." Other comments included: "I never understood why nurses just came over and turned off our baby's sounding alarms without seemingly looking at the baby"; "No one told me how difficult it would be to breastfeed a premie"; "I did not realize how different from my other children the sleep cycle would be for my premie either." These are just a few examples of information that the parents wanted. Norris and Hoyer (1993) referred to this as the medicalization of parenting, in which only passive decision making was encouraged. They concluded that use of Imogene King's framework for mutual goal setting would help parents to feel more a part of their infant's care. Barker (1995) referred to this as viewing parents as partners in their child's care.

Grief

The category of grief was first called anticipatory grief (Kenner, 1988), the rationale being that parents expressed the loss of their expected child once the reality of the neonatal problem shattered their hopes and fantasies. However, as time went on, parents continued to grieve, but in the form of anticipating that the infant would eventually die if she or he was sick enough to require special or NICU care. They continued to anticipate this death or at least that the infant would get sick again and require hospitalization after discharge. In reflecting on their perceptions, the concept seems more appropriate as grief and not anticipatory grief. The process of grief and the period of mourning begin once the infant does not meet the parents' expectations of the fantasy or ideal child. If the parents have other children, they speak of how different this child is from their others or how different the infant is from their expectations. Although the parents anticipate further problems, it is probably not anticipatory grief but rather a continuation of the grief process. There also seems to be a component of a grief for the loss of their expected parenting role. They mourn the loss of their normal, familiar role. This feeling may not be different from that of parents of normal, healthy infants, because the homecoming of those infants also requires a role adjustment. This assumption is an area still in need of further research.

Parent–Child Development

This category refers to the parents' and child's role expectations. Earlier in the chapter, role theory was examined. For anyone making a transition or entering a new level of functioning or a new stage of life, there are certain expectations about what is to come. New parents of healthy infants make adjustments in how they carry out the tasks of daily living once their newborn is at home. Each time a new member is introduced into the family, adjustments are made. When there is a problem with the infant that requires special care, parents may have to set aside their ideal expectations of what their role will be like. The hospitalization may reinforce their role or may hinder it.

Parents learn a lot about parenting by observing health care professionals. They learn what is valued. When a mother calls the unit for a progress report, she is usually told the infant's weight, amount of feedings, stooling patterns, percentage of oxygen, and how many times apnea occurred. It is not surprising that during home follow-up, parents, particularly mothers, want more information about feeding, formula, breastfeeding, elimination patterns (especially constipation), fear of the infant's losing weight (many say they have been told that if the infant loses weight, rehospitalization may be necessary), and whether the infant's breathing pattern seems normal. Nurses also may communicate to parents that the parents are not capable of caring for their infants. One family said, "I read all the literature about bonding and knew it was important to hold the baby, but we were not allowed"; "One nurse would say 'maybe in a couple of hours, maybe 4,' but that time would never come"; and "We were in the unit for 3 days before we held the baby and he was the least sick of any of the infants in the nursery." This family was from a level II unit, and the infant was experiencing some periods of apnea. Thermoregulation was not a concern in this case. The parents felt that they were not needed, not important, and certainly not capable of parenting their infant. These feelings only add to the stress of having a sick infant (Kenner, 1995).

Stress and Coping

For many families, there is no warning that a problem is pending with the infant's birth or that the infant will be sick. Therefore, there is a lack of preparation and a suddenness that come with the reality of a sick neonate. The expected feelings of joy and the months of anticipation are replaced by sharply contrasting feelings of fear, shock, and overwhelming sadness. Austin (1990) described coping methods used by families of chronically ill children as being tied to their adaptation to the situation. The McCubbin and Patterson Double ABCX Model of Family Adaptation involves the family's (1) demands, (2) adaptive resources, (3) coping, (4) definition or attitude, and (5) adaptation (Austin, 1990; McCubbin & Patterson, 1983). The stages of adaptation are (1) disbelief, (2) anger, (3) demystification, and (4) conditional acceptance. These stages resemble those of the grief process. The family experiences disbelief that there could be a problem. Even when a premature or complicated birth is expected or a neonatal problem is diagnosed in utero, many parents still do not believe that there will be a problem until the birth is over. They are usually angry that their infant is sick. Demystification is the understanding of the medical condition: that is, having the informational needs about the prognosis and plan of treatment met. The conditional acceptance is integration of the infant's problem into the family. Even if this is a time-limited condition, the illness must be incorporated into the family's attitude about the unit and the demands that are facing them.

Adaptation coping is necessary for reaching a stage of conditional acceptance. This form of coping comes about through the identification of the family's stresses from their own perspective. It also requires a determination of the resources that are available to the family. These resources might be parent support groups, parent hotlines, extended family members, friends, financial resources, or home care. Adaptation also requires a change of attitude. Information and acknowledgment of feelings before and after discharge both help to ease the transition process to home and into the role of parent. According to Austin (1990), "the change may be accomplished by introducing new information (demystifying the condition)" (p. 102). By acknowledging that other parents have been scared about assuming responsibility for their infant's care and by introducing them to successful parents, the stress is decreased and coping increased.

Graves and Ware (1990) conducted a study to compare mothers', fathers', and health care professionals' perceptions of parents' reactions to stressful stimuli during pediatric hospitalizations. They found a discrepancy between parents' perceptions and those of health care professionals (nurses and physicians). Parents expressed more stress about the uncertainty of when or whether discharge might occur. Mothers were annoyed when they were unable to meet with the physician or when the physician missed their visit. The crying of other infants was viewed as more stressful from the parents' perspective. Fathers were less stressed by their child's discomfort but more stressed by the child's crying when the parents were getting ready to leave than the health care professionals believed they were (Graves & Ware, 1990). The child's discomfort was also more stressful to fathers than mothers. This points to the need to consider the impact of the NICU stay and resultant discharge as being different for mothers and fathers. Interventions may need to be different, and yet most of the literature still speaks of parental concerns in relation to maternal concerns. These differences are in need of further research.

Continued stress, feelings of failure, and grieving for the loss of the fantasy child all have the potential for leading to maternal and paternal depression. Maternal depression has been positively associated with later child behavioral problems (Walker et al., 1989). Even after many years, mothers often still have very negative or painful memories of the NICU stay (Affleck et al., 1990). Therefore, it is imperative for the health of the family that interventions be implemented. Ehrhard (1982) conducted a case study to "investigate the physical and neurodevelopmental sequelae of an extremely premature very low birth weight infant" (p. i). When she finished her case study, she shared the information with the parents. The mother cried and stated, "Why didn't they tell me all this? I never really understood what he went through. This information helps me to understand my child and his needs." Thus while the researcher answered her research question, the parents received a lot of information as well. They got reassurance from a neonatal clinical nurse specialist that they had not caused the infant's problem and that they were not bad parents for feeling frustrated. These parents benefited by the follow-up. But these serendipitous findings are illustrative of the need for parent care both in and out of the hospital setting. Barnard and colleagues (1987) found that when follow-up was provided for mothers of premature infants, the repeated contacts and teaching sessions led to improved parent–infant interactions over time.

Social Support

Parents expressed the feeling that social support had both positive and negative facets. They meant that they saw the NICU nurses as having a lot of power and the potential to explain their infant's progress. They also believed that nurses had the potential to explain why medical treatment plans changed when there were house staff changes in teaching institutions. Nonetheless, parents did not feel that, for the most part, nurses fulfilled their role as advocate. The NICU nurses did not anticipate that the parents might be confused, and the parents readily admitted that they were too confused or intimidated by the health professionals to ask questions. They assumed that the nurses knew how they felt. They also thought that the nurses were working too many shifts in a row or too many long hours to be bothered with their seemingly trivial concerns. Some parents went so far as to describe the nurse's role as providing expert infant care but not parent care. Other parents expressed frustration over having to reorient nurses to their infant's condition. They often did not see the same nurse twice, even during a prolonged stay. Although the parents saw the potential for support, they did not feel that the support was always given. Primary nurses for continuity and mother–baby nurses for the level II parents were viewed as helpful for support.

The physician's role was viewed as being for infant care and not for the support of the family. For most families, the physician was the gatekeeper regarding what they were allowed to know about their infant. Physicians even regulated communication to parents via the nursing staff. Even after discharge, parents believed that the physician's permission was necessary to make even the smallest change in the infant's routine that had been established in the hospital. These feelings might be tied to the parents' need for structure and their attempt to continue the safety of the NICU at home. Parents also viewed nurses as gatekeepers of information (Brown & Ritchie, 1990). The nurses would let parents know when it was not appropriate, for instance, to hold the infant, but only occasionally did they say when parents could hold the infant. Once again, support for their parenting role was not always seen as readily given. Unfortunately, a side effect of this perception is the parents' sense of a lack of trust that they can provide care or a feeling that the truth about their infant's condition is being withheld from them (Brown & Ritchie, 1990).

The positive side of support was also expressed: the caring attitude by some professionals, the friendly hug, and the taking time to talk with the parents, even if it was about something other than their infant's problem. Acknowledgment of the mother's own physical discomfort conveyed a caring and supportive attitude. The availability of a phone number and the potential for a home visit were viewed as positive. Peoples-Sheps (1990) pointed out that home visits, at least in some areas, are returning. Parents often express the need for positive reinforcement and reassurance, as much as anything, once they are home. Because their infant is sick, they want this support from professionals knowledgeable in neonatal pathophysiology, the usual hospital course, and their own psychosocial needs. For many parents, the home visit provides a way to ventilate feelings that otherwise must often be suppressed around family and friends (McKim, 1989, 1993b).

Parents also believed that many times family and friends withdrew their support. As mentioned, family and friends often believe that at discharge the crisis is past. For other parents, family and friends were afraid to approach the parents for fear of doing the wrong thing. Still other times, parents felt that their family and friends wanted to tell them what they were doing wrong and how they should parent their infant. For instance, the advice several mothers got was "Don't breastfeed your premie, he will get sick. Don't allow visitors, they will only make the baby sick." The positive side of this involvement was when family and friends would tell the parents what a good job they were doing with their infant, how well they were coping, or how their feelings of inadequacy were normal for any parent. Social support differs, however, depending on whether it is professional or personal. According to Coffman and associates (1991), personal support from family and friends is related more to emotional affect and life satisfaction, whereas professional support affects personal satisfaction but not life satisfaction. Therefore, both aspects of support are important for parents, but each affects parents' attitudes about the NICU experience and their infant in very different ways.

Social support is an important aspect of coping and managing stress. If support is not provided, family functioning and health may suffer. Stewart (1989) summarized instruments that are available for measuring social support. Once social support needs are identified, a plan of action must be implemented. Because there are both positive and negative aspects of social support, it is probably more correct to term this category as social interaction. There is an interaction between at least two people, and whether it is positive or negative support is determined by the recipient (McKim et al., 1995).

The five categories of parental concerns just discussed may represent a taxonomy for transitional care follow-up. Cohen and associates (1991) suggested that a taxonomy for classification of transitional care follow-up is needed to classify appropriate intervention strategies.

INTERVENTION STRATEGIES

Many interventions are possible to alleviate a crisis situation for a family of a premature infant preparing for discharge. One such intervention, according to Kersten (1984), is to spend more time and effort preparing parents to care for their child at home by themselves. Actively listening to the parents' concerns is a first step toward effective discharge planning (Barnard et al., 1984).

The NICU nurse, in the role of primary nurse, clinical nurse specialist, or neonatal nurse practitioner, can advocate for positive parental discharge. By recognizing the need of parents for information about their infant and the required care once home, a collaborative, interdisciplinary plan of care, including discharge and follow-up, can be developed. This type of collaborative plan should include the parents' demonstrating competence and comfort with routine newborn care. Mothers, in particular, need support and reassurance, even after discharge (Bagwell et al., 1990; Kenner, 1988; Noch, 1989; Scholtes et al., 1994). The nurse needs to ensure that the parents are completely comfortable bathing, feeding, and diapering their infant, as well as administering any special care procedures, such as medication or oxygen therapy. The parents also need to be taught how the NICU infant's temperament differs from that of a normal newborn. Good discharge teaching includes all this as well as developmental information.

Parents need continuity of care, too. Many parents express the frustration of trying to build a rapport with medical staff, who change monthly, and with nurses, who change daily (McHaffie,

1989). This situation is not necessarily going to improve, as more nurses are working part time, flexible hours, or out of agencies that float them between several intensive care units.

Parents also need to be informed and reminded that even though their infant is 6 months old by chronologic age, she or he may be only 3 months old by conceptional age. Thus the infant may act more like a 3-month-old than like a 6-month-old. Tips on helping the infant adapt to home should also be included in the discharge information. Parents of former premature infants have offered such advice as leaving radios and lights on to help the infant adapt to the new environment (Simone, 1986). This need for increased stimuli may change as NICU infants begin to recognize a developmentally supportive environment (Cicco et al., 1996). Nursing research is needed in this area to determine whether NICU infants do require more lights or noise once home.

Noga (1982) found that a home visit by a community health nurse before and after the infant's discharge helped to alleviate some anxiety for the parents. Parents found it reassuring to have a professional, in addition to just friends and relatives, advise them on the infant's condition. Noga also found that parents felt more comfortable knowing that the nurse would return for visits and would be available by telephone if needed. The parents also appreciated that a medical professional saw their child before the first postdischarge pediatric check-up, which, in many cases, was up to 6 weeks after discharge. Follow-up nurses recognize that failure to use available community resources or follow professional advice may be related to coping difficulties (Klein, 1990). If this is true, avoidance of these failures may stop the cycle of stress and coping difficulties. Scheduling home visits at frequent intervals is a good strategy for assessing the family's progress (see Chapter 47, Systematic Assessment and Home Follow-Up: A Basis for Monitoring the Neonate's Integration Into the Family).

Care-by-parent units have been another way to alleviate parental anxiety and to decrease the chance for a crisis. Consolvo (1986) studied mothers who spent 36 to 48 hours in a unit caring for their infants totally during that period, with a nurse available for questioning. Consolvo's study showed no significant decrease in the mothers' anxiety, but the sample size was small, thus not allowing many differences to emerge. However, Edwards and Saunders (1990) found that when parents feel free to ask questions and express negative thoughts about themselves as parents or about their infants, their anxiety and concomitant stress diminish. As previously stated, programs such as in Utah for parents of medically fragile infants seem to help ease the transition home and increase their confidence (Scholtes et al., 1994).

Some NICUs have a modified version of this type of care known as a transition unit. This area usually has less staff, and parents are expected to provide more of the care. The irony is that parents feel very afraid of doing this. It may be their first attempt at being on their own with their infant. They need reassurance, discharge teaching, and role modeling; however, when NICUs are busy, the least experienced nurses are assigned to the transition unit. Also, as a result of the changing health care environment and hospital budget cuts, many transitional units are being supplemented with nonlicensed patient care assistants (PCAs) to help decrease the number of registered nurses needed and thus decreasing costs. The rationale is that these infants are "growers" who require minimal care. Nevertheless, some of these infants get sick again, many times owing to inept assessments that have allowed a minor problem to get out of hand. It would not be considered a good idea to assign a beginning-level nursing student to the most inexperienced clinician to learn nursing care, and yet this is precisely what is done with parents. Parents need confident, well-seasoned clinicians who value the need for parental education. Parenting is not a natural function, especially with a fragile neonate. Parents need reassurance; they need to gain self-confidence; they need someone who will recognize their needs without their having to verbalize them; and they need to know what to expect of their infant. If the infant is premature, what is the normal pattern of sleep? How long will it take for the infant's head to look like that of a full-term neonate? These are only a couple of examples of behavioral characteristics that parents need to know to understand their infant's developmental pattern of growth. State modulation and developmentally supportive environments are other areas that should be explored with parents. (See Chapter 48, Neonatal Sleep–Wake States, and Chapter 49, Assessment and Management of Neonatal Neurobehavioral Development.)

Parents' failure to identify their role in relation to their infant's role can lead to long-term problems. Froman and Owen (1989) developed a tool for measuring "infant care self-efficacy." This refers to the parents' belief that they can "accomplish some particular behavior" (p. 200). In this instance, it is the provision of infant care. The instrument has six categories by which parents can evaluate their confidence: (1) health knowledge, (2) diet knowledge, (3) safety knowledge, (4) health skills, (5) diet skills, and (6) safety skills (Froman & Owen, 1989). Of these categories, the researchers found that behaviors that are performed by parents with and for their infants, such as playing, holding, changing a diaper, and recognizing safety hazards, are all very important dimensions of self-efficacy. Behaviors such as recognizing a medical problem, treating problems such as constipation, or knowing the exact immunization schedule are less important, because this information could be obtained from health care professionals. "Self-efficacy theory suggests that estimates of efficacy are based upon reinforcement history and vicarious learning" (Froman & Owen, 1989, p. 208). For health care professionals, this implies a need to truly provide family care and not just have it appear in the mission statement of the hospital or unit.

Family Care

Another facet of discharge preparation that can be addressed in a care-by-parents or transition unit is the concept of the family as a unit. The father and siblings are often forgotten during discharge preparation. More research is needed to determine what concerns fathers have and supports they need to prepare for their infant's discharge. Also, is information given differently to fathers than to mothers? Some fathers have expressed the feeling that they were given factual, detailed information on the infant's condition, whereas the mother received very little direct information from either the nursing or the physician staff (Bagwell et al., 1990; Kenner, 1988; McKim, 1993a). Most fathers want to participate in care and decision making, both within the unit and in anticipation of the discharge (Consolvo & Wade, 1989).

Siblings must also adjust to the infant, who may not seem real to them until they are able to visit the infant in the NICU. Wolterman (1990) found that siblings who participated in a NICU sibling visitation program exhibited less negative behaviors during the infant's hospitalization and after discharge. These behaviors centered on the siblings' own interactions with the mother, their interactions with the NICU infants, and their own behaviors during daily activities. (See Chapter 7, Sibling Adaptation to the Neonate.) Unfortunately, many units are afraid to allow sibling visitation owing to the upsurge in rubella and varicella. Therefore, sibling adjustment may be postponed until the infant goes home. Thus the home health visitor may be the one to help the family recognize the need for siblings to make role transitions, too.

Communication

Communication is a key element to successful relationships. It is a new focus for medical care. Classes and seminars in "bedside manner" are being conducted in medical schools across the United States. One reason for this is consumer pressure to have physicians display a caring attitude. Another factor is that malpractice cases are brought against physicians more often when there has been a breakdown in communication between the physician and the patient. It is harder to sue a "friendly, trustworthy" physician than one who may be viewed as efficient but not concerned or personable.

Nurses are expert communicators. The art of nursing has revolved around the ability to convey care and personal attention to the client. Unfortunately, because of today's health care crisis, nursing shortages have resulted in staff mixes and use of unskilled personnel, coupled with economic constraints resulting in shortened hospital stays; nurses are also falling into the trap of assembly line health care delivery. However, nurses have the advantage of being able to identify and assess a family's needs and to convey these needs to other health care team members. Being an advocate for the family is an essential part of preparing a family for discharge. Follow-up, in essence, is allowing an open line of communication among health care professionals, the health care delivery system, and the family. It allows a partnership to develop between the health care team and the family. It gives the family back some control. Follow-up moves the family away from the learned helplessness acquired in the hospital to a more participative role. Nurses are often sought out by families wanting to ventilate feelings and concerns, as long as the family feels that the nurses care enough to be concerned. Parents need to be able to openly express their concerns about their infant's appearance and about their feelings of helplessness without fear of being judged as bad parents; these are two factors that Miles (1989) found to be stressful for NICU parents. Nonverbal cues can get in the way of communication. The nurse's expertise, knowledge, and use of medical terminology without explanations all convey the nurse's need to be in control. Someone has to be in control, but relinquishing some control to the family does not lessen one's credibility as a professional. It conveys to the family that they have a role in their infant's care and that they are important too.

Another facet to this communication system is the other health care team members. Nurses cannot afford to withhold information that might help the physicians, social workers, and financial counselors who work with the family. Nurses need to convey information and be the coordinator of the assessment data that is received. Application of the nursing process may sound trite, but it is important in terms of not only collecting data but also using the data to identify problems, make nursing diagnoses, and develop a plan of care before and after discharge.

Long-Term Implications for the Family Unit

The breakdown of communication or of family functioning can lead to a less-than-optimal environment for the infant and child to grow. Studies have documented that the infant of very low birth weight, in particular, is at risk for child abuse, neglect, nonorganic failure to thrive, and developmental and behavioral problems (Brown et al., 1989; Klein, 1990; Tobey & Schraeder, 1990). Tobey and Schraeder (1990) found that 5-year-olds who had been infants of very low birth weight had more numerous and worse than expected behavioral problems in comparison with the general population of 5-year-olds. They also found that the caregivers of these infants experienced more daily stress than did the average caregiver. Gennaro and Stringer (1991) found that maternal stress or anxiety is related to the use of health care services. The concern is that maternal stress, if not addressed, may lead to infant neglect.

Collaboration between pediatric medical follow-up, parent support or psychosocial assessments at home, and obstetrical follow-up for the mother is essential. Each health care professional has something to contribute to the family's overall well-being. It is essential not to compete but to work with other professionals for the good of the family. This means that turf issues must be settled behind the scenes. It also means that each profession must share information that it receives from the family. It is not unusual during a home visit for the family to say, "I did not tell the OB [or pediatrician] about my concern over changing from cloth diapers to disposables because I did not want to bother him about that. Yet I am afraid to make even the smallest change in my baby's routine set up by the hospital." These statements demonstrate the need for a discharge protocol for the family.

Miles and Holditch-Davis (1995) and Wereszczak and associates (1997) found in a retrospective research study that the the NICU stay has long-lasting effects on mothers of premature infants. When the children are 3 years old, these mothers are experiencing what these researchers term compensatory parenting. This parenting style is overcompensation for feeling sorry for or guilty about having an infant in the NICU. They reported trying to provide special experiences and more stimulation to foster development with these children. At the same time they have shielded their children from other life situations to protect them from further hurt (Miles & Holditch-Davis, 1995). These researchers suggest that prospective research is needed to determine when or how this parenting style evolves. The other research that is needed is testing of interventions during and after the infants' NICU stay and continuing until preschool to determine what helps mothers coping with their special infants.

CONCLUSION

The interventions discussed have been shown to have some effect in decreasing parental anxiety and thus lessening the crisis situation of the transition from the NICU to home. More research is needed to help determine whether there is a specific way to alleviate the crisis situation for a family taking home a premature infant. Existing studies also must be replicated to demonstrate that the interventions are as effective as the original research suggests. A specific research question to be considered is whether all parents of premature infants need as extensive interventions as described or whether only parents of extremely ill or premature infants need such interventions. None of the existing studies address which group of parents are more at risk for crisis problems. The results of such a study might show that all parents, not only the parents of extremely ill or premature infants, need these types of interventions.

The box is an abbreviated discharge protocol concerning parents of premature infants and the crisis situation that they face when taking their child home from a NICU.

DISCHARGE PROTOCOL

PROBLEM/GOAL	INTERVENTION	RATIONALE
Problem: Increased anxiety related to parents' lack of knowledge in caring for their infant at the time of NICU discharge. **Goal:** To decrease parental anxiety by providing information regarding infant's care, problems, needs, temperament, and developmental status. *RATIONALE:* Increasing parents' knowledge of the care, problems, needs, temperament, and developmental status of their premature or sick infant will help decrease parental anxiety and thus decrease the chance for a crisis situation.	**Diagnostic**	
	1. Assess the parents' knowledge base concerning the care, problems, needs, temperament, and developmental stage of their infant.	To determine a baseline of information regardng the parents' knowledge of their infant's care requirements, problems, needs, temperament, and developmental stage.
	2. Assess parents' educational level.	To determine the level of complexity of the information that is to be given to the parents.
	3. Assess the level of anxiety that the family is experiencing at present.	Anxiety affects the amount of information that is absorbed and retained by the parents.
	4. Evaluate any outside factors that would increase the parents' anxiety besides the discharge of the infant to home.	To be aware that outside factors can affect parental anxiety over bringing the child home.
	Therapeutic	
	1. Confirm the parents' perceptions of their infant's behavior, problems, needs, temperament, and developmental status by asking them to repeat to you what has been told to them previously.	To help alleviate parental anxiety by confirming that the parents have properly interpreted the information given to them.
	2. Have the parents care for their infant daily during the infant's stay in the NICU, increasing the parents' responsibilities as the infant becomes stronger and healthier. By the time the infant is ready to be discharged, the parents are doing most of the care, with little nursing intervention.	Parental anxiety is relieved as the parents feel more comfortable and competent in caring for the infant.
	3. Provide parents with a nonthreatening environment in which to ask questions concerning the care, needs, problems, temperament, and developmental status of their infant.	A nonthreatening environment helps parents express concerns, feelings, and questions more freely.
	4. Provide the parents with a quiet, distraction-free environment to be with their infant prior to discharge.	A quiet, distraction-free environment helps parents bond with their infant and provides time for the parents and infant to become acquainted with each other.
	Educational	
	1. Instruct parents in the care and needs of their premature or sick infant.	Every infant is different and has special care requirements and needs.
	2. Instruct the parents on the infant's specific medical problems and expected outcomes related to the infant's past and present condition.	Knowledge of their infant's condition helps the parents understand and be prepared for problems if they occur once the infant is discharged from the NICU.
	3. Discuss with the parents the temperament of the infant in comparison with that of a normal, healthy infant.	By being informed of the differences between a premature or sick infant and a normal, healthy infant, the parents can better understand their infant and thus prepare themselves for these differences once the child arrives home.
	4. Demonstrate a developmental test with the infant for the parents.	Demonstrating what the infant can and cannot do for her or his age helps parents to understand at what stage their infant is developmentally.
	5. Provide parents with written material concerning the care, needs, problems, temperament, and developmental status of their infant.	Written material reinforces what has been taught to the parents and can be used as a quick reference by the parents when questions arise.
Problem: Alterations in coping related to decrease in social supports. **Goal:** To provide for social supports after NICU discharge. *RATIONALE:* When their infant is discharged from a NICU, parents often feel isolated from friends and family, who view the crisis as being over and thus become less available for support.	**Diagnostic**	
	1. Assess parental support system when the infant is admitted to the NICU.	To be aware that a lack of support for the parents while the infant is in the NICU will probably result in a lack of support when the infant is discharged.
	2. Assess community resources for a possible parent support system.	Community groups are often of great support to parents who have no other support system available to them.
	Therapeutic	
	1. Encourage parents to use the people who are their main support to help them through the crisis of having their infant in a NICU.	To make parents aware that they will need extra support in a time of crisis.

Protocol continued on following page

DISCHARGE PROTOCOL *(Continued)*

PROBLEM/GOAL	INTERVENTION	RATIONALE
	2. Encourage the support person to visit the infant in the NICU.	To help the support person to better understand what the parents are experiencing and to become acquainted with the infant. If the support person knows the infant, she or he will be more likely to visit and help with the infant once the child has been discharged home.
	3. Discuss with the parents their need for continuing support once the infant has been discharged.	To help parents realize their need for support once they have their infant at home so that they are able to verbalize this to their support system before discharge.
	4. Introduce the parents to the home follow-up nurse or community health nurse before their infant's discharge.	This gives the parents and home follow-up nurse or community health nurse time to establish a rapport. This also gives the follow-up nurse or community health nurse time to become acquainted with the infant before discharge.
	5. Have the follow-up nurse or community health nurse visit the family 1 week and 4 weeks after discharge.	Parents feel more comfortable at discharge knowing that they are going to be visited by a nurse at their home in the first week home from the hospital.
	6. Provide parents with a phone number of the NICU and follow-up nurse for any questions after discharge.	Parents often forget questions at the time of discharge or may have questions once they are home with the infant.
	Educational	
	1. Establish a parent support group that meets weekly and at a regularly scheduled time. Encourage parents to attend the weekly meetings so that they may discuss their fears, feelings, and needs with other parents in a nonthreatening environment.	To help parents in similar situations gain strength and reassurance from each other, and to help parents increase their support systems.
Problem: Grief related to the parents' perceived loss of their infant. **Goal:** To help parents overcome their fear of losing their child. *RATIONALE:* Parents of premature infants often have a fear of losing their child and thus have a grief reaction prior to the event happening.	**Diagnostic**	
	1. Explore the parents' feelings concerning their infant and their infant's failure.	To detect any unvoiced fears about their child.
	2. Assess parents' perception of the cause of the infant's prematurity or illness.	Guilt and self-blame often accompany grief.
	Therapeutic	
	1. Provide support to parents during the infant's stay in the NICU.	To help parents feel at ease and thus feel more comfortable in expressing their fears and concerns.
	2. Provide a nonjudgmental attitude toward parents when they are expressing their concerns and fears.	A nonjudgmental attitude toward parents helps them express their feelings and fears freely.
	3. Provide parents with information concerning their infant and her or his needs and problems.	Information regarding the infant and the infant's needs and problems helps relieve parental anxiety.
	4. Communicate to the family that they may experience a grief reaction when taking the infant home or after taking the infant home.	To prepare families for the possibility of a grief reaction once they are home and to reassure them that this is common.

REFERENCES

Affleck, G., Tennen, H., Rowe, J., & Higgins, P. (1990). Mothers' remembrances of newborn intensive care: A predictive study. *Journal of Pediatric Psychology, 15*(1), 67–81.

Austin, J. K. (1990). Assessment of coping mechanisms used by parents and children with chronic illness. *American Journal of Maternal Child Nursing, 15*(2), 98–102.

Bagwell, G. A., Kenner, C., Dohme, J., et al. (1990). *Parent transition from a special care nursery to home: A replicative study.* Unpublished master's thesis, University of Cincinnati College of Nursing and Health.

Baird, S. F. (1986). Crisis intervention strategies in nursing assessment and strategies for the family at risk. In S. H. Johnson (Ed.), *High-risk parenting* (2nd ed., pp. 299–311). Philadelphia: J. B. Lippincott.

Barker, J. G. (1995). Parents as partners in the NICU. *Neonatal Network, 14*(1), 9–10.

Barnard, K. E., Hammond, M. A., Sumner, G. A., et al. (1987). Helping parents with preterm infants: Field test of a protocol. *Early Child Development and Care, 27*, 255–290.

Barnard, K. E., Snyder, C., & Spietz, A. (1984). Supportive measures for high-risk infants and families. In B. S. Raff (Ed.), *Social support and families of vulnerable infants* (pp. 290–329). White Plains, NY: March of Dimes Birth Defects Foundation.

Benner, P., & Wrubel, J. (1989). *The primacy of caring: Stress and coping in health and illness.* Menlo Park, CA: Addison-Wesley.

Bidder, R. T., Crowe, E. A., & Gray, O. P. (1974). Mothers' attitudes to preterm infants. *Archives of Disease in Children, 49*(10), 766–770.

Brown, J., & Ritchie, J. A. (1990). Nurses' perceptions of parent and nurse roles in caring for hospitalized children [Review]. *Children's Health Care, 19*(1), 28–36.

Brown, L. P., Brooten, D., Kumar, S., et al. (1989). A sociodemographic profile of families of low birth weight infants. *Western Journal of Nursing Research, 11*(5), 520–532.

Caplan, G., Mason, E. A., & Kaplan, D. (1977). Four studies of crisis in parents of prematures. In J. L. Schwartz & L. H. Schwartz (Eds.), *Vulnerable infants: A psychosocial dilemma* (pp. 89–107). New York: McGraw-Hill.

Censullo, M. (1986). Home care of the high-risk newborn. *Journal of Obstetric, Gynecologic, and Neonatal Nursing, 15*(2), 146–153.

Cicco, R., Greer, M., White, R., et al. (1996). *Making NICUs more developmentally appropriate for infants. Parents and families.* Paper presented at the Physical and Developmental Environment of the High Risk Neonate, University of South Florida College of Medicine, Clearwater Beach, FL.

Cobiella, C. W., Mabe, P. A., & Forehand, R. L. (1990). A comparison of two stress-reduction treatments for mothers of neonates hospitalized in a neonatal intensive care unit. *Children's Health Care, 19*(2), 93–100.

Coffman, S., Levitt, M. J., & Deets, C. (1991). Personal and professional support for mothers of NICU and healthy newborns. *Journal of Obstetric, Gynecologic, and Neonatal Nursing, 20*(5), 406–415.

Cohen, S. M., Arnold, L., Brown, L., & Brooten, D. (1991). Taxonomic classification of transitional follow up care nursing interventions with low birth weight infants. *Clinical Nurse Specialist, 5*(1), 31–36.

Consolvo, C. A. (1986). Relieving parental anxiety in the care-by-parent unit. *Journal of Obstetric, Gynecologic, and Neonatal Nursing, 15*(2), 154–159.

Consolvo, C. A., & Wade, J. (1989). Special touches in perinatal care. *Critical Care Nurse, 9*(1), 67–69.

Cowett, R. M. (1990). Introduction. In R. M. Cowett & W. W. Hay, Jr. (Eds.), *The micropremie: The next frontier. Report of the 99th Ross Conference on Pediatric Research* (pp. 1–3). Columbus, OH: Ross Laboratories.

Edwards, L. D., & Saunders, R. B. (1990). Symbolic interactionism: A framework for the care of parents of preterm infants. *Journal of Pediatric Nursing, 5*(2), 123–128.

Ehrhard, E. M. (1982). *The sequelae of an infant born at 24–25 weeks gestation.* Unpublished master's thesis, University of Cincinnati College of Nursing and Health.

Froman, R. D., & Owen, S. V. (1989). Infant care self-efficacy. *Scholarly Inquiry for Nursing Practice: An International Journal, 3*(3), 199–215.

Gennaro, S., & Stringer, M. (1991). Stress and health in low birthweight infants: A longitudinal study. *Nursing Research, 40*(5), 308–311.

Graves, J. K., & Ware, M. E. (1990). Parents' and health professionals' perceptions concerning parental stress during a child's hospitalization [Review]. *Children's Health Care, 19*(1), 37–42.

Harrison, H., & Kositsky, A. (1983). *The premature baby book.* New York: St. Martin's Press.

Kemp, V. H., & Page, C. K. (1987). Maternal prenatal attachment in normal and high-risk pregnancies. *Journal of Obstetric, Gynecologic, and Neonatal Nursing, 16*(3), 179–184.

Kenner, C. (1995). The transition to parenthood. In L. P. Gunderson & C. Kenner (Eds.), *Care of the 24–25 week gestational age infant: Small baby protocol* (2nd ed., pp. 171–184). Petaluma, California: NICU Ink.

Kenner, C. A. (1988). *Parent transition from the newborn intensive care unit (NICU) to home.* Unpublished doctoral dissertation, Indiana University, Indianapolis.

Kenner, C., Flandermeyer, A., & Thornburg, P. (1996). Parenting in the NICU (pp. 93–108). In J. Zaichkin (Ed.), *Newborn intensive care: What every parent needs to know.* Petaluma, CA: NICU Ink.

Kersten, E. (1984). A premature infant joins the family: The OHN as a health team member. *Occupational Health Nursing, 32*(10), 530–533.

Klein, M. J. A. (1990). The home health nurse clinician's role in the prevention of nonorganic failure to thrive. *Journal of Pediatric Nursing, 5*(2), 129–135.

Lazarus, R. S., & Folkman, S. (1984). *Stress, appraisal, and coping.* New York: Springer.

McCain, G. C. (1990). Family functioning 2 to 4 years after preterm birth. *Journal of Pediatric Nursing, 5*(2), 97–104.

McCubbin, H. H., & Patterson, J. M. (1983). The family stress process: The Double ABCX Model of Adjustment and Adaptation. *Marriage Family Reviews, 6,* 7–37.

McHaffie, H. E. (1989). Mothers of very low birth weight babies: Who supports them? *Midwifery, 5*(3), 113–121.

McKim, E. (1989). *The support needs of mothers of premature infants.* Presented at the Third International Nursing Research Symposium, McGill University School of Nursing, Montreal, Quebec, Canada.

McKim, E. (1993a). The information and support needs of mothers of premature infants. *Journal of Pediatric Nursing, 8*(4), 233–244.

McKim, E. M. (1993b). The difficult first week at home with a premature infant. *Public Health Nursing, 10*(2), 89–96.

McKim, E. M., Kenner, C., Flandermeyer, A., et al. (1995). The transition to home for mothers of healthy and initially healthy newborns. *Midwifery, 11,* 184–194.

Mercer, R. T. (1981). A theoretical framework for studying factors that impact on the maternal role. *Nursing Research, 30*(2), 73–77.

Mercer, R. T. (1986). Predictors of maternal role attainment at one year postbirth. *Western Journal of Nursing Research, 8*(1), 9–32.

Mercer, R. T., & Ferketich, S. L. (1990). Predictors of family functioning eight months following birth. *Nursing Research, 39*(2), 39–82.

Mercer, R. T., Nichols, E. G., & Doyle, G. C. (1989). *Transitions in a woman's life: Major life events in developmental context.* New York: Springer.

Miles, M. S. (1989). Parents of critically ill premature infants: Sources of stress. *Critical Care Quarterly, 12*(3), 69–74.

Miles, M. S., & Holditch-Davis, D. (1995). Compensatory parenting: How mothers describe parenting their 3-year-old, prematurely born children. *Journal of Pediatric Nursing, 10*(4), 243–253.

Noch, L. (1989). *Needs of mothers of premature infants after discharge from the NICU.* Unpublished master's thesis, University of Cincinnati College of Nursing and Health.

Noga, K. M. (1982). High-risk infants: The need for nursing follow-up. *Journal of Obstetric, Gynecologic, and Neonatal Nursing, 11*(2), 112–115.

Norris, D. M., & Hoyer, P. J. (1993). Dynamism in practice: Parenting within King's framework. *Nursing Science Quarterly, 6*(2), 79–85.

Peoples-Sheps, M. D. (1990). Perinatal home visiting returns. *Nursing Outlook, 38*(2), 54–55.

Rubin, R. (1973). Cognitive style in pregnancy. In M. H. Browning & E. P. Lewis (Eds.), *Maternal and newborn care: Nursing interventions* (pp. 22–33). New York: The American Journal of Nursing Company.

Rubin, R. (1984). *Maternal identity and the maternal experience* (pp. 52–69). New York: Springer.

Scholtes, P. F., Sherman, J., Griffin, M., et al. (1994). Management of medically fragile infants and children. *Physician Executive, 20*(9), 41–43.

Sheehan, F. (1981). Assessing postpartum adjustment: A pilot study. *Journal of Obstetric, Gynecologic, and Neonatal Nursing, 10*(1), 19–22.

Simone, J. A. (1986). Psychosocial dynamics of high-risk newborn care: The experience of families and the staff's experience. In N. S. Streeter (Ed.), *High-risk neonatal care* (pp. 39–56). Rockville, MD: Aspen.

Sims-Jones, N. (1986). Back to the theories: Another way to view mothers of prematures. *American Journal of Maternal Child Nursing, 11*(6), 394–397.

Stern, M., & Hildebrandt, K. A. (1986). Prematurity stereotyping: Effects on mother–infant interaction. *Child Development, 57*(2), 308–315.

Stewart, M. J. (1989). Social support instruments created by nurse investigators. *Nursing Research, 38*(5), 268–275.

Tobey, G. Y., & Schraeder, B. D. (1990). Impact of caretaker stress on behavioral adjustment of very low birth weight preschool children. *Nursing Research, 39*(2), 84–89.

Trause, M. A., & Kramer, L. I. (1983). The effects of premature birth on parents and their relationship. *Developmental Medicine and Child Neurology, 25*(4), 459–465.

Ventura, S. J., Martin, J. A., Taffell, S. M., et al. (1994). Advance report of final natality statistics, 1992. *Monthly Vital Statistics Report, 43*(5), 20–22.

Walker, L. S., Oritz-Valdes, J. A., & Newbrough, J. R. (1989). The role of maternal employment and depression in the psychological adjustment of chronically ill, mentally retarded, and well children. *Journal of Pediatric Psychology, 14*(3), 357–370.

Wereszczak, J., Miles, M. S., & Holditch-Davis, D. (1997). Maternal recall of neonatal intensive care unit. *Neonatal Network, 16*(4), 33–40.

Wolterman, M. C. K. (1990). *Validation of an instrument to study behaviors in siblings following sibling visitation on a neonatal intensive care unit.* Unpublished doctoral dissertation, University of Cincinnati.

Zimpelmann, D. G. (1990). *The adaptive process of the preterm infant–mother dyad.* Unpublished master's thesis, University of Cincinnati College of Nursing and Health.

CHAPTER 51

Home Care

LYNDA HUTT HALL

RESEARCH AGENDA

What is the impact of high technology in the home on family functioning?

Is home care for respiratory technology dependent children cost effective?

Does home care case management have a positive impact on home care quality and cost effectiveness?

What are the long-term financial and emotional costs to families participating in home care for their technology-dependent child?

Is there a relationship between home care and child abuse and neglect?

What ethical issues arise surrounding home care of technology-dependent infants, and what consideration should be given to these issues?

For the family of a sick newborn, the time that the infant spends in a neonatal intensive care unit (NICU) is stressful. Even though parents often have feelings of inadequacy and helplessness about their ability to care for their child, they anxiously await the time when they can take their child home. For many of these families, home care represents a desirable alternative to prolonged costly hospitalization and family separation.

Dramatic advances in medical technology have contributed to increased survival of infants with chronic medical conditions needing long-term care. Of the estimated 4 million infants born in the United States annually, more than 250,000 require some form of special care (Tooley, 1988). The incidence of low birth weight (less than 2500 g) for 1992 remains at the highest level since 1978 (Ventura et al., 1994). It continues to be well documented that low birth weight is a principle predictor of infant survival and potential morbidity (Centers for Disease Control and Prevention [CDC], 1993; McCormick et al., 1992).

Although the majority of infants requiring ongoing care—preterm and full-term infants with birth asphyxia, sepsis, respiratory distress, major congenital anomalies, metabolic problems, and hyperbilirubinemia—are also hospitalized for special care, home health care has become one alternative method of health care delivery for infants and children.

DEVELOPMENT OF HOME CARE

Home health care options for neonates and infants have grown in response to rising hospital costs, emotional need of families, and technologic advances. The trend toward home-based care has been influenced most by developmental philosophy, technologic advances, family emotional health, and cost efficiency. The factor that has created the greatest pressure to expand the home care industry is cost efficiency.

U.S. health care expenditures increased from $12.7 billion in 1950 to $820 billion in 1992. Third-party payers are unable to sustain the high costs of maintaining medically fragile infants in acute care facilities. These infants quickly exhaust insurance benefits and hospital resources. Institutions faced with unsustainable expenses are eagerly seeking more cost-effective systems to provide quality care (Schoumacher, 1991). Home care is a less expensive alternative (Vladick, 1994).

Financial savings related to neonatal home care have been well documented. In 1976, Pinney and Cotton described a home management program for infants with bronchopulmonary dysplasia; this program had resulted in a savings of $18,000 per patient. Donn (1982) documented the cost effectiveness of home management of patients with bronchopulmonary dysplasia. This study reported an average per-patient savings of $60,690. Brooten and associates (1986) demonstrated that early hospital discharge of infants of very low birth weight to follow-up home care provided by a hospital-based nurse specialist could realize a net savings of $18,560 for each infant. Thilo and colleagues (1987) found substantial cost savings for families and health insurance carriers when infants were discharged from NICUs with home oxygen therapy. This group reported a savings of $33,370 per patient.

In a home phototherapy study, Eggert and associates (1985) found home phototherapy to be feasible, safe, effective, and cost effective. They compared costs between home and in-hospital phototherapy. The results indicated home phototherapy provided a potential savings of $73,152 over a year after treating 254 infants (Eggert et al., 1985). A study in 1986 also concluded that home phototherapy is effective, safe, and cost effective, showing a savings of $430 per patient treated by home phototherapy in comparison with hospital phototherapy (Grabert et al., 1986).

In 1991, Fields and colleagues (1991b) evaluated home care costs and the cost effectiveness of home care for respiratory technology–dependent children. The study, conducted in a Medicaid Model Waiver Program in Maryland, compared the difference between the established Medicaid reimbursements for a long-term care institution and actual Medicaid reimbursements for home care. The mean annual home care costs were $109,836 (with a standard deviation of $20,781) for ventilator-dependent children and a mean cost of $63,650 (Standard Deviation: $12,350) for oxygen-dependent children with tracheostomies. The home care costs, in comparison with standard Medicaid long-term institutional care, represented an annual savings of approximately $79,000 per ventilator-dependent patient and $83,000 per oxygen-dependent patient with a tracheostomy (Fields et al., 1991b).

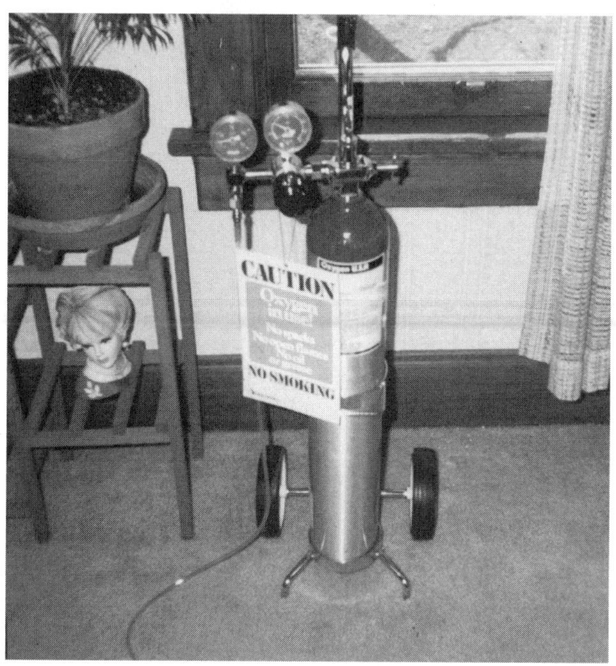

FIGURE 51–1. Oxygen tank for use in home.

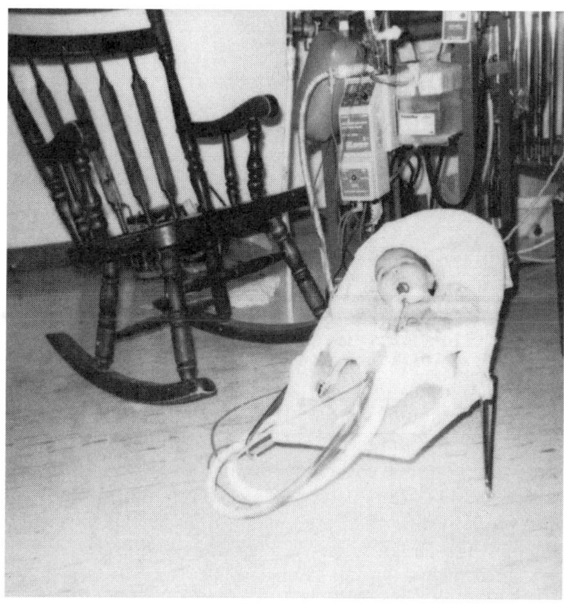

FIGURE 51–2. Home mechanical ventilation.

Several studies of home care for technology-dependent children have shown home care to be more cost effective than institutional care. Home care may save up to $300,000 per year with an average savings of 50 percent of institutional costs (Burr et al., 1983; Eigen & Zander, 1990; Frates et al., 1985; Goldberg et al., 1984).

The emotional aspect of home care for infants has been addressed by many investigators. The process of parent–infant bonding is dramatically altered when a child is hospitalized in a NICU. The authoritarianistic setting and the confusion of an acute care unit create barriers to the normal bonding activities of parents and neonate. Parents often feel as if the hospitalized infant belongs to the hospital staff. Parents feel ownership of their infant only after they are able to take the child home (Klaus & Kennell, 1982).

Prolonged infant hospitalization has been shown to be associated with failure to thrive, with child abuse, and with parental feelings of inadequacy (Desmond et al., 1980; Hayes, 1980; Jeffcoate et al., 1979; Larson, 1980). When early discharge can be facilitated, parents begin to resolve negative feelings surrounding the birth of their child. Home care can restore to some parents a positive self-image and allows them to regain feelings of control over their lives and the life of their child. The process of bonding and attachment is enhanced by uniting parents and their child in the home. Families often take pride in their accomplishments as the infant grows and develops. If medical and nursing treatments are required, parents may develop an increased sense of satisfaction from their involved loving care in the home. Family members can become accomplished in oxygen administration, gavage feedings, respiratory treatments, dressing changes, and various other tasks that are rewarding to them.

Since the 1980s, concern has been expressed regarding the adverse developmental consequences for children of prolonged institutional care. In the past, it was believed that acute care facilities offered major advantages in terms of available services for a child with special care requirements. As more investigations were conducted, a greater appreciation of the deleterious effects of prolonged hospitalization on development have been noted (Bock et al., 1983; Burr et al., 1983; Frates et al., 1985; Goldberg et al., 1984; Kohrman, 1990). Improvements in developmental performance and in social interactions have been documented after discharge to home care with consistent caregivers (Burr et al., 1983; Eigen & Zander, 1990; Field, 1979; Frates et al., 1985; Goldberg et al., 1984; Schreiner et al., 1987).

Technologic advances have made neonatal and infant care in the home not only possible but also safe and efficient. Procedures that were previously limited to in-hospital settings can now be performed in the home. Oxygen administration, respiratory care, mechanical ventilation (Figs. 51–1 to 51–3), phototherapy, intravenous therapy, and alternative modes of nutritional support are just a few of the modalities available to children in the home environment.

Manufacturers of health care products are making available supplies and equipment that make home care feasible. Monitor

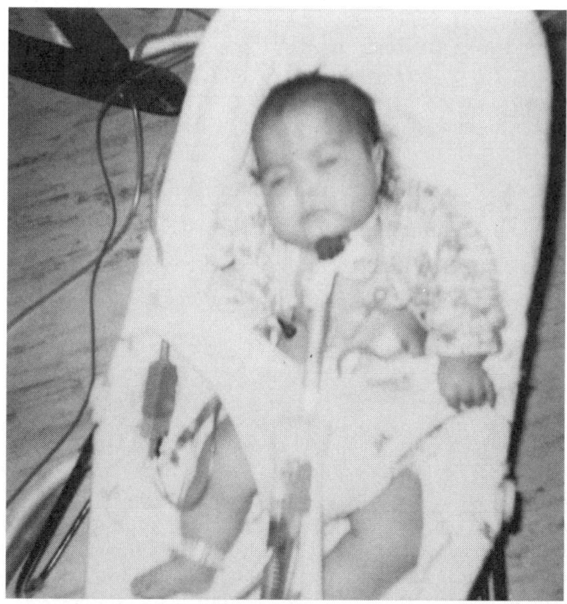

FIGURE 51–3. Home mechanical ventilation and tracheostomy.

manufacturers, oxygen supply companies, and intravenous product suppliers have developed designs specific to home care. Portable equipment has become a major market focus for the health care product industry.

As technology for home therapy expands, the need for additional home care agencies and support personnel becomes essential. Home care systems have been established in response to the demand for increasingly complex and highly technical care in the home. Entrepreneurial endeavors, proprietary home health care agencies, and hospital-based programs have been introduced into the field of home care to provide the resources and the services necessary to meet the increasing need.

In attempts to shift costs from the expensive in-patient setting to the home, hospitals are creating home care services. Neonatal home care programs are being developed to address comprehensive discharge planning, parental and family education and skills development, cardiopulmonary resuscitation instruction, and appropriate follow-up. Home follow-up and program evaluation are essential elements of neonatal home care programs. Brooten and associates (1986) described one model of home follow-up of very low birth weight infants. Early discharge of these infants with home follow-up by perinatal nurse specialists was concluded to be safe, to be cost effective, and to provide potential benefits to society in regard to potential reduction in child abuse and foster placement.

In 1991, Fields and colleagues (1991a) described an independent community-based care management model. Children in this report received home care coordinated by a community-based consortium of public and private organizations that was developed to provide case management for respiratory-disabled children in the home or alternative living facilities. This model offered maximized regional experience and expertise, case management with no financial self-interest in coordinating services, improved regional quality assurance of home care, and decreased reliance on tertiary care centers, allowing easier access to community-based resources.

As the home care industry rapidly expands, issues concerning quality of care are being addressed. In 1988, the Joint Commission on Accreditation of Healthcare Organizations (JCAHO) developed accreditation standards for home care providers, These standards are comprehensive, focusing on patient care, safety, infection control, quality assurance, management, administration, and governance. Specific standards apply to equipment management services, equipment selection, setup and maintenance, and client education. Standards pertaining to related medical supplies that are delivered to and used in the home environment have also been established. The JCAHO accreditation is awarded to home care companies that demonstrate compliance with recommended standards of practice (JCAHO, 1988).

TYPES OF HOME CARE

Home care, for most practical purposes, is classified as short-term, long-term, or hospice care. Other programs involve respite care, day care, and foster care.

Short-Term Care

Short-term care is considered by many health care services to be less than 6 months in duration. Short-term care of an infant at home may include phototherapy for hyperbilirubinemia, administration of supplemental oxygen to treat respiratory distress, home monitoring for apnea of the premature infant, medication administration for various neonatal conditions, and alternative feeding methods such as gavage for nutritional support. These treatment modalities are usually attended to by the primary caregivers in the home. Parents and families are carefully instructed in the use of any equipment placed in the home to administer health care. Extensive teaching before hospital discharge must convey the precise reasons for the therapy, the necessity for close observation of the infant by the caregivers, and the importance of communication and supervision by the primary care physician. In situations of short-term home care, the condition is usually self-limiting, and the home therapy can be discontinued at a predetermined end point.

Long-Term Care

The point at which care becomes long-term is determined by the nature of the health care needs of the individual. The time frame for long-term care is also arbitrarily set by the providers of extended care and the insurers paying for the care. In general, long-term care indicates that the duration of the condition and the need for care will exceed 6 months. Long-term home care addresses situations for children with disease processes such as bronchopulmonary dysplasia, short bowel or short gut syndrome, congenital heart disease, physical and cosmetic defects, neurologic and metabolic disorders, and numerous other prolonged pathologic conditions.

Upon discharge, these children may require home care services performed by professional home care agencies or programs. Families gradually become integrated into the health care routine. As the condition of an infant changes, the family's responsibility changes. The primary care physician must be closely involved and should be able to rely comfortably on the caregiver's judgment for making assessments and alterations in the home care plan. Long-term home care requires open communication among the family, community physicians, tertiary resources, community health care providers, home medical equipment providers, and financial providers. Many hospital records are now incorporating discharge notes, especially nursing case management notes or orders for the actual discharge and home care follow-up plan. These notes are a good vehicle for communication among the community health care providers and the discharging hospital.

Hospice Care

In spite of dramatic developments in medical expertise and technology, a significant number of neonates who are admitted to special care units do not survive. Infant mortality in the United States has declined dramatically since 1960, but this trend leveled off in the 1990s (Stricklin, 1993). Congenital anomalies are the leading cause of infant mortality in the United States and are also a major contributor to childhood morbidity, long-term disability, and loss of years of potential life (Lynberg & Khoury, 1990; National Center for Health Statistics, 1991; National Institutes of Health, 1992). The proportion of infant deaths attributed to birth defects has remained significantly high. Of 38,957 reported infant deaths in 1986, birth defects were listed as the underlying cause of death in 8005 (20.5 percent) (Massachusetts Medical Society, 1989). The 1993 provisional data from the National Center for Health Statistics indicated a 20.3 percent rate of mortality secondary to congenital anomalies (National Center for Health Statistics, 1994).

Acquired immunodeficiency syndrome (AIDS) has become one of the leading causes of death in American children from any single infectious disease agent. Among the deaths of children in the 1- to 4-year age group in 1990, human immunodeficiency virus (HIV) infection constitutes the eighth leading cause of death (Chin, 1994). This HIV catastrophic phenomenon is contributing directly to the need for increased availability of hospice care for infants and children. For an in-depth discussion of HIV and AIDS in infants and children, refer to Chapter 42, Neonatal

Acquired Immunodeficiency Syndrome: Human Immunodeficiency Virus Infection.

When it becomes clear that an infant will no longer benefit from a rescue mode of acute intervention, plans for health care should focus on physical and emotional comfort. The transition from acute care to palliative care involves concepts of hospice.

Hospice care is a philosophy of caring when cure is no longer a reasonable expectation. This care is not strictly a kind of terminal care but rather an effort to maximize current quality of life without giving up all interest in a cure (Corr & Corr, 1985). Hospice provides comfort measures and focuses on alleviation of symptoms. Whether the infant is terminally or chronically ill, the ultimate goal is to provide an environment that comforts the child and supports the family.

Hospice home care can be provided by a variety of models. Programs have been developed to use parents as primary caregivers and hospital-based personnel as facilitators and resource support. Terminal care can be shifted from hospital-based medical management to community-supported home nursing. Essential to the success of these types of programs, however, is the family's desire and their confidence in their ability to care for the child at home. In addition, they must be assured of regularly scheduled home visits and the availability of program personnel to respond when needed (Lauer & Camitta, 1980). Community caregivers with hospital coordination constitute a successful support system for families who elect to care for their dying child or a child with a disabling disease or condition for which no curative therapy is known (Martin, 1985).

Institutions dedicated to the care of the terminally ill have become an important alternative care approach and an accepted part of the health care field in the United States. Hospice facilities caring for children are currently increasing in number, but access to hospice care still has several barriers. Most facilities require a physician's certification that the child will die within 6 months. It is very often difficult to predict the remaining time that a child has left. Another serious barrier is the lack of financial reimbursement for care or the inadequacy of the reimbursement to cover the cost of hospice care (Rhymes, 1990).

Respite Care

At the time of the infant's discharge from the hospital, many parents do not perceive a need for relief or respite care. If comprehensive discharge teaching has been accomplished, parents often feel anxious and ready to assume responsibility for their child. Over the course of time, however, parents find that many of their expected support systems are unavailable to assist with a sick infant. Relatives, friends, and babysitters often feel inadequate and are unable to assume the responsibility of caring for an infant with special needs.

The daily routine for parents may be time consuming and exhausting. Practical problems arise that were not issues during hospitalization. Family and friends outside of the household cannot appreciate the constant strain that is experienced by the immediate family. Social activities become restricted and ungratifying. Even routine outings such as grocery shopping become cumbersome. The child is often too fragile to take to the store, and appropriate child care is often scarce. The resulting fatigue and frustration can threaten the quality of care provided for the child and other family members.

Social and emotional support can be provided to families in a variety of ways. Respite or relief care can be sought from willing family members, friends, the community, and health care facilities.

The Albert Einstein Medical Center (New York, NY) recognized the need for respite care for the families of infants discharged from their unit. The center established a registered nurse babysitting program. This program focuses on the babysitting needs of high-risk infants and serves to encourage auxiliaries and support groups to help underwrite the expense of a registered babysitting service in other communities (Hurt et al., 1988).

Use of homemaker home health aides has been successful in providing assistance for families caring for high-risk infants in the home. The National Home-Caring Councils (NHC), supported with funds from the March of Dimes Birth Defects Foundation, formulated a program to provide persons to help families cope with problems and to perform light housekeeping, babysitting, and respite care (Raff, 1986).

Parents need to maintain time for themselves. Privacy and recreation for parents are essential if the parents are to meet the challenge of caring for a sick infant at home successfully. Various community services are making available relief care for overburdened families. Families should be encouraged to seek out and take advantage of any available family or community source of respite care.

Day Care

Models of special day care centers are emerging across the country. These facilities offer a protected environment, medical technology, and professional nursing care in a day care setting. One such facility is Kangaroo Kids Center in Santa Ana, California. This center, established in 1989, offers a comprehensive program for medically fragile children in a day care center. Open 16 hours each day, Kangaroo Kids Center addresses the child's nursing care needs as well as the developmental and psychosocial needs of the entire family (Delaney & Zolondick, 1991).

A similar model of day care is offered by the Community Health Programs at The Children's Hospital in Denver, Colorado. KidStreet, a day care for medically fragile children, opened in August 1992. This center offers day care for children 6 weeks to 6 years of age who need the services of medicine, nursing, occupational therapy, speech/language therapy, and psychosocial support for families. As a result of the successful provision of cost-effective, safe, high-technology day care, a second center was opened in February 1995 (The Children's Hospital Practice Update, 1995).

Day care for medically fragile, technology-dependent infants is a concept with great potential for future growth. This new alternative offers a much needed care delivery system to special-needs infants and their families. This avenue of care also presents nurses with a challenge and an opportunity to expand professional knowledge and nursing expertise.

Foster Care

Parents and families of infants with complex medical conditions and complex health care needs may find themselves unable to assume the responsibility of caring for their child. The child's health status requires monitoring, compliance with medical and developmental protocols, and timely interventions. These demands are often beyond the capabilities of birth families.

The number of low birth weight infants and infants with developmental delays born to teenagers, substance-using mothers, and homeless women continues to grow rapidly (Lima & Seliger, 1990). Because of the circumstances surrounding the birth and the dysfunctional dynamics of these families, many infants are assumed to be at high risk for abuse, neglect, and abandonment. For these infants and children, medical foster care is an option.

Medical foster care for medically fragile infants can be provided through a variety of programs. The In-Home Support Project was developed by the Bienvenidos Children's Center, Inc., in eastern Los Angeles County (Lima & Seliger, 1990). This program, in coordination with the Los Angeles County Department of Children's Services and community-based agencies, helps parents become more competent and self-assured in appropriately caring for their medically fragile child in their home.

Another type of medical foster care is offered by the Medical Foster Parent Program of the Children's Home and Aid Society of Illinois and La Rabida Children's Hospital and Research Center in Chicago. This program is designed to locate families and facilitate foster care for medically dependent children under the custody or guardianship of the Illinois Department of Children and Family Services. These children are medically ready for discharge, but their families are either unable or unwilling to care for them (Yost et al., 1988).

Medical foster care poses a unique challenge for health care providers, child welfare professionals, and foster families. The successful development and management of medical foster services depend on the ability of all related community systems to be committed, flexible, creative, and aggressive in arriving at solutions that will facilitate the transition of these children from hospital to home care.

CRITERIA FOR HOME CARE

The decision to facilitate early discharge from hospital care to home care must be based on standards that are safe and that provide effective ongoing therapy. Criteria for discharge to home care must be met by the infant, the family, the home equipment, and the follow-up health care system.

Infant Criteria

The infant's home health care needs must be assessed as to technical feasibility and medical requirement. Nutritional support must be evaluated. How does the infant feed and how frequently? How often does the infant require gavage feedings and which feeding techniques are required? Pharmacologic support assessment must be evaluated. What medication does the infant need and how often? What are the desired and adverse effects of these drugs? Does the infant require supplemental oxygen, respiratory therapy treatments, or chest physical therapy? The assessment of the level of care required must be matched to the ability and skills of the home care providers. It must be determined before discharge that care in the home will be safe and meet the needs of the infant and family.

The specific criteria for discharge of special groups of children, such as those with bronchopulmonary dysplasia, short bowel or gut syndrome, neurologic disease, cardiac disease, and other pathologic conditions, are addressed in the preceding chapters.

Family Criteria

The assessment of the family's commitment to home care is perhaps the most critical factor determining the success or failure of home health care. After extensive discharge teaching, skills development, and repetitive occasions of caregiving, the family must want the child at home and under their care. They must be willing and able to devote the time and energy required to meet the physical and emotional needs of the child. These factors are essential for the well-being of the family unit.

To prepare families for the discharge of their sick or high-risk infant, NICU personnel must begin teaching them as soon as the neonate is admitted to the unit. (See Chapter 47, Systematic Assessment and Home Follow-Up: A Basis for Monitoring the Neonate's Integration Into the Family, for assessment and management in preparation for discharge.) Once the family is confident and capable of meeting the needs of the infant, a home assessment should be completed. Basic facilities such as heat, water, telephone, electricity, and transportation must be available. Appropriate support systems must be set up in the home, including the technology necessary for the delivery of care (Fig. 51–4). The operation of phototherapy lights, oxygen delivery systems, portable suction equipment (Fig. 51–5), respiratory and cardiac monitoring systems, ventilators, and numerous other devices must be thoroughly understood by the caregivers. Clear instructions need to be given to the family members by the providers of the home care technology. Ideally, the parents should bring the equipment to the hospital, or the equipment company can help transport it to the hospital before discharge. The rationale is that the parents can be taught on their own equipment. If there is a problem, it can usually be identified before the infant's discharge. The parents should spend at least 24 hours providing total care before discharge (Burstein, 1995). This time under health professionals supervision helps the family gain confidence in their caregiving abilities. They can also be reassured that they have the proper equipment.

Home Equipment Criteria

The most common equipment needs for neonates are cardiopulmonary monitoring, oxygen, suction, and feeding implements. The first decision that the family needs help in making is how to select a home care equipment company. Most hospital discharge planners or the nurse responsible for the discharge has recommendations. Burstein (1995) outlined the criteria for selecting a home care pulmonary equipment company. These criteria (Table 51–1) can be used for other types of equipment suppliers as well.

Once the supplier has been selected and the equipment that will be necessary identified, parent education can begin. This education should include neonatal cardiopulmonary resuscitation (CPR). The parents should be given written instructions to take home and a checklist for the CPR procedure that can be clearly posted. If parents cannot read, visual charts outlining the steps should be made available.

A cardiopulmonary monitor is the most common equipment needed in the home. Infants who should be placed on this type of monitoring are those whose sibling died of sudden infant death syndrome (SIDS) or who are at risk for SIDS. These infants are usually monitored until age 6 to 12 months (Burstein, 1995). An infant on home oxygen or one who has neurologic impairment is at risk for apneic or bradycardic episodes. Most of these monitors have built-in impedance pneumography capabilities that allow

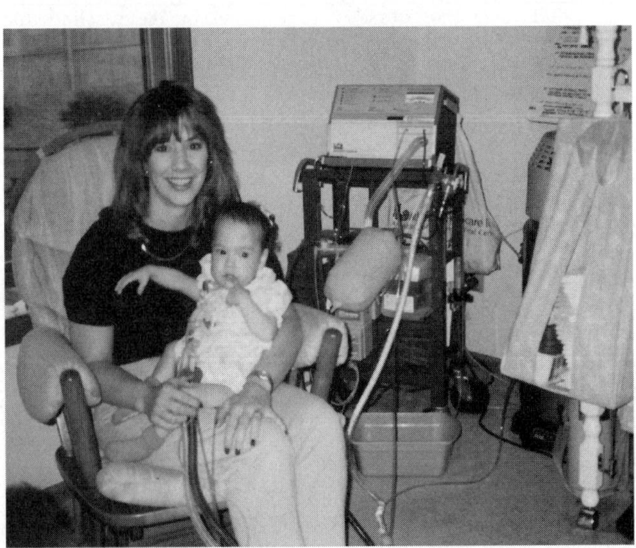

FIGURE 51–4. Home care setup.

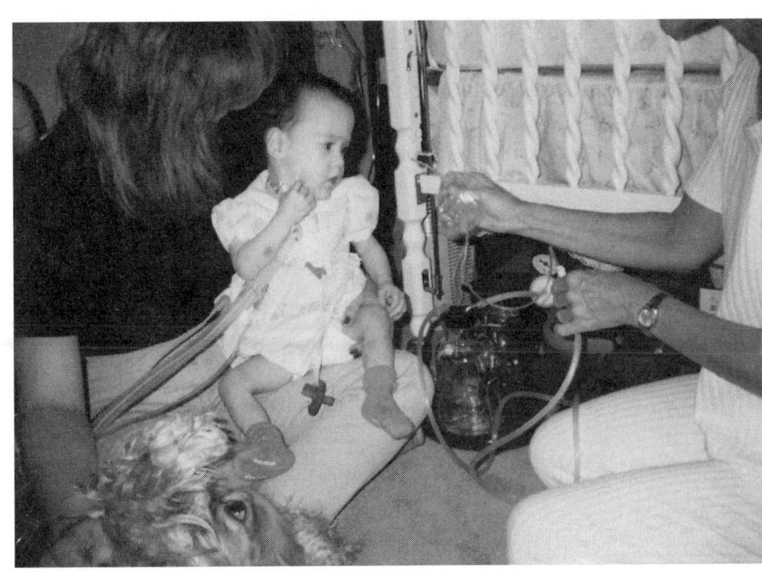

FIGURE 51–5. Portable suction.

strips to be watched or viewed by home care nurses. In some instances, these can be sent via computer modems. The parents should be told that when there is an episode of apnea or bradycardia, they must mark on the strip the infant's color, activity, and what they had to do, if anything, to stop the episode (Burstein, 1995). Burstein (1995) made two important points about this type of monitor. For infants on mechanical ventilation, chest excursion that is detected by the monitor as breathing does not allow the alarm to sound until the heart rate is affected, as in the NICU. Also, for infants who have tracheostomies, the monitoring is to identify episodes in which breathing may stop as a result of mucus plugs or thickened secretions. Yet the survival instinct of the infant, to struggle to breathe, will not allow the respiratory monitor alarm to sound as movement is detected. It is the cardiac portion of the monitor that at a much later stage detects bradycardia. Parents need to understand these delays and how to respond.

Suctioning equipment is needed for patients with tracheostomies. This equipment requires electricity and running water. One type of suctioning equipment must be portable and battery powered for trips to and from the clinic and other excursions out of the home. It should have a regulator valve to adjust the amount of suction. If the valve is not present, negative pressure can be very great and cause mucosal trauma to the nasopharyngeal and tracheal tissues. The battery-powered suction machines can be recharged much like portable phones with a direct A/C adapter into a wall outlet or via a cigarette lighter adapter (Burstein, 1995). Most run about 2 hours without recharging. The recharging process takes about 12 hours. The other type of suctioning equipment can be a stationary set-up. Parents should be taught clean suctioning technique, which is used as long as there is no danger of cross-contamination with other infectious agents in the home, as may be the case when siblings are ill. In the hospital, nosocomial infections and cross-contamination are very real possibilities. The parents should also be taught sterile technique, which should be used only when there is illness in the home that may put the infant at risk for cross-contamination.

TABLE 51–1 Criteria for Selecting a Home Care Pulmonary Equipment

Accreditation by the Joint Commission on Accreditation of Healthcare Organizations (JCAHO)
Location: within an hour's driving radius of home
Availability of equipment and supplies required for care
Experience with equipment required for care
24-hour on-call service for emergencies
Professional home care clinicians or staff*
Record system available to communicate with physician
Availability of backup equipment on site
Experience with similar clinical situations
Acceptance of assignment on insurance benefits

* Some areas may require professional services to be contracted. Contracted professionals must be available on 24-hour on-call basis.

From Burstein, L. (1995). Home care. In S. L. Barnhart & M. P. Czervinske (Eds.), *Perinatal and pediatric respiratory care* (p. 661). Philadelphia: W. B. Saunders.

Suctioning should be taught according to the physician/practitioner's orders. Usually this is done on an as-needed basis. Signs that indicate the need for suctioning are the same as those used by health professionals in the NICU: restlessness, decreased color, coughing, increased respiratory effort, or sounds of congestion. In general, suctioning is necessary every 2 to 4 hours. Parents should keep a log of the timing of the suctioning and the type of secretions obtained. In addition to the suctioning equipment, parents will need a 50–pound per square inch (PSI) portable air compressor and possibly compressed oxygen with portable reservoir. Portable or stationary oxygen devices vary in size and the amount of time that they will last. They are classified as sizes AA through K; G, H, and K are large and stationary, whereas the others are portable. The oxygen tanks for these devices differ from those of liquid oxygen in that they can be stored and will not leak if the shut off valve is left on. They are larger and are filled under high pressure so they are more difficult to move. There is slight danger from pressure if they are accidentally dropped or damaged. The liquid oxygen is more portable and smaller in size. It does not require external electricity or battery-powered sources. The cylinder is small and filled under very little pressure. The liquid oxygen must be moved from the base of the chamber to a portable reservoir. It is more costly than gas pressure oxygen cylinders.

These infants often also need an oxygen concentrator. The concentrator is like the old-fashioned mix-box used in the NICU to mix air and oxygen to achieve the desired oxygen concentration. It separates oxygen from nitrogen in room air and collects oxygen (Burstein, 1995). The concentrations that are possible with these home devices are between 45 and 95 percent (Burstein, 1995). They cannot deliver very low flow rates such as 0.5 L/minute. They are electrically powered. Portable units are needed outside the home. A back-up gas oxygen cylinder is necessary for electrical failures and for excursions outside the home. It is beyond the scope of this chapter to detail the exact procedure for the suctioning and care of the tracheostomy tube. The equipment needed for an infant with a tracheostomy is listed in Table 51–2.

Humidification of the airway is necessary for infants with artificial airways, regardless of whether they are on oxygen. If the airway is not humidified, mucous membranes may dry and crack, creating areas that may become infected. Humidification can be provided by volume jet nebulizers with a 50-PSI portable air compressor. Humidification levels of 35 to 100 percent can generally be achieved (Burstein, 1995). This compressor should be capable of providing high- or low-pressure aerosol. This capability is important if the infant requires a mist tent at night but during the day is connected to a tracheostomy collar or other airway devices. Some companies suggest use of a heat and moisture exchanger (HME), which can be used for travel and is used by itself and not in conjunction with other humidifying devices. It can be attached to the airway without intermediate equipment (Burstein, 1995).

Mechanical ventilation is another area of home care. Information on home use of ventilators can be obtained from the National Center for Home Mechanical Ventilation. The specific type of ventilator is ordered by the physician or practitioner on the basis of infant's need. The decision also takes into consideration the family's lifestyle. If the family anticipates movement from home to other areas or other relatives' homes, a portable unit may be best. All portable units must have an internal and external battery. An emergency back-up unit must be available; whether it be housed in the home or at immediate dispatch from the equipment company does not matter as long as it is available for times when there are equipment failures with the portable device. Battery back-up is necessary, too. Usually a 12-volt battery with 74-amp/hour potential is suggested; such a battery can go about 18 to 20 hours without recharge.

These areas of home care monitoring are the most common. Specific instructions on which equipment is necessary and how to use it in each situation should be obtained from a home health care agency who is to provide care, the hospital equipment vendors, and the home health care equipment vendors. Nurses who are responsible for discharge should be very familiar with the advantages and disadvantages of the equipment that the family will need. The family's lifestyle and capabilities also have to be considered when an infant is sent home on equipment.

TABLE 51–2 Equipment Supply List for Tracheostomy Patient

Apnea–bradycardia monitor
Electrodes (2 pairs)
Lead wire (2 pairs)
Belts (2 each)
Tracheostomy tubes (same size) (4 per month)
Tracheostomy tubes (one size smaller) 1 each
Velcro tracheostomy ties (2 boxes per month)
Twill tape (1 roll)
Free-standing suction machine (1 each)
Portable suction machine
Suction connecting tubing (4 per month)
Suction catheters (4 cases per month)
DeLee traps (6 each)
50-PSI portable air compressor
Jet nebulizers (4 per month)
Corrugated aerosol tubing (100-ft roll)
Tracheostomy collars (4 per month)
Liquid oxygen with portable reservoir (as needed)
Oxygen connecting tubing (4 each)
Sterile water (2 to 3 cases per month)
Normal saline, 3-ml vials (2 boxes month)
Heat and moisture exchangers (1 to 2 boxes per month)
Scissors (2 pairs)
Nonsterile gloves (2 boxes per month)
Manual resuscitation bags (2 each)
Sterile cotton-tipped applicators (2 boxes per month)
Hydrogen peroxide (2 bottles per month)
Stethoscope

Adapted from Burstein, L. (1995). Home care. In S. L. Barnhart & M. P. Czervinske (Eds.), *Perinatal and pediatric respiratory care* (p. 668). Philadelphia: W. B. Saunders.

Follow-Up System Criteria

Criteria for home care cannot be complete without accurate assessment of the availability of follow-up after discharge. Environmental conditions and social supports are two of the strongest influences on the ability of the parents to nurture their child in the home (Lang et al., 1988).

The establishment of home health visits may be accomplished by hospital-based programs that provide home health services. Community-funded home health care agencies are often available to provide some home follow-up. The departments of public health and other publicly funded agencies can be of assistance with home care follow-up.

The visiting resource person must be appropriately knowledgeable about the physical and emotional needs of the family. To be effective, the home visitor should be sensitive to cultural and ethnic differences and incorporate knowledge about them into the follow-up plan.

Public Law 99-457 regarding education of the handicapped mandates that services be available for NICU graduates. It is important that these children be referred to early intervention programs to promote the most positive development possible. Any infant is eligible who has a developmental delay, is at risk for a developmental problem, or has a condition with a high probability for developmental problems, such as Down syndrome (Stepanek, 1996). Resources for information in early intervention services include National Early Childhood Technical Assistance System (NEC°TAS), 137 East Franklin Street, Suite 500, Chapel Hill, NC 27514, 919-962-2001, or Technical Assistance for Parents Program (TAPP), 95 Berkley Street, Suite 104, Boston, MA 02116, 617-482-2915 (Stepanek, 1996).

PSYCHOLOGICAL IMPACT OF HOME CARE

As has been previously discussed, home care of sick neonates offers both economic and psychological advantages. The experience of caring for a sick neonate in the home, however, may also have negative consequences for the family.

The usual family stresses that accompany the birth of a child become magnified when families are faced with a sick infant. Fatigue, financial concerns, and sibling reactions are just a few of the issues that new parents may need to confront. If the infant requires special care, many parents may be burdened with feelings of unresolved guilt, anger, or fear concerning the illness of their newborn.

Many infants leave NICUs before complete health has been achieved. Some documented negative observations related to caring for sick infants in the home include increased parental stress, increased incidence of child abuse, parental detachment, and inappropriate parental coping behaviors. Home care issues have an impact on the parents, the infant, and the siblings.

Impact on Parents

Stress exhibited by parents of infants on home oxygen therapy and home apnea monitoring has been documented (Cain et al., 1980; Johnson, 1979; Vohr et al., 1988; Wasserman, 1984; Young et al., 1988). Parents are often fatigued, irritated, and frustrated owing to unanticipated demands and limitations of the new child. Upon the infant's discharge from the hospital, parents may fear life-threatening events related to equipment failure in the home, exposures to contagious diseases, or unrecognized disease progression. In spite of comprehensive discharge teaching, many caregivers doubt their ability to maintain the level of care they have observed in the security of the NICU. Parents are concerned about mobility and the technical aspects of care.

Once the child is home, it becomes immediately obvious that the child is different from other children. The impact of incorporating a sick child into the daily life of a family is not fully realized. The presence of a nurse and technical equipment signifies the loss of privacy for the family. This is also a constant reminder of additional medical expenses.

After the child has been in the home for a period of time, new emotional experiences begin to take place. Frequently, the primary caregiver begins to feel isolated and overwhelmed with responsibilities. Relationships between family members often become altered. Friendships begin to change because of the increased time and energy demands in the home. Pre-existing problems may worsen, and the family's plans and goals may need to be altered. Issues such as family planning often need to be reevaluated. Career plans are frequently interrupted. The financial responsibility for a sick child can be devastating to an already burdened family.

Family dynamics have been noted to change dramatically when children in the home require health care support personnel. An unusual phenomenon was reported by Byers and Fabian (1988) of the University of Colorado Children's Hospital Home Care Program: Skilled caregivers have observed that some parents and families become so dependent on home care personnel that they are unable or unwilling to participate in the child's care. Byers and Fabian (1988) termed this phenomenon the *parent drop-out syndrome*.

Many families have unresolved feelings of chronic sorrow and grieving that are incapacitating. They cannot attach, or they withdraw from attaching, to the sick infant. When some parents are confronted with the actual care of their child, they become overwhelmed and resistant to learning the necessary care techniques.

The financial impact of home care on the family must be evaluated before the child is discharged. Although it has been shown that home care can result in significantly lower costs over hospitalized care, the family does not necessarily benefit directly from the cost saving. This concept is explained in detail later in this section.

Most third-party payers save money by placing a child in the home. In addition, health care institutions are encouraged to facilitate early discharge to decrease uncompensated services and make resources available for new admissions. Therefore, there is considerable incentive for private and public payers to encourage home care rather than hospitalized care. Some families feel pressured into taking their children home before they are ready. These feelings often result in parental abuse and neglect of the ill child or the siblings (Leonard et al., 1989).

Families incur incremental costs as a result of undertaking home care of the chronically ill and handicapped infant. Often, the actual costs to the family are hidden or overlooked. Direct and indirect costs can become an enormous burden. Direct costs include such items as physician care, equipment, durable supplies and goods, home renovations, transportation, and home health services. Indirect costs include the time spent transporting and in caregiving activities, time away from work, forgone leisure time, and forgone income of the caregiver. The provision of room and board is a usual hidden cost (Jacobs & McDermott, 1989).

Occasionally, families believe that there are no other alternatives to home care. For technology-dependent children, some options include hospital transitional wards, rehabilitation or chronic care hospitals, pediatric skilled nursing facilities, specialized community group care, and foster care. In reality, some of these families have no family or friends to help, so they have no options other than those just listed.

The long-term nature of a prognosis not only affects cost but also influences quality-of-life issues. Children who are technology dependent—those who need medical technology to compensate for the loss of a normal body function—might spend their entire lives in an institution if home care is not available. Parents are faced with securing financial resources to pay for expenses incurred. Families whose insurers either refuse to fund home care or do so at an inadequate level often need to pursue lawsuits or negotiations of acceptable levels of health care services. Sometimes parents whose insurance does pay for many of the home care expenses do not realize that the maximum lifetime benefits may be used up during this period. This situation means that the family is left with no future insurance coverage and often no potential for getting another company to insure them. Nurses need to be aware of this and make families aware that they need to check their maximum policy benefits with their insurance company. After personal insurance, income, and savings are consumed and community funds and volunteer services are exhausted, parents frequently make decisions to reduce particular services. It has been observed that when services are reduced, parental stress increases. This results in parental inability to cope and thus compromises family functioning. Ultimately, the well-being of the sick child is compromised (Office of Technology Assessment, 1987).

In 1990, Quint and colleagues published a study investigating the psychosocial impact on the family providing home care for ventilator-dependent children. They found that the severity of the psychosocial impact on the family was maintained at a steady state over time. They also noted that the primary caregiver's coping abilities became reduced when the duration of the child's assisted ventilation was greater than 2 years. The combination of the amount of time spent in the sustained caretaker role and the long-term outlook of continued ventilator dependency may contribute to burnout and exhaustion (Quint et al., 1990). Patterson and Leonard (1994) noted that fathers talked more extensively about the economic impact of having a medically fragile child, whereas mothers talked more about caregiving and relationship aspects of home care. Fathers coped by working harder and engaging in more hobbies and leisure activities. Mothers coped by talking about their concerns and seeking support (Patterson & Leonard, 1994).

Many studies of ventilator-dependent children living at home have reported that strains in relationships between parents and professionals add to the already high levels of stress experienced by these families. Issues of control, distrust, perceived lack of competence, undesirable personal habits, and unprofessionalism of health care professionals contributed to strained relationships (Patterson et al., 1994).

Parents who take medically fragile children home and assume their care need support. They need support from family, friends, health care professionals, and most important, from the community.

Impact on the Infant

Ongoing technical home care can have a lasting impact on the child recipient. Often, these children are considered "special" by their parents. They become characterized as "spoiled." Many have difficulty with social interaction long after there has been total resolution of the initial health problem. Children who were monitored at home for apnea have been reported to have more separation anxiety as toddlers. They have been noted to exhibit problems with motor skills, attention span, hyperactivity, poor coordination, and speech during early school years (Wasserman, 1984).

If parents continue to perceive their child as fragile and limited, the child is at great risk for the "vulnerable child syndrome." This syndrome, described by Green and Solnet in 1964, is an imagined vulnerability of healthy children by parents who need to view them as fragile and sickly. These children grow to perceive themselves as fragile and become psychosocially handicapped. This syndrome includes behaviors such as prolonged separation anxiety, prolonged infantile behaviors, psychosomatic disorders, and underachievement in school (Gorski, 1988).

An increased incidence of child abuse and neglect has been reported to be associated with caring for the high-risk infant. In 1967, Elmer and Gregg linked prematurity with later child abuse. In 1971, Klein and Stern reported that 23.5 percent of battered children in their study had been born prematurely. Other investigators have shown child abuse and neglect to be significant problems for premature or sick infants (Du Hamel et al., 1974).

Infants discharged from NICUs behave in unexpected and frustrating patterns once they are in the home. Premature infants exhibit intervals of behavioral disorganization in relation to sleep, arousal, alertness, fussing, feeding, and newborn activity. Other infants may exhibit difficult behaviors owing to the physical limitation of their pathology. Interactional defects are also noted to develop, which may be independent of their medical complications (Minde, 1984). Parenting of these premature or sick infants is a heavy burden, even for the most stable parents who have good support and are well off financially.

Home care of the difficult infant intensifies the frustration, guilt, and responsibilities that parents feel about their child. When parents lack coping mechanisms and support systems, these children often become victims of abusive behaviors by the caregivers.

Impact on Siblings

Negative sibling reactions to the home care of a sick neonate can become problematic. Parents report sibling behaviors of anxiety, jealousy, decreased attention span, enuresis, encopresis, and speech regression. Some siblings express feelings of isolation, rejection, and anger. Frequently, parents are so consumed by the demands of the sick child that the healthy siblings feel neglected and deprived. Antisocial behaviors can be a consequence of this perceived lack of attention by adolescent siblings.

COMMUNITY RESOURCES

The successful integration of a high-risk infant into the home and community requires a well-coordinated interface between hospital-based programs and local community resources. The discharge planning process discussed in Chapter 50 is the vehicle for linking the child and the family to the community.

Various sources of support are available to families involved in home care. Programs arise from local home care agencies, support groups, and national volunteer agencies, as well as city, state, and federal agencies. Many communities have private agencies that offer services such as equipment rentals, supplies, and support services for varying fees.

Numerous support groups have been organized to assist families. These include the American Cleft Palate Association, the Down Syndrome Congress, the Osteogenesis Imperfecta Foundation, the Turner Syndrome Support Group, and Parents of Prematures and High Risk Infants (PPHRI). The Lifetime Foundation provides education concerning parenteral and enteral nutrition in the home.

National volunteer programs such as the Easter Seals Society and March of Dimes Birth Defects Foundation have local chapters that assist with specialized care of children. Most areas have specialized infant programs that may be state, city, or privately funded and that provide a wide range of services (Headlee, 1988).

State and federal governments have legislated support services for children. The Maternal Child Health Division of the Department of Health and Human Services in most states provides assistance for infants whose families meet established criteria. Crippled Children's Services vary from state to state but usually include diagnostic, treatment, and maintenance programs. Each county has a public health department that offers public health nursing home visits free of charge. Some health departments offer home care services, immunizations, and well-child clinics. Regional centers funded by state health departments provide comprehensive care for infants and young children (Headlee, 1988).

In 1981, the United States Congress enacted a law allowing the transfer of public funds from hospital care to home care through the creation of a State Medicaid Home and Community-Based Waiver Program. The crucial aspect of the Model Waiver Program is the waiving of consideration of parental income, and the consideration of the child's income becomes the only financial eligibility factor. This waiver allowed Medicaid eligibility criteria to include middle- and upper-income families either who reached their maximum private insurance benefits or whose insurance would not reimburse for home care. Each state is required to plan cooperative involvement with nursing, medicine, health, welfare groups, and organizations to provide services and advocacy for disabled children (The Omnibus Budget Reconciliation Act of 1981 [OBRA], 1981).

In April 1988, a task force on technology-dependent children was appointed by the Secretary of Health and Human Services (HHS). The task force defined technology-dependent children as "those who require medical technology to compensate for the loss of a body function, and who are in need of substantial and complex daily nursing care to avert death or further disability" (*Report to Congress,* 1988). The task force recognized that the most important aspect of appropriate home care was case management. Case management, as defined by the task force, "is a process of care coordination which promotes the effective and efficient organization and utilization of medical, social, educational, and other resources to achieve or maintain the maximum potential of the child in the most appropriate and the least restrictive environment" (*Report to Congress,* 1988). The task force also recommended that case management should be community based, family centered, and directed through a case manager for each technology-dependent child and family. In light of this recommendation, the community-based case management model for home care is becoming a desirable alternative to tertiary care case management.

With the advent of Public Law 99-457, developed as Part H of the Individuals with Disabilities Act, new resources may yet be made available to support some aspects of home care. Although this legislation is not designed to support medical services per se, some educational and allied health services required by chronically ill children may be covered. This legislation is a potential valuable support that may allow more families to care for chronically ill children at home (Struk, 1994).

COORDINATION OF FOLLOW-UP CARE

The success of caring for a sick or high-risk infant in the home lies within a comprehensive and well-coordinated follow-up plan. Meticulous attention must be paid to the implementation of the plan before discharge. Every infant who is committed to home care requires a specialized and personalized program designed to maximize the quality of home care. These specific needs are discussed in previous chapters.

The responsibility for continued health care in the home rests with the regional center and the community-based physician. Cooperation and communication between the tertiary staff and the primary care physician must be established early in the hospitalization. This provides an opportunity for the primary physician to become acquainted with the infant's needs and allows an opportunity for primary care input. During this period, the roles and responsibilities for follow-up care must be identified and clarified (Hurt, 1984).

Many tertiary centers have discharge teams composed of physicians, consultants, advanced practice nurses, specialists, and other multidisciplinary personnel who, in conjunction with the primary pediatrician and the family, formulate a written home health care plan. The home care plan must include the specific health care needs of the child; the technology, personnel, and supplies required to provide the necessary care; and the psychosocial and financial needs of the family (Fig. 51–6). The plan must identify the responsibilities and the mechanisms of accountability for all persons involved (Goldberg & Monahan, 1989). The tertiary center should coordinate the specific home care activities and special follow-up evaluations. Most regional centers routinely hold regularly scheduled clinics that provide specialized medical care and ongoing assessments.

Once the child is in the home, health care becomes a community-oriented case management process, in which the primary care pediatrician or nurse practitioner assumes the role of coordinator. The physician implements, evaluates, and subsequently modifies the care plan with the assistance of the family and home care personnel. A home care team that consists of the physician, the parents, the community health care providers, the home medical equipment providers, and the sponsors of the funds, if any, to support the home care usually evolves. The tertiary center then becomes an important resource for support and consultation (Goldberg & Monahan, 1989).

The primary physician or pediatrician performs a number of important services that cannot be performed by the referral center. Emergency care; coordination of community resources, home equipment vendors, and health care personnel; and follow-up become the responsibilities of the community-based physician. Home health nursing services and hospital-based nursing personnel assist with the ongoing aspects of home care. The pediatrician tends to the pediatric needs of the child, including immunizations, developmental assessments, and minor acute illnesses. The pediatrician also serves as a link between the family and the tertiary center and is a support resource for the family (Ward & Keens, 1988).

Regularly scheduled home visits by nursing personnel, frequent telephone contacts with the family, and regularly scheduled office visits contribute to the success of the home care program. Parental support can be enhanced by physician–parent and nurse–parent conferences. Consultations with social workers and psychiatric services should be made available periodically for the family members. Referrals to parent support groups and community support services are helpful for the families involved in home care of the sick child.

Complex home care of technology-dependent children continues to be a rapidly expanding field. It has become increasingly important for pediatricians, primary care physicians, and home health nursing personnel to keep abreast of advances in all aspects of post-NICU home care.

IMPLICATIONS FOR PROFESSIONAL NURSING

The need for a more comprehensive approach to home care of the high-risk and medically fragile infant becomes the context for the role of professional nursing. Demographics, reimbursement structures, and a growing concern for a morally just and efficient system of home care contribute to this particular nursing responsibility. In view of the existing nature of home care for high-risk children, nurses can make significant contributions by participating actively in the delivery of health services specifically aimed at the enhancement of accessibility, management, and continuity of home care for children. The nursing profession should take opportunities to address the issues of allocation of resources, effectiveness of care, cost containment, and accountability.

Nursing researchers need to address the clinical problems of the medically fragile child that are amenable to nursing intervention: that is, mobility, nutrition, growth, and development. Standards of care for technology-dependent children in the home must be studied and evaluated. Qualifications for home health care providers need to be researched for documented efficiency and effectiveness. Nursing research is needed to document the contribution of nursing care to the health and well-being of chronically ill children and their families in the home setting.

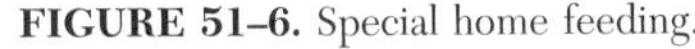

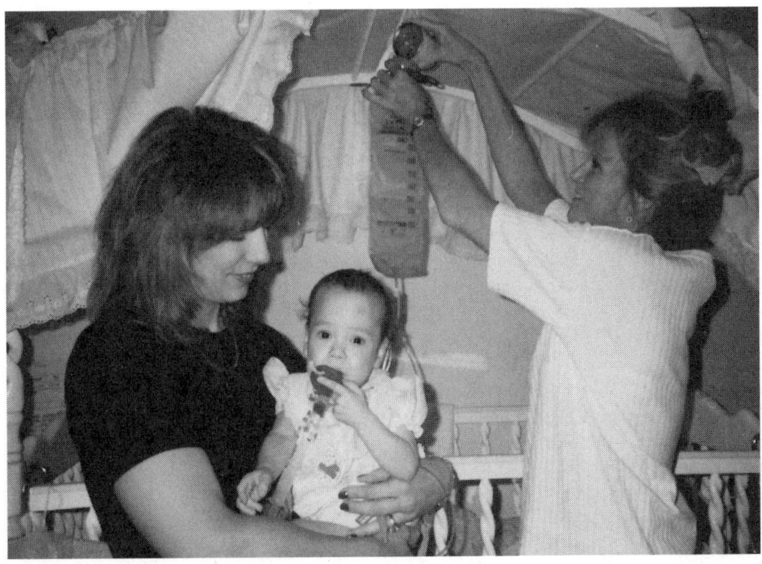

FIGURE 51–6. Special home feeding.

Critical examinations regarding the cost effectiveness of the home care setting for high-risk infants must be conducted. To accomplish this, standardized cost analysis and comparisons that include hidden costs such as respite care for parents must be established. Research must be undertaken to identify and develop resources appropriate for home care.

Policy makers and officials face difficult choices when attempting to maintain quality nursing care standards by reimbursing for professional care. These choices are often made without data demonstrating the improvements in the quality of care that result from expert nursing interventions. Nursing research must develop effective methods for measuring and demonstrating the quality of home health care provided by unskilled, skilled, or a combination of both types of care. The cost effectiveness of advanced practice nurses supervising or managing a caseload of patients in home care must be documented in more populations than just the low birth weight infants. Multivariate techniques that allow criteria evaluation and support the determination of what combination of criteria best predicts quality of care in the home must be developed.

SUMMARY

Home health care has become recognized as an alternative method of health care delivery for infants and children. By providing care in the home for sick or high-risk infants, hospitalizations can be shortened. The overall financial costs are significantly less, and the psychosocial problems of prolonged hospitalization and separation of infant and parents are reduced in number and severity.

Technologic advances have made neonatal home care not only feasible but also safe and efficient. Medical equipment specifically designed for home use in conjunction with the development of skilled home health services has made possible varying levels of home care. Home care of neonates and children ranges from home monitoring to high-technology care such as mechanical ventilation.

In spite of the many benefits of home care, significant negative consequences can result for the family and the patient. The emotional and financial costs to the family must be carefully assessed before a family is committed to health care in the home. Appropriate community resources must be identified and coordinated to provide support systems for home care families. Once the child is in the home, successful implementation of the home care plan requires careful and consistent follow-up by well-educated home care professionals.

CONCLUSION

To ensure the success of any neonatal or pediatric home care program, careful consideration must be given to medical, social, and financial issues. The tertiary center must provide extensive counseling to the family. It should provide an early and comprehensive teaching program for the parents and incorporate the parents into the decision-making process (Cicco et al., 1996). Health care personnel must foster family independence while providing support and direction.

Manufacturers and vendors must continually update equipment, supplies, and services that focus on care outside of the hospital setting. Funders and third-party providers must structure more comprehensive insurance coverage to create adequate funding for home care of children. Social policy should be formulated to minimize the total cost of home care and not just the cost of publicly provided services. Medical, financial, ethical, and humanitarian issues must be accurately and continually assessed to ensure the safety and well-being of children who are receiving health care in the home.

REFERENCES

Bock, R. H., Lierman, C., Ahmann, E., et al. (1983). There's no place like home. *Children's Health Care, 12*(2), 93–96.

Brooten, D., Kumar, S., Brown, L. P., et al. (1986). A randomized clinical trial of early hospital discharge and home follow-up of very-low-birth weight infants. *New England Journal of Medicine, 315*(15), 934–939.

Burstein, L. (1995). Home care. In S. L. Barnhart, & M. P. Czervinske (Eds.), *Perinatal and pediatric respiratory care* (pp. 658–679). Philadelphia: W. B. Saunders.

Burr, B. H., Guyer, B., Tordes, I. D., et al. (1983). Home care for children on respirators. *New England Journal of Medicine, 309*(21), 1319–1323.

Byers, J. E., & Fabian, A. M. (1988). The parent drop-out syndrome. *Caring, 7*(6), 36–38.

Cain, L. P., Kelly, D. H., & Shannon, D. C. (1980). Parents' perception of the psychological and social impact of home monitoring. *Pediatrics, 66*(1), 37–41.

Centers for Disease Control and Prevention [CDC]. (1993). Infant mortality, United States, 1990. *Morbidity and Mortality Weekly Report, 42*(9), 161–165.

Chin, J. (1994). The growing impact of HIV/AIDS pandemic on children born to HIV-infected women. *Clinics in Perinatology, 21*(1), 1–14.

Cicco, R., Greer, M., White, R., et al. (1996, January). *Making NICUs more developmentally appropriate for infants. Parents and families.* Paper presented at The Physical and Developmental Environment of the High Risk Neonate. Clearwater Beach, FL: University of South Florida College of Medicine.

Corr, C. A., & Corr, D. M. (1985). Pediatric hospice care. *Pediatrics, 76*(5), 774–780.

Delaney, N., & Zolondick, K. (1991). Day care for technology-dependent infants and children: A new alternative. *Journal of Perinatal and Neonatal Nursing, 5*(1), 80–85.

Desmond, M. M., Vorderman, A., & Salinas, M. (1980). The family and the premature infant after neonatal intensive care. *Texas Medicine, 76*(1), 60–69.

Donn, S. (1982). Cost effectiveness of home management of bronchopulmonary dysplasia [Letter]. *Pediatrics, 70*(2), 330–331.

Du Hamel, T. R., Lin, S., Skelton, A., & Hantke, C. (1974). Early parental perceptions and the high-risk neonate. Preliminary results of an early parent education program. *Clinical Pediatrics, 13*(12), 1052–1056.

Eggert, L. D., Pollary, R. A., Folland, D. S., & Jung, A. L. (1985). Home phototherapy treatment of neonatal jaundice. *Pediatrics, 76*(4), 579–584.

Eigen, H., & Zander, J. (1990). Home mechanical ventilation of pediatric patients: American Thoracic Society. *American Review of Respiratory Diseases, 141*(1), 258–259.

Elmer, E., & Gregg, G. S. (1967). Developmental characteristics of abused children. *Pediatrics, 40*(4), 596–602.

Field, T. M. (1979). *Infants born at risk.* New York: SP Medical and Scientific Books.

Fields, A. I., Coble, D. H., Pollack, M. M., & Kaufman, J. (1991a). Outcome of home care for technology-dependent children: Success of an independent, community-based case management model. *Pediatric Pulmonology, 11*(4), 310–317.

Fields, A. I., Rosenblatt, A., Pollack, M. M., & Kaufman, J. (1991b). Home care cost-effectiveness for respiratory technology-dependent children. *American Journal of Diseases of Children, 145*(7), 729–733.

Frates, R. C., Splaingard, M. L., Smith, E. D., & Harrison, G. M. (1985). Outcome of home mechanical ventilation for children. *Journal of Pediatrics, 106*(5), 850–856.

Goldberg, A. I., Faure, E. A., Vaughn, C. J., et al. (1984). Home care for life-supported persons: An approach to program development. *Journal of Pediatrics, 104*(5), 785–795.

Goldberg, A. I., & Monahan, C. A. (1989). Home health care for children assisted by mechanical ventilation: The physician's perspective. *Journal of Pediatrics, 114*(3), 378–383.

Gorski, P. A. (1988). Fostering family development after preterm hospitalization. In R. A. Ballard (Ed.), *Pediatric care of the ICN graduate* (pp. 27–32). Philadelphia: W. B. Saunders.

Grabert, B. E., Wardell, C., & Harburg, S. K. (1986). Home phototherapy. *Clinical Pediatrics, 25*(6), 291–294.

Green, M., & Solnet, A. J. (1964). Reactions to the threatened loss of a child: A vulnerable child syndrome. *Pediatrics, 34,* 56–66.

Hayes, J. (1980). Premature infant development: The relationship of neonatal stimulation, birth condition, and home environment. *Pediatric Nursing, 6*(6) 33–36.

Headlee, J. (1988). Community and agency resources. In R. A. Ballard (Ed.), *Pediatric care of the ICN graduate* (pp. 329–330). Philadelphia: W. B. Saunders.

Hurt, H. (1984). Continuing care of the high-risk infant [Review]. *Clinics in Perinatology, 11*(1), 3–17.

Hurt, H., Brodsky, N., Bealt, L., & Hopper, P. (1988). Special baby-sitters for special babies. *Perinatology/Neonatology, 12*(2), 32–34.

Jacobs, P., & McDermott, S. (1989). Family caregivers' costs of chronically ill and handicapped children: Method and literature review [Review]. *Public Health Reports, 104*(2), 158–163.

Jeffcoate, J. A., Humphrey, M. E., & Lloyd, J. K. (1979). Disturbance in parent–child relationship following preterm delivery. *Developmental Medicine and Child Neurology, 21*(3), 344–352.

Johnson, S. (1979). The premature infant. In S. Johnson (Ed.), *High-risk parenting: Nursing assessment and strategies for the family at risk* (pp. 94–116). Philadelphia: J. B. Lippincott.

Joint Commission on Accreditation of Health Care Organizations [JCAHO]. (1988). *Standards for accreditation of home care.* Chicago: Author.

Klaus, K. H., & Kennell, J. H. (1982). *Maternal-infant bonding.* St. Louis: C. V. Mosby.

Klein, M., & Stern, L. (1971). Low birthweight and the battered child syndrome. *American Journal of Diseases of Children, 122*(1), 15–18.

Kohrman, A. (1990). Psychological issues in pediatric home care. In M. Mehlman & S. Younger (Eds.), *Issues in high technology home care: A guide for decision making.* Owings Mills, MD: National Health Publishing.

Lang, M. D., Behle, M. B., & Ballard, R. A. (1988). The transition from hospital to home. In R. A. Ballard (Ed.), *Pediatric care of the ICN graduate* (pp. 12–16). Philadelphia: W. B. Saunders.

Larson, C. P. (1980). Efficacy of perinatal and postpartum home visits on child health and development. *Pediatrics, 66*(2), 191–197.

Lauer, M. E., & Camitta, B. M. (1980). Home care for dying children: A nursing model. *Journal of Pediatrics, 97*(6), 1032–1035.

Leonard, B. J., Brust, J. D., & Choi, T. (1989). Providing access to home care for disabled children: Minnesota's Medicaid Model Waiver Program. *Public Health Reports, 104*(5), 465–472.

Lima, L., & Seliger, J. (1990). Early intervention keeps medically fragile babies at home. *Children Today, 19*(1), 28–32.

Lynberg, M. C., & Khoury, M. J. (1990). *Contribution of birth defects to infant mortality among racial/ethnic minority groups, United States, 1983.* CDC Surveillance Summary, 39(ss-3), 1–12. Atlanta: Centers for Disease Control.

Martin, B. B. (1985). Home care for terminally ill children and their families. In C. A. Corr & D. M. Corr (Eds.), *Hospice approaches to pediatric care* (pp. 65–86). New York: Springer.

Massachusetts Medical Society. (1989). Birth defects. *Morbidity and Mortality Weekly Report, 38*(37), 634.

McCormick, M. C., Brooks-Gunn, J., & Workman-Daniels, K. (1992). The health and development status of very low-birth-weight children at school age. *Journal of American Medical Association, 267*(16), 2204–2208.

Minde, K. K. (1984). The impact of prematurity on the behavior of children and on their families [Review]. *Clinics in Perinatology, 11*(1), 227–244.

National Center for Health Statistics. (1991). *National hospital discharge survey.* Unpublished tabulation.

National Center for Health Statistics. (1994). Annual summary of births, deaths, marriages, and divorces, United States, 1993. *Monthly Vital Statistics Report, 42*(13).

National Institutes of Health. (1992). *An evaluation and assessment of the state of the science. Pregnancy, birth and the infant.* Washington, DC: U.S. Government Printing Office.

Office of Technology Assessment. (1987). *Technology-dependent children: Hospital v. home care. A technical memorandum.* Washington, DC: Author.

Patterson, J., & Leonard, B. (1994). Caregiving and children. In E. Kahana, D. Biegel, & M. Wykle (Eds.), *Family caregiving across the lifespan.* Newbury Park, CA: Sage.

Patterson, J. M., Jernell, J., Leonard, B. J., & Titus, J. C. (1994). Caring for medically fragile children at home: The parent–professional relationship. *Journal of Pediatric Nursing, 9*(2), 98–106.

Pinney, M. A., & Cotton, E. K. (1976). Home management of bronchopulmonary dysplasia. *Pediatrics, 58*(6), 856–859.

Quint, R. D., Chesterman, E., Crain, L. S., et al. (1990). Home care for ventilator-dependent children. Psychosocial impact on the family. *American Journal of Diseases of Children, 144*(11), 1238–1241.

Raff, B. S. (1986). The use of homemaker–home health aides' perinatal care of high-risk infants. *Journal of Obstetric, Gynecologic, and Neonatal Nursing, 15*(2), 142–145.

Report to Congress and the Secretary by the Task Force on Technology-Dependent Children (1988). Washington, DC: U.S. Department of Health and Human Services, Health Care Financing Administration.

Rhymes, J. (1990). Hospice care in America. *Journal of the American Medical Association, 264*(3), 369–372.

Schreiner, M. S., Donar, M. E., & Kettrick, R. G. (1987). Pediatric home mechanical ventilation. *Pediatric Clinics of North America, 34*(1), 47–60.

Schoumacher, R. A. (1991). Saving money with home care [Editorial]. *American Journal of Diseases of Children, 145*(7), 725.

Stepanek, J. A. (1996). Early intervention services for the high-risk infant. In E. Ahman (Ed.), *Home care for the high-risk infant* (2nd ed., pp. 279–281). Gaithersburg, MD: Aspen Publishers, Inc.

Stricklin, M. L. (1993). *The cost effectiveness of maternal-child home health care.* Paper presented to Clinton Health Care Reform Task Force, 1993, Visiting Nurse Associations of America.

Struk, C. M. (1994). Women and children: Infant mortality, urban programs, and home care. *Nursing Clinics of North America, 29*(3), 395–408.

The Children's Hospital Practice Update (1995). KidStreet. *The Children's Hospital Update, 3*(2).

The Omnibus Budget Reconciliation Act of 1981 [OBRA]. Public Law No. 97-35, Section 2176, 95 Stat 351.

Thilo, E. H., Comito, J., & McCulliss, D. (1987). Home oxygen therapy in the newborn. Costs and parental acceptance. *American Journal of Diseases of Children, 141*(7), 766–768.

Tooley, W. (1988). Preface. In R. A. Ballard (Ed.), *Pediatric care of the ICN graduate* (p. xii). Philadelphia: W. B. Saunders.

Ventura, S. J., Martin, J. A., Taffel, S. M., et al. (1994). Advance report of final natality statistics, 1992. *Monthly Vital Statistics Report, 43*(5, Suppl.).

Vladick, B. D. (1994). From the Health Care Financing Administration: Medicare home health initiative. *Journal of American Medical Association, 271,* 1566.

Vohr, B. R., Chen, A., Garcia Coll, C., & Oh, W. (1988). Mothers of preterm and full term infants on home apnea monitors. *American Journal of Disease of Children, 142,* 229–231.

Ward, S., & Keens, T. (1988). Ventilatory management at home. In R. A. Ballard (Ed.), *Pediatric care of the ICN graduate* (pp. 166–176). Philadelphia: W. B. Saunders.

Wasserman, A. L. (1984). A prospective study of the impact of home monitoring on the family. *Pediatrics, 74*(13), 323–329.

Yost, D. M., Hochstadt, N. J., & Charles, P. (1988). Medical foster care: Achieving permanency for seriously ill children. *Children Today, 17*(5), 22–26.

Young, L., Creighton, D., & Sauve, R. S. (1988). The needs of families of infants discharged home with continuous oxygen therapy. *Journal of Obstetric, Gynecologic, and Neonatal Nursing, 17*(3), 187–193.

SUGGESTED READINGS

Ballard, R. A. (1988). *Pediatric care of the ICN graduate.* Philadelphia: W. B. Saunders.

Burstein, L. (1995). Home care. In S. L. Barnhart & M. P. Czervinske (Eds.), *Perinatal and pediatric respiratory care* (pp. 658–679). Philadelphia: W. B. Saunders.

Byers, J., & Fabian, A. (1988). The parent drop-out syndrome. *Caring, 7*(6), 36–38.

Corr, C. A., & Corr, D. M. (1985). *Hospice approaches to pediatric care.* New York: Springer.

Goldberg, A. I., Gardner, G., & Gibson, L. E. (1994). Home care: The next frontier of pediatric practice. *Journal of Pediatrics, 125*(5), 686–690.

Hurt, H., & Guest, E. (1984). Symposium on continuing care of the high-risk infant. *Clinics in Perinatology, 11*(1).

Appendix

NEONATAL BILL OF RIGHTS*

1. The infant has the right to be treated as a human being with feelings and emotions.
2. The infant has the right to receive considerate and respectful care.
3. The infant has the right to receive affection, love, and understanding.
4. The infant has the right to receive the best medical care available regardless of race, color, creed, or financial ability to pay.
5. The infant's parents have the right to receive from the physician information necessary to give informed consent.
6. The infant has the right to confidentiality in all communications and records relating to his [or her] care.
7. The infant and family have the right to information concerning other health care and educational institutions.
8. The infant has the right to be as comfortable and free from pain as possible.
9. The infant has the right to receive nutritional support regardless of the expected outcome of his [or her] disease.
10. The infant has the right to die with dignity and honor.

NURSES ASSOCIATION OF THE AMERICAN ASSOCIATION OF OBSTETRICS AND GYNECOLOGY (NAACOG) STANDARDS†

Standard I: Nursing Practice

Universal Nursing Practice Standard

Comprehensive nursing care for women and newborns focuses on helping individuals, families, and communities achieve their optimum health potential. This is best achieved within the framework of the nursing process.

Neonatal Nursing Practice Standard

Comprehensive nursing care for women and newborns focuses on helping individuals, families, and communities achieve their optimum health potential. This is best achieved within the framework of the nursing process.

Standard II: Health Education and Counseling

Universal Nursing Practice Standard

Health education for the individual, family, and community is an integral part of comprehensive nursing care. Such education encourages participation in and shared responsibility for health promotion, maintenance, and restoration.

Neonatal Nursing Practice Standard

Health education for the newborn, family, and community is an integral part of comprehensive nursing care. Such education encourages participation in and shared responsibility for health promotion, maintenance, and restoration.

Standard III: Policies, Procedures, and Protocols

Universal Nursing Practice Standard

Written policies, procedures, and protocols clarify the scope of nursing practice and delineate the qualifications of personnel authorized to provide care to women and newborns within the health care setting.

Neonatal Nursing Practice Standard

Written policies, procedures, and protocols clarify the scope of nursing practice and delineate the qualifications of personnel authorized to provide care to newborn within the health care setting.

Standard IV: Professional Responsibility and Accountability

Universal Nursing Practice Standard

Comprehensive nursing care for women and newborns is provided by nurses who are clinically competent and accountable for professional actions and legal responsibilities inherent in the nursing role.

*Developed by Maria Elena E. Tice, RN, BSN, Nurse Instructor NICU/NBN, Scott and White Memorial Hospital, Temple, TX. Published in *Neonatal Network*, 9(3), 72, 1990. Reprinted with permission.

†From NAACOG. (199). *NAACOG Standards for the Nursing Care of Women and Newborns* (4th ed.). Washington, DC: Author. Reprinted with permission.

Standard V: Utilization of Nursing Personnel

Universal Nursing Practice Standard

Nursing care for women and newborns is conducted in practice settings that have qualified nursing staff in sufficient numbers to meet patient care needs.

Standard VI: Ethics

Universal Nursing Practice Standard

Ethical principles guide the process of decision making for nurses caring for women and newborns at all times and especially when personal or professional values conflict with those of the patient, family, colleagues, or practice setting.

Standard VII: Research

Universal Nursing Practice Standard

Nurses caring for women and newborns utilize research findings, conduct nursing research, and evaluate nursing practice to improve the outcomes of care.

Standard VIII: Quality Assurance

Universal Nursing Practice Standard

Quality and appropriateness of patient care are evaluated through a planned assessment program using specific, identified clinical indicators.

DOCUMENTATION OF TYPICAL POSTPARTUM ASSESSMENT

Vital Signs

Blood Pressure: Normal range is 100 to 140/60 to 90. If >140/90, recheck in other arm with patient lying in left lateral position.

Pulse: 60 to 90/minute.

Respiration: 16 to 24/minute.

Temperature: Remains <100.4°F.

Report: Blood pressure (BP) < 100/60 accompanied by weakness, dizziness, and any other signs of compromised cardiovascular functioning. Also report BP if >140/90 and accompanied by hyperreflexia, headache, dizziness, edema, blurred vision, or spots in visual field. Report any BP, pulse, or respiration outside the normal range and accompanied by signs and symptoms of hypovolemia, hypertension, or shock. Report temperature if >100.4°F.

Breasts

Warm, tender, edematous with leaking milk. Skin intact. In breastfeeding mothers, assess signs of milk production.

Report: Inflammation with reddened area extending away from nipple and or accompanied by flu-like symptoms, dimpling, or open lesions. Report if there are no signs of milk production.

Nipples

Skin intact and without cracks, fissures, or blisters. The patient may complain of tenderness but does not complain of nipple pain.

Report: Signs and symptoms of infection.

Elimination

Bladder

Nonpalpable immediately after voiding; the patient denies complaints of dysuria, urgency and frequency, and hematuria.

Report: Dysuria, urgency, frequency, hematuria.

Bowel

Bowel sounds are audible in all four quadrants. The patient may have had at least one bowel movement since delivery. If no bowel movement, instruct the patient to increase bulk foods and fluids.

Report: Distended abdomen, pain in abdomen, no bowel sounds, or severe diarrhea. Patient to report if no bowel movement in 1 week.

Hemorrhoids

No visible bleeding or complaints of bleeding; only slight edema present, and no complaints of excessive pain. Note size and number of hemorrhoids.

Report: Excessive bleeding or pain.

Lochia

May be rubra (bright red), serosa (pink or brown), or alba (creamy white). Amount may be scant (no lochia on pad; only on toilet paper after wiping), or may be small (less than a 1-inch stain on pad), moderate (1- to 4-inch stain on pad), or heavy (greater than 4-inch stain on pad) within 1 hour. Fleshy odor with clots smaller than a lemon.

Report: Foul odor, clots larger than a lemon, or amount greater than a 4-inch stain on pad within 1 hour.

Fundus

Palpated without pain midline and below umbilicus. Firm to palpation. The patient may have cramping, especially if breastfeeding.

Report: Boggy fundus that firms with massage, fundus above umbilicus with distended bladder, and excessive pain or tenderness. Patient to call physician if nontender uterus does not begin involution within 1 week.

Incision

Episiotomy or repaired perineal laceration are well approximated, with mild to moderate drainage and redness extending <2 cm from episiotomy or incision.

Abdominal incision edges are well approximated, with minimal edema and/or redness and minimal serous drainage. If staples are present, may be removed by order of physician and Steri-Strips applied.

Report: Gaping episiotomy/perineal tear or separated abdominal incision, marked discoloration or firmness >2 cm from site, excessive tenderness, and/or purulent drainage.

Edema

Inspect all areas of the skin for edema, paying particular attention to dependent body parts, such as feet and ankles. Palpate edematous areas, noting location, tenderness, and extent of edema. Assess for pitting edema by pressing edematous area firmly with thumb for 5 to 10 seconds:

1/2-cm indentation = trace
1-cm indentation = 1+
2-cm indentation = 2+
3-cm indentation = 3+
4-cm indentation = 4+

Report: Edema that has increased since delivery of infant if accompanied by increased BP or by headache, blurring of vision, spots in visual field, and/or hyperreflexia.

Homans' Sign (Calf Tenderness)

Dorsiflex foot and determine whether there is pain in calf on dorsiflexion. There should be no pain.

Report: Pain or questionable finding.

Deep Tendon Reflexes

Assess quadriceps reflex (patellar):

sluggish response = 1+
normal response = 2+
brisk response = 3+
hyperactive response = 4+

If greater than a 3+ response, assess for clonus. Sharply dorsiflex the foot and maintain this position for a moment and release briskly. If no rhythmic movement is seen or felt, clonus is not present. If clonus is present, rhythmic movements will be felt when the foot is dorsiflexed and seen as it returns to a neutral position.

Report: Sluggish or hyperactive response; presence of clonus.

Sleep/Rest

Assess visually for the appearance of fatigue. Ask how much sleep and rest the mother is getting. Determine whether support systems are in place.

Report: If the mother is exhausted with no support person and is thereby jeopardizing physical care of self or infant.

Diet

Twenty-four hour diet assessment adequately represented by food pyramid: 2 to 4 servings of milk, 2 to 3 servings meat, 3 to 5 servings vegetables, 2 to 4 servings fruit, 6 to 11 servings grain. The mother should eat three meals per day and drink 48 to 64 ounces of fluid per day. Exception: Breastfeeding mothers should consume 96 ounces of fluid per day, including 16 ounces with each feeding.

Adaptation to Mother Role/Bonding and Family Adaptation

Assess the mother's feelings for infant. Observe verbal and nonverbal cues. She should verbalize feelings of confidence with infant care; hold and cuddle infant; be able to maintain eye contact; talk appropriately and affectionately to infant; be able to comfort crying infant and attend to infant's basic needs. Assess family adaptation and interaction.

Report: Absence of parental attachment behaviors.

Psychosocial Assessment

Perform abuse assessment screen: mental/emotional status, including flat affect, uncontrolled crying, severe mood swings, agitation, whether easily distracted, and depression. Assess family history of mental/emotional disorders.

Report: Symptoms of postpartum depression or emotional distress that jeopardizes safety of self or infant.

Text continued on page 1012

DATE								
ASPECT OF CARE:	Day 1	M/U	Day 2	M/U	Day 3	M/U	Day 4	M/U
FAMILY TEACHING / DISCHARGE PLANNING	MD/RN communications with family Social Service referral - - - - - - - - -		- - - - - - - - - - - - - - - - - →		SS referral completed			
RESPIRATORY	Increased frequency of assessment as required - - - - - - - - - - - - - - -		- - - - - - - - - - - - - - - - - →		Improved respiratory status or return to baseline		As per gestational age NeoMAP	
CARDIAC	Increased frequency of assessment as required - - - - - - - - - - - - - - -		- - - - - - - - - - - - - - - - - →		Baseline status maintained - - -		- - - - - - - - - - - - - - - - →	
NUTRITION/FLUIDS ☐ Parenteral	Initiate IV access as required : adequate fluid, electrolyte, hydration status - - - - - - - - - - - - - - - - - -		- - - - - - - - - - - - - - - - - -		- - - - - - - - - - - - - - - - - - →		Baseline weight maintained or increase in growth parameter	
☐ Enteral	Initiate NPO status as required - - - -		- - - - - - - - - - - - - - - - - -		- - - - - - - - - - - - - - - - - -		- - - - - - - - - - - - - - - - →	
ELIMINATION	Appropriate for intake - - - - - - - - - -		- - - - - - - - - - - - - - - - - -		- - - - - - - - - - - - - - - - - -		- - - - - - - - - - - - - - - - →	
THERMOREGULATION	Provide for/monitor increased thermoregulation needs - - - - - - - -		- - - - - - - - - - - - - - - - - →		Requires less assistance with thermoregulation /return to baseline - - - - - - - - - - - -		- - - - - - - - - - - - - - - - →	
NEURO/NEURO BEHAVIOR	Observe for change in activity tolerance/increase in stress signals - -		- - - - - - - - - - - - - - - - - →		Infant displays improved activity, tolerance, and stabilization of stress response - - - - - - - - -		- - - - - - - - - - - - - - - - →	
DIAGNOSTIC STUDIES	CBC ☐ Urine Wellcogen ☐ Blood culture ☐ Urine culture ☐ CSF culture ☐ CXR ☐		Check results. Notify MD/ARNP. ☐ Drug serum level and report time collected ____________		Check results of cultures and studies pending.		Report final culture. Results to MD/ARNP.	
MEDICATIONS	As per MD/ARNP order - - - - - - - -		- - - - - - - - - - - - - - - - - →		D/C antibiotic pending cx results as ordered. Reorder antibiotics if continued.		☐ Continue antibiotics. Return to GA NeoMAP.	
PROCEDURES	As per MD/ARNP order - - - - - - - - -		- - - - - - - - - - - - - - - - - -		- - - - - - - - - - - - - - - - - -		- - - - - - - - - - - - - - - - →	

ADDRESSOGRAPH

FIGURE A–1. Sepsis overlay NeoMAP. M, met; U, unmet. (With permission from The Center for Case Management, Inc., South Natick, MA, and Florida Hospital Medical Center, Orlando, FL.)

PHOTOTHERAPY Last bili ____ Date ____

Single☐ Double☐ Wallaby☐
Start if bili > ____
Start date ____ end date ____
Restart if bili > ____ date ____

	GESTATIONAL AGE												
	DATE												
	DAY												
ASPECT OF CARE:		M	U	M	U	M	U	M	U	M	U	M	U
FAMILY TEACHING / DISCHARGE PLANNING	Medical/nursing staff communicates with family: ☐ Jaundice information given to parent(s)/caretakers ☐ Home phototherapy alternatives considered ☐ Home health agency referral												
RESPIRATORY	Monitor per routine or more often as patient condition warrants.												
CARDIAC	Monitor per routine or more often as patient condition warrants.												
NUTRITION/FLUIDS ☐ Parenteral ☐ Enteral	Maintain adequate hydration/nutritional intake as ordered.												
ELIMINATION	Elimination appropriate for intake.												
THERMOREGULATION	Neutral thermal environment maintained within acceptable range.												
NEURO/NEURO BEHAVIOR	Facilitate visual interaction by removing eye covering while protecting eyes from light source minimum x1/shift.												
DIAGNOSTIC STUDIES	Monitor bili level minimum once in 24 hours while receiving phototherapy. Monitor bili level and additional lab values as ordered. Report to MD/ARNP.												
MEDICATIONS	As per MD/ARNP order.												
PROCEDURES	Limit interruptions to phototherapy: not to exceed $1^1/_2$ hours/12 hours. Maintain optimal skin exposure with diaper off (face mask acceptable). Bili meter measurement each shift. Maintain at least minimum therapeutic range.												

ADDRESSOGRAPH

FIGURE A–2. Phototherapy overlay NeoMAP. M, met; U, unmet. (With permission from The Center for Case Management, Inc., South Natick, MA, and Florida Hospital Medical Center, Orlando, FL.)

Page No._____ 7 DAYS

Gestational Age
Date:
NeoMAP Day:

Aspect of Care	Descriptors of Interventions
Family Teaching/ Discharge Planning	**Family Contact daily** **If family visit, progress noted toward family teaching goals.** Social Services referral as per guidelines. Date:__________
Respiratory	FIO_2____ via N/C ☐ Oxyhood ☐ Isolette ☐ START____ D/C____ ABG q____ DUE____ CPT q____ START____ D/C____ VENT: START____ D/C____ IMV____ PIP/PEEP:____ INV I:E: START____ D/C____ WEANING ORDERS: HFV: START____ D/C____ ETT/TRACH Size: ____ AEROSOL TX____ START____ D/C____ CPAP: START____ D/C____ MODE: ET ☐ NASAL ☐ CHEST TUBES: SURFACTANT TX: DOSES____ OSC BED: START____ D/C____ SITE:____ @CM H_20 START____ D/C____ OXIMETER: START____ D/C____ ET/TCO_2: START____ D/C____ SITE:____ @CM H_20 START____ D/C____ **Optimal gas exchange/perfusion at minimal settings** ☐FIO_2 > .21 ≤ 30 days START____ STOP ____ ☐N/C @ .21/____LPM START____ STOP ____
Cardiac	**Optimal perfusion.** **Heart rate within normal limits.**
Nutrition/Fluids	NPO Total Fluids____ cc/hr IV FLUID____ @ cc/hr ADDITIVES:____ ____________________
Parenteral	**Patent UAC/UVC ≤ 14 days with no associated complications** UAC level____ Start____ D/C____ UVC level____ Start____ D/C____ **Patent PIV ≤ ____ days with no associated complications** PIV ____ Start____ D/C____ CVL ____ Start____ D/C____ PAL ____ Start____ D/C____ Dressing chg.____ **If HAF ≤ 50 days.** HAF Rate____ Start____ D/C____ Lipids ___% Rate____ Start____ D/C____ **Adequate fluid/electrolyte and hydration status.**
Enteral	FORMULA TYPE____ AMT/FREQ/SCHEDULE/TECHNIQUE: METHOD: ☐ COG: START____ STOP____ ☐GAVAGE: START____ STOP____ 1st Feed Date:____ ☐ TPR: START____ STOP____ ☐NIPPLE: START____ STOP____

FIGURE A–3. 26 Weeks and Less NeoMAP. (With permission from The Center for Case Management, Inc., South Natick, MA, and Florida Hospital Medical Center, Orlando, FL.)

Illustration continued on following page

	Consider gavage/TPR feed start prior to 26 days. **Nipple feed prior to 71 days.** **Total nipple feeds within 90 days. Date:**__________			
Elimination	**cc/Kg output within acceptable range while on continuous fluids.** **Specific gravity within acceptable range and/or no less than 6 wet diapers in 24 hours.**			
Thermal regulation	**Neutral thermal environment maintained within acceptable range while in Isolette.** ISOLETTE: Change Due______ **Temperature maintained within normal limits.**			
Neuro/Neuro behavior	**Individualized developmental support and protective measures implemented.** **Evaluate oral motor readiness and progress 32-34 weeks**______; **Suck/swallow synchrony completed 36-38 weeks**______; Progress toward all nipple feeds.			
Diagnostic Studies	Radiology DATE/TYPE ______ Diagnostic Studies DATE/TYPE ______ **Results monitored, abnormals reported & appropriate action taken.** **Consider cardiac evaluation if > 3 days** ☐**PPV and/or** ☐**murmur** LABS PENDING:			
Medications	(see culture/antibiotics table below) As per MD/ARNP order; renewed as per hospital protocol.			
Consults/Procedures	As per MD/ARNP order.			

DATE SENT	CULTURE	24°	48°	72°	ANTIBIOTICS
					START____ STOP____
					START____ STOP____
					START____ STOP____
					START____ STOP____

*BEFORE PERFORMING THE ABOVE ROUTINES, A **PHYSICIAN'S ORDER** MUST BE RECEIVED FOR THOSE ACTIVITIES REQUIRING AN ORDER.*

*Statements in **bold print** denote desired outcome.*

6/4/93

Clinical Coordinator Analysis

Primary Clinical Coordinator: __________

Associate Clinical Coordinator: __________

Date reviewed: ______ Completed by: ______

Variances Identified: Action Taken:

Notes: __________

VARIANCES

DATE	TIME	SOURCE	VARIANCE	CAUSE	ACTION	RESOLVED	INITIALS

Name/Initials: 1._________/___ 2._________/___ 3._________/___ 4._________/___ 5._________/___ 6._________/___
7._________/___ 8._________/___ 9._________/___ 10._________/___ 11._________/___ 12._________/___

CODE-VARIANCE SOURCE: 1. Event not applicable 2. Unpredicted event

A. Patient/Family
   3. Patient Condition
   4. Patient/Family Decision
   5. Patient/Family Availability
   6. Patient/Family Cognition
   7. Mother's condition

B. Caregiver/clinician
   10. Physician's Order
   11. Caregiver Decision
   12. Caregiver Action

C. Hospital
   20. Information/Data Availability
   21. Supplies/Equipment Availability
   22. Department Overbooked/Closed
   23. Delayed/Incorrect Medication/Fluids
   24. Bed Availability

D. Community
   30. Placement/Home Care Delay
   31. Transportation Delay
   32. Community Other

6/4/93

FIGURE A–3 *Continued*

Page No.______ 7 DAYS

Gestational Age						
Date:						
NeoMAP Day:						

Aspect of Care	Descriptors of Interventions						
Family Teaching/ Discharge Planning	**Family Contact daily** **If family visit, progress noted toward family teaching goals on Discharge Planning Summary.** Social Services referral as per guidelines. Date:________________						
Respiratory	FiO_2 ____ via N/C ☐ Oxyhood ☐ Isolette ☐ START____ D/C____ ABG q______ DUE______ CPT q______ START_____ D/C_____ VENT: START_____ D/C_____ IMV_______ PIP/PEEP:_______ INV I:E: START_____ D/C_____ WEANING ORDERS: HFV: START_____ D/C_____ ETT/TRACH Size: __________ AEROSOL TX____________________ START_____ D/C_____ CPAP: START_____ D/C_____ MODE: ET ☐ NASAL ☐ CHEST TUBES: SURFACTANT TX: DOSES________ OSC BED: START_____ D/C_____ SITE:____________________ @CM H_20 START_____ D/C_____ OXIMETER: START_____ D/C_____ ET/TCO_2: START_____ D/C_____ SITE:____________________ @CM H_20 START_____ D/C_____ **Optimal gas exchange/perfusion at minimal settings** ☐**FiO_2 > .21 ≤ 7 days** START__________ STOP __________ ☐N/C @ .21/______LPM START__________ STOP __________						
Cardiac	**Optimal perfusion without pressor agents.** **Heart rate within normal limits.**						
Nutrition/Fluids Parenteral	NPO ( ) Total Fluids_______________ cc/hr IV FLUID RATE__________________cc/hr **Patent UAC/UVC ≤ 7 days with no associated complications** UAC level_________ Start_____ D/C______ UVC level_________ Start_____ D/C______ **Patent PIV ≤ 6 days with no associated complications** PIV _________ Start_____ D/C______ CVL _________ Start_____ D/C______ PAL _________ Start_____ D/C______ Dressing chg.__________ **If HAF ≤ 5 days.** HAF Rate_____ Start_____ D/C_____ Lipids __% Rate_____ Start_____ D/C______ **Adequate fluid/electrolyte and hydration status.**						
Enteral	FORMULA TYPE____________________ METHOD: COG: START_____ STOP______ GAVAGE: START______ STOP______ **Consider gavage/TPR feed start prior to 4 days.** TPR: START_____ STOP______ NIPPLE: START______ STOP______ **Nipple feed prior to 6 days.** **Initial feed** ________ **All nipple feeds**_________ **Total nipple feeds within 14 days.** **Developmentally supportive feeding plan/DSF record in progress ( )**						

Elimination	**cc/Kg output within acceptable range while on continuous fluids.** **Specific gravity within acceptable range and/or no less than 6 wet diapers in 24 hours.**
Thermal regulation	**Neutral thermal environment maintained within acceptable range while in Isolette.** Isolette Change Due________ **Temperature maintained within normal limits.**
Neuro/Neuro behavior	**Individualized developmental support and protective/comfort measures implemented.** **Evaluate oral motor readiness and progress 32-34 weeks**______________; **Suck/swallow synchrony completed 36-38 weeks**______________; **Progress toward all nipple feeds with subsystem stability.**
Diagnostic Studies	Radiology DATE/TYPE ______ Diagnostic Studies DATE/TYPE ______ **Results monitored, abnormals reported & appropriate action taken.** **Consider cardiac evaluation if > 3 days ☐PPV and/or ☐murmur** LABS PENDING:
Medications	See culture/antibiotics table below. As per MD/ARNP order; renewed as per hospital protocol.
Consults/Procedures	As per MD/ARNP order.

DATE SENT	CULTURE	24°	48°	72°	ANTIBIOTICS
					START______ STOP______
					START______ STOP______
					START______ STOP______
					START______ STOP______

*BEFORE PERFORMING THE ABOVE ROUTINES, A **PHYSICIAN'S ORDER** MUST BE RECEIVED FOR THOSE ACTIVITIES REQUIRING AN ORDER.*

*Statements in **bold print** denote desired outcome.*

Clinical Coordinator Analysis

Primary Clinical Coordinator: ______

Associate Clinical Coordinator: ______

Date reviewed: ______ Completed by: ______

Variances Identified: ______ Action Taken: ______

Notes: ______

4/96

FIGURE A–4. 33 to 35 Weeks NeoMAP. (With permission from The Center for Case Management, Inc., South Natick, MA, and Florida Hospital Medical Center, Orlando, FL.)

Illustration continued on following page

VARIANCES

DATE	TIME	SOURCE	VARIANCE	CAUSE	ACTION	RESOLVED	INITIALS

Name/Initials: 1.________/____ 2.________/____ 3.________/____ 4.________/____ 5.________/____ 6.________/____
7.________/____ 8.________/____ 9.________/____ 10.________/____ 11.________/____ 12.________/____

CODE-VARIANCE SOURCE: 1. Event not applicable 2. Unpredicted event

A. Patient/Family
- 3. Patient Condition
- 4. Patient/Family Decision
- 5. Patient/Family Availability
- 6. Patient/Family Cognition
- 7. Mother's condition

B. Caregiver/clinician
- 10. Physician's Order
- 11. Caregiver Decision
- 12. Caregiver Action

C. Hospital
- 20. Information/Data Availability
- 21. Supplies/Equipment Availability
- 22. Department Overbooked/Closed
- 23. Delayed/Incorrect Medication/Fluids
- 24. Bed Availability

D. Community
- 30. Placement/Home Care Delay
- 31. Transportation Delay
- 32. Community Other

4/96

FIGURE A–4 *Continued*

Page No.______ 7 DAYS

Gestational Age				
Date:				
NeoMAP Day:				

Aspect of Care	Descriptors of Interventions
Family Teaching/ Discharge Planning	**Family Contact daily** **If family visit, progress noted toward family teaching goals on Discharge Planning Summary.** Social Services referral as per guidelines. Date:________
Respiratory	FiO_2____ via N/C ☐ Oxyhood ☐ Isolette ☐ START____ D/C____ ABG q____ DUE____ CPT q____ START____ D/C____ VENT: START____ D/C____ IMV____ PIP/PEEP:____ INV I:E: START____ D/C____ WEANING ORDERS: HFV: START____ D/C____ ETT/TRACH Size: ____ AEROSOL TX____ START____ D/C____ CPAP: START____ D/C____ MODE: ET ☐ NASAL ☐ CHEST TUBES: SURFACTANT TX: DOSES____ OSC BED: START____ D/C____ SITE:____ @CM H_20 START____ D/C____ OXIMETER: START____ D/C____ ET/TCO_2: START____ D/C____ SITE:____ @CM H_20 START____ D/C____ **Optimal gas exchange/perfusion at minimal settings** ☐**$FiO_2 > .21 \le 7$ days** START____ STOP ____ ☐N/C @ .21/____LPM START____ STOP ____
Cardiac	**Optimal perfusion without pressor agents.** **Heart rate within normal limits.**
Nutrition/Fluids	NPO ( ) Total Fluids____ cc/hr IV FLUID RATE____ cc/hr
Parenteral	**Patent UAC/UVC $\le$ 5 days with no associated complications** UAC level____ Start____ D/C____ UVC level____ Start____ D/C____ **Patent PIV $\le$ 7 days with no associated complications** PIV ____ Start____ D/C____ CVL ____ Start____ D/C____ PAL ____ Start____ D/C____ Dressing chg.____ **If HAF $\le$ 6 days.** HAF Rate____ Start____ D/C____ Lipids ___% Rate____ Start____ D/C____ **Adequate fluid/electrolyte and hydration status.**
Enteral	FORMULA TYPE____ METHOD: COG: START____ STOP____ GAVAGE: START____ STOP____ **Consider gavage/TPR feed start prior to 3 days.** TPR: START____ STOP____ NIPPLE: START____ STOP____ **Nipple feed prior to 4 days.** **Initial feed** ____ **All nipple feeds**____ **Total nipple feeds within 9 days.** **Developmentally supportive feeding plan/DSF record in progress ( )**

FIGURE A–5. 36 to 38 Weeks NeoMAP. (With permission from The Center for Case Management, Inc., South Natick, MA, and Florida Hospital Medical Center, Orlando, FL.)

Illustration continued on following page

Elimination	**cc/Kg output within acceptable range while on continuous fluids.** **Specific gravity within acceptable range and/or no less than 6 wet diapers in 24 hours.**						
Thermal regulation	**Neutral thermal environment maintained within acceptable range while in Isolette.** Isolette Change Due ______ **Temperature maintained within normal limits.**						
Neuro/Neuro behavior	**Individualized developmental support and protective/comfort measures implemented.** **Evaluate oral motor readiness and progress.** **Suck/swallow synchrony completed 36-38 weeks______________;** **Progress toward all nipple feeds with subsystem stability.**						
Diagnostic Studies	Radiology DATE/TYPE ______ Diagnostic Studies DATE/TYPE ______ **Results monitored, abnormals reported & appropriate action taken.** **Consider cardiac evaluation if > 3 days ☐PPV and/or ☐murmur** LABS PENDING:						
Medications	(see culture/antibiotics table below) As per MD/ARNP order; renewed as per hospital protocol.						
Consults/Procedures	As per MD/ARNP order.						

DATE SENT	CULTURE	24°	48°	72°	ANTIBIOTICS
					START______ STOP______
					START______ STOP______
					START______ STOP______
					START______ STOP______

BEFORE PERFORMING THE ABOVE ROUTINES, A ***PHYSICIAN'S ORDER*** *MUST BE RECEIVED FOR THOSE ACTIVITIES REQUIRING AN ORDER.*

Statements in ***bold print*** *denote desired outcome.*

4/96

Clinical Coordinator Analysis

Primary Clinical Coordinator: ______________________

Associate Clinical Coordinator: ______________________

Date reviewed: ______________ Completed by: ______________

Variances Identified: ______________ Action Taken: ______________

Notes: ______________________

VARIANCES

DATE	TIME	SOURCE	VARIANCE	CAUSE	ACTION	RESOLVED	INITIALS

Name/Initials: 1.________/____ 2.________/____ 3.________/____ 4.________/____ 5.________/____ 6.________/____
7.________/____ 8.________/____ 9.________/____ 10.________/____ 11.________/____ 12.________/____

CODE-VARIANCE SOURCE: 1. Event not applicable 2. Unpredicted event

A. Patient/Family
- 3. Patient Condition
- 4. Patient/Family Decision
- 5. Patient/Family Availability
- 6. Patient/Family Cognition
- 7. Mother's condition

B. Caregiver/clinician
- 10. Physician's Order
- 11. Caregiver Decision
- 12. Caregiver Action

C. Hospital
- 20. Information/Data Availability
- 21. Supplies/Equipment Availability
- 22. Department Overbooked/Closed
- 23. Delayed/Incorrect Medication/Fluids
- 24. Bed Availability

D. Community
- 30. Placement/Home Care Delay
- 31. Transportation Delay
- 32. Community Other

4/96

FIGURE A–5 *Continued*

Page No.______ 7 DAYS

Gestational Age							
Date:							
NeoMAP Day:							

Aspect of Care	Descriptors of Interventions
Family Teaching/ Discharge Planning	**Family Contact daily** **If family visit, progress noted toward family teaching goals on Discharge Planning Summary.** Social Services referral as per guidelines. Date:__________________
Respiratory	FIO_2_____ via N/C ☐ Oxyhood ☐ Isolette ☐ START_____ D/C_____ ABG q_______ DUE_______ CPT q_______ START______ D/C______ VENT: START______ D/C______ IMV________ PIP/PEEP:________ INV I:E: START______ D/C______ WEANING ORDERS: HFV: START______ D/C______ ETT/TRACH Size: ___________ AEROSOL TX________________________ START______ D/C______ CPAP: START______ D/C______ MODE: ET ☐ NASAL ☐ CHEST TUBES: SURFACTANT TX: DOSES__________ OSC BED: START______ D/C______ SITE:________________________ @CM H_20 START______ D/C______ OXIMETER: START______ D/C______ ET/TCO_2: START______ D/C______ SITE:________________________ @CM H_20 START______ D/C______ **Optimal gas exchange/perfusion at minimal settings** ☐ $FIO_2 > .21$ START___________ STOP ___________ ☐ N/C @ .21/______LPM START___________ STOP ___________
Cardiac	**Optimal perfusion without pressor agents.** **Heart rate within normal limits.**
Nutrition/Fluids	NPO ( ) Total Fluids_________________ cc/hr IV FLUID RATE_____________________ cc/hr
Parenteral	**Patent UAC/UVC ≤ 3 days with no associated complications** UAC level___________ Start______ D/C______ UVC level___________ Start______ D/C______ **Patent PIV ≤ 6 days with no associated complications** PIV ___________ Start______ D/C______ CVL ___________ Start______ D/C______ PAL ___________ Start______ D/C______ Dressing chg._____________ **If HAF ≤ 5 days.** HAF Rate______ Start______ D/C______ Lipids ___% Rate______ Start______ D/C______ **Adequate fluid/electrolyte and hydration status.**
Enteral	FORMULA TYPE__________________________ METHOD: COG: START______ STOP________ GAVAGE: START________ STOP_______ **Consider gavage/TPR feed start prior to 4 days.** TPR: START______ STOP________ NIPPLE: START________ STOP_______ **Nipple feed prior to 5 days.** **Initial feed** __________ **All nipple feeds**__________ **Total nipple feeds within 9 days.** **Developmentally supportive feeding plan/DSF record in progress ( )**

Elimination	**cc/Kg output within acceptable range while on continuous fluids.** **Specific gravity within acceptable range and/or no less than 6 wet diapers in 24 hours.**				
Thermal regulation	**Neutral thermal environment maintained within acceptable range while in Isolette.** Isolette Change Due ______ **Temperature maintained within normal limits.**				
Neuro/Neuro behavior	**Individualized developmental support and protective/comfort measures implemented.** **Evaluate oral motor readiness** **Suck/swallow synchrony completed** **Progress toward all nipple feeds with subsystem stability.**				
Diagnostic Studies	Radiology DATE/TYPE ______ Diagnostic Studies DATE/TYPE ______ **Results monitored, abnormals reported & appropriate action taken.** **Consider cardiac evaluation if > 3 days ☐PPV and/or ☐murmur** LABS PENDING:				
Medications	(see medications table below) As per MD/ARNP order; renewed as per hospital protocol.				
Consults/Procedures	As per MD/ARNP order.				

DATE SENT	CULTURE	24°	48°	72°	ANTIBIOTICS
					START______ STOP______
					START______ STOP______
					START______ STOP______
					START______ STOP______

*BEFORE PERFORMING THE ABOVE ROUTINES, A **PHYSICIAN'S ORDER** MUST BE RECEIVED FOR THOSE ACTIVITIES REQUIRING AN ORDER.*

*Statements in **bold print** denote desired outcome.*

Clinical Coordinator Analysis
Primary Clinical Coordinator: ______
Associate Clinical Coordinator: ______
Date reviewed: ______ Completed by: ______
Variances Identified: Action Taken:
Notes: ______

4/96

FIGURE A–6. 39 to 41 Weeks NeoMAP. (With permission from The Center for Case Management, Inc., South Natick, MA, and Florida Hospital Medical Center, Orlando, FL.)

Illustration continued on following page

VARIANCES

DATE	TIME	SOURCE	VARIANCE	CAUSE	ACTION	RESOLVED	INITIALS

Name/Initials: 1.________/____ 2.________/____ 3.________/____ 4.________/____ 5.________/____ 6.________/____
7.________/____ 8.________/____ 9.________/____ 10.________/____ 11.________/____ 12.________/____

CODE-VARIANCE SOURCE: 1. Event not applicable 2. Unpredicted event

A. Patient/Family
- 3. Patient Condition
- 4. Patient/Family Decision
- 5. Patient/Family Availability
- 6. Patient/Family Cognition
- 7. Mother's condition

B. Caregiver/clinician
- 10. Physician's Order
- 11. Caregiver Decision
- 12. Caregiver Action

C. Hospital
- 20. Information/Data Availability
- 21. Supplies/Equipment Availability
- 22. Department Overbooked/Closed
- 23. Delayed/Incorrect Medication/Fluids
- 24. Bed Availability

D. Community
- 30. Placement/Home Care Delay
- 31. Transportation Delay
- 32. Community Other

4/96

FIGURE A–6 *Continued*

Page No.______ 7 DAYS

Gestational Age
Date:
NeoMAP Day:

Aspect of Care	Descriptors of Interventions
Family Teaching/ Discharge Planning	**Family Contact daily** **If family visit, progress noted toward family teaching goals on Discharge Planning Summary.** Social Services referral as per guidelines. Date:______________
Respiratory	FiO_2____ via N/C ☐ Oxyhood ☐ Isolette ☐ START____ D/C____ ABG q______ DUE______ CPT q______ START_____ D/C_____ VENT: START_____ D/C_____ IMV_______ PIP/PEEP:_______ INV I:E: START_____ D/C_____ WEANING ORDERS: HFV: START_____ D/C_____ ETT/TRACH Size: __________ AEROSOL TX____________________ START_____ D/C_____ CPAP: START_____ D/C_____ MODE: ET ☐ NASAL ☐ CHEST TUBES: SURFACTANT TX: DOSES_________ OSC BED: START_____ D/C_____ SITE:____________________ @CM H_20 START_____ D/C_____ OXIMETER: START_____ D/C_____ ET/TCO_2 : START_____ D/C_____ SITE:____________________ @CM H_20 START_____ D/C_____ **Optimal gas exchange/perfusion at minimal settings** ☐**$FiO_2 > .21 \leq 7$ days.** START__________ STOP __________ ☐N/C @ .21/______LPM START__________ STOP __________
Cardiac	**Optimal perfusion without pressor agents.** **Heart rate within normal limits.**
Nutrition/Fluids	NPO ( ) Total Fluids_______________ cc/hr IV FLUID RATE__________________ cc/hr
Parenteral	**Patent UAC/UVC ≤ days with no associated complications** UAC level__________ Start______ D/C______ UVC level__________ Start______ D/C______ **Patent PIV ≤ 4 days with no associated complications** PIV __________ Start______ D/C______ CVL __________ Start______ D/C______ PAL __________ Start______ D/C______ Dressing chg.____________ **If HAF ≤ 4 days.** HAF Rate______ Start______ D/C______ Lipids ___% Rate______ Start______ D/C______ **Adequate fluid/electrolyte and hydration status.**
Enteral	FORMULA TYPE_____________________ METHOD: COG: START______ STOP_______ GAVAGE: START______ STOP______ **Consider gavage/TPR feed start prior to 3 days.** TPR: START______ STOP_______ NIPPLE: START______ STOP______ **Nipple feed prior to 5 days.** **Initial feed** ________ **All nipple feeds**________ **Total nipple feeds within 6 days.** **Developmentally supportive feeding plan/DSF record in progress ( )**

FIGURE A–7. 42 to 44 Weeks NeoMAP. (With permission from The Center for Case Management, Inc., South Natick, MA, and Florida Hospital Medical Center, Orlando, FL.)

Illustration continued on following page

Elimination	**cc/Kg output within acceptable range while on continuous fluids.** **Specific gravity within acceptable range and/or no less than 6 wet diapers in 24 hours.**						
Thermal regulation	**Neutral thermal environment maintained within acceptable range while in Isolette.** Isolette Change Due______ **Temperature maintained within normal limits.**						
Neuro/Neuro behavior	**Individualized developmental support and protective/comfort measures implemented.** **Evaluate oral motor readiness** **Suck/swallow synchrony completed** **Progress toward all nipple feeds with subsystem stability.**						
Diagnostic Studies	Radiology DATE/TYPE ______ Diagnostic Studies DATE/TYPE ______ **Results monitored, abnormals reported & appropriate action taken.** **Consider cardiac evaluation if > 3 days ☐PPV and/or ☐murmur** LABS PENDING:						
Medications	(see medications table below) As per MD/ARNP order; renewed as per hospital protocol.						
Consults/Procedures	As per MD/ARNP order.						

DATE SENT	CULTURE	24°	48°	72°	ANTIBIOTICS
					START______ STOP______
					START______ STOP______
					START______ STOP______
					START______ STOP______

*BEFORE PERFORMING THE ABOVE ROUTINES, A **PHYSICIAN'S ORDER** MUST BE RECEIVED FOR THOSE ACTIVITIES REQUIRING AN ORDER.*

*Statements in **bold print** denote desired outcome.*

4/96

Clinical Coordinator Analysis

Primary Clinical Coordinator: ______

Associate Clinical Coordinator: ______

Date reviewed: ______ Completed by: ______

Variances Identified: ______ Action Taken: ______

Notes: ______

VARIANCES

DATE	TIME	SOURCE	VARIANCE	CAUSE	ACTION	RESOLVED	INITIALS

Name/Initials: 1.________/___ 2.________/___ 3.________/___ 4.________/___ 5.________/___ 6.________/___
7.________/___ 8.________/___ 9.________/___ 10.________/___ 11.________/___ 12.________/___

CODE-VARIANCE SOURCE: 1. Event not applicable 2. Unpredicted event

A. Patient/Family
  3. Patient Condition
  4. Patient/Family Decision
  5. Patient/Family Availability
  6. Patient/Family Cognition
  7. Mother's condition

B. Caregiver/clinician
  10. Physician's Order
  11. Caregiver Decision
  12. Caregiver Action

C. Hospital
  20. Information/Data Availability
  21. Supplies/Equipment Availability
  22. Department Overbooked/Closed
  23. Delayed/Incorrect Medication/Fluids
  24. Bed Availability

D. Community
  30. Placement/Home Care Delay
  31. Transportation Delay
  32. Community Other

4/96

FIGURE A–7 *Continued*

CRITICAL PATHWAYS

Critical pathways are not a new concept. They are have become the buzz word with health care reform. They are a method for multidisciplinary identification and measurement of patient outcomes. They allow for anticipating the normal course of events or progress that a patient with a specific problem should follow. They are management plans that have a time frame for achievement of "milestones" according to a sequence of multidisciplinary interventions. All multidisciplinary teams may use the same plan because it is reflective of holistic care and not nursing versus medical care. This tool may be referred to as clinical pathways, care maps, or multidisciplinary action, plans to name a few (Ignatavicius & Hausman, 1995*). The salient features of any of these tools are patient outcomes, timelines, collaboration, and comprehensive care aspects. Because these are generally developed by different disciplines, there is a built-in "ownership" by health professionals responsible for managing the care versus turf issues over certain aspects of the care. These pathways help meet the Joint Commission on Accreditation of Healthcare Organizations (JCAHO) requirements for documentation or tracking of a patient's continuum of care. Ignatavicius and Hausman (1995, p. 36) outlined highlights of JCAHO Requirements:

Highlights of JCAHO Continuum of Care Requirements for 1995

- Have a process to facilitate patients' access to the appropriate clinical service and caregiver(s), based on assessed need.
- Perform an assessment before accepting patients into a given service or setting.
- Ensure as part of the admissions process that patients and families are appropriately informed about the care that will be provided.
- Assure continuity of care—a logical progression of service from assessment and diagnosis through planning and treatment.
- Assure that all care is coordinated by the health professionals in the various settings.
- Refer, transfer, or discharge the patient to the appropriate provider if assessment data indicate that a patient needs another level of care.
- Consider all the patient's care needs in the discharge plan to assure continuity of care.
- Make sure there is an exchange of appropriate patient and clinical information when patients are admitted, referred, transferred, or discharged.
- Assure that decisions to provide or deny care or service are based on the needs of the patient.

If an institution or unit is trying to develop a critical pathway, there are educational and motivational steps that must precede this process. Ignatavicius and Hausman (1995, p. 25) outlined a method for starting the development and facilitating the implementation processes of this tool:

Clinical Pathway Program

1. Educate and obtain support from staff and physicians.
2. Form the interdisciplinary teams:
   A. Steering committee and pathway-specific group
   B. A group to identify potential obstacles to implementation
3. Data collection: Determine patient population, Diagnostic Related Groups, International Code of Diseases–9 code to focus on those who are:
   A. High volume
   B. High cost
   C. High risk
   D. Difficult to manage
4. Use continuous quality improvement methods and tools to select
   A. Pareto charts
   B. Statistical process control chart
5. Determine which ICD-9 code is most predictable.
6. Determine staff interest.
7. Select pathways to develop.
8. Develop format for pathway.
9. Select interdisciplinary clinical experts for pathway team.
10. Collect clinical pathway data:
    A. Medical record review for practice patterns
    B. Literature review
    C. Comparison with other institutions
    D. Practice guidelines
11. Write the pathway:
    A. Review by staff
    B. Review as necessary
12. Develop variance analysis system:
    A. Information needed to measure compliance with the pathway
    B. Outcomes measurement
    C. Clinical and financial measurements
13. Present pathway to hospital committees for approval; incorporate revisions.
14. Develop implementation plan.
15. Provide in-service staff.
16. Use pilot pathway for 3 to 6 months; revise as needed.
17. Monitor variances:
    A. Develop automated data collection if possible
    B. Present variance data to staff and physicians

*Ignatavicius, D. D., & Hausman, K. A. (1995). *Clinical pathways for collaborative practice.* Philadelphia: W. B. Saunders.

REGIONAL NURSERY DIRECTORS' RECOMMENDATIONS FOR INFANTS DISCHARGED LESS THAN 48 HOURS AFTER UNCOMPLICATED VAGINAL DELIVERY AND INFANTS DISCHARGED LESS THAN 72 HOURS AFTER UNCOMPLICATED C-SECTION

It is the goal of this committee that all health care professionals have the means necessary to provide optimal care for mother–infant dyad without financial constraints and without compromising the quality of care.

It is our recommendation that all infants as described above should have an assessment after discharge, at 2 to 5 days of age, as directed by their primary care physician. A pathway flow chart has been developed for follow-up of these infants and is enclosed. This pathway is recommended as a guideline for care in this region.

Home care content should be consistent in the region and include, at a minimum, the following:

1. Physical assessment, including rectal/axillary temperature.
2. Parental interaction evaluation.
3. Home environment assessment with assessment of equipment available to the mother for care of her infant.
4. All infants should be weighed (visiting nurse must have a scale).
5. Documentation of the future follow-up appointment with primary care physician/visiting nurse.
6. Evaluation and documentation of pulse, respirations, and capillary refill.
7. Check for femoral pulses and respiratory effort (e.g., retractions, grunting).
8. Careful history of output since discharge from hospital, including urine and stool. Specific and complete feeding history, including type, times, and volume of feeding.

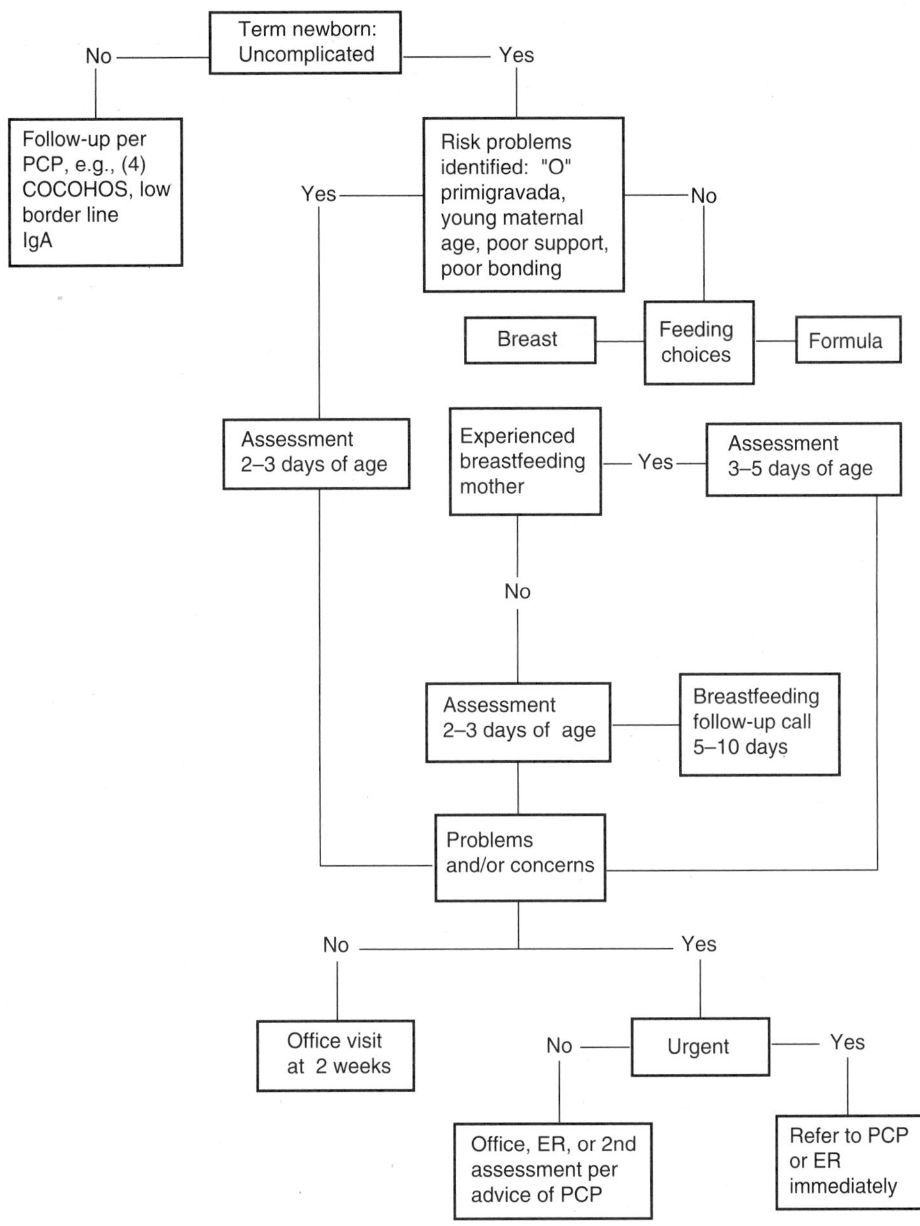

FIGURE A–8. Clinical pathway for follow-up of infants of uncomplicated vaginal full-term delivery. (From Ignatavicius, D. D., & Hausman, K. A. [1995]. *Clinical pathways for collaborative practice.* Philadelphia: W. B. Saunders.)

9. Visiting nurse must have inpatient information from hospital stay of mother and infant during home visit.
10. Forms should be the same, or similar in format, for all visiting nurses, and the forms sent to the primary care physician should be consistent.
11. The forms for metabolic screens have number, date, and time
12. General education of the family.

Credentialing:* of home care nurses should include the following:

1. The Consortium for Advancement of Perinatal Practice (CAPP). Mother and Baby I and II programs or equivalent.
2. Not less than 2000 hours of newborn care experience over 3 years' time.
3. Basic Cardiac Life Support (BCLS) certified. Neonatal Resuscitation Certification recommended, not required.
4. Skill in drawing blood, specifically for metabolic screens and bilirubin.
5. Cross-training in mother and infant care.
6. One third of continuing educational time related to mother and infant.
7. Five supervised home visits.

The third-party payors must provide the home care nurses with the means to obtain prenatal, intrapartum, postpartum, and nursery in-patient information that is available at the time of the home visit.

Postdischarge assessment as described above should be a reimbursable professional service. This assessment should be provided by physicians, nurses, or a hospital perinatal service. Home assessment visits should be a part of all hospital perinatal services.

All home care forms in the region should be consolidated into one user-friendly form for nurse, physicians, and third-party payors.

A regional data base is needed to evaluate the impact of early discharge. This should include information on emergency room visits and readmissions before the infant is 28 days of age and all visits to the primary care physician's office before the infant is 2 weeks of age.

*Didactic content and clinical skills verification for the professional nurse providing perinatal home care is based on standards published by the Association of Women's Health, Obstetric, and Neonatal Nurses (AWHONN).

Index

Note: Page numbers in *italics* refer to illustrations; page numbers followed by "t" refer to tables.

B

C

D

H

I

J

K

L

Q

R

U

V

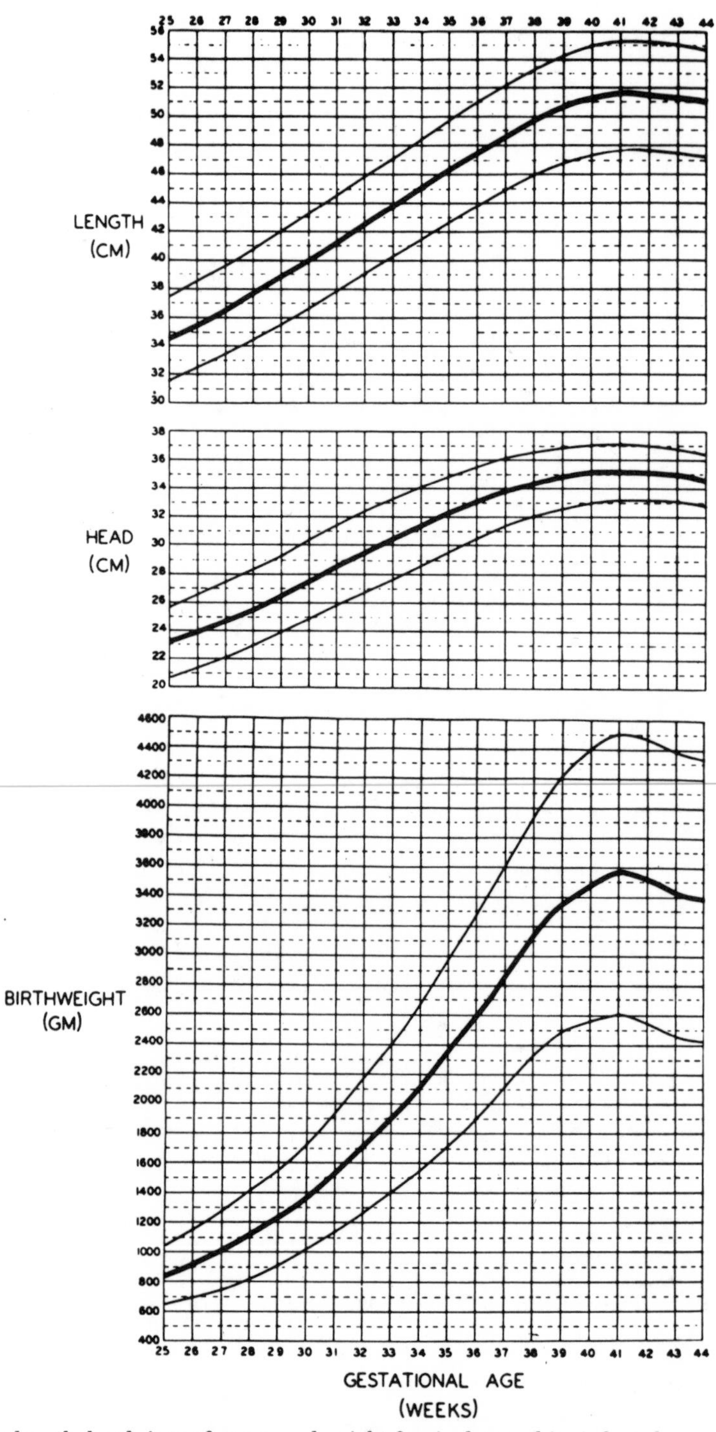

Intrauterine growth curves for length, head circumference, and weight for singleton white infants born at sea level (mean ±2 standard deviations). (Composite of graphics from Usher, R., & McLean, F. [1969]. Intrauterine growth of liveborn Caucasian infants at sea level: Standard obtained in 7 dimensions of infants born between 25 and 44 weeks of gestation. *Journal of Pediatrics, 74,* 901.)